Disorders of Voluntary Muscle

Disorders of Voluntary Muscle

Edited by

Sir John Walton
TD, MD, DSc, FRCP

Dr de l'Univ (Hon) (Aix-Marseille)
DSc (Hon) (Leeds) DSc (Hon) (Leicester)
Hon FACP

Professor of Neurology and Dean of Medicine, University of
Newcastle upon Tyne; Consultant Neurologist, Newcastle
Area Hospitals

FOURTH EDITION

CHURCHILL LIVINGSTONE
EDINBURGH LONDON MELBOURNE AND NEW YORK 1981

CHURCHILL LIVINGSTONE
Medical Division of Longman Group Limited

Distributed in the United States of America by
Churchill Livingstone Inc., 19 West 44th Street, New York,
N.Y. 10036, and by associated companies, branches and
representatives throughout the world.

First edition 1964
Second edition 1969
Third edition 1974
Fourth edition 1981

ISBN 0 443 01847 2

British Library Cataloguing in Publication Data
Disorders of voluntary muscle. – 4th ed.
  1. Muscles – Diseases
  I. Walton, John Nicholas
  616.7′4   RC925   80-41271

Filmset and printed in Great Britain by BAS Printers Limited, Over Wallop, Hampshire

Preface to the Fourth Edition

Since the appearance of the third edition of this book in 1974, there have been so many developments in the field of neuromuscular disease that extensive alterations and modifications in the structure of the volume have become necessary. In the last two editions new material on the clinical effects and on the pathology of neuronal and peripheral nerve disorders was included as these conditions so often enter into the differential diagnosis of primary muscle disease. In this edition a short section on the involvement of human muscle by parasites has been added to the chapter on inflammatory disorders of muscle, and a completely new chapter on drug-induced neuromuscular disorders has been added. The first two chapters in the last edition on anatomy and physiology of the motor unit have now been replaced by a single and much expanded opening chapter. The book has been reset in a totally different format from that of the previous editions and this has allowed extensive revision and restructuring of many of the chapters with complete rewriting of others; the great majority of the illustrations have been replaced and many new ones have been added. Acknowledgements, where necessary, to original sources of illustrations are given in the individual chapters.

Inevitably, as in previous editions, the reader will find evidence of some duplication and overlap between different chapters in that many diseases, and particularly the muscular dystrophies and spinal muscular atrophies, are commented upon in several chapters but from different points of view and with varying emphasis upon their clinical, pathological, biochemical and physiological characteristics. This has proved necessary in order that each individual chapter can stand as a comprehensive essay upon the topic to which it is devoted; I hope and believe that as a result the book will be no less useful, and may even be more so, as a work of reference.

Sadly, since the last edition was published, one much valued contributor, Dr L. A. Liversedge, has died. Because of the increasing pressure of other commitments or for other pressing personal reasons, Sir Kenneth Blaxter, Professor A. J. Buller, Dr Allan Downie, Dr H. W. Kloepfer, Dr J. Maclagan, Dr Brian McArdle, Dr C. M. Pearson, Dr A. T. Richardson, Dr K. F. A. Ross and Professor H. A. Sissons asked to be relieved of their authorship. We welcome as new contributors Dr A. Argov, Dr K. E. Åström, Mr R. Bradley, Dr Andrew Engel, Dr P. R. W. Fawcett, Dr B. F. Fell, Dr D. M. Lewis, Dr P. D. Lewis, Dr Christopher Pallis, Dr R. M. A. P. Ridge, Dr R. L. Van de Velde and Dr D. Wray. Much new material from other publications has been reproduced and referred to in this edition and I am grateful to the authors, editors and publishers concerned (whose permission is acknowledged in the individual chapters) for allowing us to include this material. And I am again especially grateful to the staff of Churchill Livingstone, to Mrs Heather Russell who has given invaluable editorial assistance, and to my secretary, Miss Rosemary Allan, for their patient and willing cooperation and for their forbearance during the production of this edition.

Newcastle upon Tyne, 1981   J.W.

Preface to the First Edition

The last fifteen years have seen a world-wide awakening of interest in diseases of muscle and during this period several outstanding books upon this subject have been published. At first sight, therefore, a new text-book devoted to this group of disorders may seem to be superfluous. However, the excellent work on *Diseases of Muscle* by Adam, Denny Brown and Pearson, now in its second edition, approaches the subject primarily from the pathological standpoint, while the three-volume work on *Structure and Function of Muscle* edited by Geoffrey Bourne, consists of a series of comprehensive essays of encyclopaedic scope, invaluable for reference by the research worker but perhaps too weighty for the general reader. Furthermore, the volume on *Neuromuscular Disorders*, embodying the proceedings of the 1958 meeting of the Association for Research in Nervous and Mental Disease, is primarily a commentary upon research in this field, while the recent work *Muscular Dystrophy in Man and Animals* edited by Bourne and Golarz, surveys only the problem of muscular distrophy.

In designing the present volume, therefore, it has been my aim and that of the other twenty-four contributors, each an acknowledged expert in the field, to give an up-to-date and comprehensive yet concise view of disorders of muscle from several standpoints. The book is aimed primarily at the clinician, whether he be a general physician, paediatrician or neurologist, a post-graduate student studying for a higher examination or any doctor wishing to expand his knowledge of this group of disorders. The first section of the book is devoted to a consideration of modern views of the structure and function of muscle, the second to the changes, both structural and biochemical, which may occur in disease, and the third contains a series of essays on the clinical and genetic aspects of muscle disease in man with a chapter describing the related disorders which occur in animals; the final section deals with electrical methods of investigation of muscular disease. Throughout, references are given not only to original sources of information but also to current research.

In the preparation of this volume I am indebted to the contributors; I am sure that many of them, like myself, are grateful for the help they have obtained from previous publications, pre-eminent among which are the four volumes to which I have referred above. More detailed acknowledgements of sources of material contained in this volume are given, where necessary, at the end of individual chapters. I wish personally to thank Mr J. Rivers, Mr A. S. Knightley and the staff of J. and A. Churchill Ltd for all the patience and understanding they have shown during the process of publication and, as always, I am deeply indebted to my secretary, Miss Rosemary Allan, for her unfailing willingness and efficiency.

Newcastle upon Tyne, 1964   J.W.

Contributors

ADAMS R. D.
MA, MD, AM (Hon), DSc(Hon), MD(Hon)
Former chief of Neurology service, Massachusetts General
Hospital. Senior Consultant in Neurology, Massachusetts
General Hospital. Emeritus Bullard Professor of
Neuropathology, Harvard University

ARGOV Z.
MD
Department of Neurology, Hadassah University Hospital,
Jerusalem, Israel

ÅSTRÖM K. E.
MD, PhD
Formerly Professor of Pathology, Karolinska Institute,
Stockholm, Sweden

BARWICK D. D.
MB, FRCP (Ed)
Consultant Neurologist (Clinical Neurophysiology),
Regional Neurological Centre, Newcastle General Hospital,
Newcastle upon Tyne; Clinical Lecturer in Neurology,
University of Newcastle upon Tyne

BRADLEY R.
BVetMed, MSc, MIBid, MRCVS
Senior Research Officer, Ministry of Agriculture, Fisheries
and Food, Pathology Department, Central Veterinary
Laboratory, New Haw, Weybridge

BRADLEY W. G.
MA, BSc, DM, FRCP
Professor of Neurology, Tufts University School of
Medicine, Boston, Massachusetts, Associate Neurologist in
Chief, New England Medical Center Hospital

BROWN J. C.
MD, FRCP, FRCP(Ed)
Consultant Neurologist, Norfolk Area Health Authority and
United Cambridge Hospitals

CAMPBELL M. J.
MB, FRCP(Lond)
Consultant Neurologist to Avon A.H.A., Bristol Royal
Infirmary, and Clinical Lecturer in Medicine to University of
Bristol

CÖERS C.
MD
Professor of the Free University of Brussels. Chief of the
Department of Neurology, Hôpital Breugmann, Brussels

CURRIE S.
MA, MD, BChir, FRCP
Consultant Neurologist, St James's University Hospital,
Leeds. Clinical Lecturer, University of Leeds.

DUBOWITZ V.
BSc, PhD, MD, FRCP, DCH
Professor of Paediatrics, Institute of Child Health and Royal
Postgraduate Medical School, University of London. Co-
Director, Jerry Lewis Muscle Research Centre, and
Honorary Consultant Physician, Hammersmith Hospital

EMERY A. E. H.
MD, PhD, DSc, FRCP(E), MFCM, FRS(E)
Professor of Human Genetics, University of Edinburgh

ENGEL A. G.
MD
Professor of Neurology, Mayo Medical School; Consultant
in Neurology, Mayo Clinic, Rochester, Minnesota

FAWCETT P. R. W.
BSc, MBBS, MRCP
Senior Registrar in Neurology (Clinical and Applied
Neurophysiology), Newcastle University Hospital Group,
Newcastle upon Tyne

FELL B. F.
PhD, MRCVS
Head of the Department of Experimental Pathology, Rowett
Research Institute, Bucksburn, Aberdeen

FOSTER J. B.
MD, FRCP
Neurologist to Regional Neurological Centre, Newcastle
AHA(T). Honorary Reader in Neurology, University of
Newcastle upon Tyne

GARDNER-MEDWIN D.
MD, FRCP
Consultant Paediatric Neurologist, Newcastle General
Hospital, Newcastle upon Tyne

GERGELY J.
MD, PhD
Director, Department of Muscle Research, Boston
Biomedical Research Institute; Biochemist, Massachusetts
General Hospital; and Associated Professor, Department of
Biological Chemistry, Harvard Medical School

HENSON R. A
MD, FRCP
Physician, Neurological Department. Chairman, Section of

Neurological Sciences, The London Hospital. Physician, National Hospitals for Nervous Diseases, (Maida Vale), London

HUDGSON P.
MD, BS, FRCP, FRACP
Consultant Neurologist, Northern Regional Health Authority and Newcastle Area Health Authority (Teaching). Senior Lecturer in Neurology, University of Newcastle upon Tyne

JOHN H. A.
BScm PhD
Research Fellow, Institute of Animal Genetics, West Mains Road, Edinburgh

JOHNS R. J.
MD
Massey Professor and Director, Department of Biomedical Engineering. Professor of Medicine, John Hopkins University and Hospital, Baltimore, Maryland

JONES K.
BSc, PhD
Reader, Institute of Animal Genetics, West Mains Road, Edinburgh

KAKULAS B. A.
MD(Hon Athens), MD(WA), FRACP, FRCPA, FRCPath
Professor of Neuropathology, University of Western Australia. Head of Neuropathology Department, Royal Perth Hospital, Western Australia

LENMAN J. A. R.
MB, ChB, FRCP(Ed), FRS(Ed)
Reader in Neurology, Dundee University. Honorary Consultant Neurologist, Tayside Area Health Board, Dundee

LEWIS D. M.
PhD, MB, BChir, BA
Reader in Physiology, University of Bristol

LEWIS P. D.
BSc, MD, MRCP, MRCPath
Senior Lecturer in Neuropathology, Royal Postgraduate Medical School. Consultant Neurologist, Hammersmith Hospital, London

LIVERSEDGE the late L. A.
BA, BSc, MD, FRCP
Former Consultant Neurologist, Manchester Royal Infirmary; former Director University Department of Neurology, Manchester

MASTAGLIA F. L.
MD, FRACP, FRCP
Associate Professor of Medicine (Neurology), University of Western Australia, Perth. Consultant Neurologist, Queen Elizabeth II Medical Centre, Perth

McCOMAS A. J.
BSc, MB, BS, FRCP(C)
Professor of Medicine (Neurology), McMaster University Medical Centre, Ontario, Canada

PALLIS C. A.
DM, FRCP
Reader in Neurology, Royal Postgraduate Medical School. Consultant Neurologist, Hammersmith Hospital, London

PENNINGTON R. J. T.
PhD, DSc, FRSE
Member of Medical Research Council External Scientific Staff. Honorary Reader in Neurochemistry, University of Newcastle upon Tyne. Honorary Senior Neurochemist, Regional Neurological Centre, Newcastle upon Tyne

PRICE H. M.
MD, MPH
Director of Anatomic Pathology, Valley Medical Center, Fresno, California. Associate Chief of Laboratories, Valley Medical Center, Fresno, California and Associate Clinical Professor of Pathology, School of Medicine, University of California, San Francisco

RIDGE R. M. A. P.
BSc, PhD
Lecturer in Physiology, University of Bristol

SIMPSON J. A.
MD, FRCP, FRCP(Ed), FRCP(Glas), FRS(Ed)
Professor of Neurology, University of Glasgow, Physician in charge, Department of Neurology, Institute of Neurological Sciences, Glasgow

THOMAS, P. K.
DSc, MD, FRCP
Professor of Neurology, University of London, Royal Free Hospital School of Medicine and the Institute of Neurology, Queen Square, London

TIZARD J. P. M.
MA, BM, BCh(Ox), FRCP(Lond), DCH(Eng)
Professor of Paediatrics, University of Oxford

VAN de VELDE R. L.
PhD
Chief, Special Anatomic Pathology Section, Cedars-Sinai Medical Center, Los Angeles, California

WALTON J. N.
TD, MD, DSc, FRCP, Dr de l'Univ(Hon) (Aix-Marseille), DSc(Hon) (Leeds), DSc(Hon) (Leicester), Hon FACP
Professor of Neurology and Dean of Medicine, University of Newcastle upon Tyne. Consultant Neurologist, Newcastle Area Hospitals

WOOLF the late A. L.
MD, MRCP, FCPath
Former Consultant Pathologist, Midland Centre for Neurosurgery and Neurology, Smethwick

WRAY D.
BA, MSc, DPhil
Lecturer in Pharmacology, Royal Free Hospital School of Medicine, University of London

WYNN-PARRY C. B.
MA, DM, ECR, FRCP, FRCS
Director of Rehabilitation, Royal National Orthopaedic Hospital, Stanmore. Honorary Consultant in Applied Electrophysiology, National Hospital for Nervous Diseases, Queen Square, London

ZAIMIS E.
MD, FRCP
Professor of Pharmacology and Head of the Department of Pharmacology, Royal Free Hospital School of Medicine, University of London

Contents

The anatomy and physiology of the motor unit

INTRODUCTION

The motor unit is the physiological and anatomical unit of reflex and willed contraction in vertebrate skeletal muscle. The concept was introduced as 'the motoneurone axon and its adjunct muscle fibres' by Liddell and Sherrington (1925) and subsequently defined by Sherrington (1925) thus: 'The term 'motor unit' includes, together with the muscle fibres innervated by the unit, the whole axon of the motoneurone from its hillock in the perikaryon down to its terminals in the muscle'. The motor neurone soma and dendrites were therefore excluded. More recent work has clearly indicated that many properties of the muscle fibres

innervated by a motor axon are determined and sustained by influences, including activity patterns, deriving from the motor neurone soma. Because motor neuronal activity is determined by synaptic input to the soma and dendrites, it seems proper to widen any discussion of the motor unit to include at least some of these factors, and we have done so in this chapter.

In the mammal, under normal conditions the motor unit behaves in an all-or-none manner, which means that an action potential in the motor axon produces an effectively synchronous contraction of all the muscle fibres it supplies. We are here concerned with the large motor neurones innervating muscle fibres that make up the mass of the muscle and develop tension at the muscle insertion (i.e. extrafusal muscle fibres). The small motor neurones innervating muscle spindles (i.e. intrafusal muscle fibres) will only be touched on in this chapter.

THE MOTOR NEURONE

It has long been known that the anterior horns of the spinal cord contain many types of neurone: the motor cells innervating the extrafusal muscle fibres (α-motor neurones) are relatively large, and are arranged in well-defined columns which extend through many spinal segments and which appear as rounded clusters in transverse sections. This arrangement is particularly clear when the cells are studied in reconstructions from short runs of serial sections (Fig. 1.1). The smaller neurones of the anterior horns are more diffusely arranged, and are thought to include both internuncial neurones and motor neurones to the intrafusal

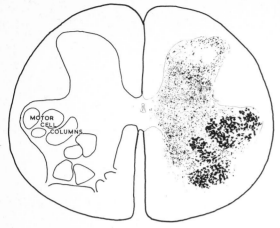

Fig. 1.1   Cell chart showing the grouping of the large motor neurones of the anterior horns of the grey matter of the 5th lumbar segment of a normal spinal cord (from Sharrard, 1955, by courtesy of H.A. Sissons: Disorders of Voluntary Muscle, 3rd edn.)

fibres of the muscle spindles (γ-motor neurones).

Sharrard (1955), from a study of the loss of anterior horn cells in the spinal cords of patients with residual paralysis from poliomyelitis, was able to determine the representation of particular muscles, or groups of muscles, in the cell columns at various segmental levels. Sharrard concluded, with regard to the muscles of the lower limbs, that flexor muscles are supplied by columns situated medial and caudal to those supplying the corresponding extensor muscles. Some muscles are supplied by long cell columns, others by short ones. The arrangement of the cell columns, and the somewhat selective and focal involvement of the anterior horns in poliomyelitis, is responsible for certain characteristic patterns of muscle paralysis in this condition. Other methods of locating the motor neurones of particular muscles have been used in experimental animals, such as chronic nerve section with later histological identification of motor neurone somata showing consequent chromatolysis and, more recently, by retrograde transport of horseradish peroxidase injected into the muscle and later made visible in the motor neurone somata (for example, in the cat; see Burke, Strick, Kanda, Kim and Walmsley, 1977). Figure 1.2 is an example produced by the latter technique applied to the hindlimb muscles of the mouse: α- and γ-motor neurones are clearly separable.

In the peripheral nerves, motor nerve fibres appear as relatively large myelinated fibres, approximately 6–20 μm in diameter in man and the larger laboratory animals. Since the study by Eccles and Sherrington (1930) of muscles and muscle nerves in cats where the appropriate dorsal root ganglia had been removed, with consequent disappearance of sensory nerve fibres, it has been apparent that muscle nerves contain many sensory fibres. Some of the sensory nerve fibres are myelinated fibres of small calibre, although some of them are large: the motor fibres of the muscle spindles, which originate from the smaller neurones of the anterior horns of the cord, are also of relatively small calibre. It has been concluded, both from animal studies (Boyd and Davey, 1968) and from observations in man (Feinstein, Lindegård, Nyman and Wohlfart, 1955), that about half of the large fibres are motor to the extrafusal fibres, the remainder being sensory. This proportion varies widely in nerves supplying different muscles, and therefore estimates of the number of motor units in a muscle derived from total axon counts may be wildly inaccurate.

Eccles and Sherrington (1930) described branching of motor nerve fibres along the course of muscle nerves in de-afferented animals. The number of α-motor axon profiles in sections of the nerve cut near the muscle can be up to 40 per cent greater than in sections cut more centrally (Wray, 1966). In the muscle biopsy material of Cöers and Woolf (1959), studied by the supravital methylene blue staining technique, the greatest degree of ramification of axons was found in the intramuscular nerve bundles, i.e. distal to the point where the nerve enters the muscle. At this point the nerve fibres are greatly reduced in diameter. The branching always occurs at a node of Ranvier. Each terminal ramification of a nerve fibre ends on a single motor end-plate. In most muscles these are located in a narrow zone across the muscle at the level of entry of the motor nerve, but in some long muscles, like sartorius, more than one transverse band is present (see Ch. 8). The divisions of each axon may extend quite widely throughout the muscle, and muscle fibres of a particular motor unit may be distributed within a part of the muscle or throughout the whole of some small muscles. This is discussed further, later in this chapter.

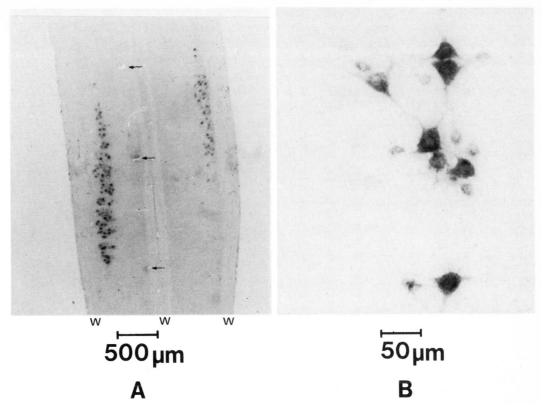

w   w   w

500 μm   50 μm

A   **B**

Fig. 1.2 Spinal motor neurones of the mouse labelled by injection of horseradish peroxidase into the muscles innervated. The HRP is then transported retrogradely into the motor neurone somata. A. Horizontal section of spinal cord at the level L2 to L4 (mouse has only six lumbar segments). Lesions indicating caudal limits of segments indicated by arrows. Top is cranial. White matter (w) is visible in the centre of the section and at either edge. Somata stained in the right ventral horn innervate anterior tibial, extensor digitorum longus and brevis and the peroneal muscles. In the left ventral horn the stained motor neurones innervate triceps surae and the deep posterior muscles. Section thickness 50 μm. Calibration bar represents 500 μm. B. A small group of motor neurons innervating soleus muscle. 7α and 9γ somata are visible. Section thickness 50 μm. Calibration bar represents 50 μm (illustration by courtesy of Mr S. McHanwell, unpublished data)

The structure of the motor end-plate is discussed in detail in Chapters 3 and 8. Each motor end-plate is a composite structure, belonging partly to the motor nerve and partly to the muscle fibre. The terminal axon loses its myelin sheath a few micrometres from the end-plate, and is covered only by attenuated Schwann cells which appear to be contiguous with the structures of the endomysial connective tissue sheath surrounding the muscle fibre. Inside the endomysium the axon ramifies within the end-plate to form a complex structure which lies in hollows—synaptic gutters—in the sarcoplasm. The actual area of contact, or synapse, between the axon and the muscle fibre is hardly visible in the light microscope, but appears on electron-microscopic examination to be a double membrane which is folded in

a complex manner (Palade, 1954; Robertson, 1956). Numerous nuclei are present in the motor end-plate, some lying within the sarcoplasm of the muscle, while others belong to adjacent Schwann cells or other connective tissue cells.

After acetylcholine was found to be the neuro-muscular chemical transmitter, cholinesterase was demonstrated in the subneural apparatus of the end-plate.

There is another connection made by many α-motor axons, and this is by intramedullary collateral branches on to spinal interneurones. The interneurones, called Renshaw cells, in turn make synaptic contact on to motor neurones of synergistic muscles. Activity in any of the collateral loops temporarily inhibits the motor neurones upon which the loop terminates. The functions of the

Renshaw loop are probably to stabilise the mean discharge frequency of motor neurone pools and to prevent the motor neurones from discharging nerve impulses at rates greatly in excess of those effective in the muscle fibres they innervate. There is evidence that their organisation is related to motor unit type: for instance, in a recent study, horseradish peroxidase was injected into the somata of motor neurones with muscle fibres which had been assigned a motor unit type (discussed below). Collateral outbulgings from the motor axons, presumably giving rise to collaterals contacting Renshaw cells, varied in number, depending on the type of motor unit (Cullheim and Kellerth, 1978).

SENSORY RECEPTORS IN MUSCLE

Limb muscles are rich in sensory innervation, the nerve fibres terminating as free nerve endings, paciniform endings associated with connective tissue, Golgi tendon organs and muscle spindles. The latter two types of ending are known to be important in reflex actions of muscle and will be discussed briefly.

Golgi tendon organs consist of the encapsulated endings of large myelinated axons (Group Ib), located at the musculotendinous junction. They lie in series with the muscle fibres and provide information to the central nervous system concerning muscle tension. Passive stretch applied to the muscle is a relatively ineffective stimulus within the physiological range of muscle lengths, but active muscular contraction is very effective, and a study by Houk and Henneman (1967) showed how specific individual tendon organ responses can be in relation to muscle contraction. They found, in the soleus muscle of the cat, that each tendon organ was sensitive to contraction in a group of 3–25 muscle fibres closely connected to it, and that contraction of one or two of these fibres could make the tendon organ discharge. Any one of 4–15 motor units could drive each tendon organ, this being due to the fact that the muscle fibres of a particular motor unit are not closely grouped together. As there are about 50 Golgi tendon organs in this muscle, there is the possibility that each tendon organ may have specific reflex effects

on small numbers of motor units, although this has not been tested. The general reflex effect of Golgi tendon organs is inhibitory upon contraction of the muscle in which they lie.

The muscle spindle is the most complex receptor found in muscle. The following account of its structure is largely based on the description by Boyd (1962). Basically, the spindle consists of one or more (usually at least two) afferent nerve fibre terminals supported by small, specialised muscle fibres, and enclosed within a well-defined capsule. One of the sensory terminals (the primary ending) is derived from a large myelinated afferent (Group Ia), and some of these afferent fibres have the largest diameters of any nerve fibres in the body. The ending is distributed to all the small intrafusal muscle fibres (2–12, but usually about 6) of the spindle in the mid-capsular or equatorial region. Branches of the ending spiral round each intrafusal fibre. Other endings (the secondary endings) are derived from rather smaller myelinated afferents (Group II), and are often selectively distributed to the smaller intrafusal fibres within the capsule, where they also appear as spirals. These spirals are arranged juxta-equatorially. Frequently, branches terminate on large intrafusal fibres also, but these endings are small and not obviously spiral.

The larger and smaller intrafusal fibres are called **nuclear bag** and **nuclear chain** fibres respectively, because of the grouping of their nuclei which, in both fibre types, are concentrated in the equatorial region of the spindle. In a transverse section, the profiles of several nuclei are seen in the nuclear bag fibres, whereas one only is seen in nuclear chain fibres, the nuclei lying in a single file or chain.

The functional complexity of the spindle is partly due to the presence of the two types of sensory endings. The primary ending is generally more sensitive to the velocity of stretch than is the secondary ending, although both provide information on static muscle length. A useful source of information on the physiology of muscle spindles is the monograph by Matthews (1972). However, the factor that makes the spindle highly complex is the presence of a specific motor supply to the intrafusal fibres, activity in which has marked effects upon spindle sensitivity. The specific motor supply is by small myelinated fibres (γ-motor) which are the axons of the small motor neurones mentioned previously. In some mammalian spindles a proportion of the motor supply is by branches from α-motor axons otherwise innervating the larger, tension-producing, extrafusal muscle fibres that make up the mass of the muscle. This type of innervation is conventionally referred to as β-innervation. This is confusing, as all sizes of α-motor neurones may supply spindles. Such an arrangement is the exclusive source of intrafusal motor supply in all the lower vertebrate spindles so far examined.

The motor supply to the mammalian muscle spindle may be divided into two parts on functional grounds, depending on whether motor activity predominantly affects spindle sensitivity to the rate of change of muscle length (velocity) or to static length. The two groups are called dynamic and static fusimotor functions respectively. There has been much controversy concerning the relationship between this functional division and what was seen anatomically in the spindle. This is a complex subject beyond the scope of the present discussion, but at least some resolution of the problems may have been achieved by the recent discovery that nuclear bag fibres are of two types, differing in their motor supply and contractile properties (*see* Barker, 1974 for structural differences; Boyd, 1976 for mechanical properties). They were first separated on the basis of their histochemistry (Ovalle and Smith, 1972). Previously, attempts had been made to match the physiological duality of dynamic and static fusimotor fibres with a proposed anatomical duality of separate γ-supplies to nuclear bag and nuclear chain intrafusal fibres. This idea turned out to be wrong, but it now seems likely that such an anatomical duality does exist in that dynamic fusimotor fibres terminate exclusively on one sort of nuclear bag fibre, and static fusimotor fibres terminate on the second sort of nuclear bag and also on nuclear chain fibres. There is still argument about how exclusive are these separate connections, but the general explanation is probably correct.

A major reflex effect of Ia afferents is excitation of the muscle in which they lie, and this is the basis of the stretch reflex where a muscle stretched in a decerebrate animal contracts against the stretching force. Many Ia afferent connections in the spinal cord are monosynaptic on to homonymous α-motor neurones. This is also true of at least some Group II afferents from spindles (Kirkwood and Sears, 1974). The reflex effects of Group II afferents are less well understood.

As in the case of the Golgi tendon organs, there is some evidence that individual spindles may be especially affected (their discharge being reduced) by the contraction of particular motor units (Binder, Kroin, Moore, Stauffer and Stuart, 1976), and certainly it would seem likely that motor units contributing β-innervation to particular spindles have a close functional connection with those spindles. At present there is nothing known about reflex effects at this refined level. There is some indication that γ-motor neurones are recruited in a fixed order during increasing voluntary effort (Burke, Hagbarth and Scuse, 1978) as are motor units (discussed later in this Chapter).

SOME PHYSIOLOGICAL PROPERTIES OF WHOLE MUSCLE

Later in this Chapter it will be shown that motor unit properties are spread over a wide range of tensions and contraction speeds. Anatomically distinct muscles often differ from one another in the proportions of motor unit types of which they are composed. A wider and more rigorous investigation can be made of a muscle than is possible for a single motor unit. Differences between muscles are therefore important in that the experimenter can infer motor unit action from a study of a single whole muscle which is believed to contain one dominant type of motor unit.

Tonic muscle

The remainder of this Chapter will be concerned with twitch muscle, which is the dominant skeletal muscle type in the mammal. However, in some sites, such as the extrinsic muscles of the eye (Hess and Pilar, 1963) the muscles of the middle ear (Erulkar, Shelanski, Whitsel and Ogle, 1969) and possibly the larynx (Rossi and Cortesina, 1965), another skeletal muscle type occurs and makes a significant contribution to the muscle contraction. This will be referred to as tonic muscle, although it is sometimes called slow muscle. All the muscles listed above are innervated by cranial nerves, and tonic muscle does not appear to occur in other parts of the body, although many of the intrafusal fibres of muscle spindles have comparable properties. Tonic muscle is striated although its microscopic structure is less well organised than that of twitch striated muscle. One important structural difference between the two types is that a normal adult twitch muscle fibre receives innervation from one axon giving rise to a single end-plate usually situated in the middle third of the muscle fibre; the tonic fibre is innervated by a number of end-plates, probably derived from several axons and distributed over the whole length of the muscle. The end-plates of tonic muscle fibres are smaller and have a simpler organisation with fewer terminals and less infolding of the muscle membrane. In parallel with this finding the release of transmitter is smaller at the tonic end-plate and does not result in a regenerative muscle action potential which propagates all along the fibre. In the tonic fibre, only a local end-plate (or junction) potential follows a single nerve impulse, and activation of the muscle fibre depends on depolarisation of the membrane at a number of end-plate sites with local decremental spread, even with tetanic stimulation. There appears to be a basic difference in membrane properties between the two fibre types, because tonic fibres do not respond with an action potential even when the membrane is stimulated directly by intracellular current injection. The contraction of twitch muscle will be described in detail below. Tonic muscle differs functionally in that typically no mechanical response can be recorded in response to a single nerve volley. Repetitive stimulation is necessary to elicit tension or shortening, and the extent of contraction depends on the rate of stimulation up to 200–300 stimuli per second. Even when maximally activated, tonic muscle develops less tension and shortens more slowly than twitch muscle, showing that there are also differences in the internal organisation and biochemistry of the two muscle types.

It is of interest to note that tonic muscle occurs in the extraocular muscles which have to perform very rapid movements. They are therefore mixed with twitch fibres which, to anticipate a later section, are the fastest-contracting in the body. It is not clear what advantage is derived from having muscles which are a mixture of the fastest and slowest in the body. Tonic muscle occurs more frequently in non-mammalian vertebrates and for a more detailed description of its properties the reader is referred to Hess (1970).

General structure of twitch muscle fibres

The structure of muscle is described in detail in Chapter 2, but some of those factors which influence function will be recalled here. The unit of structure is the muscle fibre, a syncytium of cells surrounded by the sarcolemma, by which the inner contractile elements are electrically activated. The sarcolemma consists of the plasma membrane of the muscle cells and a basement membrane of collagen and reticulum fibres of the endomysial connective tissue. Capillary blood vessels run through this fine sheath, which is continuous with the denser fibrous tissue subdividing the muscle into the fascicles which can be seen by the naked eye. The fibres are uniform over much of their length, but usually taper rapidly at their ends, although rounded or expanded ends are found. The ends are the regions of the fibre to which tendinous connections are made. Here, the collagenous connective tissue makes firm attachments to the outer membrane of the muscle fibre and tension is transmitted to the tendon, aponeurosis or periosteum. The maximum force of a muscle therefore depends on the number of muscle fibres connected to the tendon or, because fibres vary in their size, on the total cross-sectional area of the muscle. More strictly, tension depends on the number of myofilaments in the cross-section. The myofilaments (see below) are the sites for force development, and are present at higher density in fast- than slow-twitch muscle. In a multipennate muscle, a large number of short muscle fibres are obliquely inserted into a tendon which runs along much of the length of a muscle. This arrangement allows maximal potential for tension development for a given bulk of muscle.

The muscle fibre is subdivided longitudinally into units called sarcomeres, in mammals each being about 2.8 μm long when the muscle is at rest. Each sarcomere is able to shorten at a given velocity and the total shortening velocity of a muscle fibre is the sum of the velocities of its sarcomeres. Thus, a fibre which is 200 mm long will shorten twice as rapidly as one 100 mm long, if they are composed of similar sarcomeres (intrinsic differences between fast- and slow-twitch muscle will be described below). For a muscle to shorten as rapidly as possible it should, therefore, consist of long muscle fibres. Clearly, a compromise is necessary, as a muscle must develop sufficient force to achieve the tasks imposed upon it.

Muscle fibres range from a few to many centimetres in length. In cross-section, fibres are often polygonal and irregular, and are best measured by their areas. It is convenient, however, to represent a fibre by an estimated diameter, and the irregularity in normal muscle is not great enough to make such a measure inappropriate. In various vertebrate species the diameter of muscle fibres varies from about 10–100 μm. There is considerable variation between different species and groups, and within any species there is further variation between different muscles (*see* Schiefferdecker, 1909; Sissons, 1963; 1965). In man, small muscles, such as those of the eye, and the small hand muscles, have smaller fibres than the large muscles of the limbs and trunk. Some approximate values for normal adult muscles are given in Table 1.1, the information being taken from the literature already quoted, and from H.A. Sissons's material. The values are for fibre diameter as seen in paraffin

Table 1.1 Fibre diameter in various human muscles

Muscle	Approximate values for mean diameter of Muscle Fibres (μm)
Extrinsic muscles of eye	15
Platysma	20
Sternomastoid	30–35
Pectoralis major	40–45
Brachioradialis	30–35
First lumbrical	20
First dorsal interosseus	25
Biceps brachii	30–40
Sartorius	30–35
Gastrocnemius	40–50
Erector spinae	40–50

sections of formalin-fixed tissue, and are 25–30 per cent less than those for the fresh unfixed tissue.

In addition to differences between different muscles in the same individual, quite appreciable variations in mean fibre diameter are found when the same muscle is studied in different individuals (Sissons, 1963; 1965). This variation is probably attributable, in part, to differences in build and muscular development of the individuals concerned: it is, of course, an obstacle to any assessment of relatively minor changes of muscle diameter in pathological material. There are also differences in size between fibres of different histochemical type (*see below*). Figure 1.3 illustrates the variation in area between fibres from one muscle of a cat, which had been frozen for sectioning in a cryostat to minimise shrinkage. The total fibre population is shown in the top left histogram; the other three histograms show subdivisions based on histochemical fibre type. There are clear differences between the mean areas of the histochemical types, but there is a lot of overlap due to variation within the fibre-type populations. Figure 1.3 also shows how the mean diameters of the three fibre types increase with body size.

At birth, all fibres are thinner and shorter than in the adult. Growth in both dimensions occurs during postnatal development and in adult life when additional demands are placed on a muscle. Equally, atrophy will occur if a muscle is unused. Longitudinal growth occurs at the ends of the fibres by the addition of sarcomeres, the length of which remains constant throughout life (Westerman *et al.*, 1973). In the adult, sarcomeres will be laid down if unusual stretch is applied to the muscle (Goldspink, Tabary, Tabary, Tardieu and Tardieu, 1974). Lateral growth probably occurs by laying down new myofibrils which have an approximately constant diameter. No great change in the number of fibres occurs in postnatal development.

Details of the biochemical basis of contraction are given in Chapter 4, but a summary is necessary to understand the remainder of this chapter. The surface action potential initiates a regenerative depolarisation, which propagates down the transverse (T) tubules penetrating the whole muscle fibre inwards from the sarcolemma in the regions

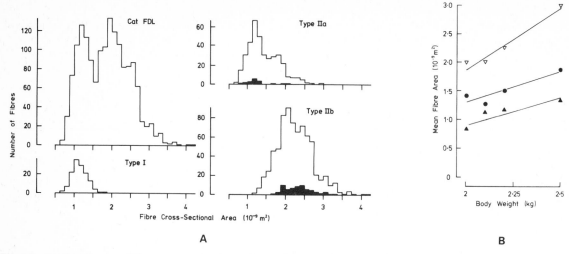

Fig. 1.3 (A) Distribution of fibre cross-sectional areas from a frozen section of a cat fast-twitch muscle. Top left: areas of about 1600 fibres. The other three histograms show the same fibres divided into three histochemical types. The shaded areas indicate fibres which do not fit exactly into the histochemical types. (B) Variation of fibre area with body weight in the cat. Types I (▲), IIa (●) and IIb (▽) have different mean areas, but all increase with body weight (from Edjtehadi and Lewis, 1979)

of the ends of the thick filaments. The activity of the T tubules excites longitudinal elements of the sarcoplasmic reticulum (SR) which run between the myofibril bundles. The specialised regions where the T tubules approach the SR are known as triads and a special coupling is necessary at this junction. The SR releases Ca^{++} which allows interaction of myosin and actin molecules in the thick and thin filaments. Both types of filament have active sites and, in the presence of free Ca^{++}, cross-bridges form between the active sites on thick and thin filaments. The cross-bridges are thought to change shape and cause the filaments to slide over each other. After the change is complete, the cross-bridge breaks and a new cross-bridge can form between a new pair of active sites. Cycles of bridge formation, bending and breaking are responsible for muscle shortening or tension development. A fuller description of the biophysics of muscle contraction has been clearly presented by Wilkie (1976).

The abilities to develop force and to shorten may be studied separately by isometric and isotonic recording. In the former, tension is recorded with the muscle held at constant length (although some shortening of the fibres will occur, together with lengthening of any tendon or other connective tissue elements included in the prep-

aration). Isotonic recording involves measurement of muscle length during contraction under constant load. Usually measurements are made at a number of loads from zero to near the maximum which the muscle can move, which is the maximum isometric tension. Isometric recording is the only technique which has been used extensively for studying the contraction of motor units. Isotonic recording is more difficult and may be considered to be invalid on the grounds that fibres of the shortening motor unit would be subjected either to the frictional forces or to the inertial load of adjacent inert fibres.

Contractions in the body are much more complex. For example, in performing one action a muscle may begin to contract isometrically until it develops sufficient force to move the load imposed on it. Additional force will be required to accelerate the load (either external or that of the moving part of the body). There may be a brief isotonic phase, but a controlled deceleration to end the action usually intervenes. During parts of many movements, antagonist muscles may be active and the agonist will have to produce force to oppose their action. However, the complex action of natural contractions may be predicated from the simplified responses which have been studied under experimental conditions. In the subsequent paragraphs, isometric and isotonic contractions will be described in more detail, together with the environmental factors which modify the response.

In these descriptions it will be necessary to distinguish between fast-twitch and slow-twitch muscle (see Fig. 1.8), remembering that these are both types of twitch muscle which contain predominantly fast-twitch and slow-twitch motor units respectively, but which are not always pure in this respect. Slow-twitch muscles are best known in quadrupedal mammals which have to support the weight of the body continuously during standing. Soleus, one of the heads of triceps surae, has usually been selected as an example of slow-twitch muscle, and in maintaining extension of the ankle it prevents flexion of this joint. Lateral gastrocnemius is the direct synergist of soleus and is a fast-twitch muscle. It has been used to compare reflex activation of the two types. However, gastrocnemius develops much more force than soleus and has a large number of slow-twitch motor units within itself. For these reasons, flexor digitorum longus (FDL) or extensor digitorum longus (EDL) have been chosen as better muscles for comparison of contractile properties with those of soleus.

The isometric twitch of fast-twitch muscle is some three times briefer than that of slow-twitch muscle. Similarly, the sarcomeres of fast muscle shorten three times as rapidly in isotonic contractions. These differences are consistent between species, even though there are absolute differences. In general, the smaller the animal the more rapid its muscles, so that the twitch of mouse soleus has approximately the same time course as that of cat FDL. These differences are reflected, for example, in the frequency of leg movement in running or in the respiratory rate of different species. Hill (1956) has suggested that such differences depend on the size of the animal. The short bones of a mouse will be subjected to smaller inertial forces during acceleration and can be accelerated more rapidly than those of a cat, without imposing stresses which could result in tearing or fracture.

Close (1971) developed the idea that isotonic shortening velocity is inversely related to isometric twitch contraction time. As indicated above, this is true when a broad range of animals is considered.

This relationship is not unexpected, because both characteristics of muscle depend on biochemical reactions of the actin–myosin cross-bridges. Bárány (1967) demonstrated that actomyosin ATPase activity is related to shortening velocity. Shortening velocity is probably limited by the rate at which cross-bridges can break, and the rate of development of tension depends on the rate of formation of cross-bridges. However, the contraction time of an isometric twitch depends not only on the latter factor but also on the extent and rates of release and removal of Ca^{++}. There is the possibility of dissociation of the two factors in the twitch, and this has been shown to happen in extraocular muscles (Close and Luff, 1974). These muscles have isometric twitch contraction times which are less than half those of fast-twitch limb muscles. However, eye and limb muscles have approximately the same sarcomere isotonic shortening velocities. Here, the difference between the twitches must lie largely in a difference in the time course of raised intrafibrillar Ca^{++}.

In man, posture does not depend on continuous activity of extensor muscles of the limbs, because the centre of gravity of the body at rest is almost directly above the pivots of the joints of the lower limb. Correspondingly, there is a relatively small difference between the contraction speed of soleus and gastrocnemius in man (Buller, Dornhorst, Edwards, Kerr and Whelan, 1959). There are differences between forelimb and hindlimb muscles, perhaps corresponding to differences in mass and inertial load. Most human muscles probably contain both fast- and slow-twitch motor units, but in different proportions throughout the body. In this way, differences between muscles in man may be compared to the differences between FDL and gastrocnemius, two predominantly fast-twitch muscles in the cat. It would be interesting to know more about the paravertebral muscles, some of which are tonically active.

The isometric twitch

The response of a muscle to a single stimulus is the twitch. Isometric twitches are illustrated later in Figure 1.8, which also shows the difference between fast- and slow-twitch muscle. The characteristic differences are seen in both the contraction and the relaxation phases. The tensions of the two muscles illustrated are approximately similar, but this is coincidental and depends on the size of the muscle chosen. However, if a proper comparison is made it is found that the tension per unit cross-sectional area is some 50 per cent higher in fast- than in slow-twitch muscle, which results in part from a greater density of myofibrils in the fibres of the former (Engel and Stonnington, 1974). The time course and the tension of the twitch may be influenced by a number of physiological factors such as muscle length, activity, temperature and adrenaline.

Increasing muscle length prolongs the twitch, the effect being greater on relaxation than on contraction. Length also affects twitch tension. There is an optimal length (close to natural resting length in the body) at which tension is maximal. If the muscle is shortened or lengthened it is able to develop less tension. This effect is considered in more detail in relation to tetanic tension.

The previous contractile history of a muscle affects its twitch. This is most clearly seen by eliciting a twitch before and after a brief tetanus. In fast-twitch muscle the post-tetanic twitch may be twice as large as the rested one. The increase of tension is accompanied by a corresponding increase in the rate of development of tension, so that the time course of the twitch is changed very little. Post-tetanic potentiation is possibly a consequence of the failure to activate the central myofibrils of a muscle fibre in a single twitch of rested muscle. In some way, a preceding tetanus may potentiate spread of activation from the surface membrane along the T tubules towards the centre of the fibre. In a slow-twitch muscle the effect of a preceding tetanus is a decrease in the twitch tension accompanied by a proportional decrease in the contraction and relaxation phases. Thus, the post-tetanic changes in fast and slow muscle are not exact mirror images. Smaller but similar effects are brought about by changing the rate at which a twitch is elicited. Little difference is seen between a rested twitch and one elicited once every 20 s, but at higher rates of stimulation, fast muscle is potentiated and slow-twitch muscle depressed.

If tetanic stimulation is continued, a decrease of tension is seen in both types of muscle and is referred to as fatigue. Fatigue is more rapid and pronounced in fast- than in slow-twitch muscle: a hundred or so brief tetani may reduce the tension of a fast-twitch muscle to zero but have little effect on a slow-twitch muscle. Fatigue reduces tetani, although less rapidly than twitches, and also impairs neuromuscular transmission. Slow-twitch muscle is resistant to fatigue for a number of reasons. Because its contraction is slower, biochemical reactions proceed at a lower rate in maintaining tension, that is, its contraction is more efficient. In addition, slow muscle has a better energy supply, with a higher capillary density and resting blood flow. The densities of mitochondrial oxidative enzymes and myoglobin are greater. (Compare the lower density of myofibrils: there is a reciprocal relationship between the two, so that the number of mitochondria per myofibril is higher in slow-twitch muscle). A caveat is necessary here; this comparison of the fatigue resistance of fast- and slow-twitch muscles depends on examples which classically have been chosen for detailed study. Fast and slow muscle have, in the past, been described as white and red (the colours depend largely on myoglobin content). However, it is now clear that speed of contraction and resistance to fatigue are not rigidly linked. It is possible to have a fast red muscle, that is, a fast-contracting muscle with a good ability to resist fatigue. Some jaw muscles are of this type, and at the motor unit level it has been shown to be a general phenomenon.

Temperature effects are important because many muscles are subjected to a wide range of temperatures. At rest in a cool environment the temperature in the muscles of the limb may be in the low thirties whereas, on maximal exercise, muscle temperature will be over 40°C. As the main source of heat, their temperature will be above that of the body. As muscle is warmed, its contractile properties will speed up, resulting in a reduction of the times of twitch contraction and twitch relaxation, and an increase in the speed of shortening. Many of the biochemical processes have a Q_{10} of more than two, so that a temperature change of the magnitude described above will result in an approximately two-fold increase in speed. Both fast and slow muscle show similar changes in their speeds of response, but their twitch tensions will be affected differently. An increase of temperature potentiates the twitch of slow muscle a little, but causes a fall in the fast-twitch by up to about one-third. This decrease may be caused by an increasing failure to activate the central regions of the muscle fibre as biochemical reactions speed up.

Finally, the effect of adrenaline on muscle must be considered. This is a β-effect and so is not produced by noradrenaline. At maximal physiological levels of adrenaline, an effect is clearly seen in slow-twitch muscle only, in which the twitch contraction and relaxation times are shortened with a decrease of tension. Fast muscle requires a five times greater adrenaline concentration to produce a maximal response. The effect is then to produce a potentiation of the twitch with prolongation of its time course. Adrenaline produces effects similar in direction to those of a preceding tetanus but, in contrast, the effects of adrenaline are more on the time course of the twitch than on the tension.

Isometric tetani

When stimuli are delivered at an interval less than the time course of the twitch, the tension builds up, giving rise to an unfused tetanus (Fig. 1.4). Decrease of the stimulus interval causes tetanic tension to increase up to a maximum when the stimulus interval is about one-tenth of the twitch duration. For example, a muscle with a twitch contraction time of 40 ms will have a total twitch duration of about 120 ms, and will produce maximal tetanic tension at a stimulus interval of 12 ms or 85 pulses/s. A sigmoidal relation exists between tension and stimulation frequency within the two limits. Stimulation at a frequency above that necessary to produce maximal tension has the further effect of increasing the rate of tension development (or the rate of shortening in an isotonic contraction). The rate of tension development (or shortening velocity) becomes maximal at a stimulus frequency some three times higher than that necessary for maximal tension (Buller and Lewis, 1965a). At even higher rates of stimulation, tension falls because of intermittent failure of the muscle action potential (Wedensky inhibition) but these rates are entirely unphysiological, as indeed

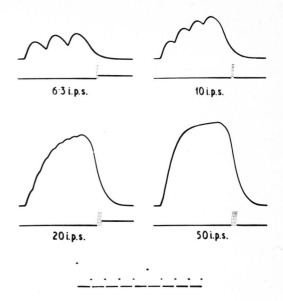

Fig. 1.4 The genesis of tetanus in a cat slow muscle (soleus). The stimulus frequencies are shown in impulses per second below each pair of traces. The lower trace of each pair indicates (by a series of dots) the peak tension developed by the contraction. Each dot represents 20 g (approximately 0.2N). Note the twitch/tetanus ratio of 0.22. Time marker: 100 ms between successive marks (by courtesy of A.J. Buller: Disorders of Voluntary Muscle, 3rd edn.)

are those necessary to produce the maximal rate of tension development.

However, in man and animals there is evidence for short bursts or pairs of high-frequency stimuli. Such short intervals produce very marked effects. Muscle fibres have a refractory period of about 1–2 ms (fast and slow respectively). At longer intervals, two stimuli produce a twitch-like contraction which becomes maximal at about twice twitch tension with a stimulus interval of 3–5 ms. Beyond 10 ms the muscle response declines again. The effect of the short interval lasts over several hundred milliseconds. If a stimulus is interposed in an unfused tetanic train, not only will there be an immediate increase in tension but also the tetanic tension will be higher than a control tetanus for hundreds of milliseconds (Burke, Rudomin and Zajac, 1976). These effects are probably a consequence of incomplete activation of the muscle fibre by a single muscle action potential in the mammal. The tension response is not just related to stimulus frequency, but it will also depend on the preceding stimulation patterns.

The length–tension relationship: muscle stiffness

Tetanic tension, like twitch tension, depends on muscle length. It is useful to consider the total tension in a muscle to be the sum of two components, the passive and active tensions (Fig. 1.5).

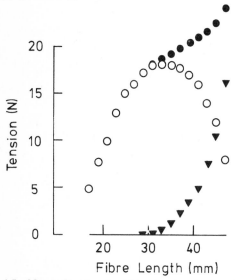

Fig. 1.5 Muscle fibre length and tension, in cat soleus. ▼: tension in inactive muscle (passive tension). ○: additional tension developed when the muscle was stimulated at 100/s (active tension). ●: total tension in stimulated muscle (passive + active tension)

The passive tension is the tension in an unstimulated muscle and it rises approximately exponentially with muscle length. It is present in an isolated muscle fibre because of the sarcolemma, but is increased in the whole muscle by parallel connective tissues. The relative magnitude of the passive tension depends on the amounts of connective tissue, so that a strong muscle sheath would produce a large effect, but it always becomes important at long muscle lengths. The active tension is taken as the difference between the total tension in a stimulated muscle and the passive tension. As it has its origin in the interaction of actin and myosin molecules in the thin and thick filaments of the myofibrils, active tension depends on the degree of overlap between the filaments and therefore on muscle length. At the optimal length, the active sites on the filaments are in maximal register and tension is greatest

(Gordon, Huxley and Julian, 1966). The shape of the active tension curve depends on the distribution of active sites on the muscle filaments, which is similar for all mammalian muscles when referred to the individual sarcomere. Thus the width of the length–tension curve depends simply on the number of sarcomeres in series, that is, on the muscle fibre length.

If a muscle is held at an abnormal length, sarcomeres are removed or laid down (at the ends of the fibre) as appropriate. In this way the muscle adjusts its length so that the sarcomeres always perform around their optimal length (Crawford, 1961; Goldspink et al., 1974).

Although active tension decreases at long lengths, this change is more than compensated for by the exponential increase in passive tension. Passive tension resists extension as well as active tension, although it cannot be responsible for muscle shortening unless the load on the muscle decreases. The shape of the muscle tension–length curve gives the muscle a response to unexpected loads on the muscle. A sudden increase in load initially will increase muscle length, but the length change will cause an increase in muscle tension which in turn will resist further increase in length. The muscle response therefore anticipates the stretch reflex, and, because it occurs immediately without conduction delays, it is important. This form of negative feedback seems to be small if the length–tension diagram of Figure 1.5 is considered alone. However, a much larger effect is seen with smaller dynamic changes. The dynamic response of a muscle may be measured from the tension oscillations produced by small length changes, the ratio of the tension change to the length change being the dynamic stiffness. Dynamic stiffness may be more than ten times greater than the stiffness measured from static tension–length curves. Moreover, dynamic stiffness is proportional to the tension developed by the muscle: the stronger a contraction, the stiffer the muscle and so the more it is able to resist a sudden change of load. This proportionality occurs because much of the dynamic stiffness is located in the cross-bridges of active muscle.

The resistance of a muscle to extension also depends on the velocity at which it is extended. Figure 1.6 shows that, during active extension of a muscle, the tension increases above the final rest level, and that the degree of overshoot increases with the velocity of extension. Thus, the more rapidly a sudden additional load is applied to an active muscle, the greater will be its response. It should be noted that, if the extension is too rapid, the extra tension may collapse and even fall below the final rest level. This collapse occurs at lower velocities when tetani are elicited at the lower rates of weak physiological contractions (Fig. 1.6a, b; Joyce, Rack and Westbury, 1969).

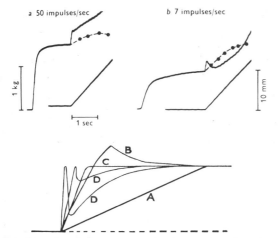

Fig. 1.6   The tension response of active muscle to forced extension. The lower diagram represents a muscle stimulated tetanically. Once a steady isometric tension had been established, the active muscle was extended at different velocities (A-D, superimposed traces: Gasser and Hill, 1924). In the upper part of the Figure are experimental records from cat soleus. The same velocity of extension was applied in the two records, but the muscle was being stimulated at a high rate in *a* and a low rate in *b* (Joyce, Rack and Westbury, 1969)

Thus, in many ways the direct response of the muscle to extension parallels and anticipates muscle reflexes. In some situations the muscle response may be small compared with the reflex, for example, in stretch of extensors of the decerebrate cat (Matthews, 1969). Elsewhere the muscle responses may dominate, for example in the control of biting force of the conscious monkey (Goodwin, Hoffman and Luschei, 1978).

The fully fused tetanus is relatively little affected by the other factors which produce large changes in the twitch. A fall of temperature results in a maximal fall of less than 10 per cent of tetanic tension. At physiological levels, adrenaline has no effect on isometric tension or isotonic shortening velocity. Preceding activity reduces tetanic tension only when there is already considerable fatigue of the twitch.

Most physiological contractions lie between twitches and fully fused tetani and are very susceptible to external factors: any influence which changes the amplitude *or* the duration of the twitch will change the unfused tetanus. Therefore, although adrenaline has a relatively small effect on twitch tension it will produce a marked decrease of the unfused tetanus of slow muscle because of the shortening of contraction and relaxation times. One action which might not be anticipated is that of muscle length on the unfused tetanus. The optimum length for twitch tension is close to that for tetanic tension, but an unfused tetanus is maximal at much longer lengths (Rack and Westbury, 1969: Fig. 1.7). This follows from the fact that, at long lengths, although twitch tension is less than at shorter lengths, the twitch is prolonged and more effective summation occurs. As a consequence, physiological (unfused) contractions show an increase of active tension with length up to much longer limits than would be anticipated from studies of twitches or fully fused tetani.

Electromyographic (EMG) studies in man show that when a motor unit of one of the intrinsic

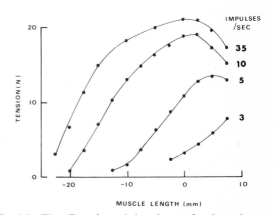

Fig. 1.7   The effect of muscle length on unfused tetani. Mean tetanic tension of cat soleus has been measured at a number of muscle lengths: each curve represents tetani elicited at a different frequency (indicated on the right). Note how the peak (optimum length) of the curve is shifted towards long lengths at lower frequencies of stimulation. Twitch contractions would have an optimum near 0 mm, which is the length at which the muscle is held when the cat is in a normal standing posture (from Rack and Westbury, 1969)

muscles of the hand is recruited it begins to fire at about 8/s, which just produces fusion (Milner-Brown, Stein and Yemm, 1973c). Increase in firing rate occurs with increasing effort up to a level at which it is impossible to distinguish individual units, but it would seem that the whole range of the ascending portion of the sigmoid tension–frequency curve is used. At moderate levels of contraction, motor units will be producing unfused tetani. The whole muscle response is smooth because motor neurones discharge asynchronously, and the peaks of one motor unit contraction will, on average, cancel out the troughs of another. Experimentally, the same result may be achieved by dividing into fine parts the ventral root supplying a muscle.. Each division is stimulated at the same frequency as, but out of phase with, the others, thus smoothing an unfused contraction. As few as five subdivisions is sufficient to smooth the response and this technique has been used to elicit several of the results of Figure 1.7.

Neural influence on muscle. The differences between fast and slow muscle are not fixed. The differences are not present at birth, and alteration of the innervation of a muscle will change its contraction (Fig. 1.8). This was first demonstrated by Buller, Eccles and Eccles (1960b) who showed that a fast muscle became slow-contracting when innervated by a nerve which originally had supplied a slow muscle. Later investigations demonstrated that many aspects of the contraction were changed by cross-innervation or other neural modifications (*see below*). Isotonic shortening velocity (Close, 1969), rate of isometric tension development (Buller and Lewis, 1965b), the effect of temperature or a tetanus on the twitch (Buller and Pope, 1977) can be modified. Biochemically, myosin ATPase activity (Bárány and Close, 1971; Buller, Mommaerts and Seraydarian, 1971), myosin light chains (Sréter, Gergely, Salmons and Romanul, 1973) and oxidative enzymes (Pette, Smith, Staudte and Vrbová, 1973) can also be

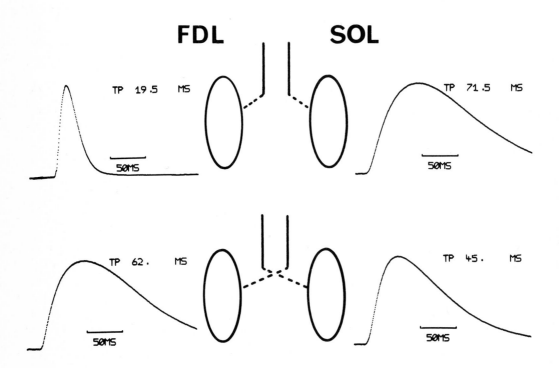

Fig. 1.8   Fast and slow twitch muscles, and the effects of reinnervation. Diagrams represent self-reinnervation (above) and cross-reinnervation (below). Beside each diagram is an isometric twitch myogram from the corresponding cat muscle, with the twitch time to peak or contraction time indicated as 'TP'. The self-reinnervated muscle contractions are identical with those of normal muscle. FDL is fast-twitch and soleus is slow-twitch (after Buller, 1972)

modified, as can muscle blood supply (Hudlická, Brown, Cotter, Smith and Vrbová, 1977).

The original experiments brought about changes in muscle characteristics by cross-reinnervation, but at the same time it was shown that reduction of motor neurone activity prevented normal postnatal maturation (Buller, Eccles and Eccles, 1960a). The importance of activity in determining muscle properties was clearly demonstrated by Salmons and Vrbová (1969), who stimulated a fast muscle nerve at 10 pulses/s (a rate characteristic of slow motor neurones) over several weeks. The activity pattern can act directly on muscle, and direct stimulation of denervated muscle will change its properties (Lømo, Westgaard and Dahl, 1974). These experiments demonstrate that activity, of itself, will modulate muscle properties, but do not exclude the possibility that the nerve also releases a trophic chemical (Buller *et al.*, 1960b). Many authors regard a hypothesis regarding a trophic chemical as redundant, but there is indirect evidence of such a factor (Drachman, 1974; McComas, Upton and Jorgensen, 1974). A good review of trophic effects on muscle has been presented by Rosenthal (1977), but since then, more direct evidence of a chemical trophic action has been found. Gilliatt, Westgaard and Williams (1978) have demonstrated that prolonged pressure block of baboon nerves induces muscle hypersensitivity to acetylcholine, as would be expected from the inactivity following failure of propagation of nerve action potentials. The degree of hypersensitivity was, however, less than that produced by denervation, arguing for the lack of something more than activity in this latter case. Mathers and Thesleff (1978) found a similar quantitative difference between the level of hypersensitivity induced by denervation and tetrodotoxin nerve block. The latter produces a smaller change, which is also of later onset.

A reciprocal interaction between muscle and nerve is seen. Motor neurone properties are dependent on contact with the muscle (Kuno, Miyata and Mũnos-Martinez, 1974) and axon conduction velocity depends on the type of muscle innervated (Lewis, Bagust, Webb, Westerman and Finol, 1977).

METHODS OF STUDY OF MOTOR UNITS

The methods of functional isolation of single motor units may be divided into two general classes. One class consists of methods that are essentially random, while the methods of the other class involve some element of selection. Clearly, methods of the first class should be used whenever possible, and if, as is often the case in human studies, the selective methods must be used, the results originating from such techniques must be interpreted with caution.

A number of random methods are available for use in experimental animals. Glass micro-electrodes may be used to penetrate single motor neurones: this method was first reported by Devanandan, Eccles and Westerman (1965), and has been much extended by Burke and his colleagues, as described later in this chapter. The micro-electrode may be used both to record the electrical properties and activity of the penetrated motor neurone soma and to stimulate it. The current needed to stimulate is so small that adjacent motor neurones are not activated and therefore the peripheral nerve axon and the muscle fibres of that motor neurone will respond in isolation and their properties can be studied. The somata of γ-motor neurones are more difficult to maintain with a penetrating microelectrode, and the method is therefore selective for α-motor neurones, but within the latter class there seems to be no further selection.

The alternative method of random isolation used in animals involves dissection of motor axons, either in peripheral nerves or in ventral roots. The former is more difficult technically because of extensive connective tissue holding the axons together. It also has the disadvantage that an apparent motor unit may derive from a branch of an axon (*see below*) rather than from the whole neurone. There seems to be little or no branching of motor axons within the spinal column. The ventral roots have little connective tissue; it is therefore easy to tease them into fine bundles with watchmakers' forceps. The bundles will not necessarily contain only one axon, because the experimental technique involves denervating all muscles in a limb or region except one, so that the bundle may contain many axons if only one of these supplies the muscle under study. This method of ventral root splitting was first described in the isolation of motor units by Denslow and Gutensohn (1950) and has been the one used most extensively. Even in young kittens (with small axons) the proportion of α- to γ-axons obtained by ventral root splitting (Bagust, Lewis and Westerman, 1974) is similar to that estimated histologically.

In man, non-selective methods can be applied in the nerve, and include micro-electrode penetration or dissection of axons (Burke, Hagbarth, Löfstedt and Wallin, 1976). The techniques have been used to study sensory axons from muscle, and could be applied to motor unit studies but would be liable to isolate branches of axons. Micro-electrodes guided through needles inserted through the skin to a nerve have been used to record from single axons. Used directly, these could give information about motor neurone activity, but the recorded action potentials could also be used to trigger recordings of muscle activity in the same way that EMG potentials have been used (see below) but with the advantage of non-selectivity. Small electrodes have been implanted in animals in the roots (Prochazka, Westerman and Ziccone, 1977) and in parts of the central nervous system, and could be used for examining motor units.

Needle exploration of muscle is a technique commonly employed in man, and wire electrodes have been implanted into muscles of other animals. These electrodes are usually employed to record EMG activity of motor units. The needles are threaded with one or more insulated wires and electrical activity is recorded between pairs of wires, or between one wire and the needle, either at the tip or through side holes in the needle. It will be shown later that most muscle fibres of a motor unit are surrounded by fibres of other motor units: a muscle electrode must therefore record from fibres of more than one motor unit. During weak contractions an electrode may have only one active motor unit within its recording territory, and useful information about the patterns of that unit's activity can be obtained. During strong contractions the muscle electrode will record from several or many motor units and the information will be confused. Later motor units will be shown

to be recruited in a specific order: those motor units which can be recorded cleanly at low levels of total activity will therefore be low threshold motor units. The recorded EMG provides useful information about motor neuronal patterns of activity, but the possibility of bias must always be considered.

A later development has been to use the EMG potentials to enable the mechanical properties of the muscle fibres of the motor unit to be studied. To do this, total muscle tension is averaged, and each sweep of the averager is triggered by a clear EMG spike (Stein, French, Mannard and Yemm, 1972). Depending upon the extent of general activity of the muscle after a number of sweeps have been averaged a myograph of the motor unit contraction will be obtained. The contractions recorded will be part of an unfused tetanus (Milner-Brown, Stein and Yemm, 1973a) because of the frequency of discharge of motor neurones. In some individuals, motor units are synchronised to some extent, and the average myograms will be the response of several units. Obviously, motor unit myograms recorded in this way will be subject to the same bias as the original EMG spikes.

A needle electrode may also be used for stimulating within the muscle. This technique was first described by Buchthal and Schmalbruch (1970). Sometimes the needle stimulates fibre fascicles but, if correctly placed, it will stimulate a nerve branch and, if the nerve action potential propagates into all other branches of the axon, it will stimulate a motor unit (Stephens and Taylor, 1975). It is possible that antidromic action potentials will not be able to invade large branches, in which case not all of the motor unit will be recorded. This method is also liable to be selective. It is true that the needle can be introduced randomly, but the probability of a motor axon being selected must depend on the extent of its branches. Therefore, the larger the motor unit the higher will be the probability of its being stimulated.

Finally, motor units have been examined by stimulating a muscle nerve electrically. The threshold of an axon in a nerve depends on two factors. One factor is the anatomical position of the axon within the nerve, and its relation to the stimulating electrode. This factor is likely to be random in relation to the axonal properties. The second factor, however, will introduce bias. Motor units with large tensions have large-diameter axons and these will have low thresholds to electrical stimulation. The relative magnitude of the two factors will determine the degree of bias.

In this last type of motor unit isolation, the electrical stimulus is increased above threshold, so that motor units are recruited and successive increments of response can be measured. The increments are assumed to be the responses of motor units. There are some problems with this assumption. First, two motor axons may have very similar thresholds. To distinguish between two such motor units, the stimulus must be increased in very small steps and held at each new value for several responses in order to test for all-or-none behaviour. Such rigorous testing is difficult in man and some apparent motor units will be double. A second problem is that the latency of a response depends on stimulus strength, so that the EMG of a motor unit will occur later after the stimulus, when the stimulus is at threshold, than when the stimulus is increased. Such a change in timing might be interpreted as recruitment of a new motor unit or, conversely, if small changes of the EMG are ignored, the recruitment of small motor units will be missed. The second problem becomes more serious after a number of units have been recruited. The method is therefore limited to the first half dozen motor units which can be stimulated, with a possible increased chance of bias. The mean muscle motor unit amplitude can be calculated from these observations. It has been commented that mean values vary greatly from subject to subject. Such variability is to be expected from a small sample (a few per cent of the total number in a muscle) particularly as most muscles have a skewed distribution of motor unit sizes (*see below*). The ratio of the maximal muscle response to the mean motor unit response gives an estimate of the number of motor units in the muscle. An additional source of error in this estimate could be non-linear summation of motor unit responses. If the chosen response were the muscle twitch, there is evidence for non-linear summation (Brown and Matthews, 1960; Lewis, Luck and Knott, 1972). Usually the EMG has been chosen as the muscle response (Sica and McComas, 1971a) on the

assumption that motor unit EMG potentials summate linearly. However, there is evidence of non-linearity in the summation of the motor unit EMG when the muscle response is near maximal (Parry, Mainwood and Chan, 1977). Such non-linear behaviour would lead to an underestimate of the number of motor units. Despite the numerous problems of interpretation, this last method has been applied extensively and can yield useful information if the possible sources of error are taken into account.

MECHANICAL PROPERTIES OF MOTOR UNITS

We have seen in the preceding sections that whole muscles in animals and man differ widely in the contraction times of the isometric twitch and in their rate of tension development during a tetanus. In addition, there are large differences in the properties of maximal tetanic tension developed at different frequencies of stimulation, and in the stimulus frequencies required to give fused tetani. Differences also exist in the ratio of twitch tension to maximal tetanic tension (twitch–tetanus ratio) between different muscles. These different properties of whole muscles are interrelated to various extents.

In the preceding section, the methods used to study single motor unit properties are described. These methods have shown that the majority of muscles studied in animals and man contain a mixture of motor units with varying properties, so that the mechanical characteristics of each muscle are determined precisely by the range of properties and the proportions of the various motor units it contains. Considerable effort has been devoted to attempts at classifying motor units into a limited number of types. This can be done, to a certain extent, on the basis of histochemical differences between muscle fibres and, since the introduction of the method of glycogen depletion, this has been extended to single motor units. Histochemical classifications will be discussed briefly later in this Chapter, and are dealt with more extensively in Chapter 8. Attempts to use mechanical differences have not been entirely straightforward, largely because in many muscles the mechanical properties of motor units are distributed continuously between extremes, often with a skewed distribution, and sometimes with more than one peak in the distribution histogram. Under these conditions it is often not clear where the limits lie between one type and the next, although in some muscles discontinuous distributions are found, which simplifies this problem. The other source of difficulty has been in relating the mechanical characteristics to the histochemical profiles of motor units in such a way that clear types emerge by convergence of these two sources of information. There is some progress here, and this will be discussed later in this Chapter. However, at present it is difficult to escape from the impression that not all motor units will conform to a rigid classification.

When considering the mechanical properties of motor units we are, at present, concerned only with isometric properties. Because of the problems of frictional and inertial loading by the whole muscle on the shortening occurring in that fraction represented by the single motor unit, there is no information on the separate isotonic properties of motor units.

Homogeneity of muscle fibre properties within motor units

It is generally considered that, at least in muscles without polyneuronal innervation of the fibres, all the muscle fibres within a motor unit have very similar mechanical properties. One reason for believing this to be the case is that the isometric twitch of a motor unit consists of a smooth development and relaxation of tension, with one clear peak and no secondary humps. This is true even in small units consisting of few fibres. On the other hand, many muscles consist of motor units displaying a wide variety of contraction times, so that in extreme cases some units take as long to reach peak twitch tension as others take to complete their twitch and relax. Therefore, there could not be an indiscriminate mixture of the muscle fibres present in the muscle within its motor units. The same argument applies for other motor unit properties in which a wide variation is found within muscles. The ranges of these properties are discussed below.

So far, there has been no detailed measurement of the narrowness of this homogeneity. This would be difficult to obtain, as it would necessitate stimulating individually and recording the twitches of a number of single muscle fibres in a motor unit with known mechanical properties. However, there is one study that provides strong support for the generally held view of homogeneity of contraction characteristics among muscle fibres of a motor unit. Emonet-Dénand, Laporte and Proske (1971) found that a quarter of the motor axons innervating the first superficial lumbrical muscle in the cat also innervated the second superficial lumbrical. Thus, single motor units were split between the two muscles. It was found that the contraction times of the two parts of each motor unit were, in most cases, the same or very similar, even though the contraction times of these split units spanned a wide range (45–85 ms). As we shall see, histochemical studies also indicate that motor units are largely or completely homogeneous in their muscle fibre content.

The picture of motor unit homogeneity may not be as simple in muscles where fibres are innervated polyneuronally (Ridge and Thomson, 1978; Thomson, 1978). Polyneuronal innervation is very uncommon or non-existent in normal adult mammalian limb muscles, although it is common in fetal and neonatal muscle and occurs at least transitorily in re-innervated adult muscle. It also occurs in adults in some muscles of the head, and is common in limb muscles of lower vertebrates.

Contraction time and unit size

In the triceps surae of the cat. There are wide ranges of motor unit sizes and contractile properties in many individual muscles and, presumably, this underlies the fact that the same muscle may be called upon to exert a wide range of effects in life. For example, in his study of the characteristics of motor units in triceps surae of the cat, Burke (1967) stimulated single units by intracellular current injection of motor neurone somata. He found that the units could be divided into two distinct groups on the basis of their contraction times; a fast group (designated F) with contraction times of 30 ms or less, and a slow group (designated S) with contraction times of

40 ms or more. All the units found in soleus were of the S type, those in gastrocnemius being of F and S types in a ratio of about 3:1. The distribution of motor unit tetanic tensions for F and S units overlapped but, in the data presented, 43 F units developed tension greater than 0.2 N (maximal 2.1 N), whereas all the S units (28) and only nine F units developed tensions less than 0.2 N⋆.

Thus, on the basis of the contraction time of its units, soleus muscle in the cat is a pure muscle (slow), whereas gastrocnemius is mixed (faster). As we shall see, the histochemical profiles of muscle fibres in the two muscles lead to the same conclusion. In addition, there are differences in resistance to fatigue between the whole muscles and between the different motor units found in them. Slow muscles, such as soleus, have a richer blood supply with a greater density of capillaries, and the muscle fibres have more numerous mitochondria (Gauthier, 1969) and are less easily fatigued (McPhedran, Wuerker and Henneman, 1965). The resistance to fatigue of individual motor units in the cat was studied by Burke and his colleagues (Burke, Levine, Tsairis and Zajac, 1973; Burke, Levine, Salcman and Tsairis, 1974). By subjecting each unit to a repeating regime of tetanic stimulation, it was found that some units took much longer to fatigue than others. The slow units in gastrocnemius, and most of the slow units in soleus, showed little or no fatigue even after an hour of the stimulation regime (S units). The fast units, on the other hand, fell into two classes, one being much more fatigue-resistant than the other (FR and FF respectively).

These differences in motor unit populations between the two muscles (and the differences in whole-muscle properties that they underlie) should lead us to expect at least a partial segregation in the functional roles of the two muscles, and recent EMG and force measurements in medial gastrocnemius and soleus of the cat *in situ* provide good evidence of this (Walmsley, Hodgson and Burke, 1978). In this study, force transducers were chronically implanted on to the

tendons of medial gastrocnemius and soleus, and the EMG was continuously monitored via implanted electrodes. The cats were then allowed to recover from the anaesthetic and walked, ran and jumped naturally. It was found that both muscles were involved in locomotion from slow walking to fast running, and were active at the same part of the step cycle, although there was some difference between the two: force production by soleus was fairly constant throughout this range of activity, whereas that of gastrocnemius altered three-fold. The greatest differences in function between the two muscles were shown when the cat was standing quietly or jumping vertically. When the cat was standing, soleus developed tensions (11.7–13.7 N) not much lower than those developed during locomotion (and at times probably representing recruitment of all the units firing near-maximally), whereas gastrocnemius made a minor contribution (about 5 N). When the cat jumped, gastrocnemius developed its full isometric tetanic tensions (and sometimes up to 15 per cent more than this—as much as 81 N). Thus, this study confirmed, and provided measurements of, the predominantly phasic activity of medial gastrocnemius in rapid movements, and demonstrated the role of soleus in posture and slow walking. As the authors point out, the different characteristics of the motor unit populations of these two muscles match the division of labour between the muscles during natural function. Other motor unit properties to be discussed in this Chapter will reinforce this view. Evidence that any pure fast muscles exist in the cat hind limb has not yet been produced. For instance, in flexor digitorum longus muscle (FDL) which is a fast-contracting muscle, although there is no clear secondary peak in the distribution histogram of either unit contraction time or tetanic tension, both show a skewed distribution (highly skewed towards long times in the case of contraction time) and quite wide ranges (Olson and Swett, 1966; Goslow, Stauffer, Nemeth and Stuart, 1972; Bagust, Knott Lewis, Luck and Westerman, 1973), although less wide than those reported in gastrocnemius (Wuerker, McPhedran and Henneman, 1965). These skewed distributions contrast with the symmetrical distributions found in soleus (Bagust, 1974). The fibres in FDL are not homogeneous histochemi-

⋆The newton (N) is the SI unit of force, and is defined as the force required to accelerate a mass of 1 kg to a velocity of 1 m/s in 1 s. In more practical terms, 0.981 N is the force exerted by gravity on a 100 g weight. Therefore, a tension of 0.2 N is approximately equal to 20 g.

cally, and the muscle is therefore not pure. The distributions of units in FDL and soleus are shown in Figure 1.9.

virtually pure fast muscle, whereas soleus is mixed (slow). Mean values for the contraction times ($\pm$SD) of these groups were: EDL fast,

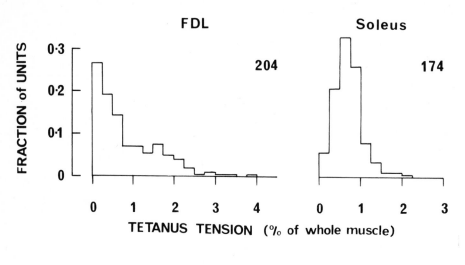

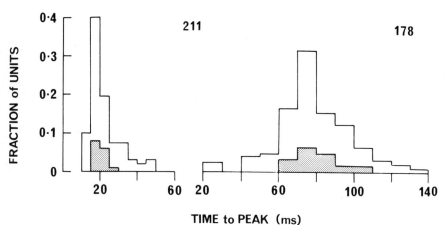

Fig. 1.9 Distributions of motor unit tetanic tensions (upper) and contraction times (lower) in cat fast (FDL—left) and slow (soleus—right) twitch muscles. Pooled data from about 25 cats. The stippled areas indicate the contraction times of the muscles from which the motor units were isolated functionally. Number of units shown on each histogram (data from Bagust, Knott, Lewis, Luck and Westerman, 1973; Bagust, 1974; Finol, Lewis and Webb, unpublished)

Motor units in other muscles. The distribution of motor units in limb muscles of the rat provides an interesting contrast to that in the cat. Motor unit properties in soleus and extensor digitorum longus (EDL) were examined by Close (1967), who found that EDL contained one group of units with short and symmetrically distributed contraction times (with one intermediate type of unit, slower than the others), whereas soleus had two groups of units, neither of which was the same as those in EDL. Therefore, in the rat, EDL is a

10.8$\pm$1.07 ms; soleus intermediate, 17.4$\pm$1.7 ms, and slow, 38.0$\pm$3.7 ms.

These rat muscles are faster-contracting than their homologues in the cat and, as well as being smaller, contain fewer motor units (soleus contains about 27 slow and three intermediate units; EDL contains about 40 fast units). The distributions of the tetanic tensions developed by the three types of unit overlapped completely.

The mouse has even faster-contracting muscles. Hitherto, very little information has been published on motor units or histochemistry of muscle fibres in the mouse. It is important that this deficiency is removed as soon as possible because the mouse is becoming an important laboratory animal in neurobiology, largely due to the availability of various mutants with clearly defined neurological lesions; the resulting clinical signs include muscular dystrophies and locomotor and postural disorders.

A range of mechanical properties of motor units has been found in muscles other than the limb muscles of the cat and rat. For example Andersen and Sears (1964) found, in cat intercostal muscles, that unit contraction times fell into two groups, with mean contraction times of 24.6 and 47 ms. By contrast, the deep and superficial lumbrical muscles of the cat have a small number of motor neurones with a fairly wide range of contraction times, but the distribution appears to be continuous, and fast and slow groups could not be differentiated (Bessou, Emonet-Dénand and Laporte, 1963; Appelberg and Emonet-Dénand, 1967). The range of contraction times (15–45 ms, superficial lumbrical) is here rather less than in the intercostal and considerably less than in triceps surae. It is interesting that these units do not conform to the classification applied in triceps surae on the basis of mechanical properties and resistance to fatigue (Kernell and Sjöholm, 1975). With respect to sensitivity to fatigue, the fast units seemed analogous to FF units in gastrocnemius, while the slow units seemed analogous to FR units in gastrocnemius. However with respect to tetanic 'sag' and post-tetanic effects, the slow lumbrical units resembled gastrocnemius S units, and some of the contraction times were as long. A correlative study with unit glycogen depletion and muscle fibre histology in this muscle could be very useful. Single motor units have been examined in rat segmental tail muscles (Steg, 1964; Andrew and Part, 1972). A wide range of contraction times was found and, in this case, the units fell into two groups. The slow units had a mean contraction time of 50.9 ± 7.1 (SD) ms, and the fast units 16.2 ± 1.9 ms.

In the baboon's forearm, Eccles, Phillips and Wu Chien-ping (1968) found in extensor digitorum communis an unusually narrow range of motor unit contraction times and twitch tensions (they did not measure tetanic tensions). Units were small, only 8.7 per cent of the sample developing twitch tensions greater than 50 mN. In 97 per cent of the units, contraction time fell between 15 and 35 ms. Perhaps this rather uniform set of small motor units has evolved to serve fine manipulative movements.

Muscles containing a range of motor unit contraction times and tetanic tensions have been described in frog (Knott, 1971; Luff and Proske, 1976), *Xenopus* toad (Ridge and Thomson, 1977) and snake (Hammond and Ridge, 1978).

Motor units in man. Motor unit contraction times have been measured in certain muscles of man. Sica and McComas (1971) recorded twitch contractions in extensor hallucis brevis. A wide range was found (35–98 ms), with a fairly narrow range of twitch tensions. Although the range of contraction times was continuous this distribution had two peaks, one at 46–50 ms, and the other between 86 and 94 ms. The fast distribution was skewed towards long contraction times, and the slow peak was roughly symmetrically placed in the slow population. In the first dorsal interosseus muscle there is also a wide range of motor unit contraction times (30–100 ms) and twitch tensions (about 1–100 mN; Milner-Brown *et al.*, 1973a). The distribution of contraction times did not show a clear separation into two peaks, although it is possible that those units with contraction times greater than 70 ms were drawn from a separate population. Over 80 per cent of the units had contraction times shorter than 70 ms. Remarkably similar ranges were found by Yemm (1977) in jaw muscles (masseter and temporalis). Motor units in human gastrocnemius have been shown recently to have two peaks in the distribution of contraction times, one major one between 60 and 80 ms, and a smaller one between 100 and 120 ms (Garnett, O'Donovan, Stephens and Taylor, 1978; 1979). The total range for all units was 40–110 ms. On examining the resistance to fatigue of the units, a close parallel emerged with the unit populations in cat gastrocnemius. Slow units were uniformly fatigue-resistant and showed weak tetanic tensions, whereas the fast group contained fatigue-resistant (FR) units with low tetanic tensions, and easily fatigued units (FF) with high tetanic tensions. A similar picture concerning resistance to fatigue of units had been observed previously in the first dorsal interosseus muscle by Stephens and Usherwood (1975). Here, the slow units with small twitch tensions were much less easily fatigued than the fast units with larger twitch tensions. Interestingly, within the fast group, resistance to fatigue was inversely and significantly related to twitch force.

A word of caution is appropriate concerning comparisons of contraction times between human and animal muscle. Human muscle is likely to be at a temperature below 37°C, especially in muscles of the extremities, whereas muscles in experimental mammals are generally controlled at 37°C. Since the Q_{10} (temperature coefficient) for contraction times is a little over two (Ranatunga, 1977), human muscles and motor units may be significantly slowed as a result of reduced temperature. Ideally, in experiments on man a small thermistor should be inserted into the muscle and temperature measured directly.

Fusion frequencies

The range of speeds of contraction found in different muscles and motor units may be important in the natural functioning of muscle, especially as the maximum rate of tension development is inversely related to contraction time (*see* Buller and Lewis, 1965a). In general, the fastest-contracting muscles are those which in nature move small inertial loads—for example, the extraocular muscles and muscles moving the digits. There are also other characteristics of muscles related to contraction time that are of obvious functional importance. We have seen already that slow-contracting units are resistant to fatigue, whereas some fast units are much less resistant. Another is the fact that the proportion of maximal tetanic tension developed during a tetanus at low stimulus frequency is greater in slow muscles than it is in fast. As one would expect, this is also true at the motor unit level (Andersen and Sears, 1964). For example, Burke (1967) found that the slow-contracting group of units in the triceps surae of the cat had median fusion frequencies (the median of frequencies required to produce a smooth tension plateau in individual units) of 25 shocks/s,

compared with 85 shocks/s for the fast-contracting group. Because tension development is maximal during a fused tetanus, this means that slow units, tonically active in life, are maximally effective at lower motor neuronal firing frequencies than are fast units, and this will hold proportionately at frequencies less than those required for fusion. This would seem to be an economical design.

HISTOCHEMICAL PROPERTIES OF MUSCLE FIBRES

By cutting frozen sections, and by using specific staining reactions leading to coloured or black products (*see* Ch. 8), it is possible to demonstrate the presence and approximate relative activities of various enzymes in muscle, and there are standard histological staining methods for the fuels glycogen and fat. If serial or semi-serial sections are cut and processed separately in different ways, a histochemical profile of individual muscle fibres in the muscle may be built up. Various muscles from a range of animals have been studied in this way. The methods commonly used so far are not quantitative in biochemical terms, but they are very useful for making comparisons between fibres. In most cases, intensity of staining has been assessed subjectively by eye and expressed on a three-point scale of dark, medium and light (or equivalent synonyms). Recently, attempts have been made to reduce subjectivity by using microphotometric measurements. For example, Spurway (1978) has applied an extensive range of histochemical reactions to mouse muscle, and measured mean light absorbance of individual fibre sections. Although this is a desirable new development, there are problems of interpretation attributable, for instance, to uneven distribution of reaction product in the fibre section, particulate as opposed to even staining, and lack of knowledge of the relationship between staining intensity and enzyme activity in the various reactions used. Since the introduction of the technique of glycogen depletion, such studies have been extended to the muscle fibres of individual motor units, and it has been possible to relate the histochemical profiles thus obtained to other properties of the motor unit, such as its mechanical characteristics and resistance to fatigue. It should be remembered that this technique depends upon detectable levels of glycogen in all the fibres of the undepleted muscle, and that the stimulation regimes used to deplete glycogen are effective for all the fibres in the muscle being studied. Strictly, controls to show that these factors are applicable should be undertaken in each study where they are feasible: where they are not feasible, due caution should be exercised in the assessment of the results.

The biochemistry and histology of muscle are dealt with in some detail in other chapters in this book (Ch. 4 and Ch. 8). A useful section on fibre histochemistry and other properties is given in a review by Close (1972). An extensive review of muscle histochemistry is given by Khan (1976), in which particular regard is paid to the underlying biochemistry. Here, a few of the results for muscle fibres in whole muscles will be described briefly, one of our aims being to illustrate some of the problems involved. The work on motor units will be considered in rather more detail. The discussion will be confined to normal mammalian skeletal muscle throughout.

Whole muscles

In animals. Studies on the distribution of lipids and glycogen have shown differences between fibres (e.g. George and Naik, 1957). However, for attempts to classify mammalian muscle fibres, the results of examination of specific enzyme levels have been more extensively used, partly because substrate levels are often inconstant by comparison. For example, Stein and Padykula (1962) examined the distribution of glycogen, succinic dehydrogenase (SDH), adenosine triphosphatase (ATPase) and esterase in the gastrocnemius and soleus muscles of the rat. On the basis of differences in staining intensity they classified the muscle fibres into three groups: A, B and C. Type A was usually rich in glycogen, the other two varying in this respect. SDH is a mitochondrial enzyme involved in the major energy-supplying pathway of muscle in oxidative metabolism. The staining intensity for SDH formed the basis of the classification. Type A fibres were low in SDH activity, types B and C were high, but type C appeared separate from B because the stain was concentrated around the edge of the fibre immediately below the sarcolemma. Differences between the fibre types for ATPase (incubated at pH 9.4, and considered to be myosin ATPase activity) and esterase, were not consistent, but there was a predominance of high ATPase activity in type A in unfixed sections, the pattern being different in fixed sections. Low esterase activity predominated. In type B predominant activities were low for ATPase and high for esterase and, in type C, high for both. This study brings out the following points, which apply also in varying degrees to other histochemical studies in muscle. First, a clear separation on the basis of one reaction (in this case SDH) is not necessarily reflected directly or inversely in other enzyme levels studied: secondly, the actual methods used (in this case for ATPase) markedly affect the results obtained. These points have been accentuated by the two studies employing microphotometric measurement (Spurway, 1978; Edjtehadi and Lewis, 1979). Edjtehadi and Lewis studied FDL of the cat, and measured and subjectively assessed levels of ATPase (with alkaline and acid pre-incubation, discussed further on p. 24), phosphorylase and SDH. The enzyme reaction intensities of the muscle fibres were distributed continuously, although peaks found in their distributions allowed all the fibres to be fitted into three classes if SDH was excluded, and if reasonable latitude was allowed on the basis of the continuous distributions. However, attempting to incorporate the SDH intensities produced a minimum of six classes, due to the fact that SDH intensity fell into two classes unrelated to the three defined by the other stains. Edjtehadi and Lewis suggested that SDH was separately controlled. In their paper they draw parallels with mechanical measurements which certainly support the idea that some, at least, of the histological data are quantitatively related to data obtained by mechanical recording. A similar but simpler parallel exists in cat soleus, where Henneman and Olson (1965) found only one fibre type by histochemistry, which was similar to one of three types they found in gastrocnemius. The three types of fibre in gastrocnemius stained differently for mitochondrial ATPase. Type A fibres were large and pale, containing few mitochondria. These were the commonest fibres. Type C fibres were small and dark, loaded with ATPase. Type B fibres were intermediate in size and in staining intensity, and the mitochondria were most densely distributed away from the centres of the fibre sections. Type C fibres had the greatest density of capillaries around them, with type B next and type A least. Type C appeared well equipped for sustained activity and it was this type alone that occurred in soleus. Because this classification is effectively based on mitochondrial densities it exactly parallels that of Stein and Padykula (1962).

The distribution of the enzyme phosphorylase has been studied in muscle. Phosphorylase catalyses the breakdown of glycogen, and is important in the only major energy-producing pathway available when oxygen is limited, as in prolonged maximal activity which reduces muscle blood flow. This pathway allows active muscle to produce lactic acid and incur an oxygen debt which is paid off in the liver. Dubowitz and Pearse (1960) found that, in a number of human, rat and pigeon muscles, phosphorylase activity of individual fibres varied inversely with their oxidative enzyme activities (especially DNP-diaphorase (DNPD) and lactic and succinic dehydrogenase). In general, small red fibres (red because of a high myoglobin content) possessed high oxidative enzyme levels, whereas large fibres showed high phosphorylase levels. However, this finding does not indicate a completely general rule, because some muscle fibres may have high activity for both enzymes (Edgerton and Simpson, 1969) or low activity for both (Prewitt and Salafsky, 1970).

The third type of enzyme used to classify muscle fibres histochemically is adenosine triphosphatase (ATPase) which, under the right conditions, is believed to be myosin ATPase, the enzyme property of the contractile protein myosin. In adult mammalian muscles there are known to be two myosin isoenzymes with different biochemical activities, and separately isolated from fast- and slow-contracting muscle (Bárány, 1967). Presumably, the isoenzyme present in the muscle determines the speed of isotonic shortening, and, in part at least, the contraction time of the isometric twitch. In an important study of various muscles in guinea pigs, ATPase levels, assessed both histochemically and biochemically, were related to whole-muscle contraction times (Barnard, Edgerton, Furukawa and Peter, 1971). The authors proposed that the muscle fibres could be classified into three groups: fast-twitch red, fast-twitch white and slow-twitch red. Because of the distribution of oxidative and glycolytic enzymes which were examined in addition to ATPase, these groups were subsequently named fast glycolytic, fast oxidative glycolytic and slow oxidative (Peter, Barnard, Edgerton, Gillespie and Stempel, 1972), later conveniently abbreviated to FG, FOG and SO respectively. This would appear to relate well to the tripartite classification in the cat of FF, FR and S, based on mechanical properties and resistances to fatigue and described earlier in this Chapter. This is discussed further in the next section. The guinea pig soleus muscle was found to be 100 per cent SO, with other muscles being mixtures of the three types.

The two myosin ATPases show different labilities to extreme pH values, and pre-incubation of sections at about pH 4.5 and 9.5 produce differences in ATPase staining between fibres. By relating biochemical measurements and histochemistry, Guth and Samaha (1969) showed in the cat that fast muscles had high myosin ATPase activity, measured biochemically, that was relatively stable in alkali and labile in acid compared with slow muscle. Histochemistry showed that high-activity, alkali-stable and acid-labile fibres predominated in sections of fast muscle, whereas the low-activity, alkali-labile and acid-stable fibres predominated in slow muscle. Guth and Samaha demonstrated a further subdivision of the high-activity fibres by diameter and susceptibility to formaldehyde fixation. Fibres with large diameters predominated in superficial parts of fast muscles, and their myosin ATPase activity was inhibited by formaldehyde. Fibres with smaller diameters were found mainly in deeper parts of fast muscles, and their myosin ATPase activity was not inhibited by formaldehyde. In the cat, soleus consisted almost exclusively of low-activity fibres. Histochemistry was also performed on muscles of rat and rabbit. In these, the same three fibre types occurred, but the solei contained a small number of fibres that had high activity which was formaldehyde-resistant. Thus, for soleus of the cat, fibres were of one group on the basis of

ATPase staining, and this is consistent with physiological unit analysis, which showed cat soleus to be a pure muscle (Burke, 1967). There was at least qualitative consistency also for the mixed solei of rat (Close, 1967) and rabbit (Bagust, 1979). In further work, Guth, Samaha and Albers (1970) named the three groups A, B and C. These groups are the same as those of Stein and Padykula (1962) in terms of SDH activity. The two types of myosin were labelled α and β. Alpha had high activity, and was labile in acid. Beta had low activity and was labile in alkali. It was proposed that in rat, B fibres contained β-myosin, C fibres contained α-myosin, and A fibres contained both α- and β-myosin. However, an important fact emerged subsequently, described in a paper by Yellin and Guth (1970). They found differences in rat and cat with regard to the parallelism between distribution of α- and β-myosin and SDH. In cat, A fibres contained α-myosin only, and C fibres contained α and β. This is a clear example of histochemistry revealing what are probably fundamental differences with functional importance between fibre types, but where it is not possible to make general classifications because of some independence between different factors in different species.

Davies and Gunn (1972) carried out a histochemical survey of diaphragm muscle from a number of different mammalian species. They stained for myosin ATPase (the sections being fixed in cacodylate-buffered formaldehyde), SDH (indicating aerobic metabolism) and phosphorylase (indicating anaerobic metabolism). They interpreted their results as showing two fibre types on the basis of ATPase staining—high activity and low activity; however, the division on the basis of aerobic and anaerobic metabolism was not simple. The fibres with high ATPase activity (presumably fast) were either mainly aerobic, mainly anaerobic, or showed a combined metabolism (possibly equivalent to a new type, FG and FOG respectively). The fibres with low ATPase activity (presumably slow) were either mainly aerobic, or showed a combined activity (possibly equivalent to SO and a new type). No physiological correlates in diaphragm beyond the presence of fast and slow units (Andersen and Sears, 1964) are yet available.

In man. In human muscle, a two-way classification of fibre types has been most generally applied. Dubowitz (1960) divided fibres into types I and II on the basis of oxidative enzyme and phosphorylase staining intensities, and Engel (1962) showed the correlated differences in ATPase staining in alkaline conditions. Type I fibres (red) have high oxidative enzyme content and low phosphorylase and ATPase, and type II fibres (pale) have a low oxidative enzyme content, high phosphorylase and ATPase. In a survey of 36 different human muscles (Johnson, Polgar, Weightman and Appleton, 1973) the relative numbers of the two fibre types are given. All the muscles examined had both fibre types (with the exception of soleus in one autopsy specimen which contained type I exclusively) but the proportions varied, and the authors discuss the results in relation to muscle function. Soleus contained the highest proportion of type I and orbicularis oculi the lowest. The muscles came from six male adults at autopsy, and there was no indication of muscle disease in any of them. In spite of this, there are wide variations in the proportions of types I and II in the same-named muscle throughout the six specimens, and this variation is analysed in the paper. It is obviously important to use this type of data when comparing the histochemistry of muscle suspected of showing pathological change.

There have been indications that human muscle should have a tripartite classification applied to it. Wachstein and Meisel (1955) found in rat, rabbit and human muscle that SDH activity was low in large fibres, high in small fibres, and that there were fibres intermediate between these. Brooke and Kaiser (1970) divided the Group II fibres of man (and rat and rabbit) into three subgroups (A, B and C) on the basis of the effects of pre-incubation at different pHs. Group IIA fibres showed almost complete inhibition of ATPase below pH 4.5. These fibres had the lowest oxidative enzyme levels and the largest diameters. IIB fibres showed partial inhibition of ATPase below pH 4.3 and had levels of oxidative enzymes and fibre diameters intermediate between those of Group I and IIA. Group IIC fibre ATPase activity was maximally inhibited below pH 3.9. These fibres were relatively infrequent, and had diameters within the range for IIA, from which they have not been separated generally. The differing diameters and levels of oxidative enzymes lead one to suspect that this tripartite classification may be equivalent to the FF, FR and S, and FG, FOG and SO classifications in animals, the equivalent order being IIB, IIA and I. This view is strengthened by the recent findings of Garnett *et al.* (1979), discussed below.

The examples discussed above give one the impression that there is no unifying classification based on histochemical profiles of muscle fibres from various muscles in various animals, because the quantities measured are not always interrelated in any unvarying way. The clearest separation probably resides in the two types of myosin, and recent developments may clarify this. Immunological staining techniques are now available (Gauthier, Lowey and Hobbs, 1978) and can be made as specific as the biochemical purification of the myosin isoenzymes allows (Weeds, 1978). However, it is known that activity patterns artificially imposed on muscle can alter the properties of the myosin ATPase and the activity levels of other enzymes. It therefore seems likely that some degree of variation in these properties, and in functional characteristics resulting from them, will occur in different muscles depending on their roles—and even in the same muscles, consequent upon variations in life styles between individuals of the same species. Therefore, there might be at least some degree of continuous plasticity within muscle fibres. Some evidence for such changes will be discussed later in this chapter.

Motor units

Edström and Kugelberg (1968) introduced the method of glycogen depletion of single motor units. In this, a regime of tetanic stimulation leads to depletion of the glycogen stores in the responding muscle fibres, so that they can be identified by a lack of staining in periodic acid Schiff's reagent (PAS) for glycogen. In other serial or semi-serial sections, a histochemical profile of the fibres can be built up. The method thus allows an examination of the degree of histochemical homogeneity of muscle fibres within a motor unit, and, if the unit is studied physiologically before depletion, the relationships between physiological properties and the histochemical profile of the fibres. Edström and Kugelberg studied a small sample of units in the anterior tibial muscle of the rat. Their stimulation regime, when applied to the whole muscle, caused depletion in all the type A fibres, all but 10 per cent of the B fibres, and was ineffective with C fibres. (In later work, total muscle depletion was obtained by combining stimulation with reduction of blood flow through the muscle). They studied the resistance to fatigue of each unit, and found a correlation between relative resistance to fatigue and oxidative enzyme staining levels. One interesting and rather puzzling finding was of a few histochemically foreign fibres in some units that were otherwise homogeneous. The A fibre units contained about two per cent B fibres, and the B units about one per cent A fibres. It is most unlikely that these resulted from inadvertent stimulation of two units. The authors suggested a possible explanation: that a small number of muscle fibres were innervated by two motor axons, one of which went to a unit predominantly made up of one fibre type and the second to the other type. This isolated observation of unit heterogeneity in histochemistry has not yet been confirmed.

So far, the most complete examination of single unit histochemistry has been carried out in Burke's laboratory, on cat muscle: Burke *et al.* (1973): gastrocnemius; Burke *et al.* (1974): soleus. In gastrocnemius, all but a very small proportion (three out of 112) of the units were classifiable into three groups, on the basis of contraction time, the shape of the record of an unfused tetanus and susceptibility to fatigue. The shape of the unfused tetanus resulting from stimulation at a specific test frequency either showed a maximum during the first few oscillations, which then declined a little (called 'sag'), or the maximum was sustained (no 'sag'). The slow units (S) were very resistant to fatigue and showed no 'sag'. The fast units, on the other hand, fell into two classes, one being much more resistant to fatigue than the other (denoted FR and FF respectively). All the fast units showed 'sag'. Mean unit size was in the order FF > FR > S. These data are presented in Figure 1.10. All three types showed post-tetanic potentiation of twitch tension in this muscle. Using glycogen depletion, a representative sample of 28 units was studied histochemically. The units studied fell clearly into

ing one unit intermediate between FF and FR, which also had a number of intermediate staining

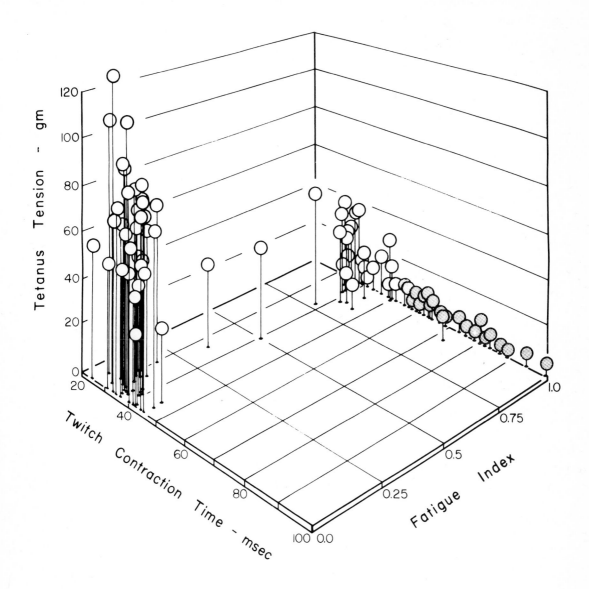

Fig. 1.10 Separation of motor units into three principal groups. Cat medial gastrocnemius muscle (3 animals). Units with 'sag' (see text), open spheres (FF units with low fatigue index; FR units with high fatigue index). Units without sag, stippled spheres (S units). (From Burke *et al.*, 1973). Soleus units (Burke *et al.*, 1974), which are not on this graph, overlap with gastrocnemius S units, but there are more with tetanic tension greater than 10 g (0.1 N)

three groups on the basis of a battery of different stains. The histochemical divisions conformed to the physiological types without exception, includ-

properties. Tests were made of the uniformity of histochemical profile within units, and no aberrant fibres were found.

Both fast types of unit stained intensely for 'myofibrillar ATPase' (alkaline pH), whereas S units showed light staining. As one might expect, FF units showed low oxidative enzyme activity (DPND and SDH) whereas FR were higher in this respect. It would seem reasonable to equate FF to FG, FR to FOG and S to SO.

In soleus, six units were identified by glycogen depletion. In some respects these were similar to type S units in gastrocnemius. They were resistant to fatigue, low in myofibrillar ATPase and high in oxidative enzymes. However, they were not the same in every respect. The mean unit tetanic tension was higher, many showed post-tetanic depression of twitch tension, and the fibres showed intense staining for ATPase in acid pH. In this last characteristic, the soleus S units were quite different from gastrocnemius S units, and re-sembled FF units. The interpretation of this latter ATPase staining is not clear, but some of it at least could be related to sarcoplasmic reticular ATPase. Another difference was in their calculated tetanic tensions per unit cross-sectional area of fibre. In the gastrocnemius S units this was calculated to be 0.06 N/mm^2, whereas in soleus units it was $0.17–0.23 \text{ N/mm}^2$. Some doubt attaches to the very low value for the S units in gastrocnemius, as the equivalent muscle fibres in FDL of the cat have a mean estimated value of 0.29 N/mm^2 (Edjtehadi and Lewis, 1979). It should be noted that these S units are difficult to deplete of their glycogen, and Burke *et al.* (1974) noted in soleus some fibres that stained lightly with PAS and which may or may not have belonged to the unit under study. Once any such doubts have entered for the soleus S units, they begin to be raised for the gastrocnemius S units too, unless specifically excluded. In neither study are controls mentioned where whole-muscle depletion was shown with the stimulation regimes used for the units, and so such doubts cannot be totally excluded.

In their recent study of motor unit types in human gastrocnemius *in situ*, Garnett *et al.* (1979) analysed histochemically five units depleted of glycogen after mechanical study, and a sixth unit in a perfused peroneus longus muscle was in-cluded. Of these, three were type S and consisted of type I fibres, and one was type FF and consisted of IIB fibres. Another F unit was of IIB, and an FR unit was correlated with type I fibres in the biopsy sample, but this last result is most unlikely to be correct, is probably artefactual and should be treated with circumspection. By difference the implication is that type FF units probably consist of IIA fibres. The histochemical segregations were on the basis of myosin ATPase staining (pH 9.4) for types I and II, and succinic dehydrogenase levels for types I and IIB (high and low respectively). It is a pity that the position of the FF units is undecided; the difficulty in the experiments was to keep large units separated long enough to obtain glycogen depletion.

AXON CONDUCTION VELOCITY AND MOTOR UNIT MECHANICAL PROPERTIES

In adult cats, motor axons going to slow red extensor muscles have a smaller average diameter than those going to fast white extensors (Eccles and Sherrington, 1930; Boyd and Davey, 1968), and the expected differences in conduction vel-ocity exist in cat (Eccles, Eccles and Lundberg, 1958; Kuno, 1959; Boyd, 1965; Burke, 1967) and also in rabbit and rat (Ridge, 1967). At the level of individual motor units there are several reports of statistically significant relationships between axon conduction velocity, contraction time and tetanic tension (normalised or otherwise). On the other hand there are reports where such relationships have been looked for and were found to be lacking, or were less clear than claimed by others. As there is much interest in the association of properties of motor neurones with the muscle fibres they innervate, it is worth discussing briefly the present picture regarding axon conduction velocity and the contraction properties of motor units.

In the deep lumbrical muscle of the cat, which is small and contains 4–10 motor units with a range of contraction times, unit axon conduction vel-ocities are linearly and inversely related to unit contraction time, with very little scatter (Bessou *et al.*, 1963). Conduction velocity was directly related to maximal tetanic tension developed by the unit, although this was not linear but dished,

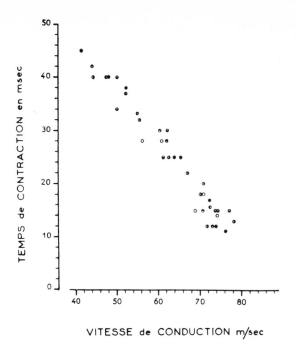

Fig. 1.11   The relation between motor axon conduction velocity and motor unit contraction time for a sample of motor units in the first deep lumbrical muscle of the hind foot. The data are pooled from six cats (from Bessou, Emonet-Dénand and Laporte, 1963)

increments in tension being smaller with increasing conduction velocity at low velocities than high. The relationship between conduction velocity and contraction time is reproduced in Fig. 1.11. Therefore, in this muscle, large units are fast-contracting and are innervated by large, fast-conducting axons, whereas small units contract slowly and are innervated by small, slowly conducting axons, these relations extending over the complete range of motor units present in the muscle. The same picture emerged from unit analysis in the larger (20–30 motor units) superficial lumbrical muscle (Appelberg and Emonet-Dénand, 1967), and subsequently it was strengthened by the finding that, where motor units were split between first and second superficial lumbricals, unit tetanic tension fell on the same line relating conduction velocity to tetanic tension of unsplit units, provided that the tension components in the separate muscles were summed for each unit (Emonet-Dénand *et al.*, 1971). Motor unit contraction times, tetanic tensions and axon conduction velocities have been shown to be interrelated also in some muscles of lower verte-

brates (frog; Luff and Proske, 1976; *Xenopus* toad; Thomson, 1978; snake; Hammond and Ridge, 1978).

In soleus of the cat, which on mechanical and histochemical grounds is a pure muscle in terms of its motor unit composition, there is a linear relationship between axon conduction velocity and unit tetanic tension (McPhedran *et al.*, 1965; Bagust, 1974). The relationships were clear within the muscle of one animal (although, even then, scatter was greater than in the data on the lumbrical muscles), but became obscured when data from several cats were pooled. This may be the reason why Mosher, Gerlach and Stuart (1972) found neither of these relationships in cat soleus, because their analyses were exclusively of pooled data.

The situation in the fast limb muscles of the cat, all of which contain mixed populations of motor units, is not clear: some studies show relationships, while others do not, and there is no obvious reason for the disagreement. For instance, Bagust *et al.* (1973) showed clearly significant relationships between conduction velocity and contraction time (inverse linear), and between conduction velocity and normalised tetanic tension (direct logarithmic; unit tetanic tension was normalised to per cent whole muscle tetanic tension) in FDL. This was irrespective of further division on the basis of motor unit types, and it was shown that the sample of motor units was representative of the whole muscle population. In the medial head of gastrocnemius, Wuerker et al. (1965) found that unit tetanic tension varied with conduction velocity, but not simply. Small units showed a relationship, while large units had fast-conducting axons but did not show a relationship within the group. We have seen already that the motor units of gastrocnemius can be assigned to three groups on the basis of histochemical staining alone (FG, FOG and SO), or a combination of mechanical characteristics, resistance to fatigue and histochemical staining (FR, FF and S). The question arises whether the relationships between axon conduction velocity, unit contraction time and size exist within groups (as apparently they do in soleus S units—at least in single muscles) or only between groups. Proske and Waite (1976) examined this question as it relates to tetanic tension (normalized and plotted on a linear scale) in gastrocnemius and found that it was possible to plot a significant straight line through the points for S units, but that FF and FR units neither fell on this line, nor did they approximate to different lines of their own. The data were pooled from five experiments and there is, therefore, the possibility that large samples from individual animals would show up relationships in these groups.

Let us now examine some of the reports where relations between axon conduction velocity and other unit parameters have been sought, but have not been found. Eccles et al. (1968) studied motor units in the extensor digitorum communis of the baboon's forearm. They could find no relationship between axon conduction velocity and either twitch tension or contraction time. It is, of course, possible that unit tetanic tensions might have been related to conduction velocity. Andrew and Part (1972) could find no correlation between axon conduction velocity and unit tetanic tension in rat soleus, although they did find an inverse relationship between conduction velocity and unit contraction time. Data were pooled from several

animals and, in view of the results for cat soleus, it is possible that a real relationship within the muscle was obscured by this. It is interesting that, in the much smaller tail muscles, conduction velocity and unit tetanic tension were found to be related.

Several papers from Stuart's group have been concerned with attempts to find relationships between axon conduction velocity, unit contraction time and tetanic tension in various cat hind limb muscles, and have found either no correlations (Mosher et al., 1972; Gerlach, Stauffer, Goslow and Stuart, 1976—in soleus, anterior tibial, plantaris, FHL and flexor digitorum brevis) or weak correlations (Reinking, Stephens and Stuart, 1975—in medial gastrocnemius). One possible explanation of the discrepancies between these results and those we have discussed previously was put forward by Stuart's group: namely, that their animals were not caged for any significant time before the experiment. The implication is that there may be some degree of plasticity in muscle fibre properties depending on usage of motor units, which would be affected by the individual life style of the animal. This may well be the case, as marked effects on whole muscle have been seen following imposed stimulation patterns. A valuable approach to this problem might be to carry out experiments such as those of Proske and Waite (1976) on separate groups of cats, reared in different environments or exposed to different exercise regimes. In these experiments, one would attempt to separate units under standard conditions on the basis of contraction properties and resistance to fatigue, and then examine for conduction velocity relations within groups.

Factors underlying differences in unit tetanus tension

One might think that the tetanic tension of a unit would be related to the number of muscle fibres it contained, and that the size (and conduction velocity) of a motor neurone axon would be related to the number of branches it made and hence to the number of muscle fibres in the motor unit. The tension developed by the unit would depend on the number of muscle fibres it contained if these were all roughly the same in cross-sectional area. This idea seems to hold approximately in soleus muscle, which contains one type of motor unit with a relatively narrow range of muscle fibre diameters. Obviously, in a muscle containing more than one type of motor unit, whether such a simple idea holds good will depend upon the different sorts of units having fibres of similar sizes, one to another, and having fibres developing similar tensions per unit cross-sectional area. If either or both of these requirements is not met, then a more complex set of relationships will prevail. There is considerable variation in the mean fibre cross-sectional area for units of different types. For example, in gastrocnemius of the cat, fibres of S units are generally the smallest; and of those slow units plotted, mean cross-sectional areas ranged from about 1000 to 2300 μm^2 (Burke and Tsairis, 1973). However, the diameters of muscle fibres in soleus are generally larger than they are in FDL (Westerman *et al.*, 1974*). In addition, there appears to be a range of tension output per unit cross-sectional area. All this militates against unit tetanic tensions being related simply to the number of divisions made by the innervating axon, at least in muscles containing mixed populations of motor units.

RECRUITMENT OF MOTOR UNITS

During an increasing voluntary contraction, the number of motor units active in the muscle is increased progressively, as is their frequency of firing (Adrian and Bronk, 1929).

We have seen how skeletal muscles contain motor units of differing mechanical properties and resistance to fatigue. If this variability is to be useful functionally, one would expect to find differences in the way that the different types of motor unit are recruited during natural or seminatural activity such as voluntary force development or movement, and reflex-induced muscle responses. Further, there might be detectable motor neurone properties underlying such functional subtleties, which might influence threshold and firing frequency. There is a growing body of

knowledge concerning unit recruitment, much of it obtained from human subjects. The degree to which unit recruitment is flexible rather than stereotyped is not yet clear, and we may expect interesting developments in this field. Intracellular recording from motor neurones in the spinal cord of experimental animals has proved to be a very powerful method, contributing vastly to knowledge of the functional basis of movement and postural control. In the following brief account we will deal with only some of the aspects of this large subject that specifically concern individual motor units. In our discussion we will start with motor neurones, go on to reflex effects and excitability, and finish by describing motor unit recruitment in human subjects.

In animals

Single motor unit activity has been recorded in muscle *in situ*, activity being induced by reflex or cortical stimulation, or by natural voluntary recruitment of units. Early examples of such work are the studies of Adrian and Bronk (1929), Gordon and Holbourn (1949) and Gordon and Phillips (1953). In the last-mentioned study, motor unit twitches of different contraction times were recorded in tibialis anterior of the cat, and it was noticed that units deep in the muscle, which were slower than the more superficial ones, had lower thresholds for central excitation. This fact has often been observed since, and differences in the potency of reflex input on to motor neurones has been found by intracellular recording from motor neurone somata (e.g. Kuno, 1959). The concept of tonic and phasic motor units was first put forward by Granit and his co-workers (Granit, Henatsch and Steg, 1956; Granit, Phillips, Skoglund and Steg, 1957) on the basis of their firing pattern when responding reflexly to muscle stretch or some other stimuli. The tonic units responded with prolonged discharges, whereas the phasic units responded with one or two spikes only. Eccles *et al.* (1958) found that the action potential of motor neurones innervating slow muscles had a longer after-hyperpolarisation than those innervating fast muscles, and this may well limit their firing frequency and account in part for the fact that this is low in reflexly activated tonic units.

*In this paper and others (Buller *et al.*, 1960a and b; Buller and Lewis, 1965a and b; Bagust *et al.*, 1973) FDL has been called incorrectly FHL.

After-potential duration was inversely related to axon conduction velocity, and Kuno (1959) found in cat triceps surae motor neurones that these two were related continuously, together with strength of antidromic inhibition (presumably by axon collaterals and Renshaw cells), rather than showing a clear break into tonic and phasic. Kernell (1966) found, in a sample of lumbosacral motor neurones in the cat, that input resistance and conduction velocity were related inversely. Measurements showed that the lower input resistance of somata with large axons was probably due to a large soma and large dendritic trunks. Presumably as a result of higher input resistance, the somata with axons of lower conduction velocities required weaker stimulating currents applied through the intracellular electrode to cause repetitive firing. The idea that variations in cell size may be a fundamental property of motor neurones used in their functional organisation, and may dictate unit sensitivity and hence order of recruitment, was formulated most clearly by Henneman, Somjen and Carpenter (1965a). They studied the order of recruitment of motor units in triceps surae of decerebrate cats in response to muscle stretch, and related this to the amplitude of impulses recorded from filaments of ventral root, and hence indirectly to axon size (which was considered to be related to cell size). They found that, in general, the order of recruitment of the units was inversely related to their cell size: small cells were recruited as a result of small stretches of the muscle, and as the stretch was increased so the cell size of the units recruited increased also. The order in which the units fell silent as stretch was reduced was the reverse of their recruitment order. In a subsequent paper (1965b) the same authors presented further evidence to support the 'size principle' relating motor neurone size inversely to excitability. This derived from other forms of reflex excitation. The order held also for inhibition. The idea was therefore put forward that excitability, and hence recruitment order, within a motor neurone pool was determined by the size of the motor neurone in the pool, smaller motor neurones being more excitable and therefore more easily recruited than larger cells. Because motor neurone size may also be related to motor unit size, this means that smaller units in a muscle will

generally be more active than large ones, which will be recruited only occasionally when large muscle responses are required. The idea of a fixed order of recruitment, whether related to size or some other property, still persists, but there are many reports contrary to its universal applicability. Henneman et al. (1965a, b) obtained their data by recording pairs of units in small ventral root filaments. Wyman, Waldron and Wachtel (1974) re-examined this phenomenon in decerebrate cats, but recorded activity of pairs of units within the muscle with bipolar needle electrodes. Reflex activity was obtained by stretching the muscle tendon and applying various noxious stimuli to the leg. Similar experiments were performed in temporalis muscle, by passive movement of the jaw, and unit activity was also recorded in throat muscles in anaesthetised cats during spontaneous breathing. In these experiments, only about one-third of the pairs of units studied showed a consistent difference in threshold between the two units. Therefore, under these conditions, the majority of motor units were not arranged in a fixed recruitment order. Wyman et al. speculate on the possibility that a fixed order is more apparent in neighbouring motor neurones, which could account for the much higher proportion of fixed-order pairs found by Henneman et al., recording in small filaments of ventral root where the adjacent axons probably derive from neighbouring motor neurones. However, more recently, Henneman's group has supported the view of a rigid excitatory hierarchy among motor neurones of cat triceps surae by experiments in which the total monosynaptic reflex was assessed and each unit threshold related to it during reflex responses to stimuli of varying strength. Each motor unit threshold was very constant, so that the total monosynaptic reflex output (O_T) could be described by the equation $O_T = O_1 + O_2 + O_3 + --- O_x$, where O_x is the threshold in terms of percentage maximum reflex response at which the highest-ranking cell discharged in the particular reflex response. This they described as a law of combination (Henneman, Clamann, Gillies and Skinner, 1974). Various inhibitory influences did not alter this ranking, but rather shifted the excitability of the whole motor neurone pool (Clamann and Henneman, 1976). It should be noted that the ranking order was derived for monosynaptic input only.

Burke, Rymer and Walsh (1976) recorded intracellularly from motor neurones of cat medial gastrocnemius. They examined the relative sizes of EPSPs produced by stimulating homonymous and heteronymous group Ia afferents from antagonistic ankle flexor muscles. They also typed the motor units, and observed that the largest EPSPs and IPSPs were found in motor neurones innervating type S motor units. They were somewhat smaller for those innervating FR and intermediate fast units, and smallest for FF units. Thus, for these spinal reflex inputs, motor neurone sensitivity (assuming a roughly constant firing threshold) is based on motor unit type. In the same muscle, Kanda, Burke and Walmsley (1977) found that, by stimulating the sural nerve, they could inhibit some motor units that were very sensitive to muscle stretch or vibration, while stimulating other units that were relatively insensitive to stretch or vibration; that is, the order of sensitivity to a Ia input could be the reverse of that to a cutaneous input. Obviously, the presence of such a system argues against sensitivity being exclusively a function of some intrinsic property of motor neurones such as cell size or input resistance, and implies that different input pathways have different orders of efficacy on the motor neurones. There are other examples leading to the same conclusion (e.g. Burke, Jankowska and ten Bruggencate, 1970; Kernell and Sjöholm, 1975).

In summary, the animal work leads one to conclude that there is a hierarchy of excitability in the motor neurone pool to a particular individual muscle, at least for some specific reflex or other input under standard conditions. This hierarchy may be based on some intrinsic property of the motor neurone. For other inputs, the hierarchy can be different, and this must be brought about via the distribution and potency of the synapses serving a particular input. Presumably, therefore, it would be possible for descending inhibitory or excitatory pathways, for instance, to alter the motor neurone hierarchy of excitation for a given reflex input when other conditions changed. We will now see to what extent the same general picture emerges from the results obtained with human subjects.

In man

There are several reports of an orderly recruitment of motor units during voluntary isometric contractions of increasing force in hand and forearm muscles (Milner-Brown et al., 1973a; Tanji and Kato, 1973; Freund, Büdingen and Dietz, 1975), jaw muscles (Yemm, 1977) and the tibialis anterior muscle of the leg (Desmedt and Godaux, 1977). By using their spike-triggered averaging method, Milner-Brown et al. were able to measure twitch tensions of the individual units in first dorsal interosseus muscle, and they found that unit twitch tension varied nearly linearly as a function of the level of force at which the unit was recruited. This relationship showed some scatter, as one would expect. The graph is shown in Figure 1.12. The larger units, recruited at higher threshold, tended to have shorter contraction times. The increasing size of each additional unit recruited was therefore proportional to the tension in the muscle at the time of recruitment. Relative fineness of control was, therefore, nearly constant throughout the complete range of tensions. However, increasing tension was dependent on increasing unit firing frequency as well as recruitment of

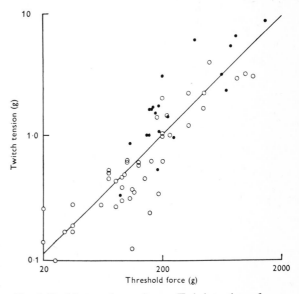

Fig. 1.12 Motor unit recruitment. Twitch tensions of motor units in one human subject plotted against the muscle force at which each unit was recruited. First dorsal interosseus muscle during voluntary effort. Both axes have log. scales (from Milner-Brown, Stein and Yemm, 1973b)

units; the latter became relatively more important as tension increased (Milner-Brown *et al.*, 1973b). The authors discuss the question of frequency coding versus recruitment and the interested reader is referred to this discussion. Tanji and Kato (1973) used fine EMG electrodes in abductor digiti minimi and found an orderly recruitment of units when the subject increased tension in tracking a linear target ramp voltage. Motor units with larger APs (presumably larger units) tended to be recruited at the higher tensions. If the contraction was carried out more quickly, motor units were recruited at lower tensions, but the order was not altered. In first dorsal interosseus and extensor indicis, Freund *et al.* (1975) found an orderly recruitment of units with smoothly increasing voluntary contraction, each unit having a threshold force for recruitment. When the subject was instructed to apply force in small-step increments, a particular unit would show a threshold for transient activity and then, at a higher tension, another threshold for sustained activity. This they called the tonic threshold. The order for both these thresholds was the same as for the threshold force for recruitment during a smooth contraction: however, the high-threshold units had a large force range below tonic threshold, in which they showed transient activity, whereas low-threshold units had a large force range above tonic threshold, where they acted tonically. This change of behaviour was arranged as a continuum throughout the unit population, so that there was no line of division between tonic and phasic units (in contrast to the observations of Gydikov and Kosarov (1974) who concluded that there were tonic and phasic units in biceps brachii). This is particularly interesting, as muscle fibres of types I and II (on the basis of ATPase staining) occur in this muscle in roughly equal proportions. The thresholds were related directly to axon conduction velocity. The findings are therefore consistent with the size principle. Yemm (1977) found the recruitment of units in masseter and temporalis to be orderly and nearly linearly related to twitch tension, as in the first dorsal interosseus (Milner-Brown *et al.*, 1973a). The range of unit contraction times was also similar. Desmedt and Godaux (1977) examined the EMG in tibialis anterior with a selective electrode, and for smooth

force developed while tracking a ramp signal at various rates, the units were recruited in a consistent order. They found the same order for rapid ballistic forces, even though units were firing at very high frequencies and starting before the muscle developed tension.

Taken together, these experiments show that for very disparate muscles, and for the same muscles doing very different jobs, consistently ordered recruitment patterns can be found.

However, there are a number of reports indicating that recruitment order can be changed under certain conditions. For instance, if motor unit firing patterns are made visible to the subject, he can learn to alter recruitment order during minimal voluntary contractions (Harrison and Mortensen, 1962) or bring in individual units at will (Basmajian, 1963). In tibialis anterior, Grimby and Hannerz (1968) reported changes in recruitment order depending on the velocity of voluntary contraction (although more recently Desmedt and Godaux (1977) have found the opposite in this muscle). The order could also be different in phasic flexion reflex responses to electrical stimulation of the plantar surface of the foot (Hannerz and Grimby, 1973) or for voluntary twitch contractions (Hannerz, 1974). In the short toe extensor muscle, Grimby and Hannerz (1977) and Borg, Grimby and Hannerz (1978) studied unit EMGs. They divided the units found, effectively into tonic, intermediate and phasic groups. In individual subjects, the distribution of unit axon conduction velocities was different for the three types of unit, although there was extensive overlapping. The mean conduction velocity of axons going to tonic units was lowest, to phasic highest, and between these for the intermediate units. They speculated that tonic units were made up of type I muscle fibres, and phasic units of type II, the two types of muscle fibre existing in about equal proportions in this muscle. There is evidence from glycogen depletion studies in human subjects undergoing various intensities of bicycle ergometer and isometric exercise that, in quadriceps, there is a selective depletion in fibres with low levels of myofibrillar ATPase and high levels of oxidative enzymes (type I) at lower exercise levels, whereas at high levels both type I and type II are depleted (Gollnick, Karlsson, Piehl and

Saltin, 1974; Gollnick, Piehl and Saltin, 1974). Of course, this is consistent with a fixed order of recruitment. Borg *et al.* (1978) found that there was selective activation of phasic units if the muscle was relaxed before a twitch contraction and an effort was made to make the twitch as fast as possible (one should note that some of these units may have been unusual because of nerve regeneration following damage caused by previous EMG studies). Stephens, Garnett and Buller (1978) found that, in the first dorsal interosseus muscle, recording with intramuscular EMG electrodes and tension measurement showed an orderly recruitment of units studied in pairs during increasing voluntary contraction. However, in every subject tested, at least one example was found where the recruitment order within the pair was reversed on electrical stimulation of the skin of the finger via ring electrodes on either side of the distal interphalangeal joint. When stimulation ceased, the previous order returned, but it took several minutes to do so. In a subsequent communication (Garnett and Stephens, 1978) it was reported that such electrical stimulation differentially affected low and high recruitment units, the threshold of the former being raised and the latter lowered, the tension separating the two groups being at 6 per cent of maximal voluntary force.

Thus, at first sight one is faced with two conflicting pictures—one of a rigidly determined recruitment order which shows itself regardless of the type of movement being performed, and the other of an order of recruitment which can be altered depending on circumstances. What is known at present suggests that motor units are organised in such a way that, in the absence of sufficiently powerful distracting input, this organisation shows itself in a reproducible recruitment order during voluntary muscular effort, and possibly during some other forms of activity. This order may well be related to some underlying physical property of the motor neurones, such as their input resistances: indeed, it would seem to be economical of synaptic input for the system to be designed in this way in relation to its most common mode of operation. However, there are other input routes present where the synapses are arranged to bring about an organised change of the recruit-ment order, either in direct response to that input route, or in response to the commonest path when operating in the presence of activity in the new input route. One therefore has an economically designed basic mode of action which, when necessary, is overridden and subject to transient rearrangement. Speculation subsequently concerns which of the other routes, or which natural or imposed situations, cause such a rearrangement, and what are the functional details of the transient orders resulting.

DEVELOPMENT

Polyneuronal innervation

It appears that, in some mammals at least, motor unit organisation within muscles is not complete at birth, but continued sorting between motor neurones and muscle fibres extends into the first few weeks of life. Many or all muscle fibres at first receive innervation from more than one motor neurone, but subsequently a selective and progressive withdrawal takes place so that, finally, only one axonal contact remains on each muscle fibre. This was first shown in rat diaphragm by Redfern (1970), who recorded end-plate potentials with intracellular micro-electrodes. The preparation was curarised at a level that paralysed the muscle, but allowed the appearance of subthreshold end-plate potentials. Redfern found that, on progressively increasing the strength of stimulus applied to the phrenic nerve, the end-plate potential increased in size in discrete steps, due to the progressive summation of units with higher thresholds. At birth there were 2–4 such units at each end-plate, the number becoming fewer during the second week of life. By 16–18 days this reduced to one, as in the adult. Redfern interpreted this as a transient polyneuronal innervation, although strictly it could have been attributable to axon branching above the stimulating electrodes. However, Redfern's interpretation proved to be correct, as polyneuronal innervation was demonstrated in a different way by Bagust, Lewis and Westerman (1973). They showed that, in young kittens, if a ventral root containing axons to soleus or FDL was split into two roughly equal filaments, then the muscle tension generated on tetanically stimulating the filaments separately was greater when added together than that generated on stimulating the two filaments simultaneously. This indicated that axons in both filaments overlapped on the muscle fibres to an extent related to the tension deficit. Records from these two demonstrations of polyneuronal innervation in young rats and kittens are shown in Figure 1.13.

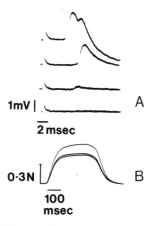

Fig. 1.13 Polyneural innervation in muscles of young animals. (A) Ten-day-old rat diaphragm muscle. Intracellular recordings from one muscle fibre during a progressively increasing stimulus strength applied to the phrenic nerve. The mammalian Ringer solution contained tubocurarine and 10 mM Ca^{++}. Note that the number of units recruited in the end-plate potential increases from 0 (lowest record) to 3 (top record). (from Redfern, 1970) (B) Three-day-old kitten—soleus muscle. The ventral roots were split into two divisions. Each of the smaller myograms was produced by stimulating each division separately. The larger myogram was produced by stimulating both together. Note the tension deficit between the larger myogram and the sum of the smaller myograms (from Bagust, Lewis and Westerman, 1973)

Further support for the overlap of motor units was obtained by showing that post-tetanic potentiation of twitch tension induced by stimulating one filament was apparent on applying single shocks to the other. Therefore, there must have been some muscle fibres receiving innervation from axons in both filaments. Of course, the explanation could have been that some axons branched near the soma (i.e. central to the ventral root): that this was not the case was shown by axon counts in nerves to FDL★ and soleus in kittens of

★See footnote to page 31

different ages, and in adult cats (Westerman *et al.*, 1974; adult values quoted from Boyd and Davey, 1966). These showed a slight increase in total motor axons with age, rather than any decrease. Polyneuronal innervation was greatest in the youngest kittens examined (3 days), less at 2 weeks and small or absent at 6 weeks of age. Over the same period the mean motor unit tetanic tension, relative to that of the whole muscle, decreased. One would expect this as the polyneuronal innervation reduced, and in rat soleus this appears to account for the total change in relative unit size (Brown, Jansen and van Essen, 1976). However, in kittens an additional factor is operating: at birth not all the motor axons have arrived at their muscle destinations, and innervation is not complete until about 2 months after birth (Nyström, 1968a). Therefore, some muscle fibres must be re-allocated to the new axons on their arrival. In the more peripheral lumbrical muscles of the rat, the picture was found to be complicated by yet another factor (Betz, Caldwell and Ribchester, 1979). Here, the estimated number of muscle fibres per motor unit was high at birth and remained nearly constant for about 10 days. The constancy was due to two processes having opposite effects. These were the elimination of some synaptic contacts, and the formation of other synapses on newly developing muscle fibres. After this period, no new muscle fibres were formed, and the number of muscle fibres per motor unit decreased as the final elimination proceeded. The polyneuronal innervation in kittens (Riley, 1976) and young rats (Bennett and Pettigrew, 1974; Riley, 1977) was shown by silver staining to be largely at a single end-plate site on each muscle fibre. The withdrawal process is associated with some ultrastructural features at the end-plate, such as vesicle aggregation and the engulfing of terminals by Schwann cells, similar to those associated with denervation (Rosenthal and Taraskevich, 1977—rat diaphragm; but *see* Korneliussen and Jansen, 1976, for rather different results in rat soleus. For an example of ultrastructural changes following denervation *see* Fukami and Ridge, 1971). Rosenthal and Taraskevich found that transmission from such a withdrawing terminal ceased abruptly, without any detectable progressive reduction that would lead to decaying end-plate amplitudes. It is not known with certainty, or in detail, what factors determine the withdrawal of supernumerary neuromuscular contacts, but it is not connected with motor neurone death, which occurs much earlier in development (e.g. Holt and Sohal, 1978). The decline in motor unit size was delayed, but not prevented, by the early surgical removal of all but a few motor axons to rat soleus (Brown *et al.*, 1976). This implies that the ultimate size of a motor unit is determined, at least in development, by some intrinsic property of the motor neurone, rather than by the availability of muscle fibres without effective neural contact. There is some evidence that muscle activity may play a part in this process. Benoit and Changeux (1975) found that tenotomy of soleus in 4-day-old rats delayed the reduction of polyneuronal innervation (presumably by reducing muscle activity, although some other result of tenotomy could have been effective); in addition, imposed activity by electrical stimulation of the sciatic nerve increased the rate of elimination in rat soleus (O'Brien, Östberg and Vrbová, 1978).

Changes in mechanical properties

It has been known for many years that limb muscles in many laboratory mammals contract slowly at birth, and differentiate into fast and slow during the first few weeks after birth (*see* Banu, 1922). The time course of changes in contraction time and other isometric mechanical characteristics with age in kittens has been described in detail by Buller *et al.* (1960a) and Buller and Lewis (1965b), and changes in force–velocity characteristics with age in rats by Close (1964). In kittens, fast and slow muscles at birth have contraction times of about 80 ms, although the muscles are different in their twitch: tetanus ratios (that for soleus being much lower than that for FDL★). Their tetani have similar, but not identical, maximum rates of rise of tension. During the six weeks after birth the maximum rates of rise separate to their adult values (FDL being 4–5 times faster than soleus) and the fast muscles attain their adult twitch contraction times (about 20 ms). Slow muscles (soleus and crureus) also show some speeding during the first four weeks (to a con-

★See footnote to page 31.

traction time of about 50 ms) but then a slowing appears, the adult value of about 80 ms being reached after 12 weeks or so.

Some of the underlying motor unit changes were studied by Bagust *et al.* (1974) in kittens aged about 2 and 6 weeks. Even at the age of 2 weeks there were marked differences between the two muscles in the distributions of unit contraction times and tetanic tensions. In FDL, both these distributions were skewed towards larger values, whereas in soleus both were more nearly symmetrically distributed. Similar patterns exist in adults (Bagust, Knott, Lewis, Luck and Westerman, 1973; Bagust, 1974). One can therefore conclude that, at two weeks, motor units were already differently organised in the two muscles. In addition it was found that linear relationships existed between axon conduction velocity and unit tetanic tensions for each of the two muscles at both ages. This shows that the motor unit organisation apparent at two weeks and older is associated with a parallel or causative neuronal organisation. Between two and six weeks the mean unit contraction time for FDL fell from 33.8 to 21.6 ms, whereas that for soleus changed very little (55.3–52.5 ms), in agreement with the whole-muscle study.

Changes in histochemistry

Studies of muscle histochemistry have also revealed changes occurring in developing young animals. In adult guinea pigs, the soleus is a histochemically pure muscle. In fetuses 10 days before birth, and in newborn animals, there are approximately even numbers of type I and type II muscle fibres (based on staining intensities including those for myosin ATPase and SDH). During maturation the proportion of type II falls and by six weeks the adult pattern is achieved, only type I being present (Karpati and Engel, 1967). Nyström (1968b) reported that, in hind limb muscles of newborn kittens, all the fibres are histochemically similar but that, by 14 days, differences had appeared between fibres in the levels of phosphorylase, glycogen, lipid and oxidative enzyme levels. By three weeks, both gastrocnemius and soleus contained at least two types of muscle fibre, but subsequently the two muscles showed separate development, gastroc-nemius further differentiating while soleus approached homogeneity. The adult pattern was largely attained by the 6–7th week. Differentiation followed by simplification was also found by Hammarberg (1974) in kittens, but he detected some differentiation in fibres of gastrocnemius and tibialis anterior in newborn animals. Using the histochemical divisions introduced by Brooke and Kaiser (1970—*see* the section on histochemistry in this Chapter), Brooke, Williamson and Kaiser (1971) found in rats that fibres first differentiated into types I and IIC. Later, IIB and IIA appeared, with an associated decrease of IIC, as if IIC fibres were being transformed. In the rat soleus, as in kittens, there is little, if any, increase in the number of muscle fibres after birth. Any major change in the proportions of histochemical fibre types must therefore be due to transformation of fibres. Kugelberg (1976) made a detailed study of the transformation of motor units in the soleus muscle of developing rats. He measured single unit contraction times, and by means of glycogen depletion and histochemistry derived innervation ratios and cross-sectional areas, and carried out ATPase and SDH staining on single units. He observed that between five and 34 weeks, the proportion of type II fibre units, with contraction times ranging from 15–26 ms, decreased from 33 to 10 per cent, whereas type I fibre units, with contraction times in the range 27–40 ms, increased from 67 to 90 per cent. This was paralleled by approximately the same relative changes in the number of type II and type I fibres in the whole muscles. At five weeks, transitional units between type II and type I were found. These were intermediate in terms of contraction time, ATPase and SDH activity, and fibre area. He concluded that whole units were converting from type II to I, presumably as a result of a change in motor neurone characteristics.

In newborn and young pigs of increasing body weight, Davies (1972) studied the histochemistry of fibres in the long back muscle (longissimus dorsi) and in the diaphragm, using reactions for myosin ATPase, SDH and phosphorylase. In longissimus dorsi the number of fibres did not change, but the proportion of fibres low in ATPase (type I) increased as body weight increased.

Adult pigs are unusual in comparison with other animals so far studied, in that fibres of a particular type occur in groups within muscles, rather than being interspersed with fibres of other types. The histochemical appearance of these muscles is, therefore, more like that of re-innervated muscles of other animals, where the fibres are 'type-grouped' (*see* the section following), than that of normal muscles of other animals with a 'mosaic' appearance. In newborn pigs, the type I fibres occurred singly, but in longissimus dorsi the group size increased with body weight until, in large animals, the mean group size was 3.2 fibres. As the total number of fibres remained constant, it seems likely that some fibres, particularly those surrounding existing type I fibres, were transforming to type I. Assuming motor unit homogeneity in pigs, this could result either from selective reinnervation or suppression of innervation of fibres, or from selective transformation of those motor units with fibres lying in contact with existing type I fibres. The latter process seems complex, but the former is not known to occur in other developing animals after the disappearance of polyneuronal innervation.

A recent immunocytochemical study of myosin isoenzymes has shown that fast and slow isoenzymes co-exist within individual fibres in rat diaphragm and EDL at early ages when polyneuronal innervation is present. However, by 21 days, when polyneuronal innervation has disappeared, the isoenzymes have become segregated into different muscle fibres, as they are in the adult (Gauthier *et al.*, 1978). Recently, however, the distribution of fibres containing slow muscle myosin has been studied in perinatal rats using immunohistochemical methods (Rowlerson, 1979). At three days before birth the myotubes containing slow myosin are concentrated within the deep parts of the muscle, which is broadly similar to the distribution of fibres containing slow myosin in the adult muscle.

RE-INNERVATION

Self-reinnervation

Nerve sprouting. Following muscle nerve section in mammals there is often very effective regeneration of the nerve, with re-establishment of functional neuromuscular contacts. However, the composition, distribution and properties of the reconstituted motor units often differ from those of the original units, and in this section we will examine some of the differences found experimentally. A discussion of some current ideas about factors governing the re-establishment of neuromuscular contacts is given by Jansen, Thompson and Kuffler (1978), and McComas (1977), in a recent book, relates experimental work to human pathology involving re-innervation.

It has long been known that, when a muscle is partly denervated, the remaining intact axons may extend their innervation territories, so that tension development by the muscle when stimulated via the nerve may even be completely restored (*see* Weiss and Edds, 1945). This process is due to terminal and preterminal sprouting by the remaining axons (Hoffman, 1951) and is independent of any regeneration of the sectioned nerves that may occur subsequently. Recently, this phenomenon has been studied in mouse (Brown and Ironton, 1978) and rat (Thompson and Jansen, 1977) muscle. In peroneus tertius of the mouse (a small muscle) the whole muscle was found to be capable of attaining full innervation again if three or more of the 11 or so units originally present remained intact after the partial denervation. When subsequent regeneration of the sectioned axons took place, some of the fibres innervated by the three units were relinquished and innervated by regenerated axons, but the three units remained larger than normal, and some muscle fibres were innervated by more than one motor unit. Such polyneuronal innervation following regeneration of innervation had been reported previously by Guth (1962) who found that it was transient. McArdle (1975) found, in the rat, that the polyneuronal innervation was nearly eliminated by 60 days (down to 3 per cent). This contrasts with the picture in the frog, where regeneration following crush of the nerve to cutaneus pectoris led to an increase of about three-fold (about 25–70 per cent) in the number of polyneuronally innervated end-plate sites (Rotshenker and McMahon, 1976). Most, or possibly all, frog muscles show considerable polyneuronal innervation under normal conditions. If the additional polyneuronal innervation following regeneration does persist, rather than just being eliminated much more slowly, then it would be interesting to know whether a similar persistence occurs in mammalian muscles with some normal polyneuronal innervation (e.g. cat cricothyroideus; Hunt and Kuffler, 1954), or whether this is a difference between frogs and mammals.

Mechanical factors. When a muscle is re-innervated by its own nerve following section, there is a period of polyneuronal innervation followed by an organised elimination, the result being a motor unit organisation similar to, but not identical with, that previously evolved during development. For instance, Bessou, Laporte and Pagès (1966) found that, in cat superficial lumbrical muscles, the regeneration following nerve section led to re-establishment of the relationships between motor unit contraction time and tension with axon conduction velocity, but with more scatter than in the normal. Bagust and Lewis (1974) studied motor unit properties in self-re-innervated fast and slow muscles of cats and found, similarly, that many of the inter-relationships of motor unit properties were re-established, except that the distribution of motor unit tensions in soleus was skewed towards larger values (normally the distribution is symmetrical) and the variance in the distribution was greater than normal in both muscles, due to the added presence of larger and smaller units. The period of re-innervation was about 207 days, so any transient polyneuronal innervation was probably eliminated. There does not appear to be any other later reorganisation on a significant scale, as recent experiments on animals kept for several years after nerve section produced essentially similar results (Lewis and Owens, 1979).

To what extent the reorganisation of the motor units is appropriate to the functioning of the muscle is an important question. Some data available at present indicate a very debased functioning of re-innervated muscle. Milner-Brown, Stein and Lee (1974) found, in human patients who had suffered severance of the ulnar nerve, that even following good re-innervation of the first dorsal interosseus muscle, where motor unit tensions were normal, the ordered recruit-

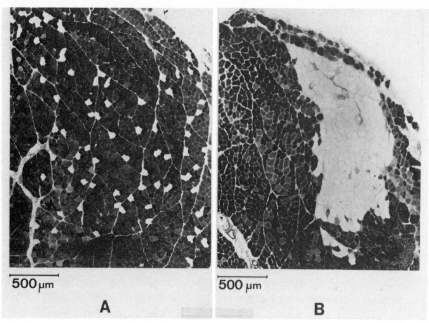

Fig. 1.14   A. Cross-section of rat anterior tibial muscle. PAS preparation, showing the scattered distribution of the PAS-negative (glycogen-depleted) muscle fibres in 3/4 of one normal motor unit. B. Cross-section of rat anterior tibial muscle after transection and union of the motor nerve. PAS preparation, showing the compact, partly fascicular delineated distribution of muscle fibres in one re-innervated motor unit with increased number of fibres and diminished innervation field (photographs kindly provided by Professor E. Kugelberg of the Karolinska Institute, Stockholm)

ment of motor units from small to large during increasing voluntary effort was lost and did not return. As one would expect, this led to reduced manual dexterity. In this study it was not known to what extent axons and muscle fibres were matched or mismatched, and animal experiments in which motor unit properties and reflex recruitment orders are studied following nerve regeneration might be useful. Of course, the loss of the normal recruitment order could have been caused by disorganisation of synaptic input to the motor neurones due, for instance, to poor sensory regeneration. It is interesting that Milner-Brown *et al.* (1974) found that, where regeneration took place down physically continuous, unsevered paths to the muscle (in relieved pressure or entrapment neuropathies), the normal recruitment order was re-established. Presumably, in this case the original organisation was largely restored by accurate regrowth of the axons. It is well known that nerve crush causes far less consequent disorganisation in the regenerating nerve than does nerve section (*see* Aitken, Sharman and

Young, 1947).

One of the most marked and apparently fully persistent differences between normally organised muscle and muscle with regenerated innervation following nerve section, is in the way muscle fibres of individual units are distributed. To appreciate this, we must first examine what is known about the distribution of the muscle fibres of single motor units within normal adult muscles.

Distribution of single motor unit fibres within muscles

Normal muscles. It is well known that, in many muscles of several mammalian species including man, the muscle fibres of a single motor unit may be widely distributed throughout the muscle, or may be more localised within the muscle, but in either circumstance are intermingled with fibres of other units (intra- or extracellular recording: Denslow and Gutensohn, 1950; Buchthal, Guld and Rosenfalck, 1957; Krnjevic and Miledi, 1958; Norris and Irwin, 1961).

The most complete and easily interpretable information on this has been obtained by the use of the glycogen depletion method by several groups of workers (e.g. Edström and Kugelberg, 1968; Brandstater and Lambert, 1973; Burke *et al.*, 1974). An example of a transverse section of a muscle showing this is given in Figure 1.14A.

Although this appears to be the most common distribution pattern, there are some possible exceptions in normal muscle. As previously mentioned, the pattern of histochemical staining in pig muscle is unusual in that fibres are grouped (Davies, 1972), but there is no direct information on the distribution of muscle fibres in motor units. Grouping has also been observed in human extensor digitorum brevis in necropsy material from eight subjects. There was no history of muscle abnormality in the subjects, and four other limb muscles examined in each showed a mosaic distribution of fibres (Jennekens, Tomlinson and Walton, 1971a). It is possible that the wearing of shoes causes small recurrent damage to the innervation of this muscle, with consequent regeneration and the appearance of type-grouping, as discussed below.

Re-innervated muscles. Muscle fibre type-grouping is well known in re-innervated muscle, and Kugelberg, Edström and Abbruzzese (1970) studied the distribution of single units in denervated and partly denervated muscle after self-reinnervation. In the former, the number of muscle fibres per motor unit was within normal limits, but the unit territories were reduced, the packing density of the fibres of a unit therefore being increased. The type-grouping is illustrated in Figure 1.14B. In the partly denervated muscles, the number of muscle fibres per motor unit with surviving innervation was up to seven times greater than normal, and the denervated fibres that had been incorporated into the now expanded surviving units were generally within the expected previous territory of each unit. Therefore, in this case also, the packing density of fibres within these units was increased. From this it would seem that axon sprouts are more likely to make contact with adjacent denervated fibres than with distant ones, and any fibre thus brought into the motor unit

transforms to the type of that motor unit if it was initially different.

Increased type-grouping has been seen in various muscles from aged human subjects at autopsy (Jennekens, Tomlinson and Walton, 1971b). This is probably due to neural degeneration followed by axonal sprouting. It is known that the number of motor units in extensor digitorum brevis in man decreases with age (Campbell and McComas, 1970).

Cross-innervation

As described in the section on whole muscle, cross-innervation between fast-twitch and slow-twitch muscles leads to remarkable changes in the muscle properties, and the first demonstration of this by Buller *et al.* (1960b) in the cat is probably the most direct and exciting illustration of the long-term influence of motor neurones on the muscle fibres they innervate. The mechanical properties of the slow muscle innervated by the nerve previously of a fast muscle came to resemble, in many respects, those of a fast muscle, and *vice versa*. Although the mechanical and histochemical properties of the whole muscles after cross-innervation have been intensively studied, little has been published on identified single units. Obviously, large changes must occur, some related to the fact that re-innervation of the muscle has taken place, and others specifically to cross-innervation. Cross-innervation between FDL and soleus in the cat led to abnormal distributions of motor unit tetanic tensions in both muscles, some being larger than normal while others were very small (Bagust, Finol, Lewis, Webb and Westerman, 1974). This is similar to the picture in self-reinnervated muscles. In addition, the normal association of short contraction times with large motor unit tetanic tensions was not seen in the cross-innervated muscles; indeed, in soleus muscle this relationship was reversed.

ACTIVITY, TRAINING AND EXERCISE

There is abundant evidence that many properties of whole muscle are largely determined by its nerve, and this has been summarised succinctly in a recent article by Rosenthal (1977). Such evidence comes from the effects of denervation on mechanical properties of muscle (e.g. Lewis, 1972) and on the distribution of acetylcholine sensitivity along the muscle fibre surface (e.g. Miledi, 1960), and the effects of cross-innervation on mechanical (e.g. Buller *et al*, 1960b), histochemical (e.g. Guth *et al.*, 1970) and biochemical (e.g. Buller *et al.*, 1971) properties. There is now little doubt (*but see* Mann and Salafsky, 1970) that these effects are largely mediated by the activity patterns imposed on the muscle, because changing these can alter the muscle properties. For instance, chronically immobilising a rat limb reduced the aggregate EMG activity in the soleus muscle, and the pattern of EMG activity was also changed from a predominantly tonic to a more phasic one. This was paralleled by a shift in the mechanical properties towards those of a fast muscle (Fischbach and Robbins, 1969). Conversely, a more generalised effect of muscle slowing was found in limb muscles following contralateral limb de-afferentation (Olson and Swett, 1969) which presumably increased activity generally in the fully innervated limb. Long-term stimulation of fast muscle by chronically implanted stimulating electrodes (Salmons and Vrbová, 1969) caused interesting changes in rabbit: histochemically and biochemically determined enzyme activities (Pette *et al.*, 1973), mechanical properties and myosin type (Salmons and Sréter, 1976) shifted to those typical of slow muscle. Tenotomy has also been used as a method of reducing muscle activity, but it is not suitable for this because considerable muscle atrophy results (McMinn and Vrbová, 1964) without much change in EMG activity patterns or contraction characteristics (Nelson, 1969) in the tenotomised muscle. In the now overloaded antagonist muscles, compensatory hypertrophy occurs, but though interesting this is apparently largely due to non-neural factors (Gutmann, Schiaffino and Hanslikova, 1971).

These major changes in whole-muscle properties, coupled with the known importance of innervation in the developmental differentiation of mammalian fast and slow muscles (e.g. Buller *et al.*, 1960a), and its probable importance in transformation in developing soleus (Kugelberg, 1976), make one wonder how plastic is the motor unit composition of particular adult muscles when either there are changes in life style within individuals or there are differences in life style between individuals of a species. So far there has been no systematic study of this problem at the motor unit level, although there are strong indications of differences between groups of cats brought up under different conditions. For instance, a group of relatively sedentary cats not only had smaller muscles developing less tension than those of more active litter-mates, but there were also differences in contraction speed. The changes were complex, involving an increase in twitch time to peak of fast muscle and an increase of isotonic shortening velocity in slow muscle. At the motor unit level, a population of less active cats had motor units with a smaller range of twitch contraction times in both fast and slow muscle (D.M. Lewis, H. Finol and S. Webb, unpublished work). A properly controlled comparison along these lines could be very valuable. In whole muscles, exercise-training in guinea pig has been found to have effects. The trained muscles were found to have reduced glycogen and phosphorylase depletion following a standard stimulation regime, when compared with untrained muscles (Edgerton, Barnard, Peter, Simpson and Gillespie, 1970). Training also led to an increase in mitochondrial protein content, rate of oxygen consumption and the capability to maintain a higher level of isometric tension over a 60-min period of contraction. There was also an increase in the percentage of 'red fibres' reported, which would imply the transformation of some motor units, if unit homogeneity persists in these conditions. However, there was no hypertrophy, no significant changes in contraction time, tetanic fusion frequency, twitch:tetanus ratio, maximum rate of rise of tetanic tension or proportion of myosin ATPase in dark and light fibres (Barnard, Edgerton and Peter, 1970a, b). A full-scale comparison of motor units in trained and untrained muscle might well be interesting.

MUSCLE EFFECTS ON MOTOR NEURONES

We have seen that motor neurone activity influences the properties of the muscle fibres innervated. This now appears to be a two-way relationship, the motor neurone depending on activity in the muscle fibres. For instance, the duration of the after-hyperpolarisation of the action potential in soleus motor neurones of the cat was found to be reduced by transection of the thoracic spinal cord, or by conduction block of the muscle nerve with tetrodotoxin applied in a cuff round the nerve (Czéh, Gallego, Kudo and Kuno, 1978). This could be prevented by daily stimulation of the sciatic nerve, and was not dependent on sensory nerve activity because stimulation central to the cuff was ineffective, and chronic section of the lumbosacral dorsal roots alone did not lead to shortening of the after-hyperpolarisation (Kuno, Miyata and Muñoz-Martinez, 1974). At present it is not known how this interesting effect is mediated. Possibly a chemical messenger travels up the motor axon to the motor neurone soma from the muscle.

ACKNOWLEDGEMENTS

We thank those authors and publishers who have allowed us to reproduce their material in our illustrations. Each is acknowledged in the appropriate place. We have incorporated some parts of the two chapters in earlier editions that this chapter replaces in the present edition; we thank Professors A. J. Buller and H. A. Sissons for this. Finally, we thank Miss Hilary Lee and Mrs Avril Lear for typing the manuscript and Mrs Barbara Colfer for the photography.

REFERENCES

Adrian, E.D. & Bronk, D.W. (1929) The discharge of impulses in motor nerve fibres. II. The frequency of discharge in reflex and voluntary contraction. *Journal of Physiology*, **67**, 119–151.

Aitken, J.T., Sharman, M. & Young, J.Z. (1947) Maturation of regenerating nerve fibres with various peripheral connections. *Journal of Anatomy*, **81**, 1–22.

Andersen, P. & Sears, T. A. (1964) The mechanical properties and innervation of fast and slow motor units in the intercostal muscles of the cat. *Journal of Physiology*, **173**, 114–129.

Andrew, B.L. & Part, N.J. (1972) Properties of fast and slow motor units in hind limb and tail muscles of the rat. *Quarterly Journal of Experimental Physiology*, **57**, 213–225.

Appelberg, B. & Emonet-Dénand, F. (1967) Motor units of the first superficial lumbrical muscle of the cat. *Journal of Neurophysiology*, **30**, 154–160.

Bagust, J. (1971) Motor unit studies in cat and rabbit solei. *Ph.D. Thesis, University of Bristol.*

Bagust, J. (1974) Relationships between motor nerve conduction velocities and motor unit contraction characteristics in a slow twitch muscle of the cat. *Journal of Physiology*, **238**, 269–278.

Bagust, J. (1979) The effects of tenotomy upon the contraction characteristics of motor units in rabbit soleus muscle. *Journal of Physiology*, **290**, 1–10.

Bagust, J., Finol, H.J., Lewis, D.M., Webb, S. & Westerman, R.A. (1974) Motor units of cross-reinnervated fast and slow twitch muscles. *Journal of Physiology*, **239**, 45–46P.

Bagust, J., Knott, S., Lewis, D.M., Luck, J.C. & Westerman, R.A. (1973) Isometric contractions of motor units in a fast twitch muscle of the cat. *Journal of Physiology*, **231**, 87–104.

Bagust, J. & Lewis, D.M. (1974) Isometric contractions of motor units in self-reinnervated fast and slow twitch muscles of the cat. *Journal of Physiology*, **237**, 91–102.

Bagust, J., Lewis, D.M. & Westerman, R.A. (1973) Polyneuronal innervation of kitten skeletal muscle. *Journal of Physiology*, **229**, 241–255.

Bagust, J., Lewis, D.M. & Westerman, R.A. (1974) The properties of motor units in a fast and a slow twitch muscle during post-natal development in the kitten. *Journal of Physiology*, **237**, 75–90.

Banu, G. (1922) *Recherches Physiologiques sur le Developpement Neuromusculaire.* Paris.

Bárány, M. (1967) ATPase activity of myosin correlated with speed of muscle shortening. *Journal of General Physiology*, **50**, 197–218.

Bárány, M. & Close, R.I. (1971) The transformation of myosin in cross-innervated rat muscles. *Journal of Physiology*, **213**, 455–474.

Barker, D. (1974) The morphology of muscle receptors. In *Handbook of Physiology* Vol. 3, Ed. C.C. Hunt, pp. 1–190 (Springer: Berlin).

Barnard, R.J., Edgerton, V.R. & Peter, J.B. (1970a) Effect of exercise on skeletal muscle. I. Biochemical and histochemical properties. *Journal of Applied Physiology*, **28**, 762–766.

Barnard, R.J., Edgerton, V.R. & Peter, J.B. (1970b) Effect of exercise on skeletal muscle. II. Contractile properties. *Journal of Applied Physiology*, **28**, 767–770.

Barnard, R.J., Edgerton, V.R., Furukawa, T. & Peter, J.B. (1971) Histochemical, biochemical and contractile properties of red, white and intermediate fibers. *American Journal of Physiology*, **220**, 410–414.

Basmajian, J.V. (1963) Control and training of individual motor units. *Science*, **141**, 440–441.

Bennett, M.R. & Pettigrew, A.G. (1974). The formation of synapses in striated muscle during development. *Journal of Physiology*, **241**, 515–545.

Benoit, P. & Changeux, J.P. (1975) Consequences of tenotomy in the evolution of multi-innervation in developing rat soleus muscle. *Brain Research*, **99**, 354–358.

Bessou, P., Emonet-Dénand, F. & Laporte, Y. (1963) Relation entre la vitesse de conduction des fibres nerveuses motrices et le temps de contraction de leurs unités motrices. *Comptes rendus hebdomadaires des seances de l'Academie des Sciences, Series D, Science Naturelles*, **256**, 5625–5627.

Bessou, P., Laporte, Y. & Pagès, B. (1966) Etude de la relation entre le temps de contraction d'unités motrices et la vitesse de conduction de leurs fibres motrices dans les muscles réinnervés. *Comptes rendus hebdomadaires des seances de l'Academie des Sciences, Series D, Science Naturelles*, **263**, 1486–1489.

Betz, W.J., Caldwell, J.H. & Ribchester, R.B. (1979) Postnatal development of motor units and muscle fibres in rat lumbrical muscles. *Journal of Physiology*, **289**, 52P.

Binder, M.D., Kroin, J.S., Moore, G.P., Stauffer, E.K. & Stuart, D.G. (1976) Correlation analysis of muscle spindle responses to single motor unit contractions. *Journal of Physiology*, **257**, 325–336.

Borg, J., Grimby, L. & Hannerz, J. (1978) Axonal conduction velocity and voluntary discharge properties of individual short toe extensor motor units in man. *Journal of Physiology*, **277**, 143–152.

Boyd, I.A. (1962) The structure and innervation of the nuclear bag muscle fibre system and the nuclear chain muscle fibre system in mammalian muscle spindles. *Philosophical Transactions of the Royal Society, Series B*, **245**, 81–136.

Boyd, I.A. (1965) Differences in the diameter and conduction velocity of motor and fusimotor fibres in nerves to different muscles in the hind limb of the cat. In *Studies in Physiology*, Eds D.R. Curtis & A.K. McIntyre (Springer: Berlin).

Boyd, I.A. (1976) The mechanical properties of dynamic nuclear bag fibres, static nuclear bag fibres and nuclear chain fibres in isolated cat muscle spindles. *Progress in Brain Research*, **44**, 33–50.

Boyd, I.A. & Davey, M.R. (1966) The composition of peripheral nerves. In *Control and Innervation of Skeletal Muscle*, Ed. B.L. Andrew, pp. 35–52 (University of St. Andrews: Dundee).

Boyd, I.A. & Davey, M.R. (1968) *Composition of Peripheral Nerve* (Livingstone: Edinburgh).

Brandstater, M.E. & Lambert, E.H. (1973) Motor unit anatomy: type and spacial arrangement of muscle fibers. In *New Developments in Electromyography and Clinical Neurophysiology*, Ed. J.E. Desmedt, pp. 14–22 (Karger: Basel).

Brooke, M.H. & Kaiser, K.K. (1970) Muscle fiber types—how many and what kind? *Archives of Neurology*, **23**, 369–379.

Brooke, M.H., Williamson, E. & Kaiser, K.K. (1971) The behavior of four fiber types in developing and re-innervated muscle. *Archives of Neurology*, **25**, 360–366.

Brown, M.C. & Ironton, R. (1978) Sprouting and regression of neuromuscular synapses in partially denervated mammalian muscle. *Journal of Physiology*, **278**, 325–348.

Brown, M.C., Jansen, J.K.S. & Van Essen, D. (1976) Polyneuronal innervation of skeletal muscles in new-born rats and its elimination during maturation. *Journal of Physiology*, **261**, 387–422.

Brown, M.C. & Matthews, P.B.C. (1960) An investigation into the possible existence of polyneuronal innervation of individual skeletal muscle fibres in certain hind-limb muscles of the cat. *Journal of Physiology*, **151**, 436–457.

Buchthal, F., Guld, C. & Rosenfalck, P. (1957) Multielectrode study of the territory of a motor unit. *Acta physiologica scandinavica*, **39**, 83–104.

Buchthal, F. & Schmalbruch, H. (1970) Contraction times and fibre types in intact human muscle. *Acta physiological scandinavica*, **79**, 435–452.

Buller, A.J. (1972) The neural control of some characteristics of skeletal muscle. In *Modern Trends in Physiology*, 1, Ed. C.B.B. Downman, pp. 72–85 (Butterworth: London).

Buller, A.J., Dornhorst, A.C., Edwards, R., Kerr, D. & Whelan, R.F. (1959) Fast and slow muscles in mammals. *Nature*, **183**, 1516–1517.

Buller, A.J., Eccles, J.C. & Eccles, R.M. (1960a) Differentiation of fast and slow muscles in the cat hind limb. *Journal of Physiology*, **150**, 399–416.

Buller, A.J., Eccles, J.C. & Eccles, R.M. (1960b) Interaction between motoneurones and muscles in respect of the characteristic speeds of their responses. *Journal of Physiology*, **150**, 417–439.

Buller, A.J. & Lewis, D.M. (1965a) The rate of tension development in isometric tetanic contractions of mammalian fast and slow skeletal muscle. *Journal of Physiology*, **176**, 337–342.

Buller, A.J. & Lewis, D.M. (1965b) Further observations on the differentiation of skeletal muscles in the kitten hind limb. *Journal of Physiology*, **176**, 355–370.

Buller, A.J., Mommaerts, W.F.H.M. & Seraydarian, K. (1971) Neural control of myofibrillar ATPase activity in rat skeletal muscle. *Nature*, **233**, 31–32.

Buller, A.J. & Pope, R. (1977) Plasticity in mammalian skeletal muscle. *Philosophical Transactions of the Royal Society, Series B*, **278**, 295–305.

Burke, D., Hagbarth, K.-E., Löfstedt, L. & Wallin, B.G. (1976) The responses of human muscle spindle endings to vibration of non-contracting muscles. *Journal of Physiology*, **261**, 673–693.

Burke, D., Hagbarth, K.-E. & Scuse, N.F. (1978) Recruitment order of human spindle endings in isometric voluntary contractions. *Journal of Physiology*, **285**, 101–112.

Burke, R.E. (1967) Motor unit types of cat triceps surae muscle. *Journal of Physiology*, **193**, 141–60.

Burke, R.E., Jankowska, & ten Bruggencate, G. (1970) A comparison of peripheral and rubrospinal synaptic input to slow and fast twitch motor units of triceps surae. *Journal of Physiology*, **207**, 709–732.

Burke, R.E., Levine, D.N., Salcman, M. & Tsairis, P. (1974) Motor units in cat soleus muscle: physiological, histochemical and morphological characteristics. *Journal of Physiology*, **238**, 503–514.

Burke, R.E., Levine, D.N., Tsairis, P. & Zajac, F.E. (1973) Physiological types and histochemical profiles in motor units of the cat gastrocnemius. *Journal of Physiology*, **234**, 723–748.

Burke, R.E., Rudomin, P. & Zajac, F.E. (1976) The effect of activation history on tension production by individual muscle units. *Brain Research*, **109**, 515–529.

Burke, R.E., Rymer, W.Z. & Walsh, J.V. (1976) Relative strength of synaptic input from short-latency pathways to motor units of defined type in cat medial gastrocnemius. *Journal of Neurophysiology*, **39**, 447–458.

Burke, R.E., Strick, P.L., Kanda, K., Kim, C.C. & Walmsley, B. (1977) Anatomy of medial gastrocnemius and soleus motor nuclei in cat spinal cord. *Journal of Neurophysiology*, **40**, 667–680.

Burke, R.E. & Tsairis, P. (1973) Anatomy and innervation ratios in motor units of cat gastrocnemius. *Journal of Physiology*, **234**, 749–765.

Campbell, M.J. & McComas, A.J. (1970) *5th Symposium on current research in muscular dystrophy and related diseases* (Muscular Dystrophy Group of Great Britain: London).

Clamann, H.P. & Henneman, E. (1976) Electrical measurement of axon diameter and its use in relating motoneuron size to critical firing level. *Journal of Neurophysiology*, **39**, 844–851.

Close, R. (1964) Dynamic properties of fast and slow skeletal muscles of the rat during development. *Journal of Physiology*, **173**, 74–95.

Close, R. (1967) Properties of motor units in fast and slow skeletal muscles of the rat. *Journal of Physiology*, **193**, 45–55.

Close, R. (1969) Dynamic properties of fast and slow skeletal muscle of the rat after nerve cross-union. *Journal of Physiology*, **204**, 331–346.

Close, R. (1971) Neural influences on physiological properties of fast and slow limb muscles. In *Contractility of Muscle Cells and Related Processes*, Ed. R.J. Podolsky (Prentice-Hall: Hemel Hempstead).

Close, R. (1972) Dynamic properties of mammalian skeletal muscles. *Physiological Reviews*, **52**, 129–197.

Close, R. & Luff, A.R. (1974) Dynamic properties of inferior rectus muscle of the rat. *Journal of Physiology*, **236**, 259–270.

Cöers, C. & Woolf, A.L. (1959) *The Innervation of Muscle: A Biopsy Study* (Blackwell: Oxford).

Crawford, G.N.C. (1961) Experimentally induced hypertrophy of growing voluntary muscle. *Proceedings of the Royal Society, Series B*, **154**, 130–138.

Cullheim, S. & Kellerth, J.-O. (1978) A morphological study of the axons and recurrent axon collaterals of cat α motoneurones supplying different functional types of muscle unit. *Journal of Physiology*, **281**, 301–313.

Czéh, G., Gallego, R., Kudo, N. & Kuno, M. (1978) Evidence for the maintenance of motoneurone properties by muscle activity. *Journal of Physiology*, **281**, 239–252.

Davies, A.S. (1972) Postnatal changes in the histochemical fibre types of porcine skeletal muscle. *Journal of Anatomy*, **113**, 213–240.

Davies, A.S. & Gunn, H.M. (1972) Histochemical fibre types in the mammalian diaphragm. *Journal of Anatomy*, **112**, 41–60.

Denslow, J.S. & Gutensohn, O.R. (1950) Distribution of muscle fibres in a single motor unit. *Federation Proceedings*, **9**, 31.

Desmedt, J.E. & Godaux, E. (1977) Ballistic contractions in man: characteristic recruitment pattern of single motor units of the tibialis anterior muscle. *Journal of Physiology*, **264**, 673–693.

Devanandan, M.S., Eccles, R.M. & Westerman, R.A. (1965) Single motor units of mammalian muscle. *Journal of Physiology*, **178**, 359–367.

Drachman, D.B. (1974) The role of acetylcholine as a neurotrophic transmitter. *Annals of the New York Academy of Sciences*, **228**, 160–176.

Dubowitz, V. (1960) A comparative histochemical study of oxidative enzyme and phosphorylase in skeletal muscle. *Histochemie*, **2**, 105–117

Dubowitz, V. & Pearse, A.G.E. (1960) Reciprocal relationship of phosphorylase and oxidative enzymes in skeletal muscle. *Nature*, **185**, 701–702.

Eccles, J.C., Eccles, R.M. & Lundberg, A. (1958) The action potentials of the alpha motoneurones supplying fast and slow muscles. *Journal of Physiology*, **142**, 275–291.

Eccles, J.C. & Sherrington, O.M. (1930) Numbers and contraction values of individual motor-units examined in some muscles of the limb. *Proceedings of the Royal Society, Series B*, **106**, 326–357.

Eccles, R.M., Phillips, C.G. & Wu, Chien-ping (1968) Motor innervation, motor unit organisation and afferent innervation of m. extensor digitorum communis of the baboon's forearm. *Journal of Physiology*, **198**, 179–192.

Edgerton, V.R., Barnard, R.J., Peter, J.B., Simpson, D.R. & Gillespie, C.A. (1970) Response of muscle glycogen and phosphorylase to electrical stimulation in trained and untrained guinea pigs. *Experimental Neurology*, **27**, 46–56.

Edgerton, V.R. & Simpson, D.R. (1969) The intermediate muscle fiber of rats and guinea pigs. *Journal of Histochemistry and Cytochemistry*, **17**, 828–838.

Edjtehadi, G.D. & Lewis, D.M. (1979). Histochemical reactions of fibres in a fast twitch muscle of the cat. *Journal of Physiology*, **287**, 439–453.

Edström, L. & Kugelberg, E. (1968) Histochemical composition, distribution of fibres and fatiguability of single motor units. Anterior tibial muscle of the rat. *Journal of Neurology, Neurosurgery and Psychiatry*, **31**, 424–433.

Emonet-Dénand, F., Laporte, Y. & Proske, U. (1971) Contraction of muscle fibres in two adjacent muscles innervated by branches of the same axon. *Journal of Neurophysiology*, **34**, 132–138.

Engel, A.G. & Stonnington, H.H. (1974) Morphological effects of denervation of muscle. A quantitative ultrastructural study. *Annals of the New York Academy of Sciences*, **228**, 68–88.

Engel, W.K. (1962) The essentiality of histo- and cytochemical studies in the investigation of neuromuscular disease. *Neurology (Minneapolis)*, **12**, 778–784.

Erulkar, S.D., Shelanskl, M.L., Whitsel, B.L. & Ogle, P. (1969) Studies of muscle fibers of the tensor tympani of the cat. *Anatomical Record*, **149**, 279–298.

Feinstein, B., Lindegård, B., Nyman, E. & Wohlfart, G. (1955) Morphologic studies of motor units in normal human muscles. *Acta Anatomica*, **23**, 127–142.

Fischbach, G.D. & Robbins, N. (1969) Changes in contractile properties of disused soleus muscles. *Journal of Physiology*, **201**, 305–320.

Freund, H.J., Büdingen, H.J. & Dietz, V. (1975) Activity of single motor units from human forearm muscles during voluntary isometric contractions. *Journal of Neurophysiology*, **38**, 933–946.

Fukami, Y. & Ridge, R.M.A.P. (1971) Electrophysiological and morphological changes at extrafusal endplates in the snake following chronic denervation. *Brain Research*, **29**, 139–145.

Garnett, R.A.F., O'Donovan, M.J., Stephens, J.A. & Taylor, A. (1979) Motor unit organisation of human medial gastrocnemius. *Journal of Physiology*, **287**, 33–43.

Garnett, R., O'Donovan, M.J., Stephens, J.A. & Taylor, A. (1978) Evidence for the existence of three motor unit types in normal human gastrocnemius. *Journal of Physiology*, **280**, 65P.

Garnett, R. & Stephens, J.A. (1978) Changes in the recruitment threshold of motor units in human first dorsal interosseus muscle produced by skin stimulation. *Journal of Physiology*, **282**, 13P.

Gasser, H.S. & Hill, A.V. (1924) The dynamics of muscular contraction. *Proceedings of the Royal Society of London, Series B*, **96**, 398–437.

Gauthier, G.F. (1969) On the relationship of ultrastructural and cytochemical features to colour in mammalian skeletal muscle. *Zeitschrift für Zellforschung und Microskopische Anatomie*, **95**, 462–482.

Gauthier, G. F., Lowey, S. & Hobbs, A.W. (1978) Fast and slow myosin in developing muscle fibres. *Nature*, **274**, 25–29.

George, J.C. & Naik, R.M. (1957) Studies on the structure and physiology of the flight muscles of bats : 1. The occurrence of two types of fibers in the pectoralis muscle of the bat (Hipposideros speoris), their relative distribution, nature of the fuel store and mitochondrial content. *Journal of Animal Morphology and Physiology*, **4**, 96–101.

Gerlach, R.L., Stauffer, E.K., Goslow, G.E. & Stuart, D.G. (1976) Relation between nerve axon size and muscle unit size and speed in motor units of cat hind limb muscles. *Electromyography and Clinical Neurophysiology*, **16**, 177–190.

Gilliatt, R.W., Westgaard, R.H. and Williams, I.R. (1978) Extra-junctional sensitivity of inactive muscle fibres in the baboon during prolonged nerve pressure block. *Journal of Physiology*, **280**, 449–514.

Goldspink, G., Tabary, C., Tabary, J.C., Tardieu, C. & Tardieu, G. (1974) Effect of denervation on the adaptation of sarcomere number and muscle extensibility to the functional length of the muscle. *Journal of Physiology*, **236**, 733–742.

Gollnick, P.D., Karlsson, J., Piehl, K. & Saltin, B. (1974) Selective glycogen depletion in skeletal muscle fibres of man following sustained contractions. *Journal of Physiology*, **241**, 59–67.

Gollnick, P.D., Piehl, K. & Saltin, B. (1974) Selective glycogen pattern in human muscle fibres after exercise of varying intensity and at varying pedalling rates. *Journal of Physiology*, **241**, 45–57.

Goodwin, G.M., Hoffman, D. & Luschei, E.S. (1978) The strength of the reflex response to sinusoidal stretch of monkey jaw closing muscles during voluntary contraction. *Journal of Physiology*, **279**, 81–111.

Gordon, A.M., Huxley, A.F. & Julian, F.J. (1966) The variation in isometric tension with sarcomere length in vertebrate muscle fibres. *Journal of Physiology*, **184**, 170–192.

Gordon, G., & Holbourn, A.H.S. (1949) The mechanical activity of single motor units in reflex contractions of skeletal muscle. *Journal of Physiology*, **110**, 26–35.

Gordon, G. & Phillips, C.G. (1953) Slow and rapid components in a flexor muscle. *Quarterly Journal of Experimental Physiology*, **38**, 35–45.

Goslow, G.E., Stauffer, E.K., Nemeth, W.C. & Stuart, D.G. (1972) Digit flexor muscles in the cat; their action and motor units. *Journal of Morphology*, **137**, 335–352.

Granit, R., Henatsch, H.D. & Steg, G. (1956) Tonic and phasic ventral horn cells differentiated by post-tetanic potentiation in cat extensors. *Acta physiologica scandinavica*, **37**, 114–126.

Granit, R., Phillips, Skoglund, S. & Steg, G. (1957) Differentiation of tonic from phasic alpha ventral horn cells by stretch, pinna and crossed extensor reflexes. *Journal of Neurophysiology*, **20**, 470–481.

Grimby, L. & Hannerz, J. (1968) Recruitment order of motor units on voluntary contraction : changes induced by proprioceptive afferent activity. *Journal of Neurology, Neurosurgery and Psychiatry*, **31**, 565–573.

Grimby, L. & Hannerz, J. (1977) Firing rate and recruitment order of toe extensor motor units in different modes of voluntary contraction. *Journal of Physiology*, **264**, 865–879.

Guth, L. (1962) Regeneration of interrupted nerve fibers into partially denervated muscle. *Experimental Neurology*, **6**, 129–141.

Guth, L. & Samaha, F.J. (1969) Qualitative differences between actomyosin ATPase of slow and fast mammalian muscle. *Experimental Neurology*, **25**, 138–152.

Guth, L., Samaha, F.J. & Albers, R.W. (1970) The neural regulation of some phenotypic differences between the fibre types of mammalian skeletal muscle. *Experimental Neurology*, **26**, 126–135.

Gutmann, E., Schiaffino, S. & Hansliková, V. (1971) Mechanism of compensatory hypertrophy in skeletal muscle of the rat. *Experimental Neurology*, **31**, 451–464.

Gydikov, A. & Kosarov, D. (1974) Some features of different motor units in human biceps brachii. *Pflugers Archiv für die Gesamte Physiologie*, **347**, 75–88.

Hammarberg, C. (1974) The histochemical appearance of developing muscle fibres in the gastrocnemius, soleus and anterior tibial muscles of the kitten, as viewed in serial sections stained for lipids and succinic dehydrogenase. *Acta neurologica scandinavica*, **50**, 285–301.

Hammond, G.R. & Ridge, R.M.A.P. (1978) Properties of twitch motor units in snake costocutaneous muscle. *Journal of Physiology*, **276**, 525–533.

Hannerz, J. (1974) Discharge properties of motor units in relation to recruitment order in voluntary contraction. *Acta physiologica scandinavica*, **91**, 374–384.

Hannerz, J. & Grimby, L. (1973) Recruitment order of motor units in man : significance of pre-existing state of facilitation. *Journal of Neurology, Neurosurgery and Psychiatry*, **36**, 275–281.

Harrison, V.F. & Mortensen, O.A. (1962) Identification and voluntary control of single motor unit activity in the tibialis anterior muscle. *Anatomical Record*, **144**, 109–116.

Henneman, E., Clamann, H.P., Gillies, J.D. & Skinner, R.D. (1974) Rank order of motoneurones within a pool : law of combination. *Journal of Neurophysiology*, **37**, 1338–1349.

Henneman, E. & Olsen, C.B. (1965) Relations between structure and function in the design of skeletal muscles. *Journal of Neurophysiology*, **28**, 581–598.

Henneman, E., Somjen, G. & Carpenter, D.O. (1965a) Functional significance of cell size in spinal motoneurones. *Journal of Neurophysiology*, **28**, 560–580.

Henneman, E., Somjen, D. & Carpenter, D.O. (1965b) Excitability and inhibitability of motoneurones of different sizes. *Journal of Neurophysiology*, **28**, 599–620.

Hess, A. (1970) Vertebrate slow muscle fibers. *Physiological Reviews*, **50**, 40–62.

Hess, A. & Pilar, G. (1963) Slow fibres in the extra-ocular muscles of the cat. *Journal of Physiology*, **169**, 780–798.

Hill, A.V. (1956) The design of muscles. *British Medical*

Bulletin, **12**, 165–166.

Hoffman, H. (1951) Fate of uninterrupted nerve fibres regenerating into partially denervated muscles. *Australian Journal of Experimental Biology and Medical Science*, **29**, 211–219.

Holt, R.K. & Sohal, G.S. (1978) Elimination of multiple innervation in the developing avian superior oblique muscle. *American Journal of Anatomy*, **151**, 313–318.

Houk, J. & Henneman, E. (1967) Responses of Golgi tendon organs to active contractions of the soleus muscle of the cat. *Journal of Neurophysiology*, **30**, 466–481.

Hudlická, O., Brown, M., Cotter, M., Smith, M. and Vrbová, G. (1977) The effect of long-term stimulation of fast muscles on their blood flow, metabolism and ability to withstand fatigue. *Pflugers Archiv für die Gesamte Physiologie*, **369**, 141–149.

Hunt, C.C. & Kuffler, S.W. (1954) Motor innervation of skeletal muscle: multiple innervation of individual muscle fibres and motor unit function. *Journal of Physiology*, **126**, 293–303.

Jansen, J.K.S., Thompson, W. & Kuffler, D.P. (1978) The formation and maintenance of synaptic connections as illustrated by studies of the neuromuscular junction. *Progress in Brain Research*, **48**, 3–19.

Jennekens, F.G., Tomlinson, B.E. & Walton, J.N. (1971a) The sizes of the two main histochemical fibre types in five limb muscles in man. An autopsy study. *Journal of the Neurological Sciences*, **13**, 281–292.

Jennekens, F.G., Tomlinson, B.E. & Walton, J.N. (1971b) Data on the distribution of fibre types in five human limb muscles: an autopsy study. *Journal of the Neurological Sciences*, **14**, 245–257.

Johnson, M.A., Polgar, J., Weightman, D. & Appleton, D. (1973) Data on the distribution of fibre types in thirty six human muscles. An autopsy study. *Journal of the Neurological Sciences*, **18**, 111–129.

Joyce, G. C., Rack, P.M.H. and Westbury, D.R. (1969). The mechanical properties of cat soleus muscle during controlled lengthening and shortening movements. *Journal of Physiology*, **204**, 461–474.

Kanda, K., Burke, R.E. & Walmsley, B. (1977) Differential control of fast and slow twitch motor units in the decerebrate cat. *Experimental Brain Research*, **29**, 57–74.

Karpati, G. & Engel, W.K. (1967) Neuronal trophic function: a new aspect demonstrated histochemically in developing soleus muscle. *Archives of Neurology*, **17**, 541–545.

Kernell, D. (1966) Input resistance, electrical excitability and size of ventral horn cells in cat spinal cord. *Science*, **152**, 1637–1640.

Kernell, D. & Sjöholm, H. (1975) Recruitment and firing rate modulation of motor unit tension in a small muscle of the cat's foot. *Brain Research*, **98**, 57–72.

Khan, M.A. (1976) Histochemical characteristics of vertebrate striated muscle-review. *Progress in Histochemistry and Cytochemistry*, **8**, 1–48.

Kirkwood, P.A. & Sears, T.A. (1974) Monosynaptic excitation of motoneurones from secondary endings of muscle spindles. *Nature*, **252**, 243–244.

Knott, S. (1971) A study of stretch receptors and motor units in frog muscle. *Ph.D. Thesis, University of Bristol.*

Korneliussen, H. & Jansen, J.K.S. (1976) Morphological aspects of the elimination of polyneuronal innervation of skeletal muscle fibres in newborn rats. *Journal of Neurocytology*, **5**, 591–604.

Krnjevic, K. & Miledi, R. (1958) Motor units in the rat diaphragm. *Journal of Physiology*, **140**, 427–439.

Kugelberg, E. (1976) Adaptive transformation of rat soleus motor units during growth. *Journal of the Neurological Sciences*, **27**, 269–289.

Kugelberg, E. Edström, L. & Abbruzzese, M. (1970) Mapping of motor units in experimentally re-innervated rat muscle. *Journal of Neurology, Neurosurgery and Psychiatry*, **33**, 319–329.

Kuno, M. (1959) Excitability following antidromic activation in spinal motoneurones supplying red muscles. *Journal of Physiology*, **149**, 374–393.

Kuno, M., Miyata, Y. & Mŭnos-Martinez, E.J. (1974) Differential reactions of fast and slow alpha-motoneurones to axotomy. *Journal of Physiology*, **240**, 725–739.

Kuno, M., Miyata, Y. & Mŭnos-Martinez, E.J. (1974) Properties of fast and slow alpha motoneurones following motor re-innervation. *Journal of Physiology*, **242**, 273–288.

Lewis, D.M. (1972) The effect of denervation on the mechanical and electrical responses of fast and slow mammalian muscle. *Journal of Physiology*, **222**, 51–75.

Lewis, D.M., Bagust, J., Webb, S.N., Westerman, R.A. & Finol, H.J. (1977) Axon conduction velocity modified by re-innervation of mammalian muscle. *Nature*, **270**, 745–746.

Lewis, D.M., Luck, J.C. & Knott, S. (1972) A comparison of isometric contractions of the whole muscle with those of motor units in a fast-twitch muscle in the cat. *Experimental Neurology*, **37**, 68–85.

Lewis, D.M. & Owens, R. (1979) Motor units in mammalian skeletal muscle after long periods of re-innervation. *Journal of Physiology*, **296**, 111P.

Liddell, E.G.T. & Sherrington, C.S. (1925) Recruitment and some other factors of reflex inhibition. *Proceedings of the Royal Society, Series B*, **97**, 488–518.

Lømo, T., Westgaard, R.H. & Dahl, H.A. (1974) Contractile properties of muscle: control by pattern of muscle activity in the rat. *Proceedings of the Royal Society, Series B*, **187**, 99–103.

Luff, A.R. & Proske, U. (1976) Properties of motor units of the frog sartorius muscle. *Journal of Physiology*, **258**, 673–685.

Mann, W.S. & Salafsky, B. (1970) Enzymic and physiological studies on normal and disused developing fast and slow cat muscles. *Journal of Physiology*, **208**, 33–47.

Mathers, D.A. & Thesleff, S. (1978) Studies on neurotrophic regulation of murine skeletal muscle. *Journal of Physiology*, **282**, 105–114.

Matthews, P.B.C. (1969) Evidence that the secondary as well as the primary endings of the muscle spindles may be responsible for the tonic stretch reflex. *Journal of Physiology*, **204**, 365–395.

Matthews, P.B.C. (1972) *Mammalian Muscle Receptors and their Central Action* (Arnold: London).

McArdle, J.J. (1975) Complex end-plate potentials at regenerating neuromuscular junction of the rat. *Experimental Neurology*, **49**, 629–638.

McComas, A.J. (1977) *Neuromuscular Function and Disorders* (Butterworth: London, Boston).

McComas, A.J., Upton, A.R.M. & Jorgensen, P.B. (1974) Serial studies of sick motoneurons: the silent synapse. In *Recent Advances in Myology*, Eds W.G. Bradley, D Gardner-Medwin & J.N. Walton, pp. 84–90 (American Elsevier: New York).

McMinn, R.M.H. & Vrbová, G. (1964) The effect of

tenotomy on the structure of fast and slow muscle in the rabbit. *Quarterly Journal of Experimental Physiology*, **49**, 424–429.

McPhedran, A.M., Wuerker, R.B. & Henneman, E. (1965) Properties of motor units in a homogeneous red muscle (soleus) of the cat. *Journal of Neurophysiology*, **28**, 71–84.

Miledi, R. (1960) The acetylcholine sensitivity of frog muscle fibres after complete or partial denervation. *Journal of Physiology*, **151**, 1–23.

Milner-Brown, H.S., Stein, R.B. & Lee, R.G. (1974) Pattern of recruiting human motor units in neuropathies and motor neurone disease. *Journal of Neurology, Neurosurgery and Psychiatry*, **37**, 665–669.

Milner-Brown, H.S., Stein, R.B. & Yemm, R. (1973a) The contractile properties of human motor units during voluntary isometric contractions. *Journal of Physiology*, **228**, 285–306.

Milner-Brown, H.S., Stein, R.B. & Yemm, R. (1973b) The orderly recruitment of human motor units during voluntary isometric contractions. *Journal of Physiology*, **230**, 359–370.

Milner-Brown, H.S., Stein, R.B. & Yemm, R. (1973c) Changes in firing rate of human motor units during linearly changing voluntary contractions. *Journal of Physiology*, **230**, 371–390.

Mosher, C.G., Gerlach, R.L. & Stuart, D.G. (1972) Soleus and anterior tibial motor units of the cat. *Brain Research*, **44**, 1–11.

Nelson, P.G. (1969) Functional consequences of tenotomy in hind limb muscles of the cat. *Journal of Physiology*, **201**, 321–333.

Norris, F.H. & Irwin, R.L. (1961) Motor unit area in a rat muscle. *American Journal of Physiology*, **200**, 944–946.

Nyström, B. (1968a) Fibre diameter increase in nerves to 'slow-red' and 'fast-white' cat muscles during postnatal development. *Acta neurologica scandinavica*, **44**, 265–294.

Nyström, B. (1968b) Histochemistry of developing cat muscles. *Acta neurologica scandinavica*, **44**, 405–439.

O'Brien, R.A.D., Ostberg, A.J.C. & Vrbová, G. (1978) Observations on the elimination of polyneuronal innervation in developing mammalian skeletal muscle. *Journal of Physiology*, **282**, 571–582.

Olson, C., & Swett, C.P. (1966) A functional and histochemical characterization of motor units in a heterogeneous muscle (flexor digitorum longus) of the cat. *Journal of Comparative Neurology*, **128**, 475–498.

Olson, C.B. & Swett, C.P. (1969) Speed of contraction of skeletal muscle. The effect of hypoactivity and hyperactivity. *Archives of Neurology*, **20**, 263–270.

Ovalle, W.K. & Smith, R.S. (1972) Histochemical identification of three types of intrafusal muscle fibers in the cat and monkey based on the myosin ATPase reaction. *Canadian Journal of Physiology and Pharmacology*, **50**, 195–202.

Palade, G.E. (1954) Electron microscopic observations of interneuronal and neuromuscular synapses. *Anatomical Record*, **118**, 335–336.

Parry, D.J., Mainwood, G.W. & Chan, T. (1977) The relationship between surface potentials and the number of active motor units. *Journal of the Neurological Sciences*, **33**, 283–296.

Peter, J.B., Barnard, R.J., Edgerton, V.R., Gillespie, C.A. & Stempel, K.E. (1972) Metabolic profiles of three fiber types of skeletal muscle in guinea pigs and rabbits. *Biochemistry*, **11**, 2627–2633.

Pette, D., Smith, M.E., Staudte, H.W. & Vrbová, G. (1973) Effects of long-term electrical stimulation on some contractile and metabolic characteristics of fast rabbit muscle. *Pflugers Archiv für die Gesamte Physiologie*, **338**, 257–272.

Prewitt, M.A. & Salafsky, B. (1970) Enzymic and histochemical changes in fast and slow muscles after cross innervation. *American Journal of Physiology*, **218**, 69–74.

Prochazka, A., Westerman, R.A. & Ziccone, S.P. (1977) Ia afferent activity during a variety of voluntary movements in the cat. *Journal of Physiology*, **268**, 423–448.

Proske, U. & Waite, P.M.E. (1976) The relation between tension and axonal conduction velocity for motor units in the medial gastrocnemius muscle of the cat. *Experimental Brain Research*, **26**, 325–328.

Rack, P.M. & Westbury, D.R. (1969) The effects of length and stimulus rate on tension in the isometric cat soleus muscle. *Journal of Physiology*, **204**, 443–460.

Ranatunga, K.W. (1977) Changes produced by chronic denervation in the temperature-dependent isometric contractile characteristics of rat fast and slow twitch skeletal muscles. *Journal of Physiology*, **273**, 255–262.

Redfern, P.A. (1970) Neuromuscular transmission in new-born rats. *Journal of Physiology*, **209**, 701–709.

Reinking, R.M., Stephens, J.A. & Stuart, D.G. (1975) The motor units of cat medial gastrocnemius: problem of their categorisation on the basis of mechanical properties. *Experimental Brain Research*, **23**, 301–313.

Ridge, R.M.A.P. (1967) The differentiation of conduction velocities of slow twitch and fast twitch muscle motor innervation in kittens and cats. *Quarterly Journal of Experimental Physiology*, **52**, 293–304.

Ridge, R.M.A.P. & Thomson, A.M. (1977) Xenopus motor units co-innervated with spindles. *Journal of Physiology*, **276**, 34–35P.

Ridge, R.M.A.P. & Thomson, A.M. (1978) Polyneuronal innervation in amphibian skeletal muscle. *Journal of Physiology*, **277**, 2P.

Riley, D.A. (1976) Multiple axon branches innervating single endplates of kitten soleus muscle. *Brain Research*, **110**, 158–161.

Riley, D.A. (1977) Spontaneous elimination of nerve terminals from the endplates of developing skeletal myofibers. *Brain Research*, **134**, 279–285.

Robertson, J.D. (1956) The ultrastructure of a reptilian myoneural function. *Journal of Biophysical and Biochemical Cytology*, **2**, 381–394.

Rosenthal, J. (1977) Trophic interactions of neurons. Chapter 21, *Handbook of Physiology, The Nervous System I*. pp. 775–801 (American Physiological Society: Washington).

Rosenthal, J.L. & Taraskevich, P.S. (1977) Reduction of multiaxonal innervation at the neuromuscular junction of the rat during development. *Journal of Physiology*, **270**, 299–310.

Rossi, G. & Cortesina, G. (1965) Multimotor end-plate muscle fibres in the human vocalis muscle. *Nature*, **206**, 629–630.

Rotshenker, S. & McMahon, U.J. (1976) Altered patterns of innervation in frog muscle after denervation. *Journal of Neurocytology*, **5**, 719–730.

Rowlerson, A. (1979) Differentiation of muscle fibre types in fetal and young rats studied with a labelled antibody to slow myosin. *Journal of Physiology*, **301**, 19P.

Salmons, S. & Sréter, F.A. (1976) Significance of impulse activity in the transformation of skeletal muscle type. *Nature*, **263**, 30–34.

Salmons, S. & Vrbová, G. (1969) The influence of activity on some contractile characteristics of mammalian fast and slow muscles. *Journal of Physiology*, **201**, 535–549.

Schiefferdecker, P. (1909) *Muskeln and Muskelkerne* (Barth: Leipzig).

Sharrard, W.J.W. (1955) The distribution of the permanent paralysis in the lower limb in poliomyelitis. *Journal of Bone and Joint Surgery*, **38B**, 540–558.

Sherrington, C.S. (1925) Remarks on some aspects of reflex inhibition. *Proceedings of the Royal Society, Series B*, **97**, 519–545.

Sica, R.E.P. & McComas, A.J. (1971) Fast and slow twitch units in a human muscle. *Journal of Neurology, Neurosurgery and Psychiatry*, **34**, 113–120.

Sissons, H.A. (1963) *Investigation of muscle fibre size. Research in Muscular Dystrophy*. Ed. by the Members of the Research Committee of the Muscular Dystrophy Group (Pitman Medical: London).

Sissons, H.A. (1965) *Further investigations of muscle fibre size. Research in Muscular Dystrophy*. Ed. by the Members of the Research Committee of the Muscular Dystrophy Group (Pitman Medical: London).

Spurway, N.C. (1978) Objective typing of mouse ankle-extensor muscle fibres based on histochemical photometry. *Journal of Physiology*, **277**, 47–48P.

Sréter, F.A., Gergely, J., Salmons, S. & Romanul, F. (1973) Synthesis by fast muscle of myosin light chains characteristic of a slow muscle in response to long-term stimulation. *Nature*, **241**, 17–18.

Steg, G. (1964) Efferent muscle innervation and rigidity. *Acta physiologica scandinavica*, **61**, Suppl. 225, 1–53.

Stein, J.M. & Padykula, H.A. (1962) Histochemical classification of individual skeletal muscle fibers of the rat. *American Journal of Anatomy*, **110**, 103–124.

Stein, R.B., French, A.S., Mannard, A. & Yemm, R. (1972) New methods for analysing motor unit function in man and animals. *Brain Research*, **40**, 187–192.

Stephens, J.A., Garnett, R. & Buller, N.P. (1978) Reversal of recruitment order of single motor units produced by cutaneous stimulation during voluntary muscle contraction in man. *Nature*, **272**, 362–364.

Stephens, J.A. & Taylor, A. (1975) Human motor unit contractions studied by controlled intramuscular microstimulation. *Journal of Physiology*, **252**, 8P.

Stephens, J.A. & Usherwood, T.P. (1975) The fatiguability of human motor units. *Journal of Physiology*, **250**, 37–38P.

Tanji, J. & Kato, M. (1973) Recruitment of motor units in voluntary contraction of finger muscle in man. *Experimental Neurology*, **40**, 759–770.

Thompson, W. & Jansen, J.K.S. (1977) The extent of sprouting of remaining motor units in partly denervated immature and adult rat soleus muscle. *Neuroscience*, **2**, 523–535.

Thomson, A.M. (1978) Motor unit properties of a toe muscle of Xenopus laevis. *Ph.D. Thesis, University of Bristol*.

Wachstein, M. & Meisel, E. (1955) The distribution of demonstrable succinic dehydrogenase and mitochondria in tongue and skeletal muscle. *Journal of Biophysical and Biochemical Cytology*, **1**, 483–488.

Walmsley, B., Hodgson, J.A. & Burke, R.E. (1978) The forces produced by medial gastrocnemius and soleus muscles during locomotion in freely moving cats. *Journal of Neurophysiology*, **41**, 1203–1216.

Weeds, A. (1978) Myosin: polymorphism and promiscuity. *Nature*, **274**, 417–418.

Weiss, P. & Edds, M.V. (1945) Spontaneous recovery of muscle following partial denervation. *American Journal of Physiology*, **145**, 587–607.

Westerman, R.A., Lewis, D.M., Bagust, J., Edjtehadi, G. & Pallot, D. (1974) Communication between nerves and muscles: postnatal development in kitten hindlimb fast and slow twitch muscle. In *Memory and Transfer of Information*, Ed. H.P. Zippel, pp. 255–291 (Plenum: New York).

Wilkie, D.R. (1976) Muscle. The Institute of Biology: *Studies in Biology No. 11* (Edward Arnold: London).

Wray, S.H. (1966) Quoted by Gilliatt, R.W. in: Axon branching in motor nerves. In *Control and Innervation of Skeletal Muscle*, Ed. B.L. Andrew, pp. 53–63 (The University of St. Andrews).

Wuerker, R.B., McPhedran, A.M. & Henneman, E. (1965) Properties of motor units in a heterogeneous pale muscle (m. gastrocnemius) of the cat. *Journal of Neurophysiology*, **28**, 85–99.

Wyman, R.J., Waldron, I. & Wachtel, G.M. (1974) Lack of fixed order of recruitment in cat motoneuron pools. *Experimental Brain Research*, **20**, 101–114.

Yellin, H. & Guth, L. (1970) The histochemical classification of muscle fibers. *Experimental Neurology*, **26**, 424–432.

Yemm, R. (1977) The orderly recruitment of motor units of the masseter and temporalis muscles during voluntary isometric contractions in man. *Journal of Physiology*, **265**, 163–174.

Ultrastructure of the skeletal muscle fibre

INTRODUCTION

By exceeding the limited resolution of light optics, electron microscopy has made it possible to define cell structure in proportions compatible with the macromolecular world of the biochemist and physiologist, thereby allowing a closer correlation between structure and function. This is vividly exemplified by studies of the subcellular organisation of the skeletal muscle cell where the findings have profoundly influenced the theories of muscle contraction. This chapter outlines the main concepts of vertebrate skeletal muscle ultrastructure, with emphasis on mammalian tissue, and also cites briefly important functional concepts.

A muscle fibre is any of the many cylindrical multinucleated cells that are bound together within a connective tissue framework to form a skeletal muscle. The length of the fibre may vary from several millimeters to centimeters and its

diameter from 10 to 100 microns depending on the animal species and the particular muscle. Each fibre is bounded by a membrane system referred to as the sarcolemma. Along the sarcolemma there is a region adapted for functional contact with a motor nerve, called the motor end-plate or myoneural junction. The major portion of the cell volume is occupied by a highly ordered fibrillar contractile system designed for unidirectional shortening during contraction. Superimposed on the contractile components are two tubular networks, the sarcoplasmic reticulum and the T system, which play an important part in the activation and subsequent deactivation of the contractile elements during contraction. In addition to these highly specialised structures, the sarcoplasm (cytoplasm) of the muscle fibre also contains organelles common to other cells (i.e. mitochondria, Golgi apparatus, lipid droplets, lipofuscin, glycogen granules and ribosomes).

SURFACE OF THE MUSCLE FIBRE

Plasma membrane and basement membrane

If a freshly dissected muscle fibre is gently pinched with a fine forceps the myoplasm will retract, leaving a structureless, transparent, tubular casing (Bowman, 1840; Speidel, 1937; Mauro and Adams, 1961). In histological preparations this sheath is difficult to see because it is so thin and stains poorly. By electron microscopy (Figs 2.1, 2.2a, 2.9 and 2.10) it can be resolved into an inner *plasma membrane, a basement membrane,* and groups of small collagen fibrils lying adjacent to, or penetrating, the basement membrane (Mauro and

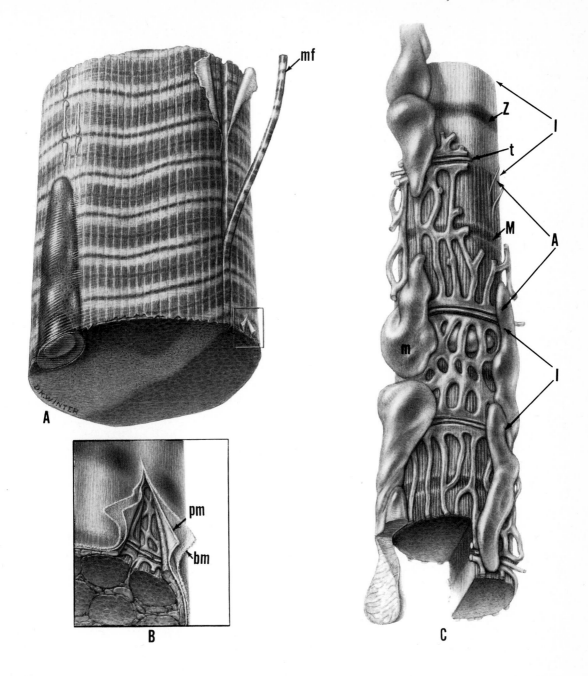

Fig. 2.1 Structural organisation of the human skeletal muscle fibre. A. Longitudinal segment of a muscle fibre as seen with a light microscope. The striped appearance of this cell is the net result of the precise alignment of its banded myofibrillar components (*mf*. myofibril). B. By electron microscopy the membranous components of the sarcolemmal sheath can be identified. Within the fibre, between the myofibrils, there are elements of the sarcoplasmic reticulum and the T system (*bm*, basement membrane; *pm*, plasma membrane). C. The isolated myofibril whose banded appearance is the result of the disposition of the thick and thin myofilaments (see text). Embracing the myofibril is the membrane-limited tubular network of the *sarcoplasmic reticulum* and the *T system*. Near the junction of the A and I bands the components of these two tubular systems form a complex called the *triad*, which is composed of an intermediate transverse tubule of the T system bounded on each side by a transverse cisterna of the sarcoplasmic reticulum (*t*, transverse tubule of T system; *I*, I band; *A*, A band; *M*, M line; *Z*, Z line; and *m*, mitochondrion)

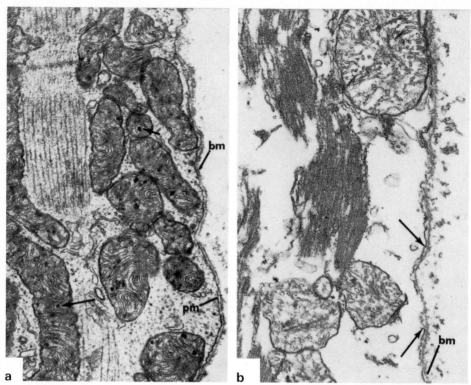

Fig. 2.2 A. Longitudinal section, margin of a normal skeletal muscle fibre showing plasma membrane (*pm*) and outer basement membrane (*bm*). Note the small dense matrix granules within the mitochondria (*arrows*), and the variability in configuration of the cristae. Electron micrograph, ×28 400. B. Margin of a muscle fibre, 15 min after focal cold injury. The mitochondria are swollen. The plasma membrane (*arrows*) is fragmented and by 24 h this membrane will no longer be evident. The basement membrane (*bm*) remains intact to form the so-called 'sarcolemmal tube' within which regeneration will eventually take place. Electron micrograph, × 19 900

Adams, 1961). The term *sarcolemma*, as used by some histopathologists and biologists, identifies the tubular sheath visible by light microscopy. Other biologists have insisted on using sarcolemma to correspond to the plasma membrane only (Bennett, 1960).

In muscle tissue subjected to conventional fixatives for electron microscopy the plasma membrane is about 7.5 nm thick and at high magnifications displays a trilaminal structure. This triple-layered appearance, which is characteristic of most cell membranes, led Robertson (1958, 1959) to propose the unit-membrane model of biological membranes. Since then our concepts of the molecular organisation of cellular membranes have been modified by the use of various other techniques, including freeze-etching, spin-labelling, X-ray diffraction and

differential colorimetry as discussed in an informative review by Oda (1976). Most notable of the new concepts has been the fluid mosaic model of Singer and Nicolson (1972) based on ultrastructural techniques using ferritin-conjugated antibodies to visualise the distribution of specific antigens on the surface of membranes. Oda (1976) proposes a model of membrane structure which seems to take into account features of both the unit-membrane model and the fluid mosaic model.

Across the plasma membrane the bioelectrical potential of the muscle fibre is maintained. When the surface membrane potential is altered by an excitatory stimulus, a wave of excitation is thought to spread within the fibre over an apparent extension of the plasma membrane—the T system (see below). Other cell components derived from the surface membrane are the small 'pinocytotic' vesicles which collect in the sarcoplasm adjacent to the plasma membrane. These vesicles seem to be formed by invaginations of the plasma membrane and may play a part in transporting materials into and out of the cells (cf. Bennett, 1960).

The basement membrane is a uniform, moderately dense, structureless lamella that is much thicker than the plasma membrane. One of its functions seems to be that of a microskeleton helping to maintain the shape and stability of individual cells (Pease, 1958). Basement membranes are not seen around single myoblasts in regenerating or developing muscle, but only around the mature multinucleated fibre (Price, Howes and Blumberg, 1964; Pryzbylski and Blumberg, 1966). The basement membrane appears to be relatively resistant to trauma and remains (without the plasma membrane) to form the 'sarcolemmal tube' (Figs 2.2b and 2.3) which guides the growth of regenerating fibres (Allbrook, 1962; Price *et al.*, 1964).

Myoneural junction

At the myoneural junction (Fig. 2.4) the cell surface exhibits a specialised structural configuration which seems to be uniformly similar in most of the mammalian skeletal muscle fibres examined so far (Reger, 1958; Andersson-Cedergren, 1959; Couteaux, 1960; Zacks, 1964; Padykula and Gauthier, 1970; Engel and Santa, 1971; Jerusalem, Engel and Gomez, 1974). There is a depression in the fibre surface which is characterised by a series of parallel running gutters or *synaptic troughs*. The muscle surface bordering on these troughs shows a series of deep narrow infoldings referred to as *junctional folds*. Lying within each synaptic trough is an unmyelinated terminal nerve branch of the motor nerve. Overlying the troughs may be a thin layer of Schwann cell cytoplasm. An amorphous material lines the junctional folds as well as the space separating the opposing plasma membranes of the muscle fibre and the terminal axon. This material is continuous with (and resembles) the basement membrane layers covering the adjacent muscle fibre and Schwann cell surfaces.

The cytoplasm of the terminal axon contains mitochondria and numerous *synaptic vesicles*. These synaptic vesicles resemble the vesicles seen in synaptic endings of the central nervous system (DeRobertis, 1958). Several experiments have demonstrated the role of synaptic vesicles in the transmission of nerve impulses (DeRobertis, 1959;

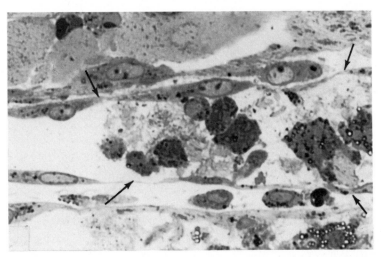

Fig. 2.3 Longitudinal section. Centre of a freeze lesion of muscle 3–4 days following injury. Portions of three 'sarcolemmal tubes' can be seen (*arrows* indicate margins of tube within centre of photograph). The sarcolemmal tube is formed by the basement membrane (see Fig. 2.2B). Within the tubes, in addition to necrotic sarcolemmal debris, are two main cell types: rounded macrophages containing many lipid droplets; and at the periphery of the tubes, spindle-shaped mononuclear myoblasts. The myoblasts may be satellite cells (Fig. 2.9) which were not affected by the injurious agent, or which had migrated into the damaged zone from the more viable parts of the muscle fibre to initiate the regeneration. Light micrograph, ×775

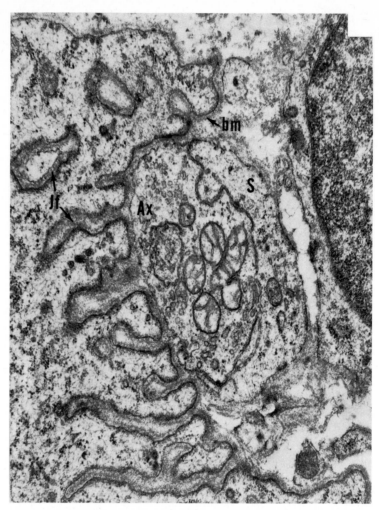

Fig. 2.4   Portion of a motor end-plate in human quadriceps femoris. The surface of the muscle fibre exhibits numerous junctional folds (*jf*), some of which show branching. The terminal axon (*Ax*) is covered by an extension of Schwann cell cytoplasm (*S*). The axoplasm contains numerous synaptic vesicles and mitochondria. Lining the junctional folds and filling the space between the surface of the muscle fibre and the surface of the terminal axon is basement material that is continuous with the basement membrane (*bm*) overlying the adjacent muscle fibre and Schwann cell surfaces, ×33 000

Pellegrino de Iraldi and De Robertis, 1963; Clark, Hurlfut and Mauro, 1972). That the transmitter substance is acetylcholine has been indicated by a variety of experiments (Jones and Kwanbunbumpen, 1970; Katz and Miledi, 1972; Clark *et al.*, 1972). The junctional sarcoplasm contains many mitochondria, numerous glycogen granules, ribonucleoprotein particles, and small vesicles.

Studies on neuromuscular junctions of rat diaphragm demonstrate that differences exist between motor neurones serving type I and type II fibres. In type II fibres, axonal vesicles are abundant and junctional folds are long and closely spaced. In type I fibres, axonal vesicles are less numerous and junctional folds are relatively short and sparse (Padykula and Gauthier, 1970). In man, Engel and Santa (1971) using histomorphometric analysis of eight components of the end-plate from intercostal muscle of individuals without known muscle disease, concluded that a degree of variability existed among different individuals and even along portions of the same end-plate. They inferred no statistically significant differences according to fibre type.

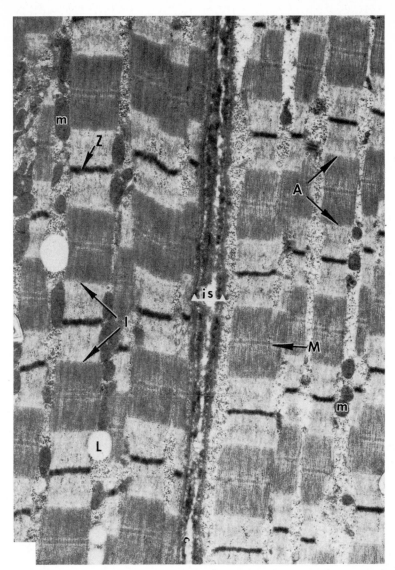

Fig. 2.5 Longitudinal section of two adjacent muscle fibres of human quadriceps femoris. The fibres are separated by an intercellular space (is). Myofibrils depict typical band pattern. A dense *Z line* divides each *I band*. A *sarcomere* is that portion of a myofibril bounded by two successive Z lines. In the centre of each sarcomere is the dense *A band* which is bisected by an *H zone*, the latter having a central *M line*. Note the disposition of the mitochondria (m), and the numerous glycogen particles dispersed within the interfibrillar spaces. Electron contrast variation in the two fibrils may reflect fibre type differences. Refer to text for difficulties in interpreting fibre types in human muscle, × 13 000

CONTRACTILE SYSTEM

The myofibril

By light microscopy the muscle fibres can be resolved into numerous thin, parallel, longitudinal contractile units termed *myofibrils* which have a diameter of approximately 1 μm (Fig. 2.1). Each myofibril exhibits a repetitive dark and light banding which lies in phase with similar dark and light bands of adjacent myofibrils to form the typical striated pattern of the muscle fibre. The band pattern varies with the state of muscle contraction and is best demonstrated in a resting or passively stretched fibre. The dark band is anisotropic (or doubly refractile) under the polarising microscope and is called the *A band*. The light band is isotropic and is called the *I band*. Each I band is divided by a thin dense *Z line*. In the centre of each A band is a pale *H zone* which is bisected by an *M line*. The structural unit lying between two successive Z lines is a *sarcomere*.

By electron microscopy the band pattern of the myofibrils is seen to be the result of an overlapping array of *thick* and *thin myofilaments* (Figs. 2.5 and 2.6). This, as well as other concepts of the fine structural organisation of the contractile system, is derived largely from the research of H. E. Huxley (1957; 1963; 1965). He predicted the existence of a double array of filaments from X-ray diffraction studies on living and glycerinated muscle and later confirmed and elaborated upon this concept with detailed electron-microscopic observations. His investigations were largely on rabbit psoas muscle; however, subsequent observations on other vertebrates, including man (van Breeman, 1960; Price, 1963; Price, Howes, Hutson, Fitzgerald, Blumberg, Pearson and Sheldon 1965; Shafiq, Gorycki, Goldstone and Milhorat, 1966) indicate a similar basic design of the contractile system.

The dimensions of the thick and thin myofilaments vary somewhat depending on the preparative methods for electron microscopy (Page and

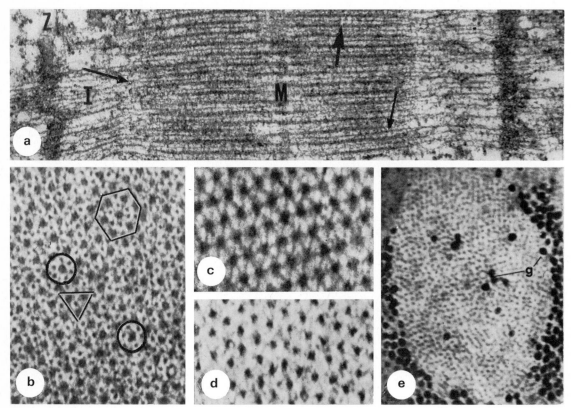

Fig. 2.6 Human quadriceps femoris. A. Thin longitudinal section. The band pattern of the sarcomere is a result of the arrangement of the thick and thin filaments. The thick filaments (*thick arrow*) determine the extent of the A band. The thin filaments (*thin arrows*) forming the *I band* extend half way into the A band in the relaxed fibre. *M*, M line, *Z*, Z line. Electron micrograph, ×44 000. B. Cross-section through A band of myofibril. Interdigitating thick and thin filaments form a double hexagonal pattern. The thick filaments are arranged in a primary hexagonal array (as in hexagon). Six thin filaments surround each thick filament forming a secondary hexagonal array (as in circles). Also, each thin filament is positioned in the centre of a triangle formed by three adjacent thick filaments (as in triangle). Electron micrograph, ×124 000. C. Cross-section through M line depicting cross-bridges connecting thick filaments in this region. These cross-bridges are not to be confused with the cross-bridges linking thick and thin filaments in other regions of the A band (see text). Electron micrograph, ×128 000. D. Cross-section through H zone of relaxed myofibril showing only thick filaments. Electron micrograph, ×80 000. E. Cross-section through I band. Only thin filaments are found in this band. Note the dense glycogen granules (*g*) dispersed around the filaments. Electron micrograph, ×64 400

Huxley, 1963). The thick filaments are confined to the A band and consequently determine its length which appears to have a constant value of 1.5–1.6 μm in vertebrates (Page, 1966). The thin myofilaments originate at the Z line, form the I band and penetrate, between thick filaments, into the A band to the edge of the H zone. Unlike the thick filaments, the length of the thin filaments varies in the muscles of different vertebrates (from approximately 1.00–1.25 μm), but their length is constant in each muscle (Page, 1966). The diameters of the thick and thin filaments are 15–18 nm and 5–6 nm respectively. Although the filament diameters are relatively uniform, the ends of the thick filaments are tapered and their centres (or M line regions) appear to be slightly thicker.

The high degree of order and spatial orientation of the filaments is best appreciated in transverse sections through the A band where they are arranged in a double hexagonal array (Fig. 2.6b). The thick filaments are disposed so that each one forms the corner of a primary hexagon. A secondary hexagon is formed by the six thin filaments that surround each thick filament. In addition, in vertebrate striated muscle, each of these thin filaments is positioned so that it lies in the centre of a triangle formed by three adjacent thick filaments. In arthropod muscle, each thin filament is located midway on a line joining two thick filaments (Smith, 1966). Cross-sections through the I band and H zone in the *relaxed* fibre reveal only thin and thick filaments, respectively (Figs 2.6c, d, e).

Another significant structural feature is a system of cross-bridges linking the thick and thin filaments (Huxley, 1957, 1963, and 1969). The cross-bridges are small, regularly spaced, lateral projections arising from the entire length of a thick filament except for a short central region which includes the M line and adjacent portions of the H zone. Low-angle X-ray diffraction patterns indicate that these thick filament projections are arranged in a helical fashion, with groups of cross-bridges occurring at intervals of 14.3 nm along the length of the filaments with a helical repeat of 42.9 nm (Huxley and Brown, 1967; Huxley, 1969). The number of cross-bridges in each group is not absolutely certain. At first it was thought to be two (Huxley and Brown, 1967), but it is more likely to be three, as implied by various studies

indicating that the myosin molecules in a thick filament are related by a three-fold rotation axis (Squire, 1973; Luther and Squire, 1978) and that there are three myosin molecules to each 14.3 nm repeat unit.

In the middle of the A band is the 0.15–0.2 μm long M region where the thick filaments do not have crossbridges (Huxley, 1963; 1965), and at the centre of the M region is the M band where there is a system of small interconnecting rods between adjacent thick filaments, which may be responsible for stabilising the hexagonal pattern of thick filaments in the A band (Fig. 2.6c). Recent studies by Luther and Squire (1978) have given us a better insight into the three-dimensional substructure of the M band. They noted that the interconnecting rods often demonstrate a thickened region halfway along their length, which has been attributed to longitudinally orientated M filaments which are, in turn, interconnected at points by a series of finer rodlets. This observation both supported and elaborated upon the three-dimensional model proposed by Knappeis and Carlsen (1968) but conflicted with another model proposed by Pepe (1975). Differences in the longitudinal substructure pattern of the M band as a function of species muscle and muscle fibre type have been reported by Sjöström and Squire (1977).

Molecular components of the myofilaments

Selective chemical extractions of thick and thin filaments combined with light, interference, and electron microscopy indicate that the thick filaments are primarily composed of myosin and the thin filaments of actin (Hasselbach, 1953; Hanson and Huxley, 1953; Perry and Corsi, 1958). This has been supported by studies employing fluorescein or mercury-labelled antibodies (Holtzer, Marshall and Finck, 1957). Furthermore, there is convincing evidence that the interaction between the contractile proteins, actin and myosin, is modulated by at least two other proteins, tropomyosin and troponin, which are located on the thin filaments.

Each thick filament is an assembly of several hundred myosin molecules. The myosin molecule consists of two globular units, each about 7.0 nm in diameter, attached to a double stranded α-

helical rod approximately 140 nm long and 2 nm in diameter (Lowey, Slayter, Weeds and Baker, 1969).

Following trypsin digestion, each myosin molecule breaks into the more rapidly sedimenting, heavy meromyosin (HMM) and light meromyosin (LMM), which retains the solubility characteristics of native myosin (Szent-Gyorgyi, 1953). LMM forms about two-thirds of the rod-like tail of myosin, and HMM comprises the rest of the rod-like portion and the globular heads of myosin (Rice, 1961; Huxley, 1963; Zobel, 1967). The actin-combining sites (i.e. cross-bridges) and ATPase properties of myosin are associated with HMM (Szent-Gyorgyi, 1953; Huxley, 1963).

Papain can further cleave HMM into two smaller fragments, termed subfragment-1 (S-1) and subfragment-2 (S-2) (Kominz, Mitchell, Lihei and Kay, 1965). HMM S-1 retains the ATPase and actin-binding properties and appears as globular fragments in electron microscopy (Lowey et al., 1969). LMM can aggregate at physiological ionic strength into large filaments which are probably analogous in structure to the backbone of the thick filaments, while the adjacent linear segment, HMM S-2, does not form aggregates, either with itself or LMM, and is completely soluble at physiological ionic strength (Lowey et al., 1969; Huxley, 1971). This suggests that weak interactions are likely to occur in vivo when HMM S-2 is compelled to lie next to neighbouring myosin molecules (Lowey et al., 1969). Thus, HMM S-2 may form a 'flexible joint' or 'hinge' at the point where HMM S-2 and LMM connect and enables the whole HMM segment of myosin to bend away flexibly from the axis of the thick filament (Lowey et al., 1969), a factor important in the sliding-filament theory of contraction (see below).

Actin may be isolated as a monomer (G-actin) that undergoes polymerisation to F-actin under appropriate conditions (Straub, 1942). In electron micrographs of negatively stained F actin filaments polymerised from a solution of the protein (possibly containing tropomyosin or other contaminant proteins), the resultant structures are identical in appearance to the thin filaments isolated from muscle (Hanson and Lowy, 1963; Huxley, 1963, 1965). The filaments are formed by the double-helical arrangement of two chains of globular monomeric sub-units. The sub-unit repeat in each chain is 5.46 nm and the length of each turn of the helix is 36.5 nm.

By electron microscopy, the tropomyosin molecule has a rod-like configuration, 40 nm in length and 2–3 nm in width (Rowe, 1964; Kung and Tsao, 1965). X-ray diffraction and optical rotary dispersion studies of tropomyosin are consistent with a coiled-coil α-helical form (Cohen and Holmes, 1963; McCubbin, Kouba and Kay, 1967; Chang and Tsao, 1962; Ooi, 1967). Tropomyosin also crystallises as an orthorhombic lattice with a unit cell of about 40 nm (Hodge, 1959; Huxley, 1963; Higashi and Ooi, 1968), and the similarity of this structure to the Z line resulted in the suggestion that tropomyosin may be located, at least in part, within the Z line (Huxley, 1963). Coexistence of tropomyosin and actin in a single myofibrillar structure was suggested to others by the stoichiometric interaction of tropomyosin with actin (Laki, Maruyama and Kominz, 1962; Martonosi, 1962; Hanson and Lowy, 1963; Maruyama, 1964). This latter concept was supported by the observation that fluorescent-labelled antitropomyosin stained the thin filaments throughout the sarcomere, while the Z line was not stained or only intermittently stained (Pepe, 1966; Endo, Lonomura, Masaki, Ohtsuki and Ebashi, 1966). Furthermore, the thin filament has a 40 nm periodicity in electron micrographs (Hanson and Lowy, 1963; 1964) and by X-ray diffraction (Worthington, 1959) that is not attributable to actin, but corresponds with the periodicity of tropomyosin crystals (Huxley, 1963; Hodge, 1959; Higashi and Ooi, 1968). The significance of this was further clarified when electron microscopy demonstrated the presence of ferritin-labelled antitroponin at 40 nm intervals along the thin filaments (Ohtsuki, Masaki, Lonomura and Ebashi, 1967) and also that troponin is evident at 40 nm periods along the tropomyosin lattice in co-crystals of troponin and tropomyosin (Higashi and Ooi, 1968). Thus, the elongated tropomyosin probably lies in a groove between two actin monomers and the 40 nm periodicity along the thin filaments probably represents the spacing of a troponin complex along the tropomyosin in the thin filament.

As already indicated, the protein troponin is in close juxtaposition with tropomyosin within the thin filament. Native tropomyosin contains troponin, which promotes the association of tropomyosin into aggregates (Ebashi and Kodama, 1966). Troponin, unlike tropomyosin, does not seem to bind strongly to actin, yet the troponin–tropomyosin complex enhances F-actin polymerisation (Ebashi and Kodama, 1966). Although troponin was initially thought to be a single globular protein, it is now known to be a complex of at least three proteins which together with tropomyosin, play a primary part in the regulation of muscular contraction (Ebashi, Ebashi and Kodama, 1967; Ebashi and Endo, 1968; Tonomura, Watanobe and Morales, 1969; Wilkinson, Terry, Cole and Trayer, 1972; Weber and Murray, 1973; Cummins and Perry, 1978). One component, which is highly negatively charged, contains a high-affinity calcium-binding site and is believed to be the *calcium receptor* of the contractile apparatus, activating actinomyosin ATPase; a second component is thought to serve as an *interaction inhibitor*, along with tropomyosin, to inhibit actinomyosin ATPase; and a third component serves as a *tropomyosin-binding protein* to bind the troponin complex to tropomyosin.

The ultrastructural and chemical characteristics of the Z line are not as well understood as those of the other components of the myofibril. Most investigators favour the concept that the thin actin filaments terminate at the Z line rather than passing through it. Several workers have advanced evidence indicating that there are thin interconnecting Z filaments, arranged in a complex tetragonal pattern, joining the actin filaments on opposite sides of the Z line (Knappeis and Carlsen, 1962; Reedy, 1964). A membranous interconnection has also been envisaged (Franzini-Armstrong and Porter, 1964). More recently a model has been proposed suggesting that within the Z line there is an interlinking of looping strands which emanate from the actin filaments of adjacent sarcomeres (Kelly, 1967a). As discussed above, tropomyosin was at one time thought to be located in the Z line, but further evidence tended to disprove this. In addition, it has been shown that both Z-line and M-line material can be simultaneously and selectively removed from glycerinated muscles, and under proper ionic conditions, the extracted fraction can be used to restore Z lines (Stromer, Harshorne and Rice, 1967). The extracted fractions appeared to be deficient in tropomyosin and another extract of natural actomyosin, known to contain tropomyosin, had greatly reduced ability to reconstitute Z lines. In the congenital disorder, nemaline myopathy, it was found that there is an excess production of Z-line material (Price, Gordon, Pearson, Munsat and Blumberg, 1965); and a chemical assay of tissue from this disorder has failed to demonstrate an excess of tropomyosin (Ebashi, 1967). Close chemical identity of the Z line filaments with actin has been suggested by experimental studies with the drug plasmocid which, in low doses, was seen to dissolve selectively Z lines and I bands (Price, Pease and Pearson, 1962). Yet the only protein shown to be definitely associated with the Z line is α-actinin (Ebashi, 1967; Suzuki, Saito, Sabo and Nonami, 1978).

Internal structure of the myofilaments

A number of attempts, using a variety of muscles, has been made to define the internal molecular organisation of the myosin filament (Baccetti, 1965, 1966; Gilev, 1966; Pepe, 1966, 1967, 1971; Pepe and Drucker, 1972; Craig and Offer, 1976; Sjöström and Squire, 1977). Two main alternative theories have emerged, one by Pepe and the other by Squire. Pepe's model is based on the assumption that the myosin filament heads are arranged on two-stranded 6/1 helices, with a pitch of 86.4 nm. This model is in keeping with the symmetry of myosin filaments as proposed by Huxley and Brown (1967). There has been some doubt cast on the validity of the Huxley and Brown model, however (Squire 1971, 1972; Tregear and Squire, 1973) and evidence has been obtained which suggests that the symmetry of the filaments may be that of a three-stranded filament of 129.6 nm pitch (Squire, 1972).

The features of Squire's (1971 and 1973) model assume that in vertebrate skeletal muscle there are antiparallel overlaps between myosin rods of 130 nm and 43 nm and a three-stranded 9/1 helix having projections with 129.6 nm pitch. The model agrees well with known proportions by weight of actin and myosin in this type of muscle (Tregear and Squire, 1973). The Squire model also suggests that molluscan thick filaments and vertebrate smooth muscles are constructed similarly, the differences being due to differences in core proteins (Squire, 1973). The packing arrangement of myosin molecules suggested by the model fits neatly with observations concerning shape, diameter, variable density of myosin filament cross-sections (Squire, 1973) and longitudinal tilt of the myosin rods as shown by King and Young (1972). Many questions about the molecular architecture still remain to be answered. For a review of some of the basic questions needing elucidation see Sjöström and Squire (1977).

Another approach to illuminate details of the filaments involved the use of negative staining to observe the sub-units of mechanically separated muscle filaments, and to observe artificial myosin filaments grown from myosin solutions (Huxley, 1963; 1969; 1971). These studies led Huxley to conclude that the molecular components of the filaments maintain a strict structural polarity. The myosin molecules within the thick filaments of one-half of an A band have one orientation and this appears to be reversed in the other half of the A band; hence the tails of the myosin molecules (or the LMM) point toward the centre of the A band (or H zone) and the head of the myosin molecule (or HMM) forms the cross-bridges that interact with actin. In turn, all the actin monomers of each F-actin filament appear to be polarised in the direction of the Z line. Thus, the interacting sites of the myosin and actin molecules are arranged so that they always have the same relative orientation to each other. If a sliding force is developed at each interacting site (see below), all the components of the force in the overlap region should add up in parallel and in the same direction, and the sites are arranged so that the direction of force is reversed in each half sarcomere: this results in the drawing together of the actin filaments at the centre of the A band (Huxley, 1969).

Structural changes during contraction

Observations on single muscle fibres by A. F. Huxley and Niedergerke (1954), using an in-terference microscope, and on isolated myofibrils by H. E. Huxley and Hanson (1954), with phase microscopy revealed that, during the contraction or passive stretching of a muscle fibre, the length of the A band and the distance between the Z line and the edge of the H zone remained constant, while the lengths of the H zone and the I band respectively shortened or lengthened. Therefore, these investigators concluded that changes in muscle length were probably the result of a sliding mechanism involving overlapping filaments whose lengths remained unchanged. Electron microscopy and X-ray diffraction studies extended these observations to the myofilament level where they have shown that contraction results from a *sliding-filament* system involving the actin and myosin myofilaments (Huxley, 1957, 1963; Elliott, Lowy and Millman, 1967; Huxley and Brown, 1967). During contraction the opposing sets of thin filaments within a sarcomere slide toward each other in between the thick filaments of the A band. Thus, at full contraction the H band is obliterated and the I bands are narrowed, with a drawing of the Z lines toward the A bands in each sarcomere. No significant shortening of either the thick or thin filaments appears to take place. As mentioned above, there is a parallel structural polarisation of the actin and myosin filaments so that their respective molecular sub-units are orientated in opposite directions in each half of a given sarcomere, thus ensuring that the individual thin filaments in each half of a sarcomere slide in one direction only. The movement of the actin filaments continuously past the myosin filaments is thought to be the result of a repetitive sequence in which a given cross-bridge attached to a specific site of the actin molecule pulls the thin filament a short distance, detaches, oscillates back, and re-attaches at another point on the actin filament. As indicated by Huxley (1969, 1971), this mechanism assumes that the sliding force is the result of a precise structural change in a protein complex involving the globular part of HMM, actin, and other components (such as tropomyosin and troponin), and is associated with the splitting of a molecule of ATP. Furthermore, this force-generating system must be able to work equally well over the increased distance between the thick and thin filaments that develops as a muscle contracts. Lowey and colleagues (1969) have proposed that the design of the myosin molecule allows it readily to adjust its length to that required for interaction within actin. To them it appears that the structural role of LMM is to maintain the organisation of the thick filament, and the linear HMM S-2 portion of a myosin molecule can be 'hinged out' by bending at the HMM-LMM junction and thus allow the HMM S-1 globular component of HMM to attach to actin while maintaining a constant orientation. They further maintain that structural studies of whole muscle by antibody-staining techniques, electron microscopy, and X-ray diffraction (Reedy, Holmes and Tregear, 1965; Pepe, 1966, 1967; Huxley and Brown, 1967; Huxley, 1969) provide additional evidence to support this concept. Detailed discussions of the possible nature of the physico-chemical forces that develop with the generation of a pull by a cross-bridge may be found in papers by A. F. Huxley (1957), Davies (1963), Elliott, Lowy and Millman (1967), Huxley and Brown (1967), Huxley (1969, 1971), Huxley and Haselgrove (1977), and Eisenberg and Hill (1978).

SARCOPLASMIC RETICULUM AND THE T SYSTEM

Structural features

In 1902 Veratti demonstrated, within silver-impregnated preparations of skeletal muscle, a reticulum of delicate black strands interwoven around the myofibrils. This structure was neglected for about 50 years and was later re-identified in early electron micrographs as an interfibrillary membranous system (Bennett and Porter, 1953). Technological improvements made it possible to show that this smooth membranous system formed a complex network of tubules (or cisternae) within the interfibrillar regions throughout the fibre (Porter and Palade, 1957; Andersson-Cedergren, 1959; Reger, 1961; Fawcett and Revel, 1961; Revel, 1962). This tubular network has been divided into two parts: the *sarcoplasmic reticulum*, and the *T system* (or transverse tubular system) (Andersson-Cedergren, 1959).

The organisation of the sarcoplasmic reticulum and the T system is intimately related (Figs 2.7 and

2.8), although the extent of their development and organisation may vary greatly in different muscles. In general, the tubules of the sarcoplasmic reticulum closely embrace a myofibril over its entire length and circumference in the form of a loosely woven network of interconnecting longitudinal and lateral tubules, which have a repetitive pattern related to the underlying sarcomeres, and which interconnect with identical tubular systems surrounding adjacent myofibrils. The configuration of the sarcoplasmic reticulum appears to be conducive to the changes of the interfibrillar space that accompany contraction. When the sarcomeres are shortened during contraction, the reticulum components appear to be shorter and wider, and when the sarcomeres are longer, the reticulum is more elongated and slender (Franzini-Armstrong and Porter, 1964). Individual transverse tubular elements of the T system extend about the myofibrils interrupting the components of the sarcoplasmic reticulum at regular intervals. At each point of interruption a complex called a *triad* is formed. The triad consists of a slender transverse T-system tubule interposed between two transverse tubular components of the SR, called *terminal cisternae*, which frequently contain dense granular material (Figs. 2.1 and 2.8). In the skeletal muscle of man, as well as in other mammals and some other vertebrates, the triads are located near the junction of the A and I bands. This results in two triads per sarcomere. However, in the muscles of certain animals such as the frog and in the white body muscles of fish, as in most cardiac muscle fibres, only one triad per sarcomere is seen, located at the Z line.

Although most of the tubules of the T system run transversely in the fibre, longitudinal branches have been observed in some vertebrates (Revel, 1962; Page, 1965; Huxley, 1964; Peachey, 1965). However, this situation is more common in muscles of invertebrates (Smith, 1966).

Published electron micrographs of fish body-muscle fibres and fibres from the ventricles of mammalian hearts clearly illustrate that the membranes forming the T system are confluent with the plasma membrane, thereby delimiting a compartment within the fibre that is continuous with the extracellular space (Simpson and Oertelis, 1962; Franzini-Armstrong and Porter, 1964;

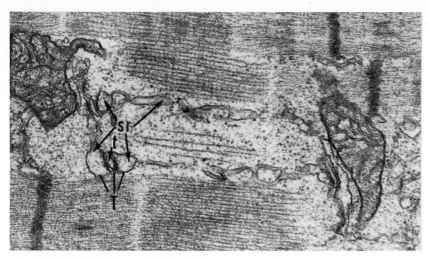

Fig. 2.7   Human quadriceps femoris. Tangential section along the longitudinal surface of myofibril showing parts of the sarcoplasmic reticulum (*sr*) and the T system (*t*). The triad (*T*) consists of the transverse tubule of the T system bounded by the lateral cisternae of the sarcoplasmic reticulum, ×40 300

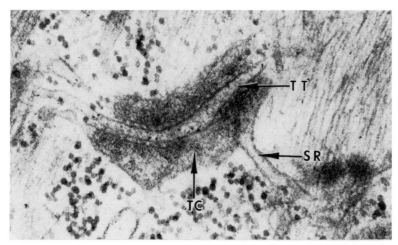

Fig. 2.8   Human quadriceps femoris. Higher magnification of a triad. The T tubule (TT)) is separated from the electron-dense lateral cisternae (TC) of the sarcoplasmic reticulum (SR) by a narrow space, ×86 650

Sommer and Johnson, 1968). In frog muscle, direct continuity has not been readily seen, but functional continuity between the space of the transverse tubular system and the extracellular space has been shown by the diffusion of molecular tracers into the fibre (Endo, 1964a, b; Hill, 1964; Huxley, 1964; Page, 1964). Physiological conductance studies on frog muscle have also yielded results that could be explained only by the presence of a space interposed between the external medium and the sarcoplasm (Hodgkin and Horowicz, 1960; Adrian and Freygang, 1962).

Although numerous observations show close juxtaposition between the plasma membrane and the T system in higher forms of life, morphological proof of direct continuity is still lacking. This continuity may be difficult to demonstrate, due to the fact that the connection between the plasma membrane and the T-system tubules occurs too irregularly around the fibre circumference, or it may be a result of the unusual lability of the T system in fixation (Fawcett and Revel, 1961; Franzini-Armstrong and Porter, 1964).

In contrast to the 'exteriorised' T system, the

sarcoplasmic reticulum appears to be a separate intracellular fluid-containing compartment with no connections to the extracellular space, the sarcoplasmic matrix, or the T system. Several authors have compared the sarcoplasmic reticulum to the smooth-surfaced endoplasmic reticulum of other cells (*cf*. Smith, 1966). In one of the vacuolar myopathies, periodic paralysis, a diffuse dilatation of the sarcoplasmic reticulum occurs without affecting the T system (Shy, Wanko, Rowley and Engel, 1961; Howes, Price, Pearson and Blumberg, 1966).

Activation of contraction and muscular relaxation

The mechanism by which the depolarisation of the surface membrane leads to the simultaneous activation of the deep as well as superficial myofibrillar contractile units of a muscle fibre has been a subject of much concern to physiologists. After due consideration of rates and distances involved, Hill pointed out 20 years ago (1948; 1949) that in fast-acting skeletal muscle fibres, in contrast to slow-contracting smooth muscle, the diffusion rates would be too slow to carry an activating substance from the plasma membrane to all the contractile elements within a fibre: a process, not a substance, must transmit a signal for contraction into the cell to account for the rapid sequence of events that results in contraction. The identification of the sarcoplasmic reticulum by electron microscopy led logically to the supposition that this membrane system might be the route along which excitation is conducted inwards from the surface membrane (Porter and Palade, 1957; see Smith, 1966). The membranes forming the triad were implicated by experiments showing that a localised contraction of sarcomeres can be elicited in single fibres when the sarcolemma is stimulated with micro-electrodes in regions corresponding to the location of triads (Huxley and Straub, 1958; Huxley and Taylor, 1958). The T-system membranes are thought to be the most likely membranous component of the triad by which the excitatory impulses are conveyed inwards (Andersson-Cedergren, 1959; Franzini-Armstrong and Porter, 1964).

Further laboratory findings have led to the concept that the contractile state of the myofibrils is influenced by the selective release and accumulation of calcium ions from the sarcoplasmic reticulum. Contraction of isolated viable muscle fibres has been produced experimentally by increasing their internal calcium concentration with micro-injection methods (Kamada and Kinosita, 1943; Heilbrunn and Wiercinski, 1947; Podolsky, 1962). Studies of cell fractions containing vesicular fragments of the sarcoplasmic reticulum and the T system have shown that these vesicular particles can take up calcium ions from a surrounding medium containing calcium, magnesium, ATP and oxalate, and effect relaxation of isolated myofibrils (Parker and Gergely, 1960; Ebashi and Lipmann, 1962; Hasselbach, 1964a, b and c; Maruyama, 1965). Although in cell fractionation studies the vesicles of the sarcoplasmic reticulum cannot be separated from those of the T system, indirect calculations suggest that most of the vesicles are from the sarcoplasmic reticulum rather than the T system (Huxley, 1964; Page, 1964; Peachey, 1965). In addition, *in vivo* localisation at the ultrastructural level using histochemical and autoradiographic techniques indicates that the calcium ions withdrawn from the sarcoplasm during relaxation are primarily concentrated in the terminal cisternae of the reticulum (Hasselbach, 1964a, b and c; Constantin, Franzini-Armstrong and Podolsky, 1965; Winegrad, 1965). See chapter 4 and several reviews (Sandow, 1970; Fuchs, 1974; and Endo, 1977) for more comprehensive discussions of the role of calcium in muscle contraction.

In the light of the above findings it is reasonable to assume that excitation of the T system somehow leads to the release of calcium ions from the cisternae of the sarcoplasmic reticulum and the liberated calcium then initiates contraction. Therefore, the structural features of the triad assume new importance. The width of the gap separating the surface membranes of the T system and sarcoplasmic reticulum is stated to range from 7.5 to 15 nm (Smith, 1966). The membrane of the lateral cisternae of the triad facing the T system is frequently scalloped (Revel, 1962; Franzini-Armstrong and Porter, 1964; Walker and Schrodt, 1965; Kelly, 1967b). In attempting to understand the structure of this specialised region, these junctions have been likened to the synaptic gap in certain nervous system synapses (*cf.* Smith, 1966), and have been compared with the junctional complexes formed by membrane systems of other cells (Fahrenbach, 1965; Peachey, 1965; Walker and Schrodt, 1965; Kelly, 1967b; Franzini-Armstrong, 1974). In a model proposed by Kelly and Cahill (1969) the SR scallops reach the T system membrane with which they form localised points of either tight or very close junction. An amorphous material was found between the SR projections and the T-system membrane in the triads of frog twitch fibres by Franzini-Armstrong (1970) who referred to the SR projections and the amorphous material as *SR feet*. It has also been proposed that some substance fills the space between the SR feet, thus forming a functional barrier between the junctional area and the rest of the sarcoplasm (Walker and Schrodt, 1965; Kelly, 1967b, 1969). However, a study using ferritin and imferon molecules as tracers in 'skinned' muscle fibres indicated that at least 50 per cent of the T-system surface is freely accessible to the sarcoplasm, that 30 per cent of the remainder of the T-system surface is covered by SR feet, and 20 per cent in the centre of the junction may or may not be accessible (Franzini-Armstrong, 1975).

In brief, depolarisation of the plasma membrane of a muscle fibre may result in the following sequence of events: (1) conduction of excitation along the membranes of the T system; (2) release of calcium ions from the cisternae of the SR by some unknown mechanism which links the depolarisation of the T system with the release of calcium; (3) diffusion of the calcium ions within the sarcoplasm, saturating the calcium-binding component of troponin; (4) reversal of a pre-existing inhibitory effect of the troponin–tropomyosin complex on actinomyosin ATPase; (5) dephosphorylation of ATP with simultaneous activity at the actin–myosin cross-bridges resulting in contraction; and (6) active re-accumulation of calcium ions by sarcoplasmic reticulum with resultant removal of calcium from binding sites on troponin and inhibition of actinomyosin ATPase by the troponin–tropomyosin complex, allowing relaxation.

MITOCHONDRIA (SARCOSOMES)

Mitochondria are compartmentalised membranous sacs formed by two separate membranes which have different structural, biochemical, and physical properties. A smooth outer limiting membrane is separated by a narrow space from an inner membrane whose surface area is increased by numerous infoldings, or *cristae*, that project into a large central chamber containing dense amorphous matrix material. The complex functional role of the mitochondria is well covered in several reviews (Novikoff, 1961; Lehninger, 1964, 1967; Green, 1965; Parsons, 1965). The mitochondria are the primary intracellular site of Krebs' tricarboxylic acid cycle activity, fatty acid, oxidation, electron transport, and oxidative phosphorylation. Biochemical and biophysical studies indicate that the enzymatic components of many, if not all, of these metabolic systems are arranged in an orderly pattern within the membranes of the mitochondria. The best documented example is the finding that the electron-carrier enzymes are located in the inner mitochondrial membrane, together with those enzymes necessary to utilise the energy resulting from electron transport to regenerate ATP from ADP and phosphate. Electron micrographs of negatively stained mitochondrial membranes show that the inner surface of the inner membrane is studded by regularly spaced 'elementary particles' composed of a knob-like structure, approximately 9 nm in diameter, linked by a stem to the body of the membrane (Fernandez-Moran, Oda, Blair and Green, 1964). These particles may represent molecules of the coupling enzymes that form ATP at the expense of electron transport (Kagawa and Racker, 1966). Thus, it is apparent that the metabolic functions of the mitochondria are dependent not only on the presence of specific enzymes, but also on the proper sequential arrangement of these enzymes (within the mitochondrial membranes). In several human myopathies it has been proposed that dysfunction may be related to alterations in the membrane-linked enzymatic assembly lines of mitochondria rather than to specific enzymatic deficiencies (*see* Price, 1967). Additional findings show that normal mitochondria contain a distinctive DNA which is different from that in the cell nucleus, that they can synthesise proteins from amino acids and may carry genetic information influencing cytoplasmic inheritance and differentiation (*see* Lehninger, 1967).

The shape of the mitochondria varies; this may reflect a specific metabolic state or possibly the direct influence of adjacent structures such as the myofibrils. The cristae can be orientated perpendicular or parallel to the long axis of the mitochondria or may form a localised concentric pattern (Fig. 2.2). The configuration and number of cristae, as well as the size and number of mitochondria, are an indication of the rate of oxidative metabolism within a given muscle. This is dramatically illustrated by the complex mitochondria seen in the hyperactive cricothyroid muscle of the bat's larynx (Revel, 1962), and in the heart muscle of the canary which has a rate of 1000 per min (Slautterback, 1965). Mitochondria are more abundant in so-called type I fibres which depend on oxidative phosphorylation as a primary source of energy and less so in type II fibres whose energy is derived mainly from glycolysis (*see* below).

Mitochondria are distributed in several specific locations within the muscle fibre. This possibly reflects a localised need for the energy-carrying ATP molecules that these organelles supply (Palade, 1956; Lehninger, 1967). One location is the interfibrillar sarcoplasm, where the mitochondria may be found either as isolated profiles symmetrically positioned in relation to the Z lines or aligned end-to-end in a single column running parallel to adjacent myofibrils for several sarcomere lengths. In the I band areas, mitochondria may seem to extend transversely across the myofibril, but serial sections have shown that many of these seemingly simple profiles are portions of a mitochondrion that may partly encircle the myofibril (Andersson-Cedergren, 1959). Mitochondrial clusters are also seen adjacent to the plasma membrane, often intimately associated with nuclei of the muscle fibre, or grouped at the motor end-plate region.

GOLGI COMPLEX

The Golgi complex is relatively inconspicuous in mature skeletal muscle fibres. It often consists of a group of flattened tubular channels in the cytoplasm near the poles of the nuclei. In a mononuclear myoblast or immature multinucleated muscle fibre it is usually more complex; the flattened sacs are often associated with prominent small vesicles and large vacuoles (Price, Howes and Blumberg, 1964; Przybylski and Blumberg, 1966).

PARTICULATE COMPONENTS OF THE SARCOPLASM

The sarcoplasmic matrix is dispersed between the myofibrils, around the sarcoplasmic reticulum, the mitochondria and nuclei, and beneath the plasma membrane; it appears as a less dense background material in electron micrographs. In living muscle, the matrix represents a continuous aqueous fluid phase containing soluble proteins such as myoglobin (Bennett, 1960).

Glycogen particles (Figs. 2.5 and 2.6e) appear as discrete granules varying from 25 to 40 nm in diameter and are distributed throughout the sarcoplasm between myofibrils and beneath the plasma membrane. The number of granules may be dependent on the metabolic demands of the cell.

Lipid droplets are large, homogeneous, circular bodies which may have either a smooth or scalloped margin, and are primarily composed of triglycerides or fatty acids (Fawcett, 1966). The intracellular location and number of lipid bodies is related to the metabolic needs of the fibre. They often lie close to mitochondria, probably providing a ready source of fuel (Lehninger, 1967), and seem more abundant in fibres (type I) whose energy demands are more dependent on oxidative enzymic activity.

Lipofuscin droplets have a constant irregular density pattern, but usually contain a small homogeneous droplet indistinguishable from lipid (Fig. 2.10). They are observed most often in fibres from older individuals or in fibres which may be undergoing partial degenerative change. It has been proposed that these structures are altered lysosomes in which oxidised cephalin and other materials have accumulated (Novikof, 1961). Acid phosphatase, one of the hydrolytic enzymes commonly found in lysosomes, has been identified histochemically within lipofuscin droplets in skeletal muscle (Gordon, Price and Blumberg, 1967).

Ribonucleoprotein particles (ribosomes), small dense granules about 15 nm in diameter, are sparse in mature skeletal muscle fibres, usually free and only rarely seen attached to a membrane. However, in developing and regenerating skeletal muscle fibres, numerous free clusters (or polyribosomes) are seen and are usually intimately associated with very fine filaments (Price *et al.* 1964; Pryzbylski and Blumberg, 1966). These RNP particles are probably sites of protein synthesis, and the fine filaments associated with them are thought to be precursors of the myofilaments that become organised into myofibrils.

NUCLEUS

The oval nuclei are located in the periphery of the muscle fibre, lying with their long axes parallel to the adjacent plasma membrane. The nuclear envelope is composed of two membranes, and continuity of the outer membrane with elements of the sarcoplasmic reticulum has been noted in cardiac and skeletal muscle (Moore and Ruska, 1957; Peachey, 1965). The nuclear envelope also displays an occasional 'pore complex' as described by Watson (1959). These pores seem to be more apparent in the nuclei of regenerating fibres (Price *et al.*, 1964).

SATELLITE CELL

With the electron microscope it is possible to identify discrete mononuclear cells wedged between the basement membrane and plasma membrane of mature skeletal muscle fibres (Fig. 2.9). The close relationship to the muscle fibre makes it impossible to resolve the plasma membrane of such cells with the limited resolution of the light microscope, in which they would appear to be a regular peripheral muscle nucleus. These cells

were called *satellite cells* by Mauro (1961), who was the first to observe them and suggest that they may be dormant myoblasts which could become activated during muscle regeneration. Further discussion of the possible functional significance of these cells may be found in the published proceedings of a symposium on muscle regeneration and myogenesis (Mauro, Shafiq and Milhorat, 1970).

FIBRE TYPES

Cytochemical studies have demonstrated the existence of two main groups of fibres within skeletal muscle (*see* Ch. 8). Fibres with high mitochondrial enzymic activity, low phosphorylase activity, abundant fat droplets, and usually a smaller diameter are referred to as type I fibres: fibres with a reverse pattern of enzymic activity, fewer fat droplets, and a tendency to have a larger diameter are called type II fibres.

Although the basic ultrastructure of the muscle fibre has been extensively investigated in vertebrates, correlation between fine structure and histochemical fibre type remains controversial in man. For other vertebrates, the distinction seems clearer. It is now fairly well established that ultrastructural differences exist between type I (red) and type II (white) fibres in pigeons (Ashhurst, 1969; James and Meek, 1974) in chickens (Shafiq, Askanas and Milhorat, 1972), in mice (Shafiq, Gorycki and Milhorat, 1969), in rats (Pellegrino and Franzini-Armstrong, 1965; Landon, 1970; Padykula and Gauthier, 1970; Schiaffino, Hanzlikova and Pierobon, 1970), the cat (Peachey, 1966), and in the guinea pig (Eisenberg and Kuda, 1976). As would be expected from histochemical studies, mitochondria are more numerous and lipid droplets more abundant in type I fibres, while the sarcoplasmic reticulum is more extensive and glycogen content greater in type II fibres. It is also reported that Z bands are wider in type I than in type II fibres.

In man, however, these differences are less distinct. Shafiq, Gorycki, Goldstone and Milhorat (1966), reported that type I and II fibers differed only in the size and number of mitochondria while Ogata and Murata (1969) concluded that size and shape were more important. Payne, Stern, Curless

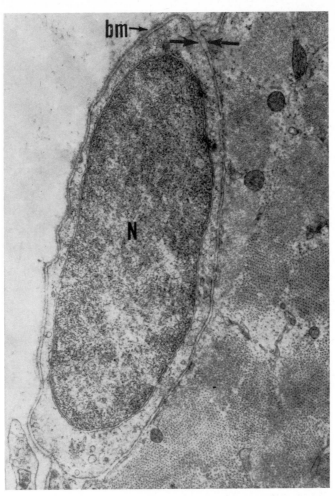

Fig. 2.9 Cross-section, human quadriceps femoris. Mononuclear satellite cell located beneath basement membrane (*bm*) of mature muscle fibre. Plasma membranes (*opposing arrows*) of satellite cell and muscle fibre are easily distinguished in this electron micrograph, but by light microscopy the nucleus of the satellite cell could not be distinguished from a typical peripheral muscle fibre nucleus (as in Fig. 2.10). Electron micrograph, ×17 000

and Hannapel (1975) found that type I fibers had the most numerous mitochondria, type IIA less numerous and IIB the least numerous and smallest mitochondria. Their study was based on human subjects with fibre deficiency disease involving at least one fibre type. Quantitative analysis of the volume fraction of several normal fibre components led Cullen and Weightman (1975) to the conclusion that no single ultrastructural feature studied by them could be used to distinguish fibre types reliably. Their data were based on morphometric analysis of mitochondria, membrane systems, volume of sarcoplasmic reticulum, lipid components and width of the Z lines. By using two

such components, only about 50 per cent of their fibres could be classified. Similar conclusions were reached in a study by Jerusalem, Engel and Peterson (1975). According to Sjöström and Squire (1977) cryo-ultramicrotomy studies of muscle fibres have demonstrated that distinct differences occur in the A band and M zone of muscle which are distinctive for species and fibre type. Thornell, Sjöström and Rinqvist, 1967, using cryo-ultramicrotomy—in conjunction with histochemical techniques on alternating ultrathin and 1 μm thick sections, have shown that differences in the M zone structure of different fibre types exist.

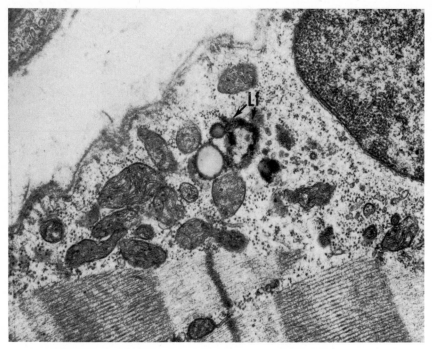

Fig. 2.10 Longitudinal section, human quadriceps femoris. Portion of muscle fibre nucleus and typical paranuclear cluster of mitochondria at margin of a fibre. Lipofuscin deposit (*Lf*) with homogeneous lipid droplet is found adjacent to mitochondria. Small glycogen particles are dispersed through sarcoplasm, ×22 000

INTRAFUSAL FIBRES OF THE MUSCLE SPINDLE

Electron-microscopic studies have enhanced our knowledge of the nuclear-chain and nuclear-bag intrafusal muscle fibres of mammalian muscle spindles (Landon, 1966; Adal, 1969; Corvaja, Marinozzi and Pompeiano, 1969; Corvaja and Pompeiano, 1970; Rumpelt, 1969; Barker, Stacey and Adal, 1970; Barker, Harker, Stacey and Smith, 1972; Scalzi and Price, 1971, 1972).

In general, the organisation of the myofilaments within myofibrils appears to be the same as that of the extrafusal muscle fibres. One exception appears to be the absence of a distinct M line in the myofibrils of nuclear-bag fibres of sheep, cat, rat, and human muscle spindles (Adal, 1969; Corvaja *et al.*, 1969; Corvaja and Pompeiano, 1970; Rumpelt, 1969; Barker *et al.*, 1972; Scalzi and Price, 1971, 1972). In preliminary observations of monkey muscle spindles, however, the nuclear-bag and nuclear-chain fibres have M lines of comparable density (Scalzi and Price, 1972).

As implied by their labels, the nuclei of the nuclear-chain fibres are aligned in a chain-like fashion within the mid-portion (or sensory region) of the fibre and, in the nuclear-bag fibre, the nuclei are clumped into a bag-like arrangement near the equator of the fibre.

Nuclear-chain fibres (Fig. 2.11) can be further characterised by their organisation and sensory innervation. There are 3–7 nuclear chain fibres per spindle and these usually do not extend the length of the receptor (Boyd, 1962; Bridgeman, Shumpert and Eldred, 1969). Adjacent nuclear-chain fibres 'pair' or form areas of close apposition (Fig. 2.12) (Adal, 1969; Corvaja *et al.*, 1969) and serial longitudinal sections from adult and newborn cats have indicated that these zones of close apposition involve the total complement of nuclear-chain fibres within a spindle (Scalzi and Price, 1969, 1971). At the zones of close apposition, the plasma membranes of adjacent nuclear-chain fibres are separated by a 10–18 nm space. These opposing plasma membranes have been thought to be held together by junctional complexes described as

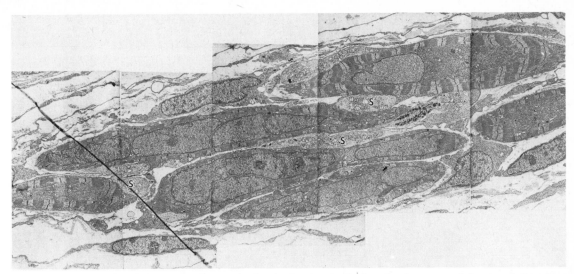

Fig. 2.11 Composite of several electron micrographs showing in a longitudinal section the pattern of close association of nuclear-chain fibres. Detailed higher power micrographs of various select areas, in a section such as this, showed that the nuclear-chain fibres were enclosed in a common continuous external lamina (or basement membrane) (Scalzi and Price, 1971). Some nuclear-chain fibres share common sensory nerves (S), ×1938 (reproduced with permission from Scalzi and Price, *J. Ultrastruct. Res.*, **36**, 375, 1971)

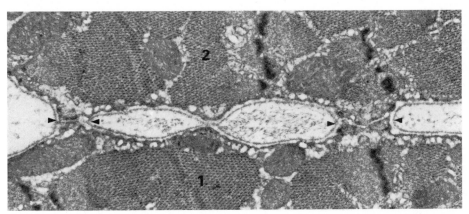

Fig. 2.12 Sites of close apposition between adjacent nuclear-chain fibres (1 and 2). The external lamina is continuous (arrows), ×14 287 (reproduced with permission from Scalzi and Price, *J. Ultrastruct. Res.*, **36**, 375, 1971)

zonulae adherentes (Corvaja *et al.*, 1969). In some of the zones of close apposition, one or more sensory nerve twigs cross between the adjacent nuclear-chain fibres (Fig. 2.13) (Scalzi and Price, 1971). Basement membrane material (or external lamina) is adjacent to all the nuclear-chain fibres except in the zones of close apposition (Fig. 2.12); and serial sections have indicated that the whole complement of nuclear-chain fibres within a spindle may be contained in a single external laminal sac (Scalzi and Price, 1971). This organ-isation of nuclear-chain fibres suggests that they may function as a morphological unit and not as independent fibres (Scalzi and Price, 1971).

There are 1–2 nuclear-bag fibres per spindle. They have a larger diameter than the nuclear-chain fibres and they usually extend the length of the receptor (Boyd, 1962; Rumpelt, 1969). Unlike the nuclear-chain fibres, the nuclear-bag fibres do not form zones of close apposition nor do they appear to share a common external lamina with each other or with nuclear-chain fibres. Also, the

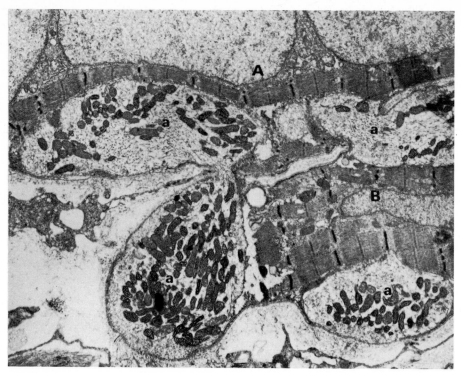

Fig. 2.13   Two branches of a single sensory nerve (a) which was followed in serial electron micrographs and shown to be shared by adjacent nuclear-chain fibres (A and B), ×7708 (reproduced with permission from Scalzi and Price, *J. Ultrastruct. Res.*, **36**, 375, 1971)

nuclear-bag fibres do not share cross sensory innervations between other nuclear-bag fibres or nuclear-chain fibres (Adal, 1969; Corvaja *et al.*, 1969; Scalzi and Price, 1969, 1971). Serial electron micrographs of longitudinal sections have shown that the annulospiral sensory innervation pattern, seen by light microscopy (Ruffini, 1898), is a more complex nerve network with numerous interconnecting links having more of a 'cage-like' configuration than a simple annulospiral appearance (Scalzi and Price, 1971).

Studies of muscle spindles in the hand muscles of monkeys have provided some interesting variations (Scalzi and Price, 1972). Serial longitudinal sections suggest that cross sensory innervation may exist between nuclear-chain and nuclear-bag fibres. However, the possibility exists that the fibre identified as a nuclear-chain fibre with cross sensory innervation to a nuclear-bag fibre is a so-called 'intermediate-type' fibre described by Barker *et al.* (1972).

CONCLUSION

The application of electron-microscopic techniques to the study of striated muscle has increased our understanding of the arrangement and function of the fibrillar proteins which form the contractile system, and has disclosed the features of the sarcoplasmic reticulum and the T system, yielding further insight into the possible mechanisms effecting contraction and relaxation. In addition, new features about the specialised intrafusal fibres of the muscle spindle have been uncovered. Identification of the satellite cell throws a new light on the phenomenon of muscle regeneration. Some progress has been made in outlining the ultrastructural characteristics of the various muscle fibre types; however, more detailed and sophisticated electron-microscopic studies are needed to define the subtle as well as the obvious differences in the membrane systems and contractile elements of these different fibres. This information should lead to an even better understanding of the basic physiological and biochemical properties of muscle, and it would also serve as a foundation for further studies of the perplexing problems presented by the various neuromuscular diseases discussed in other parts of this text.

ACKNOWLEDGEMENTS

This review was supported in part by grants from the Muscular Dystrophy Association of America, Inc. The authors are indebted to Drs H. Scalzi and E. L. Howes, Jr for co-operation in obtaining several plates from previous projects cited in this review.

REFERENCES

Adal, M.N. (1969) The fine structure of the sensory region of cat muscle spindles. *Journal of Ultrastructure Research*, **26**, 332.

Adrian, R.H. & Freygang, W.H. (1962) The potassium and chloride conductance of frog muscle membrane. *Journal of Physiology*, **163**, 61.

Allbrook, D. (1962) An electron microscopic study of regenerating skeletal muscle. *Journal of Anatomy (London)*, **96**, 137.

Andersson-Cedergren, E. (1959) Ultrastructure of motor end plate and sarcoplasmic components of mouse skeletal muscle fiber. *Journal of Ultrastructure Research*, **1** (Supplement).

Ashhurst, D.E. (1969) The fine structure of pigeon breast muscle. *Tissue and Cell*, **1**, 485.

Baccetti, B. (1965) Nouvelles observations sur l'ultra-structure du myofilament. *Journal of Ultrastructure Research*, **13**, 245.

Baccetti, B. (1966) Perplessita'e conferme sul problema della struttura del filamenti musolasi miosinici. *Bolletino della Società italiana di triologia sperimentale*, **42**, 1181.

Barker, D., Stacey, M.J. & Adal, M.N. (1970) Fusimotor innervation in the cat. *Philosophical Transactions of the Royal Society, Series B*, **258**, 315.

Barker, D., Harker, D., Stacey, M.J. & Smith, C.R. (1972) Fusimotor innervation. In *Research in Muscle Development and the Muscle Spindle*, Eds B.Q. Banker, R.J. Przbylski, J.P. VanDerMeule & M. Victor, p. 227 (Excerpta Medica: Amsterdam).

Bennett, H.S. (1960) The structure of striated muscle. In *The Structure and Function of Muscle*, Ed. G.H. Bourne, Vol. I, Ch. 6 (Academic Press: New York).

Bennett, H.S. & Porter, K.R. (1953) An electron microscope study of sectioned breast muscle of the domestic fowl. *American Journal of Anatomy*, **93**, 61.

Bowman, W. (1840) On the minute structure and movements of voluntary muscle. *Philosophical Transactions of the Royal Society of London. Series B*, **130**, 457.

Boyd, J.A. (1962) The structure and innervation of the nuclear chain muscle fiber system in mammalian muscle spindles. *Philosophical Transactions of the Royal Society, Series B*, **245**, 81.

Bridgeman, C.F., Shumpert, E.E. & Eldred, E. (1969) Insertions of intrafusal fibers in muscle spindles of the cat and other mammals. *Anatomical Record*, **164**, 391.

Chang, Y.S. & Tsao, T.C. (1962) Conformational changes of rabbit tropomyosin in different solvents. *Science Sinica*, **11**, 1353.

Clark, A.W., Hurlfut, W.P. & Mauro, A. (1972) Changes in the fine structure of the neuromuscular junction of the frog caused by black widow spider venom. *Journal of Cell Biology*, **52**, 1.

Cohen, C. & Holmes, K.C. (1963) X-ray diffraction evidence for α-helical coiled-coils in native muscle. *Journal of Molecular Biology*, **6**, 423.

Constantin, L.L., Franzini-Armstrong, C. & Podolsky, R.J. (1965) Localization of calcium-accumulating structures in striated muscle fibers. *Science*, **147**, 158.

Corvaja, N., Marinozzi, V. & Pompeiano, O. (1969) Muscle spindles in the lumbrical muscle of the adult cat. Electron microscopic observations and functional considerations. *Archives italiennes de biologie*, **107**, 365.

Corvaja, N. & Pompeiano, O. (1970) The differentiation of two types of intrafusal fibers in rabbit muscle spindles. *Pflügers Archiv für die Gesamte Physiologie*, **317**, 187.

Couteaux, R. (1960) Motor end-plate structure. In *The Structure and Function of Muscle*, Ed. G.H. Bourne, Vol. I, Structure (Academic Press: New York).

Craig, R. & Offer, G. (1976) Axial arrangement of cross-bridges in thick filaments of vertebrate skeletal muscle. *Journal of Molecular Biology*, **102**, 325.

Cullen, M.J. & Weightman, D. (1975) The ultrastructure of normal human muscle in relation to fiber type. *Journal of the Neurological Sciences*, **25**, 43.

Cummins, P. & Perry, S.V. (1978) Troponin I from human skeletal and cardiac muscles. *Biochemistry Journal*, **171**, 251.

Davies, R.E. (1963) A molecular theory of muscle contraction: calcium-dependent contractions with hydrogen bond formation plus ATP-dependent extensions of part of the myosin-actin cross-bridges. *Nature* **199**, 1068.

DeRobertis, E. (1958) Submicroscopic morphology and function of the synapse. *Experimental Cell Research*, **5**, 347 (Supplement).

DeRobertis, E. (1969) Submicroscopic morphology of the synapse. *International Review of Cytology*, **8**, 61.

Ebashi, S., cited by Pearson *et al.* (1967) *Annals of Internal Medicine*, **67**, 636.

Ebashi, S., Ebashi, F. & Kodama, A. (1967) Troponin as the Ca^{++}-receptive protein in the contractile system. *Journal of Biochemistry*, **62**, 137.

Ebashi, S. & Endo, M. (1968) Calcium ion and muscle contraction. *Progress in Biophysics and Biophysical Chemistry*, **18**, 123.

Ebashi, S. & Kodama, A. (1966) Interaction of troponin with F actin in the presence of tropomyosin. *Journal of Biochemistry*, **59**, 425.

Ebashi, S. & Lipmann, F. (1962) Adenosine triphosphate-linked concentration of calcium ions in a particulate fraction of rabbit muscle. *Journal of Cell Biology*, **14**, 389.

Eisenberg, B.R. & Kuda, A.M. (1976) Discrimination between fiber populations in mammalian skeletal muscle by using ultrastructural parameters. *Journal of Ultrastructure Research*, **54**, 76.

Eisenberg, E. & Hill, T.L. (1978) A cross bridge model of muscle contraction. *Progress in Biophysics and Molecular Biology*, **33**, 55.

Elliott, G.F., Lowy, J. & Millman, B.M. (1967) Low-angle X-ray diffraction studies of living striated muscle during contraction. *Journal of Molecular Biology*, **25**, 31.

Endo, M. (1964a) Staining of a single muscle fiber with fluorescent dyes. *Journal of Physiology*, **172**, 11P.

Endo, M. (1964b) Entry of a dye into the sarcotubular system of muscle. *Nature*, **202**, 1115.

Endo, M. (1977) Calcium release from the sarcoplasmic reticulum. *Physiological Reviews*, **57**, 71.

Endo, M., Nonomura, Y., Mosaki, T., Ohtsuki, I. & Ebashi, S. (1966) Localization of native tropomyosin in relation to striation patterns. *Journal of Biochemistry*, **60**, 605.

Engel, A.G. & Santa, T. (1971) Histometric analysis of the ultrastructure of the neuromuscular junction in myasthenia gravis and in the myasthenic syndrome. *Annals of the New York Academy of Sciences*, **183**, 46.

Fahrenbach, W.H. (1965) Sarcoplasmic reticulum: ultrastructure of the triadic junction. *Science*, **147**, 1308.

Fawcett, D.W. (1966) *The Cell, Its Organelles and Inclusions*. (W.B. Saunders Co.: Philadelphia).

Fawcett, D.W. & Revel, J.P. (1961) The sarcoplasmic reticulum of a fast-acting fish muscle. *Journal of Biophysical and Biochemical Cytology*, **10**, 89 (Supplement).

Fernandez-Moran, H., Oda, T., Blair, P.V. & Green, D.E. (1964) A macromolecular repeating unit of mitochondrial structure and function. *Journal of Cell Biology*, **22**, 63.

Franzini-Armstrong, C. (1970) Studies of the triad. I. Structure of the junction in frog twitch fibers. *Journal of Cell Biology*, **47**, 488.

Franzini-Armstrong, C. (1971) Studies of the triad. II. Penetration of tracers into the junctional gap. *Journal of Cell Biology*, **49**, 196.

Franzini-Armstrong, C. (1974) Freeze fracture of skeletal muscle from the tarantula spider. Structural differentiation of sarcoplasmic reticulum and transverse tubular system membranes. *Journal of Cell Biology*, **61**, 501.

Franzini-Armstrong, C. & Porter, K.R. (1964) Sarcolemmal invaginations constituting the T-system in fish muscle fibers. *Journal of Cell Biology*, **22**, 675.

Fuchs, F. (1974) Striated muscle. *Annual Review of Physiology*, **36**, 461.

Gilev, V.P. (1966) the ultrastructure of myofilaments. II. Further investigations of the thick filaments of crab muscles. *Biochemica et biophysica acta*, **112**, 340.

Gordon, G.B., Price, H.M. & Blumberg, J.M. (1967) Electron microscopic localization of phosphatase activities within striated muscle fibers. *Laboratory Investigation*, **16**, 422.

Green, D.E. (1965) An introduction to membrane biochemistry. *Israel Journal of Medical Science*, **1**, 1187.

Hanson, J. & Huxley, H.E. (1953) Structural basis of the cross-striations in muscle. *Nature*, **172**, 530.

Hanson, J. & Huxley, H.E. (1957) Quantitative studies on the structure of cross-striated myofibrils. II. Investigations by biochemical techniques. *Biochemica et biophysica acta*, **23**, 250.

Hanson, J. & Lowy, J. (1963) The structure of F-actin and of actin filaments isolated from muscle. *Journal of Molecular Biology*, **6**, 46.

Hanson, J. & Lowy, J. (1964) The structure of actin filaments and the origin of the axial periodicity in the I-substance of vertebrate striated muscle. *Proceedings of the Royal Society, Series B*, **160**, 449.

Hasselbach, W. (1953) Elektromikroskopische untersuchungen an muskelfibrillen bei totaler und partieller extraktion des L-myosins. *Zeitschrift für Naturforschung*, **86**, 449.

Hasselbach, W. (1964a) Relaxing factor and the relaxation of muscle. *Progress in Biophysics and Molecular Biology*, **14**, 167.

Hasselbach, W. (1964b) ATP-driven active transport of calcium in the membranes of the sarcoplasmic reticulum. *Proceedings of the Royal Society, Series B*, **160**, 501.

Hasselbach, W. (1964c) Relaxation and the sarcotubular calcium pump. *Federation Proceedings*, **23**, 09.

Hasselbach, W. & Makinose, M. (1962) The calcium pump of the relaxing vesicles and the production of a relaxing substance. *Conference on the Biochemistry of Muscle Contraction*, Dedham, Mass.

Heilbrunn, L.V. & Wiercinski, F.J. (1947) The action of various cations on muscle protoplasm. *Journal of Cellular and Comparative Physiology*, **29**, 15.

Higashi, S. & Ooi, T. (1968) Crystals of tropomyosin and native tropomyosin. *Journal of Molecular Biology*, **34**, 699.

Hill, A.V. (1948) On the time required for diffusion and its relation to processes in muscle. *Proceedings of the Royal Society of Medicine*, **B135**, 446.

Hill, A.V. (1949) The abrupt transition from rest to activity in muscle. *Proceedings of the Royal Society of Medicine*, **B136**, 399.

Hill, D.K. (1964) The space accessible to albumin within the striated muscle fibers of the toad. *Journal of Physiology*, **175**, 275.

Hodge, A.J. (1959) Fibrous proteins of muscle. In *Biophysical Science—A Study Program*, Eds J.L. Oncley, F.O. Schmitt, R.C. Williams, M.D. Rosenberg & R.H. Bolt, p. 409 (Wiley: New York).

Hodgkin, A.L. & Horowicz, P. (1960) The effect of sudden changes in ionic concentrations on the membrane potential of single muscle fibers. *Journal of Physiology*, **153**, 370.

Holtzer, H., Marshall, J.M. Jr. & Finck, H. (1957) An analysis of myogenesis by the use of fluorescent actomyosin. *Journal of Biophysical and Biochemical Cytology*, **3**, 705.

Howes, E.L., Price, H.M., Pearson, C.M. & Blumberg, J.M. (1966) Hypokalemic periodic paralysis. *Neurology (Minneapolis)*, **16**, 242.

Huxley, A.F. (1957) Muscle structure and theories of contraction. *Progress in Biophysics*, **7**, 257.

Huxley, A.F. & Niedergerke, R. (1954) Structural changes in muscle during contraction: interference microscopy of living muscle fibers. *Nature*, **173**, 971.

Huxley, A.F. & Straub, R.W. (1958) Local activation and interfibrillar structures in striated muscle. *Journal of Physiology*, **143**, 40.

Huxley, A.F. & Taylor, R.E. (1958) Local activation of striated muscle fibers. *Journal of Physiology* **144**, 426.

Huxley, H.E. (1957) The double array of filaments in cross-striated muscle. *Journal of Biophysical and Biochemical Cytology*, **3**, 631.

Huxley, H.E. (1963) Electron microscope studies of natural and synthetic protein filaments from striated muscle. *Journal of Molecular Biology*, **7**, 281.

Huxley, H.E. (1964) Evidence for continuity between the central elements of the triads and extracellular space in frog sartorius muscle. *Nature*, **202**, 1067.

Huxley, H.E. (1965) The fine structure of striated muscle and its functional significance. *Harvey Lectures*, **60**, 85.

Huxley, H.E. (1965) Structural evidence concerning the mechanism of contraction in striated muscle. In *Muscle*, Eds W.M. Paul, E.E. Daniel, C.M. Kay & G. Monckton, p. 3 (Pergamon Press: Oxford).

Huxley, H.E. (1969) The mechanism of muscular contraction. *Science*, **164**, 1356.

Huxley, H.E. (1971) The structural basis of muscular contraction. *Proceedings of the Royal Society, Series B*, **178**, 131.

Huxley, H.E. & Brown, W. (1967) The low-angle X-ray diagram of vertebrate striated muscle and its behaviour during contraction and rigor. *Journal of Molecular Biology*, **30**, 383.

Huxley, H.E. & Hanson, J. (1954) Changes in the cross-striations of muscle during contraction and stretch and their structural interpretation. *Nature*, **173**, 973.

Huxley, H.F. & Haselgrove, J.C. (1977) The structural basis of contraction in muscle and its study by rapid x-ray diffraction methods. In *Myocardial Failure*, Eds G. Reicker et al. (Springer-Verlag: Berlin).

James, N.T. & Meek, G.A. (1974) A serological analysis of mitochondrial volumes in muscle fibers. *Proceedings of the Royal Microscopical Society*, **9**, 97.

Jerusalem, F., Engel, A.G. & Gomez, M.R. (1974) Duchenne dystrophy. II. Morphometric study of motor end-plate fine structure. *Brain*, **97**, 123.

Jerusalem, F., Engel, A.G. & Peterson, H.A. (1975) Human muscle fiber fine structure. Morphometric data on controls. *Neurology (Minneapolis)*, **25**, 127.

Jones, S.F. & Kwanbunbumpen, S. (1970) The effects of nerve stimulation and hemicholinium on synaptic vesicles at the mammalian neuromuscular junction. *Journal of Physiology*, **207**, 31.

Kagawa, Y. & Racker, E. (1966) Partial resolution of the enzymes catalyzing oxidative phosphorylation. X. Correlation of morphology and function in submitochondrial particles. *Journal of Biological Chemistry*, **211**, 2475.

Kamada, T. & Kinosita, H. (1943) Disturbances initiated from naked surface of muscle protoplasm. *Japanese Journal of Zoology*, **10**, 469.

Katz, B. & Miledi, R. (1972) the statistical nature of the acetylcholine potential and its molecular components. *Journal of Physiology*, **224**, 665

Kelly, D.E. (1967a) Models of muscle Z-band fine structure based on a looping filament configuration. *Journal of Cell Biology*, **34**, 827.

Kelly, D.E. (1967b) Fine structural analysis of muscle triad junctions. *Journal of Cell Biology*, **35**, 66A.

Kelly, D.E. (1969) The fine structure of skeletal muscle triad junctions. *Journal of Ultrastructure Research*, **29**, 37.

Kelly, D.E. & Cahill, M.A. (1969) Skeletal muscle triad junction fine structure; new observations regarding dimples of the sarcoplasmic reticulum terminal cisternae. *Journal of Cell Biology*, **43**, 66A.

King, M.V. & Young, M. (1972) Evidence for flexibility of the helical rod section of the myosin molecules. *Journal of Molecular Biology*, **65**, 519.

Knappeis, G.E. & Carlsen, F. (1962) The ultrastructure of the Z-disc in skeletal muscle. *Journal of Cell Biology*, **13**, 323.

Knappeis, G.E. & Carlsen, F. (1968) The ultrastructure of the m-line in skeletal muscle. *Journal of Cell Biology*, **38**, 202.

Kominz, D.R., Mitchell, E.R., Nihei, R. & Kay, C.M. (1965) The papain digestion of skeletal myosin A. *Biochemistry*, **4**, 2373.

Kung, T.H. & Tsao, T.C. (1965) Electron microscopical studies of tropomyosin and paramyosin. *Science Sinica*, **14**, 1383.

Laki, K., Maruyama, K. & Kominz, D.R. (1962) Evidence for the interaction between tropomyosin and actin. *Archives of Biochemistry and Biophysics*, **98**, 323.

Lamvik, M.K. (1978) Muscle thick filament mass measured by electron scattering. *Journal of Molecular Biology*, **122**, 55.

Landon, D.N. (1966) Electron microscopy of muscle spindles. In *Control and Innervation of Skeletal Muscle*, Ed. B.L. Andrews, p. 96 (Livingstone: Edinburgh).

Landon, D.N. (1970) The influence of fixation upon the fine structure of the Z-disc of rat striated muscle. *Journal of Cell Science*, **6**, 257.

Lehninger, A.L. (1964) *The Mitochondrion* (W.A. Benjamin: New York).

Lehninger, A.L. (1967) Cell organelles: the mitochondrion. In *The Neurosciences*, Eds G.C. Quarton, T. Melnechuls & F.O. Schmitt (Rockefeller Univ. Press: New York).

Lowey, S., Slayter, H.S., Weeds, A.G. & Baker, H. (1969) Substructure of the myosin molecule. I. Subfragments of myosin by enzymic degradation. *Journal of Molecular Biology*, **42**, 1.

Luther, P. & Squire, J. (1978) Three-dimensional structure of the vertebrate muscle M-region. *Journal of Molecular Biology*, **125**, 313.

McCubbin, W.D., Kouba, R.F. & Kay, C.M. (1967) Physicochemical studies on bovine cardiac tropomyosin. *Biochemistry*, **6**, 2417.

Martonosi, A. (1962) VII. Ultracentrifugal analysis of partially polymerized actin solutions. *Journal of Biological Chemistry*, **237**, 2795.

Maruyama, K. (1964) Interaction of tropomyosin with actin. A flow birefringence study. *Archives of Biochemistry and Biophysics*, **105**, 142.

Maruyama, K. (1965) The biochemistry of the contractile elements of insect muscle. In *The Physiology of Insects*, p. 451, Ed. M. Rockstein (Academic Press: New York).

Mauro, A. (1961) Satellite cell of skeletal muscle fibers. *Journal of Biophysical and Biochemical Cytology*, **9**, 493.

Mauro, A. & Adams, R. (1961) The structure of the sarcolemma of the frog skeletal muscle fiber. *Journal of Biophysical and Biochemical Cytology*, **10**, 177 (Supplement).

Mauro, A., Shafiq, S.A. & Milhorat, A.T. (1970) *Regeneration of Striated Muscle and Myogenesis* (Excerpta Medica: Amsterdam).

Moore, D.H. & Ruska, H. (1957) Electron microscope study for mammalian cardiac muscle cells. *Journal of Biophysical and Biochemical Cytology*, **3**, 261.

Novikoff, A.B. (1961) Mitochondria (Chondriosomes). In *The Cell*, Eds J. Brachet & A.E. Mirsky, Vol. 2, Ch. 5 (Academic Press: New York and London).

Oda, T. (1976) Molecular organization of cellular membranes. In *Recent Progress in Electron Microscopy of Cells and Tissues*, Eds E. Yamoda et al. (University Park Press: Baltimore).

Ogata, T. & Murata, F. (1969) Cytological features of 3 fiber types in human striated muscle. *Tohoku Journal of Experimental Medicine*, **99**, 225.

Ohtsuki, I., Masaki, T., Nonomura, Y. & Ebashi, S. (1967)

Periodic distribution of troponin along the thin filament. *Journal of Biochemistry*, **61**, 817.

Ooi, T. (1967) Tryptic hydrolysis of tropomyosin. *Biochemistry*, **6**, 2433.

Padykula, H.A. & Gauthier, G.F. (1970) The ultrastructure of the neuromuscular junctions of mammalian red, white and intermediate skeletal muscle fibers. *Journal of Cell Biology*, **46**, 21.

Page, S. (1964) The organization of the sarcoplasmic reticulum frog muscle. *Journal of Physiology*, **175**, 10P.

Page, S. (1965) A comparison of the fine structure of frog slow and twitch muscle fibers. *Journal of Cell Biology*, **26**, 477.

Page, S.G. (1966) IEG #4, Memo #79 as cited by C. Pellegrino & C. Franzini-Armstrong (1969).

Page, S.G. & Huxley, H.E. (1963) Filament lengths in striated muscle. *Journal of Cell Biology*, **19**, 369.

Palade, G.E. (1956) Electron microscopy of mitochondria and other cytoplasmic structures. In *Enzymes : Unit of Biological Structure and Function*, Ed. O.H. Gaebler (Academic Press: New York).

Parker, C.J. & Gergely, J. (1960) Soluble relaxing factor from muscle. *Journal of Biological Chemistry*, **235**, 3449.

Parsons, D.F. (1965) Recent advances correlating structure and function in mitochondria. *International Review of Experimental Pathology*, **4**, 1.

Payne, C.M., Stern, L.Z., Curless, R.G. & Hannapel, L.K. (1975) Ultrastructural fiber typing in normal and diseased human muscle. *Journal of the Neurological Sciences*, **25**, 99.

Peachey, L.D. (1965) The sarcoplasmic reticulum and transverse tubules of the frog's sartorius. *Journal of Cell Biology*, **25**, 209.

Peachey, L.D. (1966) Fine structure of two fiber types in cat extra-ocular muscles. *Journal of Cell Biology*, **31**, 84A.

Pease, D.C. (1958) The basement membrane: substratum of histological order and complexity. *Fourth International Conference on Electron Microscopy*, Vol. 1, p. 140 (Berlin).

Pellegrino, C. & Franzini-Armstrong, C. (1965) An electron microscopic study of denervation atrophy in red and white skeletal muscle fibers. *Journal of Cell Biology*, **17**, 327.

Pellegrino de Iraldi, A. & DeRobertis, E. (1963) Action of reserpine, iproniazid and pyrogallol on nerve endings of the pineal gland. *International Journal of Neuropharmacology*, **2**, 231.

Pepe, F.A. (1966) Some aspects of the structural organisation of the myofibril as revealed by antibody-staining methods. *Journal of Cell Biology*, **28**, 505.

Pepe, F.A. (1967) The myosin filament. II. Interaction between myosin and actin filaments observed using antibody staining in fluorescent and electron microscopy. *Journal of Molecular Biology*, **27**, 227.

Pepe, F.A. (1971) Structure of the myosin filament of striated muscle. In *Progress in Biophysics and Molecular Biology*, Eds J.A.V. Butler & D. Noble (Pergamon Press: New York), **22**, 77.

Pepe, F.A. (1975) Structure of muscle filaments from immunohistochemical and ultrastructural studies. *Journal of Histochemistry and Cytochemistry*, **23**, 543.

Pepe, F.A. & Drucker, B. (1972) The myosin filament. IV. Observation on the internal structural arrangement. *Journal of Cell Biology*, **52**, 255.

Perry, S.V. & Corsi, A. (1958) Extraction of proteins other than myosin from isolated rabbit myofibril. *Biochemistry Journal*, **68**, 5.

Podolsky, R.J. (1962) Local activation of striated muscle

fibrils. *Proc. Int. Union Physiol. Sc. II, XXII, Int. Congress (Leiden)* p. 902.

Porter, K.R. & Palade, G.E. (1957) Studies on the endoplasmic reticulum. III. Its form and distribution in striated muscle cells. *Journal of Biophysical and Biochemical Cytology*, **3**, 269.

Price, H.M. (1963) The skeletal muscle fiber in the light of electron microscope studies. *American Journal of Medicine*, **35**, 589.

Price, H.M. (1967) Mitochondrial myopathies in man? A review of the evidence. In *Exploratory Concepts in Muscular Dystrophy and Related Disorders*, Ed. A.T. Milhorat (Excerpta Medica: New York).

Price, H.M., Howes, E.L. & Blumberg, J.M. (1964) Ultrastructural alterations in skeletal muscle fibers injured by cold. II. Cells of the sarcolemmal tube: observations on 'discontinuous' regeneration and myofibril formation. *Laboratory Investigation*, **13**, 1279.

Price, H.M., Pease, D.C. & Pearson, C.M. (1962) Selective actin filament and Z-band degeneration induced by plasmocid. An electron microscopic study. *Laboratory Investigation*, **11**, 549.

Price, H.M., Gordon, G.B., Pearson, C.M., Munsat, T.L. & Blumberg, J.M. (1965) New evidence for excessive accumulation of Z-band material in nemaline myopathy. *Proceedings of the National Academy of Sciences* (U.S.A.), **45**, 1398.

Price, H.M., Howes, E.L., Sheldon, D.B., Hutson, O.D., Fitzgerald, R.T. Blumberg, J.M. & Pearson, C.M. (1965) An improved biopsy technique for light and electron microscopic studies of human skeletal muscle. *Laboratory Investigation*, **14**, 194.

Pryzbylski, R.J. & Blumberg, J.M. (1966) Ultrastructural aspects of myogenesis in the chick. *Laboratory Investigation*, **15**, 836.

Reedy, M. (1964) The structure of actin filaments and the origin of the axial periodicity in the I-substance of vertebrate striated muscle. *Proceedings of the Royal Society, Series B*, **160**, 114.

Reedy, M.K., Holmes, K.C. & Tregear, R.T. (1965) Induced changes in orientation of the cross-bridges of glycerinated insect flight muscle. *Nature*, **207**, 1276.

Reger, J.F. (1958) The fine structure of neuromuscular synapses of gastrocnemii from mouse and frog. *Anatomical Record*, **130**, 7.

Reger, J.F. (1961) The fine structure of neuromuscular junctions and the sacroplasmic reticulum of extrinsic eye muscles of Fundulus Heteroclitus. *Journal of Biophysical and Biochemical Cytology*, **10**, 111.

Revel, J.P. (1962) The sarcoplasmic reticulum of the bat and cricothyroid muscle. *Journal of Cell Biology*, **12**, 571.

Rice, R.V. (1961) Conformation of individual macromolecular particles from myosin solutions. *Biochemica et Biophysica Acta*, **52**, 602.

Robertson, J.D. (1958) The ultrastructure of cell membranes. *Anatomical Record*, **130**, 440.

Robertson, J.D. (1959) The ultrastructure of cell membranes and their derivatives. *Biochemical Society Symposia*, **16**, 3.

Rowe, A.J. (1964) The contractile proteins of skeletal muscle. *Proceedings of the Royal Society, Series B*, **160**, 437.

Ruffini, A. (1898) On the minute anatomy of the neuromuscular spindles of the cat, and on their physiological significance. *Journal of Physiology*, **23**, 190.

Rumpelt, H.J. (1969) Zur Morphologie der Bauelementa non Muskelspindelm bei Mensch und Ratte. *Zeitschrift für*

Zellforschung und mikroskopische Anatomie, **102**, 601.

Sandow, A. (1970) Skeletal muscle. *Annual Review of Physiology*, **32**, 87.

Scalzi, H.A. & Price, H.M. (1969) Ultrastructure of the sensory region of the mammalian muscle spindle. *Journal of Cell Biology*, **43**, 124a.

Scalzi, H.A. & Price, H.M. (1971) The arrangement and sensory innervation of the intrafusal fibers in the feline muscle spindle. *Journal of Ultrastructure Research*, **36**, 375.

Scalzi, H. & Price, H.M. (1972) Electron microscopic observations of the sensory region of the mammalian muscle spindle. In *Research in Muscle Development and the Muscle Spindle*, Eds B.Q. Banker, R.J. Przbylski, J.P. VanDer-Meuller & M. Victor, p. 254 (Excerpta Medica: Amsterdam).

Schiaffino, S., Hanzlikova, V. & Pierobon, S. (1970) Relations between structure and function in rat skeletal muscle fibers. *Journal of Cell Biology*, **47**, 107.

Shafiq, S.A., Askanas, V. & Milhorat, A.T. (1972) Fiber type involvement in muscular dystrophy. In *Research In Muscle Development and The Muscle Spindle*, Eds B. Banker et al, pp. 18–31 (Excerpta Medica: Amsterdam).

Shafiq, S.A., Gorycki, M. Goldstone, L. & Milhorat, A.T. (1966) Fine structure of fiber types in normal human muscle. *Anatomical Record*, **156**, 283.

Shafiq, S.A., Gorycki, M.A. & Milhorat, A.T. (1969) An electron microscopic study of fiber types in normal and dystrophic muscles of the mouse. *Journal of Anatomy*, **104**, 281.

Shy, G.M., Wanko, T., Rowley, P.T. & Engel, A.G. (1961) Studies in familial periodic paralysis. *Experimental Neurology*, **3**, 53.

Simpson, F.O. & Oertelis, S.J. (1962) The fine structure of sheep myocardial cells; sarcolemmal invaginations and the transverse tubular system. *Journal of Cell Biology*, **12**, 91.

Singer, S.J. & Nicolson, G.L. (1972) The fluid mosaic model of the structure of cell membranes. *Science*, **175**, 720.

Sjöström, M. & Squire, J.M. (1977a) Cryo-ultramicrotomy and myofibrillar fine structure: A review. *Journal of Microscopy*, **111**, 239.

Sjöström, M. & Squire, J.M. (1977b) Fine structure of the A-band of human skeletal muscle fibers from ultra-thin cryo-sections negatively stained. *Journal of Molecular Biology*, **109**, 49.

Slautterback, D.B. (1965) Mitochondria in cardiac muscle cells of the canary and some other birds. *Journal of Cell Biology*, **24**, 1.

Smith, D.S. (1966) the organisation and function of the sarcoplasmic reticulum and T-system of muscle cells. *Progress in Biophysical and Molecular Biology*, **16**, 109.

Sommer, J.R. & Johnson, E.A. (1968) Purkinje fibers of the heart examined with the peroxidase reaction. *Journal of Cell Biology*, **37**, 570.

Speidel, C.C. (1937) Studies of living muscle. I. Growth, injury and repair of striated muscle as revealed by prolonged observations of living fibers in living frog tadpoles. *American Journal of Anatomy*, **62**, 179.

Squire, J.M. (1971) General model for the structure of all myosin containing filaments. *Nature*, **233**, 457.

Squire, J.M. (1972) General model of myosin filament structure. II. Myosin filaments and cross-bridge interactions in vertebrate striated and insect flight muscles. *Journal of Molecular Biology*, **72**, 125.

Squire, J.M. (1973) General model of myosin filament structure. III. Molecular packing arrangements in myosin filaments. *Journal of Molecular Biology*, **72**, 291.

Straub, F.B. (1942) Actin. In *Studies of the Institute of Medical Chemistry. University of Szeged.*, **2**, 3.

Stromer, M.H., Hartshorne, D.J. & Rice, R.V. (1967) Removal and reconstitution of Z-line material in striated muscle. *Journal of Cell Biology*, **35**, C23.

Suzuki, A., Saito, M. Sato, H. & Nonami, Y. (1978) Effects of materials released from myofibrils by C.A.F. (CA^{2+}-activated factor) on Z-disk reconstruction. *Agricultural and Biological Chemistry*, **42**, 2111.

Thornell, E., Sjöström, M. & Rinqvist, M. (1976) Attempts to correlate histochemical and ultrastructural features of individual skeletal muscle fibers. *Journal of Ultrastructure Research*, **57**, 224.

Tonomura, Y., Watonobe, S. & Morales, M.F. (1969) Conformational changes in the molecular control of muscle contraction. *Biochemistry*, **8**, 2171.

Tregear, R.T. & Squire, J.M. (1973) Myosin content and filament structure in smooth and striated muscle. *Journal of Molecular Biology*, **77**, 279.

Van Breeman, V.L. (1960) Ultrastructure of human muscle. I. Observations on normal striated muscle fibers. *American Journal of Pathology*, **37**, 215.

Veratti, E. (1902) Richerche sulle fine struttura della fibra musculare striata. *Memoirce Reale Istituto Lombardo*, **19**, 87.

Walker, S.M. & Schrodt, G.R. (1965) Continuity of the T system with the sarcolemma in rat skeletal muscle fibers. *Journal of Cell Biology*, **27**, 671.

Watson, M.L. (1959) Further observations on the nuclear envelope of the animal cell. *Journal of Biophysical and Biochemical Cytology*, **6**, 147.

Weber, A. (1966) Energised calcium transport and relaxing factors. In *Current Topics on Bioenergetics*, Ed. D.R. Sanadi, Vol. 1, p. 203 (Academic Press: New York).

Weber, A. & Murray, J.M. (1973) Molecular control mechanisms in muscle contraction. *Physiological Reviews*, **53**, 612.

Wilkinson, J.M., Perry, S.V., Cole, H.A. & Trayer, I.P. (1972) The regulatory proteins of the myofibril. Separation and biological activity of the components of inhibitory-factor preparations. *Biochemistry Journal*, **127**, 215.

Winegrad, S. (1965) Autoradiographic studies of intracellular calcium in frog skeletal muscle. *Journal of General Physiology*, **48**, 455.

Worthington, C.R. (1959) Large axial spacings in striated muscle. *Journal of Molecular Biology*, **1**, 398.

Zacks, S.I. (1964) *The Motor Endplate*. (W.B. Saunders: Philadelphia).

Zobel, C.R. (1967) An electron-microscopic investigation of heavy meromyosin. *Biochemica et Biophysica Acta*, **140**, 222.

General physiology and pharmocology of neuromuscular transmission

INTRODUCTION

In 1850 Pelouze and Bernard made an observation which marked the first step towards our understanding of neuromuscular transmission. They noticed that while stimulation of motor nerves in animals killed by toxic doses of a variety of substances still produced muscle contractions, this was not the case with animals poisoned with curare. Their own description was: 'sur l'animal encore chaud et mort depuis une minute les nerfs sont inertes comme sur un animal qui serait froid et mort depuis longtemps'. However, it was not until comparatively recently that sufficient information became available to allow coherent theories on the mechanism of transmission to be developed. The most important discovery during this period was the demonstration by Dale and his co-workers (Dale and Feldberg, 1934; Dale, Feldberg and Vogt, 1936; Brown, Dale and Feldberg, 1936), that transmission at the neuromuscular junction is brought about by the action of acetylcholine. 'Our observations', they said, 'seem to us to be compatible with a form of chemical transmission, in which the direct stimulant of the muscle fibre at its end-plate, acetylcholine, is liberated by arrival of the nerve impulses at the nerve ending, and destroyed during the refractory period by a local concentration of cholinesterase'. Curare has been an invaluable tool in such studies, which have also shed light on how curare itself exerts its action. Many disciplines have contributed, but it is to pharmacological analyses, fine structural studies, biochemistry and the development of valuable electrophysiological techniques that progress is primarily due.

For many years the terms 'end-plate' (*plaque terminale*) introduced by Rouget in 1862 and 'motor end-plate' (*motorische Endplatte*) introduced by Krause in the following year referred to all anatomical structures which participate in the complex known as the 'neuromuscular junction': the motor nerve ending, the Schwann cell and the postsynaptic membrane. Now, however, the term end-plate is used to designate the postsynaptic membrane only.

The nerve endings are invariably found in surface depressions of the muscle membrane (synaptic 'gutters' or 'troughs'). In this 'subneural' structure, selective staining has shown elongated ribbon-shaped lamellae (*see* review by Couteaux, 1960). Using the electron microscope, Palade (1954), Palay (1954) and Robertson (1954) showed that the subneural lamellae are narrow 'infoldings' of the muscle membrane. This area of the membrane, considerably greater than the presynaptic, contains large accumulations of mitochondria and small granules which give it the appearance of a differentiated zone of the muscle fibre. Furthermore, the use of specific histochemical staining has shown that these junctional folds are rich in cholinesterase enzyme (Koelle and Friedenwald, 1949; Couteaux, 1955).

The regularity of postsynaptic folds of the sarcolemmal membrane and their orientation at right angles to the long axis of the axonal terminal has facilitated the recognition of structural relationships between intra-axonal constituents and the sarcolemmal folds. Birks, Katz and Miledi (1960) noted that each thickening of the axonal membrane was usually situated opposite a post-synaptic fold and was associated with aggregations of synaptic vesicles within the axon terminal. In the rat diaphragm, Hubbard and Kwanbunbumpen (1968) found localised thickenings of axolemmal membrane opposite 60 per cent of post-synaptic folds. Synaptic vesicles touched or fused with axolemma at these points. Heuser and Reese (1973) described in greater detail axolemmal thickenings in the frog. They considered that the axon terminal, when sectioned longitudinally, can be differentiated into 'synaptic units', each unit being centred upon a 100 nm wide band of dense material lining the plasma membrane. This dense band lies at right angles to the long axis of the terminal and is invariably located just above a postsynaptic fold of sarcolemma. Synaptic vesicles cluster about the dense band. Tongues of Schwann cell cytoplasm are found at regular intervals between axon and sarcolemma; and where axonal membrane contacts Schwann cell process, the membrane is coated by filamentous dense material. Freeze-fracture studies by Heuser, Reese and Landis (1974) have confirmed the presence of bands of thickened axolemmal membrane which are the sites of fusion of synaptic vesicles with the membrane. These are probably sites of transmitter release, corresponding to the 'active zones' of Couteaux and Pécot-Dechavassine (1970) (*see* Fig. 3.1).

For a long time, both the electrical and chemical theories of transmission at the neuromuscular junction had their firm supporters; today, however, it is universally agreed that transmission at this site is chemical and mediated by acetylcholine (ACh), the substance which Dale *et al.* (1936) were the first to demonstrate in the fluid perfusing the leg of an anaesthetised cat while its sciatic nerve was stimulated electrically. The mediation of synaptic transmission by a specific chemical substance is fundamentally different from the process occurring when impulses are conducted along a continuous structure, in which case the essential factor for the spread of excitation is a flow

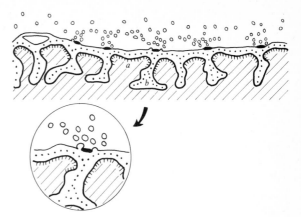

Fig. 3.1 Interpretative diagram of part of the subneural apparatus of the frog motor end-plate, to show the spatial relationships between sites of transmitter release and receptor concentrations. In the terminal axon, the presynaptic vesicles become aligned in stacks apposing the mouths of the postsynaptic folds (Birks *et al.*, 1960). Traced from micrographs of frog muscle endplates (Couteaux and Pécot-Dechavassine, (1968). The striations along the postsynaptic membrane represent its 'thickened' zone, rich in the receptors. In the mammalian white fibres, the folds are usually more closely spaced than here, so that the crests are narrower and apical. Dense bars on the presynaptic membrane represent the ridges seen in freeze-etch preparations. Dotted lines show the extent of the stainable cleft substance, and, it is presumed, of the AChE (From Porter, C.W. and Barnard, E.A. (1975). The density of cholinergic receptors at the endplate postsynaptic membrane: ultrastructural studies in two mammalian species. *J. Membrane Biol.* **20**, 31–49)

of electric current between adjacent parts.

The possibility of electrical transmission was excluded because the characteristic features of electrical synaptic transmission could not be found. Thus, Del Castillo and Katz (1956) consistently failed to demonstrate the propagation of electrotonic changes in either direction across the neuromuscular junction, thus proving that no direct 'cable-like' connection between the two synaptic membranes exists. Furthermore, the striking contrast between the small presynaptic spike and the large synaptic potential makes it improbable that the trans-synaptic flow of current would be adequate to evoke that large postsynaptic response. Moreover, transmission is vulnerable to agents that have no effect on nervous conduction. In 1954, Del Castillo and Katz demonstrated that no resting potential changes in the muscle fibre can be detected, even when the induced changes in the resting potential of the presynaptic axon are large enough to change the rate of the miniature end-plate potentials. Thus, on the electrical theory of transmission it is not possible to explain the amplification observed. On the other hand, just such a large amplification is actually produced at the neuromuscular junction by acetylcholine (*see* review by Katz, 1958). Finally, at the neuro-muscular junction, there is a *delay* between the arrival of an impulse at the motor nerve ending and its further propagation in the muscle fibre. For the neuromuscular junction of mammals, the delay has been estimated to be of the order of 0.5 ms (Eccles, Katz and Kuffler, 1941). In contrast, when acetylcholine is applied directly to the end-plate area there is no appreciable delay, suggesting that the chemical reaction involving acetylcholine at the postsynaptic membrane does not contribute significantly to the delay recorded when the muscle responds to nerve stimulation.

RELEASE OF ACETYLCHOLINE

The nerve ending

Besides ACh, the cholinergic neurones contain choline-acetylase, the specific enzyme in charge of the synthesis of ACh, and acetylcholinesterase (AChE), the enzyme which hydrolyses the trans-mitter. All three are found along the whole length of every cholinergic neurone, but the con-centration is highest at the nerve endings. Thus, although some ACh is synthesised in all parts of a cholinergic neurone, most of it is produced in close proximity to the sites from which it is released by nerve impulses. According to MacIntosh (1959) the most likely explanation for the presence of ACh and the two enzymes in the proximal parts of the neurones is that the enzymes are synthesised in the cell body and from there are carried to the nerve endings by the axoplasmic current stream-ing down each fibre.

Choline, necessary for the synthesis of ACh, is a normal constituent of the extracellular fluid. According to Birks and MacIntosh (1957), how-ever, the amounts of choline available inside the presynaptic axon may be very small; they sug-gested, therefore, the existence of a specific carrier mechanism transporting choline from the extra-cellular space into the intracellular sites of acety-lation. Their suggestion was based on the de-

monstration that in autonomic ganglia perfused either with Locke's solution or plasma, and in the presence of hemicholinium, the rate of ACh output falls off very rapidly. Schueler (1955) designated as 'hemicholiniums' a series of quater-nary bases which exhibit a kind of toxicity suggestive of some interference with cholinergic mechanisms. MacIntosh, Birks and Sastry (1956) found that hemicholinium was competing in some way with choline and therefore suggested that the drug might act as an inhibitor of choline transport.

Much of the recent data concerning the 'neurochemistry of cholinergic transmission' can be found in the excellent review by MacIntosh and Collier (1976) and also in the book entitled '*Acetylcholine Synthesis in Neurons*' by S. Tuček (1978).

The miniature end-plate potential

Fatt and Katz (1952), recording with intracellular electrodes from the end-plate region of a resting amphibian muscle, detected a local spontaneous activity which was intermittent and random, and at an intensity well below the firing threshold of the muscle fibre. The frequency of these dis-charges was low (about one per second) and, because of their size (0.5 mV), which is one per cent of that of the normal end-plate response, they were called 'miniature' end-plate potentials (mepps). Simple pharmacological tests convinced Katz and his co-workers (*see* review by Katz, 1958) that these spontaneous discharges were the result of a random impact of ACh on the end-plate region. While curare reduced their size, both their amplitude and duration were increased by neostig-mine; thus the effects of these drugs on the miniature end-plate potentials were similar to their known effects on the end-plate response produced by a nerve impulse, or on the de-polarisation elicited by the local application of ACh. Statistical tests indicated that the events were quantal in nature: in other words, that ACh was released, both by the nerve impulse and spontaneously, in 'packets' made up of about an equal number of ACh molecules. Katz and his colleagues demonstrated also that the *size* of the quantum of ACh which is liberated from the nerve terminals is remarkably constant and unaffected by any experimental procedures, whether by drugs, changes in ionic environment, temperature or osmotic differences. On the other hand, the *frequency* at which the quanta of ACh are liberated can be easily and markedly affected by factors which change the physiological conditions of the nerve endings. That the nerve endings are responsible for the release of ACh producing the miniature end-plate potentials is shown by the fact that they are abolished by nerve degeneration. Moreover, Brooks (1954) has shown that ACh is released from the isolated guinea-pig diaphragm in the absence of nerve stimulation. A comparable resting release has been found in the rat diaphragm by Straughan (1960) and by Krnjević and Mitchell (1961).

Synaptic vesicles

A consistent feature of chemical synapses is the cleft, 20–50 nm wide, that separates the pre-synaptic nerve terminals from the postsynaptic membrane. The internal architecture of nerve terminals shows elements such as mitochondria, neurofilaments, microtubules and synaptic ve-sicles. In mammalian nerve terminals these ve-sicles are bound by a unit membrane and normally are electron-lucent. In the rat the average volume of a synaptic vesicle was calculated to be about 5.2×10^4 nm^3 with an external diameter of about 45 nm and a wall 4–5 nm thick (Hubbard, 1973). In the frog the mean external diameter of vesicles in resting nerve terminals is 52 nm (Heuser and Reese, 1973). Only a few such vesicles are found in the axon above the ending or in the other cellular structures around the synapse; in fact, their high con-centration at the nerve endings helps to distinguish the axonal cytoplasm from that of the surrounding cell.

There are essentially two hypotheses which try to explain how ACh, present in the nerve ending, crosses the presynaptic membrane to reach the postsynaptic receptors. One hypothesis, proposed by Del Castillo and Katz (1955) and by Katz (1969; 1971) considers that the transmitter is packed inside the synaptic vesicles, which, having migrated to strategic synaptic sites, fuse more or less with the cytoplasmic membrane of the axon terminal, and discharge their contents into the synaptic cleft by a process which is currently called *exocytosis*. Subsequently the vesicle membrane is pinched off and returned to the interior of the cell. In a resting nerve the release of the vesicle contents occurs at a slow random rate which is greatly increased by the arrival of a suitable stimulus (Heuser and Reese, 1973; Heuser *et al.*, 1974). Throughout the years, the vesicular theory of transmitter release received much support from both biochemistry and morphology.

More recently, however, this hypothesis has been under attack from various angles. For example, there are now several reports in the literature (for details and references *see* the reviews by MacIntosh and Collier, 1976; Osborne, 1977; Marchbanks, 1977; Tauc, 1977) which suggest that the transmitter exists free in the cytoplasm from which it is released by some membrane mechanism (gating theory), the vesicles serving only to store transmitter. A serious difficulty with the vesicular theory is that vesicles isolated from nerve endings have consistently been proved to contain ACh that exchanges only very slowly with a relatively free (cytoplasmic) pool of ACh, from which the more recently formed (and therefore more strongly labelled), ACh released by nerve stimulation evidently originates. Another major difficulty concerning fusion of vesicle and axonal membranes and the recycling of vesicle membranes is the fact that the chemical composition of the vesicle and plasma membranes is very different so that there could be problems over their linkage. Moreover, the newly synthesised transmitter, or transmitter that is newly captured, appears to be preferentially released. In a recent publication, Bernard Katz (1977) himself sums up the situation as follows:

'That transmitter substances are discharged from many, and possibly from most, chemical nerve terminals in the form of discrete multi-molecular packets is probably no longer questioned. What is not quite so widely accepted is the proposition that the release of the packet occurs by exocytosis, that is, by the discharge of the diffusible contents of a synaptic vesicle into the external cleft, rather than by diffusion of solute from the cytoplasm through a transient membrane gate. It seems to me that the evidence for the 'vesicular hypothesis' has been considerably strengthened during the past decade, even in the case of cholinergic endings. The com-bination of improved ultrastructural studies, with electron-microscopic and freeze-etch techniques, along-side microphysiological recording during various stages of synaptic activity, has resulted in many new interesting findings. Moreover, there are now several recent estimates of the number of acetylcholine (ACh) molecules contained in a quantal packet. These have been obtained by chemical and pharmacological assay of impulse-evoked ACh release, by measuring the ionophoretic dose-equivalent of a miniature end-plate potential, and by using ACh-noise analysis to determine the minimum number of effective molecular collisions needed to produce a quantal action. The different values seem to converge on to the same order of magnitude, greater than 1000 and less than 10 000, and one would no longer be very hard-pressed to fit this amount inside a 50 nm vesicle. But while all this is consistent and compatible with the vesicular hypothesis, it is far from proving it, and indeed it is difficult to envisage how to proceed without clear and specific intravesicular markers, or some unforeseen advance in technique which would make the process visible without prior fixation.'

Calcium ions and acetylcholine release

Calcium ions have an important role in controlling ACh release. Fatt and Katz (1952) have shown that the end-plate potential, recorded with internal micro-electrodes, diminishes stepwise with reduced calcium concentration. Furthermore, Del Castillo and Stark (1952) found that, in the isolated frog sciatic-sartorius preparation, there is a positive relationship between the magnitude of the end-plate potential and the calcium content in the surrounding fluid. Calcium had no effect on either the time-course of the end-plate potential or the sensitivity of the end-plate region to ACh, nor any direct anticurare action. Their results suggested that the amount of ACh released by a single maximal nerve volley is a function of the calcium ion concentration. Hubbard (1961) demonstrated that, over a range of calcium concentrations from 1.5 to 10 mM, the frequency of the miniature end-plate potentials was proportional to the logarithm of the calcium concentration. MacIntosh (1959) has suggested that calcium ions, entering the nerve terminals during the impulse, release ACh by disrupting the ACh-retaining vesicles. The basis of this suggestion was the demonstration by Hodgkin and Keynes (1957) that during activity in the squid nerve fibres there is a sharp rise in calcium influx, while during rest the calcium that has entered is slowly pumped out. Other observations have shown that there is a considerable delay between a

brief depolarising pulse and the release of ACh by the nerve endings. Katz and Miledi (1967) tried to find out at what stage the external calcium ions come into play. Their findings suggest the following sequence: depolarisation of the axon terminal opens a 'gate' to calcium; calcium moves to the inside of the axon membrane; calcium becomes involved in a reaction which causes the rate of transmitter release to increase; and it is this which contributes a large part of the synaptic delay. Katz and Miledi concluded that the utilisation of external calcium ions at the neuromuscular junction is restricted to a brief period which barely outlasts the depolarisation of the nerve ending, and which precedes the transmitter release itself. Thus, transmitter release is a calcium-dependent process and stimulation in the absence of extracellular calcium completely abolishes the release that is normally associated with a nerve impulse. The most direct evidence that the calcium is required inside the cell has come from experiments with a giant synapse in the squid, where Miledi (1973) has shown that it is possible to inject calcium into the presynaptic terminal and, even in the absence of external calcium, internal application of calcium promotes transmitter release.

Using the squid giant axon as a model system, Baker and his colleagues have shown that the concentration of ionised calcium in axoplasm is maintained at a very low level—about 0.1 μM—despite the presence of a calcium concentration of about 10 000 μM in the external medium. As the intracellular concentration of ionised calcium is initially extremely low, a very small net entry serves to produce a relatively large rise in concentration. It seems to be this change that produces the trigger for initiating transmitter release, although the precise mechanism by which calcium initiates secretion is still unknown (further details and references are to be found in Professor Baker's review 'Calcium and the Control of Neuro-secretion', 1977).

The Schwann cell

The motor nerve fibres are myelinated, but towards their terminals they lose the myelin sheath and become shrouded by the Schwann cells which thereby separate the axon terminal from the surrounding tissues. The Schwann cell, however, is absent at the synaptic region between the nerve endings and the motor end-plate. Within the cleft can be seen the basement membrane, which follows the contours of the muscle surface. Schwann cell lamellae cover the terminal, sending finger-like processes around it, thereby creating regularly spaced subdivisions.

Very little is really known about the physiological role of Schwann cells. They are closely linked with the process of myelination. With electron microscopy, Robertson (1961) found that, during certain stages of myelination, spiral membrane structures are regular features of Schwann cells. These 'growth spirals' seem characteristic of growing Schwann cells, and are probably crucial for the synthesis of new membrane material for myelin formation.

This is probably not the only role of the Schwann cell, because there is also evidence that it is associated with an ACh system. The Schwann cytoplasm is quite distinct from the normal nerve terminal and, while showing granular and vesicular inclusions of various sizes, it does not contain the 'vesicles' characteristic of the axon terminal (Birks, Katz and Miledi, 1959). Nevertheless it has been suggested that, following denervation, ACh may be liberated from the Schwann cell. Katz and Miledi (1959) found that junctional transmission was abolished and spontaneous miniature end-plate potentials disappeared from the frog sartorius muscle several days after section of its nerve; a low-rate activity, however, was later resumed. This reappearance of activity was not associated with any significant changes in the sensitivity of the muscle to externally applied ACh; the well-known hypersensitivity state developed later. It was also found that, several days after motor nerve section, Schwann cells replaced the axon in its synaptic position: it was therefore suggested that these cells may be responsible for the release of the ACh quanta and the reappearance of the activity observed at the denervated end-plates (Birks *et al.*, 1959; Miledi, 1960a). Miledi and Slater (1968), using intracellular microelectrodes and electron microscopy, studied normal and denervated end-plates in the rat diaphragm, and were able to demonstrate a good correlation between the ultrastructure of the end-plate region and the presence or absence of miniature potentials. After prolonged denervation, the Schwann cell was seldom in contact with the muscle fibre and there were no miniature end-plate potentials. Conversely, when miniature end-plate potentials were recorded, there were many 'Schwann-muscle' contacts. This indicates that there is a connection between the Schwann cell and miniature potentials at denervated end-plates, and that the Schwann cell is the source of the packages of ACh or of a similar substance which produce miniature end-plate potentials in denervated muscle. There is also evidence that cholinesterase enzymes (Koelle, 1951) are present in these cells.

The mode of release of packets of ACh from the Schwann cell is different from the mechanism at nerve endings. Thus, depolarisation of the Schwann cell by K^+ ion or by electrical pulses (Dennis and Miledi, 1974) does not cause an increase in release of packets of ACh (unless the pulses are so strong that they cause membrane breakdown). The dependence of release from Schwann cells on intracellular Ca^{++} ion (Bevan, Grampp and Miledi, 1976; Ito and Miledi, 1977) also contrasts with that at nerve endings. By the use of calcium ionophores which increase the intracellular level of ionised Ca^{++}, the release of ACh packets was actually depressed, while at nerve endings ACh release was increased by calcium ionophores.

Much work still needs to be done on the Schwann cell to clarify its physiological role.

POSTSYNAPTIC RESPONSE

The acetylcholine receptor

The effect of ACh at the neuromuscular junction is produced by its interaction with specific chemoreceptor molecules in the postsynaptic cell membrane. The existence of special properties of skeletal muscle fibres in the region of their innervation has been known since the beginning of this century. For example, Langley (1906) assumed the presence of a 'receptive substance' around motor nerve terminals where a localised sensitivity exists for various chemical agents, such as nicotine. Gradually, the term receptor has become accepted to indicate a site where a transmitter, hormone, or drug exerts its effects.

Biochemical studies of receptors are difficult because the receptors are usually present in minute amounts and because the function they perform is often difficult to define after they have been removed from the membrane. The ACh receptor is the best studied receptor pharmacologically, electrophysiologically, biochemically and immunologically.

The ACh receptor is probably closely associated in the membrane with an entity which has been called by Albuquerque, Barnard, Chiu, Lapa, Dolly, Jansson, Daly and Witkop (1973) the 'ionic conductance modulator' or 'ICM'. The molecular nature of this entity and its morphological relationship to the ACh recognition site are as yet not fully known. It could be part of the ACh receptor molecule or a separate molecule that is closely associated with the receptor through non-covalent bonds. The ICM may be the ionic channel (a component that traverses the membrane through which ions pass) or an ionophore (a small molecule which shuttles across the membrane to transport ions), as well as any of the structures that link these entities to the ACh receptor.

The main components involved in the post-synaptic response to ACh appear to be three: a) the ACh receptor; b) the ionic conductance modulator which is defined by its capacity to change drastically and reversibly the Na^+ and K^+ permeability of the membrane in which it is located; c) AChE (acetylcholinesterase), known to be highly concentrated at the neuromuscular synapse.

The number of AChE molecules was the first macromolecular quantitative parameter to be established for the end-plate (for references *see* Barnard, 1974). DFP (diisopropylfluorophosphate), labelled either with ^{32}P or with 3H was used. It was found that the number of AChE molecules present at the end-plate is constant for a given muscle fibre type and size, being in the overall range (for different adult muscles) of $0.3–4.0 \times 10^7$ active centres per end-plate.

Only recently have receptor molecules for ACh been identified. Their isolation has been helped greatly by the discovery of snake toxins that bind specifically and with high affinity to ACh receptors

(Lee, 1972). Once occupied by toxin, the receptors cannot react with ACh, and this accounts for the paralysing action that results from the bite of certain snakes. One of the most useful toxins has been α-bungarotoxin, obtained from *Bungarus* snakes. The toxin can be radioactively labelled without losing its activity. Such labelled toxin is then bound to receptors, and the complex can be isolated and chemically characterised. Many of the studies have been made on the receptor-rich electric organs of the fish *Electrophorus* and *Torpedo*.

The conclusion that there may be two binding sites for α-bungarotoxin (α-BuTX) is supported by studies with the perhydro derivative of histrionicotoxin, a toxic substance isolated from the Colombian arrow-poison frog *Dendrobates histrionicus* (Albuquerque *et al.*, 1973). This toxin also blocks neuromuscular transmission, and reduces the rate of binding of α-bungarotoxin. When, however, perhydrohistrionicotoxin and tubocurarine were given together, α-bungarotoxin binding was almost completely blocked. Albuquerque and his colleagues, in discussing these results, propose that α-bungarotoxin might combine with two separate sites: one, the ACh receptor proper, which is curare-sensitive, and the other, it is proposed, the 'ionic conductance modulator' that mediates the permeability change which follows receptor activation. This latter site is thought to be blocked by perhydrohistrionicotoxin.

The idea that the entity with which the transmitter combines and the 'conductance modulator' are distinct structures, and therefore susceptible to selective blockade, is also suggested by the work of Kasai and Changeux (1971) on microsac preparations from the electroplax of *Electrophorus electricus*. The same concept appears in the suggestion by Magazanik and Vyskočil (1973) that desensitisation may involve, not the receptors proper, but a later stage in the transduction process.

Eric Barnard and his colleagues have selected the vertebrate motor end-plate as a model synapse. The results of their work, together with that from other laboratories, has led to the construction of an end-plate model showing the spatial arrangement of transmitter release in relation to ACh receptor and AChE concentrations. According to them, the vertebrate motor end-plate is at present the most promising case for a molecular analysis of synaptic function. This distinction arises from its accessibility to electrophysiological and pharmacological studies as well as to chemical analyses (for further details and references *see* Barnard, Dolly, Lang, Lo and Shorr, 1979).

Already, detailed molecular information on the ACh receptor has come in the past eight years or so from biochemical studies on receptors isolated from the electroplax of electric fishes (for details and references *see* Eldefrawi and Eldefrawi, 1977; Heidmann and Changeux, 1978). This source has the advantage of yielding much greater concentrations of the receptor than do mammalian skeletal muscles. In vertebrate skeletal muscles, the ACh receptors can be analysed either at the end-plate or after denervation, extrajunctionally. In chronic denervation, the number of receptors per fibre increases to an extent which varies with muscle type, reaching up to 40-fold.

The precise localisation and the numbers of the toxin-binding receptor sites in innervated muscles were determined (after labelling by radioactive α-toxin), by electron microscope (EM) autoradiography in two mammalian species; they are on the postsynaptic membrane, and virtually exclusively at the crests of the junctional folds, at a density there of 25 000–30 000 sites per μm^2 of membrane. They are thus concentrated immediately opposite the 'active zones' for transmitter release that occur at intervals on the nerve terminal membrane (Barnard, Dolly, Porter and Albuquerque, 1975; Porter and Barnard, 1975) (see Fig. 3.1).

The localisation of the receptors can be visualised more sharply, although without the quantitative aspect, by peroxidase-labelling cytochemistry in the electron microscope. α-BuTX linked to peroxidase, either by direct chemical coupling or by the labelled-antibody sandwich technique, is used for this purpose. Staining of end-plates at the crests of their postsynaptic folds has been shown (Engel, Lindstrom, Lambert and Lennon, 1977) but with staining also on the opposing presynaptic membrane in all cases, as well as in the cleft, on Schwann cell processes, and even on the membranes of nuclei in muscle cells (Bender, Ringel, Engel, Vogel and Daniels, 1976; S.H. Chung and E.A. Barnard, unpublished data).

In specimens stained for *brief* periods, some presynaptic stain is present, but it is not continuous and is especially noticeable at the 'active zones' for transmitter release. Schwann cell processes are negative. The cleft is free of product. The crests of the postsynaptic folds are uniformly positive and the depths negative, in agreement with EM autoradiographic evidence. It is still difficult to be certain about the origin of the presynaptic staining, but the evidence mentioned suggests that it could be due to actual receptors there. However, Porter and Barnard (1976) found earlier, using collagenase pretreatment or 3H-α-toxin treatment and denervation in order to remove the axon terminal, that in EM autoradiographic analysis any presynaptic labelled sites were below the error limit of the technique and were likely—if present—to be less than 10 per cent of the total. The latter level would still be compatible with the staining seen in the most sensitive peroxidase method, so the evidence does not exclude these presynaptic ACh receptors, *at a very low level*.

Isolation. Denervated cat leg muscles are a relatively rich source of the ACh receptor; a sarcolemmal membrane preparation from these muscles contains α-BuTX binding sites which show, also, binding of cholinergic agonists and antagonists at affinities similar to those found pharmacologically (Barnard, Coates, Dolly and Mallick, 1977).

The ACh receptor from these muscles (fresh) has been extracted in 1.5 per cent Triton X-100 containing protease inhibitors (to prevent its degradation). In the most recent form of this method, Barnard and his colleagues adsorb the receptor to an α-toxin immobilised on a gel, with elution by carbamylcholine; final purification takes advantage of the glycoprotein nature (Brockes and Hall, 1975) of this receptor, by binding to immobilised 'Lens culinaris' lectin and elution by glycosides (Shorr, Dolly and Barnard, 1978). The final specific activity achieved is 10 000–12 000 nmoles α-toxin binding sites per gram protein. This is the same as others have obtained for receptors isolated from electroplax. Moreover, the same procedure applied to the electric organ of *Torpedo marmorata* also gave a final specific activity in that range.

Properties and composition of the muscle ACh receptor. The pure ACh receptor from cat (or rabbit) denervated muscle binds nicotinic cholinergic ligands (Dolly and Barnard, 1974, 1977) with affinities quite similar to those observed (Barnard *et al.*, 1977) with membrane fragments from denervated muscle. When the ligands are at their saturating concentrations (e.g. 10^{-4}M d-tubocurarine), no 3H-toxin binding is detectable.

The ACh recognition unit of the denervated mammalian muscle receptor consists of a single sub-unit type, a glycoprotein of 41 000 MW, or of that as the main component plus a small additional complement of heavier sub-units (Shorr *et al.*, 1978). The latter are at such a low level that it has not yet been possible to decide if they are strongly bound minor impurities or a small additional component of heavier subunits. Barnard and his colleagues however, stress that this composition refers to the oligomeric protein that binds ACh or α-toxin, the ACh recognition unit. The molecular weight of the oligomer itself is around 250 000.

The receptor assembly in the synaptic membrane may contain other types of sub-units required for the ion channel or for other features of that assembly. The evidence cited does not exclude these, since they could—especially in the extra-synaptic receptor of denervated muscle—conceivably be readily detached upon extraction, leaving the ACh-binding capacity unchanged.

End-plate potential

Resting potential. The muscle cell membrane with its complex pattern of polysaccharide, muco- and lipo-protein, separates aqueous solutions having the same total osmotic pressure but radically different compositions. The extracellular fluid has high concentrations of Na^+ and Cl^- and a low concentration of K^+. On the other hand, the intracellular fluid is rich in K^+ and protein, but its content of Na^+ and Cl^- ions is low. This unequal distribution of inorganic ions across the muscle fibre membrane gives rise to an electrical potential difference (about 90 mV, inside negative) between the interior of the cell and its environment. This potential difference can be measured by inserting a fine-tipped, electrolyte-filled, glass micro-electrode into the muscle fibre.

The maintenance of these concentration differences depends upon the net movement of ions against their electrochemical potential gradients. These, in turn, develop because the cell uses metabolically derived energy to transport Na^+ out of it and K^+ into it, actively. On the other hand, passive diffusion across the membrane is slow. The demonstration that the muscle loses K^+ and gains Na^+ on stimulation and that these exchanges reverse during the recovery period led Dean (1941) to suggest that there must be a 'pump', possibly located in the fibre membrane, which can pump out the Na^+ and pump in the K^+. Everybody agrees that this process requires expenditure of energy which must be supplied by cell metabolism, but much is to be done if we are to achieve an understanding of the way in which the transport system is coupled to the cellular metabolism (Hodgkin, 1958; Hoffman, 1961).

At the neuromuscular junction a non-propagated end-plate potential precedes the action potential of the muscle fibre. In the presence of just sufficient curare to prevent contraction, a nerve volley continues to set up an electrical change in the muscle (Eccles *et al.*, 1941), *the synaptic potential*, which is attributable to the depolarisation of the motor end-plate by ACh and which is generally called the 'end-plate potential' (Göpfert and Schaefer, 1938). In the cat the latent period of this potential in the soleus muscle is about 0.5 ms, rising to a summit in 0.8 ms and then decaying in a roughly exponential manner. The average time for its half decay is about 3 ms (Eccles *et al.*, 1941). The synaptic potential is a non-propagated local response, an electrotonic potential that falls off exponentially with increasing distance from the post-junctional region. Its outstanding characteristic is that it is a graded response and can therefore be modified; consequently the amplitude of the end-plate potential may vary as a result either of a change in the amount of ACh liberated at the nerve endings or a change in the sensitivity of the end-plate to the depolarising action of ACh. For example, on increasing the concentration of curare the amplitude of the response is reduced. Thus, the stronger the stimulus, the greater the degree of depolarisation of the postsynaptic membrane leading to a greater synaptic potential. This is in contrast to the propagated response which is an all-or-nothing event and consequently can be blocked but not otherwise modified. Furthermore, the synaptic potential has no refractory period; thus additional potentials can sum with it. The moment this summated effect reaches a critical level of depolarisation it triggers the electrically propagated all-or-nothing action potential which travels along the fibre, leaving a period of refractoriness behind it. Moreover, it is possible to block selectively Na channels necessary for the action potential with TTX, but leave the end-plate potential completely unchanged, which further suggests that the ACh-induced changes producing the end-plate potential are completely separate from the sodium channels which generate the action potential. Takeuchi (1963a, b) demonstrated that the principal conductance change produced by ACh at the end-plate concerns sodium and potassium ions with chloride playing a negligible part.

Krnjević and Miledi (1958), by means of iontophoretic application of ACh, obtained, in the isolated rat diaphragm preparation, close approximation to nervous transmission; the application of ACh, in amounts as small as 1.5×10^{-17} moles, was followed by depolarisation of the end-plate membrane with a time-course almost as fast as that of the end-plate potential produced by the nerve impulse. However, even with the most refined micro-iontophoretic techniques, conditions cannot be as favourable as when ACh is liberated by the nerve endings.

Kuffler (1943) was the first to demonstrate that normal adult skeletal muscle fibres are sensitive to ACh in the regions of the neuromuscular junction only. Miledi (1960b), however, recording intracellularly from rat diaphragm fibres while ACh was applied iontophoretically, found that the chemosensitive properties of the muscle fibre membrane extend well beyond the neuromuscular junction but that the sensitivity falls off at either side of this region, becoming several thousand times smaller a few hundred microns away. He concluded, therefore, that the density of 'extra-junctional' ACh receptors decreases with distance from the synapse.

Supersensitivity to ACh is particularly marked in chronically denervated muscle. Brown (1937)

demonstrated that denervated mammalian muscle becomes about one thousand times more excitable to ACh administered by close-arterial injection. In cats, Perry and Zaimis (1953; *cited in* Zaimis and Head, 1976) found that, during the action of a depolarising drug, the rate of loss of K^+ from denervated cat muscles, previously loaded with $K^{42}Cl$, was almost three times that of normal muscles. They concluded, therefore, that during denervation the sensitivity of the muscle membrane beyond the end-plate region is sufficient to allow a response after ACh has been brought into contact with it. More direct evidence was obtained by Axelsson and Thesleff (1959) and Miledi (1960c), who applied ACh iontophoretically to single fibres and found that, after denervation, the rest of the membrane developed pharmacological properties similar to those of the end-plate region.

Noise analysis

The smallest physiological unit of ACh released by the nerve ending is a quantum, which in skeletal muscles usually produces a potential change of less than 1 mV. A quantum is made up of more than 1000 molecules (see below). Because the signals are so small, conventional recording techniques cannot resolve the events associated with the interactions of ACh molecules with individual receptors. Katz and Miledi (1972) overcame this difficulty by analysing the electrical 'noise' produced by ACh.

Using the conventional intracellular recording technique, with a single microelectrode inserted into the end-plate region of the muscle fibre and iontophoretic application of a steady dose of ACh, Katz and Miledi observed not only a steady depolarisation but also an excess of voltage noise. The basic phenomenon is illustrated in Figure 3.2.

It was quite reassuring to find that the 'extra noise' was associated with ACh-induced potential changes but did not occur when similar potential changes were produced by direct electric current.

To analyse the elementary events that make up the noise, Katz and Miledi used a method based on a theory developed more than 30 years ago for telephone communication (Rice, 1944). The underlying assumption is that the steady synaptic depolarisation results from the opening and closing of individual ionic channels, or gates, as the

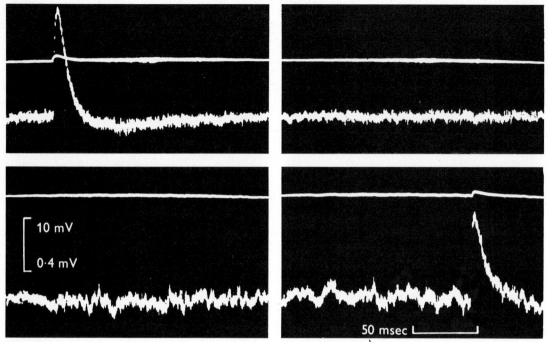

Fig. 3.2   Intracellular recording from an end-plate in frog sartorius at 21°C. In each block, the upper trace was recorded on a low-gain DC channel (scale 10 mV); the lower was simultaneously recorded on a high-gain condenser coupled channel (scale 0.4 mV). The top row shows controls (no ACh); the bottom row shows membrane noise during ACh application, by diffusion from a micropipette. In the bottom row of records, the increased distance between the low and high gain traces is due to upward displacement of the DC trace because of ACh-induced depolarisation. Two spontaneous mepps are also seen (from Katz, B. & Miledi, R. (1972). The statistical nature of the acetylcholine potential and its molecular components. *J. Physiol.* **224**, 665–699)

ACh molecules collide with receptors. Since collision with receptors is a random process, the number of channels open at any one time is not constant. Therefore, the conductance varies with the number of open channels. This, in turn, creates fluctuations in the synaptic current (and potential). A steady ACh-induced depolarisation means that many channels are open at any one time. From the fluctuations around the mean depolarisation, one can determine certain properties of the elementary components (also called 'shot' events).

Three main parameters can be extracted by noise analysis. These are the amplitude of the elementary shot effect (*a*), its time course (*τ*) and the number of channels opened per second at any given time (*n*). For simplicity, Katz and Miledi assumed that the channel opening reaches its peak (*a*) instantaneously and declines exponentially with a time constant *τ*. To obtain the amplitude of the voltage change that occurs as a result of a single

channel opening, the mean depolarisation (V) and the variance of the membrane potential ($\bar{E}^2$) must be measured*. For example, for a 10 mV depolarisation (V), the standard deviation of the noise was found to be of the order of 30–50 μV. From the equation

$$\bar{E} = \frac{Va}{2}$$

the amplitude *a* of the elementary shot event ($2\,\bar{E}^2/V$) was then calculated to be 0.18–0.5 μV in a frog muscle fibre with a resting potential of 90 mV and miniature end-plate potentials (mepps) of 0.5 mV amplitude. In this case *a* is some three orders of magnitude smaller than the mepp, which suggests that a mepp is produced by the synchronous opening of one or a few thousand ion channels. Assuming each ion channel is opened as a

*For a detailed discussion of the methods of noise analysis, *see* the more recent reviews by Katz and Miledi (1976) and Wray (1980a).

result of an effective interaction between one or a small number of receptors and of ACh molecules, the mepp requires the simultaneous action of a few thousand ACh molecules. Each released packet contains around 10^4 ACh molecules (Kuffler and Yoshikami, 1975).

The depolarisation which follows the channel opening then decays passively with a time constant, τ, which should be the same as the membrane time constant. The time course of the elementary event can be determined from a study of the frequency components present in the noise (Anderson and Stevens, 1973; Katz and Miledi, 1972). Analysis of the frequency components of the variance of the noise (the 'power spectrum') shows a typical shape which indeed depends on the time constant of decay, τ. An example of this is shown in Figure 3.3: the power spectrum, S, is flat at lower frequencies, and falls off at higher frequencies. The frequency at which the spectrum falls to one-half maximum ('half-power frequency', f_c) is of considerable significance, because

it is related to the decay time constant, τ, of the elementary event by

$$\tau = \frac{1}{2\pi f_c}.$$

The power spectrum is given by

$$S = \frac{S_o}{1+(f/f_c)^2}$$

where f is frequency and S_o is the maximum value of S (i.e. on the flat part of the curve). Therefore, by fitting the theoretical curve to the observed power spectrum, the half-power frequency can be determined, and hence τ, the time constant of decay of the elementary event can be found. As can be seen in Figure 3.3, which is for cat tenuissimus muscle at 38°C, the experimental points fit the theoretical curve (Wray, 1980b). For instance, cat tenuissimus muscle at 37°C typically has a half-power frequency, f_c, of around 80 Hz. Therefore the time constant, τ, is 2.0 ms in this case.

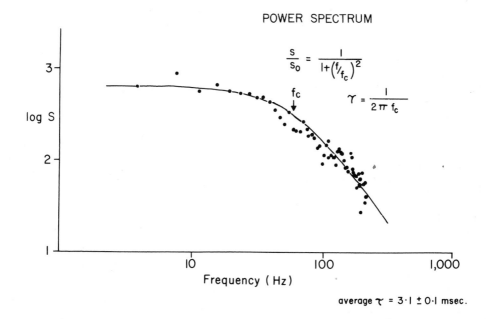

average $\tau = 3.1 \pm 0.1$ msec.

Fig. 3.3 This Figure shows a power spectrum of intracellular voltage noise recorded at an end-plate of cat tenuissimus muscle (temperature 38°C) during the application of 1 μM acetylcholine in the perfusing solution. Noise variance power density is plotted against frequency on log-log axes. The theoretical curve is shown fitted by eye to the experimental points and hence the decay constant τ determined. The mean value during the experiment was $\tau = 3.1 \pm 0.1$ ms. Eserine (3 μM) was present to prevent hydrolysis of acetylcholine, and tetrodotoxin (250 nM) was present to prevent action potentials (from Wray, D. (1980b). Prolonged exposure to acetylcholine: noise analysis and channel inactivation in cat tenuissimus muscle. *J. Physiol.*, in press)

When depolarisation (i.e. voltage change) is measured, the derived time course, τ, is the time constant for passive decay of charge from the membrane. This is longer than the time course of the underlying *current* pulse which charged the membrane in the first place. Therefore, the time course of the underlying *current* pulse cannot be measured easily by simply recording intracellular voltage: one has to measure current directly. Two methods have been used to examine fluctuations of the ionic current during the ACh response: (1) focal extracellular recording, and (2) voltage-clamping with intracellular feedback current. For the latter method, two microelectrodes have to be inserted into the muscle fibre near to each other at the end-plate region. One microelectrode records the intracellular voltage, while the other passes current into or out of the muscle fibre. Electronic circuitry controls the current passed by the latter electrode so that the intracellular voltage is held constant. When ACh reaches the postsynaptic membrane and causes an increase in permeability, current starts to flow into the fibre. This current begins to flow out again passively, but in so doing, starts to depolarise the membrane. The voltage recording electrode detects this, so the electronic circuitry causes current to pass via the other electrode, to prevent depolarisation and hence passive flow of current outwards. The current flows into the microelectrode instead, where it can be measured. The intracellular voltage is clamped at a constant value. The voltage clamp technique for noise analysis was first used by Anderson and Stevens (1973). The power spectrum of the noise can be recorded, and, just as for voltage noise, the time constant of decay of an individual current pulse can be determined from the spectrum. The time constant, τ, can be obtained from the 'half-power' frequency, just as for voltage noise. In this case, the time constant now gives the duration of the current pulse—i.e. channel lifetime. The duration of the elementary current flow is found to be $\simeq 1$ ms at room temperature.

Having determined a and τ, one can calculate n, the number of events in any given time:

$$n = \frac{V}{a\tau}$$

For a depolarisation of 20 mV in the cat's tenuissimus muscle the frequency of opening of channels by ACh is $\simeq 30 \times 10^7$/s.

Uses of noise analysis

The lifetime of the channel opened by ACh has been extensively measured by the technique of noise analysis (Katz and Miledi, 1971, 1972; Anderson and Stevens, 1973; Ben-Haim, Dreyer and Peper, 1975; Dreyer, Muller, Peper and Sterz, 1976; Colquhoun, Large and Rang, 1977; Cull-Candy, Miledi and Trautmann, 1979). There is some variation between species, with values around 1.1 ms at a temperature of 23°C and membrane potential of –75 mV, at normal end-plates.

Channel lifetime depends on temperature—as temperature is lowered by 10°C, the lifetime increases by a factor of around 2.5–3.3. The lifetime also depends on membrane potential—as membrane potential is hyperpolarised by 100 mV, the channel lifetime increases by a factor of around 2.2 (19°C).

The conductance of the channel opened by ACh has also been widely studied by noise analysis in these papers. There is little variation with species, temperature and membrane potential, with values of around 23 pS at normal end-plates.

From these values of channel conductance and lifetime, one finds that, while open, each channel passes a quantity of charge around 1.5×10^{-15} coulombs, equivalent to the passage of 10^4 univalent ions—and all this is initiated by just a few ACh molecules acting at the receptor.

An important discovery by Anderson and Stevens (1973) was that, at 8°C, the lifetime of a single channel was found to be identical to the decay constant of a miniature end-plate current, or a nerve-evoked end-plate current—even at different membrane potentials. Therefore the decay of end-plate current is determined by the rate of channel closing. Thus the nerve-released ACh must disappear (by hydrolysis and diffusion) from the synaptic cleft in a time much less than the channel open time. At higher temperatures (22°C), the decay of end-plate currents is slower than the channel lifetime by a factor of about 1.4 (Katz and

Miledi, 1973a; Colquhoun *et al.*, 1977). Therefore, at higher temperatures, some ACh remains in the cleft after some channels have closed, and continues to open channels, so prolonging the end-plate current.

The enzyme acetylcholinesterase is present in the synaptic cleft in roughly equal molecular numbers to the number of ACh receptors (Barnard, Wieckowski and Chiu, 1971; Porter, Barnard and Chiu, 1973). The receptor and the acetylcholinesterase are distinct molecules (Changeux, 1975). The effect of the acetylcholinesterase enzyme is made clear after it has been inhibited by a cholinesterase inhibitor such as neostigmine. Then one finds that miniature end-plate currents (mepcs) are prolonged by around 2–6 times, while the channel lifetime, from noise analysis, is unchanged (Katz and Miledi, 1973a). In this case, ACh molecules persist in the synaptic cleft, and so can act repeatedly, causing channels to open. Under normal conditions, in the absence of cholinesterase inhibitors, ACh is quickly removed by hydrolysis.

Noise analysis has also been used to help elucidate the action of a variety of drugs on the postsynaptic membrane. For instance, some alcohols shorten channel lifetime, while others lengthen it (Gage, 1976). Local anaesthetics (Katz and Miledi, 1975; Ruff, 1977) seem to act at the postsynaptic membrane by blocking channels while they are open—a mechanism which appears to be shared by barbiturates (Adams, 1976), and some antagonists such as atropine (Katz and Miledi, 1973b; Feltz, Large and Trautmann, 1977).

In the case of tubocurarine, noise analysis has shown that this competitive antagonist does not markedly affect the elementary event produced by a single channel but simply reduces the frequency of opening (Katz and Miledi, 1972), as may be expected for a competitive antagonist. However, even for tubocurarine, evidence has begun to accumulate for a more complicated picture, also involving channel blocking (Katz and Miledi, 1978; Colquhoun, Dreyer and Sheridan, 1979).

For denervated muscle fibres, ACh receptors are no longer located just at the end-plate, but are spread throughout the fibre (Axelsson and Thesleff, 1959). Noise analysis (Dreyer *et al.*, 1976;

Dreyer, Walther and Peper, 1976; Neher and Sakmann, 1976a) shows that, in denervated muscle, the lifetime of the channels is about 3–5 times longer than that of normal end-plate channels, while the conductance of these channels is around 70 per cent of normal. Channel lifetime for denervated muscle has similar temperature and voltage dependence to that of normal end-plate channels, while channel conductance is relatively independent of these parameters.

It is now possible to record the opening of individual channels using a rather blunt microelectrode in contact with a small patch of membrane (Neher and Sakmann, 1976b). The current which flows through this small patch of membrane can be recorded, and it is found that ACh, and other depolarising drugs, produce tiny pulses of current, with many of the properties expected or assumed in noise analysis. So, for instance, the conductance and lifetime of channels are roughly similar to the values obtained from noise analysis. The action of local anaesthetics (to block channels) has also been confirmed by these techniques (Neher and Steinbach, 1978). However, these authors use collagenase and non-specific proteases to treat the muscle before recording. This treatment may well remove surface proteins involved in the function of ion channels and so introduce artefacts into the recordings.

Noise analysis has been applied to human (intercostal) muscle (Cull-Candy *et al.*, 1979). The channel lifetime (1.5 ms) and channel conductance (22pS at 23°C) and −80 mV resting potential are very similar to values obtained in cat, rat, mouse and frog muscle. In muscle from myasthenic patients, it is found that the channel lifetime and conductance are similar to those of normal muscle. The voltage dependence of the channel lifetime is similar in normal and myasthenic muscle. In myasthenia gravis, there is evidence of a decreased number of ACh receptors at the postsynaptic membrane—for instance, binding of the snake toxin α-bungarotoxin is decreased in myasthenics as well as the amplitude of mepps (Ito, Miledi, Vincent and Newsom Davis, 1978). Indeed, estimates of the channel properties from noise analysis show that a packet of transmitter opens about 1500 channels at normal end-plates, while at myasthenic end-plates a packet opens only about

600 channels (Cull-Candy *et al.*, 1979). The size of the packet of transmitter released from myasthenic terminals is at least as large as the packet of ACh released from normal human nerve terminals.

Depolarising neuromuscular blocking drugs

For many years the only well-known neuromuscular blocking drug was curare, which has the property of being sufficiently like ACh to have an affinity for the specific receptors normally reacting to ACh at the neuromuscular junction, but is so unlike ACh that it cannot activate the receptors. In 1937, however, it was demonstrated for the first time that competition with ACh is not the only mechanism by which a substance can produce a neuromuscular block. Bacq and Brown reported in that year that ACh itself can produce an interruption of neuromuscular transmission if made to accumulate under the influence of an anticholinesterase drug. Almost ten years later, synthetic substances were discovered whose action can be regarded as similar to that of ACh, except that their action persists for much longer.

As a consequence of the observation made by W.D.M. Paton that octamethylene-bistrimethylammonium chloride (prepared by Harold King) was remarkably effective in causing neuromuscular block, a number of bisquaternary ammonium salts were synthesised by Zaimis (1950). They are all polymethylene bistrimethyl-ammonium di-iodides of the general type: $I[(CH_3)_3N(CH_2)_n{-}N(CH_3)_3]I$ where n indicates the number of methylene groups in the chain and may have any value from 2 to 13 or 18. At the same time, Barlow and Ing (1948a, b) independently prepared the dibromides, with the exception of the hexamethylene member. The name 'methonium compounds' was approved by the British Pharmacopoeia Commission for the members of the polymethylene bistrimethylammonium series, and it is under this name, preceded by the appropriate numerical prefix, that they have since been known.

One of the most remarkable properties of the members of this series, and especially of decamethonium, was the very great variation in their activity depending on the species of animal on which they were tested. Variation of this sort has been described for many other onium salts, but in the case of decamethonium its magnitude was unprecedented, and sufficient for great activity to be found in the cat but only slight activity in the rat.

The early pharmacological experiments described by Paton and Zaimis (1948a, b; 1949a, b; 1950; 1951a, b) demonstrated that although decamethonium possessed some of what were classically regarded as 'curarising' properties (i.e. it paralysed neuromuscular transmission leaving nervous conduction unaltered; it permitted the muscle to respond to direct stimulation; it prevented the effect of a close-arterial injection of ACh; it did not interfere with the release of ACh), there were also important differences. For example: (1) a phase of potentiation of the muscle twitch with fasciculations of the muscle and repetitive responses to single nerve volleys preceded the block; (2) tetanisation of the motor nerve or injection of ACh or potassium neither diminished nor deepened the block; (3) during a partial block, tetanisation of the muscle gave rise to a well-sustained contraction; (4) sensitivity to decamethonium varied greatly according to species; in order of decreasing sensitivity, the order was cat–man–rabbit–monkey–mouse–rat. Using the same tests, the variation in sensitivity with tubocurarine was much smaller, the order being rat–mouse–rabbit–cat; (5) the action of decamethonium was not antagonised by anticholinesterase drugs; (6) previous administration of tubocurarine reduced the effectiveness of decamethonium; (7) penta- and hexamethonium provided effective antagonists and the antagonism appeared to be by competitive inhibition; (8) decamethonium elicited a contraction of the frog's rectus abdominis muscle, and did not antagonise the contraction elicited by ACh; (9) decamethonium could also elicit a twitch of the cat's tibialis muscle if a small dose was given by close-arterial injection.

It was concluded, therefore, that decamethonium produced neuromuscular block by initiating some active response in the end-plate or muscle fibre and that the differences between tubocurarine and decamethonium were so striking as to indicate the possibility of a fundamental divergence in their mode of action.

An analysis of these stimulant effects by Zaimis (1951) established that they cannot be attributed to the weak anticholinesterase activity of decamethonium, and emphasised the similarities between decamethonium and ACh. The strongest evidence for its active ACh-like action was obtained from denervated cat muscle. The close-arterial injection of decamethonium into the tibialis anterior muscle, denervated by the section of its nerve supply 15–20 days previously, produced a double mechanical response consisting of a quick initial contraction followed by a prolonged contracture. The quick response was accompanied by an outburst of action potentials, greatly in excess of any previous spontaneous activity; this outburst of action potentials was cut short with the onset of slow contracture during which no more rapid action potentials could be detected. ACh, in doses similar to those of decamethonium (2–10 μg) produced the same effect. The conclusion was therefore drawn that decamethonium possesses many of the properties of ACh at the neuro-muscular junction, but differs from it in being a stable substance unaffected by the local enzyme.

End-plate depolarisation by decamethonium and suxamethonium in vivo. Burns and Paton (1951) using the gracilis muscle of the cat and recording with external electrodes, demonstrated that this resemblance of deca-methonium to ACh rests in the ability of deca-methonium to cause a persistent depolarisation of the end-plate region. They showed, moreover, that all the principal features of block by deca-methonium can be reproduced with ACh in the presence of an anticholinesterase drug. The depolarisation produced by decamethonium, although limited to the end-plate region, always extended slightly beyond the area in which end-plate potentials could be recorded. The extent of this spatial distribution increased with time. After an initial transient increase of excitability which was associated with random spontaneous fascicu-lations, the end-plate region depolarised by deca-methonium became inexcitable to direct stimu-lation, although the muscle remote from the end-plate region remained normally excitable. Burns and Paton concluded that the inexcitability of the muscle membrane around the point at which the end-plate potential is set up was a principal cause of the neuromuscular block produced by deca-methonium. Successive doses of decamethonium produced progressively smaller depolarisations, even if time was allowed for full recovery from each dose. It was suggested, therefore, that a new mechanism of block was present, namely a de-crease in the electrical excitability of the memb-rane of the end-plate region as a result of the persisting depolarisation. Similar results were obtained with suxamethonium, another de-polarising drug introduced by Bovet and Bovet-Nitti in 1955. Using the same method of recording, Paton and Waud (1962) demonstrated that when suxamethonium was given to a cat to produce between 90 and 100 per cent block for a period up to one hour, the end-plates do indeed remain depolarised throughout, but that the peak de-polarisation falls to a steady level of about half the maximum.

Effect of decamethonium, suxameth-onium and acetylcholine on the electri-cal properties of single mammalian muscle cells. More recently the electrical properties of single mammalian muscle cells were studied in the presence of concentrations of decamethonium or suxamethonium similar to those required to produce neuromuscular block (Zaimis and Head, 1976). The tenuissimus muscle of the cat was chosen for these experiments because cat and human skeletal muscles are very similar in their responses to neuromuscular blocking drugs. Moreover, the tenuissimus muscle is very similar in its physiological characteristics and its re-sponses to neuromuscular blocking drugs to the well studied tibialis anterior muscle (Paton and Zaimis, 1952; Zaimis, 1953; Maclagan, 1962). On a practical level, the muscle is thin and covered by a layer of connective tissue which is easily removed; the muscle is thus readily accessible and can be dissected easily, so that it can be isolated together with its nerve for *in vitro* experiments.

Experiments were first performed *in vivo* using slow intravenous infusions of tritiated deca-methonium (Fig. 3.4). The results showed that a plasma concentration of 1–1.4 μmol/l deca-methonium was sufficient to maintain an 80–90 per cent degree of block. This is similar to the

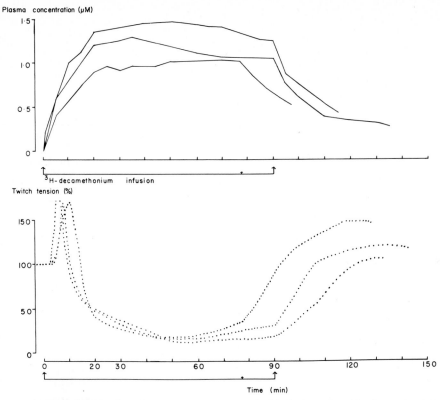

Fig. 3.4 Cat; anaesthetised with chloralose. Lower trace: neuromuscular blockade produced in three animals by tritiated decamethonium (slow intravenous infusion, 5–7 μg/kg per min). The graphs show the twitch tension of indirectly elicited maximal contractions of the tenuissimus muscle expressed as a percentage of the control value. Upper trace: plasma concentrations of tritiated decamethonium during the infusion, measured by liquid scintillation counting (from Zaimis, E. and Head, S. (1976) Depolarising neuromuscular blocking drugs. In *Handbook of Experimental Pharmacology, XLII, Neuromuscular Junction*, pp. 365–419 (Ed. E. Zaimis). Berlin: Springer Verlag)

concentration of radioactive decamethonium found necessary by Creese and Maclagan (1972) to maintain a neuromuscular block in the tibialis anterior muscle of the cat.

For the *in vitro* work (recording the muscle contractions or measurement of the electrical properties of single muscle cells) great care was taken to ensure that the muscle was rapidly dissected and that adequate oxygenation and a steady temperature were maintained. After dissection the muscle was placed within a few seconds into a beaker containing about 100 ml of oxygenated Krebs solution at 37°C. Within 30 s the muscle was transferred to a recording chamber (volume 2–3 ml) situated in a Faraday cage. Oxygenated Krebs solution at 37.5°C $\pm$ 0.5°C flowed through the chamber at a rate of 12–15 ml/min for the whole duration of the

experiment.

With the tenuissimus muscle *in vitro* it was found that at a concentration of 1 μmol/l, both decamethonium and suxamethonium produced an 80–98 per cent neuromuscular block. Thus it was established that similar concentrations give rise to the same degree of neuromuscular block in both the *in vivo* and *in vitro* preparations. Application of either decamethonium or suxamethonium was maintained for 30 min. In all preparations the neuromuscular block became maximal in about 10 min. In three out of four experiments the neuromuscular block was well maintained during the exposure of the muscle to either decamethonium or suxamethonium.

In order to test the extent to which the depolarisation was sustained during continued application of decamethonium or suxamethonium, changes in membrane potential and input resistance at the end-plate region of single surface muscle cells of the tenuissimus muscle were recorded using intracellular microelectrodes.

Membrane potential. Prolonged application of 1 μmol/l suxamethonium or decamethonium produced a depolarisation at the end-plate region. The drugs were always applied in a continuously flowing solution. From a value of about –85 mV the membrane potential decreased to about –42 mV in the presence of either drug. Contraction of the muscle did not occur when the membrane potential reached the threshold value for action potential generation of –55 mV (Boyd and Martin, 1956). It appears that the rate of depolarisation at this concentration is too slow to initiate an action potential. When a higher concentration of decamethonium was used (6 μmol/l), causing a faster initial depolarisation, action potentials were generated and contraction of the muscle occurred.

The replacement of the normal Krebs solution with a solution containing 1 μmol/l decamethonium or suxamethonium caused an almost immediate depolarisation at an initial rate of 100 to 200 mV/min, over a period of 15–20 s. This rapid phase of depolarisation was followed by a slower one, maximal depolarisation being reached in about 5–8 min.

In four experiments with decamethonium and five with suxamethonium the depolarising drug was applied continuously for 30 min. During this period a depolarisation of about 43 mV was well maintained in four out of nine fibres. In the other five fibres while depolarisation tended to diminish with time, it was still substantial after 30 min. In the preparation which showed the largest repolarisation the membrane was still depolarised by 28 mV after 30 min of continuous application of decamethonium. A maintained depolarisation could be recorded for periods of up to 50 min during continuous application of decamethonium. The time course of the depolarisation was the same as with the continuous recording. In conclusion, there was a good correlation between (a) neuromuscular block measured *in vivo* and *in vitro* by means of indirectly elicited contraction of the tenuissimus muscle and (b) the changes in memb-

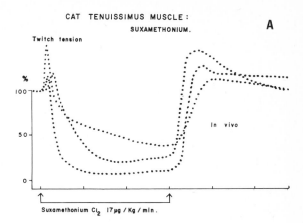

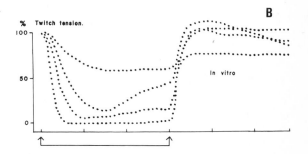

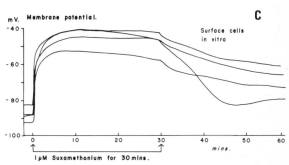

Fig. 3.5 Comparison of the effects of suxamethonium on the tenuissimus muscle: A, recording of muscle contractions *in vivo*; B, recording of muscle contractions *in vitro*; C, recording of membrane potential from single muscle fibres *in vitro* (from Zaimis, E. and Head, S. (1976) Depolarising neuromuscular blocking drugs. In *Handbook of Experimental Pharmacology, XLII, Neuromuscular Junction*, pp. 365–419 (Ed. E. Zaimis). Berlin: Springer Verlag)

rane potential at the end-plate region. Figure 3.5 illustrates this correlation for suxamethonium.

Input resistance. Electrotonic potentials were produced by the passage into the fibre of pulses of current of constant duration and magnitude from a second microelectrode inserted 70 μm away from the recording electrode. Thus not only membrane potential but also the electrotonic potentials were measured through the recording electrode. From the electrotonic potentials the input resistance of the fibre can be calculated.

Measurements of input resistance were made for both short and prolonged applications of decamethonium and suxamethonium. Input resistance decreased on applying either drug, and this decrease lasted as long as the drug was present in the bathing solution. Only after the removal of the drug did input resistance begin to return towards its previous level.

Effect of acetylcholine on membrane potential. Concentrations of ACh similar to those of decamethonium and suxamethonium had no effect on the resting potential of the tenuissimus muscle. In the presence of an anticholinesterase drug, however, the same concentration of ACh induced a depolarisation of the end-plate region. When the membrane potential reached about −60 mV, muscle contractions occurred and the microelectrode was expelled. The addition of tetrodo-

toxin to the bathing fluid prevented the muscle from contracting. The following procedure was thus adopted: an end-plate region was first located in normal Krebs solution; this solution was then replaced by one containing 250 nmol/l tetrodotoxin. Five minutes later this second solution was replaced by one containing the same concentration of tetrodotoxin and in addition eserine at a concentration of 3 μmol/1; after another 5 min ACh was added at a concentration of 1.1 μmol/l. This final solution was allowed to flow over the muscle preparation for up to 30 min. Figure 3.6 shows that in six experiments ACh produced substantial depolarisation from a resting potential of −85.7 ± 2.0 mV (mean ± SE of mean) to a potential in the presence of ACh of −51.7 ± 3.0 mV. In three of these experiments the drug was applied for 30 min. While depolarisation tended to diminish with time, it was still substantial at the end of the drug application. Complete recovery of the membrane potential occurred only on removal of ACh from the bathing solution.

Noise analysis and depolarising drugs. The technique of noise analysis provides a quantitative

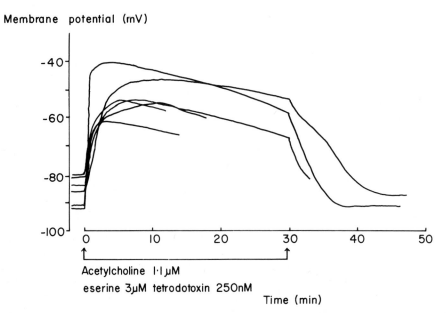

Fig. 3.6 Cat; isolated tenuissimus muscle. Depolarisations produced by acetylcholine (1.1 μmol/l in the presence of eserine, 3 μmol/l, and tetrodotoxin, 250 nmol/l) and recorded from the end-plate region of surface muscle cells in different preparations (from Zaimis, E. and Head, S. (1976) Depolarising neuromuscular blocking drugs. In *Handbook of Experimental Pharmacology, XLII, Neuromuscular Junction*, pp. 365–419 (Ed. E. Zaimis). Berlin: Springer Verlag)

tool for the further investigation of how the postsynaptic membrane responds to long applications of these drugs.

Noise analysis gives information on the frequency of opening of channels by depolarising drugs (Wray, 1980a, 1980b). Figure 3.7 shows the maintained depolarisation produced by 1 µM ACh during a 15-minute application (cat tenuissimus muscle, 37°C). It can be seen from the Figure that the number of channels opened per second falls quite slowly. The maximum number of channels opened per second was $7 \times 10^7/s$ in this experiment, falling to $5 \times 10^7/s$ after 15 min. In other words, desensitisation proceeds only slowly. When frequency of channel opening is studied for the depolarising drugs suberyldicholine, suxamethonium and decamethonium in the same concentration, similar slow de-

sensitisation is seen.

On the other hand, when ACh is applied by iontophoresis (Axelsson and Thesleff, 1958), the response of the postsynaptic membrane declines within seconds. However, the response of the postsynaptic membrane is very dependent on concentrations of applied drug, and probably the iontophoretic recordings produce high concentrations of ACh at the receptors. Desensitisation is more rapid at higher concentrations (Katz and Thesleff, 1957). It is important to take into account that the conditions of neuromuscular block, *in vivo*, by depolarising drugs, are similar to those of *in vitro* bath application at micromolar concentrations (Zaimis and Head, 1976), but not iontophoretic applications with their much higher concentrations.

Thus the evidence shows that neuromuscular

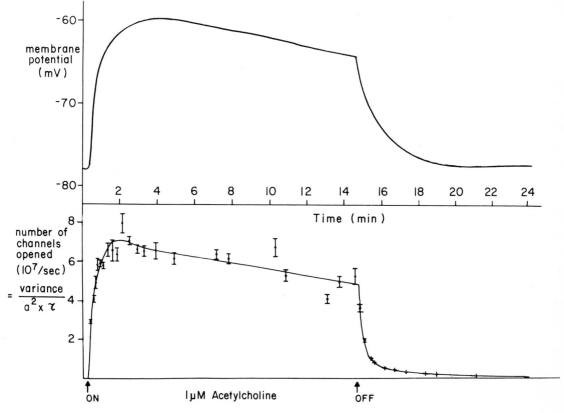

Fig. 3.7 This figure shows recording of membrane potential (upper part of figure), and frequency of opening of channels (lower part of figure) computed from the noise variance. Continuous intracellular recording was made at an end-plate of cat tenuissimus muscle (38°C). Eserine (3 µM) was present to prevent hydrolysis of acetylcholine, and tetrodotoxin (250 nM) was present to prevent action potentials. Elementary event: average magnitude a = 0.127 ± 0.004 µV, decay time constant (from power spectrum) $\tau = 3.1 \pm 0.1$ ms (from Wray, D. (1978a). End-plate voltage noise during prolonged application of acetylcholine in cat tenuissimus muscle. *J. Physiol.* **278**, 4–5P)

block does not take place by desensitisation of the ACh-receptors. All the information on depolarisation, input resistance, and noise shows that the end-plate remains sensitive to a depolarising drug as long as it is present. Rather, neuromuscular block arises because the depolarisation itself causes a failure of the action potential to be initiated at the end-plate region. The increase in Na ion permeability, vital to the action potential, can no longer occur. The end-plate chemosensitive channels behave normally, but the electrically sensitive Na channels of the action potential are inactivated by maintained depolarisation.

Noise analysis has shown that channel lifetime differs markedly for different depolarising drugs (Katz and Miledi, 1973c; Colquhoun, Dionne, Steinbach and Stevens, 1975; Dreyer et al., 1976; Neher and Sakmann, 1976a; Colquhoun et al., 1977). The channel lifetimes are (at 20°C, −75 mV) suberyldicholine: 1.6–3.3 ms; acetylcholine: 1.1 ms; acetylmonoethylcholine: 0.66 ms; carbachol: 0.3–0.4 ms; decamethonium: 0.5 ms; nicotine: 0.22 ms; acetylthiocholine: 0.12 ms. On the other hand, the single channel conductance is around the same value for these depolarising drugs.

The depolarising drugs acetylcholine, suberyldicholine, suxamethonium and decamethonium all produce large depolarisations of around 20 mV (cat tenuissimus muscle, 37°C) when exposed to similar concentrations of a depolarising drug (around 1 μM). However, the channel lifetime varies widely, and this is reflected in a corresponding variation in the size of the elementary voltage a. How do these drugs then produce a similar depolarisation (20 mV)? To study this, the action of these drugs in cat tenuissimus muscle was compared. Intracellular voltage noise was recorded at the end-plate region (Wray, 1978b, 1980b), and the depolarising drug was applied during continuous bath perfusion. The magnitude of a was in the order: decamethonium (0.012 ± 0.005 μV) < suxamethonium (0.033 ± 0.019 μV) < acetylcholine (0.086 ± 0.017 μV) < suberyldicholine (0.133 ± 0.050 μV); this suggests that the channel lifetime would also show the same trend. The frequency of channel opening also varies between the different depolarising drugs (at the same concentration, 1–2 μM). Indeed the number of channels opened per second was in the order: decamethonium (220 ± 90) × 10^7/s > suxamethonium (150 ± 89) × 10^7/s > acetylcholine (39 ± 11) × 10^7/s > suberyldicholine (17 ± 9) × 10^7/s. Thus, in spite of its transient channel lifetime, decamethonium produces large depolarisations because it opens channels more often than, for instance, suberyldicholine. Depolarisation produced by these drugs is similar because the smaller the value of the elementary voltage, a, the larger the frequency of channel opening (at similar molar concentrations). However, the underlying mechanism, at the molecular level, for this striking correlation between the frequency of channel opening and the channel lifetime is not really clear.

Desensitisation. Thesleff (1955a, b) questioned the existence of a block due solely to depolarisation and put forward the view that a major part of the block produced by decamethonium or suxamethonium was due to desensitisation even in the intact animal. Using various isolated muscle preparations he found that during the application of either ACh, decamethonium or suxamethonium the motor end-plate region became depolarised, but after a few seconds this initial depolarising effect disappeared and the muscle membrane repolarised. This development of repolarisation in the continued presence of the depolarising drug was called desensitisation (or 'receptor inactivation' by Nastuk, Manthey and Gissen, 1966) and was defined by Elmqvist and Thesleff (1962) as 'a condition in which application of a depolarising drug has made chemoreceptors of the end-plate refractory to chemical stimulation'. Since then this phenomenon of desensitisation has been widely studied and discussed (for further details, see Michelson and Zeimal, 1973; Rang, 1975; Ginsborg and Jenkinson, 1976). Reading through the literature, however, one becomes aware that 'desensitisation' means different things to different scientists. For example, there are pharmacologists and clinicians who describe as a 'desensitisation' blockade, an interruption of neuromuscular transmission which is easily antagonised by anticholinesterase drugs or by a tetanus, and potentiated by tubocurarine. Others use the term desensitisation to refer to the reduced sensitivity to ACh produced by drugs competing with it. These last two instances, however, are quite different from the phenomenon described as desensitisation by Thesleff and his colleagues.

The phenomenon of desensitisation has been the subject of much discussion in recent years. A great many factors have been suggested as being likely to influence the rate of its development. The concentration of the drug, however, appears to be one of the most important factors. Fatt (1950) was the first to describe a decrease in sensitivity of the motor end-plate after the application of ACh and to state that the rate of its development is concentration-dependent. In 1955, Del Castillo and Katz pointed out that 'with the ionophoretic applications, complications occur because nearby and more distant receptors within a single end-plate are not equally affected by the discharge of ACh from a point source. With a given dose, receptors at very close range may be saturated, or even damaged, by the momentary attainment of an excessive concentration, while more distant receptors are acted upon more slowly and at a lower concentration'. They added, 'this situation differs from the normal process of transmission and also from the more conventional methods of drug application in which the whole receptor area is subject to a uniform dose'. Axelsson and Thesleff themselves (1958) concluded that the degree of desensitisation and the speed of its onset were graded and increased with the applied concentration of ACh. Moreover, Thesleff (1959) pointed out that the duration of the initial depolarisation is inversely related to drug concentration.

Differences in drug concentration might therefore explain the very substantial differences between the results of our own experiments and those of Thesleff and his group. Using the same species (cat) and the same isolated muscle (tenuissimus) we were able to demonstrate a well-maintained depolarisation to ACh, decamethonium and suxamethonium, while in the experiments of Thesleff and his colleagues, depolarisation was short-lived and desensitisation was put forward as the mechanism behind the neuromuscular block. In our experiments the concentration of the depolarising drug was very similar to that necessary to produce an almost complete block in the intact animal. In this way unnecessarily large concentrations were avoided. In contrast, in the studies of Thesleff and his colleagues the depolarising drugs were applied either ionophoretically or in concentrations much larger than those necessary to produce an interruption of neuromuscular transmission.

Moreover, we have always found that desensitisation is not a normal phenomenon in the whole animal or man. At the end of periods in excess of two hours, during which the muscles were kept paralysed with a continuous infusion of suxamethonium, the neuromuscular block still exhibits the well-known characteristics of a depolarisation block. Thus, anticholinesterase drugs are ineffective or deepen the block, while tubocurarine antagonises it (Douglas and Paton, 1954; Cannard and Zaimis, 1959; Zaimis, 1959, 1962; Maclagan, 1962; Paton and Waud, 1962).

Scientists are interested in desensitisation because of the belief that the phenomenon may lead to an understanding of drug effects at molecular level. But they have to produce the right 'atmosphere' for desensitisation to flourish: i.e. high concentrations of the depolarising drug, long or repeated applications, incubation of the receptor material with ACh or other ACh-like substances. In other words, it is almost a 'hand-made' event, an experimental tool which can be useful in certain studies. Its importance in the intact animal or man is only marginal and it is a great pity that occasionally the terms 'depolarising' and 'desensitising' are used as synonyms when describing the actions of a neuromuscular blocking drug.

REFERENCES

Adams, P.R. (1976) Drug blockade of open end-plate channels. *Journal of Physiology*, **260**, 531.

Albuquerque, E.X., Barnard, E.A., Chiu, T.H., Lapa, A.J., Dolly, J.O., Jansson, S.-E., Daly, J. & Witkop, B. (1973) Acetylcholine receptor and ion conductance modulator sites at the murine neuromuscular junction: Evidence from specific toxin reactions. *Proceedings of the National Academy of Sciences of the United States of America*, **70**, 949.

Anderson, C.R. & Stevens, C.F. (1973) Voltage clamp analysis of acetylcholine produced end-plate current fluctuations at frog neuromuscular junction. *Journal of Physiology*, **235**, 655.

Axelsson, J. & Thesleff, S. (1958) The desensitising effect of acetylcholine on mammalian motor end-plate. *Acta physiologica scandinavica*, **43**, 15.

Axelsson, J. & Thesleff, S. (1959) A study of supersensitivity in denervated mammalian skeletal muscle. *Journal of Physiology*, **147**, 178.

Bacq, Z.M. & Brown, G.L. (1937) Pharmacological experiments on mammalian voluntary muscle, in relation to the theory of chemical transmission. *Journal of Physiology*, **89**, 45.

Baker, P.F. (1977) Calcium and the control of neuro-secretion. *Science Progress (Oxford)*, **64**, 95–115.

Barlow, R.B. & Ing, H.R. (1948a) Curare-like action of poly-methylene bis-quaternary ammonium salts. *Nature*, **161**, 718.

Barlow, R.B. & Ing, H.R. (1948b) Curare-like action of poly-methylene bis-quaternary ammonium salts. *British Journal of Pharmacology*, **3**, 298.

Barnard, E.A. (1974) Neuromuscular junction—enzymatic destruction of acetylcholine. In *The Peripheral Nervous System*, Ed. J.I. Hubbard, p. 201 (Plenum: New York).

Barnard, E.A., Coates, V., Dolly, J.O. & Mallick, B. (1977) Binding of α-bungarotoxin and cholinergic ligands to acetylcholine receptors in the membrane of skeletal muscle. *Cell Biology International Reports*, **1**, 99.

Barnard, E.A., Dolly, J.O., Lang, B., Lo, M. & Shorr, R.G. (1979) Application of specifically acting toxins to the detection of functional components common to peripheral and central synapses. In *Advance in Cytopharmacology*, Eds B. Ceccarelli & F. Clementi, Vol. 3, p. 409 (Raven Press: New York).

Barnard, E.A., Dolly, J.O., Porter, C.W. & Albuquerque, E.X. (1975) The acetylcholine receptor and the ionic conductance modulation system of skeletal muscle. *Experimental Neurology*, **48**, 1.

Barnard, E.A., Wieckowski, J. & Chiu, T.H. (1971) Cholinergic receptor molecules and cholinesterase molecules at mouse skeletal muscle junction. *Nature*, **234**, 207.

Bender, A.N., Ringel, S.P., Engel, W.K., Vogel, Z. & Daniels, M.P. (1976) Immunoperoxidase localisation of alpha bungarotoxin: a new approach to myasthenia gravis. *Annals of the New York Academy of Sciences*, **274**, 20.

Ben-Haim, D., Dreyer, F. & Peper, K. (1975) Acetylcholine receptor: modification of synaptic gating mechanism after treatment with a disulfide bond reducing agent. *Pflügers Archiv für die Gesamte Physiologie*, **355**, 19.

Bevan, S., Grampp, W. & Miledi, R. (1976) Properties of spontaneous potentials at denervated motor end-plates of the frog. *Proceedings of the Royal Society, Series B*, **194**, 195.

Birks, R., Katz, B. & Miledi, R. (1959) Electron-microscopic observations on degenerating nerve-muscle junctions of the frog. *Journal of Physiology*, **146**, 45P.

Birks, R., Katz, B. & Miledi, R. (1960) Physiological and structural changes at the amphibian myoneural junction, in the course of nerve degeneration. *Journal of Physiology*, **150**, 145.

Birks, R.I. & MacIntosh, F.C. (1957) Acetylcholine metabolism at nerve endings. *British Medical Bulletin*, **13**, 157.

Bovet, D. & Bovet-Nitti, F. (1955) Succinylcholine chloride, curarising agent of short duration of action. Pharmaco-dynamic activity and clinical application. *Scientia medica Italica*, **3**, 484.

Boyd, I.A. & Martin, A.R. (1956) The end-plate potential in mammalian muscle. *Journal of Physiology*, **132**, 74.

Brockes, J.P. & Hall, Z.W. (1975) Acetylcholine receptors in normal and denervated rat diaphragm muscle. II. Comparison of junctional and extrajunctional receptors. *Biochemistry*, **14**, 2100.

Brooks, V.B. (1954) The action of botulinum toxin on motor-nerve filaments. *Journal of Physiology*, **123**, 501.

Brown, G.L. (1937) The actions of acetylcholine on denervated mammalian and frog's muscle. *Journal of Physiology*, **89**, 438.

Brown, G.L., Dale, H.H. & Feldberg, W. (1936) Reactions of the normal mammalian muscle to acetylcholine and to eserine. *Journal of Physiology*, **87**, 394.

Burns, B.D. & Paton, W.D.M. (1951) Depolarisation of the motor end-plate by decamethonium and acetylcholine. *Journal of Physiology*, **115**, 41.

Cannard, T.H. & Zaimis, E. (1959) The effect of lowered muscle temperature on the action of neuromuscular blocking drugs in man. *Journal of Physiology*, **149**, 112.

Changeux, J.-P. (1975) The cholinergic receptor protein from fish electric organ. In *Handbook of Psychopharmaco-logy*, Eds L.L. Iversen, S.D. Iversen & S.H. Snyder, Vol. 6, p. 235 (Plenum: New York).

Colquhoun, D., Dionne, V.E., Steinbach, J.H. & Stevens, C.F. (1975) Conductance of channels opened by acetyl-choline-like drugs in muscle end-plate. *Nature* **253**, 204.

Colquhoun, D., Dreyer, F. & Sheridan, R.E. (1979) The actions of tubocurarine at the frog neuromuscular junction. *Journal of Physiology*, **293**, 247.

Colquhoun, D., Large, W.A. & Rang, H.P. (1977) An analysis of the action of a false transmitter at the neuro-muscular junction. *Journal of Physiology*, **266**, 361.

Couteaux, R. (1955) Localisation of cholinesterases at neuro-muscular junctions. *International Review of Cytology*, **4**, 335.

Couteaux, R. (1960) Motor end-plate structure. In *Structure and Function of Muscle*, Ed. G.H. Bourne, Vol. 1, p. 337 (Academic Press: New York & London).

Couteaux, R. & Pécot-Dechavassine, M. (1968) Particularités structurales du sarcoplasme sous-neural. *Comptes rendus hebdomadaires des séances de l'Académie des sciences*, **266**, 8.

Couteaux, R. & Pécot-Dechavassine, M. (1970) Vésicules synaptiques et poche au niveau des 'zones actives' de la jonction neuromusculaire. *Comptes rendus hebdomadaires des séances de l'Académie des sciences*, **271**, 2346.

Creese, R. & Maclagan, J. (1972) Uptake of ^{3}H-deca-methonium in cat muscle fibres. *V. International Congress* on Pharmacology, San Francisco, p. 864.

Cull-Candy, S.G., Miledi, R. & Trautmann, A. (1979) End-plate currents and acetylcholine noise at normal and myasthenic human end-plates. Journal of Physiology, **287**, 247.

Dale, H.H. & Feldberg, W. (1934) Chemical transmission at motor nerve endings in voluntary muscle. Journal of Physiology, **81**, 39P.

Dale, H.H., Feldberg, W. & Vogt, M. (1936) Release of acetylcholine at voluntary motor nerve endings. Journal of Physiology, **86**, 353.

Dean, R.B. (1941) Theories of electrolyte equilibrium in muscle. Biological Symposia, **3**, 331.

Del Castillo, J. & Katz, B. (1954) The failure of local-circuit transmission at the nerve-muscle junction. Journal of Physiology, **123**, 7.

Del Castillo, J. & Katz, B. (1955) On the localisation of acetylcholine receptors. Journal of Physiology, **128**, 157.

Del Castillo, J. & Katz, B. (1956) Biophysical aspects of neuro-muscular transmission. Progress in Biophysics and Biophysical Chemistry, **6**, 121.

Del Castillo, J. & Stark, L. (1952) The effect of calcium ions on the motor end-plate potential. Journal of Physiology, **116**, 507.

Dennis, M.J. & Miledi, R. (1974) Electrically induced release of acetylcholine from denervated Schwann cells. Journal of Physiology, **237**, 431.

Dolly, J.O. & Barnard, E.A. (1974) Affinity of cholinergic ligands for the partially purified acetylcholine receptor from mammalian skeletal muscle. FEBS Letters, **46**, 145.

Dolly, J.O. & Barnard, E.A. (1977) Purification and characterisation of an acetylcholine receptor from mammalian skeletal muscle. Biochemistry, **16**, 5053.

Douglas, W.W. & Paton, W.D.M. (1954) The mechanisms of motor end-plate depolarisation due to a cholinesterase-inhibiting drug. Journal of Physiology, **124**, 325.

Dreyer, F., Muller, K.-D., Peper, K. & Sterz, R. (1976) The M. omohyoideus of the mouse as a convenient mammalian muscle preparation. Pflügers Archiv für die gesamte Physiologie des Menschen und der Tiere, **367**, 115.

Dreyer, F., Walther, Chr. & Peper, K. (1976) Junctional and extrajunctional acetylcholine receptors in normal and denervated frog muscle fibres: noise analysis experiments with different agonists. Pflügers Archiv für die gesamte Physiologie des Menschen und der Tiere, **366**, 1.

Eccles, J.C., Katz, B. & Kuffler, S.W. (1941) Nature of the 'end-plate potential' in curarised muscle. Journal of Neuro-physiology, **4**, 362.

Eldefrawi, M.E. & Eldefrawi, A.T. (1977) Acetylcholine receptors. In Receptors and Recognition, Series A, Eds P. Cuatrecases & M.F. Greaves, Vol. 4, p. 197 (Chapman and Hall: London).

Elmqvist, D. & Thesleff, S. (1962) Ideas regarding receptor desensitisation at the motor end-plate. Revue canadienne de biologie, **21**, 229.

Engel, A.G., Lindstrom, J.M., Lambert, E.H. & Lennon, V.A. (1977) Ultrastructural localisation of the acetylcholine receptor in myasthenia gravis and in its experimental autoimmune model. Neurology (Minneapolis), **27**, 307.

Fatt, P. (1950) Electromotive action of acetylcholine at the motor end-plate. Journal of Physiology, **111**, 408.

Fatt, P. & Katz, B. (1952) Spontaneous subthreshold activity at motor nerve endings. Journal of Physiology, **117**, 109.

Feltz, A., Large, W.A. & Trautmann, A. (1977) Analysis of atropine action at the frog neuromuscular junction. Journal

of Physiology, **269**, 109.

Gage, P.W. (1976) Generation of end plate potentials. Physiological Reviews, **56**, 177.

Ginsborg, B.L. & Jenkinson, D.H. (1976) Transmission of impulses from nerve to muscle. In Handbook of Experimental Pharmacology, XLII, Neuromuscular Junction, Ed. E. Zaimis, p. 229 (Springer-Verlag: Berlin).

Göpfert, H. & Schaefer, H. (1938) Uber den direkt und indirekt erregten Aktionsstrom und die Funktion der motorischen Endplatte. Pflügers Archiv für die gesamte Physiologie des Menschen und der Tiere, **239**, 597.

Heidmann, T. & Changeux, J.-P. (1978) Structural and functional properties of the acetylcholine receptor protein in its purified and membrane-bound states. Annual Review of Biochemistry, **47**, 317.

Heuser, J.E. & Reese, T.S. (1973) Evidence for recycling of synaptic vesicle membrane during transmitter release at the frog neuromuscular junction. Journal of Cell Biology, **57**, 315.

Heuser, J.E., Reese, T.S. & Landis, D.M.D. (1974) Functional changes in frog neuromuscular junctions studied with freeze-fracture. Journal of Neurocytology, **3**, 109.

Hodgkin, A.L. (1958) Ionic movements and electrical activity in giant nerve fibres. Proceedings of the Royal Society, Series B, **148**, 1.

Hodgkin, A.L. & Keynes, R.D. (1957) Movements of labelled calcium in squid giant axons. Journal of Physiology, **138**, 253.

Hoffman, J.F. (1961) Molecular mechanism of active cation transport. In Biophysics of Physiological and Pharmacological Actions, Ed. A.M. Shanes, p. 3 (American Association for the Advancement of Science: Washington).

Hubbard, J.I. (1961) The effect of calcium and magnesium on the spontaneous release of transmitter from mammalian motor nerve endings. Journal of Physiology, **159**, 507.

Hubbard, J.I. (1973) Microphysiology of vertebrate neuro-muscular transmission. Physiological Reviews, **53**, 674.

Hubbard, J.I. & Kwanbunbumpen, S. (1968) Evidence for the vesicle hypothesis. Journal of Physiology, **194**, 407.

Ito, Y. & Miledi, R. (1977) The effect of calcium-ionophores on acetylcholine release from Schwann cells. Proceedings of the Royal Society, Series B, **196**, 51.

Ito, Y., Miledi, R., Vincent, A. & Newsom Davis, J. (1978) Acetylcholine receptors and end-plate electrophysiology in myasthenia gravis. Brain, **101**, 345.

Kasai, M. & Changeux, J.-P. (1971) In vitro excitation of purified membrane fragments by cholinergic agonists. II. The permeability change caused by cholinergic agonists. Journal of Membrane Biology, **6**, 24.

Katz, B. (1958) Microphysiology of the neuromuscular junction. A physiological 'quantum of action' at the myoneural junction. Bulletin of the Johns Hopkins Hospital, **102**, 275.

Katz, B. (1969) The Release of Neural Transmitter Substances (University Press: Liverpool).

Katz, B. (1971) Current views on the mechanism of quantal transmitter release. Proceedings of the International Union of Physiological Sciences, **8**, 246.

Katz, B. (1977) Prologue. In Synapses, Eds G.A. Cottrell & P.N.R. Usherwood, p. 1 (Blackie: Glasgow & London).

Katz, B. & Miledi, R. (1959) Spontaneous subthreshold activity at denervated amphibian end-plates. Journal of Physiology, **146**, 44P.

Katz, B. & Miledi, R. (1967) The timing of calcium action

during neuromuscular transmission. *Journal of Physiology*, **189**, 535.

Katz, B. & Miledi, R. (1971) Further observations on acetylcholine noise. *Nature*, **232**, 124.

Katz, B. & Miledi, R. (1972) The statistical nature of the acetylcholine potential and its molecular components. *Journal of Physiology*, **224**, 665.

Katz, B. & Miledi, R. (1973a) The binding of acetylcholine to receptors and its removal from the synaptic cleft. *Journal of Physiology*, **231**, 549.

Katz, B. & Miledi, R. (1973b) The effect of atropine on acetylcholine action at the neuromuscular junction. *Proceedings of the Royal Society, Series B*, **184**, 221.

Katz, B. & Miledi, R. (1973c) The characteristics of 'end-plate noise' produced by different depolarising drugs. *Journal of Physiology*, **230**, 707.

Katz, B. & Miledi, R. (1975) The effect of procaine on the action of acetylcholine at the neuromuscular junction. *Journal of Physiology*, **249**, 269.

Katz, B. & Miledi, R. (1976) The analysis of end-plate noise—a new approach to the study of acetylcholine/receptor interaction. In *Motor Innervation of Muscle*, Ed. S. Thesleff, p. 31 (Academic Press: London & New York).

Katz, B. & Miledi, R. (1978) A re-examination of curare action at the motor end-plate. *Proceedings of the Royal Society, Series B*, **203**, 119.

Katz, B. & Thesleff, S. (1957) A study of the 'desensitisation' produced by acetylcholine at the motor end-plate. *Journal of Physiology*, **138**, 63.

Koelle, G.B. (1951) The elimination of enzymatic diffusion artifacts in the histochemical localisation of cholinesterases and a survey of their cellular distributions. *Journal of Pharmacology and Experimental Therapeutics*, **103**, 153.

Koelle, G.B. & Friedenwald, J.S. (1949) A histochemical method for localising cholinesterase activity. *Proceedings of the Society for Experimental Biology and Medicine*, **70**, 617.

Krause, W. (1863) Über die Endigung der Muskelnerven. *Zeitschrift für Rationelle Medicin*, **18**, 136.

Krnjević, K. & Miledi, R. (1958) Acetylcholine in mammalian neuromuscular transmission. *Nature*, **182**, 805.

Krnjević, K. & Mitchell, J.F. (1961) The release of acetylcholine in the isolated diaphragm. *Journal of Physiology*, **155**, 246.

Kuffler, S.W. (1943) Specific excitability of the end-plate region in normal and denervated muscle. *Journal of Neurophysiology*, **6**, 99.

Kuffler, S.W. & Yoshikami, D. (1975) The number of transmitter molecules in a quantum: an estimate from iontophoretic application of acetylcholine at the neuromuscular synapse. *Journal of Physiology*, **251**, 465.

Langley, J.N. (1906) On nerve endings and on special excitable substances in cells. *Proceedings of the Royal Society, Series B*, **78**, 170.

Lee, C.Y. (1972) Chemistry and pharmacology of polypeptide toxins in snake venoms. *Annual Review of Pharmacology*, **12**, 265.

MacIntosh, F.C. (1959) Formation, storage and release of acetylcholine at nerve endings. *Canadian Journal of Biochemistry and Physiology*, **37**, 343.

MacIntosh, F.C., Birks, R.I. & Sastry, P.B. (1956) Pharmacological inhibition of acetylcholine synthesis. *Nature*, **178**, 1181.

MacIntosh, F.C. & Collier, B. (1976) Neurochemistry of cholinergic terminals. In *Handbook of Experimental Pharmacology, XLII, Neuromuscular Junction*, Ed. E. Zaimis, p. 99 (Springer-Verlag: Berlin).

Maclagan, J. (1962) A comparison of the responses of the tenuissimus muscle to neuromuscular blocking drugs *in vivo* and *in vitro*. *British Journal of Pharmacology*, **18**, 204.

Magazanik, L.G. & Vyskočil, F. (1973) Desensitisation at the motor end-plate. In *Drug Receptors*, Ed. H.P. Rang, p. 105 (Macmillan: London).

Marchbanks, R.M. (1977) Turnover and release of acetylcholine. In *Synapses*, Eds G.A. Cottrell & P.N.R. Usherwood, p. 81 (Blackie: Glasgow & London).

Michelson, M.J. & Zeimal, E.V. (1973) *Acetylcholine—An Approach to the Molecular Mechanism of Action* (Pergamon Press: Oxford).

Miledi, R. (1960a) Properties of regenerating neuromuscular synapses in the frog. *Journal of Physiology*, **145**, 190.

Miledi, R. (1960b) Junctional and extra-junctional acetylcholine receptors in skeletal muscle fibres. *Journal of Physiology*, **151**, 24.

Miledi, R. (1960c) The acetylcholine sensitivity of frog muscle fibres after complete or partial denervation. *Journal of Physiology*, **151**, 1.

Miledi, R. (1973) Transmitter release induced by injection of calcium ions into nerve terminals. *Proceedings of the Royal Society, Series B*, **183**, 421.

Miledi, R. & Slater, C.R. (1968) Electrophysiology and electron-microscopy of rat neuromuscular junctions after nerve degeneration. *Proceedings of the Royal Society, Series B*, **169**, 289.

Nastuk, W.L., Manthey, A.A. & Gissen, A.J. (1966) Activation and inactivation of postjunctional membrane receptors. *Annals of the New York Academy of Sciences*, **137**, 999.

Neher, E. & Sakmann, B. (1976a) Noise analysis of drug induced voltage clamp currents in denervated frog muscle fibres. *Journal of Physiology*, **258**, 705.

Neher, E. & Sakmann, B. (1976b) Single-channel currents recorded from membrane of denervated frog muscle fibres. *Nature*, **260**, 799.

Neher, E. & Steinbach, J.H. (1978) Local anaesthetics transiently block currents through single acetylcholine-receptor channels. *Journal of Physiology*, **277**, 153.

Osborne, M.P. (1977) Role of vesicles with some observations on vertebrate sensory cells. In *Synapses*, Eds G.A. Cottrell & P.N.R. Usherwood, p. 40 (Blackie: Glasgow & London).

Palade, G.E. (1954) Electron microscope observations of interneuronal and neuromuscular synapses. *Anatomical Record*, **118**, 335.

Palay, S.L. (1954) Electron microscope study of the cytoplasm of neurons. *Anatomical Record*, **118**, 336.

Paton, W.D.M. & Waud, D.R. (1962) Drug-receptor interactions at the neuromuscular junction. In *Curare and Curare-like Agents*, Ed. A.V.S. De Reuck, Ciba Foundation Study Group No. 12, p. 34 (Churchill: London).

Paton, W.D.M. & Zaimis, E. (1948a) Curare-like action of polymethylene bis-quaternary ammonium salts. *Nature*, **161**, 718.

Paton, W.D.M. & Zaimis, E. (1948b) Clinical potentialities of certain bis-quaternary salts causing neuromuscular and ganglionic block. *Nature*, **162**, 810.

Paton, W.D.M. & Zaimis, E. (1949a) The properties of polymethylene bis-trimethylammonium salts. *Journal of*

Physiology, **108**, 55P.

Paton, W.D.M. & Zaimis, E. (1949b) The pharmacological actions of polymethylene bis-trimethylammonium salts. *British Journal of Pharmacology*, **4**, 381.

Paton, W.D.M. & Zaimis, E. (1950) Actions and clinical assessment of drugs which produce neuromuscular block. *Lancet*, **2**, 568.

Paton, W.D.M. & Zaimis, E. (1951a) The action of d-tubocurarine and of decamethonium on respiratory and other muscles in the cat. *Journal of Physiology*, **112**, 311.

Paton, W.D.M. & Zaimis, E. (1951b) Paralysis of autonomic ganglia by methonium salts. *British Journal of Pharmacology*, **6**, 155.

Paton, W.D.M. & Zaimis, E. (1952) The methonium compounds. *Pharmacological Reviews*, **4**, 219.

Pelouze, T.J.P. & Bernard, C. (1850) Recherches sur le curare. *Comptes rendus hebdomadaires des séances de l'Académie des sciences*, **31**, 533.

Porter, C.W. & Barnard, E.A. (1975) The density of cholinergic receptors at the end-plate postsynaptic membrane: ultrastructural studies in two mammalian species. *Journal of Membrane Biology*, **20**, 31.

Porter, C.W. & Barnard, E.A. (1976) Ultrastructural studies on the acetylcholine receptor at motor end-plates of normal and pathologic muscles. *Annals of the New York Academy of Sciences*, **274**, 85.

Porter, C.W., Barnard, E.A. & Chiu, T.H. (1973) The ultra-structural localisation and quantitation of cholinergic receptors at the mouse end-plate. *Journal of Membrane Biology*, **14**, 383.

Rang, H.P. (1975) Acetylcholine receptors. *Quarterly Review of Biophysics*, **7**, 283.

Rice, S.O. (1944) Mathematical analysis of random noise. *Bell System Technical Journal*, **23**, 282.

Robertson, J.D. (1954) Electron microscope observations on a reptilian myoneural junction. *Anatomical Record*, **118**, 346.

Robertson, J.D. (1961) New unit membrane organelle of Schwann cells. In *Biophysics of Physiological and Pharmacological Actions*, Ed. A.M. Shanes, p. 63 (American Association for the Advancement of Science: Washington).

Rouget, M. (1862) Note sur la terminaison des nerfs moteurs dans les muscles chez reptiles, les oiseaux et les mammifères. *Comptes rendus hebdomadaires des séances de l'Académie des sciences*, **55**, 548.

Ruff, R.L. (1977) A quantitative analysis of local anaesthetic alteration of miniature end-plate currents and end-plate current fluctuations. *Journal of Physiology*, **264**, 89.

Schueler, F.W. (1955) A new group of respiratory paralyzants. I. The hemicholiniums. *Journal of Pharmacology and Experimental Therapeutics*, **115**, 127.

Shorr, R.G., Dolly, J.O. & Barnard, E.A. (1978) Composition of acetylcholine receptor protein from skeletal muscle. *Nature*, **274**, 283.

Straughan, D.W. (1960) The release of acetylcholine from mammalian motor nerve endings. *British Journal of Pharmacology*, **15**, 417.

Takeuchi, N. (1963a) Some properties of conductance changes at the end-plate membrane during the action of acetylcholine. *Journal of Physiology*, **167**, 128.

Takeuchi, N. (1963b) Effects of calcium on the conductance change at the end-plate membrane during the action of transmitter. *Journal of Physiology*, **167**, 141.

Tauc, L. (1977) Turnover and release of acetylcholine. In *Synapses*, Eds G.A. Cottrell & P.N.R. Usherwood, p. 64 (Blackie: Glasgow & London).

Thesleff, S. (1955a) Neuromuscular block caused by acetylcholine. *Nature*, **175**, 594.

Thesleff, S. (1955b) The mode of neuromuscular block caused by acetylcholine, nicotine, decamethonium and succinylcholine. *Acta physiologica scandinavica*, **34**, 218.

Thesleff, S. (1959) Interactions between neuromuscular blocking agents and acetylcholine at the mammalian motor end-plate. *Atti Congresso Societa Italiana di Anestesiologa*, p. 37.

Tuček, S. (1978) *Acetylcholine Synthesis in Neurones* (Chapman & Hall: London).

Wray, D. (1978a) End-plate voltage noise during prolonged application of acetylcholine in cat tenuissimus muscle. *Journal of Physiology*, **278**, 4P.

Wray, D. (1978b) Frequency of opening of channels by depolarising drugs. *Journal of Physiology*, **284**, 149P.

Wray, D. (1980a) Noise analysis and channels at the post-synaptic membrane of skeletal muscle. *Progress in Drug Research*, **24** (In press).

Wray, D. (1980b) Prolonged exposure to acetylcholine: noise analysis and channel inactivation in cat tenuissimus muscle. *Journal of Physiology* (In press).

Zaimis, E. (1950) The synthesis of methonium compounds, their isolation from urine and their photometric determination. *British Journal of Pharmacology*, **5**, 424.

Zaimis, E. (1951) The action of decamethonium on normal and denervated mammalian muscle. *Journal of Physiology*, **112**, 176.

Zaimis, E. (1953) Motor end-plate differences as a determining factor in the mode of action of neuromuscular blocking substances. *Journal of Physiology*, **122**, 238.

Zaimis, E. (1959) Mechanisms of neuromuscular blockade. In *Curare and Curare-like Agents*, Eds D. Bovet, F. Bovet-Nitti & G.S. Marini-Bettolo, p. 191 (Elsevier: Amsterdam).

Zaimis, E. (1962) Experimental hazards and artefacts in the study of neuromuscular blocking drugs. In *Curare and Curare-like Agents*, Ed. A.V.S. De Reuck, Ciba Foundation Study Group No. 12, p. 75 (Churchill: London).

Zaimis, E. & Head, S. (1976) Depolarising neuromuscular blocking drugs. In *Handbook of Experimental Pharmacology, XLII, Neuromuscular Junction*, Ed. E. Zaimis, p. 365 (Springer-Verlag: Berlin).

Biochemical aspects of muscular structure and function

INTRODUCTION*

In order to write a chapter on the biochemistry of muscle one really ought to write a textbook of biochemistry, because muscle has so many features in common with the biochemistry of any other tissue in the organism. A certain selection is, therefore, necessary and this article will deal with those biochemical processes in muscle that have a more or less close relationship with the contraction of muscle. In few other tissues is the relationship between structure and biochemistry as close as it is in muscle, for the ultimate aim of the processes, biochemical, biophysical or physiological, in muscle is to induce a structural change resulting in

contraction or its reversal, relaxation.

Throughout this article, therefore, close attention will be paid to the relationships between structure and function, particularly as this is manifested in the localisation of various biochemical constituents in relation to the morphological elements of muscle.

As proteins constitute 75–80 per cent of the dry weight of muscle, a good starting point might be a brief discussion of proteins in general, and their role as enzymes in particular. This will be followed by a discussion of metabolic processes in muscle, and a survey of the myofibrillar proteins will lead to problems of contraction and relaxation.

PROTEINS AND ENZYMES†

General

Proteins consist of one or more polypeptide chains, which in turn are made up of amino acids linked together by peptide bonds. Additional linkages within, or between, the polypeptide chains may involve disulphide (–S–S–) crossbridges, as for example in insulin (Sanger, 1956) or ribonuclease (Hirs, Moore and Stein, 1960). If a protein consists of more than one chain (or sub-unit) these may have been synthesised originally as separate entities (myosin, discussed below, is an example) or may have come into being by proteolytic scission of an originally single chain

*Readers interested in obtaining more information on topics covered in this chapter and on related matters may wish to consult the following chapters: Gergely, 1976; Mannherz and Goody, 1976; Perry, 1979; Squire, 1975; Tada, Yamamoto and Tonomura, 1978; Taylor, 1979; Tonomura and Inoue, 1975; and Trentham, Eccleston and Bagshaw, 1976.

†A number of recent texts and monographs can be consulted for further background. Among them are Lehninger, A.L., *Biochemistry*, 2nd edition, New York: Worth, 1975; Stryer, L., *Biochemistry*, San Francisco: Freeman, 1975; Metzler, D.E., *Biochemistry. The Chemical Reactions of Living Cells*, New York: Academic Press, 1977; Fersht, A., *Enzyme Structure and Mechanism*, Reading: W.H. Freeman, 1977.

(as in insulin (Steiner, 1969)). The linear sequence of the amino acids is referred to as the primary structure, and this is now readily determined for most known proteins. The pioneering work of Sanger (1952) and Moore and Stein (1951, 1954) was rapidly followed up; and the introduction of rapid analytical (Spackman, 1967) and sequencing (Edman and Begg, 1967) methods made progress during the past 10 years even more rapid.

Three-dimensional structure

Broadly speaking, proteins can be classified into two groups, globular and fibrous, those belonging to the former having shapes rather close to spherical, those to the latter having a high length-to-width (axial) ratio. The three-dimensional structure of proteins is determined by the way the polypeptide chains are folded. This is referred to as secondary and tertiary structure. Secondary structure is defined by the regulation in the relationship of neighbouring amino acid residues, while the overall shape of the chain, including bends and turns, reflects the tertiary structure stabilised by interactions among residues at some distance within the chain. In proteins that consist of more than one chain the interaction of these sub-units determines the quaternary structure.

One of the most important secondary structures is the α helix (Pauling, Corey and Bronson, 1951); in this case the polypeptide coils up so that there are 3.6 residues per turn, and hydrogen bonds are formed between $-C=O$ and $HN-$ groups on residues n and $n+4$, respectively.

In the case of β structures the polypeptide chains are extended and hydrogen bonds are formed between neighbouring β structures, running either in parallel or antiparallel direction, resulting in pleated β sheets. An important feature in protein structure is the reverse turn (sometimes called β turn) permitting the peptide chain to change direction.

The relative amounts of α-helical and β structures and of structures that lack readily perceived regularity* differ from protein to protein. The

---

*These structures are sometimes called random coil structures; this, however, is misleading because they lack the mobility of true randomly coiled polymers. 'Disordered structure' may be more appropriate.

packing of these structural elements into the complete structure is determined by the interaction of the sidechains on α-helical or β structures. As X-ray studies on protein crystals based on the pioneering work by Kendrew (1963) and Perutz (1963) produce more and more accurate pictures of the detailed structure of functionally important proteins, helpful schemes emerge for classifying proteins in terms of the interactions of the recognisable structural units (see e.g. Levitt and Clothia, 1976).

X-ray data are supplemented by studies of proteins in solution to determine their size and shape, and also to establish relationships between chemical and physical structure. This is helpful when X-ray data are not available. One of the most important physiochemical tools is optical rotatory dispersion and circular dichroism (see Fasman, 1967). Certain relationships have been noted from an early stage. Thus there seems to be a good inverse relationship between the content of proline—one of the amino acids—and the α-helical content of proteins (Cohen and Szent-Györgyi, 1957). Methods to establish more extensive correlations between amino acid sequence and α-helicity, disordered and β structure (e.g. Schiffer and Edmundson, 1967, 1968; Nagano, 1973; Wu and Kabat, 1973) have been refined and efforts are still continuing (Chou and Fasman, 1978). It should be noted that the structure of proteins allows for considerable motion within a polypeptide chain and in the relative position of interacting chains. The importance of such flexibility will be discussed below in relation to myosin and actin–myosin interaction.

Enzymes

Definition. Proteins provide the structural framework of cells and, as we shall see, the working elements of muscle; myofibrils are, according to our present knowledge, made up entirely of proteins. Another important role of proteins is to act as enzymes: that is, they are regulators of the rate at which metabolic processes take place in the cells. A protein which has an enzymatic function possesses a certain area—the so-called active site—which has a definite relationship in its chemical nature to the compounds whose reaction it is supposed to regulate, this regulation occurring through the formation of the so-called enzyme substrate complex. In some cases a covalent bond is formed between a group on the enzyme and the substrate or an intermediate. An instructive example of correlating detailed structural and functional information with a view to explaining enzyme action is found in the review article of Quicho and Lipscomb (1971). Another interesting enzyme is myosin, one of the proteins of the myofibrils to be discussed below, which is both an enzyme and a structural element.

Coenzymes, metals. The enzymatic function of the proteins is often intimately linked to the presence of other substances of smaller molecular weight, known as coenzymes; metal ions also play an important part in many of the enzymatic reactions. Coenzymes, as a rule, are derivatives of the vitamins, as was clearly shown by Peters and his colleagues for vitamin B_1 in relation to pyruvate metabolism (Peters, 1936). The co-enzyme role of most vitamins is clear, although the precise function of vitamin C and vitamin E has not yet been clarified.

Specific examples of enzyme-ion–coenzyme interactions will be given below in connection with a discussion of various metabolic reactions. It is well to remember that, in view of the important part that vitamins and inorganic ions, all constituents of the diet, play in biochemical reactions, nutritional deficiencies can clearly lead to extremely complex biochemical lesions and hence to disorders of function.

Regulation of enzyme activity. This concept has become of great interest during the past 15 years or so, as more and more reactions have been discovered in which the concentration of specific metabolites exerts a profound effect on the rate of the reaction (Atkinson, 1966; Newsholme and Start, 1973). The simplest type of regulation is that created by the substrate concentration, usually discussed in the framework of Michaelis-Menten kinetics. Similarly, one may consider competitive inhibition by the product of the reaction.

Another type of regulatory effect depends on the combination of a small molecule—called effector, modifier or moderator—with the enzyme, which changes its catalytic activity toward the substrate. The word 'allosteric' has been used to indicate separate interaction sites for modifier and substrate or product (Monod, Changeux and Jacob, 1963). In many cases multi-subunit enzymes are involved. Yet another type of regulation can be described as biosynthetic, in which the products of a reaction affect the biosynthesis of the enzyme catalysing the reaction, or even that of another enzyme involved in a reaction further removed in the metabolic chain. Among these the phosphorylation of enzymes by protein kinases, some of which require cyclic AMP for activity, has emerged as being of prime importance. Various instances of this type of regulation are relevant to muscle metabolism and contraction and will be discussed in more detail later in this Chapter. It now appears that hormones often act through a pathway involving cyclic AMP, which in this context has been termed *second messenger*. Another messenger that appears to have an almost ubiquitous role is the calcium ion. Numerous examples have been reviewed by Atkinson (1966) and Holtzer and Duntze (1971), and more recently by Krebs and Beavo (1979); for a novel aspect of regulation *see* Frieden (1979).

ENERGY METABOLISM

Carbohydrate metabolism

General. Glucose entering the muscle cell is stored in the form of glycogen which is broken down according to the energy requirements of the muscle. the breakdown may occur, depending on the conditions, either essentially anaerobically—that is, without oxygen—going as far as lactic acid, or it may continue with the participation of oxygen to complete the breakdown to CO_2 and water. In muscles where sudden demands on energy may arise, the anaerobic pathway is predominant and the lactic acid formed is carried by the blood stream to the liver where it is partly oxidised, partly resynthesised to glycogen (Cori, 1941). In other muscles, such as cardiac muscle, where there is a slower but steady activity the complete oxidative breakdown plays a greater part.

Differences between enzyme patterns of the so-called red and white muscles have also been noted. The difference in colour does not always correspond to differences in the myoglobin content, but it appears that the red fibres contain more mitochondria, and hence oxidative enzymes (Slater, 1960), while the white ones have a higher phosphorylase content (Dubowitz and Pearse, 1960). Many detailed studies have been carried out in recent years on other enzymatic differences among various muscle types. Most muscles are fairly heterogeneous with respect to red and white fibres and thus one can speak of red and white muscles in a more or less statistical sense (Stein and Padykula, 1962). Physiologically, most red muscles are characterised by a slower but more prolonged contraction in comparison with the faster, pale or white ones (Ranvier, 1874). For more details on muscle and fibre types see Chapters 2 and 8.

Anaerobic pathway. Figure 4.1 shows the reactions involved in carbohydrate metabolism in the absence of oxygen. Under these conditions the end product is lactic acid, the compound that, before the discovery of the role of the high-energy phosphates such as ATP, was considered to be the key substance in muscle contraction. A detailed description of all the steps in this evidently complex scheme would be beyond the scope of this article, but a few important points may be singled out for discussion.

Glycogen metabolism. As pointed out above, enzymes regulate the metabolism by increasing the rate of chemical reactions. In case a chemical reaction is reversible—that is, it can proceed either

Fig. 4.1 Pathway of anaerobic glycolysis in muscle. For details *see* Chapter 16 in Lehninger, *Biochemistry*, New York: Worth, 2nd edition, 1975

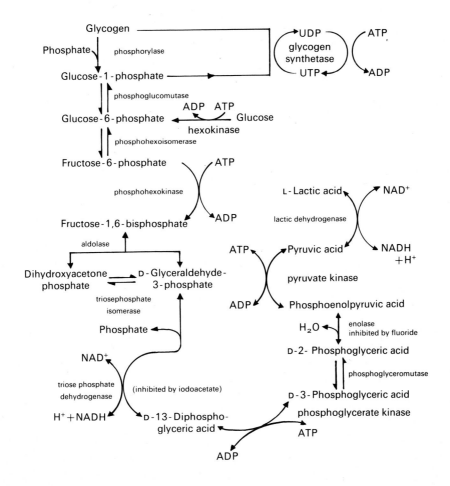

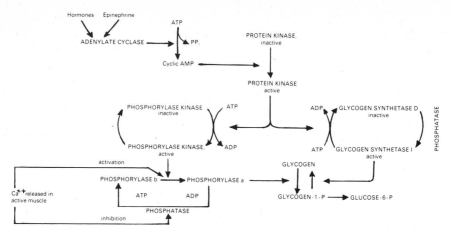

Fig. 4.2 Regulation of glycogen phosphorylase and synthetase system. For details *see* text

from the left to the right or the right to the left (e.g. A + B⇌C + D)—enzymes accelerate both rates and the direction of the reaction would be determined by the availability of the compounds that react. Thus, if those on the left-hand side of the equation are in abundance, the reaction will proceed to the right—if those on the right, the reaction will proceed to the left. It has been rather puzzling that muscle, under similar chemical conditions, can either build up glycogen or break it down. Changes in the activity of a single enzyme under these conditions would affect both pathways equally, and hence would not produce a net change in the amount of glycogen. During recent years it has become clear that in this case two different enzyme systems are involved, one used for the building up of the glycogen store and another for its breakdown (Fig. 4.2). The breakdown of glycogen involves the enzyme phosphorylase, the reaction being:

Glycogen + phosphate → glucose-1-phosphate

Phosphorylase is itself a complicated enzyme system whose structure, function and regulation have been clarified through extensive research taking its origin in the work of the Coris (Cori and Cori, 1945). As it now appears (*see* e.g. Fischer, Heilmeyer and Haschke, 1971; Krebs, 1972) phosphorylase can exist in an inactive form, phosphorylase *b*, and an active form, phosphorylase *a*. The *b*→*a* transformation is effected by ATP-dependent phosphorylation catalysed by

phosphorylase kinase, while the reconversion of phosphorylase *a* to *b* is catalysed by phosphorylase phosphatase. Phosphorylase kinase contains four different kinds of sub-units, one of which has recently been identified (Cohen, Burehall, Foulkes, Cohen, Vanaman and Nairn, 1978) with the ubiquitous Ca^{++}-binding protein, calmodulin, first discovered in brain homogenate (Cheung, 1971). This subunit is presumably the site of binding of the activating Ca^{++}. Phosphorylase kinase also exists in an active and an inactive form, and again inactivation is brought about by phosphorylation, catalysed in this case by a cyclic AMP dependent protein kinase. The production from ATP of cyclic AMP—now recognised as a key mediator in many regulatory processes (*see* e.g. Robinson, Butcher and Sutherland, 1971; Bitensky and Gorman, 1973)—is catalysed by an enzyme, adenyl cyclase, which is under the influence of hormones (glucagon) and neurohumoral agents (e.g. epinephrine). The regulation of the phosphorylase system also involves phosphatase inhibitors which are subject to control by a cAMP-dependent kinase (Cohen, 1978).

It has long been known that stimulation, and hence muscle activity itself, brings about activation of phosphorylase and in fatigued muscle the enzyme is again inactive (Cori, 1956). It should be pointed out that the problem of fatigue is a complex one; it can be due to neuromuscular factors, to accumulation of lactic acid, or the depletion of fuel stores (Christensen, 1960;

Edholm, 1960). Differences in the fatigability of various fibre types have recently been discussed (Burke, Levine, Tsairis and Zajac, 1973).

The conversion of glucose into glycogen depends on a distinct enzyme system—glycogen synthetase—involving UTP and the coenzyme uridine diphosphate glucose (UDPG) (Leloir and Cardini, 1962). Glycogen synthetase is another enzyme that exists in two interconvertible forms of differing activity, D and I. The D form is inhibited by physiological concentration of ATP and (Friedman and Larner, 1963) results from the phosphorylation of the I form by the same cyclic AMP dependent protein kinase that is involved in the regulation of the phosphorylase system (see Krebs, 1972). The D form depends on glucose-6-phosphate for activity and—in contrast to the I form—is inactive under physiological conditions, but may become active as glucose-6-P accumulates. The conversion of the inactive phosphorylated form to the active form is catalysed by phosphatases; these in turn are regulated by inhibitors (not shown in Fig. 4.2) which themselves are subject to control by cyclic AMP dependent kinase (Cohen, 1978; Krebs and Beavo, 1979).

Stimulation of muscle produces an increase in vivo of phosphorylase a relative to phosphorylase b. Similar changes can be produced by epinephrine, which also produces increased levels of cyclic AMP. An important factor in the regulation of the phosphorylase system is Ca^{++}. Ca^{++} ions, in the concentration required for activation of the actomyosin system (see below) also activate phosphorylase kinase (Oszwa, Hosoi and Ebashi, 1967; Heilmeyer, Meyer, Haschke and Fischer, 1970). Thus stimulation of phosphorylase activity via the cyclic AMP dependent phosphorylation reaction is coupled to inhibition of glycogen synthetase and vice versa. Insulin, which has long been known to promote glycogen storage, enhances glucose transport across the cell membrane (Park, Bornstein and Post, 1955) and also affects the activity of glycogen synthetase (Shen, Villar-Palasi and Larner, 1970). It now seems well established that insulin reacts with a specific binding site in the membrane (Cuatrecasas, 1972). In vivo the phosphorylase system occurs as a glycogen complex and many regulatory features are affected by this interaction (Haschke, Heilmeyer, Meyer and Fischer, 1970; Heilmeyer et al., 1970; Meyer, Heilmeyer, Haschke and Fischer, 1970).

The above discussion of the synthesis and breakdown of glycogen is somewhat simplified. Actually, both processes are catalysed by additional enzymes, corresponding to the fact that glycogen is a branched structure of glucose chains, and the making or splitting of a glucose-glucose bond, or glycosidic bonds, requires different enzymes depending on the position of the glycosidic bond. A genetically determined lack of any one of these enzymes leads to various disorders of carbohydrate metabolism discussed elsewhere in this book.

Fructose phosphokinase (phosphohexokinase). This enzyme, which catalyses the phosphorylation of fructose-6-phosphate before its breakdown into two trioses, plays a key role in the regulation of the glycolytic process (see e.g. Mansour, 1972) in that, as was first shown by Cori (1942) in muscle, the rate-limiting step in the reaction glycogen → lactic acid is that catalysed by phosphofructokinase. The binding to the enzyme of various modifiers, the concentration of which varies with rest or activity, regulates its activity. Thus, ATP is not only a substrate of fructose phosphokinase but, at higher concentrations, an inhibitor. This effect is relieved by inorganic phosphate. Thus, at high ATP levels the activity of the enzyme is shut off, while muscle activity leading to liberation of inorganic phosphate releases the flow of energy. Among other modifiers of the enzyme to be found are 3'-5' (cyclic)AMP, 5'-AMP, citrate, glucose-6-P and β-glycero-P; the control of the enzyme by some of these substances furnishes instances of allosteric effectors (Mansour, 1972; Pettigrew and Frieden, 1979). The precise way in which an increase in cyclic AMP elicited by epinephrine leads to an increased activity of the enzyme (see Mansour, 1972) has not been fully clarified.

ATP synthesis. The reaction involving glyceraldehyde-3-phosphate oxidation and NAD*

---

*NAD, nicotinamide adenine dinucleotide, is the name of the coenzyme related to the vitamin nicotinic acid; DPN, for diphosphopyridine nucleotide, is the earlier accepted name for it.

in the breakdown scheme of glycogen leads to the esterification of a phosphate residue; eventually it is transferred to adenosine diphosphate (ADP) to form adenosine triphosphate (ATP). The phosphate residue that participated in the phosphorolytic breakdown of glycogen also ends up as ATP, through the phosphoenolpyruvate-ADP reaction. Thus in the anaerobic breakdown of one glucose unit of glycogen there is a net formation of three molecules of ATP. If glucose were the starting material, only two moles of ATP would be formed from glucose because of the ATP requirement in the formation of glucose-1-phosphate via the hexokinase reaction.

Glyceraldehyde phosphate, as already mentioned, reduces NAD. Under anaerobic conditions the reduction of NAD has to be reversed through its reaction with pyruvic acid resulting in the formation of lactic acid and the reoxidised form of NAD. The glycolytic process, therefore, does not involve a net change in the state of oxidation or reduction.

Isoenzymes. Several enzymes have been found to exist in multiple forms, so-called isoenzymes. Among the earliest systems discovered is lactic dehydrogenase. It exists in various electrophoretically distinct forms, which apparently represent the aggregation of two types of units in five different combinations, the total number of subunits being four (Appela and Markert, 1961; Cahn, Kaplan, Levine and Swilling, 1962). One type is characteristic of cardiac, and slow skeletal, the other of fast skeletal muscle (Brand, Everse and Kaplan, 1962; Brody, 1968). Throughout embryonic development the cardiac form predominates in skeletal muscles, too. Among the biochemical changes accompanying the changes in physiological characteristics of a muscle on cross-innervation, that is interchanging the nerve of a fast muscle with that of a slow muscle (see below), is the shift in the ratio of the two kinds of lactic dehydrogenase sub-units (Mommaerts, Buller and Seraydarian, 1969). The change is more conspicuous in the fast → slow than in the slow → fast transformation. In certain forms of animal (Kaplan and Cahn, 1962) and human (Dreyfus, Demos, Schapira and Schapira, 1962; Wieme and Herpol, 1962; Brody, 1968) muscular dystrophies the cardiac form is predominant in skeletal muscle. It appears, however, that this change in pattern is more likely to be a response to muscle damage than a specific feature of dystrophy (Dawson and Kaplan, 1965). Myosin, the key structural enzymatic component of the myofibril also exists in isozymic forms (see below).

Aerobic metabolism. The anaerobic path of the breakdown of carbohydrates is linked to the oxidative pathway at the point of pyruvate. If there is oxidative breakdown of pyruvate the NADH formed in the reduction of glyceraldehyde phosphate cannot react with pyruvate, but will have to be oxidised too. Both the metabolism of pyruvate and the oxidation of NADH are catalysed by several enzyme complexes located in distinct structural elements or compartments in mitochondria.

Mitochondria. Recent years have seen considerable advances in our knowledge of the architecture of these elements. It should be noted that mitochondria are more numerous in the slow muscle fibres although some fast fibres too have a high mitochondrial control. Membranes consisting of lipoproteins play a major part in mitochondrial structure and function. There is an outer membrane separated by a gap from an inner membrane. There are a large number of protrusions from the inner membrane to the interior of the mitochondrion—the so-called cristae. The inner membrane encloses the matrix. Most of the enzymes of the mitochondrion are localised in these cristae. According to electron-microscopic observations, spherical particles appear to be attached to the cristae by thin stalks (Fernandez-Moran, 1962; Parsons, 1963). The precise relationship of these elementary particles to the various enzyme complexes (see below) has been the subject of very active research: for summaries of somewhat opposing views see, e.g. Green (1966) and Racker (1965). There is general agreement that the inner membranes contain the enzymes for electron transfer for oxygen and the machinery for phosphorylation of ADP to ATP.

According to current views, the structure of lipoprotein membranes involves protein molecules embedded in a semi-liquid lipid bilayer (see e.g. Bangham, 1972; Guidotti, 1972; Singer, 1972) forming a mosaic structure. Some of the proteins extend across the membrane, some are exposed to one on the other side and others are fully embedded and not accessible on either side. This model significantly deviates from the classical Davson-Danielli-Robertson model envisaging a laminar arrangement of protein-lipid-protein components. These concepts of membrane structure have an important bearing on other membrane systems and processes (see Active Transport and Sarcoplasmic Reticulum, below).

Krebs cycle. The enzymatically catalysed reaction sequence leading to the complete breakdown of pyruvic acid is known as the Krebs cycle or tricarboxylic acid cycle, the latter name taking its origin from the various organic acids containing three carboxyl groups that participate in the cycle. Pyruvate is oxidised to acetate, or rather a complex of acetate and a coenzyme so far not mentioned, coenzyme A (Lipmann, 1941), in which the acetyl residue becomes linked to an SH group. This is only one instance of the many reactions in which functionally important SH groups take part and they will recur again in the discussion of the contractile proteins. Acetyl-CoA interacts with a member of the Krebs cycle, oxaloacetic acid, to form citric acid.

The complex sequence of reactions following this condensation is outlined in Figure 4.3. In the course of these reactions both NAD and NADP★, another coenzyme, differing from NAD by the presence of an additional phosphate group, are reduced and the removal of two molecules of CO_2 and water results in the complete breakdown of the acetate residue that entered the cycle and in the regeneration of the oxaloacetic acid.

Terminal electron transport and oxidative phosphorylation. Coenzymes reduced in the operation of the citric acid cycle, as well as the NADH formed in the reactions leading from glucose to pyruvate, are finally reoxidised through a long chain of reactions catalysed by various enzymes

*NADP: nicotinamide adenine dinucleotide phosphate or, according to earlier nomenclature, triphosphopyridine nucleotide (TPN).

whose active groups are flavins and iron-containing compounds, the cytochromes. In addition, the participation of coenzyme Q, non-haem Fe and Cu has been shown (see Sanadi and Wohlrab, 1966). These enzymes form what is known as the respiratory chain and are localised in the mitochondria. They undergo cyclic reduction and reoxidation, with the formation of three ATPs for each pair of electrons. Succinate, one of the Krebs cycle intermediates, reacts directly with a flavoprotein; the rest of the electron flow is the same as when NAD participates.

The precise relationship between electron flow and the combination of inorganic phosphate with various acceptors and finally the re-phosphorylation of ADP is one of the most active fields of research. During recent years considerable progress has been made with the use of specific inhibitors to pinpoint the enzymatic reactions in which this phosphorylation takes place. Efforts directed at the identification of high-energy intermediates as phosphorylated compounds have so far been unsuccessful, and it is more generally accepted that the hypothetical energy-rich intermediates have to be replaced by H^+ concentration gradients whose energy would eventually be channelled into the formation of ATP from ADP and inorganic phosphate (Mitchell, 1977). The precise nature of the transformation of osmotic into chemical energy is still being debated. There are indications that the energy is required to release tightly bound ATP which would be spontaneously formed into P_i and ADP (Boyer, 1977). The energy derived from electron flow can also be used—instead of synthesising ATP—either to drive electrons backward or for the transport of various ions.

It is possible to separate electron flow from phosphorylation by means of various reagents, including various antibiotics. This is the so-called uncoupling of oxidation from phosphorylation. While in the normal process of oxidative phosphorylation roughly three phosphates are transformed into ATP for each oxygen atom used, uncouplers can actually increase the oxygen uptake but reduce phosphorylation practically to zero. If, as has been suggested for thyroxine (Hoch and Lipmann, 1954; Maley and Lardy, 1955), uncoupling can occur in certain pathological conditions, the

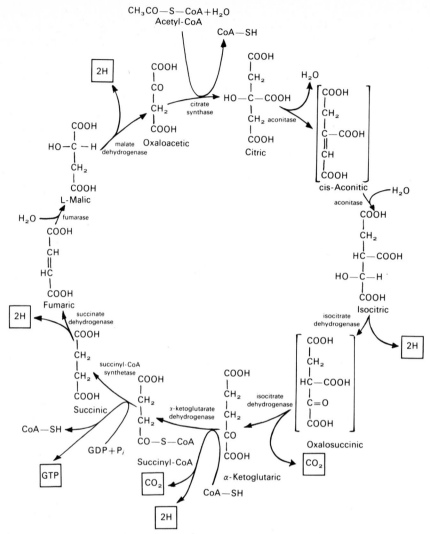

Fig. 4.3 The tricarboxylic acid cycle (reproduced with permission from Lehninger, A.L. (1975) *Biochemistry*, 2nd edition New York: Worth)

consumption of oxygen would not lead to the production of ATP, and, in effect, part of the energy would be converted into useless heat. An interaction between oxidative phosphorylation and muscle contraction is established by virtue of the fact that with a tightly coupled physiologically operating oxidation-phosphorylation system, the formation of ADP in muscle contraction, by furnishing an acceptor for phosphorylation, may serve as a regulating link between the energy-conserving and energy-producing process (Siekevitz, 1959; Chance, Mauriello and Aubert, 1960).

Fatty acid oxidation

The oxidation of fatty acids is an important source of energy in both skeletal and cardiac muscle (Fritz, Davis, Holtrop and Dundee, 1958). Detailed modern enzymatic studies of the breakdown of fatty acids (Lynen and Ochoa, 1953; Green, 1954), the hydrolytic product of neutral fats, have fully confirmed the ideas expressed by Knoop as early as 1904 on the basis of results obtained on whole animals. Accordingly, fatty acids are broken down by the repeated pair-wise removal of carbon residues starting at the COOH end of the fatty acid molecule and leading to the formation of an acetate residue or propionic acid residue, in even or odd-numbered fatty acids, respectively. Actually, both the acetate and propionate residue appear linked to the coenzyme CoA mentioned earlier in connection with the operation of a citric acid cycle. Acetyl-CoA enters the citric acid cycle in exactly the same way as that formed from the oxidation of pyruvic acid and originating in glucose. Propionyl-CoA is converted into succinate, another intermediate in the citric acid cycle, by a path involving an ATP-dependent carboxylation (Flavin and Ochoa, 1957). It should be added that the further flow of electrons involved in the re-oxidation of the reduced NAD and NADP is the same as that in the metabolism of carbohydrates discussed above.

High-energy compounds

General. The fact that ATP belongs to a class of phosphate compounds known as high-energy phosphates should be briefly discussed. This statement means that in the reaction of ATP with water, which is catalysed by various enzymes, part of the energy liberated accompanying liberation of inorganic phosphate is available for doing useful work or for driving a reaction that would not occur spontaneously. This type of energy is called free energy by the physical chemists. Space does not permit me to enter into a detailed discussion of the concept of free energy. Suffice it to say from a qualitative point of view that the various phosphate compounds can, broadly speaking, be grouped into two classes, high- and low-energy compounds, depending on the amount of energy that becomes available for work upon cleaving the phosphate bond (Burton, 1957). The concept that phosphate bonds are carriers in energy transformation and biosynthesis was originally proposed by Lipmann (1941). In the class of high-energy compounds we have ATP, acetyl phosphate, 1-phosphoglycerol-3-phosphate, phosphenolpyruvate, creatine phosphate; low-energy phosphates are glycero-1-phosphate, glucose-6-phosphate, fructose-6-phosphate, glucose-1-phosphate.

The distinction between the two classes of compounds is often somewhat blurred because the actual amount of free energy available depends on the concentration of the reactants and products of the reaction, and the so-called standard free energy

of reaction (ΔF^0), usually listed in tables, refers to a hypothetical state when all the reactants are present in the concentration of 1 mole per litre. A useful way of thinking about this so-called standard free-energy change of a reaction is in terms of the relationship of standard free-energy change with the equilibrium constant (K) of the reaction, given by

$$\Delta F^0 = -RT \ln K$$

Compounds that do not contain phosphate bonds are also often referred to as having a high-energy character, e.g., acetyl-CoA, if their hydrolysis liberates the same free energy as does a high-energy phosphate. In considering biological energy transduction involving macromolecular systems, as in the case of muscle, some useful distinctions can and should be made among various types of free energy definitions. The recent papers by Hill and his colleagues, particularly Hill and Simmons (1976), should be consulted in this context.

Reactions of ATP. Both the bond between the terminal and the middle phosphate and that between the middle phosphate and that nearest to the ribose ring of ATP are of a high-energy character. There are several enzyme systems, phosphotransferases, in the cell which provide essentially equi-energetic transfer of phosphate from one compound to another. One is the so-called creatine kinase, discovered by Lohman (1934) and later purified by Kuby, Noda and Lardy (1954), which catalyses the reaction:

$$CrP + ADP \rightleftharpoons Cr + ATP$$

Another enzyme present in muscle, myokinase (Colowick and Kalckar, 1943; Kalckar, 1943; Noda and Kuby, 1957) catalyses the transfer of phosphate from ATP to AMP resulting in the formation of two ADP molecules, thus making, by the reverse reaction, further utilisation of energy available.

In addition to the reactions of ATP involving transfer of phosphates there are enzymes in muscle that lead to the deamination of the purine ring (Schmidt, 1928; Lee, 1957). No evidence exists that ATP itself can be deaminated, but both ADP and AMP can serve as substrates of deaminase.

Furthermore, *in vivo* it seems that the NH_2 group attached to the purine ring of the ATP molecule undergoes rapid exchange. This exchange, however, is not a simple reversal of the deamination reaction but seems to proceed by a pathway involving adenylosuccinate (Newton and Perry, 1960). The precise significance of these reactions in the metabolism of muscle and in the mechanism of muscle contraction is not yet understood*.

Energetics of muscle contraction

Views on the ultimate source of the energy released by muscle in the course of contraction have undergone considerable changes over the years. The lactic acid era (Meyerhof, 1930) gave way to phosphagen (Eggleton and Eggleton, 1927a, b), as creatine phosphate was then called, particularly under the weight of evidence adduced by Lundsgaard (1930) showing the disappearance of creatine phosphate from exhausted muscle, even under conditions when no lactic acid appeared (for a review *see* Needham, 1956). In the middle 1950s doubts were cast on the immediate participation of ATP and CrP in the elementary event of muscle contraction (Mommaerts, 1954; 1955; Fleckenstein Janke, Davies and Krebs, 1954), but it has now been shown quite convincingly that 0.5–0.6 μmole of ATP are hydrolysed per gram of muscle during a single contraction (Cain, Infante and Davies, 1962). Fenn (1923; 1924) showed more than 50 years ago that the total energy output of the muscle is increased as it shortens to do work (*see also* Mommaerts, 1970). Hill (1949) originally partitioned the energy released by muscle during contraction into three terms, one corresponding to activation, another to shortening, and a third to mechanical work. The existence of a heat term which is dependent only on shortening appears doubtful in the light of recent work (Hill, 1964a, b, c, d; Wilkie, 1966). The correlation of each of these terms with chemical changes has been the subject of research in several laboratories (Cain *et al.*, 1962; Mommaerts, Seraydarian and Marechal, 1962; Carlson, Hardy and Wilkie, 1963; Marechal and Mommaerts, 1963).

*For an excellent historical review see Needham (1971); for recent reviews see Kushmerick (1977) and Homsher and Kean (1978).

It appears that there is good evidence for extra breakdown of CrP and ATP corresponding to work done (*see* e.g. Kushmerick and Davies, 1969). The chemical equivalent of the activation heat and shortening heat has yet to be established (Gilbert, Kretzschmar, Wilkie and Woledge, 1971; Woledge, 1971; Gilbert, Kretzschmar and Wilkie, 1972). Comparison of mechanical work and thermal and chemical changes has been complicated by the fact that different investigators use different experimental materials. In addition, the problems arising out of the suggestion made recently that some unknown chemical reaction(s) could be—in part—responsible for the production of heat and work (Gilbert *et al.*, 1972; Woledge, 1972; Homsher, Kean, Wallner and Garibian-Sarlan, 1979) have to be resolved. In contrast, the very recent work of Rall, Homsher and Mommaerts (1973) indicates that by proper energy book-keeping and some redefinition of terms all three types of heat terms can be accounted for by the breakdown of ATP and CrP. It should be kept in mind that some of the chemical changes may be associated (*see below*) with the Ca^{++} movement controlling excitation and relaxation (Davies, Kushmerick and Larson, 1967). For further discussion of this point see Homsher and Kean (1978). New developments in this area may be expected from the application of the powerful ^{31}P-nuclear magnetic resonance technique to contracting, living muscle (*see* e.g. Dawson, Gadian and Wilkie, 1977).

ACTIVE TRANSPORT AND MEMBRANE POTENTIAL

Active transport (Andersen and Ussing, 1960) is a process playing an important part in the function of all cells. In muscle, in particular, it is an essential process in maintaining the excitability of muscle which depends on the presence of an ionic gradient between the inside of the muscle cell and the outside medium; it is also involved in the operation of the Ca^{++} pump of the sarcoplasmic reticulum (*see below*). By active transport, in general, one means the process which utilises negative free energy from some other source to transport ions, or other types of molecules, against the so-called gradient of the electrochemical potential: that is, transport in the direction which is the opposite to that in which movement would take place in the absence of the second process that is accompanied by a decrease in free energy. Recent theoretical formulation of this problem has furnished useful insights into the coupling process (Hill, 1975a; Hill and Simmons, 1976).

It seems that the ionic composition of the muscle, taking into consideration the potential difference (about 90 mV) existing between the inside of the muscle and the extracellular medium, is such that the chloride and potassium concentration practically correspond to this potential (Horowicz, 1961) (Table 4.1). The fact that the sodium concentration is much lower inside the muscle than outside, particularly in view of the negativity of the inside of the muscle, means that there must exist a constant process of 'pumping out' of sodium from the muscle. The fact that sodium inside the muscle is in a dynamic steady state has been amply proved by experiments with radioactive sodium isotopes.

The operation of the sodium pump has been observed in other cells, such as nerve and red blood cells, and it has been shown that the sodium transport depends on an ATPase which presumably is located in the membrane, whose activity shows an interesting dependence on the sodium and potassium concentration (Post, Merritt, Kinsolving and Albright, 1960; Skou, 1960, 1971). Enzymes of this type have been demonstrated in heart muscle (Schwartz, 1962) and also in skeletal muscle (Samaha and Gergely, 1965). It is now well established that the Na^+, K^+-activated ATPase is the site at which cardiac glycosides in heart muscle act (for a review *see* Akera and Brody, 1978).

In view of the fact that ionic shifts take place in the process of excitation, further biochemical studies on this enzyme system in muscle would furnish interesting insights into the intimate molecular mechanism of excitation coupling.

MYOFIBRILLAR PROTEINS

We have to turn now to the discussion of the proteins that are constituents of contractile machinery itself. They account for 50–60 per cent of the muscle proteins (*see* e.g. Helander, 1957) As discussed in Chapter 2, high-resolution electron microscopy has shown that the myofibrils consist of two distinct sets of filaments and the evidence obtained by Huxley and Hanson (1957) and by Hasselbach (1953) suggested that one set of

Table 4.1 Comparisons of concentrations for various ions and electrical potentials in isolated sartorius muscle

Concentrations

Membrane

Inside	Outside
140 mM, K^+	2.5 mM, K^+
3.6 mM, Cl^-	120 mM, Cl^-
9.2 mM, Na^+	120 mM, Na^+
152 m-equiv., A^-	

Potentials

V = resting membrane potential = -94 mV.

$$V_K = \frac{RT}{F} \ln \frac{(K)_o}{(K)_i} = -101 \text{ mV.}$$

$$V_{Cl} = \frac{RT}{F} \ln \frac{(Cl)_i}{(Cl)_o} = -88 \text{ mV.}$$

$$V = \frac{RT}{F} \ln \frac{(Na)_o}{(Na)_i} = +64 \text{ mV.}$$

Note. $(\ )_o$ and $(\ )_i$ indicate concentrations outside and inside the fibre, V is the internal potential, F Faraday's constant, R the gas constant, and T the absolute temperature, and A^- stands for negatively charged ions other than Cl^-. (Copied, with permission, from Horowicz, 1961.)

Table 4.2 Composition of myofibrils in rabbit skeletal muscle

Protein	Quantities % of myofibrillar protein	Role	Location
Myosin	60	Contraction	Thick filaments
Actin	20	Contraction	Thin filaments
Tropomyosin	4	Regulation	Thin filaments
Troponin	3	Regulation	Thin filaments
α-actinin	1.5	Structure?	Z-band
C protein	⎫	?	Thick filaments
M protein	⎬ 11.5	Structure?	M-zone
Desmin	⎪	?	?
Connectin	⎭	?	?

In part after Ebashi, Endo and Ohtsuki, 1969.

filaments consists of the protein myosin, and the other of actin. Subsequent work has shown that a number of other proteins are also associated with the two sets of filaments and the Z band, some of which play an important part in the regulation of muscle contraction. The proteins found in rabbit myofibrils are listed in Table 4.2.

Myosin

Extraction, solubility. Myosin amounts to 55–60 per cent of the myofibrillar proteins (Hanson and Huxley, 1957). It can be extracted from muscle at about pH 6.5 with a minimal contamination of actin. Raising the pH and prolonging the time of extraction leads to the extraction of both actin and myosin in the form of actomyosin which will be discussed in more detail below. The solubility of myosin increases with ionic strength: about 0.6 is the ionic strength used for extraction. Myosin is insoluble at ionic strengths less than 0.2, when a formation of aggregates occurs. This property is used for the precipitation or, as it is often somewhat loosely termed, crystallisation of myosin (Szent-Györgyi, 1945).

Structure, subunits. Myosin is among the largest proteins whose structure has been well characterised. At present it seems to be an established fact that its molecular weight is about 500 000 and its length is of the order of 150 nM (*see* e.g. Dreizen, Gershman, Trotta and Stracher, 1967; Young, 1969). Considerable insight into the structure has been obtained by the extension of studies involving the treatment of myosin with proteolytic enzymes (Gergely, 1950, 1953; Perry, 1951; Mihalyi and Szent-Györgyi, 1953; Szent-Györgyi, 1953; Gergely, Gouvea and Karibian, 1955). Trypsin and chymotrypsin produce two types of fragments, one with a molecular weight of the order of 350 000, the so-called heavy meromyosin (HMM), the other light meromyosin (LMM), with a molecular weight of the order of 130–150 000 (Szent-Györgyi, 1953). Light meromyosin has an almost 100 per cent α-helix content. Further tryptic or chymotryptic digestion of heavy meromyosin produces smaller fragments with a molecular weight of 110 000, named HMM-S-1 (Mueller and Perry, 1962; Young, Him-

melfarb and Harrington, 1965) having ATPase activity and ability to combine with actin (*see below*). Lowey and her colleagues (Lowey, 1964; Lowey, Goldstein and Luck, 1966) have shown that a highly α-helical fragment can also be isolated from HMM. More recent work has shown that the originally isolated S-2 represents a degraded form of the α-helical rod portion of HMM, and that a longer S-2 can be obtained (Highsmith, Kretzchmar, O'Konski and Morales, 1977; Weeds and Pope, 1977; Sutoh, Sutoh, Karr and Harrington, 1978). Urea and guanidine treatment lead to the appearance of another type of subunit, whose molecular weight is about 200 000 (Kielley and Harrington, 1960). It seems now well established that there are two of these chains—so-called heavy chains—in each myosin molecule (Lowey and Cohen, 1962). This view is supported by physicochemical evidence (Lowey and Cohen, 1962; Lowey, Slayter, Weeds and Baker, 1969) and by studies of binding of nucleotides (Schliselfeld and Bárány, 1968; Lowey and Luck, 1969; *see*, however, Young, 1967) and the ATP-analogue inorganic pyrophosphate (Nauss, Kitagawa and Gergely, 1969) to myosin and its fragments, but most elegantly by direct electron microscopic observations (Fig. 4.4). The use of rotating shadow-cast specimens has made it possible to demonstrate that myosin is a two-headed structure, each head corresponding to what on proteolytic digestion appears as the HMM-S-1 fragment. LMM and the α-helical fragment (HMM-S-2) obtainable from HMM together form the rigid rodlike part of the myosin molecule. This rod can be isolated by papain digestion (Lowey *et al.*, 1969) or by mild treatment with CNBr (Young, Blanchard and Brown, 1968), and it appears that it can be broken down in a preferential way into small fragments by further proteolysis (Bálint *et al.*, 1968; Biró, Szilágyi and Bálint, 1972).

Beginning with the work of Tsao (1953), small myosin components dissociated by urea or high pH, of molecular weight 16 000–29 000, have been described (Locker, 1956; Kominz and Maruyama, 1960; Kominz and Lewis, 1964; Dreizen et al., 1967). These small subunits or, as they are now generally termed, light chains, can also be dissociated by elevated temperature, 5 M guanidine, or

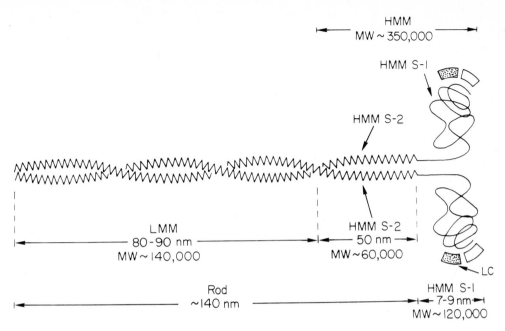

Fig. 4.4 Schematic representation of the structure of the myosin molecule, based chiefly on Lowey *et al.* (1969). The rod portion of the molecule has a coiled-coil α-helical structure. Hinge regions postulated in the mechanism of contraction (Huxley, 1969) are at the junction of HMM S-1 and HMM S-2 and of HMM S-2 and LMM. It should be noted that HMM S-1 has one chief polypeptide chain while the other fragments have two. Note the light chains (LC) in the head region. The scheme suggests the presence of two different subunits in each HMM S-1. For details *see* text

succinylation (Oppenheimer, Bárány, Hamoir and Fenton, 1967). The evidence seems good that the light chains are associated with the HMM portion (*see* Fig. 4.4).

Myosins from different types of muscle contain a different set of light chains. Myosin in a fast-twitch muscle contains three types of light chains, designated as LC_1, LC_2 and LC_3 in order of increasing speed of migration on SDS polyacrylamide gel electrophoresis. LC_1 and LC_3 are also referred to as A1 and A2, respectively, A indicating that they are removable by mild alkali. Myosin in cardiac and slow-twitch muscle contains only two types of light chains whose mobilities are similar to, but distinguishable from, those of LC_1 and LC_2 respectively, of fast muscle myosin (Lowey and Risby, 1971; Sarkar, Sreter and Gergely, 1971; Frank and Weeds, 1974). The fast (or white) skeletal muscle light chain of 18 000 daltons can be dissociated by treatment with Ellman's thiol reagent (5,5′-dithio bis-2-nitrobenzoic acid (DTNB) without significant loss of ATPase activity (Gazith, Himmelfarb and Harrington, 1970; Weeds and Lowey, 1971).

Further alkali treatment liberates two light chains having apparent molecular weights on SDS gels of about 25 000 and 16 000, LC_1 and LC_3 respectively. The three chains have distinctive chemical features although there are common sequences in the alkali light chains (Weeds, 1969; Weeds and Frank, 1972). On the basis of the sequence studies the true molecular weight of LC_1 is 21 000.

Myosin isozymes. Each molecule contains two LC_2s. In fast muscle myosin the sum of LC_1 + LC_3 is two per molecule but they occur in a ratio of about 1.4 : 0.6, suggesting that some myosin molecules contain pairs of either LC_1 or LC_3 (Sarkar, 1972). Recent work (Holt and Lowey, 1977) utilising antibodies specific for either LC_1 or LC_3 has succeeded in demonstrating the existence of such homodimers containing either a pair of LC_1 or a pair of LC_3; more recently (Hoh and Yeoh, 1979), evidence has also been obtained for the existence of molecules containing one LC_1 and one LC_3. In slow and cardiac muscle myosin it appears that there are a pair of LC_1s and a pair of

LC₂s per molecule. The possible functional role of light chains will be discussed in connection with ATPase activity.

ATPase activity. Myosin is itself an enzyme able to hydrolyse the terminal phosphate of ATP producing ADP and inorganic phosphate as first shown by Engelhardt and Ljubimova (1939). This reaction is stimulated by Ca^{++} and inhibited by Mg^{++} ions (Szent-Györgyi, 1945). Stimulation of myosin-ATPase by K^+ in the presence of EDTA is probably due to the removal of traces of Mg^{++} by the chelator (Muhlrad, Fabian and Biro, 1964; Offer, 1964). As we shall see, the combination of actin with myosin greatly increases its activity in the presence of Mg^{++}. ATPase activity is entirely restricted to the heavy meromyosin fraction (Szent-Györgyi, 1953; Gergely *et al.*, 1955) and can be recovered in the even smaller HMM-S-1 fragments discussed above. This suggests that the rod-like part has a structural role, the globular parts constituting the functional end of the myosin molecule.

The ATPase activity of myosin in fast white muscle is considerably higher than that of myosin in slow red muscles (Bárány, Bárány, Reckard and Volpe, 1965; Sreter, Seidel and Gergely, 1966). Bárány (1967) has shown that in general, good correlation exists between the ATPase activity of myosin and the speed of shortening of the muscle from which it has been isolated independently of the species or the type of muscle (smooth or striated). Myosin of slow muscles shows considerable lability at pH 9, not present in myosin of slow muscles (Sreter *et al.*, 1966; Seidel, 1967).

Regulation by light chains. The light chains may play a part in determining the character of the ATPase because the ATPase activity of hybrid reconstituted myosin seems to reflect the origin of the light chains (Dreizen and Richards, 1972; Wagner and Weeds, 1977). So far the regulatory role of a light chain has been most clearly demonstrated in molluscan myosin, the interaction of which with actin is regulated by Ca^{++}-binding to myosin (Szent-Györgyi, Szentkiralyi and Kendrick-Jones, 1973; Lehman and Szent-Györgyi, 1975) (for regulation in vertebrate muscle, *see below*). Removal of a certain type of

molluscan light chain leads to loss of Ca^{++} sensitivity; this light chain can be replaced by the LC₂ which seems to play no functional role in vertebrate myosin (Kendrick-Jones, Szentkiralyi and Szent-Györgyi, 1976).

Light chains in the LC₂ mobility class (fast, slow skeletal, cardiac) seem to be related by their ability to undergo phosphorylation by a kinase (Pires, Perry and Thomas, 1974; Yagi, Yazawa, Kakiuchi, Ohshima and Uenishi, 1978) whose activator is the ubiquitous Ca-binding protein calmodulin, also known as the calcium-dependent regulatory protein (for recent reviews *see* Wolf and Brostrom, 1979; Wang and Weisman, 1979). The function of the light chains in skeletal muscle is not clear. A light chain that can undergo phosphorylation has been implicated in the regulation of smooth muscle contraction (Sherry, Gorecka, Aksoy, Dabrowska and Hartshorne, 1978), although this issue is not yet finally settled (*see e.g.* Ebashi, Mikawa, Hirata and Nonomura, 1978). A regulatory role for LC₂ in cardiac muscle has also been suggested (Malhotra, Huang and Bhan, 1979). Although no direct regulatory function for LC₂ has been found in skeletal muscle, its phosphorylation and dephosphorylation *in vivo* during contraction and relaxation, respectively, have recently been reported (Bárány, Bárány, Gillis and Kushmerick, 1979).

It is less clear what possible part the two different non-phosphorylatable light chains—LC₁ and LC₂—may play, although differences in actin-activated ATPase of HMM-S-1, depending on which of the two is present, have been reported (Wagner and Weeds, 1977). It should be kept in mind that differences do exist in the heavy chain, as reflected in the absence of methylation of one of the histidine residues (*see below*), in the appearance of negatively stained aggregates of light meromyosin obtained from different types of myosin (Nakamura, Sreter and Gergely, 1971) and in the peptide pattern obtained on limited proteolysis (Balint, Sreter, Wolf, Nagy and Gergely, 1975).

Relation of myosin to myofilaments. As shown in Chapter 2, the electron microscope picture of a myofibril shows that myosin filaments have a diameter of about 10 nm. A consideration of the dimensions of the myosin molecule and the number of myosin molecules present in a sarcomere (Huxley, 1960) would suggest that a given myosin filament is a bundle of many myosin molecules per cross section; the rigid rod-like part of the myosin molecules makes up the body of these filaments and the enzymatically active globular end would correspond to the bridges seen in electron micrographs between myosin and actin filaments.

Huxley (1963) has demonstrated in myosin solutions at low ionic strength the formation of regular aggregates with the sidewise apposition of the rod-like part of the myosin molecules, and the globular ends appearing on the side of the aggregates. The formation of the aggregates proceeded in two directions leaving a central zone free of lateral projections quite reminiscent of the appearance of the thick filaments of myofibrils seen in the electron micrographs of muscle itself. Kaminer and Bell (1966) and Josephs and Harrington (1966) have shown that the form and size of the aggregates greatly depend on such factors as pH and ionic strength.

The electron microscopic investigation of negatively stained aggregates of LMM or of the whole rod portion of myosin under various conditions may also furnish useful insight into the forces responsible for the self-assembly of myosin molecules into thick filaments (King and Young, 1972; Cohen, Lowey, Harrison, Kendrick-Jones and Szent-Györgyi, 1970; Nakamura et al., 1971). Similarly, investigations of the aggregation properties of myosin in solution appear to throw new light on the mechanism of filament formation (Herbert and Carlson, 1971; Harrington and Burke, 1972; Harrington, Burke and Barton, 1972). Electron-microscopic and X-ray data suggest that the cross-bridges on the myosin aggregates and thick filaments are arranged on the surface in a helical fashion, the rod portions forming the core at levels separated by 14.3 nm (Huxley and Brown, 1967; Huxley, 1969). The number of cross-bridges at each level has not been definitely settled (for a review see Squire, 1975). The original estimate was two, and it was suggested that the two are diametrically opposed (Huxley and Brown, 1967) (Fig. 4.5). A number of four has been suggested, but the most likely value is three. The precise way in which the myosin rods

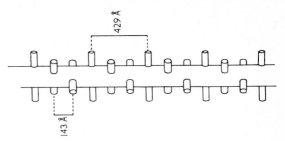

Fig. 4.5   Arrangement of heavy meromyosin projections (cross-bridges) on myosin filaments assuming a two-strand helix (copied with permission from Huxley and Brown, 1967)

are packed in the core is still not settled. Comparative studies (Wray, 1979), the use of fluorescent antibodies (Pepe, 1967a, b), and advances in electron-microscopic techniques (Pepe and Dowben, 1977) play an important part in producing new ideas in this area.

The idea that the myosin molecule contains hinges permitting segmental flexibility has greatly helped to connect information on the molecular structure of myosin, thick filament ultrastructure and theories of contraction. This will be discussed further below. At this point it should be mentioned that electron-microscopic and physicochemical evidence and the loci of proteolytic susceptibility suggest regions of flexibility at the junction of the globular heads and the rod (S-1/S-2) and within the rod itself at the junction of S-2 and light meromyosin (cf. Fig. 4.3) (Mendelson, Morales and Botts, 1973; Thomas, Seidel, Hyde and Gergely, 1975; Highsmith et al., 1977; Elliott and Offer, 1978; Sutoh et al., 1978).

Chemical aspects

Methylated amino acids. The chemistry of myosin exhibits some interesting features in that three kinds of unusual amino acids have been found in white skeletal muscle myosin of adult rabbits, 3-methyl histidine, ε-N-iminomethyl lysine and ε-N-trimethyl lysine. All these occur in the HMM-S-1 globular portion which, as discussed above, carries a site for ATPase activity and the combination with actin (Kuehl and Adelstein, 1969; Trayer, Harris and Perry, 1968; Hardy and Perry, 1969; Huszar and Elzinga, 1969).

There are one 3-methyl histidine residue and 2 moles of 3-methyl lysine in each heavy chain

(Huszar and Elzinga, 1971; Huszar, 1972). It is interesting to note that the 3-methyl histidine content of myosin varies according to the source. Myosin from slow skeletal muscle and cardiac muscle myosin contains essentially no methylated histidine (Johnson, Lobley and Perry, 1969; Kuehl and Adelstein, 1970). It also appears that fetal myosin, at least in the rabbit, contains no methylated histidine. Although fetal rabbit myosin contains a 13-residue peptide in which the histidine that is methylated in the adult can be located, this peptide differs at two sites from the corresponding methylated chain. An analogous tridecapeptide is found in rabbit cardiac muscle myosin which, in addition to lacking methylation of histidine, contains some residues that are different (Huszar, 1972). In contrast to differences in methylation at the single histidine locus, the 3-methyl lysine peptides appear to be present both in adult and fetal types of myosin. Clearly, more information is needed to establish a correlation between the functional properties of myosin and methylated amino acids. In the meantime, many interesting questions await answers. For example, is the lack of methylation in slow or cardiac muscle myosin due to lack of the methylating enzyme or is it due to changes in the primary amino acid sequence in the vicinity of the groups to be methylated? It should be pointed out that it seems likely that the methylated residues both in myosin and in actin (see below) are not incorporated into the chain as such, but methylation occurs after the polypeptide chain is synthesised (Hardy, Harris, Perry and Stone, 1970; Krzysik, Vergnes and McManus, 1971) by transfer of the methyl group from S-adenosyl methionine (Asatoor and Armstrong, 1967; Hardy and Perry, 1969).

Thiol groups. It has long been known that the ATPase activity of myosin depends on the integrity of SH groups (Barron and Singer, 1945; Bailey and Perry, 1947). Kielley and Bradley (1956) were the first to show that there are at least two classes of SH groups involved in ATPase activity. SH groups are also involved in the reaction with actin (Bailey and Perry, 1947; Bárány and Bárány, 1959). Schaub and his colleagues (Schaub and Perry, 1969; Schaub, Watterson and Wagner, 1975; Schaub, Watterson,

Walser and Waser, 1978) have shown that the reactivity of these, and other, -SH groups depends on the conformation of the myosin molecule which in turn changes during the ATPase cycle. Analysis of the N-terminal sequence of the myosin heavy chain (Starr and Offer, 1973) indicates that there are two kinds of heavy chains in fast muscle myosin preparations. Their relation to the two kinds of alkali light chains is not clear because HMM-S-1 contains only one kind of alkali light chain and fragments of both types of heavy chain (Wager and Weeds, 1977). Recently it was shown that the two SH groups whose modification affects ATPase activity are located within a decapeptide (Elzinga and Collins, 1977) which can be localised in a 20 000 dalton proteolytic fragment adjacent to the rod portion of myosin (Bálint, Wolf, Tarcsalvi, Gergely and Sreter, 1978). Harrington and his colleagues have stressed the proximity of the so-called $-SH_1$ and $-SH_2$ in the three-dimensional structure of myosin (Reisler, Burke, Himmelfarb and Harrington, 1974; Burke, Reisler and Harrington, 1976) and adduced evidence for changes in their distance on the contact of myosin with ADP or ATP. The sensitivity to proteolytic enzymes of the region is regulated by divalent cations (Biro *et al.*, 1972; Bálint *et al.*, 1975) and involves their binding to the DTNB light chain (Bagshaw, 1977; Weeds and Pope, 1977; Bagshaw and Kendrick-Jones, 1979).

Actin

Molecular weight; polymerisability. The discovery of actin by Straub (1942) in Szent-Györgyi's laboratory has opened up a new epoch in the biochemistry of muscle. What in the early literature was described as myosin turned out to be the complex of two proteins, myosin and actin. Actin itself can be extracted from acetone-dried muscle powder with distilled water. It is present in the watery extract as a globular protein—G actin. The molecular weight, as recently determined by physicochemical methods, is of the order of 46 000 (see Young, 1969). Johnson, Harris and Perry (1967) arrived at an estimate of 48 000 on the basis of the content in the unusual amino acid 3-methyl histidine. Quite recently, the determination of the amino acid sequence of actin has been completed;

the calculated molecular weight is 41 785 (Elzinga, Collins, Kuehl and Adelstein, 1973).

On addition of various salts, in a concentration of about 0.1 M for monovalent cations, and about 1 mM for divalent cations, a G-actin solution undergoes a drastic change: its viscosity increases and it exhibits birefringence of flow, suggesting the presence of large, asymmetric molecules. These are so-called F actin, for fibrous actin, particles produced through polymerisation of the globular units (Straub, 1942). The average molecular weight of F actin is of the order of 3 million (Gergely and Kohler, 1957) and its length 10 μm or longer, in contrast to actin filaments *in vivo* which have a length of 1 μm per half sarcomere (Hama, Maruyama and Noda (1965). The difference has been attributed to a protein, similar in aminoacid composition to actin, β actinin (Maruyama, 1965a, b).

The polymerisation reaction is probably of importance in the process by which actin filaments are laid down *in vivo*, but it is unlikely (Martonosi, Gouvea and Gergely, 1960b) that the polymerisation-depolymerisation cycle plays a significant part in the mechanism of muscle contraction (*see* e.g. Hayashi, 1967).

Chemistry. G actin contains tightly bound ATP and Ca (Straub and Feuer, 1950; Maruyama and Gergely, 1961)—each 1 mole per mole of actin—which can undergo rapid exchange with ATP (Martonosi, Gouvea and Gergely, 1960a) or added Ca (Bárány, Finkelman and Therattil-Antony, 1962), respectively, as shown by radioactive tracer experiments. Both the ATP and the Ca normally bound to actin can be exchanged by other nucleotides and metals, respectively (Martonosi, 1962b; Drabikowski and Strzelecka-Golaszewska, 1963; Iyengar and Weber, 1964; Oosawa, Asakura, Asai, Kasai, Kobayashi, Mihashi, Ooi, Taniguchi and Nakano, 1964). The polymerisation process is accompanied by the dephosphorylation of ATP to ADP (Straub and Feuer, 1950; Mommaerts, 1952), which remains firmly bound to actin, but in contrast to the firmly bound ATP of G actin the bound nucleotide of F actin is not available for rapid exchange reaction. Rapid exchange of ADP bound to F actin and ATP and other nucleoside triphosphates, accompanied by

liberation of inorganic phosphate, has been obtained by ultrasonic treatment (Asakura, 1961; Asakura, Taniguchi and Oosawa, 1963; Kakol and Weber, 1965). Slower exchange of ADP bound to F actin with either ADP or ATP has been demonstrated (Moos, Estes and Eisenberg, 1966; Kitagawa, Drabikowski and Gergely, 1967, 1968). It should be emphasised that the splitting of ATP by actin during polymerisation is not a typical enzymatic process in the sense that a small amount of protein can split an unlimited amount of substrate, but there is a stoichiometric relationship between the amount of actin present and the amount of phosphate liberated. Globular actin preparations that contain bound ADP and can undergo polymerisation without the splitting of ATP (Pragay, 1957; Grubhofer and Weber, 1961; Hayashi and Rosenbluth, 1962) have also been obtained. Actin that is free of either tightly bound Ca or ATP with the ability to polymerise and to react with myosin has been prepared by Oosawa and his colleagues (Kasai, Nakano and Oosawa, 1964). It seems likely that the chief function of bound metal and nucleotide is to stabilise the structure of the actin molecule rather than to participate directly in interactions with myosin or with other actin molecules (Nagy and Jencks, 1962; Lehrer and Kerwar, 1972).

With the availability of the amino acid sequence of actin it will be possible to localise those residues that may play a functional role in the structure and function of actin. SH groups are essential both for ATP binding and polymerisation and for combination with myosin (Kuschinsky and Turba, 1951; Drabikowski and Gergely, 1963; Bailin and Bárány, 1967). Of the five -SH groups (Elzinga and Collins, 1972) three are reactive in the native molecule (Lusty and Fasold, 1969) without preventing polymerisation of combination with myosin. The cysteine adjacent to the (Cys 373) C-terminal phenylalanine (Elzinga and Collins, 1972) contains the most reactive -SH group. This group reacts selectively with Cu^{++} (Lehrer, Nagy and Gergely, 1972) and a spin label attached to it can serve as an indicator of conformational change in actin (Stone, Prevost and Botts, 1970; Burley, Seidel and Gergely, 1971; 1972). The reactivity of Cys 373 increases upon the combination of actin with HMM subfragment-1, suggesting either the proximity of the groups to the myosin head or at least some coupling between the region Cys 373 and that directly involved in binding to myosin (Duke, Takashi, Eu and Morales, 1976). As suggested by Elzinga and Collins (1972) the region containing the single 3-methyl histidine residue and a tyrosine residue readily methylated by the reagent tetranitromethane may be involved in the polymerisation process. It appears so far (*see* Elzinga and Collins, 1972) that actins isolated from various sources (Carsten and Katz, 1964; Bridgen, 1971; 1972) including non-muscular contractile systems (Weihing and Korn, 1972) have similar chemical structures. It appears that amino acid replacements in actin are of a very conservative nature, i.e. preserving the character (charge hydrophobicity) of the residue, even if species far from each other on the evolutionary scale are compared. However, differences in the amino acid sequence of actins in different cell types, skeletal muscle, cardiac muscle, brain and platelets have been found in the same organisms. Gel electrophoretic differences among actins depend on a few residues at the N terminus; and while the differences correlate with certain broad groupings, the full genetic variety is not revealed by this technique but requires sequence analysis (Elzinga, Maron and Adelstein, 1976; Vanderkerckhoue and Weber, 1978). Refinements in recognising differences among closely related proteins may lead to new insights in the delineation of proteins in diseased muscles. It is also clear that the 3-methylhistidine-containing peptides in actin differ in their sequence from the 3-methylhistidine-containing peptides in myosin, thereby rendering a previously suggested evolutionary relation between myosin and actin unlikely (Huszar and Elzinga, 1971).

Structure and relation to myofilaments. Electron-microscopic studies by Hanson and Lowy (1963) have beautifully demonstrated that F actin consists of a double helix of globular actin units, which was shown by Rice (1961) and Rice, Brady, Depue and Kelly (1966) to be a right-handed helix. Actin filaments directly isolated from muscle also have the same structure. Thus it appears that each thin filament in the myofibril consists of a single F actin molecule. This is in contrast to the multi-molecular structure of the myosin filament as discussed above. The participation of other proteins in the actin filaments will be discussed below.

Actomyosin

Natural actomyosin—reaction with ATP. In view of the separate localisation of actin and myosin in distinct filaments the interaction of these proteins as a possible underlying process of muscle contraction is of great interest. As mentioned above, the early work on fibrous muscle proteins was done on solutions which according to our present knowledge would be considered to be the combination of actin and myosin, viz. actomyosin. The striking physical changes that took place on adding ATP to what then was still called myosin (Needham, Chen, Needham and Lawrence, 1941) became interpreted in the light of subsequent discoveries as a dissociation of actomyosin by ATP into actin and myosin (Szent Györgyi, 1945). The discovery and isolation of the pure proteins, myosin and actin, made it possible to study their combination.

Reconstituted actomyosin. On mixing myosin and actin there is a considerable increase in viscosity and birefringence of flow, both being reversed on addition of ATP. This was interpreted as the dissociation of actomyosin into actin and myosin (Szent-Györgyi, 1945) and could be confirmed on the basis of light-scattering measurements and ultracentrifuge experiments (Gergely, 1956; Weber, 1956). The combining ratio of actin and myosin is 1:4 on a weight basis (Spicer and Gergely, 1951) roughly corresponding to a ratio of one myosin head for each G actin unit. This combining ratio has been confirmed more recently by various techniques (for a summary *see* Seidel and Gergely, 1972).

Most of the physicochemical studies on actomyosin were carried out at high ionic strength (0.6) because of the problems of solubility. On the other hand, it is at lower ionic strength, of the order of 0.05 to 0.15, more closely corresponding to that prevailing in the muscle cell itself, that the most interesting properties of the actin-myosin interaction come to light. Under these conditions myosin ATPase is changed into what we might call the actomyosin enzyme characterised by a high rate even in the presence of Mg in contrast to the inhibition of the myosin enzyme (Szent-Györgyi, 1945). Thus actin acts as a powerful modifier of the ATPase activity of myosin, immediately suggesting interesting possibilities from the point of view of physiological regulation of energy release. It should be noted that, for quantitative studies on myosin–actin interaction, active fragments of myosin (HMM and HMM-S-1) have been widely used because complications arising out of the aggregation thereby of myosin molecules are avoided (for the most recent review *see* Taylor, 1979).

The acceleration of the Mg-moderated myosin ATPase by actin is usually interpreted, following Lymn and Taylor (1971), as being due to the accelerated breakdown, upon combination with actin, of the myosin-product complex. The resulting actomyosin complex would be dissociated by ATP yielding a myosin-ATP complex, which in turn would catalyse the formation of the myosin-$ADP.P_i$ complex. The latter would be ready for another cycle of interaction with actin. This proposal will be discussed further below in connection with the molecular mechanism of muscle contraction.

Actomyosin is not soluble at low ionic strength but forms a fine suspension which, on addition of ATP, undergoes a characteristic reaction consisting of the aggregation of the particles into a network which eventually shrinks. This process is known as super-precipitation. If an actomyosin solution in 0.6 M KCl is extruded in distilled water a fine thread is formed which contracts on adding ATP. Thus the contractile protein not only splits ATP enzymatically, as first shown by Engelhardt and Ljubimova (1939), but itself undergoes a change and Szent-Györgyi (1945) considered the above phenomenon to be a model of muscle contraction. Under certain conditions it is possible to reverse or prevent the super-precipitation of actin and myosin. This can be done by lowering the temperature to 0°C (Gergely and Spicer, 1951) or in the presence of Mg by properly adjusting the pH and ATP concentration. The change in actomyosin suspension occurring in the latter case has been termed clearing by Spicer (1952).

Hasselbach (1952) was the first who suggested that the differences in the appearance of actomyosin corresponding to the so-called sol and gel state represented different states of aggregation of actin and myosin.

Under the same conditions of ionic strength, it has been possible to show (Maruyama and Gergely, 1962) that clearing can give place to super-precipitation as the hydrolysis of ATP proceeds, and concomitantly with this physical change there is an increase in ATPase activity. If super-precipitation can be considered as a model of contraction it is not too far-fetched to consider clearing as an analogue of relaxation. This will be discussed in more detail in connection with the mechanism of the control of contraction and relaxation.

A conformational change in actin accompanying superprecipitation has been suggested by Oosawa *et al.* (1964) on the basis of increased exchange of the Ca bound to actin. Szent-Györgyi and Prior (1965; 1966) found an increased exchange of the actin-bound nucleotide in superprecipitated actomyosin. In view of the fact that nucleotide exchange in F actin alone can occur (*see above*) and is accelerated by sonic or mechanical treatment (Kakol and Weber, 1965), and in view of the relation of the kinetics of the nucleotide exchange to that of hydrolysis of ATP, it is more likely that the exchange accompanying superprecipitation reflects a secondary distortion of actin rather than an event underlying superprecipitation (Kitagawa, Martonosi and Gergely, 1965; Moos *et al.*, 1966).

Work utilising quasi-elastic light scattering of laser light by actin filaments (Ishiwata and Fujime, 1972; Oosawa, Fujime, Ishiwata and Mihashi, 1972) has redirected attention to the possibility of conformational changes in actin. Electron spin resonance, particularly saturation transfer spectroscopy, has furnished recent evidence of motion within actin filaments that undergoes a change upon combination with HMM and S-1 (Thomas, Seidel and Gergely, 1979).

Myofibrils and glycerol-extracted fibres. In addition to the study of actomyosin after reconstitution, studies on systems of somewhat higher complexity have also yielded interesting results. Glycerol-extracted muscle fibres or fibre bundles (Szent-Györgyi, 1949) or myofibrils contain actomyosin in their essentially undisturbed configuration. However, these preparations do not contain the excitatory mechanism of the intact cells not do they contain the energy supply necessary for contraction. It was found, however, that on the addition of ATP single glycerinated fibres contract, or, depending on the experimental conditions, develop tension. Myofibrils exhibit ATPase activity (for a recent study *see* Goodno, Wall and Perry, 1978) that has the characteristic feature of Mg^{++} activation observed on reconstituted and natural actomyosin, and their contraction results in a readily observable syneresis.

Chelators and Ca^{++}. Bozler (1954) and, independently, Watanabe (1955) found that ethylenediaminotetra-acetic acid (EDTA), a chelating agent, inhibits the ATP-induced contraction of glycerinated fibres; it was later found that the ATPase activity of myofibrils is also inhibited by EDTA (Perry and Grey, 1956); this was based on the action of EDTA on myofibrils and actomyosin at low ionic strength is the removal of free Ca^{++} ions which appear to be essential for maintaining the associated state of actin and myosin (Ebashi, 1961; Weber and Winicur, 1961). Particularly helpful in this area was the introduction of the use of EDTA analogues by Ebashi, Ebashi and Fujie (1960). One of these analogues, EGTA*, has a higher affinity to Ca^{++} than to Mg^{++}, thus eliminating the complications arising from the simultaneous binding of both divalent cations present in most of the systems under study. The inhibitory effect of the so-called super-optimal concentration of ATP on ATPase and contraction (Hasselbach and Weber, 1953; Perry and Grey, 1956) may also be due to the removal of Ca^{++} (Weber, 1959; Seidel and Gergely, 1963) although binding of ATP to a regulatory site has not been completely excluded (Ebashi *et al.*, 1978).

Regulatory proteins

It was first shown by Ebashi and Ebashi (1964)

*EGTA: 1,2-bis-(2-dicarboxymethylaminoethoxy)-ethane.

that the Ca^{++} requirement—or sensitivity to EGTA—depends on the presence of protein factors other than actin and myosin. Natural actomyosin, unless subjected to special purification procedures (Schaub, Hartshorne and Perry, 1967) contains these EGTA-sensitising factors while reconstituted actomyosin made with highly purified actin is insensitive to EGTA. These EGTA-sensitising factors have been resolved into several components and are usually referred to as the regulatory proteins of the myofibril. They consist of tropomyosin—a protein known and characterised for many years which, however, until recently has lacked a role—and the later-discovered troponin, a term coined by Ebashi and his colleagues; troponin is now recognised to be a complex of several protein components.

Tropomyosin. Tropomyosin can be extracted from an ethanol-treated muscle preparation (Bailey, 1948). It shows a very strong tendency to aggregation at lower ionic strength and its true physical characteristics can be obtained only by increasing the ionic strength (Bailey, 1954). Tropomyosin consists of two sub-units, each having a molecular weight of about 33 000, which can be separated under denaturing conditions (Woods, 1967). Tropomyosin is notable for its high α-helical content. In this respect it is very similar to the light meromyosin fraction of myosin (Cohen and Szent-Györgyi, 1957), and the two sub-units are thought to be arranged in a coiled-coil fashion (Cohen and Holmes, 1963). Tropomyosin is characterised by a very high proportion of polar amino acid residues which may account for its tendency to be a stubborn contaminant of actin preparations. Various methods have been developed to obtain actin free of tropomyosin (Martonosi, 1962; Drabikowski and Gergely, 1962; Spudich and Watt, 1971). Tropomyosin preparations contain two different sub-units (α and β) distinguishable by their electrophoretic mobility on SDS-polyacrylamide gels that form $\alpha\alpha$ and $\alpha\beta$ dimers (Yamaguchi, Greaser and Cassens, 1974; Cummins and Perry, 1973). The ratio of the two kinds of sub-units differs in different types of muscle (e.g. only α is found in heart muscle, and the ratio of α/β also varies according to the fibre type (Cummins and Perry,

1978) or the stage of ontological development (Roy, Sreter and Sarkar, 1979). The aggregation of tropomyosin at low ionic strength can occur both in the form of true three-dimensional crystals and so-called paracrystalline aggregates (Caspar, Cohen and Longley, 1971; Cohen, Caspar, Parry and Lucas, 1971). Various forms are observed in the electron microscope that greatly contribute to our understanding of the size and shape of the molecules and the factors responsible for the interaction among the molecules. This may explain their role in muscle structure and function, particularly with regard to the interaction with troponin (see below). During the past eight years or so the amino acid sequence of the tropomyosin sub-units has been established (Stone, Sodek, Johnson and Smillie, 1974; Stone and Smillie, 1978). The hydrophobic (non-polar) residues are alternately separated by three and two polar residues. This pattern results in the formation of the hydrophobic ridges on each of the two helices, and the interaction of these hydrophobic regions forms the basis of the coiled-coil structure. Crick (1953) originally proposed such a 'knobs-into-holes' pattern for interacting α-helices. The helix-helix interaction in tropomyosin is further stabilised by ionic interactions among polar residues (Stone, Sodek, Johnson and Smillie, 1974; Parry, 1975). Tropomyosin alone does not account for the Ca^{++} requirement of actomyosin ATPase activity. Ebashi and Ebashi (1964) initially assumed that a 'native tropomyosin' existed, but now it is well established that another moiety, troponin, is also involved (Ebashi and Kodama, 1965, 1966; Ebashi and Nonomura, 1967; Ebashi and Endo, 1968).

Troponin

Sub-units. Troponin was at first considered to be a homogeneous protein and various molecular weights have been suggested (see e.g. Hartshorne and Dreizen, 1972). The work of Hartshorne and his colleagues (Hartshorne and Mueller, 1968; Hartshorne, Theiner and Mueller, 1969) and Schaub and Perry (1969) has shown that troponin can be separated into at least two components; in addition, Greaser and Gergely (1971), by applying SDS polyacrylamide gel electrophoresis, have

shown that three components having molecular weights of 37 000, 24 000 and 20 000 are necessary for reconstruction of troponin activity. This activity is defined as the conferring of Ca^{++}-sensitivity on actomyosin in the presence of tropomyosin. Although Perry, Cole, Head and Wilson (1972) and Drabikowski, Nowak, Barylko and Dabrowska (1972) have reported reconstitution of activity without the 37 000 dalton component there seems to be a growing consensus concerning the requirement for three troponin components (Ebashi, 1972; Ebashi, Ohtsuki and Mihashi, 1972; Eisenberg and Kielley, 1972; Hitchcock and Szent-Györgyi, 1973). The three troponin components are referred to in decreasing order of molecular weight as Tn-T, Tn-I and Tn-C (Greaser, Yamaguchi, Brekke, Potter and Gergely, 1972), the letters indicating that the three separate components have the ability to combine with tropomyosin, inhibit actomyosin ATPase activity regardless of the presence of Ca^{++} (cf. Wilkinson, Perry, Cole and Trayer, 1972), and bind Ca^{++} respectively. The three troponin sub-units occur in a 1:1:1 ratio, there being one troponin complex for each tropomyosin molecule. The amino acid sequence of the sub-units has been determined (Tn-C: Collins, Potter, Horn, Wilshire and Jackman, 1973; Collins, Greaser, Potter and Horn, 1977; Tn-I: Wilkinson and Grand, 1975; Tn-T: Pearlstone, Carpenter, Johnson and Smillie, 1976); and the molecular weights are 18 000, 21 000 and 30 503 for Tn-C, Tn-I and Tn-T, respectively.

Ca^{++} binding. When Ca^{++} activates the actin-myosin interaction it binds to troponin via the TnC sub-unit. There are four Ca-binding sites in a TnC molecule, falling into two classes differing in their binding constants (Potter and Gergely, 1974): about $2.5 \times 10^7 M^{-1}$ and $4 \times 10^5 M^{-1}$. The higher affinity sites competitively bind Mg^{++} ($K5 \times 10^3 M^{-1}$); the other two are specific for Ca^{++}.

Ca^{++}-binding studies on TnC show an enhancement of its affinity for Ca^{++} upon interaction with TnI, either in the TnC-TnI complex or in whole troponin. Effects of this interaction (Drabikowski, Barylko, Dabrowska, Nowak and Szpacenko, 1974; van Eerd and Kawasaki, 1974; Winter,

Head and Perry, 1974) are also reflected in other physicochemical properties that have recently been studied in various laboratories, suggesting conformational changes induced in TnC by other sub-units and probably *vice versa*.

An important relationship between TnC and the family of proteins first found in fish muscle able to bind Ca++—parvalbumins or muscle Ca++-binding proteins—and more recently discovered in muscles of higher species (Lehky, Blum, Stein and Fischer, 1974; Pechere, 1974) has emerged. The functional role of the parvalbumins is not clear and they differ from the myofibril-bound TnC in that they appear free in the cytoplasm; their molecular weight is about half that of TnC. X-ray and amino acid sequence studies have suggested certain repeating features within the parvalbumin molecules, attributable to gene duplication or triplication (Kretsinger, 1972). Two Ca++ binding sites have been identified, each involving a 'loop' flanked by a pair of α helices (Kretsinger and Nockolds, 1973). Kretsinger and his colleagues predicted that there would be similarities between paravalbumins and TnC, and Collins and his colleagues (1973) have shown that extensive homologies exist between the amino acid sequences of TnC and parvalbumin. By comparison with the parvalbumin sequence there are four regions that would be likely candidates for the four Ca++-binding sites in TnC referred to above. Structural homologies between the light chains of myosin and parvalbumin and TnC have also been found (Collins, 1974; Weeds and McLachlan, 1974). Interestingly, with the exception of the regulatory light chain in molluscan muscle (*see below*), none of the other light chains contains a specific Ca++-binding site (*see e.g.* Bagshaw and Kendrick-Jones, 1979).

Recently it has been possible to study the interaction of Ca++ with enzymatically and chemically (cyanogen Br) produced fragments of TnC. (Drabikowski, Grabarek and Barylko, 1977; Leavis, Rosenfeld, Gergely, Grabarek and Drabikowski, 1978; Weeks and Perry, 1978). From these studies it appears that the high-affinity sites are in the C terminal half of the molecule (sites III and IV) while the low-affinity Ca++-specific sites (I and II) are in the α terminal half. Ca++-binding to sites III and IV produces major conformational

changes in the structure of TnC, while the changes occurring upon binding to site I and II are more subtle (Potter, Seidel, Leavis, Lehrer and Gergely, 1976; Levine, Mercola, Coffman and Thornton, 1977; Seamon, Hartshorne and Bothner-By, 1977; Johnson, Collins and Potter, 1978). Yet it appears that the binding of Ca++ to the latter (Ca++-specific) sites plays a crucial part in the regulation of actin-myosin interaction (Potter and Gergely, 1974) which is also reflected in the kinetics of Ca++ exchange (Johnson, Charlton and Potter, 1979).

Protein-protein interactions. The ability of Tn-T to combine with tropomyosin has been demonstrated by ultracentrifugal (Greaser *et al.*, 1972; Greaser and Gergely, 1973) and electron-microscopic (Cohen, Caspar, Johnson, Nauss, Margosian and Parry, 1972) studies. This interaction is thought to serve as a permanent anchor for the troponin complex, while the binding of other sub-units to tropomyosin and actin is Ca++-regulated (*see below*). It has been suggested that the binding site for TnT in tropomyosin is located in the region of residues 197-217 (McLachlan and Stewart, 1976) at about one third of the length of the tropomyosin molecule from the C terminus. Recent comparative studies have, however, thrown some doubt on this localisation (Cote, Lewis, Pato and Smillie, 1978).

The use of fragments to determine those regions of the sub-units that are involved in protein-protein interaction appears promising for all three troponin sub-units (Jackson, Amphlett and Perry, 1975; Syska, Wilkinson, Grand and Perry, 1976; Leavis *et al.*, 1978; Weeks and Perry, 1978).

Phosphorylation. Phosphorylation of the Tn-I and Tn-T sub-units has been reported (Cole and Perry, 1975; England, 1976; Frearson, Solaro and Perry, 1976; Syska *et al.*, 1976; Moir, Cole and Perry, 1977). Their functional role is at present not clear. The same applies to the recently reported phosphorylation of tropomyosin (Mak, Smillie and Bárány, 1978).

Hanson and Lowy (1963) were the first to suggest that tropomyosin is situated as two long strands in the two grooves of the F actin double

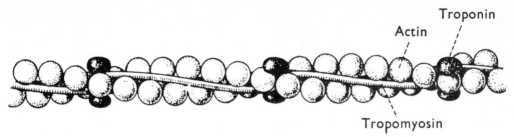

Fig. 4.6   A model for the fine structure of the thin filament. It should be noted that Ebashi and his colleagues merely had evidence for the periodic distribution of the troponin complex along the thin filaments; the relation of troponin to tropomyosin is hypothetical (reproduced with permission from Ebashi *et al.*, 1969)

helix. This has since been borne out by various electron-microscopic and X-ray studies (Moore, Huxley and DeRosier, 1970; Hanson, 1968). Ebashi *et al.* (1969) proposed that troponin would be attached to the tropomyosin strands, separated by periods of 40 nm (Fig. 4.6). Such a periodicity has been revealed before in electron-microscopic studies (*see* e.g. Hanson, 1968).

Molluscan muscle.   Molluscan muscles contain a protein with a chemical composition very close to that of tropomyosin, which seems to be the chief constituent of a fibrous structure, seen in the electron microscope, that was given the name paramyosin (Schmitt, Bear, Hall and Jakus, 1947). The terms paramyosin and tropomyosin A have been used interchangeably in the literature for this protein. Paramyosin has been implicated in the so-called catch mechanism (Ruegg, 1958, 1961; Johnson, Kahn and Szent-Györgyi, 1959). However, the idea that catch tension is attributable to direct interaction between actin and myosin (Nauss and Davies, 1966) has gained strength from recent experiments with purified catch muscle proteins (Szent-Györgyi, Cohen and Kendrick-Jones, 1971). Recent work suggests that the phosphorylation of paramyosin may be involved in the regulation of the catch state (Cooley, Johnson and Krause, 1979). The mechanism of the regulation of the interaction between actin and myosin depends on the direct action of Ca^{++} on myosin and does not involve troponin. The existence of a Ca^{++}-dependent mechanism regulating the interaction of myosin and actin but not involving the troponin system was first shown in molluscan muscle (Kendrick-Jones, Lehman and Szent-Györgyi, 1970; Lehman, Kendrick-

Jones and Szent-Györgyi, 1972; Lehman and Szent-Györgyi, 1975). This new type of regulation depends on the presence of a regulatory sub-unit in myosin which is structurally related to the myosin light chains found in vertebrate muscle. The phosphorylatable light chain of rabbit muscle can replace the regulatory light chain of molluscan muscle (Trinick and Lowey, 1977). The myosin-linked regulation appears to be widespread among invertebrates (Lehman and Szent-Györgyi, 1975) and many contain both the myosin- and actin-linked systems.

Additional myofibrillar proteins

During the last few years a number of myofibrillar proteins have been described, but their function and location have not been completely elucidated. It is also not clear in every case whether one is really dealing with a new protein or whether previously known proteins appear in modified form.

α **actinin and** β **actinin.**   Both these proteins have amino acid compositions similar to that of actin (Ebashi, Ebashi and Maruyama, 1964; Ebashi and Ebashi, 1965; Maruyama, 1965b). Although α actinin has been described as promoting superprecipitation of actomyosin (Ebashi and Ebashi, 1965), this effect has been questioned by Briskey and his colleagues (Briskey, Seraydarian and Mommaerts, 1967a, b; Seraydarian, Briskey and Mommaerts, 1967). Evidence is accumulating for the localisation of α actinin in the Z band (Goll, Mommaerts and Seraydarian, 1967; Goll, Mommaerts, Reedy and Seraydarian, 1969). The ability of α actinin to cross-link F actin (Maruyama and

Ebashi, 1965; Briskey et al., 1967a) may play a part in linking the actin filaments in the Z band. In view of these facts and since immunochemical techniques have revealed the presence of tropomyosin in the I band but not in the Z band (Pepe, 1966) the disease of muscle—nemaline myopathy—in which rod-like bodies appear to be connected with the Z bands (Shy, Engel, Somers and Wanko, 1963; Price, Gordon, Pearson, Munsat and Blumberg, 1965) requires reinterpretation in molecular terms. Originally the rod-like bodies were thought to consist of tropomyosin but this now seems unlikely and the presence of α actinin in these structures has been demonstrated (Sugita, Masaki, Ebashi and Pearson, 1974).

Another constituent of the Z band has been identified as desmin (M_r 50 000), the sub-unit of the so-called 10 nm filaments (Granger and Lazarides, 1978). Filaments in the 10 nm class have been found in a variety of cells and are considered part of the so-called cytoskeleton (see Goldman, Milsted, Schloss, Starger and Verna, 1979). Quite recently yet another protein, distinct from previously known ones, has been reported as a specific component of the Z band (Ohnishi and Maruyama, 1979).

M line constituents. The identity of the M line protein (Morimoto and Harrington, 1972), which would play a part in linking the thick filaments in the middle of the sarcomere (Pepe, 1972) has not been settled. While the presence of creatine kinase in the M line has been demonstrated (Turner, Walliman and Eppenberger, 1973) its structural role is not clear, and the role of another component (5S protein) (Trinick and Lowey, 1977) also remains to be elucidated.

C protein. The C protein may have a structural role in the architecture of thick filaments (Offer, 1972; Offer, Moos and Starr, 1973) and in regulating the interaction of myosin cross-bridges with actin (Starr and Offer, 1978).

Continuous filaments. It has been suggested that fibrillin and connectin filaments are running from Z band to Z band across the entire sarcomere (Guba, Harsanyi and Vajda, 1968). Such filaments have also been described by Hoyle and his colleagues (Hoyle, 1967; Hoyle, McNeil

and Selverston, 1973) although their role in the contraction process is not clear at present. Recent reports (Maruyama, Matsubara, Natori, Nonomura, Kimura, Ohashi, Murakami, Handa and Eguchi, 1977) on an elastic protein filament network in muscle (connectin) together with the information on 10 nm filaments may well produce a renewed interest in the function of continuous filaments in muscle.

Non-muscle contractile systems. This may be an appropriate place to call attention to the fact, now generally recognised, that all cells contain myosin, actin and other components of the myofilaments and that a variety of cell functions—including cell motility and probably cell division—depend on these proteins (Clarke and Spudich, 1977; Goldman et al., 1979). An important difference between muscle and other tissue is that in the latter the myofibrillar proteins do not form the conspicuous structures found in muscle and that the supramolecular complexes have a more fleeting existence. Detailed coverage of non-muscle cellular 'contractile' proteins is outside the scope of this Chapter.

CONTROL OF CONTRACTION AND RELAXATION

History—relaxing factor

An observation by Marsh (1951) that suspensions of fresh myofibrils in the presence of ATP could not be packed by centrifugation as readily as after some standing at room temperature, or as myofibrils that were washed several times, led him to the discovery of a factor in muscle that inhibited the ATP-dependent syneresis and ATPase of myofibrils (Marsh, 1952) and, as shown by Bendall (1952) inhibited the contraction and tension development of glycerinated fibres. This factor became known as the relaxing factor. It has also been referred to under such names as grana, microsomes, and Marsh-Bendall factor[*]. There is now general agreement that the component responsible for the activity of relaxing factor preparations consists of fragments of the so-called sarcoplasmic reticulum.

[*]The early stages of this problem are well covered in the review by A. Weber (1966).

Sarcoplasmic reticulum

Localisation. *In situ* the sarcoplasmic reticulum* appears to consist of two types of elements which can be best distinguished with reference to the so-called triad structure seen in electron micrographs (Porter and Palade, 1957). It seems assured now that the central element of the triad communicates, as the transverse tubule, with the surface of the muscle cell, and is continuous with the muscle plasma membrane (Simpson and Oertelis, 1962; Nelson and Benson, 1963; Franzini-Armstrong and Porter, 1964; Huxley, 1964). The two lateral elements correspond to longitudinally running sacs, the sarcoplasmic reticulum proper. The connection of the central element to the membrane suggests that it is closely linked to the excitation process, particularly in the light of the experiments by Huxley and Taylor (1958) showing the localised effect of microelectrodes applied to the surface of muscle cells. The excitability appeared to be at the site where the triad was located.

Fragmented sarcoplasmic reticulum. The recognition of the particulate nature of the Marsh-Bendall factor (Kumagai, Ebashi and Takeda, 1955; Ebashi, 1957) and the discovery of ATPase activity identifiable with the so-called Kielley-Meyerhof enzyme (Kielley and Meyerhof, 1948; 1950) opened up new vistas for the study of its mechanism of action. These particulate preparations contain fragments of the sarcoplasmic reticulum that form closed vesicles (for recent reviews *see* Tada, Yamamoto and Tonomura, 1978; Hasselbach, 1979). The vesicular character of these preparations is apparent in electron micrographs of sectioned (Nagai, Makinose and Hasselbach, 1960) and negatively stained material (Ikemoto, Sreter, Nakamura and Gergely, 1968).

Ca⁺⁺-uptake, ATPase and phosphorylation. In the presence of ATP there is considerable Ca^{++}-uptake by the fragment of the sarcoplasmic reticulum, and this process is promoted by a number of anions such as oxalate, phosphate and

*An excellent collection of papers on the sarcoplasmic reticulum and its history is found in the supplement to the August 1961 issue of the *J. Biophys. Biochem. Cytol.* (volume 10, number 4, part 2).

pyrophosphate (Ebashi, 1961; Hasselbach and Makinose, 1961; Ebashi and Lipmann, 1962; Martonosi and Feretos, 1964). A lower Ca^{++}-uptake has been found in fragmented sarcoplasmic reticulum from slow muscle (Sreter and Gergely, 1964). It is presumed that the splitting of ATP is the energy source for the active transport of Ca^{++} into the inside of the sarcoplasmic reticulum. *In situ* Ca-accumulation in the presence of precipitant has been demonstrated electron-microscopically in the terminal sacs of the reticulum (Hasselbach, 1964; Costantin, Franzini-Armstrong and Podolsky, 1965; Pease *et al.*, 1965). Ca deposits and ATPase have also been demonstrated electron-microscopically in the vesicles of fragmented sarcoplasmic reticulum (Ikemoto *et al.*, 1968). A value of 2.0 for the $\Delta Ca/\Delta ATP$ ratio is most likely under physiological conditions (*see* Hasselbach, 1979), while at 0°C the ratio is 1.0 (Sumida and Tonomura, 1974). A change in the Ca^{++} affinity of the protein appears to be correlated with the translocation of Ca^{++} from the low concentration outside compartment into the high concentration interior (Ikemoto, 1976).

Demonstration of the Ca^{++}-dependent formation of an acid-stable phosphorylated enzyme from ATP (Makinose, 1966; Yamamoto and Tonomura, 1967) implied in the ADP-ATP exchange described earlier (Ebashi and Lipmann, 1962; Hasselbach and Makinose, 1963) has opened up the way for the elucidation of the mechanism of an ATPase-coupled Ca^{++}-transport process (for a recent review *see* Tada *et al.*, 1978; DeMeis and Vianna, 1979; Hasselbach, 1979). The calcium pump can run in reverse, i.e. ATP is synthesised on the efflux of calcium from a Ca-loaded vesicle (Makinose, 1971; Makinose and Hasselbach, 1971). This synthesis of ATP involves the formation of a phosphoprotein intermediate from inorganic phosphate, the osmotic energy of Ca^{++} being converted into chemical energy. A limited amount of ATP can be formed also by leaky vesicles (*see* DeMeis and Vianna, 1979).

Proteins. Several protein components of the sarcoplasmic reticulum have been characterised. The ATPase moiety has a molecular weight of about 100 000 and contains the sites at which phosphorylation occurs (Martonosi, 1969; MacLennan, 1970). The spherical particles seen in electron micrographs of negatively stained preparations have been attributed to this component (Migala, Agostini and Hasselbach, 1973; Thorley-Lawson and Green, 1973; Stewart and MacLennan, 1974). It also contains three types of Ca^{++}-binding sites (Ikemoto, 1975). One has high affinity for Ca^{++} ($K \sim 10^6\ M^{-1}$) and is identifiable with the transport site. The second exhibits medium affinity for Ca^{++} at low temperature, but may become a second high-affinity site at temperatures over 20°. The third site, $K \sim 10^3\ M^{-1}$, may be an inhibitory site. Binding of Ca^{++} to the latter shows the rotational motion of the enzyme (Hidalgo, Thomas and Ikemoto, 1978). Current work in several laboratories is directed at determining the chemical structure of the ATPase/Ca-transport protein. Phosphorylation occurs at an aspartic acid residue (Bastide, Meissner, Gleischer and Post, 1973). Phosphorylation of the same residue occurs in another transport enzyme, viz. Na-K ATPase, and the two adjacent residues are also identical in the two enzymes. Tryptic digestion of the ATPase proteins has led to the formation of well-defined fragments. Some progress (Allen and Green, 1978) has been made towards the determination of their amino acid sequences and assignment of functional characteristics. Thus two fragments have been termed ionophoric, suggesting their involvement in the Ca^{++} translocation process while the ATPase site has been located in another. The state of some of the -SH groups of the ATPase protein appear to be influencing the activity. Conversely, the -SH groups fall into certain classes on the basis of their reactivity to thiol reagents; moreover, these reactivities change depending on the occupancy of various Ca^{++}-binding sites (Ikemoto, Morgan and Yamada, 1978; see also Tada et al., 1978).

Calsequestrin is another protein capable of binding Ca^{++} (Ikemoto, Bhatnagar and Gergely, 1971; MacLennan and Wong, 1971; Ikemoto, Bhatnagar, Nagy and Gergely, 1972). Various other proteins including a proteolipid (MacLennan, Yip, Iles and Seeman, 1972) and also a high-affinity Ca^{++}-binding protein (Ostwald and MacLennan, 1974) are also present but their functional and structural role has yet to be determined. A protein with a molecular weight of 22 000 has been described in cardiac sarcoplasmic reticulum (Tada, Kirchberger and Katz, 1975). This protein, named phospholamban, is phosphorylated by a cyclic AMP-dependent protein kinase, and in view of the reported stimulation of calcium transport by the kinase (Tada, Kirchberger, Repke and Katz, 1974) a regulatory role for phospholamban as a mediator of the effect of catecholamines in cardiac muscle has been suggested (for a detailed discussion see Tada et al., 1978).

Lipid-protein interaction. Early experiments showing that phospholipase destroys the ATPase and relaxing activity of elements of the sarcoplasmic reticulum (Kielley and Meyerhof, 1950; Ebashi, 1957) pointed to the involvement of phospholipids in its structure and function. Phospholipase-C-treated fragments of the sarcoplasmic reticulum that have lost their ATPase and Ca-accumulating ability again become active on the addition of phospholipids (Martonosi, 1963; Martonosi, Donley and Halpin, 1968). It is now clear that the sarcoplasmic reticulum represents a membrane-bound enzyme system carrying out the ATPase-linked Ca^{++}-transport function. An interesting feature of the sarcoplasmic reticulum is the ability of self-assembly of membrane structures from components solubilised with desoxycholate (Martonosi, 1968; MacLennan, Seeman, Iles and Yip, 1971) or Triton X-100 (Ikemoto, Bhatnagar and Gergely, 1971). These reconstituted vesicles have ATPase activity but no Ca^{++} transport capacity. Racker (1972) has reported the reconstitution of a Ca^{++} transport system from a desoxycholate solubilised ATPase preparation and soy bean phospholipids.

While many details of this transport process remain to be elucidated, it is apparent that the interaction involving the replacement of lipids with the lipid moiety determines many properties of the ATPase-transport protein. The ATPase activity depends on certain properties of the lipid moiety (Warren, Toon, Birdsall, Lee and Metcalfe, 1974), and temperature-induced changes in the motion activity of the ATPase reflect changes in the fluidity of the lipid (Inesi, Millman and Eletr, 1973; Hidalgo, Ikemoto and Gergely, 1976; Hidalgo et al., 1978).

Various mechanistic models have been proposed for the Ca^{++}-transport process involving movements within the protein or in relation to the lipid in which it is embedded (Shamoo, Scott and Ryan, 1977). Some schemes suggest changes in a monomer$\rightleftharpoons$oligomer equilibrium of the ATPase. This process, too, would require changes in the protein-lipid interaction.

Biosynthesis. A counterpart of *in vitro* reconstitution studies have been those concerned with the biosynthesis of the sarcoplasmic reticulum both *in vivo* and in culture *in vitro* (MacLennan, Zubrzyck, Jorgensen and Kalnis, 1978; Martonosi, Roufa and Boland, in press). These studies show that, in the process of the sarcoplasmic reticulum membrane assembly, the insertion of the ATPase protein is the last step. The precise details of how proteins that extend through the lipid layer of the membrane become incorporated are, in general, still not fully understood (Wickner, 1979).

Calcium storage and release *in vivo*. The ability of the terminal cisternae of the sarcoplasmic reticulum *in situ* to accumulate calcium has been mentioned above. The release of Ca^{++} into the sarcoplasm of living muscle following stimulation has been demonstrated with the use of intracellular murexide (Jobsis and O'Connor, 1966) or utilising the Ca-dependent luminescence of aequorin (Ridgway and Ashley, 1967). The key role of Ca^{++} in the excitation-contraction coupling mechanism is also supported by Winegrad's autoradiographic work, showing movement of calcium from the region of the terminal sacs of the reticulum toward the actin-myosin overlap zone during excitation and in the opposite direction during relaxation (Winegrad, 1965; 1968). Recent reports (Meissner, 1975) showing that a fraction of the sarcoplasmic reticulum rich in components originating in the terminal sac, which is adjacent to the T tubule, is also enriched in calsequestrin but low in ATPase protein, supports the concept of the storage function of the former and a differential distribution of functional components in the sarcoplasmic reticulum.

The role of the transverse (T) tubular system in transmitting the excitation process to the interior of the muscle cell has already been mentioned. Evidence is now mounting that the action potential is propagated along the T system and, in a way that is not yet fully understood, causes the release of Ca^{++} from the sarcoplasmic reticulum proper (for a review of this problem *see* Endo, 1977; Peachey, 1972). A recently proposed scheme involves a depolarisation-induced movement of electrical charges that would open up Ca^{++} channels (Schneider and Chandler, 1973; Adrain, 1978; Kovas, Rios and Schneider, 1979).

Whether, particularly in cardiac muscle and red muscle, mitochondria in which accumulation of Ca^{++} and other ions has been demonstrated (DeLuca and Engstrom, 1961; Brierley, Bachman and Green, 1962; Vasington and Murphy, 1962; Carafoli, Gazzotti, Schwerzman and Niggli, 1977) may play a part in the regulation of contraction and relaxation in addition to their function of oxidative ATP synthesis is an interesting possibility, the elucidation of which will require further work. The so-called regenerative release of Ca^{++} from sarcoplasmic reticulum demonstrated *in vitro* (Endo, Tanaka and Ogawa, 1970; Ford and Podolsky, 1970), *vis.* stimulation of Ca^{++} release by small amounts of Ca^{++} insufficient to activate the actomyosin system, is doubtful in skeletal muscle (Costantin and Taylor, 1973) but may play a part in cardiac muscle (Fabiato and Fabiato, 1979).

SYNTHESIS OF MUSCLE PROTEINS

General

In view of the important role of proteins in muscle some problems of protein synthesis, an area which has recently been the subject of very active research, deserve a brief discussion. There is no reason to believe that fundamental processes of the proteins differ in muscle from those taking place in other tissues. It is quite clear from a number of studies that the proteins in muscle are in a dynamic state of equilibrium. It would also appear that, in wasting muscle diseases such as muscular dystrophy, an imbalance exists and the destructive processes take the upper hand (Simon, Gross and Lessel, 1962). Evidently an understanding of the normal processes of protein synthesis is of great importance in understanding the pathological problems discussed elsewhere in this volume.

According to generally accepted views the first step in protein synthesis is the so-called activation of amino acids (Hoagland, 1958), described by the following reaction:

amino acid + ATP → amino-acyl-AMP + pyrophosphate

Each activated amino-acyl-AMP can attach itself to a so-called soluble (or transfer) ribonucleic acid (tRNA) molecule (Hoagland, 1958); there is a specific tRNA for each amino acid. The instructions for the synthesis of a specific protein are contained in what is known as the messenger RNA (Brenner, Jacob and Mieselson, 1961) which in turn is determined (transcription) by the genetic information contained in the DNA in the chromosomes (Crick, Barnett, Brenner and Watts-Tobin, 1962). The messenger RNA enters into a combination with the so-called ribosome particles, which are free in the cytoplasm or are attached to an intracellular membrane system, the endoplasmic reticulum, and it is on this template that the tRNA amino acids are assembled into the polypeptide chain with the release of the tRNA molecules.

During recent years many details of the process of protein synthesis, both in prokaryotes (bacteria) and in eukaryotes (higher organisms) (Lucas-Lenard and Lipmann, 1971; Weissbach and Ochoa, 1976; Ochoa and deHaro, 1979) have been clarified. It would seem that all protein chains are initiated by formyl methionyl-tRNA (Adams and Capecchi, 1966), but in most finished proteins the formyl, and often also the methionyl group, is removed by appropriate enzymes (Adams, 1966). Initiation factors are involved, together with GTP, in the binding of the first amino acid tRNA to the so-called small, 40S, ribosomal sub-unit. Other factors are responsible for the binding of the mRNA to be translated. This occurs with the formation of an 80S ribosomal complex coupled to GTP hydrolysis. There are two sites on the ribosome, A and P. The attachment of the initial aminoacyl-tRNA takes place at the P site. The attachment of subsequent aminoacyl tRNAs occurs at the A site and requires an elongation factor

and GTP. The latter is hydrolysed as a peptide band is formed between the two amino acid residues. The peptide now on site A is then transferred to the P site. This step requires catalysis by another elongation factor and is accompanied by the hydrolysis of another GTP molecule. The now empty A site is ready for the binding of the next amino acyl tRNA and another cycle of peptide band formation begins. When the peptide chain is completed, which is signalled by a termination code on the mRNA, the chain is released in a process again involving GTP and a release factor.

Biosynthesis in muscle

As shown by Rich and his colleagues (Warner, Rich and Hall, 1962; Warner, Knopf and Rich, 1963) several ribosomes are attached to a single messenger RNA molecule to form a polyribosome or polysome. Because the length of the messenger RNA is proportional to the length of the polypeptide chain encoded in the messenger, the number of ribosomes per polysome is also proportional to the chain length. For example, in the synthesis of the polypeptide chain of haemoglobin with a molecular weight of 17 000, a ribosomal pentamer is involved. Polysome fractions isolated from embryonic muscle by means of the sucrose gradient technique have been used for in vitro synthesis of myofibrillar proteins. These studies have shown that the heavy and light chains of myosin, actin and tropomyosin sub-units are coded by monocistronic mRNAs (Heywood and Rich, 1968; Sarkar and Cooke, 1970; Low, Vournakis and Rich, 1971). Many of the mRNAs coding for myofibrillar proteins have been purified recently (Modal, Sutton, Chen and Sarkar, 1974; Heywood, Kennedy and Bester, 1975; Hunter and Garrels, 1977). Myofibrillar proteins furnish good examples of post-translational modification of the peptide chain. Thus N termini of all myofibrillar proteins are blocked (acetylated), and myosin and actin contain methylated residues (methylated histidines in myosin and actin, methylated lysines in myosin). The phosphorylation of certain residues discussed above represents another type of modification. It should be emphasised that, with the exception of the smooth muscle myosin light chain phosphorylation, the functional significance of these modifications is not clear.

Regulation

The problem of the control of protein synthesis is of great importance in muscle. Some muscle diseases, as mentioned above, are probably due to a change in the steady state involving protein synthesis and destruction (Goldberg and St. John, 1976). There is also the well-known hypertrophy of muscle in response to work, resulting in increased protein synthesis in general (Goldberg, 1968) and in increased synthesis of specific enzymes, such as creatine phosphokinase (Kendrick-Jones and Perry, 1965; 1967); the response of uterine muscle to stretch (Csapo, Erdo, de Mattos, Gramss and Moscowitz, 1965); the changes in muscle protein synthesis in response to hormones; and the whole field of neurotrophic relations (Gutmann, 1976). An unsolved problem is that of the chemical signal for the increase in protein synthesis in work-induced hypertrophy. Creatine has been suggested as a possible mediator (Morales, Ingwall, Stockdale, McKay, Brivio-Haugland and Kenyon, 1974). A recent report indicates the involvement of an RNA-like molecule in the hypertrophy of various organs including those, e.g. heart, that contain muscle tissue (Hammond, Wizben and Markert, 1979). These responses, as well as the unfolding of the genetically programmed sequence of protein-synthetic steps during embryonic differentiation, are instances of regulated genetically controlled processes in which it is quite likely that transcriptional control plays a key role. In addition to the transcriptional control known in prokaryotes, translational control is important in eukaryotes (Patterson and Bishop, 1977). It has been suggested that mRNAs are stored as protein-bound complexes in the form of nonpolysomal messenger ribonucleoprotein particles which are activated for translation of the mRNAs during the terminal differentiation of muscle cells (Dym, Kennedy and Heywood, 1979). The eukaryotes, with more stable mRNAs than prokaryotes, control at the translational level (Ochoa and deHaro, 1979). This also involves phosphorylation, catalysed by cyclic AMP-independent protein kinase, of one of the initiation factor sub-units. There are several kinases that are activated in different ways, which are also involved. Another mechanism operates through degradation of mRNA. While these processes in general are well understood, many questions relating to the specificity of control remain to be solved. One of these questions concerns the need for a specific initiation factor when, for example, muscle messenger RNA is translated on erythroblast ribosomes (Rourke and Heywood, 1972).

EFFECT OF CHANGES IN ACTIVITY AND INNERVATION

Starting with the work of Eccles and his colleagues (Eccles, Eccles and Lundberg, 1958; Buller, Eccles and Eccles, 1960), several authors have reported that when a fast muscle is cross-reinnervated by a nerve that originally supplied a slow muscle, it acquires properties characteristic of a slow muscle; reciprocal changes take place in a slow muscle that has been cross-reinnervated by a fast muscle nerve. Changes in contractile speed are accompanied by corresponding changes in both the myosin ATPase activity (Buller, Mommaerts and Seraydarian, 1969; Bárány and Close, 1971) and the protein sub-unit pattern (Sreter, Gergely and Luff, 1974; Weeds, Trentham, Kean and Buller, 1974). Changes have also been observed in the pattern of metabolic enzymes (Dubowitz, 1967; Romanul and Van Der Meulen, 1967; Guth, Watson and Brown, 1968; Weeds et al., 1974) and in the activity of the sarcoplasmic reticulum.

The work of Salmons and Vrbová (1969) shows that, even with undisturbed nerve-muscle connections, changes in physiological parameters can be brought about if the pattern of neural activity reaching the muscle is changed. When the motor nerve is stimulated continuously over a period of weeks, imposing on the fast muscle a pattern of activity similar to that normally reaching a slow muscle, a marked slowing of the time course of isometric contraction and relaxation ensues. Such stimulation also produces changes in the sub-units pattern of myosin, the ATPase activity of myosin, the staining pattern of LMM paracrystals, and the

Ca^{++} uptake of the sarcoplasmic reticulum. The changes correspond to an essentially constant fast→slow transformation. The biochemical changes in myosin are paralleled by changes in the histochemical ATPase reaction as well as by changes in the glycolytic oxidative enzyme pattern (Sreter, Gergely, Salmons, and Romanul, 1973; Pette, Smith, Staudte and Vrbová, 1973; Romanul, Sreter, Salmons and Gergely, 1974; Salmons and Sreter, 1976; Heilmann and Pette, 1979).

The change-over in the muscle type is attributable to the transformation of the existing fibres by the switching-on of normally inactive genes and the switching-off of those that had been active, rather than to the destruction of the original fibre population and its replacement by new fibres. This is shown by the fact that early in the course of the transformation of fast muscle, antibodies against both fast and slow myosins react with the same fibre (Rubinstein, Mabuchi, Pepe, Salmons and Sreter, 1978), while in normal fast muscle only the antibody against fast myosin reacts (Arndt and Pepe, 1975; Weeds, Hall and Spurway, 1975). After complete transformation, again only one type of antibody reacts—that reacting with slow myosin. The same conclusion has been reached from SDS-gel electrophoretic studies on single fibres showing the transient presence in the sarcoplasmic reticulum of both fast and slow type myosin light chains (Pette and Schnez, 1977). Other interventions leaving the nerve-muscle connection intact are also able to change the muscle type, as judged by histochemical and biochemical criteria. Thus, sectioning of the peroneal nerve caused changes in the ipsilateral soleus from slow to fast type (Guth and Wells, 1976). Removal of the gastrocnemius and soleus muscle in the rat caused the ipsilateral plantaris to change from the relatively fast to the slow type (Samaha and Theis, 1976).

Clearly, the fact that the changes in the activity pattern, with an undisturbed nerve-muscle connection, can alter the physiological and biochemical properties of a muscle raises many interesting questions concerning the so-called trophic effects of the motor nerve (Gutmann, 1976). More work will be required to differentiate genuine neural effects related to the type of nerve from those effects originating in the neural activity pattern.

THEORIES OF CONTRACTION AND RELAXATION

Sliding model

It is well established that myosin and actin are localised in distinct filaments in the myofibril. Furthermore, during contraction the length of the individual filaments does not change, but rather their relative position, which leads to what is summed up in the term sliding of interdigitating model of muscle contraction (Hanson and Huxley, 1955; Huxley, 1960). The classical experiments of Gordon, Huxley and Julian (1966) on single fibres, establishing a direct relation between overlap speed of shortening independent of overlap, not only support the sliding filament model but also the concept of independent force generators (see the thoughtful analysis of A.F. Huxley, 1976; 1979) identifiable with actin-myosin links in the overlap zone.

Molecular mechanisms

The question arises, how does the interaction between actin and myosin located in different structural elements lead to tension development and to shortening of the sarcomere? X-ray work on living muscle points to the movement of the bridges projecting from the myosin filaments as the molecular event underlying contraction (Huxley and Brown, 1967). Pepe's work (1966; 1967a, b) with the use of antibody staining techniques has revealed considerable changes within the thick filament structure during shortening, indicative of flexibility in some part—presumably the rod portion—of the myosin molecule. Flexibility of the rod portion would also account for the fact that the interaction between myosin and actin filaments results in the production of constant force per cross-bridge and the separation among filaments increases with decreasing sarcomere length (see Huxley, 1968, 1969). As mentioned above, various lines of experimental evidence support such flexibility in myosin. While most authors consider a direct interaction between the nearly globular portions (subfragment-1) of myosin and actin as the key to contraction, a less direct type—perhaps longer range—interaction involving electrostatic and Van der Waals forces has also been suggested (for discussions *see* A.F. Huxley, 1974, 1979, H.E. Huxley, 1979; Noble and Pollack, 1977). The arrow-head structures resulting from the interaction of HMM or S-1 with actin (Huxley, 1963) can be explained in terms of a regular attachment of the individual myosin heads to the actin globules, each head making a precise angle with the actin filament axis (Moore *et al.*, 1970). It appears reasonable to assume that the tendency of the myosin heads to align themselves in actin in this fashion represents an important driving force in the mechanism of muscle contraction. Recent refinements of the X-ray diffraction technique have made it possible to correlate changes in the diffraction in living contracting muscles with static and dynamic tension measurements and to interpret them in molecular terms (H.E. Huxley, 1979; Podolsky, 1979).

The precise mode of the force development by muscle has, however, still not finally been settled. A.F. Huxley (1957) originally proposed a mechanism in which thermal energy stored in some portion of the connecting bridges played an important part. A later proposal (Huxley and Simmons, 1971) involved attachment of myosin heads to actin via elastic connections, with the possibility of a tension-dependent equilibrium among several stable positions (Fig. 4.7). Eisenberg and Hill (1978) locate the elasticity in the band between the myosin head and actin and assume a rigid connecting link. The details of the way in which various intermediate stages in the hydrolysis of ATP can be correlated with configurational states on the myosin head with respect to actin are currently under investigation in several laboratories; studies utilising ATP-analogues are particularly promising (for recent reviews *see* Lymn, 1979; Taylor, 1979). The original mathematical analysis given by Huxley (1957) accounted for a number of mechanical and energetic features of muscle. More recent developments in muscle energetics and mechanics and our knowledge of the details of the molecular apparatus have prompted refinements in the theoretical models, such as those by T.L. Hill and his colleagues (Hill, 1974; Hill, 1975b; Hill, Eisenberg, Chen and Podolsky, 1975; Eisenberg and Hill, 1978; Eisenberg, Hill and Chen, 1980) describing in terms of

statistical mechanics, thermodynamics and kinetics the actin-myosin nucleotide system and serving as a framework for future theoretical and experimental interpretations.

Regulation

The key role of Ca^{++} in the regulation of the actin-myosin *in vitro* interaction has been discussed above, together with the role of the sarcoplasmic reticulum in the modulation of the free sarcoplasmic Ca^{++} concentration during contraction and relaxation. The question remains of how the *in vivo* interaction of Ca^{++} with the contractile apparatus fits the picture. There is the by now classical physiological evidence that injection of Ca^{++} into muscle cells produces contraction (Heilbrunn and Wiercinski, 1947). Podolsky and

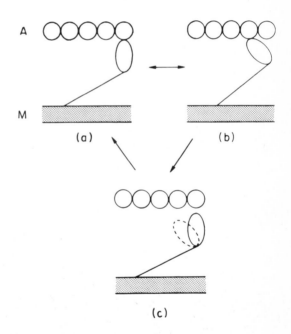

Fig. 4.7 Model of interaction of the myosin head with actin based on Huxley (1969), Huxley and Simmons (1971). (a) Attachment of myosin to actin, (b) Tilting of myosin head, (c) Detachment produced by ATP followed by its hydrolysis. On the basis of *in vitro* kinetic studies the myosin species present in (a) + (b) carries the ADP-P product complex. Whether the dissociated myosin head can oscillate between the perpendicular or tilted position or whether it is locked in the perpendicular position is not finally settled. Similarly, the precise point at which the product leaves the actin-myosin complex requires clarification. The attached head may oscillate between positions (a) and (b). For details *see text*

Costantin (1964), working on muscle stripped of its outer membrane, could by local application of Ca^{++} elicit contraction which, owing to the presence of Ca-accumulating reticular elements, spontaneously gave way to relaxation.

Activation by Ca^{++} would correspond to the removal of the inhibitory effect of the tropomyosin-troponin system in the interaction of actin and myosin observed *in vitro*. The molecular basis of this process appears to lie in a movement, deduced from X-ray and combined electron microscopic and optical diffraction studies, of the tropomyosin molecules located in the grooves of the actin filaments into positions where they would not interfere with the attachment of myosin heads (Haselgrove, 1972; Huxley, 1972; Spudich, Huxley and Finch, 1972; Parry and Squire, 1973). Whether or not such a movement relieves a steric block—and this has recently been questioned (O'Brien, Morris, Seymour and Couch, 1978)— the interaction of one tropomyosin molecule with seven actin molecules might account for the cooperative effects noted by Weber and her colleagues (Bremel and Weber, 1972; Bremel, Murray and Weber, 1972). The question of how the interaction of one or two Ca^{++} ions with one troponin complex per tropomyosin molecule can produce such a change in position might be answered on the basis of studies of the components of the myofilaments and their *in vitro* interactions (Hitchcock, Huxley and Szent-Györgyi, 1973; Margossian and Cohen, 1973; Potter and Gergely, 1975; Leavis, Rosenfeld, Gergely, Grabarek and Drabikowski, 1978). The question whether Ca^{++}

merely promotes the formation of cross-bridges between myosin and actin filaments (Podolsky and Teichholz, 1972) or whether Ca^{++} ions exert a direct influence on the movement of the myosin cross-bridges is still being debated (Julian, 1971; Julian and Sollins, 1972). The fact that Ca^{++} concentrations sufficient to activate cross-bridge formation also play a part in activating the phosphorylase system (Ozawa *et al.*, 1967) (for recent reviews *see* Cohen, 1978; Krebs and Beavo, 1979), thereby mobilising energy from glycogen, provides an interesting example of the close interweaving of various processes that underlie muscle contraction and its control. Other aspects of control that may play a part in the modulation of the activity of muscle, particularly of cardiac, on a longer time scale have been measured in connection with the phosphorylation of various protein components.

CONCLUSION

This brief survey of the biochemical features of muscle and their relation to structural problems is of necessity incomplete, but it should give an impression of the complexity of the processes involved. It clearly shows that a large number of sites at which defects may lead to serious disturbances of muscle function. Further elucidation of the gaps in our knowledge of the normal function of muscle is, therefore, of crucial importance for the understanding of the manifold disorders that are the subject of this volume.

REFERENCES

Adams, J.M. (1966) On the release of the formyl group from nascent protein. *Journal of Molecular Biology*, **33**, 571.

Adams, J.M. & Capecchi, M.R. (1966) N-formymethionyl-sRNA as the initiator of protein synthesis. *Proceedings of the National Academy of Sciences* (U.S.A.), **55**, 147.

Adrian, R.H. (1978) Charge movement in the membrane of striated muscle. *Annual Review of Biophysics and Bioengineering*, **7**, 85.

Akera, T. & Brody, T.M. (1978) The role of Na$^+$, K$^+$ ATPase in the inotropic action of digitalis. *Pharmacological Reviews*, **29**, 187.

Allen, G. & Green, N.M. (1978) Primary structure of cysteine-containing peptides from the calcium ion transporting adenosine triphosphatase of rabbit sarcoplasmic reticulum. *Biochemical Journal*, **173**, 393.

Andersen, B. & Ussing, H.H. (1960) Active transport. In *Comparative Biochemistry*, Eds M. Florkin & H.S. Mason, p. 371 (Academic Press: New York).

Appela, E. & Markert, C.L. (1961) Dissociation of lactate dehydrogenase into sub-units with guanidine hydrochloride. *Biochemical and Biophysical Research Communications*, **6**, 171.

Arndt, I. & Pepe, F. (1975) Antigenic specificity of red and white muscle myosin. *Journal of Histochemistry and Cytochemistry*, **23**, 159.

Asakura, S. (1961) F actin adenosine triphosphatase activated under sonic vibration. *Biochimica et biophysica acta* **52**, 65.

Asakura, S., Taniguchi, M. & Oosawa, F. (1963) The effect of sonic vibration on exchangeability and reactivity of the bound adenosine triphosphatase of F actin. *Biochimica et biophysica acta*, **74**, 140.

Asatoor, A.M. & Armstrong, M.D. (1967) 3-methylhistidine, a component of actin. *Biochemical and Biophysical Research Communications*, **26**, 168.

Atkinson, D.E. (1966) Regulation of enzyme activity. *Annual Review of Biochemistry*, **35**, 85.

Bagshaw, C.R. (1977) On the location of the divalent metal binding sites and the light chain sub-units of vertebrate myosin. *Biochemistry*, **16**, 59.

Bagshaw, C.R. & Kendrick-Jones, J. (1979) Characterization of homologous divalent metal ion binding sites of vertebrate and molluscan myosins using electron paramagnetic resonance spectroscopy. *Journal of Molecular Biology*, **130**, 317.

Bailey, K. (1948) Tropomyosin: A new asymmetric protein component of the muscle fibril. *Biochemical Journal*, **43**, 271.

Bailey, K. (1954) Structure Proteins II. Muscle. In *The Proteins*, Eds H. Neurath & K. Bailey, Vol. 2, p. 951 (Academic Press: New York).

Bailey, K. & Perry, S.V. (1947) The role of sulfhydryl groups in the interaction of myosin and actin. *Biochimica et Biophysica Acta*, **1**, 506.

Bailin, G. & Barany, J. (1967) Studies on actin-actin and actin-myosin interactions. *Biochimica et Biophysica Acta*, **140**, 208.

Balint, M., Sreter, F.A., Wolf, I., Nagy, B. & Gergely, J. (1975) The substructure of the heavy meromyosin. The effect of Ca^{2+} and Mg^{2+} on the tryptic fragmentation of heavy meromyosin. *Journal of Biological Chemistry*, **250**, 6168.

Bálint, M., Szilagyi, L., Fekete, G., Blasso, M. & Biro, N.A. (1968) Studies on proteins and protein complexes of muscle by means of proteolysis. Fragmentation of light meromyosin by trypsin. *Journal of Molecular Biology*, **37**, 317.

Balint, M., Wolf, I., Tarcsalvi, A., Gergely, J. & Sreter, F. (1978) Location of SH-1 and SH-2 in the heavy chain segment of heavy meromyosin. *Archives of Biochemistry and Biophysics*, **190**, 793.

Bangham, A.D. (1972) Lipid bilayers and biomembranes. *Annual Review of Biochemistry*, **41**, 753.

Bárany, M. (1967) Activity of myosin correlated with speed of muscle shortening. *Journal of General Physiology*, **50**, 197.

Bárany, M. & Bárány, K. (1959) Studies on 'active centres' of I-myosin. *Biochimica et Biophysica Acta*, **35**, 293.

Bárany, M. & Close, R.I. (1971) The transformation of myosin in cross-reinnervated rat muscle. *Journal of Physiology*, **213**, 458.

Bárány, M., Bárány, K., Reckard, T. & Volpe, A. (1965) Myosin of fast and slow muscles of the rabbit. *Archives of Biochemistry and Biophysics*, **109**, 185.

Bárány, M., Finkelman, F. & Therattil-Antony, T. (1962) Studies on the bound calcium of actin. *Archives of Biochemistry and Biophysics*, **98**, 28.

Barron, E.S.G. & Singer, T.P. (1945) Studies on biological oxidations. XIX. Sulfhydryl enzymes in carbohydrate metabolism. *Journal of Biological Chemistry*, **157**, 221.

Bastide, F., Meissner, G., Gleischer, S. & Post, R.L. (1973) Similarity of the active site of phosphorylation of the ATPase for transport of sodium and potassium ions in kidney to that for transport of calcium ions in the sarcoplasmic reticulum of muscle. *Journal of Biological Chemistry*, **248**, 8385.

Bendall, J.R. (1952) Effect of the 'Marsh Factor' on the shortening of muscle fibre models in the presence of adenosine triphosphate. *Nature*, **170**, 1058.

Bozler, E. (1954) Relaxation in extracted muscle fibers. *Journal of General Physiology*, **38**, 149.

Brand, L., Everse, J. & Kaplan, N.O. (1962) Structural characteristics of dehydrogenase. *Biochemistry*, **1**, 423.

Biró, N.A., Szilagyi, L. & Bálint, M. (1972) Studies on the helical segment of the myosin molecule. *Cold Spring Harbor Symposia on Quantitative Biology*, **37**, 55.

Bitensky, M.W. & Gorman, R.E. (1973) Cellular responses to cyclic AMP. *Progress in Biophysics and Molecular Biology*, **26**, 409.

Boyer, P.F. (1977) Oxidative phosphorylation and photophosphorylation. *Annual Review of Biochemistry*, **46**, 955.

Bremel, R.D. & Weber, A. (1972) Cooperative behaviour within the functional unit of the actin filament in vertebrate skeletal muscle. *Nature*, **238**, 97.

Brenner, S., Jacob, F. & Mieselson, M. (1961) Unstable intermediate carrying information from genes to ribosomes for protein synthesis. *Nature*, **190**, 576.

Bridgen, J. (1971) The amino acid sequence around four cysteine residues in trout actin. *Biochemical Journal*, **123**, 591.

Bridgen, J. (1972) The reactivity and function of thiol groups in trout actin. *Biochemical Journal*, **126**, 21.

Brierley, G.P., Bachman, E. & Green, D.E. (1962) Active transport of inorganic phosphate and magnesium ions by beef heart mitochondria. *Proceedings of the National Academy of Sciences of the United States of America*, **48**, 1928.

Briskey, E.J., Seraydarian, K. & Mommaerts, W.F.H.M (1967a) The modification of actomyosin by α-actinin III. The interaction between α-actinin and actin. *Biochimica et biophysica acta*, **133**, 424.

Briskey, E.J., Seraydarian, K. & Mommaerts, W.F.H.M. (1967b) The modification of actomyosin by α-actinin II. The effect of actinin upon contractility. *Biochimica et biophysica acta*, **133**, 412.

Brody, I.A. (1964) The significance of lactate dehydrogenase isozymes in abnormal human skeletal muscle. *Neurology (Minneapolis)*, **14**, 1091.

Brody, I.A. (1968) Histochemistry of lactate dehydrogenase isozymes in intact muscle. *Annals of the New York Academy of Sciences*, **151**, 587.

Buller, A.J., Eccles, J.C. & Eccles, R.M. (1960) Interactions between motor neurones and muscles in respect of the characteristic speeds of their responses. *Journal of Physiology*, **150**, 417.

Buller, A.J., Mommaerts, W.F.H.M. & Seraydarian, K. (1969) Enzymatic properties of myosin in fast and slow twitch muscles of the cat following cross-innervation. *Journal of Physiology*, **205**, 581.

Burke, R.E., Levine, D.N., Tsairis, P. & Zajac, F.E. III. (1973) Physiological types and histochemical profiles in motor units of the cat gastrocnemius. *Journal of Physiology*, **234**, 723.

Burke, M., Reisler, E. & Harrington, W.F. (1976) Effect of bridging the two essential thiols of myosin on its spectral and actin-binding properties. *Biochemistry*, **15**, 1923.

Burley, R., Seidel, J.C. & Gergely, J. (1971) The stoichiometry of the reaction of the spin labeling of F actin and the effect of orientation of spin labeled F actin filaments. *Archives of Biochemistry and Biophysics*, **146**, 597.

Burley, R., Seidel, J.C. & Gergely, J. (1972) The effect of divalent metal binding on the electron spin resonance spectra of spin labeled actin. Evidence for a spin-spin interaction involving Mn^{2+}. *Archives of Biochemistry and Biophysics*, **150**, 792.

Burton, K. (1957) In *Energy Transformation in Living Matter*, Eds H.A. Krebs & H.L. Kornberg (Springer: Berlin).

Cahn, R.D., Kaplan, N.O., Levine, L. & Swilling, E. (1962) Nature and development of lactic dehydrogenase. *Science*, **136**, 962.

Cain, D.F., Infante, A.A. & Davies, R.E. (1962) Chemistry of muscle contraction. *Nature*, **196**, 214.

Carafoli, E., Gazzotti, P., Schwerzman, K. & Niggli, V. (1977) Mitochondrial calcium binding proteins. In *Calcium Binding Proteins and Calcium Function*, Eds R.A. Corradino, E. Carafoli, R.H. Kretsinger, D.H. MacLennan & F.L. Siegal, p. 454 (North Holland: Amsterdam).

Carlson, F.D., Hardy, D.J. & Wilkie, D.R. (1963) Total energy production and phosphocreatine hydrolysis in the isotonic twitch. *Journal of General Physiology*, **46**, 851.

Carsten, M.E. & Katz, A.M. (1964) Actin: a comparative study. *Biochimica et biophysica acta*, **89**, 534.

Caspar, D.L.D., Cohen, C. & Longley, W. (1971) Tropomyosin: crystal structure polymorphism and molecular interactions. *Journal of Molecular Biology*, **41**, 87.

Chance, B., Mauriello, G. & Aubert, X.M. (1960) ADP arrival in muscle mitochondria following a twitch. In *Muscle as a Tissue*, Eds K. Rodahl & S.M. Horvath, p. 128 (McGraw Hill: New York).

Cheung, W.Y. (1971) Cyclic 3',5'-nucleotide phosphodiesterase. Evidence for and properties of a protein activator. *Journal of Biological Chemistry*, **246**, 2859.

Chou, P.Y. & Fasman, G.D. (1978) Prediction of the secondary structure of proteins from their amino acid sequence. *Advances in Enzymology*, **47**, 45.

Christensen, E.H. (1960) Fatigue of the working individual. In *Structure and Function of Muscle*, Ed. G.H. Bourne, Vol. II, p. 455 (Academic Press: New York).

Clarke, M. & Spudich, J.A. (1977) Nonmuscle contractile proteins. The role of actin and myosin in cell motility and shape determination. *Annual Review of Biochemistry*, **46**, 797.

Cohen, P. (1978) The role of cyclic AMP-dependent protein kinase in the regulation of glycose metabolism in mammalian skeletal muscle. In *Current Topics in Cell Regulation 1*, **14**, 117, Eds B.L. Horecker & E.R. Stadtman (Academic Press: New York).

Cohen, P., Burchell, A., Foulkes, G., Cohen, P.T.W., Vanaman, T.C. & Nairn, A.C. (1978) Identification of the Ca^{2+}-dependent modulator protein of the fourth sub-unit of rabbit skeletal phosphorylase kinase. *Federation of European Biochemical Society Letters*, **92**, 287.

Cohen, C., Caspar, D.L.D., Johnson, J.P., Nauss, K., Margossian, S.S. & Parry, D. (1972) Tropomyosin-troponin assembly. *Cold Spring Harbor Symposia on Quantitative Biology*, **37**, 287.

Cohen, C., Caspar, D.L.D., Parry, D.A.D. & Lucas, R.M. (1971) Tropomyosin crystal dynamics. *Cold Spring Harbor Symposia on Quantitative Biology*, **36**, 205.

Cohen, C. & Holmes, K.C. (1963) X-ray diffraction evidence for α helical coiled coils in native myosins. *Journal of Molecular Biology*, **6**, 423.

Cohen, C., Lowey, S., Harrison, R.G., Kendrick-Jones, J. & Szent-Györgyi, A.G. (1970) Fragments from myosin rods. *Journal of Molecular Biology*, **47**, 605.

Cohen, C. & Szent-Györgyi, A.G. (1957) Optical rotation and helical polypeptide chain configuration in α proteins. *Journal of the American Chemical Society*, **79**, 248.

Cole, H.A. & Perry, S.V. (1975) The phosphorylation of troponin 1 from cardiac muscle. *Biochemical Journal*, **149**, 525.

Collins, J.H. (1974) Homology of myosin light chains, troponin C and parvalbumin deduced from comparison of their amino acid sequences. *Biochemical and Biophysical Research Communications*, **58**, 301.

Collins, J.H., Greaser, M., Potter, J.D. & Horn, M. (1977) Determination of the amino acid sequence of troponin C from rabbit skeletal muscle. *Journal of Biological Chemistry*, **252**, 6356.

Collins, J.H., Potter, J.D., Horn, M., Wilshire, G. & Jackman, N. (1973) Structural studies on rabbit skeletal muscle troponin C: evidence for gene replications and homology with calcium binding proteins from carp and hake muscle. *Federation of European Biochemical Society Letters*, **36**, 268.

Colowick, S.P. & Kalckar, H.M. (1943) The role of myokinase in transphosphorylations I. The enzymatic phosphorylation of hexoses by adenyl pyrophosphate. *Journal of Biological Chemistry* **48**, 117.

Cooley, L.B., Johnson, W.H. & Krause, S. (1979) Phosphorylation of paramyosin and its possible role in the catch mechanism. *Journal of Biological Chemistry*, **254**, 2195.

Cori, C.F. (1942) Phosphorylation of carbohydrates. In *A Symposium on Respiratory Enzymes*, p. 175 (University of Wisconsin Press: Madison).

Cori, C.F. (1941) Phosphorylation of glycogen and glucose. *Biological Symposia*, **5**, 131.

Cori, C.F. (1956) In *Enzymes: Units of Biological Structure and Function*, Ed. O.H. Gaebler, p. 573 (Academic Press: New York).

Cori, G.T. & Cori, C.F. (1945) The enzymatic conversion of phosphorylase a to b. *Journal of Biological Chemistry*, **158**, 321.

Costantin, L., Franzini-Armstrong, C. & Podolsky, R. (1965) Localization of calcium accumulating structures in striated muscle fibers. *Science*, **147**, 158.

Costantin, L.L. & Taylor, S.R. (1973) Graded activation in frog muscle fibers. *Journal of General Physiology*, **61**, 424.

Crick, F.H.C., Barnett, L., Brenner, S. & Watts-Tobin, J.R. (1962) General nature of the genetic code for proteins. *Nature*, **192**, 1227.

Csapo, A., Erdos, T., de Mattos, C.R., Gramss, E. & Moscowitz, C. (1965) Stretch induced uterine growth, protein synthesis and function. *Nature*, **207**, 1378.

Cote, G.F., Lewis, W.S., Pato, M.D. & Smillie, L.B. (1978) Platelet tropomyosin; lack of binding to skeletal muscle troponin and correlation with sequence. *Federation of European Biochemical Society Letters*, **94**, 131.

Crick, F.H.C. (1953) The packing of α helices: simple coiled coils. *Acta crystallographica*, **6**, 689.

Cuatrecasas, P. (1972) Isolation of the insulin receptor of live and fat cell membrane. *Proceedings of the National Academy of Sciences of the United States of America*, **69**, 318.

Cummins, P. & Perry, S.V. (1973) D-3-hydroxybutyrate

dehydorgenase from rhodopseudomonas spheroides. *Biochemical Journal*, **133**, 765.

Cummins, P. & Perry, S.V. (1978) Troponin I from human skeletal and cardiac muscles. *Biochemical Journal*, **171**, 251.

Dabrowska, R., Sherry, J.M.F., Aromatario, D.K. & Hartshorne, D.J. (1978) Modulator protein as a component of the myosin light chain kinase from chicken gizzard. *Biochemistry*, **17**, 253.

Davies, R.E., Kushmerick, M.J. & Larson, R.E. (1967) Activation and the heat of shortening of muscle. *Nature*, **214**, 148.

Dawson, M.J., Gadian, D.G. & Wilkie, D.R. (1977) Contraction and recovery of living muscle studied by ^{31}P nuclear magnetic resonance. *Journal of Physiology*, **267**, 303.

Dawson, D.M. & Kaplan, N. (1965) Factors influencing the concentration of enzymes in various muscles. *Journal of Biological Chemistry*, **240**, 3215.

DeLuca, H.G. & Engstrom, G.W. (1961) Calcium uptake by rat kidney mitochondria. *Proceedings of the National Academy of Sciences of the United States of America*, **47**, 1744.

DeMeis, L. & Vianna, A.L. (1979) Energy interconversion by the Ca^{2+}-dependent ATPase of the sarcoplasmic reticulum. *Annual Review of Biochemistry*, **48**, 275.

Drabikowski, W., Barylko, B., Dabrowska, R., Nowak, E. & Szpacenko, A. (1974) Studies on the properties of Tn-C component of troponin and its effect on the interaction between the constituents of thin filament. In *Calcium Binding Proteins*, Eds W. Drabikowski, H. Strzelecka-Golaszewska & E. Carafoli, p. 69 (Elsevier: Amsterdam).

Drabikowski, W. & Gergely, J. (1962) The effect of the temperature of extraction on the tropomyosin content in actin. *Journal of Biological Chemistry*, **237**, 3412.

Drabikowski, W. & Gergely, J. (1963) The role of sulfhydryl groups in the polymerization and adenosine triphosphate binding of G actin. *Journal of Biological Chemistry*, **238**, 640.

Drabikowski, W., Grabarek, Z. & Barylko, B. (1977) Degradation of the TnC component of troponin by trypsin. *Biochimica et biophysica acta*, **490**, 216.

Drabikowski, W., Nowak, E., Barylko, B. & Dabrowska, R. (1972) Troponin—its composition an interaction with tropomyosin and F actin. *Cold Spring Harbor Symposia on Quantitative Biology*, **37**, 245.

Drabikowski, W. & Strzelecka-Golaszewska, H. (1963) The exchange of actin-bound calcium with various bivalent cations. *Biochimica et biophysica acta*, **71**, 486.

Dreizen, P., Gershman, L.C., Trotta, P.P. & Stracher, A. (1967) Myosin sub-units and their interactions. *Journal of General Physiology*, **50**, 85.

Dreizen, P. & Richards, D. (1972) Studies on the role of light and heavy chains in myosin adenosine triphosphatase. *Cold Spring Harbor Symposia on Quantitative Biology*, **37**, 29.

Dreyfus, J.C., Demos, J., Schapira, F. & Schapira, G. (1962) La lacticodes hydrogenase musculaire chez le myopathe: Persistence apparante du type foetal. *Comptes rendus hebdomadaire des séances de l'Academie des Sciences*, **254**, 4384.

Dubowitz, V. (1967) Cross-innervated mammalian skeletal muscle. Histochemical, physiological and biochemical observations. *Journal of Physiology*, **193**, 481.

Dubowitz, V. & Pearse, A.G.E. (1960) Reciprocal relationship of phosphorylase and oxidative enzymes in skeletal muscle. *Nature*, **185**, 701.

Duke, J., Takashi, R., Eu, K. & Morales, M.F. (1976) Reciprocal reactivities of specific thiols when actin binds to myosin. *Proceedings of the National Academy of Sciences of the United States of America*, **73**, 302.

Dym, H.P., Kennedy, D.S., & Heywood, S.M. (1979) Subcellular distribution of the cytoplasmic myosin heavy chain mRNA. *Differentiation*, **12**, 145.

Ebashi, S. (1957) Kielley-Meyerhof's granules and the relaxation of glycerinated muscle fibers. In *Conference on the Chemistry of Muscle Contraction*, p. 89 (Igaku Shoin Ltd: Tokyo).

Ebashi, S. (1961) Calcium binding activity of vesicular relaxing factor. *Journal of Biochemistry*, **50**, 236.

Ebashi, S. (1972) Separation of troponin into three components. *Journal of Biochemistry*, **72**, 787.

Ebashi, S. & Ebashi, F. (1964) A new protein component participating in the superprecipitation of myosin B. *Journal of Biochemistry*, **55**, 604.

Ebashi, S. & Ebashi, F. (1965) α-actinin: a new structural protein from striated muscle I. Preparation and action on actomyosin ATP interactions. *Journal of Biochemistry*, **58**, 7.

Ebashi, S., Ebashi, F. & Fujie, Y. (1960) The effect of EDTA and its analogues on glycerinated muscle fibers and myosin adenosine triphosphatase. *Journal of Biochemistry*, **47**, 54.

Ebashi, S., Ebashi, F. & Maruyama, K. (1964) A new protein factor promoting contraction of actomyosin. *Nature*, **203**, 645.

Ebashi, S. & Endo, M. (1968) Calcium ion and muscle contraction. *Progress in Biophysics and Molecular Biology*, **18**, 123.

Ebashi, S., Endo, M. & Ohtsuki, I. (1969) Control of muscle contraction. *Quarterly Review of Biophysics*, **2**, 351.

Ebashi, S. & Kodama, A. (1965) A new protein factor promoting aggregation of tropomyosin. *Journal of Biochemistry*, **58**, 107.

Ebashi, S. & Kodama, A. (1966) Interaction of troponin with F actin in the presence of tropomyosin. *Journal of Biochemistry*, **59**, 425.

Ebashi, S. & Lipmann, F. (1962) Adenosine triphosphate linked concentration of calcium ions in a particulate fraction of rabbit muscle. *Journal of Cell Biology*, **14**, 389.

Ebashi, S., Mikawa, T., Hirata, M. & Nonomura, Y. (1978) The regulatory role of calcium in muscle. *Annals of the New York Academy of Sciences*, **307**, 451.

Ebashi, S. & Nonomura, Y. (1967) Regulatory structural proteins of muscle. Abstract, *VIIth International Congress of Biochemistry*, Symposium VI, p. 329.

Ebashi, S., Ohtsuki, I. & Mihashi, K. (1972) Regulatory proteins of muscle with special reference to troponin. *Cold Spring Harbor Symposia of Quantitative Biology*, **37**, 215.

Eccles, J.C., Eccles, R.M. & Lundberg, A. (1958) The action potentials of the α motor neurones supplying fast and slow muscle. *Journal of Physiology*, **142**, 275.

Edholm, O.G. (1960) Some effects of fatigue, temperature and training in muscular contraction in man. In *The Structure and Function of Muscle*, Ed. G.H. Bourne, Vol. II, p. 449 (Academic Press: New York).

Edman, P. & Begg, G. (1967) A protein sequenator. *Journal of Biochemistry*, **1**, 80.

Eggleton, P. & Eggleton, G.P. (1927a) The inorganic phosphate and a labile form of organic phosphate in the gastrocnemius of the frog. *Biochemical Journal*, **21**, 190.

Eggleton, P. & Eggleton, G.P. (1927b) The physiological

significance of phosphagen. *Journal of Physiology*, **63**, 155.

Eisenberg, E. & Hill, T.L. (1978) A crossbridge model of muscle contraction. *Progress in Biophysics and Molecular Biology*, **13**, 55.

Eisenberg, E., Hill, T.L. & Chen, Yi-der (1980) A crossbridge model of muscle contraction; quantitative analysis. *Biophysical Journal*, **29**, 195.

Eisenberg, E. & Kielley, W.W. (1972) Reconstitution of active troponin-tropomyosin complex in the absence of urea from its four column purified components. *Federation Proceedings. Federation of American Societies for Experimental Biology*, **31**, 502.

Elliott, A. & Offer, G. (1978) Shape and flexibility of the myosin molecule. *Journal of Molecular Biology*, **123**, 505.

Elzinga, M. & Collins, J. (1972) The amino acid sequence of rabbit skeletal muscle actin. *Cold Spring Harbor Symposia on Quantitative Biology*, **37**, 1.

Elzinga, M. & Collins, J.H. (1977) Amino acid sequence of a myosin fragment that contains SH-1, SH-2 and N$^\tau$-methylhistidine. *Proceedings of the National Academy of Sciences of the United States of America*, **74**, 4281.

Elzinga, M., Collins, J.H., Kuehl, W.M. & Adelstein, R.S. (1973) The complete amino acid sequence of rabbit skeletal muscle actin. *Proceedings of the National Academy of Sciences of the United States of America*, **70**, 2687.

Elzinga, M., Maron, B.J. & Adelstein, R.S. (1976) Human heart and platelet actins are products of different genes. *Science*, **191**, 94.

Endo, M. (1977) Calcium release from the sarcoplasmic reticulum. *Physiological Reviews*, **57**, 71.

Endo, M., Tanaka, M. & Ogawa, Y. (1970) Calcium-induced release of calcium from the sarcoplasmic reticulum of skinned skeletal muscle fibers. *Nature*, **228**, 34.

Engelhardt, W.A. & Ljubimova, M.N. (1939) Myosins and adenosinetriphosphatase. *Nature*, **144**, 668.

England, P. (1976) Studies on the phosphorylation of the inhibitory sub-unit of troponin during modification of contraction in perfused heart. *Biochemical Journal*, **160**, 295.

Ernster, L. & Lee, C.-P. (1964) Biological oxidoreductions. *Annual Review of Biochemistry*, **33**, 729.

Fabiato, A. & Fabiato, F. (1979) Calcium and cardiac excitation-contraction coupling. *Annual Review of Physiology*, **41**, 473.

Fasman, D.G., Ed. (1967) *Poly-α-amino Acids*, Chapters 6 and 7 (Dekker: New York).

Fenn, W.O. (1923) A quantitative comparison between the energy liberated and the work performed by isolated sartorius muscle. *Journal of Physiology*, **58**, 175.

Fenn, W.O. (1924) The relation between the work performed and the energy liberated in muscular contraction. *Journal of Physiology*, **58**, 373.

Fernandez-Moran, H. (1962) Cell membrane ultrastructure. Low temperature electron microscopy and X-ray diffraction studies of lipoprotein components in lamellar systems. *Circulation*, **26**, 1039.

Fischer, E.H., Heilmeyer, L.M.G., Jr. & Haschke, R.H. (1971) Phosphorylase and the control of glycogen degradation. In *Current Topics in Cellular Regulation*, Vol. IV Eds B.L. Horecker & E.R. Stadtman, p. 211 (Academic Press: New York).

Flavin, M. & Ochoa, S. (1957) Metabolism of propionic acid in animal tissues I. Enzymatic conversion of propionate to succinate. *Journal of Biological Chemistry*, **229**, 965.

Fleckenstein, A., Janke, J., Davies, R.E. & Krebs, H.A.

(1954) Chemistry of muscle contraction. *Nature*, **174**, 1081.

Ford, L.E. & Podolsky, R.J. (1970) Regenerative calcium release within muscle cells. *Science*, **167**, 58.

Frank, G. & Weeds, A.G. (1974) The amino acid sequence of some alkali light chains of rabbit skeletal muscle myosin. *European Journal of Biochemistry*, **44**, 317.

Franzini-Armstrong, C. & Porter, K.R. (1964) Sarcolemmal invaginations and the T system in fish skeletal muscle. *Nature*, **202**, 355.

Frearson, N., Solaro, R.J. & Perry, S.V. (1976) Changes in phosphorylation of the light chain of myosin in perfused rabbit heart. *Nature*, **264**, 801.

Frieden, C. (1979) Slow transitions and hysteretic behavior in enzymes. *Annual Review of Biochemistry*, **48**, 1079.

Friedman, D.L. & Larner, J. (1963) Studies on UDPG-α-glucan transglucosylae III. Interconversion of two forms of muscle UDPG-α-glucan transglucosylase by a phosphorylation-dephosphorylation reaction sequence. *Biochemistry*, **2**, 669.

Fritz, I.B., Davis, D.G., Holtrop, R.H. & Dundee, H. (1958) Fatty acid oxidation by skeletal muscle during rest and activity. *American Journal of Physiology*, **194**, 379.

Gazith, J.S., Himmelfarb, S. & Harrington, W.F. (1970) Studies on the sub-unit structure of myosin. *Journal of Biological Chemistry*, **245**, 15.

Gergely, J. (1950) Relation of ATPase and myosin. *Federation Proceedings. Federation of American Societies for Experimental Biology*, **9**, 176.

Gergely, J. (1953) Studies on myosin-adenosine triphosphatase. *Journal of Biological Chemistry*, **200**, 543.

Gergely, J. (1956) The interaction between actomyosin and adenosine triphosphate. Light scattering studies. *Journal of Biological Chemistry*, **220**, 917.

Gergely, J. (1966). Contractile proteins. *Annual Review of Biochemistry*, **35**, 691.

Gergely, J., Gouvea, M.A. & Karibian, D. (1955) Fragmentation of myosin by chymotrypsin. *Journal of Biological Chemistry*, **212**, 165.

Gergely, J. & Kohler, H. (1957) Light scattering studies on the stepwise formation and dissociation of actomyosin. In *Conference on the Chemistry of Muscular Contraction*, p. 14 (Igaku Shoin Ltd: Tokyo).

Gergely, J. & Spicer, S.S. (1951) On factors affecting the reversible superprecipitation of actomyosin. *Biochimica et biophysica acta*, **6**, 456.

Gilbert, C., Kretzschmar, K.M. & Wilkie, D.R. (1972) Work and phosphocreatine splitting during muscular contraction. *Cold Spring Harbor Symposia on Quantitative Biology*, **37**, 613.

Gilbert, C., Kretzschmar, M., Wilkie, D.R. & Woledge, R.C. (1971) Chemical change and energy output during muscular contraction. *Journal of Physiology*, **218**, 163.

Goldberg, A.L. (1968) Protein synthesis during work induced growth of skeletal muscle. *Journal of Cell Biology*, **36**, 653.

Goldberg, A.L. & St. John, A.C. (1976) Intracellular protein degradation in mammalian and bacterial cells. *Annual Review of Biochemistry*, **45**, 933.

Goldman, R.D., Milsted, A., Schloss, J.A. Starger, J. & Yerna, M.J. (1979) Cytoplasmic fibers in mammalian cells: cytoskeleletal and contractile elements. *Annual Review of Physiology*, **41**, 703.

Goll, D., Mommaerts, W.F.H.M., Reedy, M.K. & Seraydarian, K. (1969) Studies on α-actinin-like proteins liberated during trypsin digestion of α-actinin and of myofibrils. *Biochimica et biophysica acta.* **175**, 174.

Goll, D., Mommaerts, W.F.H.M. & Seraydarian, K. (1967) Is α-actinin a constituent of the Z band of the muscle fibril. *Federation Proceedings. Federation of American Societies for Experimental Biology*, **26**, 1349.

Goodno, C.C., Wall, C.M. & Perry, S.V. (1978) Kinetics and regulation of adenosine triphosphatase. *Biochemical Journal*, **175**, 813.

Gordon, A.M., Huxley, A.F. & Julian, F.J. (1966) The variation in isometric tension with sarcomere lengths in vertebrate muscle fibers. *Journal of Physiology*, **184**, 170.

Granger, D.L. & Lazarides, E. (1978) The existence of an insoluble Z disc scaffold in chicken skeletal muscle. *Cell*, **15**, 1253.

Greaser, M. & Gergely, J. (1971) Reconstitution of troponin activity from three protein components. *Journal of Biological Chemistry*, **246**, 4226.

Greaser, M. & Gergely, J. (1973) Purification and properties of the components from troponin. *Journal of Biological Chemistry*, **248**, 2125.

Greaser, M., Yamaguchi, M., Brekke, C., Potter, J. & Gergely, J. (1972) Troponin subunits and their interactions. *Cold Spring Harbor Symposia on Quantitative Biology*, **37**, 235.

Green, D.E. (1954) Fatty acid oxidation in soluble systems of animal tissues. *Biological Reviews*, **29**, 330.

Green, D.E. (1966) The mitochondrial electron transfer system I. In *Comprehensive Biochemistry*, Eds M. Florkin and E.H. Stotz, Vol. 14, p. 309 (Elsevier: Amsterdam).

Grubhofer, N. & Weber, H.H. (1961) Uber adenin-nucleotide und die function und binding der nucleotidphosphate in G und F actin. *Zeitschrift für Naturforschung*, **16**, 435.

Guba, F., Harsanyi, V. & Vajda, E. (1968) The muscle protein fibrillin. *Acta biochimica et biophysica Acadamiae scientiarum hungaricae*, **3**, 353.

Guidotti, G. (1972) Membrane proteins. *Annual Review of Biochemistry*, **41**, 731.

Guth, L., Watson, P.K. & Brown, W.C. (1968) Effects of cross reinnervation on some chemical properties of red and white muscles of rat and cat. *Experimental Neurology*, **20**, 52.

Guth, L. & Wells, J.B. (1976) Physiological and histochemical properties of the soleus muscle after denervation of its antagonists. *Experimental Neurology*, **51**, 310.

Gutmann, E. (1976) Neurotrophic relations. *Annual Review of Physiology*, **38**, 177.

Hama, H., Maruyama, K. & Noda, H. (1965) Direct isolation of F actin from myofibrils and its physicochemical properties. *Biochimica et biophysica acta*, **102**, 149.

Hammond, G.L., Wizben, E. & Markert, C.L. (1979) Molecular signals for initiating protein synthesis in organ hypertrophy. *Proceedings of the National Academy of Sciences of the United States of America*, **76**, 2455.

Hanson, J. (1968) X-ray diffraction studies of muscle, *Quarterly Review of Biophysics*, **1**, 177.

Hanson, J. & Huxley, H.E. (1955) The structural basis of contraction in striated muscle. *Symposium of the Society of Experimental Biology*, **9**, 228.

Hanson, J. & Huxley, H.E. (1957) Quantitative studies on the structure of cross-striated myofibrils II. Investigations by biochemical techniques. *Biochimica et biophysica acta*, **23**, 250.

Hanson, J. & Lowy, J. (1963) The structure of F actin and of

elements isolated from muscle. *Journal of Molecular Biology*, **6**, 46.

Hardy, M., Harris, I., Perry, S.V. & Stone, D. (1970) ε-n-monomethyllysine and trimethyl-lysine in myosin. *Biochemical Journal*, **117**, 44P.

Hardy, M.F. & Perry, S.V. (1969) In vitro methylation of muscle protein. *Nature*, **223**, 300.

Harrington, W.F. & Burke, M. (1972) Geometry of the myosin dimer in high salt media I. Association behaviour of rod segments from myosin. *Biochemistry*, **11**, 1448.

Harrington, W.F., Burke, M. & Barton, J.S. (1972) Association of myosin to form contractile systems. *Cold Spring Harbor Symposia on Quantitative Biology*, **37**, 77.

Hartshorne, D.J. & Dreizen, P. (1972) Studies on the sub-unit composition of troponin. *Cold Spring Harbor Symposia on Quantitative Biology*, **37**, 225.

Hartshorne, D.J. & Mueller, H. (1968) Fractionation of troponin into two distinct proteins. *Biochemical and Biophysical Research Communications*, **31**, 647.

Hartshorne, D.J., Theiner, M. & Mueller, H. (1969) Studies on troponin. *Biochimica et biophysica acta*, **175**, 320.

Haschke, R., Heilmeyer, M., Meyer, F. & Fischer, F. (1970) Control of phosphorylase activity in a muscle glycogen particle I. Isolation and characterization of the protein-glycogen complex. *Journal of Biological Chemistry*, **245**, 6642.

Haselgrove, J.C. (1972) X-ray evidence for a conformational change in the actin-containing filaments of vertebrate striated muscle. *Cold Spring Harbor Symposia on Quantitative Biology*, **37**, 341.

Hasselbach, W. (1952) Die unwandlung von aktomyosin-ATPase in L-myosin-ATPase durch aktivatoren und die resultierenden aktiverungseffeke. *Zeitschrift für Naturforschung*, **7b**, 163.

Hasselbach, W. (1953) Elektronmikroskopische untersuchungen a muskelfibrillen totale und particuller extraction des L-myosins. *Zeitschrift für Naturforschung*, **86**, 449.

Hasselbach, W. (1964) Relaxation and the sarcotubular calcium pump. *Federation Proceedings. Federation of American Societies for Experimental Biology*, **23**, 909.

Hasselbach, W. (1979) The sarcoplasmic calcium pump. A model of energy transduction. In *Biological Membranes. Current Topics in Chemistry*, **78**, 1.

Hasselbach, W. & Makinose, M. (1961) Die calciumpumpe der erschlaffungs grana des muskels und ihre abhangigheit von der ATP spaltung. *Biochemische Zeitschrift*, **333**, 518.

Hasselbach, W. & Makinose, M. (1963) Uber den mechanismus des calcium transportes durch die membranen des sarkoplasmiatschen reticulums. *Biochemische Zeitschrift*, **339**, 94.

Hasselbach, W. & Weber, H.H. (1953) Der einfluss des M-B-faktors auf die kontraktion des fasermodells. *Biochimica et biophysica acta*, **11**, 160.

Hayashi, T. (1967) Reactivities of actin as a contractile protein. *Journal of General Physiology*, **50**, 119.

Hayashi, T. & Rosenbluth, R. (1962) Actin polymerization by direct transphosphorylation. *Biochemical and Biophysical Research Communications*, **8**, 20.

Heilbrunn, L.V. & Wiercinski, F.J. (1947) The action of various cations on muscle protoplasm. *Journal of Cellular and Comparative Physiology*, **29**, 15.

Heilmann, C. & Pette, D. (1979) Molecular transformations in sarcoplasmic reticulum of fast twitch muscle by electro-stimulation. *European Journal of Biochemistry*, **93**, 437.

Heilmeyer, M., Meyer, F., Haschke, R. & Fischer, E. (1970) Control of phosphorylase activity in a muscle glycogen particle II. Activation by calcium. *Journal of Biological Chemistry*, **245**, 6649.

Helander, E. (1957) On quantitative muscle protein determination, sarcoplasm and myofibrillar protein content of normal and atrophic skeletal muscles. *Acta physiologica scandinavica*, **41**, supplement 141.

Herbert, T.J. & Carlson, F.D. (1971) Spectroscopic study of the self association of myosin. *Biopolymers*, **10**, 2231.

Heywood, S.M., Kennedy, D.S. & Bester, A.J. (1975) Stored myosin messenger in embryonic chick muscle. *Federation of the European Biochemical Society Letters*, **53**, 69.

Heywood, S.M. & Rich, A. (1968) *In vitro* synthesis of native myosin, actin and tropomyosin from embryonic chick polysomes. *Proceedings of the National Academy of Sciences of the United States of America*, **59**, 590.

Hidalgo, C., Ikemoto, N. & Gergely, J. (1976) Role of phospholipids in the Ca-dependent ATPase of the sarcoplasmic reticulum. Enzymatic and electron spin resonance studies with phospholipid replaced membrane. *Journal of Biological Chemistry*, **250**, 7219.

Hidalgo, C., Thomas, D.D. & Ikemoto, N. (1978) Effect of the lipid environment on protein motion and enzymatic activity of the sarcoplasmic reticulum Ca ATPase. *Journal of Biological Chemistry*, **253**, 6879.

Highsmith, S., Kretzchmar, K.M., O'Konski, C.T. & Morales, M.F. (1977) Flexibility of the myosin rod, light meromyosin and myosin subfragment 2 in solution. *Proceedings of the National Academy of Sciences of the United States of America*, **74**, 4986.

Hill, A.V. (1949) Work and heat in a muscle twitch. *Proceedings of the Royal Society, Series B*, **136**, 220.

Hill, A.V. (1964a) The effect of load on the heat of shortening of muscle. *Proceedings of the Royal Society, Series B*, **159**, 297.

Hill, A. V. (1964b) The efficiency of mechanical power development during muscular shortening and its relation to load. *Proceedings of the Royal Society, Series B*, **159**, 319.

Hill, A.V. (1964c) The effect of tension in prolonging the active state in a twitch. *Proceedings of the Royal Society, Series B*, **159**, 589.

Hill, A.V. (1964d) The variation of total heat production in a twitch with velocity of shortening. *Proceedings of the Royal Society, Series B*, **159**, 596.

Hill, T.L. (1974) Theoretical formalism for the sliding filament model of contraction of striated muscle. Part I. *Progress in Biophysics and Molecular Biology*, **28**, 267.

Hill, T.L. (1975a) Free energy and the kinetics of biochemical diagrams including actin transport. *Biochemistry*, **14**, 2127.

Hill, T.L. (1975b) Theoretical formalism for the sliding filament model of contraction of striated muscle. Part II. *Progress in Biophysics and Molecular Biology*, **29**, 105.

Hill, T.L., Eisenberg, E., Chen, Y. & Podolsky, R.J. (1975) Some self-consistent two-state sliding filament models of muscle contraction. *Biophysical Journal*, **15**, 335.

Hill, T.L. & Simmons, R.M. (1976) Free energy levels and entropy production in muscle contraction and in related solution systems. *Proceedings of the National Academy of Sciences of the United States of America*, **73**, 336.

Hirs, C.H.W., Moore, S. & Stein, W.H. (1960) The sequence of the amino acid residues in performic acid-oxidized ribonuclease. *Journal of Biological Chemistry*, **235**, 633.

Hitchcock, S.E., Huxley, H.E. & Szent-Györgyi, A.G. (1973) Calcium sensitive binding of troponin to actin-tropomyosin: a two site model for troponin action. *Journal of Molecular Biology*, **80**, 825.

Hitchcock, S.E. & Szent-Györgyi, A.G. (1973) Calcium dependent interaction of troponin with actin and tropomyosin. *Biophysical Journal*, **13**, 79a.

Hoagland, M.B. (1958) Enzymatic reactions between amino acids and ribonucleic acid as intermediate steps in protein synthesis. In *Proceedings of the Fourth International Congress of Biochemistry*, Symposium VIII.

Hoch, F.L. & Lipmann, F. (1954) The uncoupling of respiration and phosphorylation by thyroid hormones. *Proceedings of the National Academy of Sciences of the United States of America*, **40**, 909.

Hodges, R.S., Sodek, J., Smillie, L.B. & Jurasek, L. (1972) Tropomyosin: amino acid sequence and coiled-coil structure. *Cold Spring Harbor Symposia on Quantitative Biology*, **37**, 299.

Hoh, J.F.Y. & Yeoh, G.P.S. (1979) Rabbit skeletal myosin isozymes from fetal, fast-twitch and slow-twitch muscles. *Nature*, **280**, 321.

Holt, J.C. & Lowey, S. (1977) Distribution of alkali light chains in myosin: isolation of isozymes. *Biochemistry*, **16**, 4398.

Holtzer, H. & Duntze, W. (1971) Metabolic regulation by chemical modification of enzymes. *Annual Review of Biochemistry*, **40**, 345.

Homsher, E. & Kean, C.J. (1978) Skeletal muscle energetics and metabolism. *Annual Review of Physiology*, **40**, 931.

Homsher, E., Kean, C.J., Wallner, A. & Garibian-Sarlan, V. (1979) The time course of energy balance in an isometric tetanus. *Journal of General Physiology*, **73**, 553.

Horowicz, P. (1961) Influence of ions on the membrane potential of muscle fibres. In *Biophysics of Physiological and Pharmacological Actions*, Ed. A.M. Shanes, p. 217 (American Association for the Advancement of Science: Washington).

Hoyle, G. (1967) Diversity of striated muscle. *American Zoologist*, **7**, 435.

Hoyle, G., McNeil, P.A. & Selverston, A.I. (1973). Ultrastructure of barnacle giant muscle fibers. *Journal of Cell Biology*, **56**, 74.

Hunter, T. & Garrells, J.I. (1977) Characterization of the mRNAs for α, β an γ actin. *Cell*, **12**, 767.

Huszar, G. (1972) Amino acid sequences around the two ε-n-trimethyllysine residues in rabbit. *Journal of Biological Chemistry*, **247**, 4057.

Huszar, G. & Elzinga, M. (1969) ε-n methyl lysine in myosin. *Nature*, **223**, 834.

Huszar, G. & Elzinga, M. (1971) The amino acid sequence around the single 3-methyl histidine residue in rabbit skeletal muscle myosin. *Biochemistry*, **10**, 229.

Huxley, A.F. (1957) Muscle structure and theories of contraction. *Progress in Biophysics*, **7**, 255.

Huxley, A.F. (1976) Muscular contraction: review lecture. *Journal of Physiology*, **243**, 1.

Huxley, A.F. (1979) *Reflections on Muscle* (University Liverpool Press: Liverpool).

Huxley, A.F. & Simmons, R.M. (1971) Proposed mechanism of force generation in striated muscle. *Nature*, **233**, 533.

Huxley, A.F. & Taylor, R.E. (1958) Local activation of striated muscle fibres. *Journal of Physiology*, **144**, 426.

Huxley, H.E. (1960) Muscle cells. In *The Cell*, Eds J.

Brachet & A.E. Mirsky, Vol. IV, p. 365 (Academic Press: New York).

Huxley, H.E. (1963) Electron microscope studies on the structure of natural and synthetic protein filaments from striated muscle, *Journal of Molecular Biology*, **7**, 281.

Huxley, H.E. (1964) Evidence for continuity between the central elements of the triads and extracellular space in frog sartorius muscle. *Nature*, **202**, 1067.

Huxley, H.E. (1968) Structural difference between resting and rigor muscle. Evidence from intensity changes in the low angle equatorial X-ray diagram. *Journal of Molecular Biology*, **37**, 3542.

Huxley, H.E. (1969) The mechanism of muscle contraction. *Science*, **164**, 1356.

Huxley, H.E. (1972) Structural changes in the actin- and myosin-containing filaments during contraction. *Cold Spring Harbor Symposia on Quantitative Biology*, **37**, 361.

Huxley, H.E. (1979) Structure. In *Molecular Basis of Force Development in Muscle*, Ed. N.B. Ingels, Jr., p. 1 (Palo Alto Medical Research Foundation: Palo Alto).

Huxley, H.E. & Brown, W. (1967) The low angle X-ray diagram of vertebrate striated muscle and its behaviour during contraction and rigor. *Journal of Molecular Biology*, **1**, 30.

Huxley, H.E. & Hanson, J. (1957) Quantitative studies on the structure of cross-striated myofibrils. I. Investigations by interference microscopy. *Biochimica et biophysica acta*, **23**, 229.

Ikemoto, N. (1975) Transporting and inhibitory Ca^{2+}-binding sites on the ATPase enzyme isolated from sarcoplasmic reticulum. *Journal of Biological Chemistry*, **250**, 7219.

Ikemoto, N. (1976) Behaviour of the Ca^{2+}-transport sites linked with the phosphorylation reaction of ATPase purified from the sarcoplasmic reticulum. *Journal of Biological Chemistry*, **251**, 7275.

Ikemoto, N., Bhatnagar, G. & Gergely, J. (1971) Fractionation of solubilized sarcoplasmic reticulum. *Biochemical and Biophysical Research Communications*, **44**, 1510.

Ikemoto, N., Morgan, J. & Yamada, S. (1978) Controlled conformational states of the Ca^{2+}-transport enzyme of sarcoplasmic reticulum. *Journal of Biological Chemistry*, **253**, 8027.

Ikemoto, N., Bhatnagar, G., Nagy, B. & Gergely, J. (1972) Interaction of divalent cations with the 55000 dalton protein component of the sarcoplasmic reticulum. Studies of fluorescence and circular dichroism. *Journal of Biological Chemistry*, **247**, 7835.

Ikemoto, N., Sreter, F., Nakamura, A. & Gergely, J. (1968) Tryptic digestion and localisation of Ca-uptake and ATPase activity in fragments of sarcoplasmic reticulum. *Journal of Ultrastructure Research*, **23**, 216.

Idemoto, N., Sreter, F.A., Nakamura, A. & Gergely, J. (1968) Tryptic digestion and localization of Ca-uptake and ATPase activity in fragments of sarcoplasmic reticulum. *Journal of Ultrastructure Research*, **23**, 216.

Inesi, G., Millman, M. & Eletr, S. (1973) Temperature induced transitions of function structure in sarcoplasmic reticulum membranes. *Journal of Molecular Biology*, **81**, 483.

Ishiwata, S. & Fujime, S. (1972) Effect of calcium ions on the flexibility of reconstituted thin filaments of muscle studied by quasi-elastic scattering of laser light. *Journal of Molecular Biology*, **68**, 511.

Iyengar, M.R. & Weber, H.H. (1964) The relative affinities of nucleotides to G actin and their effects. *Biochimica et biophysica acta*, **86**, 543.

Jackson, P., Amphlett, G.W. & Perry, S.V. (1975) The primary structure of troponin T and the interaction with tropomyosin. *Biochemical Journal*, **151**, 85.

Jobsis, F.F. & O'Connor, M.J. (1966) Calcium release and reabsorption in the sartorius muscle of the toad. *Biochemical and Biophysical Research Communications*, **25**, 246.

Johnson, J.D., Charlton, S.C. & Potter, J.D. (1979) A fluorescence stopped-flow analysis of Ca^{2+}-exchange with troponin C. *Journal of Biological Chemistry*, **254**, 3497.

Johnson, J.D., Collins, J.H. & Potter, J.D. (1978) Dansylaziridine-labelled troponin C. A fluorescent probe of Ca^{2+}-binding for the Ca^{2+}-specific regulatory sites. *Journal of Biological Chemistry*, **253**, 6451.

Johnson, P., Harris, C.I. & Perry, S.V. (1967) 3-methylhistidine in actin and other muscle proteins. *Biochemical Journal*, **105**, 361.

Johnson, P., Lobley, G.E. & Perry, S.V. (1969) Distribution and biological role of 3-methyl histidine in actin and myosin. *Biochemical Journal*, **115**, 993.

Johnson, W.H., Kahn, J. & Szent-Györgyi, A.G. (1959) Paramyosin and contraction of catch muscle. *Science*, **130**, 160.

Josephs, R. & Harrington, W.F. (1966) Studies on the formation and physical chemical properties of synthetic myosin filaments. *Biochemistry*, **5**, 3474.

Julian, F.J. (1971) The effect of calcium on the force-velocity relation of briefly glycerinated frog muscle fibres. *Journal of Physiology*, **218**, 117.

Julian, F.J. & Sollins, M.R. (1972) Regulation of force and speed of shortening in muscle contraction. *Cold Spring Harbor Symposium of Quantitative Biology*, **37**, 635.

Kakol, I. & Weber, H.H. (1965) Reaktinen und relative affinitaten zwischen rerschiedenen nucleotiden und F actin unter ultraschall. *Zeitschrift für Naturforschung*, **20**, 977.

Kalckar, H.M. (1943) The role of myokinase in transphosphorylation II. *Nature*, **213**, 862.

Kaminer, B. & Bell, A. (1966) Myosin filamentogenesis: effects of pH and ionic concentration. *Journal of Molecular Biology*, **20**, 391.

Kaplan, N.O. & Cahn, R.D. (1962) Lactic dehydrogenase and muscular dystrophy in the chicken. *Proceedings of the National Academy of Sciences of the United States of America*, **48**, 2123.

Kasai, M., Nakano, F. & Oosawa, F. (1964) Polymerization of actin free from nucleotides and divalent cations. *Biochimica et biophysica acta*, **94**, 494.

Kendrew, J.C. (1963) Myoglobin and the structure of proteins. *Science*, **139**, 1259.

Kendrick-Jones, J., Lehman, W. & Szent-Györgyi, A.G. (1970) Regulation in molluscan muscle. *Journal of Molecular Biology*, **54**, 313.

Kendrick-Jones, J. & Perry, S.V. (1965) Enzymic adaptation to contractile activity in skeletal muscle. *Nature*, **208**, 1068.

Kendrick-Jones, J. & Perry, S.V. (1967) Biochemical adaptation in muscle. In *Exploratory Concepts in Muscular Dystrophy and Related Disorders*, Ed. A.T. Milhorat, p. 64 (Excerpta Medica: Amsterdam).

Kendrick-Jones, J., Szentkiralyi, E.M. & Szent-Györgyi, A.G. (1976) Regulatory light chains in myosin. *Journal of Molecular Biology*, **104**, 747.

Kielley, W.W. & Bradley, J.B. (1956) The relationship between sulfhydryl groups and the activation of myosin adenosine triphosphatase. *Journal of Biological Chemistry*, **218**, 643.

Kielley, W.W. & Harrington, W.F. (1960) A model for the myosin molecule. *Biochimica et biophysica acta*, **41**, 401.

Kielley, W.W. & Meyerhof, O. (1948) Studies on adenosinetriphosphatase of muscle. II. A new magnesium-activated adenosinetriphosphatase. *Journal of Biological Chemistry*, **176**, 591.

Kielley, W.W. & Meyerhof, O. (1950) Studies on adenosinetriphosphatase of muscle III. The lipoprotein nature of the magnesium-activated adenosine triphosphatase. *Journal of Biological Chemistry*, **183**, 391.

King, M.V. & Young, M. (1972) Evidence for flexibility of the helical rod section of the myosin molecule. *Journal of Molecular Biology*, **65**, 519.

Kitagawa, W., Drabikowski, W. & Gergely, J. (1967) Factors affecting the binding of ADP to F actin. *Journal of General Physiology*, **50**, 1083.

Kitagawa, S., Drabikowski, W. & Gergely, J. (1968) The exchange and release of the bound nucleotide of F actin. *Archives of Biochemistry and Biophysics*, **125**, 706.

Kitagawa, S., Martonosi, A. & Gergely, J. (1965) Release of actin bound $C^{14}ATP$ and superprecipitation of actomyosin. *Federation Proceedings. Federation of American Societies for Experimental Biology*, **24**, 598.

Kominz, D.R. & Lewis, M.S. (1964) The 3S component of myosin. In *Biochemistry of Muscle Contraction*, Ed. J. Gergely, p. 19 (Little Brown: Boston).

Kominz, D.R. & Maruyama, K. (1960) The 3S fragments of rabbit and crayfish myosin obtained by copper cyanide treatment. *Archives of Biochemistry and Biophysics*, **90**, 52.

Kovas, L., Rios, E. & Schneider, M.E. (1979) Calcium transients and intra-membrane charge movement in skeletal muscle fibers. *Nature*, **279**, 391.

Krebs, E.G. (1972) Protein kinases. In *Current Topics in Cellular Regulation*, Eds B.L. Horecker & E.R. Stadtman, p. 99 (Academic Press: New York).

Krebs, E.G. & Beavo, J.A. (1979) Phosphorylation-dephosphorylation of enzymes. *Annual Review of Biochemistry*, **48**, 923.

Krebs, H.A. & Johnson, W.A. (1937) The role of citric acid in intermediate metabolism in animal tissue. *Enzymologia*, **4**, 148.

Kretsinger, R.H. (1972) Gene triplication deduced from the tertiary structure of a muscle calcium binding protein. *Nature*, **85**, 240.

Kretsinger, R.H., & Kockolds, C.E. (1973) Carp muscle calcium binding protein II. Structure determination and general description. *Journal of Biological Chemistry*, **248**, 3313.

Krysik, B., Vergnes, J.P. & McManus, I. (1971) Enzymatic methylation of skeletal muscle contractile proteins. *Archives of Biochemistry and Biophysics*, **146**, 34.

Kuby, S.A., Noda, L. & Lardy, H.A. (1954) Adenosinetriphosphatecreatine transphosphorylase I. Isolation of the crystalline enzyme from rabbit muscle. *Journal of Biological Chemistry*, **209**, 191.

Kuehl, W.M. & Adelstein, R.S. (1969) Identification of ε-n-monomethyllysine and ε-n-trimethyllysine in rabbit skeletal myosin. *Biochemical and Biophysical Research Communications*, **37**, 59.

Kuehl, W.M. & Adelstein, R.S. (1970) The absence of 3-methylhistidine in red, cardiac and fetal myosin.

Biochemical and Biophysical Research Communications, **39**, 956.

Kumagai, H., Ebashi, S., & Takeda, F. (1955) Essential relaxing factor in muscle other than myokinase and creatine phosphokinase. *Nature*, **176**, 166.

Kuschinsky, G. & Turba, F. (1951) Uber die rolle der SH-gruppen bei vorgangen am aktomyosin, myosin and aktin. *Biochimica et biophysica acta*, **6**, 426.

Kushmerick, M.J. (1977) Energy balance in muscle contraction: a biochemical approach. In *Current Topics in Bioenergetics*, Ed. D.R. Sanadi, p. 1 (Academic Press: New York).

Kushmerick, M.J. & Davies, R.E. (1969) The chemical energetics of muscle contraction II. The chemistry, efficiency and power of maximally working sartorius muscles with an appendix-free energy and enthalpy of ATP hydrolysis in the sarcoplasm. *Proceedings of the Royal Society, Series B*, **174**, 315.

Leavis, P.C., Rosenfeld, S., Gergely, J., Grabarek, Z. & Drabikowski, W. (1978) Proteolytic fragments of troponin C. Localization of high and low affinity Ca^{2+}-binding sites and interactions with troponin I and troponin T. *Journal of Biological Chemistry*, **253**, 5452.

Lee, Y.-P. (1957) 5'-adenylic acid deaminase. I. Isolation of the crystalline enzyme from rabbit skeletal muscle. *Journal of Biological Chemistry*, **227**, 987.

Lehman, W. & Szent-Györgyi, A.G. (1975) Distribution of actin control and myosin control in the animal kingdom. *Journal of General Physiology*, **66**, 1.

Lehky, P.L., Blum, H.E., Stein, E.A. & Fischer, E.H. (1974) Isolation and characterization of parvalbumins from the skeletal muscle of higher vertebrates. *Journal of Biological Chemistry*, **249**, 4332.

Lehman, W., Kendrick-Jones, J. & Szent-Györgyi, A.G. (1972) Myosin-linked regulatory systems: Comparative studies. *Cold Spring Harbor Symposia on Quantitative Biology*, **37**, 319.

Lehrer, S.S. & Kerwar, G. (1972) The intrinsic fluorescence of actin. *Biochemistry*, **11**, 1211.

Lehrer, S.S., Nagy, B. & Gergely, J. (1972) The binding of Cu^{2+} to actin without loss of polymerizability. The involvement of the rapidly reacting SH groups. *Archives of Biochemistry and Biophysics*, **150**, 164.

LeLoir, L.F. & Cardini, L.E. (1962) UDPG-glycogen transglucosylase. In *Enzymes*, Eds P.D. Boyer, H. Lardy and K. Myrback, Vol. VI, p. 317 (Academic Press: New York).

Levine, B.A., Mercola, D., Coffman, D. & Thornton, J.M. (1977) Calcium binding by TnC. A proton magnetic resonance study. *Journal of Molecular Biology*, **115**, 743.

Levitt, M. & Clothia, C. (1976) Structural patterns in a globular proteins. *Nature*, **261**, 552.

Lipmann, F. (1941) Metabolic generation and utilization of phosphate bound energy. *Advances in Enzymology*, **1**, 99.

Lipmann, F. (1954) Development of the acetylation problem, a personal account. *Science*, **120**, 855.

Locker, R.H. (1956) The dissociation of myosin by heat coagulation. *Biochimica et biophysica acta*, **20**, 514.

Lohman, K. (1934) Uber die enzymatische aufspaltung der kreatin-phosphorsaure: zugleich ein beitrag zum chemiismus der muskelkontraktion. *Biochemische Zeitschrift*, **271**, 264.

Low, R.B., Vournakis, J.N. & Rich, A. (1971) Identification of separate polysomes active in the synthesis of the light and heavy chains of myosin. *Biochemistry*, **10**, 1813.

Lowey, S. (1964) Meromyosin substructure: isolation of a helical sub-unit from heavy meromyosin. *Science*, **145**, 597.

Lowey, S. & Cohen, C. (1962) Studies on the structure of myosin. *Journal of Molecular Biology*, **4**, 293.

Lowey, S., Goldstein, L. & Luck, S. (1966) Isolation and characterization of a helical sub-unit from heavy meromyosin. *Biochemische Zeitschrift*, **345**, 248.

Lowey, S. & Luck, S.M. (1969) Equilibrium binding of adenosine diphosphate to myosin. *Biochemistry*, **8**, 3195.

Lowey, S. & Risby, D. (1971) Light chains from fast and slow muscle myosin. *Nature*, **234**, 81.

Lowey, S., Slayter, H.S., Weeds, A.G. & Baker, H. (1969) Substructure of the myosin molecule I. Subfragments of myosin by enzymic degradation. *Journal of Molecular Biology*, **42**, 1.

Lucas-Lenard, J. & Lipmann, F. (1971) Protein biosynthesis. *Annual Review of Biochemistry*, **40**, 409.

Lundsgaard, E. (1930) Untersuchungen uber muskelkontraktionen ohne milchsaurebildung. *Biochemische Zeitschrift*, **217**, 162.

Lusty, C.J. & Fasold, H. (1969) Characterisation of sulfhydryl groups of actin. *Biochemistry*, **8**, 2933.

Lymn, R.W. (1979) Kinetic analysis of myosin and actomyosin ATPase. *Annual Review of Biophysics and Bioengineering*, **8**, 145.

Lymn, R.W. & Taylor, E.W. (1971) Mechanism of adenosine triphosphate hydrolysis by actomyosin. *Biochemistry*, **10**, 4617.

Lynen, F. & Ochoa, S. (1953) Enzymes of fatty acid metabolism. *Biochimica et biophysica acta*, **12**, 299.

MacLennan, D.H. (1970) Purification and properties of an adenonsine triphosphatase from sarcoplasmic reticulum. *Journal of Biological Chemistry*, **245**, 4508.

MacLennan, D.H., Seeman, P., Iles, G.H. & Yip, C.C. (1971) Membrane formation by the adenosine triphosphatase of sarcoplasmic reticulum. *Journal of Biological Chemistry*, **246**, 2702.

MacLennan, D.H. & Wong, P.T.S. (1971) Isolation of a calcium-sequestering protein from sarcoplasmic reticulum. *Proceedings of the National Academy of Sciences of the United States of America*, **68**, 1231.

MacLennan, D.H., Yip, C., Iles, G.H. & Seeman, P. (1972) Isolation of sarcoplasmic reticulum proteins. *Cold Spring Harbor Symposia on Quantitative Biology*, **37**, 469.

MacLennan, D.H., Zubrzycka, E., Jorgensen, A.O. & Kalnis, V.I. (1978) Assembly of sarcoplasmic reticulum. In *The Molecular Biology of Membranes*, Eds S. Fleischer, Y. Hatefi, D.H. MacLennan & H. Tzagaloff, p. 309 (Plenum Press: New York).

Mak, A., Smillie, L.B. & Barany, M. (1978) Specific phosphorylation at serine 283 of a tropomyosin from rabbit skeletal and cardiac muscle. *Proceedings of the National Academy of Sciences of the United States of America*, **75**, 3588.

Makinose, M. (1966) Die phosphorylierung der membran des sarkoplasmatischen retikulum unter den bedingungen des aktiven Ca-transportes. *Proceedings of Second International Biophysics Congress*, p. 276.

Makinose, M. (1971) Calcium efflux-dependent formation of ATP from ADP and orthophosphate by the membranes of the sarcoplasmic reticulum vesicles. *Federation of European Biochemical Society Letters*, **12**, 269.

Makinose, M. & Hasselbach, W. (1971) ATP synthesis by the reverse of the sarcoplasmic reticulum pump. *Federation of European Biochemical Society Letters*, **12**, 271.

Maley, G.F. & Lardy, H.A. (1955) Efficiency of phosphorylation in selected oxidations by mitochondria from normal and thyrotoxic rat livers. *Journal of Biological Chemistry*, **215**, 377.

Malhotra, A., Huang, S. & Bhan, A. (1979) Subunit function in cardiac myosin: effect of removal of LC_2 ($18\,000\ M_r$) on enzymatic properties. *Biochemistry*, **18**, 461.

Mannherz, H.G. & Goody, R.S. (1976) Proteins of contractile systems. *Annual Review of Biochemistry*, **45**, 427.

Mansour, T.E. (1972) Phosphofructokinase. In *Current Topics in Cellular Regulation*, Eds B.L. Horecher & E.R. Stadtman, p. 1 (Academic Press: New York).

Marechal, G. & Mommaerts, W.F.H.M. (1963) The metabolism of phosphocreatine during an isometric tetanus in the frog sartorius muscle. *Biochimica et biophysica acta* **69**, 53.

Margossian, S.S. & Cohen, C. (1973) Troponin subunit interactions. *Journal of Molecular Biology*, **81**, 409.

Marsh, B.B. (1951) A factor modifying muscle syneresis. *Nature*, **167**, 1065.

Marsh, B.B. (1952) The effects of adenosine triphosphate on the fibre volume of a muscle homogenate. *Biochimica et biophysica acta* **9**, 247.

Martonosi, A. (1962a) Studies on actin VII. Ultracentrifugal analysis of partially polymerized actin solutions. *Journal of Biological Chemistry* **237**, 2795.

Martonosi, A. (1962b) The specificitiy of the interaction of ATP with G actin. *Biochimica et biophysica acta*, **57**, 163.

Martonosi, A. (1963) The activating effect of phospholipids on the ATPase activity and calcium uptake of fragmented sarcoplasmic reticulum. *Biochemical and Biophysical Research Communications*, **13**, 273.

Martonosi, A. (1968) Sarcoplasmic reticulum V. The structure of sarcoplasmic reticulum membranes. *Biochimica et biophysica acta*, **150**, 694.

Martonosi, A. (1969) The protein composition of sarcoplasmic reticulum membranes. *Biochemical and Biophysical Research Communications*, **36**, 1039.

Martonosi, A., Donley, J. & Halpin, R.A. (1968) Sarcoplasmic reticulum III. The role of phospholipids in the adenosine triphosphatase activity of Ca^{2+} transport. *Journal of Biological Chemistry*, **243**, 61.

Martonosi, A. & Feretos, R. (1964) Sarcoplasmic reticulum I. The uptake of calcium by sarcoplasmic reticulum fragments. *Journal of Biological Chemistry*, **239**, 648.

Martonosi, A., Gouvea, M.A. & Gergely, J. (1960a) The interaction of C^{14}-labelled adenine nucleotides with actin. *Journal of Biological Chemistry*, **235**, 1700.

Martonosi, A., Gouvea, M.A. & Gergely, J. (1960b) G-F transformation of actin and muscular contraction. *Journal of Biological Chemistry*, **235**, 1707.

Martonosi, A., Roufa, D., Ha, D.B. & Boland, R. (1980) The biosynthesis of sarcoplasmic reticulum. (In press).

Maruyama, K. (1965a) A new protein factor hindering network formation of F actin in solution. *Biochimica et biophysica acta*, **94**, 208.

Maruyama, K. (1965b) Some physico-chemical properties of β-actinin. Actin factor isolated from striated muscle. *Biochimica et biophysica acta*, **102**, 542.

Maruyama, K. & Ebashi, S. (1965) α-actinin. A new structural protein from striated muscle. II. Action on actin. *Journal of Biochemistry*, **58**, 13.

Maruyama, K. & Gergely, J. (1961) Removal of bound calcium of G actin by ethylenediaminotetra-acetate

(EDTA). *Biochemical and Biophysical Research Communications*, **6**, 245.

Maruyama, K. & Gergely, J. (1962) Interaction of actomyosin with adenosine triphosphate at low ionic strength I. Discussion of actomyosin during the clear phase. *Journal of Biological Chemistry*, **237**, 1095.

Maruyama, K., Matsubara, S., Natori, R., Nonomura, Y., Kimura, S., Ohashi, K., Murakami, F., Handa, S. & Eguchi, G. (1977) Connectin, an elastic protein of muscle, characterization and function. *Journal of Biochemistry*, **82**, 317.

McLachlan, A.D. & Stewart, M. (1976) The 14-fold periodicity in α-tropomyosin and the interaction with actin. *Journal of Molecular Biology*, **103**, 271.

Meissner, G. (1975) Isolation and characterization of two types of sarcoplasmic reticulum vesicles. *Biochimica et biophysica acta*, **389**, 51.

Mendelson, R.A., Morales, M.F. & Botts, J. (1973) Segmental flexibility of the S-1 moiety of myosin. *Biochemistry*, **12**, 2250.

Meyer, F., Heilmeyer, M., Haschke, R. & Fischer, E. (1970) Control of phosphorylase activity in a muscle glycogen particle. I. Isolation and characterisation of the protein-glycogen complex. *Journal of Biological Chemistry*, **245**, 3153.

Meyerhof, O. (1930) *Die Chemischen Vorgange in Muskel und ihr Zusammenhang mit Arbeitsleistung und Warmebildung* (Springer: Berlin).

Migala, A., Agostini, B. & Hasselbach, W. (1973) Tryptic fragmentation of the calcium transport system in the sarcoplasmic reticulum. *Zeitschrift für Naturforschung*, **28**, 178.

Mihalyi, E. & Szent-Györgyi, A.G. (1953) Trypsin digestion of muscle proteins III. Adenosinetriphosphatase activity and actin-binding capacity of the digested myosin. *Journal of Biological Chemistry*, **201**, 211.

Mitchell, P. (1966) Cheiosmatic coupling in oxidative and photosynthetic phosphorylation. *Biological Reviews*, **41**, 445.

Mitchell, P. (1977) Vectorial chemiosmotic processes. *Annual Review of Biochemistry*, **46**, 996.

Moir, A.J.G., Cole, H.A. & Perry, S.V. (1977) The phosphorylation sites of troponin T from white skeletal muscle and the effects of interaction with troponin C on their phosphorylation by phosphorylase kinase. *Biochemical Journal*, **161**, 371.

Mommaerts, W.F.H.M. (1952) The molecular transformation of actin. III. The participation of nucleotides. *Journal of Biological Chemistry*, **198**, 469.

Mommaerts, W.F.H.M. (1954) Is adenosine triphosphate broken down during a single muscle twitch? *Nature*, **174**, 1081.

Mommaerts, W.F.H.M. (1955) Investigation of the presumed breakdown of adenosine triphosphate and phosphocreatine during a single muscle twitch. *American Journal of Physiology*, **182**, 585.

Mommaerts, W.F.H.M. (1970) What is the Fenn effect? *Naturwissenschaften*, **57**, 326.

Mommaerts, W.F.H.M., Buller, A.J. & Seraydarian, K. (1969) The modification of some biochemical properties of muscle by cross-innervation. *Proceedings of the National Academy of Science of the United States of America*, **64**, 128.

Mommaerts, W.F.H.M., Seraydarian, K. & Marechal, G. (1962) Work and chemical changes in isotonic muscle contraction. *Biochimica et biophysica acta*, **57**, 1.

Mondal, H., Sutton, A., Chen, V.J. & Sarkar, S. (1974) Purified mRNA for myosin heavy chain: size and polyadenylic acid content. *Biochemical and Biophysical Research Communications*, **56**, 988.

Monod, J., Changeux, J.P. & Jacob, F. (1963) Allosteric proteins and cellular control systems. *Journal of Molecular Biology*, **6**, 306.

Moore, P.B., Huxley, H.E. & DeRosier, D.J. (1970) Three dimensional reconstruction of F actin, thin filaments and decorated thin filaments. *Journal of Molecular Biology*, **50**, 279.

Moore, S. & Stein, W.H. (1951) Chromatography of amino acids on sulfonated polystyrene resins. *Journal of Biological Chemistry*, **192**, 663.

Moore, S. & Stein, W.H. (1954) Procedures for the chromatographic determination of amino acids on 4% cross linked sulfonated polystyrene. *Journal of Biological Chemistry*, **211**, 893.

Moos, C., Estes, J.E. & Eisenberg, E. (1966) Exchange of F actin bound nucleotide in the presence and absence of myosin. *Biochemical and Biophysical Research Communications*, **23**, 347.

Morales, M.F., Ingwall, J.S., Stockdale, F.E., McKay, R., Brivio-Haugland, R. & Kenyon, G.L. (1974) Creatine and muscle protein synthesis. In *Exploratory Concepts in Muscular Dystrophy*, Ed. A.T. Milhorat, p. 212 (Elsevier: Amsterdam).

Morimoto, K. & Harrington, W.F. (1972) Isolation and physical chemical properties of an M-line protein from skeletal muscle. *Journal of Biological Chemistry*, **247**, 3052.

Mueller, H. & Perry, S.V. (1962) The degradation of heavy meromyosin by trypsin. *Biochemical Journal*, **85**, 431.

Muhlrad, A., Fabian, F. & Biro, N.A. (1964) On the activation of myosin ATPase by EDTA. *Biochimica et biophysica acta*, **89**, 186.

Nagai, T., Makinose, M. & Hasselbach, W. (1960) The physiological relaxing factor produced by the muscle grana. *Biochimica et biophysica acta*, **43**, 223.

Nagano, K. (1973) Logical analysis of the mechanism of protein folding. I. Prediction of helices, loops and β-structures from primary structure. *Journal of Molecular Biology*, **75**, 401.

Nagy, B. & Jencks, W.P. (1962) Optical rotatory dispersion of G actin. *Biochemistry*, **1**, 987.

Nakamura, A., Sreter, F.A. & Gergely, J. (1971) Comparative studies of light meromyosin in paracrystals derived from red, white and cardiac muscle myosin. *Journal of Cell Biology*, **49**, 883.

Nauss, K.M. & Davies, R.E. (1966) Changes in inorganic phosphate and arginine during the development, maintenance and loss of tension in the anterior byssus retractor muscle of mytilus edulis. *Biochemische Zeitschrift*, **345**, 173.

Nauss, K., Kitagawa, S. & Gergely, J. (1969) Pyrophosphate binding to and ATPase activity of myosin and its proteolytic fragments—implications for the substructure of myosin. *Journal of Biological Chemistry*, **244**, 755.

Needham, D.M. (1956) Energy production in muscle. *British Medical Bulletin*, **12**, 194.

Needham, D.M. (1971) *Machina Carnis* (University of Cambridge Press: Cambridge).

Needham, J., Chen, S.L., Needham, D.M. & Lawrence, A.S.G. (1941) Myosin birefringence and adenylpyrophosphate. *Nature*, **147**, 766.

Neison, D.A. & Benson, E.S. (1963) On the structural

continuities of the transverse tubular system of rabbit and human myocardial cell. *Journal of Cell Biology*, **16**, 297.

Newsholme, E.A. & Start, C. (1973) *Regulation in Metabolism* (John Wiley: London).

Newton, A.A. & Perry, S.V. (1960) The incorporation of ^{15}N into adenine nucleotides and their formation from inosine monophosphate by skeletal muscle preparations. *Biochemical Journal*, **74**, 127.

Noble, M.I. & Pollack, G.H. (1977) Molecular mechanisms of contraction. *Circulation Research*, **40**, 333.

Noda, L. & Kuby, S.A. (1957) Adenosine triphosphate-adenosine monophosphate transphosphorylase (Myokinase). *Journal of Biological Chemistry*, **226**, 541.

O'Brien, E.J., Morris, E.P., Seymour, J.V. & Couch, J. (1978) Structure of myosin thin filaments. *Proceedings of VI international Biophysics Congress*, p. 311.

Ochoa, S. & deHaro, C. (1979) Regulation of protein synthesis in eukaryotes. *Annual Review of Biochemistry*, **48**, 549.

Offer, G.W. (1964) The antagonistic action of magnesium ions and ethylene-diamine-tetraacetate on myosin A ATPase (potassium activated). *Biochimica et biophysica acta*, **89**, 566.

Offer, G. (1972) C-protein and the periodicity in the thick filaments of vertebrate skeletal muscle. *Cold Spring Harbor Symposia on Quantitative Biology*, **37**, 87.

Offer, G., Moos, C. & Starr, R. (1973) A new protein of the thick filaments of vertebrate skeletal myofibrils. *Journal of Molecular Biology*, **74**, 653.

Ohnishi, K. & Maruyama, K. (1979) A new structural protein located in the Z lines of chicken skeletal muscle. *Journal of Biochemistry*, **85**, 1103.

Oosawa, F., Asakura, S., Asai, H., Kasai, M., Kobayashi, S., Mihashi, K., Ooi, F., Taniguchi, M. & Nakano, E. (1964) Structure and function of actin polymers. In *Biochemistry of Muscle Contraction*, Ed. J. Gergely, p. 158 (Little Brown: Boston).

Oosawa, F., Fujime, S., Ishiwata, S. & Mihashi, K. (1972) Dynamic properties of F actin and thin filament. *Cold Spring Harbor Symposia on Quantitative Biology*, **37**, 277.

Oppenheimer, H., Bárány, K., Hamoir, G. & Fenton, J. (1967) Succinylation of myosin. *Archives of Biochemistry and Biophysics*, **120**, 108.

Ostwald, T.J. & MacLennan, D.H. (1974) Isolation of a high affinity calcium-binding protein from sarcoplasmic reticulum. *Journal of Biological Chemistry*, **249**, 974.

Ozawa, E., Hosoi, K. & Ebashi, S. (1967) Reversible stimulation of muscle phosphorylase b kinase by low concentrations of calcium ions. *Journal of Biochemistry*, **61**, 431.

Park, C.R., Bornstein, J. & Post, R.L. (1955) Effect of insulin on free glucose content of rat diaphragm *in vitro*. *American Journal of Physiology*, **182**, 12.

Parry, D.A.D. (1975) Analysis of the primary sequence of α-tropomyosin from rabbit skeletal muscle. *Journal of Molecular Biology*, **98**, 519.

Parry, D.A.D. & Squire, J.M. (1973) Structural role of tropomyosin in muscle regulation. Analysis of X-ray diffraction patterns from relaxed and contracting muscles. *Journal of Molecular Biology*, **75**, 33.

Parsons, D.F. (1963) Mitochondrial structure: two types of sub-units on negatively stained mitochondrial membranes. *Science*, **140**, 985.

Patterson, B.M. & Bishop, J.O. (1977) Changes in the mRNA population of chick myoblasts during myogenesis *in vitro. Cell*, **12**, 751.

Pauling, L., Corey, R.B. & Bronson, H.R. (1951) The structure of proteins: Two hydrogen bonded helical centrifugations of the polypeptide chain. *Proceedings of the National Academy of Sciences of the United States of America*, **37**, 205.

Peachey, L. (1972) Electrical events in the T system of frog skeletal muscle. *Cold Spring Harbor Symposia on Quantitative Biology*, **37**, 479.

Pearlstone, J.R., Carpenter, M.R., Johnson, P. & Smillie, L.B. (1976) Amino acid sequence of tropomyosin binding component of rabbit skeletal muscle troponin. *Proceedings of the National Academy of Sciences of the United States of America*, **73**, 1902.

Pease, D.C., Jenden, D.J. & Howell, J.N. (1965) Calcium uptake in glycerol-extracted rabbit psoas muscle fibres. *Journal of Cellular and Comparative Physiology*, **65**, 141.

Pechere, J.-F. (1974) Isoltmand d'une parvalbumine due muscle du carpin. *Compte rendus hebdomadaire des séances de l'Academie des Sciences*, **278**, 2577.

Pepe, F.A. (1966) Some aspects of the structural organisation of the myofibril as revealed by antibody-staining methods. *Journal of Cell Biology*, **28**, 505.

Pepe, F.A. (1967a) The myosin filament. I. Structural organisation from antibody staining observed in electron microscopy. *Journal of Molecular Biology*, **27**, 203.

Pepe, F.A. (1967b) The myosin filament II. Interaction between myosin and actin filaments observed during antibody staining in fluorescent and electron microscopy. *Journal of Molecular Biology*, **27**, 227.

Pepe, F.A. (1972) The myosin filament: immunochemical and ultrastructural approaches to molecular organisation. *Cold Spring Harbor Symposia on Quantitative Biology*, **37**, 97.

Pepe, F.A. & Dowben, P. (1977) The myosin filament V. Intermediate voltage electron microscopy and optical diffraction studies of the substructure. *Journal of Molecular Biology*, **113**, 199.

Perry, S.V. (1951) The adenosinetriphosphatase activity of myofibrils isolated from skeletal muscle. *Biochemical Journal*, **48**, 257.

Perry, S.V. (1979) The regulation of contractile activity in muscle. *Biochemical Society Transactions*, **7**, 593.

Perry, S.V. & Grey, T.C. (1956) A study of the effects of substrate concentration and certain relaxing factors on magnesium-activated myofibrillar adenosine triphosphatase. *Biochemical Journal*, **64**, 184.

Perry, S.V., Cole, H.A., Head, J.F. & Wilson, F.J. (1972) Localisation and mode of action in the inhibitory protein complex of the troponin complex. *Cold Spring Harbor Symposia on Quantitative Biology*, **37**, 251.

Perutz, M.F. (1963) X-ray analysis of hemoglobin. *Science*, **140**, 863.

Peters, R.A. (1936) The biochemical lesion in vitamin B deficiency. *Lancet*, **80**, 1161.

Pette, D. & Schnez, U. (1977) Co-existence of fast and slow type myosin light chains in single muscle fibers during transformation as induced by long-term stimulation. *Federation of European Biochemical Society Letters*, **83**, 128.

Pette, D., Smith, M.E., Staudte, H.W. & Vrbová, G. (1973) Effects of long-term electrical stimulation on some contractile and metabolic characteristics of fast rabbit muscle. *Pflügers Archiv für die gesamte Physiologie des Menschen und der Tiere*, **338**, 257.

Pettigrew, D.W. & Frieden, C. (1979) Rabbit muscle

phosphofructokinase. A model for regulatory kinase behaviour. *Journal of Biological Chemistry*, **254**, 1876.

Pires, E., Perry, S.V. & Thomas, M.A.W. (1974) Myosin light chain kinase. A new enzyme from striated muscle. *Federation of European Biochemical Society Letters*, **41**, 292.

Podolsky, R.J. (1979) Dynamics. In *Molecular Basis of Force Development in Muscle*, Ed. N.B. Ingels, Jr., p. 27 (Palo Alto Medical Research Foundation: Palo Alto).

Podolsky, R.J. & Costantin, L.L. (1964) Regulation by calcium of the contraction and relaxation of muscle fibres. *Federation Proceedings. Federation of American Societies for Experimental Biology*, **23**, 933.

Podolsky, R.J. & Teichholz, L.E. (1970) The relation between calcium and contraction kinetics in skinned muscle fibers. *Journal of Physiology*, **211**, 19.

Porter, K.R. & Palade, G.E. (1957) Studies on the endoplasmic reticulum III. Its form and distribution in striated muscle cells. *Journal of Biophysics and Biochemical Cytology*, **3**, 269.

Post, R.L., Merritt, C.R., Kinsolving, C.R. & Albright, C.D. (1960) Membrane adenosine triphosphatase as a participant in the active transport of sodium and potassium in the human erythrocyte. *Journal of Biological Chemistry*, **235**, 1796.

Potter, J.D. & Gergely, J. (1974) Troponin, tropomyosin and actin interactions in the Ca^{2+} regulation of muscle contraction. *Biochemistry*, **13**, 2697.

Potter, J.D., Seidel, J.C., Leavis, P., Lehrer, S.S. & Gergely, J. (1976) The effect of Ca^{2+}-binding on troponin C. Changes in spin label mobility, extrinsic fluorescence and SH reactivity. *Journal of Biological Chemistry*, **251**, 7551.

Pragay, D. (1957) Aktin fraktionen, aktin polymerisation. *Naturwissenschaften*, **44**, 397.

Price, H.M., Gordon, J.M., Pearson, C.M., Munsat, T.C. & Blumberg, J.M. (1965) New evidence for excessive accumulation of Z band material in nemaline myopathy. *Proceedings of the National Academy of Sciences of the United States of America*, **54**, 1398.

Quicho, F.A. & Lipscomb, A.N. (1971) Carboxypeptidase A: A protein and an enzyme. In *Advances in Protein Chemistry*, Eds C.B. Anfinsen, J.T. Edsall & F.B. Richards, p. 1 (Academic Press: New York).

Racker, E. (1965) *Mechanisms in Bioenergetics* (Academic Press: New York).

Racker, E. (1972) Reconstitution of a calcium pump with phospholipids and a purified Ca^{2+}-adenosine triphosphatase from sarcoplasmic reticulum. *Journal of Biological Chemistry*, **247**, 8198.

Rall, J., Homsher, E. & Mommaerts, W.F.H.M. (1973) Heat production and phosphocreatine hydrolysis with unloaded shortening in rana pipiens semi-tendinosus muscles. *Federation Proceedings. Federation of American Societies for Experimental Biology*, **32**, 730.

Ranvier, L. (1874) De quelques faits relatifs a l'histologie et la physiologie des muscles stries. *Archives of Physiology of Normal Pathology* (Deuxieme Serie), 1.

Reisler, E., Burke, M., Himmelfarb, S. & Harrington, W.F. (1974) Spacial proximity of two essential SH groups of myosin. *Biochemistry*, **13**, 3837.

Rice, R.V. (1961) Conformation of individual macromolecular particles from myosin solutions. *Biochimica et biophysica acta*, **52**, 602.

Rice, R.V., Brady, A.C., Depue, R.H. & Kelley, R.E. (1966) Morphology of individual macromolecules and their ordered aggregates by electron microscopy. *Biochemische Zeitschrift*, **345**, 370.

Ridgway, E.B. & Ashley, C.C. (1967) Calcium transients in single muscle fibers. *Biochemical and Biophysical Research Communications*, **29**, 229.

Robinson, G.A., Butcher, R.W. & Sutherland, E.W. (1971) *Cyclic AMP* (Academic Press: New York).

Romanual, F.C. & Van der Meulen, J.P. (1967) Slow and fast muscles after cross innervation. *Archives of Neurology*, **17**, 387.

Romanul, F.C.A., Sreter, F.A., Salmons, S. & Gergely, J. (1974) The effect of a changed pattern of activity on histochemical characteristics of muscle fibers. In *Exploratory Concepts in Muscular Dystrophy*, Ed. A.T. Milhorat, p. 344 (Elsevier: Amsterdam).

Rourke, A. & Heywood, S.M. (1972) Myosin synthesis and specificity of eukaryotic intiation factors. *Biochemistry*, **11**, 2061.

Roy, R., Sreter, F.A. & Sarkar, S. (1979) Changes in tropomosin sub-units and myosin light chains during development of chicken and rabbit striated muscle. *Developmental Biology*, **69**, 15.

Rubinstein, N., Mabuchi, K., Pepe, F., Salmons, S. & Sreter, F. (1978) Use of type-specific antimyosins to demonstrate the transformation of individual fibers in chronically stimulated rabbit fast muscles. *Journal of Cell Biology*, **79**, 252.

Ruegg, J.C. (1958) Interaction of ATP and invertebrate tropomyosin. *Proceedings of IVth International Congress of Biochemistry. Supplement to International Abstracts of Biological Sciences*, page 85.

Ruegg, J.C. (1961) On the tropomyosin-paramyosin system in relation to viscous tone of lamellibranch 'catch' muscle. *Proceedings of the Royal Society, Series B*, **154**, 224.

Salmons, S. & Sreter, F.A. (1976) Impulse activity in the transformation of skeletal muscle type. *Nature*, **263**, 30.

Salmons, S. & Vrbova, G. (1969) The influence of activity on some contractile characteristics of mammalian fast and slow muscle. *Journal of Physiology*, **201**, 535.

Samaha, F.J. & Gergely, J. (1965) Na^+ and K^+ stimulated ATPase in human striated muscle. *Archives of Biochemistry and Biophysics*, **109**, 76.

Samaha, F.J. & Theis, W.H. (1976) Actomyosin changes in muscle with altered function. *Experimental Neurology*, **51**, 310.

Sanadi, D.R. & Wohlrab, H. (1976) Chemical reactions in oxidative phosphorylation. In *Chemical Mechanisms in Bioenergetics*, Ed. D.R. Sanadi, p. 123 (American Chemical Society: Washington).

Sanger, F. (1952) The arrangement of amino acids in proteins. *Advances in Protein Chemistry*, **7**, 1.

Sanger, F. (1956) The structure of insulin. In *Currents in Biochemical Research*, Ed. D.E. Green, p. 434 (Interscience Publishers: New York).

Sarkar, S. (1972) Stoichiometry and sequential removal of light chains of myosin. *Cold Spring Harbor Symposia on Quantitative Biology*, **37**, 14.

Sarkar, S. & Cooke, P. (1970) *In vitro* synthesis of light and heavy polypeptide chains of myosin. *Biochemical and Biophysical Research Communications*, **41**, 918.

Sarkar, S., Sreter, F.A. & Gergely, J. (1971) Light chains of myosins from fast, slow and cardiac muscles. *Proceedings of the National Academy of Sciences of the United States of America*, **68**, 946.

Schaub, M.C., Hartshorne, D.J. & Perry, S.V. (1967) The

adenosine triphosphatase activity of desensitised actomyosin. *Biochemical Journal*, **104**, 263.

Schaub, M.C. & Perry, S.V. (1969) The relaxing protein system of striated muscle. Resolution of the troponin complex into inhibitory and calcium ion sensitising factors and their relationship to tropomyosin. *Biochemical Journal*, **115**, 993.

Schaub, M.C., Watterson, J.G. & Wagner, P.G. (1975) Radioactive labeling of specific thiol groups as influenced by ligand binding. *Hoppe-Seyler's Zeitschrift für physiologische Chemie*, **356**, 325.

Schaub, M.C., Watterson, J.G., Walser, J.T. & Waser, P.G. (1978) Hydrolytically induced allosteric change in the heavy chain of intact myosin involving non-essential thiol groups. *Biochemistry*, **17**, 246.

Schiffer, M. & Edmundson, A.B. (1967) Use of helical wheels to represent the structures of proteins and to identify segments with helical potential. *Biophysical Journal*, **7**, 121.

Schiffer, M. & Edmundson, A.B. (1968) Correlation of amino acid sequence and conformation to tobacco mosaic virus. *Biophysical Journal*, **8**, 29.

Schliselfeld, L.H. & Bárány, M. (1968) The binding of ATP to myosin. *Biochemistry*, **7**, 3206.

Schmidt, G. (1928) Uber fermentative desaminerung in muskel. *Hoppe-Seyler's Zeitschrift für physiologische Chemie*, **179**, 234.

Schmitt, F.O., Bear, R.S., Hall, C.E. & Jakus, M.A. (1947) Electron microscope and X-ray diffraction studies of muscle structure. *Annals of the New York Academy of Sciences*, **47**, 799.

Schneider, M.F. & Chandler, W.K. (1973) Voltage dependent charge movement in skeletal muscle: a possible step in excitation-contraction coupling. *Nature*, **242**, 244.

Schwartz, A. (1962) A sodium- and potassium-stimulated adenosine triphosphatase from cardiac tissue I. Preparation and properties. *Biochemical and Biophysical Research Communications*, **9**, 301.

Seamon, K.B., Hartshorne, D.J. & Bothner-by, A.A. (1977) Ca^{2+} and Mg^{2+} conformations of TnC as determined by ^1H and ^{19}F nuclear magnetic resonance. *Biochemistry*, **16**, 4039.

Seidel, J.C. (1967) Studies on myosin from red and white skeletal muscles of the rabbit II. Inactivation of myosin from red muscle under mild alkaline conditions. *Journal of Biological Chemistry*, **242**, 5623.

Seidel, J.C. & Gergely, J. (1963) Studies on myofibrillar adenosine triphosphatase with calcium-free adenosine triphosphate I. The effect of ethylene-diaminotetra-acetate, calcium, magnesium and adenosine triphosphate. *Journal of Biological Chemistry*, **238**, 3648.

Seidel, J.C. & Gergely, J. (1972) Conformational changes in myosin. *Cold Spring Harbor Symposia on Quantitative Biology*, **37**, 187.

Seraydarian, K., Briskey, E.J. & Mommaerts, W.F.H.M. (1967) The modification of actomyosin by α-actinin I. A survey of experimental conditions. *Biochimica et biophysica acta*, **133**, 399.

Shamoo, A.E., Scott, T.L. & Ryan, T.E. (1977) Active calcium transport via coupling between the enzymatic and the inophoric sites of $Ca^{2+} + Mg^{2+}$-ATPase. *Journal of Supramolecular Structure*, **6**, 345.

Shen, L.C., Villar-Palasi, C. & Larner, J. (1970) Hormonal alteration of protein kinase sensitivity to 3,5'-cyclic AMP. *Journal of Physical Chemistry and Physics*, **2**, 536.

Sherry, J.M.F., Gorecka, A., Aksoy, M.O., Dabrowska, R. & Hartshorne, D.J. (1978) Roles of calcium and phosphorylation in the regulation of the activity of gizzard myosin. *Biochemistry*, **17**, 4411.

Shy, G.M., Engel, W.K., Somers, J.E. & Wanko, T. (1963) Nemaline myopathy: new congenital myopathy. *Brain*, **86**, 793.

Siekevitz, P. (1959) Oxidative phosphorylation in muscle mitochondria and its possible regulation. *Annals of the New York Academy of Sciences*, **72**, 500.

Simon, E.J., Gross, G.S. & Lessell, I.M. (1962) Turnover of muscle and liver proteins in mice with hereditary muscular dystrophy. *Archives of Biochemistry*, **96**, 41.

Simpson, F.O. & Oertelis, S.J. (1962) The fine structure of sheep myocardial cells: sarcolemmal invaginations and the transverse tubular system. *Journal of Cell Biology*, **12**, 91.

Singer, S.J. (1972) A fluid lipid-globular protein mosaic model of membrane structure. *Annals of the New York Academy of Sciences*, **195**, 16.

Skou, J.C. (1960) Further investigation of a Mg^{++}-Na^+-activated adenosine triphosphatase, possibly related to the active, linked transport of Na^+ and K^+ across the nerve membrane. *Biochimica et Biophysica Acta*, **42**, 6.

Skou, J.C. (1971) Sequence of steps in the (Na + K)-activated energy system in relation to sodium and potassium transport. In *Current Topics in Bioenergetics*, Ed. D.R. Sanadi, Vol. 4, p. 357 (Academic Press: New York).

Slater, E.C. (1960) Biochemistry of sarcosomes. In *The Structure and Function of Muscle*, Ed. G.H. Bourne, Vol. II, p. 105 (Academic Press: New York).

Slayter, H.S. & Lowey, S. (1967) Substructure of the myosin molecule as visualised by electron microscopy. *Proceedings of the National Academy of Sciences of the United States of America*, **58**, 1611.

Spackman, D.H. (1967) Accelerated methods. In *Methods in Enzymology*, Ed. C.H.W. Hirs, Vol. XI, p. 3 (Academic Press: New York).

Spicer, S.S. (1952) The clearing response of actomyosin to adenosine triphosphate. *Journal of Biological Chemistry*, **199**, 289.

Spicer, S.S. & Gergely, J. (1951) Studies on the combination of myosin with actin. *Journal of Biological Chemistry*, **188**, 179.

Spudich, J.A., Huxley, H.E. & Finch, J.T. (1972) Regulation of skeletal muscle contraction II. Structural studies of the interaction of the tropomyosin-troponin complex with actin. *Journal of Molecular Biology*, **72**, 619.

Spudich, J.A. & Watt, S. (1971) The regulation of rabbit skeletal muscle contraction I. Biochemical studies of the interaction of the tropomyosin-troponin complex with actin and the proteolytic fragments of myosin. *Journal of Biological Chemistry*, **246**, 4866.

Squire, J.M. (1975) Muscle filament structure and muscle contraction. *Annual Review of Biophysics and Bioengineering*, **4**, 137.

Sreter, F.A. & Gergely, J. (1964) Comparative studies of Mg^{++} activated ATPase activity and Ca-uptake of fractions of white and red muscle homogenates. *Biochemical and Biophysical Research Communications*, **16**, 438.

Sreter, F.A., Gergely, J. & Luff, A.L. (1974) The effect of cross reinnervation on the synthesis of myosin light chains. *Biochemical and Biophysical Research Communications*, **56**, 84.

Sreter, F.A., Gergely, J., Salmons, S. & Romanul, F. (1973)

Synthesis by fast muscle of myosin light chains characteristic of slow muscle in reponse to long-term stimulation. *Nature*, **241**, 17.

Sreter, F.A., Seidel, J.C. & Gergely, J. (1966) Studies on myosin from red and white skeletal muscle of the rabbit. I. adenosine triphosphate activity. *Journal of Biological Chemistry*, **241**, 5772.

Starr, R. & Offer, G. (1973) Polarity of the myosin molecule. *Journal of Molecular Biology*, **81**, 17.

Starr, R. & Offer, G. (1978) Interaction of C protein with heavy meromyosin and subfragment 2. *Biochemical Journal*, **71**, 813.

Stein, J.M. & Padykula, H.A. (1962) Histochemical classification of individual skeletal muscle fibers of the rat. *American Journal of Anatomy*, **110**, 103.

Steiner, D.F. (1969) Proinsulin and the biosynthesis of insulin. *New England Journal of Medicine*, **280**, 1106.

Stewart, P.S. & MacLennan, D.H. (1974) Surface particles of sarcoplasmic reticulum membranes. Structural features of the ATPase. *Journal of Biological Chemistry*, **249**, 985.

Stone, D.B., Prevost, S.C. & Botts, J. (1970) Studies on spin labeled actin. *Biochemistry*, **9**, 3937.

Stone, D. & Smillie, L.B. (1978) The amino acid sequence of rabbit skeletal α-tropomyosin. The NH_2-terminal half and complete sequence. *Journal of Biological Chemistry*, **253**, 1137.

Stone, D., Sodek, J., Johnson, P. & Smillie, L.B. (1974) Tropomyosin: Correlation of amino acid sequence and structure. In *Proteins of the Contractile System* Vol. 31 Proceedings of the IX Federation of European Biochemical Society Meeting. Ed. N.A. Biro, p. 125 (Akad. Kiado: Budapest).

Straub, F.B. (1942) Actin. In *Studies for the Institute of Medical Chemistry, University of Szeged*, Vol. II, p. 3.

Straub, F.B. & Feuer, G. (1950) Adenodinetriphosphate: the functional group of actin. *Biochimica et biophysica acta*, **4**, 455.

Sugita, H., Masaki, T., Ebashi, S. & Pearson, C. (1974) Staining of nemaline rod by fluorescent antibody against 10s-actin. *Proceedings of the Japan Academy*, **50**, 237.

Sumida, M. & Tonomura, Y. (1974) Reaction mechanism of the Ca^{2+} dependent ATPase of sarcoplasmic reticulum from skeletal muscle. X. Direct evidence for Ca^{2+} transport coupled with formation of a phosphorylated intermediate. *Journal of Biochemistry*, **75**, 283.

Sutoh, K., Sutoh, K., Karr, T. & Harrington, W.F. (1978) Isolation and physicochemical properties of a high molecular weight subfragment 2 of myosin. *Journal of Molecular Biology*, **126**, 1.

Syska, H., Wilkinson, J.M., Grand, R.J.A. & Perry, S.V. (1976) The relationship between biological activity and primary structure of troponin I from white skeletal muscle of the rabbit. *Biochemical Journal*, **153**, 375.

Szent-Györgyi, A. (1945) Studies on Muscle. *Acta physiologica scandinavica*. Supplement XXV.

Szent-Györgyi, A. (1949) Free energy relations and contraction of actomyosin. *Biological Bulletin. Marine Biological Laboratory, Woods Hole, Mass.* **96**, 140.

Szent-Györgyi, A.G. (1953) Meromyosins, the sub-units of myosin. *Archives of Biochemistry*, **42**, 305.

Szent-Györgyi, A.G., Cohen, C. & Kendrick-Jones, J. (1971) Paramyosin and the filaments of molluscan 'catch' muscles. *Journal of Molecular Biology*, **56**, 239.

Szent-Györgyi, A.G. & Prior, G. (1965) Exchange of nucleotide bound to actin in superprecipitated actomyosin.

Federation Proceedings, Federation of American Societies for Experimental Biology, **24**, 2583.

Szent-Györgyi, A.G. & Prior, G. (1966) Exchange of adenosine diphosphate bound to actin in superprecipitated actomyosin and contracted myofibrils. *Journal of Molecular Biology*, **15**, 515.

Szent-Györgyi, A.G., Szentkiralyi, E.M. & Kendrick-Jones, J. (1973) The light chains of scallop myosin as regulatory sub-units. *Journal of Molecular Biology*, **74**, 179.

Tada, M., Kirchenberger, M.A., Li, H-C. & Katz, M. (1975) Interrelationships between calcium and cyclic AMP in the mammalian heart. In *Calcium Transport in Contraction and Secretion*, Eds E. Carafoli, F. Clementi, W. Drabikowski & A. Margreth, p. 373 (North Holland: Amsterdam)

Tada, M., Kirchberger, A., Repke, D.I. & Katz, A.M. (1974) Stimulation of calcium transport in cardiac sarcoplasmic reticulum by adenosine 3′:5′-monophosphate-dependent protein kinase. *Journal of Biological Chemistry*, **249**, 6174.

Tada, M., Yamamoto, T. & Tonomura, Y. (1978) Molecular mechanism of active calcium transport by sarcoplasmic reticulum. *Physiological Reviews*, **58**, 1.

Taylor, E.W. (1979) Mechanism of actomyosin ATPase and the problem of muscle contraction. *Critical Reviews in Biochemistry*, **6**, 103.

Thomas, D.D., Seidel, J.C. & Gergely, J. (1980) Rotational dynamics of spin labelled F actin and in the sub-millisecond time range. *Journal of Molecular Biology* (In press).

Thomas, D.D., Seidel, J.C., Hyde, J.S. & Gergely, J. (1975). Motion of the S-1 segment in myosin: Its proteolytic fragments and its supramolecular complexes: saturation transfer electron spin resonance. *Proceedings of the National Academy of Sciences of the United States of America*, **72**, 1729.

Thorley-Lawson, D.A., & Green, N.M. (1973) Studies on the location and orientation of proteins on the sarcoplasmic reticulum. *European Journal of Biochemistry*, **40**, 403.

Tonomura, Y. & Inoue, A. (1975) Energy transducing mechanisms in muscle. In *International Review of Science*, Series I. 'Energy Transducing Mechanisms', Ed. E. Racker, p. 121 (Butterworth: London).

Trayer, I.P., Harris, C.I. & Perry, S.V. (1968) 3-methyl histidine and adult and fetal forms of skeletal muscle myosin. *Nature*, **217**, 452.

Trentham, D.R., Eccleston, J.F. & Bagshaw, C.R. (1976) Kinetic analysis of ATPase mechanisms. *Quarterly Review of Biophysics*, **9**, 217.

Trinick, J. & Lowey, S. (1977) M-protein from chicken pectoralis muscle: isolation and characterisation. *Journal of Molecular Biology*, **113**, 343.

Tsao, T.-C. (1953) Fragmentation of the myosin molecule. *Biochimica et biophysica acta*, **11**, 368.

Turner, D.C., Walliman, T. & Eppenberger, H. (1973) A protein that binds specificially to the M-line of skeletal muscle is identified as the muscle form of creatine kinase. *Proceedings of the National Academy of Sciences of the United States of America*, **70**, 702.

Vanderkerckhoue, J. & Weber, K. (1978) At least six different actins are expressed in higher mammals: an analysis based on the amino acid sequence of the amino terminal peptide. *Journal of Molecular Biology*, **126**, 783.

van Eerd, J.P. & Kawasaki, Y. (1974) The effect of Ca^{2+} on the organisation of the troponin-tropomyosin system. In *Calcium Binding Proteins*, Eds W. Drabikowski, H.

Strzelecka-Golaszewska & E. Carafoli, p. 153 (Elsevier: Amsterdam).

Vasington, F.D. & Murphy, J.V. (1962) Ca++ uptake by rat kidney mitochondria and its dependence on respiration and phosphorylation. *Journal of Biological Chemistry*, **237**, 2670.

Wagner, P.D. & Weeds, A.G. (1977) Studies on the role of myosin alkali light chains. Recombination and hybridisation of light chains and heavy chains in subfragment 1 preparations. *Journal of Molecular Biology*, **109**, 455.

Wang, J.H. & Wiesman, D.H. (1980) Calmodulin and its role in the messenger system. *Current Topics in Cell Regulation* (in press).

Warner, J.R., Knopf, P.M. & Rich, A. (1963) A multiple ribosomal structure in protein synthesis. *Proceedings of the National Academy of Sciences of the United States of America*, **49**, 122.

Warner, J.R., Rich, A. & Hall, C.E. (1962) Electron microscopic studies of ribosomal clusters synthesising hemoglobin. *Science*, **138**, 1399.

Warren, G.B., Toon, P.A., Birdsall, N.J.M., Lee, A.G. & Metcalfe, J.C. (1974) Reversible lipid titrations of the activity of pure adenosine triphosphatase-lipid complexes. *Biochemistry*, **13**, 5501.

Warren, G.B., Toon, P.A., Birdshall, N.J.M., Lee, A.G. & Metcalfe, J.C. (1974) Reconstitution of a calcium pump using defined membrane components. *Proceedings of the National Academy of Sciences of the United States*, **71**, 622.

Watanabe, S. (1955) Relaxing effects of EDTA on glycerol treated muscle fibers. *Archives of Biochemistry and Biophysics*, **45**, 559.

Weber, A. (1956) The ultracentrifugal separation of L-myosin and actin in an actomyosin sol under the influence of ATP. *Biochimica et biophysica acta*, **19**, 345.

Weber, A. (1959) On the role of calcium in the activity of adenosine 5′-triphosphate hydrolysis by actomyosin. *Journal of Biological Chemistry*, **234**, 2764.

Weber, A. (1966) Energized calcium transport and relaxing factors. In *Current Topics in Bioenergetics*, Ed. D.R. Sanadi, Vol. 1, p. 203 (Academic Press: New York).

Weber, A. & Winicur, S. (1961) The role of calcium in the superprecipitation of actomyosin. *Journal of Biological Chemistry*, **236**, 3198.

Weeds, A.G. (1969) Light chains of myosin. *Nature*, **223**, 1362.

Weeds, A.G. & Frank, G. (1972) Structural studies on the light chains of myosin. *Cold Spring Harbor Symposia on Quantitative Biology*, **37**, 9.

Weeds, A.G. & Hartley, B.S. (1967) A chemical approach to the substructure of myosin. *Journal of Molecular Biology*, **24**, 307.

Weeds, A.G. & Lowey, S. (1971) Substructure of the myosin molecule II. The light chains of myosin. *Journal of Molecular Biology*, **61**, 701.

Weeds, A.G. & McLachlan, A.D. (1974) Structural homology of myosin alkali light chains, troponin C and carp calcium binding protein. *Nature*, **252**, 646.

Weeds, A.G. & Pope, B. (1977) Studies on the chymotryptic digestion of myosin. Effects of divalent cations on proteolytic susceptibility. *Journal of Molecular Biology*, **111**, 129.

Weeds, A.G., Hall, R. & Spurway, N.C.S. (1975) Characterisation of myosin light chains from histochemically identified fibers of rabbit psoas muscle.

FEBS Letters, **49**, 320.

Weeds, A.G., Trentham, D.R., Kean, C.J.C. & Buller, A.J. (1974) Myosin from cross-reinnervated cat muscles. *Nature*, **247**, 135.

Weeks, R.A. & Perry, S.V. (1978) Characterisation of a region of the primary sequence of troponin C involved in calcium ion dependent interaction with troponin I. *Biochemical Journal*, **173**, 449.

Weihing, R.T. & Korn, E.D. (1972) Acanthamoeba actin. Composition of the peptide that contains 3-methylhistidine and a peptide that contains N-methylhistidine. *Biochemistry*, **11**, 1538.

Weissbach, H. & Ochoa, S. (1976) Soluble factors required for eukaryotic protein synthesis. *Annual Review of Biochemistry*, **45**, 914.

Wickner, W. (1979) The assembly of proteins into biological membranes: the membrane tissue tissue hypothesis. *Annual Review of Biochemistry*, **48**, 23.

Wieme, R.J. & Herpol, J.E. (1962) Origin of lactate dehydrogenase isoenzyme pattern found in the serum of patients having primary muscular dystrophy. *Nature*, **194**, 287.

Wilkinson, J.M. & Grand, R.J.A. (1975) The amino acid sequence of TnI from rabbit skeletal muscle. *Biochemical Journal*, **149**, 493.

Wilkinson, J.M., Perry, S.V., Cole, H.A. & Trayer, I.P. (1972) The regulatory proteins of the myofibril. Separation and biological activity of the components of inhibitory factor preparations. *Biochemical Journal*, **127**, 215.

Winegrad, S. (1965) Autoradiographic studies on intracellular calcium in frog skeletal muscles. *Journal of General Physiology*, **48**, 455.

Winegrad, S. (1968) Intracellular calcium movements of frog skeletal muscle during recovery from tetanus. *Journal of General Physiology*, **51**, 65.

Winter, M.R.C., Head, J.F. & Perry, S.V. (1974) Conformational changes and complex formation by troponin C. In *Calcium Binding Proteins*, Eds W. Drabikowski, H. Strzelecka-Golaszewsak & E. Carafoli, p. 109 (Elsevier: Amsterdam).

Woledge, R.C. (1971) Heat production and chemical change in muscle. *Progress in Biophysics and Molecular Biology*, **22**, 37.

Woledge, R.C. (1972) Calorimetric studies relating to the interpretation of muscle heat experiments. *Cold Spring Harbor Symposia on Quantitative Biology*, **37**, 629.

Wolf, D.J. & Brostrom, C.O. (1979) Properties and functions of the calcium-dependent regulatory proteins. *Advances in Cyclic Nucleotide Research*, **11**, 27.

Woods, E.F. (1967) Molecular weight and sub-unit structure of tropomyosin B. *Journal of Biological Chemistry*, **242**, 2859.

Wray, J.S. (1979) Structure of the backbone in myosin filaments of muscle. *Nature*, **277**, 37.

Wu, T.T. & Kabat, E.H. (1973) An attempt to evaluate the influence of neighboring amino acids (n − 1) and (n +1) on the backbone conformation of amino acid (n) in proteins. Use of predicting three-dimensional structures of the polypeptide backbone of other proteins. *Journal of Molecular Biology*, **75**, 13.

Yagi, K., Yazawa, M., Kakiuchi, S., Ohshima, M. & Uenishi, K. (1978) Identification of an activator protein for myosin light chain kinase as the Ca2+-dependent modulator protein. *Journal of Biological Chemistry*, **253**, 1338.

Yamaguchi, M., Greaser, M. & Cassens, R.G. (1974)

Interactions of troponin sub-units with different forms of tropomyosin. *Journal of Ultrastructure Research*, **33**, 48.

Yamamoto, T. & Tonomura, Y. (1967) Reaction mechanism of the Ca^{2+}-dependent ATPase of sarcoplasmic reticulum from skeletal muscle. *Journal of Biochemistry*, **62**, 558.

Young, M. (1967) On the interaction of adenosine diphosphate with myosin and its enzymically active fragments. Evidence for three identical catalytic sites per myosin molecule. *Journal of Biological Chemistry*, **242**, 2790.

Young, M. (1969) The molecular basis of muscle contraction. *Annual Review of Biochemistry*, **38**, 913.

Young, D.M., Blanchard, M.H. & Brown, D. (1968) Selective non-enzymic cleavage of the myosin rod: Isolation of the coiled coil-rope section from the C terminus of the molecule. *Proceedings of the National Academy of Sciences of the United States of America*, **61**, 1087.

Young, D.M., Himmelfarb, S. & Harrington, H.E. (1965) On the structural assembly of the polypeptide chains of heavy meromyosin. *Journal of Biological Chemistry*, **240**, 2428.

Pathological reactions of the skeletal muscle fibre in man

INTRODUCTION

Myopathology comprises all known structural changes and functional derangements of muscle and also the scientific study of the causes and mechanisms of its diseases. It deals primarily with the muscle fibre and its tendinous attachments, for these represent the only unique component of the musculature. All other structural elements of muscle, namely the connective tissue sheathing, the blood vessels and the various neural elements, are shared by many other tissues. These latter at times bear the brunt of primary pathological processes within muscle, but when this happens the muscular abnormality is usually part of a more widespread or systemic disease.

The myopathologist assumes responsibility for describing the changes in muscle fibres in disease and for distinguishing them from such deviations from the normal state as occur for example in maturational delay, ageing or stress. These changes are of importance in verifying clinical diagnoses, in correlating structural changes with physiology and chemistry, in explaining symptoms, in understanding disease processes, and in drawing reasonable hypotheses as to the aetiology and pathogenesis of disease.

In classical myopathology, as in general pathology, a traditional approach has been to delineate stereotyped patterns of histological change such as hyalinisation, granular degeneration, vacuolation and fat-fanerosis, that are common to diseases in many organs. This practice, and the concepts that are derived therefrom, have become obsolete for two reasons: (1) their relation to artefactual and post-mortem changes is not always clear; (2) the terminology is inexact and such alterations cannot be correlated with changes in the specific organelles of cells in particular disease processes.

The introduction of electron microscopy in pathology has provided new insight into the morphological bases of disease. The high power of resolution of this instrument has enabled pathologists to perceive alterations in greater detail and, for the first time, to relate them to specific nuclear and cytoplasmic elements. Furthermore, in electron microscopy, in order to obtain faithful preservation of structure, improved methods for fixation and preparation have had to be developed (which have also been useful in light microscopy).

We shall describe in this Chapter the primary pathological alterations of the muscle fibre by whatever histological technique seems most appropriate for their demonstration, arrange them in meaningful patterns (reaction patterns) and discuss their possible nature and significance. The list of changes is, of course, tentative and future research in this field, which at present is very active, will without doubt reveal hitherto unknown patterns of change and modify the classification of those already known. Nevertheless, we hope that this list of recognised changes will, for the time being, serve the purposes of myopathology as specified above.

We are well aware that the mere listing of pathological reactions as presented here is artificial. In the living cell, pathogenetic mechanisms and reaction patterns do not exist in isolation but interact in the most intricate fashion. Moreover, the types of change to be described below can be linked only in a general way to specific diseases. Although one type of structural modification may be especially common in one disease (for instance nemaline bodies in nemaline disease) there are really no subcellular changes that are absolutely pathognomonic. In other words, any one of the following histological changes can occur in several different diseases and different changes may be seen in any given condition. It will be obvious to the reader that the muscle fibre, like other cells, reacts in stereotyped ways, and that these ways and the range of reaction patterns are limited.

We will endeavour here to describe only the most frequently observed morphological changes in muscle fibres. The various constellations of morphological change and their temporal ordering, which constitute the pathology of specific muscle diseases, will be found in other Chapters.

TECHNOLOGIES IMPORTANT TO MYOPATHOLOGY

A century of research on the pathological changes in muscle as seen with the light microscope has produced a wealth of information (Adams, 1975). Only in recent years have new tools, notably the electron microscope, been introduced in myopathological research. Because of the high power of resolution of this instrument, previously unknown types of reactions have been seen and details have been added to those already known (Mair and Tomé, 1972; Neville, 1973; Price, 1973; Åström and Adams, 1979; *see also* Ch. 9). The critical evaluation of this new material is of central importance in contemporary myopathology.

Histochemical methods for the demonstration of particular enzymes have also shed light on a number of obscure aspects of disease (Dubowitz and Brooke, 1973). The phosphorylase technique

has confirmed the deficiency of this enzyme in McArdle's disease. The use of the ATPase technique has permitted the subdividing of individual motor units into fast phasic and slower tonic types and has shown that the type II fibres atrophy more readily with disuse and the type I fibres are earlier affected in myotonic dystrophy and certain other congenital myopathies. Histochemical typing has been particularly useful in disclosing the group atrophy of partial denervation after there has been collateral regeneration of nerve fibres. It is our impression, however, that the histochemical techniques have revealed more of the altered physiological function to which muscle is subjected as a result of disease, than of the nature of pathological processes *per se*. For this reason, and also because there is another chapter devoted to histochemistry, fibre typing will not be emphasised here.

Radionuclide and fluorescent tagging of molecules in the end-plate and within the muscle fibre have also been added to the technical armamentarium of the myopathologist, especially when combined with electron microscopy. This method has been particularly useful in diseases such as myasthenia gravis, which previously had an uncertain morphological basis. Scanning electron microscopy, freeze-fracturing and morphometric techniques are also beginning to be applied to the muscle fibre.

SOME FEATURES OF NORMAL MUSCLE THAT ARE OF IMPORTANCE TO PATHOLOGISTS

In order to understand the possible pathological reactions of the muscle fibre, certain of its anatomical and histological properties must be kept in mind.

First, there is the biological fact that the human organism is born with nearly all the muscle fibres it is destined to have (some new fibres continue to form in the post-natal period according to Adams and DeReuck, 1973). Their formation from myoblasts, which fuse to form myotubes and then differentiate into the thin but fully constructed fibre, takes place mostly during intrauterine life. Growth of the fibres is their most important postnatal developmental activity and takes place throughout childhood. As far as we know, fibres, once formed in early life, must survive the lifetime of the human organism, and, if totally destroyed, are never restored. Premature senescence might conceivably be the basis of disease.

Second, there is the enormous size and multi-nucleation of the muscle cell or fibre. No other cell in the animal or human organism approaches it in dimensions. Some muscle cells attain a width of 0.1 mm and a length of many centimetres. There are thousands of nuclei in a single cell, and each nucleus controls only a small region of the fibre. This fact, and the great length in proportion to width, allow certain muscle diseases to destroy only one segment of the fibre, leaving the rest of it intact and ready to regenerate, like a cut earthworm, from the surviving sound portions. The surviving segment may thus become separated from its nerve supply, which normally joins the muscle fibre near its equator.

A third anatomical fact, of unquestionable significance to pathology, relates to the highly intricate and complex structure of the muscle cell. Within its irritable cytoplasmic membrane (sarcolemma) are contained the myofibrils with their thick and thin myofilaments of myosin, actin, tropomyosin and meromyosin; these account both for the characteristic striations and for the contractile process. In addition, in the intervening sarcoplasm, reside the endoplasmic reticulum (in a particular distribution with respect to the Z discs), the mitochondria and other organelles, with their rich contents of enzymes, the myoglobin and the globules of fat and glycogen. Certain of these subcellular structures, such as myofibrils, do not occur in other cells and it might be expected that certain diseases peculiar to muscle depend on an affinity between them and the noxious agents to which the musculature is susceptible.

A fourth histological peculiarity, perhaps of less clear relevance to pathology, is the investment of each muscle fibre by a thin sheath of connective tissue. This sheath is composed of delicate strands of reticulin and in places contains collagenous and elastic tissue; heavier bands of these same tissues constitute the perimysium which envelops fascicles, thus offering support and serving also to coordinate the contracting forces of aggregates of fibres. This arrangement, while mechanically advantageous, may nevertheless work to the detriment of the muscle fibre for, in the event of an inflammatory reaction, hyperplasia of these connective tissue sheaths, or oedema, may compress muscle fibres and even cause infarction, should blood vessels be simultaneously occluded. This latter phenomenon of ischaemia may also result from diseases which directly affect the blood vessels.

A fifth histological fact of pertinence to pathology derives from the close relationship between nerve and muscle. In no other organ is there found such a highly specialised functional zone between nerve fibre and parenchymal cell, nor is such evident functional and trophic influence exerted by the nervous system. Indeed, the muscle cell appears to be incapable of effective, organised activity when deprived of innervation, and cannot survive independently for more than a few months or years. The intricacies of this functional control of the musculature by the nervous system become manifest in many diseases which paralyse the numerous muscle fibres that are governed by single motor cells of the spinal cord (the motor units). These diseases constantly remind us that all reflex, postural and volitional movement consists of the combined contraction of motor units which are activated and regulated by nerves and sensory end-organs lying within muscle. These motor functions of the nervous system depend on segmental and suprasegmental influences which converge on the anterior horn cells and are transmitted to the muscle fibre via their axons and myoneural junctions. The latter are of central importance and consist of the branching nerve fibre ending (telodendrion) and a heavily-nucleated, specialised part of the muscle fibre (the end-plate). Conduction of the nerve impulse across this junction is effected by acetylcholine which is liberated from the synaptic vesicles of the nerve ending, and the intensity and duration of its action is modified by the cholinesterase of the end-plate and by certain cations such as Na^+, K^+, Ca^+ and Mg^+, which also determine the irritability of the sarcolemma. These chemical substances may be quantitatively altered by derangements of the endocrine organs, liver, and kidneys.

The last and perhaps least understood histological structures, from the pathological viewpoint, are the tendon fibrils. These latter attach to each end of the muscle cell, and the power of muscular contraction is transmitted through them to the skeleton, resulting in movement. Relatively little is known of the pathological reactions of tendinous tissue.

The aforementioned histological qualities are common to all the hundreds of millions of muscle fibres that constitute the musculature. However, it must not be assumed that all the fibres possess identical structure merely because they look alike under the light microscope. Indeed, a number of differences between the fibres of different muscles throughout the body and between those of any one muscle have been recognised. For example, it has been shown that the large fibres (type II or 'white fibres') possess a rich content of phosphorylase, and the thin ones (type I or 'red fibres') a great abundance of oxidative enzymes (Dubowitz and Brooke, 1973). Fibres of the latter type also have a larger ratio of capillaries to muscle cell. Fibres also vary with respect to their content of myoglobin, glycogen and fat, upon which depend some of the well-known differences in colour. Moreoever, the disposition of connective tissue and blood vessels varies in different muscles, accounting for greater or lesser vulnerability to ischaemia. Then there are the relationships between the numbers of nerve and muscle fibres, revealed in the size of the motor units; these ratios vary greatly, being as low as $1:c\,30$ for the external ocular muscles and as high as $1:c\,1500$ for the gastrocnemius. Finally, there are subtle differences between muscles with respect to their conductional capacity expressed by such qualities as ease of depolarisation, duration of refractory period and frequency of discharge. All these and other differences undoubtedly underlie the highly individual topography of many diseases of the musculature of man, the particular distribution of biochemical disturbances and the action of pharmacological agents.

When considering the important volumetric aspects of the muscle fibre in man and animals one must know something about the natural growth and maturational aspects of the muscle fibre and the effects upon it of age. It may be said that each muscle possesses fibres of a certain size and these vary in different epochs of life. Beginning at birth, fibres (ranging from 7 to 14 μm in diameter) gradually grow until late adolescence or early adult life, when maximal size is attained. During adult years the variations in fibre size between individual muscles are considerable. Those of the ocular muscles average 17.5–20 μm in diameter, the forearm and lower leg muscles 50–60 μm in diameter, and the glutei, paravertebral, and shoulder muscles 70–85 μm, depending on the physical condition of the subject. However, the range in size of fibres within any muscle is wide; in heavy muscles it is from 10–15 μm up to 100 μm. Groups of fibres below 40 μm in diameter are nearly always pathological.

In later life there is a loss of some fibres and a gradual increase in range of size of residual ones, at least until advanced years when diameters again diminish. Data on these points are to be found in the articles of Halban (1894), Wohlfart (1942), Banker, Victor and Adams (1957), Greenfield, Shy, Alvord and Berg (1957) and Sissons (1965), but in most instances, especially in the younger age group, they are based on too few cases to serve as a reliable guide in pathological diagnosis. More precise data concerning the biometrics of human muscle at all ages from mid-fetal life to senility are to be found in the article by Moore, Rebeiz, Holden and Adams (1971), in which are plots of the growth curves for seven muscles. The most rapid growth occurs in the first years of life with a plateau being reached by adulthood, and there is a slight decline in the senile period.

Augmentation in volume during growth is presumably attributable to direct action of growth hormone, and the atrophy after pituitary destruction (Simmonds' disease) is probably the negative effect. At puberty the male sex hormone stimulates muscle fibre growth. Thereafter the masculine fibre exceeds the feminine one in volume as well as strength and endurance, particularly in certain muscles such as the biceps brachii. After castration of the male the fibre size reverts to its prepubertal dimension (Papanicolau and Falk, 1938). Cortisone also causes atrophy and probably interferes with normal growth (see p. 161).

Concerning that aspect of muscle fibre volume related to the trophic influence of the nerve fibre, it appears that the degree of activation of muscle by the nerve impulses governs the size of the muscle fibre. The muscle fibre atrophies when activated little (disuse atrophy) and hypertrophies when activated excessively (work hypertrophy). No other cell manifests such clear volumetric change in response to the needs of the organism. This influence of activity also holds true for the heart muscle fibre. The source of the neurotrophic factor has puzzled investigators. There is no doubt that complete denervation causes a much greater degree of atrophy than complete disuse, as when a tendon is cut. Thus, lack of nerve contact does more than merely halt muscle work; presumably the additional trophic influence comes through the neuromuscular junction. On the basis of studies of embryonic muscle, Drachman (1965) suggested that acetylcholine is the neuronal trophic substance.

For a time there was disagreement as to whether muscle activity, e.g. work enlargement, resulted in an increased number of fibres (numerical increase) or an increase in size of existing fibres (volumetric increase). Morpurgo (1897) and other workers finally showed that the latter mechanism was correct. Similarly, in underuse atrophy (whether from isolating a spinal segment, splinting a limb or cutting a tendon) a volumetric, not a numerical, reduction occurs over a period of weeks but seldom exceeds 25–30 per cent of normal (contrasting with the 75–80 per cent loss of bulk in denervation atrophy). As stated above, histochemical studies reveal a greater reduction in the type II white, phosphorylase-rich fibres, the ones involved principally in fast-twitch or phasic reactions. In work hypertrophy, a volumetric increase occurs only if the muscle is required to overcome ever-increasing resistance per unit of time. Stated in another way, hypertrophy appears to be proportional to the intensity of contraction and not to duration of effort. By such a training programme, Denny-Brown (1961) succeeded in increasing the range in size of soleus fibres in the dog from 38–87 µm to 51–93 µm. Enlargement was accompanied by an increased number of myofibrils per fibre (1087–1206 in the control, compared with 1679–2063 in the conditioned animal) and in the amount of sarcoplasm. Adequate data are lacking on myofibril counts in disuse atrophy, but presumably they are decreased.

Inanition and cachexia are said to induce volumetric changes not essentially different in degree from disuse. Indeed, it is not clear in most of the studies of cachexia whether the operative factor was inactivity, cachexia, denervation, some other effect of disease or even age. Marin and Denny-Brown (1962) in a survey of 12 cases of cachexia, all except two of whom had malignant tumours, stressed the thinning of fibres and granulo-fatty degeneration. However, such studies have not taken into account the changes in muscle associated with activity and age (see Tomlinson, Walton and Rebeiz, 1969).

PATHOLOGICAL CHANGES IN STRIATED MUSCLE FIBRES

Changes in volume, number and shape

An important parameter of disease in skeletal muscle is volumetric change without qualitative alterations of structure. This may take the form of diminution in size of individual fibres (hypoplasia or atrophy) or an increase (hyperplasia or hypertrophy). Being a much less obvious change, particularly in its milder forms, the pathologist who does not habitually use an eyepiece micrometer tends to overlook this aspect of disease. Alterations of size may occur in all fibres without selectivity or in fibres of one enzymatic type only. The recognition of the latter is possible only when the morphometric analysis is made on histochemically stained preparations (Brooke and Engel, 1969 a, b, c, d; Johnson, Polgar, Weightman and Appleton, 1973; Johnson, Sideri, Weightman and Appleton, 1973).

Atrophy

Denervation atrophy. If deprived of innervation, muscle fibres atrophy at a calculated rate (Fig. 5.1)⋆. In several species of animals, including man, volumetric decrease proceeds at an even pace over a period of 120 days to a point where the weight is only 20–30 per cent of normal i.e. 70–80 per cent reduction). As the vessels and connective tissues undergo only slight changes and retain their natural appearance and bulk (they make up 10–25 per cent of muscle weight), this means that

---

⋆ Unless otherwise noted, all Figures in Chapter 5 are phase micrographs from sections of osmicated, epon-embedded material, which have been stained with paraphenylene diamine.

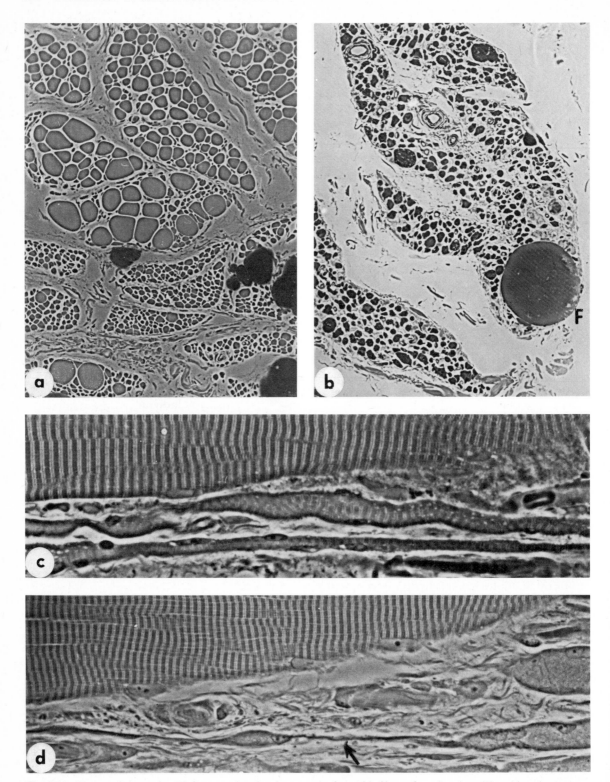

Fig. 5.1★   Denervation atrophy. (a) Cross-section showing groups of atrophic fibres of varying sizes. The widened spaces between the fibres contain connective tissue and a few fat cells (black), ×220. (b) Cross-section showing advanced degree of atrophy. Shrunken fascicles of fibres are separated by connective tissue. F = fat cell, ×220. (c) Two longitudinally cut atrophic fibres with preserved striation. Note the relative increase of sarcolemmal nuclei in the thinner fibre at bottom of picture, ×1180. (d) An atrophic fibre is reduced to a thin thread (arrow), ×735

the sarcous substance is reduced to about 5–10 per cent of its normal volume. The denervated muscle fibre loses volume, as a fibre normally does during inactivity. Re-innervation during this stage restores fibre bulk and strength of contraction. However, if regrowth of nerve does not occur within a few months or a year or more, the thin fibres pass a point of no return and will degenerate. It is as if muscle fibres are removed because they are useless to the body.

Under the light microscope the thin, atrophic fibres appear excessively nucleated (Fig. 5.1c), owing to the fact that the normal number of nuclei are crowded into a smaller volume of sarcoplasm. The nuclei are at first slightly enlarged and the residual myofibrils are intact. As the atrophy increases, the undulating course of the thin fibres (a change due to retraction of excised tissue), when observed in longitudinal sections, may result in an illusion of segmental interruption in continuity and agglutination of sarcolemmal nuclei. Gradually the muscle nuclei shrink and acquire a deep basophilia. Clumps of these dark nuclei may persist after all visible sarcoplasm has vanished.

Electron-microscopic studies of denervation in animals (Wechsler and Hager, 1961; Pellegrini and Franzini, 1963: Pellegrini and Franzini-Armstrong, 1969) and in man (Afifi, Aleu, Goodgold and MacKay, 1966; Shafiq, Milhorat, and Gorycki, 1967; Szliwowski and Drachman, 1975) demonstrate a loss of myofilaments in the periphery of myofibrils, a gradual reduction in the number of myofibrils, and possibly a selective degeneration of I-bands and Z-lines.

Following denervation in animals there is concomitant breakdown of myofibrils, an increase of hydrolytic enzymes, and lysosome-like elements (Pellegrini and Franzini, 1963). These latter findings suggest that sarcoplasmic material is being digested within autophagic vacuoles. However, the question whether the breakdown of myofibrils is taking place inside or outside the lysosomal system has not been settled (*see* Bird, 1975).

The fate of the denervated fibre is still a controversial topic and the literature which has accumulated on this subject is reviewed in the monograph of Gutmann (1962) and his Czechoslovakian school. Hyaline and vacuolar degeneration, fibrosis and fat-cell replacement are reported to occur within a few months in the denervated muscle of animals, yet in man thin fibres may survive for years. Usually it is in isolated, large fibres that the degenerative changes are most conspicuous, as though the active, innervated fibres had suffered injury (Fig. 5.2d). This dystrophic aspect of denervation atrophy occurs at a variable interval after the onset of denervation, differing possibly from one animal to another and in different muscles in any one animal. Its nature remains uncertain, and even the exhaustive studies of Gutmann have not clarified our understanding of it.

These degenerative changes also introduce a practical problem in pathological diagnosis, that of differentiating atrophy from dystrophy. After many years of denervation, when numerous muscle fibres have been replaced by fat and fibrous tissue, the distinction between the late stages of these two processes becomes increasingly uncertain; even when many fibres remain, distinction may be difficult. In the chronic polyneuropathies such as Charcot-Marie-Tooth disease (Fig. 5.2d), for example, there are scattered giant fibres among surviving units, giving an overall impression of random fibre enlargement and atrophy. Further, some of the large fibres exhibit central nucleation, hyalinisation, occasionally degeneration and phagocytosis, suggestive of a dystrophic process. Haase and Shy (1960) have interpreted these changes as primary. We would insist, however, that their observations do no more than call attention to the late secondary changes common to all denervated fibres and do not imply, either that there is a primary myopathic process in these diseases or, conversely, that dystrophies are due to denervation (*see* Drachman, Murphy, Nigam and Hills, 1967). Part of the confusion in the histological picture in denervating diseases relates to the reaction of muscle fibres with residual intact innervation. They undergo hypertrophy, sometimes striking, so that if one makes a graph of their diameters, the usual symmetrical Gaussian curve is now replaced by one with two or three peaks. Schwartz, Sargent and Swash (1976) have suggested that longitudinal splitting of muscle fibres caused by overload of poorly innervated hypertrophic fibres can also account for some of the

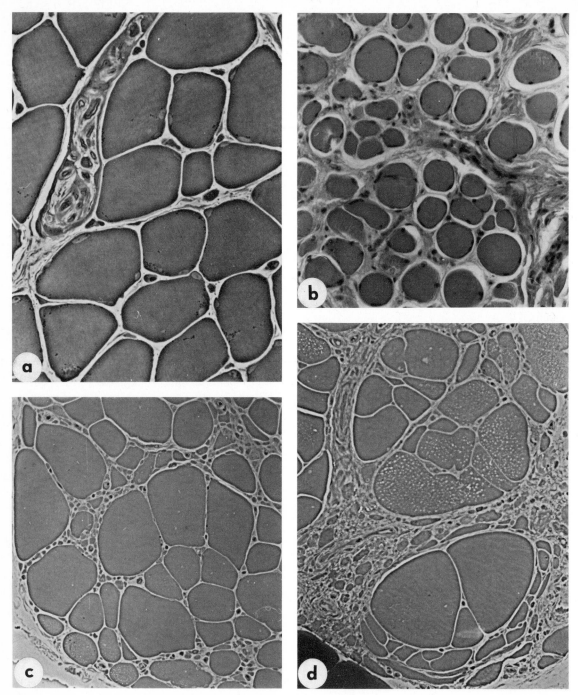

Fig. 5.2 Cross-sections showing variations in size and shape of fibres in different muscle diseases. (a) Fibres of normal polygonal shape but of reduced diameter from a case of nemaline myopathy. A normal nerve twig is seen in the upper, left part of the figure, ×545. (b) Section of thigh muscle in Duchenne dystrophy showing rounded shape and variation in diameter in muscle fibres. Endomysial connective tissue is relatively increased due to disappearance of muscle fibres. H and E, ×200. (c) Fibres of rounded shape and a variation of their diameters from case of polymyositis. Interstitial spaces contain inflammatory cells, ×220. (d) Dystrophic aspect of denervation atrophy illustrated by a section from a case of Charcot-Marie-Tooth disease. Group atrophy is seen in lower part of picture. Vacuolation in some fibres, especially the larger ones, is a sign of degeneration, ×220

'myopathic' changes in denervation atrophy.

When all of the muscle fibres suffer denervation atrophy simultaneously, as may occur in poliomyelitis or acute polyneuritis, the atrophic process is distributed diffusely throughout the muscle (Fig. 5.1b). However, even in this circumstance some fibres are thinner than others. It often happens, however, that the disease singles out one axon or nerve cell at a time, as in one of the progressive polyneuropathies or in motor neurone disease. Atrophy then expresses itself in a pattern determined by the distribution of the motor units (Fig. 5.1a). It is here that fibre-type grouping is most informative.

The residual healthy fibres of sound units rapidly increase in size, many coming to exceed 100 μm in diameter (Adams, 1968). The work hypertrophy of partly denervated muscle, expressed also in increased anabolic activity and decreased catabolism (Goldberg, 1967), is one explanation of gigantism in muscle fibres.

Re-innervation of muscle fibres after denervation is further described on page 199.

There are, then, two standard pathological pictures of denervation atrophy—that of diffuse atrophy of all motor units (Fig. 5.1b) and the multiple, successive atrophy of single units (Fig. 5.1a). In both, the fascicular atrophy expresses itself as groups of uniformly small fibres with dark clustered nuclei and only slight change in the connective tissue. For the pathologist, one of the main difficulties is the differentiation of diffuse denervation from disuse atrophy, cachexia, and senility. Whereas generalised denervation atrophy, when advanced, is obvious enough, its earlier stages, with muscle fibres only moderately reduced in volume, may be indistinguishable from the change of disuse and cachexia. Here one must appeal for final proof of denervation to histochemical stains of muscle to show large fields of one type of reinnervated fibres ('type-grouping') or to anatomical and physiological examination of the nerve or spinal cord, where the lesions causing the denervation should be demonstrable. Moreover, some of the necroses of muscle affect compact groups of fibres which, upon regeneration, may present as islands of atrophic fibres, simulating the muscle atrophy of motor unit disease.

Hypoplasia (hypotrophy) of muscle is another cause of small fibres. It has been known for many years that some children from birth or from an early age are weak and hypotonic ('floppy'), have a retarded motor development, poor reflexes and generally thin skeletal muscles. The condition is relatively non-progressive. With advancing age, strength and muscle size may slowly increase, but the musculature is always relatively subnormal. Biopsy or chance autopsy may reveal a universal smallness of normally structured muscle fibres, as though some factor essential to maturation and growth were lacking. The ailment differs from the hypoplasia resulting from the lack of normal development of motor neurones (*see* Zelena, 1962).

Walton (1957) called the condition 'benign congenital hypotonia'; eventually, the children he was studying recovered almost completely. Further study of this group of patients with congenitally weak, hypotonic muscles shows them to be suffering from a heterogeneous group of diseases. Using modern histological techniques, especially histochemical staining and electron microscopy, myopathologists have more recently been able to distinguish several more or less well-defined entities (Table 5.1). In one of the diseases (myotubular myopathy) it has been suggested that the fibres have retained their fetal character, i.e. their development has been arrested (*see* p. 195). In other cases the size of the fibres is not reduced, however; as the bulk of the muscles is diminished, there is probably a reduction in the number of fibres.

Some of the congenital hypotonias such as central core disease, nemaline myopathy, and the mitochondrial myopathies are distinguished additionally by special morphological features of the fibres, and these features have become the basis of subdivision. Nevertheless, further study has shown that there are many combinations of these structural alterations of organelles (Bethlem, Arts and Dingemans, 1978); hence, any one type of change is non-specific.

Clearly, many more observations are needed before nosology can be established, the relations between the different conditions clarified, and the significance of the structural changes and their functional equivalents ascertained.

Table 5.1 Congenital hypotonia: some reported causes

Benign congenital hypotonia	Walton (1957)
Central core disease (p. 179)	Shy and Magee (1956); Isaacs, Heffron and Badenhorst (1975); Saper and Itabashi (1976); Radu, Rosu-Serbu, Ionescu and Radu (1977)
Myotubular myopathy (p. 195)	Spiro, Shy and Gonatas (1966); Sher, Rimalovski, Athanassiades and Aronson (1967); Campbell, Rebeiz and Walton (1969); PeBenito, Sher and Cracco (1978)
Type I fibre hypotrophy and central nuclei	Engel, Gold and Karpati (1968); Kinoshita, Satoyoshi and Matsuo (1975)
Congenital fibre type disproportion	Dubowitz and Brooke (1973); Brooke (1974)
Congenital neuromuscular disease and external ophthalmoplegia	Bender and Bender (1977)
Nemaline myopathy (p. 186)	Shy, Engel, Somers and Wanko (1963); Conen, Murphy and Donohue (1963); Kuitunen, Rapola, Noponen and Donner (1972); Sreter, Åström, Romanul, Young and Jones (1976)
Megaconial and pleoconial ('mitochondrial') myopathies	Shy, Gonatas and Perez (1966)
Multicore disease	Engel, Gomez and Groover (1971); Heffner, Cohen, Duffner and Daigler (1976); Lake, Cavanagh and Wilson (1977); Bonnette, Roelofs and Olson (1974)
Congenital neuromuscular disorders with rods, cores, miniature cores and focal loss of cross-striations	Bethlem, Arts and Dingemans (1978)
Fingerprint body myopathy	Engel, Angelini and Gomez (1972); Fardeau, Tomé and Derambure (1976); Curless, Payne and Brimmer (1978)
Reducing-body myopathy	Brooke and Neville (1972); Tomé and Fardeau (1975)
Sarcotubular myopathy	Jerusalem, Engel and Gomez (1973)
Lysis of myofibrils in type I fibres	Cancilla, Kalyanaraman, Verity, Munsat and Pearson (1971)
Neuromuscular disease with trilaminar muscle fibres	Ringel, Neville, Duster and Carroll (1978)
Zebra body myopathy	Lake and Wilson (1975)
Target fibre disease	Schotland (1967)
Arthrogryposis multiplex	Banker, Victor and Adams (1957)
Congenital myopathy with subsarcolemmal masses	Sahgal and Sahgal (1977)
Diaphragmatic paralysis with type I fibre atrophy	DeReuck, Hooft, DeCoster, van den Bossche and Cuvelier (1977)

Other causes of congenital and neonatal hypotonia and hypoplasia of muscle include well-known entities such as Werdnig-Hoffmann's infantile spinal atrophy (Pearn and Wilson, 1973; Dubowitz, 1975), congenital forms of muscle dystrophy (Banker et al., 1957; Gubbay, Walton and Pearce, 1966; Zellweger, Afifi, McCormick and Mergner, 1967), dystrophia myotonica (Dyken and Harper, 1973; Zellweger and Ionasescu, 1973), myasthenia gravis (McLean and McKone, 1973; Whiteley, Schwartz, Sachs and Swash, 1976), neonatal myasthenia gravis (Namba, Brown and Grob, 1970), acid maltase deficiency (Engel, 1970a; Engel, Gomez and Seybold, 1973) and polymyopathies with developmental brain abnormalities and brain damage (Fenichel, 1967; Curless, Nelson and Brimmer, 1978).

Other conditions with small muscle fibres. Small, diffusely basophilic fibres with large, heavily stained sarcolemmal nuclei and sparse myofibrils represent a regenerative process (p. 199). This is particularly prominent after an attack of paroxysmal myoglobinuria (*see* Fig. 5.7d), in polymyositis (*see* Fig. 5.7b, c), and in the Duchenne type of progressive muscular dystrophy. In still other diseases, small fibres seem to preserve their eosinophilia, myofibrillar structure and natural nucleation without any indication of the cause of their atrophy. This is as striking in the muscular dystrophies and in some cases of polymyositis as is hypertrophy, with its tendency to central nucleation (Fig. 5.2b). Whether the small fibres are caused by splitting of the hypertrophied ones (as asserted by Wohlfart) has not been decided.

The diseases listed in Table 5.1 and in the above list do not exhaust the conditions that seem to interfere with muscular development. Mongolism and the other chromosomal trisomy states are associated with thinness of muscle and hypotonia.

In Werner's disease, which involves weight loss, weakness, baldness, cataracts, greying of hair, wrinkling of skin, diabetes, and arteriosclerosis, the muscles are thin and feeble. The reduction of the fibre girth is presumably related to some unspecified endocrine or metabolic defect. Willi-Präder syndrome (amentia, hypotonia, hypogonadism and obesity) and a variety of other metabolic and developmental diseases of the nervous system of childhood are associated with poorly developed musculature; their nature has not been ascertained.

In Cushing's disease and with chronic corticosteroid therapy (Müller and Kugelberg, 1959; Perkoff, Silber, Tyler, Cartwright and Wintrobe, 1959) there is proximal weakness of limb muscles, particularly of the thighs. Random biopsies reveal an atrophic myopathy. Such muscles are notably abnormal because of the presence of many thin fibres 10–30 μm in diameter with normal-appearing sarcoplasm and myofibrils and a relative increase in sarcolemmal nuclei, many of which are centrally located. Only a few degenerating fibres may be seen and the interstitial tissue and vessels are unaltered. In addition, there are clear central zones, impoverished of myofibrillar material, in a few of the fibres. The pathological picture can be distinguished from denervation atrophy only with difficulty, but the peripheral nerves and spinal cord are normal.

Enlargement of muscle fibres. In evaluating hypertrophy in transverse sections prepared for light microscopy, only those fibres in which the myofibrils are visible should be measured. In biopsied material many of the fibres are slightly swollen, rounded and with vitreous sarcoplasm, attributable to contraction bands or to physical alterations induced by incision. They are most prominent at the cut surfaces of the specimens. The occurrence of fibres of similar appearance, scattered throughout the specimen, is also a well-recognised feature of Duchenne dystrophy but its significance is controversial. One hypothesis holds that this is the first stage of necrosis, as indeed it may be in certain instances. Another is that it is expressive only of the unusually irritable state of the muscle fibres in this disease, a view which the authors favour.

True enlargement or hypertrophy of muscle fibres may result from the operation of a number of factors. As mentioned above, excessive activity regularly increases the diameter of fibres (work hypertrophy). Within hours or days, the anabolic activities of overworked muscle increase in proportion to the catabolic processes; within a few weeks the transverse diameters are augmented by as much as 30 per cent and the number of myofibrils by as many as 600. There are probably also more myofilaments in each myofibril. In addition it has been pointed out that, in muscles which have been partially denervated, or in which a portion of the fibres have been destroyed by disease, the healthy innervated ones show a similar hypertrophy, probably also a result of overwork.

Some degree of enlargement also occurs in the uninjured parts of fibres undergoing regeneration after segmental necrosis.

Of more obscure nature is the enlargement of muscle fibres in certain forms of muscular dystrophy: this enlargement may precede the first hint of degeneration. In the more advanced stages of muscular dystrophy, where there has been considerable loss of fibres, some of those remaining surpass the normal fibres in size, probably as a result of work hypertrophy. Studies of mouse dystrophy, where the hypertrophy is prevented by denervation, bear out this supposition that it is a reaction of intact fibres to overwork. The muscle fibres of the acromegalic and pituitary giant are also larger than normal.

Changes in shape of muscle fibres. Well-fixed and embedded microscopic sections of normal skeletal muscle, cut transversely, reveal the polygonal shape of the fibres (Fig. 5.2a). Together they form a virtual mosaic. It would seem that intramuscular pressures impart this angularity, for the fibres become manifestly more rounded when their number is depleted by disease (Fig. 5.2). Nevertheless, this is not a complete explanation, because partial denervation and atrophy do not efface the angularity. Contraction bands, biopsy trauma, and early necrosis all cause swelling and rounding of the fibres.

Once segments of muscle fibres have been destroyed, especially if the sarcolemma is breached, regeneration by budding and by the

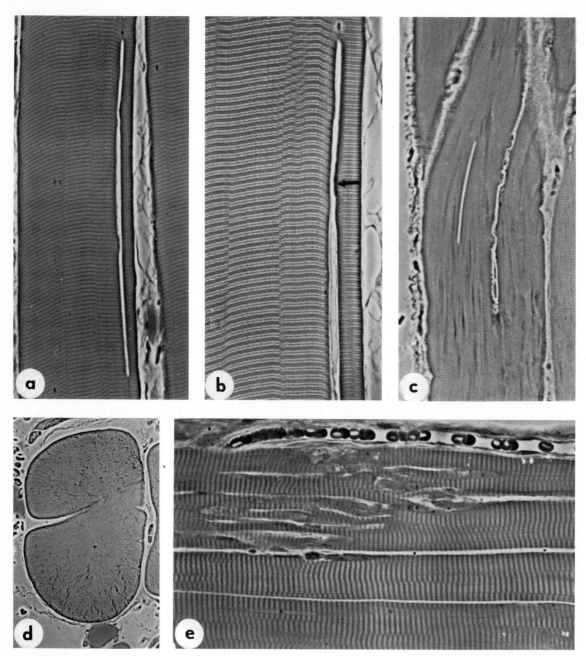

Fig. 5.3 Four longitudinal and one cross-section illustrating splitting of muscle fibres. (a) Longitudinal splitting after focal necrosis, which has partly divided a fibre into a thick and thin portion in the plane of sectioning, ×350. (b) Higher magnification of previous figure showing that the split contains a capillary. Note also the sarcolemmal nucleus in the thin portion facing the cleft (arrow), ×700. (c) Split containing capillary penetrating from interstitial spaces, ×450. (d) Cross-section showing partial splitting of fibre, ×545. (e) Splitting and indentations of fibre after a focal necrosis, which has remodelled the surface of the fibre, ×700

fusion of liberated myoblasts results in the unin-jured fibre appearing to have split. Although this may be seen to a slight degree in healthy muscle, probably as a consequence of minor injury, it is a special feature of all the necroses of muscle. Not infrequently, five or six of these small regenerating 'shoots' occupy the same region to form a compact bundle. The latter appearance may be misin-terpreted as indicating denervation atrophy of a part of a motor unit. This type of regeneration may be the basis of a slight increase in the total number of fibres in a muscle with advancing age (Adams and DeReuck, 1973).

Focal necrosis, sequestration and extrusion of necrotic remnants from autophagic vacuoles (Fig. 5.3) can also result in altered structure; there are indentations of the surface and localised splitting of fibres (Swash, Schwartz and Sargeant, 1978; Swash and Schwartz, 1977).

Changes in numbers of fibres. Disap-pearance of fibres. In the strict sense, numerical reduction of the normal complement of fibres within a muscle stands as the most incon-trovertible evidence of a primary myopathic process. It implies, essentially, a destruction of fibres in their entirety and, if severe, results in a proportionate weakening of contractile power. In contrast, denervation and disuse atrophy are for a long time manifested only by volumetric reduction in fibre size and not by a numerical reduction.

The biological factor(s) responsible for any given muscle acquiring a certain average comple-ment of muscle fibres is unknown. As remarked elsewhere, the size of the fibre population in each muscle is subject to individual variations. One suspects that hypoplasia (also called hypotrophy), may be the result of a series of developmental anomalies. This is an aspect of myopathology which has been relatively unexplored.

Assuming that segmental necrosis is regularly followed by regeneration and restoration of fibre structure in such diseases as paroxysmal idiopathic myoglobinuria and idiopathic polymyositis, one wonders why this regenerative process fails in muscular dystrophy. Certainly this would be expected if the necrosis involved the muscle fibre in its entirety, so that no regeneration could occur. However, it may be that when a given fibre is assaulted repeatedly by necrotising factors, its recuperative powers become exhausted. This feature of necrotising diseases of muscle has not been considered to any great extent.

Denervation in itself, if re-innervation is pre-vented, leads to the eventual disappearance of the atrophic fibres (Fig. 5.1d), a process which we prefer to designate as delayed denervative myo-pathy. The part played by injury is not known but it seems to hasten the process in animals.

The most extreme degrees of numerical de-pletion are seen only in the advanced stages of a dystrophic muscular disease. Here virtually all the fibres disappear and are replaced by lipocytes.

Changes in dystrophic fibres. This brings us to one of the most important problems in myopathology—the sequence of changes leading to fibre death in the muscular dystrophies.

Muscle dystrophy of Duchenne type is the one most often discussed because the changes in volume, shape and number of fibres (Fig. 5.2b) and degeneration are so striking. The latter, and some regenerative changes, are more prominent than those seen in the other dystrophies. In contrast, atrophy of fibres in haphazard distri-bution with normal-sized and large ones, and a decrease in the number of fibres, constitute the common picture of all the muscular dystrophies. Enlargement of fibres is prominent and, in our experience, accounts more often for the early enlargement (hypertrophy) of muscle in Duchenne dystrophy than does infiltration of fat cells (pseudo-hypertrophy). It is difficult to determine which, if any, of these changes are primary and which ones are the most significant.

In childhood Duchenne dystrophy, the pro-minent segmental necrosis, phagocytosis and abortive regeneration probably explain the rel-atively rapid pace of the disease. Although rarely approaching in severity that which occurs in polymyositis or paroxysmal myoglobinuria, nevertheless it exceeds that seen in all the other types of dystrophy. Other pathological findings are: (1) vitreous and swollen appearance of many muscle fibres, a change which seems not to progress to phagocytosis; (2) forking or branching of fibres; (3) central nucleation; (4) nuclear chains; (5) sarcoplasmic basophilia; (6) enlargement of sarcolemmal nuclei with prominent nucleolation; (7) infiltration of fat cells and increase in endomysial connective tissue.

The inter-relationships of these histological changes and their significance remain uncertain. We do not know whether the small fibres result from abiotrophy or represent the end-stage of segmental necrosis and regeneration. Because healthy regenerating fibres in other diseases eventually resume their normal size, whereas those in muscular dystrophy remain small, this probably means some kind of interference with a normal trophic function. Forking or branching of thin fibres, emphasised by Wohlfart (1955) as a frequent process in all the muscular dystrophies, could also be a regenerative response to segmental injury. This explanation is supported by the occurrence of the same phenomenon in chronic polymyositis. Small fibres with even, homogeneous basophilia (easily distinguished from basophilic mottling of the crush artefact), an increase in number and size of sarcolemmal nuclei, and prominent nucleolation and sparsity of myofibrils, represent a regenerative reaction to injury of the muscle fibre and are secondary to the necrotic process. Enlargement and central nucleation are in some way associated, for the inward migration of nuclei is more frequent in all conditions which induce hypertrophy. Whether the enlargement is a work hypertrophy of healthy surviving fibres or is the primary change in dystrophy has not been settled. Studies of the earliest stages in the Duchenne type of dystrophy, where the overall diameter of the muscle fibre is increased, favour the idea of Erb (1891), that enlargement is an early primary change (see Bell and Conen, 1967). Rarely, as in some cases of the late Becker type of dystrophy, described by Walton and Gardner-Medwin (1968), remarkable muscle hypertrophy may precede the degenerative stage by several years. Denervation causes it to disappear in both human (Tyler, 1950) and in mouse dystrophy (Banker and Denny-Brown, 1959).

Electron-microscopic studies of the dystrophic muscle fibre (Lapresle, Fardeau and Milhaud, 1965; Fardeau, 1970; Mair and Tomé, 1972) have failed to reveal a characteristic sequence of subcellular changes. There are only focal alterations of sarcomeres, modifications of Z material, zones of sarcoplasm containing disorganised myofilaments, variable alterations of mitochondria, dilated endoplasmic reticulum, and the presence of lysosomes and lipopigment between myofibrils and near the poles of muscle nuclei. These ultrastructural studies have done little more than add details to the known pathology without elucidating the nature of the basic process. More recently, Cullen and Fulthorpe (1975) concluded that the central process in Duchenne dystrophy is the formation of contraction clumps due to the inability of sarcomeres to relax. Mokri and Engel (1975) found focal wedge-shaped lesions (with the base towards the surface of the fibre) and disruptions in the overlying sarcolemmal membrane. They suggest that these gaps are focal disintegrations of the sarcolemma and are the initial change in the dystrophic fibre (see below, p. 175).

The end-stage of all dystrophic muscle diseases is the disappearance of muscle fibres and this, presumably, causes the progressive paralysis. Muscle is ultimately reduced to fat and connective tissue and might even be unrecognisable were it not for the presence of a few stray, surviving fibres and muscle spindles.

Fibrosis may be secondary to loss of fibres, and the fat cell infiltration to the reduced number and volume of fibres. All pathologists agree that the degenerating muscle cell itself is never transformed into a fibroblast or fat cell as was formerly suggested. There is no pathological evidence of injury to nerve cells, to nerve fibres, or to intramuscular blood vessels.

Because all the muscular dystrophies are genetically determined, one must continue to search for the ways in which the gene produces degeneration of the muscle fibre. The primary change still eludes the pathologist. Is fibre necrosis the essential pathological step, or may fibres merely waste away? Perhaps both the atrophic and necrotic processes proceed in parallel, the latter being only the expression of the more intense phase of the atrophic one. Our own observations of chronic end-stage polymyositis reveal nearly all the changes considered characteristic of dystrophy. Thus, one may conclude that many of the alterations believed to be specific for dystrophy relate more to the chronicity of the disease than to its type. It is only by systematic study of large numbers of variably affected muscles at different stages of the disease that some of these problems can be settled.

It is a conventional practice to group the following conditions under the heading of muscle dystrophy: early, childhood type (Duchenne); facioscapulohumeral (Landouzy-Dejerine); limb-girdle (Erb) and distal varieties; myotonic (Steinert) and various forms of progressive ophthalmoplegia, with or without dysphagia. This grouping is indiscriminate and misleading because it implies a common pathogenesis which is far from established. The features that these diseases share as a group are genetic origin, primary involvement of striated muscles, and slow progressivity and chronicity. However, there are also considerable differences as regards clinical pattern of involvement, life profile of the disease and other features. The slowly advancing adolescent and adult types (facioscapulohumeral, the limb-girdle and the distal forms) exhibit relatively little necrosis of muscle fibres and, at any one stage, the aforementioned variations in fibre size and central nucleation, fibrosis, and fat infiltration are extremely variable from one disease to another in any given muscle. Most conspicuously different are the muscle fibres in myotonic dystrophy, where necrosis is a rarity, rows of centrally positioned nuclei are more marked than in any other dystrophies, and spiral annulets (ringbinden) and peripheral masses of sarcoplasm filled with unorganised myofibrils, are features that clearly set this disease apart from the other dystrophies (see Fig. 5.11). Also, in myotonic dystrophy non-muscular tissues are more clearly involved: there may be testicular atrophy, cataracts, loss of hair follicles, and a mild degree of mental retardation. The prominent mitochondrial changes in the muscle fibres of the ocular and oculopharyngeal forms are also indicative of separate disease processes (see p. 188).

Destructive (necrotic) lesions

Lethal injury to cells signifies a disturbance of homeostasis of such severity that the cell cannot maintain its integrity. Its death is followed by a series of processes including autolysis, phagocytosis with removal of dead cytoplasmic ele-

ments, and repair. Mechanisms for maintaining cellular integrity and repair of injury, are, of course, immensely complex but all of them are dependent upon circulation and energy, i.e. availability of ATP. It is possible that lack of oxygen, substrate and enzymes might lead to necrosis. Viewed in another way, it would seem that under the conditions of disease the nutritional and metabolic needs of the fibre exceed the supply of substrates.

The most extreme form of myonecrosis follows severe ischaemia where all or part of the muscle fibres, without regard to their level of contractile activity, are destroyed. In addition, the interstitial tissues undergo necrosis or at least injury. However, there are lesser degrees of substrate deficiency, where the level of activity becomes a factor. An example is McArdle's disease, where the muscle fibre functions adequately and remains sound under conditions of minimal activity, but suffers injury and even destruction during exertion, because of its inability to mobilize its reserve of glycogen for glucose metabolism.

When the problem of myonecrosis is examined in greater detail, one may observe at least four types: (1) a focal destruction of the muscle fibre in a small, circumscribed zone (subfibre), that does not extend to the whole cross-sectional area of the fibre at any point; (2) segmental necrosis of the entire transverse diameter, usually over a span of several sarcomeres, and with preservation of the adjacent basement membrane; (3) regional tissue necrosis of muscle fibres as well as the interstitial tissue, such as occurs with occlusion of an artery and, less commonly, venous stasis, trauma, intense inflammation, injection of chemical agents; (4) contraction clots.

Focal subfibre destruction. We will define focal subfibre necrosis as an irreversible destruction of sarcoplasmic elements in a small zone, which does not involve a complete cross-sectional area of a muscle fibre (Figs. 5.4 and 5.5). In focal subfibre degeneration, the continuity of the fibre is not disrupted; myofibrils are intact lateral to the lesion (Fig. 5.4a). The necrotic material is not removed by invading macrophages as in segmental necrosis, but is enclosed and digested by autolytic enzymes within membrane-bound vacuoles (se-

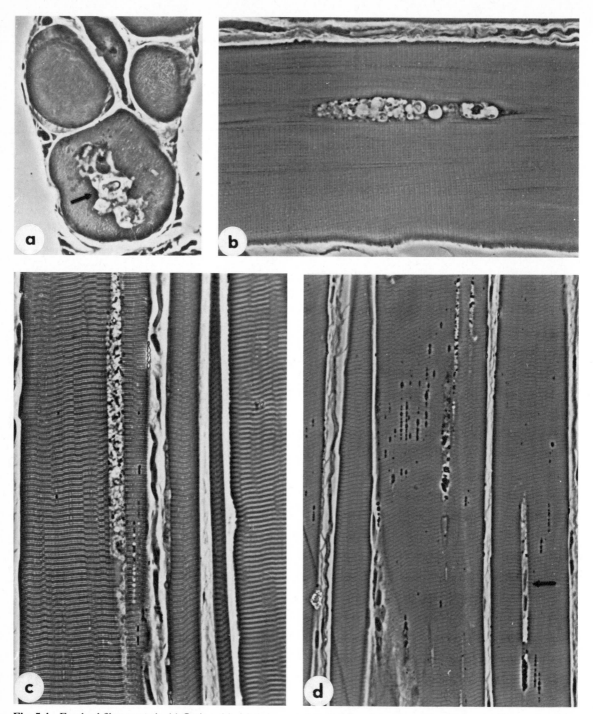

Fig. 5.4 Focal subfibre necrosis. (a) Cavity with debris in central part of fibre (arrow) resulting from a confluence of smaller, autophagic vacuoles, ×545. (b) Autophagic vacuoles have merged, forming a longitudinal cavity in a muscle fibre, ×700. (c) Focal necrosis that has resulted in an elongated cavity, which extends over many sarcomeres in this longitudinal section, ×545. (d) Fibre in the centre with two longitudinal cavities containing remnants of degenerative products. The longitudinal rows of lipofuscin bodies in this fibre indicate the location of former autophagic cavities. The split in the fibre to the right (arrow) contains capillary and connective tissue, which shows that it is connected with the interstitial space, ×350

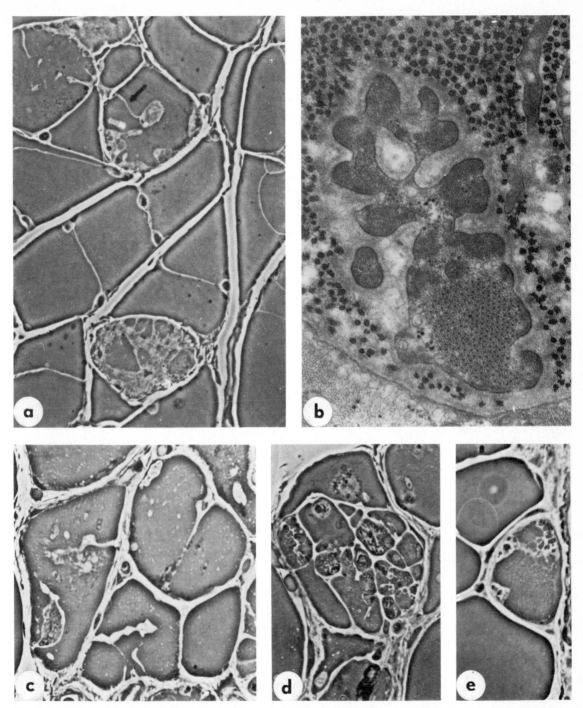

Fig. 5.5 Disfiguration of muscle fibre after focal necrosis. (a) The fibre in the lower part of the figure is split into smaller components, which are embedded in connective tissue. In the upper part of the figure, a centrally located vacuole in a fibre communicates with the outside through a thin channel (arrow), ×700. (b) Fragment of a muscle fibre with scalloped borders. It contains only one myofibril (or part thereof). Electron micrograph, ×42 400. (c) Communication between autophagic vacuoles and interstitial space resulting in splitting of fibres, ×545. (d) A fibre is split into many smaller parts, ×700. (e) peripheral destruction giving the muscle fibre a 'moth-eaten' appearance, ×545

condary lysosomes). Adjacent autophagic vacuoles may merge (Figs. 5.4a and 5.4b), forming larger lesions. The lesions may be situated at the surface near the sarcolemma or deeper within the fibre. A characteristic feature is that larger lesions may extend in a longitudinal direction over many sarcomeres (Fig. 5.4c). The end-products are either extruded into the extracellular space or converted into lipofuscin granules which remain within the muscle fibre (Fig. 5.4d). Muscle fibres appear to be unable to repair themselves completely after focal destruction, and unlike segmental necrosis, myoblasts play no part (Schutta, Kelly and Zacks, 1969). The affected fibres are indented, split, subdivided and their borders serrated, as if 'motheaten' (Figs. 5.3 and 5.5). The remodelling after focal necrosis may possibly weaken the affected fibres but apparently does not destroy them.

Segmental necrosis of muscle fibres. Muscle fibres, like nerve fibres, are capable of undergoing partial destruction, which usually permits cell survival. The uninjured parts are often able to repair the necrotic segment. This phenomenon, which we call segmental necrosis, occurs in a variety of diseases and hence is a fundamental and characteristic, though non-specific, reaction.

The zone of altered sarcoplasm may be limited to as little as one or two sarcomeres but more often 20–30 sarcomeres or more are destroyed (Fig. 5.6). Very occasionally the lesion extends along the entire length of the fibre. Usually the altered sarcous substance has a highly refractile vitreous appearance and appears brightly eosinophilic or acidophilic in the common stains. The fragility of the coagulated sarcoplasm is shown by its tendency to fracture, particularly in the tranverse plane, revealing Bowman's discs. This appearance, while clearly abnormal, may be difficult to distinguish from the artefact resulting from the crushing or cutting of fibres, which is always prominent in biopsy material, and from contraction bands or sarcoplasmic clumps (Fig. 5.8). For this reason one should always search for infiltration of leucocytes and signs of myophagia (Fig. 5.6). These reactive changes corroborate the antemortem nature of at least part of the morphological change under consideration.

Regardless of the cause of the fibre necrosis (a point of fundamental importance), after a few days the necrotic parts of the fibre are always seen to have become heavily infiltrated with pleomorphic histiocytes (Fig. 5.6c), some of which continue to divide within the fibre. Many of the sarcolemmal nuclei in the injured segments are shrunken and pyknotic.

The electron microscopy of segmental necrosis has shown destruction of all organelles and myofilaments, which are converted to amorphous debris; myelin-like bodies, vacuoles and other non-specific changes, evidence surely of a profound disturbance of the intrinsic metabolic mechanism of the muscle fibre, may also be seen. The sarcolemmal membrane is usually destroyed over the affected segments, whereas the basement membrane tends to be preserved.

Two experimental studies of acute necrosis examined by electron microscopy are of particular interest. Price, Howes and Blumberg (1964) in cold-injury noted contraction bands, which progressed to retraction clots, and the various membranous structures within the fibre were variably susceptible to injury. Mitochondria were the most sensitive organelles, but all others also degenerated rapidly. Stenger, Spiro, Scully and Shannon (1962), in a study of ischaemic lesions in muscle of the dog, also saw early alterations in membranous structures. However, in contrast to Price et al., they found that the myofibrils were most resistant to injury, maintaining their integrity as a kind of skeleton up to 24 h after ischaemia. Later there were dissolutions of I bands and degenerations of the Z lines but, even at this stage, the A bands, H discs and M lines showed 'striking preservation of structure'.

Among human studies of segmental necrosis, the findings of which differ little from those in experimental animals, may be mentioned those of Schutta et al. (1969), Kahn and Meyer (1970), Ghatak, Erenberg, Hirano and Golden (1973) and Martinez, Hooshmand and Faris (1973).

Emphasis here has been placed on the alterations of the muscle fibre, but invariably there are changes in the interstitial tissue and blood vessels. Endomysial fibroblasts adjacent to the necrotic segments enlarge, but actual proliferation does not occur unless there is collapse of several muscle

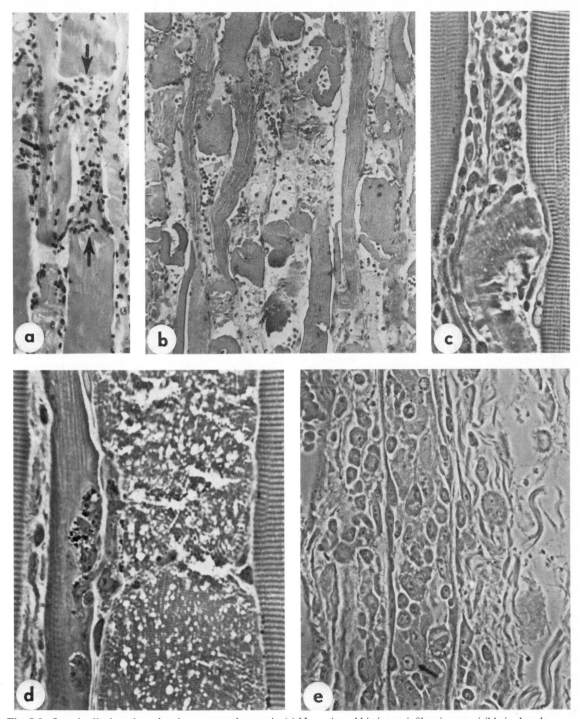

Fig. 5.6 Longitudinal sections showing segmental necrosis. (a) Necrosis and histiocyte infiltration are visible in sharply demarcated, collapsed segment of a muscle fibre from a case of polymyositis (arrows). Hyperplastic sarcolemmal nuclei in the fibre to the left (arrow) reflect regeneration. This is an example of isomorphic muscle necrosis and regeneration. H and E, ×360. (b) Severe destruction with fragmentation of fibres, oedema and infiltration of cells in specimen from case of alcoholic myopathy, ×200. (c), (d) and (e) from another case of polymyositis. (c) Necrotic segment is invaded by macrophages. The swollen retraction cap has indented adjacent fibres, which are normal, ×545. (d) The wide fibre in the centre is necrotic but has not been invaded by macrophages. The thin fibre to the left contains four macrophages, ×545. (e) Necrotic segment containing macrophages and myelocytes (arrow). The latter have large nuclei with nucleoli. The fibre is surrounded by inflammatory cells, ×545

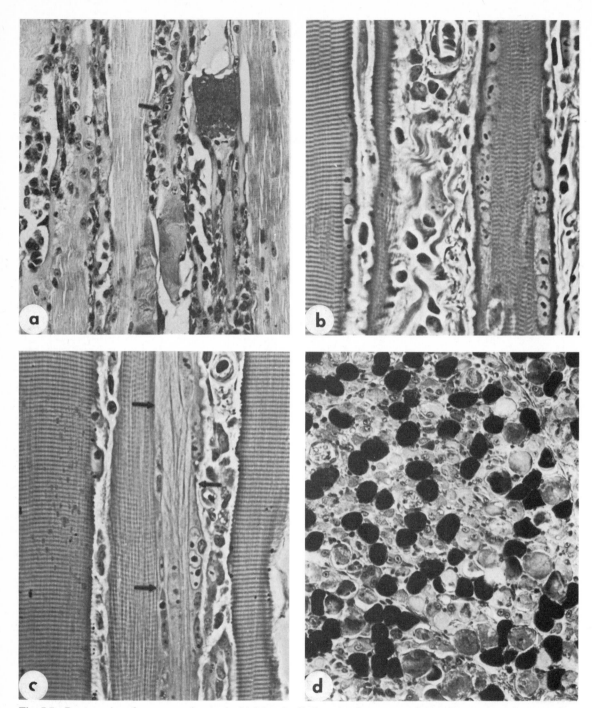

Fig. 5.7   Regeneration after segmental necrosis. (a) A longitudinal section from a case of alcoholic myopathy showing a thin regenerating fibre, which contains rows of hyperplastic sarcolemmal nuclei (arrow). The sarcoplasm is bluish in the section, which was stained with H and E. To the right is a necrotic fibre, ×240. (b) and (c) longitudinal sections from a case of polymyositis. (b) A regenerating fibre to the right of the midline with rows of hyperplastic nuclei with prominent nucleoli. Interstitial tissue with blood vessels and inflammatory cells is in the centre, ×545. (c) Regenerating fibre (arrows) containing collections of large nuclei with prominent nucleoli and single myofibrils, which appear to have recently formed, ×545. (d) Cross-section of gastrocnemius muscle from case of Meyer-Betz's paroxysmal rhabdomyolysis with myoglobinuria. The dark figures have survived injury and the pale ones with nucleolated sarcolemmal nuclei are regenerating. PTH-stain, ×225

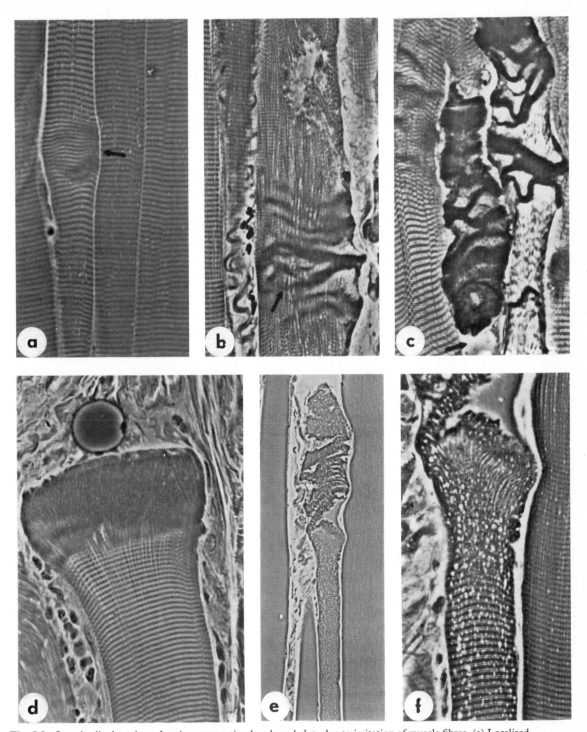

Fig. 5.8 Longitudinal sections showing contraction bands and clots due to irritation of muscle fibres. (a) Localised contraction node (arrow)—probably a reversible change, ×500. (b) 'Shredded' appearance of the fibre on the left side (arrow) representing a moderate degree of irritation; striation is still visible in the lighter areas between the dark bands. The fibre shows severe damage due to contraction. Contracted material is condensed into dark bands, ×500. (c) Contraction bands and localised disruption (arrow) of sarcous substance. ×600. (d) Retraction cap at end of severed fibre in a case of subacute polymyositis. Above the cap is connective tissue and one fat cell. A few inflammatory cells are seen to the left of the fibre, ×545. (e) A fibre showing the following changes (from bottom to top): vacuolation, retraction cap, necrosis, ×220. (f) Retraction cap and vacuolation seen at higher magnification. The swollen cap has indented an adjacent fibre, ×600

fibres and, even then, it is not prominent. The cellularity of the small vessels increases and the adventitial cells and pericytes are prominent. All these changes are of the type seen in cell necrosis in other organs and may be regarded as secondary. Incomplete regeneration, leaving a reduced population of muscle fibres, results in fibrosis, narrowing of the lumens of blood vessels and an increase in lipocytes.

In single episodes of segmental necrosis, regeneration is remarkably complete and, within a few weeks, the muscle appears to be completely restored. The regenerative process can be readily followed in lesions of different age. Surviving sarcolemmal nuclei enlarge and, once outside the sarcolemma, proliferate (Fig. 5.7). The nuclei at the junction of the healthy and necrotic segments also increase in number and size. The large size and prominence of the nucleoli of the myoblast nuclei distinguish them from histiocytes (Fig. 5.6e). Single, isolated muscle cells (myoblasts) may be seen in mitosis, but once these cells fuse to form myotubes, further division ceases. Regeneration of muscle fibre after segmental necrosis will be described further on page 199.

Severe segmental necrosis of striated muscle, while occurring in many muscle diseases, for practical reasons may be reduced to two groups.

Zenker's degeneration. This is the best known of the primary necroses of muscle. It may complicate a variety of infective diseases, such as typhoid fever, and has been observed often in muscles such as the rectus abdominis, the adductor muscles of the thighs, diaphragm, biceps brachii, pectoralis major and gastrocnemius. Portions of single fibres or groups of fibres undergo vitreous or waxy degeneration, long recognised as characteristic. However, more typically, large numbers of adjacent fibres occupying a broad field seem to have been affected simultaneously. This feature, together with the relative sparing of endomysium and blood vessels, the lack of inflammation, and the regular sequence of myophagia and regeneration, serve to identify this so-called toxic, necrotic process.

The cause of Zenker's degeneration is not understood. The common incrimination of a toxin is too ambiguous to satisfy the discriminating student of muscle disease. Its occurrence in both bacterial and viral diseases suggests a metabolic failure under conditions of stress.

Rhabdomyolysis with myoglobinuria. Extensive necrosis of muscle fibres from any cause, even if only one or two muscles are involved (as in crush injury) results in liberation of myoglobin into the bloodstream. The low renal threshold of this muscle pigment permits it to appear in the urine within a few hours. Aciduria favours the formation of myoglobin casts and often leads to tubular, 'lower nephron' nephrosis, which may be fatal. 'Myoglobinuria' is a misnomer, because it focuses attention on the appearance of myoglobin in urine. The original lesion is necrosis of skeletal muscle fibres with liberation of myoglobin, contractile proteins, enzymes, potassium and other elements into the blood, and the appearance of myoglobin in the urine is a secondary event.

The syndrome of myoglobinuria, described by Meyer-Betz in 1911, may have several different causes, but often none can be identified. In the idiopathic or Meyer-Betz syndrome the segmental necrosis of muscle fibres may follow either an unusual exertion or an infection. In biopsies, portions of many fibres are seen to contain altered sarcoplasm in various stages of disintegration. This sarcoplasm may appear waxy or fragmented or may take the form of strands or coagulated amorphous, flocculated masses. Myofibrillar structure is lost within a few hours; the sarcous material is eosinophilic in haematoxylin and eosin and reddish in phosphotungstic acid stains. Histochemical methods demonstrate an increase in bound lipids and phosphatides. Unlike McArdle's disease, in which myonecrosis and myoglobinuria may also occur after strenuous exercise, no excess of glycogen is present in either normal or diseased fibres. A peculiar property of the degenerating sarcoplasm is its affinity for calcium, which it binds within hours. The latter is easily detected even in the haematoxylin–eosin stains by a deep bluish basophilia of the calcium–protein precipitate. If the patient survives, as more than 75 per cent do, the necrotic remnants are phagocytosed and brisk regenerative activity follows within a few days (Fig. 5.7d). The muscle may be restored to a normal state although, in several cases, clumps of sarcolemmal nuclei with little or no sarcoplasm about them and a mild replacement fibrosis, remain.

In a number of patients with different types of segmental necrosis, a fetal type of myoglobin has been identified. At first Perkoff, Hill, Brown and Tyler (1962), who observed this feature in childhood muscular dystrophy, thought that it was peculiar to that disease, but it appears that fetal myoglobin is to be found in the regenerative phase of all forms of muscle necrosis.

Segmental necrosis with myoglobinuria in diseases in which the aetiology is known (cf. Rowland and Penn, 1972; Robotham and Haddow, 1976) differs only slightly from the idiopathic forms. As was stated above, it may be prominent in some cases of McArdle's disease, following a deficiency of phosphorylase (Pearson, Rimer and Mommaerts, 1961), and in phosphofructokinase and carnitine palmityl transferase deficiencies (DiMauro and Melis-DiMauro, 1973; Hostetler, Hoppel, Romine, Sipe, Gross and Higginbottom, 1978; Reza, Kar, Pearson and Kark, 1978). Intense physical exertion in untrained subjects can also lead to necrosis of muscle fibres. When affected muscle fibres lie in a tight compartment such as that in the pretibial region of the leg, the entire muscle mass may undergo ischaemic necrosis (anterior tibial syndrome). The violent activity of severe convulsions and crushing of muscle in accidental injury may have similar effects. Haff disease, an epidemic myoglobinuria due to a virus or toxin, has been noted in Eastern Europe. In the acute form of alcoholic myopathy, muscle necrosis (Fig. 5.6b) and myoglobinuria may develop after prolonged periods of drinking (Hed, Lundmark, Fahlgren and Orell, 1962; Ekbom, Hed, Kirstein and Åström, 1964). In exceptional circumstances the condition may be accompanied by renal failure and/or heart failure. Perkoff, Hardy and Velez-Garcia (1966) found that, during an alcoholic debauch, there may be a failure of lactic acid production under conditions of ischaemic work such as that which occurs in McArdle's disease. Among other toxins with a lethal effect upon segments of muscle fibres may be mentioned the poison of Malayan sea snakes, heroin, when administered intravenously (Kendrick, Hull and Knochel, 1977), and phencyclidine

(Cogen, Rigg, Simmons and Domino, 1978).

In polymyositis (Fig. 5.6c–e) one important component of the myopathology is necrosis of muscle fibres. This change appears, in serial sections, to bear a topographical relationship to foci of inflammatory cells. Denny-Brown (1960) prefers, with some justification, to set apart those cases in which degeneration of scattered muscle fibres or of groups of muscle fibres represents the only significant pathological change, which he called 'necrotising myopathy.' Myoglobinuria with renal failure has been described in a few cases of polymyositis (Sloan, Franks, Exley and Davison, 1978); myoglobin may be detected in the sera of patients with acute polymyositis before therapy (in 74.1 per cent of the cases of Kagen, 1977).

The muscle fibre may also undergo segmental necrosis in trichinosis and toxoplasmosis. The organisms penetrate the fibre and may be harboured for long periods. The trichina causes segmental necrosis of some fibres but becomes encysted in others. Eosinophilic and neutrophilic leucocytes and histiocytes may be seen in the necrotic sarcoplasm and in the endomysial tissue. The cysts ultimately calcify. Toxoplasma pseudocysts lie inertly in the muscle fibre. On rupture, however, necrosis of muscle fibre occurs with an inflammatory response.

Other myopathies have also been associated with segmental necrosis and myoglobinuria. Approximately a quarter of the published cases of myoglobinuria are said to have muscular dystrophy; however, as Berenbaum, Birch and Moreland (1953) and Pearson, Beck and Blahd (1957) point out, this chronic myopathy does not possess the usual microscopic features of muscular dystrophy, and is more likely to be a consequence of recurrent segmental necrosis of muscle fibres. This use of the term 'dystrophy' only attests to the fact that it has many different meanings in myology. Some pathologists use it to refer to any process that leads ultimately to cell death, even the terminal phase of denervation atrophy (Lapresle et al., 1965).

Progressive muscular dystrophy, particularly of the childhood Duchenne type, has been proposed as a special type of necrotising segmental myopathy where successive injuries of scattered fibres ultimately lead to their death. However, the myopathological findings fail to support this hypothesis fully, because the relation of the necrotic process to atrophy and hypertrophy with central nucleation remains to be settled. As already mentioned, we endorse the view that the muscular dystrophies involve a number of different pathogenetic mechanisms, all genetically determined.

Segmental necrosis may, of course, occur without myoglobinuria. This means only that the necrotising process is less acute and severe, involving usually only single or small groups of fibres, as in muscular dystrophy (Pearce and Walton, 1962). Acute destruction of at least 200 g muscular tissue, according to Berenbaum et al. (1953), is required to produce measurable myoglobinuria. Lesser degrees of destruction are undetectable, either in blood or urine. Recurrent muscle fibre destruction will eventually lead to chronic wasting and atrophy.

Finally, it should be pointed out that, in the many diseases leading to segmental necrosis, the pathogenesis surely must differ in each of them. After all, the necrosis is the end stage of various toxic, ischaemic, inflammatory, and metabolic processes. The morphologies of the initial phases of the pathological processes that result in necrosis are virtually unknown at present. One would expect a different sequence for each disease.

Focal destruction of muscle tissue. Here, necrosis of muscle fibres is but a part of a more extensive lesion involving interstitial tissue and blood vessels. The reaction to muscle fibre necrosis is the same as that described above, but it is accompanied by vigorous proliferation of endomysial fibroblasts, vascular reactions, and sometimes inflammation. As these do not differ from those in other organs, they will not be described further.

Vascular injury to muscle is the most thoroughly studied of the various types of focal destruction of muscular tissue. It may be caused either by venous or by arterial occlusion or haemorrhage. Arterial occlusion has a variable pathological influence on the different muscles of the body, according to the pattern of distribution or arrangement of vessels (different for each muscle). The net effect is infarct necrosis (pan-necrosis of muscle fibres, supporting tissues and small vessels) with the conventional

reactive changes. Lesser degrees of ischaemia may, however, injure the muscle fibres out of proportion to the connective tissue, and it is these effects which have been described inadequately. Venous occlusion, which adds an element of congestion and often of haemorrhage, has a more devastating effect than arterial occlusion, at least in some muscles. Swelling and oedema and hydropic change in the fibres may be prominent. The picture of infarct necrosis resembles the more diffuse necroses but differs with respect to the prominent reactions of endomysial and perimysial connective tissues and blood vessels. Nevertheless, it must be remembered that the characteristic quality of this type of disease is always the focal lesion in the artery or vein. The vascular lesion may be atherosclerosis with thrombosis, bland or septic embolism, polyarteritis nodosa or some other type of vasculitis, such as giant-cell arteritis or phlebitis. The problem in pathology is the satisfactory visualisation of the vascular lesion, which is often separated topographically from the myopathic change. Polyarteritis nodosa, a condition which involves the intramuscular vessels with striking regularity, is the lesion most frequently sought in muscle biopsies and fortunately is often easily identified by the concurrence of infarct necrosis, haemorrhage and denervation atrophy (secondary to lesions of the peripheral nerve) even when typical necrotising arteritis is not seen.

Trauma also elicits various combinations of necrosis of muscle fibres, interstitial tissue and blood vessels.

Regeneration after vascular or traumatic necrosis is described on page 200.

Contraction bands. Various pathogenic agents, but most particularly incision and other types of trauma, can briefly excite contraction of myofibrils. This reaction may involve only a short segment of the fibre (Fig. 5.8). The effect of these excitatory changes has been noted in humans and studied, particularly, in experimental animals (see Adams, 1975, for full description and bibliography). It is known that any type of external irritation of a certain degree—for instance from touching, probing, electrical stimulation, heat and cold—may be a sufficient stimulus (Fig. 5.8a). The ensuing changes may be reversible, but prolonged irritation above a certain strength produces extreme degrees of contraction, visible as alterations of sarcous substance. The affected segment of a fibre may have a 'shredded' appearance, with dark bands alternating with lighter areas in which striation is still visible (Fig. 5.8b). In the more severe lesions the dark bands are separated from lighter areas which contain amorphous material, fragments, and what appears to be fluid (Fig. 5.8b, c). The dark bands, called retraction bands or clots, consist of material which appears to be coagulated. The bands are largely perpendicular to the long axis of the fibre.

Contraction clots do not occur in smooth muscles or in regenerating and immature fibres, which lack myofibrils (Speidel, 1938). They are evidently caused by myofibrillar contractions, which are severe enough to produce internal ruptures and 'clotting'.

At the border of a zone of injury a retraction cap may appear on the severed end of the unaffected part of the fibre (Fig. 5.8d, e), causing a swelling which can indent adjacent fibres (Speidel, 1939). It is likely that this cap helps to seal the severed end of the preserved part of the fibre, thus preventing leakage of sarcoplasm.

One or two days after injury, the segment with retraction clots will be invaded by macrophages which remove the necrotic fragments. The 'cleaned' region is then repaired in the usual fashion and the integrity of the fibre is restored. However, it is possible that healing may be incomplete and that the broken fibre ends freely in the connective tissue (Fig. 5.8d).

Manipulations during biopsy procedures in humans may produce contraction bands. Certain fixatives will likewise produce such reactions in biopsies, especially if the specimen was not attached to a clamp or a stick. It is possible that certain diseased muscles are more irritable and prone to contraction bands than others.

Contraction clots occur, not only after trauma, but also in the course of disease, especially polymyositis (Fig. 5.8e, f) and in Duchenne dystrophy (Cullen and Fulthorpe, 1975), but, as was remarked above, their significance is still a matter of some debate.

Special degenerative lesions

Degeneration is here defined as any condition that alters special elements of the structure and impairs the function of the muscle fibre, but does not lead to necrosis. Unlike subfibre necroses, degenerations within a muscle fibre have several different features: selective loss of organelles, disturbance of architecture, disfiguration of organelles and inclusions of structured and non-structured elements. These changes will, somewhat arbitrarily, be subdivided into three groups.

Degenerations of single organelles

Destruction of sarcolemmal membrane. Interest has recently been focused on possible damage or defects in the surface membrane of the muscle fibre as a possible cause of muscle damage in general and in muscle dystrophy in particular (Jerusalem, 1976; Rowland, 1976; Pickard, Gruemar, Verrill, Isaacs, Robinow, Nance, Myers and Goldsmith, 1978). Mokri and Engel (1975) found disruptions of the sarcolemma over foci of necrosis in Duchenne dystrophy. The meaning of such findings is uncertain. Destruction of the membrane may be artefactual or secondary to contraction bands, or a part of a necrotic process and not a cause of it. Using a freeze-fracture technique, Schotland, Bonilla and Van Meter (1977) found (in biopsies from 8 cases of Duchenne dystrophy) a different type of membranous abnormality—a non-uniform distribution and depletion of particles on both sides of the sarcolemma. One cannot exclude the possibility that these changes were produced artificially, possibly in biochemically abnormal membranes. On the other hand, apparent structural integrity does not eliminate the possibility of a biochemical defect, perhaps one that causes the sarcolemma to be abnormally permeable.

Selective destruction of myofibrils and myofilaments. Depletion of myofilaments and the reduction in size of remaining fibrils occur in atrophy of various causes. Glycogen usually fills widened spaces beneath the sarcolemma and between remaining myofibrils.

Non-fibrillar areas at the periphery of muscle fibres may have the appearance of clear, rather homogeneous zones under the light microscope. These so-called sarcoplasmic masses (*see* Fig. 5.11) have been seen in many diseases but are especially prominent in myotonic dystrophy, where they form concentric zones around a core of normal-looking myofibrils (*see* p. 180 and Fig. 5.11a, b). Electron microscopy shows that a sarcoplasmic mass contains not only sarcoplasm but also glycogen granules, normal and degenerating mitochondria, tubules and other organelles and frequently some remaining (or newly created) myofilaments and myofibrils, which may have an abnormal orientation, occasionally into spiral annulets—the so-called ringbinden (Schröder and Adams, 1968). Sarcolemmal nuclei are increased in number, are in disarray and the cytoplasmic enzyme content of the faintly fibrillar sarcoplasmic masses is enriched.

Patchy loss of myofibrils in type I fibres may feature in certain diseases, such as the congenital myopathy described by Cancilla, Kalyanaraman, Verity, Munsat and Pearson (1971).

In contrast to complete disappearance of myofibrils and filaments, a selective destruction of parts of filaments has also been reported. Thus, lysis of myosin has been claimed to occur in miscellaneous human muscle diseases (Carpenter, Karpati, Rothman and Watters, 1976; Yarom and Shapira, 1977; Sher, Shafiq and Schutta, 1979). Partial destruction of myofilaments has also been observed under experimental conditions. For instance, Stenger *et al.* (1962) found in the experimental animal a disruption and dissolution of the thin filaments in the I band and a granular degeneration of the Z line. The A bands and H discs were well preserved.

Depletion of mitochondria. The number of mitochondria is normally adjusted to the functional demands placed on the muscle fibre and probably to other biological factors. The number may vary within wide limits. Continuous destruction and removal of mitochondria appears to be part of a constant, normal turnover in every living fibre. Depletion of mitochondria may be part of a pathological process. Accurate assessment of number and volume can be made reliably, but has not been attempted systematically in any of the myopathies.

Destruction of nuclei. Pyknosis of nuclei undoubtedly occurs in relation to segmental necrosis. However, it is hard to assess this parameter of disease in light-microscopic sections of muscle in human disease. The relations of nuclear necrosis to a pattern of changes in surrounding organelles has not been established. The only definite destructions are seen in zones of segmental necrosis or in a zone of tissue necrosis. Darkness of staining and clustering or rowing of nuclei are observed in ageing muscle fibres and in myotonic dystrophy.

Disarray of the architecture of the muscle fibre. A striking quality of the normal skeletal muscle fibre, as seen under the microscope, is its precise, regular structure. The observer especially notes how the thick and thin myofilaments interdigitate and form regular, repeated patterns in the sarcomeres, which are separated by the straight Z lines. The filaments are embedded in the sarcoplasm, which in the electron microscope lacks structure and is very lightly stained. Although the sarcoplasm appears to be amorphous, it is clear that correct structure and normal function of the muscle are dependent not only upon the composition and organisation of myofilaments, but also upon the precise molecular composition and architecture of the sarcoplasm in which the myofilaments are embedded. Filaments and sarcoplasm must constitute an integrated functional and morphological unit.

It seems reasonable that certain types of injury and genetic abnormality can result in a disturbance the precise architecture of the muscle fibre.

Streaming of the Z line. The Z line, which normally is straight and of even thickness, appears in some preparations to 'stream' into the adjacent sarcomeres. Isolated instances of streaming in otherwise normal muscle fibres usually represent either an artefact or a normal phenomenon; streaming is not, in itself, a reliable indicator of disease. However, one can never dismiss the possibility that in certain cases it may signify an early pathological disturbance of molecular architecture. For this reason it must always be

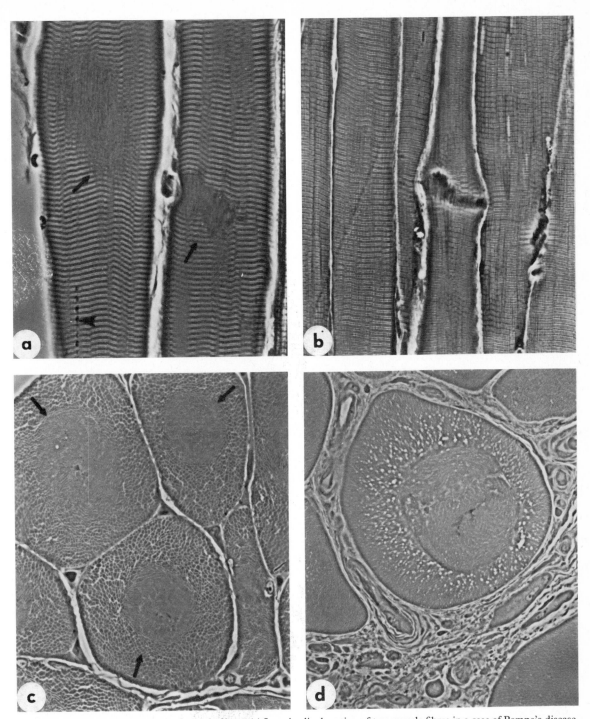

Fig. 5.9 Disarray of architecture of muscle fibres. (a) Longitudinal section of two muscle fibres in a case of Pompe's disease showing smudging of normal striation within irregularly shaped areas (arrows) (*see also* Fig. 5.10). The row of lipofuscin granules (arrowhead) indicates the location of a former autophagic vacuole, ×545. (b) Minicore of a type seen in 'multicore disease'. The fibre is swollen at the site of the change, ×545. (c) Central cores or targets (arrows) in a case of denervation atrophy. The condensed myofibrils in the centre are surrounded by a peripheral zone with normal-looking myofibrils, ×545. (d) A hypertrophic fibre from a case of Charcot-Marie-Tooth disease containing a central core or target of compacted myofibrils. The latter are surrounded by a zone of vacuolar degeneration. The connective tissue in the lower part of the fibre contains some thin, atrophic fibres, ×545

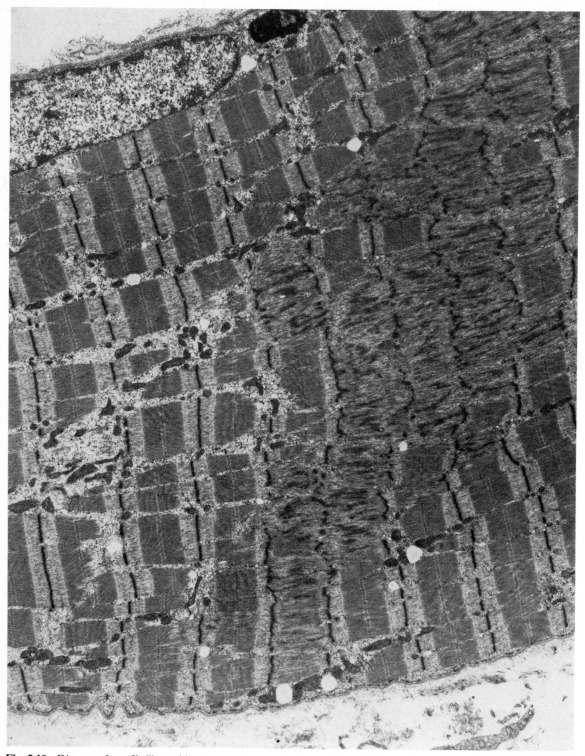

Fig. 5.10   Disarray of myofibrillar architecture seen in an early phase of Pompe's disease (same specimen as for Fig. 5.9a). Electron micrograph, ×8750

evaluated in the context of other findings and measured quantitatively (Meltzer, Kuncl, Click and Yang, 1976).

Disarray of myofibrils. This is an abnormality of striation, in which the normal, regular pattern of muscle is disturbed irregularly in spots. This results in the appearance of smudging. Such changes have been observed in a number of different diseases. They have also been seen in normal subjects, although less commonly than the streaming of Z lines (Meltzer *et al.*, 1976). Our illustrations (Figs. 5.9a and 5.10) are from a case of Pompe's disease (adult form).

Central core formation. As first noted by Shy and Magee (1956) in a rare type of myopathy, each muscle fibre contains one or more zones of a dense, amorphous, relatively hyalinised sarcous substance. In the longitudinal plane these foci are shaped like thin cylinders. In Gomori's trichrome stain (in which myofibrils normally have a reddish colour) the myofibrils in the cores are condensed, that is, more tightly packed, and bluish. Under polarised light and by the phase contrast microscope the dense zones are seen to contain myofibrils with preserved cross-striation. The cores react positively to the PAS stain and negatively for phosphorylase and oxidative enzymes (Engel, Foster, Hughes, Huxley and Mahler, 1961; Seitelberger, Wanko and Gavin, 1961).

Electron microscopy of cores has revealed such features as condensation of myofibrils, irregularity of Z lines, reduced number of mitochondria, and sarcotubular formations (Afifi, Smith and Zellweger, 1965; Gonatas, Perez, Shy and Evangelista, 1965; Dubowitz and Roy, 1970). Neville and Brooke (1973) have more recently claimed that the cores may be either structureless (they are disorganised as described above) or structured, with normal striation. Even in the latter group, however, they found that the core was in a state of contraction, which seems at least in part to reflect some disturbance of the functional state. It would seem, therefore, that the difference between the two groups may be more a matter of degree than a qualitative difference.

This peculiar disfigurative change is believed to be determined by a genetic factor, for it has been seen in several members of a family in successive generations. The significance of this core effect has not been determined. Shy and Magee (1956) and Engel *et al.* (1961) argue convincingly that the consistency of the change favours its being the mark of a distinctive disease. However, a similar core effect occurs occasionally in normal or denervated muscle (*see below and* Fig. 5.9c, d).

Apart from this curious alteration of parts of the muscle fibres, the only other morphological abnormality is excessive variation in size of the muscle fibres. The diameter of the fibres of the large limb muscles in such conditions may come to an average of 80 μm or more (slightly more than average) but some fibres attain a size of 240 μm. Little or no degeneration or loss of fibres may be observed and there is no explanation for the mild persistent weakness noted in some cases. The sarcolemmal nuclei remain in their customary position and there is no cellular reaction to the central condensation of protoplasm.

Target fibres. The term 'target fibre' (Engel, 1961) refers to the ringed or bull's eye appearance of certain muscle fibres viewed in transverse sections of histochemical preparations. A dark, inner core consists of a compaction of myofibrils, which lack the cross-striations and the mitochondrial oxidative enzyme activity usually found in myofibrils. The core is surrounded by a densely stained area and an outer zone of more normal myofibrils. In longitudinal direction the targets may, like central cores, extend over many sarcomeres. Biopsy and freezing of unfixed fibres seems to favour their occurrence. In osmiumstained sections the fibrils within the target zones appear homogenised and condensed (Fig. 5.9c, d). Target fibres are most commonly seen in denervation atrophy (Mittelbach, 1966) but may occur also in other conditions. Engel (1961) noted target fibres in 60 per cent of biopsies of muscle of denervation diseases, but also in several cases of periodic paralysis. They are not usually found in denervation of animal muscle fibres.

The morphology of central cores and target zones is similar; they may be expressions of the same pathogenetic mechanism. The nature of this mechanism and the significance of these changes are not known.

Minicores. These structures were first described by Engel, Gomez and Groover (1971) in what they called multicore disease (*see* Table 5.1 and p. 160). They differ from the cores of central core disease in that they are shorter (Fig. 5.9b), more heavily stained in osmicated preparations and more numerous. A single fibre may contain many minicores. Electron microscopy shows mostly a disorganisation of tissue and very little destruction within the minicores. Their significance is unknown.

Striated annulets (ringbinden, ring bundles, anneaux des fibrilles). This curious disorientation of the most peripheral (subsarcolemmal) myofibrils, from their longitudinal orientation to one of encircling the shaft of the fibre, was described long ago. Although observed many times in experimental animals, most descriptions are based on human material.

It is our impression that two types of ring bundles can be identified. In type I the fibre is structurally normal except for the disorientation of a peripheral packet of myofibrils, which encircle the longitudinally arranged ones (Fig. 5.11c). Sarcolemmal nuclei are in the usual position with reference to the myofibrils, in that their long axes are parallel to one another. No islands of clear sarcoplasm are present.

Type II is but a part of a profound disorder of myofibrillar organisation in which the sarcoplasm, especially peripheral, lacks myofibrils or retains only scattered disorganised ones (Fig. 5.11a) (Schröder and Adams, 1968). Occasionally a packet of circular myofibrils can be seen deep in the sarcoplasm. Some fibres may have lost all their myofibrils. The electron microscope reveals thin and thick actin and myosin filaments, Z bands, and endoplasmic reticulum, without any semblance of organisation. Such ring bundles, according to Schröder and Adams (1968) represent a profound derangement of contractile elements, presumably due to a failure in the biosynthetic processes of the cells. Thus, it happens that a sarcoplasmic mass (region of sarcoplasm devoid of myofibrils) and myofibrillar derangement may or may not coincide. In some specimens, nearly every fibre shows clear zones of sarcoplasm, but no ring bundles.

The significance of these myofibrillar disrup-

tions has long been disputed. Whereas Schäffer (1893) assumed them to be artefacts induced by incision and by the action of strong fixatives on irritable muscle, causing contraction bands and outright rupture of the myofibrils, a view with which we earlier concurred (Adams, Denny-Brown and Pearson, 1953), Heidenhain (1918), Wohlfart (1951) and Greenfield *et al.* (1957) insisted that they are a valid ante-mortem sign of disease.

The position which we would now take is that the type I ring bundles are probably artefactual. This type of change may be found in biopsies from cases of pseudotetany, tetanus, myotonia, and a variety of other conditions. It is probably not significant, being caused by the biopsy procedure, for it is rarely seen in post-mortem material from younger persons. On the other hand, the type II ring bundles stand as part of an intrinsic pathological process. It is in myotonic dystrophy (Fig. 5.11a) that they are found with such regularity (Heidenhain, 1918) as to have been accepted with sarcoplasmic masses (Wohlfart, 1951) as characteristic of this disease. The view that they are not due to fixatives has been established by their demonstration under polarised light in unfixed fresh frozen tissue (Engel, 1962b). Wohlfart (1955) also noted the increasing incidence of ring bundles with age, especially in the eye muscles and, as already mentioned, listed them among the senile changes (*see also* Hübner, 1977).

Other alterations in muscle fibres. We include in this group non-destructive modifications of parts of the muscle fibre resulting in malformations of organelles (e.g. mitochondria), the proliferation of organelles, accumulation of substances (e.g. glycogen) and the formation of new structures.

Biochemical inclusions. Glycogen, a normal component of muscle, increases when there is a deficiency of certain enzymes, usually genetically determined, necessary for intracellular metabolism of carbohydrates. This may lead to abnormal accumulations of glycogen granules beneath the sarcolemma and between myofibrils. Some of the accumulations are surrounded by

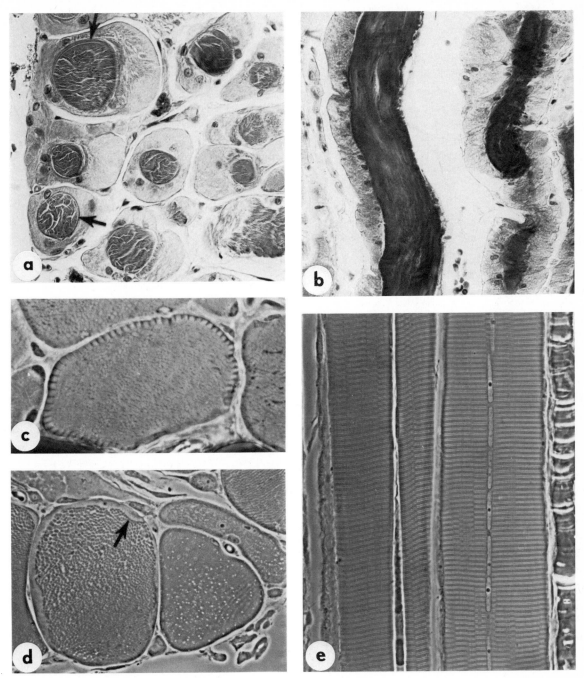

Fig. 5.11 Muscle fibres of normal appearance surrounded by sarcoplasmic masses in cross-section (a) and longitudinal section (b) from a case of myotonic dystrophy. Arrows point to ring bundles of Type II (see text). Lillie's allochrome, ×435 and 340. (c) Ring bundles of Type I (see text), ×870. (d) Sarcoplasm at periphery of fibre (arrow) devoid of myofibrils resulting from previous destruction, ×545. (e) 'Rowing' of centrally located sarcolemmal nuclei in hypertrophic fibre in ageing muscle, ×545.

newly formed membranes; others lie free in the sarcoplasm. It is noteworthy that the techniques usually employed by pathologists distort the natural appearance of glycogen stores in the muscle fibre, for much of the glycogen is water-soluble and removed during fixation, and in the haematoxylin and eosin-stained sections only clear vacuoles remain. This appearance differs from that of periodic paralysis only by the greater degree of vacuolisation. Fortunately, carmine and PAS stains usually show some of the remaining glycogen, even when special fixatives have not been used, so that there is little difficulty in diagnosis. The glycogen granules are most readily studied in electron micrographs of osmium-stained sections.

The striated muscle fibre regularly exhibits change in at least three of the glycogenoses, Cori's Type II, IV, and V (Ch. 18). In the best-known of this family of diseases, Type II of Cori, now known as Pompe's disease, in which skeletal muscles, heart and other organs are involved in various combinations owing to a deficiency of α-1–4 glucosidase, fine aggregates of glycogen accumulate in the centre of the fibre, displacing the myofibrils (Figs. 5.12 and 5.13). As the glycogen accumulates it obliterates the myofibrillar structure, leaving the muscle fibre a nondescript bag containing rows of longitudinally oriented vacuoles, rounded basophilic refractile bodies and granules. Some of the impregnated fibres enlarge to as much as twice their normal size. The peripherally placed sarcolemmal nuclei usually retain their natural appearance. Every muscle is involved and hence biopsy diagnosis is usually easy. The weakness and hypotonia are presumably ascribable to loss of contractile elements in the glycogen-impregnated fibres.

The characteristic abnormality in Type V, McArdle's disease, is the absence or reduction of phosphorylase in muscle fibres (Pearson et al., 1961). The accumulation of glycogen, the failure of the muscle fibres to contract and to relax under conditions requiring strenuous work, and even the necrosis of fibres, are all secondary. In severe cases blebs, filled with granulated material, are seen around the margins of fibres. In cross-sections such blebs may encircle two-thirds of the fibre, and in longitudinal sections they take the form of spindles, measuring up to 200 μm in length

(Fig. 5.12a, b). Myofibrils are pressed away from the sarcolemma and the 'thickened' appearance of the latter is due to a thin band of sarcoplasm, which remains between it and the glycogen. Usually the sarcolemmal nuclei remain inactive. Here and there single muscle fibres have disappeared and have been replaced by connective tissue. However, this does not prove that glycogen deposit alone has resulted in necrosis. The mild progressive myopathy accounts for the persistent weakness noted in some cases.

Further chemical and pathological studies of this group of diseases are needed. Its boundaries are far from clear. Some of the cases of physiological contracture induced by exercise which we have studied have had no defect of phosphorylase, as shown by standard histochemical techniques. Presumably, some other enzymatic defect is responsible. Tarui, Okuno, Ikura, Tanaka, Suda and Nishikawa (1965), Satoyoshi and Kowa (1967), Layzer, Rowland and Ranney (1967) and Layzer and Rowland (1971) have demonstrated contracture in patients with phosphofructokinase and phosphohexoseisomerase deficiency.

Normal muscle contains droplets of lipid. They are seen as tiny vacuoles in sections from paraffin-embedded material but are best studied in electron micrographs.

A lipid-storage disease is based on an enzymatic defect, which prevents the utilisation of fatty acids and results in the abnormal accumulation of lipid. A deficiency of carnitine has now been established as one of the causes of excess of lipid aggregates in skeletal muscle. In routine microscopic preparations the lipid appears as vacuoles within the sarcoplasm (Engel and Angelini, 1973). The broader subject of 'lipid storage myopathies' has been reviewed by Angelini (1976) and Bradley, Tomlinson and Hardy (1978).

Lipid inclusions of other types have also been found in striated muscle. Examples are cases of ceroid lipofuscinosis (Haltia, Rapola and Santavuori, 1973; Carpenter, Karpati, Andermann, Jacob and Andermann, 1977) and Fabry's disease (Tomé, Fardeau and Lenoir, 1977). Carpenter et al. consider the study of skin and muscle biopsy material under the electron microscope to be a reliable procedure for the diagnosis of all forms of lipofuscinosis.

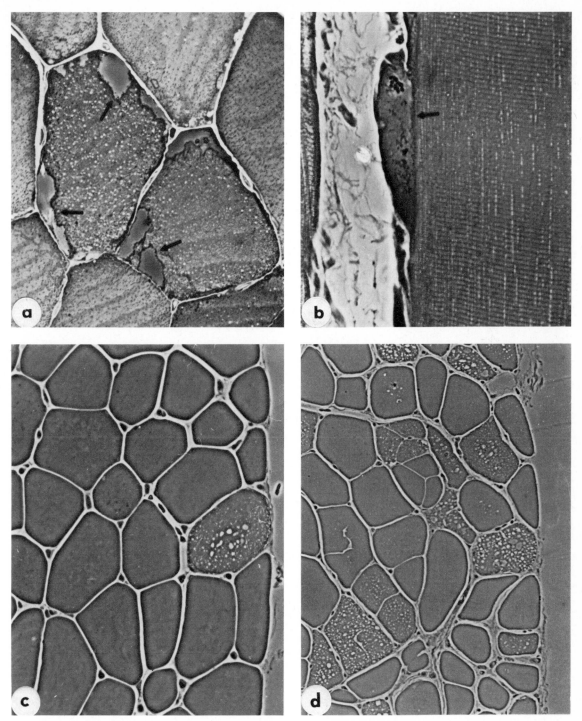

Fig. 5.12 Glycogen storage diseases. (a) and (b) from a case of McArdle's disease. (a) Glycogen accumulated peripherally in two cross-sectioned fibres (arrows). The collections have a homogeneous, greyish appearance, ×545. (b) Longitudinal section showing subsarcolemmal collection of glycogen (arrow), ×545. (c) and (d) from a case of the adult form of Pompe's disease. (c) At an earlier stage of the disease only one fibre (shown) in many blocks of the biopsy appeared to be affected, i.e. was vacuolated, ×350. (d) In a second biopsy, taken several years later, many fibres are vacuolated. The unaffected fibres have a normal appearance, ×220.

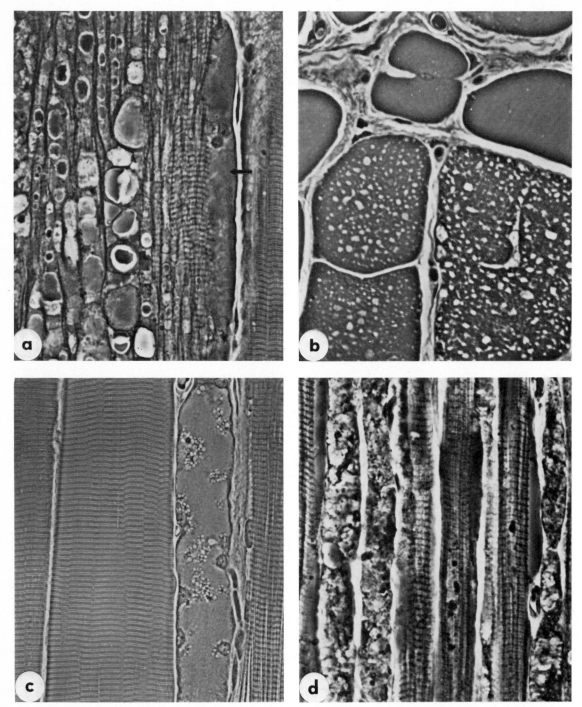

Fig. 5.13 Pompe's disease. (a), (b), and (c) are from an adult case (same biopsy as in Fig. 5.12 (c) and (d)). (a) Longitudinal section of a severely affected fibre in which vacuoles of glycogen and debris (lysosomal) are located between a few remaining intact myofibrils. Glycogen has also accumulated beneath the sarcolemma (arrow), ×545. (b) Characteristic vacuolation in cross-section. Partial splitting of fibre in the upper part of the picture is due to previous focal necrosis, ×545. (c) Longitudinal section showing severe destruction in a fibre, which contains fluid and macrophages. Adjacent fibre appears normal, ×545. (d). Longitudinal section from infantile case of Pompe's disease. There is vacuolation and severe destruction of fibres. Note also subsarcolemmal bags with glycogen, ×545

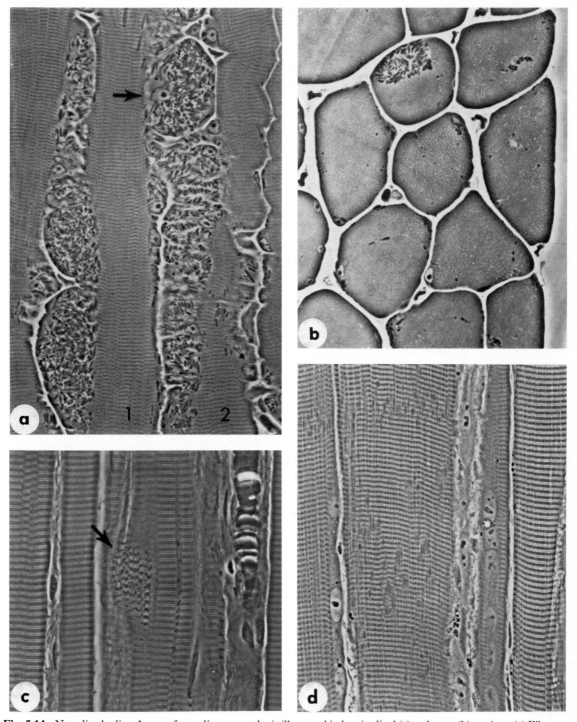

Fig. 5.14 Nemaline bodies. A case of nemaline myopathy is illustrated in longitudinal (a) and cross (b) sections. (a) Fibre no. 1 contains three huge subsarcolemmal aggregates of nemaline bodies. The two rounded collections on the left side are separated from each other by a cleft. A sarcolemmal nucleus (arrow) is visible in the third collection in the upper right part of the fibre. Fibre no. 2 has a large collection in its left side. Nemaline bodies within these masses have a haphazard orientation. Those in the interior of the fibres tend to have a longitudinal direction. Except for the collections of rod-like bodies the muscle fibres appear to be unaffected, ×545. (b) Nemaline bodies seen in one large collection in one fibre and singly or in smaller groups in others, ×640. (c) Longitudinal section of muscle in spinal atrophy showing local swelling of fibre with rod-like bodies, *cf*. electron micrograph in Fig. 5.15, ×700. (d) Rod-like bodies scattered in a muscle fibre in a case of polymyositis, ×545

Inclusions of formed elements. We include here structured elements, which have little or no resemblance to the organelles of the normal muscle fibre. Some of them probably originate in organelles which, in the course of degeneration, become distorted beyond recognition. Others may represent *de novo* formations.

Nemaline bodies (Fig. 5.14) were first seen in a new type of myopathy, which was termed nemaline myopathy because of the presence of thread- or worm-like particles beneath the sarcolemma (Conen, Murphy and Donohue, 1963; Shy, Engel, Somers and Wanko, 1963). In this condition the rod-shaped structures (about 0.3–0.7 μm in diameter and 1.5–5.0 μm in length) occur singly or in aggregates, often arranged irregularly or in palisades and usually without reference to the axis of the fibre (Fig. 5.14a, b). When single and situated deep within the fibre, the rods are orientated parallel to the myofibrils. Under the electron microscope the rod-shaped bodies have some resemblance to the Z lines. This has led to the postulation of a disorder of the muscle protein of which Z line material is believed to be composed.

Although the rod-shaped bodies identify this disease, there are usually other changes as well, such as smallness of many of the fibres, greater than normal variation in size and some degenerative signs (Sreter, Åström, Romanul, Young and Jones, 1976). Necrosis of fibres and phagocytosis was prominent in the cases described by Price, Gordon, Pearson, Munsat and Blumberg (1965), but not in others. These findings correlate with the clinical finding of slender muscles, corresponding in this respect to congenital hypoplasia. Weakness and hypotonia, which are early clinical features, resemble those seen in amyotonia congenita of Oppenheim (p. 159). In later life, some fibre loss occurs in proximal limb and trunk muscle. The specificity of the nemaline bodies is negated by the fact that they are found (in smaller numbers) in other human muscle diseases and in experimental animals (Fig. 5.14c, d; Fig. 5.15).

Cytoplasmic bodies may be seen with the light microscope (Engel, 1962a; Adams and Rebeiz, 1966) but are best observed under the electron microscope. They are spherical bodies with an average diameter of 4 μm. The centre is dense and homogeneous, whereas the peripheral zone contains radiating, fine fibrils. The structures appear to be composed of a collection of contracted myofilaments (Engel, 1962a; Kinoshita, Satoyoshi and Suzuki, 1975; Cullen and Fulthorpe, 1975) but it is possible that they also contain material derived from Z discs (MacDonald and Engel, 1969). Cytoplasmic bodies are non-specific. they have been found in several different diseases.

Tubular aggregates, structures that are best seen with the electron microscope (Ch. 9), are groups of tightly packed, longitudinally orientated tubules, that lie among the myofibrils and cause little, if any, destruction of cytoplasmic elements. They probably represent a new growth of membranes, derived, in our opinion, from the SR system.

Tubular aggregates appear regularly in all types of periodic paralysis (Dyken, Zeman and Rausche, 1969; Bradley, 1969; Meyers, Gilden, Rinaldi and Hansen, 1972; Engel, Bishop and Cunningham, 1970; Schiffer, Giordana, Monga and Mollo, 1976) but have been seen in a variety of unrelated conditions.

So-called honeycomb structures, zebra bodies, filamentous, fingerprint and reducing bodies, and laminated bodies (Payne and Curless, 1976) have been observed in patients with muscular symptoms. Some of them are said to be characteristic of specific diseases and in some instances the disease has been named after the specific body (Table 5.1). Their significance is unknown. It seems unlikely that they figure in the pathogenesis of any particular disease.

Mitochondrial abnormalities. It was first proposed by Luft, Ikkos, Palmieri, Ernster and Afzelius (1962) that a meaningful association may exist between clinical symptoms and the abnormal structure and function of mitochondria in skeletal muscles. The concept of 'mitochondrial myopathy' has, since then, become firmly entrenched in the literature and is the source of confusion. Logically it should mean that a disturbance in mitochondrial structure is the mechanism whereby a muscle fibre becomes diseased. However, abnormal mitochondria may also represent a secondary or compensatory reaction. Thus, in severely degenerated muscles, impairment of oxidation or 'respiratory control' may be secon-

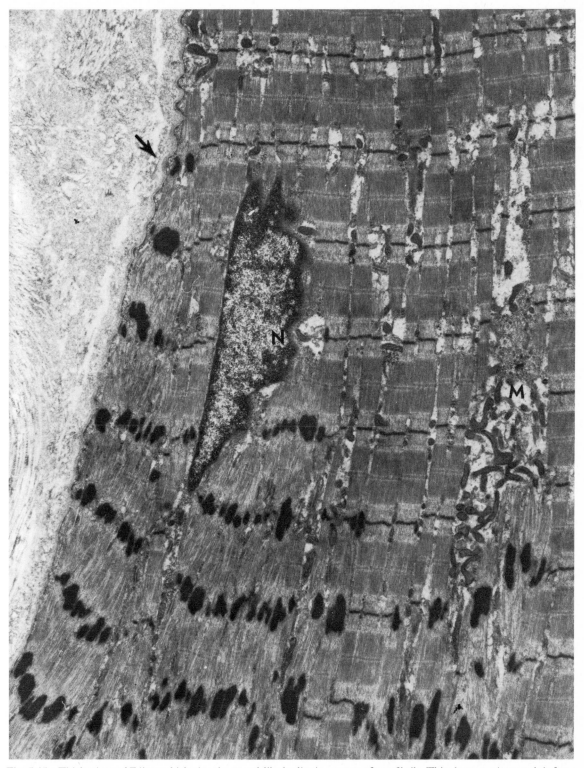

Fig. 5.15   Thickenings of Z lines which give rise to rod-like bodies in a group of myofibrils. This electron micrograph is from the same case as the phase micrograph in Fig. 5.14 (c). Arrows have equivalent positions in the two pictures. N=sarcolemmal nucleus. M = mitochondria, ×10 725

dary to the degenerative process (Peter, Stempel and Armstrong, 1970). It is also conceivable that a pathogenetic factor, operating inside or outside the muscle, may cause degenerative changes in mitochondria and in other parts of the muscle fibre as a collateral 'epiphenomenon': in other words, these changes are signs of, but not a cause of, disease (Askanas, Engel, Britton, Adornato and Eiben, 1978). Even when primary, a mitochondrial change is not always associated with myopathy, and need not have led to degeneration within the fibre. Indeed, in some cases of reported 'mitochondrial myopathy' the patient did not have a muscle disease at all, or had at most only a general feeling of fatigue. For instance, in the case described by Luft et al. (1962) the clinical picture was dominated by non-muscular symptoms. It is stated in their paper that 'muscular strength was decreased but paresis was not present', and there was no destructive process in the muscle fibres (light microscopy in this case was carried out by one of us, KEÅ). Finally, one should remember that biopsies are taken more often from skeletal muscles than from other organs (one reason being the ease of the operation). Hence, it is possible that interest is focused on the muscles and that more universal affections are overlooked. It is known, in fact, that in some cases of so-called mitochondrial myopathy abnormalities are found not only in muscle mitochondria but also in other organs. Mitochondrial disease, rather than myopathy, would be a more appropriate eponym in such cases.

Abnormal appearance of mitochondria has been noted in many established disease entities, for instance muscular dystrophy, which lack signs of disturbance of the cellular respiratory system. The changes appear here to be secondary and of no pathogenetic significance. Apart from such cases there remains a series of reports of clinical cases— beginning with that of Luft et al. (1962)—from which emerges the picture of true mitochondrial diseases, especially myopathies.

We will use the term mitochondrial disease to refer to a condition in which an alteration of mitochondria is the only consistent change and in which symptoms, signs, laboratory data, and morphological findings are best explained by specific disturbed functions of mitochondria (see DiMauro, Schotland, Bonilla, Lee, Gambetti and Rowland, 1973). It follows that, in a case of suspected mitochondrial myopathy, clinical assessment should ideally include biochemical investigation of the organelles, which have been isolated from the biopsy specimen.

Reports of cases of suspected mitochondrial diseases may tentatively be put into five groups. Biochemical findings of interest are listed in Table 5.2.

(1) Hypermetabolism of non-thyroid origin. This has been reported in only two cases.

(2) A group of proximal myopathies.

(3) Ophthalmoplegic myopathies (see Ch. 14). At least three syndromes with ophthalmoplegia have been recognised: I. progressive external ophthalmoplegia, first described by von Graefe in 1856 and identified as myopathy by Kiloh and Nevin (1951); II. oculopharyngeal myopathy, first described by Taylor in 1915 and recognised as myopathy by Victor, Hayes and Adams in 1962; III. the Kearns-Sayre syndrome, described as a clinical entity in 1958 by Kearns and Sayre, and by Kearns in 1965.

(4) A syndrome of retarded somatic growth, varying symptoms of disordered functioning of central nervous system and skeletal muscles and a lactic acidosis (Suzuki and Rapin, 1969; Hackett, Bray, Ziter, Nyhan and Creer, 1973; Tarlow, Lake and Lloyd, 1973; Tsairis, Engel and Kark, 1973; Shapira, Cederbaum, Cancilla, Nielsen and Lippe, 1975; Hart, Chang, Perrin, Neerunjun and Ayyar, 1977; Askanas et al., 1978; see also Table 5.2).

(5) Non-muscular diseases (see Table 5.2).

Because the pathology in muscle is the same in all, a single description will suffice for the group. In all the muscle diseases called mitochondrial, the specific pathologic alteration is not, as a rule, revealed under the light microscope. In exceptional cases the sarcolemma is separated from the myofibrils by granular material, which proves on electron microscopy to be attributable to groups of mitochondria. The mitochondria-laden fibres react intensely to stains for oxidative enzymes, and they have been called 'ragged-red fibres' because of the red appearance of the mitochondrial aggregates in Gomori-stained sections (Olson, Engel, Walsh and Einaugler, 1972).

Table 5.2 'Mitochondrial diseases': biochemical findings.
M=mitochondria; B=blood

(1) Hypermetabolism of non-thyroid origin

Luft, Ikkos, Palmieri, Ernster and Afzelius (1962)	M: loose coupling of oxidative phosphorylation
Afifi, Ibrahim, Bergman, Abu Haydar, Mire, Bahuth and Kaylani (1972); DiMauro, Bonilla, Lee, Schotland, Scarpa, Conn and Chance (1976)	M: loose coupling

(2) Myopathies

Hülsmann, Bethlem, Meijer, Fleury and Schellens (1967)	M: loose coupling of oxidative phosphorylation
Spiro, Prineas and Moore (1970)	M: loose coupling; normal function of cytochrome and electron transport systems
Hudgson, Bradley and Jenkison (1972); Worsfold, Park and Pennington (1973);	M: poor coupling of oxidative phosphorylation
Bradley, Tomlinson and Hardy (1978) (3 reports on family with facioscapulohumeral myopathy)	B: severe lactic acidosis during terminal illness of one member of family
Black, Judge, Demers and Gordon (1975)	M: lack of respiratory control with α-glycerophosphate
Schotland, DiMauro, Bonilla, Scarpa and Lee (1976)	M: decreased respiratory control with NAD and FAD-linked substrates
Morgan-Hughes, Darveniza, Kahn, Landon, Sherratt, Land and Clark (1977)	M: loose coupling; deficiency or reducible cytochrome b B: probably partially compensated lactic acidosis B: abnormal lactic acidosis after exercise
Sengers, ter Haar, Trijbels, Willems, Daniels and Stadhouders (1975) (also cardiomyopathy and cataracts; 3 families)	
Rawles and Weller (1974) (also sideroblastic anaemia; family history)	B: excessive production of lactic acid; acidosis
Larsson, Linderholm, Müller, Ringqvist and Sörnäs (1964) (paroxysmal myoglobinuria; family history; mitochondria not examined)	B: lactic acidosis; abnormal glycolysis

(3) Ophthalmic myopathies

Progressive external ophthalmoplegia

DiMauro, Schotland, Bonilla, Lee, Gambetti and Rowland (1973)	M: lack of respiratory control with α-glycerophosphate
Sulaiman, Doyle, Johnson and Jennett (1974)	B: increased lactate and pyruvate, decreased ketone bodies and free fatty acids after exercise
Carroll, Zwillich, Weil and Brooke (1976) (case 2)	Reduced ventilatory response to hypoxia and hypercapnia
Reske-Nielsen, Lou and Lowes (1976)	B: lactic acidaemia

Kearns-Sayre syndrome

Carroll *et al.* (1976) (cases 1, 3, 4)	Reduced ventilatory response to hypoxia and hypercapnia
Berenberg, Pellock, DiMauro, Schotland, Bonilla, Eastwood, Hays, Vicale, Behrens, Chutorian and Rowland (1976)	M: decreased respiratory rate and defective ATPase stimulation in one patient; no abnormality in three patients

(4) Syndrome: retarded growth, muscle weakness, central nervous system disease and lactic acidosis

van Wijngaarden, Bethlem, Meijer, Hülsmann and Feltkamp (1967)	M: loose coupling of oxidative phosphorylation
van Biervliet, Bruinvis, Ketting, de Bree, van der heiden, Wadman, Willems, Brookelman, van Haelst and Monnens (1977)	M: deficiency of cytochrome aa₃ and b
Spiro, Moore, Prineas, Strasberg and Rapin (1970)	M: reduction of cytochrome b; abnormal in sensitivity to antimycin A; loose coupling B: note, no mention of lactic acid level

(5) Non-muscular diseases

Zellweger's disease: Goldfischer, Moore, Johnson, Spiro, Valsamis, Wisniewsky, Ritch, Norton, Rapin and Gartner (1973)	M: (liver and cortical astrocytes): defect in electron transport prior to the cytochromes
'Kinky hair disease': French, Sherard Lubell, Brotz and Moore (1972); Ghatak, Hirano, Poon and French (1972)	M: (brain, liver and muscles): cytochrome a+a₃ diminished

Under the electron microscope the mitochondria are usually found to be enlarged and have an abnormal, often bizarre appearance. They contain stacks of parallel lamellae, concentric rings of membranes, paracrystalline bodies and granular material (Ch. 9).

The abnormal mitochondria are usually increased in number and may form large aggregates at the periphery of fibres. It is striking that many affected fibres are of normal size and shape and are otherwise of normal appearance except for a frequent and characteristic finding of collections of glycogen and fat within the muscle fibres, which may raise the possibility of storage disease. Nevertheless, destruction of fibres may occur, especially in the cranial muscles. As the number of fibres diminishes there is replacement by interstitial fibrous tissue and lipocytes. In contrast, trunk and limb muscles in such cases are hardly affected, if at all.

Autopsy examinations have shown that the central nervous system is not involved in the progressive external ophthalmoplegia of von Graefe, Kiloh and Nevin (Beckett and Netsky, 1953; Schwartz and Liu, 1954) nor in the oculopharyngeal form of Taylor (Rebeiz, Caulfield and Adams, 1969). Likewise, one member of such a family with facioscapulohumeral myopathy (Table 5.2) had no signs of disease in the central nervous system except for an acute infarct (Bradley et al., 1978). Of particular interest in the latter case is that the mitochondrial changes were restricted to the skeletal muscles. These data support the conclusion that muscular changes and symptoms in this group of diseases are of myogenic and not of neurogenic origin. On the other hand, a spongiform encephalopathy has been found in autopsied cases of the Kearns-Sayre syndrome (Kearns and Sayre, 1958; Daroff, Solitaire, Pincus and Glaser, 1966; Castaigne, Laplane, Escourolle, Augustine, de Recondo, Martinez Lage and Villaneuva Eusa, 1971; Berenberg, Pellock, DiMauro, Schotland, Bonilla, Eastwood, Hays, Vicale, Belirens, Chutorian and Rowland, 1976). In this syndrome abnormal mitochondria have been noted, not only in skeletal muscles, but also in other organs, such as the Purkinje cells of the cerebellum (Gonatas, Evangelista and Martin, 1967). The lesions in the central nervous system

explain symptoms such as ataxia, mental retardation and abnormal electroencephalographic patterns, which are common in the Kearns-Sayre syndrome.

With regard to pathogenesis, one can only speculate that abnormality of one or several genes (hereditary or acquired) may result in deficiency of one or several mitochondrial enzymes and/or impairment of the function of the respiratory chain in forming ATP. Multiple gene damage could explain the combinations of symptoms resulting from dysfunction of skeletal muscles and other organs. It is possible that the morphological changes in the mitochondria are only secondary, i.e. that they represent an attempt on the part of muscle cells to compensate for the deficiency of an enzyme situated in mitochondria. Lactic acidosis in blood and accumulation of glycogen and fat in muscles with abnormal mitochondria also reflect a functional disturbance of the muscle fibres' oxidative functions.

Vacuoles may be seen as small holes in muscle fibres, but fine details regarding their contents, surrounding membranes, if any, and relationship to the sarcotubular system are demonstrable only with the electron microscope (*see* Ch. 9).

Vacuolation ('hydropic degeneration' in the classical literature) is another non-specific feature of myopathies. The expression 'vacuolar myopathy' has little meaning in pathology, because the associated changes are so heterogeneous, and there must be many different causes and pathogenetic mechanisms.

True vacuoles are surrounded by membranes. The latter are probably formed from the system of normal membranous structures, which occupy a major part of the volume of the muscle fibres (*see* Ch. 2 for ultrastructure of the normal fibre). Probably most of the membranes around vacuoles come from the T tubules and the sarcoplasmic reticulum (Bird, 1975). Other less likely sources are the Golgi apparatus, which is small in muscle fibres, and the perinuclear membranes.

Following focal necrosis (*see* Fig. 5.4 and p. 165), the degenerate material is walled off from the remaining healthy muscle fibre by a membrane, which forms an autophagic vacuole (also called a secondary lysosome). The sequestered material is

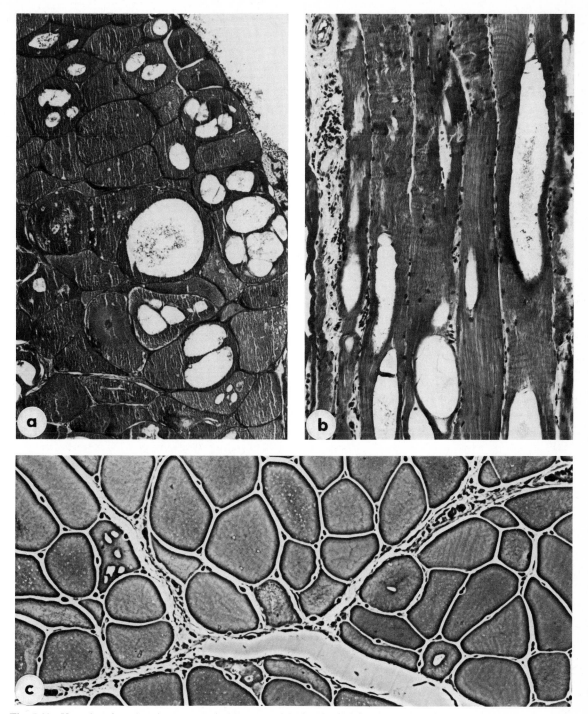

Fig. 5.16   Vacuoles of varying sizes are seen in (a) cross and (b) longitudinal sections of muscle fibres in a case of hypokalaemic periodic paralysis. Large vacuoles have expanded some muscle fibres leaving only a thin rim of muscle tissue at the periphery. H and E, ×225. (c) Lesser degree of vacuolation noted in biopsy from a case of hyperkalaemic periodic paralysis. ×295

digested by autolytic enzymes. End-products in the vacuoles are eventually extruded into the extracellular space, but some products may remain as lipofuscin bodies (Fig. 5.4d).

Autophagic vacuoles have been seen in different muscle diseases but are especially prominent in Pompe's disease (Fig. 5.12 and 5.13), periodic paralysis syndromes (Fig. 5.16) and in chloroquine-induced myopathy (Engel, 1973). We are at present studying two cases of middle-aged men with progressive weakness, in which multiple autophagic vacuoles were prominent findings. The classification of these cases is so far undecided.

Multifocal hydropic change in muscle fibres is a characteristic feature of familial hypokalaemic periodic paralysis (Fig. 5.16). In this disease as many as a quarter of all muscle fibres may be vacuolated. The vacuoles range in size from less than five to more than 25 μm, and in many places several may appear to have coalesced. Their longitudinal dimension varies from five to 200 μm, and one fibre may contain vacuoles at several non-aligned points. The myofibrils and sarcoplasm, being displaced laterally, must curve around the vacuoles. Within the cleared zone a fine pre-cipitated material, which stains with carmine and in the periodic-acid-Schiff (PAS) reaction, may be seen.

In some cases, biopsies taken between attacks have disclosed entirely normal muscle structure. However, the idea that the vacuolisation occurs only during attacks is patently refuted by the finding of extreme degrees of this feature in patients who have not suffered a manifest attack of even mild weakness for 20 years. Such instances indicate that this morphological change may be the principal finding in a late, chronic, progressive stage of this myopathy. Such pronounced vacuolisation led to necrosis of single muscle fibres in the family studied by Gruner and Porte (1959). Many attacks of paralysis, then, seem to initiate a mild progressive myopathy. The necrotic seg-ments of the fibre may be restored, after phagocy-totic removal, by regeneration. Incomplete res-toration of damaged fibres may lead to a slightly reduced population of muscle fibres and mild endomysial fibrosis. The creation of com-munications between vacuoles and the extracel-lular space, with indentation of the surface membrane, will result in remodelling and splitting of fibres (Engel, 1970b).

A similar vacuolar change is said to accompany occasionally the paralysis of hyperaldosteronism and the normokalaemic periodic paralysis de-scribed by Tyler, Stephens, Gunn and Perkoff (1951), and by Poskanzer and Kerr (1961).

The paramyotonia of Eulenberg and the related adynamia episodica hereditaria of Gamstorp (1956), where transient paralysis may be induced by potassium and is relieved by a high dietary intake of carbohydrate, are states which might be re-garded as the obverse of hypokalaemic periodic paralysis. Multifocal vacuolisation has been obser-ved (Fig. 5.16c), but only rarely, as might be expected, for the water content of the fibre is said to be reduced. Full details of the changes in muscle are not known. Drager, Hammill and Shy (1958) noted zones of clear sarcoplasm, devoid of myofib-rils in some muscle fibres in their cases of paramyotonia and Gamstorp (1956) observed similar alterations in one of her three cases of hereditary episodic adynamia, together with ring bundles, which are more often seen in myotonic dystrophy.

The cause and the pathogenesis of the vacuoles in periodic paralysis have been discussed in numerous publications. Shy, Wanko, Rowley and Engel (1961) demonstrated intracellular oedema by direct measurement. The associated reduction in serum potassium is presumably caused by a movement of this cation into the muscle fibre, but no explanation has been found for the intracellular migration of either the potassium or water. The paralysis, which attends the biochemical change, should probably not be ascribed to the mechanical effect of the vacuolisation *per se*, for loss of function greatly exceeds that which would be expected if all the vacuolated muscle fibres were powerless to contract. It is more likely that the paralysis is due to a change in the electrical properties of the sarcolemma or its inward exten-sion into the transverse tubule, or in the SR system (Shy *et al.*, 1961; Engel, 1970b).

The vacuoles then, must be regarded as a consequence of the disease and not a cause of the paralytic attacks. With regard to the origin of these vacuoles, Shy *et al.* (1961) postulated that they are formed from local dilatations and coalescence of

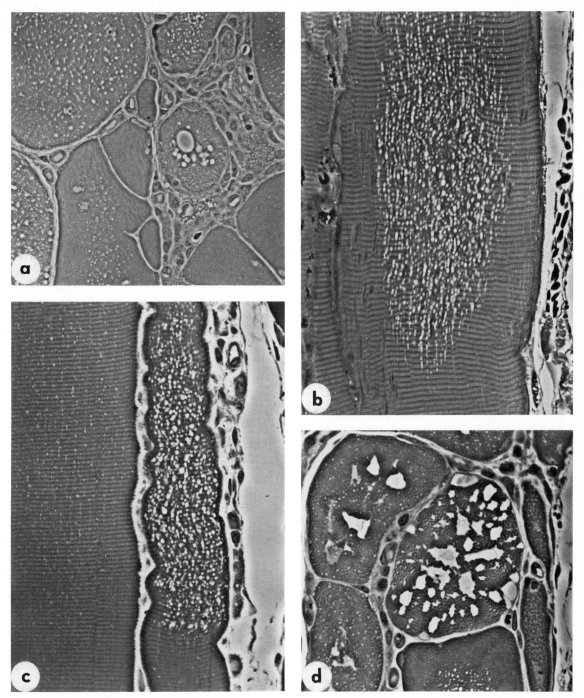

Fig. 5.17 Multiple small vacuoles in various muscle diseases. (a) Cross-sectioned fibres in a case of Charcot-Marie-Tooth disease containing many small vacuoles, surrounded by a membrane. They are seen mostly in large fibres and are most numerous in the central regions of fibres. Compare this Figure with those in Figs. 5.2 (d) and 5.9 (d), which are from the same patient, ×545. (b) Longitudinal section from a case of neurogenic atrophy showing many small vacuoles in the central part of the fibre, ×545. (c) Longitudinal section of muscle fibre in a case of polymyositis (same as (d)); note vacuolation near zone of necrosis (not shown in the picture), ×545. (d) Cross-section of muscle from a case of polymyositis showing vacuolation of fibres, ×545

SR tubules. Engel (1970b) traced the earliest stage of vacuolisation to proliferation and dilatation of SR and T systems. The mature vacuoles were found to be in communication with the extracellular space via the T tubules.

As stated above, a small part of glycogen in the muscle fibres is normally enclosed in membrane-bound vacuoles where it is broken down by lysosomal enzymes (acid maltase). The deficiency of this enzyme in Pompe's disease (Hers, 1963) leads to accumulation of glycogen in membrane-bound bags. Proliferation of such bags is a characteristic feature of this type of glycogen storage disease, which is an example of the so-called lysosomal diseases (Hers, 1965). Thus, Pompe's glycogen storage disease is characterised by two types of lysosomal vacuoles—the glycogen-filled vacuoles and the autophagic vacuoles with debris, which were described on page 182 (Figs 5.12 and 5.13).

Multiple small vacuoles occur in various other conditions (Fig. 5.17). We have seen them *inter alia*, in denervation atrophy and polymyositis. Of particular interest is one of our patients with Charcot-Marie-Tooth's disease, in the muscle of whom we found late dystrophic changes of denervation (Fig. 5.2d), target phenomena (Fig. 5.9d) and multiple vacuoles (Figs. 5.9d and 5.17a). Electron microscopy showed that the vacuoles were membrane-bound and had the appearance of lysosomes.

Crescent formations. The term 'thyroid myopathy', which draws attention to the association of disease of the thyroid gland and disorders of muscle, came to medical attention through the original reports of Hoffmann (1893) and Debré and Semelaigne (1935). With regard to muscle pathology, most textbooks refer to an article by Askanazy (1898), which described and illustrated a widespread necrotising myopathy in cases of thyrotoxicosis. His findings, however, have never been corroborated. It seems probable that Askanazy's cases were complicated by infection and other disease processes, which could have caused a Zenker's type of necrosis. Only in the ophthalmic Graves' disease have consistent structural alterations been found. In the eye muscle, infiltration of fat cells is the most obvious change,

but degeneration of muscle fibres, a variable regenerative reaction and infiltration of lymphocytes and mononuclear histiocytes also occur. Conventional histological stains have not usually disclosed any definitive muscular lesion in either thyrotoxic myopathy or hypothyroidism, apart from a slight volumetric decrease in the former and increase in the latter. In one specimen (from a 71-year-old woman, who died in myxoedemic coma without ever having received thyroid treatment), Åström, Kugelberg and Müller (1961) discovered accumulations of mucoid material within some skeletal muscle fibres. The earlier literature contains a few reports of similar findings in severe protracted cases of hyperthyroidism.

The paper by Asbøe-Hansen, Iversen and Wichman (1952) on 'crescent formation', deserves special comment. In all 10 cases of exophthalmic goitre, in nine out of 10 cases of thyrotoxicosis without exophthalmos, and in one out of seven cases of myxoedema, these authors observed in muscle biopsy sections curious deposits of semilunar or crescent form (in cross-sections) or spindle form (in longitudinal sections) beneath the sarcolemma. The myofibrils were pushed aside. The chemical composition of the deposits could not be ascertained. Their demonstration required a basic lead acetate fixative. Water solubility and extractability by hyaluronidase, and the staining properties of the material suggested that it contained mucopolysaccharide.

No other worker has seen these crescents, nor have we been able to find them, using the same method of fixation and staining. Their occurrence in both hyper- and hypothyroidism, two diseases of almost diametrically opposite functional and biochemical properties, must raise some doubts as to whether they reflect a basic pathologic process. Clearly, these myopathies merit further study.

Nuclear alterations. Nuclear number and position within the fibre have already been mentioned in several contexts. Atrophy or hypoplasia of fibres results in a population of nuclei that is larger in proportion to the volume of visible sarcoplasm without an actual increase in numbers. In addition, in muscle hypertrophy the nuclei are more widely spaced (and sometimes central in position) without an actual decrease in number. True nuclear hyperplasia probably signifies necrosis with regeneration in most instances; in the earlier phases of this process the nuclei enlarge and acquire a prominent nucleolus (Fig. 5.7).

One special form of hyperplasia is that in which there are rows of sarcolemmal nuclei ('rowing phenomenon'; see Fig. 5.11e). Usually the end of one nucleus touches the end of the adjacent one and as many as 15–20 nuclei lie like this. The nuclei tend to be small and hyperchromatic. The phenomenon of 'rowing' is seen most consistently in myotonic dystrophy, together with disorganisation of myofibrils and sarcoplasmic masses, but it occurs to a lesser degree in many other diseases and in ageing muscle. In the latter, as well as in denervation atrophy, extreme degrees of atrophy may reduce the muscle fibre to a bag of pyknotic nuclei so tightly clustered as to resemble, in haematoxylin–eosin stains, a particle of calcium.

Intranuclear inclusions have been described under several different conditions. One of the authors reported in 1965 a case of inclusion body myopathy in which a progressive generalised paralysis seemed to be attributable to a viral infection (Adams, Kakulas and Samaha, 1965). Electron micrographs obtained later revealed aggregates of virus particles within the sarcoplasm. Other inclusions within nuclei proved, on electron-microscopic examination, to be caused by unfolding of the nuclear membrane. Within this type of inclusion are cytoplasmic organelles such as glycogen particles. Schröder and Adams (1968) illustrated such inclusions in their communication on the ultrastructure of muscle fibres in myotonic dystrophy and congenital myotonia, and the inclusions have been seen in other atrophic and degenerative myopathies.

It has also been reported that nuclei may contain nemaline-like bodies (Jenis, Lindquist and Lister, 1969; Engel, 1975) and filamentous inclusions (Oteruelo, 1976).

Arrested development of muscle fibres

Spiro, Shy and Gonatas (1966) described the case of a 12-year-old boy with a congenital, progressive muscle disease. The resemblance of the muscle fibres in biopsies to the myotubular state of development persuaded them that an arrest in development had occurred—a kind of muscle retardation. Since then approximately 30 similar cases have been reported under names such as myotubular, centronuclear and pericentronuclear myopathy (see Table 5.1 for references).

The muscle fibres are usually fairly thin, but they are never as small as true embryonal fibres. Most nuclei are centrally situated. A few fibres show mild signs of degeneration and discrete alterations of internal architecture. Loss of fibres is not observed. Histochemical studies suggest that, in many cases, central nucleation is confined to small type I fibres (Engel, Gold and Karpati, 1968).

The idea of arrest of muscle development in the fetus is interesting. It recalls the earlier postulation of Krabbe (1949) that the weak, hypotonic child with the amyotonia congenita syndrome of Oppenheim (1900) might be suffering from a congenital muscular hypoplasia. However, central nucleation is a common finding in many myopathic disorders.

Senile and non-specific changes

In surveying skeletal muscle tissue it is important to consider that such tissue may be acted upon in a variety of ways by ageing and by many pathological conditions, some of which have no relation to the disease under consideration. With regard to the latter, surveys of the musculature, in random post-mortem examinations, have disclosed a surprising number of instances of single fibre necrosis and phagocytosis and aggregates of lymphocytes. Wallace, Lattes, Malia and Ragen (1958) and Pearson (1959) have confirmed that this type of change may be found in autopsy material, where death has been sudden and traumatic or due to some disease not known to affect the muscle fibres or endomysial tissue. These findings indicate that minor muscle fibre injury is continually occurring during everyday life. The pathologist must exercise caution in accepting such changes as expressions of specific muscle diseases.

Our own studies of seven muscles from 134 random autopsies (Moore et al., 1971) reveal in late life incidence (over 80 per cent) of group atrophy and single-fibre atrophy and of nuclear aggregates, especially in leg muscles, and a lesser number of specimens with more extensive necrosis of fibres and vacuolisation.

Pigmentary atrophy, the homologue of brown atrophy of heart muscle, appears to be one of the most reliable indices of ageing, though similar impregnation of sarcoplasm near muscle nuclei by lipofuscin accompanies vitamin E deficiency, even in relatively young animals. A longitudinal row of lipofuscin pigments may also be a residue of previous focal destruction (*see* p. 168 and Fig. 5.4d).

Regarding other aspects of ageing, only a few facts are available. Assuming that nearly all the muscle fibres in the human organism have formed before birth and that all natural, postnatal modifications of structure consist essentially of growth, i.e., increase in size, the fate of such long-enduring fibres becomes a matter of great interest. Do old muscle fibres, like old neurones, ultimately waste away and disappear? Is there a sequence of disfigurative change which might constitute a 'senile myopathy'? We believe that both questions may be answered affirmatively. The range of fibre size increases in the ageing muscle because of increasing numbers of isolated small fibres. Tightly agglutinated knots of dark sarcolemmal nuclei, probably the terminal phase of the atrophic process, and group atrophy, perhaps attributable to senile loss of motor nerve cells, are also present, especially in the leg muscles.

Fibre wasting, with loss of myofibrils and lipfuscin increase, has been noted in normal eye muscles in late life, and has been called senescent atrophy (Rebeiz *et al.*, 1969). Moreover, in the ocular muscles peripheral myofibrils disappear, leaving faintly fibrillar sarcoplasmic masses; spiral annulets or ringbinden occur in some fibres and increase with each decade of life, as first pointed out by Wohlfart (1955) and confirmed by Hübner (1977).

Inflammation

In essence, the problem here is how certain microbes, protozoa, and parasites (Clostridia, Trichinae, Cysticercae, Toxoplasmas, sarcocysts), the toxins they elaborate, or the autoallergic inflammation which they trigger, can affect the muscle fibres. Some organisms, such as Trichinae,

exhibit an almost specific affinity for sarcoplasm. However, the most frequent and puzzling of the inflammatory diseases of muscles are not those caused by visible organisms but the cases of so-called idiopathic polymyositis. As shown by Walton and Adams (1958), nearly half of the latter cases bear some relation to one or other of the connective tissue diseases, and a dermatitis is frequently conjoined.

The relatively benign course of the disease, in many instances, has prevented an extensive study of post-mortem material. Biopsies of muscle have tended to yield only an incomplete idea of the pathological process. Thus, sections often give negative findings in the face of active disease, or reveal only one element of the process.

One component of the myopathology of this condition is necrosis of muscle fibres, which appears in random sections to bear an uncertain topographical relationship to foci of inflammatory cells or to visible changes in vessels or connective tissue. Necrosis may be extremely widespread in the severe and acute cases. More often, segments of single fibres are destroyed (Fig. 5.6). In less severe lesions, it is often the peripheral fibres of fasciculi that bear the brunt of the affection. Some of the surviving fibres, especially in cases of lupus erythematosus, are vacuolated.

Aggregates of inflammatory cells (lymphocytes, mononuclear leucocytes, plasma cells) constitute the most obvious component of the lesion. Without this finding the diagnosis is always in doubt (the mere presence of aggregates of histiocytes (myophagia) should not be mistaken for it (Walton and Adams, 1958)). The inflammatory cells must bear a relationship to some component(s) of the muscle fibres. However, because of the haphazard and incomplete sampling of lesions by the average biopsy, necrosis of muscle may be the only change, or inflammatory cell infiltration may appear to stand alone. When present, inflammatory changes are often most evident in close proximity to small blood vessels, especially small veins. Occlusion of arteries or veins is not found in adult cases except in rare instances, where a vasculitis such as polyarteritis has complicated the picture, or in lupus erythematosus, where thrombo-embolic lesions may have occurred. According to Banker and Victor (1966) some of the childhood cases of dermatomyositis have a special attribute: the major pathological feature is inflammation of vessels and thrombosis leading to infarction of muscle tissue, small peripheral nerves and other organs such as the gastrointestinal tract. Electron microscopy of the muscle changes in childhood dermatomyositis has been described by Carpenter *et al.* (1976) and by Banker (1975). The manner in which the myonecrosis, focal inflammation and connective tissue reaction are related can be demonstrated only in serial sections. In a study of the stereology of the lesion, segmental necrosis was invariably seen to be contiguous to a focus of perivenous lymphocytes and monocytes (Rebeiz, Kakulas and Adams, unpublished observations). The lesions should be viewed as consequences of the operation of a single factor which varies in extent and intensity. The details of the early phases of the injury are unknown. Once destroyed, the necrotic parts of the muscle fibre are removed by macrophages and the regenerative cycle described below commences. Necrosis may recur, and the terminal phases of the lesion result in atrophy of fibres, loss of fibres, and fibrosis.

The cause is indeterminate. Two types of virus-like particles have been seen in muscle biopsies from patients with polymyositis (Chou, 1968; Chou and Gutmann, 1970; Mastaglia and Walton, 1970; and Tang, Sedmak, Siegesmund and McCreadie, 1975), but their pathogenicity is unproved. An allergic inflammation of the autoimmune type has also been postulated, a theory strengthened by the common association with other diseases of connective tissue. Kakulas (1966) has shown that activated lymphocytes from animals sensitised to sarcoplasm cause degeneration of striated fibres in tissue culture (Ch. 11). Human lymphocytes from patients with polymyositis have been shown to have the same effect. These findings support the view that the condition is due to lymphocyte-mediated delayed hypersensitivity. In carcinomatous polymyositis, which is still indistinguishable from the idiopathic variety both clinically and pathologically, the neoplasm in some obscure way sets off the autoimmune process.

Idiopathic polymyositis is further described in Chapter 15.

Myopathies without established changes in muscle fibres

There are many clinically recognisable diseases of muscle with a severe and often fluctuant course, sometimes fatal, in which the pathologist can identify no characteristic specific change in the muscle fibres *per se*. Some of these diseases, such as tetanus with its fatal neurogenic and myogenic spasms and contractures, and acute botulism, have revealed nothing of their nature after the most careful study under the light microscope. Furthermore, there are some diseases of muscle, such as the myopathies of hyper- and hypothyroidism, of Addison's disease, of renal acidosis and in Milkman's disease, where pathological study has been too limited to determine the morphological status of the fibre.

The generalised contractures of unknown type, vaguely grouped as the 'stiff-man syndrome', have not been fully elucidated clinically, electromyographically or pathologically. At times this disease may seem localised in onset, but it is soon evident that other muscles share the abnormality.

In myasthenia gravis, the primary abnormality appears to be at the neuromuscular junction (Santa, Engel and Lambert, 1972), specifically the acetylcholine receptors on the motor end-plate (Bender, Ringel and Engel, 1976). Doubts still exist concerning pathological changes within the fibres themselves. Whereas, in many fatal cases of this disease, the only visible change is the mild disuse atrophy, in others isolated necrosis of single muscle fibres and a few aggregates of lymphocytes and monocytes have been found. When unusually prominent, as they may rarely be, the question of polymyositis or of Zenker's necrosis secondary to the terminal infection or a myopathy associated with neoplasia (e.g. malignant thymoma) always arises. In a few cases, as also noted by others, there has been unmistakable evidence of group atrophy, indicative of denervation. The occasional collections of lymphocytes in muscle in such cases (so-called lymphorrhages) probably indicate an autoimmune process.

Mass lesions in muscle

Muscle masses fall mainly into two categories,

namely tumours and exuberant connective tissue regeneration.

The muscle cell itself seldom undergoes neoplastic transformation, as is true of many highly organised post-mitotic cells, but when it does the tumour always take the form of the highly malignant rhabdomyosarcoma. These, and secondary tumours of muscles, are of concern to surgery and general pathology.

The benign muscle masses of non-neoplastic type comprise a special and relatively neglected group of disorders, even though their clinical presentation is often perplexing.

Rupture of a muscle tendon represents one type of mass lesion. Usually it has been recognised by its onset (a snap during exertion) and by the typical gross deformity in the profile of a muscle with weakening of its force upon all attempts at contraction. Reports on the pathology have been meagre. Biopsy may reveal only normal muscle or zones of injured muscle fibre replaced by connective tissue.

After extensive destruction of muscle tissue, whether from a vascular lesion, haemorrhage, or inflammation, the regenerating muscle fibres and connective tissue may produce one or more firm lumps in the muscle substance. During contraction they become hard, but still have more or less the feel of normal muscle. The mass may reach enormous proportions. We have observed more than a dozen cases where the presenting symptom was a muscle mass of this type. Operation revealed a network of interlacing strands of connective tissue and regenerating muscle cells. The appearance was not that of a malignant tumour and the health of the patients and the remainder of their musculature were normal several years later. This type of lesion may follow a mild injury and the enlarging muscle may raise fears of pseudo-hypertrophic muscular dystrophy. Probably some of these pseudotumours represent a desmoid reaction. The latter most often occurs in the rectus abdominis of the post-parturient woman, and consists of large masses of hyperplastic connective tissue engulfing muscle fibres.

Another similar problem is an inflammatory pseudohypertrophy of muscles. This may involve the sternomastoid and anterior scalene muscles which become swollen and painful, first on one side, then on the other. Great overgrowth of connective tissue, giant muscle fibres measuring up to 200 μm in diameter, and atrophic fibres are mixed with infiltrations of inflammatory cells, remnants of necrotic fibres and cellular blood vessels.

Finally, a persistent and tender lump in a muscle can be due to some type of localised spasm or possibly to an intramuscular rupture. Here one becomes involved in the confusing problem of differentiating fibrositis and myositis from emotional tension with tender spots in muscles. Over the years we have received biopsy material from cases in which the only finding has been an extreme state of contraction of muscle fibres resembling artefactual change. Of course, one cannot always be sure that the offending lump was sampled in the biopsy. These cases deserve more thorough clinical, physiological and pathological study.

RESTORATION OF MUSCLE FIBRES AFTER DENERVATION AND INJURY

Experimentally induced muscle destruction and repair has been studied in animals for more than 100 years and the observations of the early workers were at times remarkably detailed, extensive and accurate. Almost everything we know about muscle repair has resulted from experimental studies.

The lesions have been produced in innumerable ways, for example by mechanical injury of all kinds, heating, freezing, electricity and other means. Most of the lesions have been unpredictable in size and location because the injury was inflicted imprecisely. Cellular reactions have been difficult to interpret because destruction involved, to a variable degree, different elements of muscle. There is a need for studies in which precise lesions of known dimension have been produced in predetermined locations. Another major drawback in the analysis has been that most of the microscopic examinations have sampled only a few brief phases of a continuous process. Conclusions concerning the complete sequence have had to be extrapolated from a series of static pictures. The work of Speidel (1938, 1939) is an exception because it was carried out on living animals (tadpoles). However, he made no attempt to describe the cytological events.

Observations on experimental animals, which go back to the work of Sherrington and his school, have also contributed greatly to our understanding of the motor unit and the effects of denervation upon skeletal muscle fibres.

Restoration of fibres after denervation and re-innervation

The thin, denervated striated muscle fibres (p. 155 regain their normal size if they are re-innervated within a certain time interval. The mode of restoration is dependent upon how re-innervation is accomplished. Denervated muscle fibres may have become re-innervated in one of two ways. In the first, the central part of the damaged nerve grows out and its axons re-establish connections with the same muscle fibres which had been denervated originally. In a favourable case there are no losses of nerve and muscle fibres and the motor units are restored completely. Re-innervation of this type is likely to occur especially if the nerve was not completely severed (as in crush injury) and the lesion was situated distally, near the corresponding muscle. This type of re-innervation is less likely to occur if the nerve was completely severed and the lesion was located proximally; it does not occur at all after injury to motor cell bodies and roots. Second, denervation of scattered motor units in a muscle allows collateral regeneration from adjacent axons. This results in a regrouping of muscle fibres, so that fewer neurones and axons serve the same number of muscle fibres. This regrouping is seen especially in chronic neuropathies and in motor neurone disease.

Kugelberg, Edström and Abbruzzese (1970) have shown that the muscle fibres within one motor unit (which are histochemically uniform) are normally scattered, so that the fibres on a cross-section of muscle appear to be isolated from each other, forming a checkerboard-like pattern. Thus, primary denervation of one motor unit results in atrophy of scattered muscle fibres and not in compact group atrophy, as was formerly believed. Only successive episodes of denervation of several

motor units, after collateral re-innervation has regrouped the fibres, may result in the typical group atrophy (called neurogenic atrophy): then the affected fibres in a given cluster are of the same histochemical type, because they belong now to one motor unit. In conclusion, neurogenic atrophy and re-innervation may result in various rearrangements of muscle fibre patterns, which are best studied in histochemical preparations.

Muscle fibres permanently deprived of innervation ultimately degenerate through a series of stages described on page 157.

Regeneration after destruction of fibres

Regeneration after a necrotising lesion of muscle is fundamentally different from that which follows denervation. In the latter case the atrophic fibre is thin but has retained its general shape and internal structure and has all the necessary metabolic machinery for renewed growth after re-innervation. On the other hand, the necrotic fibre, usually certain segments of it (segmental destruction, see p. 168, has lost its continuity and is usually broken into two or more pieces. Regeneration after necrosis involves multiplication of nuclei, creation of new sarcoplasm of organelles, and fusion and alignment into an integrated unit (Fig. 5.7).

The regenerative power of muscle after segmental necrosis is tremendous. After an acute attack of rhabdomyolysis with myoglobinuria one can see in repeated biopsies that the devastating destruction of muscle fibres is followed by swift removal of necrotic sarcoplasm and complete reconstitution of muscle within 3–4 weeks.

However, if an entire fibre is destroyed, there would seem to be no possibility of a new one being formed from pluripotential mesodermal cells, a process which for the most part ceases before birth. Regeneration after destruction can take place only if parts of the affected fibre remain intact.

Two types of regeneration occur after segmental necrosis—'continuous' and 'discontinuous'. In continuous regeneration, or 'budding', the regeneration begins at the healthy end of a severed fibre. Sarcolemmal nuclei migrate into the junctional zone, and myoblasts that have migrated outside the fibre may fuse with it (Sloper and

Pegrum, 1967). The nuclei are large, with prominent nucleoli, and the surrounding cytoplasm is stained bluish in haematoxylin–eosin preparations because of increase of ribonucleoprotein. Aggregates of nuclei may resemble multinucleated giant cells (muscle giant cells).

In many instances, one finds evidence that the regenerative process results in a series of muscle sprouts, sometimes forming a compact cluster of 5–6 or more. In cross-section they fit together like the pieces of a mosaic. The parent fibre, from which they have formed, is usually enlarged. The ends of these shoots are difficult to follow; some end in connective tissue, probably rendering their contractile force ineffective.

In 'discontinuous' or 'embryonal' regeneration, mononuclear myoblasts lying free in the tissue align in a single row, fuse and form myotubes, which will grow and mature into fibres of adult type. This formation of new segments is reminiscent of the original creation of muscle in fetal life.

Once a myotube forms, the new fibre can be traced through several stages (Fig. 5.7). At an early stage, the rows of heavily nucleated myocytes are surrounded by RNA-rich, slightly basophilic sarcoplasm and a small complement of thick, non-striated protomyofibrils. Later, the thin new fibres are distinguished from the normal ones only by their smaller size, the faint basophilia of their sarcoplasm, their smaller complement of large myofibrils (protofibrils), the large size and central position of their nuclei with prominent nucleoli and increased numbers of ribosomes and microtubules. Later, the nuclei become peripheral and the myofibrils increase in number. The fibre may thus reconstitute itself completely within a few weeks. On the other hand, the regenerative process may stop short: the new muscle nuclei undergo degeneration and the sarcoplasm withers.

The origin of the myoblasts is still a matter of conflicting opinion. The peri-endomysial connective tissue can be excluded as a source (Walker, 1963). The majority are known to originate within the muscle fibre. There are two hypothetical explanations of their origin; one is that they are derived from sarcolemmal nuclei (Hay, 1971; Reznik, 1969; 1973); the other is that they come from so-called satellite cells (Church, 1969). We favour the former view, that near an injured region sarcolemmal nuclei with some cytoplasm envelop themselves with membrane, become sequestered from the remainder of the fibre (Reznik, 1969) and appear as satellite cells (Mauro, 1961), i.e. cells that are situated between the basement membrane and the sarcolemma of the fibre. The satellite cells then divide and the daughter cells develop into myoblasts, which migrate outside the fibre. The alternative hypothesis postulates that the satellite cells are created during fetal life and exist in normal adult muscle (Schmalbuch and Hellhammer, 1976) although in a dormant state. Awakened by injury, they divide and give rise to myoblasts. According to this hypothesis the sarcolemmal nuclei do not participate in regeneration after necrosis.

The effectiveness of regeneration depends upon whether or not the scaffolding of basement membranes and supporting tissues remains intact and the basic pathologic process subsides. The preservation of these structures is needed for so-called isomorphic regeneration, in which the orientation of regenerating fibres parallels that of the original fibres. The sarcolemma usually disappears over necrotic segments and its destruction probably facilitates the migration of phagocytes into the softened, necrotic muscle, and of satellite cells out of the fibre. The removal of dead tissue is a pre-requisite for swift and complete repair.

Isomorphic regeneration with more or less complete reconstitution of muscle is usually seen after segmental necrosis, where supporting tissues are relatively uninjured. Fibroblastic and vascular reactions are minimal. Only in trauma, haemorrhage, infection, infarction and other crude injury does one see complete disorientation of regenerating fibres and vigorous proliferations of fibroblasts and vessels. This so-called anisomorphic regeneration may give rise to a kind of tumefaction of muscle—a local pseudotumour (see p. 197).

It is largely unknown how small, focal lesions involving only parts of a fibre are being repaired. No cells invade the damaged fibre at the site of the lesion. The dead material is digested in a phagic vacuole but it is not known how the fibre repairs the defect.

Repeated biopsies have shown that some degenerative lesions, such as vacuoles in periodic paralysis and tubular aggregates, are reversible, but how these structures disappear and the affected fibres reconstitute themselves is not known.

CONCLUSIONS

We have tried to isolate and define the different types of changes which have been observed in skeletal muscles, and to arrange them in a logical system. This list of basic alterations, defined as exactly as modern methods permit, serves as a kind of 'language' in describing the constellation of changes which occur in diseases, in normal muscles subjected to stress and in the course of ageing.

These structural changes are not to be taken as the equivalents of disease, for a full definition of the pathology of a disease comprises many parameters other than the morphological ones. It should include: (1) all the visible structural changes in muscle; (2) their topography in the entire muscular system; (3) the presence or absence of involvement of cardiac muscle and non-muscular tissues (nervous system, eye, skin, connective tissues etc.); and (4) the chronology of the changes, best expressed by the sequence of the functional disorders they produce during life. The myopathologist with access to a small specimen only from one muscle, obtained in a single instant in the life-profile of a disease, cannot be depended upon even to provide the first component in the array of data necessary for the diagnosis of disease. To ascertain the topography of a disease in muscle a complete post-mortem study must be made; alternatively, as is more often the case, this must be determined by clinical examination and physiological testing. The same is true of data concerning involvement of other tissues. The chronology can be divulged only by the history of the illness or by a succession of examinations.

The clinician must keep these points in mind when he sends a biopsy specimen to the pathology laboratory. If he expects more than a cursory description of one or a few morphological changes, he must send with the specimen all other data concerning these aspects of the disease.

Following injury, the muscle fibre reacts in many respects like other living cells in the body. However, the range of its structural alterations is larger than those of any other cell in the body, and there are a number of modifications that are unique because of the special features of anatomy and physiology, discussed in the Introduction.

With regard to the meaning of the structural changes in the muscle fibre, one should first realise that such changes usually, if not always, are secondary effects of a more fundamental abnormality, which can be revealed only by biochemical or immunological methods. These secondary structural changes together constitute a heterogeneous group. Some of them are a direct consequence of the original defect. For example, the primary defect in McArdle's disease—deficiency of the enzyme muscle phosphorylase—causes morphological changes resulting from excessive accumulation of glycogen under the sarcolemma and between myofibrils. Likewise, one can conjecture that a primary genetic error in the production of protein may lead to the appearance of abnormal structures such as nemaline bodies and tubular aggregates. Other changes in muscle fibres are more strictly reparative and compensatory reactions, which have the purpose of reducing the damaging effect of the original injury, and of repairing defects after destruction. Necrotic and reparative processes which follow the death of tissue are examples of such lesions. In the case of mitochondrial myopathies, the overgrowth of mitochondria appears to represent an attempt on the part of the muscle fibres to compensate for the deficiency of respiratory enzymes.

Recent histological techniques permit the structural changes in skeletal muscles to be described in greater detail and new types of reaction patterns to be discovered. In addition, one can expect that, in the near future, other methodological developments will enable the myopathologist to discern hitherto undescribed morphological alterations and to improve the definition of those already known. More important, one can look forward to a more complete understanding of their nature and their relation to causative factors. Without doubt, the major problems with regard to aetiology and pathogenesis for most muscle diseases remain to be solved. Essential for the solution of these problems are first, a clear definition of structural changes at all stages of evolution of the disease and second, an understanding of their pathogenesis, meaning and interrelationship.

ACKNOWLEDGEMENTS

We thank Mr L. Cherkas for help with the photography. This study was supported in part by Grant N.S. 07596 from the National Institute of Neurological Diseases and Stroke.

REFERENCES

Adams, R.D. (1968) The giant muscle fibre; its place in myopathology. In *Modern Neurology : Papers in Tribute to D. Denny-Brown*, Ed. S. Locke, pp. 225–240 (Little Brown and Co: Boston).

Adams, R.D. (1975) *Diseases of Muscle : A Study in Pathology*. 3rd Edn. (Harper and Row: Hagerstown, Maryland).

Adams, R.D. & DeReuck, J. (1973) Metrics of muscle. In *Basic Research in Myology. Proceedings of the Second International Congress on Muscle Diseases*, Ed. B.A. Kakulas, Vol. I. Ch. 1, p. 3 (Excerpta Medica: Amsterdam).

Adams, R.D. & Rebeiz, J.J. (1966) Histopathologie der Myotonischen Erkrankungen. In *Progressive Muskeldystrophie, Myotonie, Myasthenie Symposium*, Ed. E. Kuhn, p. 191 (Springer-Verlag: New York).

Adams, R.D., Denny-Brown, D. & Pearson, C.M. (1953) *Diseases of Muscle : A Study in Pathology*. 1st Edn. (Hoeber: New York).

Adams, R.D., Kakulas, B.A. & Samaha, F.A. (1965) A myopathy with cellular inclusions. *Transactions of the American Neurological Association*, **90**, 213.

Afifi, A.K., Smith, J.W. & Zellweger, H. (1965) Congenital nonprogressive myopathy: central core disease and nemaline myopathy in one family. *Neurology (Minneapolis)*, **15**, 371.

Afifi, A.K., Aleu, F.P., Goodgold, J. & Mackay, B. (1966) Ultrastructure of atrophic muscle in amyotrophic lateral sclerosis. *Neurology (Minneapolis)*, **16**, 475.

Afifi, A.K., Ibrahim, Z.M., Bergman, R.A., Abu Haydar, N., Mire, J., Bahuth, N. & Kaylani, I. (1972) Morphologic features of hypermetabolic mitochondrial disease. A light microscopic, histochemical and electron microscopic study. *Journal of the Neurological Sciences*, **15**, 271.

Angelini, C. (1976) Lipid storage myopathies. A review of metabolic defect and of treatment. *Journal of Neurology (Berlin)*, **214**, 1.

Asbøe-Hansen, G., Iversen, K. & Wichman, B. (1952) Malignant exophthalmos: muscular changes and thyrotropin content in serum. *Acta Endocrinologica*, **11**, 376.

Askanas, V., Engel, W.K., Britton, D.E., Adornato, B.T. & Eiben, R.M. (1978) Reincarnation in cultured muscle of mitochondrial abnormalities. *Archives of Neurology*, **35**, 801.

Askanazy, M. (1898) Pathologisch-anatomische Beiträge zur Kenntniss des Morbus Basedowii, inbesondere über die dabei aufretende Muskelerkrankung. *Deutsche Archiv für Klinische Medizin*, **16**, 118.

Åström, K.E. & Adams, R.D. (1980) The pathologic reactions of the skeletal muscle fibre. In *Handbook of Clinical Neurology : Diseases of Muscle*, Eds S.P. Ringel & H.L. Klawans (American Elsevier: New York).

Åström, K.E., Kugelberg, E. & Müller, R. (1961) Hypothyroid myopathy. *Archives of Neurology*, **5**, 472.

Banker, B.Q. (1975) Dermatomyositis of childhood. Ultrastructural alterations of muscle and intramuscular blood vessels. *Journal of Neuropathology and Experimental Neurology*, **34**, 66.

Banker, B.Q. & Denny-Brown, D. (1959) A study of denervated muscle in normal and dystrophic mice. *Journal of Neuropathology and Experimental Neurology*, **18**, 517.

Banker, B.Q. & Victor, M. (1966) Dermatomyositis (systemic angiopathy) of childhood. *Medicine*, **45**, 261.

Banker, B.Q., Victor, M. & Adams, R.D. (1957) Arthrogryposis multiplex due to congenital muscular dystrophy. *Brain*, **80**, 210.

Beckett, R.S. & Netsky, M.G. (1953) Familial ocular myopathy and external ophthalmoplegia. *Archives of Neurology and Psychiatry*, **69**, 64.

Bell, C.D. & Conen, P.E. (1967) Change in fibre size in Duchenne muscular dystrophy. *Neurology (Minneapolis)*, **17**, 902.

Bender, A.N. & Bender, M.B. (1977) Muscle fibre hypotrophy with intact neuromuscular junctions. A study of a patient with congenital neuromuscular disease and ophthalmoplegia. *Neurology (Minneapolis)*, **27**, 206.

Bender, A.N., Ringel, S.P. & Engel, W.K. (1976) The acetylcholine receptor in normal and pathologic states. Immune peroxidase visualisation of alpha-bungatoxin binding at a light and electron microscopic level. *Neurology (Minneapolis)*, **26**, 477.

Berenbaum, M.C., Birch, C.A. & Moreland, J.D. (1953) Paroxysmal myoglobinuria. *Lancet*, **1**, 892.

Berenberg, R.A., Pellock, J.M., DiMauro, S., Schotland, D.L., Bonilla, E., Eastwood, A., Hays, A., Vicale, C.T., Behrens, M., Chutorian, A. & Rowland, L.P. (1976) Lumping or splitting? 'Ophthalmoplegia-Plus' or Kearns-Sayre syndrome. *Annals of Neurology*, **1**, 37.

Bethlem, J., Arts, W.F. & Dingemans, K.P. (1978) Common origin of rods, cores, miniature cores, and focal loss of cross-striations. *Archives of Neurology*, **35**, 555.

van Biervliet, J.P.G.M., Bruinis, I., Ketting, D., De Bree, P.K., van der heiden, C., Wadman, S.K., Willems, J.L., Brookelman, H., van Haelst, U. & Monnens, L.A.H. (1977) Hereditary mitochondrial myopathy with lactic acidemia, a de Toni-Fanconi-Debré syndrome and a defective respiratory chain in voluntary striated muscles. *Pediatric Research*, **11**, 1088.

Bird, J.W. (1975) Skeletal muscle lysosomes. In *Lysosomes in Biology and Pathology*, Eds J.T. Dingle & R.T. Dean, Vol. 4, Ch. 4, p. 75 (North Holland: Amsterdam).

Black, J.T., Judge, D., Demers, L. & Gordon, S. (1975) Ragged-red fibres. A biochemical and morphological study. *Journal of the Neurological Sciences*, **26**, 479.

Bonnette, H., Roelofs, R. & Olson, W.H. (1974) Multicore disease: report of a case with onset in middle age. *Neurology (Minneapolis)*, **24**, 1039.

Bradley, W.G. (1969) Ultrastructural changes in adynamia episodica hereditaria and normokalemic familial periodic paralysis. *Brain*, **92**, 379.

Bradley, W.G., Tomlinson, B.E. & Hardy, M. (1978) Further studies of mitochondrial and lipid storage myopathies. *Journal of the Neurological Sciences*, **35**, 201.

Brooke, M.H. (1974) Congenital fibre type disproportion. In *Clinical Studies in Myology. Proceedings of the Second International Congress on Muscle Diseases*, Ed. B.A. Kakulas, Vol. 2, Ch. 3, p. 147 (Excerpta Medica: Amsterdam).

Brooke, M.H. & Engel W.K. (1969a) The histographic analysis of human muscle biopsies with regard to fibre types. 1. Adult male and female. *Neurology (Minneapolis)*, **19**, 221.

Brooke, M.H. & Engel, W.K. (1969b) The histographic analysis of human muscle biopsies with regard to fibre types. 2. Diseases of the upper and lower motor neuron. *Neurology (Minneapolis)*, **19**, 378.

Brooke, M.H. & Engel, W.K. (1969c) The histographic analysis of human muscle biopsies with regard to fibre types. 3. Myopathies, myasthenia gravis, and hypokalemic periodic paralysis. *Neurology (Minneapolis)*, **19**, 469.

Brooke, M.H. & Engel, W.K. (1969d) The histographic analysis of human muscle biopsies with regard to fibre types. 4. Children's biopsies. *Neurology (Minneapolis)*, **19**, 591.

Brooke, M.H. & Neville, H.E. (1972) Reducing body myopathy. *Neurology (Minneapolis)*, **22**, 829.

Campbell, M.J., Rebeiz, J.J. & Walton J.N. (1969) Myotubular, centronuclear or peri-centronuclear myopathy? *Journal of the Neurological Sciences*, **8**, 425.

Cancilla, P.A., Kalyanaraman, K., Verity, M.A., Munsat, T. & Pearson, C.M. (1971) Familial myopathy with probable lysis of myofibrils in Type I fibres. *Neurology (Minneapolis)*, **21**, 579.

Carpenter, S., Karpati, G., Rothman, S. & Watters, G. (1976) The childhood type of dermatomyositis. *Neurology (Minneapolis)*, **26**, 952.

Carpenter, S., Karpati, G., Andermann, F., Jacob, J.C. & Andermann, E. (1977) The ultrastructural characteristics of the abnormal cytosomes in Batten-Kufs' disease. *Brain*, **100**, 137.

Carroll, J.E., Zwillich, C., Weil, J.V. & Brooke, M.H. (1976) Depressed ventilatory response in oculocraniosomatic neuromuscular disease. *Neurology (Minneapolis)*, **26**, 140.

Castaigne, P., Laplane, D., Escourolle, R., Augustine, P., de Recondo., J., Martinez Lage, G.J. & Villaneuva Eusa, J.A. (1971) Ophthalmoplegie externe progressive avec spongiose des noyaux du tronc cérébral. *Revue Neurologique (Paris)*, **124**, 454.

Chou, S.M. (1968) Myxovirus-like structures and accompanying nuclear changes in chronic polymyositis. *Archives of Pathology*, **86**, 649.

Chou, S.M. & Gutmann, L. (1970) Picornavirus-like crystals in subacute polymyositis. *Neurology (Minneapolis)*, **20**, 205.

Church, J.C.T. (1969) Satellite cells and myogenesis; a study in the fruit bat web. *Journal of Anatomy*, **105**, 419.

Cogen, F.C., Rigg, G., Simmons, J.L. & Domino, E.F. (1978) Phencyclidine-associated acute rhabdomyolysis. *Annals of Internal Medicine*, **88**, 210.

Conen, P.E., Murphy, E.G. & Donohue, W.C. (1963) Light and electron microscopic studies of 'myogranules' in a child with hypotonia and muscle weakness. *Canadian Medical Association Journal*, **89**, 983.

Cullen, M.J. & Fulthorpe, J.J. (1975) Stages in fibre breakdown in Duchenne muscular dystrophy. *Journal of the Neurological Sciences*, **24**, 179.

Curless, R.G., Nelson, M.B. & Brimmer, F. (1978) Histological patterns of muscle in infants with developmental brain abnormalities. *Developmental Medicine and Child Neurology*, **20**, 159.

Curless, R.G., Payne, C.M. & Brimmer, F.M. (1978) Fingerprint body myopathy: a report of twins. *Developmental Medicine and Child Neurology*, **20**, 793.

Daroff, R.B., Solitaire, G.B., Pincus, J.H. & Glaser, G.H. (1966) Spongiform encephalopathy with chronic progressive external ophthalmoplegia. Central ophthalmoplegia mimicking ocular myopathy. *Neurology (Minneapolis)*, **16**, 161.

Debré, R. & Semelaigne, G. (1935) Syndrome of diffuse muscular hypertrophy in infants causing athletic appearance; its connection with congenital myxedema. *American Journal of Diseases of Children*, **50**, 1351.

Denny-Brown, D. (1960) The nature of polymyositis and related muscular diseases. *Transactions of the College of Physicians—Philadelphia*, **28**, 14.

Denny-Brown, D. (1961) Experimental studies pertaining to hypertrophy, regeneration and degeneration. *Research Publications of the Association for Research in Nervous and Mental Disease*, **38**, 147.

De Reuck, J., Hooft, C., De Coster, W., van den Bossche & Cuvelier, C. (1977) A progressive congenital myopathy. Initial involvement of the diaphragm with type I muscle fibre atrophy. *European Neurology*, **15**, 217.

DiMauro, S. & Melis-DiMauro, P.M. (1973) Muscle carnitine palmityl transferase deficiency and myoglobinuria. *Science*, **182**, 929.

DiMauro, S., Schotland, D.L., Bonilla, E., Lee, C.P., Gambetti, P. & Rowland, L.P. (1973) Progressive ophthalmoplegia, glycogen storage and abnormal mitochondria. *Archives of Neurology*, **29**, 170.

DiMauro, S., Bonilla, E., Lee, C.P., Schotland, D.L., Scarpa, A., Conn, H., Jr. & Chance, B. (1976) Luft's disease. Further biochemical and ultrastructural studies of skeletal muscle in the second case. *Journal of the Neurological Sciences*, **27**, 217.

Drachman, D. (1965) Pharmacological denervation of skeletal muscle in chick embryos treated with botulinus toxin. *Transactions of the American Neurological Association*, **90**, 241.

Drachman, D.B., Murphy, S.R., Nigam, M.P. & Hills, J.R. (1967) Myopathic changes in chronically denervated muscles. *Archives of Neurology*, **16**, 14.

Drager, G.A., Hammill, J.F. & Shy, G.M. (1958) Paramyotonia congenita. *Archives of Neurology and Psychiatry*, **80**, 1.

Dubowitz, V. (1975) Infantile spinal muscular atrophy. In *Handbook of Clinical Neurology: System Disorders and Atrophies*, Eds P.J. Vinken, & G.W. Bruyn, Vol. 22, Ch. 4, p. 81 (North Holland: Amsterdam).

Dubowitz, V. & Brooke, M.H. (1973) *Muscle Biopsy: A Modern Approach* (Saunders: Philadelphia).

Dubowitz, V. & Roy, S. (1970) Central core disease of muscle: clinical, histochemical and electron microscopic studies of an affected mother and son. *Brain*, **93**, 133.

Dyken, P.R. & Harper, P.S. (1973) Congenital dystrophia myotonica. *Neurology (Minneapolis)*, **23**, 465.

Dyken, M., Zeman, W. & Rausche, T. (1969) Hypokalemic

periodic paralysis. *Neurology (Minneapolis)*, **19**, 691.

Ekbom, K., Hed, R., Kirstein, L. & Åström, K.E. (1964) Muscular affections. *Archives of Neurology*, **10**, 440.

Engel, A.G. (1970a) Acid maltase deficiency in adults: studies in four cases of a syndrome which may mimic muscular dystrophy or other myopathies. *Brain*, **93**, 599.

Engel, A.G. (1970b) Evolution and content of vacuoles in primary hypokalemic periodic paralysis. *Mayo Clinic Proceedings*, **45**, 774.

Engel, A.G. (1973) Vacuolar myopathies: multiple etiologies and sequential structural studies. In *The Striated Muscle*, Eds C.M. Pearson, & F.K. Mostofi, p. 301 (Williams and Wilkins: Baltimore).

Engel, A.G. & Angelini C. (1973) Carnitine deficiency of human skeletal muscle with associated lipid storage myopathy: a new syndrome. *Science*, **173**, 899.

Engel, A.G., Angelini, C. & Gomez, M.R. (1972) Fingerprint body myopathy, a newly recognized congenital muscle disease. *Mayo Clinic Proceedings*, **47**, 377.

Engel, A.G., Gomez, M.R. & Groover, R.V. (1971) Multicore disease. *Mayo Clinic Proceedings*, **46**, 666.

Engel, A.G., Gomez, M.R. & Seybold, M.E. (1973) The spectrum and diagnosis of acid maltase deficiency. *Neurology (Minneapolis)*, **23**, 95.

Engel, W.K. (1961) Muscle target cells: A newly recognized sign of denervation. *Nature*, **191**, 389.

Engel, W.K. (1962a) The essentiality of histo- and cytochemical studies of skeletal muscles in the investigation of neuromuscular disease. *Neurology (Minneapolis)*, **12**, 778.

Engel, W.K. (1962b) Chemocytology of striated annulets and sarcoplasmic masses in myotonic dystrophy. *Journal of Histochemistry and Cytochemistry*, **10**, 229.

Engel, W.K. (1975) Abundant nuclear rods in adult-onset rod disease. *Journal of Neuropathology and Experimental Neurology*, **34**, 119.

Engel, W.K., Bishop, D.W. & Cunningham, G.G. (1970) Tubular aggregates in type II muscle fibres; ultrastructural and histochemical consideration. *Journal of Ultrastructure Research*, **31**, 507.

Engel, W.K., Gold, G.N. & Karpati, G. (1968) Type I fibre hypotrophy and central nuclei. A rare congenital muscle abnormality with a possible experimental model. *Archives of Neurology*, **18**, 435.

Engel, W.K., Foster, J.B., Hughes, B.P., Huxley, H.E. & Mahler, R. (1961) Central core disease—An investigation of a rare muscular abnormality. *Brain*, **84**, 167.

Erb, W. (1891) Dystrophia muscularis progressiva; Klinische und pathologischanatomische Studien. *Deutsche Zeitschrift für Nervenheilkunde*, **1**, 13.

Fardeau, M. (1970) Ultrastructural lesions in progressive muscular dystrophies. A critical study of their specificity. In *Muscle Diseases. International Congress Series No. 199*, Eds N. Canal, G. Scarlatti, & J.N. Walton, p. 98 (Excerpta Medica: Amsterdam).

Fardeau, M., Tomé, F.M. & Derambure, S. (1976) Familial fingerprint body myopathy. *Archives of Neurology*, **33**, 724.

Fenichel, G.M. (1967) Abnormalities of skeletal muscle maturation in brain-damaged children. *Developmental Medicine and Child Neurology*, **9**, 419.

French, J.H., Sherard, E.S., Lubell, H., Brotz, M. & Moore, C.L. (1972) Trichopoliodystrophy. I. Report of a case and biochemical study. *Archives of Neurology*, **26**, 229.

Gamstorp, I. (1956) Adynamia episodica hereditaria. *Acta Paediatrica Scandinavica*, Supplement, 108, **45**, 1.

Ghatak, N.R., Erenberg, G., Hirano, A. & Golden, G.S. (1973) Idiopathic rhabdomyolysis in children. *Journal of the Neurological Sciences*, **20**, 253

Ghatak, N.R., Hirano, A., Poon, T.P. & French, J.H. (1972) Trichopoliodystrophy. II. Pathological changes in skeletal muscle and nervous system. *Archives of Neurology*, **26**, 60.

Goldberg, A.F. (1967) Protein synthesis in tonic and phasic skeletal muscles. *Nature*, **216**, 1219.

Goldfischer, S., Moore, C.L., Johnson, A.B., Spiro, A.J., Valsamis, M.P., Wisniewsky, H.K., Ritch, R.H., Norton, W.T., Rapin, I. & Gartner, L.M. (1973) Peroxisomal and mitochondrial defects in the cerebro-hepato-renal syndrome. *Science*, **182**, 62.

Gonatas, N.K., Evangelista, I. & Martin, J. (1967) A generalized disorder of nervous sytem, skeletal muscle and heart resembling Refsum's disease and Hurler's syndrome. Part 2 (Ultrastructure). *American Journal of Medicine*, **42**, 169.

Gonatas, N.K., Perez, M.C., Shy, G.M. & Evangelista, I. (1965) Central 'core' disease of skeletal muscle. Ultrastructural and cytochemical observations in two cases. *American Journal of Pathology*, **47**, 503.

Greenfield, J.G., Shy, G.M., Alvord, E.C. & Berg, L. (1957) *An Atlas of Muscle Pathology in Neuromuscular Diseases* (Livingstone: Edinburgh).

Gruner, J. & Porte, A. (1959) Les lesions musculaires de paralysie periodique familiale. *Revue Neurologique*, **101**, 501.

Gubbay, S.S., Walton, J.N. & Pearce, G.W. (1966) Clinical and pathological study of a case of congenital muscular dystrophy. *Journal of Neurology, Neurosurgery and Psychiatry*, **29**, 500.

Gutmann, E. (1962) *The Denervated Muscle* (Publishing House of Czechoslovak Academy of Science: Prague).

Haase, G.R. & Shy, G.M. (1960) Pathological changes in muscular biopsies from patients with peroneal muscular atrophy. *Brain*, **83**, 631.

Hackett, T.N. Jr., Bray, P.F., Ziter, F.A., Nyhan, W.L. & Creer, K.M. (1973) A metabolic myopathy associated with chronic lactic acidemia, growth failure and nerve deafness. *Journal of Pediatrics*, **83**, 426.

Halban, J. (1894) Die Dicke der quergestreiften Muskelfasern und ihre Bedeutung. *Anatomische Hefte*, **3**, 267.

Haltia, M., Rapola, J. & Santavuori, P. (1973) Infantile type of so-called neuronal ceroid-lipofuscinosis. Histological and electron microscopic studies. *Acta Neuropathologica (Berlin)*, **26**, 157.

Hart, Z.W., Chang, C.H., Perrin, E.V., Neerunjun, J.S. & Ayyar, R. (1977) Familial poliodystrophy, mitochondrial myopathy and lactic acidemia. *Archives of Neurology*, **34**, 180.

Hay, E.P. (1971) Skeletal muscle regeneration. *New England Journal of Medicine*, **284**, 1033.

Hed, R., Lundmark, C., Fahlgren, H. & Orell, S. (1962) Acute muscular syndrome in chronic alcoholism. *Acta Medica Scandinavica*, **171**, 585.

Heffner, R., Cohen, M., Duffner, P. & Daigler G. (1976) Multicore disease in twins. *Journal of Neurology, Neurosurgery and Psychiatry*, **39**, 602.

Heidenhain, M. (1918) Über progressive Veränderungen der Muskulatur bei Myotonia atrophica. *Beiträge zu Pathologische Anatomie und zu Allgemeine Pathologie*, **64**, 198.

Hers, F.L. (1963) Alpha-glucosidase deficiency in

generalized glycogen storage disease (Pompe's disease). *Biochemical Journal*, **86**, 11.

Hers, F.L. (1965) Inborn lysosomal diseases. *Progress in Gastroenterology*, **48**, 625.

Hoffmann, J. (1893) Ueber chronische spinale muskelatrophie im Kindesalter auf familiärer Basis. *Deutche Zeitschrift für Nervenheilkunde*, **3**, 427.

Hostetler, K.Y., Hoppel, C.L., Romine, J.S., Sipe, J.C., Gross, S.R. & Higginbottom, P.A. (1978) Partial deficiency of muscle carnitine palmityltransferase with normal ketone production. *New England Journal of Medicine*, **298**, 553.

Hübner, G. (1977) Ringbinden der quergestreiften Muskulatur. Ein Beitrag zur Aussagekraft derartiger Struktur an einem unausgewählten Sektionsmaterial. *Acta Neuropathologica (Berlin)*, **38**, 27.

Hudgson, P., Bradley, W.G. & Jenkison, M. (1972) Familial 'mitochondrial' myopathy. A myopathy associated with disordered oxidative metabolism in muscle fibres. Part I. Clinical, electrophysiological and pathological findings. *Journal of the Neurological Sciences*, **16**, 343.

Hülsmann, W.C., Bethlem, J., Meijer, A.E.F.H., Fleury, P. & Schellens, J.P.M. (1967) Myopathy with abnormal structure and function of muscle mitochondria. *Journal of Neurology, Neurosurgery and Psychiatry*, **30**, 519.

Isaacs, H., Heffron, J.J. & Badenhorst, M. (1975) Central core disease. A correlated genetic, histochemical, ultramicroscopic and biochemical study. *Journal of Neurology, Neurosurgery and Psychiatry*, **38**, 1177.

Jenis, E.H., Lindquist, R.R. & Lister, R.C. (1969) New congenital myopathy with crystalline intranuclear inclusions. *Archives of Neurology*, **20**, 281.

Jerusalem, I. (1976) Hypotheses and recent findings concerning aetiology and pathogenesis of the muscular dystrophies. *Journal of Neurology*, **213**, 155.

Jerusalem, F., Engel, A.G. & Gomez, M.R. (1973) Sarcotubular myopathy. A newly recognized, benign, congenital, familial muscle disease. *Neurology (Minneapolis)*, **23**, 897.

Johnson, M.A., Polgar, J., Weightman, D. & Appleton, D. (1973) Data on distribution of fibre types in thirty-six human muscles. An autopsy study. *Journal of the Neurological Sciences*, **18**, 111.

Johnson, M.A. Sideri, G., Weightman, D. & Appleton, D. (1973) A comparison of fibre size, fibre type constitution and spatial fibre type distribution in normal human muscle and in muscle from cases of spinal muscular atrophy and from other neuromuscular disorders. *Journal of the Neurological Sciences*, **20**, 345.

Kagen, L.J. (1977) Myoglobinemia in inflammatory myopathies. *Journal of American Medical Association*, **237**, 1448.

Kahn, L.B. & Meyer, J. S. (1970) Acute myopathy in chronic alcoholism. A study of 22 autopsy cases with ultrastructural observations. *American Journal of Clinical Pathology*, **53**, 516.

Kakulas, B.A. (1966) *In vitro* destruction of skeletal muscle by sensitized cells. *Nature*, **210**, 1115.

Kearns, T.P. (1965) External ophthalmoplegia, pigmentary degeneration of the retina and cardiomyopathy: a newly recognized syndrome. *Transactions of the American Ophthalmologic Society*, **63**, 559.

Kearns, T.P. & Sayre, G.P. (1958) Retinitis pigmentosa, external ophthalmoplegia and complete heart block; unusual syndrome with histologic study in one of two cases. *Archives of Ophthalmology*, **60**, 280.

Kendrick, W.C., Hull, A.R. & Knochel, J.P. (1977) Rhabdomyolysis and shock after intravenous amphetamine administration. *Annals of Internal Medicine*, **86**, 381.

Kiloh, I.G. & Nevin, S. (1951) Progressive dystrophy of the external ocular muscles. *Brain*, **74**, 9.

Kinoshita, M., Satoyoshi, E. & Matsuo, N. (1975) 'Myotubular myopathy' and type I fibre atrophy in a family. *Journal of the Neurological Sciences*, **26**, 575.

Kinoshita, M., Satoyoshi, E. & Suzuki, Y. (1975) Atypical myopathy with myofibrillar aggregates. *Archives of Neurology*, **32**, 417.

Krabbe, K. (1949) Les lèsions embryonnaires à la lumière des défectuosités mammaires et pectorales de la syndactylie et de la microdactylie. *Acta psychiatrica et neurologica*, **24**, 539.

Kugelberg, E., Edström, L. & Abbruzzese, M. (1970) Mapping of motor units in experimentally reinnervated rat muscle. *Journal of Neurology, Neurosurgery and Psychiatry*, **33**, 319.

Kuitunen, P., Rapola, J., Noponen, A.L. & Donner, M. (1972) Nemaline myopathy. Report of 4 cases and review of the literature. *Acta Paediatrica Scandinavica*, **61**, 353.

Lake, B.D. & Wilson, J. (1975) Zebra body myopathy. Clinical, histochemical and ultrastructural studies. *Journal of the Neurological Sciences*, **24**, 437.

Lake, B.D., Cavanagh, N. & Wilson, J. (1977) Myopathy with minicores in siblings. *Neuropathology and Applied Neurobiology*, **3**, 159.

Lapresle, J., Fardeau, M. & Milhaud, M. (1965) Étude des ultrastructures dans les dystrophies musculaires progressives. *Proceedings of the Fifth International Congress of Neuropathology. International Congress Series No. 100*, p. 602 (Excerpta Medica: Amsterdam).

Larsson, L.E., Linderholm, H., Müller, R., Ringqvist, T. & Sörnäs, R. (1964) Hereditary metabolic myopathy with paroxysmal myoglobinuria due to abnormal glycolysis. *Journal of Neurology, Neurosurgery and Psychiatry*, **27**, 361.

Layzer, R.B. & Rowland, L.P. (1971) Cramps. *New England Journal of Medicine*, **285**, 31.

Layzer, R.B., Rowland, L.P. & Ranney, H.M. (1967) Muscle phosphofructokinase deficiency. *Archives of Neurology*, **17**, 512.

Luft, R., Ikkos, D., Palmieri, G., Ernster, L. & Afzelius, B. (1962) A case of severe hypermetabolism of nonthyroid origin with a defect in the maintenance of mitochondrial respiratory control. A correlated clinical, biochemical and morphological study. *Journal of Clinical Investigation*, **41**, 1776.

Macdonald, R.D. & Engel, A.G. (1969) The cystoplasmic body: another structural anomaly of the Z disc. *Acta Neuropathologica (Berlin)*, **14**, 99.

Mair, W.G.P. & Tomé, F.M.S. (1972) *Atlas of the Ultrastructure of Diseased Human Muscle* (Williams and Wilkins: Baltimore).

Marin, O & Denny-Brown, D. (1962) Changes in skeletal muscle associated with cachexia. *American Journal of Pathology*, **41**, 23.

Martinez, A.J., Hooshmand, H. & Faris, A.A. (1973) Acute alcoholic myopathy: Enzyme histochemistry and electron microscopic findings. *Journal of the Neurological Sciences*, **20**, 245.

Mastaglia, F.L. & Walton, J.N. (1970) Coxsackie virus-like particles in skeletal muscle from a case of polymyositis.

Journal of the Neurological Sciences, **11**, 593.

Mauro, A. (1961) Satellite cell of skeletal muscle fibres. *Journal of Biophysical and Biochemical Cytology*, **9**, 493.

McLean, W.T. & McKone, R.C. (1973) Congenital myasthenia gravis in twins. *Archives of Neurology*, **29**, 223.

Meltzer, H.Y., Kuncl, R.W., Click, J. & Yang, V. (1976) Incidence of Z band streaming and myofibrillar disruptions in skeletal muscle from healthy young people. *Neurology (Minneapolis)*, **26**, 853.

Meyer-Betz, F. (1911) Beobachtungen an einem eigenartigen mit Muskellähmungen verbundenen Fall von Hämoglobinurie. *Deutsche Archiv für Klinische Medizin*, **85**, 127.

Meyers, K.R., Gilden, D.H., Rinaldi, F.J. & Hansen, J.L. (1972) Periodic muscle weakness, normokalemia, and tubular aggregates. *Neurology (Minneapolis)*, **22**, 269.

Mittelbach, F. (1966) 'Die Begleitmyopathie bei neurogenen Atrophien'. *Monographien aus dem Gesamtgebiet der Neurologie und Psychiatrie*. Heft 113. (Springer: Heidelberg).

Mokri, B. & Engel, A.G. (1975) Duchenne dystrophy: electron microscopic findings pointing to a basic or early abnormality in the plasma membrane of the muscle fibre. *Neurology (Minneapolis)*, **25**, 1110.

Moore, M.J., Rebeiz, J.J., Holden, M. & Adams, R.D. (1971) Biometric analyses of normal skeletal muscle. *Acta Neuropathologica (Berlin)*, **19**, 51.

Morgan-Hughes, J.A., Darveniza, P., Kahn, S.N., Landon, D.N., Sherratt, R.M., Land, J.M. & Clark, J.B. (1977) A mitochondrial myopathy characterized by a deficiency in reducible cytochrome b. *Brain*, **100**, 617.

Morpurgo, B. (1897) Ueber Activitäts-Hypertrophie der willkürlichen Muskeln. *Virchows Archiv für Pathologische Anatomie*, **150**, 522.

Müller, R. & Kugelberg, E. (1959) Myopathy in Cushing's syndrome. *Journal of Neurology, Neurosurgery and Psychiatry*, **22**, 314.

Namba, T., Brown, S.B. & Grob, D. (1970) Neonatal myasthenia gravis: report of two cases and review of the literature. *Pediatrics*, **45**, 488.

Neville, H.E. (1973) Ultrastructural changes in muscle disease. In *Muscle Biopsy: A Modern Approach*, Eds V. Dubowitz and M.H. Brooke, p. 383 (Saunders: Philadelphia).

Neville, H.E. & Brooke, M.H. (1973) Central core fibres: structured and unstructured. In *Basic Research in Myology. Proceedings of the Second International Congress on Muscle Diseases*, Ed. B.A. Kakulas, Vol. I, p. 497 (Excerpta Medica: Amsterdam).

Olson, W., Engel, W.K., Walsh, G.O. & Einaugler, R. (1972) Oculocraniosomatic neuro-muscular disease with 'ragged-red' fibres. *Archives of Neurology*, **26**, 193.

Oppenheim, H. (1900) Ueber allgemeine und localisierte Atonie der Muskulatur (Myatonia) in frühen Kindesalter. *Monatschrift für Psychiatrie and Neurology*, **8**, 232.

Oteruelo, F.T. (1976) Intranuclear inclusions in a myopathy of late onset. *Virchows Archiv; Abteilung B: Zell-Pathologie*, **20**, 319.

Papanicolau, G.N. & Falk, E.A. (1938) General muscular hypertrophy induced by androgenic hormone. *Science*, **87**, 238.

Payne, C.M. & Curless, R.G. (1976) Concentric laminated bodies. Ultrastructural demonstration of muscle fibre type specificity. *Journal of the Neurological Sciences*, **29**, 311.

Pearce, G.W. & Walton, J.N. (1962) Progressive muscular dystrophy: the histopathological changes in skeletal muscle obtained by biopsy. *Journal of Pathology and Bacteriology*, **83**, 535.

Pearn, J.H. & Wilson, J. (1973) Acute Werdnig-Hoffman disease. Acute infantile spinal muscular atrophy. *Archives of Diseases in Childhood*, **48**, 425.

Pearson, C.M. (1959) The incidence and type of pathological alterations observed in muscle in a routine autopsy survey. *Neurology (Minneapolis)*, **9**, 757.

Pearson, C.M., Beck, W.S. & Blahd, W.H. (1957) Idiopathic paroxysmal myoglobinuria. *Archives of Internal Medicine*, **99**, 376.

Pearson, C.M., Rimer, D.G. & Mommaerts, W.F.H.M. (1961) A metabolic myopathy due to absence of muscle phosphorylase. *American Journal of Medicine*, **30**, 502.

PeBenito, R., Sher, J.H. & Cracco, J.B. (1978) Centronuclear myopathy: clinical and pathologic features. *Clinical Pediatrics*, **17**, 259.

Pellegrini, C. & Franzini, C. (1963) An electron microscopic study of denervation atrophy in red and white skeletal muscle fibres. *Journal of Cell Biology*, **17**, 327.

Pellegrini, C. & Franzini-Armstrong, C. (1969) Recent contributions of electron microscopy to the study of normal and pathological muscle. *International Review of Experimental Pathology*, **7**, 139.

Perkoff, G.T., Hardy, P. & Velez-Garcia, E. (1966) Alcoholic myopathy. *New England Journal of Medicine*, **274**, 1277.

Perkoff, G.T., Hill, R.L., Brown, D.M. & Tyler, F.M. (1962) The characterization of adult human myoglobin. *Journal of Biological Chemistry*, **237**, 2820.

Perkoff, G.T., Silber, R., Tyler, F.H., Cartwright, G.E. & Wintrobe, M.M. (1959) Myopathy due to the administration of therapeutic amounts of 17-hydroxycorticosteroids. *American Journal of Medicine*, **26**, 891.

Peter, J.B., Stempel, K. & Armstrong, J. (1970) Biochemistry and electron microscopy of mitochondria in muscular and neuromuscular diseases. In *Muscle Diseases. Proceedings of an International Conference on Muscle Diseases. International Congress Series* No. 199, Eds N. Canal, G. Scarlato & J.N. Walton, p. 228 (Excerpta Medica: Amsterdam).

Pickard, N.A., Gruemer, H-D., Verrill, H.L., Isaacs, E.R., Robinow, M., Nance, W.E., Myers, E.C. & Goldsmith, B. (1978) Systemic membrane defect in the proximal muscular dystrophies. *New England Journal of Medicine*, **299**, 841.

Poskanzer, D. & Kerr, D.N.S. (1961) A third type of periodic paralysis with normokalemia and favourable response to sodium chloride. *American Journal of Medicine*, **31**, 328.

Price, H.M. (1973) Ultrastructural pathologic characteristics of skeletal muscle fibre: an introductory survey. In *The Striated Muscle*, Eds C.M. Pearson & F.K. Mostofi, p. 144 (Williams and Wilkins: Baltimore).

Price, H.M., Howes, E.L. & Blumberg, J.M. (1964) Ultrastructural muscle fibres injured by cold I. The acute degenerative changes. *Laboratory Investigation*, **13**, 1264.

Price, H.M., Gordon, G.B., Pearson, C.M., Munsat, T.L. & Blumberg, J.M. (1965) New evidence for excessive accumulation of Z-band material in nemaline myopathy. *Proceedings of the National Academy of Science*, **54**, 1398.

Radu, H., Rosu-Serbu, A.M., Ionescu, V. & Radu, A. (1977) Focal abnormalities in mitochondrial distribution in muscle. *Acta Neuropathologica (Berlin)*, **39**, 25.

Rawles, J.M. & Weller, R.O. (1974) Familial association of metabolic myopathy, lactic acidosis and sideroblastic anemia. *American Journal of Medicine*, **56**, 891.

Rebeiz, J.J., Caulfield, J.B. & Adams, R.D. (1969) Oculopharyngeal dystrophy—a presenescent myopathy. In *Progress in Neuro-Ophthalmology, International Congress Series* No. 176, p. 12 (Excerpta Medica: Amsterdam).

Reske-Nielsen, E., Lou, H.C. & Lowes, M. (1976) Progressive external ophthalmoplegia. Evidence for a generalised mitochondrial disease with a defect in pyruvate metabolism. *Acta Ophthalmologica*, **54**, 553.

Reza, M.J., Kar, N.C., Pearson, C.M. & Kark, R.A.P. (1978) Recurrent myoglobinuria due to muscle carnitine palmityl transferase deficiency. *Annals of Internal Medicine*, **88**, 610.

Reznik, M. (1969) Origin of myoblasts during skeletal muscle regeneration. Electron microscopic observations. *Laboratory Investigation*, **20**, 353.

Reznik, M. (1973) Current concepts of skeletal muscle regeneration. In *The Striated Muscle*, Eds C.M. Pearson & F.K. Mostofi, p. 185 (Williams and Wilkins: Baltimore).

Ringel, S.P., Neville, H.E., Duster, M.C. & Carroll, J.E. (1978) A new congenital neuromuscular disease with trilaminar muscle fibres. *Neurology (Minneapolis)*, **28**, 282.

Robotham, J.L. & Haddow, E. (1976) Rhabdomyolysis and myoglobinuria in childhood. *Pediatric Clinics of North America*, **23**, 279.

Rowland, L.P. (1976) Pathogenesis of muscular dystrophies. *Archives of Neurology*, **33**, 315.

Rowland, L.P. & Penn, A.S. (1972) Myoglobinuria. *Medical Clinics of North America*, **56**, 1233.

Sahgal, V. & Sahgal, S. (1977) A new congenital myopathy. A morphological, cytochemical and histochemical study. *Acta Neuropathologica (Berlin)*, **37**, 225.

Santa, T., Engel, A.G. & Lambert, E.H. (1972) Histometric study of neuromuscular junction ultrastructure. I. Myasthenia gravis. *Neurology (Minneapolis)*, **22**, 71.

Saper, J.R. & Itabashi, H.H. (1976) Central core disease—a congenital myopathy. *Diseases of the Nervous System*, **37**, 649.

Satoyoshi, E. & Kowa, H. (1967) A myopathy due to glycolytic abnormality. *Archives of Neurology*, **17**, 248.

Schäffer, J. (1893) Beiträge der Histologie und Histogenese der quergestreiften Muskelfasern des Menschen und einiger Wierbelthiere. *Sitzungsgeschichte der Kaiserlichen Akademie der Wissenschaft in Wien; matematische-naturwissenschaftiche Classe*, **102**, 1.

Schiffer, D., Giordana, M.T., Monga, G. & Mollo, F. (1976) Histochemistry and electron microscopy of muscle fibres in a case of congenital paramyotonia. *Journal of Neurology*, **211**, 125.

Schmalbruch, H. & Hellhammer, U. (1976) The number of satellite cells in normal human muscle. *Anatomical Record*, **185**, 279.

Schotland, D. (1967) Congenital target fibre disease. *Transactions of the American Neurological Association*, **92**, 107.

Schotland, D.L., Bonilla, E. & van Meter (1977) Duchenne dystrophy: alteration in muscle plasma membrane structure. *Science*, **196**, 4293.

Schotland, D.L., Di Mauro, S., Bonilla, E., Scarpa, A. & Lee, C.P. (1976) Neuromuscular disorder associated with a defect in mitochondrial energy supply. *Archives of Neurology*, **33**, 475.

Schröder, M. & Adams, R.D. (1968) Ultrastructural morphology of the muscle fibre in myotonic dystrophy.

Acta Neuropathologica (Berlin), **10**, 218.

Schutta, H.S., Kelly, A.M. & Zacks, S.I. (1969) Necrosis and regeneration of muscle in paroxysmal idiopathic myoglobinuria: electron microscopic observations. *Brain*, **92**, 191.

Schwartz, G.A. & Liu, C.N. (1954) Chronic progressive external ophthalmoplegia: clinical and neuropathologic report. *Archives of Neurology and Psychiatry*, **71**, 31.

Schwartz, M.S., Sargent, M. & Swash, M. (1976) Longitudinal fibre splitting in neurogenic muscular disorders: its relation to the pathogenesis of 'myopathic' change. *Brain*, **99**, 617.

Seitelberger, F., Wanko, T. & Gavin, M.A. (1961) The muscle fibre in central core disease. Histochemical and electron microscopic observations. *Acta Neuropathologica (Berlin)*, **1**, 223.

Sengers, R.C.A., ter Haar, B.G.A., Trijbels, J.M.F., Willems, J.L., Daniels, O. & Stadhouders, A.M. (1975) Congenital cataract and mitochondrial myopathy of skeletal and heart muscle associated with lactic acidosis after exercise. *Journal of Pediatrics*, **86**, 873.

Shafiq, S.A., Milhorat, A.T. & Gorycki, M.S. (1967) Fine structure of human muscle in neurogenic atrophy. *Neurology (Minneapolis)*, **17**, 934.

Shapira, Y., Cederbaum, S.D., Cancilla, P.A., Nielsen, D. & Lippe, B.M. (1975) Familial poliodystrophy, mitochondrial myopathy and lactic acidemia. *Neurology (Minneapolis)*, **25**, 614.

Sher, J.H., Shafiq, S.A. & Schutta, H.S. (1979) Acute myopathy with selective lysis of myosin filaments. *Neurology (Minneapolis)*, **29**, 100.

Sher, J.H., Rimalovski, A.B., Athanassiades, T.J. & Aronson, S.M. (1967) Familial myotubular myopathy. *Journal of Neuropathology and Experimental Neurology*, **24**, 132.

Shy, G.M. & Magee, K.R. (1956) A new non-progressive myopathy. *Brain*, **79**, 610.

Shy, G.M., Gonatas, N.K. & Perez, M. (1966) Two childhood myopathies with abnormal mitochondria. I. Megaconial myopathy. II. Pleoconial myopathy. *Brain*, **89**, 133.

Shy, G.M., Engel, W.K., Somers, J.E. & Wanko, T. (1963) Nemaline myopathy: A new congenital myopathy. *Brain*, **86**, 793.

Shy, G.M., Wanko, T., Rowley, P.T. & Engel, A.G. (1961) Studies in familial periodic paralysis. *Experimental Neurology*, **3**, 53.

Sissons, H. (1965) Further observations on muscle fibre size. In *Current Research in Muscular Dystrophy. The Proceedings of the Third Symposium*, p. 107 (Pitman Medical: London).

Sloan, M.F., Franks, A.J., Exley, K.A. & Davison, A.M. (1978) Acute renal failure due to polymyositis. *British Medical Journal*, **1**, 6125.

Sloper, J.C. & Pegrum, G.D. (1967) Regeneration of crushed mammalian skeletal muscle and effects of steroids. *Journal of Pathology and Bacteriology*, **93**, 47.

Speidel, C.C. (1938) Studies on living muscles. I. Growth, injury and repair of striated muscle, as revealed by prolonged observations of individual fibres in living frog tadpoles. *American Journal of Anatomy*, **62**, 179.

Speidel, C.C. (1939) Studies of living muscle. II. Histological changes in single fibres of striated muscle during contraction and clotting. *American Journal of Anatomy*, **65**, 471.

Spiro, A.J., Prineas, J.W. & Moore, C.L. (1970) A new mitochondrial myopathy in a patient with salt craving. *Archives of Neurology*, **22**, 259.

Spiro, A.J., Shy, G.M. & Gonatas, N.K. (1966) Myotubular myopathy—Persistance of fetal muscle in an adolescent boy. *Archives of Neurology*, **14**, 1.

Spiro, A.J., Moore, C.L., Prineas, J.W., Strasberg, P.M. & Rapin, I. (1970) A cytochrome-related inherited disorder of the nervous system and muscle. *Archives of Neurology*, **23**, 103.

Sreter, F.A., Åström, K.E., Romanul, F.C.A., Young, R.R. & Jones, H.R., Jr. (1976) Characteristics of myosin in nemaline myopathy. *Journal of the Neurological Sciences*, **27**, 99.

Stenger, R.J., Spiro, D., Scully, R.E. & Shannon, J.M. (1962) Ultrastructural and physiologic alterations in ischemic skeletal muscle. *American Journal of Pathology*, **40**, 1.

Sulaiman, W.R., Doyle, D., Johnson, R.H. & Jennett, S. (1974) Myopathy with mitochondrial inclusion bodies: histological and metabolic studies. *Journal of Neurology, Neurosurgery and Psychiatry*, **37**, 1236.

Suzuki, K. & Rapin, I. (1969) Giant mitochondria in an infant with microcephaly and seizure disorder. *Archives of Neurology*, **20**, 62.

Swash, M. & Schwartz, M.S. (1977) Implications of longitudinal muscle fibre splitting in neurogenic and myopathic disorders. *Journal of Neurology, Neurosurgery and Psychiatry*, **40**, 1152.

Swash, M., Schwartz, M.S. & Sargeant, M.K. (1978) Pathogenesis of longitudinal splitting of muscle fibres in neurogenic disorders and polymyositis. *Neuropathology and Applied Neurobiology*, **4**, 99.

Szliwowski, H.B. & Drochman, P. (1975) Ultrastructural aspects of muscle and nerve in Werdnig-Hoffman disease. *Acta Neuropathologica (Berlin)*, **31**, 281.

Tang, T.T., Sedmak, G.V., Siegesmund, K.A. & McCreadie, S.R. (1975) Chronic myopathy associated with Coxsackie virus type A9. A combined electron microscopical and viral isolation study. *New England Journal of Medicine*, **292**, 608.

Tarlow, M.J., Lake, B.D. & Lloyd, J.K. (1973) Chronic lactic acidosis in association with myopathy. *Archives of Diseases of Children*, **48**, 489.

Tarui, S., Ikuno, G., Ikura, Y., Tanaka, T., Suda, M. & Nishikawa, M. (1965) Phosphofructokinase deficiency in skeletal muscle: A new type of glucogenosis. *Biochemical and Biophysical Research Communications*, **19**, 517.

Taylor, E.W. (1915) Progressive vagus—glossopharyngeal paralysis with ptosis: contribution to a group of family diseases. *Journal of Nervous and Mental Diseases*, **42**, 129.

Tomé, F.M. & Fardeau, M. (1975) Congenital myopathy with 'reducing bodies' in muscle fibres. *Acta Neuropathologica (Berlin)*, **31**, 207.

Tomé, F.M., Fardeau, M. & Lenoir, G. (1977) Ultrastructure of muscle and sensory nerve in Fabry's disease. *Acta Neuropathologica (Berlin)*, **38**, 187.

Tomlinson, B.E., Walton, J.N. & Rebeiz, J.J. (1969) The effects of aging and of cachexia upon skeletal muscle. A histopathological study. *Journal of the Neurological Sciences*, **9**, 321.

Tsairis, P., Engel, W.K. & Kark, P. (1973) Familial myoclonic epilepsy syndrome associated with skeletal muscle mitochondrial abnormalities. *Neurology (Minneapolis)*, **23**, 408.

Tyler, F.H. (1950) Studies in disorders of muscle. III. Pseudohypertrophy of muscle in progressive muscular dystrophy and other neuromuscular disease. *Archives of Neurology and Psychiatry*, **63**, 425.

Tyler, F.H., Stephens, F.E., Gunn, F.D. & Perkoff, G.T. (1951) Studies in disorders of muscles. VII. Clinical manifestations and inheritance of a type of periodic paralysis without hypopotassemia. *Journal of Clinical Investigation*, **30**, 492.

Victor, M., Hayes, R. & Adams, R.D. (1962) Oculopharyngeal muscular dystrophy. A familial disease of late life characterized by dysphagia and progressive ptosis of the eyelids. *New England Journal of Medicine*, **267**, 1267.

Walker, B.E. (1963) The origin of myoblasts and the problem of dedifferentiation. *Experimental Cell Research*, **30**, 80.

Wallace, S.L., Lattes, R., Malia, J.P. & Ragen, C. (1958) Diagnostic significance of the muscle biopsy. *American Journal of Medicine*, **25**, 600.

Walton, J.N. (1957) The limp child. *Journal of Neurology, Neurosurgery and Psychiatry*, **20**, 144.

Walton, J.N. & Adams, R.D. (1958) *Polymyositis* (Livingstone: Edinburgh).

Walton, J.N. & Gardner-Medwin, D. (1968) Second thoughts on classification of the muscular dystrophies. In *Current Research in Muscular Dystrophy. Proceedings of the Fourth Symposium* (Pitman Medical: London).

Wechsler, W. & Hager, H. (1961) Electronmikroskopische Befunde bei Muskelatrophie nach Nervendruchtrennung bei der weissen Ratte. *Beiträge der Pathologischen Anatomie*, **125**, 31.

Whiteley, A.M., Schwartz, M.S., Sachs, J.A. & Swash, M. (1976) Congenital myasthenia gravis: clinical and HLA studies in two brothers. *Journal of Neurology, Neurosurgery and Psychiatry*, **39**, 1145.

van Wijngaarden, G.K., Bethlem, J., Meijer, A.E.F.H., Hülsmann, W.C. & Feltkamp, C.A. (1967) Skeletal muscle disease with abnormal mitochondria. *Brain*, **90**, 577.

Wohlfart, G. (1942) Quantitativ-histologische Studien an der Skelettmuskulatur während der Entwicklung und bei der Atrophie nach Nervendurchschneidung. *Zeitschrift für Mikroskopisch-Anatomische Forschung*, **5**, 480.

Wohlfart, G. (1951) Dystrophia myotonica and myotonia congenita: Histopathological studies with special reference to changes in muscles. *Journal of Neuropathology and Experimental Neurology*, **10**, 109.

Wohlfart, G. (1955) Aktuelle Probleme der Muskelpathologie. *Deutsche Zeitschrift für Nervenheilkunde*, **173**, 426.

Worsfold, M., Park, D.C. & Pennington, R.J. (1973) Familial 'mitochondrial' myopathy. A myopathy associated with disordered oxidative metabolism in muscle fibres. Part 2. Biochemical findings. *Journal of the Neurological Sciences*, **19**, 261.

Yarom, R. & Shapira, Y. (1977) Myosin degeneration in a congenital myopathy. *Archives of Neurology*, **34**, 114.

Zelena, J. (1962) The effect of denervation on muscle development. In *The Denervated Muscle*, Ed. E. Gutman, p. 103 (Publishing House of Czechoslovak Academy of Sciences: Prague).

Zellweger, H. & Ionasescu, V. (1973) Early onset of myotonic dystrophy in infants. *American Journal of Diseases of Children*, **125**, 601.

Zellweger, H., Afifi, A., McCormick, W.F. & Mergner, W. (1967) Severe congenital muscular dystrophy. *American Journal of Diseases of Children*, **114**, 591.

The pathology of peripheral nerve disease

INTRODUCTION

The last 25 years have witnessed a much greater understanding of disease of the peripheral nerves. This has resulted from combined advances in the twin fields of physiology and pathology. In pathology, quantitative histological techniques, the study of single nerve fibres, and electron microscopy have been prominent developments. The basic processes underlying peripheral nerve degeneration are now well understood, although uncertainty still exists concerning a number of processes such as the 'dying back' neuropathies and 'secondary demyelination'. The pathological processes are not, however, in most cases specific to an individual disease, and the causes of most disorders remain to be elucidated.

In this chapter we propose to discuss the salient features of the pathological changes seen in peripheral nerve disorders. The clinical and electrophysiological aspects of these conditions are discussed in Chapter 21. Emphasis will be placed on the changes in the nerve trunks, because they can be biopsied. For a more detailed discussion of the pathology of the anterior horn cells and dorsal root ganglion cells in peripheral neuropathy, the reader is referred to Prineas and Spencer (1975) and to Chapter 20 of this volume.

For descriptive convenience, peripheral neuropathies can be classified in terms of the structure in the nerve that is primarily affected by the disease process, although it must be realised that a single process may simultaneously affect more than one component of the nerve. For the present purposes, therefore, the histopathological changes observed in neuropathies will be considered in terms of those alterations that result from conditions primarily affecting the axons, either directly or by an effect on the cell body, and those that result from damage to the supporting structures. The latter can be subdivided into those that affect primarily the Schwann cells, the connective tissues, or the vascular supply. Finally, there are those conditions in which the nerve fibres are affected by dysfunction in tissues external to the nerve.

ANATOMICAL CONSIDERATIONS

Nerve trunks consist of assemblies of myelinated and unmyelinated axons and their supporting structures. The extreme length of the nerve fibres is responsible for many of the diseases to which the nervous system is heir. An axon 8 μm in diameter and 1 m long may arise from a nerve cell body of 100 μm diameter. Ninety-eight per cent of the cell cytoplasm therefore lies in the one long process which is the axon. The maintenance of metabolic control of the terminal parts of the axon by the nucleus is a problem in such a system. The mechanism of this control has been elucidated in part at least in recent years. Particle movement within cells including neurones has been known for many years. Weiss and Hiscoe (1948) suggested the existence of bulk centrifugal flow of axoplasm and the existence of axonal transport systems is now well established. Two major rates of flow of protein and other material have been described, a fast flow of about 360 mm/day at 37°C, and a slow flow of 2–3 mm/day (Lasek, 1968). It is now recognised that the process is more complex. Different substances move at different rates along the axon. Many different rates of transport exist, though the transport of most substances falls into either the slow or the fast category. When any part of a cell is disconnected from the nucleus, that part eventually dies. The nerve cell is no exception to this rule. This accounts for the rapid centrifugal advance of degeneration following nerve section (Lubińska and Waryszewska, 1973) and the inverse relationship between the distal length of nerve remaining and the rate of failure of the nerve terminals (Miledi and Slater, 1970; Harris and Thesleff, 1972). The structures most closely associated with the axons are the Schwann cells, which are a type of satellite cell. These supporting cells differ in structure depending upon whether they surround myelinated or unmyelinated fibres. The former, the Schwann cells, produce the myelin sheath as will be seen below. Schwann cells investing unmyelinated axons are sometimes called Remak cells. Work in several different areas indicates the intimate interrelationship between the neurone and the satellite cell. This includes studies by Hydén on the neurones and glial cells of vestibular nuclei (Hydén, 1959), and the changes in the satellite cells of anterior horn cells following peripheral axon section (Pannese, 1964; Leech, 1967; Dixon, 1969). It has been suggested that the satellite cells are responsible for providing nutrients for the neurone, and collecting metabolic degradation products. Similarly, Singer and Salpeter (1966a, b) have suggested that the Schwann cells are responsible for passing amino acids into the axons. The role of such amino acids is not clear because there is dispute as to whether significant amounts of ribonucleic acids are present and whether protein synthesis occurs in the peripheral nerve axoplasm (see discussion by Bradley and Jaros, 1973). Nevertheless, it is likely that the Schwann cells are responsible for modulating the metabolic environment of the axons.

The origin of the myelin sheath remained in dispute until the advent of electron microscopy, when it was demonstrated that it is derived by the spiralling of the Schwann cell surface membrane around the axon. The nodes of Ranvier represent junctions between adjacent Schwann cells; electron microscopy has revealed that they possess a high degree of structural complexity (Landon and Williams, 1963), presumably related to their function in the propagation of the nerve impulse. The nodes are more widely spaced on fibres of larger diameter than on smaller fibres (Fig. 6.1). This relationship tends to become less exact in human nerves with advancing age (Lascelles and Thomas, 1966).

Whereas in each internodal segment of myelinated nerve fibres the axon is surrounded by a single Schwann cell, several unmyelinated axons are related to each Schwann or Remak cell. The structural arrangements differ slightly in human nerves, compared with those of most laboratory animals: in man, individual unmyelinated axons are usually surrounded by a separate Schwann cell process, each Schwann cell giving rise to multiple processes (Gamble and Eames, 1964).

The connective tissue of nerves is customarily subdivided into three components, the endoneurium, perineurium and epineurium, although the perineurium is perhaps not strictly classifiable as connective tissue (Ross and Reith, 1969). The endoneurium comprises the intrafascicular connective tissue, including the collagenous sheaths of myelinated nerve fibres. The perineurium is a lamellated structure bounding the individual fascicles and is composed of flattened mesothelial cells with intervening layers of collagen and elastic fibres. The perineurium is known to act as a diffusion barrier and is possibly contractile (Ross and Reith, 1969), but its precise role in the functional organisation of nerve is not yet clear. It may act in regulating the composition

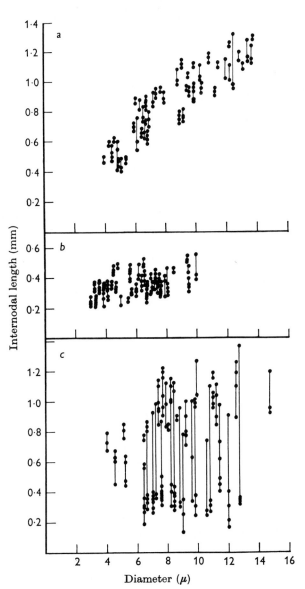

Fig. 6.1 Graphs showing relationship between internodal length and fibre diameter from normal guinea pig sciatic nerve (above), after Wallerian degeneration and regeneration (middle), and following segmental demyelination and remyelination (below). The internodal lengths of individual fibres have been plotted against the diameter of the widest internode, and the points joined by vertical lines (from Fullerton *et al.*, 1965)

of the endoneurial tissue fluid (Thomas and Olsson, 1975). The epineurium consists of collagen and elastic fibres which surround and bind together the fascicles; it contains varying quantities of fatty tissue. At the junction of the peripheral nerve trunks with the nerve roots, the epineurium becomes continuous with the outer part of the dura mater, and the perineurium divides to become continuous with the dural mesothelium and the inner part of the root sheaths (Haller and Low, 1971). The quantity of endoneurial collagen in the roots is less than in the peripheral nerves and the nerve fibres are not invested with definite collagenous sheaths (Gamble, 1964). The main vasa nervorum run in the epineurium forming a longitudinal anastomotic network, and are connected to the nutrient vessels. Arterioles and venules penetrate the perineurium and connect with a longitudinal anastomotic capillary network within the fascicles (Adams, 1943). There is evidence for the existence of a blood-nerve barrier (*see* Olsson, 1975). This shows species differences and tends to be less efficient in the roots than in the nerve trunks, a difference that has been adduced as a reason for the selective vulnerability of the roots in some pathological conditions.

DISORDERS PRIMARILY AFFECTING AXONS

Wallerian degeneration

Waller in 1850 studied the glossopharyngeal and hypoglossal nerves of the frog after section and clearly outlined the processes involved in the nerve fibre degeneration that follows axonal interruption. Subsequent studies have amplified the details of this process. When a nerve is crushed, the basal laminae (basement membranes) of the Schwann cells remain intact, allowing regeneration within the same basal laminal tubes (Haftek and Thomas, 1968). Following nerve section with loss of continuity of the Schwann cell basal laminal tubes, regeneration is more haphazard.

Within 2 min of crushing the nerve there is retraction of myelin from the nodes of Ranvier, and dilatation of Schmidt-Lantermann clefts for up to 5 mm distal to the crush in all fibres (Williams and Hall, 1971a). Histochemistry demonstrates an immediate loss of enzymes in the injured Schwann cell cytoplasm (Morgan-Hughes and Engel, 1968). Within 10 min, nodal retraction and Schmidt-Lantermann cleft dilatation has spread for a distance of up to 20 mm distal to the crush in the small fibres, and by 1 h the large fibres are involved over a similar distance (Williams and Hall, 1971a). By 1 h, the proximal and distal axon stumps adjacent to the crush show spirals and balls, a process that gradually spreads in both directions for up to 2 mm within the next 24 h (Morgan-Hughes and Engel, 1968). The immediate increase in DPNH-tetrazolium reductase and lactic dehydrogenase adjacent to the crush is due to activation of the Schwann cell cytoplasm (Morgan-Hughes and Engel, 1968), and the increase in DNA and RNA (Oderfeld-Nowak and Niemierko, 1969) is perhaps caused by the infiltration by macrophages into the area of the crush. There is a rapid increase in inorganic phosphate incorporation into acid-soluble organic phosphates throughout the distal part of the nerve within an hour (Gueuning and Graff, 1971).

By 2 h, there has been an increase in the acid phosphatase and lysosomal activity at the nodes of Ranvier immediately adjacent and distal to the crush (Holtzman and Novikoff, 1965). At 3 h, small abortive axon sprouts may be found arising from the proximal axon stump (Young, 1942), although effective regeneration does not develop until about the fifth day.

By 12 h after the crush, the distal axons begin to show signs of degeneration with the paranodal accumulation of mitochondria (Webster, 1962a; Ballin and Thomas, 1969b). The unmyelinated fibres begin to swell (Berger, 1971; Bray, Peyronnard and Aguayo, 1972) and undergo beading (Weddell and Glees, 1941). There is a diffuse increase in acid phosphatase and protease activity throughout the distal nerve (Hallpike and Adams, 1969). By 24 h, axoplasmic degeneration distal to the crush becomes evident, with increased electron density of the axoplasm, and fragmentation of the neurofilaments, microtubules and endoplasmic reticulum (Vial, 1958; Nathaniel and Pease, 1963a; Ballin and Thomas, 1969b). The rate of degeneration is somewhat variable: in general it is inversely proportional to fibre diameter. Although some unmyelinated axons are the first to degenerate (Ranson, 1912; Weddell and Glees, 1941; Lubińska and Waryszewska, 1973), others persist for longer than myelinated axons (Thomas, King and Phelps, 1972). Degeneration of unmyelinated axons (Fig. 6.2) is quite extensive by 24 h (Taxi, 1959; Roth and Richardson, 1969; Dyck and Hopkins, 1972). It is likely that the fragmentation and apparent expulsion of the unmyelinated axons from the Remak cell cytoplasm described by Taxi was due to the appearance of early axon sprouts.

By 24 h most of the myelinated fibres show the onset of degeneration of the myelin sheaths (Weddell and Glees, 1941). The myelin splits at the intra-period line and lamellae peel off at the nodes (Glimstedt and Wohlfart, 1960; Ballin and Thomas, 1969b; Williams and Hall, 1971b); the Schwann cells give rise to processes which extend over the nodes of Ranvier (Ballin and Thomas, 1969b) (Fig. 6.3). There is an increase in ribosomes in the Schwann cell cytoplasm (Nathaniel and Pease, 1963a), and of protein synthesis in the Schwann cell cytoplasm adjacent to the crush (Kreutzberg, 1967). Schwann cells begin to divide 24–28 h after the crush (Rexed and Fredriksson, 1956; Friede and Johnstone, 1966; Bradley and Asbury, 1970).

By the third day there is marked hypertrophy of the Schwann cell cytoplasm with phagocytosis of myelin debris (Glimstedt and Wohlfart, 1960; O'Daly and Imaeda, 1967). An increase in total DNA is now measurable biochemically (Seiler and Schröder, 1970). Estimates of the peak rates of division of Schwann cells in the distal nerve vary from 3 to 9 days (Abercrombie and Johnson, 1946; Rexed and Frederiksson, 1956; Friede and Johnstone, 1966; Bradley and Asbury, 1970). The maximum number of Schwann cells in the distal nerve is seen at about 15–25 days after the crush (Abercrombie and Johnson, 1946; Logan, Mannell and Rossiter, 1952). The rate and extent of Schwann cell division is greatest in nerves composed of large myelinated fibres, and is much less in nerves with only unmyelinated axons (Abercrombie and Johnson, 1946; Thomas, 1948;

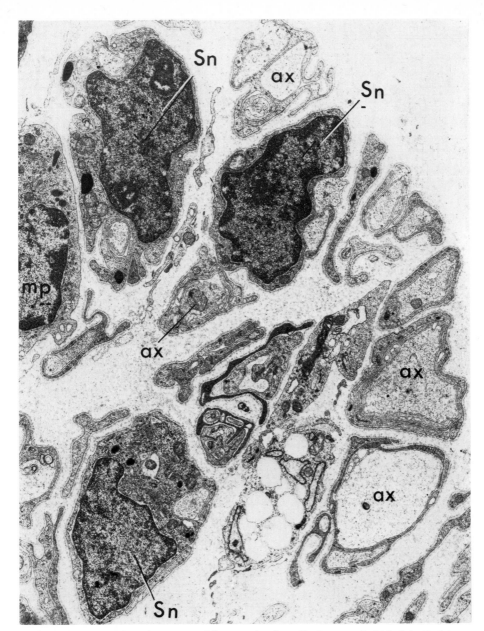

Fig. 6.2 Unmyelinated axons (*ax*) in various stages of degeneration from distal stump of rabbit abdominal vagus nerve · days after section. *Sn* Schwann cell nuclei; *mp* macrophage, ×16 600. (figure kindly provided by Dr R.H.M. King)

Abercrombie, Evans and Murray, 1959).

Degeneration of the myelin sheath progresses steadily from the third day. It becomes segmented into progressively shorter ellipsoids (Fig. 6.4A) by interruption and fusion of the myelin sheath immediately adjacent to the wider ends of the Schmidt-Lantermann incisures (Webster, 1965;

Ghabriel and Allt, 1979) and then into progressively smaller droplets (Fig. 6.4A), some of which may be seen as osmiophilic inclusions within the Schwann cell cytoplasm. Despite initial argument, there is now no doubt that most of the early breakdown of myelin is achieved by Schwann cells. The active metabolic intervention of cells is

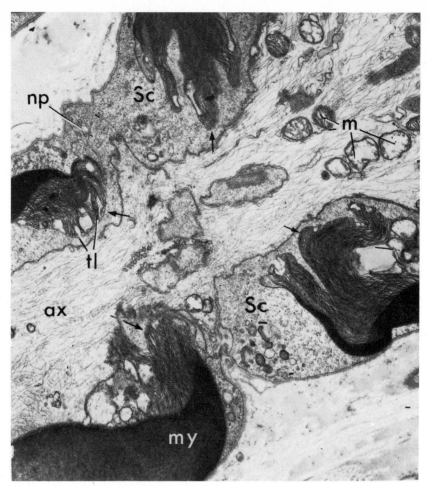

Fig. 6.3 Node of Ranvier during Wallerian degeneration of rat sural nerve 30 h after nerve section. The terminal loops (*tl*) of the myelin (*my*) have become separated from the axolemma by Schwann cell processes (arrowed). Schwann cell cytoplasm (*Sc*) has extended into the nodal gap and has displaced the Schwann cell nodal processes (*np*) away from the axolemma. The axon (*ax*) contains mitochondria (*m*), some of which display degenerative swelling, ×8740 (figure kindly provided by Dr R.H.M. King)

required for this myelin breakdown (Masurovsky and Bunge, 1971).

By the fifth day, there are many lipid-filled macrophages within the distal nerve (Williams and Hall, 1971b), and by 16 days most of the myelin sheaths have been removed, although some myelin debris may still be seen within macrophages three months after nerve degeneration (Luse and McCaman, 1957; Nathaniel and Pease, 1963b). The origin of the macrophages during Wallerian degeneration of peripheral nerve is still uncertain. Claims have been made that they are haematogenous (Olsson and Sjöstrand, 1969; Asbury, 1970; Gibson, 1979), whereas other studies favour

a local origin (Berner, Torvik and Stenwig, 1973), possibly by 'transformation' of Schwann cells (Holtzman and Novikoff, 1965). There is evidence that a large part of the cholesterol of the digested myelin is re-utilised by Schwann cells for the synthesis of new myelin sheaths (Rawlins, Hedley-Whyte, Villegas and Uzman, 1970).

If regeneration fails to occur immediately, the distal stump comes to consist of longitudinally continuous columns of Schwann cells, the bands of Büngner, that have arisen by Schwann cell proliferation within the persisting basal laminal tubes. If reinnervation of the distal stump fails to occur, the Schwann cells ultimately disappear

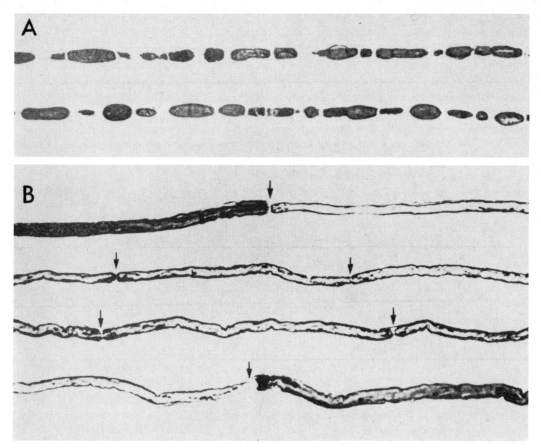

Fig. 6.4   A. Consecutive portions of degenerating myelinated nerve fibre from distal stump of rat sural nerve four days after nerve section. The myelin has broken down into osmiophilic ellipsoids of varying size. Osmium tetroxide, ×117. B. Consecutive portions of myelinated nerve fibre from proximal stump of rat sural nerve central to an amputation neuroma following a nerve transection performed two weeks before. The fibre shows a region of segmental demyelination and remyelination with five intercalated internodes bounded on either side by thicker segments of preserved myelin. The position of the nodes of Ranvier is indicated by the arrows. Osmium tetroxide, ×148 (figure kindly provided by Dr P.S. Spencer)

(Weinberg and Spencer, 1978). After a localised crush injury, regenerating axon sprouts appear in the distal stump at about the fifth day (Barton, 1962; Nathaniel and Pease, 1963b; Bray *et al.*, 1972). Regeneration of the axons of myelinated fibres takes place along the bands of Büngner, which provide the guidance pathways back to the periphery. The situation differs for regenerating unmyelinated axons, the guidance mechanisms being less precise. Evans and Murray (1954) found that, following cervical vagus crush lesions in the rabbit, unmyelinated axons grew in profusion into the recurrent laryngeal nerve, which normally contains very few unmyelinated fibres. Maturation of the myelinated fibres subsequently takes place,

with a gradual return towards normal axon diameters and myelin thickness, although this is never fully achieved even after crush injuries where most axons regain their former terminations at the periphery (Cragg and Thomas, 1964). Maturation is considerably less if contact with normal peripheral connections is not achieved (Aitken, Sharman and Young, 1947). During regeneration, the proliferated Schwann cells space themselves along the axons at intervals, comparable to the situation during normal development. If regeneration has taken place in the adult state after growth in length of the nerve has ceased, internodal length is then found to be uniformly short on fibres of all diameters (Fig. 6.1) (Vizoso and

Young, 1948; Fullerton, Gilliatt, Lascelles and Morgan-Hughes, 1965).

Following repeated Wallerian degeneration with intervening regeneration, extensive nerve fibre systems composed of groups of myelinated and unmyelinated axons with associated Schwann cells are observed (Thomas, 1970). Concentric Schwann cell proliferation with the formation of hypertrophic 'onion bulbs' does not occur. Above neuromata resulting from nerve section, giant ballooning of the myelin sheath may occur, with extensive demyelination (Fig. 6.4B) (Spencer and Thomas, 1970).

Axonal degeneration from other causes

Axons degenerate not only when they are transected mechanically, but also when they are interrupted by damage from the local application of toxic substances such as phenol (Schaumburg, Byck and Weller, 1970), by ischaemia (Blunt, 1960) or by cold injury (Denny-Brown, Adams, Brenner and Doherty, 1945). They are also lost in the neuronopathies, in which there is degeneration of the whole neurone, including the central and peripheral axons and the perikaryon. Examples are loss of primary sensory neurones produced by methyl mercury (Jacobs, Carmichael and Cavanagh, 1975), and doxorubicin (Adriamycin) (Cho, 1977) intoxication. In many other neuropathies axonal degeneration with secondary myelin disruption may also be encountered, although the site of the damage to the neurone in these disorders remains to be elucidated.

Ultrastructural changes in intact axons have been noted in a number of neuropathies in which axonal degeneration occurs, for example uraemic neuropathy (Dyck, Johnson, Lambert and O'Brien, 1971). Of particular interest is the condition of giant axonal neuropathy originally described by Asbury, Gale, Cox, Baringer and Berg (1972) and subsequently by Carpenter, Karpati, Andermann and Gold (1974), Igisu, Ohta, Tabira, Hosokawa. Goto and Kuroiwa (1975) and others. The condition is characterised by the presence of segmentally enlarged axons that contain closely packed neurofilaments, and which closely resemble those encountered in a number of

toxic neuropathies, as discussed in the next section.

In certain chronic neuropathies associated with repeated axonal degeneration, large clusters of myelinated and unmyelinated axons with associated Schwann cells may be observed (Fig. 6.5), similar to those produced experimentally by repeated crush injuries (Thomas, 1970). Such 'hyperneurotisation' of Büngner bands was noted in experimental isoniazid neuropathy by Schröder (1968).

'Dying-back' neuropathies

Since the end of the nineteenth century, neuropathologists have recognised that degeneration may be concentrated in the most distal parts of nerve fibre tracts of the central nervous system furthest from the perikarya. This is particularly striking in Friedreich's ataxia and amyotrophic lateral sclerosis. Similarly, in the peripheral nervous system, changes predominating in the distal parts have been recognised for many years (Greenfield and Carmichael, 1935). Since then, many reports have emphasised the distal predominance of a number of neuropathies involving axonal degeneration, and the term 'dying-back' has been applied to these. This has been recognized in thiamine deficiency (Swank, 1940; Denny-Brown, 1958), acrylamide neuropathy (Fullerton and Barnes, 1966 and triorthocresylphosphate (TOCP) neuropathy (Cavanagh, 1964). In some neuropathies, such as that of acute intermittent porphyria, the distal parts of the larger fibres appear to 'die back', although it is not the longest fibres which are involved (Cavanagh and Mellick, 1965).

Although the term 'dying-back' has been widely employed, more detailed analysis undertaken in recent years and reviewed by Spencer and Schaumburg (1974, 1976, 1978) has revealed that this is not strictly accurate and the term 'distal axonopathy' is preferable. The process has been examined experimentally in the neuropathies produced by acrylamide, TOCP, n-hexane and methyl n-butyl ketone. With n-hexane-induced neuropathy, massive focal accumulations of 10 nm neurofilaments are a feature. These originally develop on the proximal side of the last node of Ranvier of the parent fibre before the terminal

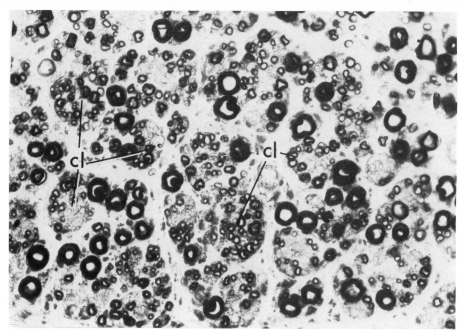

Fig. 6.5   Chronic peripheral neuropathy with conspicuous axonal degeneration and sprouting which has given rise to clusters (*cl*) of small regenerating axons. Kultschitsky's haematoxylin, ×344

arborisation of the fibre. The axonal swellings are accompanied by focal demyelination and are a prelude to Wallerian-type degeneration of the fibre distal to this level. Subsequently, such changes extend progressively to more proximal nodes. The diameter of the fibres, as well as their length, is important in determining the vulnerability of the fibres. Thus, the larger calibre fibres in the tibial nerve that supply the calf musculature are affected before the thinner fibres in the plantar nerves. The type of change varies somewhat for different toxic agents. With acrylamide neuropathy, the focal neurofilament accumulations occur only with slowly induced intoxication.

Cavanagh (1964) originally proposed that, in dying-back neuropathies, the synthetic processes that occur in the neuronal perikaryon are impaired, so that the supply of material for transport down the axon is deficient, the consequences first being noticeable at the periphery. Spencer and Schaumburg (1974, 1976, 1978) have proposed that the toxic substances interfere with those processes within the axons themselves upon which axonal integrity depends. At present it is difficult to understand how a wide range of chemically

dissimilar toxins gives rise to a substantially comparable end result. Suggestions have been made that this is related to impaired glycolysis in nerve (Spencer, Sabri, Schaumburg and Moore, 1979) or through an interference with coenzymes (Schoental and Cavanagh, 1977).

SCHWANN CELL DISORDERS AND SEGMENTAL DEMYELINATION

It is evident that some disorders primarily affect either the Schwann cells or the myelin and lead to the occurrence of segmental demyelination. The consequences of diseases affecting the Schwann cells associated with unmyelinated axons are obscure at present.

In comparison with Wallerian degeneration, segmental demyelination is a much more variable process, affecting some Schwann cells, sparing others, and very largely sparing the axons. It was first recognised by Gombault (1880) in the peripheral neuropathy due to lead. Diphtheritic neuropathy has been used to the greatest extent as an experimental model to investigate segmental demyelination, but the latter has been shown to be the salient pathological change in a number of human peripheral neuropathies.

Diphtheritic neuropathy

The mechanism by which diphtheria toxin damages Schwann cells is not entirely clear. It causes inhibition of protein synthesis (Collier and Pappenheimer, 1964a, b), and particularly inhibits the synthesis of proteolipid and basic protein during myelination (Pleasure, Feldmann and Prockop, 1973). However, it is difficult to believe that this is the mode of action upon adult Schwann cells, for there are many cells in the body with more rapid protein turnover than myelin, but which are not specifically sensitive to diphtheria toxin. Perivascular haemorrhages are found throughout the body in diphtheritic neuropathy (Hochhaus, 1891; Heinlein, 1949; Waksman, Adams and Mansmann, 1957). When found at autopsy, these may in part be due to asphyxia, although the toxin can also damage endoneurial blood vessels (Bradley and Jennekens, 1971). Nevertheless, its mode of action on Schwann cells is likely to be metabolic rather than ischaemic. The toxin becomes fixed within one hour, and is not then susceptible to neutralisation by antitoxin. There is, however, a delay thereafter of 5–50 days in patients with the disease, before the onset of symptoms and signs, and of 4–7 days in the experimental situation (Cavanagh and Jacobs, 1964). The delay seems to be inversely proportional to the dose of toxin. What is occurring during this delay period is not known.

Different parts of the peripheral nervous system are affected in different species. Waksman (1961) has suggested that this is due to deficiencies of the blood-nerve barrier in the sites of predilection in the different animals. The nerve roots are more particularly involved than the peripheral nerves in man and the rabbit (Fisher and Adams, 1955; Waksman *et al.*, 1957), the dorsal roots being more severely involved in the cat (McDonald, 1963). In the guinea pig, however, there is more widespread peripheral nerve damage, and in these animals there does not appear to be a blood-nerve barrier.

The earliest change in the peripheral nervous system which can be detected after the latent interval is an increase in the *normal* irregularities of the myelin sheaths (Webster, Spiro, Waksman and Adams, 1961). This is followed by a widening of the nodal gap (Cavanagh and Jacobs, 1964; Morgan-Hughes, 1968), the smaller fibres being affected before the larger. Myelin in the affected internodes then begins to break down starting at the Schmidt-Lantermann clefts and in the paranodal region. In some internodes the myelin sheath may degenerate up to 200–300 μm from the node, although the remainder of the sheath may remain intact, while in other fibres the whole internodal myelin may break down. Coincident with the earliest appearance of myelin breakdown, there is an accumulation of lysosomes and acid phosphatase activity at the nodal regions in the Schwann cells of the small fibres (Weller, 1965; Weller and Mellick, 1966), but not of the larger (Weller and Nester, 1972). The relative part played by the Schwann cells and macrophages in myelin destruction is as debatable in diphtheritic neuropathy as it is in Wallerian degeneration, but it is now accepted that the major part of myelin breakdown occurs within the Schwann cell cytoplasm itself. There is little or no axonal damage in most instances (McDonald, 1963), although the axoplasm may show increased osmiophilia (Allt, 1969).

The timing of the stages of degeneration in diphtheritic neuropathy can best be followed by intraneural injection of the toxin (Jacobs, Cavanagh and Mellick, 1967; Allt and Cavanagh, 1969). As in Wallerian degeneration, the smallest fibres show greater susceptibility (Cavanagh and Jacobs, 1964). By the third day small myelinated fibres show myelin breakdown, which does not begin in the large fibres until about the fifth day. From the third day onwards there is peeling back of the outer lamellae of the myelin sheaths from the nodes (Fig. 6.6A and B), producing measurable widening of the node of Ranvier. By the seventh day there is swelling of the Schwann cell cytoplasm which covers the node of Ranvier (Fig. 6.6A and B). Macrophages begin to infiltrate the nerve at this stage, phagocytosing myelin degeneration products released by Schwann cells (Webster *et al.*, 1961). By the tenth day there is extensive nodal widening. Myelin debris is seen within Schwann cell processes alongside the axon and regions of bare axon may be present (Fig. 6.6D). Some

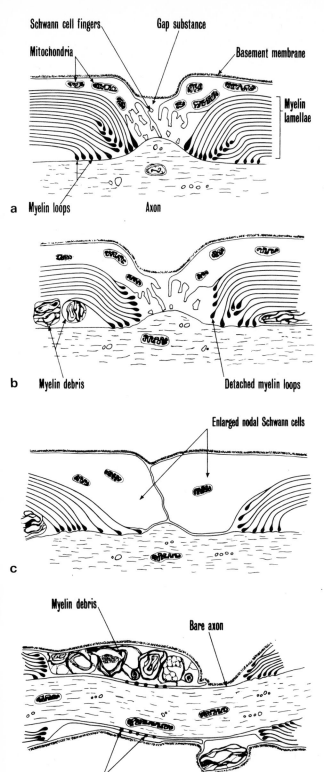

Schwann cells go through a phase of apparent inhibition of metabolic activity at this stage with loss of cellular organelles (Allt, 1969). A proportion show total degeneration, and there may be breakdown of the axolemma if this occurs (Webster *et al.*, 1961).

Although a few Schwann cells die, the majority show rapid mobilisation. They begin dividing from the third day onwards, the peak of activity being at about the seventh day (Jaobs *et al.*, 1967). The early formation of non-compacted thin myelin sheaths can be seen from the tenth day onwards in a few fibres (Webster *et al.*, 1961; Webster, 1964). In segments where damage has been limited to the paranodal region, the new myelin sheath grows in again from one or both adjacent Schwann cells. If a whole internode has been demyelinated, the area originally invested by one Schwann cell becomes the responsibility of two or more newly divided Schwann cells. The result of these intercalated myelin segments is a decrease in the internodal length of these areas, and therefore an increased variability of internodal length (Fig. 6.1).

The Guillain-Barré-Strohl syndrome

The primary pathological change in the Guillain-Barré-Strohl syndrome (acute inflammatory polyneuropathy) (Asbury, Arnason and Adams, 1969), and in its possible experimental counterpart, experimental allergic neuritis (Waksman and Adams, 1955, 1956), is segmental demyelination. If the changes are very severe, axonal degeneration also occurs. Inflammatory cells, predominantly lymphocytes, infiltrate the perivascular spaces and interstitium, particularly in the nerve roots.

Fig. 6.6 Diagram of changes at the nodes of Ranvier after local injection of diphtheria toxin into rat sciatic nerve (from Allt and Cavanagh, 1969). A. Normal node of Ranvier. B. At 3 days, outer myelin loops are detached from the axolemma and inner lamellae are disorganised. C. At 7 days the node is widened, Schwann cell 'fingers' and gap substance are absent, and the gap is replaced by swollen Schwann cell cytoplasm. D. At 10 days, there is marked nodal widening; there is much myelin debris within Schwann cell processes and the axon is bare of Schwann cell covering in places. Severed terminal myelin loops are still present attached to the axolemma

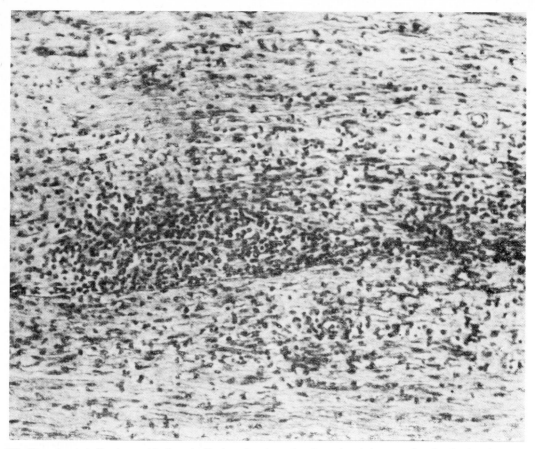

Fig. 6.7 Experimental allergic neuritis. Longitudinal section through guinea pig sciatic nerve showing focal perivenous accumulation of inflammatory cells. Haematoxylin light green, ×90

As discussed in Chapter 21, the exact aetiology of acute inflammatory polyneuropathy still remains in doubt, although it is likely to be due to a cell mediated delayed hypersensitivity reaction. In the tissues, infiltrating lymphocytes are believed to release a cytotoxic agent which damages the myelin (Fig. 6.7). Macrophages then make their appearance in the peripheral nerve, a 'macrophage inhibition factor' released by lymphocytes perhaps playing a part in this process (Caspary, Currie, Walton and Field, 1971). The macrophages, both in acute inflammatory polyneuropathy and experimental allergic neuritis, seem to play a major part in the breakdown of the myelin, for they infiltrate beneath the basal laminae of the Schwann cells and strip the myelin away from the axons (Fig. 6.8) (Lampert, 1969; Wisniewski, Terry, Whitaker, Cook and Dowling, 1969; Carpenter, 1972). The vesicular degeneration of myelin observed in acute

inflammatory polyneuropathy by Wisniewski *et al.* and by Carpenter, is perhaps a post-mortem artefact, as suggested by Prineas (1973). However, in experimental allergic neuritis Ballin and Thomas (1969a) and Schröder and Krücke (1970) found degeneration of myelin without the direct intervention of macrophages. In the peripheral nerve of animals immunised against central nervous myelin, Wisniewski, Prineas and Raine (1969) again found infiltration of the myelin sheaths by macrophages, with vesicular disruption of the myelin, and suggested that the Schwann cells were largely bystanders in this process.

Metachromatic and globoid cell leucodystrophy

There is pathological evidence that peripheral nerve myelin may be involved in several leucodystrophies, even though the symptoms and signs of central nervous involvement are more striking. Biopsies of the peripheral nervous system are less hazardous than brain biopsies and therefore offer a diagnostic test in some of these conditions. The neurones of the peripheral autonomic system may be involved and can be obtained for study by a full-thickness biopsy of the rectal mucosa. Biopsy procedures, however, have largely been superseded where specific enzyme defects are demonstrable, such as that of aryl sulphatase A in metachromatic leucodystrophy.

The changes in the peripheral nerve are most striking in metachromatic leucodystrophy (sulphatide lipidosis). As well as an increased incidence of the normal irregularities of the myelin sheaths, and segmental demyelination, there are numerous Schwann cell inclusions which stain metachromatically with basic dyes such as toluidine blue and cresyl fast violet (Dayan, 1967) (Fig. 6.9). Under the electron microscope these have a varied appearance; some are multilaminated bodies indistinguishable from myelin in the process of degradation (Webster, 1962b) (Fig. 6.10).

Globoid cell (Krabbe) leucodystrophy in man and the dog is associated with segmental demyelination in the peripheral nerves, and the accumulation of crystalline deposits and acid phosphatase activity in the Schwann cell cytoplasm. Foamy macrophages are found in the peripheral nerves, although large accumulations such as are seen in the brain do not occur (Sourander and Olsson, 1968; Bischoff and Ulrich, 1969; Dunn, Lake, Dolman and Wilson, 1969).

Hypertrophic neuropathy

The characteristic appearances of hypertrophic neuropathy were initially recognised by Gombault and Mallet (1889) and subsequently linked to a progressive hereditary polyneuropathy with an onset in childhood by Dejerine and Sottas (1893). The essential histological change is a concentric proliferation of Schwann cells around the nerve fibres (Fig. 6.11) leading to structures that in transverse section resemble cross-sections through an onion. such 'onion bulbs' were, for a long time, believed to be specific for Dejerine-Sottas

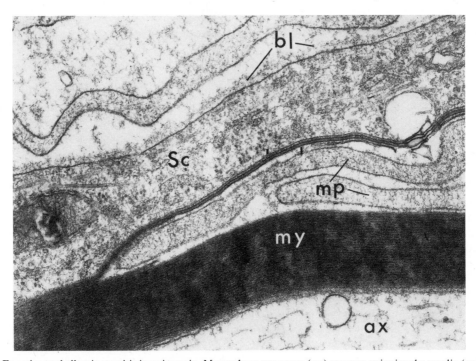

Fig. 6.8   Experimental allergic neuritis in guinea pig. Macrophage processes (*mp*) are seen stripping the myelin (*my*) away from the axon (*ax*). *Sc* Schwann cell cytoplasm; *bl* basal lamina, × 30 340 (figure kindly supplied by Dr R.H.M. King)

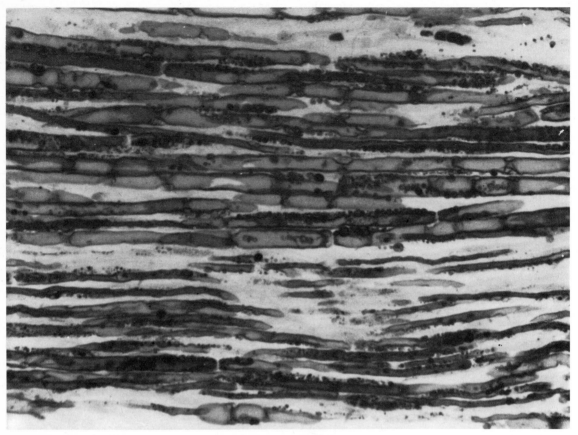

Fig. 6.9 Longitudinal section of sural nerve of a child with metachromatic leucodystrophy showing numerous coarsely granular inclusions and irregularities in the myelin sheaths. Weigert-Pal, ×332

neuropathy and were considered to result from a primary proliferation of Schwann cells. They are now realised to be a non-specific consequence of repeated demyelination and remyelination (Thomas and Lascelles, 1967; Weller, 1967; Ballin and Thomas, 1968), and are encountered in a wide variety of peripheral nerve disorders, both inherited and acquired (see Chapter 21). They have also been reproduced experimentally in a number of situations, all of which have in common the occurrence of repeated segmental demyelination and remyelination (Weller and Das Gupta, 1968; Ballin and Thomas, 1969a; Dyck, 1969). Segmental demyelination leads to Schwann cell proliferation. A surplus of Schwann cells is produced and the supernumerary cells remain alongside the nerve fibres. Their concentric arrangement is probably due to their alignment inside the basal lamina that had surrounded the original Schwann cells (Lampert and Schochet, 1968).

The peripheral nerve trunks in hypertrophic neuropathy are often enlarged. This is partly the result of the Schwann cell proliferation, but is also due to extensive endoneurial collagen formation (Webster, Schröder, Asbury and Adams, 1967) and to the accumulation of amorphous metachromatically staining material in the endoneurium.

Dyck, Lambert, Sanders and O'Brien (1971) demonstrated that, in cases of hypertrophic neuropathy of Dejerine-Sottas type, the normal relationship between myelin thickness and axon diameter is lost, suggesting that the Schwann cells are unable to maintain adequate myelination. Apart from the occurrence of demyelination and remyelination, such nerves are thus also 'hypomyelinated'. It is of interest that, in this disorder, a

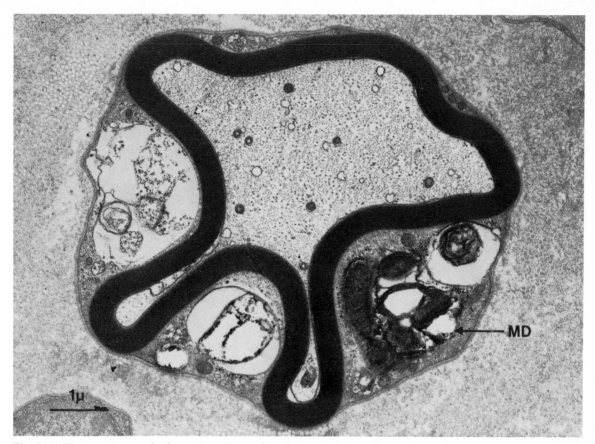

Fig. 6.10 Electron micrograph of a myelinated nerve fibre from a case of metachromatic leucodystrophy showing inclusions within the Schwann cell cytoplasm (MD)

disturbance in the metabolism of ceramide hexosides and hexoside sulphates has been reported (Dyck, Ellefson, Lais, Smith, Taylor and Van Dyke, 1970). A disturbance of lipid metabolism is known to exist in Refsum's disease (phytanic acid storage disease), in which hypertrophic changes also occur (Cammermeyer, 1956; Fardeau and Engel, 1969).

Other Schwann cell disorders

There is evidence that, in the early stages of leprous neuropathy, the *Mycobacterium leprae* selectively colonises the Schwann cells (Fig. 6.12) (Rees, Weddell, Palmer and Jamison, 1965) and segmental demyelination is known to occur in this disorder (Fig. 6.13) (Dayan and Sandbank, 1970). In more advanced stages, there is extensive involvement of the supporting tissues of the nerve.

In Tangier disease (hereditary high density lipoprotein deficiency), nerve biopsies may show a severe loss of unmyelinated and myelinated axons accompanied by a striking accumulation of lipid deposits, probably neutral lipids and cholesterol esters, within Schwann cells (Kocen, King, Thomas and Haas, 1973). The cause of the axonal degeneration is unknown, but the accumulation of lipid within Schwann cells may be related to a failure to remove the breakdown products of nerve degeneration, either because of defective removal from the cells or because of a failure of intracellular transport mechanisms (Kocen *et al.*, 1973; Dyck, Ellefson, Yao and Herbert, 1978).

Peripheral neuropathy may be a feature of the Chediak-Higashi syndrome. Lockman, Kennedy and White (1967) found that the massive lysosomes characteristic of this disorder were present within Schwann cells and suggested that they were

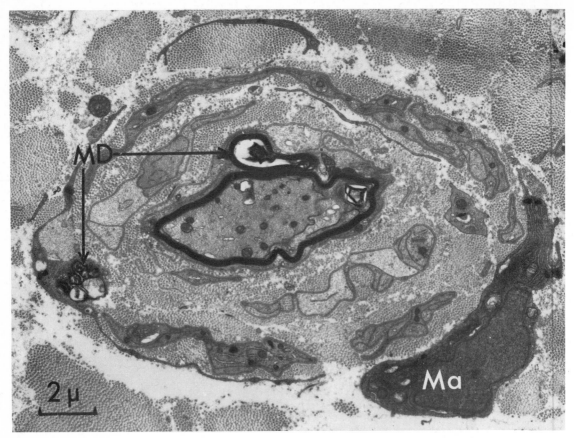

Fig. 6.11   Electron micrograph of transverse section through an 'onion bulb' formation from the sural nerve of a child with hypertrophic neuropathy of Dejerine-Sottas type. Myelin debris (MD) is present in some lamellae. The outer nucleated process is a macrophage (Ma)

involved in the genesis of the neuropathy.

Secondary axonal degeneration and secondary segmental demyelination

Most clinical diseases of peripheral nerve are of mixed nature, with segmental demyelination and axonal degeneration occurring to a varying degree (Thomas, 1971). For example, acute inflammatory polyneuropathy is *predominantly* demyelinating, whereas the neuropathy of porphyria is *predominantly* axonal in type, although both processes occur in each disease.

It is not easy to quantitate the extent of these two processes. Segmental demyelination is easily seen in single teased nerve fibres, while axonal degeneration is recognised only while myelin debris remains, unless axon regrowth occurs. The total

number of myelinated nerve fibres counted in transverse sections of the nerve cannot be relied upon to separate the two processes, for the number is decreased in demyelinating neuropathies by the presence of demyelinated segments. A total axon count would be required to demonstrate fibre loss.

It has occasionally been noted that the changes in the proximal parts of the nerves are predominantly demyelinating, whereas those in the distal parts take the form of axonal degeneration, as for example in coyotillo poisoning (Charlton and Pierce, 1969). Where there is severe segmental demyelination, such as in the familial hypertrophic neuropathies, there frequently appears to be a decrease in the total number of axons. It has often been suggested that Schwann cell disease may cause axonal degeneration (e.g. Bradley and Jennekens, 1971). Schlaepfer (1969) has suggested

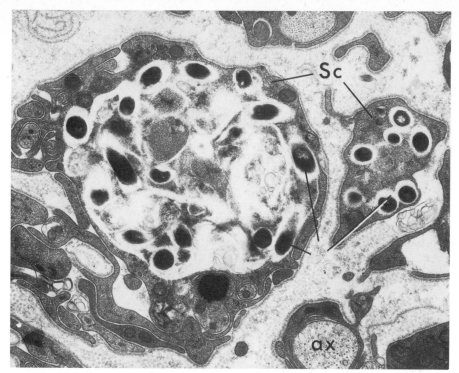

Fig. 6.12 Electron micrograph of sural nerve from a case of borderline lepromatous leprosy. The Schwann cells (Sc) contain numerous leprosy bacilli (b). ax = axon, ×12750 (figure kindly supplied by Dr R.H.M. King)

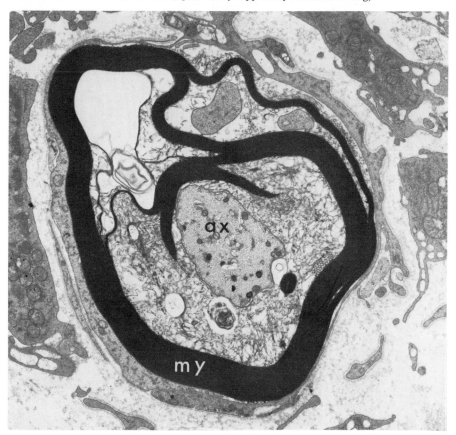

Fig. 6.13 Electron micrograph of sural nerve from a case of borderline lepromatous leprosy. Myelinated nerve fibre showing intact axon (ax) surrounded by degenerating myelin (my), ×8140 (figure kindly supplied by Dr R.H.M. King)

that in lead neuropathy the combination of these two processes could result from a toxic effect on both the capsular cells of the posterior root ganglia and the Schwann cells. Conversely, the influence of the axon upon the Schwann cell is clear. This is illustrated by the Schwann cell changes occurring in Wallerian degeneration. Jennekens, Van Spijk and Dorhout Mees (1969) found that in uraemic neuropathy some fibres show little or no segmental demyelination, while in others many of the internodes are demyelinated. Dyck *et al.* (1971) and Thomas, Hollinrake, Lascelles, O'Sullivan, Baillod, Moorhead and McKenzie (1971) confirmed this observation and suggested that an abnormality of the axons gave rise to a *secondary segmental demyelination*.

DISORDERS PRIMARILY AFFECTING NEURAL CONNECTIVE TISSUES

In a number of neuropathies, the connective tissues of the peripheral nerves are affected by a pathological process with secondary damage to the nerve fibres. This may be a direct mechanical effect, but in some circumstances it is conceivable that a disruption of the permeability barrier provided by the perineurium and vasa nervorum could influence the activity of the nerve fibres. Endoneurial oedema may be a conspicuous feature of some neuropathies. This has been studied in experimental lead neuropathy (Ohnishi, Schilling, Brimijoin, Lambert, Fairbanks and Dyck, 1977), where it is known that it is associated with an increase in intraneural pressure (Low and Dyck, 1977). Whether such increases in endoneurial pressure have any deleterious effect on the function of the nerve fibres is still uncertain. Illustrative examples of neuropathies in which there is a primary involvement of neural connective tissues are infiltrative processes such as granulomatous conditions and certain neoplasms, and neuropathies involving the deposition of extracellular material, such as amyloid, in the nerves.

Amyloidosis

A neuropathy occurs with any frequency only in the primary familial types, but is also seen in sporadic cases of primary amyloidosis, and in amyloidosis related to myelomatosis. As described in Chapter 21, there are three main familial amyloid neuropathies. In the Andrade type, amyloid is present both in the adventitia and media of small arterioles, and in masses free within the endoneurium (Fig. 6.14). It shows the characteristic staining reactions with Congo red and thioflavin T, and is composed of non-branching fibrils of 7–10 nm diameter (Coimbra and Andrade, 1971). The nerve fibres may be compressed

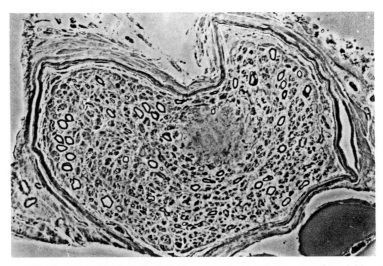

Fig. 6.14 Transverse section of nerve from a case of amyloid neuropathy showing a mass of amyloid material beneath the perineurium. Osmium tetroxide, ×1105 (figure kindly supplied by Dr P.J. Dyck)

by the endoneurial deposits (Dyck and Lambert, 1969). The most striking feature in the cases of Dyck and Lambert (1969) was the loss of un-myelinated and small myelinated nerve fibres, corresponding closely to the early loss of pain and temperature sensation and disturbances of autonomic function. Coimbra and Andrade (1971) could not confirm this dramatic loss of un-myelinated axons, but it was evident in the cases reported by Thomas and King (1973).

In the Rukavina type, amyloid is initially deposited particularly in the flexor retinaculum of the carpal tunnel, though it is also seen in the walls of small blood vessels (Mahloudji, Teasdall, Adamkiewicz, Hartmann, Lambird and McKusick, 1969). The resultant thickening of the flexor retinaculum gives rise to the carpal tunnel syndrome, which is the presenting feature of these patients. Later a more widespread neuropathy develops.

The Van Allen type (Van Allen, Frohlich and Davis, 1969) is characterised by the presence of amyloid within the nerve roots, the posterior root ganglia, and the sympathetic nerves and ganglia. Again, the blood vessel walls and interstitium are particularly affected.

The mechanism of the nerve fibre damage, apart from the occurrence of the carpal tunnel syndrome in the Rukavina type, has not been satisfactorily established. The early involvement of unmyeli-nated axons argues against an ischaemic basis. Although mechanical distortion from endoneurial deposits may be of some significance, it seems difficult to ascribe the manifestations solely to this: the larger myelinated fibres are those most susceptible to pressure and are the last to be affected. Coimbra and Andrade (1971) considered that the amyloid deposition was preceded by nerve fibre de-generation, but this observation requires verifi-cation. It seems likely that the infiltration of the posterior root ganglia and autonomic ganglia, leading to replacement of many of the neurons with amyloid, is probably the cause of the specific and marked axonal loss (Appenzeller, 1970).

Inflammatory disorders

As described in Chapter 21, two polar forms of leprous neuropathy are recognised, although intermediate forms occur, providing a continuous gradation between these extremes (Ridley and Jopling, 1966). Several studies on the path-ology of the peripheral nerves in leprosy have been published, including those by Job and Desikan (1968) and Job (1971). In lepromatous neuropathy the infected individual has a low resistance to the disease. Numerous bacilli are present in all elements of the nerves, but probably initially within Schwann cells (Fig. 6.12). At first there is little damage to nerve fibres. Later, segmental demyelination (Fig. 6.13) and axonal destruction gradually appear, large numbers of foamy mac-rophages containing bacilli are present, and extensive fibrosis develops. In tuberculoid leprosy the individual has a high resistance. In contrast to the lepromatous form, it is difficult to detect bacilli in the peripheral nerves, which show much axonal destruction and contain epithelioid and giant cells, and collections of lymphocytes. Cold abscess formation sometimes occurs. The nerves are thickened and may be compressed in anatomical tunnels.

Although the mechanism of peripheral nerve involvement in sarcoidosis is not yet understood (Matthews, 1975), occasionally the nerves are infiltrated with sarcoid granulomata. A further interesting inflammatory process affecting the connective tissues of peripheral nerve has been described by Asbury, Picard and Baringer (1972) under the name of sensory perineuritis. This consisted of a distal painful and partly remitting disturbance of the cutaneous nerves, associated pathologically with inflammatory scarring re-stricted to the perineurium, with apparent com-pression of the contained nerve fibres. It involved the component fascicles of the nerve in a random manner, leaving some entirely unaffected.

Other examples of connective tissue involvement

The commonest peripheral nerve disturbance in acromegaly is the carpal tunnel syndrome, al-though rarely a more widespread polyneuropathy may occur. The peripheral nerves have been shown to be of increased size, this being related to a proliferation of endoneurial and perineurial con-nective tissue (Stewart, 1966). This may lead to an increased susceptibility to entrapment syndromes, although tissue overgrowth external to the nerves is also presumably involved.

Thomas and Walker (1965) described patients with primary biliary cirrhosis with hypercholesterolaemia, who developed a mild sensory polyneuropathy. Xanthomatous deposits were present in the nerves, particularly in the perineurium, and were extensive enough to disorganise the neural architecture.

Deposits of glycolipid have been demonstrated within the perineurial cells in Fabry's disease (Bischoff, Fierz, Regli and Ulrich, 1968; Kocen and Thomas, 1970). They are probably unrelated to the mild peripheral neuropathy that may occur in this disorder.

NEUROPATHIES DUE TO VASCULAR DISEASE

Ischaemic neuropathy

Because of the extensive intraneural plexus of small arteries, with a number of larger feeding vessels, occlusion of a single nutrient artery will not produce ischaemia. This requires widespread occlusions or a decrease in perfusion pressure. Thus Adams (1943) occluded all the macroscopically visible feeding arteries to the sciatic nerve in the thigh of rabbits, and found damage in only two of 12 animals so treated. Dyck, Conn and Okazaki (1972), from a study of the neuropathy of necrotising angiopathies, suggested that there are watershed zones with relatively decreased supply in the

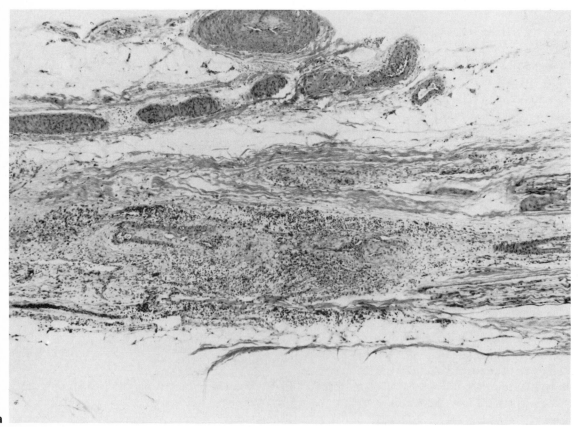

a

Fig. 6.15   Polyarteritis nodosa. a. Longitudinal section of small artery in sural nerve showing occlusion, recanalisation and a periarterial inflammatory focus (Haematoxylin and eosin, ×30). b. Higher power view of another vessel showing hyaline degeneration of vessel wall and a periarterial collection of inflammatory cells of mixed type (Haematoxylin and eosin, ×200). c. Transverse section of sural nerve showing total loss of myelinated nerve fibres from some fascicles and a patchy loss from others. Weigert-Pal, ×30

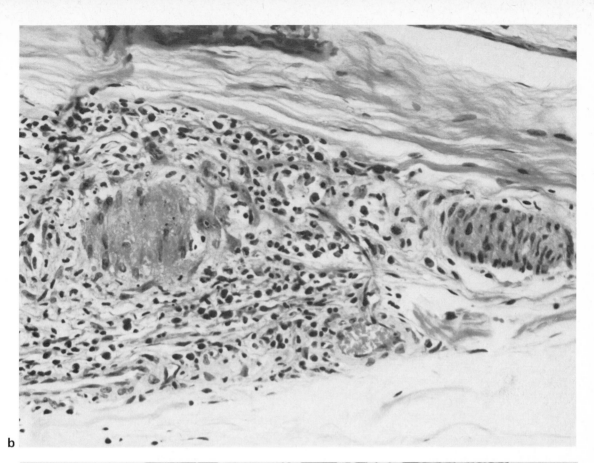

b

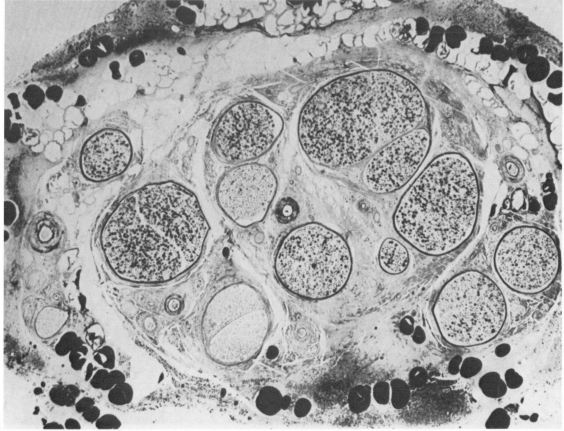

c

main nerves of the mid-upper arm and mid-thigh.

Atheromatous large artery occlusive disease is associated with a clinically mild neuropathy in which there is both segmental demyelination and axonal degeneration (Chopra and Hurwitz, 1967; Eames and Lange, 1967). This probably results both from poor perfusion due to major artery disease, and from secondary changes in the endoneurial vessels, with increased perivascular connective tissue, osmiophilic inclusions in the endothelial cell cytoplasm, endothelial proliferation, and occasional complete occlusion by fibrin. It is uncertain whether these changes are due to coexistent hypertension or micro-embolisation from proximal atheroma.

It is now clear that many of the lesions thought to be nerve infarcts in the case of diabetic proximal motor neuropathy described by Raff, Sangalang and Asbury (1968) were Renaut corpuscles. However, a probable ischaemic basis has been demonstrated for two cases of oculomotor nerve palsy in diabetic subjects (Dreyfus, Hakim and Adams, 1957; Asbury, Aldredge, Hershberg and Fisher, 1970), and it seems likely that diabetic small-vessel disease contributes to the development of focal nerve lesions in this disorder. Such vessels show an accumulation of PAS-positive

material in their walls. Electron-microscopic observations show the PAS-staining material to be reduplicated basal lamina (Bischoff, 1968). The origin of such vascular changes is at present uncertain.

Peripheral nerve lesions consequent upon a necrotising angiopathy may be seen in a variety of disorders including polyarteritis nodosa (Fig. 6.15), rheumatoid arthritis and Wegener's granulomatosis. The pattern of neural damage in these conditions has been analysed by Dyck *et al.*, (1972). Circumscribed necrosis such as occurs in brain is not encountered, but areas of nerve fibre degeneration may be observed, probably related to poor perfusion. These tend to begin centrally within fascicles, and to involve some fasciculi severely while sparing others.

NEUROPATHY DUE TO EXTRANEURAL CAUSES

Compression neuropathy

Peripheral nerves may be damaged by compression from a wide variety of causes including tumours, perineural haemorrhage, entrapment in anatomical tunnels and external compression.

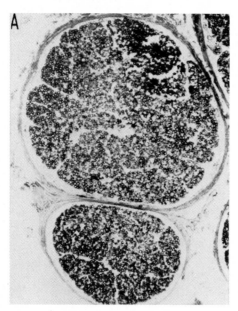 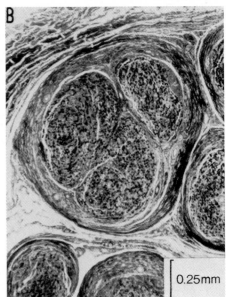

Fig. 6.16   Transverse sections of median nerve from a case of the carpal tunnel syndrome. A. Mid-forearm level. B. At level of flexor retinaculum. Haematoxylin-light green (from Thomas and Fullerton, 1963, reproduced by kind permission of the *Journal of Neurology, Neurosurgery and Psychiatry*)

Acute localised compression, if severe, may lead to axonal interruption with Wallerian degeneration below the level of the lesion. If milder, a temporary localised conduction block may be produced. Denny-Brown and Brenner (1944) showed that this was related to local demyelination with axonal preservation. The detailed pathology of this type of lesion was illuminated by the studies of Ochoa, Danta, Fowler and Gilliatt (1971). In experimental studies on hind limb nerves of the baboon, using a pneumatic cuff, they demonstrated that pressure lesions occur at the edges of the cuff. The axons were dislocated away from the site of pressure, leading to myelin damage at the nodes, which later underwent local demyelination. Recovery is associated with remyelination.

A natural model of pressure neuropathy was discovered by Fullerton and Gilliatt (1967a) in the hind feet of guinea pigs housed in cages with wire floors. The repeated trauma of the wire causes changes in these nerves, ranging from segmental demyelination at the level of the compression to complete Wallerian degeneration below the site of damage. Behse, Buchthal, Carlsen and Knappeis (1972) have studied nerve biopsies from cases of hereditary neuropathy with liability to pressure palsies. The vulnerability of the nerve fibres was related to localised regions along a proportion of the internodes where there was a 'sausage-shaped' increase in myelin thickness accompanied by axonal narrowing. A similar pathological change occurs in hereditary liability to pressure palsy, and the term, 'tomaculous neuropathy' has been suggested for this appearance (Madrid and Bradley, 1975; Bradley, Madrid, Thrush and Campbell, 1975).

Entrapment neuropathy

There are many sites throughout the body at which nerves are vulnerable to compression by other tissues in 'anatomical tunnels', such as when passing under ligaments or aponeuroses. It is normal for the nerve, at sites where it is exposed to pressure, to be slightly thickened with an increased amount of epi- and endoneurial connective tissue. When compression occurs, there is narrowing of the nerve with pallor of the superficial blood vessels. Few pathological studies of such nerves in

man are available. Thomas and Fullerton (1963) studied serial transverse sections of the median nerve in a patient with the carpal tunnel syndrome. They found evidence of demyelination at the level of the compression (Fig. 6.16). More recently, Neary and Eames (1975) and Neary, Ochoa and Gilliatt (1975) have demonstrated displacement of myelin along internodes, together with demyelination and remyelination, in relation to median and ulnar nerve entrapment. Aguayo, Nair and Midgley (1971) experimentally produced an entrapment by fitting a Silastic tube around the medial popliteal nerve of young rabbits, and allowing growth to cause compression. The outer fibres of the nerve were more affected than the inner, and there was narrowing of axons, thinning of the myelin sheaths, and segmental demyelination at the level of the compression. Distally, a few fibres underwent axonal degeneration and regeneration.

A natural animal model of an entrapment neuropathy was also discovered by Fullerton and Gilliatt (1967b) in guinea pigs, in which species combined compression of the median and ulnar nerves under the cartilaginous transverse carpal bar may develop. The changes were similar to those found in man by Thomas and Fullerton (1963), but they additionally demonstrated the occurrence of segmental demyelination in the compressed region.

CONCLUSIONS

It has not been possible in this chapter to give a comprehensive account of the pathological abnormalities in peripheral nerve disorders. Instead, an attempt has been made to define the general patterns of structural change in peripheral neuropathy and to illustrate these with appropriate examples. No consideration has been given to peripheral nerve tumours and for this the reader is referred to the review by Kramer (1970). It is evident that further elucidation of the mechanisms involved in peripheral nerve disorders are to be anticipated as the techniques of cell biology are increasingly applied to the pathological situation.

REFERENCES

Abercrombie, M., Evans, D.H.L. & Murray, J.G. (1959) Nuclear multiplication and cell migration in degenerating unmyelinated nerve fibres. *Journal of Anatomy*, **93**, 9.

Abercrombie, M. & Johnson, M.L. (1946) Quantitative histology of Wallerian degeneration. I. Nuclear population in rabbit sciatic nerve. *Journal of Anatomy*, **80**, 37.

Adams, W.E. (1943) The blood supply of nerves. II. The effects of occlusion of its regional sources of supply on the sciatic nerve of the rabbit. *Journal of Anatomy*, **77**, 243.

Aguayo, A., Nair, C.P.V. & Midgley, R. (1971) Experimental progressive compressive neuropathy in the rabbit. Histological and electrophysiological studies. *Archives of Neurology*, **24**, 358.

Aitken, J.T., Sharman, M. & Young, J.Z. (1947) Maturation of regenerating nerve fibres with various peripheral connections. *Journal of Anatomy*, **81**, 1.

Allt, G. (1969) Repair of segmental demyelination in peripheral nerves: an electron microscope study. *Brain*, **92**, 639.

Allt, G. & Cavanagh, J.B. (1969) Ultrastructural changes in the region of the node of Ranvier in the rat caused by diphtheria toxin. *Brain*, **92**, 459.

Appenzeller, O. (1970) *The Autonomic Nervous System* (North-Holland Publishing Co: Amsterdam).

Asbury, A.K. (1970) The histogenesis of phagocytosis during Wallerian degeneration: radioautographic observations, *Proceedings VIth International Congress of Neuropathology* p. 666 (Masson: Paris).

Asbury, A.K., Aldredge, H., Hershberg, R. & Fisher, C.M. (1970) Oculomotor palsy in diabetes mellitus: a clinico-pathological study. *Brain*, **93**, 555.

Asbury, A.K., Arnason, B.G. & Adams, R.D. (1969) The inflammatory lesion in idiopathic polyneuritis. Its role in pathogenesis. *Medicine*, **48**, 173.

Asbury, A.K., Gale, M.K., Cox, S.C., Baringer, J.R. & Berg, B.O. (1972) Giant axonal neuropathy—a unique case with segmental neurofilamentous masses. *Acta Neuropathologica (Berlin)*, **20**, 237.

Asbury, A.K., Picard, E.H. & Baringer, J.R. (1972) Sensory perineuritis. *Archives of Neurology*, **26**, 302.

Ballin, R.H.M. & Thomas, P.K. (1968) Hypertrophic changes in diabetic neuropathy. *Acta Neuropathologica (Berlin)*, **11**, 93.

Ballin, R.H.M. & Thomas, P.K. (1969a) Electron microscopic observations on demyelination and remyelination in experimental allergic neuritis. I. Demyelination. *Journal of the Neurological Sciences*, **8**, 1.

Ballin, R.H.M. & Thomas, P.K. (1969b) Changes at the nodes of Ranvier during Wallerian degeneration: an electron microscopic study. *Acta Neuropathologica (Berlin)*, **14**, 237.

Barton, A.A. (1962) An electron microscope study of degeneration and regeneration of nerve. *Brain*, **85**, 799.

Behse, F., Buchthal, F., Carlsen, F. & Knappeis, G.G. (1972) Hereditary neuropathy with liability to pressure palsies: electrophysiological and histopathological aspects. *Brain*, **95**, 777.

Berger, B. (1971) Etude ultrastructurale de la dégénérescence Wallérienne experimentale d'un nerf entièrement amyelinique: le nerf olfactif. I. Modifications axonales. *Journal of Ultrastructural Research*, **37**, 105.

Berner, A., Torvik, A. & Stenwig, A.F. (1973) Origin of macrophages in traumatic nerve lesions and Wallerian degeneration in peripheral nerves. *Acta Neuropathologica (Berlin)*, **25**, 228.

Bischoff, A. (1968) Diabetische Neuropathie: pathologische Anatomie, Pathophysiologie und Pathogenese auf Grund elektronen-mikroskopischer Untersuchungen. *Deutsche Medizinische Wochenschrift*, **93**, 237.

Bischoff, A., Fierz, U., Regli, F. & Ulrich, J. (1968) Periphereneurologische Störungen bei der Fabryschen Krankheit (Angiokeratoma corporis diffusum universale). Klinisch-elektronenmikoskopische Befunde bei einem Fall. *Klinische Wochenschrift*, **46**, 666.

Bischoff, A. & Ulrich, J. (1969) Peripheral neuropathy in globoid cell leukodystrophy (Krabbe's disease). Ultrastructural and histochemical findings. *Brain*, **92**, 861.

Blunt, M.J. (1960) Ischemic degeneration of nerve fibers. *Archives of Neurology*, **2**, 528.

Bradley, W.G. & Asbury, A.K. (1970) The duration of synthesis phase in neurilemma cells in mouse sciatic nerve during degeneration. *Experimental Neurology*, **26**, 275.

Bradley, W.G. & Jaros, E. (1973) Axoplasmic flow in axonal neuropathies. II. Axoplasmic flow in mice with motor neuron disease and muscular dystrophy. *Brain*, **96**, 247.

Bradley, W.G. & Jennekens, F.G.I. (1971) Axonal degeneration in diphtheritic neuropathy. *Journal of the Neurological Sciences*, **13**, 415.

Bradley, W.G., Madrid, R., Thrush, D.C. & Campbell, M.J. (1975) Recurrent brachial plexus neuropathy. *Brain*, **98**, 381.

Bray, G.M., Peyronnard, J.M. & Aguayo, A.J. (1972) An ultrastructural study of degeneration and regeneration of unmyelinated nerve fibres. *Journal of Neuropathology and Experimental Neurology*, **31**, 197.

Cammermeyer, J. (1956) Neuropathological changes in hereditary neuropathies: manifestations of the syndrome of heredopathia atactica polyneuritiformis in the presence of interstitial hypertrophic polyneuropathy. *Journal of Neuropathology and Experimental Neurology*, **15**, 340.

Carpenter, S. (1972) An ultrastructural study of an acute fatal case of the Guillain-Barré syndrome. *Journal of the Neurological Sciences*, **15**, 125.

Carpenter, S., Karpati, G., Andermann, F. & Gold, R. (1974) Giant axonal neuropathy. A clinically and morphologically distinct neurological disease. *Archives of Neurology*, **31**, 312.

Caspary, E.A., Currie, S., Walton, J.N. & Field, E.J. (1971) Lymphocyte sensitization to nervous tissues and muscle in patients with the Guillain-Barré syndrome. *Journal of Neurology, Neurosurgery and Psychiatry*, **34**, 179.

Cavanagh, J.B. (1964) Peripheral nerve changes in orthocresyl phosphate poisoning in the cat. *Journal of Pathology and Bacteriology*, **87**, 365.

Cavanagh, J.B. & Jacobs, J.M. (1964) Some quantitative aspects of diphtheritic neuropathy. *British Journal of Experimental Pathology*, **45**, 309.

Cavanagh, J.B. & Mellick, R.S. (1965) On the nature of the peripheral nerve lesions associated with acute intermittent porphyria. *Journal of Neurology, Neurosurgery and Psychiatry*, **28**, 320.

Charlton, K.M. & Pierce, K.R. (1969) Peripheral neuropathy in experimental coyotillo poisoning in goats. *Texas Reports on Biology and Medicine*, **27**, 387.

Cho, E.S. (1977) Toxic effects of Adriamycin on the ganglia of the peripheral nervous system. A neuropathological study. *Journal of Neuropathology and Experimental Neurology*, **36**, 907.

Chopra, J.S. & Hurwitz, L.J. (1967) Internodal length of sural nerve fibres in chronic occlusive vascular disease. *Journal of Neurology, Neurosurgery and Psychiatry*, **30**, 207.

Coimbra, A. & Andrade, C. (1971) Familial amyloid polyneuropathy. An electron microscopic study of the peripheral nerve in five cases. *Brain*, **94**, 199–206, 207.

Collier, R.J. & Pappenheimer, A.M. Jr. (1964a) Studies on the mode of action of diphtheria toxin. I. Phosphorylated intermediates in normal and intoxicated HeLa cells. *Journal of Experimental Medicine*, **120**, 1007.

Collier, R.J. & Pappenheimer, A.M. Jr. (1964b) Studies on the mode of action of diphtheria toxin. II. Effect of toxin on amino acid incorporation in cell-free systems. *Journal of Experimental Medicine*, **120**, 1019.

Cragg, B.G. & Thomas, P.K. (1964) the conduction velocity of regenerated peripheral nerve fibres. *Journal of Physiology*, **171**, 164.

Dayan, A.D. (1967) Peripheral neuropathy of metachromatic leucodystrophy. Observations on segmental demyelination and remyelination and the intracellular distribution of sulphatide. *Journal of Neurology, Neurosurgery, and Psychiatry*, **30**, 311.

Dayan, A.D. & Sandbank, U. (1970) Pathology of the peripheral nervous system in leprosy. *Journal of Neurology, Neurosurgery and Psychiatry*, **33**, 586.

Dejerine, J. & Sottas, J. (1893) Sur la névrite interstitielle, hypertrophique et progressive de l'enfance. *Comptes rendues mensuels des séances de la Societé de biologie et de ses finales*, **45**, 63.

Denny-Brown, D. (1958) The neurological aspects of thiamine deficiency. *Federation Proceedings*, **17**, Suppl. 2, 35.

Denny-Brown, D., Adams, R.D., Brenner, C. & Doherty, M.M. (1945) The pathology of injury to nerve induced by cold. *Journal of Neuropathology and Experimental Neurology*, **4**, 305.

Denny-Brown, D. & Brenner, G. (1944) Paralysis of nerve induced by direct pressure and by tourniquet. *Archives of Neurology and Psychiatry*, **51**, 1.

Dixon, J.S. (1969) Changes in the fine structure of satellite cells surrounding chromatolytic neurons. *Anatomical Record*, **163**, 101.

Dreyfus, P.M., Hakim, S. & Adams, R.D. (1957) Diabetic ophthalmoplegia. *Archives of Neurology and Psychiatry*, **77**, 337.

Dunn, H.G., Lake, B.D., Dolman, C.L. & Wilson, J. (1969) The neuropathy of Krabbe's infantile cerebral sclerosis. (Globoid cell leucodystrophy). *Brain*, **92**, 329.

Dyck, P.J. (1969) Experimental hypertrophic neuropathy. Pathogenesis of onion-bulb formations produced by repeated tourniquet applications. *Archives of Neurology*, **21**, 73.

Dyck, P.J. & Hopkins, A.P. (1972) Electron microscopic observations on degeneration and regeneration of unmyelinated fibres. *Brain*, **95**, 223.

Dyck, P.J. & Lambert, E.H. (1969) Dissociated sensation in amyloidosis. Compound action potential, quantitative histologic and teased fiber, and electron microscopic studies of sural nerve biopsies. *Archives of Neurology*, **20**, 490.

Dyck, P.J., Conn, D.L. & Okazaki, H. (1972) Necrotizing angiopathic neuropathy. Three-dimensional morphology of fiber degeneration related to sites of occluded vessels. *Proceedings of the Mayo Clinic*, **47**, 461.

Dyck, P.J., Ellefson, R.D., Yao, J.K. & Herbert, P.N. (1978)

Adult-onset of Tangier disease: I. Morphometric and pathologic studies suggesting delayed degradation of neutral lipids after fiber degeneration. *Journal of Neuropathology and Experimental Neurology*, **37**, 119.

Dyck, P.J., Johnson, W.J., Lambert, E.H. & O'Brien, P.C. (1971) Segmental demyelination secondary to axonal degeneration in uremic neuropathy. *Proceedings of the Mayo Clinic*, **46**, 400.

Dyck, P.J., Lambert, E.H., Sanders, K. & O'Brien, P.C. (1971) Severe hypomyelination and marked abnormality of conduction in Dejerine-Sottas hypertrophic neuropathy: myelin thickness and compound action potential of sural nerve *in vitro*. *Proceedings of the Mayo Clinic*, **46**, 432.

Dyck, P.J., Ellefson, R.D., Lais, A.C., Smith, R.C., Taylor, W.F. & Van Dyke, R.A. (1970) Histologic and lipid studies of sural nerves in inherited hypertrophic neuropathy: preliminary report of a lipid abnormality in nerve and liver in Dejerine-Sottas disease. *Proceedings of the Mayo Clinic*, **45**, 286.

Eames, R.A. & Lange, L.S. (1967) Clinical and pathological study of ischaemic neuropathy. *Journal of Neurology, Neurosurgery and Psychiatry*, **30**, 215.

Evans, D.H.L. & Murray, J.G. (1954) Regeneration of non-medullated nerve fibres. *Journal of Anatomy*, **88**, 465.

Fardeau, M. & Engel, K. (1969) Ultrastructural study of a peripheral nerve biopsy in Refsum's disease. *Journal of Neuropathology and Experimental Neurology*, **28**, 278.

Fisher, C.M. & Adams, R.D. (1955) Diphtheritic polyneuritis: a pathological study. *Journal of Neuropathology and Experimental Neurology*, **15**, 243.

Friede, R.L. & Johnstone, M.A. (1966) Responses of thymidine labeling in grey matter and nerve following sciatic transection. *Acta Neuropathologica (Berlin)*, **7**, 218.

Fullerton, P.M. & Barnes, J.M. (1966) Peripheral neuropathy in rats produced by acrylamide. *British Journal of Industrial Medicine*, **23**, 210.

Fullerton, P.M. & Gilliatt, R.W. (1967a) Pressure neuropathy in the hind foot of the guinea pig. *Journal of Neurology, Neurosurgery and Psychiatry*, **30**, 18.

Fullerton, P.M. & Gilliatt, R.W. (1967b) Median and ulnar nerve neuropathy in the guinea pig. *Journal of Neurology, Neurosurgery and Psychiatry*, **30**, 393.

Fullerton, P.M., Gilliatt, R.W., Lascelles, R.G. & Morgan-Hughes, J.A. (1965) Relation between fibre diameter and internodal length in chronic neuropathy. *Journal of Physiology*, **178**, 26P.

Gamble, H.J. (1964) Comparative electron-microscopic observations on the connective tissues of a peripheral nerve and a spinal nerve root in the rat. *Journal of Anatomy*, **98**, 17.

Gamble, H.J. & Eames, R.A. (1964) An electron microscope study of the connective tissues of human peripheral nerve. *Journal of Anatomy*, **98**, 655.

Ghabriel M.N. & Allt, G. (1979) the role of Schmidt-Lantermann incisures in Wallerian degeneration. II An electron microscope study. *Acta Neuropathologica (Berlin)*, **48**, 95.

Gibson, J.G. (1979) The origin of the neural macrophage. A quantitative ultrastructural study of cell population changes during Wallerian degeneration. *Journal of Anatomy*, **129**, 1.

Glimstedt, G. & Wohlfart, G. (1960) Electron microscopic observations on Wallerian degeneration in peripheral nerves. *Acta Morphologica Neerlando-Scandanavica*, **3**, 135.

Gombault, A. (1880) Contribution à l'étude anatomique de la névrite parenchymateuse subaiguë et chronique. Névrite segmentaire péri-axile. *Archives de Neurologie (Paris)*, **i**, 177.

Gombault, A. & Mallet, J. (1889) Un cas du tabes ayant debute dans l'enfance: autopsie. *Archives Médicales*, **1**, 385.

Greenfield, J.G. & Carmichael, E.A. (1935) The peripheral nerves in cases of subacute combined degeneration of the cord. *Brain*, **58**, 483.

Gueuning, C. & Graff, G.L.A. (1971) Métabolisme des phosphates inorganiques et organiques acidosolubles dans le nerf sciatique du rat au cours de la phase aiguë de la dégénérescence Wallérienne. *Comptes rendus des séances de la Société de biologie*, **165**, 1479.

Haftek, J. & Thomas, P.K. (1968) Electron-microscope observations on the effects of localized crush injuries on the connective tissues of peripheral nerve. *Journal of Anatomy*, **103**, 233.

Haller, F.R. & Low, F.N. (1971) The fine structure of the peripheral nerve root sheath in the subarachnoid space in the rat and other laboratory animals. *American Journal of Anatomy*, **131**, 1.

Hallpike, J.F. & Adams, C.W.M. (1969) Proteolysis and myelin breakdown: a review of recent histochemical and biochemical studies. *Histochemistry Journal*, **1**, 559.

Harris, J.B. & Thesleff, S. (1972) Nerve stump length and membrane changes in denervated skeletal muscle. *Nature*, **236**, 60.

Heinlein, H. (1949) Die Verlaufsformen der Diphtherie. *Klinische Wochenschrift*, **27**, 721.

Hochhaus, H. (1891) Ueber diphtherische Lähmungen. *Virchows Archiv für pathologische Anatomie und Physiologie und für klinische Medizin*, **124**, 226.

Holtzman, E. & Novikoff, A.B. (1965) Lysosomes in the rat sciatic nerve following crush. *Journal of Cell Biology*, **27**, 651.

Hydén, H. (1959) Biochemical changes in glial cells and nerve cells at varying activity. In *Biochemistry of the Central Nervous System*, p. 64 (Pergamon: New York).

Igisu, H., Ohta, M., Tabira, T., Hosokawa, S., Goto, I. & Kuroiwa, Y. (1975) Giant axonal neuropathy: a clinical entity affecting the central as well as the peripheral nervous system. *Neurology (Minneapolis)*, **25**, 717.

Jacobs, J.M., Carmichael, N. & Cavanagh, J.B. (1975) Ultrastructional changes in the dorsal root and trigeminal ganglion of rats poisoned with methyl mercury. *Neuropathology and Applied Neurobiology*, **1**, 1.

Jacobs, J.M., Cavanagh, J.B. & Mellick, R.S. (1967) Intraneural injection of diphtheria toxin. *British Journal of Experimental Pathology*, **48**, 204.

Jennekens, F.G.I., Van Spijk, D. Van Der Most & Dorhout Mees, E.J. (1969) Nerve fibre degeneration in uraemic polyneuropathy. *Proceedings of the European Dialysis and Transplant Association*, **6**, 191.

Job, C.K. (1971) Pathology of peripheral nerve lesions in lepromatous leprosy. A light and electron microscopic study. *International Journal of Leprosy*, **39**, 251.

Job, C.K. & Desikan, K.V. (1968) Pathologic changes and their distribution in peripheral nerves in lepromatous leprosy. *International Journal of Leprosy*, **36**, 257.

Kocen, R.S. & Thomas, P.K. (1970) Peripheral nerve involvement in Fabry's disease. *Archives of Neurology*, **22**, 81.

Kocen, R.S., King, R.H.M., Thomas, P.K. & Haas, L.F. (1973) Nerve biopsy findings in two cases of Tangier disease. *Acta Neuropathologica (Berlin)*, **26**, 317.

Kramer, W. (1970) Tumours of nerves. In *Handbook of Clinical Neurology*, Eds P.J. Vinken, & G.W. Bruyn, Vol. 8, p. 412 (North-Holland: Amsterdam).

Kreutzberg, G.W. (1967) Autoradiographic study on incorporation of Leucine-H³ in peripheral nerves during regeneration. *Experientia*, **23**, 33.

Lampert, P. (1969) Mechanism of demyelination in experimental allergic neuritis. *Laboratory Investigation*, **20**, 127.

Lampert, P.W. & Schochet, S.S. (1968) Demyelination and remyelination in lead neuropathy. Electron microscope studies. *Journal of Neuropathology and Experimental Neurology*, **27**, 527.

Landon, D.N. & Williams, P.L. (1963) Ultrastructure of the node of Ranvier. *Nature*, **199**, 575.

Lascelles, R.G. & Thomas, P.K. (1966) Changes due to age in internodal length in the sural nerve of man. *Journal of Neurology, Neurosurgery and Psychiatry*, **29**, 40.

Lasek, R. (1968) Axoplasmic transport in cat dorsal root ganglion cells as studied with ³H-L-leucine. *Brain Research*, **7**, 360.

Leech, R.W. (1967) Changes in satellite cells of rat dorsal root ganglia during central chromatolysis. *Neurology (Minneapolis)*, **17**, 349.

Lockman, L.A., Kennedy, W.R. & White, J.G. (1967) The Chediak-Higashi syndrome: electrophysiological and electron microscope observations on the peripheral neuropathy. *Journal of Pediatrics*, **70**, 942.

Logan, J.E., Mannell, W.A. & Rossiter, R.J. (1952) Chemical studies of peripheral nerve during Wallerian degeneration. 3: Nucleic acids and other protein-bound phosphorus compounds. *Biochemistry Journal*, **51**, 482.

Low, P.A. & Dyck, P.J. (1977) Increased endoneurial fluid pressure in experimental lead neuropathy. *Nature*, **269**, 427.

Lubińska, L. & Waryszewska, J. (1973) Wallerian degeneration and axoplasmic flow. *Proceedings of the Symposium on Structure and Function of Normal and Disordered Muscle and Peripheral Nerve*. Kazimierz, Poland.

Luse, S.A. & McCaman, R.E. (1957) Electron microscopy and biochemistry of Wallerian degeneration in optic and tibial nerves. *American Journal of Pathology*, **33**, 586.

McDonald, W.I. (1963) Effect of experimental demyelination on conduction in peripheral nerve. I. Clinical and histological observations. *Brain*, **86**, 481.

Madrid, R. & Bradley, W.G. (1975) The pathology of neuropathies with focal thickening of the myelin sheath (tomaculous neuropathy). *Journal of the Neurological Sciences*, **25**, 415.

Mahloudji, M., Teasdall, R.D., Adamkiewicz, J.J., Hartmann, W.H., Lambird, P.A. & McKusick, V.A. (1969) The genetic amyloidoses, with particular reference to hereditary neuropathic amyloidosis, Type II (Indiana or Rukavina Type). *Medicine*, **48**, 1.

Masurovsky, E.B. & Bunge, R.P. (1971) Patterns of myelin degeneration following rapid death of cells in cultures of peripheral nerve tissue. *Journal of Neuropathology and Experimental Neurology*, **30**, 311.

Matthews, W.B. (1975) Sarcoid neuropathy. In *Peripheral Neuropathy*, Eds P.J. Dyck, P.K. Thomas, & E.H. Lambert (Saunders: Philadelphia).

Miledi, R. & Slater, C.R. (1970) On the degeneration of rat neuromuscular junctions after nerve section. *Journal of Physiology*, **207**, 507.

Morgan-Hughes, J.A. (1968) Experimental diphtheritic neuropathy. A pathological and electrophysiological study. *Journal of the Neurological Sciences*, **7**, 157.

Morgan-Hughes, J.A. & Engel, W.K. (1968) Structural and histochemical changes in the axons following nerve crush. *Archives of Neurology*, **19**, 598.

Nathaniel, E.J.H. & Pease, D.C. (1963a) Degenerative changes in rat dorsal roots during Wallerian degeneration. *Ultrastructural Research*, **9**, 511.

Nathaniel, E.J.H. & Pease, D.C. (1963b) Regenerative changes in rat dorsal roots following Wallerian degeneration. *Ultrastructural Research*, **9**, 533.

Neary, D. & Eames, R.A. (1975) The pathology of ulnar nerve compression in man. *Neuropathology and Applied Neurobiology*, **1**, 69.

Neary, D., Ochoa, J. & Gilliatt, R.W. (1975) Sub-clinical entrapment neuropathy in man. *Journal of the Neurological Sciences*, **24**, 283.

Ochoa, J., Danta, G., Fowler, T.J. & Gilliatt, R.W. (1971) Nature of the nerve lesion caused by a pneumatic tourniquet. *Nature*, **233**, 265.

O'Daly, J.A. & Imaeda, T. (1967) Electron microscopic study of Wallerian degeneration in cutaneous nerves caused by mechanical injury. *Laboratory Investigation*, **17**, 744.

Oderfeld-Nowak, N. & Niemierko, S. (1969) Synthesis of nucleic acids in the Schwann cells as the early cellular response to nerve injury. *Journal of Neurochemistry*, **16**, 235.

Ohnishi, A., Schilling, K., Brimijoin, W.S., Lambert, E.H., Fairbanks, F. & Dyck, P.J. (1977) Lead neuropathy. I. Morphometry, nerve conduction and choline acetyl transferase transport: new finding of endoneurial edema associated with segmental demyelination. *Journal of Neuropathology and Experimental Neurology*, **36**, 499.

Olsson, Y. (1975) Blood supply to peripheral nerve and altered vascular permeability in disease. In *Peripheral Neuropathy*, Eds P.J. Dyck, P.K. Thomas & E.H. Lambert (Saunders: Philadelphia).

Olsson, Y. & Sjöstrand, J. (1969) Origin of macrophages in Wallerian degeneration of peripheral nerves demonstrated autoradiographically. *Experimental Neurology*, **23**, 102.

Pannese, E. (1964) Number and structure of perisomatic satellite cells of spinal ganglia under normal conditions or during axon regeneration and neuronal hypertrophy. *Zeitschift für Zellforschung und mikropische Anatomie*, **63**, 568.

Pleasure, D.E., Feldmann, B. & Prockop, D.J. (1973) Diphtheria toxin inhibits the synthesis of myelin proteolipid and basic proteins by peripheral nerve *in vitro*. *Journal of Neurochemistry*, **20**, 81.

Prineas, J. (1973) Demyelination in the Guillain-Barré syndrome: an electron microscopic study. *Proceedings of the 2nd International Congress on Muscle Diseases*, Perth, W. Australia (Excerpta Medica: Amsterdam).

Prineas, J. & Spencer, P.S. (1975) Pathology of the nerve cell body in disorders of the peripheral nervous system. In *Peripheral Neuropathy*, Eds P.J. Dyck, P.K. Thomas, & E. H. Lambert (Saunders: Philadelphia).

Raff, M.C., Sangalang, V. & Asbury, A.K. (1968) Ischemic mononeuropathy multiplex associated with diabetes mellitus. *Archives of Neurology*, **18**, 487.

Ranson, S.W. (1912) Degeneration and regeneration of nerve fibers. *Journal of Comparative Neurology*, **22**, 487.

Rawlins, F.A., Hedley-Whyte, E.T., Villegas, G. & Uzman, B.G. (1970) Reutilisation of cholesterol-1,2-H^3 in the regeneration of peripheral nerve. *Laboratory Investigation*, **23**, 237.

Rees, R.J.W., Weddell, G., Palmer, E. & Jamison, D.G. (1965) Experimental studies on nerve fibres in leprosy. II. The reaction of human Schwann cells toward carbon particles and leprosy bacilli. *International Journal of Leprosy*, **33**, 160.

Rexed, B. & Fredriksson, T. (1956) The frequency of Schwann cell mitoses in degenerating nerves. *Acta Societatis Medicorum Upsaliensis*, **61**, 199.

Ridley, D.S. & Jopling, W.H. (1966) Classification of leprosy according to immunity: a five group system. *International Journal of Leprosy*, **34**, 255.

Ross, M.H. & Reith, E.J. (1969) Perineurium: evidence for contractile elements. *Science*, **165**, 604.

Roth, C.D. & Richardson, K.C. (1969) Electron microscopical studies on axonal degeneration in the rat iris following ganglionectomy. *American Journal of Anatomy*, **124**, 341.

Schaumburg, H.H., Byck, R. & Weller, R.O. (1970) The effects of phenol on peripheral nerve. A histological and electrophysiological study. *Journal of Neuropathology and Experimental Neurology*, **29**, 615.

Schlaepfer, W.W. (1969) Experimental lead neuropathy: a disease of the supporting cells in the peripheral nervous system. *Journal of Neuropathology and Experimental Neurology*, **28**, 401.

Schoental, R. & Cavanagh, J.B. (1977) Mechanisms involved in the 'dying-back' process—an hypothesis implicating coenzymes. *Neuropathology and Applied Neurobiology*, **3**, 145.

Schröder, J.M. (1968) Die Hyperneurotisation Büngnerscher Bänder bei der experimentellen Isoniazid-Neuropathie: Phasenkontrast- und elekronenmikroskopische Untersuchungen. *Virchow Archiv, Abt. B. Zellpath.*, **1**, 131.

Schröder, J.M. & Krücke, W. (1970) Zur Feinstruktur der experimentellallergischen Neuritis beim Kaninchen. *Acta Neuropathologica (Berlin)*, **14**, 261.

Seiler, N. & Schröder, J.M. (1970) Beziehungen zwischen Polyaminen und Nucleinsauren. II. Biochemische und feinstrukturelle Untersuchungen am peripheren Nerven während der Wallerschen Degeneration. *Brain Research*, **22**, 81.

Singer, M. & Salpeter, M.M. (1966a) The transport of ^{3}H-L-histidine through the Schwann cell and myelin sheath into the axon, including a re-evaluation of myelin function. *Journal of Morphology*, **120**, 281.

Singer, M. & Salpeter, M.M. (1966b) Transport of tritium-labelled L-histidine through the Schwann and myelin sheaths into axons of peripheral nerve. *Nature*, **210**, 1225.

Sourander, P. & Olsson, Y. (1968) Peripheral neuropathy in globoid cell leucodystrophy (Morbus Krabbe). *Acta Neuropathologica (Berlin)*, **11**, 69.

Spencer, P.S., Sabri, M.I. Schaumburg, H.H. & Moore, C.L. (1979) Hypothesis: does a defect of energy metabolism in the nerve fiber underlie axonal degeneration in polyneuropathies? *Annals of Neurology*, **5**, 501.

Spencer, P.S. & Schaumburg, H.H. (1974) A review of acrylamide neurotoxicity. *Canadian Journal of Neurological Sciences*, **1**, 143, 152.

Spencer, P.S. & Schaumburg, H.H. (1976) Central-peripheral distal axonopathy—the pathology of dying-back polyneuropathies. *Progress in Neuropathology*, **3**, 253.

Spencer, P.S. & Schaumburg, H.H. (1978) Pathobiology of neurotoxic axonal degeneration. In *Physiology and Pathobiology of Axons*, Ed. S.G. Waxman (Raven Press: New York).

Spencer, P.S. & Thomas, P.K. (1970) The examination of isolated nerve fibres by light and electron microscopy with observations on demyelination proximal to neuromas. *Acta Neuropathologica (Berlin)*, **16**, 177.

Stewart, B.M. (1966) Hypertrophic neuropathy of acromegaly. *Archives of Neurology*, **14**, 107.

Swank, R.L. (1940) Avian thiamine deficiency. A correlation of the pathological and clinical behavior. *Journal of Experimental Medicine*, **71**, 683.

Taxi, J. (1959) Etude au microscope électronique de la dégénérescence Wallérienne des fibres nerveuses amyéliniques. *Comptes rendus hebdomadaires des séances de l'Academie des Sciences*, **248**, 2796.

Thomas, G.A. (1948) Quantitative histology of Wallerian degeneration. II. Nuclear populations in two nerves of different fibre spectrum. *Journal of Anatomy*, **82**, 135.

Thomas, P.K. (1970) The cellular response to nerve injury. 3: The effect of repeated crush injuries. *Journal of Anatomy*, **106**, 463.

Thomas, P.K. (1971) Morphological basis for alterations in nerve conduction in peripheral neuropathies. *Proceedings of the Royal Society of Medicine*, **64**, 295.

Thomas, P.K. & Fullerton, P.M. (1963) Nerve fibre size in the carpal tunnel syndrome. *Journal of Neurology, Neurosurgery and Psychiatry*, **26**, 520.

Thomas, P.K., Hollinrake, K., Lascelles, R.G., O'Sullivan, D.J., Baillod, R.A., Moorhead, J.F. & McKenzie, J.C. (1971) The polyneuropathy of chronic renal failure. *Brain*, **94**, 761.

Thomas, P.K. & King, R.H.M. (1974) Peripheral nerve changes in amyloid neuropathy. *Brain*, **97**, 395.

Thomas, P.K., King, R.H.M. & Phelps, A.C. (1972) Electron microscope observations on the degeneration of unmyelinated fibres following nerve section. *Journal of Anatomy*, **113**, 279.

Thomas, P.K. & Lascelles, R.G. (1967) Hypertrophic neuropathy. *Quarterly Journal of Medicine*, **36**, 223.

Thomas, P.K. & Olsson, Y. (1975) The microscopic anatomy and function of the connective tissue components of peripheral nerve. In *Peripheral Neuropathy*, Eds P.J. Dyck, P.K. Thomas & E.H. Lambert (Saunders: Philadelphia).

Thomas, P.K. & Walker, J.G. (1965) Xanthomatous neuropathy in primary biliary cirrhosis. *Brain*, **88**, 1079.

Van Allen, M.W., Frohlich, J.A. & Davis, J.R. (1969) Inherited predisposition to generalised amyloidosis. Clinical and pathological study of a family with neuropathy, nephropathy and peptic ulcer. *Neurology (Minneapolis)*, **19**, 10.

Vial, J.D. (1958) the early changes in the axoplasm during Wallerian degeneration. *Journal of Biophysical and Biochemical Cytology*, **4**, 551.

Vizoso, A.D. & Young, J.Z. (1948) Internodal length and fibre diameter in developing and regenerating nerves. *Journal of Anatomy*, **82**, 110.

Waksman, B.H. (1961) Experimental study of diphtheritic polyneuritis in the rabbit and guinea pig. III. The blood-nerve barrier in the rabbit. *Journal of Neuropathology and Experimental Neurology*, **20**, 35.

Waksman, B.H. & Adams, R.D. (1955) Allergic neuritis: an experimental disease of rabbits induced by the injection of peripheral nervous tissue and adjuvants. *Journal of Experimental Medicine*, **102**, 213.

Waksman, B.H. & Adams, R.D. (1956) A comparative study of experimental allergic neuritis in the rabbit, guinea pig and mouse. *Journal of Neuropathology and Experimental Neurology*, **15**, 293.

Waksman, B.H., Adams, R.D. & Mansmann, H.C. Jr. (1957) Experimental study of diphtheritic polyneuritis in the rabbit and guinea pig. Part I. Immunologic and histopathologic observations. *Journal of Experimental Medicine*, **105**, 591.

Webster, H. de F. (1962a) Transient focal accumulation of axonal mitochondria during the early stages of Wallerian degeneration. *Journal of Cell Biology*, **12**, 361.

Webster, H. de F. (1962b) Schwann cell alterations in metachromatic leukodystrophy: preliminary phase and electron microscopic observations. *Journal of Neuropathology and Experimental Neurology*, **21**, 534.

Webster, H. de F. (1964) Some ultrastructural features of segmental demyelination and myelin regeneration in peripheral nerve. In *Mechanisms of Neural Regeneration*, Eds M. Singer & J.P. Schadé, *Progress in Brain Research*, **13**, 151–172.

Webster, H. de F. (1965) The relationship between Schmidt-Lantermann incisures and myelin segmentation during Wallerian degeneration. *Annals of the New York Academy of Sciences*, **122**, 29.

Webster, H. de F., Schröder, J.M. Asbury, A.K. & Adams, R.D. (1967) The role of Schwann cells in the formation of 'onion bulbs' found in chronic neuropathies. *Journal of Neuropathology and Experimental Neurology*, **26**, 276.

Webster, H. de F., Spiro, D., Waksman, B. & Adams, R.D. (1961) Phase and electron microscope studies of experimental demyelination. II. Schwann cell changes in guinea pig sciatic nerves during experimental diphtheritic neuritis. *Journal of Neuropathology and Experimental Neurology*, **20**, 5.

Weddell, G. & Glees, P. (1941) The early stages in the degeneration of cutaneous nerve fibres. *Journal of Anatomy*, **76**, 65.

Weinberg, H.J. & Spencer, P.S. (1978) The fate of Schwann cells isolated from axonal contact. *Journal of Neurocytology*, **7**, 555.

Weiss, P. & Hiscoe, H. (1948) Experiments on the mechanism of nerve growth. *Journal of Experimental Zoology*, **107**, 315.

Weller, R.O. (1965) Diphtheritic neuropathy in the chicken. *Journal of Pathology and Bacteriology*, **89**, 591.

Weller, R.O. (1967) An electron microscope study of hypertrophic neuropathy of Dejerine and Sottas. *Journal of Neurology, Neurosurgery and Psychiatry*, **30**, 111.

Weller, R.O. & Das Gupta, T.K. (1968) Experimental hypertrophic neuropathy. An electron microscopic study. *Journal of Neurology, Neurosurgery and Psychiatry*, **31**, 34.

Weller, R.O. & Mellick, R.S. (1966) Acid phosphatase and lysosomal activity in diphtheritic neuropathy and Wallerian degeneration. *British Journal of Experimental Pathology*, **47**, 425.

Weller, R.O. & Nester, B. (1972) Early changes at the node of Ranvier in segmental demyelination: histochemical and electron microscopical observations. *Brain*, **95**, 665.

Williams, P.L. & Hall, S.M. (1971a) Prolonged *in vivo* observations of normal peripheral nerve fibres and their acute reactions to crush and deliberate trauma. *Journal of Anatomy (London)*, **108**, 397.

Williams, P.L. & Hall, S.M. (1971b) Chronic Wallerian

degeneration—an *in vivo* and ultrastructural study. *Journal of Anatomy*, **109**, 487.

Wisniewski, H., Prineas, J. & Raine, C.S. (1969) An ultrastructural study of experimental demyelination and remyelination. I. Acute experimental allergic encephalomyelitis in the peripheral nervous system. *Laboratory Investigation*, **21**, 105.

Wisniewski, H., Terry, R.D., Whitaker, J.N., Cook, S.D. & Dowling, P.C. (1969) The Landry-Guillain-Barré syndrome. A primary demyelinating disease. *Archives of Neurology*, **21**, 269.

Young, J.Z. (1942) Functional repair of nervous tissue. *Physiological Reviews*, **22**, 318.

Pathological anatomy of the intramuscular motor innervation

INTRODUCTION

Within the muscles are found the peripheral endings of the anterior horn cells and of some of the cells of the posterior root ganglia, the γ fibres providing the motor innervation of the muscle spindles, and also postganglionic fibres of the autonomic system. In this chapter we shall concern ourselves particularly with the pathology of the anterior horn cells and α-motor neurones, because the authors have little experience of abnormalities of the other types of nerve endings and it appears that there have been few reports of any such abnormalities in the literature (Kennedy, 1969; Swash, 1972; Swash and Fox, 1974, 1975a, b).

Muscle biopsy is of considerable value to neuropathology and in neurological diagnosis as it permits the microscopic investigation of a group of neurones during life. Muscle biopsy is particularly useful in the study of the neurone by means of electron microscopy in that the nerve fibres separate from one another after their emergence from the intramuscular nerve bundles; each nerve fibre may therefore be followed in isolation for long distances against the comparatively simple background of the muscle fibres, an impossible achievement in the dense network of glial and neuronal processes in the brain.

It cannot be denied that the absence of the cell body of the anterior horn cell from muscle biopsy specimens constitutes a major weakness of this method of neuronal study. On the other hand, it sharpens the acuteness with which we endeavour to interpret the changes in the nerve endings. In this interpretation we are greatly assisted by the phenomenon of 'dying back' of the neurone (see discussion in Coërs and Woolf, 1959) first described almost 100 years ago and responsible for some of the most characteristic features of disease of the peripheral nerves. The tendency for the earliest changes in the anterior horn cell to take place at, and to remain for a time localised to, the end-plate and the adjacent portion of the axon, not only greatly enhances the value of muscle biopsy but makes this *intra-vitam* examination an essential part of the investigation of any neuromuscular disease. Full demonstration of the nerve endings cannot be achieved after death so that, where post-mortem study only is possible, the most meticulous histological study of the cord may still fail to show any sign of neuronal disease.

The standing of muscle biopsy, both as a diagnostic weapon and as a research tool, has been greatly enhanced in the last three decades and this development has been made possible through the following contributions: (1) the demonstration of the zonal distribution of the intramuscular nerve endings (Coërs, 1953a); (2) the introduction into human muscle biopsy technique of vital staining of the nerve fibres and endings with methylene blue (Coërs, 1952); (3) the application to human muscle biopsies of Koelle's method of demonstration of the subneural apparatus of the end-plate by means of its cholinesterase activity (Coërs, 1953b).

The zonal distribution of the motor nerve endings

The cholinesterase technique (*see below*) clearly demonstrated that the motor end-plates are situated near the centre of each muscle fibre and are therefore confined in each fasciculus to a restricted zone (the innervation zone) (Fig. 7.1) (Coërs, 1953a). In certain muscles it was possible to localise this zone by determining the motor point by direct electrical stimulation, the innervation zone lying immediately deep to the motor point. This constituted a great advance in biopsy technique because it was now possible to decide more or less accurately the point over which the skin incision should be centred in order best to expose the nerve endings. Because of their position at the centre of the muscle fibre it followed that the end-

plates would lie on the surface only in those muscles in which the fasciculi ran parallel with the surface of the limb, while in those in which the fasciculi arose from the fascia and were inserted into a deeply situated tendon (e.g. tibialis anterior) the end-plates would be deeply situated and it would be difficult to obtain nerve endings in a specimen, except by cutting deeply into the muscle. It appears that there are some muscles (e.g. sartorius) which are formed of parallel bundles of short fibres linked together in series so that there is a corresponding series of innervation bands at intervals along the length of the muscle, but this is exceptional.

Vital staining with methylene blue

The ability of axons and their endings to take up methylene blue as a vital process was first demonstrated by Ehrlich (1882, 1886). Subsequently Dogiel (1890, 1891, 1902) and Attias (1912) used this phenomenon to demonstrate human nerve endings; they immersed the tissue to be examined in the methylene blue solution after removal (supravital staining). Later, workers using experimental animals introduced the stain by perfusion (Hines and Tower, 1928). Weddell (1941a, b) introduced it by local injection in studies of human

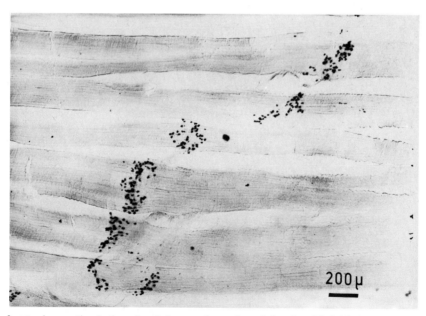

Fig. 7.1 Zone of motor innervation in the palmaris longus of a newborn infant (modified thiocholine method)

cutaneous nerve endings. The technique of local injection was subsequently applied to muscle biopsy in man (Coërs, 1952).

Vital staining with methylene blue has the great advantage over silver impregnation that it shows the end-plate with a completeness and delicacy never attained with silver (Figs. 7.2 and 7.3) it also enables the terminal axoplasmic expansions to be demonstrated and photographed, even before fixation, when they are in a living or near-living state. Under these circumstances the expansions appear fuller than after fixation and this may well prove to be of importance in controlling electron-microscopic studies.

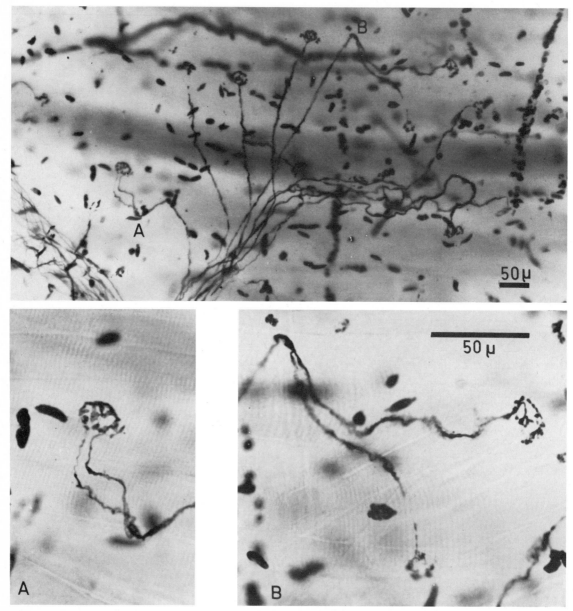

Fig. 7.2　Normal pattern of terminal motor innervation (vital staining with methylene blue. Squash preparation). A. Distal branching forming one motor arborisation. B. Collateral branching forming two motor arborisations subserving different muscle fibres

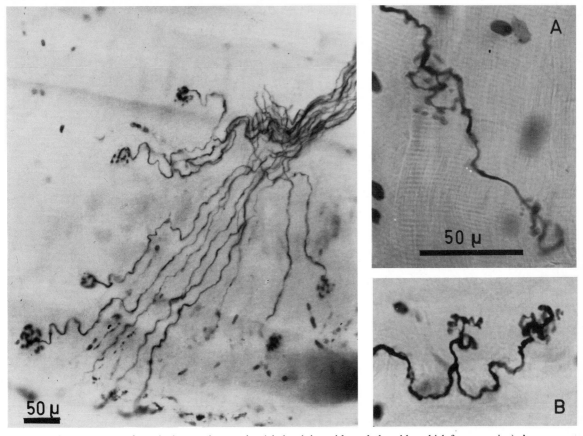

Fig. 7.3 Normal pattern of terminal motor innervation (vital staining with methylene blue, thick frozen section). A. Ultraterminal ramification subserving two different muscle fibres. B. Distal ramification forming two motor arborisations subserving the same muscle fibre

Demonstration of cholinesterase in the subneural apparatus of the end-plates

Many histochemical techniques have been applied to muscle but none shows up morphological details as well as does the demonstration of cholinesterase activity, which reveals the structure of the sub-neural apparatus of the end-plate (Fig. 7.4). This effect is apparently due to the high concentration of the enzyme in the junctional sarcolemmal folds and its precise restriction to this area.

Two methods have been used to demonstrate the enzyme—the copper thiocholine technique of Koelle (Koelle and Friedenwald, 1949; Couteaux, 1951; Coërs, 1953b; Coërs and Woolf, 1959) and the indoxyl method of Holt (Holt, 1952, 1956; Holt and Withers, 1956). We have experience only of the former method, but it may well be that the dye technique shows the subneural apparatus

more sharply; certainly it has the advantage of requiring a very short period of incubation with substrate, which may be of great value where it is intended to examine the specimen with the electron microscope (see below).

TECHNIQUE OF MUSCLE BIOPSY

Selection of muscle

The selection of muscles for biopsies suitable for study of changes in the motor nerve endings requires a knowledge of the likely distribution of the disease process in each case. It is essential to choose a muscle in which the innervation is only lightly, though definitely, affected, as the earliest stages of the pathological changes are likely to be

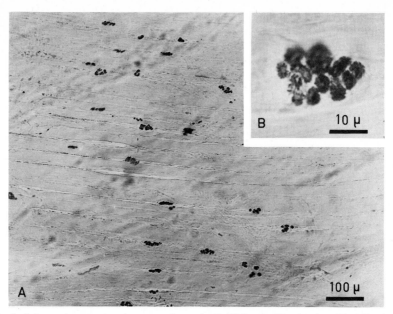

Fig. 7.4   A. Subneural apparatuses in a normal muscle. B. High magnification (modified Koelle method)

the most characteristic and, in severely affected muscles, nerve fibres may be scarce or totally absent. For these reasons, muscles which show marked weakness and wasting should not be biopsied. On the other hand a clinically unaffected forearm muscle may be more suitable, even if signs of disease are confined to the lower limbs. This is particularly likely to be the case if the disease is such that it affects all lower motor neurones, though showing itself especially at the distal ends of those with the longest axons. This applies to most peripheral neuropathies and the choice of a forearm muscle is justified if there is a complaint of paraesthesiae in the finger tips. Even in the absence of such symptoms we have often been rewarded by studying an upper extremity muscle, because demonstration of involvement of its innervation permits exclusion of lumbosacral root or cord compression as an explanation of obvious lower motor neurone disease in the legs. To demonstrate degeneration in the leg muscles by biopsy in such cases is merely to provide super-fluous evidence of what is already known. The possibility of causing a traumatic myositis by carrying out preliminary electromyography on the muscle to be biopsied must be noted. The danger lies in accepting the resultant myositis as being the primary disease (Woolf, 1962c).

There are additional advantages in studying a forearm muscle wherever possible, especially flexor carpi radialis or palmaris longus. In these two muscles the fasciculi run parallel with the overlying fascia, so that they can be exposed practically from origin to insertion simply by incising the fascia in the line of the tendon of insertion. The end-plates lie at the centre of each fasciculus and as, in these muscles, the motor nerve pierces and penetrates the muscle from a point at the centre of the muscle on its deep surface, it is clear that if the incision in the skin and fascia is centred on the motor point (determined by electrical stimulation) the innervation zones will be exposed. This by no means applies to other muscles. As mentioned above, in some muscles (e.g. flexor carpi ulnaris, tibialis anterior) the fasciculi arise superficially but plunge deeply towards the tendon of insertion so that the innervation zone is buried. In others, such as peroneus longus and gastrocnemius, the motor nerve does not penetrate the muscle from its deep surface and pass through it to the surface at almost a right angle to its long axis; in contrast, it runs parallel to the latter so that the innervation zone is also aligned in this direction and does not (for the superficial fasciculi) underlie the motor point. For these reasons also the forearm muscles mentioned are most suitable for biopsy, especially as the situation of the scar, on the inner aspect of the forearm, renders it inconspicuous. Of the two, palmaris longus is the muscle of choice because of its comparative lack of importance in normal function and the shortness of its belly, which facilitates the localisation of the nerve endings. A final advantage of palmaris longus is the frequency with which a branch of the medial antebrachial cutaneous nerve of the forearm is located deep to the line of the incision, a convenient arrangement when sensory nerve biopsy is also desirable.

The vastus internus is also recommended as the muscle of the quadriceps group with the smallest length in which the innervation zone closely underlies the motor point. The deltoid has fasciculi running parallel with the surface but they tend to be adherent to the fascia and are decidedly longer than the forearm flexors. However, it has been used successfully on many occasions and routinely by some experts. Furthermore, it is probably the muscle of choice when this type of biopsy is to be combined with chemical studies which require larger amounts of muscle than can be taken from the forearm muscles. Biceps brachii can also be used although its motor point does not correspond as sharply to the innervation zone.

In order to increase the accuracy of the sampling, it is recommended that the innervation zone be localised by electrical stimulation of the exposed muscle, this zone having a much lower threshold of excitability than other parts of the muscle.

The peroneus brevis as a muscle for nerve-ending studies

In the early years this muscle was frequently used by one of us (A.L.W.) for nerve-ending studies, when it was desirable to study the endings in a disease thought to involve them in the lower extremity only and to a minimal degree. This was particularly the case in Ekbom's syndrome and it is the analysis of the findings in this disease that prevents the recommendation of peroneus brevis in unqualified terms. In a study by Harriman, Taverner and Woolf (1970), the authors were surprised to find florid terminal axonic sprouting and expansion of the terminal arborisation of the

end-plates in all the cases with Ekbom's syndrome (restless legs) or painful paraesthesiae that were examined, together with large numbers of spherical axonic swellings in the majority of these patients. Because there was delayed conduction in the anterior tibial nerve, and changes in the muscle fibres in haematoxylin and eosin preparations in an occasional case, they were at first inclined to accept the abnormal appearances of the nerve endings as being the cause of the symptoms in these unfortunate patients. However, a comparison of the appearance of the nerve endings in many hundreds of biopsy specimens from patients with a wide variety of diseases, showed convincingly that spherical axonic swellings were much more commonly encountered in specimens taken from the peroneus brevis than from forearm muscles, and that they were rare before the fourth decade. It is, therefore, clear that these swellings may be no more than an expression of ageing in the longest neurones in the body, revealing itself markedly at their most distal extremity. Further work will be required to establish whether this ageing process is accelerated in patients with Ekbom's syndrome (which may occur in young patients), and whether the axonic swellings play a part either in slowing nerve conduction or in producing the symptoms.

Whatever may be the significance of the findings for the pathogenesis of Ekbom's syndrome they suggest that very great caution must be exercised in interpreting changes in the intramuscular nerve endings in peroneus brevis.

Operative technique

This was described in detail in Coërs and Woolf (1959) and certain modifications were given later (Woolf, 1962c). After local anaesthesia of the subcutaneous tissue, the skin and fascia are incised across the motor point, parallel to the main direction of the muscle fibres. Only a 4–5 cm length need be opened. Accurate localisation of the terminal innervation area on the exposed muscle is achieved with a sterile metallic electrode connected to the cathode of the stimulator. Currents of 0.1 ms duration are delivered at a frequency of 1 s. The nerve endings will be found at the points where a single fasciculus, and not the whole muscle, contracts when stimulated by a current too weak to produce contraction when applied to any other part of that fasciculus. The current should usually be of the order of 0.1–0.5 mA with a stabilised current stimulator, or 1–10 V with a stabilised voltage apparatus. The accuracy of this localisation can be blurred in partly denervated muscles, or in myopathy when the innervation zone is enlarged (see below). Failure to localise the terminal innervation zone may also occur in myasthenia, owing to neuromuscular block caused by repetitive stimulation. On the whole, the yield of the method is about 95 per cent. Confirmation that localisation of the terminal innervation zone was correct can usually be obtained by stroking along the fasciculus with the point of a scalpel. When this crosses the innervation zone it produces a twitching of the muscle.

Before staining the selected fasciculus with methylene blue, specimens are removed from outside the innervation zone for histological and histochemical examination. If electron microscopy is to be performed, a strip, not wider than 2 mm, is removed with a biopsy forceps across the innervation zone. Another strip may be removed within the same area for cholinesterase staining, if needed. Then the selected fasciculus is injected with a 0.02–0.05 per cent solution of methylene blue in physiological saline, using the finest needle available. The needle is introduced parallel to the direction of the fasciculus and just below its surface, and the solution is gently injected as the needle is being withdrawn. This is repeated along the length to be removed (2–3 cm), over 3–5 min, using 10–30 ml of solution. We do not normally inject local anaesthetic into the muscle before taking the specimen, but this may be done before injecting methylene blue; this does not interfere with the staining and prevents the aching pain which sometimes accompanies the injection or the removal of the specimen. One or two strips a few mm thick are removed and placed on a gauze moistened with physiological saline and oxygenated for 1 h. Immediately after oxygenation has been completed the muscle is immersed in a filtered cold aqueous saturated solution of ammonium molybdate and left at 4°C for 24 h. After washing in three changes of distilled water, the specimens are fixed in 10 per cent formol saline for 24 h. They are then cut as longitudinal frozen sections 50–100 μm thick.

One of us (A.L.W.) abandoned the preparation of frozen sections of methylene blue stained sections because this required post-fixation with formalin, which seemed to extract a certain amount of stain from the tissue and also caused some shrinkage and loss of delicacy of the structures of the end-plate, possibly accentuated by the mechanical damage of freezing and sectioning. Instead, the technique of squash preparation (Dastur, 1956) was adopted, which requires extreme delicacy of handling before fixation for 12 h in ice-cold 8 per cent ammonium molybdate, preliminary manual squashing between microscope slides under the low power of the microscope and careful dissection away of all but the innervation zone. A final preparation of about 3 × 4 mm is obtained; it is again squashed under a weight similar to that of a rocker microtome and dehydrated in alcohol. The most suitable mounting medium is DPX (Gurr). It is advisable in the dissection of the specimens to view them from both sides of the slide as the best areas of innervation may be visible only from the undersurface of the slide. The final preparations almost invariably show large numbers of well-stained end-plates which can be followed without much difficulty to their fibre of origin in the terminal nerve bundle (Fig. 7.2). This is valuable in calculating the Terminal Innervation Ratio (TIR). Furthermore, the end-plates, and especially the terminal neuronal arborisation, are shown with greater delicacy than in frozen sections. Nevertheless, thick frozen sections have the advantage of preserving the normal relationship between the subterminal nerve fibres, an appearance which is often blurred in squash preparations (Fig. 7.3). Usually about 50 subterminal axons, suitable for the calculation of TIR, will be present; occasionally more than 200 are available.

THE PATTERN OF TERMINAL MOTOR INNERVATION

We hoped originally that the outcome of our studies of terminal motor innervation would be the development of a diagnostic system in which each disease would be represented by characteristic changes in the nerve endings. While it has been possible to recognise certain broad patterns of change, some more frequently encountered in one disease than another, it must be admitted that our main contribution has been to demonstrate a remarkable plasticity in the behaviour of the peripheral extremity of the lower motor neurone. We have indeed been able to deduce, from a study of fixed preparations, a striking picture of vital reactivity on the part of the axon and its termination which had, until this time, been portrayed by most writers as a rigid structure comparable to the cables of a man-made electrical circuit. Indeed, this approach by those skilled in electronic theory may have made it more difficult for them to envisage the structural neuronal abnormalities which could underlie the changes they encountered in electromyography. During the last 25 years, neuromuscular biopsies have been performed in many centres throughout the world and a considerable amount of material is available for study.

Normal pattern

When the intramuscular nerves reach the terminal innervation band, they spread into individual fibres which run only a short course in isolation before they reach the muscle fibre and form their terminal arborisation (Figs 7.2 and 7.3). These nerve fibres may be justifiably referred to as terminal axons, in spite of the occasional branching which occurs between the terminal bundle and the muscle fibre or from the motor arborisation, at ultraterminal level. The two arborisations resulting from such a branching usually innervate the same muscle fibre (Fig. 7.3B). Less frequently they innervate two different muscle fibres (Figs 7.2B and 7.3A). This branching can be quantitatively estimated as the Terminal Innervation Ratio (TIR). In order to give a functional significance to this ratio, we must count the double end-plates on a single muscle fibre as units and consider, in arriving at the functional or true TIR, only the formation by subterminal nerve fibres of end-plates on more than one muscle fibre.

The normal value of TIR, initially based on the findings in 12 individuals who were normal both clinically and electromyographically, was 1.10±0.06 (Coërs, 1955). Additional information has been obtained from 13 neuromuscular biopsies taken from volunteer University students (Reske-Nielsen, Coërs and Harmsen, 1969; Coërs, Reske-Nielsen and Harmsen, 1973). The mean value of the TIR in this material was 1.12±0.04, the range of measured values extending from 1.05 to 1.20. These results were compared with the findings in a group of 43 biopsies taken for diagnostic purposes, in which there were no clinical or EMG indications of neuromuscular disease, nor any histological changes in the muscle tissue stained with conventional methods. The mean TIR of this group was 1.10 ± 0.05, the highest observed value being 1.20. There was no significant difference between these figures and the values obtained from the volunteer students ($p > 0.2$). Therefore it may be accepted that the pooled mean TIR from these two groups of biopsies is representative of the normal. Its value is 1.11, with a standard deviation of 0.05. Values higher than 1.26 (mean + 3 SD) can be considered to be abnormal (Coërs, Telerman-Toppet and Gérard, 1973a).

The structure and dimensions of the myoneural junction were studied in these control biopsies. The sizes of the motor end-plates were estimated by the measurement of either the diameter or the surface of the subneural apparatus. The mean diameter was 32.2 μm $\pm$ 10.5, the observed values extending from 10 up to 80 μm (Coërs, 1955). The mean value of the synaptic area of the motor end-plates, estimated by the surface of the subneural apparatus, extended from 177 to 314 μm^2 (Coërs and Hildebrand, 1965; Reske-Nielsen et al., 1969). The histograms of both the diameters and the surfaces of the motor end-plates corresponded to unimodal-normal or logarithmic-normal distribution curves and did not indicate that more than one population of motor nerve endings, which could be related to the functional heterogeneity of the muscle fibres, was present. The only correlation to be found was that the size of the motor endings was proportional to the diameter of the muscle fibre they supplied (Coërs, 1955; Anzenbacher and Zenker, 1963; Nyström, 1968; Witalinski and Loesch, 1975).

Despite marked variations in size, the structure of the motor nerve endings is fairly constant in normal muscles. However, some motor arborisations in biopsies from healthy young adults show marked irregularity of the size of terminal expansions of the telodendrion, a feature that was previously considered to indicate a regressive or dystrophic state (Coërs, 1962). Such abnormal end-plates were observed in healthy young mammals by Barker and Ip (1965) and interpreted by Tuffery (1971) as indicating an ageing process.

The effects of ageing upon the terminal motor innervation pattern constitute an important diagnostic hazard. Thus, in 1965 Woolf wrote 'More and more we have come to appreciate the extreme lability of the terminal motor innervation so that we feel that it is likely that already in the first decade of life and certainly by the end of the third, many of the terminal sprays of axons will have undergone the indelible changes of pattern which seem to follow quite minor constitutional disturbances. Coërs and Hildebrand (1965) described the striking changes that accompany diabetes mellitus and chronic alcoholism in the absence of any clinical evidence of neuropathy. Similar changes can easily be conceived to accompany other reversible metabolic and toxic disorders or minor traumata and to persist and confuse the unwary observer for years after recovery from the causal disturbance'. The fact that the muscles of healthy young adults contain some apparently abnormal end-plates must be taken into account in the interpretation of pathological findings.

Buchthal (1957) showed that there is a steady increase in the duration of motor unit action potentials with increasing age. This surely has a morphological basis which one would like to see studied in the same statistical manner as that used by Buchthal and his school. So far, we have not found a significant increase in the TIR with increasing age (Coërs et al., 1973a).

Pathological changes

Marked changes in the rather simple and uniform pattern of intramuscular motor innervation are observed in neuromuscular diseases. Most of these changes are non-specific, being found both in myopathy and in denervation. However, our accumulated experience has established that denervation produces characteristic regressive and reactive alterations of the motor nerve and its

endings that can be useful in histological diagnosis.

Regressive changes. The histological expression of an acute injury of the lower motor neurone or of its axonal process is the well-known phenomenon of Wallerian degeneration. In fact, the process of axonal fragmentation is seldom visible in biopsy material obtained in cases of acute denervation, for example, in poliomyelitis or nerve injury. This distintegration, that starts at the terminal arborisation and spreads proximally, proceeds so rapidly that, within a few days, the axonal debris, initially in the form of pale globules (when stained by methylene blue), will have disappeared from the intramuscular nerve bundles. By contrast, the postsynaptic component undergoes a change that persists for a long time, as revealed in histochemical preparations. The lamellated layer of the units of the subneural apparatus becomes pale (poorly stained) and irregular, and the stained products accumulate within the cuplets, which are normally unstained (Fig. 7.5). This change could be related to electron-microscopic observations of denervated myoneural junctions, in which the cytoplasm of the Schwann cell tends to flow into the space vacated by the degenerating terminal axoplasmic expansions, thereby usurping their synaptic position (Birks, Katz and Miledi, 1960; Johnson and Woolf, 1965). In slowly progressive denervation, the motor nerve fibres may show localised swellings or take on a reticulated appearance. The localised swellings consist of spherical or elongated enlargements along the course of otherwise normal-appearing axis cylinders (Fig. 7.6). They are occasionally observed in chronic neuropathies and more rarely in motor neurone diseases and other anterior horn cell disorders. They could represent the earliest morphological expression of an axonal disturbance. The reticulated axons are networks of very fine beaded nerve fibres wandering among the muscle fibres without making visible contact with them (Fig. 7.7). These formations are often seen in disorders of the motor neurone, particularly in Werdnig-Hoffmann's disease and in hereditary neuropathies of the Charcot-Marie-Tooth type. One may assume that they reflect an

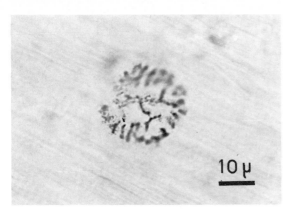

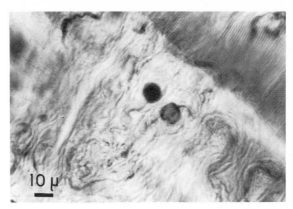

Fig. 7.5 Subneural apparatus in acute denervation in rat (modified Koelle method)

Fig. 7.6 Localized spherical swellings of motor axons in chronic denervation (vital staining with methylene blue)

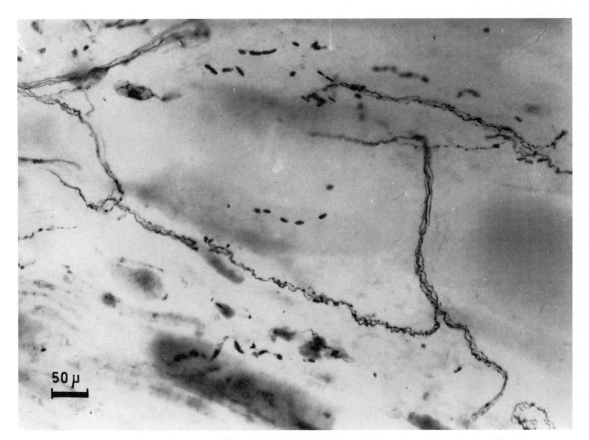

Fig. 7.7 Reticulated motor axons in a case of Charcot-Marie-Tooth disease (vital staining with methylene blue)

incapacity of growing diseased fibres to make a proper neuromuscular contact.

Non-specific changes. These changes may be observed in motor end-plates and in intramuscular nerve fibres.

In many biopsies one frequently encounters fine and beaded axons (Fig. 7.8) which could either be regenerating nerve fibres, such as are seen in muscle recovering from a nerve injury, or abnormal fibres coursing in degenerated or atrophic

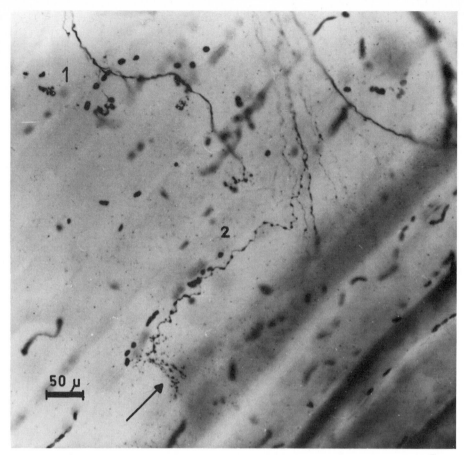

Fig. 7.8 Chronic polyneuropathy. 1. Increased collateral ramification. 2. Fine beaded motor axon ending as a plexiform network (arrow) (vital staining with methylene blue)

muscle tissue, as in the myopathies (*see* Fig. 7.16). In chronic involvement of the lower motor neurone and peripheral nerve, such finely beaded nerve fibres could be either regenerating or degenerating axis cylinders.

Some motor end-plates may present abnormally large junctional swellings (Fig. 7.9). These changes are reflected in the structure of the subneural apparatus, the units of which show marked variations in size (irregular end-plates). The motor endings may also be abnormally small and reduced to a few or even to one large terminal expansion (reduced end-plates), as if the arborisation had fused into a single mass (Fig. 7.10a). The corresponding subneural apparatuses are formed by a single large unit with a well-preserved laminated border (Fig. 7.10b). Such changes are particularly conspicuous in diabetic neuropathy (Woolf and

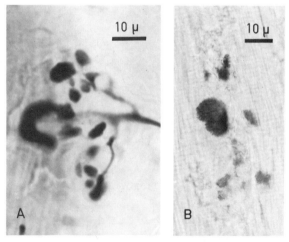

Fig. 7.9 A. Irregular motor arborisation in myotonic dystrophy (vital staining with methylene blue). B. Irregular subneural apparatus in chronic polyneuropathy (modified Koelle method)

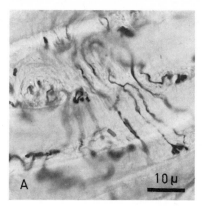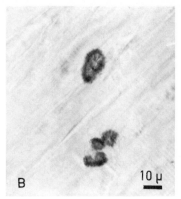

Fig. 7.10   Diabetic neuropathy. Reduced motor end-plates. A. Methylene blue. B. Modified thiocholine method

Malins, 1957), though they have also been observed in other conditions, such as alcoholic neuropathy (Coërs and Hildebrand, 1965) and coeliac disease (Cooke, Johnson and Woolf, 1966). This reduction in the size of end-plates seems to represent the earliest morphological indication of a disease process affecting motor nerve fibres. However, it must be pointed out that this apparently regressive process closely resembles the first stage of differentiation of the motor end-plate, either in normal development or in regeneration, at a time when the axoplasmic growth cone reaches the sarcoplasm and before it starts its ramification. In addition, the possibility exists that the reduction and simplification of motor end-plates is related merely to the atrophy of the muscle fibre occuring in any neuromuscular disease, in keeping with the principle that there is a correlation between the size of the muscle fibre and its motor ending. For example, it is difficult to decide whether diminutive end-plates found in nemaline and centronuclear myopathy and in familial focal loss of cross striations (Fig. 7.11) are related to delayed maturation of the myoneural junction or to the small size of muscle fibres (Coërs, Telerman-Toppet, Gérard, Szliwowski, Bethlem and Van Wijngaarden, 1976; Van Wijngaarden, Bethlem, Dingemans, Coërs, Telerman-Toppet and Gérard, 1977).

Changes related to axonal sprouting. Excessive branching of intramuscular nerve fibres may occur at various levels, collateral, terminal or ultraterminal. The result of terminal and ultrater-minal ramification, taking place distally, is usually the formation of expanded motor endings or of several motor arborisations on the same muscle fibre, and this may be observed either in denervation or myopathy, usually on hypertrophic muscle fibres (Figs. 7.12 and 7.14). In some instances, however, such expanded motor endings may be seen on normal-sized or small muscle fibres, and this is particularly the case in myotonic dystrophy (see Figs. 7.19 and 7.20), myasthenia gravis (see Fig. 7.22) and myositis (Coërs, 1965).

Collateral ramification of the proximal part of the subterminal axons and, occasionally, ultraterminal ramification result in the innervation of different muscle fibres and an increase of this process is most often observed in denervation (Figs. 7.13 and 7.14). Collateral sprouting has been noted both in experimental material (Edds, 1950; Hoffman, 1950; Hildebrand, Joffroy and Coërs, 1968; Hildebrand, Joffroy, Graff and Coërs, 1968) and in human diseases (Coërs, 1955; Wohlfart, 1957, 1960; Coërs and Woolf, 1959; Coomes, 1960; Harriman, 1961; Hatsuyama, 1964). This sprouting results in an increase of the functional (true) TIR, i.e. the number of muscle fibres innervated by a given number of subterminal axons, and therefore representing an extension of the territory of the motor unit by inclusion of muscle fibres from denervated units. The TIR was found to be significantly increased in 87 per cent of denervating diseases, reaching 97 per cent in clinically affected muscles and being 74 per cent in biopsies from clinically and histologically normal muscles in patients with peripheral

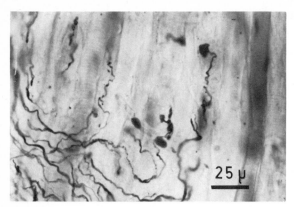

Fig. 7.11 Reduced motor endings in familial focal loss of cross-striations (vital staining with methylene blue)

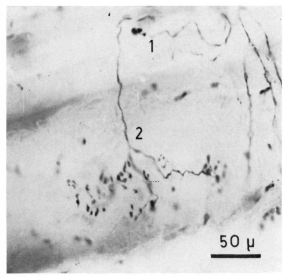

Fig. 7.12 Limb-girdle muscular dystrophy. 1. Reduced motor ending (vital staining with methylene blue). 2. Distal branching forming an expanded motor ending on a hypertrophic muscle fibre

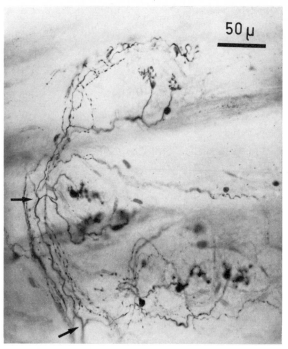

Fig. 7.14 Kugelberg-Welander disease. Collateral re-innervation (arrows) and distal branching forming several motor arborisations on hypertrophic muscle fibres. Some axons are abnormally thin and beaded (vital staining with methylene blue)

neuropathies. In muscular dystrophy the TIR was within the normal range in 82 per cent of cases, including all cases of Duchenne muscular dystrophy and congenital myopathies (Coërs, Telerman-Toppet and Gérard, 1973b, Coërs *et al.*, 1976).

PATHOPHYSIOLOGICAL AND DIAGNOSTIC IMPLICATIONS

Amyotrophic lateral sclerosis

As might be expected, the 'dying back' phenomenon is strongly in evidence in amyotrophic lateral sclerosis (ALS) and the terminal motor axons may appear to be normal right down to the end-plate or, alternatively, there may be undue slenderness of fine beading of the most distal part of the axon. The end-plate itself has an attenuated

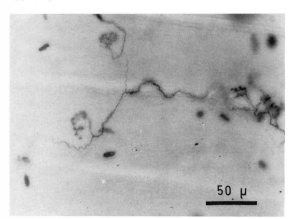

Fig. 7.13 Well-established collateral re-innervation in hypertrophic polyneuropathy (vital staining with methylene blue)

appearance, the terminal axonic expansions being small and spherical and often dark-staining, while the filaments of the terminal arborisation are unduly slender and delicate. In spite of the attenuated appearance of its constituents the arborisation may be unduly expanded, with an excessive number of terminal expansions. This appearance of the end-plates in ALS contrasts with that seen in the Guillain-Barré syndrome, where the terminal axonic expansions tend to fuse into a single irregularly shaped dark-staining mass. Eventually the attenuation of the end-plates reaches a stage when contact is lost with the muscle fibre and the axon appears to 'die back' from the periphery. Just how long this process takes is not known but it is characteristic to find many fine, beaded nerve fibres in the terminal nerve bundles, from which they emerge to form plexiform networks on the muscle fibres, not necessarily ending in a recognisable end-plate (Fig. 7.15). If these fine, beaded fibres are followed back into the larger nerve bundles they are seen to be the continuation of normal-looking fibres. The possibility that these fine, beaded sprouts are present in the more proximal parts of the motor and spinal nerves and that their unstable polarization may be related to the fasciculation found in ALS has been discussed on several occasions (Woolf, 1956, 1957, 1962; Coërs and Woolf, 1959).

The changes seen with the electron microscope in the intramuscular nerve bundles mirror the findings noted with vital staining. Thus, Schwann cells may be devoid of axons and there is an increase in FLS collagen. In accordance with the

principle of 'dying back' of the neurone, the more distal the nerve bundle the smaller chance there is of encountering axons within the Schwann cell. The lamellated bodies thought by Evans, Finean and Woolf (1965) to be granules of Doinikow, are frequently encountered in the cytoplasm of the Schwann cells.

Because of the relatively slow progression of ALS it is difficult to find, in biopsy specimens, end-plates in an early stage of degeneration. Occasionally some are seen with a broken and ill-defined presynaptic membrane, with few synaptic vesicles and rather dense, degenerate mitochondria. The secondary synaptic folds are reduced in number and shorter than usual. It is more common to encounter end-plates from which the axonal component is entirely lacking, the presynaptic position being occupied by wispy collagen fibres or granular material.

Werdnig-Hoffmann disease

In no other malady is the phenomenon of 'dying back' of the neurone so well demonstrated as in Werdnig-Hoffmann disease where the motor axons typically continue to the last millimetre of their course, only to break up into a tangle of fine, beaded fibres in the terminal nerve bundles. From this 'tangle' the emerging fibres end in a poorly formed end-plate in the more slowly progressive cases. This loss of neuromuscular connection makes it impossible to measure the TIR in most biopsies. The 'tangle' is typical of this disease and enables it to be distinguished from other causes of infantile muscular weakness and hypotonia in most instances (Woolf, 1960).

Charcot-Marie-Tooth disease

In Charcot-Marie-Tooth disease (CMT), which has a much slower and milder evolution than ALS, the process of collateral ramification is significantly more marked, the mean TIR measured in 12 cases being 2.16 ± 0.56 whereas the mean value was 1.66 ± 0.30 in 18 cases of ALS ($p < 0.05$) (Telerman-Toppet and Coërs, 1978). This difference indicates that the unaffected motor neurones in CMT have a better capacity for reinnervation of adjacent denervated muscle fibres

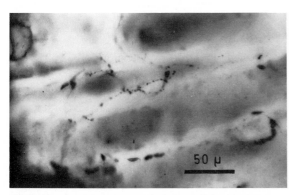

Fig. 7.15 Amyotrophic lateral sclerosis. Network of fine beaded motor fibres (vital staining with methylene blue)

than do their counterparts in ALS. The high value of TIR is reflected in an increased degree of type grouping in CMT as compared with ALS (Dubowitz and Brooke, 1973; Jennekens, Meijer, Bethlem and Van Wijngaarden, 1974; Telerman-Toppet and Coërs, 1978). Electromyographic estimation of fibre density (Schwarz, Stålberg, Schiller and Thiele, 1976) has produced results in agreement with these morphometric data, which provide evidence that both increased collateral branching and type grouping are an expression of the compensatory increase in the size of residual motor units that takes place in chronic denervation. Similarly, the formation of muscle fibre groups having the same enzymatic profile, typical of either type I or type II, suggests that reinnervation of muscle fibres by collaterals from motor neurones of a different type may lead to full conversion of their metabolic characteristics, as has been demonstrated by experimental cross-reinnervation experiments (Close, 1972).

Duchenne muscular dystrophy

The investigation of intramuscular innervation of 19 muscle biopsy specimens demonstrated that there was no reinnervation through collateral sprouting in Duchenne muscular dystrophy, as assumed by Desmedt and Borenstein (1973, 1976). The mean TIR was 1.12 ± 0.06, not significantly different from the results in controls ($P > 0.4$) and the range of individual values extended from 0.01 to 1.23 (Coërs and Telerman-Toppet, 1977).

It seems likely that the collateral sprouting represents an attempt to compensate for the loss of motor axons that characterises lower motor neurone and peripheral nerve disorders. In muscular dystrophy, such axonal loss does not take place. On the contrary, a very dense innervation persists in muscles which have been deprived of many muscle fibres and there is apparently an excess of motor axons. It is easy in methylene blue preparations to follow 'unemployed' nerve fibres running in connective tissue parallel to the longitudinal axis of the muscle and ending freely (Fig. 7.16). Eventually, these fibres make contact with a muscle fibre as a diminutive motor arborisation, sometimes several millimeters apart from the intramuscular nerve (Fig. 7.17). These nerve fibres are often abnormally thin and beaded, but do not branch excessively. This distorted pattern of motor innervation results in a very marked enlargement of the terminal innervation area and a longitudinal scatter of motor end-plates that may reach 10 mm (Fig. 7.18), whereas the terminal innervation area in the muscles of normal children does not exceed 1 mm.

This dispersion of motor endings may be explained in two ways. According to Desmedt and Borenstein (1973), focal necrosis can produce a transection of muscle fibres with the consequent formation of denervated segments. It may be assumed that 'unemployed' axons available in the vicinity of the denervated segments could be accepted and would then form ectopic end-plates. They could just as well be used to innervate regenerated muscle fibres (Desmedt and Borenstein, 1976), because regeneration is known to take place in the early stages of the disease. Another possibility could be that the dispersion of the motor end-plate is merely related to the longitudinal displacement of transected muscle fibres resulting from focal necrosis.

In any case, there is apparently no need for collateral sprouting in muscles having a redundant innervation, and this is in agreement with morphological evidence. On the other hand, this evidence indicates that if a 'neural factor' is involved in Duchenne dystrophy, as postulated by McComas, Sica and Currie (1970), it is not denervation in the conventional sense of axonal degeneration.

Limb-girdle progressive muscular atrophy and dystrophy

Measurement of TIR has been particularly useful in the differential diagnosis between juvenile spinal muscular atrophy (SMA) and limb-girdle muscular dystrophy (LGM) (Coërs and Telerman-Toppet, 1979). The clinical picture of the two conditions may be very similar, and the secondary myopathic changes in the muscle fibres may be so prominent in SMA that its neurogenic nature may be overlooked (Gardner-Medwin, Hudgson and Walton, 1967; Mastaglia and Walton, 1971). We studied 18 patients with a progressive proximal muscular atrophy and weakness without fasciculations. Only two cases could be safely diagnosed as spinal muscular atrophy according to classical criteria. Both showed extensive 'group atrophy' and a neurogenic EMG; they also had a very high TIR. A firm diagnosis of muscular dystrophy could be made in two other cases in which only myopathic changes were found in the biopsy and EMG, and both had a normal TIR. In other cases, diagnosis remained uncertain on the basis of both the histology and the EMG, because of discrepancies or inconclusive data. Some had a predominantly neurogenic EMG with marked myopathic histological changes; others had a myopathic EMG with histological changes suggesting denervation, or a mixture of neuropathic and myopathic signs in both the EMG and biopsy. In such ambiguous situations, measurement of TIR settled the diagnosis. In one case, an increased TIR conformed to the EMG pattern of denervation despite a myopathic biopsy. In one other case, a normal value of TIR confirmed the diagnosis of myopathy as suggested by the EMG, although there were numerous small dark angular fibres and small groups of atrophic fibres with a bimodal distribution of fibre diameters. In a third case, in which neither the histology nor the EMG were conclusive, an increased TIR suggested denervation.

On the whole, the TIR was more closely correlated with the EMG than histological muscle fibre changes, particularly small areas of 'group atrophy' and small angular dark fibres, and appeared to be the most accurate morphological index of denervation.

Myotonic dystrophy

A very marked distortion of the terminal motor innervation pattern takes place in this disease. Subterminal axons are intermingled, sometimes whirling around muscle fibres and being difficult to follow individually. The end-plates tend to cover a larger area than normal, while the terminal expansions are larger and often more numerous

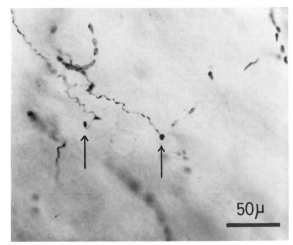

Fig. 7.16 'Unemployed' motor axons in Duchenne dystrophy (vital staining with methylene blue)

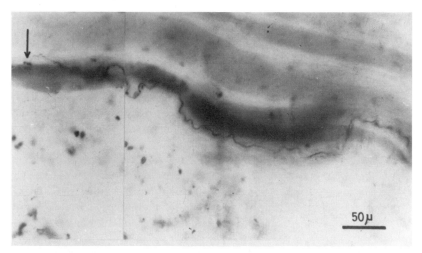

Fig. 7.17 Duchenne dystrophy. Motor nerve fibre running along an atrophic muscle fibre and ending as a diminutive motor ending (arrow) (vital staining with methylene blue)

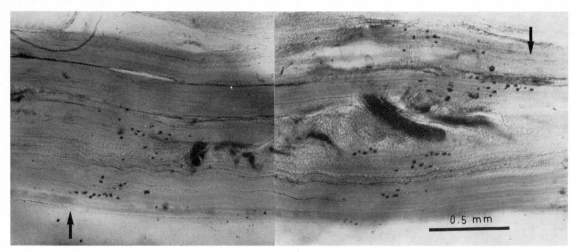

Fig. 7.18 Abnormal dispersion of motor end-plates (arrows) in Duchenne dystrophy (compare with Fig. 7.1) (modified Koelle method)

than normal (Coërs and Woolf, 1959; Woolf, 1962c) (Figs 7.19 and 7.20). There is often striking axonal sprouting, leading to the formation of several end-plates on a single muscle fibre, or to the innervation of several muscle fibres, thus increasing the TIR. More impressive, however, is the tendency for axonal sprouts to wander between muscle fibres, giving off on either side short collateral sprouts terminating upon the muscle fibres in a series of miniature synapses at intervals of about 20–50 μm, along a length of several millimetres of the fibre (Coërs and Woolf, 1959, Figures 120, 122, 229). These synapses may be clearly demonstrated with the help of techniques for the demonstration of cholinesterase (*see* Coërs and Woolf, 1959, Figures 223, 227–228; Woolf, 1962b).

A neural disorder in myotonic dystrophy has been postulated by MacDermot (1961) in view of the very marked changes in intramuscular innervation contrasting with the relative integrity of the muscle fibres, and by McComas, Campbell and Sica (1971), from electromyographic data. Caccia, Negri and Pretoparvis (1972) also found clinical and EMG evidence of peripheral nerve disturbance in two cases of myotonic dystrophy. According to Panayiotopoulos and Scarpalezos (1976, 1977) this evidence of peripheral nerve involvement is present in addition to the primary muscle disorder in some cases of myotonic dystrophy. Therefore, the increased TIR found in five

of 13 cases (Coërs *et al.*, 1973b) does not indicate that myotonic dystrophy is due to denervation, but rather that this polysystemic disease can occasionally be associated with a neuropathy.

Myasthenia gravis

The first definite indication of neural abnormality was found in a patient with congenital myasthenia, aged 6 years at the time of biopsy (Coërs and Woolf, 1954). Methylene blue preparations showed remarkably elongated, almost filamentous motor end-plates. Cholinesterase preparations disclosed a ribbon-like appearance of the subneural apparatus, corresponding to the elongated motor arborisations.

Later studies reported by Woolf, Bagnall, Bauwens and Bickerstaff (1956), Coërs and Desmedt (1959), Coërs and Woolf (1959), Woolf (1959a, b), Bickerstaff and Woolf (1960) and MacDermot (1960) have indicated that, in addition to elongated end-plates (Fig. 7.21), myasthenic muscles contained enlarged and irregular end-plates similar to those seen in other neuromuscular disorders (Fig. 7.22), whereas their elongated appearance is quite different from anything that has been seen in any other disease.

In a series of 45 cases (Coërs and Telerman-Toppet, 1976), elongated end-plates were found in 26 biopsies, more frequently in younger patients, and consequently more often in women who predominate within the younger age-group. There was no correlation between the incidence of this change and the severity of the disease, nor with the histological and histochemical appearance of the muscle fibres. Non-specific changes of motor endings were present in 38 biopsies without any correlation with clinical data, age or the histochemical pattern of the muscle fibres. In addition, a TIR exceeding the upper normal limit and suggesting denervation was found in seven biopsies, all coming from patients over the age of 50 years. Denervation in myasthenia has been postulated from the histological and histochemical changes in the muscle fibres (Fenichel and Shy, 1963; Brody and Engel, 1964). However, there is a discrepancy between the relatively small proportion of biopsies with an increased TIR and the high incidence of histochemical changes suggesting denervation found by Engel and McFarlin (1966).

The reciprocal relationship between an increased TIR, occurring in elderly patients, and the presence of elongated end-plates, which tend to be more frequent in younger patients, suggests a chronological evolution of the innervation pattern in myasthenic muscles. Elongation and simplification of the motor endings could be the primary change, followed by distal branching of motor axons forming expanded or multiple motor arborisations, that could represent a process compensating for impaired neuromuscular transmission, similar to the axonal changes obtained by local application of *Clostridium botulinum* toxin

(Duchen and Strich, 1967). Collateral branching with reinnervation of adjacent muscle fibres appears as a late and infrequent feature in myasthenia, taking place only in some elderly patients, whatever the apparent duration or severity of the disease. Another possibility could be that the presence of elongated motor endings characterises a type of myasthenia occurring preferentially in a younger age-group, contrasting with other types of myasthenia, some of which are related to denervation and affect older subjects.

Since these results were obtained, an important contribution to knowledge of the changes in myasthenic motor end-plates has been provided by Engel and his colleagues (Santa, Engel and Lambert, 1972). Quantitative ultrastructural study showed that the postsynaptic region was smaller and simpler than normal, with widening of the synaptic space, suggesting focal degeneration and regeneration of the junctional folds. The average nerve terminal area was also smaller than normal, but the synaptic vesicle and mitochondrial concentration was normal. The same changes were induced in animals by prolonged administration of anticholinesterase drugs (Engel, Lambert and Santa, 1973) and also in experimental autoimmune myasthenia gravis (Engel, Tsujihata, Lindström and Lennon, 1976) induced by immunisation with acetylcholine receptor protein (Lenon, Lindström and Seybold, 1975). Seven to 11 days after immunisation, mononuclear cell infiltration takes place in the end-plate and its vicinity, with degeneration and phagocytosis of the postsynaptic region. Subsequently, the inflammatory reaction

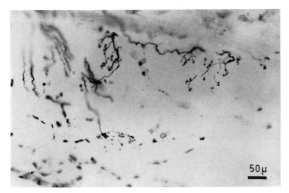

Fig. 7.19 Expanded motor endings in myotonic dystrophy (vital staining with methylene blue)

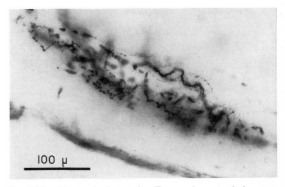

Fig. 7.20 Myotonic dystrophy. Extremely expanded motor ending (vital staining with methylene blue)

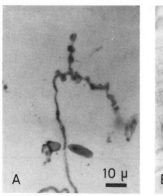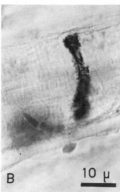

Fig. 7.21 Elongated motor end-plate in myasthenia gravis. A. Vital staining with methylene blue. B. Modified Koelle method

subsides and the intact nerve terminal innervates a simplified postsynaptic region. This experimental model of myasthenia gravis suggests that the alterations in the nerve terminals observed in myasthenic patients are secondary to the postsynaptic changes related to an autoimmune aggression. Elongation and simplification of motor endings could be the earliest consequence of this aggression, compensatory distal sprouting taking place at a later stage. It may be assumed that anticholinesterase therapy could participate in the production of the changes in motor endings, but the importance of this factor is still undetermined, as far as elongated end-plates are concerned, because they have been observed in previously undiagnosed and untreated cases (Coërs and Telerman-Toppet, 1976).

Myositis

A morphometric study of intramuscular innervation was performed in 16 cases of dermatomyositis, nine cases of polymyositis and in six cases of muscle sarcoidosis (granulomatous myopathy according to Coërs and Carbone, 1966 and Coërs, 1967) (Coërs et al., 1973b). In some biopsies, the changes in motor innervation were similar to those seen in other myopathies and involved the more distal part of the nerve fibres, forming small and irregular motor endings or abnormally expanded or multiple terminal arborisations through distal branching. In other samples, marked collateral ramification increased the TIR. Usually, the axonal branching occured in the vicinity of, or within, foci of cellular infiltration (Fig. 7.23), so that the degree of ramification differed from one part of the specimen to another. In one case of granulomatous myopathy, the TIR was 1.73 in regions with granulomatous infiltration and 1.17 elsewhere, with a mean of 1.44. The mean TIR was significantly increased in dermatomyositis and granulomatous myopathy and did not exceed normal in polymyositis. it was regarded as a reaction to axonal breakdown within the muscle, in the vicinity or within the foci of

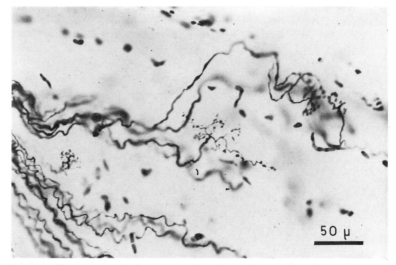

Fig. 7.22 Expanded motor endings in myasthenia gravis (vital staining with methylene blue)

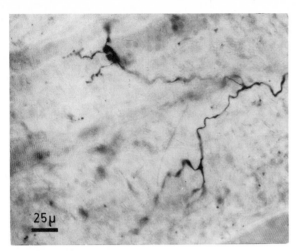

25μ

Fig. 7.23   Collateral branching in granulomatous myopathy (vital staining with methylene blue)

inflammatory cells (intramuscular denervation). The higher incidence of an increased TIR found in dermatomyositis and granulomatous myopathy, in which the cellular infiltration was more marked than in polymyositis, supports this interpretation.

CONCLUSIONS

Studies of neuromuscular biopsies have revealed the high sensitivity of the motor innervation of voluntary muscle to various noxious factors, and its remarkable capacity for regeneration. Excessive branching of intramuscular nerve fibres is common in all kinds of neuromuscular disorder, but its functional significance appears to be different in neurogenic and myogenic conditions. In denervation the axonal sprouting attempts to compensate for the loss of nerve fibres and ensures the reinnervation of denervated muscle fibres. In other diseases, the principal result of axonal ramification is the formation of expanded or multiple motor arborisations on the same muscle fibre, without extension to adjacent muscle fibres. This terminal branching may be a response to disturbed function of the muscle, as in muscular

dystrophy, or to impaired neuromuscular transmission, as in myasthenia. It can also be merely an adaptation of the size of the myoneural junction to muscle fibre hypertrophy.

The functional specificity of collateral branching is made clear by measuring the true TIR. This value has been found to be significantly increased in nearly all disorders associated with long-lasting denervation whereas it remains normal in most myopathies. This increase is also an early indication of peripheral nerve involvement, as it has been observed in a high proportion of clinically and histologically normal muscles in patients with neuropathy. This change, therefore, appears to be a very sensitive and reliable morphological index of denervation. Rarefaction of intramuscular nerve fibres and a reticulated appearance of these fibres provides additional evidence of a disease process affecting the lower motor neurone and peripheral nerves.

Other pathological changes in intramuscular axons and motor endings do not have the same specificity because they are found both in denervation and myopathy, and can be the expression of degenerative or regenerative processes. Nevertheless, elongation and simplification of motor endings are characteristic of myasthenia gravis.

ACKNOWLEDGEMENTS

This work was aided by grants from the Muscular Dystrophy Association of America, Inc., the Muscular Dystrophy Group of Great Britain, the Fonds de la Recherche Scientifique Médicale of Belgium and the Free University of Brussels.

We wish to thank the editors and publishers of the following journals for kind permission to reproduce illustrations: The Journal of the Neurological Sciences (Fig. 7.2), Archives of Neurology (Figs. 7.3, 7.7, 7.8, 7.13, 7.16, 7.18 and 7.23), Neurology (Figs. 7.12 and 7.14), and the Annals of the New York Academy of Sciences (Fig. 7.21).

REFERENCES

Anzenbacher, H. & Zenker, W. (1963) Über die Grössenbezichung der Muskelfasern zu ihren motorischen Endplatten und Nerven. *Zeitschrift für Zellforschung*, **60**, 860–871.

Attias, G. (1912) Die Nerven der Hornhaut des Menschen. *Albrecht v. Graefes Archiv für Ophthalmologie*, **83**, 207.

Barker, D. & Ip, M.C. (1965) Sprouting and degeneration of mammalian motor axons in normal and de-afferented skeletal muscle. *Proceedings of the Royal Society. Series B*, **163**, 538–554.

Bickerstaff, E.R. & Woolf, A.L. (1960) The intramuscular nerve endings in myasthenia gravis. *Brain*, **83**, 10.

Birks, R., Katz, B. & Miledi, R. (1960) Physiological and structural changes at the amphibian myoneural junction, in the course of nerve degeneration. *Journal of Physiology* **150**, 145–168.

Brody, I.A. & Engel, W.K. (1964) Denervation of muscle in myasthenia gravis. *Archives of Neurology*, **11**, 350–354.

Buchthal, F. (1957) *An Introduction to Electromyography* (Scandinavian University Books: Copenhagen).

Caccia, M.R., Negri, S. & Pretoparvis, V. (1972) Myotonic dystrophy with neural involvement. *Journal of the Neurological Sciences*, **16**, 253–269.

Close, R. (1972) Dynamic properties of mammalian skeletal muscles. *Physiological Reviews*, **52**, 129–197.

Coërs, C. (1952) The vital staining of muscle biopsies with methylene blue. *Journal of Neurology, Neurosurgery, and Psychiatry*, **15**, 211.

Coërs, C. (1953a) Contribution à l'etude de la jonction neuromusculaire II, Topographie zonale de l'innervation, motrice terminale dans les muscles striés. *Archives de Biologie*, **64**, 495.

Coërs, C. (1953b) La détection de la cholinesterase au niveau de la jonction neuromusculaire. *Revue belge de pathologie et de médicine experimentale*, **22**, 306.

Coërs, C. (1955) Les variations structurelles normales et pathologiques de la jonction neuromusculaire. *Acta neurologica et psychiatrica Belgica*, **55**, 741.

Coërs, C. (1962) Analyse critique et essai d'interprétation des anomalies de la jonction neuro-musculaire en pathologie humaine. *Mémoires de L'Académi royale médecine de Belgique*, **4**, 71.

Coërs, C. (1965) Histology of the myoneural junction in myopathies. In *Muscle*, Eds W.M. Paul, E.E. Daniel, C.M. Kay, G. Monckton, p. 453 (Pergamon Press: Oxford, New York).

Coërs, C. (1967) The histological features of muscle sarcoïdosis. *Acta Neuropathologica (Berlin)*, **7**, 242–252.

Coërs, C. & Carbone, F. (1966) La myopathie granulomateuse. *Acta neurologica et psychiatrica Belgica*, **66**, 353–381.

Coërs, C. & Desmedt, J.E. (1959) Mise en évidence d'une malformation caractéristique de la jonction neuromusculaire dans la myasthénie. *Acta Neurologica Belgica*, **59**, 539.

Coërs, C. & Hildebrand, J. (1965) Latent neuropathy in diabetes and alcoholism. *Neurology (Minneapolis)*, **15**, 19–38.

Coërs, C. & Woolf, A.L. (1954) Étude histologique et histochimique de la jonction neuromusculaire dans la myasthérie. *Comptes rendus du Congrés des Médecins Aliénistes et Neurologistes*, Liège, 19–26 July, 1954.

Coërs, C. & Woolf, A.L. (1959) *The Innervation of Muscle* (Blackwell: Oxford).

Coërs, C. & Telerman-Toppet, N. (1976) Morphological and histochemical changes of motor units in myasthenia. *Annals of the New York Academy of Science*, **274**, 6–19.

Coërs, C. & Telerman-Toppet, N. (1977) Morphological changes of motor units in Duchenne's muscular dystrophy. *Archives of Neurology*, **34**, 396–402.

Coërs, C. & Telerman-Toppet N. (1979) Differential diagnosis of limb girdle muscular dystrophy and spinal muscular atrophy. *Neurology (Minneapolis)*, **29**, 957–972.

Coërs, C., Reske-Nielsen, E. & Harmsen, A. (1973) The pattern of terminal motor innervation in healthy young adults. *Journal of the Neurological Sciences*, **19**, 351.

Coërs, C., Telerman-Toppet, N. & Gerard, J.M. (1973a) Terminal and innervation ratio in neuromuscular diseases. I Methods and Controls. *Archives of Neurology*, **29**, 210.

Coërs C., Telerman-Toppet, N. & Gerard, J.M. (1973b) Terminal innervation ratio in neuromuscular disease. II Disorders of lower motor neuron, peripheral nerve and muscle. *Archives of Neurology*, **29**, 215–222.

Coërs, C., Telerman-Toppet N., Gerard J.M., Szlioowski H., Bethlem J. & Van Wijngaarden G.K., (1976) Changes in motor innervation and histochemical congenital myopathies. *Neurology (Minneapolis)*, **26**, 1046–1053.

Cooke, W.T., Johnson, A.G. & Woolf, A.L. (1966) Vital staining and electron microscopy of the intramuscular nerve-endings in the neuropathy of adult coeliac disease. *Brain*, **89**, 663–682.

Coomes, E.N. (1960) A correlated study of intensity duration curves and terminal neuronal reinnervation of muscle. *Annals of Physical Medicine*, **5**, 243–251.

Couteaux, R. (1951) Remarques sur les méthodes actuelles de détection histochimique des activités cholinestérasiques. *Archives internationales de physiologie*, **59**, 526.

Dastur, D.K. (1956) The motor unit in leprous neuritis. A clinico-pathological study. *Bulletin of the Neurological Society (India)*, **4**, 1.

Desmedt, J.E. & Borenstein, S. (1973) Collateral innervation of muscle fibres by motor axons of dystrophic motor units. *Nature*, **264**, 500–501.

Desmedt, J.E. & Borenstein, S. (1976) Regeneration in Duchenne dystrophy. *Archives of Neurology*, **33**, 642–650.

Dogiel, A.S. (1890) Die Nerven der Cornea des Menschen. *Anatomischer Anzeiger*, **5**, 483.

Dogiel, A.S. (1891) Die nervenendkörperchen (Endkolben, W. Krause) in der Cornea und Conjunctiva Bulbi des Menschen. *Archiv für mikroskopische Anatomie*, **37**, 502.

Dogiel, A.S. (1902) Die Nervenendigungen im Bauchfell in der Sehnen den Muskelspindeln und dem Centrum tendineum des Diaphragmas bei Menschen und bei Säugethieren. *Archiv für mikroskopische Anatomie*, **59**, 1.

Dubowitz, V. & Brooke, M.H. (1973) Muscle biopsy: A modern approach. In the Series *Major Problems in Neurology* Vol. 2 (W.B. Saunders: Eastbourne).

Duchen, L.W. & Strich, S.J. (1967) Changes in the pattern of motor innervation of skeletal muscles in the mouse after local injection of *Clostridium botulinum* toxin. *Journal of Physiology*, **189**, proc. pp. 16–17.

Edds, Mc. V. Jr. (1950) Collateral regeneration of residual motor axons in partially denervated muscles. *Journal of Experimental Zoology*, **113**, 517–552.

Ehrlich, P. (1882) Zur biologischen Verwertung des Methylenblau. *Zentralblatt für die medizinischen*

Wissenschaften, **12**, 49.

Engel, W.G. & McFarlin, D.E. (1966) Discussion of paper by G.M. Fenichel. *Annals of the New York Academy of Sciences*, **135**, 68.

Engel, A.G., Lambert, E.H. & Santa, T. (1973) Study of long-term anticholinesterase therapy. Effect on neuromuscular transmission and on motor end-plate fine structure. *Neurology (Minneapolis)*, **23**, 1273.

Engel, A.G., Tsujihata, M., Lindström, J. & Lennon, V.A. (1976) The motor end-plate in myasthenia gravis and in experimental autoimmune myasthenia gravis. A quantitative ultrastructural study. *Annals of New York Academy of Science*, **274**, 60–79.

Evans, M.J., Finean, J.B. & Woolf, A.L. (1965) Ultrastructural studies of human cutaneous nerve with special reference to lamellated cell inclusions and vacuole-containing cells. *Journal of Clinical Pathology*, **18**, 188–192.

Fenichel, G.M. & Shy, G.M. (1963) Muscle biopsy experience in myasthenia gravis. *Archives of Neurology*, **9**, 237–243.

Gardner-Medwin, D., Hudgson, P. & Walton, J.N. (1967) Benign spinal muscular atrophy arising in childhood and adolescence. *Journal of the Neurological Sciences*, **5**, 121–158.

Harriman, D. (1961) The diagnostic value of motor-point muscle biopsy. In *Scientific Aspects of Neurology*, Ed. H.G. Garland, p. 37 (Livingstone: Edinburgh).

Harriman, D.G.F., Taverner, D. & Woolf, A.L. (1970) Ekbom's syndrome and burning paraesthesiae—a biopsy study. *Brain*, **93**, 393–406.

Hatsuyama, Y. (1964) Histological studies on the reinnervation of denervated muscle with special reference to collateral branching. *Journal of Japanese Orthopedic Association*, **38**, 375–393.

Hildebrand, J., Joffroy, A. & Coërs, C. (1968) Myoneural changes in experimental isoniazid neuropathy. *Archives of Neurology*, **19**, 60–70.

Hildebrand, J., Joffroy, A., Graff, G. & Coërs, C. (1968) Neuromuscular changes with alloxan hyperglycemia. *Archives of Neurology*, **18**, 633–641.

Hines, M. & Tower, S.S. (1928) Studies on the innervation of skeletal muscles. II. Of muscle spindles in certain muscles of the kitten. *Bulletin of the Johns Hopkins Hospital*, **42**, 264.

Hoffman, H. (1950) Local reinnervation in partially denervated muscle. A histopathological study. *Australian Journal of Experimental Biology and Medical Sciences*, **28**, 383–397.

Holt, S.J. (1952) A new principle for the histochemical localization of hydrolytic enzymes. *Nature*, **169**, 271.

Holt, S.J. (1956) The value of fundamental studies of staining reactions in enzyme histochemistry with reference to indoxyl methods of esterases. *Journal of Histochemistry and Cytochemistry*, **4**, 541.

Holt, S.J. & Withers, R.F.J. (1956) Cytochemical localization of esterases using odoxyl derivatives. *Nature*, **170**, 1012.

Jennekens, F.G.I., Meijer, A.E.F.H., Bethlem, J. & Van Wijngaarden, G.K. (1974) Fibre hybrids in type groups. An investigation of human muscle biopsies. *Journal of the Neurological Sciences*, **23**, 337–352.

Johnson, A.G. & Woolf, A.L. (1965) Replacement at the neuromuscular synapse of the terminal axonic expansion by the Schwann cell. *Acta Neuropathologica (Berlin)*, **4**, 436–441.

Kennedy, W.K. (1969) Innervation of human muscle spindle in patients with polyneuropathy. *Transactions of the American Neurological Association*, **94**, 59.

Koelle, G.B. & Friedenwald, J.S. (1949) A histochemical method for localizing cholinesterase activity. *Proceedings of the Society for Experimental Biology and Medicine*, **70**, 617.

Lennon, V., Lindström, J. & Seybold, M. (1975) Experimental autoimmune myasthenia (EAMG): A model of myasthenia gravis in rats and guinea pigs. *Journal of Experimental Medicine*, **141**, 1365–1375.

Mastaglia, F.L. & Walton, J.N. (1971) Histological and histochemical changes in skeletal muscles from cases of chronic juvenile and early adult spinal muscular atrophy (the Kugelberg—Welander syndrome). *Journal of the Neurological Sciences*, **12**, 15–44.

McComas, A.J., Campbell, M.J. & Sica, R.E.P. (1971) Electrophysiological study of dystrophia myotonica. *Journal of Neurology, Neurosurgery and Psychiatry*, **34**, 132–139.

McComas, A.J., Sica, R.E.P. & Currie, S. (1970) Muscular dystrophy, evidence for a neural factor. *Nature*, **226**, 1263.

MacDermot, V. (1960) The changes in the motor end-plate in myasthenia gravis. *Brain*, **83**, 24.

MacDermot, V. (1961) The histology of the neuromuscular junction in dystrophia myotonica. *Brain*, **84**, 75.

Nyström, B. (1968) Postnatal development of motor nerve terminals in 'slow-red' and 'fast-white' cat muscles. *Acta neurologica Scandinavica*, **44**, 363–383.

Panayiotopoulos, C.P. & Scarpalezos, S. (1976) Dystrophia myotonica. Peripheral nerve involvement and pathogenetic implications. *Journal of the Neurological Sciences*, **27**, 1–16.

Panayiotopoulos, C.P. & Scarpalezos, S. (1977) Dystrophia myotonica. A model of combined neural and myopathic muscle atrophy. *Journal of the Neurological Sciences*, **31**, 261–268.

Reske-Nielsen, E., Coërs, C. & Harmsen, A. (1969) Qualitative and quantitative histological study of neuromuscular biopsies from healthy young men. *Journal of the Neurological Sciences*, **10**, 369.

Santa, T., Engel, A.G. & Lambert, E.H. (1972) Histometric study of neuro-muscular junction ultrastructure I. Myasthenia gravis. *Neurology (Minneapolis)*, **22**, 71–82.

Schwarz, M.S., Stålberg, E., Schiller, H.H. & Thiele, B. (1976) The reinnervated motor unit in man. *Journal of the Neurological Sciences*, **27**, 303–312.

Swash, M. (1972) The morphology and innervation of the muscle spindle in dystrophia myotonica. *Brain*, **95**, 357–368.

Swash, M. & Fox K.P. (1974) The pathology of the human muscle spindle: effect of denervation. *Journal of the Neurological Sciences*, **22**, 1–24.

Swash, M. & Fox, K.P. (1975a) The fine structure of the spindle abnormality in myotonic dystrophy. *Neuropathology and applied Neurobiology*, **1**, 171–187.

Swash, M. & Fox, K.P. (1975b) The pathology of the muscle spindle in myasthenia gravis. *Journal of the Neurological Sciences*, **26**, 39–47.

Telerman-Toppet, N. & Coërs, C. (1978) Motor innervation and fiber type pattern in amyotrophic lateral sclerosis and in Charcot-Marie-Tooth disease. *Muscle and Nerve*, **1**, 133–139.

Tuffery, A.R. (1971) Growth and degeneration of motor end plates in normal cat hind limb muscles. *Journal of Anatomy*, **110**, 221.

Van Wijngaarden, G.K., Bethlem, J., Dingemans, K.P., Coërs, C., Telerman-Toppet, N. & Gerard, J.M. (1977)

Familial focal loss of cross striations. *Journal of Neurology*, **216**, 163–172.

Weddell, G. (1941a) The pattern of cutaneous innervation in relation to cutaneous sensibility. *Journal of Anatomy*, **75**, 346.

Weddell, G. (1941b) The multiple innervation of sensory spots in the skin. *Journal of Anatomy*, **75**, 441.

Witalinski, W. (1974) Structure of muscle fibres and motor end-plates in the intercostal muscles of Lizard, Lacerta agilis L. *Zeitschrift für mikroskopische-anatomic Forschung*, **5**, 796–808.

Witalinski, W. & Loesch, A. (1975) Structure of muscle fibres and motor end-plates in extraocular muscles of the grass snake. Natrix natrix L. *Zeitschrift für mikroskopische-anatomic Forschung*, **89**, 1133–1146.

Wohlfart, G. (1957) Collateral regeneration from residual motor nerve fibres in amyotrophic lateral sclerosis. *Neurology (Minneapolis)*, **7**, 124.

Wohlfart, G. (1960) Clinical significance of collateral sprouting of remaining motor nerve fibres in partially denervated muscles. *Journal of the Experimental Medical Sciences*, **3**, 128–133.

Woolf, A.L. (1956) Recent advances in the technique of muscle biopsy. *Journal of Clinical Pathology*, **9**, 184.

Woolf, A.L. (1957) The significance of the sprouting of intramuscular nerves. *Nederlands tijdschrift voor geneeskunde*, **101–102**, 1506.

Woolf, A.L. (1959a) Biopsy study of the pathology of the lower motor neurone. *American Journal of Physical Medicine*, **38**, 26.

Woolf, A.L. (1959b) Bie Pathologie des peripheren motorischen Neurons im Bild der Muskelbiopsie. *Deutsche Zeitschrift für Nervenheilkinde*, **179**, 423.

Woolf, A.L. (1960) Muscle biopsy in the diagnosis of the 'floppy baby': infantile hypotonia. *Cerebral Palsy Bulletin*, **2**, 19.

Woolf, A.L. (1962a, b) The theoretical basis of clinical electromyography, Parts I and II. *Annals of Physical Medicine*, **6**, 189, 241.

Woolf, A.L. (1962c) Muscle biopsy. In *Modern Trends in Neurology*, Ed. D. Williams, 3rd Edn. (Butterworth: London).

Woolf, A.L. (1965) the pathology of the intramuscular nerve-endings. *Proceedings Vth international Congress Neuropathology*, Zürich, 641–647.

Woolf, A.L., Bagnall, H.J., Bauwens, P. & Bickerstaff, E.R. (1956) A case of myasthenia gravis with changes in the intramuscular nerve endings. *Journal of Pathology and Bacteriology*, **71**, 173.

Woolf, A.L. & Malins, J.M. (1957) Changes in the intramuscular nerve endings in diabetic neuropathy: A biopsy study. *Journal of Pathology and Bacteriology*, **73**, 316.

Histochemical aspects of muscle disease

INTRODUCTION

Histochemistry is a relatively young science and found its first applications to the study of muscle as recently as the late 1950s. Yet within a mere 10 years or so it probably contributed more to our understanding of neuromuscular disorders than conventional histology in the previous 100 years. Histochemical techniques may lack the quantitative precision of biochemical methods, but they do have the distinct advantage of accurate localisation at a cytological level. It is thus possible to compare the activities of a cell with those of its neighbour and also to correlate chemical reactions with morphological structures within the cell itself.

The scope of histochemistry is wide. It is not possible in the confines of this chapter to cover all aspects in relation to muscle. I shall rather concentrate on only a few aspects of enzyme histochemistry and I shall include an appraisal of the results in normal as well as in diseased muscle.

Enzyme histochemistry has made three main contributions in the study of muscle—the recognition of fibre types in human and animal muscle and their response to disease processes and to neural and other influences; the demonstration of abnormalities in muscle fibres which appear to be normal by conventional staining methods; and the diagnosis of specific enzyme deficiencies, e.g. phosphorylase deficiency.

A mere 15 years ago histochemistry was still a research tool in the investigation of muscle disorders. Now it has become a routine procedure in most laboratories and an essential component of any diagnostic analysis by means of muscle biopsy; it provides the only method of recognising some of the congenital myopathies, selective fibre-type involvement, fibre-type grouping and other changes which would not be apparent with routine histological stains.

METHODS

Choice of biopsy material

Muscle is not a uniform homogeneous tissue. In animals, and probably also in humans, there are differences from muscle to muscle and perhaps even in the same muscle in different individuals. For comparative enzyme studies in normal muscle it is thus desirable to restrict oneself to the same anatomical groups of muscles in order not to introduce unpredictable variables.

In the assessment of diseased muscle the selection is even more critical. The muscle of choice should be one which is clinically affected, but not to such an advanced degree that all muscle tissue has degenerated beyond recognition. For example, in an early case of childhood muscular dystrophy there is no point in choosing a muscle in the upper limb which may be readily accessible but shows no histological change, and in an advanced case equal difficulty may arise from choosing a muscle completely replaced by fat. Where a disease process is fairly focal, e.g. peroneal muscular atrophy, care should be taken to select a muscle that is affected by the disease.

In general I have found the rectus femoris to be an easily accessible and useful muscle for the investigation of proximal muscle syndromes, such as infantile spinal muscular atrophy or progressive muscular dystrophy. The gastrocnemius will also show early signs in progressive muscular dystrophy. It has been my practice to do all biopsies under local anaesthesia, and to select three or four separate samples of the muscle in order not to miss focal pathological changes. The recent application of needle biopsy sampling has made the procedure less traumatic and yet it provides an adequate sample for routine diagnostic purposes.

Method of preparation

Some enzymes are able to withstand fixation, but many are destroyed by the process. In general, fresh frozen tissue has distinct advantages for enzyme study as well as for routine histological stains.

Improvements in the methods for rapid freezing of tissue and for cutting thin sections have eliminated many of the early artefacts such as disruption of muscle fibres and ice crystal formation.

The method we have favoured is rapid quenching of the specimens in liquid nitrogen ($-180°C$) (Dubowitz and Pearse, 1961). The conventional slower freezing with solid CO_2 ($-70°C$) or CO_2-acetone mixtures is more likely to result in freezing artefact such as ice crystal formation with 'holes' in the tissue.

Specimens of muscle approximately 0.5 cm³ or less are carefully orientated in a transverse or longitudinal plane on a slice of cork about 0.25 cm thick, cut from an ordinary bottle cork (about 1 cm diameter). In general, transverse sections are much more informative than longitudinal. Better orientation of the specimen in an accurate plane can be achieved by mounting it in 10 per cent tragacanth gum or 'Tissue Tek' (OCT Compound, Miles Laboratories). Relevant data can be written on the side of the cork. The specimen is then submerged in liquid nitrogen for approximately 10 s. A good indication of the end point is when the large bubbles cease and a fine stream of small bubbles appears. Submersion for too long a period causes cracking of the specimen, while if it is too short artefacts appear in the muscle.

Isopentane cooled in liquid nitrogen may be used as an alternative. It has the added advantage of even more rapid freezing in the absence of a protective layer of gas bubbles, and accordingly even less artefact. (For further details of biopsy techniques see Dubowitz and Brooke, 1973.) Needle biopsy samples are more difficult to orientate in an absolute transverse plane, but this can be achieved by mounting the specimen on to a cork, as above, under a dissecting microscope and carefully orientating it before freezing. The subsequent handling of the specimen is similar to that of open biopsies.

Specimens can be stored at $-20°C$ or lower, preferably in an airtight container to prevent drying. The cork is then mounted on a tissue holder by freezing with a few drops of water, and sections are cut in a cryostat (cold microtome) at about $-20°$ to $-30°C$. In dystrophic muscle with extensive adipose tissue, an even lower temperature may be an advantage. This can be achieved by placing solid CO_2 directly on the tissue holder of the cryostat or by using CO_2-cooled or thermoelectrically cooled holders.

Mounting the tissue on slices of cork has the additional advantage that the cork can be removed from the tissue holder of the microtome and subsequently refrozen on to it again with a few drops of water, without disturbing the specimen.

Sections can be mounted directly on coverslips. This is economical in the use of reagents and also speeds up the rate of processing. Most enzyme reactions, and special stains such as those for lipids and glycogen, can be done on frozen sections. For routine stains sections can be post-fixed for 5 min (or longer) in 5 per cent acetic ethanol. For the histological diagnosis of myopathies, haematoxylin and eosin and the Van Gieson stain have been found adequate. The Verhoeff-Van Gieson modification has an advantage in also staining the myelin of any nerves present. The modified Gomori trichrome stain (Engel and Cunningham, 1963) is useful for the detection of some of the congenital non-progressive myopathies, e.g. nemaline myopathy.

Tissue blocks can be stored at $-30°C$ in polythene containers or sealed in polythene tubing. For prolonged storage, a lower temperature $(-70°C)$ is to be preferred.

Other methods are available for preparation. Freeze-drying, for example, has the advantage of better preservation of tissue and provides the possibility of storage for an indefinite period. However, there is a limit to the size of the specimen that can be used and, with most forms of apparatus, the method is more time-consuming.

Scope

The total number of enzyme systems that can be assessed by histochemical methods has steadily increased over the past 20 years (Pearse, 1968). The following are of particular interest in relation to muscle metabolism.

Glycogen synthesis and breakdown
Phosphorylase
α-1,4-glucosidase (acid maltase)
Dextrin-1,6-glucosidase (debranching enzyme)
α-1,4-glucan: α-1,4-glucan 6-glycosyl transferase (branching enzyme)
Uridine diphosphate (UDP) glucose-glycogen glucosyltransferase
Aldolase
Phosphofructokinase.

Diaphorases and dehydrogenases
Nicotinamide-adenine dinucleotide (NAD)-tetrazolium reductase (*DPN diaphorase)

and NADP-tetrazolium reductase (*TPN diaphorase)
NAD-linked isocitrate, malate, α-glycerophosphate, lactate, alcohol, and glutamate dehydrogenases
NADP-linked isocitrate, β-hydroxybutyrate and glucose-6-phosphate dehydrogenases
Non-coenzyme-linked α-glycerophosphate and succinate dehydrogenases

Oxidases
Cytochrome oxidase.

Phosphatases
Adenosine triphosphatase, acid and alkaline phosphatases, 5-nucleotidase.

Esterases
Acetylcholinesterase, pseudocholinesterase and non-specific esterases.

In addition to methods for enzymes there are also histochemical techniques available for the assessment of various chemical radicals.

General considerations

It is pointless to try to apply new methods to the assessment of pathological tissue before one has a clear knowledge of the normal. In a study of normal muscle, one is particularly interested in the presence or absence of certain enzyme systems, the relation of the enzyme systems to known structures of the muscle, and the variation in activity of individual fibres within the muscle itself. A further extension of the methods to animal muscle allows one to compare different levels of phylogenetic development and also to investigate particular aspects under controlled conditions.

In general, it is preferable to study a group of enzymes in a particular cycle or system rather than to try to draw far-reaching conclusions from the investigation of a single enzyme.

NORMAL MUSCLE

Oxidative enzymes

These enzymes, which include the dehydrogenases, diaphorases and oxidases, are impor-

*The Commission on enzymes of IUB, 1961, 1964, recommended the replacement of these terms by nicotinamide-adenine dinucleotide (NAD) and nicotinamide-adenine dinucleotide phosphate (NADP).

tant in so far as they reflect the utilisation of various metabolic intermediaries of the Krebs' cycle and related pathways. They therefore give an indication of the possible sources of energy in muscle metabolism.

The first advance in this field was the development of a reliable method for demonstrating succinate dehydrogenase (Rutenburg, Gofstein and Seligman, 1950; Seligman and Rutenberg, 1951). This was followed by the introduction of satisfactory techniques for diphosphopyridine nucleotide (DPN) and triphosphopyridine nucleotide (TPN) diaphorases (Farber, Sternberg and Dunlap, 1956; Nachlas, Walker and Seligman, 1958a, b; Scarpelli, Hess and Pearse, 1958) and various dehydrogenases connected with the Krebs' cycle and glycolytic and related pathways (Hess, Scarpelli and Pearse, 1958).

The *dehydrogenases* are substrate-specific oxidative enzymes which transfer electrons (hydrogen) from a substrate to an acceptor. Apart from succinate dehydrogenase and non-coenzyme linked α-glycerophosphate dehydrogenase, all the remaining dehydrogenases require in addition a coenzyme—either NAD (coenzyme I) or NADP (coenzyme II)—to act as a carrier in the passage of the electrons to molecular oxygen:

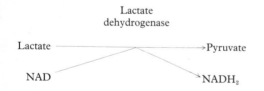

The reduced coenzymes ($NADH_2$ and $NADPH_2$) in turn are oxidised by the diaphorases (NAD-D and NADP-D) which are flavoprotein enzymes:

$NADPH_2 \longrightarrow$ NADP-D (flavoprotein)

Tetrazolium Cyt.b→Cyt.c→Cyt.a→O_2
salt

$NADH_2 \longrightarrow$ NAD-D (flavoprotein)

The principle of the methods used is to employ a soluble tetrazolium salt which intercepts the electrons at some point in the respiratory chain and is reduced to an insoluble formazan product, which precipitates at the site of the enzyme

activity. In the case of the coenzyme-linked dehydrogenases, such as lactate dehydrogenase, the final product probably demonstrates the localisation of the respective coenzyme diaphorase rather than the actual site of the dehydrogenase itself (Farber *et al.*, 1956; Blanchaer and van Wijhe, 1962). Moreover, the addition of an electron acceptor, such as phenazine methosulphate, will alter the localisation in the lactate dehydrogenase reaction in muscle (van Wijhe, Blanchaer and Jacyk, 1963).

Wattenberg and Leong (1960) described a method for demonstrating a non-coenzyme linked α-glycerophosphate dehydrogenase by using vitamin K_3 (menadione) as an intermediate electron acceptor.

The first application of these methods to human muscle was the investigation of autopsy specimens by Wachstein and Meisel (1955). They noted a variation in the succinate dehydrogenase activity of individual fibres and observed that the more reactive fibres tended to be smaller in diameter. Beckett and Bourne (1958a) found a similar variation in the activity of succinate dehydrogenase but in a parallel assessment of cytochrome oxidase (an enzyme which carries electrons from cytochrome c to oxygen) they were unable to demonstrate any correlation between the presence of this enzyme and succinate dehydrogenase.

The activities of the following oxidative enzyme systems were investigated by Dubowitz and Pearse (1960a, 1961) in biopsy specimens of human muscle: NAD and NADP-diaphorases, NAD-linked β-hydroxybutyrate, isocitrate, malate, glutamate, α-glycerophosphate, alcohol and lactate dehydrogenases; NADP-linked isocitrate and glucose-6-phosphate dehydrogenases; non-coenzyme linked succinate dehydrogenase.

Positive reactions were obtained with all the enzymes except β-hydroxybutyric dehydrogenase, which was consistently negative. The reactions for $NADH_2$-diaphorase and lactate dehydrogenase were the most intense (Fig. 8.1) and those for glucose-6-phosphate and alcohol dehydrogenases the weakest.

It was found that there was a striking variation in the activity of individual fibres (Figs 8.1 and 8.2). These fell mainly into two groups. One group of fibres, usually of smaller diameter, gave a

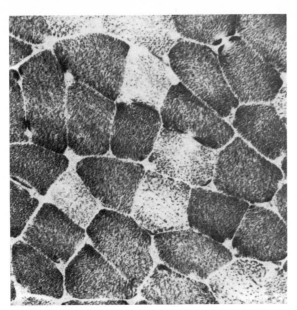

Fig. 8.1 Normal quadriceps muscle showing checkerboard pattern of dark (type I) and light (type II) fibres. NADH-TR, ×330

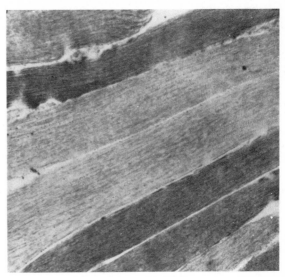

Fig. 8.2 Normal quadriceps muscle showing uniformity of enzyme activity throughout the length of the fibre in a longitudinal section. NADH-TR, ×330

stronger reaction and was found on serial section to do so consistently for all the oxidative enzymes investigated. The other group, usually of larger diameter, gave a consistently weaker reaction for all the oxidative enzyme systems tested. In addition, fibres of intermediate activity and size were present. In longitudinal section, a particular fibre gave a uniform reaction throughout its length and the granular deposits tended to be arranged in a linear fashion. Although this corresponded to the electron-microscopic distribution of the mito-chondria between the myofibrils (Bennett and Porter, 1953) there was still doubt about which of these enzymes are truly associated with mitochon-dria and which are cytoplasmic. At present only succinate, β-hydroxybutyrate and noncoenzyme-linked α-glycerophosphate dehydrogenases and the NAD and NADP diaphorases are regarded as definitely mitochondrial.

A parallel study of cytochrome oxidase accord-ing to the methods of Nachlas, Crawford, Gold-stein and Seligman (1958) and Burstone (1959) demonstrated a similar variation and a con-centration of activity in the same fibres as the other oxidative enzymes.

The above observations in human muscle brought to mind the well-known division of animal muscle into red and white fibres and the physiological distinction between slow and fast muscles. (For a detailed historical review on physiological and structural aspects of fibre types in animal muscle see Dubowitz (1968a).) Various workers have investigated the oxidative enzymes in *animal muscle*. Semenoff (1935), using the classical methylene blue technique for succinate dehydrogenase, found a variation in the activity of individual fibres in amphibian muscle. Similar observations on mammalian muscle were reported by Padykula (1952), Wachstein and Meisel (1955), Buño and Germino (1958). Nachmias and Pady-kula (1958) observed that in the soleus of the rat, which is a red muscle, the succinate dehydro-genase activity in the fibres was uniformly strong. On the other hand, in the biceps femoris and the tibialis anterior, which are mixed muscles, there was a marked variation between the fibres. In an investigation of the succinate dehydrogenase activity in the muscles of fish, frogs, birds and mammals, Ogata (1958a) recognised three types of fibres: a large white fibre with weak enzyme activity, a small red fibre strong in activity and a 'medium' fibre intermediate in size and activity. He obtained similar results with the cytochrome oxidase reaction (Ogata, 1958b) and with DPN-

and TPN-diaphorases (Ogata, 1958c). George and Scaria (1958a) carried out similar investigations in the breast and leg muscles of the pigeon and fowl and were able to correlate high oxidative enzyme activity with red muscle fibres and with a high content of mitochondria in the fibres. Stein and Padykula (1962) were able to recognise three types of fibres in the gastrocnemius of the rat on the basis of succinate dehydrogenase activity. They comprised one group with low succinate dehydrogenase activity and two groups with high activity. In the soleus there were two types, both with high activity. Similar observations have been made in the 'red' and 'white' muscles of the rat and the monkey (Bocek and Beatty 1966) and in the soleus, crureus and other muscles of the rat, rabbit and cat (Nyström, 1966; Dubowitz, personal observations).

Enzymes connected with glycogen metabolism

Phosphorylase. This cytoplasmic enzyme is of interest because it is thought to reflect the utilisation of glycogen in muscle metabolism. It effects the synthesis and destruction of α-1,4^1-glucosidic linkages by catalysing the reversible reaction:

Glucose-1-phosphate+polysaccharide prime & inorganic phosphate+glucosyl (α-1,4^1) primer (Stetten and Stetten, 1960). These glucosidic linkages form the basis of glycogen:

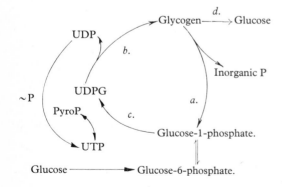

Enzymes: a=phosphorylase and debranching enzyme.
            b=UDP glucose-glycogen glucosyltransferase and branching enzyme.
            c=UDP glucose-pyrophosphorylase.
            d=α-1,4-glucosidase (acid maltase).

Although reversible in the test tube, the action of phosphorylase *in vivo* is thought to proceed from right to left in this reaction and thus to be concerned only with the breakdown of the α-1,4^1-glucosidic linkages in glycogen. The histochemical method for the demonstration of phosphorylase (Takeuchi and Kuriaki, 1955; Takeuchi, 1956) uses glucose-1-phosphate as substrate and assesses the extent of glycogen production. There were subsequently a number of improvements in the technique (Eränkö and Palkama, 1961; Sawyer, Sie and Fishman, 1965).

In an application of this method to muscle (Dubowitz and Pearse, 1960a; 1961) a variation in the activity of individual fibres was noted (Fig. 8.3). In contrast to the dehydrogenases, however, it was the larger fibres which gave the stronger reaction for phosphorylase. In serial sections there was a consistent reciprocal relationship between the content of the oxidative enzymes and that of phosphorylase in any given muscle fibre. This reciprocal relationship was present in all the samples of human muscle studied, and has been consistently verified in our subsequent investigations of both adult and infant muscle.

We concluded from these observations that, in human muscle, there were two separate fibre types which had a different source of energy for their function. Thus, the fibres with high phosphorylase content were probably mainly dependent on the intrinsic glycogen for their energy, while the fibres with the high levels of oxidative enzymes probably obtained their energy by preferential use of the substrates of the Krebs' cycle and some of the associated pathways.

A comparative study of the muscles of the rat, pigeon, toad and goldfish (Dubowitz and Pearse, 1960b), confirmed the observations of earlier authors on some of the oxidative enzymes. This study was extended to include various other dehydrogenases and also phosphorylase. Muscles of the rat and pigeon contained fibres with either high or low oxidative enzyme content. On serial section, individual fibres showed a consistent activity of the various oxidative enzymes. As in the human, there was a reciprocal relation between the phosphorylase content and the oxidative enzyme activity in individual fibres. Red muscle such as the pectoralis of the pigeon was composed almost

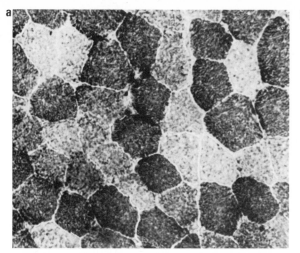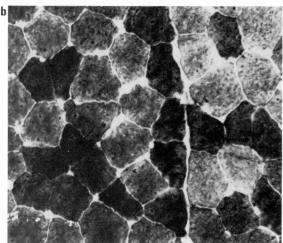

Fig. 8.3 Normal muscle showing reciprocal activity between oxidative enzyme (a) and phosphorylase (b) activity in individual fibres. Quadriceps. (a) NADH-TR, ×330; (b) phosphorylase, ×330

entirely of small fibres high in oxidative enzymes and low in phosphorylase. The fibres of high oxidative enzyme activity thus correspond to the red fibres in animals and, as the Krebs' cycle is a much better source of energy-rich phosphate bonds than the glycolytic pathway, these fibres are well adapted for sustained activity. The fibres rich in phosphorylase, on the other hand, correspond to the white or pale fibres and are designed for rapid but unsustained activity. Because of the confusion in the use of the terms 'red' and 'white' muscle in the literature, and the difficulty of designating human muscle as 'fast' or 'slow', it was thought more satisfactory to subdivide arbitrarily the muscle fibres in both human and other mammalian muscle into type I and type II fibres, based either on the reciprocal activity of oxidative enzymes and phosphorylase in individual fibres, or on the ATPase activity (*see* below).

In an application of the method for demonstrating the non-coenzyme linked mitochondrial form of α-glycerophosphate dehydrogenase, Pearse (1961) found that in rat muscle the enzyme was more strongly concentrated in the large fibres (type II fibres). This was subsequently confirmed in biopsies of human muscle but the results were not as consistent (Dubowitz, unpublished results).

Uridine diphosphate glucose-glycogen glucosyl transferase. A method has been described for the histochemical demonstration of UDPG-glycogen transferase (Takeuchi and Glenner, 1960; 1961). This enzyme is capable of synthesising glycogen from glucose-1-phosphate via the uridine diphosphate glucose (UDPG) cycle (Leloir and Cardini, 1957), according to the reactions:

Glucose-1-phoshate + uridine diphosphate $\rightleftharpoons$ UDPG + phosphate.
UDPG + saccharide primer $\rightleftharpoons$ UDP + glucosyl $(\alpha\text{-}1,4^1)$ primer

Hess and Pearse (1961) applied the histochemical technique for this enzyme to rat muscle, but it has not yet found much application in human muscle.

Branching enzyme. This enzyme, amylo $(1,4 \rightarrow 1,6)$ transglucosidase, introduces $\alpha\text{-}1,6^1$ bonds and hence side chains in the linear glucosyl $(\alpha\text{-}1,4^1)$ primer, produced by UDPG-glycogen transferase. These two enzymes are thus responsible for the synthesis of glycogen from glucose-1-phosphate.

A histochemical method for demonstrating the branching enzyme was described by Takeuchi (1958). He obtained a positive reaction in skeletal muscle. However, there has not been any more comprehensive study of this enzyme in muscle since that time.

Aldolase. Earlier methods for aldolase were unreliable, but a number of improved techniques have been published (Nepveux and Wegmann, 1962; Abe and Shimizu, 1964; Lake, 1965). In an application of these methods to human and animal muscle, we found that type I fibres gave a stronger reaction than type II. This is contrary to expectation and it is possible that the method reflects a false localisation, as in the case of lactate dehydrogenase (van Wijhe *et al.*, 1963), and is limited by the level of $NADH_2$ diaphorase in the muscle fibre. Biochemical studies have shown a higher level of aldolase in the flexor digitorum longus muscle of the cat, containing predominantly type II fibres, than in the soleus with predominantly type I (Prewitt and Salafsky, 1967).

Phosphatases

These enzymes are able to hydrolyse various organic phosphate esters with the liberation of phosphate. The non-specific alkaline phosphatase reaction has been widely studied in many tissues. Some of the pitfalls in interpretation of the results of this relatively simple method have been reviewed by Pearse (1960).

Alkaline phosphatase. This enzyme is absent from the fibres of human and animal muscle (Gomori, 1939; Rossi, Pescetto and Reale, 1954; Beckett and Bourne, 1958b). It can be demonstrated in the walls of capillaries and in the muscular and intimal coats of large vessels.

Acid phosphatase. Gomori (1941) was unable to demonstrate any acid phosphatase activity in human muscle obtained at biopsy or *post mortem*. Dempsey, Wislocki and Singer (1946) obtained a similar result, but did note that after prolonged incubation (24–72 h) with certain substrates at pH 7.0, there was a positive reaction in some of the muscle fibres. Rossi, Pescetto and Reale (1953; 1954) obtained a positive reaction in the nuclei of developing human fetal muscle as well as in adult muscle. Beckett and Bourne (1958b) were able, after prolonged incubation, to demonstrate acid phosphatase activity in the muscle fibres, the nuclei and Golgi apparatus, and also in the adipose tissue and connective tissue.

5-Nucleotidase. This is a specific phosphatase

which is able to split off the phosphate in the 5 position of the ribose ring as in adenosine-5^1-monophosphoric acid (AMP).

Newman, Feigin, Wolf and Kabat (1950) did an extensive investigation of phosphatases in various tissues using a variety of substrates. They found that with the use of adenosine-5^1-monophosphoric acid (muscle adenylic acid) or adenosine triphosphoric acid as substrates the subsequent localisation of enzyme activity in tissues differed from that of other substrates. They concluded that this reaction was due to a specific phosphatase, 5-nucleotidase, similar to that recognised chemically by Reis (1934). Its characteristic location was in the muscular walls of medium-sized arteries. In skeletal muscle a positive reaction was present in capillary endothelium. With AMP as substrate, Maengwyn-Davies, Friedenwald and White (1952) obtained a weak diffuse reaction in the muscle fibres after prolonged incubation. There was also some weak activity in the muscle nuclei and in the adventitia and media of blood vessels.

Beckett and Bourne (1958c) found that in normal muscle 5-nucleotidase activity is often entirely absent; any enzyme activity present is restricted to the connective tissue and is found in the walls of large blood vessels, in axons and the neurokeratin network of peripheral nerves, in the connective tissue sheaths of muscle spindles, and in occasional fibroblasts.

Adenosine triphosphatase (ATPase). This enzyme breaks down adenosine triphosphate to adenosine diphosphate with the release of an energy-rich phosphate bond. Recent work has shown that, by varying the pH of the substrate solution and by the use of certain activators and inhibitors, the histochemical localisation of ATPase can vary considerably (Brooke and Kaiser, 1969). This explains some of the discrepancies when comparing earlier reports.

Wachstein and Meisel (1956) noted some variation in the activity of individual muscle fibres at pH 7.2. Nachmias and Padykula (1958) observed that, at pH 9.4, variation in fibre activity was present in the rat soleus and biceps femoris. There was no apparent correlation between depth of the stain and fibre size. The intrafusal fibres of the muscle spindles showed strong activity.

Freiman and Kaplan (1960) showed that at least three different phosphatases, viz. non-specific alkaline phosphatase, ATPase and less specific polyphosphatase, can split ATP at pH 9.4. These enzymes can be distinguished by appropriate inhibitors. Gauthier and Padykula (1962) described methods for demonstrating ATPase localised to three different sites in muscle. These comprise a mitochondrial ATPase, a myosin ATPase, localised to the A bands of the myofibrils, and a third form which cytochemically forms a reticular pattern around individual myofibrils.

Stein and Padykula (1962) attempted to correlate the ATPase activity in individual muscle fibres of the rat with succinic dehydrogenase and also with non-specific esterase. On the basis of the succinic dehydrogenase (SD) activity they divided the fibres into three types—A fibres with low SD content corresponding to fast or white fibres and B and C fibres with high SD activity which were two forms of slow red fibres. Type A fibres were rich in ATPase and poor in nonspecific esterase, type B were poor in ATPase and rich in esterase, while type C had a high content of both ATPase and esterase. Engel (1962) demonstrated that in human muscle the type II fibres have a higher content of myofibrillar ATPase than the type I fibres. Subsequently Drews and Engel (1966) demonstrated a reversal of this reaction by pre-incubating with EDTA at pH 4.3. The type I fibres were then strongly reactive, and the type II weak. Brooke and Kaiser (1969) showed that this was purely an effect of the pH and not dependent on the EDTA.

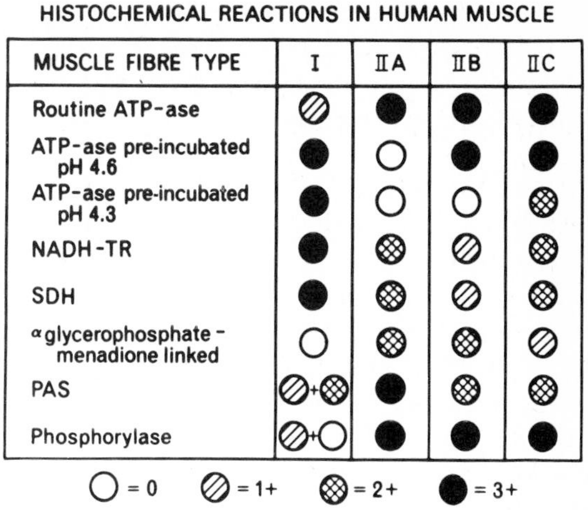

Glycogen

The early methods for demonstrating glycogen in tissue were not consistently reliable, particularly in fixed material. This may account for the relative paucity of detailed studies on muscle in the earlier literature.

Beckett and Bourne (1958d) compared various methods. They found that glycogen could be demonstrated in human muscle for 1–12 h *post mortem* and tended to disappear in 12–48 h. There was a variation in the glycogen content from one muscle to another under normal conditions.

In rat muscle, Nachmias and Padykula (1958),

HISTOCHEMICAL REACTIONS IN HUMAN MUSCLE

MUSCLE FIBRE TYPE	I	IIA	IIB	IIC
Routine ATP-ase	1+	3+	3+	3+
ATP-ase pre-incubated pH 4.6	3+	0	3+	3+
ATP-ase pre-incubated pH 4.3	3+	0	0	2+
NADH-TR	3+	2+	1+	2+
SDH	3+	2+	1+	2+
α glycerophosphate - menadione linked	0	2+	2+	1+
PAS	1+ & 2+	3+	2+	2+
Phosphorylase	1+ & 0	3+	3+	3+

○ = 0   ⊘ = 1+   ⊗ = 2+   ● = 3+

Fig. 8.4 Histochemical reactions of the different fibre types in human muscle (from Dubowitz and Brooke, 1973)

using the periodic-acid-Schiff technique, obtained better results with frozen than with fixed tissue. They observed that the fibres in the soleus showed a uniformity of glycogen content, but that in the biceps femoris the larger fibres tended to stain more strongly, but the correlation of activity to size was not a consistent one.

George and Naik (1958) found a high glycogen content in the broad fibres of the pigeon breast muscle. These fibres were low in oxidative enzyme content. Hess and Pearse (1961), on the other hand, found that in rat muscles the glycogen tended to be concentrated in the smaller fibres. In human muscle the type II fibres tend to have a higher glycogen content than type I but intermediate-staining fibres are also present (Dubowitz and Brooke, 1973) (*see* Fig. 8.4.).

Lipids

Sudanophilic stains were extensively used by the early workers investigating the nature of dark and light fibres and the interstitial granules in muscle (Bullard, 1912; Denny-Brown, 1929).

In their investigations in rat muscle, Nachmias and Padykula (1958) found a uniform fat content in the fibres of the soleus, but marked variation in the fibres of the biceps femoris, gastrocnemius and pectorals. The larger fibres were less sudanophilic than the narrow ones. There was a correlation between the greater staining of the smaller fibres and their increased mitochondrial content. George and Naik (1958) similarly noted an increased lipid content in the narrow fibres of the pigeon breast muscles. George and Scaria (1958b) found that the narrow fibres of the pigeon pectoralis muscle also had a higher lipase content than the broad fibres.

With the use of Sudan Black stain, Beckett and Bourne (1958e) noted a 'tremendous variation' in the amount of fat from one specimen to another and also between individual muscle fibres. Gauthier and Padykula (1966) used the Sudan Black stain as an index of mitochondrial content of the fibres they were studying in the diaphragm of various animals.

FIBRE TYPES

The subdivision of muscle fibres into two types (Table 8.1) on the basis of either the oxidative enzymes and phosphorylase (Dubowitz and Pearse, 1960) or myofibrillar ATPase (Engel, 1962) has found wide application in the interpretation of normal and diseased human muscle, in contrast to the more complex systems of three (Stein and Padykula, 1962) or even eight fibre types (Romanul, 1964 in animals).

Table 8.1 Histochemical activity of fibre types

Enzyme Reaction	Type I	Type II
NADH$_2$-TR	Strong	Weak
Phosphorylase	Weak	Strong
Myofibrillar ATPase	Weak	Strong

One of the problems in comparative studies has been the presence of intermediate-reacting fibres with any particular system, especially in animal muscles. Moreover, the physiologists have had difficulty in correlating physiological with histochemical data. Thus, in the extensor digitorum longus of the rat, a mixed muscle histochemically, all the motor units were fast (Close, 1967), whereas the soleus, an apparently uniform muscle on oxidative enzyme reaction, showed about 10 per cent of units faster in activity than the remaining slow ones. Edström and Kugelberg (1968) subsequently showed that the motor units of small, mitochondria-rich fibres in the rat EDL were as

fast physiologically as the motor units with mitochondria-poor fibres. This led to the introduction of a somewhat complex nomenclature of 'fast-twitch white', 'slow-twitch red' and 'fast-twitch intermediate' fibres (Barnard, Edgerton, Furukawa and Peter, 1971).

With a further extension of the ATPase reaction, by pre-incubation at pH 4.2, 4.6 and 9.4, Brooke and Kaiser (1970) were able to define three subtypes of the type II fibre (Fig. 8.4). From further correlative studies in human and animal muscle it seems likely that this subdivision into type I and type IIA, IIB and IIC fibres will account, not only for all the intermediate reacting fibres with various reactions in human muscle, but also the various physiological and histochemical permutations, with their complex nomenclature, suggested in animal muscle by Barnard *et al.* (1971) and Burke, Levine, Zajac, Tsairis and Engel (1971) (Dubowitz and Brooke, 1973).

Type I, type IIA and type IIB comprise approximately equal proportions of adult human muscle fibres, whereas type IIC fibres are normally not present in mature human muscle, but do occur in fetal muscle and under pathological conditions.

Most of the advances in the interpretation of muscle biopsies, have resulted from the recognition of these fibre types in human muscle and their selective involvement in various disease processes. In practice, only a small number of histochemical procedures is necessary for their recognition, such as the ATPase and the NADH–tetrazolium reductase reactions. Additional information may be obtained from the phosphorylase reaction and a glycogen stain (PAS) (Table 8.2).

DEVELOPING MUSCLE

The presence of different types of muscle fibres is a feature of mature muscle.

In a study of oxidative enzymes, phosphorylase and adenosine triphosphatase in developing muscle (Dubowitz, 1963a), it was found that, in full-term human infants, differentiation of the muscle into two groups of fibres was already present at birth. The enzymic activities were

Table 8.2 Muscle biopsy: routine preparations

Stain/enzyme reaction	Information
Haematoxylin and eosin	Normal/abnormal
Verhoeff–van Gieson	Connective tissue, nerves
Gomori trichrome	Nemaline rods, 'ragged red' fibres
Oil red O	Fat
PAS	Glycogen
Acid phosphatase	Degenerating fibres
RNA (methyl green pyronine)	Regenerating fibres
ATPase (pH 9.4)	Fibre types (type I light; type II dark)
ATPase (pH 4.6, 4.3)	Fibre subtypes (type IIA, B, C)
NADH-TR	Fibre types (type I dark; type II light) Structural abnormalities (cores; mitochondria)

comparable to those of adult muscle, although the muscle fibres at this stage were much smaller in diameter, and in cross-section they tended to be rounded rather than polygonal.

Developing animal muscle

Variation in enzymic activity was also noted at birth in the skeletal muscle fibres of the guinea-pig, rabbit and hamster (Dubowitz, 1963a; 1965a; 1968a). This was most striking in the guinea-pig where the muscle fibres were polygonal in shape and distinctly arranged into bundles, as in the adult muscle. The muscles of the rabbit and hamster also showed differentiation, but this was not as well developed as in the guinea-pig. In the case of the rat, the fibres were not differentiated at birth. There was a uniform activity for each of the enzymes investigated. The muscle fibres were small and rounded and not arranged in compact bundles. Differentiation occurred at about 7–10 days of age. The rate of differentiation varied from one muscle group to another. It also seemed to be influenced by nutrition and general growth, because rats from smaller litters showed faster growth and earlier differentiation of the muscle. By the age of 2 weeks the muscle fibres were well differentiated, polygonal in shape, arranged in bundles, and resembled adult muscle.

The difference in maturation of the muscle in these animals may be partly correlated with their length of gestation and degree of maturity at birth.

The guinea-pig with a 68-day gestation period has a more mature fur at birth and is more mobile than the others. The rabbit (30–32 days gestation) has a better-developed fur and is more active than the rat (gestation 21 days).

The hamster, although having a shorter gestation (16–19 days) than the rat, also appears to be more active at birth and has a better-formed fur. The rat is not very mobile in the first few days and does not develop a fur before the fourth or fifth day.

In the cat, Nyström (1966) has shown that both the gastrocnemius and the soleus initially give a uniform reaction with NADH-tetrazolium reductase. By 15 days the gastrocnemius is clearly differentiated into two fibre types, while the soleus remains of one fibre type. Cosmos (1966) has demonstrated in the developing chick that both the pectoralis and the gastrocnemius initially consist of type I fibres only and that differentiation into predominantly type II fibres in the pectoralis and a mixture of type I, type II and intermediate fibres in the gastrocnemius occurs during development.

In a study of the developing soleus and crureus muscle of the cat and rabbit (Dubowitz, unpublished results) there was a uniform reaction with NADH-tetrazolium reductase and succinate dehydrogenase, but the phosphorylase and ATPase reactions in contrast showed a subdivision into strongly and weakly reacting fibres. This suggested that in the soleus some enzymes may show variation while others do not. In the gastrocnemius, flexor hallucis longus and flexor digitorum longus, the fibres were uniform in activity, particularly with the NADH-tetrazolium reductase reaction, but by one week of age showed differentiation similar to adult muscle. The differentiation became apparent with the phosphorylase and ATPase reactions before the NADH-tetrazolium reductase. Recently Burke et al. (1971) showed, in the gastrocnemius of the cat, that fibres with high oxidative enzyme content might belong to either fast or slow motor units, and had respectively high or low ATPase activity.

Karpati and Engel (1967) have shown that the soleus of the developing guinea-pig initially gives a mixed pattern with the ATPase reaction, and subsequently becomes uniformly weak, with the exception of a small proportion of fibres.

Developing human muscle

In the developing human fetus there appear to be three distinct phases in the differentiation of the muscle into fibre types (Dubowitz, 1965b; 1968a).

In the early fetus, up to about 18 weeks' gestation, there is no clear-cut subdivision into fibre types. There may be some variation in enzyme activity, but the strongly or weakly reacting fibres tend to occur in clusters, and there is no reciprocal reaction between oxidative enzymes on the one hand and phosphorylase and ATPase on the other.

Between 18 and about 28 weeks the fibres are subdivided into type I and type II fibres with similar enzyme patterns to adult muscle. However, the type I fibres form only a small proportion (about 5–10 per cent) of the total (Fig. 8.5) and correspond in distribution to Wohlfart B fibres (Wohlfart, 1937).

After 30 weeks' gestation the muscle has a checkerboard pattern, as in mature muscle. Brooke, Williamson and Kaiser (1971) suggested that the undifferentiated fibres in human fetal muscle are type IIC fibres and that these are the precursors of both the type I and the type IIA and

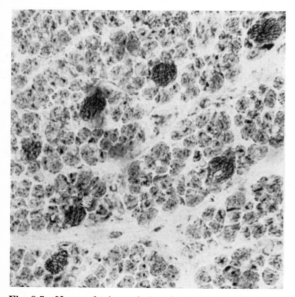

Fig. 8.5 Human fetal muscle (quadriceps) at about 21 weeks' gestation showing a small proportion of darker-staining (type I) fibres. Remaining fibres uniform in activity and still undifferentiated and correspond to type IIC fibres. NADH-TR, ×330

IIB fibres of mature human muscle. This has been supported by the extensive study of the histochemistry of human fetal muscle by Colling-Saltin (1978).

Histochemical studies on cross-innervation of fast and slow animal muscles have shown the important influence of the nervous system on the enzyme pattern of individual fibres (Dubowitz, 1966a, 1967a; Dubowitz and Newman, 1967; Romanul and van der Meulen, 1966, 1967). It seems likely that the change in enzyme patterns in developing human and animal muscle is the result of the innervation, and a direct influence from the nervous system.

DISEASED MUSCLE

Histochemical methods have been extensively used in the study of progressive muscular dystrophies, neurogenic atrophies, congenital myopathies, glycogenoses and other miscellaneous disorders.

Muscular dystrophy (Duchenne)

Oxidative enzymes and phosphorylase. In an application of the methods for oxidative enzymes and phosphorylase to progressive muscular dystrophy of the classical Duchenne ('pseudohypertrophic') type, we were unable to demonstrate any enzyme defect or gross deviation from the normal (Dubowitz and Pearse, 1961). It was of particular interest, however, that even in the pathological muscle it was possible to pick out the two muscle fibre types on histochemical grounds. Moreover, in the more advanced myopathic muscle the abnormally large muscle fibres tended to react strongly for phosphorylase and weakly for the oxidative enzymes, while the small atrophic fibres appeared to have a high oxidative enzyme content and to be poor in phosphorylase.

In progressive muscular dystrophy the abnormal enlargement of the one type and the tendency to atrophy of the other may reflect a different response on the part of the two groups of muscle fibres to the same underlying pathological or biochemical abnormality. However, the selective enlargement or atrophy of the fibre types is less

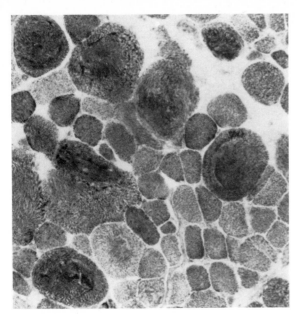

Fig. 8.6 Duchenne muscular dystrophy (aged 4½ years) showing variation in fibre size, predominance of strongly reacting (type I) fibres and presence of whorled fibres with distortion in internal structure of fibre. Quadriceps. NADH-TR, ×200.

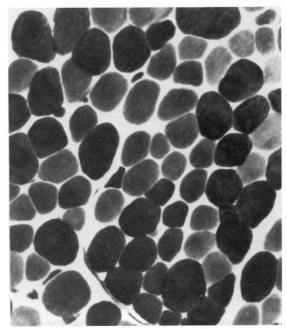

Fig. 8.7 Duchenne muscular dystrophy showing variability in fibre size and involvement of both fibre types by process of hypertrophy or atrophy. ATPase (pH 9.4), ×200

striking in the early stages of the disease and more extensive studies subsequently showed that this was not a consistent feature. An additional observation in some of the early ambulant cases was the presence of fibres with a high content of all the enzymes studied (Dubowitz, 1968a). These fibres probably correspond to type IIC fibres.

ATPase. With the routine myofibrillar ATPase reaction the distribution between fibre types is less clear-cut in many cases of Duchenne dystrophy than in the normal (Brooke and Engel, 1969). However the subdivision into fibre types is clear-cut with the ATPase reaction following pre-incubation at pH 4.3 or 4.6 (Dubowitz and Brooke, 1973).

One strikingly consistent feature of Duchenne muscular dystrophy is the distribution of weakness, with early involvement of certain proximal girdle muscles. It was hoped that a variation in the proportion of fibre types in various muscles might well explain this characteristic, but no proof of this has been established. The only fairly consistent feature histochemically in Duchenne dystrophy is a predominance of type I fibres. The structural

integrity of the intermyofibrillar network of individual fibres, as reflected by the NADH-TR reaction, is remarkably well preserved, and 'moth-eaten' or whorled fibres are relatively infrequent in comparison with some of the more benign dystrophies (Figs 8.6, 8.7).

5-Nucleotidase. The presence of proliferating connective tissue in muscular dystrophy has been noted since the first descriptions of the disease, and Duchenne (1868) suggested the name 'paralysie myosclerosique' because of it. Bourne and his co-workers studied 5-nucleotidase extensively in diseased muscle. Beckett and Bourne (1957a) noted that in dystrophies characterised by atrophy of muscle fibres and their replacement by connective tissue, there was a strong 5-nucleotidase reaction in the connective tissue and capillaries, which appeared to be invading and destroying the muscle fibres. The atrophic fibres also reacted strongly. Bourne and Golarz (1959) showed, by varying the substrate in the phosphatase reaction, that the connective tissue was also able to dephosphorylate a number of other high-energy phosphate compounds. They concluded from these observations that the fundamental defect in progressive muscular dystrophy might be in the connective tissue and not in the muscle fibre itself.

There are, however, a number of difficulties in accepting this theory without reservation. Beckett and Bourne (1957b; 1958c), in a study of 33 biopsies from patients with a 'variety of muscular and neuromuscular disorders', obtained a negative (normal) result for 5-nucleotidase in seven, and in several others the reaction was limited to large blood vessels as in controls. There was a positive result in about one-quarter, but this could not be correlated with the clinical diagnosis. Thus a positive result occurred in one case of motor neurone disease and also in one of the controls.

It is debatable whether the presence of 5-nucleotidase activity in this proliferating connective tissue confers on it the ability to dephosphorylate energy-rich compounds in the muscle fibres and thus to interfere with their function. The enzyme is present normally in the walls of capillaries and blood vessels and in peripheral nerves. In addition to an occasional positive reaction in normal perimysial connective tissue, it has also been present in the connective tissue of otherwise normal-looking muscle from some hypotonic infants and also of fetal muscle (Dubowitz, unpublished results).

Fat. In spite of the remarkable increase in endomysial and perimysial adipose tissue in many patients with muscular dystrophy, there is no firm evidence of an increase in fat in the actual muscle fibres (Adams, Denny-Brown and Pearson, 1953; Greenfield, Shy, Alvord and Berg, 1957; Beckett and Bourne, 1958c). In frozen sections from dystrophic muscle stained with Oil Red O, we observed fine droplets in relation to the muscle fibres, but concluded from phase-contrast microscopy that these were probably on the surface of the fibre and an artefact produced by the spreading of the interstitial fat during sectioning.

Muscular dystrophy carriers

Muscle biopsies from known carriers of Duchenne muscular dystrophy have shown focal changes of a 'myopathic' nature (Dubowitz, 1963b, c; Emery, 1963; Pearson, Fowler and Wright, 1963). There

does not appear to be a selective involvement of one or other fibre type by the pathological process. Histochemical studies have shown isolated fibres with core-like or 'moth-eaten' changes (Roy and Dubowitz, 1970), and Morris and Raybould (1971) showed a higher than normal incidence of these abnormal fibres in a quantitative assessment of a series of biopsies from Duchenne dystrophy carriers.

Other dystrophies

Within the classical forms of dystrophy a number of histochemical and structural changes have, in recent years, been defined which appear to be more characteristic of the particular syndromes concerned (Dubowitz and Brooke, 1973). The following are some of these more distinctive changes which are superadded to the underlying 'myopathic' changes in the biopsies.

Limb-girdle muscular dystrophy. In contrast to Duchenne dystrophy the standard ATPase reaction shows good fibre-type differentiation. There is a marked tendency to longitudinal splitting of fibres and internal nuclei are commonly present. With oxidative enzyme reactions many fibres show disruption of the intermyofibrillar network and a 'moth-eaten' appearance (Fig. 8.8). Ring fibres are common in limb-girdle dystrophy and are readily demonstrated with the PAS stain or NADH-TR reaction.

Facioscapulohumeral dystrophy. This slowly progressive form of dystrophy may show less degenerative changes in the biopsy than the Duchenne or limb-girdle types. Only a minority of cases show a myopathic picture suggestive of a dystrophy. The commonest pattern is one of focal, very small, angulated atrophic fibres in an otherwise normal-looking muscle. Some cases show a remarkable degree of inflammatory response resembling polymyositis but are, nevertheless, usually unresponsive to steroid therapy. 'Moth-eaten' fibres are also common in these cases.

Myotonic dystrophy. The distinctive features in this condition are selective atrophy of the type I

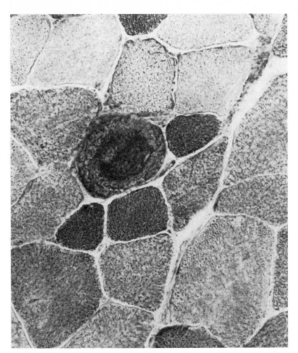

Fig. 8.8 Mild limb-girdle dystrophy of 10 years' duration in 13-year-old ambulant girl. Biopsy of biceps shows variability in fibre size affecting both fibre types and presence of whorled fibre. NADH-TR, ×330

fibres, extensive internal nuclei, and structural changes within the fibre, such as ring fibres, sarcoplasmic masses and 'moth-eaten' fibres. In the congenital form of myotonic dystrophy the muscle is usually normal in appearance apart from the presence of type I fibre atrophy.

Congenital muscular dystrophy. There is usually marked replacement by adipose tissue and also marked connective tissue proliferation. The residual muscle fibres often show a type I fibre predominance and a high incidence of structural change such as 'moth-eaten' fibres seen with the NADH-TR reaction (Fig. 8.9).

Inflammatory myopathies

In dermatomyositis and polymyositis the classical feature is the marked inflammatory response. However, this may be relatively insignificant or even absent, especially in acute childhood dermatomyositis. Degenerative changes in the muscle may, in these circumstances, also be relatively mild. Unlike the dystrophies, there are usually no hypertrophied fibres in polymyositis.

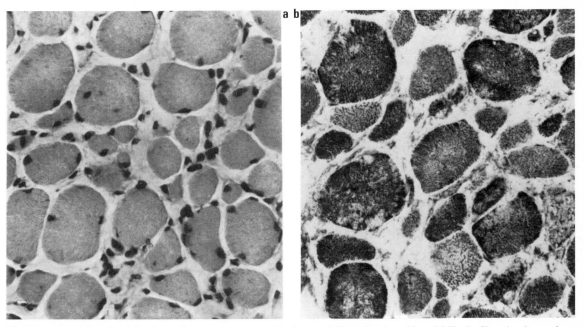

a b

Fig. 8.9 Congenital muscular dystrophy (non-progressive) in 9-year-old boy showing: (a) variability in fibre size, internal nuclei and degenerative change fibres and marked endomysial connective tissue proliferation (H and E, ×330); and (b) striking disruption of structure in individual fibres with 'moth-eaten' appearance (NADH-TR, ×330)

There is a tendency for the atrophy to have a perifascicular distribution and it affects both fibre types. This is often more conspicuous with the histochemical preparations than on routine histological staining. 'Moth-eaten' fibres are commonly present (Fig. 8.10).

Glycogen storage diseases

McArdle's disease. In 1951 McArdle described a myopathy in a 30-year-old man, due to a defect in the breakdown of muscle glycogen. Schmid and Mahler (1959) showed that it was due to a deficiency of phosphorylase in the voluntary muscle. Schmid, Robbins and Traut (1959) demonstrated that the enzyme which synthesises glycogen from glucose-1-phosphate via the uridine diphosphate glucose pathway was present in approximately half the normal amount while the level of phosphorylase was only 0.5 per cent of normal. Mommaerts, Illingworth, Pearson, Guillory and Seraydarian (1959) confirmed the absence of phosphorylase, the presence of uridine diphosphate glucose-glycogen transferase, and the excess of glycogen, in another patient with this disease. In

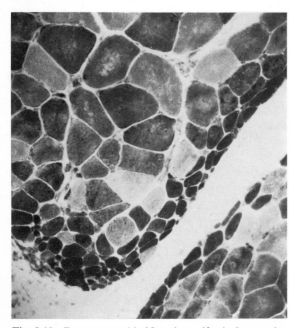

Fig. 8.10 Dermatomyositis. Note the perifascicular atrophy and the presence of 'moth-eaten' fibres. Quadriceps. NADH-TR, ×330

a further study on this patient, Pearson, Rimer and Mommaerts (1961) were able to demonstrate by histochemical methods the absence of phosphorylase and the excess of glycogen. Mellick, Mahler and Hughes (1962) reported a case of McArdle's syndrome with absence of phosphorylase in the muscle sections, but they were unable to demonstrate an excess of glycogen by routine staining methods. In a number of subsequent case reports the absence of phosphorylase has been clearly demonstrated histochemically. The excess of glycogen is not always striking, but often there are subsarcolemmal blebs or vacuoles, which may have PAS-positive granules in them. Apart from that, the histology of the biopsy may be strikingly normal, or show only focal degenerative fibres.

McArdle's disease is of great interest, not only because it is the first myopathy in which a specific biochemical abnormality has been demonstrated, but it has also provided the biochemist and the histochemist with a common ground for investigation and diagnosis.

Other glycogenoses. There are a number of other forms of glycogen storage disease which may affect voluntary muscle. (For a detailed review *see* Dubowitz and Brooke, 1973 or Dubowitz, 1978). Most of these present with hypotonia or muscle weakness in early infancy but they may also manifest at a later age, usually with a nonprogressive proximal myopathy.

The various enzymes associated with the building and breakdown of glycogen have been summarised (*see* p. 266).

The commonest form of glycogen storage disease (Type I, von Gierke's disease), due to deficiency of glucose-6-phosphatase, does not affect muscle, because this enzyme is normally absent from muscle.

Type II glycogenosis (Pompe's disease (Pompe, 1932, 1933)) leads to excessive deposition of structurally normal glycogen in cardiac and skeletal muscle, as well as in the central nervous system and other organs. It is usually fatal in early infancy, but recently mild cases with only proximal muscle weakness have been identified (Courtecuisse, Royer, Habib, Monnier, and Demos, 1965; Zellweger, Illingworth Brown, McCormick and Tu, 1965; Hudgson, Gardner-

Medwin, Worsfold, Pennington and Walton, 1968; Engel, 1970). The enzyme which is deficient is α-1,4-glucosidase (acid-maltase) and the excess glycogen deposition is probably lysosomal in distribution (Hers, 1963). The muscle shows a striking vacuolar change and there is staining of the material within vacuoles with specific stains for glycogen.

Type III glycogenosis is characterised by the presence of an abnormal form of glycogen (limit dextrin) in heart and skeletal muscle and also in the liver (Illingworth and Cori, 1952; Forbes, 1953; Krivit, Polglase, Gunn and Tyler, 1953). This is due to absence of the debranching enzyme, dextrin-1,6-glucosidase (Illingworth, Cori and Cori, 1956). Phosphorylase, present in normal amounts, can only partly degrade the outer branches of the glycogen as far as the limit dextrin, which then accumulates. The biopsy does not show the striking vacuolar change as seen in type II and the excess glycogen may not be as strikingly apparent in the stained sections.

Recent new additions to the list include a muscle glycogenosis thought to be due to an inhibitor of phosphohexose isomerase (Satoyoshi and Kowa, 1967), and one due to deficiency of phosphofructokinase (Tarui, Okuno, Ikura, Tanaka, Suda and Nishikawa, 1965; Layzer, Rowland and Ranney, 1967). Bonilla and Schotland (1970) described a histochemical method for phosphofructokinase, and were able to demonstrate absence of the enzyme in the muscle biopsy of the case reported by Layzer et al. (1967).

Until recently, histochemical studies in these glycogen storage diseases were limited to routine stains for glycogen. The application of the newer methods for demonstrating some of the enzymes associated with glycogen breakdown and synthesis may prove helpful in diagnosis and may, in association with biochemical study, provide further information on the basic defect in the various forms of disease.

The congenital myopathies

The more enthusiastic investigation of muscle biopsies in recent years has led to the recognition of a number of muscle diseases with specific structural changes, which would readily be missed on routine histological processing. These cases usually present in infancy with a floppy infant syndrome, or later with relatively non-progressive muscle weakness.

Central core disease

In 1956 Shy and Magee described 'a new congenital non-progressive myopathy' characterised histologically by amorphous areas within the muscle fibres and subsequently named central core disease (Greenfield, Cornman and Shy, 1958). Shy and Magee (1956) found that with a trichrome stain the central core stained blue, whereas the periphery stained red. The periodic-acid-Schiff reaction was more strongly positive in the core than in the rest of the muscle fibre. However, this reaction was not influenced by prior treatment with diastase so that it was probably not due to glycogen.

A patient with the same illness was extensively investigated in England by Engel, Foster, Hughes, Huxley and Mahler (1961). They found that the core region stained more deeply than the non-core region with a number of acidic as well as basic dyes. With Gomori trichrome stain, the core regions were purplish and the non-core regions red. The core regions did not stain with the periodic acid-Schiff reagent. In this biopsy of the biceps most fibres had a single central core. A second biopsy from the vastus lateralis showed multiple cores in most fibres. A specimen of the latter biopsy was examined histochemically for various enzyme activities (Dubowitz and Pearse, 1960c). In contrast to the variation in enzyme activity between individual fibres of normal muscle, all the fibres in the muscle from the patient with central core disease showed a uniform degree of activity for any particular enzyme. All the fibres reacted strongly for phosphorylase as well as the various oxidative enzymes. In contrast to the rest of the fibre the cores themselves were practically devoid of any oxidative enzyme or phosphorylase activity. The enzyme pattern in biopsies from both parents was normal and showed the usual variation between fibres and the reciprocal relation of oxidative enzymes and phosphorylase.

Bethlem and Meyjes (1960) described the histological features of a biopsy from the triceps of

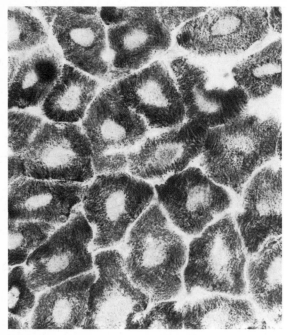

Fig. 8.11 Central core disease. Biopsy from quadriceps of 29-year-old woman showing uniformity of enzyme pattern (type I) and single central cores in practically all the fibres. NADH-TR, ×330

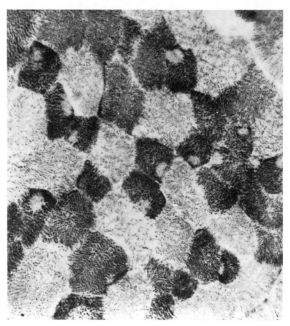

Fig. 8.12 Central core disease. Biopsy from quadriceps of 4-year-old son of patient in Fig. 8.11, showing normal distribution of fibre types and the presence of eccentric 'central' cores in a small number of type I fibres. NADH-TR, ×330

a Dutch patient with this disease. Almost all the fibres had a single central core.

In central core disease the cores are much more readily discernible with the enzyme techniques than with the routine histological stains: this provides a useful and quick screening test for central core disease in the biopsy from a patient with infantile hypotonia or a non-progressive myopathy.

The absence of any enzyme activity in the cores suggests that they are a non-functioning part of the muscle. The histochemical findings are further supported by the electron-microscopical picture which shows almost complete absence of mitochondria in the core regions (Engel *et al.*, 1961).

The biopsy from a 40-year-old woman with central core disease (Dubowitz and Platts, 1965) showed a normal subdivision of the muscle into type I and type II fibres. The cores were practically confined to type I fibres. In the biopsy from a 29-year-old woman investigated by Dubowitz and Roy (1970), 98 per cent of the fibres were type I and a centrally placed single core was present in every type I fibre (Fig. 8.11). Her 4-year-old son

had a normal subdivision into fibre types (65 per cent type I), and only 3 per cent of his type I fibres contained cores, which were eccentrically placed. (Fig. 8.12). A follow-up biopsy of his quadriceps 12 years later showed a picture identical to that of his mother, with only type I fibres throughout the biopsy and almost every fibre having a single, or occasional multiple, fairly centrally placed core (Fig. 8.13).

Engel (1961) observed 'target' fibres in adult patients with long-standing neurogenic atrophies and, in view of their striking resemblance to central cores, suggested that the latter might be due to denervation. In experimental animals I observed core-like fibres in the phase of re-innervation (Dubowitz, 1967b) suggesting that the abnormality is a feature of re-innervation rather than denervation in long-standing neurogenic atrophies.

Minicore disease (Multicore disease)

In 1971 Engel, Gomez and Groover documented two unrelated children with a benign congenital

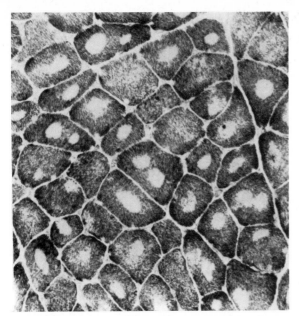

Fig. 8.13   Central core disease. Biopsy of quadriceps of same child as in Fig. 8.12 at 16 years of age, showing evolution of disease with uniformity of fibre type and centrally placed cores in almost all fibres. Compare with Fig. 8.11. NADH-TR, ×200

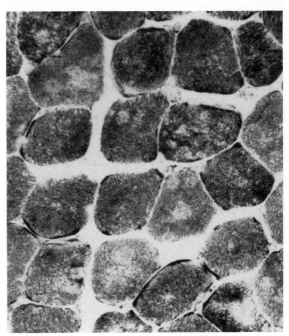

Fig. 8.14   Minicore disease (multicore disease) in deltoid muscle from a 10-year-old child showing presence of multiple small cores in many of the fibres. NADH-TR, ×330

non-progressive myopathy associated with multifocal areas of degeneration in the muscle fibres. The foci showed decrease in mitochondrial enzyme activity and also focal myofibrillar degeneration (Fig. 8.14). The condition is probably distinct from central core disease as it appears to have an autosomal recessive inheritance. As in central core disease, there is a tendency for the muscle to show type I fibre predominance and for the minicores to have a predilection for type I fibres (Dubowitz, 1978). On routine histological staining the muscle may look essentially normal, apart from some variability in fibre size and the presence of fibres with internal nuclei.

Nemaline myopathy

This is another non-progressive congenital myopathy. The characteristic rod bodies or nemaline rods were first recognised by Conen, Murphy and Donohue (1963) and Shy, Engel, Somers and Wanko (1963). The nemaline rods are devoid of enzyme activity and can be demonstrated by the Gomori trichrome or phosphotungstic acid haematoxylin stains. The nemaline rods have been

shown on electron microscopy to be in continuity with the Z bands (Price, Gordon, Pearson, Munsat and Blumberg, 1965).

Nienhuis, Coleman, Jann Brown, Munsat and Pearson (1967) noted in their cases of nemaline myopathy that all fibres were uniform in enzyme activity and showed no differentiation into fibre types. Usually there is a subdivision into fibre types but a bimodal distribution of small and large fibres with a tendency to atrophy of type I fibres which also have more involvement with rods (Fig. 8.15a). With the ATPase reactions the rod areas show up devoid of stain (Fig. 8.15b). Other cases do not show the presence of atrophic fibres.

Clinically, the condition is often very mild and non-progressive, but even these cases have a tendency to severe respiratory deficit and respiratory failure.

In a histochemical study of various muscles from an infant with nemaline myopathy who died at the age of 10 months (Shafiq, Dubowitz, Peterson and Milhorat, 1967), the muscle showed a normal subdivision into two fibre types, both of which contained the rods. Special stains showed the presence of tyrosine in the rods, confirming

a
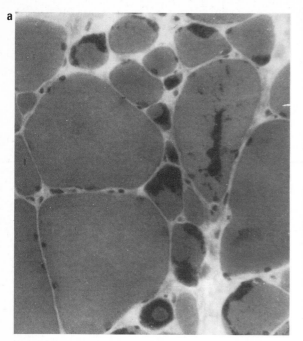

b
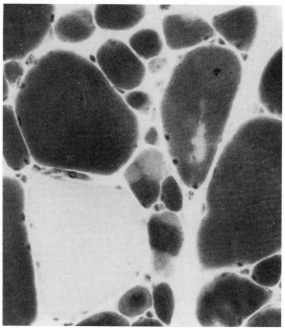

Fig. 8.15   Nemaline myopathy. Biopsy of gastrocnemius from 12-year-old boy showing (a) variation in fibre size and presence of dark (red) staining rods mainly in the smaller fibres (Gomori trichrome, × 330) and (b) absence of staining in the rods with the ATPase reaction (ATPase, pH 4.3, × 330)

their protein nature. The absence of tryptophan in the rods supported the view that they may be composed of tropomyosin, because this is the only muscle protein devoid of tryptophan. However, the composition of the rods has still not been finally established (Sugita, Masaki, Ebashi and Pearson, 1972). Recent fluorescent antibody studies have shown the presence of α-actinin in the rods as well as in the Z lines.

Mitochondrial myopathies

Ernster, Ikkos and Luft (1959) and Luft, Ikkos, Palmieri, Ernster and Afzelius (1962) first recorded a case of myopathy associated with abnormal mitochondria and hypermetabolism. Shy, Gonatas and Perez (1966) described two cases of myopathy with abnormal mitochondria, which they labelled 'megaconial' and 'pleoconial' myopathy respectively. There was no associated hypermetabolism. Similar cases were subsequently reported by van Wijngaarden, Bethlem, Meijer, Hulsmann and Feltkamp (1967) and by Price, Gordon, Munsat and Pearson (1967). In all these cases the abnormality could be suspected in the

histochemical preparations for oxidative enzymes, which show aggregates of prominent mitochondria, especially in the subsarcolemmal region.

Mitochondrial myopathy is not a single entity, but mitochondrial abnormalities have now been described in a large number of different clinical syndromes of muscle weakness, including the limb girdle and facioscapulohumeral syndromes and cases with distal weakness. Mitochondrial abnormalities are a consistent feature in the so-called oculocraniosomatic syndrome or 'ophthalmoplegia plus' (Kearns and Sayre, 1958; Drachmann, 1968; Olson, Engel, Walsh and Einaugler, 1972) in which there is external ophthalmoplegia, pigmentary retinopathy and heart block in association usually with only mild skeletal weakness and also additional neurological or somatic features.

Mitochondrial abnormality is also the predominant feature of a syndrome presenting with generalised muscle weakness and hypotonia in infancy, mainly in the second year of life (Dubowitz, 1978).

Mitochondrial myopathies are likely to be missed on routine histological staining (although they may show some increased granularity of fibres

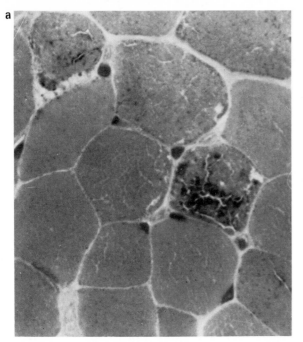
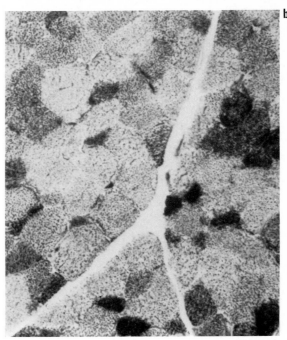

Fig. 8.16   Mitochondrial myopathy. Biopsy from rectus femoris of 2-year-old weak floppy child, showing; (a) 'ragged-red fibres' with Gomori trichrome stain (×560); and (b) isolated fibres with intense oxidative activity (NADH-TR, ×330)

even with H and E and Verhoeff-van Gieson stains) but are usually suspected from the presence of disrupted, red-staining fibres with the Gomori trichome stain ('ragged-red fibres') and from very strongly reactive fibres on oxidative enzyme preparations (Figs. 8.16, 8.17). They are confirmed on electron microscopy by the presence of abnormality in number, size and structure of the mitochondria.

It is quite likely that the structural abnormality of the mitochondria is secondary to an underlying biochemical abnormality which in most syndromes has not yet been identified. In a number of recent case studies (usually in adults able to donate biopsies of 4–5 g of muscle) there have been suggestions of deficits along the cytochrome chain.

Myotubular myopathy

In the first reported case of this non-progressive (or slowly progressive) myopathy, Spiro, Shy and Gonatas (1966) suggested the name myotubular myopathy because of the resemblance of the fibres to the myotubes of fetal muscle. A striking histological characteristic of the condition is the

centrally placed prominent nuclei, much like those of fetal muscle.

Sher, Rimalovski, Athanassiades and Aronson (1967) suggested the term centronuclear myopathy as an alternative name. Their two cases showed normal subdivision into type I and type II fibres, as in mature muscle.

The prominent central nuclei are readily seen on routine staining (Fig. 8.18a). Histochemical stud-

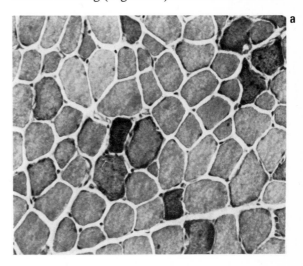

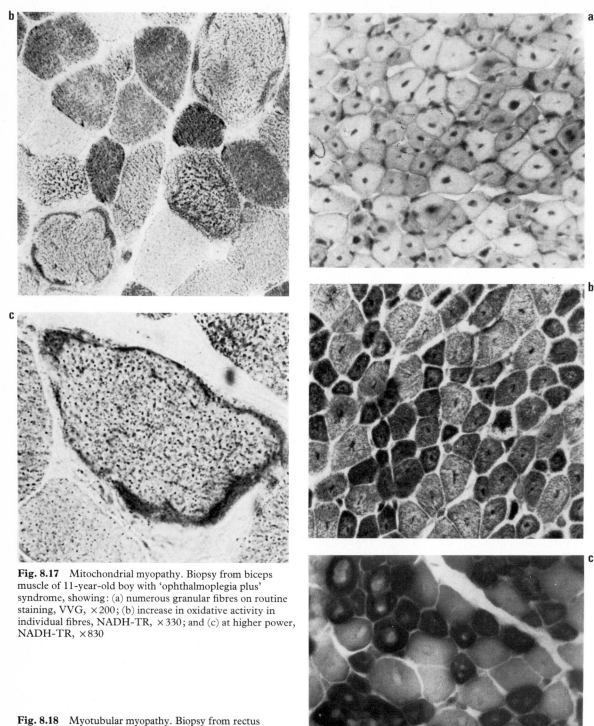

Fig. 8.17   Mitochondrial myopathy. Biopsy from biceps muscle of 11-year-old boy with 'ophthalmoplegia plus' syndrome, showing: (a) numerous granular fibres on routine staining, VVG, ×200; (b) increase in oxidative activity in individual fibres, NADH-TR, ×330; and (c) at higher power, NADH-TR, ×830

Fig. 8.18   Myotubular myopathy. Biopsy from rectus femoris of 14-year-old boy showing: (a) striking internal nuclei (VVG, ×330); (b) focal aggregation of oxidative activity at site of nuclei (NADH-TR, ×330); and (c) 'holes' in fibres at site of nuclei due to absence of myofibrillar structure (ATPase, ×330)

ies show a striking and characteristic aggregation of oxidative activity in the central region in relation to the nuclei, often with a clear halo around (Fig. 8.18b). The ATPase reaction shows a consistent absence of activity in these central zones due to absence of myofibrillar structure at the site of the nuclei (Fig. 8.18c).

Myotubular myopathy with type I fibre hypotrophy

Engel, Gold and Karpati (1968) reported an 11-month-old child with severe and progressive weakness, whose muscle had profuse central nuclei, restricted to type I fibres, which were also small in diameter. They suggested that this might represent a maturational arrest, or 'hypotrophy', of the type I fibres rather than an atrophy. Further cases with milder clinical involvement but a similar biopsy picture have been reported by Bethlem, van Wijngaarden, Meijer and Hülsmann (1969), Karpati, Carpenter and Nelson (1970), and Dubowitz (1978).

A severe X-linked form of myotubular myopathy with a high mortality among the affected males in the neonatal period has been reported in two Dutch families (van Wijngaarden, Fleury, Bethlem and Meijer, 1969; Barth, van Wijngaarden and Bethlem, 1975).

Congenital fibre type disproportion

In their histographic analysis of muscle biopsies, Brooke and Engel (1969) suggested classifying children's biopsies on the relative size of type I and type II fibres. Normally the fibre types are of approximately equal diameter. In some cases with a relatively non-progressive weakness, type I fibres were noted to be smaller than type II. Brooke (1973) subsequently delineated a fairly consistent clinical picture, usually presenting with hypotonia at birth or in early infancy and having a benign course. The only abnormality on biopsy is the disproportion in size of the fibre types, with striking and uniform atrophy of the type I fibres and normal-sized or enlarged type II fibres (Fig. 8.19).

This condition has to be distinguished from dystrophia myotonica and myotubular myopathy with type I fibre atrophy, which also present with hypotonia and weakness in early infancy (Dubowitz and Brooke, 1973) and from the early stage of infantile spinal muscular atrophy (Werdnig-Hoffmann disease) (Dubowitz, 1968b).

Infantile hypotonia

There are many causes of the floppy infant syndrome and this has been the subject of a

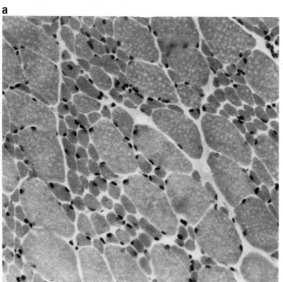 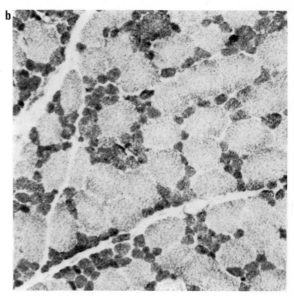

Fig. 8.19 Congenital fibre type disproportion in 4½-year-old floppy weak child, showing: (a) presence of two populations of fibres on routine staining (H and E, ×200); and (b) strikingly uniform atrophy (hypotrophy) of type I fibres (dark) in contrast to normal sized or enlarged type II fibres (NADH-TR, ×200)

separate monograph (Dubowitz, 1968b, 1980). From a practical point of view it is important to separate those cases with weakness and involvement of the lower motor neurone from the floppy infants with hypotonia of 'central' nervous origin or related to more remote disorders. In addition to electrodiagnostic investigations, which are a useful screening test for identifying a myopathic, neurogenic or normal pattern of muscle activity, muscle biopsy with detailed histochemical study is essential in this group of disorders in order to confirm the diagnosis of a spinal muscular atrophy or congenital muscular dystrophy, or to identify one of the rarer forms of congenital myopathy with specific structural abnormality. In the congenital form of dystrophia myotonica, which presents at birth with marked muscle weakness and hypotonia with associated swallowing and respiratory problems, the muscle may be essentially normal apart from a tendency to atrophy of type I fibres, and the diagnosis is more readily confirmed by clinical and electrodiagnostic assessment of the mother, who invariably has the dominantly inherited condition. In the Prader-Willi syndrome (Prader, Labhart and Willi, 1956; Prader and Willi, 1963) the infant presents with profound hypotonia and associated sucking and swallowing difficulty at birth, but with relatively good muscle power and a gradual

resolution of the hypotonia. Muscle biopsy is unlikely to be of diagnostic help as the histological and histochemical patterns are usually normal and the diagnosis has to rest on the typical clinical features.

Neurogenic atrophies

There are a large number of clinical disorders affecting the lower motor neurone, some having a proximal distribution of weakness (e.g. the spinal muscular atrophies) and others a distal distribution (e.g. peroneal muscular atrophy). Although the biopsy in all of them will reflect the denervating process, detailed histochemical studies have revealed patterns more or less distinctive for some of the syndromes.

The characteristic histological change in (longstanding) denervation of muscle is uniform atrophy of groups of muscle fibres, so-called 'largegroup atrophy' or 'small-group atrophy', in association with other fibres of normal or enlarged size (Fig. 8.20). Histochemically, the atrophic fibres are of both fibre types, thus helping to distinguish this condition from those with selective atrophy of one fibre type. The large fibres are often uniform in type, suggesting that they are reinnervated rather than normal unaffected fibres, which would have a mixed pattern (Fig. 8.20).

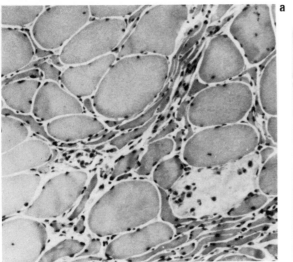 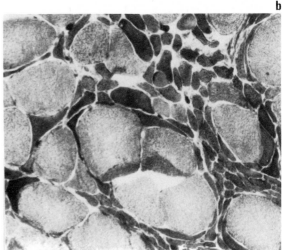

Fig. 8.20 Neurogenic atrophy. Biopsy from quadriceps of 35-year-old man with rapidly progressive motor neurone disease showing: (a) large groups of atrophic fibres and also 'myopathic changes' in some large fibres with internal nuclei and presence of necrotic (pale) fibres (H and E, ×120); and (b) mixed fibre type pattern in atrophic fibres and uniformity of enzyme reaction in large fibres (NADH-TR, ×120)

Another pattern characteristic of denervation is fibre type-grouping, where large clusters of one fibre type occur alongside clusters of fibres of the other type (Fig. 8.21). This represents a process of re-innervation of previously denervated fibres, as a result of sprouting of the terminal axons of surviving nerves. It is usually a feature of long-standing and relatively slowly progressive neuropathies and the muscle biopsy may be completely normal apart from the type grouping.

'Target' fibres are also a feature of longstanding denervation (Engel, 1961). They resemble central core disease in their oxidative enzyme pattern, except for the presence of three zones of activity— the central zone devoid of enzyme activity, the outer normal-staining region of the fibre and an intermediate darkly stained zone—in contrast to the two zones in central core disease.

Another feature suggestive of denervation is the presence of small angulated fibres with a very intense reaction for NADH-tetrazolium reductase (Fig. 8.22). These fibres vary in their ATPase activity, some being strongly reacting (cor-responding to type II) and others weakly reacting (corresponding to type I).

Spinal muscular atrophy

One of the common forms of neurogenic atrophy is spinal muscular atrophy, a genetically determined condition (usually autosomal recessive), in which

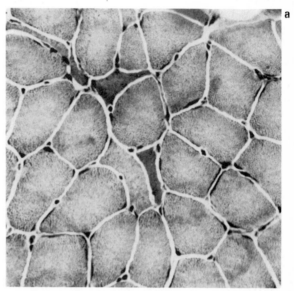

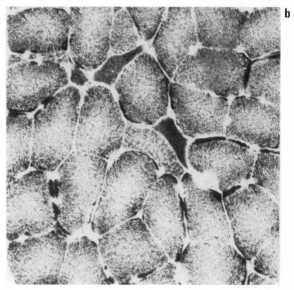

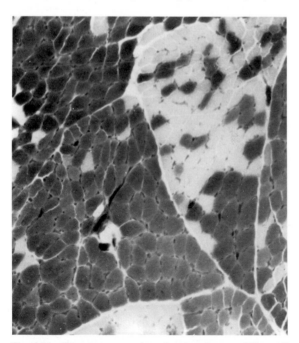

Fig. 8.21 Fibre type-grouping, showing clusters of fibres of uniform fibre type, characteristic of re-innervation. Biopsy of gastrocnemius of 5-year-old girl with mild almost non-progressive neurogenic weakness (? spinal muscular atrophy, ? peripheral neuropathy) ATPase, ×120

Fig. 8.22 Biopsy from rectus femoris of 12-year-old boy with mild slowly progressive motor neurone disease showing focal angulated atrophic fibres which have intense activity with oxidative enzyme reaction, while remaining fibres are uniform in enzyme activity, suggesting a reinnervation process. (a) VVG, ×330; (b) NADH-TR, ×330

there is degeneration of the anterior horn cells of the cord and at times, of cranial nerve nuclei. The condition ranges in severity from the very severe infantile spinal muscular atrophy (Werdnig-Hoffmann disease) at one extreme, to the very mild proximal neurogenic atrophy (Kugelberg-Welander disease) with only limited proximal weakness at the other, and an intermediate group, spanning the two extremes. Overlap in severity may occasionally be observed within a family (Dubowitz, 1964).

The biopsy in the severe infantile cases and in the cases of intermediate severity looks very similar, irrespective of the degree of weakness (Fig. 8.23). It usually shows large group atrophy; occasionally a section may show universal atrophy. The atrophic fibres are rounded and of both fibre types. This mixed pattern suggests that, even in the congenital cases, with weakness already present at birth, the process is one of denervation of previously fully mature muscle, already differentiated into fibre types, and not a maturational arrest of embryonic fibres as suggested by some authors in the past (Dubowitz, 1966b). The large fibres may occur singly or in clusters and tend to be uniform in enzyme activity, suggesting re-innervation of the muscle by sprouting of nerves of one type (Fig. 8.23). They are more often uniformly type I, but at times type II or even a mixture of the two.

In milder cases there may be less extensive atrophy and the presence of fibre type-grouping in otherwise normal-looking bundles. However, the extent of the atrophy varies considerably even in cases of equal clinical severity and it is not possible to prognosticate on the basis of the biopsy findings.

In the longstanding Kugelberg-Welander variety, the fibres may in addition show structural changes in the large fibres, such as coil fibres and disruption of the intermyofibrillar network. Some of the large fibres may also have internal nuclei,

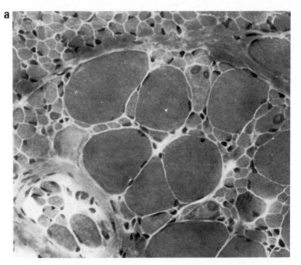

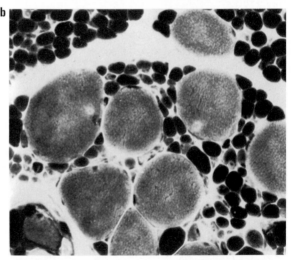

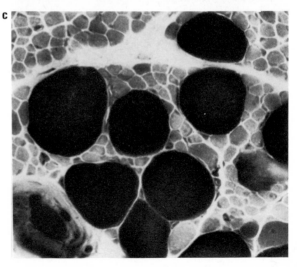

Fig. 8.23 Spinal muscular atrophy of intermediate severity in 21-month-old child. Rectus femoris shows atrophy of large groups of fibres of mixed fibre type, together with enlarged fibres of uniform enzyme type. Note muscle spindle (bottom left) with intrafusal fibres of comparable size to the atrophic fibres. Serial sections. (a) H and E, (b) ATPase pH 9.4, (c) ATPase pH 4.6, ×330

which are not a feature of the large fibres in the severe forms.

The uniformity of enzyme activity in the large fibres is almost certainly indicative of re-innervation. The influence of innervation of the fibre type has been conclusively demonstrated in recent studies of cross-innervation of slow and fast muscles in animals.

EXPERIMENTAL STUDIES

Myopathies in animals

In recent years, hereditary myopathies resembling human muscular dystrophy have been described in the mouse (Michelson, Russell and Harman, 1955), the chick (Asmundson and Julian, 1956), the hamster (Homburger, Baker, Nixon and Wilgram, 1962) and in other animals.

A number of histochemical studies have been undertaken. In the chick, Cosmos (1966) showed a delay in the maturation and change from type I to type II fibres in the affected pectoralis muscle. In the dystrophic mouse, Harman, Tassoni, Curtis and Hollinshead (1963) observed that the dystrophic muscle showed no correlation between fibre size and enzyme activity with advance of the disease, while Bajusz (1965) and Meier (1967) noted a loss of the normal checkerboard pattern.

Denervation

Humoller and his co-workers (1950, 1951, 1952) studied the effects of denervation and tenotomy on the chemical constituents of rat muscle. There have since been a number of histochemical studies along similar lines. Nachmias and Padykula (1958) noted that, in the rat, denervation produced a decrease in succinate dehydrogenase of the soleus muscle fibres, while in the biceps only the narrow fibres showed a decreased activity. There was also a reduction in glycogen and lipid in both muscles, but the ATPase content was not affected. Bajusz (1965) observed a loss of the checkerboard pattern following denervation in the mouse, comparable to his observations in the muscle of the dystrophic mouse. Smith (1965) found an early loss of phosphorylase and α-glycerophosphate and lactate dehydrogenase in denervated rat muscle, and a disappearance of the normal checkerboard pat-

tern. In a study of denervated gastrocnemius, plantaris and soleus of the rat, Romanul and Hogan (1965) observed that individual fibre types lost those enzymes normally present in higher concentration, whereas there was little or no change in enzymes normally low. As a result the enzymatic profiles of individual fibres gradually disappeared. It is difficult to correlate these results of acute and complete denervation in the experimental animal with the picture seen in human neurogenic atrophies, where the lesion is partial and there is associated re-innervation.

Tenotomy

In the rabbit, McMinn and Vrbová (1962) observed that tenotomy of the fast, pale, peroneus longus muscle produced only minimal changes, while after tenotomy the slow, red, soleus muscle showed early and extreme histological changes. In a subsequent histochemical study (McMinn and Vrbová, 1964) there was a marked reduction in succinate dehydrogenase activity of the soleus, but not in the peroneus longus. Engel, Brooke and Nelson (1966) compared the changes produced by tenotomy and denervation in the gastrocnemius and soleus of the cat.

Cross-innervation

In a fascinating series of experiments, Buller, Eccles and Eccles (1960) showed that cross-union of the nerves to the fast flexor digitorum longus (FDL) and slow soleus muscles resulted in a slowing of the contraction time of FDL and an acceleration of the contraction speed of soleus. Histochemical studies after cross-union showed a striking change in enzyme pattern (Dubowitz, 1966a, 1967a; Dubowitz and Newman, 1967; Romanul and van der Meulen, 1966, 1967). The soleus which normally contains type I fibres only (Fig. 8.24) had areas of type II fibres, while the FDL which normally has a small proportion of type I fibres and a larger number of type II fibres (Fig. 8.25) contained large areas of type I fibres, which were indistinguishable from normal soleus (Fig. 8.26).

These experiments suggest that the nervous system determines not only the contractile properties of the fast and slow muscle but also their metabolic and structural makeup. It also provides an explanation, on the basis of specific innervation by type I or type II nerve fibres, for the changing patterns of fibre types during normal development and the uniformity of fibre type in the large fibres in neurogenic atrophies.

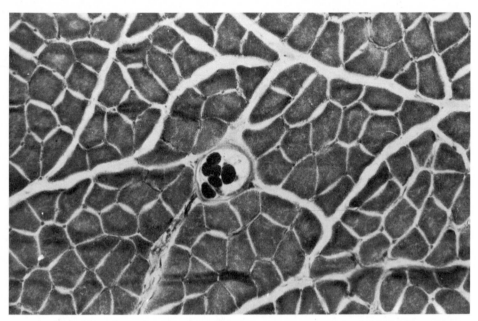

Fig. 8.24   Normal cat soleus showing uniformly strong enzyme activity. NADH-TR, ×100

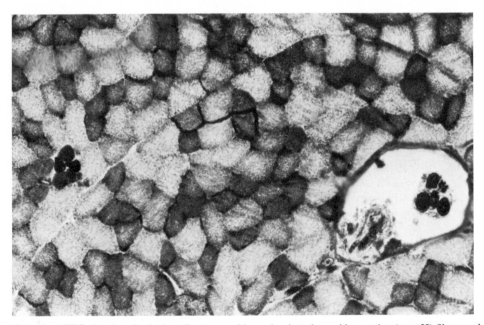

Fig. 8.25   Normal cat FDL showing checkerboard pattern, with predominantly weakly reacting (type II) fibres and small proportion of strongly reacting type I fibres. NADH-TR, ×100

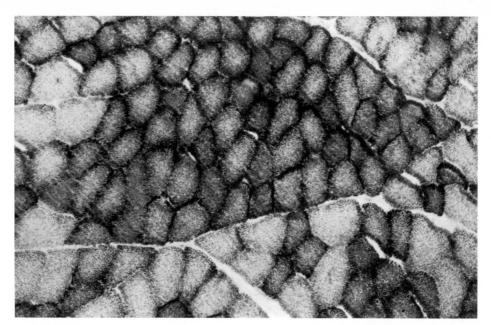

Fig. 8.26   Cat FDL after cross-innervation by nerve to soleus. Shows area of strongly reacting type I fibres indistinguishable from normal soleus. NADH-TR, ×100

Impulse activity

Salmons and Vrbová (1969) demonstrated that chronic stimulation of the intact nerve to a fast muscle at a frequency of stimuli corresponding to that of a slow muscle (10 impulses per second) caused a transformation in the physiological parameters of the fast muscle to those corresponding to a slow muscle. They postulated that the impulse frequency might be the mechanism of change in cross-innervation rather than a biochemical trophic influence, and Salmons and Sréter (1976) were subsequently able to show that the effects of cross-innervation of the slow soleus muscle by a fast nerve could be prevented by subsequent chronic stimulation of that nerve at a slow rate. Recently, Rubinstein, Mabuchi, Pepe, Salmons, Gergely and Stréter (1978) were able to demonstrate, in the rabbit fast muscle undergoing chronic stimulation, not only a conversion of the histochemical pattern but also a change of the specific myosin from the fast to the slow form by the use of type-specific fluorescein-labelled antibodies.

These animal studies have important implications for the processes of adaptation of muscle, not only under physiological conditions but possibly also in response to pathological circumstances.

Tissue culture

Histochemical studies of human muscle in tissue culture have shown a consistent and similar pattern of enzyme activity in the multinucleate myoblasts from normal and diseased muscle (Gallup, Strugalska-Cynowska and Dubowitz, 1972). The myotubes in isolated culture will develop cross-striations but show no spontaneous contractility and do not mature into fibre types. After innervation by neurones from explanted mouse spinal cord in culture, human muscle cells, both normal and dystrophic, show spontaneous synchronised contractions, the nuclei migrate peripherally, and there is further maturation in the enzyme systems (Gallup and Dubowitz, 1975).

Muscle transplantation

Minced preparations of muscle will regenerate when autotransplanted or homotransplanted in experimental animals (Carlson, 1972). When normal or dystrophic muscle is transplanted into a normal mouse (Laird and Timmer, 1966) or hamster (Jasmin and Bokdawala, 1970) it will regenerate, and the dystrophic muscle will retain its dystrophic characteristics, but when normal or dystrophic muscle is implanted into a dystrophic host there is no regeneration. In a study of the physiological characteristics of the transplanted muscle in normal and dystrophic mice, Salafsky (1971) also failed to obtain regeneration in the dystrophic host, but in the normal host both normal and dystrophic implants developed normal twitch characteristics. In a histochemical study of the regenerates in normal and dystrophic mice, we observed that the regenerates of both normal and dystrophic muscle in a normal host were similar in pattern, supporting the observations of Salafsky, whereas in the dystrophic host the muscle consistently degenerated after an initial period of regeneration (Neerunjun and Dubowitz, 1975).

CONCLUSIONS

Enzyme histochemistry has already contributed much to our understanding of normal and diseased muscle, and has established its place as an essential part of the routine investigation of every muscle biopsy. With its wider application in clinical practice, further advances in recognition and understanding of neuromuscular disorders are bound to follow.

Histochemical techniques also have an important role in the many experimental studies on the effects of various factors on the properties of normal and diseased muscle.

ACKNOWLEDGEMENTS

I am grateful to Dr M.H. Brooke and W.B. Saunders Ltd for permission to reproduce Figure 8.4; to the Editor and publishers of the Journal of Physiology for permission to reproduce Figures 8.24, 8.25 and 8.26; and to W.B. Saunders Ltd for permission to reproduce the following figures: 8.8, 8.9a, 8.9b, 8.12, 8.14, 8.15a, 8.15b, 8.16a, 8.18b, 8.18c, 8.19a, 8.19b, 8.22a, 8.22b, 8.23b and 8.23c.

Much of the work reported in this chapter was supported financially by grants from the Muscular Dystrophy Group of Great Britain, the Medical Research Council and the Muscular Dystrophy Association of America.

REFERENCES

Abe, T. & Shimizu, N. (1964) Histochemical method for demonstrating aldolase. *Histochemie*, **4**, 209.

Adams, R.D., Denny-Brown, D & Pearson, C.M. (1953) *Diseases of Muscle. A Study in Pathology*, 1st Edn. (Hoeber: New York).

Asmundson, V.S. & Julian, L.M. (1956) Inherited muscle abnormality in the domestic fowl. *Journal of Heredity*, **47**, 248.

Bajusz, E. (1965) Succinic dehydrogenase in muscular dystrophy. An experimental study on secondary changes resulting from disturbance in neuro-muscular integrity. *Experimental Medicine and Surgery*, **23**, 169.

Barnard, R.J., Edgerton, V.R., Furukawa, T. & Peter, J.B. (1971) Histochemical, biochemical and contractile properties of red, white and intermediate fibers. *American Journal of Physiology*, **220**, 410.

Barth, P.G., van Wijngaarden, G.K. & Bethlem, J. (1975) X-linked myotubular myopathy with fatal neonatal asphyxia. *Neurology (Minneapolis)*, **25**, 531.

Beckett, E.B. & Bourne, G.H. (1957a) Some histochemical observations on human dystrophic muscle. *Science*, **126**, 357.

Beckett, E.B. & Bourne, G.H. (1957b) The histochemistry of normal and abnormal human muscle. *Proceedings of the Royal Society of Medicine*, **50**, 308.

Beckett, E.B. & Bourne, G.H. (1958a) Histochemical observations on the cytochrome oxidase and succinic dehydrogenase activity of normal and diseased human muscle. *Acta Anatomica*, **33**, 289.

Beckett, E.B. & Bourne, G.H. (1958b) Acid and alkaline phosphatases in normal and diseased human muscle. *Acta Anatomica*, **35**, 326.

Beckett, E.B. & Bourne, G.H. (1958c) 5-Nucleotidase in normal and diseased human skeletal muscle. *Journal of Neuropathology and Experimental Neurology*, **17**, 199.

Beckett, E.B. & Bourne, G.H. (1958d) Some studies on the glycogen of normal and diseased human skeletal muscle, using the lead tetra acetate-Schiff and the periodic acid-Schiff techniques. *Acta Anatomica*, **34**, 235.

Beckett, E.B. & Bourne, G.H. (1958e) Some observations on normal and pathological human muscle, using a combined McManus periodic acid-Schiff reaction and Sudan black stain on gelatine sections. *Acta Anatomica*, **34**, 111.

Bennett, H.S. & Porter, K.R. (1953) An electron microscopic study of sectional breast muscle of the domestic fowl. *American Journal of Anatomy*, **93**, 61.

Bethlem, J. & Meyjes, F.E.P. (1960) Congenital, non-progressive central core disease of Shy and Magee. *Psychiatria, Neurologia, Neurochirugia*, **63**, 246.

Bethlem, J., van Wijngaarden, C.K., Meijer, A.E.F.H. &

Hülsmann, W.C. (1969) Neuromuscular disease with type 1 fiber atrophy, central nuclei and myotube-like structures. *Neurology (Minneapolis)*, **19**, 705.

Blanchaer, M. & van Wijhe, M. (1962) Distribution of lactic dehydrogenase in skeletal muscle. *Nature*, **193**, 877.

Bocek, R.M. & Beatty, C.H. (1966) Glycogen synthetase and phosphorylase in red and white muscle of rat and rhesus monkey. *Journal of Histochemistry and Cytochemistry*, **14**, 549.

Bonilla, E. & Schotland, D.L. (1970) Histochemical diagnosis of muscle phosphofructokinase deficiency. *Archives of Neurology*, **22**, 9.

Bourne, G.H. & Golarz, M.N. (1959) Human muscular dystrophy as an aberration of the connective tissue. *Nature*, **183**, 1741.

Brooke, M.H. (1973) A neuromuscular disease characterized by fiber type disproportion. In *Proceedings of II International Congress on Muscle Disease*. Ed. B.A. Kakulas, I.C.S. No. 237 (Excerpta Medica: Amsterdam).

Brooke, M.H. & Engel, W.K. (1969) The histographic analysis of human muscle biopsies with regard to fibre types. 4. Children's biopsies. *Neurology (Minneapolis)*, **19**, 591.

Brooke, M.H. & Kaiser, K.K. (1969) Some comments on the histochemical characterization of muscle adenosine triphosphatase. *Journal of Histochemistry and Cytochemistry*, **17**, 431.

Brooke, M.H. & Kaiser, K.K. (1970) Muscle fiber types: how many and what kind? *Archives of Neurology*, **23**, 369.

Brooke, M.H., Williamson, E. & Kaiser, K.K. (1971) The behavior of four fiber types in developing and reinnervated muscle. *Archives of Neurology*, **25**, 360.

Bullard, H.H. (1912) On the interstitial granules and fat droplets of striated muscle. *American Journal of Anatomy*, **14**, 1.

Buller, A.J., Eccles, J.C. & Eccles, R.M. (1960) Interactions between motor-neurones and muscles in respect of the characteristic speeds of their contraction. *Journal of Physiology*, **150**, 417.

Buño, W. & Germino, N.I. (1958) Distribution of succinic dehydrogenase in the organs of the adult albino rats. *Acta Anatomica*, **33**, 161.

Burke, R.E., Levine, D.N., Zajac, F.E., Tsairis, P. & Engel, W.K. (1971) Mammalian motor units: Physiological-histochemical correlation in three types in cat gastrocnemius. *Science*, **174**, 709.

Burstone, M.S. (1959) New histochemical techniques for the demonstration of tissue oxidase (Cytochrome oxidase). *Journal of Histochemistry and Cytochemistry*, **7**, 112.

Carlson, B.M. (1972) *The Regeneration of Minced Muscles* (Karger: Basel).

Close, R. (1967) Properties of motor units in fast and slow skeletal muscles of the rat. *Journal of Physiology*, **193**, 45.

Colling-Saltin, A. (1978) *Skelettmuskulaturens differentiering under fosterstadiet hos mämmiska: En histokemisk, ultrastrukturell och biokemisk studie*. Stockholm.

Conen, P.E., Murphy, E.G. & Donohue, W.C. (1963) Light and electron-microscopic studies of 'myogranules' in a child with hypotonia and muscle weakness. *Canadian Medical Association Journal*, **89**, 983.

Cosmos, E. (1966) Enzymic activity of differentiating muscle fibres. 1. Development of phosphorylase in muscles of the domestic fowl. *Developmental Biology*, **13**, 163.

Courtecuisse, V., Royer, P., Habib, R., Monnier, C. & Demos, J. (1965) Glycogénose musculaire par deficit d'alpha-1-4-glucosidase simulant une dystrophie musculaire progressive. *Archives Françaises de Pédiatrie*, **22**, 1153.

Dempsey, E.W., Wislocki, G.B. & Singer, M. (1946) Some observations on the chemical cytology of striated muscle. *Anatomical Record*, **96**, 221.

Denny-Brown, D. (1929) The histological features of striped muscle in relation to its functional activity. *Proceedings of the Royal Society*, **B104**, 371.

Drachmann, D.B. (1968) Ophthalmoplegia plus, the neurodegenerative disorders associated with progressive external ophthalmoplegia. *Archives of Neurology*, **18**, 654.

Drews, G.A. & Engel, W.K. (1966) Reversal of the ATPase reaction in muscle fibers by EDTA. *Nature*, **212**, 1551.

Dubowitz, V. (1963a) Enzymic maturation of skeletal muscle. *Nature*, **197**, 1215.

Dubowitz, V. (1963b) Myopathic changes in muscular dystrophy carrier. *Journal of Neurology, Neurosurgery and Psychiatry*, **26**, 322.

Dubowitz, V. (1963c) Myopathic changes in muscular dystrophy carriers. *Proceedings of the Royal Society of Medicine*, **56**, 810.

Dubowitz, V. (1964) Infantile muscular atrophy. A prospective study with particular reference to a slowly progressive variety. *Brain*, **87**, 707.

Dubowitz, V. (1965a) Enzyme histochemistry of skeletal muscle. I. Developing animal muscle. *Journal of Neurology, Neurosurgery and Psychiatry*, **28**, 516.

Dubowitz, V. (1965b) Enzyme histochemistry of skeletal muscle. II. Developing human muscle. *Journal of Neurology, Neurosurgery and Psychiatry*, **28**, 519.

Dubowitz, V. (1966a) Cross innervation of fast and slow muscle: Histochemical, physiological and biochemical studies. In *Exploratory Concepts in Muscular Dystrophy and Related Disorders*. Proceedings of the conference, New York, October, 1966. Excerpta Medica series no. 147, p. 164.

Dubowitz, V. (1966b) Enzyme histochemistry of skeletal muscle. III. Neurogenic muscular atrophies. *Journal of Neurology, Neurosurgery and Psychiatry*, **29**, 23.

Dubowitz, V. (1967a) Cross innervated mammalian skeletal muscle: histochemical, physiological and biochemical observations. *Journal of Physiology*, **193**, 481.

Dubowitz, V. (1967b) Pathology of experimentally re-innervated skeletal muscle. *Journal of Neurology, Neurosurgery and Psychiatry*, **30**, 99.

Dubowitz, V. (1968a) *Developing and Diseased Muscle: A Histochemical Study* (Heinemann: London).

Dubowitz, V. (1968b) *The Floppy Infant* (Heinemann: London).

Dubowitz, V. (1978) *Muscle Disorders in Childhood* (W.B. Saunders: London, Philadelphia and Toronto).

Dubowitz, V. (1980) *The Floppy Infant*, 2nd Edn. (Heinemann: London).

Dubowitz, V. & Brooke, M.H. (1973) *Muscle Biopsy: A Modern Approach* (Saunders: London).

Dubowitz, V. & Newman, D.L. (1967) Change in enzyme pattern after cross-innervation of fast and slow skeletal muscle. *Nature*, **214**, 840.

Dubowitz, V. & Pearse, A.G.E. (1960a) Reciprocal relationship of phosphorylase and oxidative enzymes in skeletal muscle. *Nature*, **185**, 701.

Dubowitz, V. & Pearse, A.G.E. (1960b) A comparative histochemical study of oxidative enzyme and phosphorylase activity in skeletal muscle. *Histochemie*, **2**, 105.

Dubowitz, V. & Pearse, A.G.E. (1960c) Oxidative enzymes and phosphorylase in central-core disease of muscle. *Lancet*, **2**, 23.

Dubowitz, V. & Pearse, A.G.E. (1961) Enzymic activity of normal and diseased human muscle: a histochemical study. *Journal of Pathology and Bacteriology*, **81**, 365.

Dubowitz, V. & Platts, M. (1965) Central core disease of muscle with focal wasting. *Journal of Neurology, Neurosurgery and Psychiatry*, **28**, 432.

Dubowitz, V. & Roy, S. (1970) Central core disease of muscle. Clinical histochemical and electron miscroscopic studies of an affected mother and child. *Brain*, **93**, 65.

Duchenne, G.B. (1868) Recherches sur la paralysis musculaire pseudohypertrophique ou paralysie myosclerosique. *Archives Générales de Médicine*, 6 ser., **II**, 5.

Edström, L. & Kugelberg, E. (1968) Histochemical composition, distribution of fibres and fatiguability of single motor units. Anterior tibial muscle of the rat. *Journal of Neurology, Neurosurgery and Psychiatry*, **31**, 424.

Emery, A.E.H. (1963) Clinical manifestations in two carriers of Duchenne muscular dystrophy. *Lancet*, **1**, 1126.

Engel, A.G. (1970) Acid maltase deficiency in adults: Studies in four cases of a syndrome which may mimic dystrophy or other myopathies. *Brain*, **93**, 599–616.

Engel, A.G., Gomez, M.R. & Groover, R.V. (1971) Multicore disease. *Mayo Clinic Proceedings*, **10**, 666.

Engel, W.K. (1961) Muscle target fibres, a newly recognized sign of denervation. *Nature*, **191**, 389.

Engel, W.K. (1962) The essentiality of histo- and cytochemical studies of skeletal muscle in the investigation of neuromuscular disease. *Neurology (Minneapolis)*, **12**, 778.

Engel, W.K., Brooke, M.H. & Nelson, P.G. (1966) Histochemical studies of denervated or tenotomized cat muscle: illustrating difficulties in relating experimental animal conditions to human neuromuscular disorders. *Annals of the New York Academy of Sciences*, **138**, 160.

Engel, W.K. & Cunningham, G.G. (1963) Rapid examination of muscle tissue. An improved trichrome method for fresh frozen biopsy sections. *Neurology (Minneapolis)*, **13**, 919.

Engel, W.K., Foster, J.B., Hughes, B.P., Huxley, H.E. & Mahler, R. (1961) Central core disease. An investigation of a rare muscle cell abnormality. *Brain*, **84**, 167.

Engel, W.K., Gold, G.N. & Karpati, G. (1968) Type 1 fiber hypotrophy and central nuclei. *Archives of Neurology*, **18**, 435.

Eränkö, O. & Palkama, A. (1961) Improved localization of phosphorylase by the use of polyvinyl pyrrolidine and high substrate concentration. *Journal of Histochemistry and Cytochemistry*, **9**, 585.

Ernster, L., Ikkos, D. & Luft, R. (1959) Enzymic activities of human skeletal muscle mitochondria: a tool in clinical metabolic research. *Nature*, **184**, 1851.

Farber, R., Sternberg, W.H. & Dunlap, C.E. (1956) Histochemical localization of specific oxidative enzymes. I. Tetrazolium stains for diphosphopyridine nucleotide diaphorase and triphosphopyridine nucleotide diaphorase. *Journal of Histochemistry and Cytochemistry*, **4**, 254.

Forbes, G.B. (1953) Glycogen disease. Report of a case with abnormal glycogen storage structure in liver and skeletal muscle. *Journal of Pediatrics*, **42**, 645.

Freiman, D.G. & Kaplan, N. (1960) Studies on the histochemical differentiation of enzymes hydrolysing adenosine triphosphate. *Journal of Histochemistry and Cytochemistry*, **8**, 159.

Gallup, B., Strugalska-Cynowska, H. & Dubowitz, V. (1972) Histochemical studies on normal and diseased human and chick muscle in tissue culture. *Journal of the Neurological Sciences*, **17**, 109.

Gallup. B. & Dubowitz, V. (1975) Regeneration and innervation of normal and dystrophic muscle cultured with normal and dystrophic spinal cord. *Neuropathology and Applied Neurobiology*, **1**, 205.

Gauthier, G.F. & Padykula, H.A. (1962) Cytochemical studies of the ATPases of skeletal muscle fibres. *Journal of Histochemistry and Cytochemistry*, **10**, 661.

Gauthier, G.F. & Padykula, H.A. (1966) Cytological studies of fiber types in skeletal muscle. A comparative study of the mammalian diaphragm. *Journal of Cellular Biology*, **28**, 333.

George, J.C. & Naik, R.M. (1958) Relative distribution of the mitochondria in the two types of fibres in the pectoralis major muscle of the pigeon. *Nature*, **181**, 782.

George, J.C. & Scaria, K.S. (1958a) A histochemical study of dehydrogenase activity in the pectoralis major muscle of the pigeon and certain other vertebrate skeletal muscles. *Quarterly Journal of Microscopical Science*, **99**, 469.

George, J.C. & Scaria, K.S. (1958b) Histochemical demonstration of lipase activity in the pectoralis major muscle of the pigeon. *Nature*, **181**, 783.

Gomori, G. (1939) Microtechnical demonstration of phosphatase in tissue sections. *Proceedings of the Society for Experimental Biology and Medicine*, **42**, 23.

Gomori, G. (1941) Distribution of acid phosphatase in the tissues under normal and under pathological conditions. *Archives of Pathology*, **32**, 189.

Greenfield, J.G., Cornman, T. & Shy, G.M. (1958) The prognostic value of the muscle biopsy in 'floppy infant'. *Brain*, **81**, 461.

Greenfield, J.G., Shy, G.M., Alvord, E.C. & Berg, L. (1957) *An Atlas of Muscle Pathology in Neuromuscular Diseases* (Livingstone: Edinburgh).

Harman, P.J., Tassoni, J.P., Curtis, R.L. & Hollinshead, M.B. (1963) Muscular dystrophy in the mouse. In *Muscular Dystrophy in Man and Animals*, Eds G.H. Bourne & M.N. Golarz, p. 407 (Karger: Basel).

Hers, H. (1963) α-glucosidase deficiency in generalized glycogen-storage disease (Pompe's disease). *Biochemical Journal*, **86**, 11.

Hess, R., Scarpelli, D.G. & Pearse, A.G.E. (1958) The cytochemical localization of oxidative enzymes. II. Pyridine nucleotide-linked dehydrogenases. *Journal of Biophysical and Biochemical Cytology*, **4**, 753.

Hess, R. & Pearse, A.G.E. (1961) Dissociation of uridine diphosphate glucose-glycogen transglucosylase from phosphorylase activity in individual muscle fibres. *Proceedings of the Society for Experimental Biology and Medicine*, **107**, 569.

Homburger, F., Baker, J.R., Nixon, C.W. & Wilgram, G. (1962) New hereditary disease of Syrian hamsters. primary generalized polymyopathy and cardiac necrosis. *Archives of Internal Medicine*, **110**, 660.

Hudgson, P., Gardner-Medwin, D., Worsfold, M., Pennington, R.J.T. & Walton, J.N. (1968) Adult myopathy from glycogen storage disease due to acid maltase deficiency. *Brain*, **91**, 435.

Humoller, F.L., Griswold, B. & McIntyre, A.R. (1950) Comparative chemical studies in skeletal muscle following neurotomy and tenotomy. *American Journal of Physiology*, **161**, 406.

Humoller, F.L., Griswold, B. & McIntyre, A.R. (1951) Effect of neurotomy on succinic dehydrogenase activity of muscle. *American Journal of Physiology*, **164**, 742.

Humoller, F.L., Hatch, D. & McIntyre, A.R. (1952) Cytochrome oxidase activity in muscle following neurotomy. *American Journal of Physiology*, **170**, 371.

Illingworth, B. & Cori, G.T. (1952) Structure of glycogens and amylopectins. III. Normal and abnormal human glycogen. *Journal of Biological Chemistry*, **199**, 653.

Illingworth, B., Cori, G.T. & Cori, C.F. (1956) Amylo-1,6-glucosidase in muscle tissue in generalized glycogen storage disease. *Journal of Biological Chemistry*, **218**, 123.

Jasmin, G. & Bokdawala, F. (1970) Muscle transplantation in normal and dystrophic hamsters. *Revue Canadienne de Biologie*, **29**, 197.

Karpati, G., Carpenter, S. & Nelson, R.F. (1970) Type 1 muscle fibre atrophy and central nuclei. A rare familial neuromuscular disease. *Journal of the Neurological Sciences*, **10**, 489.

Karpati, G. & Engel, W.K. (1967) Neuronal trophic function. *Archives of Neurology*, **17**, 542.

Kearns, T.P. & Sayre, G.P. (1958) Retinitis pigmentosa, external ophthalmoplegia and complete heart block. *Archives of Ophthalmology*, **60**, 280.

Krivit, W., Polglase, W.J., Gunn, F.D. & Tyler, F.H. (1953) Studies in disorders of muscle. IX. Glycogen storage disease primarily affecting skeletal muscle and clinically resembling amyotonia congenita. *Pediatrics*, **12**, 165.

Laird, J.L. & Timmer, R.F. (1966) Transplantation of skeletal muscle into a host with muscular dystrophy. *Texas Reports on Biology and Medicine*, **24**, 169.

Lake, B.D. (1965) The histochemical demonstration of fructose-I-phosphate aldolase and fructose-I-6-diphosphate aldolase, and application of the method to a case of fructose intolerance. *Journal of the Royal Microscopical Society*, **84**, 489.

Layzer, R.B., Rowland, L.P. & Ranney, H.M. (1967) Muscle phosphofructokinase deficiency. *Archives of Neurology*, **17**, 512.

Leloir, L.F. & Cardini, C.E. (1957) Biosynthesis of glycogen from uridine diphosphate glucose. *Journal of the American Chemical Society*, **79**, 6340.

Luft, R., Ikkos, D., Palmieri, G., Ernster, L. & Afzelius, B. (1962) A case of severe hypermetabolism of nonthyroid origin with a defect in the maintenance of mitochondria respiratory control: a correlated clinical, biochemical, and morphological study. *Journal of Clinical Investigation*, **41**, 1776.

McArdle, B. (1951) Myopathy due to a defect in muscle glycogen breakdown. *Clinical Science*, **10**, 13.

McMinn, R.M.H. & Vrbová, G. (1962) Morphological changes in red and pale muscle following tenotomy. *Nature*, **195**, 509.

McMinn, R.M.H. & Vrbová, G. (1964) The effect of tenotomy on the structure of fast and slow muscle in the rabbit. *Quarterly Journal of Experimental Physiology*, **49**, 424.

Maengwyn-Davies, G.D., Friedenwald, J.S. & White, R.T. (1952) Histochemical studies of alkaline phosphatases in the tissues of the rat using frozen sections. *Journal of Cellular and Comparative Physiology*, **39**, 395.

Meier, H. (1967) Histochemical observations in preclinical mouse muscular dystrophy. *American Journal of Pathology*, **50**, 691.

Mellick, R.S., Mahler, R.F. & Hughes, B.P. (1962) McArdle's Syndrome. Phosphorylase-deficient myopathy. *Lancet*, **1**, 1045.

Michelson, A.M., Russell, E.S. & Harman, P.J. (1955) Dystrophia muscularis: a heriditary primary myopathy in the house mouse. *Proceedings of the National Academy of Sciences (U.S.A.)*, **41**, 1079.

Mommaerts, W.F.H.M., Illingworth, B., Pearson, C.M., Guillory, R.J. & Seraydarian, K. (1959) A functional disorder of muscle associated with the absence of phosphorylase. *Proceedings of the National Academy of Sciences (U.S.A.)*, **45**, 791.

Morris, C.J. & Raybould, J.A. (1971) Histochemically demonstrable fibre abnormalities in normal skeletal muscle and in muscle from carriers of Duchenne muscular dystrophy. *Journal of Neurology, Neurosurgery and Psychiatry*, **34**, 348.

Nachlas, M.M., Walker, D.G. & Seligman, A.M. (1958a) A histochemical method for the demonstration of diphosphopyridine nucleotide diaphorase. *Journal of Biophysical and Biochemical Cytology*, **4**, 29.

Nachlas, M.M., Walker, D.G. & Seligman, A.M. (1958b) The histochemical localization of triphosphopyridine nucleotide diaphorase. *Journal of Biophysical and Biochemical Cytology*, **4**, 467.

Nachlas, M.M., Crawford, D.T., Goldstein, T.P. & Seligman, A.M. (1958) The histochemical demonstration of cytochrome oxidase with a new reagent for the Nadi reaction. *Journal of Histochemistry*, **6**, 445.

Nachmias, V.T. & Padykula, H.A. (1958) A histochemical study of normal and denervated red and white muscles of the rat. *Journal of Biophysical and Biochemical Cytology*, **4**, 47.

Neerunjun, J.S. & Dubowitz, V. (1975) Muscle transplantation between normal and dystrophic mice. 2. Histochemical studies. *Neuropathology and Applied Neurobiology*, **1**, 125.

Nepveux, P. & Wegmann, R. (1962) Les enzymes du métabolisme des fructose phosphates. I. Démonstration de l'activité aldolasique. Note préliminaire. *Annales d'histochimie*, **7**, 21.

Newman, W., Feigin, I., Wolf, A. & Kabat, E.A. (1950) Histochemical studies on tissue enzymes. IV. Distribution of some enzyme systems which liberate phosphate at pH 9.2 as determined with various substrates and inhibitors: demonstration of three groups of enzymes. *American Journal of Pathology*, **26**, 257.

Nienhuis, A.W., Coleman, R.F., Jann Brown, W., Munsat, T.L. & Pearson, C.M. (1967) Nemaline myopathy, a histopathologic and histochemical study, *American Journal of Clinical Pathology*, **48**, 1.

Nyström, B. (1966) Succinic dehydrogenase in developing cat leg muscles. *Nature*, **212**, 954.

Ogata, T. (1958a) A histochemical study of the red and white muscle fibres. Part I. Activity of the succinoxidase system in muscle fibres. *Acta Medicinae Okayama*, **12**, 216.

Ogata, T. (1958b) A histochemical study of the red and white muscle fibres. Part II. Activity of the cytochrome oxidase in muscle fibres. *Acta Medicinae Okayama*, **12**, 228.

Ogata, T. (1958c) A histochemical study of the red and white muscle fibres. Part III. Activity of the diphosphopyridine nucleotide diaphorase and triphosphopyridine nucleotide diaphorase in muscle fibres. *Acta Medicinae Okayama*, **12**, 233.

Olson, W., Engel, W.K., Walsh, G.O. & Einaugler, R. (1972)

oculocraniosomatic neuromuscular disease with 'ragged-red' fibres. *Archives of Neurology*, **26**, 193.

Padykula, H.A. (1952) The localization of succinic dehydrogenase in tissue sections of the rat. *American Journal of Anatomy*, **91**, 107.

Pearse, A.G.E. (1960) *Histochemistry. Theoretical and Applied*, 2nd Edn. (Churchill: London).

Pearse, A.G.E. (1961) Direct relationship of phosphorylase and mitochondrial α-glycerophosphate dehydrogenase activity in skeletal muscle. *Nature*, **191**, 504.

Pearse, A.G.E. (1968) *Histochemistry, Theoretical and Applied*, Vol. 1, p. 475, 3rd Edn. (Churchill: London).

Pearson, C.M., Fowler, W.M. & Wright, S.W. (1963) X-chromosome mosaicism in females with muscular dystrophy. *Proceedings of the National Academy of Sciences (U.S.A.)*, **50**, 24.

Pearson, C.M., Rimer, D.G. & Mommaerts, W.F.H.M. (1961) A metabolic myopathy due to absence of muscle phosphoryalse. *American Journal of Medicine*, **30**, 502.

Pompe, J.C. (1932) Over idiopatische hypertrophie van het Hart. *Nederlandsch Tijdschrift Geneesk*, **76**, 304.

Pompe, J.C. (1933) Hypertrophie idiopathique du coeur. *Annales d'Anatomie Pathologique*, **10**, 23.

Prader, A., Labhart, A. & Willi, H. (1956) 'Ein Syndrom von Adipositas, Kleinwuchs, Kryptorchismus und Oligophrenie nach myotonieartigem Zustand im Neugeborenenalter.' *Schweizerische medizinische Wochenschrift*, **86**, 1260.

Prader, A. & Willi, H. (1963) 'Das Syndrom von Imbezillitat, Adipositas, Muskelhypotonie, Hypogenitalismus, Hypogonadismus, and Diabetes Mellitus mit "Myatonie"–anamnese.' Verh. 2 *Int. Kongr. Psych. Entw.–Stor. Kindes–Alt.* Vienna, 1961, pt. 1, p. 353.

Prewitt, M.A. & Salafsky, B. (1967) Effect of cross innervation on biochemical characteristics of skeletal muscles. *American Journal of Physiology*, **213**, 295.

Price, H.M., Gordon, G.B., Munsat, T.L. & Pearson, C.M. (1967) Myopathy with atypical mitochondria in the (type 1) skeletal muscle fibers. *Journal of Neuropathology and Experimental Neurology*, **26**, 475.

Price, H.M., Gordon, G.B., Pearson, C.M., Munsat, T.L. & Blumberg, J.M. (1965) New evidence for excessive accumulation of Z-band material in nemaline myopathy. *Proceedings of the American Academy of Sciences*, **54**, 1398.

Reis, J. (1934) La nucleotidase et sa relation avec la desamination des nucleotides dans le coeur et dans le muscle. *Bulletin de la Societé de chimie biologique*, **16**, 385.

Romanul, F.C.A. (1964) Enzymes in Muscle. I. Histochemical studies of enzymes in muscle fibres. *Archives of Neurology*, **11**, 355.

Romanul, F.C.A. & Hogan, E.L. (1965) Enzymatic changes in denervated muscle. I. Histochemical Studies. *Archives of Neurology*, **13**, 263.

Romanul, F.C.A. & van der Meulen, J.P. (1966) Reversal of the enzyme profiles in fast and slow muscles by cross-innervation. *Nature*, **212**, 1369.

Romanul, F.C.A. & van der Meulen, J.P. (1967) Slow and fast muscles after cross-innervation. *Archives of Neurology*, **17**, 387.

Rossi, F., Pescetto, G. & Reale, E. (1953) La reazione istochemica per la fosfatasi acida nell studio dello sviluppo prenatale dell'uoma. *Zeitschrift für anatomie und Entwicklungsgeschichte*, **117**, 36.

Rossi, F., Prescetto, G. & Reale, E. (1954) Histochimie enzymatique pendant l'organogénèse et la différenciation embryonaire de l'homme. *Comptes rendues de l'Association des anatomistes*, **41e**, 1 (Réunion, Gênes).

Roy, S. & Dubowitz, V. (1970) Carrier detection in Duchenne muscular dystrophy. A comparative study of electron microscopy, light microscopy and serum enzymes. *Journal of the Neurological Sciences*, **11**, 65.

Rubinstein, N., Mabuchi, K., Pepe, F., Salmons, S., Gergely, J. & Sréter, F. (1978) Use of type-specific antimyosins to demonstrate the transformation of individual fibers in chronically stimulated rabbit fast muscles. *Journal of Cellular Biology*, **79**, 252.

Rutenburg, A.M., Gofstein, R. & Seligman, A.M. (1950) Preparation of a new tetrazolium salt which yields a blue pigment on reduction and its use in the demonstration of enzymes in normal and neoplastic tissues. *Cancer Research*, **10**, 113.

Salafsky, B. (1971) Functional studies of regenerated muscles from normal and dystrophic mice. *Nature*, **229**, 270.

Salmons, S. & Sréter, F.A. (1976) Significance of impulse activity in the transformation of skeletal muscle type. *Nature*, **263**, 30.

Salmons, S. & Vrbová, G. (1969) The influence of activity on some contractile characteristics of mammalian fast and slow muscles. *Journal of Physiology*, **201**, 535.

Satoyoshi, E. & Kowa, H. (1967) A myopathy due to glycolytic abnormality. *Archives of Neurology*, **17**, 248.

Sawyer, D., Sie, H. & Fishman, W.H. (1965) A technique for preparing permanent histochemical preparations of liver phosphorylase. *Journal of Histochemistry and Cytochemistry*, **13**, 605.

Scarpelli, D.G., Hess, R. & Pearse, A.G.E. (1958) The cytochemical localization of oxidative enzymes. I. Diphosphopyridine nucleotide diaphorase and triphosphopyridine nucleotide diaphorase. *Journal of Biophysical and Biochemical Cytology*, **4**, 747.

Schmid, R., Robbins, P.W. & Traut, R.R. (1959) Glycogen synthesis in muscle lacking phosphorylase. *Proceedings of the National Academy of Sciences (U.S.A.)*, **45**, 1236.

Schmid, R. & Mahler, R. (1959) Chronic progressive myopathy with myoglobinuria: demonstration of a glycogenolytic defect in muscle. *Journal of Clinical Investigation*, **38**, 2044.

Seligman, A.M. & Rutenberg, A.M. (1951) The histochemical demonstration of succinic dehydrogenase. *Science*, **113**, 317.

Semenoff, W.E. (1935) Mikrochemische Bestimmung der Aktivitat der succinodehydrase in den Organen der Rana Temporaria. *Zeitschrift für Zellforschung und mikroskopische*, **22**, 305.

Shafiq, S.A., Dubowitz, V., Peterson, H. de C. & Milhorat, A.T. (1967) Nemaline myopathy: report of a fatal case, with histochemical and electron microscopic studies. *Brain*, **90**, 817.

Sher, J.H., Rimalovski, A.B., Athanassiades, T.J. & Aronson, S.M. (1967) Familial centronuclear myopathy: A clinical and pathological study. *Neurology (Minneapolis)*, **17**, 727.

Shy, G.M., Engel, W.K., Somers, J.E. & Wanko, T. (1963) Nemaline myopathy. A new congenital myopathy. *Brain*, **86**, 793.

Shy, G.M., Gonatas, N.K. & Perez, M. (1966) Two childhood myopathies with abnormal mitochondria. *Brain*, **89**, 133.

Shy, G.M. & Magee, K.R. (1956) A new congenital non-progressive myopathy. *Brain*, **79**, 610.

Smith, B. (1965) Changes in the enzyme histochemistry of skeletal muscle during experimental denervation and reinnervation. *Journal of Neurology, Neurosurgery and Psychiatry*, **28**, 99.

Spiro, A.J., Shy, G.M. & Gonatas, N.K. (1966) Myotubular myopathy. *Archives of Neurology*, **14**, 1.

Stein, J.M. & Padykula, H.A. (1962) Histochemical classification of individual skeletal muscle fibers of the rat. *American Journal of Anatomy*, **110**, 103.

Stetten, D. & Stetten, M.R. (1960) Glycogen Metabolism. *Physiological Reviews*, **40**, 505.

Sugita, H., Masaki, T., Ebashi, S., Pearson, C.M. (1972) Protein composition of rods in nemaline myopathy (abstract). *In* Abstracts of Papers presented at *II International Congress on Muscle Diseases*, Perth, Australia. I.C.S. No. 237, p. 17 (Excerpta Medica: Amsterdam).

Takeuchi, T. (1956) Histochemical demonstration of phosphorylase. *Journal of Histochemistry and Cytochemistry*, **4**, 84.

Takeuchi, T. (1958) Histochemical demonstration of branching enzyme (amylo-1,4,→1,6-transglucosidase) in animal tissues. *Journal of Histochemistry and Cytochemistry*, **6**, 208.

Takeuchi, T. & Glenner, G.G. (1960) Histochemical demonstration of a pathway for polysaccharide synthesis from uridine diphosphoglucose. *Journal of Histochemistry and Cytochemistry*, **8**, 288.

Takeuchi, T. & Glenner, G.G. (1961) Histochemical demonstration of uridine diphosphate glucose-glycogen transferase in animal tissues. *Journal of Histochemistry and Cytochemistry*, **9**, 304.

Takeuchi, T. & Kuriaki, H. (1955) Histochemical detection of phosphorylase in animal tissues. *Journal of Histochemistry and Cytochemistry*, **3**, 153.

Tarui, S., Okuno, G. Ikura, Y., Tanaka, T., Suda, M. & Nishikawa, M. (1965) Phosphofructokinase deficiency in skeletal muscle. A new type of glycogenosis. *Biochemical and Biophysical Research Communications*, **19**, 517.

van Wijhe, M., Blanchaer, M.C. & Jacyk, W.R. (1963) The oxidation of lactate and α-glycerophosphate by red and white skeletal muscle. ii. Histochemical studies. *Journal of Histochemistry and Cytochemistry*, **II**, 505.

van Wijngaarden, G.K., Fleury, P., Bethlem, J. & Meijer, A.E.F.H. (1969) Familial 'myotubular' myopathy. *Neurology (Minneapolis)*, **19**, 901.

van Wijngaarden, G.K., Bethlem, J., Meijer, A.E.F.H., Hulsmann, W. Ch. & Feltkamp, C.A. (1967) Skeletal muscle disease with abnormal mitochondria. *Brain*, **90**, 577.

Wachstein, M. & Meisel, E. (1955) The distribution of demonstrable succinic dehydrogenase and of mitochondria in tongue and skeletal muscle. *Journal of Biophysical and Biochemical Cytology*, **1**, 483.

Wachstein, M. & Meisel, E. (1956) Histochemistry of substrate specific phosphatase at a physiological pH. *Journal of Histochemistry and Cytochemistry*, **4**, 424.

Wattenberg, L.W. & Leong, J.L. (1960) Effects of coenzyme Q_{10} and menadione on succinic dehydrogenase activity as measured by tetrazolium salt reduction. *Journal of Histochemistry and Cytochemistry*, **8**, 296.

Wohlfart, G. (1937) Uber das vorkommen verschiedener Arten von Muskelfasern in der skelett-muskulatur des menschen und einiger saugitere. *Acta psychiatrica et neurologica*, Suppl. 12.

Zellweger, H., Illingworth Brown, B., McCormick, W.F. & Jun-bi Tu. (1965) A mild form of muscular glycogenosis in two brothers with alpha-1,4-glucosidase deficiency. *Annales Paediatrici (Basel)*, **205**, 413.

Ultrastructural studies of diseased muscle

INTRODUCTION

In the third edition of this book an attempt was made to review what was known at the time of the ultrastructural changes in muscle fibres in the more important diseases of muscle. In the ensuing five years, important advances have been made which have provided valuable insights into the pathogenesis of a number of muscle diseases and into the mechanisms of certain basic reactions of the muscle fibre. As a result it has been necessary to modify some of the conclusions reached in the previous edition.

Electron-microscopic examination of human and experimental animal material has provided further information about the ultrastructural reactions of muscle fibres and about the mech-anisms of degeneration and repair in diseased muscle. In addition, several new disease entities with distinctive morphological changes in muscle fibres have been identified. It has been recognised that certain ultrastructural changes may be found not only in disease states but also in biopsy material from healthy volunteers (Reske-Nielsen and Harmsen, 1972).

Morphometric and stereological techniques have allowed a more objective interpretation of changes in muscle fibres, motor end-plates and blood vessels in naturally occurring and experimental muscle disorders (Engel, Santa, Stonnington, Jerusalem, Tsujihata, Brownell, Sakakibara, Banker, Sahashi and Lambert, 1979a). The ultrastructural characteristics of normal human muscle have also been defined in quantitative terms using these techniques (Cullen and Weightman, 1975; Payne, Stern, Curless and Hannapel, 1975). Important advances in the study of the integrity of the sarcolemma, of cellular interfaces and of the sarcotubular systems have come from the use of electron-dense extracellular markers such as horseradish peroxidase and lanthanum (Chou and Nonaka, 1977). One of the major advances of the past four years has been the application of electron-immunocytochemical techniques to label the acetylcholine receptors at the neuromuscular junction using α-bungarotoxin or antibodies conjugated to horseradish peroxidase (HRP). Such studies have greatly improved our understanding of the pathogenetic mechanisms involved in myasthenia gravis. The application of the freeze-fracture technique to the study of diseased muscle has provided information complementary to that derived from transmission electron microscopy and has led to the recognition

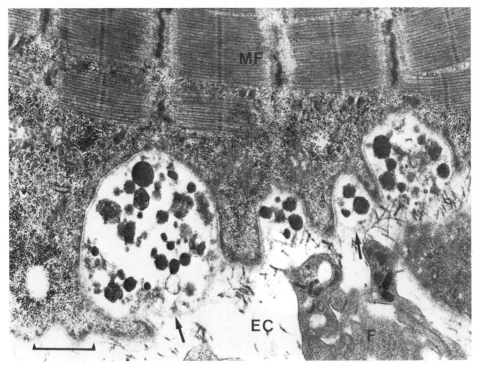

Fig. 9.1 Irregularity of the surface of a muscle fibre due to the presence of exocytotic vacuoles which contain granular and membranous debris enclosed by the basement membrane (arrows). MF: myofibrils; EC: extracellular space; F: fibroblast. Myopathy due to ε-aminocaproic acid. Bar: 1.0 μm

of differences between the surface membranes of normal and dystrophic muscle fibres. Lastly, the application of X-ray microanalysis has made it possible to study the elemental composition of various components of the muscle fibre and has added a new dimension to the study of diseased muscle (Maunder, Yarom and Dubowitz, 1977).

ULTRASTRUCTURAL REACTIONS OF THE MUSCLE FIBRE

Over the past 15 years, electron microscopists have become increasingly aware of the fact that the muscle fibre shows only a limited number of ultrastructural reactions, and that few, if any, of these are specific for a particular disease entity (Engel and MacDonald, 1970; Fardeau, 1970; Neville, 1973). In spite of this lack of specificity, students of diseased muscle have recognised that certain combinations or sequences of changes— reaction patterns—seen in certain myopathies are sufficiently distinctive to be of diagnostic value.

The more important ultrastructural reactions of the muscle fibre components and the ultrastructural correlates of some of the well-known light-microscopic reactions of the muscle fibre will now be considered.

Reactions of muscle fibre components

Surface membrane changes. The surface of muscle fibres is usually relatively smooth and under normal circumstances the plasma and basement membranes are closely applied to each other. Irregular projections of the surface of the muscle fibre may be due to the fact that it is fixed in a state of contraction, but these have also been noted frequently in various neuromuscular disorders (Neville, 1973). Papillary projections from the surface of diseased muscle fibres may be seen in fibres which are undergoing atrophy or in fibres of normal size, and may be due either to loss of fibre bulk or else may be a sequel to extrusion of degradation products from the surface of the fibre (*exocytosis*) (Fig. 9.1) (Engel and MacDonald,

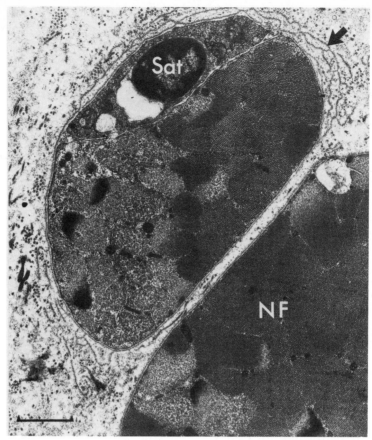

Fig. 9.2   Redundant folds of basement membrane (arrow) surrounding a small muscle fibre. An inactive satellite cell (Sat) is situated internal to the basement membrane. NF: normal muscle fibre. Congenital myotonic dystrophy. Bar: 1.0 μm

1970). Deep infoldings of the sarcolemma are seen in fibres which are undergoing longitudinal splitting, and are prominent in dystrophia myotonica (Schröder, 1970; Casanova and Jerusalem, 1979).

In atrophying fibres the basement membrane may separate from the plasma membrane forming redundant folds which may remain even after the rest of the fibre has disappeared (Fig. 9.2). Reduplication of the basement membrane is a common finding in the muscular dystrophies and other necrotising myopathies (Neville, 1973) probably being a sequel to muscle fibre regeneration (Karpati, Carpenter, Melmed and Eisen, 1974). Thickening of the basement membrane is a non-specific finding in a variety of situations (Mastaglia, McCollum, Larson and Hudgson, 1970b).

Focal or more extensive deficits in the plasma membrane are frequently observed in fibres undergoing necrosis. Focal defects have also been described in otherwise normal fibres in carefully prepared material from patients with Duchenne muscular dystrophy (*vide infra*) and it has been suggested that these may be of pathogenetic importance in the fibre necrosis which occurs in this disease (Mokri and Engel, 1975). Increased numbers of pinocytotic vesicles associated with the plasma membrane are also found in a variety of situations (Engel and MacDonald, 1970).

Nuclear reactions. The reactions of the myonuclei are relatively limited. Internally placed nuclei which are otherwise normal are commonly found in any chronic myopathic or neurogenic disorder, and are particularly prominent in dystrophia myotonica and centronuclear myopathy.

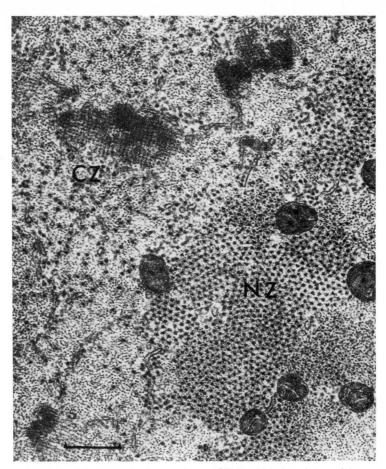

Fig. 9.3. Targetoid fibre in a case of polymyositis. A central zone (CZ) in which there is loss of the normal hexagonal arrangement of thick and thin myofilaments, disorganisation of the sarcoplasmic reticulum and loss of mitochondria borders on a normal portion of the fibre (NZ). Bar: 0.5 μm

Nuclear crowding occurs in fibres undergoing atrophy. Convolution of the nuclear membrane may also be seen in atrophying fibres and, unless serial sections are examined, may produce a false impression suggestive either of nuclear division or of nuclear inclusions resulting from invagination of cytoplasmic organelles. It is also a feature of nemaline myopathy. Other nuclear changes seen in denervated fibres consist of clumping of nuclear chromatin and a tendency for the nucleolus to become shrunken and dense (Lee and Altschul, 1963). Enlarged nuclei with dispersed chromatin and large nucleoli ('vesicular' nuclei) are seen in regenerating or hypertrophying muscle fibres (Mastaglia, 1973) and may also be a feature in Werdnig-Hoffmann disease and congenital myotonic dystrophy where a maturational arrest of muscle fibres has been postulated (Sarnat and Silbert, 1976). Various fibrillar, tubular and rod-like inclusions have been described in myonuclei in acquired and congenital myopathies. The earlier suggestion that some of these inclusions are viral in nature now seems unlikely.

Reactions of myofibrils. The orderly sarcomere pattern and regular alignment of myofibrils seen in normal muscle may be disorganised in a number of different ways in disease. Focal areas of disruption involving a single or a few adjoining sarcomeres are commonly found in a variety of disorders and their significance is uncertain. In a number of children with a congenital myopathy this was found to be the principal change in muscle fibres and the terms *multicore* and *minicore* disease

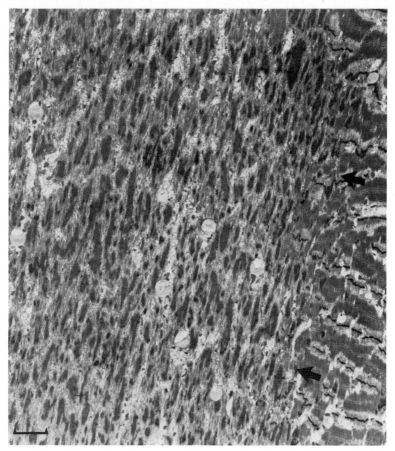

Fig. 9.4 Central core-like area (arrows) showing marked disorganisation of the sarcomere pattern of myofibrils in a muscle fibre. Mitochondrial myopathy. Bar: 2.0 μm

were applied to such cases (Engel, Gomez and Groover, 1971).

More extensive disorganisation of myofibrils in the central portions of the muscle fibres is found in *target* fibres and in *central cores*. *Target* fibres are found in denervating conditions, after re-innervation, and in some myopathies, including familial periodic paralysis and polymyositis. Within such fibres a central zone of marked myofibrillar disorganisation is separated from an outer zone of normal myofibrils by an intermediate zone in which the degree of myofibrillar disarray is relatively mild. Within the central zone there is disruption of the myofibril pattern, spreading of Z-band material, loss of mitochondria and disorganisation of the sarcoplasmic reticulum (SR) (Fig. 9.3) (Schotland, 1969).

In so-called *targetoid* fibres, which may be found both in denervating and in myopathic conditions (Dubowitz and Brooke, 1973), the intermediate zone is lacking and the appearance is similar to that seen in the variety of central core disease in which fibres contain *unstructured* cores (Fig. 9.4 and 9.5). This similarity has led to the suggestion that both of these types of change should be included under the common term *core-targetoid* fibres (Engel, Brooke and Nelson, 1966). In contrast, the type of change described in the earlier reports of central core disease was quite different and was associated with preservation of the cross-striated sarcomere pattern within the central core (Shy and Magee, 1956; Engel, Foster, Hughes, Huxley and Mahler, 1961). This appearance has since been termed a *structured* core

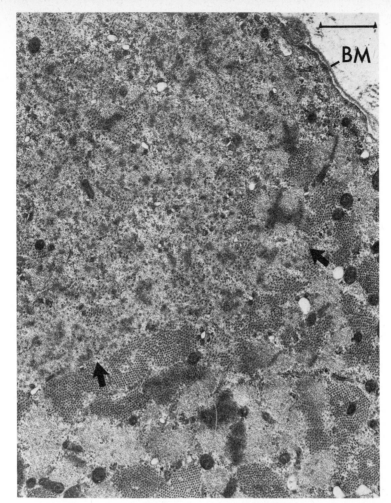

Fig. 9.5 Peripheral core-like area (arrows) showing disorganisation of the contractile elements and sarcoplasmic reticulum
and reduced numbers of mitochondria in a muscle fibre. BM:
basement membrane. Polymyositis. Bar: 1.0 μm

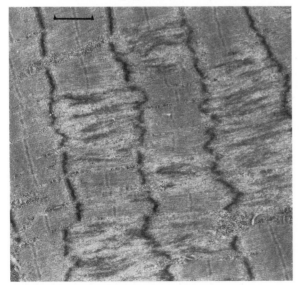

Fig. 9.6 Portion of a muscle fibre from a case of
polymyositis showing Z-line 'streaming' and focal
disorganisation of myofilaments in several sarcomeres. Bar:
1.0 μm

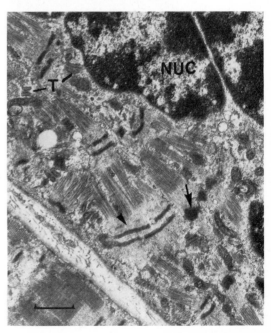

Fig. 9.7 Portion of an atrophic muscle fibre from a case of
spinal muscular atrophy showing disorganisation of
myofibrils, Z-line reduplication (arrowhead) and spreading
(arrow), displacement of triads (T) and congregation of
myonuclei (NUC). Bar: 1.0 μm

and has been differentiated from the *unstructured core* in which the sarcomere pattern within the core is disorganised (Neville, 1973). The suggestion that all of these phenomena may be related and may form part of a continuum seems a not unreasonable one (Schmitt and Volk, 1975). A common origin has recently also been proposed for central cores, miniature cores, focal loss of cross-striations, and rod bodies in muscle fibres (Bethlem, Arts and Dingemans, 1978).

The Z band shows a variety of distinctive reactions. The most frequent consists of irregularities of outline or *streaming* of the Z band material (Fig. 9.6). This type of change is commonly seen in the areas of myofibrillar disorganisation mentioned above and in a variety of other disorders. Other common changes in the Z band include zig-zag irregularities, duplication (Fig. 9.7), and *rod body* formation (Figs. 9.8 and 9.9) (Neville, 1973). The latter consist of elongated electron-dense structures derived from the Z band (Price, Gordon, Pearson, Munsat and Blumberg, 1965; Gonatas, 1966) and are the central feature of nemaline myopathy (Shy, Engel, Somers and Wanko, 1963; Hudgson, Gardner-Medwin, Fulthorpe and Walton, 1967). These structures have been shown to contain α-actinin bound to the actin filaments of the I bands (Yamaguchi, Robson, Stromer, Dahl and Oda, 1978b). Although seen most strikingly in nemaline myopathy, rod bodies originating from the Z band have also been described in a variety of other situations and are clearly a non-specific reaction of the Z band.

The so-called *cytoplasmic body* (MacDonald and

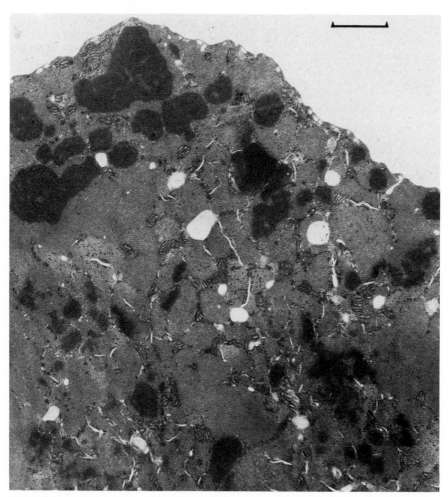

Fig. 9.8 Nemaline rods (sectioned transversely) at the periphery of a muscle fibre and to a lesser extent more centrally. Nemaline myopathy. Bar: 1.0 μm

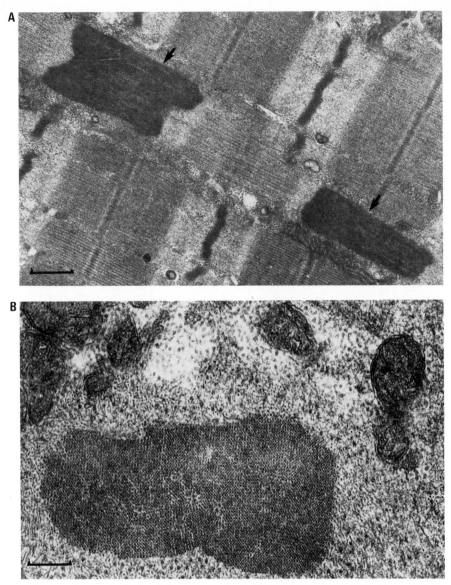

Fig. 9.9 Nemaline myopathy. A. Two small rod bodies are present in a myofibril at the level of the Z lines (arrows). Bar: 0.5 μm. B. Higher magnification of a transversely sectioned rod body showing the characteristic lattice-like appearance. Bar: 0.25 μm

Engel, 1969) probably also represents a reaction of the Z band. These structures, which may be confined to either type I (Jerusalem, Ludin, Bischoff and Hartmann, 1979) or to type II fibres (Engel and MacDonald, 1970), have an electron-dense core which in some instances is clearly seen to be derived from a Z band, and which is surrounded by a light halo of filamentous material. At times a distinctive pattern of regularly orien-

tated myofibrils is seen around the dense central core (Fig. 9.10). Cytoplasmic bodies have been observed as an occasional finding in a number of human and experimental neuromuscular disorders. They have, however, been a major change in two cases of an unusual form of chronic progressive neuromyopathy presenting with respiratory failure and weight loss which has been termed cytoplasmic body neuromyopathy (Jer-

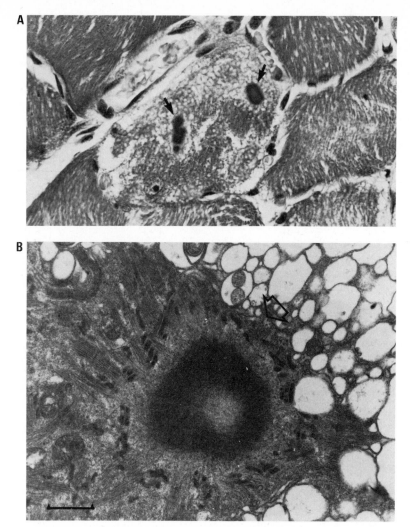

Fig. 9.10 Cytoplasmic bodies in muscle fibres in two cases of mitochondrial myopathy (arrows). A. Haematoxylin and eosin, ×640. B. Electronmicrograph showing electron-dense centre surrounded by radially orientated myofibrils and triads. Bar: 1.0 μm

usalem *et al.*, 1979), and in a large kindred with a benign late-onset form of autosomal dominant myopathy (Clark, D'Agostino, Wilson, Brooks and Cole, 1978).

Another distinctive structure which is probably derived from the myofilaments is the *filamentous body*. These consist of more-or-less circumferentially orientated filaments resembling the thick myosin filaments of the myofibrils, and are usually found in the subsarcolemmal region (Fig. 9.11). They have been described in various disorders but also in normal muscle (Mair and Tomé, 1972a).

Another non-specific change involving the

myofibrils is that seen in *ring fibres* in which one or more otherwise normal myofibrils, usually beneath the sarcolemma, are found to be circumferentially orientated (Fig. 9.12). In some such fibres the peripheral myofibrils show varying degrees of disorganisation and may be separated from the sarcolemma by a zone of sarcoplasm containing myonuclei, disorganised myofilaments and other organelles (*sarcoplasmic mass*). Such fibres may be found in a variety of situations but are particularly prominent in myotonic dystrophy, limb-girdle muscular dystrophy and in some cases of hypothyroid myopathy (Fardeau, 1970). Bundles of

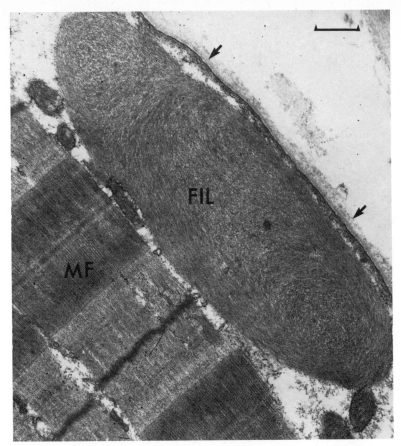

Fig. 9.11 Sub-sarcolemmal filamentous body (FIL) in an otherwise normal muscle fibre. Arrows: basement membrane; MF: myofibrils; Bar: 0.5 μm

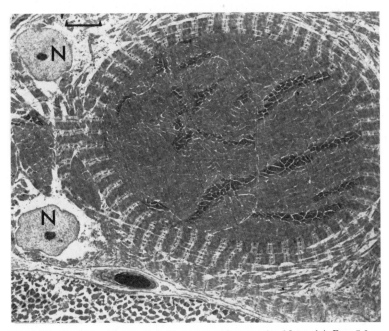

Fig. 9.12 Ring fibre from a case of hypothyroid myopathy. N: nuclei; Bar: 5.0 μm

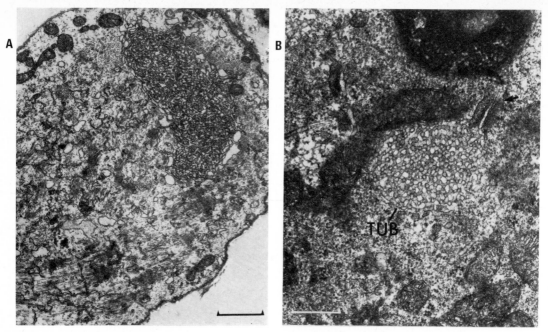

Fig. 9.13 A. Dilatation and proliferation of the sarcoplasmic reticulum in an atrophic fibre showing marked loss of myofibrils. Bar: 1.0 μm. B. Honeycomb tubular array (TUB) in close proximity to a triad (arrow) with which it appears to be in continuity. Polymyositis. Bar: 0.5 μm

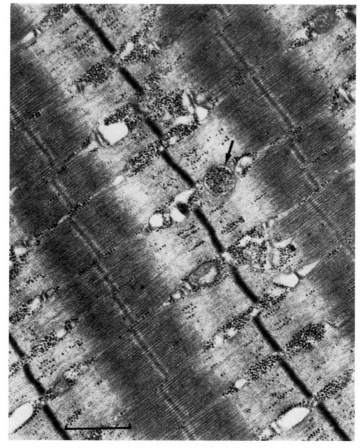

Fig. 9.14 Dilatation of transverse tubules and lateral sacs of the sarcoplasmic reticulum. Arrow: small area of autophagia. Duchenne muscular dystrophy. Bar: 1.0 μm

aberrrant myofibrils with or without evidence of myofibrillar degeneration are also found in so-called *lobulated* muscle fibres (Bethlem, Van Wijngaarden and De Jong, 1973).

Reactions of the sarcoplasmic reticulum and T system. When seen as an isolated change, and particularly when associated with vacuolation of mitochondria, dilatation of the SR is usually due to inadequate fixation. On the other hand, focal dilatation of the SR may be a genuine change which has been found in a variety of neuromuscular disorders, and is particularly prominent in the periodic paralyses (Engel and MacDonald, 1970) and in so-called *sarcotubular myopathy* (Jerusalem, Engel and Gomez, 1973). Dilatation or apparent proliferation of the SR has also been noted in regenerating fibres (Engel and MacDonald, 1970), after denervation (Schiaffino and Settembrini, 1970) (Fig. 9.13A), and in various forms of hereditary myotonia (Schröder and Becker, 1972; Casanova and Jerusalem, 1979).

Dilatation of the tubules of the T system (Fig. 9.14) has also been described in various myopathies, particularly in the muscular dystrophies and polymyositis, but this too may represent a fixation artefact. Proliferation of T tubules resulting in the formation of labyrinthine networks (Fig. 9.13B) has also been found in a variety of neuromuscular disorders, but is particularly prominent in myotonic dystrophy (Schotland, 1970) and in hypothyroid myopathy (Afifi, Najjar, Mire-Salman and Bergman, 1974). The continuity of such networks with the T system and the extracellular space has been demonstrated by the use of the electron-dense marker horseradish peroxidase (HRP) (Engel and MacDonald, 1970). Tubular networks of this type have been found in close proximity to autophagic vacuoles and it has been suggested that in certain situations the limiting membranes of such vacuoles are derived from the T system (Engel and MacDonald, 1970). Such tubular networks have also been noted at the interface between lymphoid cells and muscle fibres in polymyositis and experimental allergic myositis (Fulthorpe, 1979). It has also been suggested that the large vacuoles seen in periodic paralysis (Schutta and Armitage, 1969) and in idiopathic myoglobinuria (Schutta, Kelly and Zacks, 1969)

are derived from the T system. Displacement, distortion and reduplication of *triads* is a common accompaniment of myofibrillar disorganisation in fibres undergoing degeneration or atrophy (Fig. 9.7) (Neville, 1973).

Mitochondrial reactions. The number and size of mitochondria in muscle fibres vary considerably. Focal loss of mitochondria is a common accompaniment of myofibrillar disorganisation or breakdown in various myopathies (Engel and MacDonald, 1970). Focal increases in mitochondrial numbers have also been noted in a variety of myopathies. Peripheral aggregates of morphologically normal mitochondria (Fig. 9.15) have been found to be particularly prominent in corticosteroid myopathy (Engel, 1966a) and in hypokalaemic periodic paralysis (MacDonald, Rewcastle and Humphrey, 1969). Triangular subsarcolemmal aggregates of normal mitochondria are found in so-called *lobulated* muscle fibres which occur in facioscapulohumeral muscular dystrophy and a number of other neuromuscular disorders, and account for the characteristic histochemical appearance of these fibres in oxidative enzyme preparations (Bethlem et al., 1973).

In a separate category are cases in which mitochondria are not only copious but also show bizarre abnormalities such as increases in size, abnormal cristae and the presence of amorphous, tubular or paracrystalline inclusions (Fig. 9.16). Such changes have again been found in various forms of inherited and acquired myopathy but have been particularly prominent in the group of so-called *mitochondrial myopathies* in which they represent the most prominent and earliest morphological change seen in muscle fibres. The various types of mitochondrial inclusion have been considered in detail by a number of previous authors (Chou, 1969; Neville, 1973). Prominent electron-dense granules (Fig. 9.17), which are thought to be a calcific in nature, have been noted in mitochondria in a number of situations including glycogen storage disease of muscle (Engel and Dale, 1968) and hypothyroid myopathy (Mastaglia, Sarnat, Dawkins, Papadimitriou and Kakulas, 1980).

Vacuolation of mitochondria is an unreliable sign which is usually related to poor fixation. On

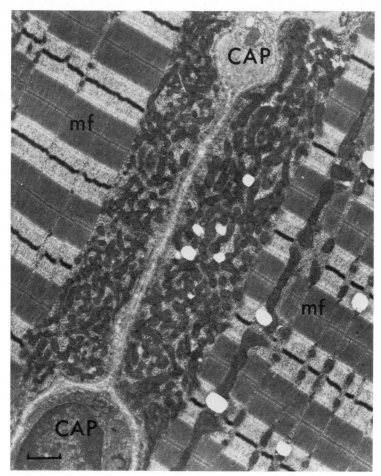

Fig. 9.15 Large sub-sarcolemmal aggregates of morphologically normal mitochondria in two muscle fibres (mf) in a case of mitochondrial myopathy. Two capillaries (CAP) indent the surface of the muscle fibres. Bar: 1.0 μm

the other hand, the type of vacuolation produced by separation of the inner and outer mitochondrial membranes ('outer chamber' or 'low amplitude' swelling) which has been seen in a case of chloroquine neuromyopathy (Mastaglia, Papadimitriou, Dawkins and Beveridge, 1977) probably represents a genuine change (Fig. 9.18). Similarly, breakdown of cristal membranes is difficult to evaluate, particularly when associated with vacuolation, but the presence of myelin-like bodies is probably a genuine sign of mitochondrial degeneration (Fig. 9.19).

Reactions of the Golgi apparatus. The Golgi apparatus is inconspicuous in normal muscle fibres but becomes more prominent after denervation (*see* Fig. 9.29A) and in regenerating muscle fibres (Mastaglia and Walton, 1971b). It has also been shown to contribute to membranes which limit autophagic vacuoles in certain situations such as acid maltase deficiency (Engel and Dale, 1968; Engel and MacDonald, 1970). Relatively little is known about its reactions in disease states.

Other distinctive changes. A number of other distinctive ultrastructural changes of uncertain origin have been recognised in muscle fibres in human neuromuscular disorders.

Tubular aggregates. These are aggregates of closely packed parallel double-walled long straight tubules which have usually been confined to type IIb and occasionally to type I fibres (Dobkin and

Verity, 1978) (Fig. 9.20A–C). They have been described as an occasional incidental finding in various situations (Mastaglia, 1973), and even in muscle from healthy young people (Reske-Nielsen and Harmsen, 1972), but have been particularly striking in patients with periodic paralysis (Grüner, 1966; Engel, Bishop and Cunningham, 1970; Bergman, Afifi, Dunkle and Johns, 1970), myotonia congenita (Schröder and Becker, 1972) and paramyotonia congenita (Julien, Vital, Vallat and Martin, 1971), and in a group of patients with exertional muscle pain and cramping (Engel et al., 1970; Lewis, Pallis and Pearse, 1971). There has been debate about the source of origin of these tubules: a recent experimental study suggests that they are derived from the SR (Schiaffino, Severin, Cantini and Sartore, 1977).

Concentric laminated bodies. These structures, which appear to be filamentous in nature, have been found in a variety of neuromuscular disorders and are clearly non-specific (Fig. 9.21A and B). It has been suggested that they are found only in type II fibres and that they may be derived from actin filaments (Payne and Curless, 1976).

Fingerprint inclusions. These consist of lamellae which often have a sawtooth-like configuration and are arranged in peculiar curvilinear patterns (Fig. 9.22A). They are non-specific, having been described in benign congenital myopathy (Engel, Angelini and Gomez, 1972), dystrophia myotonica (Tomé and Fardeau, 1973) and oculopharyngeal muscular dystrophy (Julien, Vital, Vallat, Vallat and LeBlanc, 1974). It has been suggested that they occur exclusively in type I fibres and that they are derived from degenerating mitochondria (Payne and Curless, 1977) but their origin remains uncertain.

Zebra bodies. These ladder-like filamentous structures are normally found in muscle fibres close to the region of the myotendinous junction (Mair and Tomé, 1972b). They were a frequent finding in a patient with an unusual form of slowly progressive congenital myopathy (Lake and Wilson, 1975), and we have observed them in a case of hypothyroid myopathy (Fig. 9.22B). Their significance is uncertain.

Curvilinear bodies. These structures, which appear to be basically membranous in nature, have been observed in association with lipofuscin bodies in chloroquine myopathy (Mastaglia et al., 1977; Neville, Maunder-Sewry, McDougall, Sewell and Dubowitz, 1979) and are identical to the curvilinear bodies described in cerebral glial cells and neurones in neuronal ceroid-lipofuscinosis (Rapola and Haltia, 1973) (Fig. 9.22C).

Spheroid bodies. This term has been used to describe more-or-less spherical heterogeneous bodies with both fine fibrillar and amorphous granular components, which have been a striking finding in members of a family with a slowly progressive autosomal dominant neuromuscular disorder (Goebel, Muller, Gillen and Merritt, 1978).

Satellite cells. The 'resting' satellite cell is an undifferentiated mononucleated cell with little cytoplasm and few cytoplasmic organelles (Fig. 9.23A). Identification of these cells and demarcation of cellular interfaces has been facilitated by the use of the electron-dense tracers lanthanum nitrate (Chou and Nonaka, 1977) and ruthenium red (Popiela, 1976). The number of satellite cells has been shown to be increased in Duchenne muscular dystrophy (Wakayama, Schotland, Bonilla and Orecchio, 1979) and in polymyositis (Chou and Nonaka, 1977) and evidence of 'activation' is commonly seen in these situations. Activated satellite cells are of increased size, have more cytoplasm which contains greater numbers of ribosomes, polyribosomes, rough endoplasmic reticulum, and increased numbers of caveolae, and a prominent nucleolus. The finding of primitive myofilaments and myofibrils in some cells confirms that they are undergoing transformation into myoblasts (Chou and Nonaka, 1977). Activation of satellite cells has also been noted in muscle hypertrophy (Reger and Craig, 1968) (Fig. 9.23B). Increased numbers of satellite cells have been noted in congenital myotonic dystrophy (Sarnat and Silbert, 1976) and in muscle undergoing denervation atrophy, for example in cases of Werdnig-Hoffmann disease and the Kugelberg-Welander syndrome (Van Haelst, 1970; Mastaglia

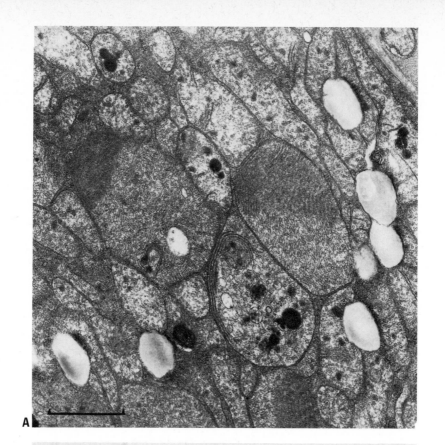

A

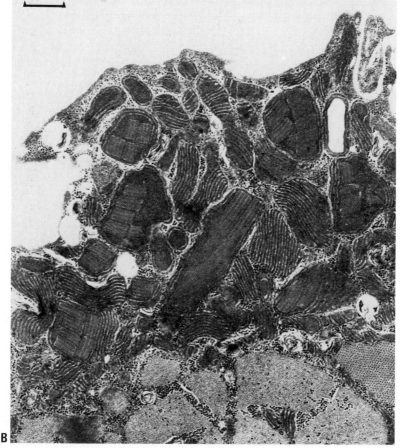

B

Fig. 9.16 Mitochondrial myopathy. A. Sub-sarcolemmal collection of pleomorphic mitochondria some of which have electron-dense inclusions and abnormal cristal configurations. Bar: 1.0μm. B. Peripheral aggregate of mitochondria with paracrystalline inclusions of various types and abnormal cristal patterns. Bar: 0.5μm. C. Abnormal mitochondrion with rectangular 'parking-lot' inclusions and coiled cristae. G: glycogen granules; Bar: 0.5μm. D. Electron-dense elongated crystalline mitochondrial inclusions. MF: myofibrils; F: fibroblast; Bar: 0.5μm

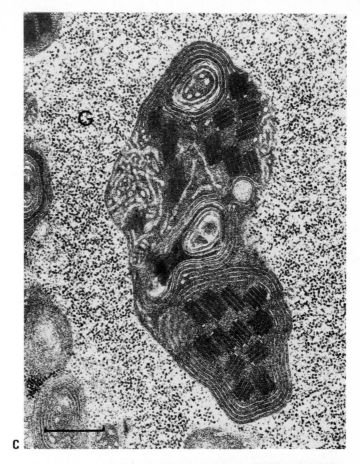

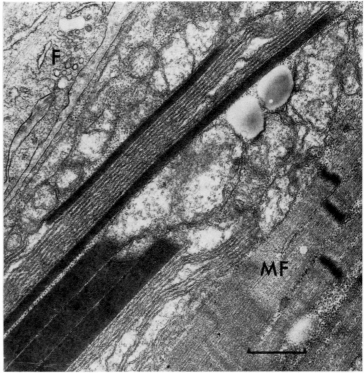

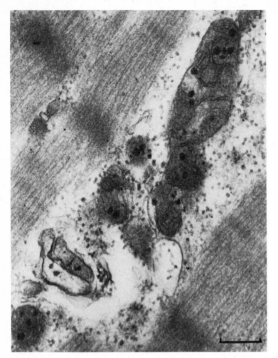

Fig. 9.17 Unduly prominent electron-dense granules of probable calcific nature within mitochondria. Hypothyroid myopathy. Bar: 0.25 μm

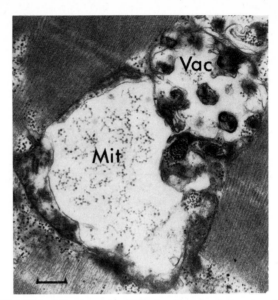

Fig. 9.18 Mitochondrion (Mit) showing vacuolation caused by separation of the inner and outer membranes (outer chamber swelling). Glycogen granules are present within the vacuole. A small autophagic vacuole (Vac) is also present. Chloroquine neuromyopathy. Bar: 0.25 μm

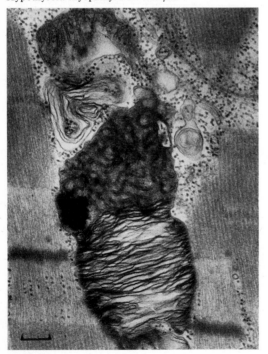

Fig. 9.19 Abnormal membranous bodies, possibly within a degenerating mitochondrion. Chloroquine neuromyopathy. Bar: 0.25 μm

and Walton, 1971a), but evidence of activation is not often seen in these situations. On the other hand, evidence of satellite cell activation is seen after acute denervation by neurectomy in the experimental animal (Schultz, 1978).

Reactions of intrafusal muscle fibres. The ultrastructural changes in intrafusal muscle fibres have been studied particularly in myotonic dystrophy, in which marked fibre splitting has been found (Swash and Fox, 1976).

Blood vessel reactions. Electron-microscopic observations have been made on the changes in muscle capillaries and other small blood vessels in a variety of disorders. Thickening of the capillary basement membrane is a common finding which is particularly prominent in diabetes (Zacks, Pegues and Elliott, 1962) as well as in polymyositis (Vick, 1971; Mastaglia and Walton, 1971b) and in a variety of other neuromuscular disorders. The normal capillary basement membrane thickness in human muscle has been found to be 150–440 nm (Vick, 1971). Lamellation of the capillary basement membrane is also seen in a number of conditions including Duchenne dystrophy and periodic paralysis (Koehler, 1977), and polymyositis (Mastaglia and Walton, 1971b).

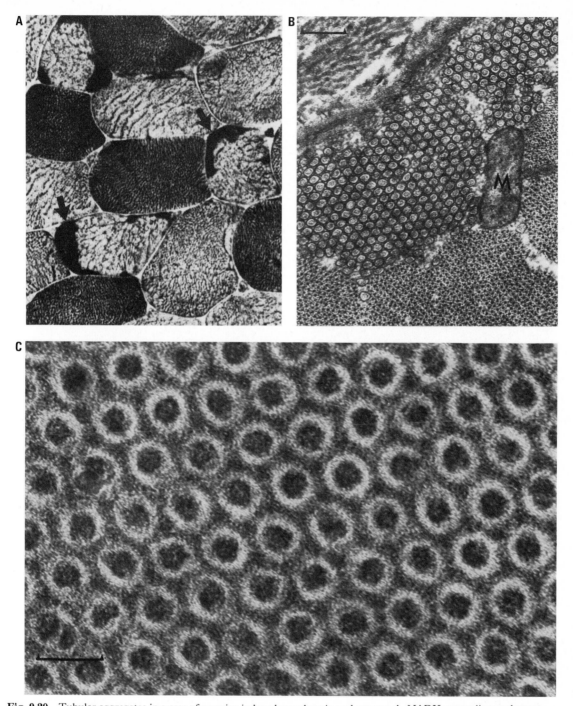

Fig. 9.20 Tubular aggregates in a case of exercise-induced muscle pain and spasms. A. NADH-tetrazolium reductase preparation showing the densely staining aggregates at the periphery of several Type 2 fibres (arrows), × 612. B. Electron micrograph showing typical appearance of double-walled tubules. M: mitochondrion; Bar, 0.25 μm. C. Higher magnification of tubules. Bar: 0.1 μm

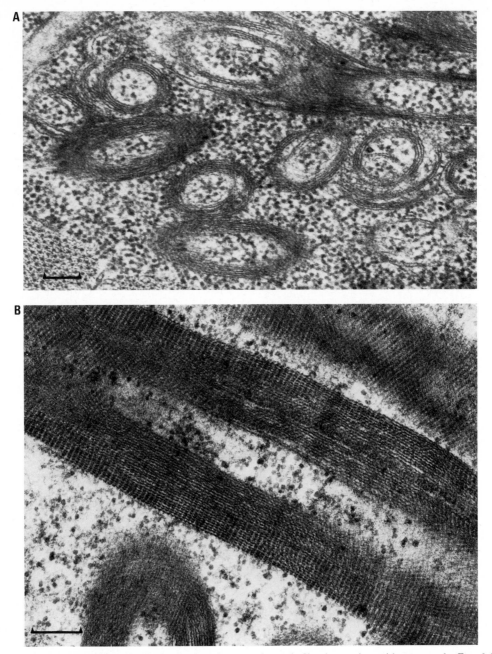

Fig. 9.21 A. Concentric laminated bodies in an otherwise normal muscle fibre in a patient with acromegaly. Bar: 0.25 μm. B. Higher magnification showing typical periodicity. Bar: 0.25 μm

An increase in size of endothelial cells and increased numbers of pinocytotic vesicles in such cells have been found in polymyositis (Mastaglia and Walton, 1971b), Duchenne dystrophy (Jerusalem, Engel and Gomez, 1974a) and in various other situations and is clearly a non-specific reaction. Degenerative changes in the endothelial cells of small vessels, such as the finding of myelin-like bodies, are also non-specific and have been noted in hypothyroid myopathy (Mastaglia et al., 1980) and in chloroquine neuromyopathy (Mastaglia et al., 1977) (Fig. 9.22D).

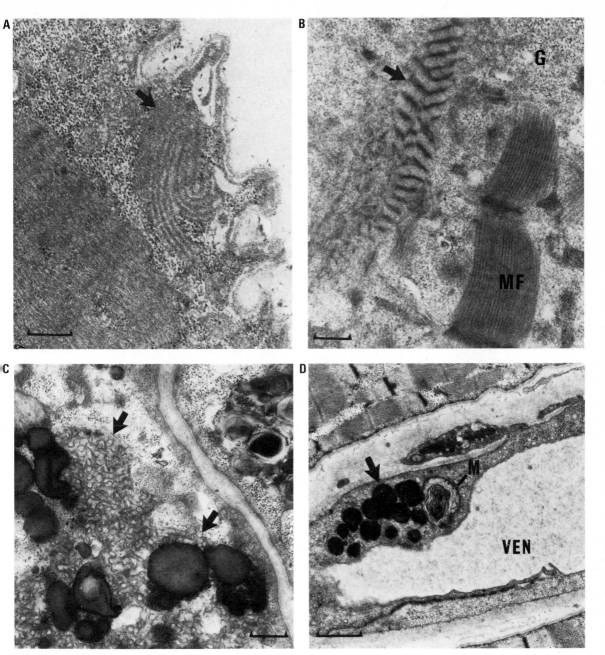

Fig. 9.22   A. Small *fingerprint body* (arrow) at the periphery of a hypercontracted fibre. Uraemic myopathy. Bar: 0.5 μm. B. *Zebra body* (arrow) in a case of hypothyroid myopathy. MF: myofibril; G: glycogen granules; Bar: 0.5 μm. C. *Curvilinear body* (arrows) at periphery of a muscle in a case of chloroquine neuromyopathy. Bar: 0.5 μm. D. Osmiophilic *myelin-bodies* (arrow) in the cytoplasm of an endothelial cell, and also within a mitochondrion (M). VEN: venule; Bar: 1.0 μm

Basic pathological reactions

   Atrophy. The most obvious change in atrophic muscle fibres, whether the atrophic process is due to denervation (Recondo, Fardeau and Lapresle, 1966, Mastaglia and Walton, 1971a), to disuse (Klinkerfuss and Haugh, 1970; Mendell and Engel, 1971; Dastur, Gagrat and Manghani, 1979), or to other causes, is a progressive reduction

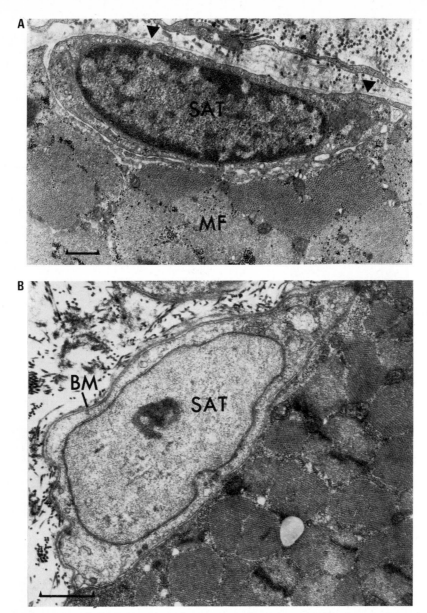

Fig. 9.23 A. Inactive satellite cell (SAT) beneath the basement membrane (arrowheads) of a normal muscle fibre (MF). Polymyositis. Bar: 0.5 μm. B. Satellite cell (SAT) with 'active' nucleus within a hypertrophied muscle fibre. BM: basement membrane. Acromegaly. Bar: 1.0 μm

in the cross-sectional area of the myofibrils and disorganisation of the contractile elements and triads. There is an increase in the surface area of the sarcotubular membranes which may proliferate to form labyrinthine structures (Fig. 9.13A), and in Golgi cisternae, ribosomes and granular endoplasmic reticulum (Stonnington and Engel, 1973; Cullen, Appleyard and Bindoff,

1978). The latter features suggest increased protein synthesis which may be related to the production of lysosomal enzymes or of new acetylcholine receptors in the plasma membrane (Cullen and Pluskal, 1977). The plasma membrane of atrophic fibres shrinks, perhaps as a result of increased endocytotic activity (Libelius, Lundqvist, Templeton and Thesleff, 1978) whereas the basement membrane becomes redundant and convoluted (Mastaglia and Walton, 1971a) (Fig. 9.2). Freeze-fracture studies have shown distinctive changes in the plasma membrane in neurogenic atrophy, the number of particles on the inner face of the membrane being significantly reduced (Ketelsen, 1975). The number of satellite cells associated with denervated atrophic fibres appears to be increased (Van Haelst, 1970; Mastaglia and Walton, 1971a), and autoradiographic studies in animals suggest that this is due to proliferation of these cells (McGeachie and Allbrook, 1978).

The factors responsible for the breakdown of the contractile elements in atrophying fibres are poorly understood. Although autophagic vacuoles and other secondary lysosomes may be seen in such fibres, they do not appear to play a part in the disassembly of the myofibrils (Cullen et al., 1978). It has been suggested that this may be brought about by extralysosomal proteases which have been isolated from muscle tissue and which have been shown to be capable of degrading a number of the myofibrillar proteins at neutral pH (Busch, Stromer, Goll and Suzuki, 1972).

Hypertrophy. The ultrastructural changes in muscle fibres undergoing hypertrophy have been studied principally in the experimental animal in situations of compensatory work hypertrophy and in the transient hypertrophy which occurs after denervation in the diaphragm. The increased cross-sectional area of the muscle fibres has been shown to be due principally to an increase in the number of myofibrils (Miledi and Slater, 1969). This is accompanied by increased synthesis of RNA and of sarcoplasmic and myofibrillar proteins, and reduced breakdown of these proteins (Goldspink, 1972). Longitudinal splitting of myofibrils once they reach a certain critical size may be one of the ways in which the number of myofibrils is increased (Goldspink, 1972). Little is known about the way in which newly synthesised myofilaments are laid down in hypertrophying muscle fibres. Satellite cells have been noted to be prominent in hypertrophic human muscle (Reger and Craig, 1968; Mastaglia, 1973) (Fig. 9.23B) and it has been suggested that these cells may be incorporated into muscle fibres to increase the complement of myonuclei. Longitudinal splitting

of muscle fibres occurs in compensatory work hypertrophy (Hall-Craggs, 1972; James, 1973) and accounts for the apparent increase in muscle fibre numbers reported in some light microscope studies (Gonyea, Ericson and Bonde-Petersen, 1977).

Autophagy. Evidence of autophagy is seen in a variety of situations in which a sub-lethal injury leads to cytoplasmic degradation and is a mechanism for disposing of damaged components in muscle fibres (Cullen et al., 1978). Autophagic vacuoles are particularly prominent in chloroquine and vincristine myopathy, and in acid maltase deficiency, but may be seen in any myopathy (Engel and MacDonald, 1970). They contain sequestered sarcoplasm, mitochondria and other organelles undergoing degradation (Fig. 9.24 and 9.25), and are bounded by single, double or multiple membranes which are derived from the SR (Cullen et al., 1978) or from the T system or Golgi apparatus (Engel and MacDonald, 1970). Small autophagic vacuoles which are usually limited by a double membrane (Fig. 9.24) coalesce to form larger vacuoles with scalloped borders. The localisation of lysosomal enzymes (such as acid phosphatase) to the contents of autophagic vacuoles indicates that they are secondary lysosomes (Engel and MacDonald, 1970), as are multivesicular bodies and lipofuscin granules. The origin of these secondary lysosomes is uncertain, as primary lysosomes cannot be positively identified morphologically in muscle fibres (Cullen et al., 1978). The contents of autophagic vacuoles become degraded progressively and are eventually extruded from the cell (exocytosis) and come to lie between the plasma and basement membranes (Fig. 9.1), or within the endomysial connective tissue. How much of the degraded material is extruded from the fibre and how much is retained in the form of residual material such as lipofuscin, is not known.

Necrosis. Although necrosis of the muscle fibre may result from a variety of exogenous or endogenous causes, certain generalisations can be made about the ultrastructural changes which accompany death of the muscle cell. The changes in the myofibrils may take several forms (Cullen et

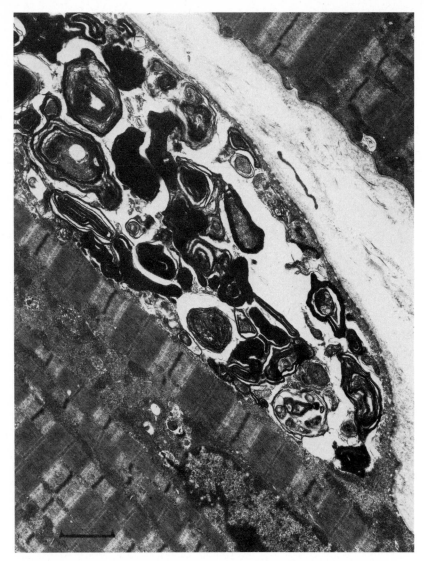

Fig. 9.24 *Myelin bodies* within an autophagic vacuole without a clearly defined limiting membrane at the periphery of a muscle fibre. Vacuolar myopathy of undetermined cause. Bar: 2.0 μm

al., 1978) First, there may be severe over-contraction of sarcomeres leading to the formation of dense contraction clumps which alternate with segments of discontinuity in the myofibrils (*see* Fig. 9.30A). This is probably the forerunner of the 'coagulative' change seen in some necrotic fibres in which the myofibrils become converted into a dense homogeneous mass in which individual filaments can no longer be identified (Fig. 9.26). Secondly, preferential loss of the Z band and I band or of the A band leading to discontinuity between individual sarcomeres (Fig. 9.27A and B)

can occur. Thirdly, there may be a total disorganisation of thick and thin myofilaments. These changes may be confined to a segment of the muscle fibre (*segmental necrosis*) and may actually co-exist at different sites in the same muscle fibre. Although attempts have been made to associate certain changes such as selective lysis of Z-I or A bands with specific aetiological agents, consistent correlations are not possible and these types of myofibrillar change appear to be quite non-specific.

It has been argued that contraction clumps

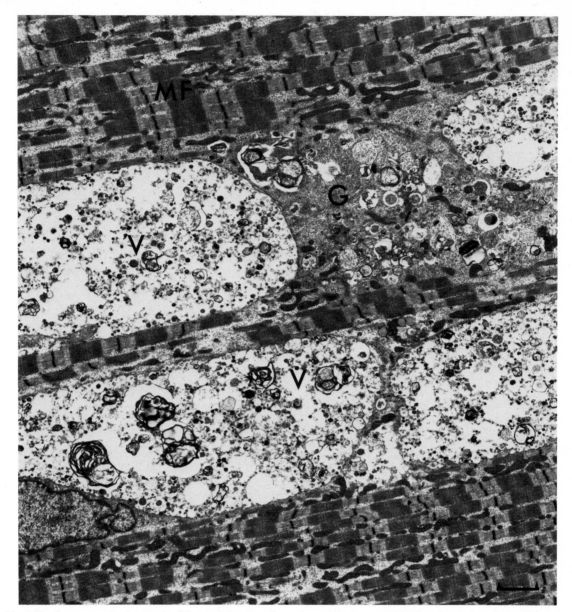

Fig. 9.25 Large autophagic vacuoles (V) containing granular and membranous material. The vacuoles have led to wide separation of the myofibrils (MF). G: glycogen. Vacuolar myopathy of undetermined cause. Bar: 2.0 μm

merely represent an artefact of tissue handling and fixation (Adams, Denny-Brown and Pearson, 1962). However, while it is true that they may be produced in this way, the fact that they are also found in carefully handled unfixed material from patients with Duchenne dystrophy, and that they sometimes contain macrophages, indicates that in certain situations they do represent a genuine pathological change (Cullen and Fulthorpe, 1975;

Cullen *et al.*, 1978). It has been suggested that the over-contraction of the myofibrils results from a sustained elevation of intracellular Ca++ levels due to a functional (or structural) breakdown of the integrity of the plasma membrane of the muscle fibre, and there is now a good deal of evidence to support this hypothesis (Oberc and Engel, 1977; Cullen *et al.*, 1978). Raised intracellular Ca++ levels could also be responsible for disassembly of

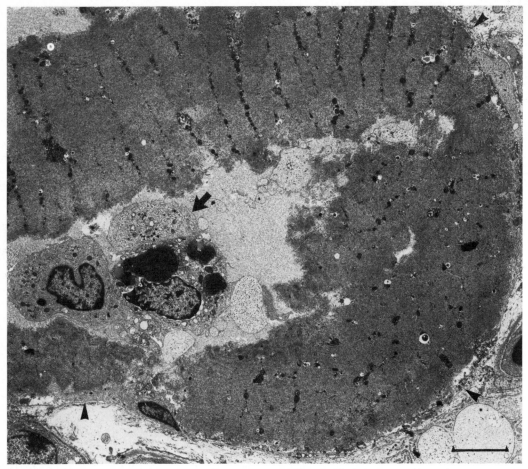

Fig. 9.26 Necrotic muscle fibre undergoing phagocytosis. The remaining myofibrils have massed together and sarcomere detail is largely lost. The mitochondria are shrunken and electron-dense. Arrow: mononuclear phagocytic cells. Arrowheads: basement membrane. Myopathy due to ε-aminocaproic acid. Bar: 5.0 μm

the myofilaments by activating the sarcoplasmic protease CANP (Busch *et al.*, 1972), leading to dissolution of the Z line and breakup of the myofibrils. The subsequent breakdown of the sarcomeres takes place in macrophages (Fig. 9.28), and lysosomes originating in the muscle fibre itself probably play little if any part.

The mitochondria in necrotic fibres become rounded and dense (Fig. 9.26), and may contain various amorphous deposits or paracrystalline inclusions. Swelling of the SR leads to the formation of vacuoles. Focal discontinuities of variable extent appear in the plasma membrane, while the basement membrane remains intact unless necrosis is due to a mechanical or other severe exogenous form of injury. The myonuclei

initially become shrunken with clumping of chromatin, and at a later stage undergo lysis (Cullen *et al.*, 1978).

Regeneration. Electron microscopy greatly clarified our understanding of the repair processes in muscle fibres after injury. After mild forms of injury which do not lead to necrosis, degradation and repair of the injured portion of the fibre occur together and new myofibrils are formed to replace those which have been broken down. The ultrastructural signs of such synthetic activity are the presence of many ribosomes and polyribosomes and a prominent Golgi apparatus (Cullen *et al.*, 1978).

When necrosis of the muscle fibre occurs,

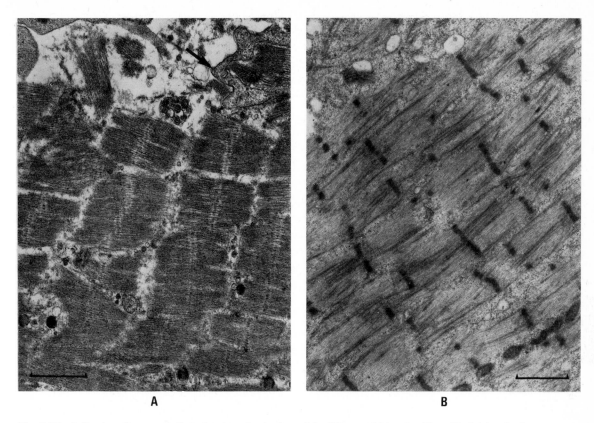

A   B

Fig. 9.27   A. Portion of a necrotic fibre showing selective loss of the Z lines and I bands with residual A bands. Arrow: processes of phagocytic cells. Polymyositis. Bar: 1.0 μm. B. Portion of a necrotic fibre showing selective loss of A bands, with residual Z lines and I bands. Myopathy due to ε-aminocaproic acid. Bar: 1.0 μm

regeneration of the damaged segment of the muscle fibre is brought about by mononucleated myoblasts which appear internal to the basement membrane of the fibre as its degenerate contents are undergoing phagocytosis and lysis. These cells generally have large nuclei with prominent nucleoli, and their cytoplasm contains many ribosomes, polyribosomes and granular endoplasmic reticulum. The myogenic nature of these cells is confirmed by the presence in the cytoplasm of newly synthesised thin (actin) and thick (myosin) filaments and assembling myofibrils. Electron microscopic and autoradiographic studies suggest that the subsarcolemmal satellite cells which are present in small numbers in mature muscle fibres (Mauro, 1961) are the major source of myoblasts (Reznik, 1969a and b; Konigsberg, Lipton and Konigsberg, 1975; Snow, 1977, 1978). Electron-microscopic observations also indicate that some myoblasts may be formed by cleavage of existing

myonuclei and their surrounding sarcoplasm from the degenerating fibre (Reznik, 1969a; Mastaglia, Dawkins and Papadimitriou, 1975). Myoblasts undergo mitotic division and fusion to form a variable number of primitive multinucleated myogenic cells (myotubes) which subsequently establish continuity with the intact ends of the necrotic fibre. This form of repair of damaged segments of muscle fibres is one of the ways in which longitudinally split or forked muscle fibres can arise (Schmalbruch, 1976; Chou and Nonaka, 1977). Myotubes contain myofilaments and developing myofibrils, numerous ribosomes and polyribosomes and microtubules which are orientated in the longitudinal axis of the developing fibre (Fig. 9.29.) Developing myofibrils at first contain relatively few myofilaments and the Z bands are wide and not sharply defined, an appearance resembling that of nemaline rods (Fig. 9.29B). The regenerate fibres become enveloped

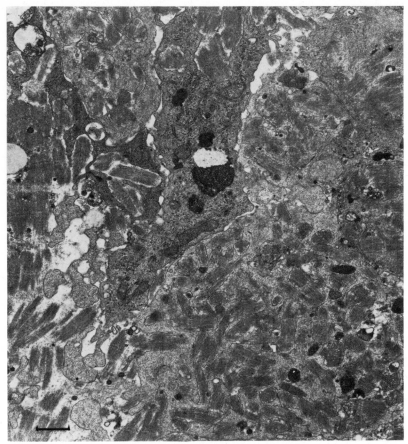

Fig. 9.28   Necrotic muscle fibre. The processes of phagocytic cells have engulfed the residual A bands of sarcomeres in which there has been selective lysis of Z lines and I bands. Polymyositis. Bar: 10.0 μm

by a new basement membrane but the original membrane may remain and may be seen lying redundant outside the new membrane.

THE MUSCULAR DYSTROPHIES

In previous editions of this book, this section encompassed the ultrastructural pathology of all the 'classical' muscular dystrophies listed in the World Federation of Neurology classification of neuromuscular disorders (1968, *see* Appendix to Ch. 13) and defined as *progressive, genetically determined, primary degenerative myopathies* (Walton, 1961). For some years before the publication of the third edition of this book (1974) and certainly since then, clinicopathological and electrophysiological evidence has been adduced to show that *some* forms of 'dystrophy' do not

conform to this definition. In particular, it has become clear that some are due to degeneration of the anterior horn cell rather than the skeletal muscle fibre or at least to changes in the latter which could not be classed as primary, necrobiotic degeneration (Bradley, 1980). These observations apply particularly to many cases diagnosed in the past as examples of limb-girdle and facioscapulohumeral dystrophy, both of which should be regarded as syndromes rather than disease entities in their own right. However we believe that the nosological integrity of Duchenne's disease as a primary, necrobiotic myopathy remains unchallenged. There can be equally little doubt about the status of myotonic dystrophy on clinical and genetic grounds. Accordingly this section will be restricted to a consideration of the ultrastructural pathology of these two conditions only, without

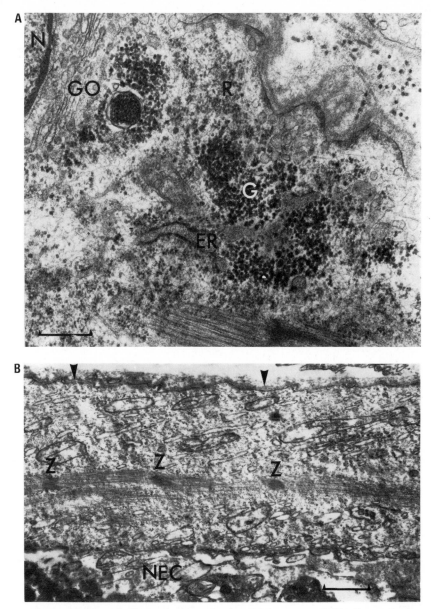

Fig. 9.29 Regenerating muscle fibres. A. Paranuclear area showing Golgi apparatus (GO), ribosomal aggregates (R), granular endoplasmic reticulum (ER), aggregates of glycogen granules (G). Thin filaments are also seen lying free in the sarcoplasm. N: nucleus. Myopathy due to ε-aminocaproic acid. Bar: 0.5 μm. B. Primitive myofibril with immature Z-lines (Z) in a regenerating fibre at the periphery of a necrotic fibre which is undergoing phagocytosis (NEC). The cytoplasm of the regenerating fibre contains many ribosomes, mitochondria and elongated sacs of endoplasmic reticulum. Arrowheads: basement membrane. Polymyositis. Bar: 1.0 μm

prejudice to any of the current hypotheses about their aetiology and pathogenesis. A discussion of the ultrastructural abnormalities underlying the facioscapulohumeral and limb-girdle syndromes will be found in sections concerning spinal muscular atrophy, mitochondrial myopathy. etc.

Duchenne muscular dystrophy (DMD)

In the five years since the third edition of this book was published, waves of enthusiasm for the so-called 'neurogenic' and 'vascular' hypotheses for the pathogenesis of DMD have reached their zeniths and have subsequently waned. Once more, attention is being directed to the muscle cell itself as a source for its own destruction, whether it be via sarcolemmal defects permitting the ingress of calcium ions (*see above*) or because of a fundamental abnormality of a structural protein. Certainly the histopathological abnormalities in skeletal muscle in DMD as revealed by the light microscope can be construed only as being due to a primary necrotising myopathy in which reconstitution of normal structure is incomplete because of ineffective regeneration (Mastaglia and Kakulas, 1969; Mastaglia, Papadimitriou and Kakulas, 1970a) (Fig. 9.30). In spite of the many technical and interpretational difficulties besetting the electron microscopy of skeletal muscle, it can now be claimed that the development of the necrobiotic lesions in DMD can be followed, stage by stage, by electron microscopy and, in some instances, that an explanation can be suggested for these lesions in terms of antecedent molecular abnormalities.

In earlier editions, it was variously suggested that the A band and the I band were the sites of the earliest degenerative changes in DMD (Pearce, 1964; Hudgson and Mastaglia, 1974). Certainly, such changes can be observed in both regions early in the natural history of the disease, in the case of the A band with myofilament loss and in the I band with Z band degeneration or 'streaming'. Indeed these features may have progressed as far as virtually complete disappearance of one or other structure in some areas with little or no cellular reaction. However, the observations of a number of workers on very carefully processed 'early' material have led to a revival of the 'leaky membrane' theory for the pathogenesis of DMD, originally favoured by many biochemists (Pennington, 1963).

The observations of Cullen and Fulthorpe (1975) on the development of hyaline degeneration in some muscle fibres in DMD led them to speculate that the degenerative changes noted could be due to an abnormal influx of calcium ions through the sarcolemma, causing hypercontraction of the affected fibre (Fig. 9.30A and B). In this study, Cullen and Fulthorpe analysed the various stages of the breakdown of muscle fibres in DMD, defining five stages leading to phagocytosis of a fibre in which contraction clumps (the

morphological substrate for the appearance of hyaline fibres) and areas of sarcoplasm devoid of contractile elements have developed (Fig. 9.30A). In stage 1, the ultrastructure of the muscle fibres appears to be normal although morphometric analysis demonstrated a 35–80 per cent increase in the relative volume of the sarcoplasm compared with normal control material (Cullen and Weightman, 1975). In stage 2, the authors noted minor abnormalities in both the A and Z bands (*see their* Fig. 7), with evidence of overcontraction of some parts of the fibre and overstretching of others. These processes proceed through stages 3 and 4 in which large 'bare' areas develop, culminating in stage 5 in which phagocytes invade the overstretched/hypercontracted fibre. In an attempt to demonstrate that the various abnormalities described in the plastic-embedded material were not artefactual, Cullen and Fulthorpe examined teased, unfixed fibres from Duchenne biopsies using differential interference microscopy and plane polarised light. By these means, they were able to show areas of hyaline change and overstretching/hypercontraction (*see their* Figs. 3 and 4). In their Discussion, Cullen and Fulthorpe suggested that excessive accumulation of Ca^{++} within the muscle fibre might be the explanation for the overstretching/hypercontraction sequence, a possibility already suggested by the biochemical observation that Ca^{++} tends to accumulate in the SR in DMD (Peter and Worsfold, 1969).

The presence of excessive calcium within the hyaline fibres has been confirmed histochemically by Bodensteiner and Engel (1978) on cryostat sections from 114 DMD biopsies. Analysis of their data revealed that non-necrotic, calcium-positive fibres were significantly more frequent in DMD than in normal and other pathological controls, that hyaline fibres were encountered 12 times more often in DMD than in all other cases, and that 43 per cent of these were calcium-positive. Calcium-positive hyaline fibres were extremely uncommon in normal controls and other myopathies. Using the potassium pyroantimonate technique for localisation of calcium at the ultrastructural level, Oberc and Engel (1977) found increased calcium precipitates in mitochondria, nuclei and SR in necrotic, degenerating and regenerating muscle fibres in Duchenne dystrophy as well as in other

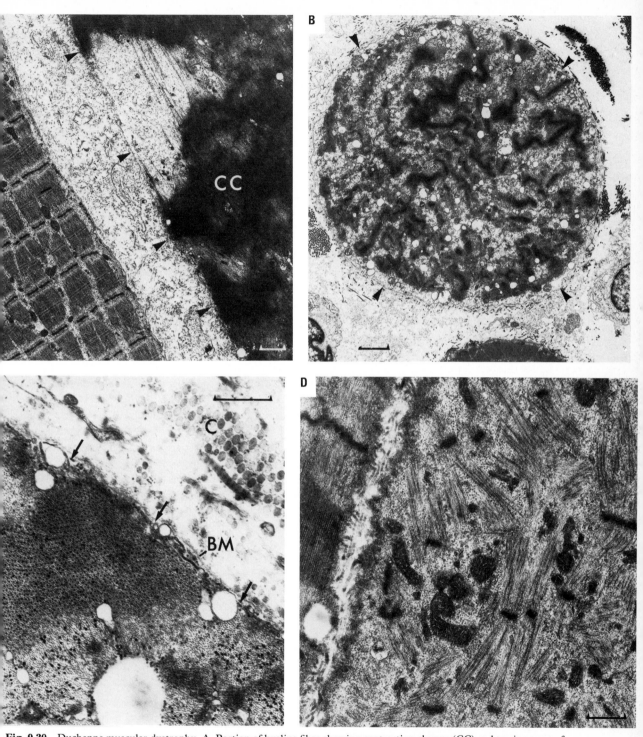

Fig. 9.30 Duchenne muscular dystrophy. A. Portion of hyaline fibre showing contraction clumps (CC) and tearing apart of the myofibrils in places. Arrowheads: basement membrane. The plasma membrane has broken down. Bar: 1.0 μm. B. Transversely sectioned necrotic fibre showing disrupted masses of myofibrils, distended sarcoplasmic reticulum, and loss of the plasma membrane. Arrowheads: basement membrane. Bar: 2.0 μm. C. Focal loss of plasma membrane (arrows) in a fibre which shows dilatation of the sarcoplasmic reticulum but which is otherwise normal. BM: basement membrane; C: collagen fibres; Bar: 0.5 μm. D. Disorganised myofibrils in what is probably an abnormal regenerating fibre. Bar: 0.5 μm

myopathies.

Further to this, a possible role for Ca^{++} ions in initiating hypercontraction and eventual necrosis of the muscle fibre has been suggested by Ebashi and Sugita (1979). In a series of studies on muscle from patients with DMD, they have shown that the earliest sign of degradation of the muscle fibres is a decrease in the regulatory proteins troponin I and C which, together with tropomyosin, regulate the interaction of actin and myosin. This alteration is produced by calcium-activated neutral protease and possibly by serine protease which is also Ca^{++}-activated.

More recent morphological studies suggest that defects in the plasma membrane of the muscle fibre may constitute a portal of entry for an abnormal influx of calcium ions which in turn precipitates over-contraction of the myofibrils. Schmalbruch (1975) and Mokri and Engel (1975) described focal defects in the plasma membrane of muscle fibres from patients with DMD. Mokri and Engel associated these defects with immediately sub-jacent wedge-shaped lesions in the fibres which otherwise appeared to be morphologically normal (Fig. 9.30C). They pointed out that the bases of the wedges or *delta* lesions were in close apposition to the plasmalemmal defects (*see their* Figs. 1–4) and they were able to demonstrate abnormal permeability of the sarcolemma to HRP in these regions, ostensibly via the plasmalemmal defects (*see their* Figs. 5, 6 and 7).

Mokri and Engel considered that the sarcolem-mal defects were unlikely to be artefactual for the following reasons:

1. similar abnormalities could not be found in the plasma membranes of their 'normal' muscle fibres prepared for electron microscopy in pre-cisely the same way;

2. the defects are unlikely to have been produced by contraction during fixation because contraction clumps can be seen in fresh dystrophic muscle viewed with differential interference microscopy (Cullen and Fulthorpe, 1975);

3. the undue permeability of the sarcolemma to HRP in the region of the plasmalemmal defects;[*]

4. the abundant ultrastructural evidence of

muscle fibre degeneration within the delta lesions, such as the presence of autophagic vacuoles, myelin whorls and focal dilatation of the SR;

5. the evident integrity of the plasmalemma overlying contraction clumps in muscle fibres in normal biopsies.

Reasoning from these observations, Mokri and Engel suggested that the membrane defects (and the associated delta lesions) in DMD were early changes and they speculated that these defects may be fundamental to the muscle cell necrosis which is the primary histopathological feature of the disease, a thesis supported more recently by Carpenter and Karpati (1979). Further support for the presence of an abnormality in the plasma membrane in DMD has been furnished by the freeze-fracture studies of Schotland, Bonilla and van Meter (1977). These workers observed an abnormal distribution and depletion of particles on both the P and E faces of the plasmalemma compared with normal control material and they suggested that this indicated a derangement of the internal molecular architecture of the membrane.

In our view the observations discussed above constitute the most important morphological contributions to our understanding of the patho-genesis of DMD in the five years since the last edition of this book appeared. There have been numerous other ultrastructural studies of muscle in DMD but these have been helpful in a negative sense only. Jerusalem, Engel and Gomez (1974a) were unable to find any significant evidence of abnormality in a morphometric study of the motor end-plates and nerve terminals in DMD and concluded that their study provided no support for the 'sick' motor neurone hypothesis (McComas, Sica and Campbell, 1971). Harriman (1976) has reached the same conclusion. Jerusalem, Engel and Gomez (1974b) and Musch, Papapetropoulos, McQueen, Hudgson and Weightman (1975) examined the fine structure of the muscle micro-vasculature in DMD and found no evidence to support the 'ischaemic' hypothesis for the patho-genesis of the disease. More recently Wyatt and Cox (1977) described what they claimed were 'specific' cytoplasmic inclusion bodies in fibro-blast cell lines from patients with DMD, an observation which has not been confirmed by Cullen and Parsons (1977) working in our laborat-

---

[*]This is supported further by the recent observation that the so-called hyaline fibres in DMD are unduly permeable to the dye Procion yellow (Bradley and Fulthorpe, 1978).

ories in Newcastle (they found similar inclusions in cultured fibroblasts derived from patients with DMD and from normal controls).

Myotonic dystrophy (Steinert's disease)

Myotonic dystrophy is now regarded as a multi-system disorder in which the numerous clinical manifestations, involving many tissues and organs, may all be attributable to what is (arguably) a common abnormality of excitable membrane function (Roses and Appel, 1975). Certainly, there is no particular reason to believe that the morphological abnormalities in skeletal muscle as revealed by the light or electron microscopes are likely to help in elucidating the pathogenesis of the condition.

The interest of morphologists seems to have been concentrated on the peripheral nervous system in the recent past. Pollock and Dyck (1976) failed to find any abnormalities in the population of myelinated fibres in the superficial and deep peroneal nerves of patients with myotonic dystrophy. In a morphometric analysis of the fine structure of those nerves, these authors were unable to find any differences between the dystrophic nerves and control material with respect to numbers of myelin lamellae, neurofilaments per unit area and microtubules per unit area of axis cylinder. In contrast, Borenstein, Noël, Jacquy and Flament-Durand (1977) reported a case of myotonic dystrophy accompanied by a hypertrophic neuropathy with typical 'onion bulb' formation, extensive endoneurial fibrosis and paracrystalline inclusions in fibroblast processes. Borenstein and colleagues pointed out that any relationship between the nerve and muscle conditions must be conjectural, although there is increasing physiological evidence for an associated neural defect (McComas, Campbell and Sica, 1971; Panayiotopoulos and Scarpalezos, 1977).

As mentioned in the previous edition, there were a number of accounts in the literature of the ultrastructural pathology of this condition in the late 1960s (Fardeau, Lapresle and Milhaud, 1965; Klinkerfuss, 1967; Samaha, Schröder, Rebeiz and Adams, 1967; Schröder and Adams, 1968). None of the ultrastructural changes described in those papers can be regarded as specific although the composite picture they represent may be characteristic (Schröder and Adams, 1968). Segmental hyaline degeneration was said to be an infrequent finding in spite of the histopathological evidence of numerous contraction clumps in longitudinal muscle sections although there was abundant evidence of myofilamentous and myofibrillar disorientation in the muscle fibres. Sarcoplasmic masses, which can be seen either at the periphery or within some muscle fibres with the light microscope, consist of disarrayed myofilaments with associated nuclei, mitochondria and other organelles (Fardeau et al., 1965; Schröder and Adams, 1968). This type of sub-sarcolemmal change has certain similarities to that seen in some cases of hypothyroid myopathy (Pongratz, Schultz, Koppenwallner and Hübner, 1979; Mastaglia et al., 1980). Circumferentially orientated myofibrils (ring-fibres or ringbinden; Fig. 9.12) may be found either deep to sarcoplasmic masses or beneath the sarcolemma and, in either case, they may represent no more than artefacts of fixation although they can also be seen in rapidly frozen as well as formalin-fixed material. Other changes, such as invagination of nuclear membranes (Johnson and Woolf, 1969), the formation of cytoplasmic 'cysts', the accumulation of lipofuscin and myelin-bodies and splitting of muscle fibres (Schröder and Adams, 1968) are unlikely to be of primary importance.

Electron microscopy has failed to disclose a structural basis for myotonia. Complex infoldings of the sarcolemma are a common finding but are not usually found in 'non-dystrophic' fibres or in myotonia congenita (Samaha et al., 1967) and are also found in a number of non-myotonic conditions (Mussini, Di Mauro and Angelini, 1970). A finding which may be more relevant to the phenomenon of myotonia is dilatation and proliferation of SR tubules (Casanova and Jerusalem, 1979) and the presence of labyrinthine tubular arrays which communicate with the extracellular space in otherwise normal fibres (Schotland, 1970; Mussini et al., 1970).

Electron-microscopic examination of the neuromuscular junctions in myotonic dystrophy has shown elongation of the synaptic region with an increased number of terminal axonic expansions and hyperplasia of secondary synaptic folds

(Allen, Johnson and Woolf, 1969). Certain changes in the end-plate zone have been likened to those resulting from denervation (Allen *et al.*, 1969).

POLYMYOSITIS AND DERMATOMYOSITIS

Electron-microscopic studies have provided information on the ultrastructural changes in muscle in polymyositis and have contributed significantly to our understanding of the pathogenesis of the inflammatory myopathies.

Muscle fibre changes

A variety of degenerative changes have been described in muscle fibres (Shafiq, Milhorat and Gorycki, 1967a, b; Rose, Walton and Pearce, 1967; Mintz, Gonzalez-Angulo, Fraga and Zavala, 1968; Chou, 1967, 1968, 1969; Mastaglia and Walton, 1971b). The most severe of these is the myofibrillar contracture which occurs in entire segments of muscle fibres and which is followed by progressive disruption of the contractile elements and phagocytosis (Fig. 9.26A). Less severe changes include areas of focal myofibrillar disorganisation (Fig. 9.6) which may take the form of *cytoplasmic bodies* (Fig. 9.10) or of targetoid areas (Figs. 9.4 and 9.5) and the formation of myelin-like bodies and autophagic vacuoles. The relationship between these latter changes and the segmental necrosis which appears to be the fundamental lesion both at light- and electron-microscopic levels is uncertain. The mechanism of breakdown of the myofibrillar apparatus in degenerating fibres has been discussed in detail by Cullen and Fulthorpe (1980). The regenerative changes in necrotic muscle fibres have been well documented by a number of authors (Shafiq, Gorycki and Milhorat, 1967; Engel and MacDonald, 1970; Mastaglia and Walton, 1971b).

Blood vessel changes

A number of changes have been described in the small intra-muscular blood vessels in polymyositis and dermatomyositis. These include thickening and reduplication of the basement membrane and swelling of endothelial cells which may contain autophagic vacuoles, multivesicular bodies (Shafiq *et al.*, 1967a; Gonzalez-Angulo, Fraga, Mintz and Zavala, 1968; Norton, 1970; Mastaglia and Currie, 1971) and tuboreticular inclusions within the endoplasmic reticulum (Norton, 1970; Hashimoto, Robinson, Velayos and Niizuma, 1971; Nick, Prunieras, Bakouche, Reignier and Nicolle, 1971; Jerusalem *et al.*, 1974b; Carpenter, Karpati, Rothman and Watters, 1976). Such inclusions are found most characteristically in the childhood form of dermatomyositis (Banker, 1975; Carpenter *et al.*, 1976; Oshima, Becker and Armstrong, 1979). They have also been described in the endothelium of cutaneous blood vessels (Landry and Winkelmann, 1972) and in lymphocytes (Nick *et al.*, 1971) in some cases of dermatomyositis, and identical structures are found in the lymphocytes of some normal subjects (White, 1972) and in endothelial cells in a variety of other conditions (Györkey, Min, Sinkovics and Györkey, 1969; Norton, 1970; Baringer, 1971). The original view that they are viral in nature (Györkey *et al.*, 1969; Hashimoto *et al.*, 1971) is now regarded as unlikely.

Attention has been drawn to the occurrence of capillary necrosis particularly in a form of dermatomyositis which occurs in children and young adults (Jerusalem *et al.*, 1974b; Carpenter *et al.*, 1976) and it has been suggested that the resulting capillary depletion causes progressive ischaemia which is responsible for the muscle fibre damage in this form of dermatomyositis (Carpenter *et al.*, 1976). Immune complex deposition has been demonstrated ultrastructurally in the walls of intramuscular blood vessels in a case of polymyositis associated with Waldenström macroglobulinaemia (Ringel, Thorne, Phanuphak, Lava and Kohler, 1979).

Inflammatory cells

Electron-microscopic observations on the inflammatory cells in the muscle lesions in polymyositis have provided support for the view that a cell-mediated immune mechanism is involved in the pathogenesis of the muscle damage. Mastaglia and Currie (1971) found 'activated', 'transformed' and dividing lymphoid cells among the peri-

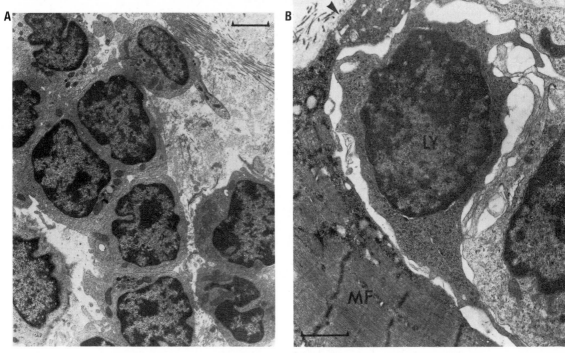

Fig. 9.31 Sub-acute polymyositis. A. Interstitial lymphoid cells. Bar: 2.0 μm. B. Lymphoid cells (LY) which have penetrated the basement membrane (arrowhead) of a muscle fibre (MF). Bar: 1.0 μm

vascular and interstitial inflammatory cells in two cases of polymyositis. They also found cells resembling lymphoid cells situated internal to the basement membrane of some muscle fibres and in some instances actually lying within the fibre, having invaginated the plasma membrane (Fig. 9.31A and B). Similar observations have since been made by Cullen and Fulthorpe (personal communication, 1980). This relationship between lymphoid cells and muscle fibres has also been seen in allogeneic muscle grafts undergoing rejection (Mastaglia, Papadimitriou and Dawkins, 1975). An interesting change found in the region of contact between the lymphoid cell and the muscle fibre is the formation of tubular arrays, probably arising from the T system and identical to the honeycomb arrays found within muscle fibres in a variety of conditions. Whether some form of physical contact between activated lymphoid cells and muscle fibres is integral to the mechanism of cell-mediated myotoxicity or whether muscle fibre damage may be effected at a distance by lymphotoxins liberated from remotely situated lymphoid cells remains to be determined.

'Virus-like' inclusions

Since the original report of myxovirus-like structures in muscle fibres in a case of chronic polymyositis (Chou, 1967; 1968), virus-like inclusions have been described in at least a further 26 cases. In a number of cases of chronic polymyositis, inclusions consisting of 5–7 nm filaments or of filamentous microtubules of variable diameter (8–25 nm) resembling myxo- or paramyxovirus nucleocapsids have been found.[*] In some cases these have been confined to myonuclei or have been present both in nuclei (Fig. 9.32A) and in the sarcoplasm (Fig. 9.32B), while in others inclusions have been found only in the sarcoplasm. Mitochondrial abnormalities and massive accumulations of membranous bodies (*myeloid bodies*) have also been found consistently in such cases. Many such patients have also had other features in

*(Adams, Kakulas and Samaha, 1965; Chou, 1967, 1968; Carpenter, Karpati and Wolfe, 1970; Hudson, Oteruelo and Haust, 1971; Sato, Walker, Peters, Reese and Chou, 1971; Yunis and Samaha, 1971; Jerusalem, Baumgartner and Wyler, 1972; Schochet and McCormick, 1973; Hughes and Esiri, 1978; Oteruelo, 1976; Ketelsen, Beckman, Zimmerman and Sauer, 1977; Carpenter, Karpati, Heller and Eisen, 1978).

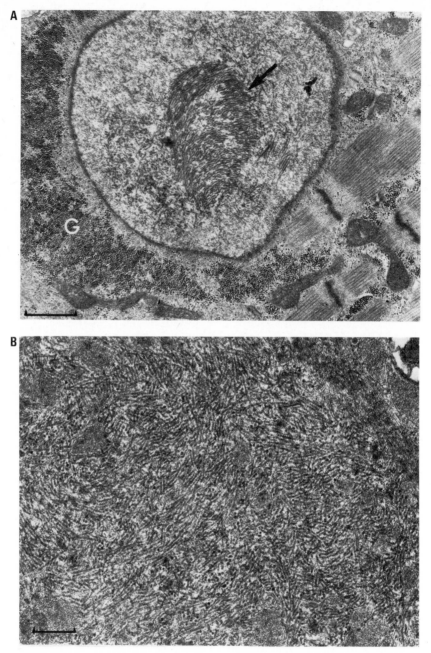

Fig. 9.32 Inclusion body myositis. Intranuclear (arrow) (A) and cytoplasmic (B) aggregates of virus-like filamentous tubules. G: glycogen granules; Bar: (A) 1.0 μm; (B) 0.5 μm

common: a very protracted clinical course; frequent involvement of distal muscle groups; and failure to respond to corticosteroid therapy. The term *inclusion body myositis* has been applied to such cases and it has been suggested that this represents a distinct form of inflammatory myop-

athy (Carpenter *et al.*, 1978).

The nature of the nuclear and sarcoplasmic inclusions in these cases is uncertain. The variable dimensions, sub-structure, and distribution within muscle fibres of the filamentous inclusions suggests that they are probably derived from several different sources. While the possibility remains that, at least in some cases, they are viral in nature, an infective agent has yet to be isolated from any such cases and serological studies have also failed to provide evidence for a myxo- or paramyxovirus infection. On the other hand, if a viral agent is present in muscle in such cases it may not necessarily be in an infective form, and its isolation may require the use of specialised co-cultivation techniques rather than the conventional tissue culture methods used for the isolation of infective viruses.

A second variety of virus-like inclusions has been described in some cases of acute or sub-acute dermatomyositis. These have been confined to the sarcoplasm and have consisted of paracrystalline arrays of 1.5–3 nm particles resembling viruses of the picorna group,* or in one case, of non-crystalline aggregates of 16–24 nm particles resembling viral ribonucleoprotein (Fig. 9.33) (Mastaglia and Walton, 1970). Attempts at viral isolation from muscle have been successful in only one of these cases in which Coxsackie A9 virus was grown (Tang et al., 1975). The finding of identical structures, often without accompanying pathological changes, in malignant hyperpyrexia (Schiller and Mair, 1974), Reye's syndrome (Alvira and Mendoza, 1975; Hanson and Urizar, 1975), idiopathic scoliosis (Webb and Gillespie, 1976) and various other situations (Schmalbruch, 1967; Caulfield, Rebeiz and Adams, 1968) raises the possibility that these structures may not be viral in nature. It has been suggested that paracrystalline arrays of this type may represent one of the forms in which glycogen may be present in muscle fibres. However, Fukuhara (1979) using the cis-platinum (II) technique has shown that they contain nucleic acids and has concluded that they may after all represent an RNA virus.

Cytoplasmic aggregates of larger 87 nm spherical particles of possible viral origin have also been described in muscle fibres in a young woman with rapidly progressive fatal polymyositis (Martinez, Hooshmand, Indolos, Mendoza and Winston,

*(Chou and Gutmann, 1970; Mastaglia and Walton, 1970; Ben-Basset and Machtey, 1972; Sato and Nakamura, 1975; Tang, Sedmak, Siegesmund and McCreadie, 1975; De Reuck, De Coster and Inderadjaja, 1977; Fukuyama, Ando and Yokota, 1977; Györkey, Cabral, Györkey, Uribe-Botero, Dreesman and Melnick, 1978).

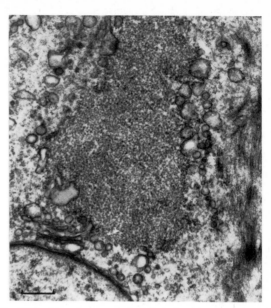

Fig. 9.33 Granular paranuclear inclusion in a regenerating muscle fibre in a case of sub-acute dermatomyositis. Bar: 0.5 μm

1974). Attempts at virus isolation from muscle in this case were also unsuccessful.

The evidence for a viral aetiology in polymyositis and dermatomyositis remains in doubt. Further studies, using not only conventional methods for virus isolation, but also techniques for the identification of viral genome within cells (Jones, Kinross, Maitland and Norval, 1979) and for the isolation of defective or *latent* virus from tissues are required to clarify the role of viruses in the pathogenesis of these diseases.

MYASTHENIC SYNDROMES

There can be few instances in the field of human pathology when it can be said with confidence that the application of new techniques has clarified the nature of a disease process with such precision as in myasthenia gravis. Certainly, it is the only disease in which the pathogenesis of an immunological disease has been elucidated primarily by the use of morphological techniques, and particularly those involving the use of the electron microscope. In view of this, it seems superfluous to do more than review in brief the various descriptions of the ultrastructural pathology of the neuromuscular junction in myasthenia antedating the immunocytochemical studies of Engel's group (*see below*).

Myasthenia gravis

A variety of abnormalities were delineated in purely descriptive studies of myasthenic motor end-plates in the past. These included focal areas of reduced density in the post-synaptic membrane (Zacks, Bauer and Blumberg, 1962), poorly developed junctional folds and secondary synaptic clefts (Zacks *et al.*, 1962; Woolf, 1966; Edwards, 1970; Fardeau and Godet-Guillain, 1970; Bergman, Johns and Afifi, 1971), the presence of dense bodies, myelin-figures and mitochondria of decreased (Edwards, 1970), or increased, density (Woolf, 1966) in nerve terminals, increased (Woolf, 1966), or decreased (Edwards, 1970) numbers of synaptic vesicles, absence of nerve terminals from some post-synaptic areas, and the presence of mycoplasma-like structures between Schwann cells in the synaptic region (Edwards, 1970).

A histometric study of end-plates on intercostal muscles from myasthenic patients (Engel and Santa, 1971; Santa, Engel and Lambert, 1972a) showed a reduction in nerve terminal area and in the area of post-synaptic membrane per nerve terminal, although the density and sizes of synaptic vesicles did not differ significantly from normal. Similar findings have been reported more recently in limb muscles (Tsujihata, Hazama, Ishii, Ide, Mori and Takamori, 1979). Bergman *et al.* (1971) suggested that the primary structural defect in myasthenia gravis may have been incomplete differentiation of the post-synaptic membrane, although the burden of physiological and morphological evidence at the time favoured a pre-synaptic defect (Thesleff, 1966; Lambert and Elmqvist, 1971; McComas, Sica and Brown, 1971; Brownell, Oppenheimer and Spalding, 1972) and any abnormalities observed in the postsynaptic membrane were thought to be secondary to reduced release of acetylcholine from the motor nerve terminals (Engel and Santa, 1971).

The concept of myasthenia gravis as an autoimmune disease was suggested first by Simpson

(1960) and has been supported indirectly by a number of clinicopathological and immunological observations since then, for example the response to immunosuppressive therapy and thymectomy, circulating antimuscle antibodies in high titre in some cases, the presence of 'lymphorrhages' in muscle and germinal centres in the lymph follicles of hyperplastic thymus glands in others. Less circumstantial evidence for an autoimmune pathogenesis has been provided by the demonstration of significantly raised titres of anti-acetylcholine receptor (AChR) immunoglobulin in the sera of approximately 80 per cent of all cases of myasthenia, irrespective of clinical type (Appel, Almon and Levy, 1975). The direct demonstration of structural pathology in the neuromuscular junction consistent with an autoimmune pathogenesis was made possible by the location of the AChR sites to the terminal expansions of the postsynaptic folds using α-bungarotoxin conjugated with horseradish peroxidase, and other techniques of a similar nature (Engel, Lindstrom, Lambert and Lennon, 1977). These techniques enabled Engel and his colleagues to study the progression of the structural lesions affecting the AChR sites in both the human disease and in experimental allergic myasthenia gravis (EAMG)[*] and to show that there were striking similarities between the two. In particular they were able to show morphological abnormalities at the tips of the post-synaptic folds both in myasthenia gravis and EAMG, these degenerating and eventually disappearing to leave a very much simplified subneural apparatus (Fig. 9.34) (Engel, Tsujihata, Lambert, Lindstrom and Lennon, 1976; Engel *et al.*, 1977). Using anti-IgG globulin and anticomplement globulin, these workers were also able to demonstrate that the early stages of the evolution of these lesions were accompanied by the deposition of both IgG and the C3 component of complement on the postsynaptic folds both in myasthenia gravis (Engel, Lambert and Howard, 1977) and in EAMG (Engel, Sakakibara, Sahashi, Lindstrom, Lambert and Lennon, 1979b). This dramatic immunocytochemical evidence at the electron-microscopic level is entirely consistent with the concept that

[*] Induced by immunisation of the experimental animal with AChR protein, Freund's adjuvant and *B. pertussis* organisms.

myasthenia gravis is a classical autoimmune disease, the basic structural lesion being mediated by circulating immunoglobulins.

Eaton-Lambert syndrome

The ultrastructural changes in motor end-plates in the Eaton-Lambert syndrome have been found to be quite distinct from those in myasthenia gravis. The postsynaptic membrane is markedly convoluted (Fukuhara, Takamori, Gutmann and Chou, 1972) with a noticeable increase in the surface area of junctional folds and secondary synaptic clefts per nerve terminal (Engel and Santa, 1971; Santa, Engel and Lambert, 1972b). The numbers and sizes of synaptic vesicles are not significantly abnormal (Santa *et al.*, 1972b). However, the electrophysiological evidence points to a presynaptic defect in acetylcholine release (Lambert and Elmqvist, 1971) and the significance of the postsynaptic changes therefore remains uncertain. Fukuhara *et al.* (1972) also found evidence of demyelination and remyelination of preterminal intramuscular nerves and of degeneration of terminal axons and have suggested that the postsynaptic changes may be secondary to repeated degeneration and regeneration of terminal axons. These workers also found atrophic changes and 'megaconial' mitochondria in some muscle fibres in this condition.

METABOLIC MYOPATHIES

An increasing number of genetically determined or acquired systemic metabolic diseases in which myopathy forms part of the clinical syndrome have been recognised. These included the periodic paralyses and other electrolyte disturbances, the glycogen storage disorders and a number of endocrine disturbances, the most important of which are thyrotoxicosis, hypothyroidism, disturbances of adrenal cortical function, and acromegaly. In addition to these disorders, we have included in this section those myopathies in which there appears to be a primary abnormality of mitochondrial structure and function, or of lipid metabolism in muscle.

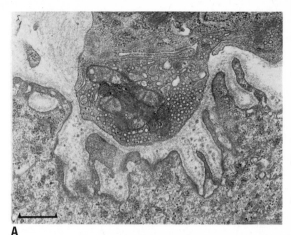

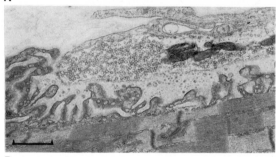

Fig. 9.34 Electron micrographs of motor end-plates in myasthenia gravis (A) and chronic experimental allergic myasthenia (B) showing marked atrophy of the postjunctional folds and widening of the synaptic space. Bar: (A) 0.5 μm; (B) 1.0 μm

Periodic paralysis syndromes

These rare disorders, which are usually familial, are associated with abrupt rises or falls in the serum potassium level (*see* Ch. 18). Hypokalaemic periodic paralysis is also a well-recognised but uncommon complication of thyrotoxicosis, particularly among Orientals, and may be the presenting manifestation of the disorder.

Electron-microscopic studies of muscle have been carried out in the hypokalaemic (Shy, Wanko, Rowley and Engel, 1961; Pearce, 1964; Engel, 1966a; Howes, Price, Pearson and Blumberg, 1966; Odor, Patel and Pearce, 1967; MacDonald *et al.*, 1969), the hyperkalaemic (adynamia episodica hereditaria) and so-called normokalaemic forms (Bradley, 1969), and in the thyrotoxic form of periodic paralysis (Engel, 1966a; Norris, Panner and Stormont, 1968;

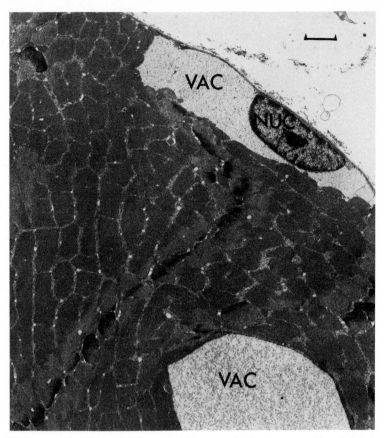

Fig. 9.35 Vacuoles (VAC) containing finely granular material in a muscle fibre in a case of hypokalaemic periodic paralysis. NUC: nucleus; Bar: 2.0 μm

Takagi, Schotland, Di Mauro and Rowland, 1973). The most characteristic ultrastructural change found in muscle fibres in each of these disorders has been a marked dilatation of the sarcotubular system which leads to the formation of the vacuoles (Fig. 9.35) which are seen with the light microscope during paralytic attacks (Pearson, 1964; Ch. 18). This dilatation is thought to arise in the terminal cisternae of the SR (Bradley, 1969) and comparable observations have been made in experimental studies of the effects of chronic hypokalaemia in the rat (Kao and Gordon, 1977; De Coster, 1979). It is known from light-microscopic observations (Pearson, 1964) that the vacuolation of muscle fibres is most striking during attacks of paralysis and that little, if any, abnormality may be seen in biopsies obtained in the interval between attacks. In contrast, dilatation of the SR and other ultrastructural changes may be found even between attacks, although these changes are more marked during an attack, or when weakness becomes established in the later stages of the disease. In one particular study of the hypokalaemic form of periodic paralysis, it was found that the numbers and sizes of vacuoles did not appear to vary appreciably during or between attacks (Gordon, Green and Lagunoff, 1970). That the function of the SR is significantly disturbed during attacks of paralysis is shown by the finding of impaired Ca^{++}-binding and Mg^{++}-ATPase activity in SR membranes from cases of thyrotoxic periodic paralysis (Takagi et al., 1973).

A number of other ultrastructural changes have been prominent in cases of periodic paralysis. These include *tubular aggregates* (*see* p. 308), which have been found in cases of hypo- and hyperkalaemic periodic paralysis (Grüner, 1966; Odor *et al.*, 1967; Engel *et al.*, 1970) and in thyrotoxic periodic paralysis (Bergman *et al.*, 1970). As mentioned previously, these structures appear to be derived from the SR (Schiaffino *et al.*, 1977). Other types of tubular proliferation which probably are also derived from the SR have been described in cases of hypokalaemic periodic paralysis (MacDonald *et al.*, 1969). The presence of apparently increased quantities of glycogen lying free in the sarcoplasm in the sub-sarcolemmal region and between myofibrils has been noted in the hypokalaemic (Howes *et al.*, 1966; Odor *et al.*, 1967), the hyperkalaemic and normokalaemic forms (Bradley, 1969) and in thyrotoxic periodic paralysis (Takagi *et al.*, 1973) and is in accord with the finding of granular PAS-positive material in the sub-sarcolemmal region in some cases (Engel, Potter and Rosevear, 1967; Brody and Dudley, 1969). In some cases this observation was supported by the finding of an increased content of glycogen measured quantitatively (Takagi *et al.*, 1973), whereas in others the glycogen content has been found to be within the normal range (Engel *et al.*, 1967).

Weller and McArdle (1971) have drawn attention to the finding of a characteristic type of basophilic granular degeneration in muscle fibres in various types of periodic paralysis, which they consider to be caused by the deposition of calcium salts (in a form resembling hydroxyapatite crystals) in association with acid mucopolysaccharide. They postulate that this intracellular deposition of calcium salts occurs initially in the SR, but have also found evidence of calcium deposition in the extracellular space.

Glycogen storage disease

Children with skeletal muscle glycogenosis usually present with infantile hypotonia, and adult patients with glycogen storage disease presenting exclusively or predominantly with myopathy are rare. In the relatively few cases of this kind reported to date, a number of different deficiencies of enzymes of the glycolytic pathway have been reported. These have included muscle phosphorylase (Engel, Eyerman and Williams, 1963), acid maltase (α-1,4-glucosidase) (Courtecuisse, Royer, Habib, Monnier and Demos, 1965; Zellweger, Brown, McCormick and Tu, 1965; Cardiff, 1966;

Smith, Amick and Sidbury, 1966; Isch, Juif Sacrez and Thiebaut, 1966; Hudgson, Gardner-Medwin, Worsfold, Pennington and Walton, 1968; Engel, 1970; Martin, De Barsy, Van Hoof and Palladini, 1973; Hudgson and Fulthorpe, 1975; Martin, De Barsy, De Schrijver, Leroy and Palladini, 1976; Schlenska, Heene, Spalke and Seiler, 1976; Karpati, Carpenter, Eisen, Aube and Di Mauro, 1977), amylo-1,6-glucosidase (Oliner, Schulman and Larner, 1961; Murase, Ikeda, Muro, Nakao and Sugita, 1973), and possibly phosphoglucomutase (Thomson, MacLaurin and Prineas, 1963). In addition, a number of familial cases have been reported in which the disorder presented with symptoms indistinguishable from those due to muscle phosphorylase deficiency and in which there were no demonstrable clinical abnormalities at rest. In two families the symptoms were shown to be due to phosphofructokinase deficiency (Tarui, Okuno, Ikura, Tanaka and Suda, 1965; Layzer, Rowland and Ranney, 1967) and in one to a disturbance of hexosephosphate isomerase activity (Satoyoshi and Kowa, 1967).

The light-microscopic changes found in muscle obtained at biopsy in these patients have been essentially similar: a vacuolar myopathy of greater or lesser severity, with accumulation of glycogen granules within the vacuoles, particularly in those lying immediately under the sarcolemma. Electron-microscopic studies have been performed in a number of these conditions. In the case of acid maltase deficiency, Hudgson *et al.*, (1968) and Engel (1970) emphasised the sequestration of glycogen within vacuoles lined by a unit membrane, believing this to be a hallmark of a lysosomal storage disorder (Figs. 9.36A and B). They also described vacuoles containing osmiophilic material and complex lipid structures, regarding these as autophagic vacuoles or secondary lysosomes, their contents being the degradation products of phospholipid membranes within the muscle cell. Engel (1970) classified the deposits of glycogen within the muscle according to the abnormal spaces in which they were stored, calling these Types 1–4 on the basis of their ultrastructural appearance :-

Type 1 spaces. These are sarcoplasmic/ intermyofibrillar deposits of glycogen which displace other subcellular organelles and which appear to occupy whole segments of affected fibres in some areas. The facile explanation for these deposits has been the rupture of overdistended 'lysosomes' and Hudgson and Fulthorpe (1975) adduced some ultrastructural evidence in support of this (*see below*). However, it has to be conceded that the majority of the glycogen appears to be sarcoplasmic in location in both the infantile and late-onset forms of acid maltase deficiency and this led Cardiff (1966) to question its status as a single-enzyme defect disease.

Type 2 spaces. Engel (1970) defined these as smooth-contoured sacs lined by continuous unit or double membranes and containing only glycogen (Figs. 9.36A and B). Many of these were quite small (<0.5 μm in diameter) and, in some instances, appeared to be the only abnormality in the muscle cell. Hudgson and Fulthorpe (1975) were able to demonstrate these structures within a satellite cell.

Type 3 spaces. Engel (1970) and Hudgson and Fulthorpe (1975) all described numerous autophagic vacuoles in material from infantile and adult cases (Type 3 spaces). These contained a variety of structures including small, dense osmiophilic bodies, lipid droplets and complex membranous structures (Fig. 9.36C). Using Barka's* technique (1964), Engel was able to demonstrate acid phosphatase activity within these spaces in material from three of his cases, supporting the concept that these structures were lysosomal in nature. In contrast, he found no evidence of acid phosphatase activity within the Type 2 spaces or on their membranes, concluding that they may have been abnormal lysosomes deficient in acid hydrolases.

Type 4 spaces. Engel defined these as transitional regions in which admixtures of two or more of the other categories could be seen.

Essentially similar abnormalities to those described above have been reported in a series of subsequent reports on cases of acid maltase deficiency by Martin *et al.* (1973, 1976), Schlenska *et al.* (1976) and Karpati *et al.* (1977). In addition,

*J. Histochem. Cytochem., 12, 229, 1964.

Martin *et al.* (1973) adduced histological and ultrastructural evidence of glycogen storage within the central and peripheral nervous systems in their infantile case, and Karpati *et al.* (1977) found electrophysiological and histochemical abnormalities suggesting denervation in material from their case, an adult male. Interestingly, Askanas, Engel, Di Mauro, Brooks and Mehler (1976) were able to demonstrate identical changes in muscle growth in tissue cultures established from the biopsy.

In McArdle's disease, glycogen accumulates mainly in the sub-sarcolemmal region (Fig. 9.36D) (Korenyi-Both, Smith and Baruah, 1977) and in debrancher enzyme deficiency in the intermyofibrillar spaces (Murase *et al.*, 1973; Di Mauro, Hartwig, Hays, Eastwood, Franco, Olarte, Chang, Roses, Fetell, Schoenfeldt and Stern, 1979).

In addition to these 'cardinal' ultrastructural features, Engel and Dale (1968), Hudgson *et al.* (1968), Engel (1970) and Hudgson and Fulthorpe (1975) all reported increased numbers of lipid droplets within the muscle fibres from their patients with adult acid maltase deficiency. Hudgson and Fulthorpe were impressed particularly by the numbers of lipid droplets in the material from their infantile cases and speculated that this may have been due to increased mobilisation of fat stores because of impaired glycogen breakdown. Certainly, hyperlipidaemia is well recognised in other forms of glycogenosis (Types I, III and VI), possibly because of the chronic hypoglycaemia associated with these conditions (Jakovics, Khachadurian and Hsia, 1966) and this mechanism was suggested as a causal factor for the lipid storage myopathy developing in Type I glycogenosis (von Gierke's disease) (Yamaguchi, Santa, Inove and Omae, 1978a). In this context it is also of interest that mixed glycogen and lipid storage in the presence of structurally abnormal mitochondria has been reported in a child with an improving congenital myopathy (Jerusalem, Angelini, Engel and Groover, 1973), and in glycogen storage disease associated with structurally and functionally abnormal mitochondria in a patient with progressive external ophthalmoplegia (Di Mauro, Schotland, Bonilla, Lee, Gambetti and Rowland, 1973).

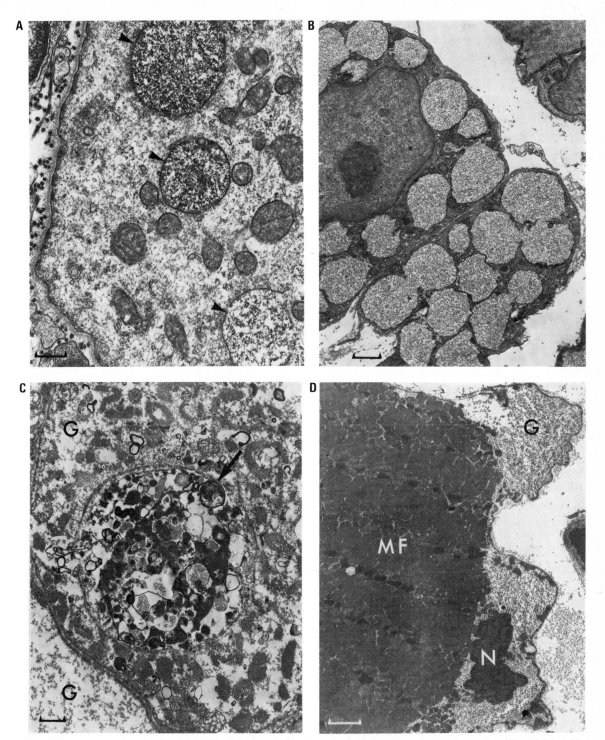

Fig. 9.36 Glycogen storage disease. A. Membrane-bound aggregates of glycogen (arrowheads) in a muscle fibre. Adult acid-maltase deficiency. Bar: 0.5 μm. B. Large membrane-bound collections of glycogen in two interstitial cells. Infantile acid-maltase deficiency (Pompe's disease). Bar: 1.0 μm. C. Autophagic vacuole (arrow) containing sequestered glycogen and other granular and membranous debris in a muscle fibre in which there is also excessive accumulation of free glycogen (G) in the sarcoplasm (some of which has been lost during preparation of the section) leading to separation of the myofibrils. Adult acid maltase deficiency. Bar: 1.0 μm. D. Sub-sarcolemmal and perinuclear accumulation of glycogen (G) in a case of McArdle's disease. N: nucleus; MF: myofibrils; Bar: 2.0 μm

Engel and Dale (1968) described a coiled inclusion in one muscle fibre in their case of late-onset adult muscular dystrophy and Engel (1970) found giant mitochondria with crystalloid inclusions in one of his four cases. Hudgson and Fulthorpe (1975) and Korenyi-Both *et al.* (1977) described concentrically lamellated inclusions in material from patients with the adult form of acid maltase deficiency and McArdle's disease respectively. The former authors likened these to the inclusions in the muscle fibres of patients with abnormal carbohydrate tolerance, described by Fisher, Gonzalez, Khurana and Danowski (1972), and of a patient with mucopolysaccharidosis (Afifi, der Kaloustian, Bahuth and Mire-Salman, 1974a).

Myopathies associated with abnormalities of oxidative metabolism

The next group of myopathies we wish to deal with in this section are those in which there appears to be a primary abnormality in oxidative metabolism. The first patient in whom such an abnormality was defined was a 35-year-old woman who showed severe hypermetabolism which was manifestly not due to thyroid overactivity (Ernster, Ikkos and Luft, 1959; Luft, Ikkos, Palmieri, Ernster and Afzelius, 1962; Ernster and Luft, 1963). Histological examination of a biopsy specimen from sartorius muscle showed absence of the sub-sarcolemmal myofibrils in up to 50 per cent of the muscle fibres and occasional sub-sarcolemmal aggregations of PAS-positive granules. Quantitative assay of mitochondrial function in this muscle showed loose 'coupling' of oxidative phosphorylation and this condition is now known as Luft's disease. Ernster and Luft (1963) first suggested that patients with this condition had two sub-populations of mitochondria, one consisting of normal-sized organelles and the other of enlarged ones, each having defective respiratory control. The recent electron-cytochemical studies of Bonilla, Schotland, Di Mauro and Lee (1977) support this concept.

The first description of structurally abnormal mitochondria in muscle disease *per se* appeared in 1966 when Shy, Gonatas and Perez described two types of abnormal mitochondria in two children suffering from congenital myopathies, one of which they termed 'megaconial myopathy' and the other 'pleoconial myopathy'. In the first the mitochondria were grossly enlarged, bizarre in appearance and contained large, often crystalline inclusions of various shapes. In the second there was a significant increase in the population of mitochondria which contained numerous cristae which were, in some instances, arranged in concentric circles instead of interdigitating in the normal manner. Some of these mitochondria also contained round, densely staining osmiophilic inclusions. No other definite abnormalities were found in this material. Interestingly the clinical features in the patient with pleoconial myopathy and in one of his sibs clinically resembled those of the cases of sodium chloride-responsive familial periodic paralysis described by Poskanzer and Kerr (1961). A similar clinical presentation with salt craving and periodic attacks was described by Spiro, Prineas and Moore (1970) and their patient had both 'megaconial' and 'pleoconial' mitochondrial abnormalities in biopsy muscle. Subsequently, Price, Gordon, Munsat and Pearson (1967) reported the presence of structurally abnormal mitochondria in a young adult male who complained of undue fatigability on exertion, and Coleman, Nienhuis, Brown, Munsat and Pearson (1967) described abnormal accumulation of neutral fat and unusually large mitochondria with very high oxidative enzyme activities in histochemical studies of muscle from the case studied by Price and his colleagues, and from another similar one.

Van Wijngaarden and co-workers (1967) found large, bizarre mitochondria in large numbers, particularly beneath the sarcolemma, in muscle from a 15-year-old boy who had suffered from a gradually progressive proximal myopathy, without salt craving or paralytic attacks, since the age of 4 years. Biochemical examination showed that oxidative phosphorylation was only loosely coupled in this case.

Since then there have been many reports of 'abnormal' mitochondria in a variety of clinical situations and the pattern of ultrastructural changes seems to be remarkably uniform in these. Indeed, Shafiq, Milhorat and Gorycki (1967b) described 'pleoconial' and 'megaconial' abnormalities in muscle from patients with polymyositis and denervation atrophy, and Fardeau (1970), who found 'abnormal' mitochondria in myotonic dystrophy, warned against regarding them as pathognomonic of anything! Nonetheless, Kamieniecka (1976) was able to identify several clinical syndromes which were associated consistently with mitochondrial abnormalities in a review of 17 cases drawn from 135 consecutive patients with 'myopathy' studied in Copenhagen. Local experience and a review of the recent literature is in agreement with this and, as a consequence, we suggest the following scheme for the clinical patterns associated with structurally abnormal mitochondria:

1. non-thyroidal hypermetabolism with or without myopathy (loosely coupled oxidative phosphorylation);

2. facioscapulohumeral myopathy with associated cardiomyopathy, lactate acidaemia, diabetes mellitus, cerebral degeneration (Alpers' syndrome) in some cases;

3. myopathy with paralytic attacks provoked by exercise, cold or ethanol ingestion (cytochrome b deficiency) (Morgan-Hughes, Darveniza, Kahn, Landon, Sherratt, Land and Clark, 1977) or exercise intolerance and fluctuating lactic acidaemia with a defect in the NADH-coenzyme Q reductase complex (Morgan-Hughes, Darveniza, Landon, Land and Clark, 1979);

4. progressive external ophthalmoplegia with or without limb-girdle myopathy, bulbar paresis, retinal pigmentation and cerebellar degeneration (Kearns-Sayre syndrome).

It has to be emphasised that there is considerable overlap between these clinical syndromes, and precise correlations between the metabolic errors demonstrated so far and the numerous clinical syndromes listed above is difficult, if not impossible. In view of this, it is perhaps not surprising that the ultrastructural abnormalities seen in muscle in the 'mitochondrial' myopathies are stereotyped, albeit spectacular. In addition, similar changes can be induced in the experimental animal by the *in vivo* uncoupling of oxidative phosphorylation (Melmed, Karpati and Carpenter, 1975).

The ultrastructural abnormalities seen in skeletal muscle in these conditions can be summarised as follows:

1. an increase in the population of mitochondria;

2. the presence of giant and/or bizarre forms, for example mitochondria with concentric as opposed to interdigitating cristae;

3. the presence of mitochondrial inclusions of various kinds, particularly paracrystalline or crystalline bodies which are related intimately to the cristae;

4. an increase in the number of lipid droplets and sometimes glycogen granules (occasionally within mitochondria) in muscle fibres.

These changes are illustrated in Figs. 9.16A–D.

Disorders of lipid metabolism

In the last decade it has become clear that there is a group of 'storage' disorders affecting muscle in which neutral lipid accumulates within the muscle fibre, in most cases as a result of defective transport of free fatty acids (FFA) across the mitochondrial membrane to participate in β-oxidation. There appear to be two modes of presentation, one with a relapsing and remitting myopathy and the second with exercise-induced muscle cramps, sometimes accompanied by myoglobinuria (*cf* disorders of glycolytic metabolism in muscle). In the first instance, the patients usually present in early adult life with clinical features not unlike those of polymyositis (Bradley, Hudgson, Gardner-Medwin and Walton, 1969; Engel and Siekert, 1972) and they may even show a partial response to treatment with corticosteroids (Engel and Siekert, 1972; Johnson, Fulthorpe and Hudgson, 1973). Engel and Angelini (1973) demonstrated deficiency of carnitine, a base with which FFAs combine before crossing the mitochondrial membrane, in one of their cases and this observation has been confirmed in a number of other cases with similar clinical presentations; it has also been shown that this defect may be restricted to muscle or it may be generalised, in some instances being associated with a fatal cardiomyopathy (*see* Ch. 18).

In patients with carnitine deficiency, enzyme histochemistry will demonstrate a gross increase in the population of lipid droplets, particularly in the type I fibres, an abnormality paralleled by the ultrastructural appearance of these fibres

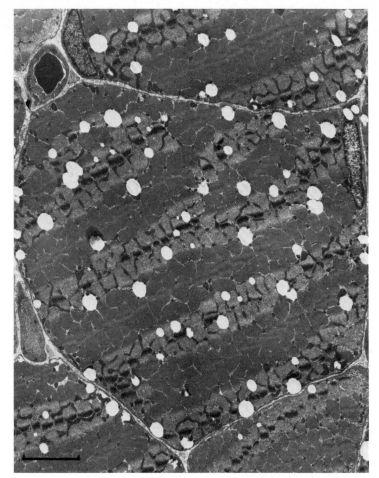

Fig. 9.37   Increased numbers of lipid droplets in muscle fibres in a case of carnitine deficiency. Bar: 5.0 μm

(Fig. 9.37). In addition, the sub-sarcolemmal mitochondrial aggregates are usually larger than normal and the individual organelles may contain inclusions. In general terms, however, their appearance is less bizarre than in the 'mitochondrial' myopathies.

Deficiency of the transferase enzyme systems, notably CPT, responsible for transporting the acyl-carnitine complex across the mitochondrial membrane, may also lead to lipid accumulation within the muscle fibre and causes recurrent episodes of exertional muscle pain, cramps and myoglobinuria. In these patients, lipid storage may be demonstrable only while the patient has symptoms, the abnormal accumulations disappearing after a period of rest (Cumming, Hardy, Hudgson and Walls, 1976).

Myopathies associated with hyperthyroidism and hypothyroidism

Hyperthyroidism. The few electron-microscopic studies of muscle from patients with thyrotoxicosis have shown only relatively minor changes and have not contributed significantly to our understanding of the mechanism of muscle dysfunction in such patients. In a study of biopsy material from two cases of thyrotoxic myopathy Engel (1966) found prominent papillary projections from the sarcolemma of muscle fibres, large sub-sarcolemmal accumulations of glycogen in some fibres, focal dilatations of transverse tubules, and degenerative changes in mitochondria, but no abnormality of the contractile elements. He suggested that the last two changes may have been relevant to the pathogenesis of thyrotoxic myopathy, the mitochondrial abnormalities suggesting the possibility of a disturbance of oxidative metabolism, and the T-tubule changes a possible disturbance of electrical excitation of muscle fibres. Similar changes were found by Gruener, Stern, Payne and Hannapel (1975) who also noted atrophy of both type I and type II fibres.

In thyrotoxic periodic paralysis, glycogen accumulation and distension of the lateral sacs of the SR have been described both during and between attacks of paralysis (Engel, 1966; Bergman et al., 1970; Takagi et al., 1973).

Hypothyroidism. There have been few ultrastructural studies of muscle in patients with hypothyroid myopathy. In general, the changes found have been more striking than those in thyrotoxic myopathy. Norris and Panner (1966) found focal areas of mitochondrial disorganisation, paracrystalline and other types of mitochondrial inclusion, and excessive amounts of glycogen in an adult with a hypertrophic myopathy associated with severe myxoedema. They also noted occasional necrotic fibres but commented that the majority of muscle fibres showed no ultrastructural abnormality. The electron-microscopic findings in the hypertrophic form of myopathy associated with congenital hypothyroidism (Kocher-Debré-Sémélaigne syndrome) have been described in a number of cases (Spiro, Hirano, Beilin and Finkelstein, 1970; Afifi, Najjar, Mire-Salman and Bergman, 1974b). Spiro et al. (1970) found focal accumulations of glycogen, distension of the SR, and sub-sarcolemmal areas devoid of myofibrils and other organelles in one patient. Afifi et al. (1974a) in a study of 10 such children, found very variable ultrastructural changes and commented upon dilatation of the SR, sub-sarcolemmal crescents which in some cases were very large, focal areas of myofibrillar disruption, ring fibres, and the presence of honeycomb-like tubular arrays which were striking in some cases. In a study of a patient with an atrophic form of hypothyroid myopathy, Godet-Guillain and Fardeau (1970) also commented upon the frequency of inclusions and other structural changes in mitochondria, the presence of focal areas of myofibrillar damage which were at times associated with autophagic vacuole formation, dilatation and proliferation of the SR, and abnormal sub-sarcolemmal areas filled with disorganised filaments (sarcoplasmic masses) and often associated with annular myofibrils. They commented upon the similarity of these changes to those found in myotonic dystrophy.

We have confirmed the above observations in a study of four cases of hypothyroid myopathy (Mastaglia et al., 1980). Degenerative changes in mitochondria, and the presence of small myeloid bodies in muscle fibres and in endothelial cells, were the most frequent findings. In addition, in two cases core-like areas of variable size, which were devoid of enzyme activity in histochemical preparations, were prominent and were found to contain finely granular material which bore a superficial resemblance to glycogen but showed unusual staining properties (Fig. 9.38). Mitochondria contained unduly prominent calcific granules (Fig. 9.17) and, in some instances, paracrystalline inclusions.

The ultrastructural findings therefore suggest that the principal effects of prolonged hypothyroidism are on mitochondria and on carbohydrate metabolism, with the accumulation of glycogen and possibly of some abnormal form of polysaccharide. These findings are in accord with experimental studies which have shown defective oxidative phosphorylation, with changes in mitochondrial morphology and numbers, in thyroidectomised animals (Gustafsson, Tata, Lindberg and Ernster, 1965; Meijer, 1972), and with the impairment of glycogenolysis which has been reported in patients with hypothyroid myopathy (Hurwitz, McCormick and Allen, 1970; McDaniel, Pittman, Oh and Di Mauro, 1977).

Myopathies associated with disturbances of ACTH and adrenal corticosteroid metabolism

Proximal muscle weakness is commonly found in cases of both Cushing's syndrome and Addison's disease and is a relatively common finding in patients on long-term corticosteroid therapy, particularly with the fluorinated steroids (see Ch. 25). There have been few studies of the ultrastructural changes in muscle in such cases (Pearce,

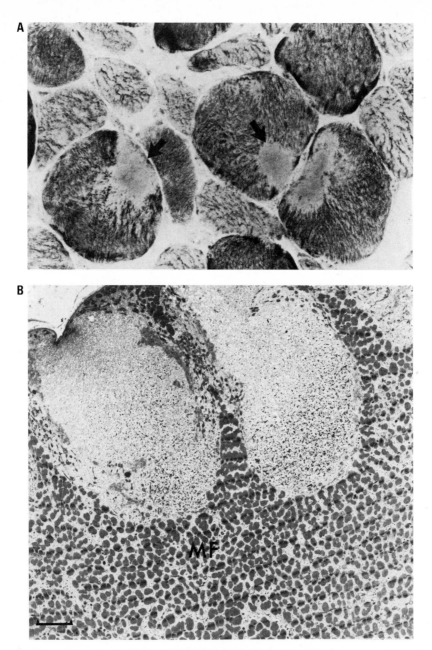

Fig. 9.38   Hypothyroid myopathy. A. Eccentric core-like areas (arrows) are present in three muscle fibres. Succinic dehydrogenase preparation. X400. B. Electron micrograph of core-like areas showing that they consist of finely granular material with varying staining properties. Similar material separates the myofibrils (MF). Bar: 5.0 μm

1964; Engel, 1966; Afifi, Bergman and Harvey, 1968). These have not shown any specific changes and have not contributed materially to our understanding of the pathogenesis of the muscle dysfunction. Focal accumulations of mitochondria and vacuolation and degeneration of these organelles

has been noted in some cases (Pearce, 1964; Engel, 1966) but it is not clear to what extent these changes were artefactual. Enlargement of muscle mitochondria and similar changes to those found in some of the human cases have also been found in experimental steroid myopathy in the rat and in the rabbit (D'Agostino and Chiga, 1966; Ritter, 1967; Afifi and Bergman, 1969; Freund-Mölbert, Ketelsen and Beckmann, 1973).

Other changes which have been described in the human and experimental myopathy include an increase in intermyofibrillar sarcoplasm, an apparent increase in glycogen (Pearce, 1964; D'Agostino and Chiga, 1966; Ritter, 1967), and neutral lipid droplets (D'Agostino and Chiga, 1966; Harriman and Reed, 1972; Freund-Mölbert et al., 1973) and thickening of the basement membrane of muscle fibres (Afifi et al., 1968; Mastaglia et al., 1970b. The accumulation of glycogen is in accord with the finding of increased glycogen synthetase activity in muscle in experimental steroid myopathy (Shoji, Takagi, Sugita and Toyokura, 1974). Necrosis and calcification of muscle fibres has been found in some of the short-term high-dose experimental animal studies (Afifi and Bergman, 1969; Freund-Mölbert et al., 1973) but is not a feature of human steroid myopathy.

The question of the differential involvement of the type II (glycolytic) fibres in human steroid myopathy and of fast-twitch (white) muscles in animals has not been adequately explored in ultrastructural studies.

It is also appropriate to include in this section a reference to the myopathy which develops in patients who have undergone bilateral adrenalectomy for Cushing's syndrome (Prineas, Hall, Barwick and Watson, 1968). A proportion of such patients develop very high serum ACTH levels with generalised skin pigmentation (Nelson's syndrome) and, subsequently, proximal limb muscle weakness. The presence of myopathy was confirmed in these patients electromyographically and Prineas and his colleagues showed histochemically and electron-microscopically that the type I fibres contained excessive amounts of neutral lipid droplets, which were almost exclusively situated beneath the sarcolemma, usually in association with sentinel mitochondria.

CONGENITAL MYOPATHIES

The difficulties encountered in the clinical classification of this heterogeneous group of disorders are discussed in detail in Chapter 17. Unfortunately, the ultrastructural study of biopsy material from 'floppy' infants and other patients with congenital myopathies has not contributed as much as was expected to the clarification of their nosology. However electron-microscopic studies have provided the morphological substrate for the provisional designation of a number of pathological entities since the mid-1950s, although some of their supposedly 'characteristic' structural abnormalities are not entirely specific. Notwithstanding, some of these have stood the test of time and will be discussed in detail below. In addition, brief accounts will be given of the numerous descriptions of single cases of families in which infantile hypotonia or congenital myopathy has been associated with unusual ultrastructural findings in muscle. These disorders will be discussed under the following headings:

1. abnormalities of the contractile apparatus;
2. abnormalities of other sarcoplasmic organelles;
3. myopathies with intracellular inclusions of various types.

Abnormalities of the contractile apparatus

The first account of a congenital myopathy with a 'specific' pathological basis was given by Shy and Magee (1956) in their description of central core disease, a benign condition usually presenting with infantile hypotonia and with a family history suggesting autosomal dominant inheritance. In this disorder, the type I muscle fibres in particular contain cores in which there are variable degrees of disruption of the normal myofibrillar architecture, the cores being termed 'structured' or 'unstructured', depending upon the degree of abnormality (Neville, 1973). In the most severely affected fibres, the cores contain no normal cytoplasmic organelles such as SR or mitochondria. Absence of the latter is reflected in the failure of the appropriate histochemical stains to demonstrate any evidence of oxidative enzyme activity within the cores (Dubowitz and Pearse, 1960; Engel et al., 1961). Since then a number of variations on the original description have been reported. Afifi, Smith and Zellweger (1965) described two members of a family in which central cores were demonstrated in biopsy specimens, but in which foci of Z band degeneration resembling that seen in nemaline myopathy were also found. Engel et al. (1971) described congenital myopathies characterised by the presence of multiple and/or miniature cores (multi- and mini-core disease respectively). In addition Radu, Rosu-Serbu, Ionescu and Radu (1977) described two cases in which the muscle fibres contained structured, unstructured and 'reversed' cores, the latter containing central agglomerations of mitochondria.

Loss of the normal ultrastructure of the contractile elements and reduction in the mitochondrial population occurs also in target and targetoid fibres (Figs. 9.3–9.5). These are seen most often in denervated fibres, and focal lesions of a similar nature have been described in patients with progressive congenital muscle weakness (Van Wijngaarden, Bethlem, Dingemans, Cöers, Telerman-Toppet and Gerard, 1977; Yarom and Shapira, 1977). This curious abnormality is accompanied by type I fibre predominance, the individual fibres being significantly reduced in diameter. The pathogenetic basis for this condition is unknown, although Van Wijngaarden and colleagues suggested that delayed development of motor nerves may have been involved on the basis of abnormalities demonstrated by supravital staining of the motor end-plates. Van Wijngaarden and colleagues (1977), in a comprehensive review of the literature, considered that several other reported cases were either identical or very similar to their own.

The next disease 'entity' to be described was *nemaline myopathy*, first reported by Conen, Murphy and Donohue (1963) under the name 'myogranular' myopathy. Subsequently, sporadic cases or families with members suffering from the disease were described by Shy et al. (1963), Engel, Wanko and Fenichel (1964), Spiro and Kennedy (1964), Price, Gordon, Pearson, Munsat and Blumberg (1965), Gonatas (1966), Gonatas, Shy and Godfrey (1966), Engel and Gomez (1967), Hudgson et al. (1967) and Shafiq, Dubowitz, Peterson and Milhorat (1967). Autopsy confirmation of the widespread distribution of nemaline rods in a patient with adult-onset symptoms diagnosed on biopsy in life has recently been provided by Brownell, Gilbert, Shaw, Garcia, Wenkeback and Lam (1978). Bender and Willner (1978), in a histochemical study of a biopsy specimen of muscle obtained from the mother of a patient with myopathy who was diagnosed on ultrastructural grounds as having nemaline myopathy, found abnormalities closely resembling those seen in the child's biopsy although the mother's muscle contained no rod bodies. They suggested that this established her status as the gene carrier.

Nemaline myopathy is characterised pathologically by the presence of tiny rod-like bodies (up to 5 μm in length and 1.5 μm in diameter) which lie within the muscle fibre; most of these bodies are concentrated in aggregates at the poles of the muscle nuclei. At the light-microscopic level these 'rod' bodies are usually brilliantly refractile with phase-contrast and interference illumination (Gonatas, 1966; Hudgson et al., 1967) and stain intensely with the modified Gomori trichrome, picro-Mallory and PTAH stains. Ultrastructurally the rod bodies are electron-dense and the larger ones correspond roughly in size to those seen in light-microscopic sections (Fig. 9.8). These larger bodies may occupy up to two sarcomeres' length of the affected fibres and, as in the light-microscopic sections, appear to be concentrated near the poles of the muscle nuclei. Moving away from the nuclei, the bodies steadily decrease in number and it becomes increasingly obvious that they are intimately related to the Z bands (Fig. 9.9A). The smallest ones, in fact, appear to be mere bulbous expansions of the Z bands (Fig. 9.9A and B).

In many illustrations, the rods appear to be 'cross-hatched' due to the presence of transverse and axial striae (Fig. 9.9B). In various reports the transverse striae have had a periodicity of approximately 14.5 nm and the axial ones a periodicity ranging from 12–18 nm. The measurements quoted by Price et al. (1965) differed significantly from those in most other descriptions of the disease, and led them to propose that the rod bodies might be composed of an altered form of tropomyosin B. Engel and Gomez (1967) found that the periodicity of the striae in the rod bodies in their material did not correspond with that of the crystal lattice of Z bands. On the basis of experiments involving glycerination of the biopsy and extraction of the filaments with Guba-Straub-ATP solution, followed by treatment of the residue with Szent-Györgyi's actin-extracting solution, they suggested that the rods might contain actin, tropomyosin B, a combination of the two, or another protein with solubility properties common to both. However, the most recent evidence available suggests that the rods are composed of α-actinin on a skeleton of actin (Ebashi, 1967; Yamaguchi et al., 1978b).

As we have pointed out in other sections of this Chapter, many so-called specific ultrastructural anomalies, previously identified with discrete clinical syndromes, can occur in a variety of naturally occurring and experimental myopathies. This is certainly the case with nemaline-like degeneration in the Z bands, which can be produced by experimental denervation or tenotomy in animals (Engel, Brooke and Nelson, 1966). Fardeau (1970) has described a similar change in myotonic dystrophy; Cape, Johnson and Pitner (1970) found rod bodies in material from a patient with polymyositis and we have seen them in various other disorders including muscular dystrophy, mitochondrial myopathy, the myopathy associated with chronic renal failure, and in spinal muscular atrophy and glycogen storage disease (Hudgson and Fulthorpe, 1975). However, we believe that rod-body formation is still the most important single structural abnormality in some congenital myopathies, particularly those associated with dysmorphogenetic states such as Marfan's syndrome (Hudgson et al., 1967).

The last entity to be considered in this section is the 'new' congenital neuromuscular disease with trilaminar fibres described recently by Ringel, Neville, Duster and Carroll (1978). In what was clearly an unusual clinical situation, the authors described an infant who was born with a marked increase in muscle tone, paucity of spontaneous movements and increased serum creatine kinase (CK) activity. Biopsy of muscle at the age of 7 weeks demonstrated numerous 'trilaminar' fibres containing three concentric zones (see their Figs 2 and 3). Electron microscopy revealed that the central zone contained densely packed mitochondria, glycogen, electron-dense material and single myofilaments, the middle zone consisted of de-

ranged myofibrils showing Z band streaming, and the outer zone resembled a sarcoplasmic mass (see their Figs 4–7). Appropriate cytochemical techniques demonstrated extrajunctional AChR between the middle and outer zones in the trilaminar fibres. The authors considered that this finding, together with the child's rigidity, was in keeping with abnormal neural influences of some kind. It is, however, a little difficult to reconcile this with the grossly elevated serum CK levels (2240 iu/l at birth and 2290 at 14 days) and the gross disruption of the cyto-architecture of the muscle fibres.

Abnormalities of other sarcoplasmic organelles

The first condition to be described under this heading was myotubular myopathy (Spiro, Shy and Gonatas, 1966), now better known as centronuclear myopathy (Sher, Rimalovski, Athanassiades and Aronson, 1967). There are now approximately 50 cases recorded in the literature, although Palmucci, Bertolotto, Monga, Ardizzone and Schiffer (1978) have questioned the validity of some of these cases, pointing out that the mere presence of internal nuclei in fibres otherwise resembling myotubes is not sufficient to justify the diagnosis. Nevertheless, there does appear to be a substantial measure of agreement about the histochemical and ultrastructural characteristics of the disease.

In this condition, which appears to be genetically determined (with variable mode of inheritance) and slowly progressive, the majority of the muscle fibres (up to 85 per cent in the cases described by Spiro and colleagues) resemble fetal muscle fibres, being of small diameter and containing central nuclei. Histochemical studies (Sher et al., 1967; Kinoshita and Cadman, 1968) have shown that oxidative enzyme activity may be either increased or decreased in the central region of the fibres, and that myofibrillar adenosine triphosphatase activity is usually absent centrally (Sher et al., 1967). Electron-microscopic studies (Spiro et al., 1966; Sher et al., 1967; Kinoshita and Cadman, 1968) have demonstrated that, in addition to the presence of central nuclei, the central region of the fibres is usually devoid of myofibrils. Sher and her co-workers also found a small number (less than 1 per cent) of centrally situated mitochondria which were vacuolated and contained myelin whorls. In contrast, Campbell, Rebeiz and Walton (1969) found large numbers of similarly placed mitochondria in material from a case of myotubular myopathy studied in this department.

The aetiology and pathogenesis of this condition is unknown, although Spiro and associates (1966) suggested that it may develop as a result of 'maturation arrest' because of the structural resemblances between the myopathic fibres and those seen in fetal skeletal muscle. In 1969, Bethlem, Van Wijngaarden, Meijer and Hülsmann suggested a neurogenic basis for the condition in their discussion of the fourth reported case and, more recently, Serratrice, Pellissier, Faugere and Gastaut (1978) supported this suggestion. They considered that their histochemical evidence particularly favoured a neurogenic aetiology, their material showing a type I fibre preponderance and atrophy. The authors likened the latter feature to the appearance of type I fibre hypotrophy with internal nuclei (Engel, Gold and Karpati, 1968) in which a neurogenic basis has also been suggested. In this context, it may also be relevant that De Reuck, Hooft, De Coster, Van den Bossche and Cuvelier (1977) described type I fibre atrophy particularly in respiratory muscles in a child with severe neonatal respiratory distress. They considered that a neurogenic basis for the muscle disorder was the most attractive of the possible hypotheses. However, Palmucci et al. (1978) claimed that centronuclear myopathy is likely to be a histopathological syndrome produced by several unrelated disease entities, a suggestion mooted previously by Bradley, Price and Watanabe (1970).

In 1973, Jerusalem, Engel and Gomez described a new, benign congenital disorder in two brothers born of a consanguineous marriage. They called this condition *sarcotubular myopathy* and reported that it was characterised histopathologically by microvacuolar degeneration affecting the type II more than the type I fibres (*see their* Figs 3 and 4), and which was segmental in distribution in longitudinal sections. Electron micrographs of the affected fibres showed that they contained rows of membrane-bound spaces, some of which were coalescing and some were in close relationship to tubular profiles (*see their* Fig. 7). Appropriate electron-cytochemical techniques showed that the vacuoles probably originated from the SR rather than the T system. The authors concluded that segmental vacuolation of the SR with selective affection of type II fibres was the characteristic morphological abnormality and they differentiated this from the non-specific dilatation of the SR which occurs in many necrobiotic myopathies and in the periodic paralyses.

Myopathies with intracellular inclusions

The presence of inclusion bodies of various kinds within mitochondria in patients with mitochondrial myopathy and other conditions has already been discussed. In this section, we propose to consider a number of congenital myopathies with inclusions in other compartments of the muscle cell.

Jenis, Lindquist and Lister (1969) described a fatal congenital myopathy in which they were able to demonstrate eosinophilic crystalline inclusions within the myonuclei, with similar smaller bodies within the sarcoplasm and arising from the Z bands of the muscle fibres. Multiple passage of material from this case through suckling mice and rhesus monkey and human embryonal kidney in tissue culture failed to adduce any evidence of viral infection, but electron microscopy of the intranuclear and sarcoplasmic inclusions indicated that they possessed a crystal lattice not unlike that of nemaline rods (*see their* Fig. 7 particularly). The authors were unable to reach any definite conclusions about the fundamental nature of this condition and particularly about its relationship to other congenital myopathies including nemaline disease. As far as we are aware, no similar case has been described subsequently.

Brooke and Neville (1972) reported two unrelated cases of a progressive congenital myopathy which also had a fatal termination. In each case, light microscopy of biopsy muscles revealed scattered sub-sarcolemmal inclusions which were eosinophilic with haematoxylin and eosin, and red in the modified trichrome preparation. Further histochemical studies demonstrated that the bodies contained both RNA and sulphydryl groups in high concentration, the latter observation prompting the authors to call them 'reducing bodies'. Electron microscopy showed that these bodies were densely eosinophilic, porous structures up to about 10 μm in length. They were not membrane-bound, contained beaded fibrillar material in places and the pores often contained glycogen (see their Figs 13 and 10). Speculating on the possible origin of these structures, the authors considered the possibility that they were derived from an RNA virus. They noted, in addition, that the presence of sulphydryl groups in high concentration in skeletal muscle is most unusual, although the sulphydryl-containing amino acid, homocysteine, is produced during the transmethylation of guanidoacetate to creatine.

As far as we know, no other cases of this kind have been reported, although Sahgal and Sahgal (1977) described a non-progressive congenital myopathy characterised by the presence of subsarcolemmal inclusions reacting strongly for sulphydryl groups, particularly in type I fibres. However, these inclusions contained granular and filamentous material only at the ultrastructural level and did not resemble the 'reducing bodies' of Brooke and Neville (1972) in any other respect.

At about the same time as the description of reducing-body myopathy appeared, Engel et al. (1972) described another curious inclusion in a child with non-progressive weakness since infancy. These inclusions were observed first by phase-contrast microscopy of semithin Epon sections, and were described as being oval or irregularly circular in shape, invariably subsarcolemmal in situation, often near the muscle nuclei and from 7–10 μm in length. Ultrastructurally they were composed of complex, convoluted lamellae arranged in 'fingerprint' patterns (see their Fig. 5). In each inclusion the lamellae were spaced 30 nm apart and were studded with sawtooth-like projections 6.5 nm wide and 16 nm high, with a period varying from 14.5–16 nm. Predigestion of the muscle with RNase and amylase, disruption of the membranous components of the muscle fibres by glycerination and selective extraction of the myosin and actin filaments, M bands and Z bands did not alter the appearance of these structures. 'Finger-print' inclusions have been reported in several other cases of congenital myopathy (Fardeau, Tomé and

Derambure, 1976), dystrophia myotonica (Tomé and Fardeau, 1973) and oculopharyngeal dystrophy (Julien et al., 1974). In addition, we have seen a similar structure in material from a patient with uraemic myopathy (Fig. 9.22A).

More recently, Fardeau's group (1978) reported a family with a genetically determined myopathy (autosomal dominant inheritance) with affection of skeletal, pharyngeal and respiratory musculature, cardiomyopathy and lens opacities. The biopsies from affected members of the family revealed what the authors described as 'rubbing out' of the intermyofibrillar network in the type I fibres, electron microscopy showing that this was associated with the deposition of electron-dense granular and filamentous material in the sarcoplasm of the fibres. In some areas, this material was arranged in a meshwork around the myofibrils, although it did not appear to have any structural relationship with the Z band or indeed with any of the other components of the contractile apparatus.

The final condition cited in this section is the recently reported myofibrillar inclusion-body myopathy or cytoplasmic-body neuromyopathy presenting with respiratory insufficiency and weight loss (Clark et al., 1978; Jerusalem et al., 1979). In this condition the type I fibres contain numerous typical cytoplasmic bodies (Jerusalem et al., 1979—see their Fig. 4). The nature of this condition remains obscure, although some cases are familial with an autosomal dominant form of inheritance.

CONCLUSIONS

Although the electron-microscopic examination of diseased muscle has made a number of positive contributions to our understanding of the pathogenesis of muscle diseases, it has become increasingly apparent that the extent of this contribution is limited and that electron microscopy on its own will not provide the answer to certain fundamental problems. Certainly, the electron microscope will not provide a solution to the aetiology of Duchenne dystrophy, much less to that of any of those diseases where the fundamental defect lies outside the muscle cell, even with the technical sophistication conferred by such innovations as electron-probe and X-ray diffraction analysis.

Notwithstanding the point made in previous editions, that the morphological study of suitably prepared biopsy specimens of muscle from patients with certain muscle diseases (such as nemaline myopathy) can point the way to a rational approach by the biochemist and the molecular biologist, the major contributions are likely to continue to come from the combined use of electon microscopy with other available techniques, for example phase-contrast optics, histochemistry, quantitative biochemical techniques and immunocytochemistry.

ACKNOWLEDGEMENTS

The work discussed above was carried out with the aid of grants from the Medical Research Council, the Muscular Dystrophy Associations of America, Inc. and the Muscular Dystrophy Group of Great Britain. We wish to acknowledge the invaluable technical assistance of Miss M. Jenkison and Mr J. Fulthorpe and the advice and criticism of many colleagues, especially Professor Sir John Walton and Dr Michael Cullen who kindly provided some of the illustrations. We are indebted to the Elsevier Publishing Co. for permission to reproduce Fig. 9.10B, 9.16B and C, 9.19, 9.22C and D, 9.29B and 9.33 from the *Journal of the Neurological Sciences.* Dr A.G. Engel kindly provided Figs. 9.34A and B and permission to reproduce these was granted by the New York Academy of Sciences to whom we wish to express our thanks.

The manuscript for this Chapter was typed by Mrs I. Gibbs and Mrs C.K. Wood whose continued loyalty and efficient services are greatly appreciated. We are also very grateful to Dr Margaret J. Hudgson who compiled and checked the references.

REFERENCES

Adams, R.D., Denny-Brown, D. & Pearson, C.M. (1962) *Diseases of Muscle: A Study in Pathology*, 2nd Edn. (New York: Hoeber).

Adams, R.D., Kakulas, B.A. & Samaha, F.J. (1965) A myopathy with intracellular inclusions. *Transactions of the American Neurological Association*, **90**, 213.

Afifi, A.K. & Bergman, R.A. (1969) Steroid myopathy. A study of the evolution of the muscle lesion in rabbits. *Johns Hopkins Medical Journal*, **124**, 66.

Afifi, A.K., Bergman, R.A. & Harvey, J.C. (1968) Steroid myopathy. Clinical, histologic and cytologic observations. *Johns Hopkins Medical Journal*, **123**, 158.

Afifi, A.K., Smith, J.W. & Zellweger, H. (1965) Congenital non-progressive myopathy. Central core disease and nemaline myopathy in one family. *Neurology (Minneapolis)*, **15**, 371.

Afifi, A.K., der Kaloustian, V.M., Bahuth, W.B. & Mire-Salman, J. (1974a) Concentrically-laminated membranous inclusions in myofibres of Dyggve-Melchior-Clausen Syndrome. *Journal of the Neurological Sciences*, **21**, 335.

Afifi, A.K., Najjar, S.S., Mire-Salman, J. & Bergman, R.A. (1974b) The myopathology of the Kocher-Debré-Sémélaigne syndrome. *Journal of the Neurological Sciences*, **22**, 445.

D'Agostino, A.N. & Chiga, M. (1966). Corticosteroid myopathy in rabbits: A light and electron microscopic study. *Neurology (Minneapolis)*, **16**, 257

Allen, D.E., Johnson, A.G. & Woolf, A.L. (1969). The intramuscular nerve endings in dystrophia myotonica–a biopsy study by vital staining and electron microscopy. *Journal of Anatomy*, **105**, 1.

Alvira, M.M. & Mendoza, M. (1975) Reye's syndrome: A viral myopathy? *New England Journal of Medicine*, **292**, 1297.

Appel, S.H., Almon, R.R. & Levy, N. (1975) Acetylcholine receptor antibodies in myasthenia gravis. *New England Journal of Medicine*, **293**, 760.

Askanas, V., Engel, W.K., Di Mauro, S., Brooks, B.R. & Mehler, M. (1976) Adult onset acid maltase deficiency. *New England Journal of Medicine*, **294**, 573.

Banker, B.Q. (1975) Dermatomyositis of childhood. Ultrastructural observations of muscle and intramuscular blood vessels. *Journal of Neuropathology and Experimental Neurology*, **34**, 46.

Baringer, J.R. (1971) Tubular aggregates in endoplasmic reticulum in herpes-simplex encephalitis. *New England Journal of Medicine*, **285**, 943.

Ben-Bassat, M. & Machtey, I. (1972) Picornavirus-like structures in acute dermatomyositis. *American Journal of Clinical Pathology*, **58**, 245.

Bender, A.N. & Engel, W.K. (1976) Light-cored dense particles in mitochondria of a patient with skeletal muscle and myocardial disease. *Journal of Neuropathology and Experimental Neurology*, **35**, 46.

Bender, A.N. & Willner, J.P. (1978). Nemaline (rod) myopathy: the need for histochemical evaluation of affected familes. *Annals of Neurology*, **4**, 37.

Bergman, R.A., Johns, R.T. & Afifi, A.K. (1971) Ultrastructural alterations in muscle from patients with myasthenia gravis and Eaton-Lambert syndrome. *Annals of the New York Academy of Sciences*, **183**, 88.

Bergman, R.A., Afifi, A.K., Dunkle, L.M. & Johns, R.T. (1970). Muscle pathology in hypokalaemic periodic paralysis with hyperthyroidism. *Annals of the New York Academy of Sciences*, **126**, 100.

Bethlem, J., Arts, W.F. & Dingemans, K.F. (1978) Common origin of rods, cores, miniature cores and focal loss of cross-striations. *Archives of Neurology*, **35**, 555.

Bethlem, J. Van Wijngaarden, G.K. & De Jong, J. (1973) The incidence of lobulated fibres in the FSH type of muscular dystrophy and the limb-girdle syndrome. *Journal of the Neurological Sciences*, **18**, 351.

Bethlem, J., van Wijngaarden, G.K., Meijer, A.E.F.H. & Hülsmann, W.C. (1969) Neuromuscular disease with type I fiber atrophy, central nuclei and myotube-like structures. *Neurology (Minneapolis)*, **19**, 705.

Bodensteiner, J.B. & Engel, A.G. (1978) Intracellular calcium accumulation in Duchenne dystrophy and other myopathies: A study of 567,000 muscle fibers in 114 biopsies. *Neurology (Minneapolis)*, **28**, 439.

Bonilla, E.,Schotland, D.L., Di Mauro, S. & Lee, C.-P. (1977) Luft's disease: An electron cytochemical study. *Journal of Ultrastructure Research*, **58**, 1.

Borenstein, S., Noël, P., Jacquy, J. & Flament-Durand, J. (1977) Myotonic dystrophy with nerve hypertrophy. *Journal of the Neurological Sciences*, **34**, 87.

Bradley, W.G. (1969) Ultrastructural changes in adynamia episodica hereditaria and normokalaemic familial periodic paralysis. *Brain*, **92**, 379.

Bradley, W.G. (1980) The limb-girdle syndromes. In *Handbook of Clinical Neurology*. Vol. 40, Eds P.J. Vinken & G.W. Bruyn (Elsevier/North-Holland: Amsterdam).

Bradley, W.G. & Fulthorpe, J.J. (1978). Studies of sarcolemmal integrity in myopathic muscle. *Neurology (Minneapolis)*, **28**, 670.

Bradley, W.G., Price, D.L. & Watanabe, C.K. (1970) Familial centronuclear myopathy. *Journal of Neurology, Neurosurgery and Psychiatry*, **33**, 687.

Bradley, W.G., Hudgson, P., Gardner-Medwin, D. & Walton, J.N. (1969) Myopathy with abnormal lipid metabolism in skeletal muscle. *Lancet*, **1**, 495.

Brody, I.A. & Dudley, A.W. (1969) Thyrotoxic hypokalemic periodic paralysis. Muscle morphology and functional assay of sarcoplasmic reticulum. *Archives of Neurology*, **21**, 1.

Brooke, M.H. & Neville, H.E. (1972) Reducing body myopathy. *Neurology (Minneapolis)*, **22**, 829.

Brownell, A.K.W., Gilbert, J.J., Shaw, D.T., Garcia, B., Wenkeback, G.F. & Lam, A.K.S. (1978) Adult onset nemaline myopathy. *Neurology (Minneapolis)*, **28**, 1306.

Brownell, B., Oppenheimer, D.R. & Spalding, J.M.K. (1972) Neurogenic muscle atrophy in myasthenia gravis *Journal of Neurology, Neurosurgery and Psychiatry*, **35**, 311.

Busch, W.A., Stromer, M.H., Goll, D.E. & Suzuki, A. (1972) Ca²⁺-specific removal of Z lines from rabbit skeletal muscle. *Journal of Cell Biology*, **52**, 367.

Campbell, M., Rebeiz, J.J. & Walton, J.N. (1969) Myotubular, centronuclear or pericentrinuclear myopathy? *Journal of the Neurological Sciences*, **8**, 425.

Cape, C.A., Johnson, W.M. & Pitner, S.E. (1970) Nemaline structures in polymyositis. *Neurology (Minneapolis)*, **20**, 494.

Cardiff, D.R. (1966) A histochemical and electron microscopic study of skeletal muscle in a case of Pompe's disease (glycogenosis II). *Pediatrics*, **37**, 249.

Carpenter, S. & Karpati, G. (1979) Duchenne muscular dystrophy. Plasma membrane loss initiates muscle cell necrosis unless it is repaired. *Brain*, **102**, 147.

Carpenter, S., Karpati, G. & Wolfe, L. (1970) Virus-like filaments and phospholipid accumulation in skeletal muscle. *Neurology (Minneapolis)*, **20**, 889.

Carpenter, S., Karpati, G., Heller, I. & Eisen, A. (1978) Inclusion body myositis: A distinct variety of idiopathic inflammatory myopathy. *Neurology (Minneaplis)* **28**, 78.

Carpenter, S., Karpati, G., Rothman, S. & Watters, G. (1976) The childhood type of dermatomyositis. *Neurology (Minneapolis)*, **26**, 952.

Casanova, G. & Jerusalem, F. (1979) Myopathology of myotonic dystrophy. *Acta Neuropathologica (Berlin)*, **45**, 231.

Caulfield, J.B., Rebeiz. J.J. & Adams, R.D. (1968) Viral involvement of human muscle. *Journal of Pathology and Bacteriology*, **96**, 232.

Chou, S.M. (1967) Myxovirus-like structures in a case of human chronic polymyositis. *Science*, **158**, 1453.

Chou, S.M. (1968) Myxovirus-like structures and accompanying nuclear changes in chronic polymyositis. *Archives of Pathology*, **86**, 649.

Chou, S.M. (1969) 'Megaconial' mitochondria in a case of chronic polymyositis. *Acta neuropathologica (Berlin)*, **12**, 68.

Chou, S.M. & Gutmann, L. (1970). Picornavirus-like crystals in subacute polymyositis. *Neurology (Minneapolis)*, **20**, 205.

Chou, S.M. & Nonaka, I. (1977) Satellite cells and muscle regeneration in diseased human skeletal muscles. *Journal of the Neurological Sciences*, **34**, 131.

Clark, J.R., D'Agostino, A.N., Wilson, J., Brooks, R.R. & Cole, G.C. (1978) Autosomal dominant myofibrillar inclusion body myopathy–clinical, histologic, histochemical and ultrastructural characteristics. *Neurology (Minneapolis)* **28**, 399.

Coleman, R.F., Nienhuis, A.W., Brown, W.J., Munsat, T.L. & Pearson, C.M. (1967) New myopathy with mitochondrial enzyme hyperactivity. *Journal of the American Medical Association*, **199**, 624.

Conen, P.E., Murphy, E.G. & Donohue, W.L. (1963) Light and electron microscopic studies of 'myogranules' in a child with hypotonia and weakness. *Canadian Medical Association Journal*, **89**, 983.

Courtecuisse, V., Royer, P., Habib, R., Monnier, C. & Demos, J. (1965) Glycogenose musculaire par deficit d'alpha-1,4-glucosidase simulant une dystrophie musculaire progressive. *Archives françaises de pediatrie*, **22**, 1153.

Cullen, M.J. & Fulthorpe, J.J. (1975) Stages in fibre breakdown in Duchenne muscular dystrophy. *Journal of the Neurological Sciences*, **24**, 179.

Cullen, M.J. & Fulthorpe, J.J. (1980) Z and I band loss and A band phagocytosis in polymyositis (submitted for publication).

Cullen, M.J. & Parsons, R. (1977) Inclusion bodies in muscular dystrophy. *Lancet*, **2**, 929.

Cullen, M.J. & Pluskal, M.J. (1977) Early changes in the ultrastructure of denervated rat skeletal muscle. *Experimental Neurology*, **56**, 115.

Cullen, M.J. & Weightman, D. (1975) The ultrastructure of normal human muscle in relation to fibre type. *Journal of the Neurological Sciences*, **25**, 43.

Cullen, M.J., Appleyard, S.T. & Bindoff, L. (1978) Morphologic aspects of muscle breakdown and lysosomal activation. *Annals of the New York Academy of Sciences*, **317**, 440.

Cumming, W.J.K., Hardy, M., Hudgson, P. & Walls, J. (1976) Carnitine palmityl transferase deficiency. *Journal of the Neurological Sciences*, **30**, 347.

Dastur, D.K., Gagrat, B.M. & Manghani, D.K. (1979) Fine structure of muscle in human disuse atrophy: Significance of proximal muscle involvement in muscle disorders. *Neuropathology and Applied Neurobiology*, **5**, 85.

De Coster, W.J.P. (1979) Experimental hypokalaemia: ultrastructural changes in rat gastrocnemius muscle. *Archives of Neurology*, **45**, 79.

De Reuck, J., De Coster, W. & Inderadjaja, N. (1977) Acute viral polymyositis with predominant diaphragm involvement. *Journal of the Neurological Sciences*, **33**, 453.

De Reuck, J., Hooft, C., De Coster W., Van den Bossche, H. & Cuvelier, C. (1977) A progressive congenital myopathy. *European Neurology*, **15**, 217.

Di Mauro, S., Schotland, D.L., Bonilla, E., Lee, C.-P., Gambetti, P. & Rowland, L.P. (1973) Progressive ophthalmoplegia, glycogen storage and abnormal mitochondria. *Archives of Neurology*, **29**, 170.

Di Mauro S., Hartwig, G.B., Hays, A., Eastwood, A.B., Franco, R., Olarte, M., Chang, M., Roses, A.D., Fetell, M., Schoenfeldt, R.S. & Stern, L.Z. (1979) Debrancher deficiency: Neuromuscular disorder in 5 adults. *Annals of Neurology*, **5**, 422.

Dobkin, B.H. & Verity, M.A. (1978) Familial neuromuscular disease with type 1 fiber hypoplasia, tubular aggregates, cardiomyopathy and myasthenic features. *Neurology (Minneapolis)*, **28**, 1135.

Dubowitz, V. & Brooke, M.H. (1973) *Muscle Biopsy: A Modern Approach* (W.B. Saunders: London).

Dubowitz, V. & Pearse, A.G.E. (1960) Oxidative enzymes and phosphorylase in central core disease of muscle. *Lancet*, **2**, 23.

Ebashi, S. (1967) Quoted by C.M. Pearson. In: Skeletal muscle. Basic and clinical aspects and illustrative new diseases. *Annals of Internal Medicine*, **67**, 614.

Ebashi, S. & Sugita, H. (1979) The role of calcium in physiological and pathological process of skeletal muscle. In *Current Topics in Nerve and Muscle Research*, Eds A.J. Aguayo & G. Karpati, pp. 73–84 (Excerpta Medica: Amsterdam).

Edwards, W. (1970) Ultrastructural changes in human motor endplate in myasthenia gravis. (Abst.) *Proceedings of the Sixth International Congress of Neuropathology*, Paris, p. 751.

Engel, A.G. (1966) Thyrotoxic and corticosteroid-induced myopathies. *Mayo Clinic Proceedings*, **41**, 785.

Engel, A.G. (1970) Acid maltase deficiency in adult life. *Brain*, **93**, 599.

Engel, A.G. & Angelini, C. (1973) Carnitine deficiency of human skeletal muscle with associated lipid storage. *Science*, **179**, 899.

Engel, A.G. & Dale, A.J.D. (1968) Autophagic glycogenosis of late onset with mitochondrial abnormalities; Light and electron microscopic observations. *Mayo Clinic Proceedings*, **43**, 233.

Engel, A.G. Gomez, M.R. (1967) Nemaline (Z disc) myopathy: Observations of the origin, structure and solubility properties of the nemaline structures. *Journal of Neuropathology and Experimental Neurology*, **26**, 601.

Engel, A.G. & MacDonald, R.D. (1970) Ultrastructural reactions in muscle disease and their light-microscopic correlates. In *Muscle Diseases*, Eds J.N. Walton, N. Canal & G. Scarlato (Excerpta Medica: Amsterdam).

Engel, A.G. & Santa, T. (1971) Histometric analysis of the ultrastructure of the neuromuscular junction in myasthenia gravis and the myasthenic syndrome. *Annals of the New York Academy of Sciences*, **183**, 46.

Engel, A.G. & Siekert, R.G. (1972) Lipid storage myopathy responsive to prednisone. *Archives of Neurology*, **27**, 174.

Engel, A.G., Angelini, C. & Gomez, M.R. (1972) Fingerprint body myopathy. *Mayo Clinic Proceedings*, **47**, 377.

Engel, A.G., Gomez, M.R. & Groover, R.V. (1971) Multicore disease: A recently recognized congenital myopathy associated with multifocal degeneration of muscle fibres. *Mayo Clinic Proceedings*, **46**, 666.

Engel, A.G., Lambert, E.H. & Howard, F.M. (1977) Immune complexes (IgG and C3) at the motor end-plate in myasthenia gravis. *Mayo Clinic Proceedings*, **52**, 267.

Engel, A.G., Potter, C.S. & Rosevear, J.W. (1967) Studies on carbohydrate metabolism and mitochondrial respiratory activities in primary hypokalemic periodic paralysis. *Neurology (Minneapolis)*, **17**, 329.

Engel, A.G., Lindstrom, J.M., Lambert, E.H. & Lennon, V.A. (1977). Ultrastructural localisation of acetylcholine receptors in myasthenia gravis and in its experimental auto-immune model. *Neurology (Minneapolis)*, **27**, 307.

Engel, A.G., Tsujihata, M., Lambert, E.H., Lindstrom, J.M. & Lennon, V.A. (1976) Experimental autoimmune myasthenia gravis. *Journal of Neuropathology and Experimental Neurology*, **35**, 569.

Engel, A.G., Sakakibara, H., Sahashi, K., Lindstrom, J., Lambert, E.H. & Lennon, V.A. (1979b). Passively transferred experimental autoimmune myasthenia gravis. *Neurology (Minneapolis)*, **29**, 179.

Engel, A.G., Santa, T., Stonnington, H.H., Jerusalem, F., Tsujihata, M., Brownell, A.K.W., Sakakibara, H., Banker, B.Q., Sahashi, K. & Lambert, E.H. (1979a). Morphometric study of skeletal muscle ultrastructure. *Muscle and Nerve*, **2**, 229.

Engel, W.K., Bishop, D.W. & Cunningham, G.G. (1970). Tubular aggregates in Type II muscle fibres: Ultrastructural and histochemical correlation. *Journal of Ultrastructure Research*, **31**, 507.

Engel, W.K., Brooke, M.H. & Nelson, P.G. (1966). Histochemical studies of denervated or tenotomized muscle. *Annals of the New York Academy of Sciences*, **138**, 160.

Engel, W.K., Eyerman, E.L. & Williams, H.E. (1963) Late onset type of skeletal muscle phosphorylase deficiency: A new familial variety with completely and partly affected subjects. *New England Journal of Medicine*, **268**, 135.

Engel, W.K., Gold, N. & Karpati, G. (1968) Type I fiber hypotrophy and central nuclei. *Archives of Neurology*, **18**, 435.

Engel, W.K., Wanko, T. and Fenichel, G.M. (1964) Nemaline myopathy: A second case. *Archives of Neurology*, **11**, 22.

Engel, W.K., Foster, J.B., Hughes, B.P., Huxley, H.E. & Mahler, R. (1961) Central core disease: An investigation of a rare muscle cell abnormality. *Brain*, **84**, 167.

Ernster, L. & Luft, R. (1963) Further studies on a population of human skeletal muscle mitochondria lacking respiratory control. *Experimental Cell Research*, **32**, 26.

Ernster, L., Ikkos, D. & Luft, R. (1959) Enzymic activities of human skeletal muscle mitochondria: A tool in clinical metabolic research. *Nature*, **184**, 1851.

Fardeau, M. (1970) Ultrastructural lesions in progressive muscular dystrophies. A critical study of their specificity. In *Muscle Diseases*, Proceedings of an International Congress (Excerpta Medica: Amsterdam).

Fardeau, M. & Godet-Guillain, J. (1970). Étude ultrastructurale des plaques motrices due muscle squelettique et de leurs modifications pathologiques. (Abst.). *Proceedings of the Sixth International Congress of Neuropathology*, Paris, p. 746.

Fardeau, M., Lapresle, J. & Milhaud, E. (1965) Contribution a l'étude des lesions elementaires du muscle squelettique: Ultrastructure des masses sarcoplasmiques laterales (observées dans un cas de dystrophie myotonique). *Comptes rendus des séances de la Société de biologie et des filiales*, **159**, 15.

Fardeau, M., Tomé, F.M.S. & Derambure, S. (1976) Familial fingerprint body myopathy. *Archives of Neurology*, **33**, 724.

Fardeau, M., Godet-Guillain, J., Tomé, F.M.S., Collin, H., Gaudeau, S., Boffety, Cl.L. & Vernant, P. (1978) Une nouvelle affection musculaire. *Revue neurologique*, **131**, 411.

Fisher, E.R., Gonzalez, A.R., Khurana, R.C. & Danowski, T.S. (1972) Unique, concentrically laminated, membranous, inclusions in myofibers. *American Journal of Clinical Pathology*, **48**, 239.

Freund-Mölbert, E., Ketelsen, U.-P. & Beckmann, R. (1973) Ultrastructural study of experimental steroid myopathy. In *Basic Research in Myology* Ed. B.A. Kakulas, pp. 595–604 (Excerpta Medica: Amsterdam).

Fukuhara, N. (1979) Electron microscopical demonstration of nucleic acids in virus-like particles in the skeletal muscle of a traffic accident victim. *Acta neuropathologica (Berlin)*, **47**, 55.

Fukuhara, N., Takamori, M., Gutmann, L. & Chou, S.M. (1972) Eaton-Lambert syndrome. Ultrastructural study of the motor end-plates. *Archives of Neurology*, **27**, 67.

Fukuyama, Y., Ando, J.T. & Yokota, J. (1977) Acute fulminant myoglobinuric polymyositis with picornavirus-like crystals. *Journal of Neurology, Neurosurgery and Psychiatry*, **40**, 755.

Fulthorpe, J.J. (1979) Experimental allergic myositis. M. Phil. Thesis, Sunderland Polytechnic, UK.

Godet-Guillain, J. & Fardeau, M. (1970) Hypothyroid myopathy. Histological and ultrastructural study of an atrophic form. In: *Muscle Diseases*, Eds J.N. Walton, N. Canal & G. Scarlato, pp. 512–513 (Excerpta Medica: Amsterdam).

Goebel, H.H., Muller, J., Gillen, H.W. & Merritt, A.D. (1978). Autosomal dominant 'spheroid body' myopathy. *Muscle and Nerve*, **1**, 14.

Goldspink, D. (1972) Postembryonic growth and differentiation of striated muscle. In: *Structure and Function of Muscle*, Vol. 1. G.H. Bourne, p. 179, (Academic Press: New York and London).

Gonatas, N.K. (1966) The fine structure of the rod-like bodies in nemaline myopathy and their relation to the Z discs. *Journal of Neuropathology and Experimental Neurology*, **25**, 409.

Gontas, N.K., Sky, G.M. & Godfrey, E.H. (1966). The origin of nemaline structures. *New England Journal of Medicine*, **274**, 535.

Gonyea, W., Ericson, G.L. & Bonde-Petersen, F. (1977) Skeletal muscle fiber splitting induced by weight-lifting exercise in cats. *Acta physiologica Scandinavica*, **99**, 105.

Gonzalez-Angulo, A., Fraga, A., Mintz, G. & Zavala, B. (1968) Sub-microscopic alterations in capillaries of skeletal muscles in polymyositis. *American Journal of Medicine*, **45**, 873.

Gordon, A.M., Green, J.R. & Lagunoff, D. (1970). Studies on a patient with hypokalaemic familial periodic paralysis. *American Journal of Medicine*, **48**, 185.

Gruener, R., Stern, L.Z., Payne, C. & Hannepel, L. (1975) Hyperthyroid myopathy. *Journal of the Neurological Sciences*, **24**, 339.

Grüner, J.E. (1966) Anomalies du réticulum sarcoplasmique et prolifération des tubules dans le muscle d'une paralysie périodique familiale. *Comptes rendus des séances de la Société de biologie et des filiales*, **26**, 555.

Györkey, F., Min, F.-W., Sinkovics, J.G. & Györkey, P. (1969) Systemic lupus erythematosus and myxovirus. *New England Journal of Medicine*, **280**, 333.

Györkey, F., Labral, G.A., Györkey, P., Uribe-Botero, G., Dressman, G.-R. and Melnick, J.L. (1978). Coxsackie virus aggregates in muscle cells of a polymyositis patient. *Intervirology*, **10**, 69.

Hall-Craggs, E.C.B. (1972) The significance of longitudinal fibre division in skeletal muscle. *Journal of the Neurological Sciences*, **15**, 27.

Hanson, P.A. & Urizar, R.E. (1975) Reye's syndrome–virus or artifact in muscle *New England Journal of Medicine*, **293**, 505.

Harriman, D.G.F. (1976) A comparison of the fine structure of motor end-plates in Duchenne dystrophy and human neurogenic diseases. *Journal of the Neurological Sciences*, **28**, 233.

Harriman, D.G.F. & Reed, R. (1972) The incidence of lipid droplets in human skeletal muscle in neuromuscular disorders. *Journal of Pathology*, **106**, 1.

Hashimoto, K., Robinson, L., Velayos, E. & Niizuma, K. (1971) Dermatomyositis. Electron microscopic, immunological, and tissue culture studies of paramyxovirus-like inclusions. *Archives of Dermatology*, **103**, 120.

Howes, E.L., Price, H.M., Pearson, C.M. & Blumberg, J.M. (1966) Hypokalemic periodic paralysis: Electron microscopic changes in the sarcoplasm. *Neurology (Minneapolis)*, **16**, 242.

Hudgson, P. & Fulthorpe, J.J. (1975) The pathology of type II skeletal muscle glycogenosis. A light and electronmicroscopic study. *Journal of Pathology*, **116**, 139.

Hudgson, P., Gardner-Medwin, D., Fulthorpe, J.J. & Walton, J.N. (1967) Nemaline myopathy. *Neurology (Minneapolis)*, **17**, 1125.

Hudgson, P., Gardner-Medwin, D., Worsfold, M., Pennington, R.J.T. & Walton, J.N. (1968) Adult myopathy from glycogen storage disease due to acid maltase deficiency. *Brain*, **91**, 435.

Hudson, A.J., Oteruelo, F.T. & Haust, M.D. (1971) Unusual generalised myopathy of late onset. Clinical and morphological study. In *Actualités de Pathologie Neuromusculaire*, Eds G. Serratrice & H. Roux, pp. 140–142 (L'Expansion Scientifique Francaise: Paris).

Hughes, J.T. & Esiri, M.M. (1978) Ultrastructural studies in human polymyositis. *Journal of the Neurological Sciences*, **25**, 347.

Hurwitz, L., McCormick, D. & Allen, V.I. (1970) Reduced muscle α-glucosidase (acid maltase) activity in hypothyroid myopathy. *Lancet*, **1**, 67.

Isch, F., Juif, J.-G., Sacrez, R. & Thiebaut, F. (1966) Glycogenose musculaire; à forme myopathique par deficit en maltase acide. *Pédiatrie*, **21**, 71.

Jakovics, S., Khachadurian, A.K. & Tsia, D.Y.Y. (1966) The hyperlipidemia in glycogen storage disease. *Journal of Clinical Laboratory Medicine*, **68**, 769.

James, N.T. (1973) Compensatory hypertrophy in EDL of the rat. *Journal of Anatomy*, **116**, 57.

Jenis, E.H., Lindquist, R.R. & Lister, R.C. (1969) New congenital myopathy with crystalline intramuscular inclusions. *Archives of Neurology*, **20**, 281.

Jerusalem, F., Baumgartner, G. & Wyler, R. (1972) Virus-ahnliche Einschlusse bei chronischen neuro-muskularen Prozessen. Electronenmikroskopische Biopsiebefunde von 2 Fallen. *Archiv für Psychiatrie und Nerven-Krankheiten*, **215**, 418.

Jerusalem, F., Engel, A.G. & Gomez, M.R. (1973) Sarcotubular myopathy. *Neurology (Minneapolis)*, **23**, 897.

Jerusalem, F., Engel, A.G. & Gomez, M.R. (1974a) Duchenne dystrophy. II Morphological study of motor end-plate fine structure. *Brain*, **97**, 123.

Jerusalem, F., Engel, A.G. & Gomez, M.R. (1974b). Duchenne dystrophy. I. Morphometric study of the muscle microvasculature. *Brain*, **97**, 115.

Jerusalem, F., Angelini, C., Engel, A.G. & Groover, R.V. (1973) Mitochondria-lipid-glycogen (MLG) disease of muscle. *Archives of Neurology*, **29**, 162.

Jerusalem, F., Ludin, H., Bischoff, A. & Hartmann, G. (1979) Cytoplasmic body neuromyopathy presenting as respiratory failure and weight loss. *Journal of the Neurological Sciences*, **41**, 1.

Johnson, A.G. & Woolf, A.L. (1969) Abnormal sarcolemmal nuclei encountered in several cases of dystrophia myotonica. *Acta neuropathologica (Berlin)*, **12**, 183.

Johnson, M.A., Fulthorpe, J.J. & Hudgson, P. (1973) Lipid storage myopathy. A clinicopathologically recognizable entity. *Acta Neuropathologica (Berlin)*, **24**, 97.

Jones, K.W., Kinross, J., Maitland, N. & Norval, M. (1979) Normal human tissues contain RNA and antigens related to infectious adenovirus Type 2. *Nature*, **277**, 274.

Julien, J., Vital, C.L., Vallat, J.-M. & Martin, F. (1971) Paramyotonie d'Eulenburg. *Journal of the Neurological Sciences*, **13**, 447.

Julien, J., Vital, C.L., Vallat, J.-M., Vallat, M. & Le Blanc, M. (1974) Oculopharyngeal muscular dystrophy–a case with abnormal mitochondria and 'fingerprint' inclusions. *Journal of the Neurological Sciences*, **21**, 165.

Kamienicka, Z. (1976) Myopathies with abnormal mitochondria. *Acta neurologica Scandinavica*, **55**, 57.

Kao, I. & Gordon, A.M. (1977) Alteration of skeletal muscle cellular structures by potassium depletion. *Neurology (Minneapolis)*, **27**, 855.

Karpati, G., Carpenter, S., Melmed, C. & Eisen, A.A. (1974) Experimental ischaemic myopathy. *Journal of the Neurological Sciences*, **23**, 129.

Karpati, G., Carpenter, S., Eisen, A., Aube, M. & Di Mauro, S. (1977) The adult form of acid maltase (α-1,4-glucosidase) deficiency. *Annals of Neurology*, **1**, 276.

Ketelsen, U.-P. (1975) On the ultrastructure of the atrophic muscle cell. *Pathologia Europea*, **10**, 73.

Ketelsen, U.-P., Beckmann, R., Zimmerman, H. & Sauer, M. (1977) Inclusion body myositis. A 'slow virus' infection of skeletal musculature? *Klinische Wochenschrift*, **55**, 1063.

Kinoshita, M. & Cadman, T.E. (1968) Myotubular myopathy. *Archives of Neurology*, **18**, 265.

Klinkerfuss, G.H. (1967) An electron microscopic study of myotonic dystrophy. *Archives of Neurology*, **16**, 181.

Klinkerfuss, G.H. & Haugh, M.J. (1970) Disuse atrophy of muscle. *Archives of Neurology*, **22**, 309.

Koehler, J. (1977) Blood vessel structure in Duchenne muscular dystrophy. 1. Light and electron microscopic observations in resting muscle. *Neurology (Minneapolis)*, **27**, 861.

Konigsberg, U.R., Lipton, B.H. & Konigsberg, I.R. (1975) The regenerative response of single mature muscle fibres isolated *in vitro*. *Developmental Biology*, **45**, 260.

Korenyi-Both, A., Smith, B.H. & Baruah, J.K. (1977). McArdle's syndrome. Fine structural changes in muscle. *Acta neuropathologica* **40**, 11.

Lake, B.D. & Wilson, J. (1975) Zebra body myopathy. Clinical, histochemical and ultrastructural studies. *Journal of the Neurological Sciences*, **24**, 437.

Lambert, E.H. & Elmqvist, D. (1971) Quantal components of end-plate potentials in the myasthenic syndrome. *Annals of the New York Academy of Sciences*, **183**, 183.

Landry, M. & Winkelmann, R.K. (1972) Tubular cytoplasmic inclusion in dermatomyositis. *Mayo Clinic Proceedings*, **47**, 479.

Layzer, R.B., Rowland, L.P. & Ranney, H.M. (1967) Muscle phosphofructokinase deficiency. *Archives of Neurology*, **17**, 512.

Lee, J.C. & Altschul, R. (1963) Electron microscopy of the nuclei of denervated skeletal muscle. *Zeitschrift für Zellforschung und mikroscopische Anatomie*, **61**, 168.

Lewis, P.D., Pallis, C. & Pearse, A.G.E. (1971) 'Myopathy' with tubular aggregates. *Journal of the Neurological Sciences*, **13**, 381.

Libelius, R., Lundqvist, I., Templeton, W. & Thesleff, S. (1978) Intracellular uptake and degradation of extracellular tracers in mouse skeletal muscle *in vitro*: effect of denervation. *Neuroscience*, **3**, 641.

Luft, R., Ikkos, D., Palmieri, G., Ernster, L. & Afzelius, B. (1962) A case of severe hypermetabolism of non-thyroid origin with a defect in the maintenance of mitochondrial respiratory control: A correlated clinical, biochemical and morphological study. *Journal of Clinical Investigation*, **41**, 1776.

MacDonald, R.D. & Engel, A.G. (1969) The cytoplasmic body: another structural anomaly of the Z discs. *Acta Neuropathologica (Berlin)*, **14**, 99.

MacDonald, R.D., Rewcastle, N.B. & Humphrey, J.G. (1969) Myopathy of hypokalaemic periodic paralysis. *Archives of Neurology*, **20**, 565.

McComas, A.J., Campbell, M.J. & Sica, R.E.P. (1971) Electrophysiological study of dystrophia myotonica. *Journal of Neurology, Neurosurgery and Psychiatry*, **34**, 132.

McComas, A.J., Sica, R.E.P. & Brown, J.C. (1971) Myasthenia gravis: Evidence of a 'central' defect. *Journal of the Neurological Sciences*, **13**, 107.

McComas, A.J., Sica, R.E.P. & Campbell, M.J. (1971) 'Sick motoneurones'. A unifying concept of muscle disease. *Lancet*, **1**, 231.

McDaniel, H.G., Pitman, C.S., Oh, S.J. & Di Mauro, S. (1977) Carbohydrate metabolism in hypothyroid myopathy. *Metabolism*, **26**, 867.

McGeachie, J. & Allbrook, D. (1978) Cell proliferation in skeletal muscle following denervation or tenotomy. *Cell and Tissue Research*, **193**, 259.

Mair, W.G.P. & Tomez, F. (1972a) *Atlas of the Ultrastructure of Diseased Human Muscle* (Churchill Livingstone: Edinburgh).

Mair, W.G.P. & Tomé, F. (1972b) The ultrastructure of the adult and developing human myotendinous junction. *Acta neuropathologica. (Berlin)*, **21**, 239.

Martin, J.J., De Barsy, Th., De Schrijver, F., Leroy, J.G. & Palladini, G. (1976) Acid maltase deficiency (Type II glycogenosis). *Journal of the Neurological Sciences*, **30**, 155.

Martin, J.J., De Barsy, Th., Van Hoof, F. & Palladini, G. (1973) Pompe's disease: An inborn lysosomal disorder with storage of glycogen. *Acta neuropathologica (Berlin)*, **23**, 229.

Martinez, A.J., Hooshmand, H., Indolos Mendoza, G. & Winston, Y.E. (1974) Fatal polymyositis: Morphogenesis and ultrastructural features. *Acta neuropathologica (Berlin)*, **29**, 251.

Mastaglia, F.L. (1973) Pathological changes in skeletal muscle in acromegaly. *Acta neuropathologica (Berlin)*, **24**, 273.

Mastaglia, F.L. & Currie, S. (1971) Immunological and ultrastructural observations on the role of lymphoid cells in the pathogenesis of polymyositis. *Acta neuropathologica (Berlin)*, **18**, 1.

Mastaglia, F.L. & Kakulas, B.A. (1969) Regeneration in Duchenne muscular dystrophy: A histological and histochemical study. *Brain*, **92**, 809.

Mastaglia, F.L. & Walton, J.N. (1970) Coxsackie virus-like particles in skeletal muscle from a case of polymyositis. *Journal of the Neurological Sciences*, **11**, 593.

Mastaglia, F.L. & Walton, J.N. (1971a). An electron microscopic study of skeletal muscle from cases of the Kugelberg-Welander syndrome. *Acta neuropathologica (Berlin)*, **17**, 201.

Mastaglia, F.L. & Walton, J.N. (1971b). An ultrastructural study of skeletal muscle in polymyositis. *Journal of the Neurological Sciences*, **12**, 473.

Mastaglia, F.L., Dawkins, R.L. & Papadimitriou, J.M. (1975) Morphological changes in skeletal muscle after transplantation. *Journal of the Neurological Sciences*, **25**, 227.

Mastaglia, F.L., Papadimitriou, J.M. & Dawkins, R.L. (1975) Mechanisms of cell-mediated myotoxicity. Morphological observations in muscle grafts and in muscle exposed to sensitized spleen cells in vivo. *Journal of the Neurological Sciences*, **25**, 269.

Mastaglia, F.L., Papadimitriou, J.M. & Kakulas, B.A. (1970a) Regeneration of muscle in Duchenne muscular dystrophy. An electron microscope study. *Journal of the Neurological Sciences*, **11**, 425.

Mastaglia, F.L., McCollum, J.P.K., Larson, P.F. & Hudgson, P. (1970b) Steroid myopathy complicating McArdle's disease. *Journal of Neurology, Neurosurgery and Psychiatry*, **33**, 111.

Mastaglia, F.L., Papadimitriou, J.M., Dawkins, R.L. & Beveridge, B. (1977) Vacuolar myopathy associated with chloroquine, lupus erythematosus and thymoma. *Journal of the Neurological Sciences*, **34**, 315.

Mastaglia, F.L., Sarnat, H.B., Dawkins, R.L., Papadimitriou, J.M. & Kakulas, B.A. (1980) Myopathies associated with hypothyroidism. In preparation.

Maunder, C.A., Yarom, R. & Dubowitz, V. (1977) Electron-microscopic X-ray microanalysis of normal and diseased human muscle. *Journal of the Neurological Sciences*, **33**, 323.

Mauro, A. (1961) Satellite cells of skeletal muscle fibers. *Journal of Biophysical and Biochemical Cytology*, **9**, 493.

Meijer, A.E.F.H. (1972) Mitochondria with defective respiratory control of oxidative phosphorylation isolated from muscle tissues of thyroidectomised rabbits. *Journal of the Neurological Sciences.*, **16**, 445.

Melmed, C., Karpati, G. & Carpenter, S. (1975) Experimental mitochondrial myopathy produced by *in vivo* uncoupling of oxidative phosphorylation. *Journal of the Neurological Sciences*, **26**, 305.

Mendell, J.R. & Engel, W.K. (1971) The fine structure of type II muscle fibre atrophy. *Neurology (Minneapolis)*, **21**, 358.

Miledi, R. & Slater, C.R. (1969) Electron microscopic structure of denervated skeletal muscle. *Proceedings of the Royal Society of London, Series B*, **174**, 253.

Mintz, G., Gonzalez-Angulo, A., Fraga, A. & Zavala, B. (1968) Ultrastructure of muscle in polymyositis. *American Journal of Medicine*, **44**, 216.

Mokri, B. & Engel, A.G. (1975) Duchenne dystrophy: Electron microscopic findings pointing to a basic or early abnormality in the plasma membrane as the muscle fibre. *Neurology (Minneapolis)*, **25**, 1111.

Morgan-Hughes, J.A., Darveniza, P., Kahn, S.N., Landon, D.N., Sherratt, R.M., Land, J.M. & Clark, J.B. (1977) A mitochondrial myopathy characterised by a deficiency in reducible cytochrome b. *Brain*, **100**, 617.

Morgan-Hughes, J.A., Darveniza, P., Landon, D.N., Land, J.M. & Clark, J.B. (1979) A mitochondrial myopathy with a deficiency of respiratory chain NADH-CoQ reductase activity. *Journal of the Neurological Sciences*, **43**, 27.

Murase, T., Ikeda, H., Muro, T., Nakao, K. & Sugita, H. Myopathy associated with Type III glycogenosis. *Journal of the Neurological Sciences*, **20**, 287.

Musch, B.C., Papapetropoulos, T.A., McQueen, D.A., Hudgson, P. & Weightman, D. (1975) A comparison of the structure of small blood vessels in normal, denervated and dystrophic human muscle. *Journal of the Neurological Sciences*, **26**, 221.

Mussini, I., Di Mauro, S. & Angelini, C. (1970) Early ultrastructural and biochemical changes in muscle in dystrophia myotonica. *Journal of the Neurological Sciences*, **10**, 585.

Neville, H.E. (1973) Ultrastructural changes in muscle disease. In *Muscle Biopsy*, Eds V. Dubowitz & M. Brooke, pp. 383–444 (Saunders: London).

Neville, H.E., Maunder-Sewry, C.A., McDougall, J., Sewell, J.R. & Dubowitz, V. (1979) Chloroquine-induced cytosomes with curvilinear profiles in muscle. *Muscle and Nerve*, **2**, 376.

Nick, J., Prunieras, M., Bakouche, P., Reignier, A. & Nicolle, M.-H. (1971) Inclusions dans les cellules endotheliales et les lymphocytes au cours d'un cas de dermatomyosite. *Revue Neurologique*, **125**, 22.

Norris, F.H. & Panner, B.J. (1966) Hypothyroid myopathy: Clinical, electromyographical and ultrastructural observations. *Archives of Neurology*, **14**, 574.

Norris, F.H., Panner, B.J. & Stormont, J.M. (1968) Thyrotoxic periodic paralysis. Metabolic and ultrastructural studies. *Archives of Neurology*, **19**, 88.

Norton, W.L. (1970) Comparison of the microangiopathy of systemic lupus erythematosus, dermatomyositis, scleroderma and diabetes mellitus. *Laboratory Investigation*, **22**, 301.

Oberc, M.A. & Engel, W.K. (1977) Ultrastructural localisation of calcium in normal and abnormal skeletal muscle. *Laboratory Investigation*, **36**, 566.

Odor, D.L., Patel, A.N. & Pearce, L.A. (1967) Familial hypokalemic periodic paralysis with permanent myopathy. *Journal of Neuropathy and Experimental Neurology*, **26**, 98.

Oliner, L., Schulman, & Larner, J. (1961) Myopathy associated with glycogen deposition resulting from generalised lack of amylo-1,6-glucosidase. *Clinical Research* 243.

Oshima, Y., Becker, L.E. & Armstrong, D.L. (1979) An electron microscopic study of childhood dermatomyositis. *Acta neuropathologica (Berlin)*, **47**, 189.

Oteruelo, F.T. (1976) Intranuclear inclusions in a myopathy of late onset. *Virchows Archiv Abteilung B. Zellpathologie*, **20**, 319.

Palmucci, L., Bertolotto, A., Monga, G., Ardizzone, G. & Schiffer, D. (1978) Histochemical and ultrastructural findings in a case of centronuclear myopathy. *European Neurology*, **17**, 327.

Panayiotopoulos, C.P. & Scarpalezos, S. (1977) Dystrophia myotonica. A model of combined neural and myopathic muscle atrophy. *Journal of the Neurological Sciences*, **31**, 261.

Payne, C.M. & Curless, R.G. (1976) Concentric laminated bodies–ultrastructural demonstration of fibre type specificity. *Journal of the Neurological Sciences*, **29**, 311.

Payne, C.M. & Curless, R.G. (1977) Fingerprint inclusions. *Journal of the Neurological Sciences*, **31**, 379.

Payne, C.M., Stern, L.Z., Curless, R.G. & Hannapel, L.K. (1975) Ultrastructural fibre typing in normal and diseased human muscle. *Journal of the Neurological Sciences*, **25**, 99.

Pearce, G.W. (1964) Tissue culture and electron microscopy in muscle disease. In *Disorders of Voluntary Muscle*, 1st Edn. Ed. J.N. Walton (Churchill: London).

Pearson, C.M. (1964) The periodic paralyses: Differential features and pathological observations in permanent myopathic weakness. *Brain*, **87**, 341.

Pennington, R.J.T. (1963) Biochemistry of dystrophic muscle. *Biochemical Journal*, **88**, 64.

Peter, J.B. and Worsfold, M. (1969) Muscular dystrophy and other myopathies: sarcotubular vesicles in early disease. *Biochemical Medicine*, **2** 364.

Pollock, M. & Dyck, P.J. (1976) Peripheral nerve morphometry in myotonic dystrophy. *Archives of Neurology*, **33**, 33.

Pongratz, D., Schultz, D., Koppenwallner, C.H. & Hübner, G. (1979) Wertigkeit der muskelbiopsie in der diagnostia der dystrophia myotonica (Curschmann-Steinert). *Klinische Wochenschrift*, **57**, 215.

Popiela, H. (1976) Muscle satellite cells in amphibians: Facilitated identification of satellite cells using ruthenium red staining. *Journal of Experimental Zoology*, **198**, 57.

Poskanzer, D.C. & Kerr, D.N.S. (1961) A third type of periodic paralysis with normokalaemia and a favourable response to sodium chloride. *American Journal of Medicine*, **31** 328.

Price, H.M., Gordon, G.B., Munsat, T.L. & Pearson, C.M. (1967) Myopathy with atypical mitochondria in type I skeletal muscle fibres. *Journal of Neuropathology and Experimental Neurology*, **26**, 475.

Price, H.M., Gordon, G.B., Pearson, C.M., Munsat, T.L. & Blumbert, J.M. (1965) New evidence for accumulation of excessive Z band material in nemaline myopathy. *Proceedings of the National Academy of Sciences of the United States of America*, **64**, 1398.

Prineas, J.W., Hall, R., Barwick, D.D. & Watson, A.J. (1968) Myopathy associated with pigmentation following adrenalectomy for Cushing's syndrome. *Quarterly Journal and Medicine*, **37**, 63.

Radu, H., Rosu-Serbu, A.M., Ionescu, V. & Radu, A. (1977) Focal abnormalities in mitochondrial distribution in muscle. *Acta neuropathologica (Berlin)*, **39**, 25.

Rapola, J. & Haltia, M. (1973) Cytoplasmic inclusions in the vermiform appendix and skeletal muscle in two types of so-called neuronal ceroid-lipofuscinosis. *Brain*, **96**, 833.

Recondo, J. de, Fardeau, M. & Lapresle, J. (1966). Étude au microscope electronique des lesions musculaires d'atrophie neurogene par atteinte de la corne anterieure (observées dans huit cas de sclerose lateral amyotrophique). *Revue Neurologique*, **114**, 169.

Reger, J.F. & Craig, A.S. (1968) Studies on the fine structure of muscle fibers and associated satellite cells in hypertrophic human deltoid muscle. *Anatomical Record*, **162**, 483.

Reske-Nielsen, E. & Harmsen, A. (1972) Electron microscopical study of muscle biopsies from healthy young people. *Acta pathologica et microbiological Scandinavica*, **80A**, 449.

Reznik, M. (1969a) Origin of myoblasts during skeletal muscle regeneration. Electron microscopic observations. *Laboratory Investigation*, **20**, 353.

Reznik, M. (1969b). Thymidine-^{3}H uptake by satellite cells of regenerating skeletal muscle. *Journal of Cell Biology*, **40**, 568.

Ringel, S.P., Neville, H.E., Duster, M.C. & Carroll, J.E. (1978) A new congenital neuromuscular disease with trilaminar muscle fibers. *Neurology (Minneapolis)*, **28**, 282.

Ringel, S.P., Thorne, E.G., Phanuphak, P., Lava, N.S. & Kohler, P.S. (1979) Immune complex vasculitis, polymyositis and hyperglobulinaemic purpura. *Neurology (Minneapolis)*, **29**, 682.

Ritter, R.A. (1967) The effect of cortisone on the structure and strength of skeletal muscle. *Archives of Neurology*, **17**, 493.

Rose, A.L., Walton, J.N. & Pearce, G.W. (1967) Polymyositis: An ultramicroscopic study of muscle biopsy material *Journal of the Neurological Sciences*, **5**, 457.

Roses, A.D. & Appel, S.H. (1975) Phosphorylation of component a in the human erythrocyte membrane in myotonic muscular dystrophy. *Journal of Membrane Biology*, **20**, 51.

Sahgal, V. & Sahgal, S. (1977) A new congenital myopathy. *Acta neuropathological (Berlin)*, **37**, 225.

Samaha, F.J., Schröder, J.M., Rebeiz, J. & Adams, R.D. (1967) Studies on myotonia. Biochemical and electron microscopic studies on myotonia congenita and myotonia dystrophica. *Archives of Neurology*, **17**, 22.

Santa, T., Engel, A.G. & Lambert, E.H. (1972a). Histometric study of neuromuscular junction ultrastructure. I. Myasthenia gravis. *Neurology (Minneapolis)*, **22**, 71.

Santa, T., Engel, A.G. & Lambert, E.H. (1972b) Histometric study of neuromuscular junction ultrastructure. II. Myasthenic syndrome. *Neurology (Minneapolis)*, **22**, 370.

Sarnat, H.B. & Silbert, S.W. (1976) Maturational arrest of fetal muscle in neonatal myotonic dystrophy. *Archives of Neurology*, **33**, 466.

Sato, T. & Nakamuna, N. (1975) Myositis and virus. *Naika (Tokyo)*, **35**, 239.

Sato, T., Walker, D.L., Peters, H.A., Reese, H.N. & Chou, S.M. (1971) Chronic polymyositis and myxovirus-like inclusions. Electron microscopic and viral studies. *Archives of Neurology*, **24**, 409.

Satoyoshi, E. & Kowa, H. (1967). A myopathy due to a glycolytic abnormality. *Archives of Neurology*, **17**, 248.

Schiaffino, S. & Settembrini, P. (1970) Studies on the effect of denervation in developing muscle. *Virchows Archiv*

Abteilung B. Zellpathologie, **4**, 345.

Schiaffino, S., Severin, E., Cautini, M. and Sartore, S. (1977) Tubular aggregates induced by anoxia in isolated rat skeletal muscle. *Laboratory Investigation*, **37**, 228.

Schiller, H.H. & Mair, W.G.P. (1974) Ultrastructural changes of muscle in malignant hyperthermia. *Journal of the Neurological Sciences*, **21**, 93.

Schlenska, G.K., Heene, R.,Spalke, G. & Seiler, D. (1976) The symptomatology, morphology and biochemistry of glycogenosis type II (Pompe) in the adult. *Journal of Neurology*, **212**, 237.

Schmalbruch, H.H. (1967) Kristalloide in menschlichen skelett-muskelfasern. *Naturwissenschaften*, **54**, 519.

Schmalbruch, H.H. (1975) Segmental fibre breakdown and defects of the plasmalemma in diseased human muscles. *Acta Neuropathologica (Berlin)*, **33**, 129.

Schmalbruch, H.H. (1976) Muscle fibre splitting and regeneration in diseased human muscle. *Neuropathology and Applied Neurobiology*, **2**, 3.

Schmitt, H.P. & Volk, B. (1975) The relationship between target, targetoid and targetoid/core fibres in severe neurogenic muscular atrophy. *Journal of Neurology*, **210**, 167.

Schochet, S.S. & McCormick, F. (1973) Polymyositis with intra-muscular inclusions. *Archives of Neurology*, **28**, 280.

Schotland, D.L. (1969) An electron microscopic study of target fibers, target-like fibers and related abnormalities in human muscle. *Journal of Neuropathology and Experimental Neurology*, **28**, 214.

Schotland, D.L. (1970) An electron microscopic investigation of myotonic dystrophy. *Journal of Neuropathology and Experimental Neurology*, **29**, 241.

Schotland, D.L., Bonilla, E. & Van Meter, M. (1977) Duchenne dystrophy: Alterations in muscle plasma membrane structure. *Science*, **196**, 1005.

Schröder, J.M. (1970) Sarcolemmal indentations resembling junctional folds in myotonic dystrophy. In *Muscle Diseases*, Eds J.N. Walton, N. Canal & G. Scarlato, pp. 109–111 (Excerpta Medica: Amsterdam).

Schröder, J.M. & Adams, R.D. (1968) The ultrastructural morphology of the muscle fibre in myotonic dystrophy. *Acta Neuropathologica (Berlin)*, **10**, 218.

Schröder, J.M. & Becker, P.E. (1972) Anomalien des T-systems und des sarkoplasmatischen reticulums bei der myotonie, paramyotonie und adynamie. *Virchows Archiv Abteilung A. Pathologische Anatomie*, **357**, 319.

Schultz, E. (1978) Changes in the satellite cells of growing muscle following denervation. *Anatomical Record*, **190**, 299.

Schutta, H.S. & Armitage, J.L. (1969) Thyrotoxic hypokalaemic periodic paralysis: A fine structure study. *Journal of Neuropathology and Experimental Neurology*, **28**, 321.

Schutta, H.S., Kelly, A.M. & Zacks, S.I. (1969) Necrosis and regeneration of muscle in paroxysmal idiopathic myoglobinuria. Electron microscopic observations. *Brain*, **92**, 191.

Serratrice, G., Pellissier, J.F., Faugere, M.C. & Gastaut, J.L. (1978) Centronuclear myopathy: Possible central nervous system origin. *Muscle and Nerve*, **1**, 62.

Shafiq, S.A., Gorycki, M.A. & Milhorat, A.T. (1967) An electron microscopic study of regeneration and satellite cells in human muscle. *Neurology (Minneapolis)*, **17**, 507.

Shafiq, S.A., Milhorat, A.T. & Gorycki, M.A. (1967a) An electron microscopic study of muscle degeneration and changes in blood vessels in polymyositis. *Journal of Pathology and Bacteriology*, **94**, 139.

Shafiq, S.A., Milhorat, A.T. & Gorycki, M.A. (1967b) Giant mitochondria in human muscle with inclusions. *Archives of Neurology*, **17**, 666.

Shafiq, S.A., Dubowitz, V., Peterson, H. de C. & Milhorat, A.T. (1967) Nemaline myopathy: Report of a fatal case with histochemical and electronmicroscopic studies. *Brain*, **90**, 817.

Sher, J.H., Rimalovski, A.B., Athanassiades, T.J. & Aronson, S.M. (1967) Familial centronuclear myopathy. *Neurology (Minneapolis)*, **17**, 721.

Shoji, S., Takagi, A., Sugita, H. & Toyokura, Y. (1974) Muscle glycogen metabolism in steroid-induced myopathy in rabbits. *Experimental Neurology*, **45**, 1.

Shy, G.M. & Magee, K.R. (1956) A new non-progressive myopathy. *Brain*, **79**, 610.

Shy, G.M. Gonatas, N.K. & Perez, M. (1966) Two childhood myopathies with abnormal mitochondria. I. Megaconial myopathy. II. Pleoconial myopathy. *Brain*, **89**, 133.

Shy, G.M., Engel, W.K., Somers, J.E. & Wanko, T. (1963) Nemaline myopathy: A new congenital myopathy. *Brain*, **86**, 793.

Shy, G.M., Wanko, T., Rowley, P.T. & Engel, A.G. (1961) Studies in familial periodic paralysis. *Experimental Neurology*, **3**, 53.

Simpson, J.A. (1960) Myasthenia gravis: a new hypothesis. *Scottish Medical Journal*, **5**, 419.

Smith, H.L., Amick, L.D. & Sidbury, J.B. (1966) Type II glycogenosis: report of a case with 4 year survival and absence of acid maltase associated with an abnormal glycogen. *American Journal of Diseases of Children*, **111**, 475.

Snow, M.H. (1977) Myogenic cell formation in regenerating rat skeletal muscle injured by mincing. *Anatomical Record*, **188**, 181.

Snow, M.H. (1978) An autoradiographic study of satellite cell differentiation into regenerating myotubes following transplantation of muscle in young rats. *Cell Tissue Research*, **186**, 537.

Spiro, A.J. & Kennedy, C. (1964) Hereditary occurrence of nemaline myopathy. *Transactions of the American Neurological Association*, **89**, 62.

Spiro, A.J., Prineas, J.W. & Moore, C.L. (1970) A new mitochondrial myopathy in a patient with salt craving. *Archives of Neurology*, **22**, 259.

Spiro, A.J., Shy, G.M., & Gonatas N.K. (1966) Myotubular myopathy. *Archives of Neurology*, **14**, 1.

Spiro, A.J., Hirano, A., Beilin, R.L. & Finkelstein, J.W. (1970) Cretinism with muscular hypertrophy (Kocher-Debré-Sémélaigne syndrome). *Archives of Neurology*, **23**, 340.

Stonnington, H.H. & Engel, A.G. (1973) Normal and denervated muscle. *Neurology (Minneapolis)*, **23**, 714.

Swash, M. & Fox, K.P. (1976) The pathology of the muscle spindle in Duchenne muscular dystrophy. *Journal of the Neurological Sciences*, **29**, 17.

Takagi, A., Schotland, D.L., Di Mauro, S. & Rowland, L.P. (1973). Thyrotoxic periodic paralysis. Function of sarcoplasmic reticulum and muscle glycogen. *Neurology (Minneapolis)*, **23**, 1008.

Tang, T.T., Sedmak, G.V., Siegesmund, K.A. & McCreadie, S.R. (1975) Chronic myopathy associated with

Coxsackie virus type A9. A combined electron microscopical and viral isolation study. *New England Journal of Medicine*, **292**, 608.

Tarui, S., Okuno, G., Ikura, Y., Tanaka, T. & Suda, M. (1965) Phosphofructokinase deficiency in skeletal muscle: A new type of glycogenosis. *Biochemical and Biophysical Research Communications*, **19**, 517.

Thesleff, S. (1966) Acetylcholine utilisation in myasthenia gravis. *Annals of the New York Academy of Sciences*, **135**, 195.

Thomson, W.H.S., MacLaurin, J.C. & Prineas, J.W. (1963) Skeletal muscle glycogenosis: An investigation of two dissimilar cases. *Journal of Neurology, Neurosurgery and Psychiatry*, **26**, 60.

Tomé, F.M.S. & Fardeau, M. (1973) 'Fingerprint inclusions' in muscle fibres in dystrophia myotonica. *Acta Neuropathologica (Berlin)*, **24**, 62.

Tsujihata, M., Hazama, R., Ishii, N., Ide, Y., Mori, M. & Takamori, M. (1979) Limb muscle end-plates in ocular myasthenia gravis. Quantitative ultrastructural study. *Neurology (Minneapolis)*, **29**, 654.

Van Haelst, U. (1970) An electron microscopic study of muscle in Werdnig-Hoffmann's disease. *Virchows Archiv Abteilung A. Pathologische Anatomie*, **351**, 291.

Van Wijngaarden, G.K., Bethlem, J, Meijer, A.E.F.H., Hulsmann, W.C. & Feltkamp, C.A. (1967) Skeletal muscle disease with abnormal mitochondria. *Brain*, **90**, 577.

Van Wijngaarden, G.K., Bethlem, J., Dingemans, K.P., Cöers, C., Telerman-Toppet, N. & Gerard, J.M. (1977) Familial focal loss of cross striations. *Journal of Neurology*, **216**, 163.

Vick, N.A. (1971) Skeletal muscle capillary basement membranes in humans. *Acta neuropathologica (Berlin)*, **17**, 1.

Wakayama, Y., Schotland, D.L., Bonilla, E. & Orecchio, E. (1979) Quantitative ultrastructural study of muscle satellite cells in Duchenne dystrophy. *Neurology (Minneapolis)*, **29**, 401.

Walton, J.N. (1961) Muscular dystrophy and its relationship to other myopathies. *Research Publications, Association for Research in Nervous and Mental Disease*, **38**, 378.

Webb, J.N. & Gillespie, W.J. (1976) Virus-like particles in paraspinal muscle in scoliosis. *British Medical Journal*, **4**, 912.

Weller, R.O. & McArdle, B. (1971) Calcification within muscle fibres in the periodic paralyses. *Brain*, **94**, 263.

White, J.G. (1972) Lymphocyte inclusions. *Annals of Internal Medicine*, **76**, 1042.

Woolf, A.L. (1966) Morphology of the myasthenic neuromuscular junction. *Annals of the New York Academy of Sciences*, **135**, 35.

Wyatt, P.R. & Cox, D.M. (1977) Duchenne's muscular dystrophy: studies in cultured fibroblasts. *Lancet*, **1**, 172.

Yamaguchi, K., Santa, T., Inove, K. & Omae, T. (1978a) Lipid storage in Von Gierke's disease. *Journal of the Neurological Sciences*, **38**, 195.

Yamaguchi, M., Robson, R.M., Stromer, M.H., Dahl, D.S. & Oda, T. (1978b) Actin filaments form the backbone of nemaline myopathy rods. *Nature*, **27**, 265.

Yarom, R & Shapira, Y. (1977) Myosin degeneration in a congenital myopathy. *Archives of Neurology*, **34**, 114.

Yunis, E.J. & Samaha, F.J. (1971) Inclusion body myositis. *Laboratory Investigation*, **25**, 240.

Zacks, S.I., Bauer, W.C. & Blumberg, J.M. (1962) The fine structure of the myasthenic neuromuscular junction. *Neuropathology and Experimental Neurology*, **21**, 335.

Zacks, S.I., Pegues, J.J. & Elliott, F.A. (1962) Interstitial muscle capillaries in patients with diabetes mellitus: A light and electron microscope study. *Metabolism*, **II**, 381.

Zellweger, H., Brown, B.I., McCormick, W.F. & Tu, J.-B. (1965) A mild form of muscular glycogenosis in two brothers with alpha-I,4-glucosidase deficiency. *Annals of Paediatrics*, **205**, 413.

Tissue culture in muscle disease

INTRODUCTION

A number of studies have shown that mononucleated cells migrating from the cut surface of vertebrate muscle fragments or released from muscle tissue by enzyme digestion will, under appropriate tissue culture conditions, divide, fuse and differentiate to form syncytial myotubes which contain muscle-specific proteins and may contract spontaneously. In mixed cultures of muscle and nerve cells, functional neuromuscular junctions may be formed. It seems very likely that myogenesis and the integration of nerve and muscle development in the whole animal involves similar processes.

There are a number of advantages in investigating myogenesis in tissue culture:

(1) the cells differentiate more rapidly and with a greater degree of synchrony than *in vivo*;

(2) the living cells are obtained in thin layers, usually only one cell thick and extended in one plane of focus upon a transparent surface and are therefore most suitable for microscopic examination and electrophysiological experiments when alive, or histochemical, immunochemical and autoradiographic experiments when fixed;

(3) the closed *in vitro* system provided by tissue culture makes it particularly easy to control environmental conditions. In the body, muscle cells are exposed to undefined complex humoral influences. The closed system is also particularly suitable for the administration of radioactive precursors, testing of drugs, growth and differentiation factors;

(4) methods for obtaining cultures of pure myogenic cells (by cloning or establishment of cell lines) make it possible to investigate myogenesis in the absence of other cells which are usually closely associated with muscle *in situ* and which may influence events.

Since the previous edition of this book, extensive studies have been made of normal and diseased cells in tissue culture. Witkowski (1977) has recently reviewed the literature concerned principally with the behaviour of diseased human and animal muscle. The present Chapter will therefore be concerned with only a brief review of the more recent investigations of cell morphology and growth pattern of human diseased muscle cells in tissue culture. The main emphasis will be on papers which have increased our basic understanding of the process of differentiation of muscle cells and especially of the intrinsic and extrinsic factors which affect muscle-cell gene expression. In many cases, resolution of the molecular events underlying differentiation has been made possible only by the technical advantages of the tissue culture system. The main research effort has been directed towards investigation of normal myogenesis but the increased knowledge of the normal differentiation process obtained using a wide range of analytical approaches has already indicated profitable areas in which to study pathological muscle in tissue culture.

TISSUE CULTURE TECHNIQUES

For details of methods the reader is referred to the monograph on tissue culture technique by Paul (1970). Culture technique with particular reference to muscle has recently been reviewed by Witkowski (1977) who discusses techniques for treatment of muscle tissue to obtain myogenic cultures, culture media and methods for the preparation of pure muscle cultures.

Two techniques have been widely used for setting up cultures of muscle cells:

(1) the explant technique, in which fragments of muscle, sometimes embedded in a thin layer of clotted plasma are immersed in tissue culture medium (Carrel, 1924) so that mononucleate myogenic cells (myoblasts) migrate from the cut surface of the fragment (explant);

(2) the disaggregation technique, in which proteolytic enzymes are used to digest away the intercellular material, reducing the muscle to a suspension of single cells which are seeded out in tissue culture (Moscona and Moscona, 1952; Rinaldini, 1959).

From the point where mononucleate cells are obtained in a monolayer on the surface of the tissue culture dishes the process of myogenesis is similar, following either method of establishing the culture. After a period of cell division, the cells align and then undergo fusion to form multinucleate syncytia which further differentiate into myotubes (Fig. 10.1).

CELL MORPHOLOGY AND GROWTH PATTERN

Cell morphology and the growth pattern of diseased muscle cells in tissue culture have been investigated by both the explant and disaggregation culture techniques. The aim of such experiments is to see whether the pathological condition still manifests itself in tissue culture. If this is the case it would suggest that the patho-

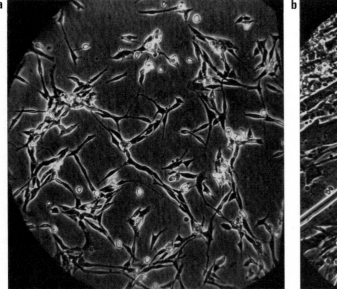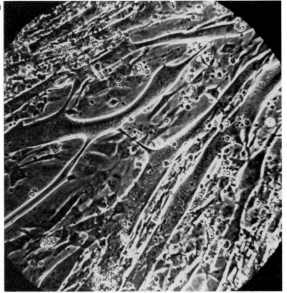

Fig. 10.1   a. Rat myoblasts on the point of fusing. Cells were disaggregated from neonatal rat muscle by trypsinisation. After 2 days of proliferation in culture, the cells were detached from the dishes by trypsinisation and the fibroblasts removed from suspension by the 'differential adhesion' method (Yaffe, 1968). The myoblasts were then allowed to attach to gelatin-coated culture dishes and grown for a further day. b. Rat myotubes, differentiated after a further 3 days (Guinness, 1973)

logical lesion is intrinsic to muscle cells. On the other hand, absence of differences between cultures of diseased and normal cells would suggest that either the disorder is not primarily myopathological, or that factors present in or absent from the culture environment have prevented full expression of the pathological process.

Explant technique

Until recently, the explant technique was the only successful method for culturing fully differentiated muscle, and was therefore extensively used to study those myopathies in which abnormalities are manifested only in late development. Muscle cells from many human neuromuscular diseases (e.g. Becker muscular dystrophy, limb-girdle dystrophy, facioscapulohumeral dystrophy, spinal muscular atrophy and myotonic dystrophy) have been grown using the technique and no abnormality has been observed in culture (Bishop, Gallup, Skeate and Dubowitz, 1971; Witkowski, Durbridge and Dubowitz, 1976).

The explant technique has been widely used to culture muscle obtained from patients with Duchenne muscular dystrophy. Earlier studies reported differences in morphology and cell migration between normal and dystrophic cells. Geiger and Garvin (1957) found that diseased muscle did not differentiate properly and cross-striations did not develop. Other investigators found more extensive growth of muscle from dystrophic patients than from normal subjects and dystrophic mononucleate cells were smaller than normal (Goyle, Kalra and Singh, 1967; 1968; Kakulas, Papadimitriou, Knight and Mastaglia, 1968).

More recent studies using the explant technique have suggested that there is no significant difference between normal and dystrophic cells in culture. Skeate, Bishop and Dubowitz (1969) found differentiated myotubes with cross-striations in both normal and dystrophic muscle. Statistical analysis by Bishop et al. (1971) showed no significant differences between normal and diseased muscle in the length, breadth or number of myotubes. Witkowski et al. (1976) found that the mononucleate cells, growth rate and degree of differentiation were similar. Morphologically similar cell features in cultures from normal and

Duchenne muscle have also been reported by Herrmann, Konïgsberg and Robinson (1960), Askanas and Engel (1975) and Ionasescu, Zellweger, Ionasescu, Lara-Brand and Cancilla (1976).

In tissue culture of muscle explants from normal fetuses and male fetuses at risk for Duchenne muscular dystrophy, no differences were found with regard to the ease with which cultures could be established and maintained, or in gross morphology or rate of growth and differentiation in culture. Yet, before culture, muscle histology was clearly abnormal in at least one of the at-risk fetuses (Emery and McGregor, 1977). The mean area of myotube nuclei in cultures of Duchenne muscle was found to be significantly larger than that of the myotube nuclei in cultures of normal muscle when measurements were made on fixed and stained preparations (Vassilipoulos, Emery and Gordon, 1977).

Disaggregation technique

The disaggregation technique has been most frequently used to prepare cultures from embryonic tissue. Hauschka (1974a) found that collagenase could be successfully used for enzymatic disaggregation of normal human embryonic skeletal muscle.

More recently, a method for preparing mononucleate cells by enzymatic digestion of human adult skeletal muscle using a mixture of collagenase and trypsin has been described by Yasin, van Beers, Bulien and Thompson (1976). Cells from muscle biopsies from patients with myotonic dystrophy, inflammatory myopathy, spinal muscular atrophy, scapuloperoneal dystrophy and denervation have been cultured (Yashin, van Beers, Nurse, Al-Ani, Landon and Thompson, 1977). No gross differences in plating efficiency, rate of myotube formation or CPK specific activity were found for the diseased cells, although a higher cell yield was obtained from muscles of patients with an inflammatory myopathy.

However, an abnormality in cellular behaviour was found in cells prepared from muscle of Duchenne patients (Thompson, Yasin, van Beers, Nurse and Al-Ani, 1977). The first sign of abnormality was detected four days after plating the cells and consisted of areas where the cells were clustered together in close proximity, rather than being more uniformly distributed in a monolayer. The nuclei and the perinuclear cytoplasm of some of the cells in the clusters seemed to be increased in size. There was, however, a proportion of myoblasts which fused to form myotubes in apparently normal fashion. With further differentiation, there were a certain number of refractile myotubes, but their distribution was again abnormal in that they spanned the gap between the cell clusters.

Conclusions

In summary, most recent reports indicate that when cultures of normal and Duchenne muscle cells are set up by the explant technique there is no dramatic difference between them in the morphology and growth pattern, suggesting that either the pathological condition is not intrinsic to muscle cells or that conditions of culture have prevented full expression of the pathological lesion. In contrast, when cultures are set up by the disaggregation technique, the Duchenne cells do not remain dispersed after plating but form clusters of cells that were apparently never seen in any control culture. This observation of clustering has been interpreted to indicate that there is a myogenic defect in Duchene muscular dystrophy.

It is worth while considering possible explanations for these contrasting observations.

The muscle biopsy used to establish a culture probably contains several cell types, including fully differentiated myotubes (muscle fibres), myoblasts, satellite cells, fibroblasts and fat cells. Biopsies from pathological muscle may contain higher proportions of some cell types compared with normal muscle biopsies. For example, muscle tissue is replaced by adipose tissue in advanced cases of Duchenne muscular dystrophy and by fibroblastic cells and connective tissue in facioscapulohumeral muscular dystrophy. The differing proportions of cells may influence the appearance of the culture and its growth patterns and this would be particularly dependent on the technique for establishing the culture. When cells are disaggregated by enzyme, all cells that survive the treatment have an equal opportunity to settle on the culture dish surface and establish the monolayer. When an explant culture is set up, only those cells which are capable of migrating from the fragment will appear in the cell monolayer. It is possible that the cells that initiate cluster formation in disaggregation cultures of Duchenne cells (Thompson et al., 1977) are a cell type that is relatively immobile, would not migrate from explants and would not therefore be seen in cultures set up by the explant technique.

Alternatively, if myogenic cells in a biopsy of Duchenne muscle were affected by the disease to different degrees, there might be selection of the less severely affected cells in the culture environment. Migration out of an explant may be beyond the capability of more severely affected cells, but when disaggregated from the tissue these may remain viable and manifest pathological conditions in the monolayer.

It may take as long for pathological changes to develop in dystrophic myotubes in tissue culture as in vivo. It cannot be ruled out that some techniques of culture, for example, the disaggregation technique, may bring the cells to the stage of showing pathological changes more rapidly.

Identification of mononucleate cells

Much attention has been given to distinguishing between different mononucleate cells in the stages of culture before the fusion of myoblasts to form myotubes.

Konigsberg (1963) has attempted to distinguish myoblasts from fibroblasts of embryonic chick using the method of 'clonal analysis', by which the cells were first separated individually by trypsinisation and then separately plated out at very low density in a culture medium. An appreciable proportion of these cells were then observed to undergo a succession of mitoses to form 'clones', or individual colonies of cells, each derived from a single separated cell. These colonies were found to be of two types:

(1) colonies of rather flattened cells that stayed separate from one another and exhibited extensive 'ruffled membranes' at their borders, which were designated 'fibroblasts' (see Fig. 10.2a);

(2) colonies of cells that were usually fusiform or

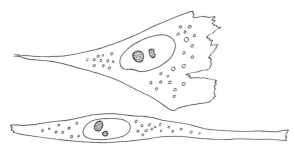

Fig. 10.2 Typical shapes assumed by fibroblasts and by myoblasts in cultures of cells from chick embryo muscle explants, as determined by Konigsberg's cloning techniques (see below); (a) typical spread-out fibroblast; (b) typical spindle-shaped myoblast

spindle-shaped with very small regions of 'ruffled membrane' confined to their ends, and which, after ceasing to divide, began fusing with each other to form syncytia in a manner characteristic of the normal pattern of myogenesis. These were designated 'myoblasts' (*see* Fig. 10.2b).

Konigsberg (1963) recorded that, in most cases, the final character of a colony could be predicted by the morphological appearance of the parent cell of the clone before it began to divide. The results show that, of the 1313 colonies that grew successfully from single cells, 96.5 per cent of the elongated fusiform-shaped cells (Fig. 10.2b) produced colonies of fusing myoblasts, and 85 per cent of the more flattened irregular-shaped cells (Fig. 10.2a) produced colonies of non-fusing cells, thereby defined as fibroblasts. Thus, one in 35 of the 'myoblast-like' cells might be expected to be a fibroblast and one in six of the 'fibroblast-like' cells could, conversely, be expected to be a myoblast, which shows that a high degree of correct designation of chick cells is possible on the basis of cell morphology.

A different approach has been used to identify cells by Goyle, Virmani and Singh (1973). The morphology of the cells growing from explanted muscle biopsies was compared with that of lipocytes growing from subcutaneous fat explants and of fibroblasts growing from fascia. The lipocytes in young cultures were elongated, narrow, highly refractile uni- or multinucleated cells with round or oval nuclei. As these cells aged, their cytoplasm tended to retract towards the nucleus and they looked round in shape. The young fibroblasts were broader cells with central spheri-

cal nuclei and, occasionally, binucleate cells were seen. The fibroblasts tended to retain their shape as the culture became older. These morphological criteria were used to identify cells migrating from muscle explants.

However, morphological criteria are evidently not a dependable means of identifying individual cells in a mixed culture, because a cell may sometimes assume uncharacteristic shapes and, therefore, at any given time a proportion of the cells in a culture will be liable to misclassification. Human myoblasts are flatter than those of rats, mice and birds and, for these, the only time to distinguish with certainty even clonal colonies of myoblasts is when they have actually shown some differentiation into myotubes. Binucleate cells can arise in cultures of fibroblasts and a cell should possess at least three morphologically normal nuclei before being classified as a myotube. Richler and Yaffe (1970) have commented on the variability of the phenotype even in cloned myogenic cells (i.e. derived from a single cell).

The culture environment may alter normal cell myogenesis from that *in vivo* in several respects. Okazaki and Holtzer (1965) emphasised the enormously faster metabolism and development of myotubes under optimum conditions *in vitro* compared with their growth *in vivo*. The pattern of development also differed in some respects; e.g. chick myotubes frequently branched *in vitro* although apparently they never do so in the whole animal.

Origin of myoblasts

The myoblasts that grow in tissue culture originate either from embryonic or adult muscle. In rapidly growing embryonic muscle *in vivo* there are large numbers of dividing myoblasts of recent mesenchymal origin. Hauschka (1974a, b) carried out cell-cloning experiments to examine proportions of myoblasts present in human fetuses of different ages. Muscle cells were prepared by enzymatic disaggregation and plated at cloning densities. The percentage of clones containing myotubes rose from 12 per cent at 31 days' gestation to 90 per cent at 172 days and the plating efficiency rose from 1 per cent to 24 per cent at 88 days' gestation.

The source of the myogenic cells from adult muscle which grow in tissue culture is still not entirely certain. Mauro (1961), in the course of an electron-microscopic study of frog muscle, discovered separate cellular elements in muscle fibres lying within the sarcolemmal membrane but separated from the muscle syncytium by their own membranes, which he named 'satellite cells'. Evidence has now accumulated from studies of muscle regeneration *in vivo* to suggest that these satellite cells are the main source from which myoblasts in regenerating muscle are derived (Ch. 5).

Evidence from tissue culture experiments also supports the role of the satellite cells in muscle regeneration. Segments of individual differentiated fibres have been dissected and cultured from muscle of the quail (Konigsberg, Lipton and Konigsberg, 1975), the rat (Bischoff, 1975) and from man (Witkowski, 1977, p. 458). During the first few hours in tissue culture, the fibre shows degenerative changes including the formation of myofibrillar contraction clots and pyknosis of most nuclei. The endomysial tube (basement lamina) remains intact along the entire length of the fibre. Those nuclei which survive are found to be contained within separate mononucleated cells closely applied to, and within, the endomysial tube. An examination of the fine structure of the mononucleate cells that survive degeneration shows them to be separate, mononucleated cells contained within the basement lamina of the degenerating fibre. These cells are identical, on the basis of their ultrastructure as well as their location, to satellite cells associated with muscle fibres in the source tissue (Konigsberg *et al.*, 1975). Regeneration activity seems to be of two types. Quail fibre mononucleate cells divide and cells migrate out from the endomysial tube to form a colony of cells which can undergo myotube formation (Konigsberg *et al.*, 1975). Rat mononucleate cells divide and remain within the endomysial tube, and the satellite-cell progeny begin to fuse to form myotubes within the endomysial tube of the original fibre. The myotubes display spontaneous contractile activity and may extend throughout the length of the endomysial tube (Bischoff, 1975).

These studies do not rule out the possibility that cell budding from muscle fibres (Reznik, 1969) and cells from the circulation outside muscle (Bayliss and Sloper, 1973; Yarom and Havivi, 1977) also contribute to the regenerative process *in vivo*.

PROTEINS CHARACTERISTIC OF MUSCLE

Protein synthesis in the dividing myoblast is geared to cell proliferation whereas, in the post-mitotic myoblasts and myotubes, synthesis of muscle-specific proteins predominates. Many investigators have taken advantage of the synchrony of development possible in culture to study the process of muscle differentiation as judged by the criterion of the synthesis of muscle-specific proteins.

In recent years, improved methods have been developed for synchronising and/or arresting myogenic cell fusion in monolayer cultures to determine the importance of fusion in triggering off the expression of muscle-specific genes. Synchronisation can be achieved by changing the composition of the culture medium, particularly the concentration and type of serum and embryo extract (Yaffe, 1971; Emerson and Beckner, 1975). Fusion can be arrested by manipulation of the Ca^{++} concentration of the culture medium using chelating agents such as EGTA (Paterson and Strohman, 1972) or Chelex (Moss and Strohman, 1976; Vertel and Fischman, 1976). Removal of the chelating agent can lead to a very rapid burst of fusion.

In some biochemical investigations it has been difficult to decide whether certain proteins are being synthesised in myotubes or in the dividing cell population (myoblasts and fibroblasts). This problem has been resolved by using drugs to kill the proliferating cells leaving cultures of pure myotubes (e.g. FUdR (Coleman and Coleman, 1968), cytosine arabinoside (Chi, Fellini and Holtzer, 1975a; Chi, Rubinstein, Strahs and Holtzer, 1975b)).

However, the exact timing of the synthesis of muscle-specific proteins such as myosin, actin, creatine phosphokinase, acetylcholine receptors, acetylcholinesterase and the sarcoplasmic reticulum Ca^{++}- and Mg^{++}-dependent ATPase has been controversial. Conclusions drawn in such investigations are very much dependent on the methods used for the detection of muscle-specific protein and these differ in their degrees of sensitivity, as indicated below.

Direct visualisation by electron microscopy

Electron-microscopic examination indicates that the formation of the myofibril involves thin filaments of actin (6–7 nm in diameter) and thick filaments of myosin (14–16 nm in diameter). There are reports of the presence of an excess of free thin filaments, presumed to be actin, suggesting that the synthesis of actin and myosin filaments precedes that of myosin (*see* Fischman, 1970). However, several classes of fine filaments have been reported in myogenic cells and microtubules 10 nm wide are abundant: these could be mistakenly identified as contractile protein filaments (Ishikawa, Bischoff and Holtzer, 1969) in the absence of confirmatory evidence, such as that afforded by the complexes which appear when glycerinated myogenic cells are treated with heavy meromyosin and negatively stained (Huxley, 1963). Such so-called arrowhead complexes formed all along the thin filaments of the nascent as well as mature myofilaments, both in mononucleated myoblasts and in multinucleated myotubes (Ishikawa *et al.*, 1969). No excess of randomly orientated, free actin filaments was detected by this method, indicating that they interacted with the myosin filaments immediately after synthesis.

Recent electron-microscopic investigation has shown that thin and thick filaments organised into myofibrils occur in fusion-blocked cells (Emerson and Beckner, 1975; Holtzer, Croop, Dienstman, Ishikawa and Somlyo, 1975; Moss and Strohmann, 1976; Vertel and Fischman, 1976).

Histochemical studies

Enzymes or substrates can be localised within individual mononucleate cells or myotubes by histochemical techniques.

Gallup *et al.* (1972) found that, during myogenesis in tissue culture, normal human undifferentiated mononucleate myoblasts have a strongly glycolytic metabolism (high phosphory-lase, high glycogen). In contrast, the myotubes have a strongly oxidative metabolism (high NADH-TR) and high myofibrillar ATPase. It is therefore of crucial importance to ensure that cultures being compared are at the same stage of differentiation. Gallup *et al.* (1972) further found that myotubes in cultures of diseased muscle from patients with Duchenne muscular dystrophy and myotonic dystrophy were enzymatically normal, and they concluded that the underlying pathological process does not affect enzymatic differentiation. In contrast, Goyle *et al.* (1973) found differences in succinic dehydrogenase, glucose-6-phosphate dehydrogenase and triglyceride content in Duchenne cultures but the data do not make it clear whether the cells examined were at the mononucleate or myotube stage.

Immunological methods

Immunological techniques have been used to investigate the synthesis of myosin during myogenesis in tissue culture using antibodies raised against the native protein (Coleman and Coleman, 1968) and against light meromyosin, which is a fragment of the tail region of the myosin heavy chain subunit (Chi *et al.*, 1975b). The early work, reporting that antibodies raised to contractile proteins from adult muscle will react with embryonic or cultured muscle, suggested that the proteins were very similar (Holtzer and Sanger, 1972). Fluorescein-labelled antibodies against skeletal light meromyosin were bound along the lateral edges of emerging and definitive thick filaments in cultured myotubes (Chi *et al.*, 1975a, b).

Masaki (1974) established that the heavy chains of myosins from chicken fast white, slow red, and cardiac muscles were immunologically distinguishable. The heavy chain of each myosin reacted with its antibody in the presence of SDS, suggesting that differences in primary sequence are involved. Investigations of muscle development *in vivo*, using these highly specific antibodies labelled with fluorescein, indicated that individual myotubes and individual myofibrils at an early stage of development contain all three myosins—fast white, slow and cardiac (Masaki and Yoshizaki,

1974). Similar immunological distinctions can be made between the light chains of different mammalian myosins, and these fluorescein-labelled antibodies indicate that fast white and slow myosin also occur together at an early stage of development (Gauthier, Lowey and Hobbs, 1978).

In contrast, Rubinstein, Pepe and Holtzer (1977), using an immunoprecipitation technique, found that embryonic chick pectoralis muscle (a fast muscle in the adult) contained only fast-type myosin, while embryonic anterior lattissimus dorsi (a slow muscle in adult) contained both types and there was a progressive decrease in the proportion of fast myosin during its development. The authors suggested that myosin similar to the adult fast type is synthesised initially in both presumptive fast and slow muscles, and only at a later stage is slow myosin synthesised, probably as a result of innervation.

These contrasting results may be due to the different immunochemical techniques used. Immunofluorescence is highly sensitive and detects both soluble and precipitable complexes, but its reliability depends crucially on the purity of the antibody. Gauthier et al. (1978) used highly purified antigens and the antibodies raised were purified by immunoadsorption and affinity chromatography. The procedure of immunoprecipitation to identify complexes, as used by Rubinstein et al. (1977), can fail to detect non-precipitable or low-affinity reactions.

Biochemical techniques

In recent years, increasingly sophisticated methods for the isolation and characterisation of proteins have been developed. Many of these procedures have been scaled down or used in conjunction with radioactive labelling to investigate the synthesis of specific proteins during myogenesis in tissue culture.

Myosin. Paterson and Strohman (1972) developed a technique capable of detecting the synthesis of very small quantities of radioactively labelled myosin. Myosin from $3–6 \times 10^6$ chick embryo cells in culture was extracted with a small volume of high-salt buffer and the total extract mixed with adult myosin and electrophoresed on SDS-acrylamide gels. The amount of radioactive myosin co-electrophoresing with the large subunit of the adult myosin was determined. Making certain assumptions, it was calculated that it was possible to detect the synthesis of as little as 75 myosin molecules per cell, or less than one-half of one thick filament per cell per hour. Myosin synthesis was measured using this technique, both in these cultures and rat embryo muscle cells (Yaffe and Dym, 1972) before, during and after a period of rapid cell fusion leading to the formation of myotubes. Before fusion, myosin synthesis was virtually undetectable, but began at a linearly increasing rate with a lag period of approximately 4 h after fusion. Cultures treated with EGTA for up to 60 h to block fusion did not synthesise myosin (Paterson and Strohmann, 1972). Emerson and Beckner (1975) also found that dividing quail myoblasts did not synthesise very much myosin heavy chain, but that during the period of fusion there was substantial synthesis. However, myosin synthesis was activated in myoblasts (which had been prevented, by EGTA, from fusing) to reach rates similar to those attained in myotubes. This activation occurred under conditions in which EGTA-inhibited myoblasts were induced to withdraw from the cell-division cycle by reducing the concentration of the serum and embryo extract components of the culture medium. Emerson and Beckner (1975) therefore concluded that the activation of myosin synthesis in myoblasts does not require fusion, but is coordinated with the withdrawal from the cell cycle.

Recent work by Moss and Strohmann (1976) and Vertel and Fischman (1976) indicated that, when post-mitotic fusion-blocked myogenic cells are maintained in culture for longer periods, they do synthesise and accumulate myosin at rates comparable to those in normally differentiated myotubes. There seems, therefore, to be a consensus that cell fusion is not a prerequisite for the activation of myosin synthesis during skeletal muscle myogenesis.

However, Holtzer and his co-workers (Chi et al., 1975a, b) used scaled-down biochemical procedures to extract myosin and actomyosin from chick cultures, and found that there were different isoenzymatic forms present at different stages of differentiation. The ratio of myosin to actin and the type of myosin light chain in replicating mononucleate cells (myoblasts and fibroblasts) was different from that in fusion-blocked myoblasts and myotubes. The authors suggested that one set of structural genes for the myosin light and heavy chains was active in dividing cells and another set in fusion-blocked myoblasts and myotubes.

Holtzer and co-workers (Chi *et al.*, 1975a, b) also reported that the molar ratios of the myosin light chains of myotube myosin and the specific Ca^{++} ATPase were similar to those of adult fast myosin (*see also* Sreter, Holtzer, Gergely and Holtzer, 1972).

John and Jones (1975) found that radioactively labelled myosin from rat myotubes in culture contained only two light chains which co-electrophoresed with the LC_1 and LC_2 light chains of adult rat fast myosin. Consistently, there was a high proportion of label in the heavy chain compared with the light chains (13:1). The adult rat myosin preparation had a heavy chain to light chain (LC_1 and LC_2) ratio of 4:1, determined by densitometry, suggesting that in myotube myosin either the overall proportion of light chains is less, or the timing of synthesis or turnover differs from that of the heavy chain. Direct analysis of myosin extracted from a large number of cells suggested that there is a reduced proportion of light chains (H.A. John and K.W. Jones, unpublished work). The specific Ca^{++}-ATPase of myotube myosin was very low 0.011 μmol ADP/mg myosin/min) compared with that for adult rat myosin (0.38 μmol ADP/mg/min). No labelled myosin could be detected in dividing cultures.

There are a number of reports suggesting that myosin or actomyosin may be affected in muscular dystrophy. Samaha and Gergely (1969) found that the Mg^{++}-ATPase activity of actomyosin from patients with Duchenne dystrophy was low and the degree of superprecipitation was lower than normal, indicating involvement of the contractile apparatus at least in the later stages of the disease. In the case of dystrophy induced by vitamin E deficiency in rabbits, the specific Ca^{++}-ATPase activity of adult myosin decreased to a lower level characteristic of fetal myosin and this was correlated with a reduction in the relative amount of the myosin light chain LC_3 (Lobley, Perry and Stone, 1971; Perrie, Smillie and Perry, 1972). John (1974; 1976) also found a reduction in the specific Ca^{++}-ATPase and in the relative amount of LC_3 in the myosin of the dystrophic mouse. Decreased myosin ATPase activity and abnormality in the light chain pattern purified from biopsies of a patient with nemaline myopathy has been reported (Sreter, Astrom, Romanul, Young and Jones, 1976).

Investigations of tissue culture myogenesis have indicated that rat myotubes *in vitro* do not contain the LC_3 light chain (John and Jones, 1975; Yablonka and Yaffe, 1976). Further investigation of the factors that control the synthesis of this myosin light chain, using the tissue culture system, may be relevant to understanding why this particular chain is affected *in vivo* in a number of dystrophic conditions.

Total protein synthesis showed a significant decrease (half of control values) in muscle cultures from patients with Duchenne muscular dystrophy, but this was not due to a difference in synthesis of myosin heavy chain, which was the same in both normal and dystrophic cultures (Ionasescu *et al.*, 1976).

The thin filament proteins: actin, tropomyosin and troponin. The technique of isoelectric focusing enabled Whalen, Butler-Browne and Gros (1976) to discover that actin exists in three forms (α, β and γ) possessing similar biochemical properties and identical molecular weights but having slightly different isoelectric points. Two of the forms (β and γ) are found in prefusion dividing cells and also in cultured non-myogenic cells. The third form (α) is the only one found in fetal muscle tissue and is predominant in myotube cultures. Thus it would seem that actin can exist in several polymorphic forms, of which one is specific to fused muscle tissue.

The high-resolution two-dimensional electrophoresis technique (O'Farrell, 1975) has been used to study protein synthesis at different stages of myogenesis in culture (Whalen *et al.*, 1976; Devlin and Emerson, 1978; Storti, Horovitch, Scott, Rich and Pardue, 1978). Whalen *et al.* (1976) found that, although a significant number of differences are found between proteins synthesised in dividing and fused calf-cell cultures, most protein species were synthesised at both stages. Storti *et al.* (1978) identified three distinct classes of proteins in *Drosophila* myogenesis: most proteins were synthesised throughout myogenesis, the synthesis of some was initiated during myogenesis and others were synthesised at specific during myogenesis. Storti *et al.* (1978) also found that three forms of actin could be identified in culture, one of which showed increased synthesis concomitant with myogenesis and was considered to be a muscle-specific form of actin.

Devlin and Emerson (1978) measured the synthesis of specific proteins by autoradiography and fluorography of two-dimensional gels using a scanning densitometer. Contractile proteins synthesised by quail muscle cell cultures were identified by co-electrophoresis with purified contractile proteins. The results showed that synthesis of myosin heavy chain, two myosin light chains, two sub-units of troponin and two subunits of tropomyosin was first detected at the time of myoblast fusion and then increased at least 500-fold to maximum rates which remained constant in myotubes. Both the kinetics of activation and the molar rates of synthesis of these contractile proteins were virtually identical. Muscle-specific actin (α) synthesis also increased at the time of myoblast fusion, but this actin was synthesised at three times the rate of the other contractile proteins. The synthesis rate of 30 other muscle cell proteins was measured, and most of these were shown to follow different patterns of regulation. The authors concluded that the synthesis of the contractile proteins is regulated coordinately during myoblast differentiation.

John (1976) found that myofibrils from the skeletal muscle of adult dystrophic mice had a Mg^{++}-ATPase activity and myosin light chain LC_3 content at an intermediate level between normal and adult fetal myofibrils. However, the content of α-tropomyosin, the type of troponin and the inhibition of Mg^{++}-ATPase due to EGTA (which reflects the functioning of the troponin–tropomyosin complex) did not differ from normal. The weight ratio of myosin heavy chain to actin was not altered in dystrophic muscle.

Creatine phosphokinase. The characteristic isoenzyme transitions of creatine phosphokinase (CPK) known to occur in developing muscle *in vivo* have been demonstrated in extracts of cultured myogenic cells. The technique of cellulose polyacetate electrophoresis followed by specific staining has been used to show that the replacement of embryonic BB-CPK in dividing cultures by MM-CPK in myotube cultures begins in fusion-blocked cells (Turner, Gmur, Siegrist, Burckhardt and Eppenberger, 1976). However, Morris, Piper and Cole (1976), using a combination of electrophoresis and a fluorimetric technique which allowed measurement of low levels of CPK isoenzymes, showed that the early increase in CPK activity during early stages of fusion is of the embryonic BB type, and only later does the adult muscle form make a major contribution to the total increase in enzyme activity. A further investigation (Morris and Cole, 1977) of increased CPK activity after incubation of cells with radioactive amino acids indicated that, while increases in MM-CPK during differentiation involved *de novo* enzyme synthesis, the early increases in BB-CPK do not, but presumably reflect activation of existing enzyme.

An elevated serum CPK level is a sensitive indicator of muscular dystrophy (Ebashi, Toyokura, Momoi and Sugita, 1959). The presence of fetal and hybrid forms of CPK in muscle in human and animal genetic dystrophies has been shown by Schapira (1967). In dystrophy induced by vitamin E deficiency in adult rabbits, fetal and hybrid forms of CPK reappear (Perry, 1971).

Weinstock and Jones (1977) investigated CPK in dystrophic chick embryo muscle cells in tissue culture. In dystrophic cultures, CPK activities increased to higher levels than those of controls, before declining. In the medium from dystrophic cultures, CPK activity increased markedly at the same time that cellular CPK was rapidly decreasing. Maximum CPK activities in the medium of dystrophic cultures were, on average, two and a half times greater than in controls. In controls there was no consistent correlation between maximum CPK in the medium, and any phase of cellular CPK activity.

Specialised membrane components. The differentiation of muscle in tissue culture involves the elaboration of several specialised membrane components, including the acetylcholine receptor (Fambrough and Rash, 1971; Patrick, Heinemann, Lindstrom, Schubert and Steinbach, 1972; Vogel, Sytkowski and Nirenberg, 1972) and acetylcholinesterase (Oh and Johnson, 1972; Fluck and Strohman, 1973). Prives and Paterson (1974) found that acetylcholine receptor, acetylcholinesterase and adenylate cyclase appeared concurrently in both control and fusion-arrested cultures, suggesting that the differentiation of skeletal muscle cell membranes involves the coordinated synthesis of discrete membrane components.

The biopsynthesis of the Ca^{++}- and Mg^{++}-dependent adenosine triphosphatase (ATPase) of the sarcoplasmic reticulum has also been used as a criterion for muscle-cell differentiation. Holland and MacLennan (1976) estimated rates of synthesis at various stages of differentiation from the incorporation of tritium-labelled leucine into the ATPase which was isolated by antibody precipitation and the enzyme separated by electrophoresis. Synthesis of the sarcoplasmic reticulum ATPase was greatly accelerated as rat myoblasts fuse and differentiate into myotubes, but synthesis also occurred in fusion-blocked cells. The concentration of the Ca^{++}-Mg^{++}-ATPase measured by selective labelling of the enzyme with ^{32}P ATP also began to increase during fusion of chick myogenic cells (Martonosi, Roufa, Boland, Reyes and Tillack, 1977).

It has been suggested that Duchenne muscular dystrophy may be due to a generalised membrane abnormality (Rowland, 1976; Bosmann, Gerston, Griggs, Howland, Hudecki, Katyare and McLaughlin, 1976) which may show itself not only in muscle tissue but in all cells. Morphological, physicochemical and biochemical changes have been described mainly in studies of the erythrocyte cell membrane (Ch. 12). Some of the proteins that have been found to be abnormal have been studied in tissue culture. For example, Mawatari, Miranda and Rowland (1976) found that the adenyl cyclase activity of fused dystrophic cultures was twice that of fused normal cultures. In normal cultures the high activity of dividing cultures fell after fusion.

Human patients with myasthenia gravis have antibodies against acetylcholine receptors in their sera, and their muscles exhibit reduced miniature end-plate potential amplitudes, a reduced sensitivity to acetylcholine and contain decreased amounts of receptor (see Heinemann, Bevan, Kullberg, Lindstrom and Rice, 1977). Human myasthenic sera reduced acetylcholine sensitivity of human myotubes in tissue culture (Bevan, Kullberg and Heinemann, 1977; Bevan, Kullberg and Rice, 1978). This reduction was thought to result from some action on ACh receptors of the antireceptor antibodies. Although the myasthenic serum reduced ACh sensitivity by about 95 per cent, this reduction was not caused by altered conductance of ACh-activated channels. When ACh receptor content was assayed by measurement of ^{125}I-labelled α-bungarotoxin binding, and acetylcholine receptor function was assayed by the sensitivity to acetylcholine iontophoresis in rat cells treated with myasthenic serum, the results suggested that the antibodies may contribute to the functional defects of neuromuscular transmission by accelerating the rate of internalisation and degradation of surface membrane ACh receptors (Appel, Anwyl, McAdams and Elias, 1977).

Conclusions

If a genetic myopathological condition is an intrinsic lesion of the muscle cell it is possible that it would be manifested as a missing or abnormal protein. However, such detectable differences found in vivo and in tissue culture should be interpreted with caution for the reasons discussed below.

It is now established that different polymorphic forms of a protein appear at different stages of muscle development. Perry (1971) has pointed out that, in some types of muscular dystrophy, certain isoenzymes are found in proportions typical of fetal tissue. The presence of fetal isoenzymes may be due to a reversion or arrest of the normal developmental process as suggested by Perry (1971). Alternatively, it may reflect the areas of regenerating tissue, presumably at a stage equivalent to that of fetal tissue, which may be present in pathological muscle. Whatever the explanation, it is possible that some differences that are detectable in proteins may be attributable to the occurrence of different polymorphic forms.

Different isoenzymatic or polymorphic forms of many proteins are also present at different stages of myogenesis in tissue culture. Furthermore, it is known that many of the proteins which were once considered characteristic of muscle cells (e.g. myosin and actin) are found in many non-myogenic cells. Obviously, methods for detecting the muscle-specific form of a protein in tissue culture cells are essential and the importance of comparing cultures at similar stages of morphological differentiation, and with similar proportions of non-myogenic cells, cannot be over-emphasised.

An important consideration is whether a protein difference found *in vivo* will still be apparent in cultured muscle cells. Acid-maltase deficiency (Pompe's disease) is a well-defined inherited metabolic myopathy caused by the absence of α-1-4 glucosidase. Askanas, Engel, Di Mauro, Brooks and Mehler (1976) found that myotubes in muscle cultures from an adult patient contained vacuoles, positive to acid phosphatase, that increased in size and number in older cultures. Ultrastructural changes in myotubes closely resembled changes found in the biopsy, with an increased number of membrane-bound vacuoles containing glycogen. Acid maltase was not detectable in these cultures when maltose was used as a substrate, but a low level of activity was detected with the artificial substrate 4-methylumbelliferyl-α-D-glucoside, suggesting that the molecular defect was the production of an abnormal enzyme rather than total absence of the enzyme.

In contrast, Roelofs, Engel and Chauvin (1972) found that phosphorylase activity reappeared in myotubes cultured from biopsies of phosphorylase-deficient muscle (McArdle's disease). The reappearance of phosphorylase seemed to be related to regeneration and not to culture conditions, as a second biopsy taken at the site of the initial one showed that regenerating fibres *in vivo* had also recovered phosphorylase activity. Similarly, Delain (1972) found that the M4 isoenzyme of lactate dehydrogenase was absent from dystrophic chick muscle and present in normal muscle *in vivo*, but was found in both normal and dystrophic cultures, suggesting that synthesis of the M4 subunit is repressed in the adult dystrophic chicken and de-repressed in culture.

Any protein, the appearance of which *in vivo* is normally correlated with the differentiation of physiologically different muscle fibres *in vivo* would be unlikely to be detectable in tissue culture, because so far no differentiation of fibre types has been obtained in tissue culture (Askanas, Shafiq and Milhorat, 1972; Askanas and Engel, 1975).

TRANSCRIPTION

During the differentiation of muscle, certain gene sequences in chromosomal DNA (the muscle-specifying genes) are transcribed into messenger RNA, which passes from the nucleus to the cytoplasm before being translated into muscle-specific proteins. To find out how this process occurs is an indispensable step towards an understanding of the nature of the controlling elements in myogenesis. Investigations of RNA metabolism in tissue culture myogenesis have helped to illuminate this process.

Although earlier investigators had been technically unable to resolve all the different classes of RNA, there was a strong indication that RNA metabolism altered during myogenesis in tissue culture.

Several workers have reported that, following cell fusion during myogenesis, there is a reduction in the rate of RNA synthesis. On the basis of autoradiographic studies, Yaffe and Fuchs (1967) suggested that a decrease in the rate of incorporation of radioactive precursors into RNA occurred as myogenic cells fused to form syncytia. Coleman and Coleman (1968) also found that, in autoradiographs, syncytial cell nuclei had fewer grains than did mononuclear cell nuclei after a 20- or 30-minute incubation in ^{3}H-uridine. Furthermore, in the mononucleate cell population, bipolar cells had a considerably lower incorporation rate than did fibroblastic cells. Coleman and Coleman (1968) also compared the rate of incorporation into acid-precipitable RNA, in cultures in which a pure population of myotubes was maintained by 5-fluorodeoxyuridine, with control cultures which contained many mononucleate cells, and found a lower rate of incorporation in the former cultures. Gallup *et al.* (1972) reported an autoradiographic investigation of RNA synthesis during myogenesis in cultures of human, chick and rat muscle. Species differences were observed in the comparative rate of incorporation by the multinucleate and mononucleate cells (synthesis was estimated by grain counts). In human cultures the multinucleates were labelled more than the mononucleates; in chick cultures they were labelled to the same extent and in rat cultures the multinucleates were less labelled than mononucleates.

Messenger RNA

A number of discoveries have led to substantial progress in investigations of messenger RNA (mRNA). The presence of polyadenylated (polyA) sequences at the 3′ end in most mRNA and its absence from ribosomal and transfer RNA provides a method for distinguishing between, and separating, these types of RNA. PolyA has the capacity to form complementary base-paired structures with polyT or polyU, and this property has been exploited in affinity chromatography to provide a highly specific and simple means of separating mRNA from other RNA species. This chromatographic technique utilises the ability of the polyA segments that are an integral part of the mRNA molecule to hybridise selectively and reversibly to synthetic oligo dT or polyU chains immobilised on a solid support such as cellulose (Aviv and Leder, 1972). Isolated mRNA can be efficiently translated into proteins in cell-free systems derived from reticulocytes (Pelham and Jackson, 1976) or wheat germ (Roberts and Paterson, 1973) before characterisation of the protein.

Most RNAs have the capacity to act as templates in the synthesis of complementary DNA copies (referred to as cDNA) using the enzyme reverse transcriptase obtained from avian myeloblastosis virus (Kacian, Spiegelman, Bank, Terada, Metafora, Dow and Marks, 1972; Verna, Temple, Fan and Baltimore, 1972). Radioactive cDNA specific for muscle mRNA has proved a most valuable probe for a variety of operations. The kinetics of hydridisation of the complementary DNA with an excess of the mRNA from which it was made indicates how many different mRNA sequences are present, while reassociation of the cDNA to an excess of the DNA of the genome can indicate approximately how many copies of each gene occur. The cDNA can also be used as a probe to detect and measure the number of molecules of the mRNA produced at different stages of differentiation in culture. Finally, the cDNA can be hybridised to mRNA in cytological preparations (the technique of *in situ* hybridisation) to reveal the distribution of mRNA in individual muscle cells at different stages in myogenesis. This technique can permit a clearer interpretation of the kinetics of mRNA synthesis, to identify the cells in which synthesis is first initiated and to determine the sites of concentration within the cell.

Thus, with the preparation of mRNA for muscle-specific proteins, it is now possible to analyse specific components of the transcriptional and translational system of the differentiating muscle cell. A major aim of such investigations has been to understand the mechanism of gene regulation during differentiation. Two mechanisms have been proposed for the regulation of new genes expressed. First, there is transcriptional control, in which changes in the pattern of RNA synthesis lead to qualitative or quantitative alterations in the pool of mRNA sequences that are available to the protein-synthesising machinery. It is implied that the concentration of a particular mRNA sequence in the cell determines, for the most part, the rate of synthesis of the corresponding protein. Second, there is translational control, in which gene expression is modulated by a mechanism that selects or activates particular mRNA sequences from a pre-existing pool of untranslated mRNA.

Transcriptional control. Cytoplasmic polyadenylated mRNA from differentiated muscle cultures, when incubated in a cell-free translation system, has been shown to direct the synthesis of actin (Paterson, Roberts and Yaffe, 1974), myosin heavy chain (Strohman, Moss, Micou-Eastwood, Spector, Przybyla and Paterson, 1977) and tropomyosin (Carmon, Neuman and Yaffe, 1978). The relative amount of the mRNA increased dramatically at cell fusion in each case. Fusion was a prerequisite for transcription at least of actin mRNA (Paterson *et al.*, 1974). In all cases, the amount of protein synthesised in the cell-free system was proportional to the rate of the protein synthesis in the cultures from which the RNA was extracted, suggesting that the synthesis of these three proteins is regulated by the respective mRNA content of the cell.

Paterson and Bishop (1977) detected changes in the sequence complexity, distribution of abundance classes and coding capacity of the total mRNA population of primary chick embryo muscle cultures during myogenesis. The change from myoblast to myotube resulted in the appearance of a new abundant class consisting of six different mRNA sequences, each present in 15 000 copies per cell, and a complete change in mRNA abundance class distribution. The increased synthesis of the major muscle structural proteins in myotubes was correlated with increased synthesis of these proteins in a cell-free system in response to total cellular RNA. The synthesis of these proteins was due to the new abundant class of mRNA found in the myotube. These findings suggested that the synthesis of the muscle-specific proteins was controlled mainly at the transcriptional level.

Translational control. Yaffe and Dym (1972) had found that when actinomycin D, at a concentration that blocks RNA synthesis, was added to cultures at, or just before, fusion, the appearance of muscle-specific proteins was not blocked immediately. This observation raised the question of possible accumulation of muscle-specific mRNA in the myoblast before fusion.

In dividing calf myoblast cultures, when myosin synthesis was very low, there was a high level of polyadenylated 26S RNA (Buckingham, Caput, Cohen, Whalen and Gros, 1974), the size of the putative mRNA for the large sub-unit of myosin (Heywood and Nwagwu, 1969). In the transition period before fusion, there was a pronounced production of 26S RNA which diminished during fusion. At fusion, the rate of turnover of the 26S and other mRNA species decreased. The authors proposed that the transition to the differentiated myotube that synthesises muscle-specific proteins is effected by the stabilisation of mRNA already being transcribed.

In a later investigation, Buckingham, Cohen and Gros (1976) demonstrated that the short-lived 26S RNA from dividing myoblasts was present in

ribonucleoprotein particles which do not enter the heavy polysomes. In contrast, the more stable 26S RNA, also initially present as a ribonucleoprotein particle, just before and in the early stages of fusion was shown to enter the heavy polysomes known to synthesise the myosin heavy chain later in fusion.

In independent studies, Heywood, Kennedy and Bester (1975) and Bag and Sarkar (1976) reported that 12-day chick embryonic leg muscle *in vivo* (at a time preceding extensive fusion) contained a considerable amount of myosin mRNA stored in ribonucleoprotein particles. When the mRNA was purified from these particles it could translate myosin heavy chain in a cell-free system.

Further evidence for the presence of untranslated mRNA comes from the studies of Yablonka and Yaffe (1976) who found that, although rat myogenic cells synthesised two myosin light chains only, polyadenylated RNA extracted from the same cells directed the synthesis of the third light chain in a cell-free system. These results suggested that the mRNA for the third light chain was present in the intact cell, but not expressed because of translational control.

Heywood and his colleagues have proposed two mechanisms by which muscle-specific protein synthesis may be controlled at a post-transcriptional level. First, the message may be kept in an inert form (stored mRNA or messenger ribonucleoprotein particle); a small RNA molecule termed translational control RNA is involved in this repression (Bester, Kennedy and Heywood, 1975). Second, muscle tissue-specific initiation factors are necessary so that mRNA may bind to ribosomes and translation of proteins may be initiated (Bester *et al.*, 1975).

Conclusions. Investigations of mRNA synthesis during muscle differentiation have been interpreted to indicate that gene expression may be controlled at either the transcriptional or translational level. There are a number of assumptions which affect these conclusions.

In experiments where the synthesis of muscle-specific proteins in cell-free systems is used as an assay of the level of translatable mRNA the following assumptions are made. First, it is assumed that all mRNA present at all culture times is in fact, translatable and that no mRNA exists in an inactive (stored) form that is not converted to an active form by the isolation procedure and/or by the translation machinery of the cell-free system. Second, it is assumed that the RNA from one culture condition does not contain inhibitors for translation that are not present in other culture conditions.

Although Buckingham *et al.* (1974; 1976) reported that cultures of calf muscle yield 26S mRNA which has many of the characteristics expected of myosin heavy chain mRNA, these investigators had not translated the mRNA in a cell-free system.

Investigations of muscle-specific mRNA have not really resolved whether the fusion of adjacent myoblasts is necessary for the transcription to begin or whether there is just enhancement of an existing low level of transcription.

John, Patrinou-Georgoulas and Jones (1977) have approached these controversial questions by direct measurement and detection of myosin heavy chain mRNA (MHCmRNA) in chick myogenic cultures by *in vitro* and *in situ* hybridisation using a cDNA copy of highly purified and characterised mRNA (Patrinou-Georgoulas and John, 1977). The technique of *in situ* hybridisation enables individual cells in mixed populations to be analysed, a valuable approach in a potentially complex situation such as tissue culture. The method is independent of morphological criteria to define cell function, so that morphologically aberrant cell types can be defined and analysed.

The majority of cells in replicating mononucleate myogenic cell cultures contained no detectable MHCmRNA. The detection of MHCmRNA in fusion-blocked mononucleate cells indicated that fusion was not a necessary event for the transcription of muscle MHCmRNA. However, the number of MHCmRNA molecules per nucleus was higher in myotubes, suggesting that fusion may enhance mRNA transcription (Fig. 10.3).

The organisation of the muscle-specific genes

Reassociation analyses of DNA have demonstrated that sequences occur in three classes: highly repetitive, moderately repetitive and non-repetitive (single copy). Paterson and Bishop (1977) found that an abundant class of myotube mRNA contains six types of mRNA molecules in exceptionally high concentration and these were responsible for the synthesis of the major myofibrillar proteins. Between 20–30 per cent of the abundant mRNA (3–5 per cent of the total mRNA population) was apparently transcribed from

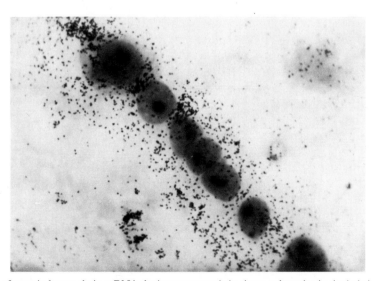

Fig. 10.3 Detection of myosin heavy chain mRNA during myogenesis in tissue culture by *in situ* hybridisation of myosin heavy chain cDNA to cytological preparations of cells

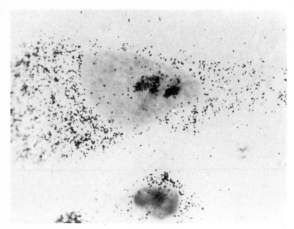

Fig. 10.4   Myotubes showing nucleolar localisation of myosin heavy chain mRNA detected by *in situ* hybridisation of myosin heavy chain cDNA

moderately repetitive DNA sequences. The remainder of the abundant, and all the less abundant mRNA, was transcribed from single-copy DNA. It therefore seems likely that there is moderate repetition of the genes of one or two of the major myofibrillar proteins. This may be repetition to meet the demand for a high concentration of these particular proteins. An alternative explanation is that there may be several almost identical polymorphic forms of a protein, the corresponding mRNAs of which differ so little that they cannot be differentiated by hybridisation kinetics.

Recent reports have shown that some genes are split into segments, each coding for part of a protein. The intervening segments are transcribed, but later excised, and the mRNA is spliced together again before translation into protein begins. This processing of the pre-mRNA takes place in the nucleus (*see* Nordstrom, Roop, Tsai and O'Malley, 1979). Little is known about the intranuclear metabolism of muscle-specific mRNA at present. However, it may be significant that nucleolar localisation of MHCmRNA was observed using *in situ* hybridisation of cDNA (Fig. 10.4), suggesting an involvement of the nucleolus in mRNA metabolism (John *et al.*, 1977). The involvement of the nucleolus in cytoplasmic expression of specific proteins has been suggested from experiments involving the irradiation of nucleoli in cell hybrids with ultra-violet microbeams (Harris, Sidebottom, Grace and Bramwell, 1969).

Ribosomal RNA

Ribosomes are a vital component in protein biosynthesis. The ribosome content of somatic cells can be regulated by control of ribosomal RNA (rRNA) transcription, by degradation of rRNA or by turnover of cytoplasmic ribosomes. Different cell types use different combinations of these mechanisms for regulation.

Myoblasts do not enter a resting state at the time of fusion but irreversibly lose the capacity for cell division and yet remain highly active in protein synthesis.

Previous studies of embryonic and cultured muscle have indicated that ribosome accumulation ceases after fusion (Hosik and Strohman, 1971). In addition, incorporation of radioactive precursors into rRNA decreased after fusion (Yaffe and Fuchs, 1967; Coleman and Coleman, 1968; Man and Cole, 1972) and myotubes formed excess 30S rRNA molecules which were degraded during processing to 28S rRNA (Clissold and Cole, 1973). These observations suggested that ribosome accumulation in myotubes was regulated by a decrease in the transcription of RNA and by degradation of rRNA during processing.

Bowman and Emerson (1977) have investigated the extent to which transcription and processing of rRNA quantitatively regulate ribosome accumulation during myoblast differentiation and have also examined the role of ribosome turnover in this regulation. The rates of accumulation of rRNA and ribosomes decreased in cultures after quail myoblasts fused. The mechanisms which regulated ribosome accumulation in myotubes were the turnover of 28S and 18S rRNA and the degradation of newly synthesised rRNA during processing.

RNA synthesis in muscle disease

There have been few investigations of RNA synthesis in diseased muscle in tissue culture.

Autoradiographic investigations of RNA synthesis (Gallup *et al.*, 1972) showed no differences in cultures from normal and Duchenne human muscle, suggesting that, in culture, diseased muscle is capable of normal RNA metabolism.

Ross and Parsons (1973) made densitometric measurements of total RNA of cells from a single biopsy from a patient and compared these with cells from a single control biopsy. They found that the total RNA content of dystrophic cells was higher than that of normal cells, but they did not state whether these measurements were made on myotubes or mononucleate cells. In earlier studies, Ross and his colleagues (*reviewed in* Ross, Jones and John, 1974) found that nucleolar dry weight determined by densitometry was found to be lower in mononucleate cells derived from mouse dystrophic muscle explants.

RNA sequence complexities of normal and dystrophic mouse tissues were measured to determine whether or not the disease process altered the transcriptional diversity of normal development (Grouse, Nelson, Omenn and Schrier, 1978). It was found that dystrophic muscles contained a 60 per cent higher concentration (per mg of total RNA) of complex, low-frequency RNA species than did control muscles, although the complexities of dystrophic and control muscles were not distinguishable. Total cellular RNAs from spinal cord, brain and liver of dystrophic mice were also found to have RNA complexities which were indistinguishable from the same tissues in normal mice.

FACTORS AFFECTING THE EXPRESSION OF MUSCLE-SPECIFIC GENES IN CULTURED CELLS

Gene expression during the differentiation of muscle is influenced by many intrinsic and extrinsic factors.

Intrinsic factors

The role of intrinsic factors in inheritance of the epigenetic state. One of the remarkable things about the differentiation of cells is that, in many cases, once a cell has been induced to take up a differentiated state it can divide repeatedly and still apparently 'remember' its particular state of differentiation. The fact that a muscle cell, for example, can reproduce itself under relatively non-specific culture conditions without converting to some other cell type, suggests that muscle cells *in vivo* are not being continuously induced by humoral influences to maintain their particular state of differentiation. It is possible that cells

remember their cell type in tissue culture by, for instance, simply continuing to translate mRNA already present in the cells at the time that they are explanted. That this is not the case is shown by the existence of myogenic cell lines which retain the ability to differentiate after a number of divisions in culture sufficient to have diluted out all the molecules originally present. In some way the differentiated state is self-replicating.

An interesting approach to understanding how the state of differentiation is 'remembered' (inheritance of the epigenetic state) has been made in experiments in which muscle cells are induced to fuse with non-muscle cells using inactivated Sendai virus. Carlsson, Ringertz and Savage (1974) found that the dormant nucleus of a chick erythrocyte was reactivated when introduced into a rat myoblast. Activation of both RNA and DNA synthesis was observed. Rat antigens characteristic of nucleoplasm and nucleoli migrated into chick erythrocyte nuclei in rat myoblast × chick erythrocyte heterokaryons. It was postulated that these antigens might represent a class of molecules instrumental in activating chick genes and that, furthermore, the erythrocyte nuclei might possibly be reprogrammed for gene expression as in the case of the rat nuclei which specified the migrating molecules. However, chick myosin could not be detected in the heterokaryons by immunological methods (Carlsson, Luger, Ringertz and Savage, 1974). In contrast, Guinness (1973) found that chick erythrocyte nuclei could be specifically reactivated by fusion into rat myotubes where they began to direct the synthesis of chicken myosin as detected by immunological methods. The latter investigation indicated that the signals controlling the muscle-specific genes present in rat muscle cells can be received and acted upon by chicken erythrocyte nuclei. This activation of an inert nucleus was trans-specific, suggesting that the signals controlling differentiated functions of cells are highly conserved in evolution, implying that essential features of the genes responsible for the control are undiverged over the period of evolutionary time separating chickens and rats.

Critical final mitosis. Terminal differentiation of myogenic cultures is characterised by cell fusion to form multinucleated myotubes, cessation of DNA synthesis with irreversible withdrawal from the cell cycle, and production of muscle-specific proteins.

There are two lines of evidence which demonstrate that, when myoblasts fuse into syncytia, the nuclei do not again divide. First, nuclei within multinucleated myotubes do not incorporate tritiated thymidine into DNA nor are mitotic figures ever observed (Stockdale and Holtzer, 1961). Second, microspectrophotometric measurements of DNA content per nucleus reveal that all the nuclei within multinucleated myotubes contain only the diploid (2N) complement of DNA (Strehler, Konigsberg and Kelley, 1963).

Holtzer and his co-workers (Bischoff and Holtzer, 1969; Holtzer, Sanger, Ishikawa and Strahs, 1972; Dienstmann and Holtzer, 1977) have postulated that the transition of a myogenic cell from an actively dividing undifferentiated cell to a post-mitotic cell capable of fusion and biochemical differentiation follows a special mitosis ('quantal' mitosis) during which, genes involved in cell proliferation are repressed and the genes needed for differentiation are switched on. The decision to differentiate is made during the phase of DNA synthesis (S) before the 'quantal' mitosis, and sets in motion the metabolic steps required for the subsequent fusion and biochemical differentiation which start during the G_1 phase after 'quantal' division. The major rearrangement of chromatin that occurs during S may make it a particularly suitable time for extensive changes in the genetic programme needed for differentiation.

Gurdon and Woodland (1968) have also proposed that a critical mitosis may precede differentiation. They argued that, only during mitosis, when the nuclear membrane disappears transiently, can proteins easily leave the nucleus, and can new proteins responsible for re-programming the genes move from the cytoplasm and bind to the decondensing chromosomes.

Holtzer and his co-workers postulated that the dividing, undifferentiated myogenic cell cannot transform into the post-mitotic myoblast without undergoing a critical 'quantal' mitosis. After this mitosis, one or both of the daughter cells is a post-mitotic myoblast. The theory predicts that myogenic cells have only one pathway open to them—either to divide or to differentiate—but not both.

The fact that the tissue culture environment can be manipulated so that cultured cells will either multiply or differentiate makes it possible to test the quantal mitosis theory. Some investigators (O'Neill and Stockdale, 1972; Buckley and Konigsberg, 1974) found that chick myogenic cultures which had ceased proliferating and in which differentiation was imminent, and which would presumably have undergone 'quantal' mitosis, could be stimulated to more DNA synthesis and cell division if they were given fresh medium. Inhibition of DNA synthesis did not prevent cell fusion (Doehring and Fischman, 1974). More recently, Nadal-Ginard (1978) found that DNA synthesis was not required to switch from growth to differentiation and that, after cell division, rat myogenic cell line myoblasts had the option either to fuse or to proliferate without intervening DNA synthesis. Furthermore, commitments to differentiation occurred in the G_1 before fusion.

In contrast, Dienstmann and Holtzer (1977) found that daily feeding did not prevent fusion and that inhibition of DNA synthesis in cells that normally would have multiplied *in vitro* did not prompt these cells to fuse.

Buckley and Konigsberg (1977) have presented data suggesting that, *in vivo*, myogenic cells do not withdraw from the cell cycle before fusion, but as a consequence of fusion. According to these investigators, the probability that a cell will fuse directly correlated to the length of time it spends in G_1 (Buckley and Konigsberg, 1974; Konigsberg, Sollmann and Mixter, 1978).

John *et al.* (1977) detected muscle-specific myosin heavy chain mRNA in myogenic cells undergoing mitosis, using the technique of *in situ* hybridisation (Fig. 10.5). If the presence of skeletal MHCmRNA in cells undergoing mitosis is a normal occurrence during myogenesis, it would suggest that withdrawal from the cell division cycle is not an inflexible pre-condition for the transcription of muscle-specific mRNAs.

The role of cyclic nucleotides. It has been suggested that the decision whether a cell continues to divide or becomes differentiated is determined by the intracellular concentration of cyclic AMP and cyclic GMP (*reviewed by* Hogan

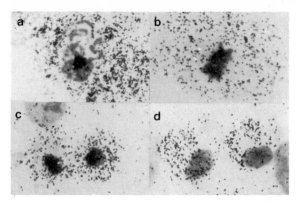

Fig. 10.5 Detection of myosin heavy chain mRNA by *in situ* hybridisation of myosin heavy chain cDNA to cells in different stages of mitosis in dividing myoblast cultures: (a) prophase; (b) metaphase; (c) telophase; (d) daughter cells

and Shields, 1974). These compounds are thought to act as chemical 'mediators' and their concentration would be determined by events at the cell membrane. High levels of cGMP and low levels of cAMP will favour rapid cell division, while low levels of cGMP and high cAMP will promote cell differentiation and slow cell division. Cyclic AMP is synthesised from its precursor ATP by an enzyme, adenylate cyclase, embedded in the outer cell membrane in close association with the receptor sites of different kinds of regulatory molecules such as hormones and prostaglandins.

Zalin and Montague (1974) observed a 10 to 15-fold spontaneous but transient increase in intracellular cAMP 5–6 h before the onset of fusion in primary chick myoblasts. This correlated with an increase in adenylate cyclase activity. When myoblast DNA synthesis and differentiation were prevented by FUdR there was no increase in cAMP in the cultures, suggesting that DNA synthesis is necessary and there is a link between the myoblast cell cycle and the transient cAMP increase. Physiological concentrations of prostaglandin E_1 added to cultures produced a similar intracellular increase in cAMP, 4 h earlier than that occurring normally, and brought forward the fusion process by a corresponding 4 h. These results suggested that cAMP is acting as a signal for muscle-cell fusion. Two inhibitors of prostaglandin synthesis produced a marked inhibition of cell fusion which it was possible to reverse by the further addition of prostaglandin E_1 (Zalin,

1977). These findings provide evidence of prostaglandin synthesis in cultures and suggest that prostaglandin E_1 is required for the generation of a transient increase in intracellular cyclic AMP, which brings about the cellular changes necessary for fusion to occur.

Cyclic AMP is known to exert control by activating an enzyme called protein kinase, which transfers a phosphate group to other enzymes (phosphorylation), thus activating them. Scott and Dousa (1978) have shown that some cAMP-dependent protein phosphorylation enzymes are tightly bound to the plasma membrane in myoblasts of the L_6 cell line.

Myoblast fusion. Cell fusion is an event which is almost unique to myogenesis and is absent from the development of any other tissue in a higher organism. In the previous sections the question of whether fusion triggers off gene expression at the transcriptional and translational level has been considered. In summary, most evidence suggests that, when fusion is blocked, muscle-specific mRNA and proteins can still be synthesised. However, under normal circumstances it does seem that fusion is accompanied by a massive increase in transcription and translation. It is, therefore, worth considering what is known about the molecular events involved in the fusion process.

Holtzer and Sanger (1972) pointed out that fusion involves cell recognition and the restructuring of the cortices of juxtaposed cells. Alterations in the cell surface, its constituent and associated proteins during cell fusion have been reported.

Cloned cells of a myoblast line showed the presence of GM_3, GM_2, GM_1 and GD_{1a} gangliosides (Whatley, Ng, Rogers, McMurray and Sanwal, 1976). The amount of GM_3, GM_2 and GM_1 gangliosides did not vary significantly during the differentiation of myoblasts to myotubes. However, the concentration of GD_{1a} transiently increased almost three-fold just before the fusion of myoblasts, and returned to the basal levels in the myotubes. Mutant myoblasts, selected for 5-azacytidine resistance and unable to fuse, produced only GM_3 and traces of GM_2. It was concluded that GD_{1a} probably participates in the fusion process.

In a comparison of the morphological and biochemical characteristics of isolated plasma membrane, Scott (1978) found little difference between undifferentiated and differentiated L_6 myoblasts.

Soluble extracts of myoblast clone L_6 agglutinated trypsin-treated glutaraldehyde-fixed rabbit erythrocytes (Novak, Haywood and Barondes, 1976). Agglutination activity of L_6 myoblasts increased three-fold as the myoblasts fused to form multinucleated myotubes, suggesting the presence of developmentally regulated lectins. Agglutination activity was blocked by thiodigalactoside lactose and related saccharides, but not by many other saccharides.

Schudt and Pette (1976) added monosaccharide components of plasma membrane oligosaccharides to fusing cultures in order to study their possible participation in aggregation or fusion. As no inhibitory effects were observed, it was assumed that monosaccharides were not involved specifically in this type of cell–cell interaction.

Treatment of fusing myoblasts with neuraminidase and phospholipases A and C revealed strong inhibition of fusion (Schudt and Pette, 1976; Trotter and Nameroff, 1976).

Indirect immunofluorescence techniques have revealed that fibronectin is distributed on cell surfaces in a fibril-like structure (Wartiovaara, Linder, Ruoslathi and Vaheri, 1974). Using high-titre anti-fibronectin, Chen, Gallimore and McDougall (1976) showed that expression of fibronectin is primarily mediated by cell contact. Fibronectin was localised in cell–cell contact areas in two-day-old fibroblast cultures, and its progressive production leads to a massive network of fibrillar fibronectin. This observation suggested that fibronectin is a surface matrix protein involved in cell adhesion and not involved in other biological roles such as growth control.

An investigation by Chen (1977) of cell surface alterations during myogenesis indicated that, in pre-fusion myoblasts, fibronectin is distributed over the cells as a diffuse network. In post-fusion myotubes the fibrillar network of fibronectin disappears completely. The very small amount of surface fibronectin detectable on some myotubes exists as small discrete patches from 1–20 per myotube.

Creatine production–a positive feed-back effector of gene expression? To explain the fact that increased muscular activity results in hypertrophy of skeletal muscle, Ingwall and her colleagues (Ingwall, Morales and Stockdale, 1972; Ingwall, Weiner, Morales, Davis and Stockdale, 1974; Ingwall, 1976) have postulated that creatine, a unique product of muscle activity, stimulates synthesis of contractile proteins and muscle-specific isoenzymes. Skeletal muscle cells in monolayer cultures, or cells still within explants, synthesised the myosin heavy chain actin and muscle CPK faster when supplied with creatine. Well-developed myotubes are stimulated more than newly formed myotubes; the effect seems to be selective for myosin, actin and muscle CPK, because the rate of total protein synthesis and non-muscle CPK was unaffected, suggesting that creatine has some role other than involvement in a system energising general protein synthesis or in cell nutrition. The results were consistent with the idea that creatine is a positive feed-back effector in a system relating muscular activity and muscle-protein synthesis. The fact that decreased muscular activity leads to atrophy may be because creatine must be maintained at certain minimal levels, and this may be relevant to some studies of muscle disease.

Extrinsic factors

Neighbouring cells. The differentiation of a myogenic cell is almost certainly influenced by neighbouring myogenic cells and fibroblasts.

Neighbouring myogenic cells. One condition which precedes fusion in culture is the progressive increase in the muscle-cell population density. Konigsberg (1961) has suggested that population density might affect the initiation of fusion by either of two mechanisms. At the higher cell densities, cell-to-cell contacts might occur more frequently, thus increasing the probability of encounters between two cells competent to fuse. Alternatively, increased cell density would accelerate any alterations of the medium generated by the metabolic activities of the cells. In this way, high cell density might facilitate the establishment of a microenvironment, in some way more favourable for the initiation of fusion.

Earlier investigations to discriminate between these two possibilities led to the observation that medium withdrawn from confluent mass cultures supported the development of high proportions of well-differentiated muscle clones (Konigsberg, 1963). Later studies (Hauschka and Konigsberg, 1966) indicated that depositing a layer of collagen on the surface of the tissue culture dish could substitute for the use of 'conditioned medium'. However, Konigsberg (1970) subsequently observed that, when single quail myoblasts were cloned in the absence of collagen, the daughter cells tended to remain in close proximity. Under these conditions of high cell density, fusion occurred earlier than when a collagen substratum was present, and resulted in the formation of a minute clone in which most of the nuclei were in syncytial association.

Further studies (Konigsberg, 1971) of quail cell microcultures of uniform diameter positioned on collagen-treated dishes indicated a diffusion-mediated, cell density-dependent control over the time of initiation of fusion. The onset of fusion was delayed either by decreasing the inoculum size or by increasing the volume of the medium. Furthermore, initiation of fusion was also delayed by continuous circulation of the medium. This delay could be circumvented by increasing the initial cell density or by using media withdrawn from cultures of fusing myoblasts. These results suggested a transmission of the effect of cell density via the medium. Whenever fusion was experimentally delayed, proliferation continued, at an undiminished rate, for longer, generating a larger cell population. This indicated that, although close proximity was a necessary condition for fusion, it was not alone a sufficient condition. Fusion may be promoted by the accumulation of cell products or by the depletion of media constituents. The fusion-promoting activity in the medium did not pass through a dialysis membrane nor a Diaflo XM 300 membrane during ultrafiltration, indicating that the molecule or molecules involved were larger than a spherical molecule with a molecular weight of 300 000. The activity was not generated by fibroblasts, cardiac muscle or liver cells.

The results of Hauschka and White (1971) also indicated a cell density effect distinct from the collagen requirement. In these studies, a con-ditioned medium factor increased that percentage of clones from early embryonic muscle which could express their myogenic potential. Activity was also measured in the presence of a collagen substratum and seemed to reside in a non-dialysable, high molecular weight fraction.

Using a method for both collection and assay of 'conditioning' factors in a defined medium devoid of both serum and embryo extract, Doehring and Fischman (1977) demonstrated that conditioned medium activity is the result both of nutrient depletion and of the addition of macromolecules, probably protein in nature, with a molecular weight greater than 10 000. The active component was not released by other cell types in tissue culture, but was secreted by muscle cells, both pre- and post-fusion.

In contrast, Yeoh and Holtzer (1977) found no evidence that increased cell density induced precocious fusion in myogenic cells. The results of testing conditioned medium prepared by the method of Doehring and Fischman (1977) were less clear. During the early stages of primary cultures in conditioned medium there was more extensive myotube formation, but these cultures degenerated after day 4 in culture.

In tissue culture, myoblasts divide several times; subsequently, some fuse and produce cell-specific proteins while others (possibly analogous to the satellite cells *in vivo*) remain as mononucleate cells. When the cells from advanced cultures are transferred to new culture dishes it is presumably these mononucleate cells that resume myogenic activity, because whole syncytial myotubes will not normally stick down afresh. Some clue as to the mechanism which underlies this difference in myoblast behaviour has been provided by Nameroff and Holtzer (1969). Embryonic myogenic cells were readily induced to mimic the behaviour of satellite cells by seeding them on a variety of cellular substrates (e.g. 5-day cultures of muscle, cartilage or liver). On such substrates presumptive myoblasts did not migrate, fuse, replicate, or synthesise contractile proteins. However, when removed from the inactivating influence of these cellular substrates and subcultured, they migrated, multiplied and fused to form typical myotubes. Nameroff and Holtzer postulated that the extra-cellular polysaccharide matrix present is responsible for the observed behaviour.

Neighbouring fibroblasts. Fibroblasts are responsible for laying down the muscle connective tissue system which involves synthesis of large amounts of collagen. *In vivo*, muscle cells come to lie in bundles enclosed by layers of connective membranes: the endomysium or basement lamina surrounding each individual myotube, the perimysium enclosing a bundle of myotubes, and the epimysium which surrounds a whole series of bundles of myotubes making up the anatomical muscle. It is now established that there are different types of collagen, and recently it has been shown (Duance, Restall, Beard, Bourne and Bailey, 1977; Bailey, Shellswell and Duance, 1979) that different connective tissue membranes of muscle contain predominantly one of the collagen types: endomysium contains type Vv; perimysium contains type III; epimysium contains type I. The possibility arises that there may be a direct relationship between the type of collagen laid down, and muscle cell differentiation. Hauschka and Konigsberg (1966) demonstrated that, when the culture dish surface was coated with rat tail type I collagen, muscle-cell growth and differentiation were promoted.

Recently, it has been shown that different collagen types are synthesised at different stages of myogenesis (Bailey *et al.*, 1979). Type I and type III collagen could not be detected until after myoblast fusion, whereas the type V collagen appeared during growth of the myoblasts before myotube formation. This suggests that the presence of type V is probably involved in the sequence of events leading to myoblast differentiation and could serve as a marker of differentiating myoblasts. However, in these experiments collagen synthesis could be due to both myogenic cells and to fibroblasts.

Ketley, Orkin and Martin (1976) found that the four different types of collagen were equally effective as substrates for chick myogenesis.

Ionasescu and co-workers found that intracellular collagen synthesis was significantly decreased and extracellular collagen synthesis significantly increased in rapidly dividing fibroblast cultures from patients with Duchenne muscular dystrophy (Ionasescu, Lara-Brand, Zellweger, Ionasescu and Burmeister, 1977).

Humoral influences. *In vivo*, muscle cells are exposed to complex humoral influences. In culture, myogenic cells cannot grow and differentiate in completely defined medium without supplementation with serum and chick embryo extract. These supplements may contain nutrients, hormones, parahormones and trophic factors which have a role in regulating muscle differentiation *in vivo*.

Serum. The type of serum used in tissue culture can affect both growth and differentiation. Fetal calf serum is considered to favour division of myogenic cells in culture, while horse serum promotes differentiation (Yaffe, 1971; Morris and Cole, 1972).

It is not usually necessary to use homologous serum for myogenic cells in culture. However, it is interesting that Morgan and Cohen (1974) found that it was necessary to use human serum to obtain extensive development of cross-striations in human myotubes. In addition, Hauschka (1974a) found that human serum alone could replace a mixture of horse serum and chick embryo extract for human fetal myogenic cultures.

The active components of serum have been identified as orosomucoid (an α-acid glycoprotein) and α_2-macroglobulin (*see* Paul, 1970). Both disappear from the medium during cultivation of cells. Each, alone, has a small effect in stimulating growth; together, they have a marked effect and can replace serum. The macroglobulin can be replaced by non-protein molecules but the acid glycoprotein cannot be so replaced. These findings suggest that glycoproteins associated with Cohn's fraction V are the important components in serum.

De La Haba, Cooper and Etling (1966) reported that fusion of chick myoblasts to form myotubes in culture was almost completely reduced in the absence of horse serum. Myotube formation was restored by addition of high concentrations of insulin to the culture medium in the absence of serum, although not to the extent obtained if serum was present. When somatotropin and insulin were both added to replace serum, an even greater degree of myotube formation took place, but somatotropin could not replace the effect of insulin.

Powers and Florini (1975) found that physiological levels of testosterone stimulated division of rat muscle cells. The effect of testosterone on isolated muscle cells indicates that the effect of male sex hormones results from a direct interaction with muscle rather than from a primary interaction with some other tissue.

Kohama and Ozawa (1978a) reported that low concentrations of chicken serum stimulated the proliferation of cultures of 12-day embryonic chick muscle cells. The activity of serum varied during the course of development. The activity of serum from the embryo was high from day 11 to day 13 of incubation and then decreased, reaching a minimum on day 16. This decrease correlated with the period of decreased cell division and increased fusion of myotubes in vivo (Herrmann, Heywood, and Marchok, 1970). Subsequently, the activity of the serum increased, reaching a peak around the day of hatching. After hatching, the activity of the serum began to decrease on day 4 and reached a minimum at day 18.

Ozawa and Kohama (1978) tested the ability of hormones or extracts from adult chicken tissues to replace or influence the activity of the serum factor. Pituitary gland extracts did not replace the serum factor in a range equivalent to normal serum concentrations of somatotropin, although high concentrations of such an extract showed a significant ability to mimic the serum. Both pituitary extract and insulin showed a potentiating effect on the serum factor when added to the medium. However, the concentrations necessary for this effect were too high to be considered physiological. Since Kohama and Ozawa (1978a) considered that chick embryo extract contained the same active factor as serum they proposed that the results obtained by De La Haba et al. (1966) and Powers and Florini (1975) might be due to the hormones having a potentiating effect on this chick embryo extract factor activity. However, testosterone did not potentiate the serum factor when tested in tissue culture (Ozawa and Kohama, 1978); nevertheless, when testosterone was injected into chickens, the activity of the serum then recovered was increased, suggesting that testosterone may play a physiological role in regulating the level of serum factor (Kohama and Ozawa, 1978b).

Chick embryo extract. Chick embryo extract (CEE) has been frequently used to supplement medium in myogenic cultures (*reviewed by* Witkowski, 1977). De La Haba, Kamali and Tiede (1975) separated CEE into two fractions: a non-filterable fraction (including molecules of molecular weight greater than 10 000) which promotes both the fusion of myoblasts to form syncytia and the further differentiation of these syncytia into myotubes, and a filterable fraction which stimulated myoblast fusion to form syncytia only. The filterable fraction promoted myotube formation if the cells were grown on a collagen substratum. The non-filterable fraction already contained a collagen-like molecule.

In contrast, Yaffe (1971) found that reduced CEE concentration caused proliferating cells to cease dividing and to undergo fusion, suggesting that a high concentration may be a non-specific stimulator of cell proliferation.

It seems likely that there may be active components found in CEE which are also present in serum used as a medium supplement. Kohama and Ozawa (1978a) reported that both CEE and chicken serum stimulated proliferation of chick muscle cultures to about the same degree.

Neuronal control of muscle development. Of all tissues, the nervous system exerts the most extended and continuous influence on muscle development and maintenance. The fact that nerve cells and muscle cells can be grown together in tissue culture makes the *in vitro* system ideal for investigating various aspects of nerve–muscle interaction in a controlled environment. Attention has been particularly concentrated on determining the relationship between innervation and the acetylcholine sensitivity of the muscle cell.

Acetylcholine is the synaptic transmitter between the motor neurones and skeletal muscle fibres of vertebrates. The amount of current generated by the fine nerve branch is too small to stimulate the much larger muscle fibre directly, but at the neuromuscular junction there is a specialised end-plate which acts as a kind of amplifier. When the nerve impulse reaches the end-plate some acetylcholine (ACh) is released, which effectively depolarises the muscle membrane by increasing the permeability to all ions; this sets off an action potential which is propagated down the muscle fibre.

Muscle cells are sensitive to iontophoretically applied ACh in the absence of nerve cells. Fambrough and Rash (1971) found that mononucleate myoblasts from chick rat embryo were not sensitive, but multinucleate myotubes were depolarised by ACh. Mononucleate cells which constructed myofibrils without cell fusion were also ACh-sensitive, suggesting that the appearance of myofibrils and ACh-sensitivity are closely linked. The ability of the cell membrane to respond to a depolarising stimulus by generating an action potential is related to an increase in the resting potential caused by the changes in membrane permeability that occur after fusion (Fambrough and Rash, 1971).

Robbins and Yonezawa (1971) proposed that the neurotransmitter in early junctions in rat cell culture was probably ACh because, in a few cases tested, D-tubocurarine (an antagonist of ACh) completely eliminated excitatory junction potentials. Fischbach (1972) found that the synapses formed between dissociated neurones from chick spinal cord and dissociated myoblasts were cholinergic, and transmitter release, which even in the youngest cultures is quantal, was regulated by Ca^{++} and Mg^{++}. The major functional differences from adult vertebrate neuromuscular junctions were: (1) slow synaptic potential time-course; (2) low end-plate potential quantum content and miniature end-plate potential frequency; (3) occurrence of spontaneous end-plate potentials; and (4) lack of functional acetylcholinesterase.

The acetylcholine receptor is a membrane protein that facilitates transmission of the action potential between nerve and muscle. These receptors are precisely located at neuromuscular junctions and were thought to be more uniformly distributed over the entire surface of muscle fibres without established innervation (reviewed by Frank, 1979). However, muscle cells cultured in the absence of nerve cells have several clusters of ACh receptors (Vogel, Sytkowski and Nirenberg, 1972; Fischbach and Cohen, 1973).

These observations led to the proposal that the receptor clusters might serve as recognition sites for cholinergic nerves innervating muscle. The clusters might act as pre-formed post-synaptic sites and a cholinergic nerve encountering such a site would form a synapse there.

However, recent evidence suggests that nerve–muscle synapses do not form at pre-existing receptor clusters. Cohen and his colleagues used fluorescein-labelled α-bungarotoxin to follow the distribution of receptors during synapse formation on myocytes cultured from Xenopus larvae (Anderson and Cohen, 1977; Anderson, Cohen and Zorychta, 1977). The fluorescent patches under nerve processes, presumably at synapses, were different in shape from those on myocytes not contacted by nerve cells. In a few cases, the distribution of receptors was followed on a single myocyte while it was contacted by a neurite. Receptor molecules already labelled with fluorescent toxin coalesced under the neurite and adjacent pre-existing fluorescent patches often disappeared. Neural clusters were thus formed by recruitment of surrounding unclustered receptors and perhaps by receptors from dispersed pre-existing clusters as well. Similar results were obtained when the ACh sensitivity profile of chick myotubes in culture was determined physiologically during innervation by explants of embryonic chick spinal cord (Frank and Fischbach, 1979). New areas of high sensitivity appeared at newly formed synapses. In no case was a synapse observed to form at a pre-existing sensitive spot. These pre-existing clusters often disappeared when they were adjacent to synapses. Because of the method used to assay ACh receptor distribution it could not be determined whether receptors were recruited from adjacent areas or represented the incorporation of new receptors into the post-synaptic membrane.

How nerves induce receptor clusters is unknown. It is interesting that a contact between a neuroblastoma cell and a muscle (L_6 line) leads to increased ACh sensitivity at the point of contact (Harris, Heinemann, Schubert and Tarakis, 1971). The evidence indicated, first, a general lowering of ACh sensitivity near the contact, followed by development of a high sensitivity at the point of contact. There were no clear signs of synaptic transmission when action potentials were evoked in the neuroblastoma cells, and a simultaneous recording taken from a muscle fibre in contact, suggesting that close contact between the neuroblastoma cell process and the developing muscle was sufficient to mediate the restriction of ACh sensitivity. The trophic effect demonstrated is exerted by the processes of neuroblastoma cells, which are derived essentially not from motor neurones but from the sympathetic system, and the enzymatic composition of which is thus characteristic of sympathetic neurones (they do not release ACh). The combination of sympathetic nerves and skeletal muscle cells does not occur naturally, but it seems that some of the trophic effects of nerve on muscle can be produced as effectively by sympathetic nerves as by motor nerves. The question arises whether the muscle cell has induced an alteration in the specificity of the nerve cell.

More recently, it has been suggested that the mere physical presence of the nerve could produce a high receptor density, because a thread or dead nerve placed on the surface of a muscle can produce a local area of sensitivity.

The architecture of nerve–muscle contacts in initially dissociated cell cultures, as revealed by silver impregnation and electron microscopy, is rather primitive in comparison to those between explants of spinal cord and attached explants of muscle, which are nearly identical to adult neuro-muscular junctions. In short-term cultures, fine neurites terminate over muscle cells in a few simple swellings or boutons, and are not covered by Schwann cells; there are no post-synaptic gutters or folds or membrane thickenings and the muscle fibres are not covered by a basal lamina (Shimada, Fischman and Moscona, 1969a). Rather simple *en plaque* endings and non-muscle nuclei, possibly Schwann cells, have been observed in older cultures (Shimada *et al.*, 1969b).

Robbins and Yonezawa (1971) observed nerve–muscle contacts in cultures of rat embryonic spinal cord with either explants of muscle or dissociated myoblasts, with some of the ultrastructural features of adult neuromuscular junctions. Excitatory junction potentials (EJPs) were obtained by stimulating the spinal cord fragment or nerve fibre and recording with an intracellular electrode in the muscle cell. EJPs were never found in cells devoid of nerve contacts and were more readily obtained in nerve-contacts myotubes with a large number of nuclei than from

myotubes consisting of only a few cells.

It is now established that the type of innervation affects gene expression during the differentiation of muscle cells. Experiments in which fast and slow muscle were cross-reinnervated suggested that patterns of impulses may be important, and this was confirmed by direct electrical stimulation of muscle via nerve *in vivo* (Salmons and Sreter, 1976).

Intermittent electrical stimulation of myotube cultures in the total absence of nerves leads to loss of sensitivity to iontophoretically applied acetylcholine and less binding of ^{125}I-labelled α-bungarotoxin in comparison with inactive fibres (Cohen and Fischbach, 1973), decreased synthesis of ACh receptors (Shainberg and Burstein, 1976) and reduced acetylcholinesterase activity (Walker and Wilson, 1975). Repetitive stimulation increased protein synthesis and particularly myosin synthesis (Brevet, Pinto, Peacock and Stockdale, 1976).

However, there is also evidence that nerve cells can produce so-called neurotrophic factors which can influence differentiation of muscle cells. Oh, Johnson and Kim (1972) found that acetylcholinesterase activity in chick muscle cultures was increased by the presence of innervating spinal cord explants. The increased activity could still be obtained if the muscle cells were on one side of a coverslip and the nerve cells on the other, indicating that a functional synapse was not necessary. Furthermore, soluble protein extracts of the spinal cord could induce the same effect, suggesting that nerve cells could produce a diffusible factor. There is evidence that proteins synthesised in the spinal cord can flow distally along the peripheral nerves *in vivo* (*see* Komiya and Austin, 1974).

Oh (1976) found that a soluble extract of adult chicken sciatic nerve enhanced the rate and degree of morphological differentiation and maturation, DNA and protein synthesis, and acetylcholinesterase activity of muscle cultures. The active factor had a native molecular weight of 25000 (Markelonis and Oh, 1978).

Medium from spinal cord explant cultures was capable of producing the same reduction in transverse membrane resistance as the coculturing of spinal cord explants with muscle (Engelhardt, Ishikawa, Mori and Shimabukuro, 1977).

Extracts of rat spinal cord added to an L_6 cloned rat muscle cell line increased the number of ACh receptors and also increased the number of clusters of receptors (Podleski, Axelrod, Ravdin, Greenberg, Johnson and Salpeter, 1978). The active component appears to be a protein with a molecular weight of about 100 000.

Komiya and Austin (1974) have reported that there is an abnormal axoplasmic flow of protein along the sciatic nerve of dystrophic mice *in vivo*.

The crucial importance of nerve influence on so many aspects of muscle structure and function suggests that an abnormal relationship between the nerve and muscle cell may be responsible for many muscle diseases. Some of the investigations of myogenesis of diseased muscle in cultures consisting of muscle cells from biopsies of patients with Duchenne muscular dystrophy showed apparently normal myogenesis. This suggests that the underlying pathological process does not affect the early stages of myogenesis. It is possible that abnormalities in myogenesis become apparent only at the stage of muscle–nerve interaction. However, the results of tissue culture experiments coupling muscle and nerve cells derived from humans and animals with neuromuscular disorders are controversial or difficult to interpret (*reviewed by* Witkowski, 1977).

FUTURE PROSPECTS

Tissue culture studies of Duchenne muscular dystrophy (DMD) have been hindered by many factors, for example, the variable nature of biopsies reflecting both technical and genetic factors, and the variable nature of culture conditions used in different laboratories. If we add to these the fact that there is no consensus about which tissue is primarily affected, it is not surprising to find that not much progress has been made in understanding this disease, either from the tissue culture standpoint, or by any other means. However, some steps may be taken to control some of the sources of variability by standardising culture conditions, but, perhaps more important, attention should be paid to the fact that tissue culture media and sera have been optimised for the growth of cells and may therefore mask the deficiencies that are being sought. In view of this, it might be instructive,

wherever possible, to culture DMD tissues in homologous sera. It should also be possible to overcome the problem of variability from genetic sources by taking advantage of cell cloning techniques. This could be done by cloning cells from individual carriers of DMD, the rationale for which follows.

Cell cloning from DMD carriers. The mammalian female possesses two X chromosomes of maternal and paternal origin respectively. Early in embryogenesis, one X chromosome in each cell enters an inactive state, bringing about a situation in which two populations of cells expressing either the paternal or the maternal X-linked genes are created (Lyon, 1962). The inactivation is irreversible *in vivo* or in tissue culture, so that descendants of the cells in the early embryo are, whatever their functions, clones, with respect to which X is active (*see* Hellkuhl and Grzeschik, 1978). The autosomes, as far as is known, are not similarly affected and provide a constant genetic background upon which the maternal or paternal X-linked genes constitute variables. In DMD carriers this implies that approximately half of the cells in the body will express the dystrophic gene while the other half will express its normal allele. Thus, if cells are cultured from such carriers and clones are established from single cells, some of these potentially will express the dystrophic gene and the others the normal allele. This should enable meaningful comparisons to be made between them, which may reflect the genetic differences of the two X chromosomes. A requirement for this approach will be some means of distinguishing cells expressing the maternal X from those expressing the paternal X in tissue culture. Thus, DMD carriers will be needed who are heterozygous for one of the X-linked markers that are expressed in culture (McKusick and Ruddle, 1977). Such individuals are fairly rare, but they do exist in certain populations. Obviously, this approach to some extent depends upon being able to culture cells in which the basic lesion of DMD is expressed. On the other hand, the objective comparisons that it will facilitate may enable a decision to be made as to which types of cells do not exhibit differences due to the expression of the diseased or normal X. This may narrow the problem of defining the tissue which sustains the basic lesion and should lead to more rapid progress than might otherwise be possible.

Another approach which should become possible in the immediate future also employs tissue culture in conjunction with genetic engineering, or gene cloning, techniques.

Genetic engineering. Gene cloning techniques have contributed revolutionary new information on gene structure. These techniques involve inserting DNA fragments from eukaryotes into suitable prokaryotic plasmid, or bacteriophage, vectors which are then grown in a host bacterium. The DNA fragments are usually either synthesised from an mRNA preparation or are obtained directly from the DNA of the eukaryotic genome by endonuclease digestion or mechanical shearing. Such techniques have immense significance for the investigation of human genetic disease, although so far there have been no direct applications to the study of neuromuscular diseases.

The main advantage of gene cloning is that it makes available relatively large quantities of specific genes for structural and functional studies. This has made it possible, for example, to compare the gene with its primary RNA transcript (HnRNA) and its translated product (mRNA). Such studies have revealed that many genes contain inserted sequences (introns) which are transcribed but are edited out of the mRNA and so not translated. Such introns may account for as much as 95 per cent of certain genes; they have been shown to sustain mutations which are not expressed in the resulting proteins. Thus, the gene is much more complex than was formerly thought, and there are correspondingly more ways in which it might mutate without inevitable alterations in protein structure. Whether such alterations in non-translated regions of some genes might cause abnormalities in their expression is not clear at present, but this does not seem unlikely. It is also implicit that processing enzymes exist which are responsible for trimming or excising the RNA sequences coded by the introns during mRNA production, which might also be a possible source of abnormality in developing systems. The significance of these new aspects of gene structure and function for understanding neuromuscular diseases is obvious and might bear upon the fact that DMD, in particular, has an unusually high spontaneous mutation rate, suggesting that its causal element(s) might have unusual features at the DNA level. Study of DMD at the DNA level will be likely to involve tissue culture, from the standpoint both of obtaining a suitable supply of DNA from patients for use in gene cloning techniques and in constructing and testing nucleic acid probes with which to detect genes of interest. A particularly useful approach to gene cloning is afforded by the facility possessed by some bacteriophages of packaging DNA during *in vitro* virus assembly (Hohn and Hohn, 1974). In such controlled reactions, eukaryotic DNA fragments linked to viral DNA are incorporated by the virus and subsequently can be cloned in a suitable host bacterium. The DNA fragments are selected on a random basis so that, if sufficient are cloned, the whole human genome can be packaged and stored on about 100 bacterial culture plates (Maniatis, Hardison, Lacy, Laver, O'Connell, Quon, Sim and Efstratiadis, 1978). Such a 'library' can be established from the DNA recovered from a single tissue culture, and offers the prospect of constructing a library of DMD DNA for comparison with normal DNA. By means of suitable techniques, DNA of the X chromosome could be selectively recovered from such a library of human DNA and used to map neuromuscular functions originating from X-linked genes. Knowledge of the genetic structure of the X chromosome by these and other methods (McKusick and Ruddle, 1977), for example cell hybridisation, cannot fail to lead to advances in our understanding of human X-linked disease, and the rapid adoption of these approaches can confidently be predicted in the immediate future.

REFERENCES

Anderson, M.J. & Cohen, M.W. (1977) Nerve-induced and spontaneous redistribution of acetylcholine receptors on cultured muscle cells. *Journal of Physiology*, **268**, 757.

Anderson, M.J., Cohen, M.W. & Zorychta, E. (1977) Effect of innervation on the distribution of acetylcholine receptors on cultured muscle cells. *Journal of Physiology*, **268**, 731.

Appel, S.H., Anwyl, R., McAdams, M.W. & Elias, S. (1977) Accelerated degradation of acetylcholine receptor from cultured rat myotubes with myasthenia gravis sera and globulins. *Proceedings of the National Academy of Sciences USA*, **74**, 2130.

Askanas, V. & Engel, W.K. (1975) A new program for investigating adult human skeletal muscle grown aneurally in tissue culture. *Neurology (Minneapolis)*, **25**, 58.

Askanas, V., Shafiq, S.A. & Milhorat, A.T. (1972) Histochemistry of cultured aneural chick muscle: morphological maturation without differentiation of fibre types. *Experimental Neurology*, **37**, 218.

Askanas, V., Engel, W.K., Di Mauro, S., Brooks, B.R. & Mehler, M. (1976) Adult-onset-acid-maltase deficiency. *New England Journal of Medicine*, **294**, 573.

Aviv, H. & Leder, P. (1972) Purification of biologically active globin messenger RNA by chromatography on oligothymidylic acid-cellulose. *Proceedings of the National Academy of Sciences USA*, **69**, 1408.

Bag, J. & Sarkar, S. (1976) Studies on a nonpolysomal ribonucleoprotein coding for myosin heavy chains from chick embryonic muscles. *Journal of Biological Chemistry*, **251**, 7600.

Bailey, A.J., Shellswell, G.B. & Duance, V.C. (1979) Identification and change of collagen types in differentiating myoblasts and developing chick muscle. *Nature*, **278**, 67.

Bayliss, L.M. & Sloper, J.C. (1973) The role of the circulating cell as a source of myoblasts in the repair of injured skeletal muscle: evidence derived from the pre-irradiation of injured tissue and the use of tritiated thymidine. In *Basic Research in Myology*, Ed. B.A. Kakulas (Excerpta Medica: Amsterdam).

Bester, A.J., Kennedy, D.S. & Heywood, S.M. (1975) Two classes of translational control RNA: their role in the regulation of protein synthesis. *Proceedings of the National Academy of Sciences USA*, **72**, 1523.

Bevan, S., Kullberg, R.W. & Heinemann, S.F. (1977) Human myasthenia sera reduce acetylcholine sensitivity of human muscle cells in tissue culture. *Nature*, **267**, 263.

Bevan, S., Kullberg, R.W. & Rice, J. (1978) Acetylcholine-induced conductance fluctuations in cultured human myotubes. *Nature*, **273**, 469.

Bischoff, R. (1975) Regeneration of single skeletal muscle fibres in vitro. *The Anatomical Record*, **182**, 215.

Bischoff, R. & Holtzer, H. (1969) Mitosis and the process of differentiation of myogenic cells in vitro. *Journal of Cell Biology*, **41**, 188.

Bishop, A., Gallup, B., Skeate, Y. & Dubowitz, V. (1971) Morphological studies on normal and human muscle in culture. *Journal of the Neurological Sciences*, **13**, 333.

Bosmann, H.B., Gerston, D.M., Griggs, R.C., Howland, J.L., Hudecki, M.S., Katyare, S. & McLaughlin, J. (1976) Erythrocyte surface membrane alterations. *Archives of Neurology*, **33**, 135.

Bowman, L.H. & Emerson, C.P. (1977) Post-transcriptional regulation of ribosome accumulation during myoblast differentiation. *Cell*, **10**, 587.

Brevet, A., Pinto, E., Peacock, J. & Stockdale, F.E. (1976) Myosin synthesis increased by electrical stimulation of skeletal muscle cell cultures. *Science*, **193**, 1152.

Buckingham, M.E., Cohen, A. & Gros, F. (1976) Cytoplasmic distribution of pulse-labelled poly(A)-containing RNA, particularly 26S RNA, during myoblast growth and differentiation. *Journal of Molecular Biology*, **103**, 611.

Buckingham, M.E., Caput, D., Cohen, A., Whalen, R.G. &

Gros, F. (1974) The synthesis and stability of cytoplasmic messenger RNA during myoblast differentiation in culture. *Proceedings of the National Academy of Sciences USA*, **71**, 1466.

Buckley, P.A. & Konigsberg, I.R. (1974) Myogenic fusion and the duration of the post-mitotic gap (G_1). *Developmental Biology*, **37**, 193.

Buckley, P.A. & Konigsberg, I.R. (1977) Do myoblasts in vivo withdraw from the cell cycle? A reexamination. *Proceedings of the National Academy of Sciences USA*, **74**, 2031.

Carlsson, S-A., Ringertz, N.R. & Savage, R.E. (1974) Intracellular antigen migration in interspecific myoblast heterokaryons. *Experimental Cell Research*, **84**, 255.

Carlsson, S-A., Luger, O., Ringertz, N.R. & Savage, R.E. (1974) Phenotypic expression in chick erythrocyte × rat myoblast hybrids and in chick myoblast × rat myoblast hybrids. *Experimental Cell Research*, **84**, 47.

Carmon, Y., Neuman, S. & Yaffe D. (1978) Synthesis of tropomyosin in myogenic cultures and in RNA-directed cell-free systems: qualitative changes in the polypeptides. *Cell*, **14**, 393.

Carrel, A. (1924) Tissue culture and cell physiology. *Physiological Reviews*, **4**, 1.

Chen, L.B. (1977) Alteration in cell surface LETS protein during myogenesis. *Cell*, **10**, 393.

Chen, L.B., Gallimore, P.H. & McDougall, J.K. (1976) Correlation between tumour induction and the large external transformation sensitive protein on the cell surface. *Proceedings of the National Academy of Sciences USA*, **73**, 3570.

Chi, J.C., Fellini, S.A. & Holtzer, H. (1975a) Differences among myosins synthesized in non-myogenic cells, presumptive myoblasts and myoblasts. *Proceedings of the National Academy of Sciences USA*, **72**, 4999.

Chi, J.C.H., Rubinstein, N., Strahs, K. & Holtzer, H. (1975b) Synthesis of myosin heavy and light chains in muscle cultures. *Journal of Cell Biology*, **67**, 523.

Clissold, P. & Cole, R.J. (1973) Regulation of ribosomal RNA synthesis during mammalian myogenesis in culture. *Experimental Cell Research*, **80**, 159.

Cohen, S.A. & Fischbach, G.D. (1973) Regulation of muscle acetylcholine sensitivity by muscle activity in cell culture. *Science*, **181**, 76.

Coleman, J.R. & Coleman, A.W. (1968) Muscle differentiation and macromolecular synthesis. *Journal of Cellular Physiology*, **72**, Supp. 1, p. 19.

De La Haba, G., Cooper, G.W. & Etling, V. (1966) Hormonal requirements for myogenesis of striated muscle in vitro: insulin and somatotropin. *Proceedings of the National Academy of Sciences USA*, **56**, 1719.

De La Haba, G., Kamali, H.M. & Tiede, D.M. (1975) Myogenesis of avian striated muscle in vitro: role of collagen in myofibre formation. *Proceedings of the National Academy of Sciences USA*, **72**, 2729.

Delain, D. (1972) Comportement des isozymes de la lacticodeshydrogenase dans les cultures de cellules musculaires de poulets normaux et dystrophiques. *Comptes Rendus de Seances de la Societe de Biologie et de ses Filiales*, **166**, 308.

Devlin, R.B. & Emerson, C.P. (1978) Coordinate regulation of contractile protein synthesis during myoblast differentiation. *Cell*, **13**, 599.

Dienstmann, S.R. & Holtzer, H. (1977) Skeletal myogenesis. Control of proliferation in a normal cell lineage.

Experimental Cell Research, **107**, 355.

Doehring, J.L. & Fischman, D.A. (1974) The in vitro cell fusion of embryonic chick muscle without DNA synthesis. *Developmental Biology*, **36**, 225.

Doehring, J.L. & Fischman, D.A. (1977) A fusion-promoting macromolecular factor in muscle conditioned medium. *Experimental Cell Research*, **105**, 437.

Duance, V.C., Restall, D.J., Beard, H., Bourne, F.J. & Bailey, A.J. (1977) The location of three collagen types in skeletal muscle. *FEBS Letters*, **79**, 248.

Ebashi, S., Toyokura, Y., Momoi, H. & Sugita, H. (1959) High creatine phosphokinase activity of sera of progressive muscular dystrophy patients. *Journal of Biochemistry (Tokyo)*, **46**, 103.

Emerson, C.P. & Beckner, S.K. (1975) Activation on myosin synthesis in fusing and mononucleated myoblasts. *Journal of Molecular Biology*, **93**, 431.

Emery, A.E.H. & McGregor, L. (1977) The fetus in Duchenne muscular dystrophy: muscle growth in tissue culture. *Clinical Genetics*, **12**, 183.

Engelhardt, J.K., Ishikawa, K., Mori, J. & Shimabukuro, Y. (1977) Neurotrophic effects on the electrical properties of cultured muscle produced by conditioned medium from spinal cord explants. *Brain Research*, **128**, 243.

Fambrough, D. & Rash, J.E. (1971) Development of acetylcholine sensitivity during myogenesis. *Developmental Biology*, **26**, 55.

Fischbach, G.D. (1972) Synapse formation between dissociated nerve and muscle cells in low density cell cultures. *Developmental Biology*, **28**, 407.

Fischbach, G.D. & Cohen, S.A. (1973) The distribution of acetylcholine sensitivity over uninnervated and innervated muscle fibres grown in cell culture. *Developmental Biology*, **31**, 147.

Fischman, D.A. (1970) The synthesis and assembly of myofibrils in embryonic muscle. *Current Topics in Developmental Biology*, **5**, 235.

Fluck, R.A. & Strohman, R.C. (1973) Acetylcholinesterase activity in developing skeletal muscle cells in vitro. *Developmental Biology*, **33**, 417.

Frank, E. (1979) Acetylcholine receptor clusters. *Nature*, **278**, 599.

Frank, E. & Fischbach, G.D. (1979) In *Neurobiology*, Eds Otsuka & Hall.

Gallup, B., Bishop, A. & Dubowitz, V. (1972) Autoradiographic studies of RNA and DNA synthesis during myogenesis in cultures of human, chick and rat muscle. *Journal of the Neurological Sciences*, **17**, 127.

Gauthier, G.F., Lowey, S. & Hobbs, A.W. (1978) Fast and slow myosin in developing muscle fibres. *Nature*, **274**, 25.

Geiger, R.S. & Garvin, J.S. (1957) Pattern of regeneration of muscle from progressive muscular dystrophy patients cultivated in vitro as compared to normal human skeletal muscle. *Journal of Neuropathology and Experimental Neurology*, **16**, 532.

Goyle, S., Kalra, S.L. & Singh, B. (1967) The growth of normal and dystrophic human skeletal muscle in tissue culture. *Neurology (India)*, **15**, 149.

Goyle, S., Kalra, S.L. & Singh, B. (1968) Further studies on normal and dystrophic human skeletal muscle in tissue culture. *Neurology (India)*, **16**, 87.

Goyle, S., Virmani, V. & Singh, B. (1973) Cytochemical studies on cells grown in vitro from explants of normal and dystrophic human skeletal muscle, subcutaneous fat and fascia. In *Basic Research in Myology*, Ed. B.A. Kakulas, pp. 582–592 (Excerpta Medica: Amsterdam).

Grouse, L.D., Nelson, P.G., Omenn, G.S. & Schrier, B.K. (1978) Measurements of gene expression in tissues of normal and dystrophic mice. *Experimental Neurology*, **59**, 470.

Guinness, F.B. (1973) Ph.D. Thesis, University of Edinburgh.

Gurdon, J.B. & Woodland, H.R. (1968) The cytoplasmic control of nuclear activity in animal development. *Biological Reviews*, **43**, 233.

Harris, A.J., Heinemann, S., Schubert, D. & Tarakis, H. (1971) Trophic interaction between cloned tissue culture lines of nerve and muscle. *Nature*, **231**, 296.

Harris, H., Sidebottom, E., Grace, D.M. & Bramwell, M.E. (1969) The expression of genetic information: a study with hybrid animal cells. *Journal of Cell Science*, **4**, 499.

Hauschka, S.D. (1974a) Clonal analysis of vertebrate morphogenesis. II. Environmental influences upon human muscle differentiation. *Developmental Biology*, **37**, 329.

Hauschka, S.D. (1974b) Clonal analysis of vertebrate myogenesis. III. Developmental changes in the muscle-colony-forming cells of the human fetal limb. *Developmental Biology*, **37**, 345.

Hauschka, S.D. & Konigsberg, I.R. (1966) The influence of collagen on the development of muscle clones. *Proceedings of the National Academy of Sciences USA*, **55**, 119.

Hauschka, S.D. & White, N.K. (1971) Study of myogenesis in vitro. In *Research in Muscle Development and the Muscle Spindle*, Eds B.Q. Banker, R.J. Przbylski, J Van der Meulen & M. Victor (Excerpta Medica: Amsterdam).

Heinemann, S., Bevan, S., Kullberg, R., Lindstrom, J. & Rice, J. (1977) Modulation of acetylcholine receptor by antibody against the receptor. *Proceedings of the National Academy of Sciences USA*, **74**, 3090.

Hellkuhl, B. & Grzeschik (1978) Partial reactivation of a human inactive X chromosome in human-mouse somatic cell hybrids. *Human Gene Mapping 4*, Ed. D. Bergsma (Karger: Basel).

Herrmann, H., Heywood, S.M. & Marchok, A.C. (1970) Reconstruction of muscle development as a sequence of macromolecular synthesis. *Current Topics in Developmental Biology*, **5**, 181.

Herrmann, H., Konigsberg, U.R. & Robinson, G. (1960) Observations on culture in vitro of normal and dystrophic muscle tissue. *Proceedings of the Society for Experimental Biology and Medicine*, **105**, 217.

Heywood, S.M. & Nwagwu, M. (1969) Partial characterisation of presumptive myosin messenger ribonucleic acid. *Biochemistry*, **8**, 3839.

Heywood, S.M., Kennedy, D.S. & Bester, A.J. (1975) Stored myosin messenger in embryonic chick muscle. *FEBS Letters*, **53**, 69.

Hogan, B. & Shields, R. (1974) Ying-Yang hypothesis of growth control. *New Scientist*, **62**, 323.

Hohn, B. & Hohn, T. (1974) Activity of empty, beadlike particles for packaging of DNA of Bacteriophage γ in vitro. *Proceedings of the National Academy of Sciences USA*, **71**, 2372.

Holland, P.C. & MacLennan, D.H. (1976) Assembly of the sarcoplasmic reticulum. Biosynthesis of the adenosine triphosphatase in rat skeletal muscle cell culture. *Journal of Biological Chemistry*, **251**, 2030.

Holtzer, H. & Sanger, J.W. (1972) Myogenesis: old views rethought. In *Research in Muscle Development and the Muscle Spindle*, Ed. B. Barnier (Excerpta Medica: Amsterdam).

Holtzer, H., Sanger, J.W., Ishikawa, H. & Strahs, K. (1972) Selected topics in skeletal myogenesis. In *The Mechanism of Muscle Contraction. Cold Spring Harbour Symposia on Quantitative Biology*, **37**.

Holtzer, H., Croop, J., Dienstman, S., Ishikawa, H. & Somlyo, A.P. (1975) Effects of cytochalasin B and colcemide on myogenic cultures. *Proceedings of the National Academy of Sciences USA*, **72**, 513.

Hosik, H.L. & Strohman, R.C. (1971) Changes in ribosomal–polysome balance in chick muscle cells during tissue dissociation, development in culture, and exposure to simplified culture medium. *Journal of Cellular Physiology*, **77**, 145.

Huxley, H.E. (1963) Electron microscope studies on the structure of natural and synthetic filaments from striated muscle. *Journal of Molecular Biology*, **7**, 281.

Ingwall, J.S. (1976) Creatine and the control of muscle-specific protein synthesis in cardiac and skeletal muscle. *Circulation Research*, **28**, sup. **1**, 115.

Ingwall, J.S., Morales, M.F. & Stockdale, F.E. (1972) Creatine and the control of myosin synthesis in differentiating skeletal muscle. *Proceedings of the National Academy of Sciences USA*, **69**, 2250.

Ingwall, J.S., Weiner, C.D., Morales, M.F., Davis, E. & Stockdale, F.E. (1974) Specificity of creatine in the control of muscle protein synthesis. *Journal of Cell Biology*, **62**, 145.

Ionasescu, V., Lara-Brand, C., Zellweger, H., Ionasescu, R. & Burmeister, L. (1977) Fibroblast cultures in Duchenne muscular dystrophy. *Acta Neurologica Scandinavica*, **55**, 407.

Ionasescu, V., Zellweger, H., Ionasescu, R., Lara-Brand, C. & Cancilla, P.A. (1976) Protein synthesis in muscle cultures from patients with Duchenne muscular dystrophy. *Acta Neurologica Scandinavica*, **54**, 241.

Ishikawa, H., Bischoff, R. & Holtzer, H. (1969) Formation of arrowhead complexes with heavy meromyosin in a variety of cell types. *Journal of Cell Biology*, **43**, 312.

John, H.A. (1974) Myosin of developing and dystrophic skeletal muscle. *FEBS Letters*, **39**, 278.

John, H.A. (1976) Myofibrillar proteins of developing and dystrophic skeletal muscle. *FEBS Letters*, **64**, 116.

John, H.A. & Jones, K.W. (1975) Tissue culture investigations of the effect of nerve on myosin structure and function. In *Recent Advances in Myology*, Eds W.G. Bradley, D Gardner-Medwin, & J.N. Walton (Excerpta Medica: Amsterdam).

John, H.A., Patrinou-Georgoulas, M. & Jones, K.W. (1977) Detection of myosin heavy chain mRNA during myogenesis in tissue culture by in vitro and in situ hybridisation. *Cell*, **12**, 501.

Kacian, D.L., Spiegelman, S., Bank, A., Terada, M., Metafora, S., Dow, L. & Marks, P.A. (1972) In vitro synthesis of DNA components of human genes for globins. *Nature New Biology*, **235**, 167.

Kakulas, B.A., Papadimitriou, J.M., Knight, J.D. & Mastaglia, F.L. (1968) Normal and abnormal human muscle in tissue culture. *Proceedings of the Australian Association of Neurology*, **5**, 79.

Ketley, J.N., Orkin, R.W. & Martin, G.R. (1976) Collagen in developing chick muscle in vivo and in vitro. *Experimental Cell Research*, **99**, 261.

Kohama, K. & Ozawa, E. (1978a) Muscle trophic factor: II Ontogenic development of activity of a muscle trophic factor in chicken serum. *Muscle and Nerve*, **1**, 236.

Kohama, K. & Ozawa, E. (1978b) Muscle trophic factor: IV Testosterone-induced increase in muscle trophic factor in chicken serum. *Muscle and Nerve*, **1**, 320.

Komiya, Y. & Austin, L. (1974) Axoplasmic flow of protein in the sciatic nerve of normal and dystrophic mice. *Experimental Neurology*, **43**, 1.

Konigsberg, I.R. (1961) Some aspects of myogenesis in vitro. *Circulation*, **24**, 447.

Konigsberg, I.R. (1963) Clonal analysis of myogenesis. *Science*, **140**, 1213.

Konigsberg, I.R. (1970) The relationship of collagen to the clonal development of embryonic skeletal muscle. In *Chemistry and Molecular Biology of Intracellular Matrix*, Ed. E.A. Balazs, Vol. 3 (Academic Press: New York).

Konigsberg, I.R. (1971) Diffusion-mediated control of myoblast fusion. *Developmental Biology*, **26**, 133.

Konigsberg, U.R., Lipton, B.H. & Konigsberg, I.R. (1975) The regenerative response of single mature muscle fibres isolated in vitro. *Developmental Biology*, **45**, 260.

Konigsberg, I.R., Sollmann, P.A. & Mixter, L.O. (1978) The duration of the terminal G_1 of fusing myoblasts. *Developmental Biology*, **63**, 11.

Lobley, G.E., Perry, S.V. & Stone, D. (1971) Structural changes in myosin induced by vitamin E dystrophy. *Nature*, **231**, 317.

Lyon, M.F. (1962) Sex chromatin and gene action in the mammalian X-chromosome. *American Journal of Human Genetics*, **14**, 135.

Man, N.T. & Cole, R.J. (1972) RNA synthesis during mammalian myogenesis in culture. *Experimental Cell Research*, **73**, 429.

Maniatis, T., Hardison, R.C., Lacy, E., Lauer, J., O'Connell, C., Quon, D., Sim, G.K. & Efstratiadis, A. (1978) The isolation of structural genes from libraries of eukaryotic DNA. *Cell*, **15**, 687.

Markelonis, G.J. & Oh, T.H. (1978) A protein fraction from peripheral nerve having neurotrophic effects on skeletal muscle cells in culture. *Experimental Neurology*, **58**, 285.

Martonosi, A., Roufa, D., Boland, R., Reyes, E. & Tillack, T.W. (1977) Development of sarcoplasmic reticulum in culture of chicken muscle. *Journal of Biological Chemistry*, **252**, 318.

Masaki, T. (1974) Immunochemical comparison of myosins from chicken cardiac, fast white, slow red, and smooth muscle. *Journal of Biochemistry (Tokyo)*, **76**, 441.

Masaki, T. & Yoshizaki, C. (1974) Differentiation of myosin in chick embryos. *Journal of Biochemistry (Tokyo)*, **76**, 123.

Mauro, A. (1961) Satellite cells of skeletal muscle fibres. *Journal of Biophysical and Biochemical Cytology*, **9**, 493.

Mawatari, S., Miranda, A. & Rowland, L.P. (1976) Adenyl cyclase abnormality in Duchenne muscular dystrophy: muscle cells in culture. *Neurology (Minneapolis)*, **26**, 1021.

McKusick, V.A. & Ruddle, F.H. (1977) The status of the gene map of the human chromosomes. *Science*, **196**, 390.

Morgan, J. & Cohen, L. (1974) Use of papain in the preparation of adult mammalian skeletal muscle for tissue. *In Vitro*, **10**, 188.

Morris, G.E. & Cole, R.J. (1972) Cell fusion and differentiation in cultured chick muscle cells. *Experimental Cell Research*, **75**, 191.

Morris, G.E. & Cole, R.J. (1977) Biosynthesis of muscle-specific creatine kinase during differentiation in vitro. *FEBS Letters*, **79**, 183.

Morris, G.E., Piper, M. & Cole, R.J. (1976) Differential

effects of calcium ion concentration on cell fusion, cell division and creatine kinase activity in muscle cell cultures. *Experimental Cell Research*, **99**, 106.

Moscona, A. & Moscona, H. (1952) The dissociation and aggregation of cells from organ rudiments of the early chick embryo. *Journal of Anatomy*, **86**, 287.

Moss, P.S. & Strohman, R.C. (1976) Myosin synthesis by fusion-arrested chick embyro myoblasts in cell culture. *Developmental Biology*, **48**, 431.

Nadal-Ginard, B. (1978) Commitment, fusion and biochemical differentiation of a myogenic cell line in the absence of DNA synthesis. *Cell*, **15**, 855.

Nameroff, M. & Holtzer, H. (1969) Interference with myogenesis. *Developmental Biology*, **19**, 380.

Nordstrom, J.L., Roop, D.R., Tsai, M.-J. & O'Malley, B.W. (1979) Identification of potential ovomucoid mRNA precursors in chick oviduct nuclei. *Nature*, **278**, 328.

Novak, T.P., Haywood, P.L. & Barondes, S.H. (1976) Developmentally regulated lectin in embryonic chick muscle and a myogenic cell line. *Biochemical and Biophysical Research Communications*, **68**, 650.

O'Farrell, P.H. (1975) High resolution two dimensional electrophoresis of proteins. *Journal of Biological Chemistry*, **25**, 4007.

Oh, T.H. (1976) Neurotrophic effects of sciatic nerve extracts on muscle development in culture. *Experimental Neurology*, **50**, 376.

Oh, T.H. & Johnson, D.D. (1972) Effects of acetyl-β-methylcholine on development of acetylcholinesterase and butyrylcholinesterase activities in cultured chick embryonic skeletal muscle. *Experimental Neurology*, **37**, 360.

Oh, T.H., Johnson, D.D. & Kim, S.V. (1972) Neurotrophic effect on isolated chick embryo muscle in culture. *Science*, **178**, 1298.

Okazaki, K. & Holtzer, H. (1965) An analysis of myogenesis in vitro using fluorescein-labelled antimyosin. *Journal of Histochemistry and Cytochemistry*, **13**, 726.

O'Neill, M.C. & Stockdale, F.E. (1972) A kinetic analysis of myogenesis in vitro. *Journal of Cell Biology*, **52**, 52.

Ozawa, E. & Kohama, K. (1978) Muscle trophic factor: III Effect of hormones and tissue extracts on muscle trophic-factor activity. *Muscle and Nerve*, **1**, 314.

Paterson, B.M. & Bishop, J.O. (1977) Changes in the mRNA population of chick myoblasts during myogenesis in vitro. *Cell*, **12**, 751.

Paterson, B. & Strohman, R.C. (1972) Myosin synthesis in cultures of differentiating chicken embryo skeletal muscle. *Developmental Biology*, **29**, 113.

Paterson, B.M., Roberts, B.E. & Yaffe, D. (1974) Determination of actin messenger RNA in cultures of differentiating embryonic chick skeletal muscle. *Proceedings of the National Academy of Sciences (U.S.A.)*, **71**, 4467.

Patrick, J., Heinemann, S.F., Lindstrom, J., Schubert, D. & Steinbach, J.H. (1972) Appearance of acetylcholine receptors during differentiation of a myogenic cell line. *Proceedings of the National Academy of Sciences USA*, **69**, 2762.

Patrinou-Georgoulas, M. & John, H.A. (1977) The genes and mRNA coding for the heavy chains of chick embryonic skeletal myosin. *Cell*, **12**, 491.

Paul, J. (1970) *Cell and Tissue Culture* (Livingstone: Edinburgh and London).

Pelham, H.R.B. & Jackson, J. (1976) An efficient mRNA-dependent translation system from reticulocyte lysates.

European Journal of Biochemistry, **67**, 247.

Perrie, W.T., Smillie, L.B. & Perry, S.V. (1972) A phosphorylated light chain component of myosin from skeletal muscle. In *The Mechanism of Muscle Contraction. Cold Spring Harbor Symposia on Quantitative Biology*, **37**.

Perry, S.V. (1971) Development and specialisation in muscle and the biochemistry of the dystrophics. *Journal of the Neurological Sciences*, **12**, 289.

Podleski, T.R., Axelrod, D., Ravdin, P., Greenberg, I., Johnson, M.M. & Salpeter, M.M. (1978) Nerve extract induces increase and redistribution of acetylcholine receptors on cloned muscle cells. *Proceedings of the National Academy of Sciences USA*, **75**, 2035.

Powers, M.L. & Florini, J.R. (1975) A direct effect of testosterone on muscle cells in tissue culture. *Endocrinology*, **97**, 1043.

Prives, J.M. & Paterson, B.M. (1974) Differentiation of cell membranes in cultures of embryonic chick breast muscle. *Proceedings of the National Academy of Sciences USA*, **71**, 3208.

Reznik, M. (1969) Origin of myoblasts during skeletal muscle regeneration. *Laboratory Investigation*, **20**, 353.

Richler, C. & Yaffe, D. (1970) The in vitro cultivation and differentiation capacities of myogenic cell lines. *Developmental Biology*, **23**, 1.

Rinaldini, L.M. (1959) An improved method for the isolation and quantitative cultivation of embryonic cells. *Experimental Cell Research*, **16**, 477.

Robbins, N. & Yonezawa, T. (1971) Developing neuromuscular junctions: first signs of chemical transmission during formation in tissue culture. *Science*, **172**, 395.

Roberts, B.E. & Paterson, B.M. (1973) Efficient translation of tobacco mosaic virus RNA and rabbit globin 9S RNA in a cell-free system from commercial wheat germ. *Proceedings of the National Academy of Sciences USA*, **70**, 2330.

Roelofs, R.I., Engel, W.K. & Chauvin, P.B. (1972) Histochemical phosphorylase activity in regenerating muscle fibres from myophosphorylase-deficient patients. *Science*, **177**, 795.

Ross, K.F.A. & Parsons, R. (1973) RNA, nucleoli and metabolism of cells grown from normal and dystrophic muscle explants. In *Basic Research in Myology*, Ed. B.A. Kakulas (Excerpta Medica: Amsterdam).

Ross, K.F.A., Jones, K.W. & John, H.A. (1974) Tissue culture in muscle disease. In *Disorders of Voluntary Muscle*, 3rd Ed. J.N. Walton (Churchill Livingstone: London).

Rowland, L.P. (1976) Pathogenesis of the muscular dystrophies. *Archives of Neurology*, **33**, 315.

Rubinstein, N.A., Pepe, F.A. & Holtzer, H. (1977) Myosin types during the development of embryonic chicken fast and slow muscles. *Proceedings of the National Academy of Sciences USA*, **74**, 4524.

Salmons, S. & Sreter, F.A. (1976) Significance of impulse activity in the transformation of skeletal muscle type. *Nature*, **263**, 30.

Samaha, F.J. & Gergely, J. (1969) Biochemical abnormalities of the sarcoplasmic reticulum in muscular dystrophy. *New England Journal of Medicine*, **280**, 184.

Schapira, F. (1967) Variations pathologiques, en rapport avec l'ontogenese, des formes moleculaires multiples de la lactico-deshydrogenase, de la creatine-kinase et de l'aldolase. *Bulletin de la Societié chimie biologique*, **49**, 1647.

Schudt, C. & Pette, D. (1976) Influence of monosaccharides, medium factors and enzymatic modification on fusion of myoblasts in vitro. *Cytobiologie (Stuttgart)*, **13**, 74.

Scott, R.E. (1978) Undifferentiated and differentiated L_6 myoblast plasma membranes. II: comparison of the morphological and biochemical characteristics of isoaleil plasma membranes. *Cell Differentiation*, **7**, 335.

Scott, R.E. & Dousa, T.P. (1978) Plasma membrane cyclic AMP-dependent protein phosphorylation system in L_6 myoblasts. *Biochimica Biophysica Acta*, **509**, 499.

Shainberg, A. & Burstein, M. (1976) Decrease of acetylcholine receptor synthesis in muscle cultures by electrical stimulation. *Nature*, **264**, 368.

Shimada, Y., Fischman, D.A. & Moscona, A.A. (1969a) Formation of neuromuscular junctions in embryonic cell cultures. *Proceedings of the National Academy of Sciences USA*, **62**, 715.

Shimada, Y., Fischman, D.A. & Moscona, A.A. (1969b) The development of nerve-muscle junctions in monolayer cultures of embryonic spinal cord and skeletal muscle cells. *Journal of Cell Biology*, **43**, 382.

Skeate, Y., Bishop, A. & Dubowitz, (1969) Differentiation of diseased human muscle in culture. *Cell and Tissue Kinetics*, **2**, 307.

Sreter, F., Holtzer, S., Gergely, J. & Holtzer, H. (1972) Some properties of embryonic myosin. *Journal of Cell Biology*, **55**, 586.

Sreter, F.A., Astrom, K.-E., Romanul, F.C.A., Young, R.R. & Jones, H.R. (1976) *Journal of the Neurological Sciences*, **27**, 99.

Stockdale, F.E. & Holtzer, H. (1961) DNA synthesis and myogenesis. *Experimental Cell Research*, **2**, 508.

Storti, R.V., Horovitch, S.J., Scott, M.P., Rich, A. & Pardue, M.L. (1978) Myogenesis in primary cell cultures from Drosophila melanogaster: protein synthesis and actin heteroglueity during development. *Cell*, **13**, 589.

Strehler, B.L., Konigsberg, I.R. & Kelley, J.E.T. (1963) Ploidy of myotube nuclei developing in vitro as determined with a recording double beam micro-spectrophotometer. *Experimental Cell Research*, **32**, 232.

Strohman, R.C., Moss, P.S., Micou-Eastwood, J., Spector, D., Przybyla, A. & Paterson, B. (1977) Messenger RNA for myosin polypeptides: isolation from single myogenic cell cultures. *Cell*, **10**, 265.

Thompson, E.J., Yasin, R., Van Beers, G., Nurse, K. & Al-Ani, S. (1977) Myogenic defect in human muscular dystrophy. *Nature*, **268**, 241.

Trotter, J.A. & Nameroff, M. (1976) Myoblast differentiation in vitro: morphological differentiation of mononucleated myoblasts. *Developmental Biology*, **49**, 548.

Turner, D.C., Gmur, R., Siegrist, M., Burckhardt, E. & Eppenberger, H.M. (1976) Differentiation in cultures derived from embryonic chicken muscle. I. Muscle-specific enzyme changes before fusion in EGTA-synchronised cultures. *Developmental Biology*, **48**, 284.

Vassilipoulos, D., Emery, A.E.H. & Gordon, N. (1977) Nuclear changes in cultured human dystrophic muscle. *Experientia*, **33**, 759.

Verma, I.M., Temple, G.F., Fan, H. & Baltimore, D. (1972) In vitro synthesis of DNA complementary to rabbit reticulocyte 10S RNA. *Nature New Biology*, **235**, 163.

Vertel, B.M. & Fischman, D.A. (1976) Myosin accumulation in mononucleated cells of chick muscle cultures. *Developmental Biology*, **48**, 438.

Vogel, Z., Sytkowski, A.J. & Nirenberg, M.W. (1972) Acetylcholine receptors of muscle grown in vitro.

Proceedings of the National Academy of Sciences USA, **69**, 3180.

Walker, C.R. & Wilson, B.W. (1975) Control of acetylcholinesterase by contractile activity of cultured muscle cells. *Nature*, **256**, 215.

Wartiovaara, J., Linder, E., Ruoslathi, E. & Vaheri, A. (1974) Distribution of fibroblast surface antigen: association with fibrillar structures of normal cells and loss upon viral transformation. *Journal of Experimental Medicine*, **140**, 1522.

Weinstock, J.M. & Jones, K.B. (1977) Creatine phosphokinase in cultured control and dystrophic chick embryo muscle. *Biochemical Medicine*, **18**, 245.

Whalen, R.G., Butler-Browne, G.S. & Gros, F. (1976) Protein synthesis and actin heterogeneity in calf muscle cells in culture. *Proceedings of the National Academy of Sciences USA*, **73**, 2018.

Whatley, R., Ng, S.K.-C., Rogers, J., McMurray, W.C. & Sanwal, B.D. (1976) Developmental changes in gangliosides during myogenesis of a rat myoblast cell line and its drug resistant variants. *Biochemical and Biological Research Communications*, **70**, 180.

Witkowski, J.A. (1977) Diseased muscle cells in tissue culture. *Biological Reviews*, **52**, 431.

Witkowski, J.A., Durbrige, M. & Dubowitz, V. (1976) Growth of human muscle in tissue culture. *In Vitro*, **12**, 98.

Yablonka, Z. & Yaffe, D. (1976) Synthesis of polypeptides with the properties of myosin light chains directed by RNA extracted from muscle cultures. *Proceedings of the National Academy of Sciences USA*, **73**, 4599.

Yaffe, D. (1968) Retention of differentiation potentialities during prolonged cultivation of myogenic cells. *Proceedings of the National Academy of Sciences USA*, **61**, 477.

Yaffe, D. (1971) Developmental changes preceding cell fusion during muscle differentiation in vitro. *Experimental Cell Research*, **66**, 33.

Yaffe, D. & Dym, H. (1972) Gene expression during differentiation of contractile muscle fibres. In *The Mechanism of Muscle Contraction. Cold Spring Harbor Symposia on Quantitative Biology*, **38**.

Yaffe, D. & Fuchs, S. (1967) Autoradiographic study of the incorporation of uridine-^{3}H during myogenesis in tissue culture. *Developmental Biology*, **15**, 33.

Yarom, R. & Havivi, Y. (1977) Acceleration of muscle regeneration by bone marrow cells. *Experientia*, **33**, 195.

Yasin, R., Van Beers, G., Bulien, D. & Thompson, E.J. (1976) A quantitative procedure for the dissociation of adult mammalian muscle into mononucleated cells. *Experimental Cell Research*, **102**, 405.

Yasin, R., Van Beers, G., Nurse, K.C.E., Al-Ani, S., Landon, D.N. & Thompson, E.J. (1977) A quantitative technique for growing human adult skeletal muscle in culture starting from mononucleated cells. *Journal of the Neurological Sciences*, **32**, 347.

Yeoh, G.C.T. & Holtzer, H. (1977) The effect of cell density, conditioned medium and cytosine arabinoside on myogenesis in primary and secondary cultures. *Experimental Cell Research*, **104**, 63.

Zalin, R.J. (1977) Prostaglandins and myoblast fusion. *Developmental Biology*, **59**, 241.

Zalin, R.J. & Montague, W. (1974) Changes in adenylate cyclase, cyclic AMP, and protein kinase levels in chick myoblasts and their relationship to differentiation. *Cell*, **2**, 103.

Experimental myopathies

INTRODUCTION

One purpose of experimental myopathology is to provide an understanding of muscle lesions which occur in human disease. Another is to explore the basic biological and pathological properties of skeletal muscle. In this way some experimental work is concerned with the basic reaction of the injured muscle fibre, while other undertakings are attempts to reproduce animal counterparts of human conditions. These studies, which complement those of the 'natural' myopathies in animals, are now responsible for much improvement in our knowledge of muscle disease in man. There are many conditions in animals which bear greater or lesser resemblance to human muscle diseases. For instance, genetically determined muscular dystrophy is a natural disorder of the mouse, mink, chicken, duck and sheep. A polymyositis-like disease occurs in the Syrian hamster. Myotonia is a natural disorder of the goat. The malignant hyperpyrexia syndrome is found in the Landrace

pig, while various nutritional myopathies are well known in farm animals. Because these are 'natural' conditions and are not experimentally induced, they will not be considered further here (but *see* Ch. 24).

The methods used to explore the basic properties of the injured muscle fibre are numerous. They include simple injury, such as that produced by cold, crush, irradiation, myotoxic chemicals or biological agents. Other methods are hormonal, nutritional or immunological. The effects of denervation represent a special separate category of voluntary muscle reaction. Denervation has gained increased attention because of the potential 'importance' of neurotrophic influences. Many aspects of denervation are considered by Gutmann (1962) and by Adams (1975).

A notable consequence of muscle fibre injury is regeneration, which always occurs if the animal survives the immediate assault. Regeneration of skeletal muscle receives wide attention and muscle fibre regeneration is a component of the histopathology of the progressive muscular dystrophies, the non-hereditary human myopathies such as polymyositis and of many of the drug-induced and toxic myopathies. In recent years the study of regeneration linked to myogenesis has become a distinct discipline (Mauro, Shafiq and Milhorat, 1970; Banker, Przybylski, Van Der Meulen, and Victor, 1972; Kakulas, 1973).

Of the attempts to reproduce models of naturally occurring human diseases in animals, the more important are the 'dystrophy-like', 'myasthenia gravis' and 'polymyositis'. Banker (1960), Adams (1975) and Kakulas (1975) have reviewed the experimental myopathies.

Myopathic conditions sometimes occur as untoward complications of drug treatment in clinical medicine (Ch. 25). This is the stimulus underlying the many laboratory studies of the drug-induced myopathies. The more important agents in this aspect are the steroid hormones and the antimalarials, but there are numerous other drugs which will cause myopathic side effects in some patients. Skeletal muscle is thus very 'sensitive' to a wide variety of drugs and poisons. This sensitivity is due both to the high metabolic and biochemical specificity of muscle and to the fact that it is required to provide much energy at short notice. As might be expected, most of the drugs which are known to produce myonecrosis clinically (Lane and Mastaglia, 1978) have also been shown to cause a comparable experimental animal myopathy. It may also be predicted that, in those instances where no animal model is yet recorded, such a copy could easily be reproduced experimentally.

The principles of myopathology, derived from the experimental study of the nutritional myopathy of the Rottnest Island Quokka (*Setonix brachyurus*) (Kakulas and Adams, 1966) allow an appreciation of the pathogenesis of all those muscle conditions in which focal necrosis is the prime event, whatever the cause. Such an understanding allows the prediction of the histopathology and natural history in these situations (Kakulas, 1975). The determining factors are the severity, the anatomical extent of the lesion and the period over which the noxious influence is active.

Although a wide range of laboratory-induced muscle diseases now exist there are, nevertheless, several conditions in man which do not have their experimental counterparts, e.g. dystrophia myotonica, and there are many other gaps in our knowledge.

Although further work on similar lines will continue to provide useful information, it is from the application of advances in molecular biology to the human myopathic problems that real solutions are most likely to be derived.

THE REACTION OF THE MUSCLE FIBRE TO VARIOUS FORMS OF SIMPLE INJURY

Necrosis

Simple injury, such as that caused by crush or freezing, has been closely studied, and the sequential microscopic changes which eventually lead to regeneration are well known. Soon after injury there is removal of debris by macrophages (myophagia). This event is soon accompanied by proliferation of spindle cells which differentiate to form myoblasts. These cells soon fuse to produce young myotubes. Thus simple injury of sarcoplasm will lead to complete regeneration of the muscle fibres and restoration of the total muscle. This phenomenon is true even in 'higher' mammals.

In simple injury, focal necrosis of the muscle fibre is seen under the light microscope as loss of the normal architectural markings, eosinophilia or basophilia and a granular, flocculated or vacuolated appearance of the necrotic sarcoplasm. With the electron microscope, swelling of mitochondria, disruption of organelles, dilatation of the sarcoplasmic reticulum and dissolution of myofibrils can be seen; Z-band streaming, myelin figures, lysosomes and other dense bodies are also observed.

The derangements seen under both types of microscope are similar, whatever the specific cause of the damage, whether this be toxic, metabolic, immunological or genetically determined.

Focal myonecrosis is also the common denominator of many of the human dystrophies, particularly the 'aggressive' or Duchenne form. It is also found in the metabolic and nutritional myopathies of comparative myopathology, the hormonal and dysionic states as described below, and in physical injury or microbial infection. However, the actual mechanism of submicroscopic injury which must precede obvious necrosis will differ according to the specific cause. For instance, destruction of the microscopic elements may be due to the accumulation of a biochemical substrate resulting from the interruption, by a toxin, of a metabolic pathway. A virus will revise the molecular genetics of the nucleus toward the production of proteins and other compounds which will lead to its own replication and to damage to the cell (see below). Necrosis may be simply attributable to mechanical damage or interference with blood supply. In immunologically induced myonecrosis it is likely that 'cytotoxins' released from sensitised T cells damage the membrane and possibly specific organelles. In many situations the fundamental mechanisms are unknown and it is likely that their discovery will depend upon advances in molecular biology.

Regeneration

In recent years, interest in regeneration has been extended to include the wider field of muscle transplantation as well as myogenesis. As a result, a new body of information is now available (Mauro et al., 1970) and some biochemical aspects of myogenesis are under investigation in vitro (Holtzer, 1974). The fusion of myoblasts, and other events including the production of young myotubes, closely resemble the fetal development of muscle. Ultrastructurally, there are a large number of ribosomal particles among fine, newly formed myofibrils. The origin of myoblasts is considered by Mauro (1961) to be from satellite cells. This suggestion is supported by Muir, Kanji and Allbrook (1965) and by Shafiq, Gorycki and Milhorat (1967). This concept has also gained more support recently, although there remains some doubt as to whether such satellite cells exist in completely normal adult muscle despite their being observed in the human dystrophies and in simple injury.

It should be noted that complete regeneration depends upon an uninjured endomysial sheath. However, this collagenous sheath is usually preserved in the natural myopathies and in the metabolic and toxic conditions, so that a framework for restoration exists (Kakulas, 1966a).

In those instances where the endomysial sheath is disrupted, as will occur in mechanical injury, and when haemorrhage is also present, scar tissue will form. This is a common finding in earlier studies of regeneration and it is this fibrous tissue proliferation which led to the earlier and now discarded belief that muscle possessed a limited regenerative potential.

PHYSICAL METHODS

Trauma

Following the classic studies of simple crush by Le Gros Clark (1946) and Le Gros Clark and Wajda (1947) regeneration after crush was investigated electron-microscopically by Allbrook (1962). These studies confirmed the earlier observations of Volkmann (1893). These pioneer observations of Le Gros Clark have since been greatly extended (Reznik, 1973). The events which follow localised crush injury to muscle in the first few hours consist of altered morphology with obscured markings. Necrosis, evident as fragmentation and disintegration of sarcoplasm, is followed by phagocytosis of debris and spindle cell proliferation. The term 'isomorphic' regeneration is applied in this case.

When the connective and supporting tissues are also destroyed, regeneration is less well orientated and results in a mixture of fibroblasts, collagen and irregularly distributed muscle fibres, an appearance which is termed 'anisomorphic' regeneration (Kakulas and Adams, 1966).

The effects of needle-induced myopathy have been studied experimentally in the rat. The lesions are characterised initially by haemorrhagic focal destruction followed by cellular infiltration, local necrosis and single fibre degeneration, regeneration and dystrophy-like changes. After several weeks the muscle returns to normal (Mumenthaler and Paakkari, 1974).

Surprisingly, major trauma to muscle has been little studied. In this instance there is often associated haemorrhage, and healing is accompanied by the formation of granulation tissue. With the destruction of the supporting tissue elements, muscle regeneration is partly obscured by the proliferation of fibroblasts and later there is collagenous fibrosis. Nevertheless, in such lesions myoblasts and tongue-like myotubes are readily identified, especially in sections stained with phosphotungstic acid haematoxylin (PTAH). The experimental findings are similar to those which occur in accidental massive injury to muscle in man (Anastas and Kakulas, 1968). Such lesions may be present clinically as tumorous masses and in this case they are the equivalent in muscle of the 'traumatic' neuroma of peripheral nerve.

X-irradiation

Skeletal muscle is relatively resistant to X-irradiation as it is a highly differentiated tissue. The effects of massive experimental X-irradiation were described in the studies of Warren (1943) who considered the vascular changes to be primary. Amino-aciduria resulting from whole-body irradiation was reported (Goyer and Yin, 1967). Khan (1974) studied radiation-induced changes in skeletal muscle under the electron microscope.

Other physical methods

Experimentally induced temperature changes are known to cause coagulative necrosis (Adams, 1975). Gutmann and Guttmann (1942) studied the effect of electrical stimulation upon the prevention of changes secondary to denervation. Nageotte (1937) reported a shredding effect in muscle fibres produced by electrically induced severe contraction *in vitro*. Muscle changes caused by electrical stimulation are described by a number of workers (Smith, Beeuwkes, Tomkiewicz, Tadaaki and Town, 1965). The lesions were produced by AC and DC electrical discharge through the fore and hind limbs of dogs. Skin and subcutaneous tissues were not injured but the skeletal muscle showed subsarcolemmal nuclear proliferation, loss of striations, vacuolisation and ultimately frank necrosis. Changes were indistinguishable regardless of the type and polarity of the discharge. Ring fibres were not found although these are reported to be easily produced by tendon-cutting (Bethlem and van Wijngaarden, 1963), which also produces target fibres (De Reuck, De Coster and Van Der Eecken, 1977). In addition to necrosis caused by burns, supercontraction of myofibrils and nuclear streaming result from electrical injury.

Examination of the ultrastructure of freeze-injured muscle fibres shows dissolution of organelles and rarefaction of myofibrils (Fig. 11.1). Such injuries in partly affected muscle fibres result

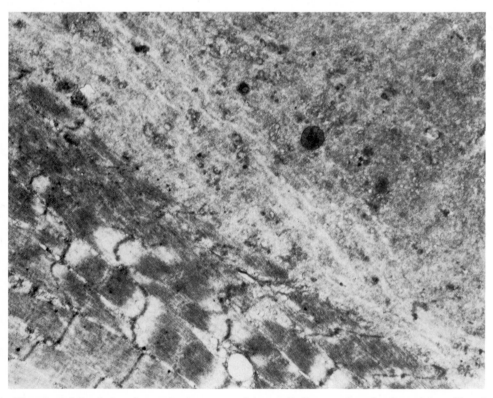

Fig. 11.1   There is total dissolution of organelles in one part of the muscle fibre two days after freeze injury. Uranyl acetate–lead citrate, ×35 000

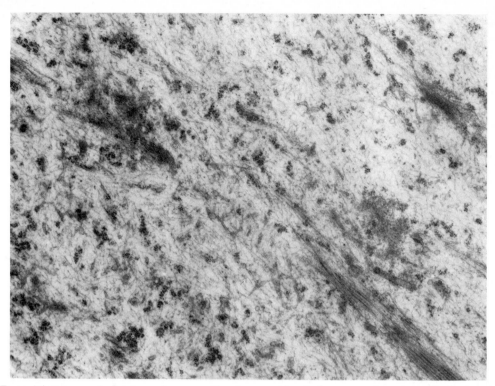

Fig. 11.2   Freeze injury to muscle showing early regenerative changes with polyribosomes and sparse myofibrils seven days after the injury. In this case regeneration is of the 'continuous' type. Uranyl acetate–lead citrate, ×54 600

in the appearance of large numbers of ribosomes as a sign of early repair (*see* Fig. 11.2).

Muscle transplantation

Muscle transplantation has attracted increasing attention in recent years and numerous reports have appeared in the current literature (Mauro *et al.*, 1970; Gutmann and Hanzlikova, 1975). Factors which affect the success of transplantation of skeletal muscle in the rat were studied by Gutmann and Hanzlikova (1975). The 'morphogenetic effects of cross-transplantation of muscle upon the epimorphic regenerative process' is considered in detail by Carlson (1974). The host reaction of muscle grafts in mice was investigated by Mastaglia, Dawkins and Papadimitriou (1974). Partridge and Sloper (1977) demonstrated a host contribution to regeneration in muscle grafts. This was found by analysis of two distinct isoenzymic forms of NADP-dependent malate dehydrogenase as genetic markers in the two strains of mice used

(CBA donors and C3H hosts). It was shown that little, if any, of the muscle formed was of donor origin.

CHEMICAL METHODS

Metabolic poisons

Powerful metabolic poisons, such as iodoacetate which blocks lactate production and causes massive Rhabdomyolysis (Fig. 11.3), are commonly used in experimental myopathology. A metabolic myopathy induced in rabbits by hypoglycaemia following administration of insulin (Tannenberg, 1939) is associated with single-fibre necrosis in both cardiac and skeletal muscle. Another agent is imidazole which accelerates the catabolism of cyclic AMP and thus causes myopathic changes in the gastrocnemius muscle of rats (Fenichel and Martin, 1974). Such chemicals usually cause pure sarcoplasmic necrosis and spare the sarcolemmal and endomysial fibrous tissue sheaths. Because of

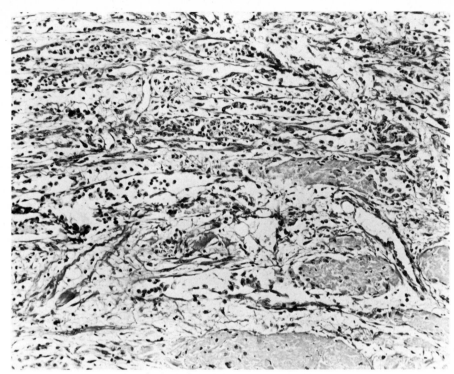

Fig. 11.3   Abdominal wall of rat injected with 0.04 mg of iodoacetate into the peritoneal cavity five days previously. There is widespread muscle fibre destruction. Recent necrosis is present (*bottom right*) and phagocytosis of debris (*above*) is in progress. Regenerative changes in the form of elongated spindle cells are conspicuous. H & E, ×120

this, in the recovery phase, connective tissue proliferation is minimal and regeneration is complete.

These experimental metabolic conditions bear a strong resemblance to some metabolic myopathies in man where, again, regeneration is complete when the cause is rectified. The same is true of the human drug-induced myopathies.

Jasmin and Gareau (1961) studied the skeletal muscle lesions produced in rats injected with diphenylenediamine. Swelling and homogenisation occurred in 24 hours and coagulation necrosis followed. The necrotic muscle segments acted as foreign bodies and gave rise to a histiocytic reaction with multinucleated giant cells. Regenerative changes occurred parallel to the severity of the lesions with regeneration *ad integrum* in less than 20 days. Mascres and Jasmin (1975) later used *p*-phenylenediamine (PPD) to investigate the inflammatory and degenerative patterns of muscle lesions in rats. Fifteen minutes after the injection of PPD, subsarcolemmal oedema was visible in the

diaphragm under the electron microscope. Enzymatic changes appeared in the first hour while pathological features were prominent after 24 hours. There was segmental necrosis adjacent to unaltered fibres and several particular types of abnormal fibres such as target, snake coils and core fibres were seen.

Recently, uraemic myopathy was produced in rats in which atrophy of type I fibres was found, but there were no structural changes (Bundschu, Pfeilsticker, Suchenwirth, Matthews and Ritz, 1974).

Extensive biochemical and morphological studies were carried out by Rubin, Katz, Lieber, Stein and Puszkin (1976) in volunteers in relation to studies of human alcoholic myopathy. Ultrastructural changes consisted of distortion of mitochondria, dilatation of the sarcoplasmic reticulum and increased amounts of fat and glycogen.

Graham, Bonilla, Gonatas and Schotland (1976) reported that core formation was observed in the muscles of rats intoxicated by triethyltin sulphate

(TET). The changes affected only the type I fibres and were observed in the soleus muscle in animals intoxicated with TET for up to 23 days. The development of core-like structures which occur after tenotomy in association with nemaline body formation and vacuolar degeneration of muscle fibres may be compared with those structures which are found after emetine intoxication and in which there are large lesions extending throughout the transverse axis of fibres, associated with loss of oxidative enzyme activity. By contrast alkyltin intoxication differs, in that in this case the central nervous system shows intramyelinic vacuolisation.

Drugs

From the knowledge derived from adverse clinical experience, a number of myotoxic drugs, particularly the antimalarials such as plasmocid and chloroquine, are often used to produce experimental lesions. Another example is dimethylsulphoxide (DMSO) (Fig. 11.4), originally introduced as an anti-inflammatory agent (Walters, Papadimitriou and Shilkin, 1967). DMSO is known specifically to injure plasma membranes and causes a myopathy in the experimental animal. Electron-microscopic examination shows fragmentation and disarray of the contractile apparatus of the muscle fibre, mitochondria are swollen and the sarcotubular system is greatly dilated forming large vacuoles which measure 5000–6000 nm in diameter. Muscle fibre necrosis with complete loss of structure and invasion by leucocytes also occurs (Fig. 11.5).

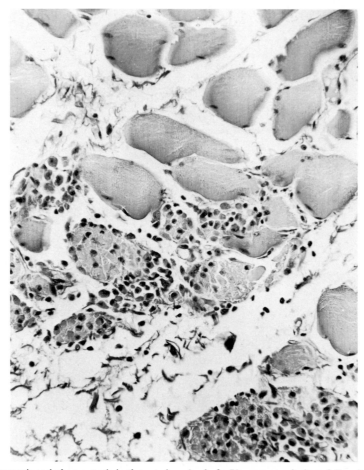

Fig. 11.4 Muscle fibre necrosis and phagocytosis in the rat given 1 ml of a 50 per cent solution of dimethylsulphoxide (DMSO) by injection 48 h previously. Van Gieson stain, × 260

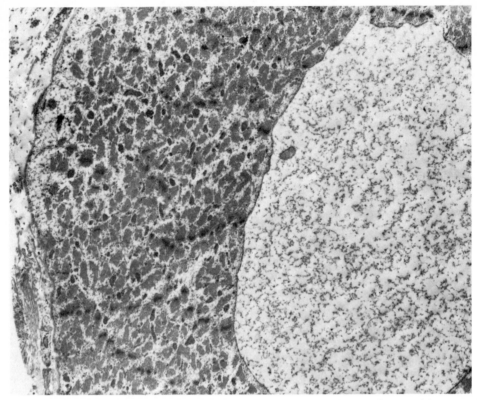

Fig. 11.5 Electron micrograph of muscle lesion due to DMSO. There is fragmentation and disarray of the contractile system (*left*) and the sarcotubular system is dilated and forms large vacuoles (*right*). Uranyl acetate–lead citrate, ×3280

The antimetabolites used in the treatment of malignant diseases are particularly potent myotoxins, e.g. the oncolytic agent vincristine sulphate frequently causes a neuromyopathy. This side effect was studied in the experimental animal by Slotwiner, Song and Anderson (1966). They describe peculiar 'spheromembranous' structures in affected muscles observed by phase microscopy. Vincristine can be seen by electron-microscopic examination to produce disarray and loss of the contractile elements of myocytes. The cytoplasmic space between the adjacent myofibrils is increased and contains remnants of myofilaments, swollen mitochondria and large aggregates of vesicles. The vesicles are arranged in a whorled fashion and probably represent altered components of the sarcoplasmic system. These vesicular aggregates are often large, measuring 1000–2000 nm in diameter, and probably represent the spheromembranous structures of phase microscopy (*see*

Fig. 11.6). Clarke, Karpati, Carpenter and Wolfe (1972) also undertook a comprehensive study of vincristine myopathy using histochemical, ultrastructural and chemical techniques.

Winer, Klachko, Baer, Langley and Burns (1966) reported a myotonic response in rats, induced by inhibitors of cholesterol biosynthesis. They suggested that desmosterol accumulation in combination with a specific drug effect may be the cause. The relationship between the experimental disorder and human myotonia is unknown.

Myotonia of the diaphragm is produced by 2,4-dichlorphenoxyacetate (2,4-D) (Rudel and Keller, 1975). The subacute skeletal myopathy induced by high doses of 2,4-D in guinea pigs has been studied recently by Danon, Karpati and Carpenter (1978). A number of histochemical changes were observed while, with the electron microscope, proliferation consisting of tubular profiles, intranuclear filaments and osmiophilic

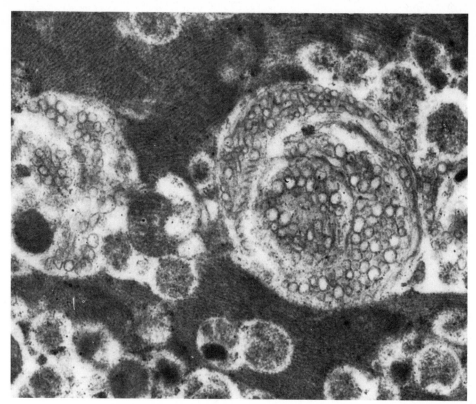

Fig. 11.6 Electron micrograph of muscle lesion in rat following six intraperitoneal injections of 0.06 mg vincristine sulphate over three days. Contractile elements are disrupted, mitochondria are swollen and whorled aggregates of dilated vesicles are present forming the spheromembranous bodies. Uranyl acetate–lead citrate, ×25 800

lattices was found, together with disintegration of myofilaments and Z lines. 25-azocholesterol continues to be used in order to produce an experimental model of myotonia (Dobosz, Mrozek and Kwiecinski, 1974).

The effects of phencyclidine on skeletal muscle have been investigated in conjunction with the effects of restraint stress. Ultrastructurally there is extensive disruption of myofibrillar architecture and Z-band streaming (Kuncl, 1974).

Emetine myopathy was studied in the rat by Bradley, Fewings, Harris and Johnson (1976). Morphological and histochemical changes were induced by increasing doses of emetine administered for up to 22 days. Necrotic hyaline and split fibres were described with focal loss of myofibrillar ATPase and other histochemical changes. The authors concluded that muscle weakness was due to a direct effect on the muscle fibres at subcellular level, with no evidence that emetine produced its

effect by denervation. Iodide-induced skeletal muscle necrosis in rats was reported by Cantin in 1967. Cramps occurred and muscle-fibre necrosis and degeneration were observed under the microscope.

Plasmocid (8-(3-diethylaminopropyl-amino)-6-methoxyquinoline dihydrochloride) is also noted for its powerful myotoxic effects. The drug was first synthesised as a potential antimalarial drug but proved too toxic for clinical use. Hicks (1950) noted that intraperitoneal injections in rats and mice produced widespread skeletal muscle lesions. The changes were necrotic, phagocytic and regenerative (Fig. 11.7).

Price, Pease and Pearson (1962) and D'Agostino (1963) reported that destruction of actin filaments and Z-line changes were found in rats as a result of plasmocid administration. Plasmocid also causes mitochondrial swelling, diminution of cristae and dilated sarcotubules.

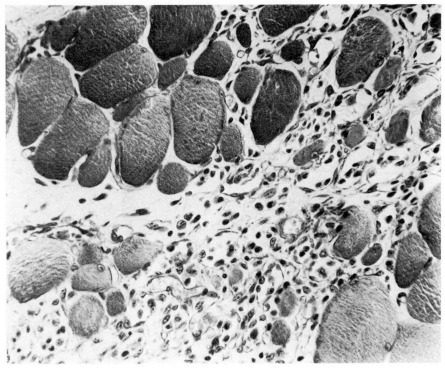

Fig. 11.7   Rectus abdominis muscle of rat four days after parenteral administration of 0.6 mg plasmocid. There is muscle fibre necrosis and macrophage activity (*centre, below*) and intact fibres (*above*). Van Gieson stain, ×260

Bowden and Goyer (1962) described widespread necrotic foci in muscles after administration of plasmocid to rats, and showed that marked increases in serum aspartate aminotransferase (SGOT) activity occurred in 8–12 hours. These workers also found on urinanalysis that the myopathy was associated with the urinary excretion of large quantities of the amino acid taurine.

Chloroquine produces focal muscle fibre necrosis in a manner similar to that induced by plasmocid, with the predominant changes being in the red fibres (Smith and O'Grady, 1966). Although the mechanism of action is unknown, Gutierrez (1966) found disturbances of lipid metabolism in turkey erythrocytes and heart muscle homogenates.

Further observations on experimental chloroquine myopathy were undertaken by Aguayo and Hudgson (1970), in which the short-term effects of chloroquine on skeletal muscle were studied in rabbits. Serum enzymes including creatine kinase were raised. In this work no evidence of vascular changes was found but there was focal necrosis and phagocytosis in skeletal and cardiac muscle.

Markand and D'Agostino (1971) studied the effects of intraperitoneal injections of colchicine in rats. The rats became paralysed one to two days after injection. The lesions in muscle, examined with the electron microscope, showed damage to all organelles but the most conspicuous finding was the accumulation of large sarcoplasmic membranous bodies. There was a good correlation between the presence of such membranous bodies and overt weakness.

The antimicrobial agent, nitroxoline, causes neuromyopathic changes in the mouse (O'Grady and Smith, 1966). Muscle changes consist of swollen fibres with central nuclei but there is little evidence of necrosis. Phosphorylase preparations showed loss of activity in affected muscle fibres.

Yamamura (1977) studied the effects of various antibiotics injected into muscle. Intramuscular injections of chloramphenicol and oxytetracycline in mice were found to produce more severe muscle damage than streptomycin, cephalosporin and aminobenzyl penicillin. Electron microscopy showed degeneration of muscle fibres, motor end-plates and peripheral nerves one day after a single injection. In animals injected on three occasions, localised fibrosis and degenerating myotubes which were attributed to peripheral nerve damage were also produced.

Selye (1965) reported 'muscular dystrophy changes' produced by injections of serotonin in experimental animals. He considered the effects to be attributable to vascular changes. Serotonin will induce muscle weakness in the rat (Patten and Oliver, 1974). Other catecholamines have been found by Felmus, Patten, Hart and Martinez (1977) to induce muscle weakness in rabbits. An experimental myopathy resembling human dystrophy was produced by the monoamine oxidase inhibitor pargyline hydrochloride, causing excessive levels of catecholamine in the tissues and urine of myopathic animals. These workers believe that their experiments support the hypothesis that catecholamines could play a pathogenetic role in some dystrophic conditions 'especially since abnormal accumulation of catecholamine in human dystrophic muscle has been observed'.

Diphenylhydantoin was shown to produce histological changes in the muscle of cats given intramuscular injections. These changes consisted of haemorrhage and necrosis with crystallisation of the diphenylhydantoin being observed in association with necrotic muscle (Serrano and Wilder, 1974).

Martin, Laskowski and Fenichel (1977) have shown that an acetylcholine-mediated myopathy may be produced in rat soleus muscle by daily injections of imidazole, a drug which accelerates the metabolism of adenosine $3',5'$ cyclic phosphate by activating the enzyme phosphodiesterase.

Clofibrate myopathy was studied in the rat by Teräväinen, Larsen and Hillbom (1977), and minor myopathic abnormalities were observed with both the light and the electron microscope. The changes consisted of necrosis and phagocytosis, with ultrastructural autolysis.

Cannabinoids were shown to produce muscle fibre necrosis and regeneration with associated myopathic changes in mice (Giusti, Ghiarotti, Passatore, Gentile and Fiori, 1977).

The above commentary lists the large number of drug-induced experimental myopathies which have been studied, and it may be expected that, with the continuing introduction of new therapeutic agents, further drug-induced myopathies will occur. In this event it is fortunate that the inherent ability of muscle to regenerate once the cause of necrosis is removed, ensures that many of these untoward effects are likely to be reversible on withdrawal of the agent.

Dysionic states

The effects of potassium deficiency as a cause of focal necrosis are well known, especially from veterinary experience (Hove and Herndon, 1955). The injurious effects of steroid hormones (considered below) are also influenced by electrolyte changes. Bajusz (1965) has shown that in the experimental animal with $NaClO_4$-induced motor disturbances, the predominantly mineralocorticoids will greatly enhance the effect while glucocorticoids are preventive. Bajusz (1965) further reports that an acute paralytic condition may be caused in rabbits by a combination of methylchlorocortisol and NaH_2PO_4 administration. The condition, which resembles familial periodic paralysis in man, is prevented by chlorides (Selye and Bajusz, 1960).

The main effect of calcium deficiency is the physiological disorder of contraction manifest as tetany. Trace element (e.g. selenium) deficiency is a well-known cause of muscle fibre necrosis in farm animals and there are several experimental studies dealing with the effect of selenium on skeletal muscle (Schwarz and Foltz, 1957).

BIOLOGICAL METHODS

Toxins

Bacterial toxins are powerful myonecrotic agents. Morita (1926) studied the effect of clostridial toxin, such as that from *Clostridium welchii*, which usually destroys connective tissue as well as causing muscle fibre necrosis. The effects of *Clostridium botulinum* were recently studied, with denervation changes being reported by Johnston and Drachman (1974).

Adams (1975) reported fatty degeneration in cardiac muscle after the administration of diphtheria toxin to guinea pigs. However, no consistent changes in skeletal muscle were observed, and he found that direct inoculation of diphtheria organisms into muscle caused lesions which did not differ from those produced by any bacterial necrosis.

Keast (1967) in his studies on the origin of lesions in neonatal mice receiving neomycin sulphate, investigated the effect of *E.coli* endotoxin, and in this way produced widespread muscle fibre necrosis (Fig. 11.8).

Tiger snake toxin causes skeletal muscle degeneration and subsequent regeneration when injected into the rat (Pluskal, Pennington, Johnson and Harris, 1975).

The oriental hornet (*Vespa orientalis*) causes a lesion of the muscle transverse-tubular system (Ishay, Lass and Sandbank, 1975). Light-microscopic examination showed that vacuoles appear in the sartorius muscle incubated in hornet venom–Ringer's solution. Under the electron microscope it was observed that these vacuoles were caused by greatly distended T-tubules and distended terminal cisternae.

Bacteria and viruses

Bacterial myositis has not been studied systematically in the laboratory but the subject is reviewed by Banker (1960) and by Adams (1975); Banker also considered parasitic infections of muscle. As might be expected, pyogenic organisms cause acute abscesses and similar lesions result from injections of turpentine into muscle.

Many viruses are capable of producing experimental myositis, including mouse encephalomyelitis (GD–VII and FA strains) and the Mitchell strain of lymphocytic choriomeningitis (Rustigan and Pappenheimer, 1949). The Coxsackie viruses (Dalldorf, 1950) are especially known to cause myositis and Type A (Field, 1960) is more active in this regard (Fig. 11.9).

Arboviruses also cause myositis. It has been demonstrated in this connection that myofibrils

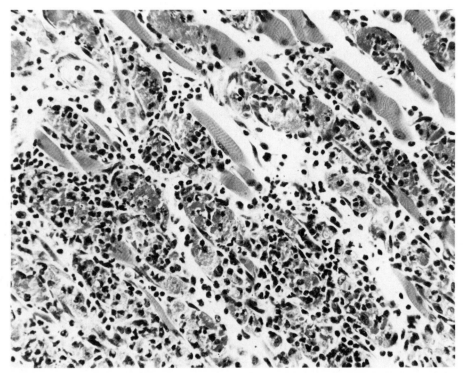

Fig. 11.8   Muscle lesion in neonatal mouse following intraperitoneal injection of 0.01 ml of 10^9 dilution of *E. coli* endotoxin 16 days previously. There is widespread muscle fibre necrosis and macrophage reaction (specimen provided by Mr D. Keast). H & E, × 300

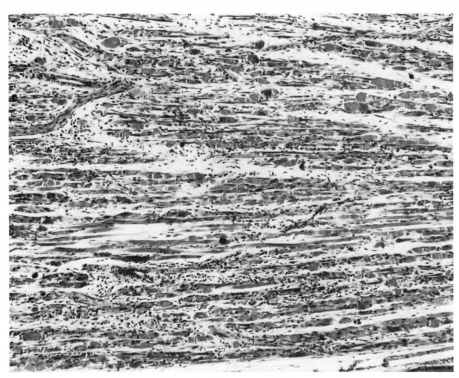

Fig. 11.9   Coxsackie virus myositis in mouse. There is widespread muscle fibre necrosis and leucocytic infiltration (specimen provided by Dr R.D. Adams). H & E, ×80

are severely damaged with accompanying dilatation of T-tubules and of the sarcoplasmic reticulum (SR), with the accumulation of mature arbovirus particles within the cisternae and vacuoles (Sato, Sakuragawa and Tsubaki, 1975).

Miranda, Gamboa, Armstrong and Hsu (1978) have studied influenza virus infection of human skeletal muscle in tissue culture. Using scanning and transmission electron microscopes, cytopathic changes, both in organelles and surface elements were observed. Cell injury and death appear to be caused by massive accumulation of virus-induced products that alter cellular metabolism *in vitro*.

Hormones

Because of the wide therapeutic use of steroid hormones, much attention has been devoted to 'cortisone' myopathy. The first reports of experimental cortisone myopathy were those of Ellis (1953, 1956) who studied cortisone-induced muscle lesions in rabbits. Muscle fibre necrosis was found and he recorded the now familiar

sequence leading to regeneration. In the cortisone-induced muscle lesions, many necrotic foci were impregnated with calcium salts and foreign body giant-cell forms were observed. Ellis (1956) found that similar myopathic changes were produced by potassium depletion but in this case myocardial necrosis was also produced. Similar lesions were observed in the mouse treated with large doses of hydrocortisone (Fig. 11.10). D'Agostino and Chiga (1966) used the electron microscope to examine cortisone-induced lesions in the diaphragm of rabbits. Granular muscle fibres were primarily involved and increased lipid content was observed. Glycogen also accumulated in both granular and agranular fibres. Bizarre mitochondria were common in the degenerating fibres.

Experimental cortisone myopathy was studied by Luca, Hategan, Anghelescu, Alexianu and Petrovici (1974). With small doses, muscle enzyme hyperactivity was observed. At high doses, enzyme hypoactivity was considered to be attributable probably to muscle degeneration. Motor innervation in cortisone myopathy was studied in

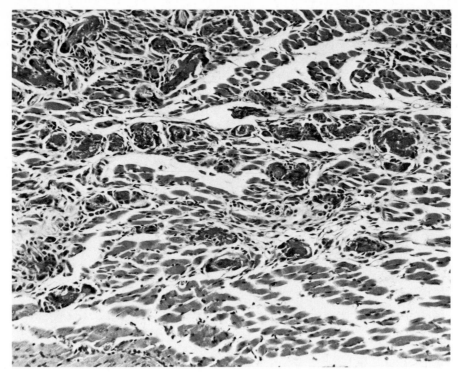

Fig. 11.10   Paravertebral muscles of mouse showing focal necrosis of sarcoplasm and impregnation with calcium salts, injected with 0.1 mg/g body weight hydrocortisone 14 days previously (specimen provided by Mr D. Keast). H & E, ×83

the rat by Pellissier and Fardeau (1975). The persistence of motor nerve endings in atrophying and necrotising muscles was demonstrated and variable changes in the different components of motor end-plates occurred.

In medical practice a number of well-defined endocrinopathies such as acromegaly, hypothyroidism (Aström, Kugelberg and Muller, 1961) and Cushing's disease may cause myopathic changes, but experimental studies of such disorders are very limited. It is known that thyroxin will induce the production of sarcoplasmic masses in the tadpole. Dobosz *et al.* (1975) have shown that there is no myosin ATPase activity in the sarcoplasmic masses.

Dietary factors

Myopathies can be induced by nutritional deficiencies such as those of vitamin E, thiamine, choline and vitamin C in guinea pigs (low protein and raw egg-white myopathies) (Banker, 1960). Disorders produced in this way are similar to the

naturally occurring myopathies of nutritional origin (*see* Ch. 24).

Vitamin E deficiency is a very potent cause of muscle fibre necrosis and the resulting myopathic effects are well known (Hadlow, 1962). In the experimental context, vitamin E deficiency provides much useful information concerning the pathogenesis of muscle lesions in dystrophic states. In this regard, the Rottnest Island quokka (*Setonix brachyurus*) has proved to be a most useful model (Kakulas, 1966).

Howell and Buxton (1975) have described α-tocopherol-responsive muscular dystrophy in guinea pigs. Muscle fibre necrosis, regeneration and cellular infiltrates were similar to those which were found in the Rottnest Island quokka with nutritional myopathy. CPK levels fell in the guinea pigs, but the animals revived after treatment with α-tocopherol.

Vitamin D deficiency results in defective calcium uptake in the sarcoplasmic reticulum, and protein deficiency will cause pseudomyopathic changes (Francis, Curry and Smith, 1974). Ward and Goldspink (1974) studied the response of different muscle fibre types to changes in the activity pattern in protein malnutrition in the mouse.

Rats placed on an iodine-deficient diet by Rosman, Schapiro and Haddow (1978) in order to produce hypothyroidism, unexpectedly developed progressive muscle weakness. The myopathy was due to a deficiency of a number of dietary constituents, only one of which was iodine. Necrosis and atrophy of cells was seen as well as variability of muscle fibre size and shape.

Circulatory disturbances

Ischaemic muscle injury was studied by Adams (1975) and the resulting pan-necrosis was considered in detail. Scully, Shannon and Dickersin (1961) examined the factors involved in recovery from experimental skeletal muscle ischaemia in dogs. Boehme and Themann (1966) reported structural and ultrastructural changes in striated human muscle caused by chronic ischaemia in amputated human legs. Electron microscopic observations disclosed fibres in which mitochondria and sarcoplasmic reticulum were well preserved and others in which degeneration of these elements was prominent. Glycogen was actually increased in some fibres. These observations were considered to be relevant to human Volkmann's ischaemic contracture.

DENERVATION

The work of Buller, Eccles and Eccles (1960) on the physiological relationship between motor nerve and muscle is well known. The denervation studies of Kugelberg, Edstrom and Abbruzzese (1970) defined the histochemical specificity of muscle fibre types within individual motor units. Peter (1973), who fully reviewed this subject, believes that the particular histochemical fibre type is governed by the physiological function of the motor unit rather than by anterior horn cell specificity. The histochemical type is thus determined by physiological demand rather than by 'immutable' motor unit specificity.

The paradoxical phenomenon of 'denervation hypertrophy' is of considerable experimental interest. New fibre formation is also associated with this phenomenon in adult animals (Sola, Christensen and Martin, 1973). There is considerable interest in the definition of trophic and developmental influences in fetal muscle under experimental conditions, and denervation is employed in such studies (Margreth, Salviati and Carraro, 1974). In the biochemistry of denervated muscle, attention was paid to protein synthesis and oxidation by Gauthier and Schaeffer (1975) and by Kark, Edgerton and Whiteman (1975).

Myographic and electroneurographic responses of leg muscles to cross-innervated sciatic nerves are reported to be normal in dystrophic mice united by parabiosis (Douglas, 1974). The investigation of neurotrophic influences has extended to the investigation of intramuscular injection of spinal cord homogenate. Such studies demonstrate enhancement of protein synthesis (Crockett and Edgerton, 1974).

The histochemistry of regenerating myofibres before and after reinnervation was undertaken to determine the role of 'trophic influences' in creating 'type specificity' of muscle fibres. It was found that differentiation of regenerated myofibres into several types begins four to five weeks after injury and is related to re-innervation. Unusual checkerboard distribution of type I and type II fibres and heterogeneous myofibres occur in the major part of a muscle which, before injury, contained type II fibres almost exclusively. Additionally, large and small regenerating myofibres had end-plates which were often abnormal. The results suggest that axons sprouting from different motor units proliferate in the same area and innervate new myofibres at random. Such modifications are quite different from the fibre-type grouping described after spontaneous or experimentally induced re-innervation of normal myofibres (Reznik, 1973; Manolov, 1974).

Denervation caused the appearance of central nuclei and muscle-fibre splitting with eventual loss of architecture in the experimental myopathy induced by paroxan and organophosphorus (Wecker and Dettbarn, 1977).

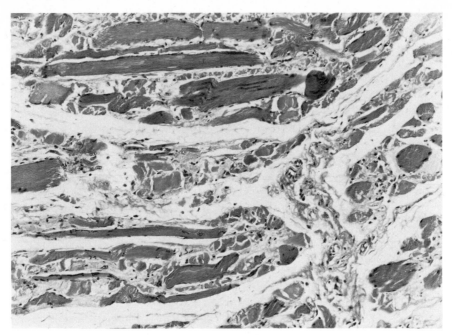

Fig. 11.11   Widespread hyaline and granular necrosis with myophagia of muscle fibres in nutritional myopathy of the Rottnest Island quokka. There is also loss of muscle fibres, fibrous tissue condensation and fat increase. The changes bear a resemblance to those found in human muscular dystrophy, ×142

EXPERIMENTAL MODELS OF HUMAN MYOPATHIES

Most of the work in this area is concerned with three human conditions, progressive muscular dystrophy, myasthenia gravis and polymyositis. The human and animal dystrophies are the subject of intensive enquiry because of their devastating clinical effects. To help achieve an understanding of these conditions the natural dystrophies in animals are studied and attempts are made to reproduce similar myopathies in the laboratory. Some of this research examines simple chemical or physical injury to muscle as outlined above. Other methods, such as microembolisation (Engel, 1973) and, more particularly, the effects of controlled deprivation of vitamin E (Kakulas and Adams, 1966) are more sophisticated.

Dystrophy

Vitamin E. Of the numerous attempts to simulate muscular dystrophy in animals, the myopathy of experimental vitamin E deficiency in the Rottnest Island quokka (*Setonix brachyurus*) more closely resembles the naturally occurring conditions than do others (Fig. 11.11). In this model there is polyfocal muscle fibre necrosis and reactive cellular changes are concerned with the removal of debris and regeneration. Using the quokka, it is possible to regulate the deficiency of vitamin E so that the changes which occur in human progressive muscular dystrophy are closely reproduced. These lesions result from chronic continuing necrosis due to marginal deficiency of the vitamin. The proximal distribution of paralysis in the animal also follows the pattern of the human condition.

The early lesions in the vitamin E deficient quokka resemble those in the early stages of Duchenne muscular dystrophy but they are more acute. There is focal necrosis, attempted regeneration and general disorganisation of muscle architecture. Apart from the lack of the very large round fibres common in the gastrocnemius in Duchenne dystrophy, the changes are very similar in both conditions. At the end of the process, the histopathology consists of a few preserved muscle fibres which are irregular in size and shape and nuclear distribution is disordered. There is also fat and connective tissue increase, which results from collapse of endomysial fibrous tissue.

Numerous studies continue to take place using dystrophic mice, chickens and hamsters. These include re-innervation experiments after experimental denervation, studies of the biochemistry of subcellular organelles and of the effects of therapeutic agents (Ashmore and Doerr, 1974; Owens, Ruth, Gottwik, McNamara and Weglicki, 1975; Park, Chou, Hill, Pinson, Bartle, Connally, Lequire, Roelofs and Olson, 1975; Wrogemann, Mezon, Boeckx, Thakar, Picard and Blanchaer, 1975). Jasmin, Bajusz and Solymoss (1975) report that verapamil will prevent hereditary cardiomyopathy in the Syrian hamsters.

Microembolisation. Engel (1973) induced focal muscle fibre necrosis in rabbits using microembolisation. The lesions appeared to be grouped, and regeneration ensued. To some extent the lesions resembled those of the naturally occurring human and animal dystrophies.

Immunological attempts to produce dystrophic changes were less successful. In early reports of the use of immunological methods the changes were considered dystrophic in character by Tal and Liban (1962). However, the lesions seemed to be more in accord with atrophy caused by chronic disuse and poor nutrition.

Myasthenia gravis

Efforts to reproduce myasthenia gravis in the laboratory have a long history. The most popular method is the immunisation of the animal using muscle extracts, crude or purified, with or without adjuvant. Many of these experiments have resulted in 'myasthenia', if it is defined as excessive fatiguability and increased sensitivity to curare (Goldstein and Whittingham, 1966; Whittingham and Mackay, 1966). Where reported, histological muscle lesions consist of focal necrosis and inflammation, otherwise the muscles are normal in appearance. Parkes (1966) failed to produce a model for myasthenia gravis by immunological methods in the rat, although muscle fibre necrosis was produced. Nevertheless, Goldstein and Whit-

tingham (1966) considered that they had produced an experimental counterpart to myasthenia gravis. A naturally occurring animal model of myasthenia in the dog is well known (Palmer, Harriman and Barker, 1974). Patrick and Lindstrom (1973) observed that repeated immunisation of rabbits with nicotinic acetylcholine receptor (AChR) purified from the electric organ of *Electrophorus electricus* produced muscular weakness and a decrementing electromyogram response to repeated nerve stimulation. The changes were reversible with anticholinesterase drugs.

Serum from rabbits immunised with antigens derived from the electrical organs of other eels have serum antibodies to AChR. This antibody is capable of blocking the depolarisation response of the electroplaque to carbamyl choline (Patrick, Lindstrom, Culp and McMillan, 1973).

More recently, experimental myasthenia has been produced in rabbits injected with isolated nicotinic acetylcholine receptor purified from the electrical organ of *Torpedo marmorata* by affinity chromatography (Heilbronn, Mattson and Stalberg, 1975). The rabbits developed flaccid paralysis within three weeks. Experimental myasthenia in monkeys produces ptosis which is reversible with edrophonium (Tarrab-Hazdai, Aharanov, Abramsky, Yaar and Fuchs, 1975). In this manner, investigators have successfully produced experimental myasthenia gravis which closely resembles the clinical disease and may be passively transferred in breast milk (Sanders, Cobb and Winfield, 1978).

Furthermore, Engel, Tsujihata, Lambert, Lindstrom and Lennon (1976) have shown morphological and electrophysiological changes at the neuromuscular junction in the rat with experimental autoimmune myasthenia gravis (EAMG); these changes closely resemble the alterations seen at the end-plate in human myasthenia gravis in the chronic phase. Thus, the ultrastructure of the neuromuscular junction in EAMG in experimental animals immunised with highly purified eel acetylcholine receptor protein and adjuvants is similar to that in human myasthenia gravis. In the early phases, mononuclear cells infiltrate the end-plate regions and there is intense degeneration in the postsynaptic area with splitting of abnormal junctional folds from the underlying muscle fibres. Macrophages remove the degenerating folds by phagocytosis. Nerve terminals are displaced. Such changes are accompanied by blocked neuromuscular transmission. In the more chronic phase in this experimental model, after day 11 nerve terminals return to the highly simplified postsynaptic regions and the inflammatory reaction subsides. Subsequently postsynaptic folds become reconstituted, but they again degenerate. Immature junctions with poorly differentiated postsynaptic regions and nerve sprouts near end-plates are also observed. Postsynaptic membrane length and miniature end-plate potential (mepp) amplitudes are decreased in all animals in the chronic phase. In another experiment Lennon, Lindstrom and Seybold (1976) demonstrated the passive transfer of EAMG by lymphoid cells.

Toyka, Drachman, Griffin, Pestronk, Winkelstein, Fischbeck and Kao (1977) report the passive transfer of myasthenia gravis to mice, with immunoglobulins derived from patients with myasthenia gravis. Typical reductions in mepp occur and the data suggest that the pathogenesis of myasthenia gravis often involves an antibody-mediated autoimmune attack on the acetylcholine receptors of the neuromuscular junction.

Employing the α-bungarotoxin radioimmunoassay methods, Lindstrom, Lennon, Seybold and Whittingham (1976) measured antibody against human muscle AChR. They also found that rat thymus contains a small amount of AChR. When the same radioimmunoassay was used with human sera they reported significant titres of anti-AChR antibody in 82 of 84 sera from 50 patients with active myasthenia gravis, whereas none of the 82 sera from patients without myasthenia gravis contained anti-AChR antibodies. Lindstrom, Seybold, Lennon, Whittingham and Duane (1976) showed that such titres of antibody correlate well with the clinical severity of the disease, including the response to treatment with corticosteroids, and also with spontaneous remission. Titres are increased in myasthenic patients with thymoma.

Engel, Lambert and Howard (1977) interpreted their experimental studies of IgG and C3 at motor end-plates in myasthenia gravis both at the sites of AChR and on degenerate material in the synaptic space as evidence that myasthenic weakness is caused by AChR destruction resulting from the autoimmune reaction.

Satyamurti, Drachman and Slone (1975) demonstrated electrophysiological and pharmacological changes typical of myasthenia gravis in rat muscle induced by the blockade of AChRs by the α-toxin of the Formosan cobra (*Naja naja atra*).

In 1960 Simpson suggested on clinical grounds that myasthenia might be an autoimmune disease. He suggested that myasthenia gravis was a multisystem disease analogous to systemic lupus erythematosus, and based his opinion on an association with other disorders affecting tissues other than muscle, including thyroid disorders and rheumatoid arthritis (Simpson, 1964, 1966).

In previous editions of this book a detailed discussion of the experimental findings in conjunction with the laboratory findings in patients with myasthenia gravis was given. However, because of the more recent work of Lindstrom and Engel, such considerations are now redundant. A very clear understanding of EAMG has emerged from the work of Lindstrom (1978), by developing the acetylcholine receptor model, and of Engel (1978), using a combination of morphological and physiological observations; the experimental disease has many features in common with natural myasthenia gravis.

Simpson (1977, 1978a, b) has reviewed the experimental data extensively and puts forward a 'personal view' of the pathogenesis and mechanism of myasthenia gravis. He re-asserts that myasthenia gravis is a disease of disordered immunity and that the neuromuscular junction is immunologically damaged. He considers that such damage is due to a breakdown in immunological tolerance and that the thymus plays a significant part in this process. He also reports a frequent association between the HL-8A antigen and myasthenia gravis but points out that there are HL-8A negative cases. Simpson suggests that this may be a marker of a defective suppressor T cell function. He summarises his views as follows. Serum antibodies and circulating T cells raised against acetylcholine receptor substance produce a good experimental model of myasthenia gravis. New methods of assay which test the affinity of end-plate receptor for toxins believed to react specifically, indicate the presence of complement-fixing humoral neuromuscular-blocking globulin in myasthenic subjects and not in normal controls.

There is some evidence that lymphocytes may attack motor end-plates. If the lymphocytes are from myasthenic donors or from electroplaque-immunised animals, the damage to end-plates reflects the difference in source; in the latter case they passively transfer a myasthenia-like disease. He concludes that AChR blockade with antibody and structural changes results from cell-mediated immunological damage to the neuromuscular junction both presynaptically and postsynaptically, and that such a mechanism would adequately account for all known clinical, electrophysiological and pharmacological phenomena of myasthenia gravis.

Engel (1978) has recently reported that there is excellent morphological evidence to indicate that both IgG and C3 bind to AChR at the end-plate in both myasthenia gravis and in EAMG. He finds that the abundance of immune complexes is proportional to the abundance of AChR that remains at the end-plate, and that impaired neuromuscular transmission is primarily caused by the AChR deficiency at the end-plate. Antibody-dependent, complement-mediated destruction of segments of the postsynaptic membrane represents one of the mechanisms which can result in AChR deficiency in both myasthenia gravis and in experimental myasthenia.

Polymyositis

A variety of experimental methods are used to produce a 'polymyositis-like' disorder in animals. These began in 1937 with Kallos and Pagel who used a passive immune method. An active immunological approach was employed by Pearson in 1956. Although noting that myositis was present, Pearson became more concerned with the polyarthritis produced by Freund's adjuvant than with the myositis. The suggestion that human polymyositis may be the result of disordered immune function was based on the presence of raised levels of serum globulins in the serum of many patients with the disease, the sometimes dramatic response to steroid hormones given for therapeutic purposes, and the known clinical association with disorders of presumed immunological aetiology, e.g. systemic lupus erythematosus (Walton and Adams, 1958).

A 'polymyositis-like' condition, subsequently

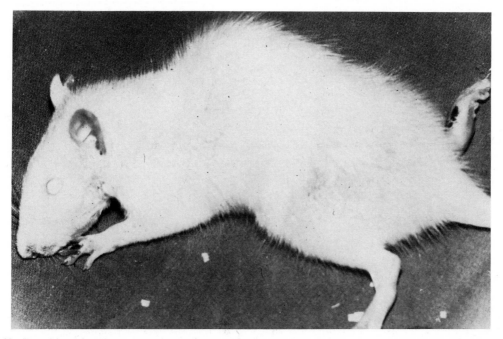

Fig. 11.12 Rat with profound muscle weakness after sensitisation to rabbit muscle and Freund's adjuvant by repeated foot-pad injections

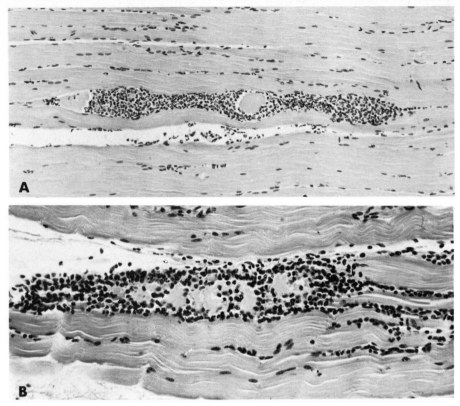

Fig. 11.13 A. Immunologically induced muscle-fibre necrosis and leucocytic infiltration in guinea pig following repeated injections of rabbit muscle and adjuvant. H & E, ×112. B. Focal muscle-fibre necrosis and round-cell collections in rat, produced by similar means. H & E, ×208

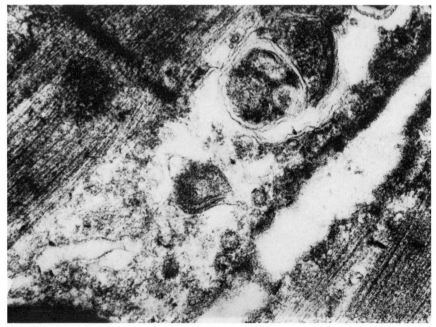

Fig. 11.14 Electron micrograph of vastus lateralis muscle of rat sensitized to rabbit muscle, showing loss of mitochondria, dilatations of sarcoplasmic reticulum, disappearance of myofilaments and presence of membranous structures. Uranyl acetate–lead citrate, ×16 000

named experimental allergic myositis (EAM), is produced in rats by immunological methods (Dawkins, 1965; Kakulas, 1966b). A rat with this immunologically induced myositis (Kakulas, 1973) is seen in Figure 11.12. Histological features include focal necrotic and inflammatory changes (Fig. 11.13). Electron microscopy provides further detail of the necrosis which affects all ultrastructural elements but especially the myofibrils. Membranous structures are also visible (Fig. 11.14).

It is also shown (Figs. 11.15 and 11.16) that *in vitro* transfer of lymphocytes from animals with EAM produces cytotoxic effects in tissue cultures of fetal rat muscle (Kakulas, 1966b). Similar experiments with slight variations in technique or animal species give essentially similar results (Webb, 1970; Currie, Saunders, Knowles and Brown, 1971).

The close relationship of the experimental disease to human polymyositis is demonstrated by the presence of *in vitro* cytotoxic effects of human lymphocytes from patients with the disease, when these cells are applied to human fetal muscle in culture (Kakulas, 1970, 1973). In muscle biopsies of patients with polymyositis, lymphocytes and plasma cells are mainly perivenular and appear to be closely related to necrotic foci (Adams, 1973).

Chou (1973) discusses the problem further in the light of the possible role of a virus as the sensitising agent which might enter the skeletal muscles at the time of a minor injury, thus penetrating single myoblasts. This observation, together with the demonstrations by Granger (1969) and Peter (1971), of a cytotoxic factor produced by lymphocytes, suggest that such a virus is possibly the antigen to which the lymphocytes are sensitised in patients with polymyositis.

Experimental studies of EAM are also directed towards determining the nature of the antigen (Esiri and MacLennan, 1975). Myofibrillar antigens appear to be more potent than those of other subcellular components of muscle (Manghani, Partridge, Smith and Sloper, 1975). These workers established that lymphocytes from myositic animals are sensitised to the outer surface of muscle cells. The macrophage-migration inhibition test was used to identify the components within the muscle fibres to which lymphocytes are also sensitised. Their studies indicate that there is lymphocyte sensitisation against the myofibrillar fraction and especially against the proteins myosin and tropomyosin. Guinea pigs injected with rabbit myofibrillar fractions and Freund's adjuvant regularly develop myositis. These animals show many more lesions in muscles than do those animals given other subcellular fractions. The lesions consist of areas of round cell infiltration and muscle fibre necrosis.

Penn (1977), in reviewing the pathogenesis of myasthenia gravis, polymyositis and dermatomyositis, concludes that the humoral arm of the defence appears to be directly responsible for the lesion in myasthenia gravis but cellular mechanisms at the thymic regulatory level are also involved. Cytotoxic T cells seem to produce the lesion of experimental myositis in which anti-muscle antibodies can be detected and those of polymyositis and dermatomyositis in which antibodies have not been convincingly shown. Childhood dermatomyositis is considered to be a probable exception in which antibodies and complement contribute to underlying vasculitis. Immunosuppressive measures can modify or prevent the disease in experimental models and Penn believes that the evidence indicates a solid rationale for their use in the human diseases, although much more information is required concerning the site of action and appropriate therapeutic planning.

Experimental malignant hyperthermia

Malignant hyperpyrexia is inducible in Pietrain pigs by the administration of halothane and succinylcholine. This allows electrophysiological studies to be undertaken as well as investigation of the mechanism of heat generation. Neither of the electrical phenomena, pseudotremor and increase in neuromuscular block, relate to the contracture while steep thermal gradients develop with increasing tissue and skin insulation. Histology and histochemistry show no specific alteration in muscle tissue (Schiller, Esslen, Weihe, Haldemann and Teelmann, 1974).

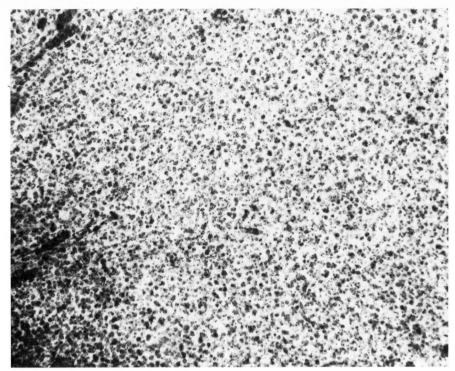

Fig. 11.15 *In vitro* destruction of muscle fibres following addition of 4×10^6 lymph-node cells of rat sensitised to rabbit muscle. Numerous enlarged debris-containing cells and few small lymphoid cells. PTAH, $\times 120$

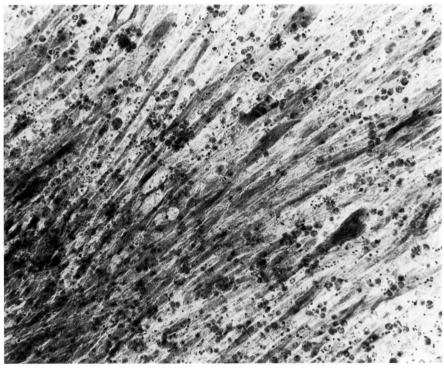

Fig. 11.16 Muscle fibres *in vitro* remain intact after addition of 4×10^6 lymph-node cells of untreated control rat. PTAH, $\times 120$

Tumours

Experimentally induced tumours are also the subject of study. In a biochemical report muscle acid proteinase, alkaline proteinase arylamidase and cathepsin C were increased and cathepsin E1 was decreased. Cathepsin A autolytic activity and trypsin inhibitory capacity were unchanged in the extensor digitorum muscle (Holmes, Dickson and Pennington, 1974).

CONCLUSIONS

The reaction of skeletal muscle to injury of various types is now well understood as a result of the large number of experimental studies and the variety of techniques which have been used, as recounted above. The most notable aspect of the pathology of injured muscle is the remarkably stereotyped character of the resulting changes, a fact which is demonstrated by the many diverse agents producing similar results. The elementary lesion in most of these conditions is focal necrosis of the muscle fibre with preservation of the endomysial sheath. If the animal survives, necrosis is always followed by a series of changes which appear to be inherent properties of skeletal muscle. These events lead to the removal of debris by macrophages and the appearance of myoblasts. Myoblasts multiply and join together to form myotubes so that eventually there is complete regeneration. The sequence is the same regardless of whether the cause is physical, chemical, drug-induced or results from some other mechanism, provided that the duration of action of the noxious influence is finite.

The variability in the microscopic appearance of myopathies in which myonecrotic changes occur is related to the severity of action of the noxious influence and the period over which it acts, rather than to any specificity derived from its cause. This fact, together with the anatomical extent of the injurious agent on the muscle mass determines the character of the eventual architectural derangement. The microscopic lesions, which appear in the experimental and human myopathies in which necrosis is manifestly the first visible feature, are governed by such factors.

By adding the inherent biological capability of muscle to regenerate after focal injury, the histopathology of the necrotising myopathies may be fully explained. However, it must be kept in mind that the regenerative potential is not infinite and, if continuously stimulated, especially in a cyclical fashion, regeneration will eventually be exhausted, muscle fibres lost and secondary fat replacement will take up the dead space. Fibrous tissue increase is merely due to the condensation of endomysial fibrous tubes from which sarcoplasm has been totally lost.

If the term *focal* is used to represent the anatomical aspect of the lesion and if the term *phasic* refers to the time factor and the prefixes *mono* and *poly* are added, the full spectrum of histopathological changes may be described precisely, and even predicted. Examples are easily found for each of these possibilities.

Thus, first, *a monofocal and monophasic disorder* results from an isolated mechanical injury to muscle. Such a lesion could result from a single insertion of a needle into muscle. The second possibility is *polyfocal* and *monophasic*. For instance, this occurs when a single sublethal dose of a powerful myotoxin (such as iodoacetate) is given. Such a lesion is widespread with *polyfocal* necrosis present, but the changes are all *in phase*. If the animal survives the insult, regeneration will also be *in phase*. The same result will appear in drug-induced myopathy where the rhabdomyolysis occurs acutely and the drug is withdrawn quickly, so that histological events are *in phase*. The effect in naturally occurring paroxysmal myoglobinuria (Meyer-Betz disease) is similar.

The third possibility is when the muscle lesion is *monofocal* and *polyphasic*. In this case the lesion is in one anatomical site but is repeated. Such would be the case with recurring mechanical injury, e.g. in some orthopaedic conditions.

The fourth of the theoretical examples is when the myopathological changes are both *polyfocal* and *polyphasic*. This is the most common combination and such changes are observed in the aggressive human dystrophies and in polymyositis. Similar lesions occur in the metabolic and nutritional myopathies, both human and experimental, where necrosis continues over a long period. The total disorganisation of muscle architecture common in these states is due to the *polyfocal* necrosis occurring in a *polyphasic* manner. Initially, regenerative changes are prominent but, because the regenerated muscle fibres undergo further necrosis, the potential for regeneration will become exhausted and muscle fibres are lost, so that fat replacement and fibrous tissue condensation occur. The 'myopathic' appearance of the few remaining muscle fibres which are found in these situations even at the 'end stages', such as irregularities in size and shape of muscle fibres, central placement of nuclei and muscle fibre splitting are non-specific and represent either attempts at compensatory hypertrophy or incomplete regeneration. 'End-stage' muscle disease of this type is found in human muscular dystrophy and in polymyositis in the terminal period. It can also be reproduced in the experimental animal, e.g. the quokka, with chronic marginal vitamin E myopathy.

It is thus shown that the experimental approach to muscle diseases provides information which is of great value in elucidating the mechanisms and pathogenesis of human skeletal muscle disorders.

These principles emphasise that simple morphological similarity of lesions is not an indication of similarity of primary cause. Muscle fibre necrosis is the common factor observed in many diverse conditions whether they are infective, toxic, immunological, metabolic, drug-induced, hormonal or genetically determined. The lesions are different only because of the variability in severity, anatomical distribution and temporal duration of the effects of these noxious agents.

Thus, when searching for causes of yet unsolved human disorders, e.g. the muscular dystrophies, these principles of myopathology show that a search for the cause of the necrosis, rather than a preoccupation with its morphological effects, is more likely to be fruitful.

ACKNOWLEDGEMENTS

The photomicrographs were prepared by Mr. H. Upenieks A.R.P.S. and gratitude is expressed to A/Professor J.M. Papadimitriou and Mrs. K.J. Mellor for the electron micrographs. The material used in Figures 11.1 and 11.2 was prepared with the assistance of Dr. Lee Yoke Sun.

REFERENCES

Adams, R.D. (1973) In *Clinical Studies in Myology*, Ed. B.A. Kakulas, p. 40 (Excerpta Medica: Amsterdam).

Adams, R.D. (1975) *Diseases of Muscle. A Study in Pathology*, 3rd Edn. (Harper & Rowe: New York).

D'Agostino, A.N. (1963) An electron microscopic study of skeletal and cardiac muscle of the rat by plasmocid. *Laboratory Investigation*, **12**, 1060.

D'Agostino, A.N. & Chiga, M. (1966) Cortisone myopathy in rabbits. A light and electron microscopic study. *Neurology (Minneapolis)*, **16**, 257.

Aguayo, A.J. & Hudgson, P. (1970) Observations on the short-term effects of chloroquine on skeletal muscle. An experimental study in the rabbit. *Journal of the Neurological Sciences*, **11**, 301.

Allbrook, D. (1962) An electron microscopic study of regenerative skeletal muscle. *Journal of Anatomy*, **96**, 137.

Anastas, N.C. & Kakulas, B.A. (1968) Muscle lesions associated with bony injuries. *Proceedings of the Australian Association of Neurologists*, **5**, 553.

Ashmore, C.R. & Doerr, L. (1974) Reinnervation of a β-fibered muscle mince by nerve from an α-fibered muscle in normal and dystrophic chicks. In *IIIrd International Congress on Muscle Diseases, International Congress Series No. 334*, Abstract 130 (Excerpta Medica: Amsterdam).

Aström, K.-E., Kugelberg, E. & Muller, R. (1961) Hypothyroid myopathy. *Archives of Neurology*, **5**, 472.

Bajusz, E. (1965) Experimental myopathies: influence of various factors as reflected by histochemical and morphological studies. In *Myopathien*, p. 121 (Georg Thieme: Stuttgart).

Banker, B.Q. (1960) Chapter VII. The Experimental Myopathies. *Research Publications. Association for Research in Nervous and Mental Diseases*, **38**, 197.

Banker, B.Q., Przybylski, R.J., Meulen, J.P. Van Der & Victor, M. (1972) Research in muscle development and the muscle spindle. *International Congress Series No. 240* (Excerpta Medica: Amsterdam).

Bethlem, J. & van Wijngaarden, G.K. (1963) The incidence of ringed fibres and sarcoplasmic masses in normal and diseased muscle. *Journal of Neurology, Neurosurgery and Psychiatry*, **26**, 326.

Boehme, D. & Themann, H. (1966) Structural and ultrastructural changes in striated human muscle caused by chronic ischemia. *American Journal of Pathology*, **49**, 569.

Bowden, D.H. & Goyer, R.A. (1962) Drug-induced muscle necrosis with massive taurinuria. *Archives of Pathology*, **74** 137.

Bradley, W.G., Fewings, J.D., Harris, J.B. & Johnson, M.A. (1976) Emetine myopathy in the rat. *British Journal of Pharmacology*, **57**, 29.

Buller, A.J., Eccles, J.C. & Eccles, R.M. (1960) Interaction between motoneurones and muscles in respect of the characteristic speeds of their response. *Journal of Physiology*, **150**, 417.

Bundschu, H.D., Pfeilsticker, H., Suchenwirth, R., Matthews, C. & Ritz, E. (1974) Experimental uremic myopathy. In *IIIrd International Congress on Muscle Diseases, International Congress Series No. 334*, Abstract 330 (Excerpta Medica: Amsterdam).

Cantin, M. (1967) Skeletal muscle lesions in iodide-treated rats. *Archives of Pathology*, **83**, 500.

Carlson, B.M. (1974) Morphogenetic effects of cross-transplanted muscles upon an epimorphic regenerative process. In *IIIrd International Congress on Muscle Diseases, International Congress Series No. 334*, Abstract 273 (Excerpta Medica: Amsterdam).

Chou, S. (1973) In *Clinical Studies in Myology*, Ed. B.A. Kakulas, p. 17 (Excerpta Medica: Amsterdam).

Clark, W.E. Le Gros. (1946) An experimental study of the regeneration of mammalian striped muscle. *Journal of Anatomy*, **80**, 24.

Clark, W.E. Le Gros & Wajda, H.S. (1947) The growth and maturation of regenerating striated muscle fibres. *Journal of Anatomy*, **81**, 56.

Clarke, J.T.R., Karpati, G., Carpenter, S. & Wolfe, L.S. (1972) The effect of vincristine on skeletal muscle in the rat. A correlative histochemical, ultrastructural and chemical study. *Journal of Neuropathology and Experimental Neurology*, **31**, 247.

Crockett, J.L. & Edgerton, V.R. (1974) Enhancement of muscle protein and tetanic tension after intramuscular spinal cord homogenate injections. In *IIIrd International Congress on Muscle Diseases, International Congress Series No. 334*, Abstract 22 (Excerpta Medica: Amsterdam).

Currie, S., Saunders, M., Knowles, M. & Brown, A.E. (1971) Immunological aspects of polymyositis. The *in vitro* activity of lymphocytes on incubation with muscle antigen and with muscle cultures. *Quarterly Journal of Medicine*, **40**, 63.

Dalldorf, G. (1950) The Coxsackie viruses. *Bulletin of the New York Academy of Medicine*, **26**, 329.

Danon, J.M., Karpati, G. & Carpenter, S. (1978) Subacute skeletal myopathy induced by 2,4-dichlorophenoxyacetate in rats and guinea pigs. *Muscle and Nerve*, **1**, 89.

Dawkins, R.L. (1965) Experimental myositis associated with hypersensitivity to muscle. *Journal of Pathology and Bacteriology*, **90**, 619.

De Reuck, J., De Coster, W. & Eecken, H. Vander (1977) The target phenomenon in rat muscle following tenotomy and neurotomy. *Acta Neuropathologica*, **37**, 49.

Dobosz, I., Mrozek, K. & Kwiecinski, H. (1974) Biochemical studies of sarcoplasmic reticulum and muscle plasma membranes on myotonic rats. In *IIIrd International Congress on Muscle Diseases, International Congress Series No. 334*, Abstract 354 (Excerpta Medica: Amsterdam).

Douglas, W.B. (1974) Myographic and electroneurographic responses of leg muscles and cross-innervated sciatic nerves in normal and dystrophic mice (129B6F$_1$ hybrid) united in parabiosis. In *IIIrd International Congress on Muscle Diseases, International Congress Series No. 334*, Abstract 19 (Excerpta Medica: Amsterdam).

Ellis, J.T. (1953) Studies on the nature and pathogenesis of muscular degeneration in cortisone-treated rabbits. *Bulletin of the New York Academy of Medicine*, **29**, 814.

Ellis, J.T. (1956) Necrosis and regeneration of skeletal muscles in cortisone-treated rabbits. *American Journal of Pathology*, **32**, 993.

Engel, A.G. (1978) The ultrastructural immunopathology of myasthenia gravis; Abstracts of the International Conference of Plasmapheresis and the Immunobiology of Myasthenia Gravis, June 22–24 1978. *Muscle and Nerve*, **1**, 337.

Engel, A.G., Lambert, E.H. & Howard, F.M. (1977) Immune complexes (IgG and C3) at the motor end-plate in myasthenia gravis. Ultrastructural and light microscopic localisation and electrophysiologic correlations. *Proceedings of Staff Meetings of the Mayo Clinic*, **52**, 267.

Engel, A.G., Tsujihata, M., Lambert, E.H., Lindstrom, J.M. & Lennon, V.A. (1976) Experimental autoimmune myasthenia gravis: a sequential and quantitative study of the neuromuscular junction ultrastructure and electrophysiologic correlations. *Journal of Neuropathology and Experimental Neurology*, **35**, 569.

Engel, W.K. (1973) Duchenne muscular dystrophy. A histologically based ischemia hypothesis and comparison with experimental ischemic myopathy. In *The Striated Muscle*, Eds C.M. Pearson & F.K. Mostifi, p. 453 (Williams & Wilkins Co: Baltimore).

Esiri, M.M. & MacLennan, I.C.M. (1975) Some immunological studies of an experimental allergic myositis in rats. In *Recent Advances in Myology*, Eds W.G. Bradley, D. Gardner-Medwin & J.N. Walton, pp. 380–386 (Excerpta Medica: Amsterdam).

Felmus, M.T., Patten, B.M., Hart, A. & Martinez, C. (1977) Catecholamine-induced muscle weakness. *Archives of Neurology*, **34**, 280.

Fenichel, G.M. & Martin, J.T. (1974) An experimental myopathy in rats produced with imidazole. In *IIIrd International Congress on Muscle Diseases, International Congress Series No. 334*, Abstract 331 (Excerpta Medica: Amsterdam).

Field, E.J. (1960) Virus infections. In *The Structure and Function of Muscle*, Ed. G.H. Bourne, Ch. 3, p. 85 (Academic Press: New York).

Francis, M.J.O., Curry, O.B. & Smith, R. (1974) Vitamin D and muscle: a defect of calcium uptake by sarcoplasmic reticulum in vitamin D deficient rabbits. In *IIIrd International Congress on Muscle Diseases, International Congress Series No. 334*, Abstract 324 (Excerpta Medica: Amsterdam).

Gauthier, G.F. & Schaeffer, S.F. (1975) Ultrastructural evidence of early subsarcolemmal protein synthesis in denervated skeletal muscle fibres. In *Recent Advances in Myology*, Eds W.G. Bradley, D. Gardner-Medwin & J.N. Walton, pp. 27–32 (Excerpta Medica: Amsterdam).

Giusti, G.V., Chiarotti, M., Passatore, M., Gentile, V. & Fiori, A. (1977) Muscular dystrophy in mice after chronic subcutaneous treatment with cannabinoids. *Forensic Science*, **10**, 133.

Goldstein, G. & Whittingham, S. (1966) Experimental autoimmune thymitis. An animal model of human myasthenia gravis. *Lancet*, **2**, 315.

Goyer, R.A. & Yin, M.W. (1967) Taurine and creatine excretion after x-irradiation and plasmocid-induced muscle necrosis in the rat. *Radiation Research*, **30**, 301.

Graham, D.I., Bonilla, E., Gonatas, N.K. & Schotland, D.L. (1976) Core formation in the muscles of rats intoxicated with triethyltin sulfate. *Journal of Neuropathology and Experimental Neurology*, **35**, 1.

Granger, G.A. (1969) In *Mediators of Cellular Immunity*, Eds H.S. Lawrence & M. Landy, Ch. 5, p. 324 (Academic Press: New York).

Gutierrez, J. (1966) Effect of the antimalarial chloroquine on the phospholipid metabolism of avian malaria and heart tissue. *American Journal of Tropical Medicine and Hygiene*, **15**, 818.

Gutmann, E. (1962) In *The Denervated Muscle*: (Prague: *Publishing House of the Czechoslovak Academy of Sciences*).

Gutmann, E. & Guttmann, L. (1942) Effect of electrotherapy on denervated muscles in rabbits. *Lancet*, **1**, 169.

Gutmann, E. & Hanzlikova, V. (1975) Factors affecting success of transplantation of skeletal muscle in the rat. In *Recent Advances in Myology*, Eds W.G. Bradley, D. Gardner-Medwin & J.N. Walton, pp. 57–63 (Excerpta Medica: Amsterdam).

Hadlow, W.J. (1962) Diseases of skeletal muscle. In *Comparative Neuropathology*, Eds Innes & Saunders, pp. 147–232 (Academic Press: New York).

Heilbronn, E., Mattson, C. & Stalberg, E. (1975) Immune response in rabbits to a cholinergic receptor protein: possibly a model for myasthenia gravis. In *Recent Advances in Myology*, Eds W.G. Bradley, D. Gardner-Medwin & J.N. Walton, pp. 486–492 (Excerpta Medica: Amsterdam).

Hicks, S.P. (1950) Brain metabolism *in vivo*. In The distribution of lesions caused by azide, malononitrile, plasmocid and dinitrophenol poisoning in rats. *Archives of Pathology*, **50**, 545.

Holmes, D., Dickson, J.A. & Pennington, R.J. (1974) Peptide hydrolases in muscle from tumour-bearing rats. In *IIIrd International Congress on Muscle Diseases, International Congress Series No. 334*, Abstract 326 (Excerpta Medica: Amsterdam).

Holtzer, H. (1974) The synthesis of contractile proteins in definitive muscle cells, precursor muscle cells and non-muscle cells. In *IIIrd International Congress on Muscle Diseases. International Congress Series No. 334*, Abstract 258 (Excerpta Medica: Amsterdam).

Hove, E.L. & Herndon, J.F. (1955) Potassium deficiency in the rabbit as a cause of muscular dystrophy. *Journal of Nutrition*, **55**, 363.

Howell, J.McC. & Buxton, P.H. (1975) α-tocopherol responsive muscular dystrophy in guinea pigs. *Neuropathology and Applied Neurobiology*, **1**, 49.

Ishay, J., Lass, Y. & Sandbank, U. (1975) A lesion of muscle transverse tubular system by oriental hornet (*Vespa orientalis*) venom; electron microscopic and histological study. *Toxicon*, **13**, 57.

Jasmin, G. & Gareau, R. (1961) Histopathological study of muscle lesions produced by paraphenylenediamine in rats. *British Journal of Experimental Pathology*, **42**, 592.

Jasmin, G., Bajusz, E. & Solymoss, B. (1975) Selective prevention by verapamil and other drugs of the hamster hereditary cardiomyopathy. In *Recent Advances in Myology*, Eds. W.G. Bradley, D. Gardner-Medwin & J.N. Walton, pp. 413–417 (Excerpta-Medica: Amsterdam).

Johnston, D.M. & Drachman, D.B. (1974) Neurotrophic regulation of dynamic properties of skeletal muscle: effects of botulinum toxin and denervation. In *IIIrd International Congress on Muscle Diseases, International Congress Series No. 334*, Abstract 21 (Excerpta Medica: Amsterdam).

Kakulas, B.A. (1966a) Regeneration of skeletal muscle in the Rottnest quokka. *Australian Journal of Experimental Biology and Medical Science*, **44**, 673.

Kakulas, B.A. (1966b) Destruction of differentiated muscle cultures by sensitized lymphoid cells. *Journal of Pathology and Bacteriology*, **91**, 495.

Kakulas, B.A. (1970) The pathogenesis of human muscle disease. In *Muscle Diseases*, Eds J.N. Walton, N. Canal, & G. Scarlato, p. 337 (Excerpta Medica: Amsterdam).

Kakulas, B.A. (1973) Observations on the etiology of polymyositis. In *The Striated Muscle*, Eds C.M. Pearson & F.K. Mostofi, pp. 485–497 (Williams & Wilkins: Baltimore).

Kakulas, B.A. (1975) Experimental muscle diseases. In *Methods and Achievements in Experimental Pathology*, Eds G. Jasmin & M. Cantin, Vol. 7, pp. 109–131 (Karger: Basel).

Kakulas, B.A. & Adams, R.D. (1966) Principles of myopathology as illustrated in the nutritional myopathy of the Rottnest quokka (*Setonix brachyurus*). *Annals of the New York Academy of Sciences*, **138**, 90.

Kallos, P. & Pagel, W. (1937) Experimentelle Untersuchungen über asthma bronchale. *Acta medica scandinavica*, **91**, 292.

Kark, R.A.P., Edgerton, V.R. & Whiteman, N. (1975) Decreased oxidation by muscle after denervation but not disuse atrophy. In *Recent Advances in Myology*, Eds W.G. Bradley, D. Gardner-Medwin & J.N. Walton, pp. 33–41 (Excerpta Medica: Amsterdam).

Keast, D. (1967) Personal communication.

Khan, M.Y. (1974) Radiation-induced changes in skeletal muscle: an electron microscopic study. *Journal of Neuropathology and Experimental Neurology*, **33**, 42.

Kugelberg, E., Edstrom, L. & Abbruzzese, M. (1970) Mapping of motor units in experimentally reinnervated rat muscle. Interpretation of histochemical and atrophic fibre pattern in neurogenic lesions. *Journal of Neurology, Neurosurgery and Psychiatry*, **33**, 319.

Kuncl, R.W. (1974) Pathologic effect of phencyclidine and restraint stress on rat skeletal muscle ultrastructure: an animal model. In *IIIrd International Congress on Muscle Diseases, International Congress Series No. 334*, Abstract 334 (Excerpta Medica: Amsterdam).

Lane, R.J.M. & Mastaglia, F.L. (1978) Drug-induced myopathies in man. *Lancet*, **2**, 562.

Lennon, V.A., Lindstrom, J.M. & Seybold, M.E. (1976) Experimental autoimmune myasthenia gravis: cellular and humoral immune responses. *Annals of the New York Academy of Sciences*, **274**, 283.

Lindstrom, J.M. (1978) The role of antibodies to the acetylcholine receptor, protein and its component peptides in experimental autoimmune myasthenia gravis in rats. Abstracts of the International Conference on Plasmapheresis and the Immunobiology of Myasthenia Gravis. In *Muscle and Nerve*, **1**, 335–336.

Lindstrom, J.M., Lennon, V.A., Seybold, M.E. & Whittingham, S. (1976) Experimental autoimmune myasthenia gravis and myasthenia gravis: biochemical and immunological aspects. *Annals of the New York Academy of Sciences*, **274**, 254.

Lindstrom, J.M., Seybold, M.E., Lennon, V.A., Whittingham, S. & Duane, D.D. (1976) Antibody to acetylcholine receptor in myasthenia gravis. Prevalence, clinical correlates, and diagnostic value. *Neurology (Minneapolis)*, **26**, 1054.

Luca, W., Hategan, D., Anghelescu, N., Alexianu, M. & Petrovici, A. (1974) Biochemical, histological and electron microscopical study of experimentally-induced cortisone myopathy. In *IIIrd International Congress on Muscle Diseases, International Congress Series No. 334*, Abstract

333 (Excerpta Medica: Amsterdam).

Manghani, D., Partridge, T., Sloper, J.C. & Smith, P. (1975) Role of myofibrillar antigens in the pathogenesis of experimental myositis, with particular reference to lymphocyte sensitization, the transfer of the disease by lymphocytes and the preferential attachment of lymphocytes from animals with experimental myositis to cultured muscle cells. In *Recent Advances in Myology*, Eds W.G. Bradley, D. Gardner-Medwin & J.N. Walton, pp. 387–394 (Excerpta Medica: Amsterdam).

Manolov, S. (1974) Regeneration of rat neuromuscular junctions. In *IIIrd International Congress on Muscle Diseases, International Congress Series No. 334*, Abstract 183 (Excerpta Medica: Amsterdam).

Margreth, A., Salviati, G. & Carraro, U. (1974) Biochemical characteristics of skeletal muscles in relation to the pattern and rate of activity. In *IIIrd International Congress on Muscle Diseases, International Congress Series No. 334*, Abstract 10 (Excerpta Medica: Amsterdam).

Markand, O.N. & D'Agostino, A.N. (1971) Ultrastructural changes in skeletal muscle induced by colchicine. *Archives of Neurology*, **24**, 72.

Martin, J.T., Laskowski, M.B. & Fenichel, G.M. (1977) Imidazole myopathy: production of the myopathy and its dependence on acetylcholine. *Neurology (Minneapolis)*, **27**, 484.

Mascres, C. & Jasmin, G. (1975) Changes in the muscle fibre induced in the rat by *p*-phenylenediamine. *Pathology and Biology*, **23**, 193.

Mastaglia, F.L., Dawkins, R.L. & Papadimitriou, J.M. (1974) A morphological study of muscle grafts in mice. In *IIIrd International Congress on Muscle Diseases, International Congress Series No. 334*, Abstract 275 (Excerpta Medica: Amsterdam).

Mauro, A. (1961) Satellite cells of skeletal muscle fibres. *Journal of Biophysical and Biochemical Cytology*, **9**, 493.

Mauro, A., Shafiq, S.A. & Milhorat, A.T. (1970) Regeneration of striated muscle, and myogenesis. *International Congress Series No. 218* (Excerpta Medica: Amsterdam).

Miranda, A.F., Gamboa, E.T., Armstrong, C.L. & Hsu, K.C. (1978) Susceptibility of human skeletal muscle culture to influenza virus infection. Part 2. Ultrastructural cytopathology. *Journal of the Neurological Sciences* **36**, 63.

Morita, H. (1926) An experimental study on the pathology of the black-leg. *Journal of the Japanese Society of Veterinary Science*, **5**, 1.

Muir, A.R., Kanju, A.H.M. & Allbrook, D. (1965) The structure of the satellite cells in skeletal muscle. *Journal of Anatomy*, **99**, 435.

Mumenthaler, M. & Paakkari, I. (1974) The needle myopathy. An experimental study. In *IIIrd International Congress on Muscle Diseases, International Congress Series No. 334*, Abstract 341 (Excerpta Medica: Amsterdam).

Nageotte, J. (1937) Sur la contraction extreme des muscles squelettiques chez les vertebres. *Zeitschrift für Zellforschung und mikroskopische Anatomie*, **26**, 603.

O'Grady, F. & Smith, B. (1966) Neuromyopathy in the mouse produced by the antimicrobial agent nitroxoline. *Journal of Pathology and Bacteriology*, **92**, 43.

Owens, K., Ruth, R.C., Gottwik, M.G., McNamara, D.B. & Weglicki, W.B. (1975) Muscular dystrophy of the chicken: distribution of subcellular organelles in zonal gradients. In *Recent Advances in Myology*, Eds W.G. Bradley, D.

Gardner-Medwin & J.N. Walton, pp. 395–400 (Excerpta Medica: Amsterdam).

Palmer, A.C., Harriman, D.G.F. & Barker, J. (1974) Myasthenia in the dog. In *IIIrd International Congress on Muscle Diseases, International Congress Series No. 334* (Excerpta Medica: Amsterdam).

Park, J.H., Chou, T.H., Hill, E.J., Pinson, R., Bartle, E., Connally, J., Lequire, V., Roelofs, R. & Olson, W. (1975) Improvement of hereditary avian muscular dystrophy by penicillamine therapy. In *Recent Advances in Myology*, Eds W.G. Bradley, D. Gardner-Medwin, & J.N. Walton, pp. 401–406 (Excerpta Medica: Amsterdam).

Parkes, J.D. (1966) Attempted production of myasthenia gravis in the rat. *British Journal of Experimental Pathology*, **47**, 577.

Partridge, T.A. & Sloper, J.C. (1977) A host contribution to the regeneration of muscle grafts. *Journal of the Neurological Sciences*, **33**, 425.

Patrick, J. & Lindstrom, J. (1973) Autoimmune response to acetylcholine receptor. *Science*, **180**, 871.

Patrick, J., Lindstrom, J., Culp, B. & McMillan, J. (1973) Studies on purified eel acetylcholine receptor and antiacetylcholine receptor antibody. *Proceedings of the National Academy of Sciences of the United States of America*, **70**, 3334.

Patten, B.M. & Oliver, K.L. (1974) Serotonin induced muscle weakness. In *IIIrd International Congress on Muscle Diseases, International Congress Series No. 334*, Abstract 335 (Excerpta Medica: Amsterdam).

Pearson, C.M. (1956) Development of arthritis, periarthritis and periosteitis in rats given adjuvants. *Proceedings of the Society for Experimental Biology and Medicine*, **91**, 95.

Pellissier, J.F. & Fardeau, M. (1974) Motor innervation study in cortisone myopathy of rabbits. In *IIIrd International Congress on Muscle Diseases, International Congress Series No. 334*, Abstract 332 (Excerpta Medica: Amsterdam).

Penn, A.S. (1977) Myasthenia gravis, dermatomyositis, and polymyositis: immunopathological diseases. In *Advances in Neurology*, Eds R.C. Griggs & R.T. Moxley, Vol. 1, pp. 41–61 (Raven Press: New York).

Peter, J.B. (1971) Cytotoxin(s) produced by human lymphocytes: Inhibition by anti-inflammatory steroids and anti-malarial drugs. *Cellular Immunology*, **2**, 199.

Peter, J.B. (1973) Skeletal muscle: diversity and mutability of its histochemical electron microscopic, biochemical and physiologic properties. In *The Striated Muscle*, Eds C.M. Pearson & F.K. Mostofi, pp. 1–18 (Williams and Wilkins: Baltimore).

Pluskal, M.G., Pennington, R.J., Johnson, M.A. & Harris, J.B. (1974) Some effects of tiger snake toxin upon skeletal muscle. In *IIIrd International Congress on Muscle Diseases, International Congress Series No. 334*, Abstract 327 (Excerpta Medica: Amsterdam).

Price, H.M., Pease, D.C. & Pearson, C.M. (1962) Selective actin filament and Z-band degeneration induced by plasmocid. An electron microscopic study. *Laboratory Investigation*, **11**, 549.

Reznik, M. (1973) Current concepts of skeletal muscle regeneration. In *The Striated Muscle*, Eds C.M. Pearson & F.K. Mostofi, 185–225 (Williams and Wilkins: Baltimore).

Rosman, N.P., Schapiro, M.B. & Haddow, J.E. (1978) Muscle weakness caused by an iodine-deficient diet: investigation of a nutritional myopathy. *Journal of*

Neuropathology and Experimental Neurology, **37**, 192.

Rubin, E., Katz, A.M., Lieber, C.S. Stein, E.P. & Puszkin, S. (1976) Muscle damage produced by chronic alcohol consumption. *American Journal of Pathology*, **83**, 499.

Rüdel, R. & Keller, M. (1975) Intracellular recording of myotonic runs in dantrolene-blocked myotonic muscle fibres. In *Recent Advances in Myology*, Eds W.G. Bradley, D. Gardner-Medwin & J.N. Walton, pp. 441–445 (Excerpta Medica: Amsterdam).

Rustigan, R. & Pappenheimer, M. (1949) Myositis in mice following intramuscular injection of viruses of the mouse encephalomyelitis group and of certain other neurotropic viruses. *Journal of Experimental Medicine*, **89**, 69.

Sanders, D.B., Cobb, E.E. & Winfield, J.B. (1978) Neonatal experimental autoimmune myasthenia gravis. *Muscle and Nerve*, **1**, 146.

Sato, T., Sakuragawa, N. & Tsubaki, T. (1974) Arbovirus myositis: initiation and multiplication of sindbis virus in mouse skeletal muscles. In *IIIrd International Congress on Muscle Diseases, International Congress Series No. 334*, Abstract 391 (Excerpta Medica: Amsterdam).

Satyamurti, S., Drachman, D.B. & Slone, F. (1975) Blockade of acetylcholine receptors. A model of myasthenia gravis. *Science*, **187**, 955.

Schiller, H.H., Esslen, E., Weihe, W.H., Haldemann, G. & Teelmann, K. (1974) Investigations on experimental malignant hyperthermia (MH) in pigs. In *IIIrd International Congress on Muscle Diseases, International Congress Series No. 334*, Abstract 129 (Excerpta Medica: Amsterdam).

Schwarz, K. & Foltz, C. (1957) Selenium as an integral part of factors against dietary necrotic liver degeneration. *Journal of the American Chemical Society*, **79**, 3292.

Scully, R.E., Shannon, J.M. & Dickersin, G.R. (1961) Factors involved in recovery from experimental muscle ischemia produced in dogs. 1. Histologic and histochemical pattern of ischemic muscle. *American Journal of Pathology*, **39**, 721.

Selye, H. (1965) Ein durch Serotonin erzeugte Muskeldystrophie. *Naturwissenschaften*, **52**, 519.

Selye, H. & Bajusz, E. (1960) The prevention of experimental myopathies by various chlorides. *Journal of Nutrition*, **72**, 37.

Serrano, E.E. & Wilder, B.J. (1974) Intramuscular administration of diphenylhydantoin; histologic follow-up studies. *Archives of Neurology*, **31**, 276.

Shafiq, S.A., Gorycki, M.A. & Milhorat, A.T. (1967) An electron microscopic study of regeneration and satellite cells in human muscle. *Neurology (Minneapolis)*, **17**, 567.

Simpson, J.A. (1960) Myasthenia gravis: a new hypothesis. *Scottish Medical Journal*, **5**, 419.

Simpson, J.A. (1964) Immunological disturbances in myasthenia gravis with a report of Hashimoto's disease developing after thymectomy. *Journal of Neurology, Neurosurgery and Psychiatry*, **27**, 485.

Simpson, J.A. (1966) Myasthenia as an autoimmune disease. *Annals of the New York Academy of Sciences*, **135**, 506.

Simpson, J.A. (1977) Myasthenia gravis—validation of a hypothesis. *Scottish Medical Journal*, **22**, 201.

Simpson, J.A. (1978a) Myasthenia gravis: a personal view of pathogenesis and mechanism, Part 1. *Muscle and Nerve*, **1**, 45.

Simpson, J.A. (1978b) Myasthenia gravis: a personal view of pathogenesis and mechanism, Part 2. *Muscle and Nerve*, **1**, 151.

Slotwiner, P., Song, S.K. & Anderson, P.J. (1966) Spheromembranous degeneration of muscle induced by vincristine. *Archives of Neurology*, **15**, 172.

Smith, B. & O'Grady, F. (1966) Experimental chloroquine myopathy. *Journal of Neurology, Neurosurgery and Psychiatry*, **29**, 255.

Smith, G.T., Beeuwkes, R., Tomkiewicz, Z.M., Tadaaki, A. & Town, B. (1965) Pathological changes in skin and skeletal muscle following alternating current and capacitor discharge. *American Journal of Pathology*, **47**, 1.

Sola, O.M., Christensen, D.L. & Martin, A.W. (1973) Hypertrophy and hyperplasia of adult chicken anterior latissimus dorsi muscles following stretch with and without denervation. *Experimental Neurology*, **41**, 76.

Tal, C. & Liban, E. (1962) Experimental production of muscular dystrophy-like lesions in rabbits and guinea pigs by an autoimmune process. *British Journal of Experimental Pathology*, **43**, 525.

Tannenberg, J. (1939) Pathological changes in the heart, skeletal musculature and liver in rabbits treated with insulin in shock dosage. *American Journal of Pathology*, **15**, 25.

Tarrab-Hazdai, R., Aharonov, A., Abramsky, O., Yaar, I. & Fuchs, S. (1975) Passive transfer of experimental autoimmune myasthenia by lymph node cells in inbred guinea pigs. *Journal of Experimental Medicine*, **142**, 785.

Teräväinen, H., Larsen, A. & Hillbom, M. (1977) Clofibrate induced myopathy in the rat. *Acta Neuropathologica (Berlin)*, **39**, 135–138.

Toyka, K.V., Drachman, D.B., Griffin, D.B., Pestronk, A., Winkelstein, J.A., Fischbeck, K.H. & Kao, I. (1977) Myasthenia gravis; study of humoral immune mechanisms by passive transfer to mice. *New England Journal of Medicine*, **296**, 125.

Volkmann, R. (1893) Ueber die Regeneration des quergestreiften Muskelgewebes beim Menschen und Säugethier. *Beiträge zur pathologischen Anatomie und zur allgemeinen Pathologie*, **12**, 233.

Walters, M. N-I., Papadimitriou, J.M. & Shilkin, K.B. (1967) Inflammation induced by dimethylsulfoxide (DMSO). 1. Ultrastructural investigation of the preinflammatory phase. *Experimental and Molecular Pathology*, **6**, 106.

Walton, J.N. & Adams, R.D. (1958) *Polymyositis*. (Livingstone: Edinburgh).

Ward, P. & Goldspink, G. (1974) Response of different fibre types to changes in activity pattern and to protein malnutrition. In *IIIrd International Congress on Muscle Diseases, International Congress Series No. 334*, Abstract 16 (Excerpta Medica: Amsterdam).

Warren, S. (1943) Effects of radiation on normal tissues. XIV. Effects on striated muscle. *Archives of Pathology*, **35**, 347.

Wecker, L. & Dettbar, W.D. (1977) Effects of denervation on the production of an experimental myopathy. *Experimental Neurology*, **57**, 94.

Whittingham, S. & Mackay, I.R. (1966) Autoimmune aspects of myasthenia gravis. *Proceedings of the Australian Association of Neurologists*, **4**, 27.

Winer, N., Klachko, D.M., Baer, R.D., Langley, P.L. & Burns, T.W. (1966) Myotonic response induced by inhibitors of cholesterol biosynthesis. *Science*, **153**, 312.

Wrogemann, K., Mezon, B.J., Boeckx, R.L., Thakar, J.H., Picard, S. & Blanchaer, M.C. (1975) Defective oxidative phosphorylation: is it responsible for muscle necrosis in muscular dystrophy? In *Recent Advances in Myology*, Eds W.G. Bradley, D. Gardner-Medwin, & J.N. Walton, pp. 441–445 (Excerpta Medica: Amsterdam).

Yamamura, S. (1977) An experimental study on the mechanism of fibrous myopathy produced by intramuscular injections of chloramphenicol. *Clinical Neurology (Tokyo)*, **17**, 344.

Biochemical aspects of muscle disease

INTRODUCTION

A muscle is essentially a chemical machine, almost unbelievably complicated, highly organised and delicately balanced. Moreover, it is integrated chemically, by a continuous exchange of substances with the blood, into the larger machine, the body. Disease is an expression of alteration in the normal chemical composition and pattern of chemical reactions. In a few instances, such as in muscle phosphorylase deficiency, there may be important alterations in only a limited field of muscle chemistry. In other muscle diseases such as the muscular dystrophies, with which this Chapter is primarily concerned, the chemical alterations may initially be limited and subtle but later become widespread and associated with the gradual deterioration of the muscle tissue. Biochemical study of the disease then becomes extremely complicated; the more fundamental changes,

those which are presumed to initiate the process of degeneration, are obscured by the numerous secondary disturbances. This is one reason why nothing is yet known of the cause of any type of muscular dystrophy. Moreover, the diagnostic value of many of the secondary changes is limited by the fact that muscle degeneration, whatever the ultimate cause, appears to have many common features.

Since the last edition of this book appeared, hundreds of papers, concerned, directly or indirectly, with the biochemistry of the muscular dystrophies have been published and the output appears to be increasing. A primary aim, of course, is to identify the genetic defects responsible for these diseases; this may provide an approach to rational therapy. Nevertheless, accurate description of the secondary changes associated with the progress of the disease may be valuable in itself, because it may point the way to treating some of these and thus delaying, halting or even reversing degeneration of the muscles.

Some of the reported studies have comprised direct investigation of biochemical changes in biopsied muscle (and sometimes other tissues) from patients. For obvious reasons, much more work has been done on laboratory animals with hereditary myopathies, particularly those in the mouse, chicken and hamster, and will be referred to frequently in this chapter. It is generally recognised that such models are not identical to any of the forms of human muscular dystrophy, but many of the secondary changes in the muscles are similar and it is possible that the underlying defects may be closely related. A useful brief review and discussion of such models has recently been published (Lunt and Marchbanks, 1978).

More details will be found in the proceedings of a meeting organised by the New York Academy of Sciences in January, 1978 (Harris, 1979). A few biochemical studies have been carried out also on muscle cultured from human patients or affected animals. Although one or two claims have been made that abnormalities can be seen in muscle cultured from patients, not everyone is convinced that the genetic defect will be manifested in the early stages of development of the muscle fibres: histological abnormalities in dystrophic muscle are not much in evidence at the fetal stage.

As well as the investigation of affected muscle, much relevant research involves studies on normal muscle alone, with special emphasis on those features, such as membrane biochemistry, which it is commonly supposed may be disturbed in dystrophic muscle. Clearly, there is a possibility that the more important alterations in disease may involve facets of muscle biochemistry not yet fully explored in normal tissue. Evidently, it is preferable that, where feasible, such studies should be carried out using human muscle because of possible inter-species differences.

One problem to be faced when reviewing the biochemistry of muscle diseases is the number of potentially important, but unconfirmed, findings in the literature. Unfortunately, in the past several such promising reports have proved on further investigation to be unfounded, and some caution is necessary in assessing new claims.

Because of the large number of studies which have now been published, it is not practicable to include a fully comprehensive bibliography. Where a choice has to be made, reference will be made to the more recent papers on a particular topic; these usually provide references to the earlier work. Apologies are offered, therefore, to those authors whose work is not quoted directly.

The material in this chapter will be, naturally, of most interest to those concerned directly or indirectly with research into muscle disease, especially muscular dystrophy. Practical clinical applications are restricted to the use of serum enzymes, notably creatine kinase, in the diagnosis of muscular dystrophy and, most important, in identification of the genetic carriers. This will be discussed fully.

MUSCLE BIOCHEMISTRY

General remarks

It is reasonable to suppose that direct analysis of affected muscle, its chemical composition and enzyme activities, is most likely to lead to understanding of the causes and progression of the muscular dystrophies.

Before outlining our existing knowledge of the biochemistry of diseased muscle, some preliminary remarks are necessary concerning the significance of the changes observed. All biochemical studies must take into account the profound histological changes occurring in the affected muscles, notably the proliferation of connective tissue and sometimes of fat, and the structural changes in the fibres. It is evident that marked alterations may occur in the overall chemical and enzymic composition of the muscle tissue merely as a result of these changes. Knowledge of such secondary alterations is hardly likely to add to our understanding of the cause and progress of the disease, and hence biochemical research must try to discriminate between these and more fundamental changes. An obvious consideration is the relative decrease in the amount of muscle fibres which results from the proliferation of connective tissue and increase in fat. Comparison of the concentration of muscle cell constituents in diseased and normal cells expressed in terms of total muscle weight is of little value unless the changes are very large indeed. Some of the early data on changes in composition of diseased muscle were vitiated by lack of a suitable reference base. A simple and reasonably satisfactory way of overcoming this problem is to use as a reference base for comparison the protein of the muscle which will dissolve in dilute alkali at room temperature. This 'non-collagen protein' excludes the alkali-insoluble collagen and elastin and is easily determined—an important requirement of a reference base. Typically it represents over 90 per cent of the total protein of normal muscle but may be less than 50 per cent when the muscle is in an advanced state of degeneration. It is used by most workers and it may be hoped that it will be adopted by all as a reference base. Any criterion which is chosen must be arbitrary to some extent, but the use of such a common procedure will facilitate comparison of results.

Second, where increases in metabolic activities of affected muscle are recorded, it must be asked whether these may be associated with an increase in connective tissue or with invading macrophages; probable instances are mentioned below. Changes will occur also in the relative amounts of vascular and nervous tissue and probably of mast cells. Finally, the presence of regenerating fibres, which have characteristic metabolic profiles, must be considered. Such difficulties as these, which stand in the way of investigations into the more fundamental biochemical defects and the biochemical changes in degenerating fibres, can best be circumvented by study of muscle in which the disease has made only minimal progress. In practice it is normally more difficult to obtain specimens of such muscle for investigation; consequently, there have as yet been few studies of this nature. When volunteered, the availability of muscle biopsies from genetic carriers, particularly from those with high serum creatine kinase activity but minimal histopathological changes, should be valuable. The importance of comparing results with those derived from normal muscle, preferably obtained from individuals of about the same age, must also be emphasised, because many workers have demonstrated that there are age variations in the amounts of enzymes and others proteins in muscle. Furthermore, in view of the recognised quantitative metabolic differences between different muscles, in particular between 'red' and 'white' muscles, it is desirable that the diseased muscle should be compared with the same muscle in the normal subject. In practice the use of abdominal muscle offers advantages in this respect.

Muscle enzymes—general

Numerous workers have measured the activity of various enzymes in biopsies of diseased muscle, particularly in those obtained from patients with Duchenne muscular dystrophy. However, not more than about 50 enzymes have yet been studied, out of hundreds possible. Nevertheless, many have already been shown to display a changed level of activity in dystrophic muscle.

Undoubtedly, many such changes will result merely from the kind of factors mentioned above and can throw little, if any, light on the nature of the disease. Others, however, may represent aspects of fundamental metabolic changes which occur during the progression of the disease.

To assess the significance of observed enzyme changes may often be difficult. Probably, many will be understood only when many other enzymes have been studied at different stages of the disease and meaningful patterns have begun to emerge.

It is a reasonable supposition, by analogy with some other hereditary diseases, that the ultimate defect resulting from the genetic aberration is a complete or partial failure to synthesise a particular enzyme, the activity of which is essential for the maintenance of normal cell structure. If a primary enzyme defect does, in fact, exist in any type of muscular dystrophy, its recognition as such might be relatively easy once its activity has been measured, because of the magnitude of the change observed and its absolute specificity for the particular disease.

Many of the enzymes which have been measured fall into broad classes, which will now be discussed.

Lysosomal enzymes

A striking feature of many myopathies (human and animal) is an increase, in the diseased muscle, of the activity of many lysosomal enzymes. (The association of such enzymes with lysosomes is based predominantly on investigations with tissues, such as liver, from which lysosomes can be isolated and studied relatively easily). These enzymes hydrolyse various cell constituents and have maximum activity *in vitro* at a low pH which is assumed to simulate conditions within lysosomes. An extensive series of reports, published by Kar and Pearson from 1972 onwards, on the levels of such enzymes in muscle diseases has confirmed earlier findings and added new observations. They have noticed some interesting differences in the degree of elevation of these enzymes in relation to the nature and progression of the disease. The increase in cathepsin (probably cathepsin D), an enzyme which attacks proteins, was general among the myopathies but was significant in severely affected muscle only (Kar and Pearson, 1972a). On the other hand, four other enzymes which degrade proteins or peptides (cathepsin A, cathepsin B1 and dipeptidyl peptidases I and II) were raised even in mildly affected muscle in various diseases (Kar and Pearson, 1976a, 1977, 1978). (It should be noted that, in these studies, cathepsin B1 was measured by the hydrolysis of benzoylarginine 2-naphthylamide; this substrate is split by at least one other peptidase in muscle (Hardy and Pennington, 1979). Other lysosomal enzymes, notably acid phosphatase, β-acetylglucosaminidase, α-fucosidase, α-mannosidase and α-glucosidase, are increased in advanced cases only (Kar and Pearson, 1972b, 1973a). Hooft, de Laey and Lambert (1966) reported increased aryl sulphatase activity at various stages of progression of Duchenne dystrophy. An increase in acid ribonuclease activity in Duchenne dystrophy was found by Abdullah and Pennington (1968).

Increased concentrations of lysosomal enzymes in genetic and nutritional myopathies in animals have been found by Tappel, Zalkin, Caldwell, Desai and Shibko (1961) and by other investigators. It can be assumed that invading macrophages, which are rich in these enzymes, will contribute to these changes. High levels are found also in muscle fibroblasts (Parsons, Parsons and Pennington, 1978). It is difficult to assess the extent of their contribution but, if one assumes that a similar response mechanism operates in various types of muscle damage, there is reason to believe that it does not fully explain the increased activities. Weinstock, Marshall and Jenkins (1962) reported that the electrophoretic behaviour of acid cathepsin from muscles of rabbits with nutritional muscular dystrophy differed from that of cathepsin from peritoneal macrophages or from connective tissue. In addition, it has been found that experimentally denervated muscle shows increased activity of this group of enzymes, but there does not appear to be any appreciable increase in macrophages during the first few days following nerve section. Further evidence that the increase in acid proteinase and cathepsin B1 in denervated muscle is not due to mononuclear cells has been provided by Maskrey, Pluskal, Harris and Pennington (1977).

The presence of regenerating muscle fibres in diseased muscle may also contribute to the increased levels of lysosomal enzymes. Iodice, Chin, Perker and Weinstock (1972) found a decrease in the activity of several cathepsins during maturation of breast muscle in the chicken. However, this again is likely to be only a partial explanation, because regeneration is not seen in denervated muscle.

It would appear likely, therefore, that muscle fibres respond in some way to damaging influences by an increase in their content of lysosomal enzymes. How this occurs and what may be its biological significance is unknown, as is its contribution to the subsequent degeneration of the fibres. Although these increased enzyme activities are relatively non-specific and undoubtedly secondary, the possibility must not be excluded that their investigation may ultimately point the way to progress in halting the course of muscular dystrophy, even while the basic cause of the disease remains unknown. It is, perhaps, of interest to compare the well-studied proliferation of lysosomes which occurs in insect intersegmental muscles when they break down during metamorphosis (Lockshin and Beaulaton, 1974). It has, indeed, been postulated by Webb (1974) that muscular dystrophy may be a disturbance of a process of 'cell death' which occurs in normal fetal development. The lysosomal alterations in ischaemic myocardium and their significance, discussed by Wildenthal (1978) may also have some common features.

Having said all this, however, it must be stressed that there is still much uncertainty regarding the nature of the function, if any, of acid hydrolases within normal muscle. The activity of these enzymes in muscle homogenates can be increased, under suitable conditions, by the use of detergents; thus they exhibit the 'latency' characteristic of lysosomal enzymes in other tissues. However, the extent to which cells other than the muscle fibres contribute to these activities is not known. Histochemical studies on normal muscle (e.g., Shannon, Adams and Courtice, 1974) have usually failed to show up lysosomal enzymes within the muscle fibres. On the other hand, in muscle affected by disease (such as muscular dystrophy in hamsters (Al-Azzawi and Stoward, 1972), denervation (Schiaffino and Hanzlikova,

1972), starvation (Bird, 1975) or ischaemia (Shannon et al., 1974), there is histochemical evidence of the appearance of lysosomes or lysosomal enzymes. Canonico and Bird (1970), however, who fractionated normal rat muscle homogenates by centrifuging on density gradients, obtained evidence for two groups of particle-bound acid hydrolases, one of which they considered to originate from the muscle fibres. Assuming the presence of lysosomal enzymes in normal muscle fibres, their intracellular location is still uncertain. The possibility that they are associated with the sarcoplasmic reticulum or Golgi apparatus rather than being contained in the familiar vesicles is discussed by Bird (1975).

Enzymes of energy metabolism

Enzymes of glycolysis and related enzymes. One of the earliest studies on enzyme levels in dystrophic muscle was carried out by Dreyfus, Schapira, Schapira and Demos (1956). Specimens of transversus abdominis from patients were compared with the corresponding normal muscle, obtained during appendicectomies. The rate of glycolysis of the dystrophic muscle was much less than normal; values ranged from 0.44 to 1.18 mmol of glucose transformed per g of non-collagen protein per hour at 38°C (average normal value, 2.85). The extent of the decrease paralleled the state of progress of the disease. Assays of individual enzymes showed that α-glucan phosphorylase, phosphoglucomutase and aldolase—each of which catalyses a step in the glycolytic pathway—had low activity. Aldolase activity, for instance, was from 1.3 to 10.5 mmol of fructose diphosphate converted per g of non-collagen protein per hour at 38°C, the average normal value being 19. In contrast, the activity of a number of other enzymes, such as cytochrome oxidase, succinate dehydrogenase, aconitase, fumarase and the aminotransferases, was not significantly different from normal. Other workers, quoted by these authors, had previously carried out similar investigations in experimental neurogenic muscular atrophy; the changes were, in general, similar. They are not, however, an invariable consequence of muscle atrophy because aldolase activity and rate of glycolysis are largely un-

impaired in myopathic mouse muscle. It is of interest, also, that di Mauro, Angelini and Catani (1967) reported that, in contrast with other glycolytic enzymes, muscle phosphorylase showed an earlier and more marked loss in progressive muscular dystrophies than in neurogenic diseases. Studies by Vignos and Lefkowitz (1959) showed that the rate of glycolysis is low in the juvenile forms but is essentially normal in the adult forms of muscular dystrophy. The latter workers found also a low activity of creatine kinase and adenosine triphosphatase in juvenile muscular dystrophy and neurogenic atrophy of muscle, but only marginal changes in adult muscular dystrophy. Many of these findings have been confirmed in extensive investigations by Heyck, Laudahn and Luders (1963), Hooft et al., (1966) and Kleine and Chlond (1967) which have also shown decreases in other enzymes in dystrophic muscle, including adenylate kinase and a number of glycolytic enzymes. The enzyme, fructose1,6-diphosphatase, which in muscle may be concerned with the control of glycolysis is, however, present in normal amounts in various kinds of muscular dystrophy (Kar and Pearson, 1972c).

Another enzyme, AMP aminohydrolase (AMP deaminase), found to be markedly decreased in dystrophic mouse muscle (Pennington, 1961) is sharply decreased in Duchenne dystrophy even at an early stage, while in other muscle diseases a low level is seen only in severely affected muscle (Kar and Pearson, 1973b). This enzyme occurs in far greater concentration in skeletal muscle than in other tissues; while its precise role is not yet clear, it is considered to be important in the control of glycolysis in muscle (Fishbein, Armbrustmacher and Griffin, 1978).

Cause of changes. It seems unlikely that the enhanced leakage of these enzymes from diseased muscle, which is described below, is an important cause of their low activities in muscle. Thus there is no increase in serum AMP deaminase in Duchenne dystrophy (Pennington, unpublished) while, conversely, aminotransferases, which are released into the blood, are not decreased in muscle. A further point to be considered is that, as shown by turnover studies with isotopes, muscle enzymes, in common with most animal proteins, are being continually replaced by the tissue. Nothing is known of the mechanisms which normally balance the rates of breakdown and resynthesis of a protein and of how these would respond if the protein leaked out of the cells. However, from what is known about the rates of synthesis of muscle enzymes (see, for example, Schapira, Kruh, Dreyfus and Schapira (1960), who reported a half-life of about 20 days for muscle aldolase), and from what can be supposed about the rates of loss of enzymes from the cells (see below) it would probably require only a relatively small acceleration in synthesis rate to compensate for the leakage. It is highly probable, therefore, that there is a decreased synthesis or possibly an accelerated destruction of these enzymes in the muscle fibres, to account for the low enzyme levels.

Work in developmental biochemistry has suggested new possibilities relating to the significance of these changes. It has become evident from the work of Dawson and Kaplan (1965), Hooft et al. (1966), Kendrick-Jones and Perry (1967) and others, that many of the enzymes concerned show a marked increase in activity in the muscles of normal animals during development. Hence, the levels of these enzymes in dystrophic muscle tend to resemble those of normal muscle at an earlier stage of development. A probable partial explanation for the lower enzyme activities in both diseased muscle and fetal muscle is that they are the result, engineered by an adaptive mechanism, of a lower level of physical activity. The increase in certain muscle enzymes during development can be correlated clearly with the use of the muscles (Dawson and Kaplan, 1965; Kendrick-Jones and Perry, 1967). Moreover, exercise can increase the concentration of muscle enzymes (Kendrick-Jones and Perry, 1965) and also of myoglobin (Pattengale and Holloszy, 1967). One can only speculate on the possible mechanisms by which muscular activity could influence the concentration of muscle enzymes. Possibly, nerve impulses facilitate the transfer from nerve to muscle of 'trophic' substances which specifically enhance the synthesis of certain muscle enzymes. Alternatively, some product of glycolysis or change in pH or O_2 tension may stimulate the synthesis of these enzymes, thus ensuring that their level would be automatically related to muscle activity.

It seems improbable, however, that muscular activity provides a complete explanation for the changes in glycolytic enzymes during development and disease. Mann and Salafsky (1970) reported that the large increases in aldolase and pyruvate kinase observed during the development of the anterior tibial muscle in the kitten were not prevented by immobilising the muscle. Other work (e.g. Riley and Allin, 1973), demonstrating that the levels of glycolytic enzymes are influenced by the pattern of nerve impulses, is of interest here also.

Isoenzymes. Certain enzymes have also been shown to display in diseased muscle an isoenzyme pattern which is abnormal for adult muscle but resembles that of immature muscle. Isoenzymes are different proteins (or contain varying proportions of the same protein sub-units) with similar enzymic properties; they are usually recognised and differentiated by electrophoresis on gels or other suitable media or by ion-exchange chromatography. Many enzymes display such multiplicity; in many instances, the isoenzyme pattern varies with the tissue of origin of the enzyme. Wieme and Lauryssens (1962) found differences between normal and diseased human muscle (muscular dystrophy and neurogenic atrophy), in the relative amounts of the five lactate dehydrogenase isoenzymes. The major component of lactate dehydrogenase in most normal muscles is the most slow-moving on electrophoresis (LDH 5). They found that, in normal muscle, it represented an average of 31.4 per cent of the total lactate dehydrogenase, but in myopathic muscle only 17.7 per cent. Numerous subsequent investigations have confirmed and extended these findings: it appears that such changes are usually, but not invariably, present in Duchenne dystrophy and many other muscle diseases (Emery, 1968; Kowalewski and Rotthauwe, 1972). As first shown by Dreyfus, Demos, Schapira and Schapira (1962), the abnormal isoenzyme pattern in diseased muscle resembles that of normal fetal muscle. The abnormal pattern has been observed at a very early stage in Duchenne muscular dystrophy, and Kowalewski and Rotthauwe (1972) could find no correlation between the extent of the change and histological or clinical features. It is possible that, in many instances, the normal mature pattern is never attained. A decreased proportion of LDH5 was reported also in muscle of some female carriers of Duchenne dystrophy (Emery, 1964), although Kowaleski and Rotthauwe (1972) could find no abnormalities in their series of carriers.

A similar phenomenon is seen in the case of creatine kinase (Goto, Nagamine and Katsuki, 1969; Tzvetanova, 1971). The 'BB' isoenzyme (found also in brain) is predominant in the early stages of muscle development; at a later stage the 'MB' (hybrid) form is much in evidence. Adult muscle contains largely the 'MM' type, sometimes with a small proportion of 'MB'. In some, but not all, muscles from a variety of muscle disorders, an increased proportion of 'MB' and the presence of 'BB' has been detected by these workers and by Cao, de Virgiliis, Lippi and Coppa (1971).

The report by Strickland and Ellis (1975), that there is an abnormal pattern of hexokinase isoenzymes in Duchenne muscle, must be placed in a different category because this abnormal pattern (which involves isoenzyme II) does not resemble that of fetal muscle. Moreoever, it was claimed that the abnormality was seen in other tissues, suggesting a generalised genetic defect. This potentially important observation still awaits confirmation, however.

Adenylate kinase is an enzyme which alters the level of adenine nucleotides and which, because of this, is considered to play a role in the control of glycolysis. The enzyme in Duchenne muscle is only partly inactivated by Ellman's reagent which, in normal muscle, blocks its activity completely (Schirmer and Thuma, 1972). It is not clear whether this is attributable to a change in isoenzyme pattern or to modification of the enzyme protein.

Fat metabolism. Relatively little attention has been paid to fat metabolism in muscular dystrophy, but Lin, Hudson and Strickland (1972) found that the oxidation of palmitate by skeletal muscle mitochondria was markedly reduced in cases of Duchenne dystrophy where the inheritance of the disease was established but, surprisingly, not in isolated cases. They also found a low activity in female carriers. In a recent paper (Lin, Hudson and Strickland, 1976) these workers have shown that a similar abnormality found in dystrophic mouse muscle is not due to a deficiency of palmityl-CoA synthetase.

The oxidation of fatty acids in muscle requires carnitine for their transfer across the mitochondrial membrane, and a specific deficiency of this compound has recently been recognised (see Chapter 18). In many muscle diseases, particularly Duchenne dystrophy, there appears to be a non-specific lowering of muscle carnitine (Borum, Broquist and Roelofs, 1977).

Oxidative phosphorylation. Mitochondria isolated from Duchenne muscle appear to have a normal ability to carry out oxidative phosphorylation, unless the disease is far advanced (Olson, Vignos, Woodlock and Perry, 1968; Peter, 1971). Vignos and Warner (1963) and Stengel-Rutkowski and Barthelmai (1973) have found a decrease in the amount of ATP and creatine phosphate (related to non-collagen N) in Duchenne muscle. However, only the former group could observe a decrease in the ATP/ADP and creatine phosphate/creatine ratios. In dystrophic mice and chickens, normal concentrations of ATP and creatine phosphate have been reported (Farrell and Olson, 1973).

In dystrophic hamsters there is a defect in oxidative phosphorylation which appears to be due to an abnormal accumulation of calcium in the mitochondria (see below).

Pentose phosphate pathway. It was observed by Heyck et al. (1963) that, in marked contrast to the fall in glycolytic enzymes there was, in human dystrophic muscle, increased activity of glucose 6-phosphate dehydrogenase and 6-phosphogluconate dehydrogenase, the first two enzymes of the pentose phosphate pathway of glucose utilisation. This is, however, a very nonspecific phenomenon, because a similar change is seen in dystrophic mouse muscle (McCaman, 1960) and various types of experimental muscle damage (reviewed by Wagner, Kauffman and Max, 1978). Various factors may be responsible for these changes. There is a relatively high level of these enzymes in connective tissue and in macrophages, and recently Wagner et al. (1978) demonstrated a high activity in regenerating muscle fibres. It appears likely that one function of this pathway is the provision of pentoses for nucleic acid synthesis.

Both glucose 6-phosphate dehydrogenase and 6-phosphogluconate dehydrogenase transfer electrons between their substrate and NADP, and it is of interest that two other NADP-linked enzymes, isocitrate dehydrogenase and glutathione reductase, also increase in dystrophic muscle (McCaman, 1960; Heyck *et al.*, 1963).

Miscellaneous. Following earlier studies suggesting that there was a deficiency of coenzyme Q in dystrophic muscle, Folkers, Nakamura, Littarru, Zellweger, Brunkhorst, Williams and Langston (1974) have reported that treatment with coenzyme Q reduced serum creatine kinase levels in two boys with preclinical Duchenne dystrophy. Coenzyme Q is involved in the electron transport chain in oxidation by mitochondria.

Ellis, Strickland and Eccleston (1973) found that biopsy specimens of Duchenne muscle converted ^{14}C glucose into fructose to a greater extent than normal muscle. The abnormality was noted also in muscle from genetic carriers of the disease. More recently, the same group (West, Ellis and Strickland, 1977) have reported that Duchenne muscle also converted more of the glucose into neutral lipid. Nevertheless, the possible contribution to these results of other cell types, particularly fat cells, must be considered.

Myotonic dystrophy. It has been recognised for many years that patients with myotonic dystrophy commonly display an excessive pancreatic insulin secretory response to glucose or to other agents. On the other hand, a degree of glucose intolerance has also been widely reported. Poffenbarger, Pozefsky and Soeldner (1976) obtained evidence against the secretion of a biologically inactive form of insulin in this disease, and their studies showed a balanced secretion of insulin and proinsulin. Insulin-binding to monocyte receptors has been found to be normal and this is considered to be good evidence that muscle insulin receptors are also normal (Kobayashi, Meek and Streib, 1977).

Protein metabolism

Proteins are the main constituents of muscle fibres and, accordingly, muscle degeneration involves large protein loss. It is not, therefore, surprising that much attention has been focused on muscle protein metabolism in muscular dystrophy. In healthy muscle fibres, as in most animal cells, the proteins are in a dynamic state, being continually broken down and resynthesised. The rate at which this occurs has been the subject of a great deal of research using mainly isotopic labelling techniques. Recent studies on man (McKeran, Halliday and Purkiss, 1978) gave a myofibril protein catabolic rate of 2.16 per cent or 1.47 per cent per day, depending upon the procedure used. There is good evidence that the individual muscle proteins turn over at different rates. The way in which protein degradation and synthesis are normally integrated to maintain a steady level of protein is still not known. Protein loss in disease could obviously result from either impairment of its synthesis or increased degradation. Meaningful study of protein synthesis in human muscular dystrophy is difficult and the picture is not clear. In a series of reports, Ionasescu and colleagues (*see* Ionasescu, 1975) have studied protein synthesis by ribosomes isolated from muscle affected by various kinds of muscular dystrophy and also from genetic carriers of Duchenne dystrophy. Increased, rather than decreased activity was generally observed, apparently not always attributable to an increase in the synthesis of collagen. These findings do not appear to have been confirmed as yet. Monckton and Marusyk (1976) assessed, by autoradiography, the incorporation of labelled leucine into isolated pieces of muscle. They found increased incorporation into sarcoplasm and decreased incorporation into myofibrils in dystrophic muscle. A possible difference in the rate of transport of the amino acid into the fibres must be taken into account when interpreting these results, however.

Actin in all muscle fibres and myosin in white fibres contain 3-methylhistidine, formed by methylation of histidine residues in the peptide chains. When these proteins are broken down in the cell, the released 3-methylhistidine is not re-utilised but is quantitatively excreted. That there is an increase in the rate of muscle protein breakdown in Duchenne muscular dystrophy is suggested by the observation (McKeran, Halliday and Purkiss, 1977) that the urinary excretion of 3-methylhistidine is increased three-fold when related to the excretion of creatinine; the latter is taken as a measure of muscle mass. The magnitude of this estimated increase in protein catabolic rate is too large to be accounted for by the net loss of muscle protein in the disease: it therefore provides indirect evidence for an increased rate of muscle protein synthesis.

An *in vitro* technique for studying protein turnover in pieces of biopsied human muscle was described by Lundholm, Bylund, Holm and Schersten (1976) and was used by them to show a decreased protein synthesis and increased protein breakdown in muscle from cancer patients. This procedure may be useful in helping to elucidate the changes in dystrophic muscle.

The evidence for hyperactive protein synthesis in dystrophic muscle is intriguing, but the extent to which it is caused by the presence of regenerating fibres has to be clarified before useful conclusions can be drawn.

Human growth hormone was shown by metabolic balance studies to provoke a protein catabolic effect in boys with Duchenne dystrophy, in contrast with its normal anabolic action (Chyatte, Rudman, Patterson, Gerron, O'Beirne, Barlow, Jordan and Shavin, 1973).

Muscle proteinases. The enzymic apparatus for the breakdown of muscle protein, and the factors which control its activity, are still not clear. A number of enzymes (peptide hydrolases) which attack proteins and smaller peptides have been identified in skeletal muscle (*see* Pennington, 1977a), but little is yet known about their participation in protein breakdown in normal and pathological states. The lysosomal cathepsins have already been mentioned, but because of their restricted intracellular distribution and low pH optimum it seems unlikely that these are responsible for the initial attack on muscle proteins, although Schwartz and Bird (1977) have reported that cathepsins B and D are able to degrade myosin and actin. A serine proteinase studied by Katunuma and co-workers shows increased activity in Duchenne muscle (Katunuma, Yasogawa, Kito,

Sanada, Kawai and Myoshi, 1978); it seems possible, however, that this enzyme may be located in mast cells in the muscle (Park, Parsons and Pennington, 1973). Another proteinase, which requires calcium for its activity, has been described and shown to be capable of attacking some myofibrillar proteins (Dayton, Reville, Goll and Stromer, 1976). It was shown by Sugita and Toyokura (1976) that troponin I and troponin C were attacked more readily than troponin T by this proteinase. They showed also that, in Duchenne muscle, the amount of troponins I and C decrease more than troponin T, and suggested that the two findings may be related. Kar and Pearson (1976b) have reported that there is increased activity of a calcium-activated neutral proteinase in homogenates of muscle from patients with Duchenne and Becker dystrophies, but not in limb-girdle dystrophy or denervating diseases. It is not clear, however, whether this is identical to the enzyme mentioned above. The current, widely accepted theory is that the calcium-requiring proteinase (Dayton *et al.*, 1976) may become activated in diseased muscle, by influx of calcium ions from the extracellular space resulting from a damaged or defective sarcolemma. The enzyme is not active at the low concentration of calcium which is present in healthy fibres.

Increased alkaline proteinase activity in Duchenne muscle was observed by Pennington and Robinson (1968). Another enzyme, dipeptidyl peptidase IV, was found to increase sharply in many muscle-wasting conditions (Kar and Pearson, 1978): on the other hand, arylamidase and dipeptidyl peptidase III, two other peptide hydrolases believed not to be associated with lysosomes, were not significantly altered (Kar and Pearson, 1976a, 1978).

Animal myopathies. Quite extensive studies have been carried out on muscle protein metabolism in the animal myopathies, especially that seen in the mouse. Although earlier studies pointed to an increased rate of muscle protein synthesis in the dystrophic mouse, Kitchin and Watts (1973) have claimed that there is no difference in the incorporation of labelled amino acid when correction is made for the size of the amino acid pool; some differences were seen in the case of individual proteins, however. A few studies on protein synthesis with isolated ribosomes have been carried out but have shown no clear picture. There is an increase in alkaline proteinase activity in muscles in the dystrophic mouse (Pennington, 1963).

The recent finding (Stracher, McGowan and Shafiq, 1978) that injection of the proteinase inhibitors leupeptin and pepstatin will delay muscle degeneration in dystrophic chickens is of considerable interest. Pepstatin has also been shown to have a beneficial effect in muscular dystrophy in the mouse (Schorr, Arnason, Aström and Darzynkiewicz, 1978). Pepstatin is an inhibitor of cathepsin D, while leupeptin inhibits both cathepsin B and the calcium-activated muscle proteinase (Toyo-oka, Shimizu and Masaki, 1978). The compounds appear to have low toxicity and may be suitable for therapeutic tests in human muscular dystrophy; in addition, they may be used to elucidate the mechanism of protein degradation in diseased muscle.

Contractile proteins

Vignos and Lefkowitz (1959) showed a decrease, relative to non-collagen nitrogen, in the amount of the main contractile protein, myosin, in dystrophic muscle: the change was more marked in adult patients than in the childhood form of muscular dystrophy. Evidence for a change in some of the properties of myosin and associated proteins in Duchenne dystrophy was brought forward by Furukawa and Peter (1971, 1972). Duchenne myosin showed a low ATPase activity and a markedly delayed superprecipitation, presumably related to the low ATPase. The trypsin-sensitive calcium-binding ability of the actomyosin (a property of the troponin component) was less than normal; this was not so in some other muscle diseases studied. On the other hand, Penn, Cloak and Rowland (1972), using immunodiffusion analysis and agarose electrophoresis, could find no abnormality in myosin in Duchenne or other forms of muscular dystrophy. A number of workers have examined the properties of myosin in animal myopathies but there is as yet no general agreement on how it differs from normal. Smoller and Fineberg (1975) reported

that there were extensive differences in composition of myosin from normal and dystrophic mice: however, Oppenheimer, Bárány and Milhorat (1964) found no difference in its behaviour in the ultracentrifuge and it also showed a similar ATPase activity and an ability to combine with actin. Morey, Tarczy-Hornoch, Richards and Brown (1967) were unable to find any difference between myosin from normal and dystrophic chick muscle. It does not seem likely, however, that the primary defect in human muscular dystrophy is in the contractile system; as is now well recognised, detectable muscle weakness only occurs when the histopathological changes are widespread.

Membranes

Sarcolemma. The long-established phenomenon of the leakage of muscle enzymes into the blood in the muscular dystrophies, particularly in Duchenne dystrophy, has commonly been associated with the idea that there is a defect in the structure of the sarcolemma, although opinion varies on whether this is a primary or secondary change (*see* Rowland, 1976). Recently, in accord with a general surge of interest in membrane biochemistry more workers have looked for experimental evidence of changes in cell membranes in muscular dystrophy. Much of their work has been concerned with erythrocyte membranes (*see below*). Biochemical investigation of the sarcolemma is less easy because of the difficulty of isolating it in pure form, as well as the low yield, which necessitates the use of relatively large quantities of muscle. Numerous procedures for preparing sarcolemma from animal muscles have been described. That of Barchi, Bonilla and Wong (1977) appears to be promising.

Peter and Fiehn (1972) found that isolated sarcolemma from patients with myotonic dystrophy had a higher content of unsaturated fatty acids in the phospholipids than normal; a decrease in cholesterol content was also observed. The possible effect of diet upon the fatty acid composition of muscle phospholipids (Alling, Bruce, Karlsson and Svennerholm, 1974) must be borne in mind, however. Peter, Fiehn, Nagatomo, Andiman, Stempel and Bowman (1974) have reported also that there were no significant abnormalities in the proportions of the various sarcolemma phospholipids in Duchenne or myotonic dystrophy, nor were there any differences in any of the sarcolemmal ATPase activities. On the other hand Dhalla, McNamara, Balasubramanian, Greenlaw and Tucker (1973), using a different procedure for isolation of the sarcolemma, found a lower Na^+, K^+-ATPase and higher Ca^{++}- and Mg^{++}-ATPases in Duchenne dystrophy.

Decreased activity of adenylate cyclase in muscle in various muscle diseases has been observed by a number of workers (e.g. Susheela, Kaul, Sachdeva and Singh, 1975). This enzyme is present in plasma membranes, although it is found also associated with the sarcoplasmic reticulum in muscle (Raible, Cutler and Rodan, 1978). In muscle cells cultured from patients with Duchenne dystrophy, the adenylate cyclase showed an abnormally low response to catecholamines and to fluoride (Mawatari, Miranda and Rowland, 1976). A specific decrease in cyclic nucleotide phosphodiesterase in Duchenne muscle has been observed by Canal, Frattola and Smirne (1975). The enzyme 5'-nucleotidase increases in many muscle diseases and the increase can be seen at an early stage in Duchenne dystrophy (Kar and Pearson, 1973c). Although earlier histochemical studies pointed to an endomysial location for this enzyme, it has been shown in several studies to be associated with isolated plasma membranes, including the sarcolemma, and appears to be located on the outer surface of the sarcolemma (Woo and Manery, 1975).

Evidence for altered membrane properties in muscular dystrophy comes from enzyme leakage studies (*see below*) and also from a decreased ability to retain injected ^{137}Cs and ^{83}Rb (Lloyd, Mays, McFarland, Zundel and Tyler, 1973); the latter was characteristic of all the muscle diseases studied but was not seen in genetic carriers of Duchenne dystrophy. A decrease in potassium content and an increase in sodium is a well-recognised characteristic of diseased muscle. In Duchenne dystrophy, at least, it is not attributable to increased aldosterone or other causes of renal wastage of potassium, because urinary excretion of sodium, potassium and aldosterone was found not to differ significantly from normal (Garst, Vignos, Hadaday and Matthews, 1977).

Recent electron-microscopic studies on the sarcolemma in diseased muscle should be mentioned here. Mokri and Engel (1975) and Schmalbruch (1975) have demonstrated focal lesions in the sarcolemma in Duchenne muscular dystrophy; the latter worker observed similar, although less prominent, changes in other muscle diseases. A more general type of change has been reported by Schotland, Bonilla and Van Meter (1977). These workers, using freeze-fracture studies, observed a depletion of particles on both sides of the muscle plasma membrane in Duchenne muscle; such particles are considered to be protein components of the membrane. In myotonic dystrophy, however, the opposite was observed (Schotland and Bonilla, 1977).

A few studies have been carried out on isolated sarcolemma in animal myopathies. De Kretser and Livett (1977) found changes in its lipid composition in the dystrophic mouse, in particular a four-fold decrease in the relative amount of free cholesterol. However, the sarcolemmal enzymes which they measured were unchanged. Sarcolemma from dystrophic chickens has been reported to show elevated adenylate cyclase (Rodan, Hintz, Sha'afi and Rodan, 1974) and increased microviscosity (Sha'afi, Rodan, Hintz, Fernandez and Rodan, 1975); similar alterations were seen in plasma membranes from liver and erythrocytes.

In studies of phospholipids in whole muscles, Hughes (1970) found an increased quantity of sphingomyelin in Duchenne muscular dystrophy, while Kunze and Olthoff (1970) observed a decrease in phosphatidylcholine and phosphatidylethanolamine in Duchenne dystrophy, but not in neurogenic muscle atrophy. These changes may be assumed to reflect membrane alterations, but no distinction is made between the different membranes in muscle.

Sarcoplasmic reticulum. An important function of the sarcoplasmic reticulum membrane system in muscle is the re-uptake of calcium following muscle contraction, thus inducing relaxation. A number of investigators have examined the ability of fragmented sarcoplasmic reticulum from diseased muscle to take up calcium *in vitro*. Sugita, Okimoto and Ebashi (1966) stated that this ability was decreased in Duchenne dystrophy and some other muscle diseases, an observation which was confirmed for Duchenne dystrophy by Samaha and Gergely (1969). Surprisingly, the latter workers found that in myotonic dystrophy, in which muscle relaxation is delayed, uptake was at least as high as normal. Decreased calcium affinity of the fragmented sarcoplasmic reticulum, which may be a better criterion of abnormality, has been observed in Duchenne dystrophy and poly-myositis (Peter, 1971). Subsequent study of the biochemistry of the sarcoplasmic reticulum in human muscle disease appears to have been sparse until a recent report by Samaha and Congedo (1977) that, in Duchenne dystrophy, the proteins of the sarcoplasmic reticulum display an abnormal pattern on acrylamide gel electrophoresis. More-over, the abnormal pattern fell into two types and these workers therefore suggested that Duchenne dystrophy may comprise two biochemically dis-tinct diseases.

There appears to be a difference between the effect of muscular dystrophy upon calcium uptake by isolated sarcoplasmic reticulum in the mouse and hamster on the one hand and in the chicken on the other. In the first two animals there is a decrease (Martinosi, 1968; Dhalla, Singh, Lee, Anand, Bernatsky and Jasmin, 1975) which is not seen in the chicken (Sylvester and Baskin, 1973).

Muscle and calcium

The suggestion that there may be an influx of calcium into diseased muscle from the extracel-lular space was mentioned earlier, in connection with the calcium-activated proteinase. Recently Bodensteiner and Engel (1978) have supported this possibility by histochemical demonstration of calcium in non-necrotic fibres in diseased muscle; this occurred more frequently in Duchenne dys-trophy than in other muscle diseases. Previously, Wrogemann and his colleagues (Wrogemann, Jacobson and Blanchaer, 1973: Wrogemann and Nylen, 1978) had shown that in the muscle of dystrophic hamsters there is an accumulation of calcium in mitochondria at an early stage of the disease. This caused, among other things, a defect in oxidative phosphorylation and could thus contribute to the death of the fibres.

Recently, a hypothesis has been put forward implicating prostaglandins in calcium accumu-lation in muscular dystrophy (Horrobin, Morgan, Karmali, Manku, Karmazyn, Ally and Pmtabaji, 1977).

Miscellaneous findings

Kar and Pearson, in a long series of studies, have measured the activity (related to non-collagen protein) of several enzymes in muscle biopsy samples obtained from various muscle diseases at different stages. Acyl phosphatase, the cellular function of which is not clear, was decreased only in advanced cases of various muscle diseases (Kar and Pearson, 1972d). Cholinesterase was increased in Duchenne dystrophy but not in other muscle diseases, whereas β-naphthyl acetate esterase was normal in all cases (Kar and Pearson, 1973d). Monoamine oxidase was also normal (Kar and Pearson, 1974); thus the reported increase in catecholamines or related compounds in Duch-enne muscle (Wright, O'Neill and Olson, 1973) does not appear to be a consequence of reduced activity of this enzyme. Glyoxalase I activity was decreased in Duchenne and limb-girdle dys-trophies only, and glyoxalase II was unaltered; phosphodiesterases I and II showed a non-specific increase which was more marked in advanced cases; lipase was increased in Duchenne dystrophy only (Kar and Pearson, 1975a, b, c).

Human muscle contains ribonucleases active at high pH, as well as acid (presumably lysosomal) ribonucleases, and alkaline ribonucleases are markedly increased in Duchenne dystrophy (Ab-dullah and Pennington, 1968).

The similarity in symptoms between the genetic muscular dystrophies and nutritional muscular dystrophy has frequently led to speculation that the former, like the latter, may involve damage by lipid peroxidation. Omaye and Tappel (1974) found increased thiobarbituric acid-reactive pro-ducts (an index of lipid peroxidation) in muscles of genetically dystrophic mice and chickens. These workers also found increased glutathione per-oxidase and glutathione reductase activities, while Bell and Draper (1976) observed an increase in glutathione and glutathione peroxidase in dys-trophic mouse muscle; this suggests a possible adaptive increase in the protective mechanism against lipid peroxidation. The postulated effectiveness of penicillamine (a sulphydryl compound) in improving the condition of genetically dystrophic chickens (Chou, Hill, Bartle, Woolley, LeQuire, Olson, Roelofs and Park, 1975) could result from its protection of lipids or possibly of protein sulphydryl groups.

With regard to muscle constituents other than enzymes, many workers have attempted to characterise the myoglobin in dystrophic muscle. This haem protein functions as an oxygen carrier in muscle. The existence of many genetic variations in haemoglobin popularised the idea that a genetic abnormality in myoglobin may underly muscular dystrophy. Variable results were obtained, however, in investigations of myoglobin in diseased muscle; these have been critically reviewed by Romero-Herrera, Lehmann, Tomlinson and Walton (1973), who have discussed possible artefacts in these studies which may account for the reported changes. The latter workers found no abnormalities in tryptic peptides or amino acids in myoglobin from a case of Duchenne muscular dystrophy and one of distal type muscular dystrophy.

Recently (Kremzner, Tennyson and Miranda, 1978) differences have been noted in the concentration of certain polyamines (putrescine, spermidine and spermine) in muscle, in human muscle diseases and in the dystrophic mouse, although the implication of these changes is not clear.

SERUM ENZYMES

Much attention has been paid to the changes in the activities of certain enzymes in the blood of patients with muscle diseases, and such changes are undoubtedly the most useful contribution to biochemical diagnosis. It would be impossible to catalogue all the individual reports here, but the main findings will be outlined.

Creatine kinase

Many of the earlier studies concerned measurement of serum aldolase, but it is now generally acknowledged that increase in the enzyme creatine kinase is the most sensitive index of muscle disease; measurement of this enzyme for the diagnosis of muscular dystrophy was introduced by the Japanese workers, Ebashi, Toyokura, Momoi and Sugita (1959). Furthermore, an increased concentration of this enzyme is rather more specific than that of most enzymes for muscle disease and, in addition, because erythrocytes contain very little creatine kinase, assays in serum are not vitiated by haemolysis of the sample—an important practical point. Creatine kinase transfers a phosphate group from creatine phosphate to ADP forming creatine and ATP, and the enzyme can be assayed by measuring the rate of the reaction in either direction. Nowadays it is normally measured in the direction of ATP and creatine formation, but some earlier studies used the opposite reaction, which proceeds at a very much slower rate. The rate of ATP and creatine formation is usually determined either by colorimetric measurement of creatine or, more commonly, by measuring ATP by means of a coupled enzyme reaction resulting in the reduction of a pyridine nucleotide, which is measured by a change in ultraviolet absorbance. Favourable conditions for the former procedure were established by Hughes (1962). In the author's experience it is the most accurate method and is normally used in our laboratory. Reagent kits for the coupled enzyme procedure are obtainable from numerous commercial sources, with many variations in detail. Consequently, it is usually necessary for each laboratory to establish its own range of normal serum creatine kinase activities.

It has been found empirically that the logarithms of serum creatine kinase values in healthy subjects show an approximately normal distribution and the confidence limits for the normal range can be determined simply by making use of this. In our laboratory, however, the distribution, even of the logarithms of the normal values, is slightly skewed; we prefer, therefore, to deduce the normal range from a cumulative frequency curve plotted on logarithmic paper (Griffiths, 1966). With this procedure, 97.5 per cent of all values for adult women do not exceed 60 units (μmol/min, measured at 37°C) per litre. Many workers (e.g. Hughes, 1962; Griffiths, 1966; Munsat, Baloh, Pearson and Fowler, 1973) have found a higher average level in men than women, presumably because of the relatively greater muscle mass of the men. Factors, other than disease, which may affect serum creatine kinase levels, are discussed below.

The most striking increases in serum creatine kinase concentration occur in Duchenne-type dystrophy; values of up to several hundred times normal are common in early cases. As in the case of aldolase, the levels decline markedly as the disease progresses (Pearce, Pennington and Walton, 1964b). There is a particularly sharp fall around the age of 10 years, probably because the patient starts to use a wheelchair at that age (Thomson, Sweetin and Elton, 1974). In adult dystrophies and myotonic dystrophy there is usually an increased level although not as high as is seen in the Duchenne type. Variable results are obtained in polymyositis; occasionally, extremely high values are found and the serum activity of this enzyme is normally raised in untreated cases. Representative data are given by Pearce et al. (1964b). Increased values in the overtly neurogenic muscle diseases appear to be more common than was once supposed (Koufen and Consbruch, 1970; Williams and Bruford, 1970). The author and his colleagues have recorded many raised values in cases of spinal muscular atrophy. Further information is given by Pennington (1977b).

The syndrome of malignant hyperpyrexia occurring under anaesthesia is associated with a myopathy, and some affected individuals and their relatives are known to have raised serum creatine kinase levels. However, there does not appear to be a good correlation between susceptibility to the condition and increased creatine kinase activity (Ellis, Clarke, Modgill, Currie and Harriman, 1975).

An important aspect of the use of serum enzymes in the detection of Duchenne muscular dystrophy is that a substantial rise may occur long before clinical symptoms are evident. The time course of such early changes in several serum enzymes was followed closely by Heyck, Laudahn and Carsten (1966). In the brother of a patient with Duchenne dystrophy they found increased activities directly after birth, peak values at 14–22 months and, subsequently, a slow decline. At 28 months there were still no clinical signs of muscular dystrophy, although the disease had been confirmed by biopsy. Undoubtedly, advantage will be taken of such early detection when an effective method of treatment is discovered; meanwhile it facilitates study of the disease at a very early stage, which should aid efforts to elucidate its cause. Recent evidence (Mahoney, Haseltine, Hobbins, Banker, Caskey and Golbus, 1977) that the enzyme level may be raised in an affected fetus may prove to be particularly important in this respect.

Genetic carriers. In many hereditary diseases it has long been recognised that clinically normal carriers of the abnormal gene may show, to a minor degree, biochemical abnormalities characteristic of the disease. It is now well established that many of the mothers who transmit the Duchenne-type dystrophy may have some increase in serum enzyme levels. Measurable differences are seen most commonly in the case of serum creatine kinase. Findings at many centres suggest that about two-thirds of all carriers have a serum creatine kinase above the normal range. The difference is often small; thus Pearce, Pennington and Walton (1964c) found that about one-half of the raised values were less than twice the upper limit of the normal range. It is, therefore, necessary to take account of factors which influence serum creatine kinase levels in normal individuals, in order to derive the maximum value from the test. It is established that they are higher in early life, at least during the first year (Pearce, Pennington and Walton, 1964a; Malo, de la Torre, Deutsch and Falcone, 1970; Gilboa and Swanson, 1976). Meltzer (1971) found that, in adults, levels tended to be highest during the second and fifth decades. Both Paterson and Lawrence (1972) and Perry and Fraser (1973), however, noted a slight increase with age in adult women. Meltzer (1971) also noted an effect of race; the mean level in Negroes was higher than that in Caucasians. Early pregnancy is associated with a lowering of creatine kinase (Blyth and Hughes, 1971; King, Spikesman and Emery, 1972). There is, however, some disagreement about the effect of contraceptive pills (Simpson, Zellweger, Burmeister, Christee and Nielsen, 1974). Numerous studies have shown that physical exercise, if sufficiently severe and prolonged, can cause marked increases in serum enzyme levels and should therefore be avoided for at least one day before the test.

A few carriers display very high serum creatine kinase levels, up to about one hundred times the normal upper limit. These differences among carriers have not, so far, been consistently related to any other features such as the degree of histopathological or electrophysiological changes, and the underlying basis of this wide variation is not clear. It cannot be explained solely by age, although there is a gradual decline with age in carriers, which indicates the importance of early carrier detection measurements (Munsat *et al.*, 1973; Moser and Vogt, 1974). It is generally considered that the pathological changes in carriers can be explained by the inactivation in each muscle cell nucleus of either the paternal (normal) or maternal (abnormal) X chromosome, according to the Lyon hypothesis. This is complicated by the multinucleate nature of the muscle fibre; it seems reasonable to assume that the degree of abnormality will be related to the proportion of abnormal X chromosomes in the fibre, although the effective range of action of each individual nucleus is unknown.

Other enzymes

Apart from creatine kinase, many other enzymes appear in increased amounts in the blood in muscular dystrophy although, in most cases, the relative rise is less. Of these, aldolase, the two aminotransferases (transaminases)—aspartate and alanine aminotransferases, commonly referred to as GOT and GPT respectively—and lactate dehydrogenase, have received the most attention. In addition, glucose phosphate isomerase (Dreyfus, Schapira and Schapira, 1958) phosphoglucomutase (Berni, Rea and Schettini, 1961), α-hydroxybutyrate dehydrogenase (Cutillo, Colletta, Lupi and Canani, 1962) and malate dehydrogenase (Chowdhury, Pearson, Fowler and Griffith, 1962) increase; a rise in malate dehydrogenase was found only in childhood dystrophy. On the other hand, β-acetylglucosaminidase and arylsulphatase A, both lysosomal enzymes, were raised in some patients with active polymyositis or dermatomyositis and certain other inflammatory diseases, but not in the muscular dystrophies (Kar

and Pearson, 1972e). Negative results have been reported for cholinesterase, 5'-nucleotidase, adenosine triphosphatase, isocitrate dehydrogenase, acid and alkaline phosphatases and γ-glutamyl transpeptidase. Myoglobinaemia has been detected in Duchenne and congenital muscular dystrophy, using a sensitive immunoelectrophoretic technique (Ando, Shimizu, Kato, Ohsawa and Fukuyama (1978). It has been found also in polymyositis and dermatomyositis, particularly when the disease is active (Kagen, 1977).

More recently (Harano, Adair, Vignos, Miller and Kowal, 1973) a consistently high level of serum pyruvate kinase has been demonstrated in Duchenne muscular dystrophy. Alberts and Samaha (1974) subsequently claimed that a higher proportion of Duchenne carriers had an increase of serum pyruvate kinase activity than of creatine kinase. We were unable to confirm this in our laboratory (Hardy, Gardner-Medwin and Pennington, 1977) and other, conflicting, reports have also appeared. Clearly, more extended studies are required to ascertain whether pyruvate kinase can usefully supplement creatine kinase estimation in carrier detection.

Zatz, Shapiro, Campion, Oda and Kaback (1978) found that pyruvate kinase levels were raised much more frequently than were those of creatine kinase in facioscapulohumeral muscular dystrophy.

Isoenzymes

Several studies (e.g. Somer, Donner, Murros and Konttinen, 1973) have shown that the increase in serum lactate dehydrogenase activity in muscular dystrophy is due mainly to an increase in the more negatively charged components (LDH 1–3), which presumably is caused by the change in the isoenzyme composition of dystrophic muscle, mentioned above. Surprisingly, however, it has been reported recently (Roses, Roses, Nicholson and Roe, 1977) that in serum from carriers of Duchenne dystrophy there is a particularly noticeable increase in the amount of LDH 5, the cathodic isoenzyme. In the last few years more attention has been given to isoenzymes of creatine kinase in the serum. There is general agreement (*see* Takahashi, Shutta, Matsuo, Takai, Takao and Imura,

1977) that, in the majority of cases of Duchenne dystrophy, the MB isoenzyme can be detected; this isoenzyme is rarely seen in normal serum. In other neuromuscular diseases MB is commonly found, but less frequently than in Duchenne dystrophy. Cardiac muscle normally contains the MB isoenzyme, but its presence in serum in Duchenne dystrophy does not appear to be related to cardiac involvement in the disease (Silverman, Mendell, Sahenk and Fontana, 1976) and probably reflects the changed isoenzyme pattern of the muscle.

Leakage of enzymes from muscle fibres

There can be little doubt that the increased amounts of the above-mentioned enzymes appearing in the blood originate largely or wholly in the muscle tissue itself, leaking out of the fibres as the latter are affected by the disease. The enzymes concerned are known to be present in high concentration in muscle. Creatine kinase, which shows a particularly sharp rise, is present in higher concentration in skeletal muscle than in other tissues; in fact, there is relatively little in many tissues, including liver and kidney. That the serum aldolase in muscular dystrophy originates in the muscle accords with the observation of the Paris workers (Dreyfus *et al.*, 1958) that the serum enzyme has no activity on fructose-1-phosphate; the liver enzyme, for instance, has high activity towards this compound as well as towards fructose 1,6-diphosphate. The fact that higher enzyme levels are seen in the earlier stages of the disease is understandable because, in this phase, there will be large numbers of fibres which are involved but still rich in enzymes.

In considering the significance of the enzyme leakage from diseased muscle it is useful to have some idea of the rate at which this occurs, in relation to the amount of enzyme in the muscle. A rough estimate may be made, although this involves some uncertainties, especially in the rate of clearance from the blood. Bär and Ohlendorf (1970) estimated the clearance rate from the rate of fall in the concentration of plasma enzymes following their rapid release into the blood after, for example, a myocardial infarction. In the case of creatine kinase they concluded that about 5 per cent of the plasma enzyme was lost per hour. However, a more recent estimate of the clearance of injected creatine kinase in the dog (Rapaport, 1975) gave a rate which was about one order greater than this. As the creatine kinase concentration in human muscle is about 500 IU/g it can be readily deduced, using the former estimate, that even in a patient with very high serum creatine kinase activity (10 000 IU/l) less than 1 per cent of the total creatine kinase in the muscle must leak out per day.

Reasons for enzyme leakage

It is not possible yet to give an adequate explanation for the release of intracellular constituents from diseased muscles. Most of the enzymes detected in increased amounts in the blood in muscle disease are major 'soluble' (sarcoplasmic) enzymes in muscle, although the mitochondrial form of aspartate aminotransferase is also found (Matsuda, Miyoshino, Miike, Nagata, Tamari, Taniguchi, Ohno and Watanabe, 1978). There are a number of possible factors involved in the release, but their relative importance cannot be stated with certainty. Clearly, enzymes and other constituents may be lost from necrotic fibres, but this is not generally considered to be the whole explanation, because high serum enzyme levels in very early stages of Duchenne dystrophy and in some genetic carriers of this disease may not be paralleled by a prominent degree of necrosis. The reported focal rupture of the sarcolemma, mentioned above, may be important; its contribution to the leakage process can better be judged when it has been studied at very early stages of Duchenne dystrophy.

An alternative possibility, that there is a general change in the structure of the sarcolemma at the molecular level, is widely held to account for the leakage. Such a mechanism might be expected to lead to a more selective passage of cell constituents, and it does appear that the leakage is a selective process. Thus, in Duchenne dystrophy the level of serum creatine kinase may be of the order of 100 times that of aldolase, whereas the activities of these enzymes in muscle are of the same order, and the blood clearance rates appear to be similar (Bär and Ohlendorf, 1970). Two of the major muscle enzymes, phosphofructokinase (Rowland, Layzer and Kagen, 1968) and AMP deaminase (Pennington, unpublished) could not be detected in serum in Duchenne dystrophy. As would be expected, molecular size appears to play some part in the selectivity. The molecular weight of aldolase (150 000) is greater than that of creatine kinase (81 000), while the weights of phosphofructokinase and AMP deaminase are very high (400 000 and 320 000 respectively).

The selective character of the increased serum enzyme levels does, therefore, point to a membrane lesion at the molecular level. One note of caution must be expressed, however, in this interpretation of the evidence. The so-called 'soluble' enzymes of muscle may bind variably to intracellular structures (see Clarke and Masters, 1976), thus introducing another complication.

Origin of increased permeability. As discussed above, the leakage of enzymes from diseased muscle fibres is at present a main pillar of support for the supposition that there is a sarcolemmal defect in muscular dystrophy. This concept has been particularly associated with the Duchenne type, where the leakage is exceptionally high. While the existence of such a disturbance in the membrane seems very probable, its immediate cause is not known and may have to await further advances in our knowledge of the structure and function of membranes. This is, at present, a very active field of research. Some workers have inclined to the belief that an inherited defect in the structure of sarcolemma is the ultimate cause of Duchenne dystrophy. The evidence from this extreme view, however, is not very convincing. As mentioned above, increased serum enzyme levels are found in many human muscle disorders and are seen also in animal myopathies. A similar phenomenon is encountered also in many other diseases; thus, enzyme leakage is a widespread, non-specific consequence of tissue damage. The very early increase in serum creatine kinase in Duchenne dystrophy has been thought to have special significance, but even the earliest reported rise, in a 20-week old fetus (Mahoney et al., 1977) was accompanied by characteristic histopathological changes in the muscles. The hypothesis of a primary membrane defect has stimulated many

workers to look for abnormalities in the more accessible plasma membranes of erythrocytes and fibroblasts. Although changes have been reported (see below) the general picture is not clear and little attention has been given to their aetiology.

Apart from a genetically determined defect in membrane structure, other possibilities are that membranes may be damaged by a circulating factor or may be affected by a disturbance in the metabolism of the fibres. An interference in energy supply to the membrane is worth considering here, as there is evidence that such interference can increase enzyme efflux; such an effect may eventually be understood in the terms of the modern fluid-mosaic concept of membrane structure. Mendell, Engel and Derrer (1972) found that ligature of the aorta in rats markedly increased many plasma enzymes, although there was little muscle necrosis. Other studies along these lines are discussed by Pennington (1977b). The influence of energy supply on enzyme leakage was examined in early in vitro studies by Zierler (1958, 1961). He found that the rate of efflux of aldolase from isolated rat peroneus longus muscle was increased by anoxia or lack of glucose, or by iodoacetate or cyanide, which interfere with energy supply. These results must be interpreted with caution, however, because the rate of aldolase efflux in vitro appears to be several orders higher than it is in vivo. More recently (Hallak and Wilkinson, 1977), erythrocytes and lymphocytes have been used to study the possible influence of energy and other factors upon enzyme efflux from cells. Studies on the influence of corticosteroids and other drugs upon enzyme efflux (Cohen, Morgan and Bozyk, 1977; Verrill, Pickard and Gruemer, 1977a; de Leiris, Peyrot and Feuvray, 1978) may also help eventually in the understanding of the phenomenon in muscular dystrophy.

It should be mentioned that marked muscle wasting is not always associated with enzyme leakage. In the protein-deficiency disease, kwashiorkor, serum creatine kinase activity is, on average, lower than normal (Reindorp and Whitehead, 1971). Rapid muscle atrophy of neurogenic origin may occur without appreciable increase in serum enzyme levels, and experimental nerve section in animals does not usually cause an appreciable rise. Furthermore, steroid myopathy seldom, if ever, produces such an increase. In these conditions, therefore, membrane integrity in this respect seems unimpaired. Nevertheless, Pellegrino and Bibbiani (1964) were able to demonstrate *in vitro* an increased permeability to aldolase in denervated muscle.

SERUM PROTEINS, INCLUDING GLYCOPROTEINS AND LIPOPROTEINS

Characteristic quantitative disturbances of the normal electrophoretic pattern of serum proteins occur in many diseases. Comprehensive investigations of human and animal myopathies have been described by Oppenheimer and Milhorat (1961). The most notable feature of their results was an increase in the α_2-globulin fraction, which was evident in every type of human myopathy which they studied. A similar change has been reported by others, for example Ionasescu and Lucal (1960), and appears to be the most consistent alteration in serum proteins in muscle disease. Oppenheimer and Milhorat (1961) suggest that the increase in the α_2-globulin peak may actually be due to an increase in conjugated non-protein constituents of the peak. In particular, sialic acid, a constituent of some glycoproteins, may be involved: these workers showed that there was a high level of this compound in the serum of muscular dystrophy cases, and the highest proportion of sialic acid in serum occurs in the α_2-globulin fraction. Their suggestion receives some support from the work of Corridori (1960), who found an increase in serum α_2-glycoprotein in many muscle diseases.

Oppenheimer and Milhorat (1961) found also that protein-bound hexose was decreased in the serum of children with muscular dystrophy, scoliosis or Perthe's disease, but not in myositis. Hexosamine showed a significant decrease in Perthe's disease only. The immediate cause of the serum glycoprotein changes in muscle disease is unknown. Changes in serum glycoproteins (most commonly, an increase in one or both of the α-globulin fractions) occur in a wide variety of conditions, including some minor ailments. As yet there is insufficient evidence to decide between various hypotheses which have been propounded to account for the changes. It is perhaps convenient to stress here, moreover, that none of these changes in serum proteins are of any diagnostic value. Apart from their lack of specificity, the mean alterations, although statistically significant, are usually not large compared with known variations in the normal values.

As well as the rise in α_2-globulin, on which there is general agreement, other changes in serum proteins have been reported by the individual groups mentioned above. Oppenheimer and Milhorat (1961) found a decrease in albumin in cases of myositis and of scoliosis and an increase in γ-globulin in the latter. Corridori (1960) found no change in the electrophoretic pattern in myasthenia gravis. In various myopathies, Ionasescu and Lucal (1960) reported decreased albumin, increased α_1- and β-globulins and normal γ-globulin. Puricelli, Cacciatore, Hermida and Toffoli de Matheos (1961) have found raised β-globulin and lowered α_1- and γ-globulin in dystrophia myotonica.

In general there has been little attempt to investigate in depth the serum protein changes brought out by the analytical data. However, Wochner, Drews, Strober and Waldmann (1966) have shown that there is a reduced amount of immunoglobulin G (IgG) in myotonic dystrophy and that catabolism of IgG is greatly accelerated. Serum concentrations and catabolic rates of IgM and IgA were normal.

Askanas (1966a, b) made use of immunoelectrophoresis to search for abnormal serum proteins in muscle diseases. Specific rabbit 'anti-Duchenne' serum gave, with most Duchenne patients, an additional arc in the β_1-globulin zone. This was tentatively identified as haemopexin which is, therefore, considered to be present in larger amounts or in altered form in the patients' serum. Seventy per cent of female carriers of Duchenne dystrophy also showed this precipitation line. Immunodiffusion plates for measuring haemopexin are now commercially available and Danieli and Angelini (1976), using this method, have also found a raised level in many Duchenne carriers.

Rather less information is available on changes in the lipoprotein bands in muscle disease. In normal serum, lipoprotein is found associated with the α- and β-globulin bands. It is notable that both Oppenheimer and Milhorat (1961) and Puricelli *et al.* (1961) found an increase in β-lipoprotein in myotonic dystrophy. According to the latter group, α-lipoprotein, on the other hand, decreases in this condition; however, Oppenheimer and Milhorat (1961) found a significant decrease in non-myotonic dystrophy only. Turning to investigations on individual lipid components, both Danowski, Wirth, Leinberger, Randall and Peters (1956) and Oppenheimer and Milhorat (1961) noted some decrease in serum cholesterol in children with muscular dystrophy. It is perhaps worth mentioning that this finding represents a biochemical difference between human muscular dystrophy and muscular dystrophy caused by vitamin E deficiency in the rabbit; in the latter case, serum cholesterol increases sharply. This, and other biochemical differences, need not necessarily rule out the idea that human muscular dystrophy is a consequence of a genetic defect in the utilisation of vitamin E—a hypothesis to which a few workers have inclined in the past. Inadequate utilisation of vitamin E in one species might not have the same effect as an inadequate supply of the vitamin in another species. However, there is at present no good evidence for any fundamental relationship between nutritional and hereditary muscular dystrophy.

A pronounced fall in serum phospholipids in muscular dystrophy has been reported by Dryer, Tammes, Routh and Paul (1956) but Oppenheimer and Milhorat (1961) found little or no change in their cases. Evidently, further studies are required to clarify this point. More recently, Wakamatsu, Nakamura, Ito, Anazawa, Okajima, Okamoto, Shigeno and Yuichiro (1970) have observed an increase in serum desmosterol, total cholesterol and triglyceride in myotonic dystrophy; these workers suggest a pathogenic role for abnormal lipid metabolism in this disease.

CREATINURIA

The urine of normal adults contains little or no creatine but its anhydride, creatinine, is excreted in considerable and quite constant amounts, (1–2 g/day). One of the earliest discovered characteristics of myopathy, reported over 50 years ago, was a marked increase in creatine excretion; extensive investigations by numerous workers have shown this to be true of almost all types of muscle disease (it may occur also in some other conditions such as fasting and hyperthyroidism). Typical data are given by Van Pilsum and Wolin (1958) whose analytical techniques were probably more specific than those used in many earlier studies. They found creatinuria in a wide variety of diseases affecting the muscles, although the exception was myasthenia gravis, and creatinuria was slight in myotonic dystrophy. In most cases there was also a decrease in urinary creatinine and an increased blood creatine, both of which findings have been reported frequently, and an increase in urinary guanidoacetic acid, a precursor of creatine in the body. (It is suggested by the authors that the rise in blood creatine may inhibit to some extent the methylation of guanidoacetic acid to form creatine). Others (e.g. Danowski, Wirth, Leinberger, Randall and Peters, 1956) have demonstrated a decreased creatine tolerance in muscular dystrophy patients.

It is now generally accepted that creatinuria is a non-specific manifestation of muscle atrophy, and that there is an obvious connection between the two. Creatine is synthesised (its synthesis involving glycine, arginine and methionine) largely in tissues other than muscle; kidney, liver and pancreas are probably the most important, although there is some doubt about their relative contributions. Most of the creatine formed is rapidly taken up by the muscle fibres and is converted reversibly, by the action of creatine kinase, to creatine phosphate (the latter represents an important reserve of energy for muscular contraction). Creatinine arises, probably spontaneously, from the creatine and creatine phosphate. If the amount of muscle is reduced because of wasting, creatine will be removed less rapidly from the blood, the blood level will be higher and more will be excreted by the kidneys. It seems likely that, in myotonic dystrophy, the production of creatine is also diminished, possibly because of endocrine disturbances; consequently creatinuria is low or absent. Myotonic subjects, like normal individuals, show creatinuria after administration of methyltestosterone (Zierler, Folk, Magladery and Lilienthal, 1949). It is of interest that dystrophic mice of the Bar Harbor strain do not show an increase in creatine excretion (Perkoff and Tyler, 1958); this disease has been shown to resemble myotonic dystrophy in other respects also.

It appears from the work of Fitch and Sinton (1964) that a contributory cause of the creatinuria of muscular dystrophy may be the inability of the remaining muscle to retain creatine normally. The half-time of the decrease in specific radioactivity of urine creatinine after intravenous injection of creatine labelled with ^{14}C was considerably decreased in patients with Duchenne and facioscapulohumeral muscular dystrophy. On the other hand, patients with amyotrophic lateral sclerosis and a myopathy of late onset showed a normal rate of decrease. The nature of the defect in the dystrophic muscle is not clear; it may represent either an alteration in cell membrane properties or a change in the intracellular binding of creatine. This is discussed by Fitch (1977).

AMINOACIDURIA

Normal individuals regularly excrete small quantities of several amino acids in the urine, although the nature and amounts show considerable variation. Qualitative or semi-quantitative data on amino acid excretion are readily obtained by paper chromatography and abnormal excretion patterns have been found in a number of diseases. A number of such investigations on dystrophy patients were reported a decade or so ago, but no consistent excretion pattern emerged. Bank, Rowland and Ipsen (1971) have determined quantitatively, by column chromatography, the concentration of 33 amino acids in the plasma and urine of patients with muscle disease. In Duchenne dystrophy, plasma amino acids were normal and there was no characteristic pattern of aminoaciduria, although excretion of taurine was frequently increased. No abnormalities were observed in a smaller number of cases of limb-girdle and facioscapulohumeral dystrophy and myotonic dystrophy. Emery and Burt (1972), however, in a larger study of patients with myotonic dystrophy,

have reported significantly increased excretion (related to creatinine) of threonine, glycine, glutamine, serine and ornithine.

The excretion of hydroxyproline is decreased in patients with muscular dystrophy: a quantitative study by Kibrick, Hashiro, Walters and Milhorat (1964) showed decreased excretion at all stages in Duchenne dystrophy. The results were less clear-cut in the case of other muscle diseases. This amino acid is found only in collagen and elastin and its reduced excretion may be related to the formation of extra connective tissue in muscular dystrophy.

OTHER CHANGES IN BODY FLUIDS

The thorough studies of Danowski and his co-workers (1965a, b) on childhood muscular dystrophy demonstrated increases in serum inorganic phosphate and calcium and a decrease in chloride. In each case the effect was small, with considerable overlap of the individual values, but the mean difference was highly significant. There was no indication that the difference from normal was any greater or less in the more advanced cases. No difference was found in serum total carbon dioxide, sodium, potassium, total protein, albumin or globulin or in fasting levels of venous whole-blood non-protein nitrogen and sugar. In a further paper, dealing with endocrine studies (Danowski, Bastiani, McWilliams, Mateer and Greenman, 1956a) these workers reported normal serum corticoids and urinary gonadotrophin and 17-oxosteroid excretion in their patients. On the other hand, the children with muscular dystrophy had serum protein-bound iodine values in the upper half of the normal range or above it; however, they were able to dispose of administered thyroxine at a normal rate. The same group (Fergus, Nichols, Horne and Danowski, 1956) also confirmed an earlier observation that the blood sugar response to adrenaline injection is subnormal in dystrophy patients. The accompanying decreases in serum inorganic phosphate, potassium and total CO_2 were also found to be less than normal. Plasma serotonin levels were found to be normal in Duchenne dystrophy (Murphy, Mendell and Engel, 1973) and there were no alterations in the urinary excretion of adrenaline, noradrenaline or 5-hydroxyindoleacetic acid (Mendell, Murphy, Engel, Chase and Gordon, 1972).

Smith, Fischer and Etteldorf (1962) investigated serum magnesium levels in muscular dystrophy. They were able to show that, although in untreated serum much less magnesium can be detected (by EDTA titration), normal values are found if the analyses are carried out after wet-ashing or on serum ultrafiltrates. This finding indicates that, in serum from the patients, magnesium is bound by an unusually high extent to some constituent of large molecular weight, presumably protein.

Some evidence has been put forward (Gross, 1977) for a difference in urinary peptides in Duchenne muscular dystrophy, but the nature and origin of this difference is obscure.

Among other reported differences, passing mention should perhaps be made of the reported urinary excretion of ribose (combined in a complex containing phosphorus) in patients with muscular dystrophy, as noted by a number of workers. It now seems clear, however, that the excretion of ribose is neither a consistent nor a specific finding in muscle disease. Thus, Walton and Latner (1954) found ribosuria in only 12 out of 89 myopathy cases, while Ronzoni, Wald, Lam and Gildea (1956) found bound ribose in the urine of both dystrophy patients and control subjects, but no free ribose in either. More recently, Kondo, Abe and Ikeda (1967) reported that about one-third of the patients with Duchenne dystrophy which they studied excreted nicotinamide-adenine dinucleotide (NAD) in the urine; this ribose-containing coenzyme was absent from the urine of normal subjects.

There are two rare familial muscle disorders in which an alteration in blood composition appears to be all-important. In hypokalaemic periodic paralysis (see Chapter 18) the attacks are associated with a rapid fall in serum potassium, which may persist for days. This fall is apparently due to a shift of the ion into the cells and probably results in hyperpolarisation of the fibres, with consequent paralysis. The underlying biochemical mechanism remains unknown. The other condition, in which attacks are precipitated by a high serum potassium, is equally obscure.

Myoglobinuria may occur in inflammatory myopathies (Kagen, 1977). It is also found in a number of metabolic disorders of muscle (see Ch. 18) as well as in certain rare muscle disorders of unknown aetiology, in which it occurs spasmodically.

BIOCHEMICAL STUDIES OF OTHER TISSUES

Erythrocytes

The past three or four years have seen a remarkable surge of interest in investigations directed at red blood cells from patients with muscle diseases, particularly Duchenne muscular dystrophy. The relatively ready availability of blood samples has doubtless been a contributory factor. Attention has been focused mainly on the plasma membrane of the erythrocyte, motivated by the possibility, discussed earlier, that there may be a general abnormality in plasma membranes in this disease. Some of these reports are contradictory, in some cases apparently because of inadequate planning and control of the studies, but probably also because of the sensitivity of red-cell ghosts to small variations, often not explicit, in the procedures used in their preparation and washing. It is possible that even circadian changes in erythrocytes, reported by a number of workers (e.g. Hartman, Ashkenazi and Epel, 1976), may have to be taken into account.

The earliest and most widely repeated study was that of Brown, Chattopadhyay and Patel (1967). These workers stated that the ATPase activity of red-cell ghosts from patients with Duchenne and other muscular dystrophies was stimulated by the cardiac glycoside, ouabain, which normally depresses the total ATPase activity by inhibiting the Na^+, K^+-activated ATPase. Numerous other groups have repeated these studies, mainly on Duchenne dystrophy, with conflicting results. Recent reports include those of Pearson (1978) and of Souweine, Bernard, Lasne and Lachanat (1978). While a few have confirmed the stimulatory effect of ouabain, others have observed only a lesser degree of inhibition by ouabain in the patients, and yet other workers have failed to find any abnormality at all. Although there are variations in experimental details between the studies, none of these appear to correlate with the differences in the findings. It is hoped that these difficulties will soon be overcome. The interest in this finding is heightened by the observation of an abnormal response to ouabain by the sarcolemmal ATPase of the myopathic hamster (Dhalla *et al.*, 1975) and mouse (de Kretser and Livett, 1977).

In a series of communications, Appel and Roses and their colleagues (*see* Roses, Herbstreith, Metcalf and Appel, 1976) have reported that red-cell membranes from patients with Duchenne muscular dystrophy, when incubated under suitable conditions with ^{32}P ATP, show a higher than normal labelling of the protein band II (a component of spectrin) obtained on polyacrylamide gel electrophoresis. A similar abnormality was found in the female carriers. In myotonic dystrophy a different abnormality was seen, notably a decrease in labelling of band III. Again, other workers have failed to confirm these observations, and further investigation of the experimental conditions is required.

It is well known that the behaviour of membrane enzymes may be affected by their lipid environment. Several attempts have been made to find abnormalities in the lipid composition of red-cell membranes in muscular dystrophy. A number of such have been reported (e.g. by Koski, Jungalwala and Kolodny, 1978) but disagreements exist; some of the reported abnormalities concern minor lipid components, which are difficult to analyse accurately. Structural changes in red-cell membranes in both myotonic dystrophy and Duchenne dystrophy have been indicated by electron spin resonance and related techniques (Butterfield, 1977; Wilkerson, Perkins, Roelofs, Swift, Dalton and Park, 1978).

Other reported biochemical abnormalities in erythrocytes in Duchenne dystrophy include an increased rate of potassium efflux (Howland, 1974) and raised phospholipase A activity (Iyer, Katyare and Howland, 1976); the latter was found also in myotonic dystrophy. Physical properties of erythrocytes have also been investigated. A change of shape has been postulated but is controversial (Matheson, Engel and Derrer, 1976); there are also reports of decreased deformability (Percy and Miller, 1975) and increased osmotic fragility (Fisher, Silvestri, Vester, Nolan, Ahmad and Danowski, 1976).

Some of the postulated erythrocyte changes, discussed, for example, by Godin, Bridges and MacLeod (1978), could be explained by an alteration in the cell's handling of calcium. Permeability of the erythrocytes to Ca^{++} is normally slight and the low intracellular Ca^{++} concentration is further maintained by an ATP-dependent Ca^{++} pump. Hodson and Pleasure (1977) found that the Ca^{++}-ATPase of erythrocyte ghosts from Duchenne patients showed increased substrate affinity, while Dise, Goodman, Lake, Hodson and Rasmussen (1977) obtained evidence that the red-cell membrane in this disease has an increased sensitivity to the influence of Ca^{++}. Erythrocytes from patients with myotonic dystrophy were found to accumulate Ca^{++} at a rate higher than that in controls (Plishker, Gitelman and Appel, 1978).

As discussed above, a change in membrane behaviour could possibly arise from interference with energy-supplying mechanisms in the cell; energy in the form of ATP is required to drive the ion pumps and possibly for other membrane functions. However, this does not appear to be the case with red-cell membranes in Duchenne and myotonic dystrophy, because the erythrocyte ATP content is increased (Danon, Marshall, Sarpel and Omachi, 1978).

There appears to be no difference in the age distribution of erythrocytes in Duchenne dystrophy (Campbell, Suelter and Puite, 1977). The possibility that changes in red-cell membranes in patients with muscle disease may result from alterations in the blood plasma does not appear to have been widely examined. This is, perhaps, surprising because it is well known that there is a ready exchange of lipids between membrane and plasma (*see* Bruckdorfer and Graham, 1976). (It may be important that this occurs also with muscle membranes (Graham and Green, 1967)). In two instances, however, that of the abnormal response of the ATPase to ouabain in Duchenne dystrophy (Siddiqui and Pennington, 1977), and the abnormality of endogenous protein phosphorylation in myotonic dystrophy (Iyer, Hoenig, Sherblom and Howland, 1977), there is evidence that plasma factors may be involved. It can be expected that there will be fairly rapid progress in resolving this and other problems in this very active area of research.

Other tissues

Skin fibroblasts can readily be grown in culture; a few investigators have recently made use of this fact to look for possible abnormalities in these cells in patients with muscle disease and, doubtless, many more studies will appear. They are of particular interest in relation to the suggestion, which occasionally has been put forward, that muscular dystrophy is fundamentally a disease of the connective tissue. Kohlschütter, Wiesmann, Herschokowitz and Ferber (1976) could find no abnormality of phospholipid or fatty acid composition in such cultures from Duchenne patients, while 1-^{14}C acetate incorporation into fibroblast lipids was normal in myotonic dystrophy (Thomas and Harper, 1978). However, alterations in the synthesis of collagen and other proteins in fibroblasts in Duchenne dystrophy have been reported (Ionasescu, Lara-Braud, Zellweger, Ionasescu and Burmeister, 1977).

Platelets from patients with Duchenne dystrophy but not from those with other neuromuscular disorders have been reported to show a decreased rate of uptake of serotonin (Murphy et al., 1973). In myotonic dystrophy, platelet aggregation displayed enhanced sensitivity to adrenaline (Bousser, Conard, Lecrubier and Samama, 1975). Lymphocytes from patients and also from carriers of Duchenne dystrophy have recently been found to show reduced cap formation (Verrill, Pickard and Greumer, 1977b), suggesting an abnormality in the plasma membranes of these cells.

The pattern of plasma enzyme elevations in disease commonly provides clues pinpointing the affected tissues. In Duchenne dystrophy the pattern can be attributed largely to damaged muscles, although Kleine (1970) has concluded that it also implicates other tissues, such as liver and heart. Two characteristic liver enzymes, γ-glutamyltransferase (Rosalki and Thomson, 1971) and sorbitol dehydrogenase (Kar and Pearson, 1973e), appear to show normal serum levels.

Danowski et al. (1956a, b) and others have, nevertheless, reported that there are occasional abnormalities in liver function tests. Gamma-glutamyltransferase levels, however, have been found to be increased in myotonic dystrophy (Alevizos, Spengos, Vassilpoulos and Stefanis, 1976).

Paulson, Engel and Gomez (1974) could find no evidence for a circulatory abnormality in Duchenne or limb-girdle dystrophy. They found, using the xenon-133 injection method, that muscle blood flow was normal at rest and during exercise-induced hyperaemia. Capillary diffusion capacity, measured with ^{51}Cr-EDTA, was at least as high as normal. These results, therefore, provided no evidence for the hypothesis that ischaemia may be important in the pathogenesis of Duchenne dystrophy.

Particular interest has been shown in the possibility of chemical alterations in the nervous system in Duchenne muscular dystrophy, in view of the theory (reviewed recently by Sica and McComas, 1978) that the muscle damage has a neural origin. Muscle, as is well known, can atrophy as a result of damage to its motor nerve. Moreover, following the work of Buller and his associates on the effect of cross-innervation in reversing the contraction time of fast and slow muscles, it is now recognised that the nervous system may exert a more discriminating control over the metabolism of muscle fibres than was previously realised. Romanul and Van Der Meulen (1966), Dubowitz and Newman (1967) and others have shown by cross-innervation and histochemical techniques that the characteristic enzyme profile of red and white fibres is influenced by their motor nerves. The relative amounts of myoglobin in the two muscle types are also altered by cross-innervation (McPherson and Tokunaga, 1967), while Guth and Watson (1967) have shown that this procedure alters the protein electrophoresis pattern of the slow muscle towards that characteristic of a fast muscle. Quantitative enzyme studies by Prewitt and Salafsky (1970) have shown that, after cross-innervation, the activity of the glycolytic enzymes, aldolase and pryuvate kinase, increases in the soleus and decreases in the flexor digitorum longus. It remains to be seen whether these effects result in some way from the different pattern of impulses from the different motor nerves, or whether they are due to passage from the nerves of 'trophic' factors which influence the synthesis of specific proteins in the muscle. The former possibility now seems more likely. The existence of trophic factors has often been suggested but direct evidence is slight. Some workers (e.g. Appeltauer and Korr, 1977) maintain that they have demonstrated a transfer of compounds from nerve to muscle; a disturbance in the passage of such 'trophic' factors could be invoked in muscular dystrophy. Confirmation and extension of these studies is required, however. The existence of such a detailed control of muscle metabolism by the nerve, whatever its mechanism, might allow for the possibility that muscle disease could result from changes in the nerve which are more subtle than those occurring in the recognised neurogenic disorders and which have, so far, escaped observation. There is scant biochemical evidence for changes in the nervous system in human muscular dystrophies. Changes in CSF proteins in adult muscular dystrophies have been observed by Kjellin and Stibler (1976), but their origin is not clear.

CONCLUSION

In conclusion, an attempt has been made in this Chapter to review the main biochemical approaches to the investigation of muscle diseases and to comment, where possible, on the implications of the findings. It has obviously been impossible to mention every published study; moreover, research is proceeding at an increasing pace and one can merely draw a line under what has been achieved up to a particular moment. Relatively little has been said about the endocrine and metabolic myopathies, which are discussed fully in Chapter 18. It has been seen that some practical success has been attained, as in the improved diagnosis of muscular dystrophy and the identification of carriers of the X-linked Duchenne gene. However, in spite of attacks on a number of fronts, biochemical research has not yet achieved a breakthrough leading to the cure of any major muscle disease, because of the complexities of the problems involved. Research on diseased muscle must at present be pursued bearing in mind the fact that understanding the disease may involve as yet undiscovered features of the chemistry of normal muscle. It is undoubtedly by the combined results of research on the normal and diseased state that these problems will eventually be solved.

ACKNOWLEDGEMENTS

I am grateful to the Medical Research Council, the Muscular Dystrophy Group of Great Britain and the Muscular Dystrophy Associations of America for financial assistance for some of the work referred to in this Chapter.

REFERENCES

Abdullah, F. & Pennington, R.J. (1968) Ribonucleases in normal and dystrophic human muscle. *Clinica Chimica Acta*, **20**, 365.

Al-Azzawi, H.T. & Stoward, P.J. (1972) *Abstracts of Sixth Symposium on Current Research in Muscular Dystrophy and Related Diseases*, Abstract No. 29 (Muscular Dystrophy Group of Great Britain, Nattrass House, 35 Macaulay Road, London SW4 OQP).

Alberts, M.C. & Samaha, F.J. (1974) Serum pyruvate kinase in muscle disease and carrier states. *Neurology (Minneapolis)*, **24**, 462.

Alevizos, B., Spengos, M., Vassilpoulos, D. & Stefanis, C. (1976) γ-glutamyl transpeptidase—elevated activity in myotonic dystrophy. *Journal of the Neurological Sciences*, **28**, 225.

Alling, C., Bruce, A., Karlsson, I. & Svennerholm, L. (1974) Effect of different dietary levels of essential fatty acids on the fatty acid composition of lecithin in rat skeletal muscle. *Nutrition and Metabolism*, **16**, 1.

Ando, T., Shimizu, T., Kato, T., Ohsawa, M. & Fukuyama, Y. (1978) Myoglobinemia in children with progressive muscular dystrophy. *Clinica Chimica Acta*, **85**, 17.

Appeltauer, G.S.L. & Korr, I.M. (1977) Further electrophoretic studies on proteins of neuronal origin in skeletal muscle. *Experimental Neurology*, **57**, 713.

Askanas, W. (1966a) Immunoelectrophoretic examination of blood serum proteins in patients with neurogenic muscular atrophy. *Life Sciences*, **5**, 1517.

Askanas, W. (1966b) Identification of the agent responsible for the abnormal immunoelectrophoretic pattern of serum in Duchenne's progressive muscular dystrophy. *Life Sciences*, **5**, 1767.

Bank, W.J., Rowland, L.P. & Ipsen, J. (1971) Amino acids of plasma and urine in diseases of muscle. *Archives of Neurology*, **24**, 176.

Bär, U. & Ohlendorf, S. (1970) Studien zur Enzymelimination. I. Halbwertszeiten einiger Zellenzyme beim Menschen. *Klinische Wochenschrift*, **48**, 776.

Barchi, R.L., Bonilla, E. & Wong, M. (1977) Isolation and characterisation of muscle membranes using surface-specific labels. *Proceedings of the National Academy of Sciences (U.S.A.)*, **74**, 34.

Bell, R.R. & Draper, H.H. (1976) Glutathione peroxidase activity and glutathione concentration in genetically dystrophic mice. *Proceedings of the Society for Experimental Biology and Medicine*, **152**, 520.

Berni, C.M., Rea, F. & Schettini, F. (1961) Demonstration of the phosphoglucomutase activity in the serum of children with progressive muscular dystrophy. *Bollettino della Società Italiana di Biologia Sperimentale*, **37**, 845.

Bird, J.W.C. (1975) Skeletal muscle lysosomes. In *Lysosomes in Biology and Pathology*, Eds J.T. Dingle & R.T. Dean, p. 75 (North Holland: Amsterdam).

Blyth, H. & Hughes, B.P. (1971) Pregnancy and serum-CPK levels in potential carriers of 'severe' X-linked muscular dystrophy. *Lancet*, **1**, 855.

Bodensteiner, J.B. & Engel, A.G. (1978) Intracellular calcium accumulation in Duchenne dystrophy and other myopathies: A study of 567,000 muscle fibres in 114 biopsies. *Neurology (Minneapolis)*, **28**, 439.

Borum, P.R., Broquist, H.P. & Roelofs, R.I. (1977) Muscle carnitine levels in neuromuscular disease. *Journal of the Neurological Sciences*, **34**, 279.

Bousser, M.G., Conard, J., Lecrubier, C. & Samama, M. (1975) Increased sensitivity of platelets to adrenaline in human myotonic dystrophy. *Lancet*, **2**, 307.

Brown, H.D., Chattopadhyay, S.K. & Patel, A.B. (1967) Erythrocyte abnormality in human myopathy. *Science*, **157**, 1577.

Bruckdorfer, K.R. & Graham, J.M. (1976) The exchange of cholesterol and phospholipids between cell membranes and lipoproteins. In *Biological Membranes*, Vol. 3, Eds D. Chapman & D.F.H. Wallach, p. 103 (Academic Press, New York).

Butterfield, D.A. (1977) Electron spin resonance investigations of membrane proteins in erythrocytes in muscle diseases. Duchenne and myotonic muscular dystrophy and congenital myotonia. *Biochimica et Biophysica Acta*, **470**, 1.

Campbell, J.C.W., Suelter, C.H. & Puite, R.H. (1977) 5′-AMP aminohydrolase activity in erythrocytes from normal and dystrophic individuals. *Clinica Chimica Acta*, **79**, 379.

Canal, N., Frattola, L. & Smirne, S. (1975) The metabolism of cyclic-3′-5′-adenosine monophosphate (cAMP) in diseased muscle. *Journal of Neurology*, **208**, 259.

Canonico, P.G. & Bird, J.W.C. (1970) Lysosomes in skeletal muscle tissue. Zonal centrifugation evidence for multiple cellular sources. *Journal of Cell Biology*, **45**, 321.

Cao, A., de Virgiliis, S., Lippi, C. & Coppa, G. (1971) Serum and muscle creatine kinase isoenzymes and serum aspartate aminotransferase isoenzymes in progressive muscular dystrophy. *Enzyme*, **12**, 49.

Chou, T., Hill, E.J., Bartle, E., Woolley, K., LeQuire, V., Olson, W., Roelofs, R. & Park, J.H. (1975) Beneficial effects of penicillamine treatment of hereditary avian muscular dystrophy. *Journal of Clinical Investigation*, **56**, 842.

Chowdhury, S.R., Pearson, C.M., Fowler, W.W. Jr. & Griffith, W.H. (1962) Serum enzyme studies in muscular dystrophy. III. Serum malic dehydrogenase 5-nucleotidase and adenosine triphosphatase. *Proceedings for the Society of Experimental Biology and Medicine*, **109**, 227.

Chyatte, S.B., Rudman, D., Patterson, J.H., Gerron, G.G., O'Beirne, I., Barlow, J., Jordan, A. & Shavin, J.S. (1973) Human growth hormone and estrogens in boys with Duchenne muscular dystrophy. *Archives of Physical Medicine and Rehabilitation*, **54**, 248.

Clarke, F.M. & Masters, C.J. (1976) Interactions between muscle proteins and glycolytic enzymes. *International Journal of Biochemistry*, **7**, 359.

Cohen, L., Morgan, J. & Bozyk, M.E. (1977) Variable effects of corticosteroid treatment on serum enzyme activities in Duchenne's muscular dystrophy. *Research Communications in Chemical Pathology and Pharmacology*, **17**, 529.

Corridori, F. (1960) Studies on the electrophoretic picture of the serum proteins and glycoproteins in progressive muscular dystrophy and myotonic dystrophy. *Rivista Sperimentale di Freniatria*, **84**, 52.

Cutillo, S., Colletta, A., Lupi, L. & Canani, M.B. (1962) The relationship between lactic and α-hydroxybutyric dehydrogenase of the serum in children with progressive muscular dystrophy. *Bollettino della Società Italiana di Biologia Sperimentale*, **38**, 691.

Danieli, G.A. & Angelini, C. (1976) Duchenne carrier detection. *Lancet*, **2**, 90.

Danon, M.J., Marshall, W.E., Sarpel, G. & Omachi, A. (1978) Erythrocyte metabolism in muscular dystrophy. *Archives of Neurology*, **35**, 592.

Danowski, T.S., Bastiani, R.M., McWilliams, F.D., Mateer, F.M. & Greenman, L. (1956) Muscular dystrophy. IV. Endocrine studies. *American Journal of Diseases of Children*, **91**, 356.

Danowski, T.S., Wirth, P.M., Leinberger, M.H., Randall, L.A. & Peters, J.H. (1956) Muscular dystrophy. III. Serum and blood solutes and other laboratory indices. *American Journal of Diseases of Children*, **91**, 346.

Dawson, D.M. & Kaplan, N.O. (1965) Factors influencing the concentration of enzymes in various muscles. *Journal of Biological Chemistry*, **240**, 3215.

Dayton, W.R., Reville, W.J., Goll, D.E. & Stromer, M.H. (1976) A Ca^{2+}-activated protease possibly involved in myofibrillar protein turnover. Partial characterisation of the purified enzyme. *Biochemistry*, **15**, 2159.

Dhalla, N.S., McNamara, D.B., Balasubramanian, V., Greenlaw, R. & Tucker, F.R. (1973) Alterations of adenosine triphosphatase activities in dystrophic muscle sarcolemma. *Research Communications in Chemical Pathology and Pharmacology*, **6**, 643.

Dhalla, N.S., Singh, A., Lee, S.L., Anand, M.B., Bernatsky, A.M. & Jasmin, G. (1975) Defective membrane systems in dystrophic skeletal muscle of the UM-X7.1 strain of genetically myopathic hamster. *Clinical Science and Molecular Medicine*, **49**, 359.

Dise, C.A., Goodman, D.B.P., Lake, W.C., Hodson, A. & Rasmussen, H. (1977) Enhanced sensitivity to calcium in Duchenne muscular dystrophy. *Biochemical and Biophysical Research Communications*, **79**, 1286.

Dreyfus, J.C., Schapira, G. & Schapira, F. (1958) Serum enzymes in the physiopathology of muscle. *Annals of the New York Academy of Sciences*, **75** (I), 235.

Dreyfus, J.C., Demos, J., Schapira, F. & Schapira, G. (1962) La lacticodéshydrogenase musculaire chez le myopathe:

persistance apparente du type foetal. *Comptes rendus hebdomadaire des séances l'Académie des sciences*, **245**, 4384.

Dreyfus, J.C., Schapira, G., Schapira, F. & Demos, J. (1956) Activités enzymatiques du muscle humain. Recherches sur la biochimie comparée de l'homme normal et myopathique et du rat. *Clinica Chimica Acta*, **1**, 434.

Dryer, R.L., Tammes, A.R., Routh, J.I. & Paul, W.D. (1956) Blood lipids in progressive muscular dystrophy. *Proceedings of the Iowa Academy of Sciences*, **63**, 398.

Dubowitz, V. & Newman, D.L. (1967) Change in enzyme pattern after cross-innervation of fast and slow skeletal muscle. *Nature*, **214**, 840.

Ebashi, S., Toyokura, Y., Momoi, H. & Sugita, H. (1959) High creatine phosphokinase activity of sera of progressive muscular dystrophy patients. *Journal of Biochemistry (Tokyo)*, **46**, 103.

Ellis, D.A., Strickland, J.M. & Eccleston, J.F. (1973) The direct interconversion of glucose and fructose in human skeletal muscle with special reference to childhood muscular dystrophy. *Clinical Science*, **44**, 321.

Ellis, F.R., Clarke, I.M.C., Modgill, M., Currie, S. & Harriman, D.G.F. (1975) Evaluation of creatinine phosphokinase in screening patients for malignant hyperpyrexia. *British Medical Journal*, **3**, 511.

Emery, A.E.H. (1964) Electrophoretic pattern of lactate dehydrogenase in carriers and patients with Duchenne muscular dystrophy. *Nature*, **201**, 1044.

Emery, A.E.H. (1968) Muscle lactate dehydrogenase isoenzymes in hereditary myopathies. *Journal of the Neurological Sciences*, **7**, 137.

Emery, A.E.H. & Burt, D. (1972) Amino acid, creatine and creatinine studies in myotonic dystrophy. *Clinica Chimica Acta*, **39**, 361.

Farrell, P.M. & Olson, R.E. (1973) Creatine phosphate and adenine nucleotides in muscle from animals with muscular dystrophy. *American Journal of Physiology*, **225**, 1102.

Fergus, E.B., Nichols, W.R., Horne, L.M. & Danowski, T.S. (1956) Muscular dystrophy. VI. Diminished blood sugar and serum electrolyte response to epinephrine. *American Journal of Diseases of Children*, **91**, 436.

Fishbein, W.N., Armbrustmacher, V.W. & Griffin, J.L. (1978) Myoadenylate deaminase deficiency. A new disease of muscle. *Science*, **200**, 545.

Fisher, E.R., Silvestri, E., Vester, J.W., Nolan, S., Ahmad, U. & Danowski, T.S. (1976) Increased erythrocytic osmotic fragility in pseudohypertrophic muscular dystrophy. *Journal of the American Medical Association*, **236**, 955.

Fitch, C.D. (1977) Significance of abnormalities in creatine metabolism. In *Pathogenesis of Human Muscular Dystrophies*, Ed. L.P. Rowland, p. 329 (Excerpta Medica: Amsterdam).

Fitch, C.D. & Sinton, D.W. (1964) A study of creatine metabolism in diseases causing muscle wasting. *Journal of Clinical Investigation*, **43**, 444.

Folkers, K., Nakamura, R., Littarru, G.P., Zellweger, H., Brunkhorst, J.B., Williams, C.W. Jr. & Langston, J.H. (1974) Effect of coenzyme Q on serum levels of creatine phosphokinase in preclinical muscular dystrophy *Proceedings of the National Academy of Sciences (U.S.A.)*, **71**, 2098.

Furukawa, T. & Peter, J.B. (1971) Superprecipitation and adenosine triphosphatase activity in myosin B in Duchenne muscular dystrophy. *Neurology (Minneapolis)*, **21**, 290.

Furukawa, T. & Peter, J.B. (1972) Muscular dystrophy and other myopathies. Troponin activity of natural actomyosin from skeletal muscle. *Archives of Neurology*, **26**, 385.

Garst, J.B., Vignos, P.J. Jr., Hadaday, M. & Matthews, D.N. (1977) Urinary sodium, potassium and aldosterone in Duchenne muscular dystrophy. *Journal of Clinical Endocrinology and Metabolism*, **44**, 185.

Gilboa, N. & Swanson, J.R. (1976) Serum creatine phosphokinase in normal newborns. *Archives of Disease in Childhood*, **51**, 283.

Godin, D.V., Bridges, M.A. & MacLeod, P.J.M. (1978) Chemical compositional studies of erythrocyte membranes in Duchenne muscular dystrophy. *Research Communications in Chemical Pathology and Pharmacology*, **20**, 331.

Goto, I., Nagamine, M. & Katsuki, S. (1969) Creatine phosphokinase isoenzymes in muscles. Human fetus and patients. *Archives of Neurology*, **20**, 422.

Graham, J.M. & Green, C. (1967) The binding of sterols in cellular membranes. *Biochemical Journal*, **103**, 16c.

Griffiths, P.D. (1966) Serum levels of ATP: creatine phosphotransferase (creatine kinase). The normal range and effect of muscular activity. *Clinica Chimica Acta*, **13**, 413.

Gross, S. (1977) Peptides in Duchenne muscular dystrophy. *Clinical Chemistry*, **23**, 299.

Guth, L. & Watson, P.K. (1967) The influence of innervation on the soluble proteins of slow and fast muscles of the rat. *Experimental Neurology*, **17**, 107.

Hallak, G.J. & Wilkinson, J.H. (1977) Action of adenosine phosphates on the release of intracellular lactate dehydrogenase from human and rat lymphocytes. *Enzyme*, **22**, 361.

Harano, Y., Adair, R., Vignos, P.J. Jr., Miller, M. & Kowal, J. (1973) Pyruvate kinase isoenzymes in progressive muscular dystrophy and in acute myocardial infarction. *Metabolism*, **22**, 493.

Hardy, M.F. & Pennington, R.J.T. (1979) Separation of cathepsin B1 and related enzymes from rat skeletal muscle. *Biochimica et Biophysica Acta* (in press).

Hardy, M.F., Gardner-Medwin, D. & Pennington, R.J.T. (1977) Serum pyruvate kinase in carriers of Duchenne muscular dystrophy. *Journal of the Neurological Sciences*, **32**, 137.

Harris, J.B. Ed. (1979) Muscular Dystrophy and other Inherited Diseases of Muscle. *Annals of the New York Academy of Sciences*, **317.**

Hartman, H., Ashkenazi, I. & Epel, B.L. (1976) Circadian changes in membrane properties of human red blood cells in vitro, as measured by a membrane probe. *FEBS Letters*, **67**, 161.

Heyck, H., Laudahn, G. & Carsten, P.M. (1966) Enzymaktivitätsbestimmungen bei Dystrophia musculorem progressiva. IV. Mitteilung. Die serumenzymkinetic im präklinischen Stadium des Typus Duchenne während der ersten Lebensjahre. *Klinische Wochenschrift*, **41**, 695.

Heyck, H., Laudahn, G. & Luders, C.-J. (1963) Fermentaktivitätsbestimmungen in der gesunden, menschlichen Muskulatur und bei Myopathien. II Mitteilung. Enzymaktivitätsveränderungen im Muskel bei Dystrophia musculorum progressiva. *Klinische Wochenschrift*, **41**, 500.

Hodson, A. & Pleasure, D. (1977) Erythrocyte cation-activated adenosine triphosphatases in Duchenne muscular dystrophy. *Journal of the Neurological Sciences*, **32**, 361.

Hooft, C., de Laey, P. & Lambert, Y. (1966) Étude comparative de l'activité enzymatique du tissu musculaire de l'enfant normal et d'enfants atteints de dystrophie musculaire progressive aux différents stades de la maladie. *Revue Française d'Etudes Cliniques et Biologiques*, **11**, 510.

Horrobin, D.F., Morgan, R., Karmali, R.A., Manku, M.S., Karmazyn, M., Ally, A. & Pmtabaji, J. (1977) The roles of prostaglandins and calcium accumulation in muscular dystrophy. *Medical Hypotheses*, **3**, 150.

Howland, J.L. (1974) Abnormal potassium conductance associated with genetic muscular dystrophy. *Nature*, **251**, 724.

Hughes, B.P. (1962) A method for the estimation of serum creatine kinase and its use in comparing creatine kinase and aldolase in normal and pathological sera. *Clinica Chimica Acta*, **7**, 597.

Hughes, B.P. (1970) Lactate dehydrogenase isoenzymes and phospholipids in normal and diseased human muscle. In *Muscle Diseases. Proceedings of the International Congress, Milan, 1969*, Eds J.N. Walton, N. Canal & G. Scarlato, p. 294 (Excerpta Medica: Amsterdam).

Iodice, A.A., Chin, J., Perker, S. & Weinstock, I.M. (1972) Cathepsins A, B, C, D and autolysis during development of breast muscle of normal and dystrophic chickens. *Archives of Biochemistry and Biophysics*, **152**, 166.

Ionasescu, V. (1975) Distinction between Duchenne and other muscular dystrophies by ribosomal protein synthesis. *Journal of Medical Genetics*, **12**, 49.

Ionasescu, V. & Lucal, N. (1960) Changes in the serum electropherogram in myopathies. *Review of Neurology*, **102**, 253.

Ionasescu, V., Lara-Braud, C., Zellweger, H., Ionasescu, R. & Burmeister, L. (1977) Fibroblast cultures in Duchenne muscular dystrophy. Alterations in synthesis and secretion of collagen and non-collagen proteins. *Acta Neurologica Scandinavica*, **55**, 407.

Iyer, S.L., Katyare, S.S. & Howland, J.L. (1976) Elevated erythrocyte phospholipase A associated with Duchenne and myotonic muscular dystrophy. *Neuroscience Letters*, **2**, 103.

Iyer, S.L., Hoenig, P.A., Sherblom, A.P. & Howland, J.L. (1977) Membrane function affected by genetic muscular dystrophy. I. Erythrocyte ghost protein kinase. *Biochemical Medicine*, **18**, 384.

Kagen, L.J. (1977) Myoglobinemia in inflammatory myopathies. *Journal of the American Medical Association*, **237**, 1448.

Kar, N.C. & Pearson, C.M. (1972a) Acid, neutral and alkaline cathepsins in normal and diseased human muscle. *Enzyme*, **13**, 188.

Kar, N.C. & Pearson, C.M. (1972b) Acid hydrolases in normal and diseased human muscle. *Clinica Chimica Acta*, **40**, 341.

Kar, N.C. & Pearson, C.M. (1972c) Fructose 1,6-diphosphatase in normal and diseased human muscle. *Clinica Chimica Acta*, **38**, 252.

Kar, N.C. & Pearson, C.M. (1972d) Acyl phosphatase in normal and diseased human muscle. *Clinica Chimica Acta*, **40**, 262.

Kar, N.C. & Pearson, C.M. (1972e) Serum β-acetylglucosaminidase and arylsulfatase A in inflammatory disorders of muscle and connective tissue *Proceedings of the Society for Experimental Biology and Medicine*, **140**, 1480.

Kar, N.C. & Pearson, C.M. (1973a) Glycosidases in normal and diseased human muscle. *Clinica Chimica Acta*, **45**, 269.

Kar, N.C. & Pearson, C.M. (1973b) Muscle adenylic acid deaminase activity. Selective decrease in early-onset Duchenne muscular dystrophy. *Neurology (Minneapolis)*, **23**, 478.

Kar, N.C. & Pearson, C.M. (1973c) 5′-Nucleotidase activity of normal and dystrophic human muscle. *Proceedings of the Society for Experimental Biology and Medicine*, **143**, 1125.

Kar, N.C. & Pearson, C.M. (1973d) Cholinesterase and esterase activity in normal and dystrophic human muscle. *Biochemical Medicine*, **7**, 452.

Kar, N.C. & Pearson, C.M. (1973e) Sorbitol dehydrogenase in muscle disease. *Lancet*, **1**, 673.

Kar, N.C. & Pearson, C.M. (1974) Monoamine oxidase activity in normal and dystrophic human muscle. *Clinica Chimica Acta*, **50**, 431.

Kar, N.C. & Pearson, C.M. (1975a) Glyoxalase enzyme system in human muscular dystrophy. *Clinica Chimica Acta*, **65**, 153.

Kar, N.C. & Pearson, C.M. (1975b) Phosphodiesterases in normal and dystrophic human muscle. *Proceedings of the Society for Experimental Biology and Medicine*, **148**, 1005.

Kar, N.C. & Pearson, C.M. (1975c) Lipase activity in normal and dystrophic human muscle. *Biochemical Medicine*, **14**, 135.

Kar, N.C. & Pearson, C.M. (1976a) Arylamidase and cathepsin A activity of normal and dystrophic human muscle. *Proceedings of the Society for Experimental Biology and Medicine*, **151**, 583.

Kar, N.C. & Pearson, C.M. (1976b) A calcium-activated neutral protease in normal and dystrophic human muscle. *Clinica Chimica Acta*, **73**, 293.

Kar, N.C. & Pearson, C.M. (1977) Early elevation of cathepsin B1 in human muscle disease. *Biochemical Medicine*, **18**, 126.

Kar, N.C. & Pearson, C.M. (1978) Dipeptidyl peptidases in human muscle disease. *Clinica Chimica Acta*, **82**, 185.

Katunuma, N., Yasogawa, N., Kito, K., Sanada, Y., Kawai, H. & Miyoshi, K. (1978) Abnormal expression of a serine protease in human dystrophic muscle. *Journal of Biochemistry (Japan)*, **83**, 625.

Kendrick-Jones, J. & Perry, S.V. (1965) Enzymatic adaptation to contractile activity in skeletal muscle. *Nature*, **208**, 1068.

Kendrick-Jones, J. & Perry, S.V. (1967) The enzymes of adenine nucleotide metabolism in developing skeletal muscle. *Biochemical Journal*, **103**, 207.

Kibrick, A.C., Hashiro, C., Walters, M. & Milhorat, A.T. (1964) Hydroxyproline excretion in urine of patients with muscular dystrophy and other muscle diseases. *Proceedings of the Society for Experimental Biology and Medicine*, **115**, 662.

King, B., Spikesman, A. & Emery, A.E.H. (1972) The effect of pregnancy on serum levels of creatine kinase. *Clinica Chimica Acta*, **36**, 267.

Kitchin, S.E. & Watts, D.C. (1973) Comparison of the turnover patterns of total and individual muscle proteins in normal mice and those with hereditary muscular dystrophy. *Biochemical Journal*, **136**, 1017.

Kjellin, K.G. & Stibler, H. (1976) Isoelectric focusing and electrophoresis of cerebrospinal fluid proteins in muscular dystrophies and spinal muscular atrophies. *Journal of the Neurological Sciences*, **27**, 45.

Kleine, T.O. (1970) Evidence for the release of enzymes from different organs in Duchenne's muscular dystrophy. *Clinica Chimica Acta*, **29**, 227.

Kleine, T.O. & Chlond, H. (1967) Enzymmuster gesunder skelett-, herz und glatter Muskelatur des Menschen sowie ihrer pathologischen Veränderungen mit besonderer Berucksichtigung der progressiven Muskeldystrophie (Erb). *Clinica Chimica Acta*, **15**, 19.

Kobayashi, M., Meek, J.C. & Streib, E. (1977) The insulin receptor in myotonic dystrophy. *Journal of Clinical Endocrinology and Metabolism*, **45**, 821.

Kohlschütter, A., Wiesmann, U.N., Herschkowitz, N. & Ferber, E. (1976) Phospholipid composition of cultivated skin fibroblasts in Duchenne's muscular dystrophy. *Clinica Chimica Acta*, **70**, 463.

Kondo, F., Abe, E. & Ikeda, M. (1967) Occasional appearance of diphosphopyridine nucleotide in urine of patients with progressive muscular dystrophy. *Tohoku Journal of Experimental Medicine*, **91**, 191.

Koski, C.L., Jungalwala, F.B. & Kolodny, E.H. (1978) Normality of erythrocyte phospholipids in Duchenne muscular dystrophy. *Clinica Chimica Acta*, **85**, 295.

Koufen, H. & Consbruch, U. (1970) Die Serum-Creatin-Phosphokinase-(CPK)-Aktivität bei amyotropher Lateralsklerose (ALS) und anderen neurogenen Muskelatrophien unter Berücksichtigung differentialdiagnosticher Aspekte. *Der Nervenarzt*, **41**, 599.

Kowalewski, S. & Rotthauwe, H-W. (1972) LDH-Isoenzyme in Muskel bei neuromuskulären Erkrankungen und bei Konduktorinnen der recessiv X-chromosomalen Muskeldystrophie (Duchenne). *Zeitschrift für Kinderheilkunde*, **113**, 55.

Kremzner, L.T., Tennyson, V.M. & Miranda, A.F. (1978) Polyamine metabolism in normal, denervated and dystrophic muscle. In *Advances in Polyamine Research*, **2**, 241.

de Kretser, T. & Livett, B.G. (1977) Skeletal-muscle sarcolemma from normal and dystrophic mice. *Biochemical Journal*, **168**, 229.

Kunze, D. & Olthoff, D. (1970) Der Lipidgehalt menschlicher Skelettmuskulatur bei primären und sekundären Myopathien. *Clinica Chimica Acta*, **29**, 455.

Leiris, de J., Peyrot, M. & Feuvray, D. (1978) Pharmacological reduction of ischaemia-induced enzyme release from isolated rat hearts. *Journal of Molecular Medicine*, **3**, 111.

Lin, C.H., Hudson, A.J. & Strickland, K.P. (1972) Fatty acid oxidation by skeletal muscle mitochondria in Duchenne muscular dystrophy. *Life Sciences (Part II)*, **11**, 355.

Lin, C.H., Hudson, A.J. & Strickland, K.P. (1976) Palmityl-CoA synthetase activity in the muscle of dystrophic mice. *Life Sciences*, **18**, 613.

Lloyd, R.D., Mays, C.W., McFarland, S.S., Zundel, W.S. & Tyler, F.H. (1973) Metabolism of ^{83}Rb and ^{137}Cs in persons with muscle disease. *Radiation Research*, **54**, 463.

Lockshin, R.A. & Beaulaton, J. (1974) Programmed cell death. Cytochemical evidence for lysosomes during the normal breakdown of the intersegmental muscles. *Journal of Ultrastructure Research*, **46**, 43.

Lundholm, K., Bylund, A., Holm, J. & Schersten, T. (1976) Skeletal muscle metabolism in patients with malignant tumour. *European Journal of Cancer*, **12**, 465.

Lunt, G.G. & Marchbanks, R.M. (Eds) (1978) *The Biochemistry of Myasthenia Gravis and Muscular Dystrophy*, p. 239 (Academic Press: London).

McCaman, M.W. (1960) Dehydrogenase activities in dystrophic mice. *Science*, **132**, 621.

McKeran, R.O., Halliday, D. & Purkiss, P. (1977) Increased myofibrillar protein catabolism in Duchenne muscular dystrophy measured by 3-methylhistidine excretion in the urine. *Journal of Neurology, Neurosurgery and Psychiatry*, **40**, 979.

McKeran, R.O., Halliday, D. & Purkiss, P. (1978) Comparison of human myofibrillar protein catabolic rate derived from 3-methylhistidine excretion with synthetic rate from muscle biopsies during L-[α-^{15}N]lysine infusion. *Clinical Science and Molecular Medicine*, **54**, 471.

McPherson, A. & Tokunaga, J. (1967) Effects of cross-innervation on the myoglobin content of tonic and phasic muscles. *Journal of Physiology*, **188**, 121.

Mahoney, M.J., Haseltine, F.P., Hobbins, J.C., Banker, B.Q., Caskey, C.T. & Golbus, M.S. (1977) Prenatal diagnosis of Duchenne's muscular dystrophy. *New England Journal of Medicine*, **297**, 968.

Malo, M.A.G., de la Torre, C.P., Deutsch, S. & Falcone, A. (1970) Étude de la créatine-phosphokinase sérique chez l'enfant de la naissance jusqu'à 13 ans. *Bulletin de la Société de Chimie Biologique*, **52**, 1467.

Mann, W.S. & Salafsky, B. (1970) Enzymic and physiological studies on normal and diseased developing fast and slow cat muscles. *Journal of Physiology*, **208**, 33.

Martinosi, A. (1968) Sarcoplasmic reticulum. VI. Microsomal Ca^{2+} transport in genetic muscular dystrophy of mice. *Proceedings of the Society for Experimental Biology and Medicine*, **127**, 824.

Maskrey, P., Pluskal, M.G., Harris, J.B. & Pennington, R.J.T. (1977) Studies on increased acid hydrolase activities in denervated muscle. *Journal of Neurochemistry*, **28**, 403.

Matheson, D.W., Engel, W.K. & Derrer, E.C. (1976) Erythrocyte shape in Duchenne muscular dystrophy. *Neurology (Minneapolis)*, **26**, 1182.

Matsuda, I., Miyoshino, S., Miike, T., Nagata, N., Tamari, H., Taniguchi, N., Ohno, H. & Watanabe, H. (1978) Mitochondrial fraction of serum glutamic-oxaloacetic transaminase in Duchenne muscular dystrophy. *Clinica Chimica Acta*, **83**, 231.

di Mauro, S., Angelini, C. & Catani, C. (1967) Enzymes of the glycogen cycle and glycolysis in various human neuromuscular disorders. *Journal of Neurology, Neurosurgery and Psychiatry*, **30**, 411.

Mawatari, S., Miranda, A. & Rowland, L.P. (1976) Adenyl cyclase abnormality in Duchenne muscular dystrophy: muscle cells in culture. *Neurology (Minneapolis)*, **26**, 1021.

Meltzer, H.Y. (1971) Factors affecting serum creatine phosphokinase levels in the general population. The role of race, activity and age. *Clinica Chimica Acta*, **33**, 165.

Mendell, J.R., Engel, W.K. & Derrer, E.C. (1972) Increased plasma enzyme concentrations in rats with functional ischaemia of muscle provide a possible model of Duchenne muscular dystrophy. *Nature*, **239**, 522.

Mendell, J.R., Murphy, D. Engel, W.K., Chase, T.N. & Gordon, E. (1972) Catecholamines and indoleamines in patients with Duchenne muscular dystrophy. *Archives of Neurology*, **27**, 518.

Mokri, B. & Engel, A.G. (1975) Duchenne dystrophy: Electron microscopic findings pointing to a basic or early abnormality in the plasma membrane of the muscle fibre. *Neurology (Minneapolis)*, **25**, 1111.

Monkton, G. & Marusyck, H. (1976) Myofibrillar incorporation of ^{3}H (G) L-leucine in progressive muscular dystrophy and motor neurone disease. *Neurology*

(*Minneapolis*), **26**, 234.

Morey, K.S., Tarczy-Hornoch, K., Richards, E.G. & Brown, W.D. (1967) Myosin from dystrophic and control chicken muscle. I. Preparation and preliminary characterisation. *Archives of Biochemistry*, **119**, 491.

Moser, H. & Vogt, J. (1974) Follow-up study of serum-creatine-kinase in carrier of Duchenne muscular dystrophy. *Lancet*, **2**, 661.

Munsat, T.L., Baloh, R., Pearson, C.M. & Fowler, W. Jr. (1973) Serum enzyme alterations in neuromuscular disorders. *Journal of the American Medical Association*, **226**, 1536.

Murphy, D.L., Mendell, J.R. & Engel, W.K. (1973) Serotonin and platelet function in Duchenne muscular dystrophy. *Archives of Neurology*, **28**, 239.

Olson, E., Vignos, P.J. Jr., Woodlock, J. & Perry, T. (1968) Oxidative phosphorylation of skeletal muscle in human muscular dystrophy. *Journal of Laboratory and Clinical Medicine*, **71**, 220.

Omaye, S.T. & Tappel, A.L. (1974) Glutathione peroxidase, glutathione reductase and thiobarbituric acid-reactive products in muscles of chickens and mice with genetic muscular dystrophy. *Life Sciences*, **15**, 137.

Oppenheimer, H. & Milhorat, A.T. (1961) Serum proteins, lipoproteins and glycoproteins in muscular dystrophy and related diseases. *Annals of the New York Academy of Sciences*, **94** (**I**), 308.

Oppenheimer, H., Bárány, K. & Milhorat, A.T. (1964) Myosin from mice with hereditary muscular dystrophy. *Proceedings of the Society for Experimental Biology and Medicine*, **116**, 877.

Park, D.C., Parsons, M.E. & Pennington, R.J.T. (1973) Evidence for mast cell origin of proteinase in skeletal muscle homogenates. *Biochemical Society Transactions*, **1**, 730.

Parsons, M.E., Parsons, R. & Pennington, R.J.T. (1978) Peptide hydrolase activities in rat muscle cultures. *International Journal of Biochemistry*, **9**, 745.

Paterson, Y. & Lawrence, E.F. (1972) Factors affecting serum creatine phosphokinase levels in normal adult females. *Clinica Chimica Acta*, **42**, 131.

Pattengale, P.K. & Holloszy, J.O. (1967) Augmentation of skeletal muscle myoglobin by a program of treadmill running. *American Journal of Physiology*, **213**, 783.

Paulson, O.B., Engel, A.G. & Gomez, M.R. (1974) Muscle blood flow in Duchenne type muscular dystrophy, limb-girdle dystrophy, polymyositis and in normal controls. *Journal of Neurology, Neurosurgery and Psychiatry*, **37**, 685.

Pearce, J.M.S., Pennington, R.J.T. & Walton, J.N. (1964a) Serum enzyme studies in muscle disease. Part I: Variations in serum creatine kinase activity in normal individuals. *Journal of Neurology, Neurosurgery and Psychiatry*, **27**, 1.

Pearce, J.M.S., Pennington, R.J.T. & Walton, J.N. (1964b) Serum enzyme studies in muscle disease. Part II: Serum creatine kinase activity in muscular dystrophy and in other myopathic and neuropathic disorders. *Journal of Neurology, Neurosurgery and Psychiatry*, **27**, 96.

Pearce, J.M.S., Pennington, R.J.T. & Walton, J.N. (1964c) Serum enzyme studies in muscle disease. Part III: Serum creatine kinase activity in relatives of patients with the Duchenne type of muscular dystrophy. *Journal of Neurology, Neurosurgery and Psychiatry*, **27**, 181.

Pearson, T.W. (1978) ($Na^+ + K^+$)-ATPase of Duchenne muscular dystrophy erythrocyte ghosts. *Life Sciences*, **22**, 127.

Pellegrino, C. & Bibbiani, C. (1964) Increase of muscle permeability to aldolase in several experimental atrophies. *Nature*, **204**, 483.

Penn, A.S., Cloak, R.A. & Rowland, L.P. (1972) Myosin from normal and dystrophic human muscle. Immunochemical and electrophoretic studies. *Archives of Neurology*, **27**, 159.

Pennington, R.J.T. (1961) 5′-Adenylic acid deaminase in dystrophic mouse muscle. *Nature*, **192**, 884.

Pennington, R.J.T. (1963) Biochemistry of dystrophic muscle. 2. Some enzyme changes in dystrophic mouse muscle. *Biochemical Journal*, **88**, 64.

Pennington, R.J.T. (1977a) Proteinases of muscle. In *Proteinases in Mammalian Cells and Tissues*, Ed. A.J. Barrett, p. 515 (North Holland: Amsterdam).

Pennington, R.J.T. (1977b) Serum enzymes. In *Pathogenesis of Human Muscular Dystrophies*, Ed. L. P. Rowland, p. 341 (Excerpta Medica: Amsterdam).

Pennington, R.J.T. & Robinson, J.E. (1968) Cathepsin activity in normal and dystrophic human muscle. *Enzymologia Biologica et Clinica*, **9**, 175.

Percy, A.K. & Miller, M.E. (1975) Reduced deformability of erythrocyte membranes from patients with Duchenne muscular dystrophy. *Nature*, **258**, 147.

Perkoff, G.T. & Tyler, F.H. (1958) Creatine metabolism in the Bar Harbor strain dystrophic mouse. *Metabolism*, **7**, 745.

Perry, T.B. & Fraser, F.C. (1973) Variability of serum creatine phosphokinase activity in normal women and carriers of the gene for Duchenne muscular dystrophy. *Neurology (Minneapolis)*, **23**, 1316.

Peter, J.B. (1971) Biochemical approaches to the study of muscle disease. *Birth Defects*, **7**, 38.

Peter, J.B. & Fiehn, W. (1972) Distinctive lipid abnormalities in sarcolemma from patients with muscular dystrophy. *Clinical Research*, **20**, 192.

Peter, J.B., Fiehn, W., Nagatomo, T., Andiman, R., Stempel, K. & Bowman, R. (1974) Studies of sarcolemma from normal and diseased skeletal muscle. In *Exploratory Concepts in Muscular Dystrophy, II*, Ed. A.T. Milhorat, p. 479 (Excerpta Medica: Amsterdam).

Plishker, G.A., Gitelman, H.J. & Appel, S.H. (1978) Myotonic muscular dystrophy: Altered calcium transport in erythrocytes. *Science*, **200**, 323.

Poffenbarger, P.L., Pozefsky, T. & Soeldner, J.S. (1976) The direct relationship of proinsulin-insulin hypersecretion to basal serum levels of cholesterol and triglyceride in myotonic dystrophy. *Journal of Laboratory and Clinical Medicine*, **87**, 384.

Prewitt, M.A. & Salafsky, B. (1970) Enzymic and histochemical changes in fast and slow muscles after cross-innervation. *American Journal of Physiology*, **218**, 69.

Puricelli, H.A., Cacciatore, J., Hermida, M.E. & Toffoli de Matheos, M. (1961) Electrophoretic investigations of the proteins and lipids of the plasma in Steinert's disease. *Acta Neuropsiquiatrica Argentina*, **7**, 293.

Raible, D.G., Cutler, L.S. & Rodan, G.A. (1978) Localisation of adenylate cyclase in skeletal muscle sarcoplasmic reticulum and its relation to calcium accumulation. *FEBS Letters*, **85**, 149.

Rapaport, E. (1975) The fractional disappearance rate of the separate isoenzymes of creatine phosphokinase in the dog. *Cardiovascular Research*, **9**, 473.

Reindorp, S. & Whitehead, R.G. (1971) Changes in serum creatine kinase and other biological measurements associated with musculature in children recovering from kwashiorkor. *British Journal of Nutrition*, **25**, 273.

Riley, D.A. & Allin, D.F. (1973) The effects of inactivity, programmed stimulation and denervation on the histochemistry of skeletal muscle fibre types. *Experimental Neurology*, **40**, 391.

Rodan, S.B., Hintz, R.L., Sha'afi, R.I. & Rodan, G.A. (1974) The activity of membrane bound enzymes in muscular dystrophic chicks. *Nature*, **252**, 589.

Romanul, F.C.A. & Van Der Meulen, J.P. (1966) Reversal of the enzyme profiles of muscle fibres in fast and slow muscles by cross-innervation. *Nature*, **212**, 1369.

Romero-Herrera, A.E., Lehmann, H., Tomlinson, B.E. & Walton, J.N. (1973) Myoglobin in primary muscular disease. I. Duchenne muscular dystrophy and II. Muscular dystrophy of distal type. *Journal of Medical Genetics*, **10**, 309.

Ronzoni, E., Wald, S.M., Lam, R.L. & Gildea, E.F. (1956) Ribosuria in muscular dystrophy. *Neurology (Minneapolis)*, **5**, 412.

Rosalki, S.B. & Thomson, W.H.S. (1971) Serum gamma-glutamyl transpeptidase in muscle disease. *Clinica Chimica Acta*, **33**, 264.

Roses, A.D., Herbstreith, M., Metcalf, B. & Appel, S.H. (1976) Increased phosphorylated components of erythrocyte membrane spectrin band II with reference to Duchenne muscular dystrophy. *Journal of the Neurological Sciences*, **30**, 167.

Roses, A.D., Roses, M.J., Nicholson, G.A. & Roe, C.R. (1977) Lactate dehydrogenase isoenzyme 5 in detecting carriers of Duchenne muscular dystrophy. *Neurology (Minneapolis)*, **27**, 414.

Rowland, L.P. (1976) Pathogenesis of muscular dystrophies. *Archives of Neurology*, **33**, 315.

Rowland, L.P., Layzer, R.B. & Kagen, L.J. (1968) Lack of some muscle proteins in serum of patients with Duchenne dystrophy. *Archives of Neurology*, **18**, 272.

Samaha, F.J. & Congedo, C.Z. (1977) Two biochemical types of Duchenne dystrophy: Sarcoplasmic reticulum membrane proteins. *Annals of Neurology*, **1**, 125.

Samaha, F.J. & Gergely, J. (1969) Biochemical abnormalities of the sarcoplasmic reticulum in muscular dystrophy. *New England Journal of Medicine*, **280**, 184.

Schapira, G., Kruh, J., Dreyfus, J.C. & Schapira, F. (1960) The molecular turnover of muscle aldolase. *Journal of Biological Chemistry*, **235**, 1738.

Schiaffino, S. & Hanzlikova, V. (1972) Studies on the effect of denervation in developing muscle. II. The lysosomal system. *Journal of Ultrastructure Research*, **39**, 1.

Schirmer, R.H. & Thuma, E. (1972) Sensitivity of adenylate kinase isozymes from normal and dystrophic human muscle to sulfhydryl reagents. *Biochimica et Biophysica Acta*, **268**, 92.

Schmalbruch, H. (1975) Segmental fibre breakdown and defects of the plasmalemma in diseased human muscle. *Acta Neuropathologica*, **33**, 129.

Schorr, E.E.C., Arnason, B.G.W., Aström, K. & Darzynkiewicz, Z. (1978) Treatment of mouse muscular dystrophy with the protease inhibitor pepstatin. *Journal of Neuropathology and Experimental Neurology*, **37**, 263.

Schotland, D.L. & Bonilla, E. (1977) Myotonic dystrophy: Alteration in the internal molecular architecture of the muscle plasma membrane. *Neurology (Minneapolis)*, **27**, 379.

Schotland, D.L., Bonilla, E. & Van Meter, M. (1977)

Duchenne dystrophy: Alteration in muscle plasma membrane structure. *Science*, **196**, 1005.

Schwartz, W.N. & Bird, J.W.C. (1977) Degradation of myofibrillar proteins by cathepsins B and D. *Biochemical Journal*, **167**, 811.

Sha'afi, R.I., Rodan, S.B., Hintz, R.L., Fernandez, S.M. & Rodan, G.A. (1975) Abnormalities in membrane microviscosity and ion transport in genetic muscular dystrophy. *Nature*, **254**, 525.

Shannon, A.D., Adams, E.P. & Courtice, F.C. (1974) The lysosomal enzymes acid phosphatase and β-glucuronidase in muscle following a period of ischaemia. *Australian Journal of Experimental Biology and Medical Science*, **52**, 157.

Sica, R.E.P. & McComas, A.J. (1978) The neural hypothesis of muscular dystrophy. *Le Journal Canadien des Sciences Neurologiques*, **5**, 189.

Siddiqui, P.Q.R. & Pennington, R.J.T. (1977) Effect of ouabain upon erythrocyte membrane adenosine triphosphatase in Duchenne muscular dystrophy. *Journal of the Neurological Sciences*, **34**, 365.

Silverman, L.M., Mendell, J.R., Sahenk, Z. & Fontana, M.B. (1976) Significance of creatine phosphokinase isoenzymes in Duchenne dystrophy. *Neurology (Minneapolis)*, **26**, 561.

Simpson, J., Zellweger, H., Burmeister, L.F., Christee, R. & Nielsen, M.K. (1974) Effect of oral contraceptive pills on the level of creatine phosphokinase with regard to carrier detection in Duchenne muscular dystrophy. *Clinica Chimica Acta*, **52**, 219.

Smith, H.L., Fischer, R.L. & Etteldorf, J.N. (1962) Magnesium and calcium in human muscular dystrophy. *American Journal of Diseases of Children*, **103**, 771.

Smoller, M. & Fineberg, R.A. (1965) Studies of myosin in hereditary muscular dystrophy in mice. *Journal of Clinical Investigation*, **44**, 615.

Somer, H., Donner, M., Murros, J. & Konttinen, A. (1973) A serum isozyme study in muscular dystrophy. Particular reference to creatine kinase, aspartate aminotransferase and lactic acid dehydrogenase isozymes. *Archives of Neurology*, **29**, 343.

Souweine, G., Bernard, J.C., Lasne, Y. & Lachanat, J. (1978) The sodium pump of erythrocytes from patients with Duchenne muscular dystrophy: effect of ouabain on the active sodium efflux and on (Na^+, K^+) ATPase. *Journal of Neurology*, **217**, 287.

Stengel-Rutkowski, L. & Barthelmai, W. (1973) Über den Muskel-Energie—Stoffwechsel bei Kindern mit progressiver Muskeldystrophie Typ Duchenne. Metabolite der Glykolyse, des Citratcyclus und energiereicher Phosphate sowie Aktivitäten der alpha-Glycerinphosphatoxidase, Succinatedehydrogenase und 6-Phosphogluconatedehydrogenase. *Klinische Wochenschrift*, **51**, 957.

Stracher, A., McGowan, E.B. & Shafiq, A. (1978) Muscular dystrophy: inhibition of degeneration *in vivo* with protease inhibitors. *Science*, **200**, 50.

Strickland, J.M. & Ellis, D.A. (1975) Isoenzymes of hexokinase in human muscular dystrophy. *Nature*, **253**, 464.

Sugita, H. & Toyokura, Y. (1976) Alteration of troponin subunits in progressive muscular dystrophy (DMP). II. Mechanism of the alteration of troponin subunits in DMP. *Proceedings of the Japan Academy*, **52**, 260.

Sugita, H., Okimoto, K. & Ebashi, S. (1966) Some

observations on the microsome fraction of biopsied muscle from patients with muscular dystrophy. *Proceedings of the Japan Academy*, **42**, 295.

Susheela, A.K., Kaul, R.D., Sachdeva, K. & Singh, N. (1975) Adenyl cyclase activity in Duchenne dystrophic muscle. *Journal of the Neurological Sciences*, **24**, 361.

Sylvester, R. & Baskin, R.J. (1973) Kinetics of calcium uptake in normal and dystrophic sarcoplasmic reticulum. *Biochemical Medicine*, **8**, 213.

Takahashi, K., Shutta, K., Matsuo, B., Takai, T., Takao, H. & Imura, H. (1977) Serum creatine kinase isoenzymes in Duchenne muscular dystrophy. *Clinica Chimica Acta*, **75**, 435.

Tappel, Z., Zalkin, H., Caldwell, K.A., Desai, I.D. & Shibko, S. (1961) Increased lysosomal enzymes in genetic muscular dystrophy. *Archives of Biochemistry*, **96**, 340.

Thomas, N.S.T. & Harper, P.S. (1978) Myotonic dystrophy: Studies on the lipid composition and metabolism of erythrocytes and skin fibroblasts. *Clinica Chimica Acta*, **83**, 13.

Thomson, W.H.S., Sweetin, J.C. & Elton, R.A. (1974) The neurogenic and myogenic hypotheses in human (Duchenne) muscular dystrophy. *Nature*, **249**, 151.

Toyo-oka, T., Shimizu, T. & Masaki, T. (1978) Inhibition of proteolytic activity of calcium activated neutral protease by leupeptin and antipain. *Biochemical and Biophysical Research Communications*, **82**, 484.

Tzvetanova, E. (1971) Creatine kinase isoenzymes in muscle tissue of patients with neuromuscular diseases and human fetuses. *Enzyme*, **12**, 279.

Van Pilsum, J.F. & Wolin, E.A. (1958) Guanidinium compounds in blood and urine of patients suffering from muscle disorders. *Journal of Laboratory and Clinical Medicine*, **51**, 219.

Verrill, H.L., Pickard, N.A. & Gruemer, H.D. (1977a) Mechanisms of cellular enzyme release. I. Alteration in membrane fluidity and permeability. *Clinical Chemistry*, **23**, 2219.

Verrill, H.L., Pickard, N.A. & Gruemer, H.D. (1977b) Diminished cap formation in lymphocytes from patients and carriers of Duchenne muscular dystrophy. *Clinical Chemistry*, **23**, 2341.

Vignos, P.J. & Lefkowitz, M. (1959) A biochemical study of certain skeletal muscle constituents in human progressive muscular dystrophy. *Journal of Clinical Investigation*, **38**, 873.

Vignos, P.J. & Warner, J.L. (1963) Glycogen, creatine and high energy phosphate in human muscle disease. *Journal of Laboratory and Clinical Medicine*, **62**, 579.

Wagner, K.R., Kauffman, F.C. & Max, S.R. (1978) The pentose phosphate pathway in regenerating skeletal muscle. *Biochemical Journal*, **170**, 17.

Wakamatsu, H., Nakamura, H., Ito, K., Anazawa, W., Okajima, S., Okamoto, S., Shigeno, K. & Yuichiro, G. (1970) Serum desmosterol and other lipids in myotonic dystrophy. A possible pathogenesis of myotonic dystrophy. *Keio Journal of Medicine*, **19**, 145.

Walton, J.N. & Latner, A.L. (1954) Ribosuria in muscular

dystrophy. *Archives of Neurology and Psychiatry*, **72**, 362.

Webb, J.N. (1974) Muscular dystrophy and muscle cell death in normal fetal development. *Nature*, **252**, 233.

Weinstock, I.M., Marshall, M. & Jenkins, H. (1962) Cathepsin activity in nutritional muscular dystrophy. *Federation Proceedings*, **21**, 320.

West, D.P., Ellis, D.A. & Strickland, J.M. (1977) Incorporation of U-^{14}C glucose into neutral lipids and sn-glycerol-3-phosphate in muscle from Duchenne muscular dystrophy and control patients. *Journal of the Neurological Sciences*, **33**, 131.

Wieme, R.J. & Lauryssens, M.J. (1962) Lactate dehydrogenase multiplicity in normal and diseased human muscle. *Lancet*, **1**, 433.

Wildenthal, K. (1978) Lysosomal alterations in ischaemic myocardium: Result or cause of myocellular damage? *Journal of Molecular and Cellular Cardiology*, **10**, 595.

Wilkerson, L.S., Perkins, R.C., Roelofs, R., Swift, L., Dalton, L.R. & Park, J.H. (1978) Erythrocyte membrane abnormalities in Duchenne muscular dystrophy monitored by saturation transfer electron paramagnetic resonance spectroscopy. *Proceedings of the National Academy of Sciences, USA*, **75**, 838.

Williams, E.R. & Bruford, A. (1970) Creatine phosphokinase in motor neurone disease. *Clinica Chimica Acta*, **27**, 53.

Wochner, R.D., Drews, G., Strober, W. & Waldmann, T.A. (1966) Accelerated breakdown of immunoglobulin G (IgG) in myotonic dystrophy: A hereditary error of immunoglobulin catabolism. *Journal of Clinical Investigation*, **45**, 321.

Woo, Y. & Manery, J.F. (1975) 5′-Nucleotidase: an ecto-enzyme of frog muscle. *Biochimica et Biophysica Acta*, **397**, 144.

Wright, T.L., O'Neill, J.A. & Olson, W.H. (1973) Abnormal intrafibrillar monoamines in sex-linked muscular dystrophy. *Neurology (Minneapolis)*, **23**, 511.

Wrogemann, K. & Nylen, E.G. (1978) Mitochondrial calcium overloading in cardiomyopathic hamsters. *Journal of Molecular and Cellular Cardiology*, **10**, 185.

Wrogemann, K., Jacobson, B.E. & Blanchaer, M.C. (1973) On the mechanism of a calcium-associated defect of oxidative phosphorylation in progressive muscular dystrophy. *Archives of Biochemistry and Biophysics*, **159**, 267.

Zatz, M., Schapiro, L.J., Campion, D.S., Oda, E. & Kaback, M.M. (1978) Serum pyruvate-kinase (PK) and creatine phosphokinase (CPK) in progressive muscular dystrophies. *Journal of the Neurological Sciences*, **36**, 349.

Zierler, K. (1958) Muscle membrane as a dynamic structure and its permeability to aldolase. *Annals of the New York Academy of Sciences*, **75** (I), 227.

Zierler, K. (1961) Potassium flux and further observations on aldolase flux in dystrophic mouse muscle. *Bulletin of the Johns Hopkins Hospital*, **108**, 208.

Zierler, K., Folk, B.P., Magladery, J.W. & Lilienthal, J.L. Jun. (1949) On creatinuria in man. The roles of the renal tubule and of muscle mass. *Bulletin of the Johns Hopkins Hospital*, **85**, 370.

Clinical examination of the neuromuscular system

INTRODUCTION

The neuromuscular disorders are those conditions in which the patient's symptoms result from abnormalities in the lower motor neurones (including the motor nuclei of the cranial nerves, the anterior horn cells of the spinal cord, the spinal motor roots, the motor fibres of the peripheral nerves), the neuro-muscular junction and the voluntary muscles themselves. Lesions or pathological processes involving the spinal cord, spinal roots or peripheral nerves commonly involve sensory as well as motor pathways, thus giving rise to pain, paraesthesiae and sensory loss which may vary in character and distribution depending upon the nature and site of the lesion or process concerned. Some such symptoms and their accompanying signs are considered in Chapters 21 and 23. This chapter will deal essentially with the clinical manifestations of motor dysfunction resulting from disease of the neuromuscular apparatus.

SYMPTOMS AND SIGNS IN NEUROMUSCULAR DISEASE

Although the neuromuscular disorders are numerous the symptoms to which they give rise are few, pain and weakness being the most frequent, and limpness, fatigue, wasting, spontaneous movements, palpable tenderness, local or diffuse swelling of nerves and/or muscles and contractures the only others of importance. Very often a definite diagnosis can and should be reached only after biochemical, electrophysiological and histological investigation. But this in no way diminishes the importance of the clinical history and examination, which will usually restrict the differential diagnosis to a few conditions and will also be of great value in indicating the best site for electromyography and muscle biopsy. These all-important investigations can be inconclusive or even misleading if a muscle in too advanced or too early a stage of the disease is chosen.

In the following catalogue of the clinical features of muscle disease, symptoms and signs are often necessarily discussed together but, as far as possible, points arising from the history are mentioned before the findings on examination. Details of methods of eliciting physical signs are generally omitted but useful accounts of these are given in de Jong (1979), Bickerstaff (1973), Bradley (1974) and 'Aids to the examination of the peripheral nervous system' (Medical Research Council, 1976). Valuable information on the examination of children will be found in André-Thomas, Chesni and Dargassies (1960), Paine and Oppé (1966), Gamstorp (1970) and Dubowitz (1978).

Family history

The familial occurrence of a disorder is of obvious diagnostic help. Sometimes, however, the course of the disease may differ greatly in different members of a family; this can be particularly striking in infantile and juvenile spinal muscular atrophy and in glycogen-storage disease of muscle, where slowly progressive proximal weakness in one sib may bear little resemblance to the severe and rapidly fatal disease in another. Better understood examples include the homozygous and heterozygous forms of the distal type of muscular dystrophy, inter-sib variation in the peroneal muscular atrophy syndrome and the subclinical myopathy of the female carriers of the gene for Duchenne dystrophy.

On the whole it is among the sex-linked and dominant conditions that the family history is most helpful; the early diagnosis of Duchenne, facioscapulohumeral and myotonic muscular dystrophy or of the periodic paralyses is much easier if others in the family have been affected. In obscure myopathies the discovery of parental consanguinity may, on the other hand, direct attention to the possibility of a rare autosomal recessive disorder. The patient's statement that there is 'no family history of muscle disease' should not be accepted without a detailed pedigree enquiry. Especially in the case of myotonic dystrophy, facioscapulohumeral dystrophy, peroneal muscular atrophy and its variants and in the congenital myopathies it is a common experience to find previously unrecognised cases when the whole family is carefully examined.

Muscle pain at rest

Painful muscular contraction is the basis of many of the commonest of all symptoms, including tension headache, low back pain and 'fibrositis'. Fear, often irrational and unconscious (such as that associated with depression and anxiety), and minor trauma may each be responsible. In a particularly sophisticated form these mechanisms may give rise to writer's cramp and other occupational neuroses. Painful muscle spasm often accompanies joint disease. Furthermore, pain may often be referred to muscle from other sites. These

banal though important conditions cannot be discussed here. *Cramp* is a transient, involuntary and painful muscular contraction which may result from unaccustomed exertion, sodium depletion, uraemia, tetany or drugs but is much more often unexplained. In spinal cord lesions, especially multiple sclerosis, *flexor spasms* due to spasticity may be very painful. In *compression of spinal roots or nerves* resulting, say, from intervertebral disc disease or peripheral nerve entrapment, pain commonly radiates along the cutaneous dermatome innervated by the sensory component of the spinal or peripheral nerve concerned, but sometimes dull aching pain is felt in the muscles innervated by their motor component. Nerve trunks may become tender or painful on palpation or stretching when one or more of their component roots is so affected, or at or near sites of entrapment. Tapping over a nerve at such a site can give, not only pain, but also paraesthesiae radiating down its cutaneous sensory distribution. *Neuralgic amyotrophy* begins with severe aching pain in the shoulder or arm followed after a few days by wasting and weakness which usually involves the serratus anterior, trapezius, deltoid, biceps or spinati. Often there is a preceding febrile illness. The pain generally clears up after a few weeks and the weakness after a few months but both may persist for several months and the weakness may be permanent. In both *poliomyelitis* and the *Guillain-Barré syndrome* the onset of muscle weakness may be preceded by pain, and in poliomyelitis there is often visible fasciculation at this stage. Other painful *polyneuropathies* are those associated with alcoholism, porphyria, arsenic poisoning and polyarteritis nodosa. In yet others including those due to deficiency of vitamin B1 or B12 the muscles are tender. In diabetic amyotrophy, usually due to a mononeuropathy of the femoral nerve, less often of the lumbar plexus, there is pain and atrophy of the quadriceps or rarely of other muscles. Myalgia is common in virus infections and varies in severity from that commonly experienced in influenza, to the more severe pain of benign myalgic encephalomyelitis and the very severe diaphragmatic pain of *Coxsackie B myalgia (Bornholm disease)*. *Polymyalgia rheumatica* affects elderly people who may be severely incapacitated by muscular pains in the arms and legs without weakness or sensory change; the ESR is always raised and the condition responds well to steroid therapy. *Polymyositis* is rarely painful but some tenderness may be found in acute and severe cases.

Pain on exertion

This is usually attributable to muscle ischaemia, illustrated by the familiar experiment of exercising the forearm muscles with a cuff at above arterial pressure around the arm and by 'intermittent claudication' resulting from atherosclerotic occlusion of the iliac or femoro-popliteal arteries. Occasionally the weakness and paraesthesiae in the leg and foot during walking, which result from intermittent ischaemia of the spinal cord or cauda equina, may cause confusion. In *McArdle's disease* (myophosphorylase deficiency), and related disorders of muscle glycolytic metabolism including phosphofructokinase deficiency, the earliest symptom is usually an aching sensation in the calves during walking, which becomes more painful if the patient perseveres and other muscles become similarly painful, often with temporary contracture, if vigorously exercised. Not infrequently, patients with this symptom are investigated enthusiastically with disappointingly negative results, and the cause of these benign exertional cramps in otherwise apparently healthy people is poorly understood. Rare causes of exertional muscle pain and cramp, often associated with myoglobinuria, include certain lipid storage myopathies and especially carnitine palmityl transferase deficiency. Sometimes cramp on exertion is a feature of muscular dystrophy, early motor neurone disease or even early spasticity but it is rarely, if ever, a presenting symptom in the absence of other signs of these disorders.

Weakness as a symptom

The disability to which muscle weakness may give rise depends not only on the muscles involved but upon the patient's way of life. Few people use any of their muscles to full capacity and sometimes quite profound weakness may go unnoticed by apparently intelligent people. It is not, therefore, surprising that difficulty in walking is a common presentation of muscle disease, as this is a form of exertion that few escape. Difficulty in running, in climbing stairs or on to bus platforms and in getting out of low chairs are the usual early symptoms of proximal limb weakness and often shoulder-girdle weakness may be equally severe but asymptomatic. Those whose occupation involves lifting weights or the arrangement of complex hairstyles may notice upper-limb weakness first. Quadriceps weakness sometimes leads to sudden falls because of the resulting instability of the knee, and muscle weakness may not even be considered once the idea of 'drop attacks' has entered the examiner's mind. Distal weakness leads to tripping over carpets, kerbs and stairs and to weakness of the hands often first described as clumsiness. Patients who complain of difficulty in walking *down* stairs often turn out to have spasticity of the legs or cerebellar ataxia.

The mode of onset and progression of the weakness are of great importance in neuromuscular disease. A rapid onset after a minor febrile illness may suggest poliomyelitis or the Guillain-Barré syndrome. It is less well known that spinal muscular atrophy, either Werdnig-Hoffmann disease or its benign variant, may present in this way and may then show further less rapid progression. Benign spinal muscular atrophy is also notable for its tendency to undergo static periods, lasting sometimes for many years, between phases of deterioration. Probably the condition called 'poliomyélite chronique' is a form of this disorder. Many of the myopathies progress steadily at rates which vary widely from one condition to another but tend to be fairly uniform among cases of each disease. The inflammatory myopathies, however, and especially polymyositis, have a wide spectrum of progression from a fulminating course of a few days to an indolent one spanning several decades. The periodic paralyses give recurring episodes of weakness which usually give rise to little confusion, especially when there is a family history. In isolated cases, thyrotoxicosis and hyperaldosteronism should be excluded. A story of remission and relapse over longer periods suggests myasthenia gravis or a relapsing peripheral neuropathy.

Weakness—the patient in action

The first stage of the examination in a suspected muscle disorder is to watch the patient in action—his posture and gait especially. The facial expression may be critical in giving the first clue to the diagnosis—myotonic dystrophy is the supreme example of this among the muscle disorders because of the variety of features which may be immediately evident—baldness, apathy, atrophy of temporal and sternomastoid muscles, masseter weakness, ptosis, drooping of the cheeks and lower lip, and cataract. In facioscapulohumeral dystrophy only the everted position of the lips and the lack of facial lines may be apparent at first. Here the facial weakness needs to be demonstrated on movement. The 'snarl' of myasthenia gravis is shown in Chapter 16 (Fig. 16.5). In facioscapulohumeral dystrophy the shoulders have a strikingly sloping posture and a very characteristic sign is the remarkable elevation of the scapula which occurs when the arm is abducted (Ch. 14, Fig. 14.5). *Winging of the scapulae at rest* is seen in serratus palsies and in limb-girdle muscular dystrophy but it must generally be brought out by putting serratus anterior into action in the other types of muscular dystrophy and in the many other conditions in which it occurs. *Kyphoscoliosis* is seen early in Friedreich's ataxia and neurofibromatosis. In the muscular dystrophies and in the spinal muscular atrophies severe degrees of kyphoscoliosis may occur but not until muscular weakness is obvious; thus it is important in the management but not in the diagnosis of these conditions. However contractures of the calf muscles and of the hip flexors may contribute significantly to the lordotic tip-toe position which patients with muscular dystrophy often adopt at a stage when the diagnosis still remains in doubt. The posture and appearance of the hands and feet are characteristic and well known in various nerve palsies, tetany, peroneal muscular atrophy and the other hereditary neuropathies, motor neurone disease and syringomyelia.

The *gait* may be very valuable in convincing the examiner that weakness is present, and in indicating its approximate distribution. Not too much more should be expected of this valuable part of the examination and it is wrong to suggest that any abnormal gait is 'pathognomonic' of a specific neuromuscular disorder. In general the 'steppage' gait of pure peripheral muscle weakness (for example in peroneal muscular atrophy) is noticeably more fluent and confident than the combination of foot-drop with ataxia seen in the sensory neuropathies and in tabes. In the spastic foot-drop of pyramidal tract disease the foot is dragged rather than lifted. Mild weakness of dorsiflexion is easily detected if patients are asked to walk on their heels. The waddling lordotic gait of proximal lower-limb weakness is even less specific. It is seen most typically in the childhood muscular dystrophies when it is often associated with a tip-toe stance. In benign spinal muscular atrophy and in polymyositis a similar gait is often seen; in the former the waddle may be even more extreme but the lordosis is often less. The gait in disorders of the hip joint such as the epiphyseal dysplasias may be deceptively similar and in young children who cannot cooperate in muscle testing, investigations may be pursued to a late stage before a radiograph reveals the true diagnosis. In early and doubtful cases of proximal weakness it is invaluable to watch the patient running and trying to hurry up stairs. Attempts to run may resemble a 'racing walk' and the hands may push on the knees or pull on the banister to help him up the stairs. These signs are usually the earliest to be detectable in Duchenne dystrophy.

Gowers' sign, illustrated in Chapter 14 (Fig. 14.1), is also valuable but, in the very early stages of proximal weakness, patients may be able to stand up fairly easily with only perhaps a brief push with a hand on one knee. Weakness of the quadriceps muscle is best shown during attempts to climb stairs or to stand up from a chair without using the arms. Much can be learned by asking a patient to sit up from the lying position; weakness of the anterior neck muscle will cause the head to lag instead of being the first part to be lifted from the couch, weakness of either hip flexion or the abdominal muscles may make the manoeuvre impossible, and localised weakness of the upper or lower abdominal muscles will cause a shift of the umbilicus from the mid position. Early paraspinal weakness can be tested in the prone position by asking him to lift the head and shoulders backwards from the couch.

For comparative studies and particularly in trials of treatment it is useful to record, not only the strength of individual muscles, but also the patient's overall disability. The following scheme, modified from Vignos and Archibald (1960), is suitable for cases of muscular dystrophy but could be adapted for other purposes if, for example, information about early loss of function in the arms or bulbar muscles were important.

Grade 0 Preclinical. All activities normal.

Grade 1 Walks normally. Unable to run freely.

Grade 2 Detectable defect in posture or gait. Climbs stairs without using the banister.

Grade 3 Climbs stairs only with the banister.

Grade 4 Walks without assistance. Unable to climb stairs.

Grade 5 Walks without assistance. Unable to rise from a chair.

Grade 6 Walks only with calipers or other aids.

Grade 7 Unable to walk. Sits erect in a chair. Able to roll a wheelchair and eat and drink normally.

Grade 8 Sits unsupported in chair. Unable to roll wheelchair or unable to drink from a glass unassisted.

Grade 9 Unable to sit erect without support or unable to eat or drink without assistance.

Grade 10 Confined to bed. Requires help for all activities.

In the early stages further quantitative information can be gained by timing the patient walking over measured distances, climbing standard stairs, standing up from the supine position or from a low chair, or from low stools of graded height. In children especially these tests are more valid than measurement of muscle strength.

Weakness—detailed muscle testing

The examination of a patient with muscular weakness must determine whether the weakness is genuine or spurious, its degree, distribution and symmetry and whether it changes after exercise.

The last point is dealt with in the section on fatiguability.

The question of the reality of the weakness is put first, not through cynicism, but because it poses a common problem. Ill patients may develop severe weakness which is easily missed unless careful muscle testing is performed. Traumatic nerve palsies following operations, and drug-induced neuropathies developing in the course of illnesses such as tuberculosis or renal failure are obvious examples, but the outstanding example of this is the myopathy associated with osteomalacia in renal failure or malabsorption, which is very commonly ignored. 'Neurasthenia' may be blamed for the weakness in myasthenia gravis or thyrotoxic myopathy. The obverse problem of spurious or hysterical weakness masquerading as neuromuscular disease is more easily dealt with because the situation invites careful neurological examination. Spasticity and extrapyramidal rigidity or akinesia may give an initial impression of weakness. Pain due to joint disease is a common pitfall in muscle testing and is especially liable to cause confusion at the hips and knees. The position is often made more complex by the genuine weakness and wasting which may develop, for example, in the quadriceps in the presence of rheumatoid disease or osteoarthritis of the knee, or in the small muscles of an arthritic hand. The diagnosis of hysterical weakness or malingering depends chiefly on the discovery of inconsistencies when all the clinical signs are considered as a whole, but a good deal can be learned in the course of manual muscle testing. There is often a momentary initial contraction of reasonable strength, followed by a sudden 'give' in the resistance, which is never found in true weakness except in the presence of pain. The other useful sign in malingering and the less sophisticated degrees of hysteria is simultaneous contraction in agonist and antagonist muscles, with a failure of synergist and stabilising muscles to contract, although they may be found to be strong when they are tested separately. Thus, in testing the quadriceps in a case of suspected hysteria, an unobtrusive hand on the hamstrings on the same side or under the opposite heel may give valuable information.

Much can be learned about the degree of severity of muscle weakness by watching the patient in action, walking, hopping, jumping, climbing stairs, getting up from the floor or from a chair, sitting up from a couch, trying to lift his arms above his head or writing his name. A great deal of time can be saved by these tests and, indeed, some muscles such as those of the abdomen and trunk cannot be satisfactorily tested by any other means. In examining children this approach may be the only one possible. However, detailed information is best acquired by manual testing of each muscle or group in turn. The proper methods for these tests are briefly summarised in Table 13.1 and are more fully described and illustrated in several texts including Daniels, Williams and Worthingham (1956), Bickerstaff (1973) and the M.R.C. memorandum (1976). A few of the more important tests are illustrated in Figures 13.1–13.5. The precise positioning of the limb and of the examiner's resistance are very important but, with practice, the methods are reliable. Usually isometric resistance is applied to the fully contracted muscle until it gives way (the 'break' test) but in some circumstances it is useful to test a muscle's strength throughout its full range of movement. It is best to palpate the contracting muscle at the same time. The results are commonly expressed on the scale in the Medical Research Council memorandum (1976).

Grade 0 No contraction.
Grade 1 Flicker or trace of contraction.
Grade 2 Active movement with gravity eliminated.
Grade 3 Active movement against gravity.
Grade 4 Active movement against gravity and resistance.
Grade 5 Normal power.

Grades 4−, 4 and 4+ may be used to indicate movement against slight, moderate and strong resistance respectively. For accurate comparative work there is no substitute for measurement, but here the difficulties of using standard methods and of eliminating gravity and friction are multiplied and it requires a good deal of skill to assess whether the patient is exerting his full strength. Non-extensive strain gauges have theoretical advantages but, in practice, a spring balance held by the examiner is often as good an instrument as any because the 'feel' of the patient's effort can be assessed at the same time. The Hammersmith myometer has been found to give reasonably accurate and reproducible measurements of muscle power in clinical practice (Edwards and McDonnell, 1974; Dubowitz, 1978).

Broadly speaking, the interpretation of the muscle weakness which is found is an exercise in

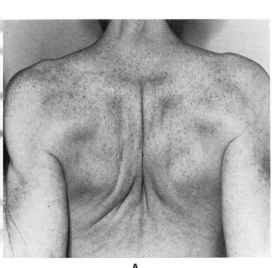
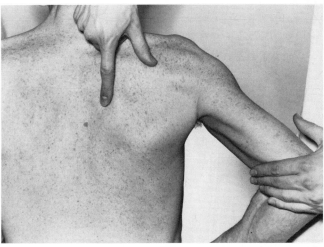

A   **B**

Fig. 13.1   A. The horizontal fibres of trapezius adduct the scapulae when the shoulders are braced backwards (normal subject). B. The rhomboids may be felt when the elbow is pushed backwards against resistance. The overlying trapezius is relaxed (normal subject)

Table 13.1   The nerve and root supply of the principal muscles with methods of testing their actions. Modified from Gray's Anatomy (1967) and M.R.C. memorandum (1976). Where any single root supplying a particular muscle is more important than the others it is printed in bold type.

Nerve	Muscle	Roots	Action tested
Accessory nerve	Trapezius	spinal root	Elevation of shoulders. Adduction of scapulae
	Sternocleidomastoid	spinal root	Tilting of head to same side with rotation to opposite side
Brachial plexus	Pectoralis major		
	Clavicular part	**C5**, C6	Adduction of elevated arm
	Sternocostal part	C6, **C7, C8**	Adduction and forward depression of arm
	Serratus anterior	C5, C6, C7	Fixation of the scapula during forward thrusting of the arm
	Rhomboids	C4, C5	Elevation and fixation of scapula
	Supraspinatus	**C5**, C6	Initiation of abduction of arm
	Infraspinatus	**C5**, C6	External rotation of arm
	Latissimus dorsi	C6, **C7**, C8	Adduction of horizontal, externally rotated arm. Coughing
Axillary nerve	Deltoid	**C5**, C6	Lateral and forward elevation of arm to horizontal
Musculocutaneous nerve	Biceps ⎫ Brachialis ⎭	C5, C6	Flexion of the supinated forearm
Radial nerve	Triceps	C6, **C7**, C8	Extension of forearm
	Brachioradialis	C5, **C6**	Flexion of semi-prone forearm
	Extensor carpi radialis longus	**C6**	Extension of wrist to radial side
Posterior interosseous nerve	Supinator	C6, C7	Supination of extended forearm
	Extensor digitorum	**C7**, C8	Extension of proximal phalanges
	Extensor carpi ulnaris	**C7**, C8	Extension of wrist to ulnar side
	Extensor indicis	**C7**, C8	Extension of proximal phalanx of index finger
	Abductor pollicis longus	**C7**, C8	Abduction of first metacarpal in plane at right angle to palm
	Extensor pollicis longus	**C7**, C8	Extension at first interphalangeal joint
	Extensor pollicis brevis	**C7**, C8	Extension at first metacarpophalangeal joint
Median nerve	Pronator teres	C6, C7	Pronation of extended forearm
	Flexor carpi radialis	C6, C7	Flexion of wrist to radial side
	Flexor digitorum superficialis	C7, **C8**, T1	Flexion of middle phalanges
	Abductor pollicis brevis (ulnar nerve rarely)	C8, **T1**	Abduction of first metacarpal in plane at right angle to palm
	Flexor pollicis brevis (more often ulnar nerve)	C8, **T1**	Flexion of proximal phalanx of thumb
	Opponens pollicis (rarely ulnar nerve)	C8, **T1**	Opposition of thumb against fifth finger
	1st and 2nd lumbricals	C8, **T1**	Extension of middle phalanges while proximal phalanges are fixed in extension
Anterior interosseous nerve	Flexor digitorum profundus (lateral part)	**C8**, T1	Flexion of terminal phalanges of index and middle fingers
	Flexor pollicis longus	**C8**, T1	Flexion of distal phalanx of the thumb

Table 13.1.—*continued*

Nerve	Muscle	Roots	Action tested
Ulnar nerve	Flexor carpi ulnaris	C7, **C8**, T1	Observe tendon during testing abductor digiti minimi
	Flexor digitorum profundus (medial part)	C7, **C8**	Flexion of distal phalanges of ring and little fingers
	Hypothenar muscles	C8, **T1**	Abduction and opposition of little finger
	3rd and 4th lumbricals	C8, **T1**	Extension of middle phalanges while proximal phalanges are fixed in extension
	Adductor pollicis	C8, **T1**	Adduction of thumb against palmar surface of index finger
	Flexor pollicis brevis (sometimes median nerve)	**C8**, T1	Flexion of proximal phalanx of the thumb
	Interossei	C8, **T1**	Abduction and adduction of the fingers
Femoral nerve	Iliopsoas (and lumbar nerves)	**L1**, **L2**, L3	Hip flexion from semi-flexed position
	Sartorius	L2, L3	Hip flexion from externally rotated position
	Quadriceps (rectus femoris and the lateral and medial vasti)	L2, **L3**, **L4**	Extension at the knee
Obturator nerve	Adductor longus magnus* brevis	**L2**, **L3**, L4	Adduction of the thigh
Superior gluteal nerve	Gluteus medius	**L4**, **L5**, S1	Abduction of the thigh. Internal rotation of the thigh
	Tensor fasciae latae	L4, L5	
Inferior gluteal nerve	Gluteus maximus	**L5**, **S1**, S2	Extension of the thigh
Sciatic nerve	Biceps femoris	L5, **S1**, S2	Flexion at the knee
	Semitendinosus	L5, **S1**, S2	
	Semimembranosus	L5, **S1**, S2	
Peroneal nerve (deep)	Anterior tibial	**L4**, L5	Dorsiflexion of the foot
	Extensor digitorum longus	**L5**, S1	Dorsiflexion of the toes
	Extensor hallucis longus	**L5**, S1	Dorsiflexion of great toe
	Extensor digitorum brevis	L5, S1	Dorsiflexion of the toes
Peroneal nerve (superfic.)	Peroneus longus Peroneus brevis	L5, S1	Eversion of the foot
Tibial nerve	Gastrocnemius	**S1**, S2	Plantar-flexion of the foot
	Soleus	S1, **S2**	
	Tibialis posterior	L4, **L5**	Inversion of plantar-flexed foot
	Flexor digitorum longus	L5, **S1**, **S2**	Flexion of toes (distal phalanges)
	Flexor hallucis longus	L5, **S1**, **S2**	Flexion of great toe (distal phalanx)
	Flexor digitorum brevis	S1, S2	Flexion of toes (middle phalanges)
	Flexor hallucis brevis	S1, S2	Flexion of great toe (proximal phalanx)
Pudendal nerve	Perineal muscles	S2, S3, S4	Tension of anal sphincter

*Adductor magnus is partly supplied by the sciatic nerve.

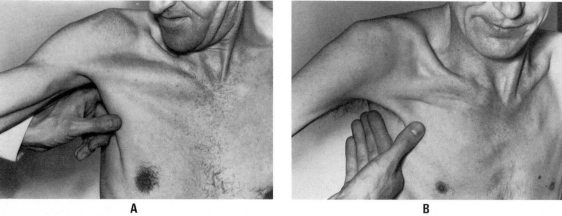

Fig. 13.2 The arm is being adducted and depressed against resistance, the sternocostal fibres of pectoralis major are clearly seen and felt. A. Normal subject, B. Becker type of muscular dystrophy.

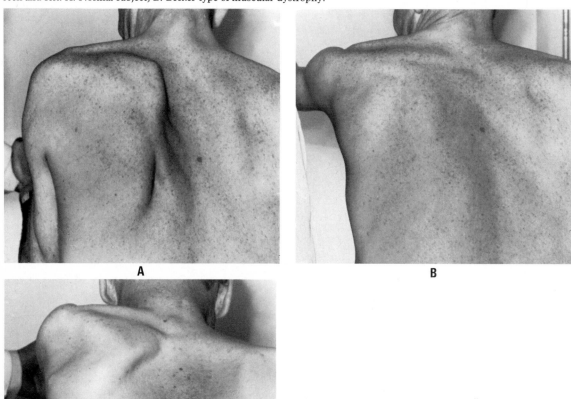

Fig. 13.3 Testing serratus anterior. The upper limb is being thrust forwards against resistance. With the elbow flexed by the side some winging of the scapula may be seen in normal subjects (A) but with the arm outstretched there is a clear difference between the normal (B) and abnormal (C) (Becker dystrophy)

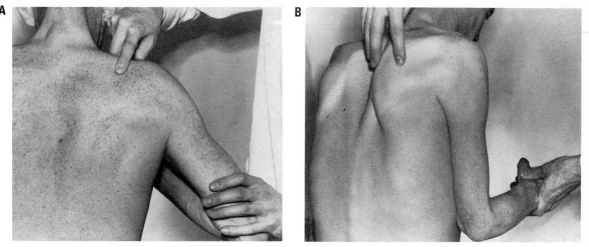

Fig. 13.4 A. Supraspinatus acts as the principal abductor with the elbow close to the trunk. Its contraction can easily be felt (normal subject). B. Infraspinatus is tested during external rotation of the arm against resistance. The wasting of the muscle can be seen and felt (Becker dystrophy)

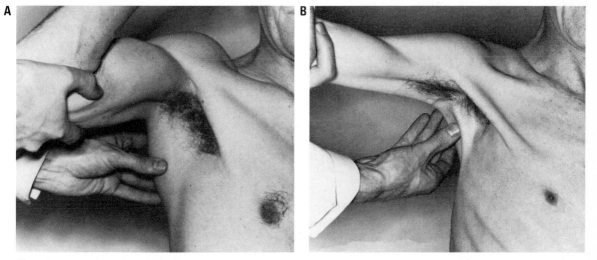

Fig. 13.5 Latissimus dorsi. The elbow of the externally rotated arm is being pushed downwards against resistance. the difference between the normal bulky muscle (A) and the wasted remnant in Becker muscular dystrophy (B) is clear

applied anatomy when the lesion is in the lower motor neurone and a matter of pattern recognition in the myopathies. The diagnosis of upper motor neurone lesions requires a combination of these two approaches and is beyond the scope of this chapter. Localised weakness in a single limb is usually neurogenic although the effects of muscle trauma such as severe ischaemia or tendon rupture may sometimes cause confusion. Details of the root and nerve supply of the principal muscles are given in Table 13.1. When localised weakness seems to fit into no anatomical pattern, polio-myelitis and early motor neurone disease should be considered. It is difficult to discuss briefly the patterns of muscular involvement in the myopathies. Nor is it proper to consider the diagnostic value of these patterns without reference to other important points such as the duration and mode of progression of the disease, the presence of other symptoms, the presence or absence of wasting or reflex change, and so on. However, the information given in Table 13.2 may be helpful as an approximate guide and a further discussion will be found in the section on differential diagnosis in

Table 13.2   An outline of some of the common patterns of muscular weakness and atrophy in various disorders

	Generalised	Mainly distal	Mainly Proximal	Symmetrical—Highly Selective	Asymmetrical
With little or no wasting	Polymyositis Myasthenia gravis Myasthenic-myopathic syndrome Periodic paralyses Hypothyroidism Addison's disease Steroid myopathy	Upper motor neurone lesions	Polymyositis Myasthenia gravis Myasthenic-myopathic syndrome Myopathy with osteomalacia Periodic paralyses Steroid myopathy Hypothyroidism Upper motor neurone lesions	Periodic paralyses	Periodic paralyses Peripheral neuropathy U.M.N. lesion
With wasting	Werdnig-Hoffmann disease Benign congenital myopathies M.N.D. (Polymyositis)	Most peripheral neuropathies Peroneal muscular atrophy M.N.D. Distal myopathy Myotonic dystrophy* Ocular myopathy (U.M.N. lesions)	Muscular dystrophy† Benign spinal muscular atrophy Thyrotoxic myopathy Glycogen-storage disease Lipid storage myopathies Myasthenic-myopathic syndrome Motor neuropathy M.N.D. Polymyositis	Muscular dystrophy† Benign spinal muscular atrophy Thyrotoxic myopathy M.N.D. Motor neuropathy Ocular myopathy Glycogen-storage disease (Poliomyelitis)	M.N.D. Poliomyelitis Peripheral neuropathy Benign spinal muscular atrophy (Limb-girdle muscular dystrophy)

M.N.D. = motor neurone disease. U.M.N. = upper motor neurone.

Unusual presentations are given in brackets. Causes of purely localised weakness have been excluded.

*In myotonic dystrophy the weakness is semi-distal, i.e. involves the forearm and the leg but not small hand muscles at first.

†'Muscular dystrophy' refers to the X-linked, limb-girdle and facioscapulohumeral types.

Chapter 14. It is of special importance to decide whether proximal muscle weakness involves all the shoulder girdle or pelvic muscles to about the same degree (as in polymyositis or thyrotoxic myopathy, for instance) or certain muscles selectively. A selective, symmetrical pattern of involvement in a chronic progressive myopathy is suggestive of muscular dystrophy, although spinal muscular atrophy and other disorders may imitate this. The exact distribution of this selective involvement may be of great help in distinguishing one form of muscular dystrophy from another, especially in the early stages. An atypical distribution of weakness and wasting in a case of apparent muscular dystrophy should arouse immediate suspicions about the diagnosis and should be regarded as an absolute indication for full investigation, including muscle biopsy.

Fatiguability

Muscular weakness which is variable in degree and is made worse by repeated contraction is characteristic of myasthenia. It must be distinguished from simple fatigue due to constant slight muscular weakness and from stiffness or pain induced by exercise. Clinical demonstration of myasthenia is usually possible if the strength of an affected muscle is compared with its contralateral equivalent before and after repeated contraction. The reverse phenomenon, weakness which improves during the first few contractions following a period of inactivity, may occur in the so-called myasthenic–myopathic or Eaton–Lambert syndrome. The clinical features of these conditions are described in Chapters 16 and 19. Although characteristic cases are easily recognised, patients do not always notice the effect of exercise. It is, therefore, wise to try the effect of intravenous edrophonium in every case of obscure muscular weakness and this should be one of the earliest investigations whenever muscular weakness is not associated with conspicuous wasting, especially if the tendon reflexes are preserved. The retention of the tendon reflexes is typical of myasthenia gravis while in the Eaton-Lambert syndrome these reflexes are lost. Another point of distinction between these conditions is the tendency for the lower limbs to be affected first in the myasthenic–myopathic syndrome while myasthenia gravis rarely presents in this way.

Atrophy

Atrophy brings patients to the doctor much less often than weakness but may do so in motor neurone disease or syringomyelia, when the small muscles of the hand are affected, and occasionally in other disorders. As a physical sign of muscle disease, however, atrophy is second in importance only to weakness. It is particularly valuable to compare the degrees of atrophy and weakness in affected muscles; this is illustrated in Table 13.2.

In most patients atrophy can be recognised by systematic inspection of the muscles but in many women and in the obese it may be difficult to assess. When asymmetry is suspected, limb girth must be measured at points equidistant from well-defined bony landmarks on the two sides. Palpation of the muscles during contraction is often helpful and occasionally soft tissue radiography is also useful, as is computed tomography (O'Doherty, Schellenger and Raptoponess, 1977). Sometimes confusion is caused by congenital absence of muscles (most commonly of the pectoralis major–Figure 13.6). Atrophy may involve only part of a muscle. This is often the case in limb-girdle dystrophy, in which localised dimples may be seen when the muscles are contracted against resistance and, in the late stages, it is usual for the uppermost third of the deltoid muscle to be wasted and fibrotic while the lower two-thirds are soft and much bulkier, even hypertrophic. A similar combination of atrophy and hypertrophy is sometimes found in the quadriceps, usually with atrophy of medial, and partial hypertrophy of lateral vasti. The other major cause of focal atrophy of a muscle is infarction. Focal atrophy

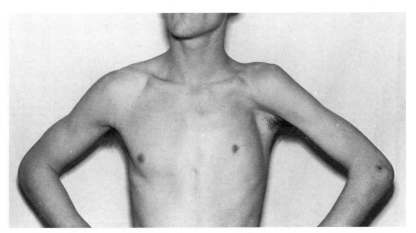

Fig. 13.6 Congenital absence of the left pectoralis major.
The patient had developed a secondary brachial plexus lesion
and the wasting of the left deltoid can be seen

may be simulated by the appearance after rupture of a tendon (e.g. long head of biceps brachii) or of the perimysial sheath.

The question of the distribution of muscle involvement is discussed in the section on weakness. In most disorders of the lower motor neurone and in many myopathies, muscle wasting and weakness go hand in hand. In motor neurone disease there tends to be proportionately more wasting and in muscular dystrophy proportionately more weakness, but these points are subtle and often not of much help. However Table 13.2 lists myopathies in which quite severe weakness may be associated with very little atrophy, and because several of these are treatable, this circumstance should be recognised as being of great significance. The most important of these conditions are myasthenia gravis, polymyositis, periodic paralysis and the myopathy of osteomalacia; careful investigation to exclude these four conditions is necessary in any case of muscle weakness in which atrophy is not prominent. Such investigations should include an edrophonium test, measurement of the evoked muscle action potentials during and after repetitive nerve stimulation, electromyography, estimation of the serum creatine kinase activity, calcium, phosphorus, alkaline phosphatase and potassium, and muscle biopsy. When the weakness is recent, atrophy may not have had time to develop. After complete traumatic denervation, clinical atrophy becomes evident after about two weeks and is maximal after about 12 weeks. Another pitfall is the atrophy which may develop after many years in myasthenia gravis, polymyositis, periodic paralysis and in McArdle's disease and other metabolic myopathies.

The reverse situation, muscular atrophy with little or no weakness, is a common feature of many wasting diseases such as tuberculosis, malnutrition and carcinomatosis and simple atrophy due to ageing. In fact, muscular atrophy in the elderly, especially in certain lower limb muscles such as soleus, is associated with histological appearances indistinguishable from those of denervation and may be due to a progressive loss of anterior horn cells in the spinal cord consequent upon ageing processes (Jennekens, Tomlinson and Walton, 1971). Some cases of thyrotoxic myopathy are masked by the generalised weight loss which occurs in this condition and it is possible that the myasthenic–myopathic syndrome of Eaton and Lambert (see Ch. 19) may sometimes go unrecognised in the general malaise and weight loss of carcinomatosis.

Muscular hypertrophy and pseudohypertrophy

It is very doubtful whether increasing muscle bulk is ever a primary pathological phenomenon. Of all the muscle diseases it is seen most strikingly in myotonia congenita, where the muscle hypertrophy may resemble that of a professional weightlifter. The strength of the muscles in this condition is consistent with their bulk and it is possible that work hypertrophy induced by the myotonia is responsible. It may even be that the bulky muscles seen in the 'pseudohypertrophic' forms of muscular dystrophy initially pass through a similar phase. Certainly the enlarged muscles seen in the earliest stages of the Duchenne type of dystrophy are relatively strong (for example the calves, deltoids and lateral vastus of quadriceps) and contain a high proportion of hypertrophied fibres. Later in the disease replacement by fat and connective tissue sometimes maintains the bulk despite loss of muscle fibres. This is the stage of pseudohypertrophy. Failure to distinguish between these two stages is perhaps responsible for the contradictory descriptions of the consistency of these muscles as 'rubbery' and 'inelastic' or 'firm' and 'doughy'. In fact they are generally firm while they are strong and soft when they are weak but, apart from establishing this fact, palpation is not of much help in the diagnosis of the 'pseudohypertrophic' muscular dystrophies. Only inspection of the muscles or measurement can make it clear whether they are abnormally bulky or not.

Enlargement of muscles is fairly common in limb-girdle muscular dystrophy and very common in the Becker type as well as in the Duchenne type. It is also a common clinical manifestation of myopathy in carriers of the Duchenne gene. It may also occur in the myopathy of hypothyroidism and occasionally in polymyositis. Nor is it pathognomonic of myopathy as it occurs in benign spinal muscular atrophy. There seem to have been no recent studies of the condition known as hypertrophia musculorum vera and its current status is uncertain (*see* Ch. 14). In de Lange's (1934) syndrome of athetosis and mental defect, muscle hypertrophy may be the result of continuous muscle spasm.

Spontaneous movement

Two closely similar forms of spontaneous movement may signify neuromuscular disease, *viz.*, fasciculation and myokymia. Both are painless contractions of small groups of muscle fibres which may cause visible movement of the overlying skin but not usually of the neighbouring joints. These points distinguish them not only from the contraction of single fibres (fibrillation) which is detectable only by electromyography or by examination of the exposed muscle which 'is involved in a confusion of very small twitches'—'without either apparent rhythm or obvious centre of activity' (Denny-Brown and Pennybacker, 1938), but also from tremor, myoclonus, chorea and other more gross movements which are unrelated to muscular disease. Both fasciculation and myokymia may be felt by the patient.

Fasciculations are brief twitches of groups or bundles of fibres which often involve the same group repetitively over short periods but may be totally irregular. They are best seen where the muscle is superficial, in the hands and especially the tongue and can often be induced by percussing or pinching the muscle. They occur in active degenerative disorders of the anterior horn cell but may be induced in normal individuals by anticholinesterase drugs. Fasciculation is a valuable clue to the diagnosis in motor neurone disease and in benign spinal muscular atrophy and should be sought particularly in the tongue, which should lie relaxed in the floor of the mouth. Absence of fasciculation, however, does not by any means exclude anterior horn cell disease. Spontaneous benign fasciculation in normal subjects is not uncommon, especially in the calf or small hand muscles. It cannot be distinguished with certainty from the pathological type, but fasciculation which is seen *only* after movement or strong contraction, and is not associated with muscle weakness, is usually benign. Rarely, fasciculation occurs in inflammatory or compressive nerve root lesions, but here its character is different, for it involves larger fasciculi and tends to occur repetitively in the same fasciculus during minimal contraction but not during complete relaxation. It corresponds to the 'giant units' in the electromyogram.

Myokymia is a slower contraction of independent small bands or strips of muscle fibres which give an undulating or rippling appearance to the overlying skin, the movement often being recognisably in the direction of the muscle fibres. The difference between the single twitch of the fasciculation and the tetanic contraction of myokymia may be evident only on electromyography in difficult cases. Myokymia is rare and is seen in some cases of thyrotoxicosis, or may be associated with cramp, hyperhidrosis, myotonia-like contractions and muscular atrophy in various combinations (Gamstorp and Wohlfart, 1959; Gardner-Medwin and Walton, 1969). The syndrome is closely related to, if not identical with, the 'syndrome of continuous muscle fibre activity and spasm' described by Isaacs in 1961, later called 'neuromyotonia' by Mertens and Zschocke (1965); but the latter is a misnomer as the phenomenon differs from true myotonia. This activity is abolished by neuromuscular block but not by proximal nerve block, which suggests that it arises in the distal part of the α-motor neurone. It may be associated with mild peripheral neuropathy (Wallis, Poznak and Plum, 1970) and there are some cases in which a familial incidence has been reported but not confirmed (Welch, Appenzeller and Bicknell, 1972). Most cases are sporadic and of unknown aetiology but the onset in two reported cases was related to exposure to dichlorophenoxyacetic acid herbicide (Wallis *et al.*, 1970) or an alcoholic debauch (Williamson and Brooke, 1972). An interesting episodic variety of myokymia involving one side of the face may occur in multiple sclerosis or as an isolated phenomenon (Matthews, 1966). The recurrent twitches of the eyelid or of particular parts of muscles, which are commonly experienced by normal people and are often called myokymia, are probably more closely related to benign fasciculations; they have no pathological significance but are often induced by fatigue.

Facial clonic spasm or hemifacial spasm is a

recurrent twitch of part, or sometimes the whole, of the musculature supplied by the facial nerve on one side. Rarely it is bilateral. The movement is stereotyped in form but irregular in timing and the former point distinguishes it from chorea and facial dyskinesia. Facial tic or habit spasm is often similar, but less rapidly repeated. Tetany, tetanus and blepharospasm due to ocular irritation or to facial spasticity should be considered in differential diagnosis. Hemifacial spasm is an intractable condition usually seen after the fifth decade. Its pathogenesis is obscure and it is thought to be due to an irritative lesion of the facial nerve or nucleus. Sometimes it is seen in geniculate herpes.

Movement induced by contraction or stimulation

Myotonia is easier to describe than to define because its pathophysiology is still incompletely understood. Denny-Brown and Nevin (1941) found that it occurred after nerve block or curarisation, and recent work suggests that it is associated with a defect of chloride conductance in the muscle fibre membrane (Adrian and Marshall, 1976). Clinically it is characterised by a failure of the muscle to relax immediately after voluntary contraction has ceased and a tendency for a dimple to persist for a few seconds after percussion of the muscle. Electromyographically a specific form of high-frequency discharge occurs after voluntary contraction or electrical or mechanical stimulation of the muscle (*see* Ch. 28). The diseases associated with myotonia and their differentiation are discussed in Chapter 14. In infants with myotonia the face and eyelids may fail to relax for several seconds after a sneeze or cry, the cry itself may sound strangled and the limbs may seem stiff. Later in life, patients complain of stiffness of the limbs, difficulty in walking or inability to relax the grip. Generally myotonia improves after repeated contraction and is worse in the cold. These effects are so striking in paramyotonia that it may be necessary to ask the patient to chill the hands in cold water before any abnormality can be demonstrated. Grip myotonia is shown by failure of relaxation lasting usually for 5–10 seconds after a tight contraction but occasionally for as long as a minute. Often the fingers and thumb remain flexed at the metacarpophalangeal joints while the other joints are extended. Percussion myotonia in the thenar eminence results not only in a dimple but in a slow tonic opposition of the thumb and gradual relaxation lasting altogether 2–10 seconds. A small tendon hammer may be used to percuss the tongue against a spatula placed over the lower teeth when a persistent dimple is again seen. There is little difficulty in recognising myotonia once the possibility of its presence has occurred to the examiner. However, percussion myotonia may be confused with *myoidema*, which is an electrically silent ridge (not a depression) induced by percussion of atrophic muscles in such wasting conditions as tuberculosis and malabsorption (Denny-Brown and Pennybacker, 1938; Salick and Pearson, 1967). Contraction myotonia can really be mistaken only for the very similar but electrically distinct phenomenon which may be associated with myokymia (Gamstorp and Wohlfart, 1959) and with the pseudomyotonia of hypothyroidism (Hoffmann's syndrome). This question is further discussed in Chapter 14. Leyburn and Walton (1959) described a method of quantitative assessment of myotonia for use in trials of treatment.

Tetany may be associated with hypocalcaemia, with alkalosis and possibly with hypomagnesaemia. It is heralded by tingling in the extremities or lips and, in the latent phase, spasms may be induced by nerve percussion (Chvostek's sign) or ischaemia (Trousseau's sign). Later, stridor and dyspnoea may occur and intermittent muscle cramp and spasm develop. Although these spasms may occur spontaneously they are increased by mechanical stimulation or contraction of the muscle because the excitability of both nerve and muscle is increased. They affect chiefly the hands, which adopt the 'main d'accoucheur' position, and the feet. More generalised involvement with opisthotonos may develop in severe cases and may be accompanied by colic and fits. Only in this advanced stage is tetany painful.

In *tetanus* the hyperexcitability of the nerves and muscles resembles that of tetany. In addition, however, there is usually an underlying state of continuous muscle spasm and this results in the well-known features of trismus, neck retraction and the risus sardonicus. This predilection for the face and neck contrasts with the carpopedal spasm of early tetany but the site of early involvement in tetanus also depends on the site of the infection. Indeed the spasm may remain localised in some cases, usually in partly immunised subjects. In the later stages the spasm becomes widespread and any movement or external stimulus induces paroxysmal and painful exacerbations. The bite of the American Black Widow spider (*Lactrodectus mactans*) may result in a similar condition of painful muscle spasm. The *stiff-man syndrome* is a poorly understood disorder in which progressive spasms usually begin in the proximal muscles and may become generalised. It is discussed further in Chapter 23.

Cramp contracture is electrically silent shortening of the muscles induced by exertion. It is seen in McArdle's disease, phosphofructokinase deficiency and in a few closely related forms of glycogen-storage disease of muscle (Lehoczky, Halasy, Simon and Harmos, 1965; Satayoshi and Kowa, 1967). Perkoff, Hardy and Velez-Garcia (1966) have shown that a similar reversible metabolic disorder with cramp contracture may occur in chronic alcoholism after heavy bouts of drinking. The exercised muscle develops aching or cramping pain and then becomes stiff and weak. Continued gentle exercise may enable some patients to enter a 'second wind' stage with lessening of the pain as they continue. More often the pain forces them to halt and if the muscle is then examined it may be found to be shortened, tense and tender. Only electromyography can distinguish this from true cramp in doubtful cases. The contracture lasts from a few minutes to several hours, depending on its severity. Very severe pain which passes off rapidly is not due to McArdle's disease.

Muscle tone

In infants hypotonia is one of the earliest and most important indications of muscle disease. The problem of diagnosis of the 'floppy infant' is dealt with in Chapter 17 and all that needs to be said here is that the cause may lie in the brain (especially the parietal lobes and cerebellum), the anterior horns or posterior columns of the spinal cord, the motor or sensory nerves, the myoneural junctions or the muscle fibres and possibly in the muscle spindles or ligaments. Hypotonia may also be a result of malnutrition, malabsorption and metabolic disorders. Part of the diagnostic problem may lie in the failure to define the precise meaning of tone and hypotonia. André-Thomas *et al.* (1960) have described methods for testing several different aspects of muscle tone, each of which may be disturbed independently. Thus the *consistency* of a muscle may be tested by wobbling it laterally with a finger, by shaking the limbs and by palpation, its *extensibilité* by slow movement of joints through their full range and its '*passivité*' by, for example, measuring the amplitude of the flapping movement when the proximal part of a limb is shaken. The *recoil* of a muscle suddenly released from a fully stretched position is another manifestation of tone. The different functions of tonic and phasic reflexes account for some of the apparent inconsistencies when tone is tested in different ways but, in general, the pathological significance of the separate manifestations is not properly understood. In muscle disease consistency and '*passivité*' are more often abnormal than '*extensibilité*'. Other useful signs of hypotonia are the hanging posture of the head and limbs when the baby is lifted supine with the hand under his back and the tendency to slip through the hands when he is held under the axillae. It is important to remember that muscle tone normally decreases from birth until the second to sixth month and gradually increases again in later childhood.

In *children* beyond the 'floppy infant' stage, hypotonia is a valuable sign before full cooperation in muscle strength tests is possible. An important example is the looseness of the shoulders in early Duchenne dystrophy.

In *adults* most myopathies and disorders of the lower motor neurone are associated with a moderate reduction in muscle tone. Because of the much more definite information given by assessment of muscle power and atrophy, the tone is rarely of much importance in diagnosis, except when it is apparently out of keeping with the other signs. Thus, in cases of combined pyramidal tract and lower motor neurone involvement as in some of the hereditary ataxias, spasticity in weak, wasted, areflexic muscles may be the only indication of the upper motor neurone lesion.

Palpation of nerves and muscles

As mentioned above, peripheral nerves may become tender to palpation at sites of entrapment (as with the ulnar nerve behind the medical epicondyle of the humerus) or when their component roots are compressed or irritated (as in the sciatic nerve in cases of sciatica due to lumbar intervertebral disc prolapse). Localised swelling or hypertrophy of peripheral nerves can occur in leprosy or neurofibromatosis, more generalised enlargement, even involving the greater auricular nerve, in cases of hypertrophic neuropathy (as in some cases of peroneal muscular atrophy and related disorders, or in recurrent demyelinating peripheral neuropathy).

The importance of palpation in the assessment of tone, atrophy, hypertrophy or weakness of muscle has already been stressed. In addition, local areas of tenderness may be discovered, an event which generally provides more satisfaction for the anxious patient than for the thoughtful physician, for the cause and site of origin of such local tenderness are rarely found. Nevertheless in certain fairly well-defined syndromes such as 'tennis elbow', which is due to a localised tendinitis at the lateral epicondyle of the humerus or in the region of the neck of the radius resulting from repetitive movement, useful treatment may result. Palpable masses in muscle are generally either areas of local spasm, post-traumatic haematomata or, less commonly, infarcts (in polyarteritis nodosa) or areas of localised nodular myositis. The differentiation between these may be difficult in acute cases. Sometimes myositis ossificans can be felt and, rarely, a local mass turns out to be a tumour either primary in muscle (rhabdomyosarcoma) or expanding from deeper structures such as an osteogenic sarcoma. Herniation of muscle fibres through a ruptured perimysial sheath (a muscle hernia) may feel deceptively like a tumour.

Reflex change

Quite different patterns of reflex changes may be found in otherwise similar disorders. In peripheral neuropathies, even in the absence of sensory loss, the tendon reflexes are usually abolished early and they are often absent in muscles which seem otherwise unaffected. In the muscular dystrophies, loss of the reflexes tends to follow closely the degree of weakness and they are absent in any muscle with easily demonstrable weakness. In motor neurone disease, however, quite marked wasting and weakness may be found in muscles with brisk reflexes, presumably because of the survival of some motor units with intact peripheral nerve conduction in the presence of corticospinal tract involvement. Polymyositis, myasthenia gravis and the myopathy of osteomalacia or hyperparathyroidism are other disorders in which the reflexes tend to be preserved in weak muscles. The tendon reflexes are valuable in the distinction between myasthenia gravis (in which they are preserved) and the myasthenic syndrome associated with carcinoma (in which they are abolished early). It is well known that in hypothyroidism, with or without myopathy, the rates of contraction and relaxation in the reflex response are characteristically slow and less often, excessively rapid responses may be observed in thyrotoxicosis.

The plantar responses are, of course, generally flexor in neuromuscular disorders. Generally speaking, the discovery of extensor plantar responses in cases of proximal muscle weakness should arouse suspicions of motor neurone disease or of those rare instances of spinal muscular atrophy in which evidence of pyramidal tract disease is sometimes found (Gardner-Medwin, Hudgson and Walton, 1967).

Contracture

Contracture is a state of shortening of a muscle not caused by active contraction. It may be acute and spontaneously reversible, as in McArdle's disease, but far more often it is the result of the rearrangement of the collagen fibrils within the muscle over a longer period. At this stage it is fully reversible by repeated stretching. Later, actual fibrosis may make it increasingly difficult to treat. Another form of contracture is the failure of a muscle to grow in length when its action is not opposed by a sufficiently powerful antagonist. Palpation of the muscle during attempts at passive movement at the affected joint will rapidly distinguish contracture from ankylosis in one case and active contraction in another although, occasionally, examination under general anaesthesia may be necessary when both are present. When the relevant muscles are inaccessible, for example at the hip joint or in the 'frozen shoulder' syndrome, these distinctions may be difficult, and indeed it is probable that the latter may pass through all three stages of muscle spasm, contracture and ankylosis. Demonstration of contractures is usually easy, but they may be missed at the shoulder if the scapula is not fixed, and at the hips if the lumbar lordosis is not first eliminated by flexing the opposite hip so that the thigh touches the abdomen.

Contractures develop in many of the chronic muscle diseases, whether neurogenic or myopathic, and are especially prominent in the syndrome of arthrogryposis multiplex congenita, in muscular dystrophy of the Duchenne type, and in poliomyelitis and the other chronic spinal muscular atrophies. In muscular dystrophy they are an important source of early difficulty in walking (see Ch. 14). In acute polymyositis they may rarely develop very rapidly within a few weeks, even in muscles with surprisingly little weakness. In progressive myosclerosis, contracture may be the major cause of disability; here, weakness may not be detectable at all, but the muscles have a woody or fibrotic consistency.

The muscles supplied by the cranial nerves

The examination of the *external ocular muscles* is a complex art which is described by Cogan (1956) and Walsh and Hoyt (1969). Only a few points of special relevance to muscle disease are mentioned here. Pareses which do not conform to the pattern of single or multiple nerve palsies suggest a local muscular disorder, but this may be caused by expanding orbital lesions as well as by inflammatory, metabolic or degenerative myopathies. Thus, in polymyositis the ocular muscles are sometimes involved, as they are in the rare orbital myositis and the closely related condition of orbital pseudotumour, which is often unilateral but sometimes bilateral, giving proptosis as well as impaired ocular movement and usually a raised erythrocyte sedimentation rate. In the ocular, oculopharyngeal and myotonic muscular dystrophies, ptosis invariably occurs before ocular pareses, and diplopia is only rarely an early symptom. Later, ocular myopathy may progress to complete external ophthalmoplegia. An isolated superior rectus palsy is commonly the earliest feature of the ophthalmic form of Graves' disease. If proptosis is not obvious in such cases it should be sought using an exophthalmometer and, in most cases, conjunctival oedema is also present. Myasthenia gravis is a great imitator of ocular palsies and should be considered wherever the diagnosis is uncertain. Maintaining upward gaze for a full minute will usually induce some ptosis in these cases but, even if it does not do so, an edrophonium test should always be tried. In children the association of bilateral facial weakness with apparently bilateral sixth nerve palsies suggests Möbius' syndrome, which may be a purely myopathic disorder (sometimes being one manifestation of myotubular myopathy) in some cases although it is certainly the result of nuclear agenesis in others. Another imitator of abducens palsy is Duane's syndrome, in which impaired abduction of the affected eye is associated with ptosis and enophthalmos during adduction. It is due to fibrosis of the external rectus muscle and may be bilateral. In some families there is dominant inheritance of this anomaly.

The *muscles of mastication* may be affected late in the course of many disorders but are often involved in the early stages of myasthenia gravis, in which the hand supporting the lower jaw is a useful clue to the diagnosis, of tetanus (trismus) and of myotonic dystrophy, in which wasting of the temporal and masseter muscles and the characteristic drooping jaw contribute to the typical facial appearance. The rare condition of so-called branchial myopathy can give bilateral masseter hypertrophy. Trismus may be of emotional origin or can occur transiently in patients receiving phenothiazines.

The facial muscles are commonly involved in myopathies and rather uncommonly in progressive muscular atrophy. A brisk jaw jerk will usually distinguish the latter. Bilateral lower motor neurone weakness, for example in the Guillain-Barré syndrome, sarcoidosis, poliomyelitis and pontine lesions may sometimes be indicated by loss of taste, but may closely resemble myopathic weakness. A distinguishing point is the inability to close the eyes in facial nerve lesions whereas this is less often seen in myopathy except in advanced facioscapulohumeral dystrophy. In young children, gross facial myopathy is usually caused by Möbius' syndrome or myotonic dystrophy. In facioscapulohumeral dystrophy the involvement may be severe or slight and is best shown by asking the patient to shut his eyes tightly, or to hold air in his mouth under pressure. In the middle and late stages of Duchenne dystrophy, facial weakness is rarely absent, though usually slight. Here the failure to retract the corners of the mouth and to blow out the cheeks are the most useful signs.

Dysarthria and dysphagia are common in myasthenia gravis and polymyositis. In the myotonic and oculopharyngeal muscular dystrophies dysphagia alone is more frequent. Bulbar involvement in poliomyelitis, motor neurone disease and acute polyneuritis are well known.

The *sternomastoid* muscles are severely wasted and weakened in dystrophia myotonica and often in such neurogenic disorders as motor neurone disease, poliomyelitis and craniovertebral anomalies involving the accessory nerve. Of the other myopathies, myasthenia gravis and polymyositis are two in which weakness of neck flexion or extension is particularly prominent. Selective trapezius weakness may occur in the limb-girdle type of muscular dystrophy and in accessory nerve lesions.

The *tongue* is chiefly important in muscle disease because of the ease with which it shows fasciculation. The significance of this in motor neurone disease and other spinal muscular atrophies has been discussed. Few of the myopathies affect the tongue. In dystrophia myotonica, lingual dysarthria is more often a sign of myotonia than of weakness. In Duchenne dystrophy the speech is often indistinct and in some cases there is enlargement of the tongue. Tongue hypertrophy is also a rare manifestation of late-onset glycogen-storage disease due to acid maltase deficiency. A curiously selective form of atrophy of the tongue in myasthenia gravis is illustrated in Chapter 16 (Figure 16.3).

Important non-muscular symptoms and signs

In polymyositis these have special importance and here Raynaud's phenomenon, dysphagia and, above all, skin changes may help in diagnosis. The rash in dermatomyositis may involve the face, trunk or limbs, but in difficult cases the eyelids and nail beds should be examined with particular care. In other obscure myopathies uveitis, erythema nodosum, or dyspnoea with pulmonary infiltration may give the clue to sarcoidosis; anaemia, proteinuria, rashes, arthropathy, pleurisy or splenomegaly to the collagen diseases; tight shiny skin over the face or fingers to systemic sclerosis; and diarrhoea or steatorrhoea, uraemia, bony tenderness or radiological abnormalities in the bones to osteomalacia or hyperparathyroidism. In all these cases the myopathy may be the presenting feature before the more usual symptoms are obvious. Rarely, this also occurs in thyrotoxic myopathy in which, however, thyroid function tests will be found to be abnormal. The same is true of the myopathy of hypothyroidism (Wilson and Walton, 1959) but in Cushing's syndrome, Addison's disease and acromegaly or hypopituitarism, the myopathy amounts to no more than an incidental part of the disease. Severe fatiguability with increased pigmentation of the skin after bilateral adrenalectomy for Cushing's disease should arouse suspicion of very high levels of circulating ACTH (Prineas, Hall, Barwick and Watson, 1968). Myoglobinuria is associated with severe necrotising myopathy in polymyositis, acute alcoholism and other intoxications, and after exercise in the anterior tibial syndrome and McArdle's disease (*see* Ch. 18). The inherited myopathies may be associated with other congenital abnormalities; these are especially prominent in the myotonic and ocular forms of muscular dystrophy (*see* Ch. 14), in nemaline myopathy (a high-arched palate, long face, protruding jaw and dental malocclusion), in a-β-lipoproteinaemia (steatorrhoea, retinal degeneration, ataxia and acanthocytosis), in ataxia telangiectasia (ataxia, conjunctival telangiectasia and recurrent infections); and in Types II and III glycogen-storage disease in which hepatic involvement and (in Type II) cardiac, cerebral and spinal cord involvement occur.

APPENDIX

The following classification of neuromuscular disorders was originally prepared for the World Federation of Neurology (1968) and is reprinted here with many changes and additions. Abbreviated references are given to some conditions not described *inextenso* in the relevant chapters in this book.

The term 'amyotrophy' is used repeatedly, not in the literal sense of 'muscular atrophy' but with the more restricted meaning of neurogenic muscular atrophy as distinct from myopathy or primary disease of muscle. As this is a classification of neuromuscular disorders, those diseases of roots and peripheral nerves which give rise solely to sensory, as distinct from motor, dysfunction are omitted. Certain doubtful entities are preceded by a question mark.

1. SPINAL MUSCULAR ATROPHIES AND OTHER DYSFUNCTIONS OF ANTERIOR HORN CELLS

A. *Genetically determined*

1. Infantile and juvenile spinal muscular atrophy
   (a) Acute infantile spinal muscular atrophy (Werdnig-Hoffmann disease) (autosomal recessive)
   (b) Arthrogryposis multiplex due to anterior horn cell disease
   (c) Pseudomyopathic familial spinal muscular atrophy (Kugelberg and Welander—autosomal recessive; X-linked—Tsukagoshi *et al.* (1970). *Neurology (Minneap.)*, **20**, 1188; dominant—Zellweger *et al.* (1972). *Neurology (Minneap.)*, **22**, 957)
   (d) Scapuloperoneal form of spinal muscular atrophy (recessive or dominant–Kaeser (1965), *Brain*, **88**, 407; X-linked, with cardiopathy—Mawatari *et al.* (1973), *Arch. Neurol.*, **28**, 55)
   (e) Distal spinal muscular atrophy (Dyck and Lambert (1968). *Arch. Neurol.*, **18**, 619; with optic atrophy and nerve deafness, Iwashita *et al.* (1970). *Arch. Neurol.*, **22**, 357).

2. Guam motor neurone disease★
3. Familial motor neurone disease (other than the Guam type) (Horton *et al.* (1976). *Neurology (Minneap.)*, **26**, 460)
4. Familial bulbar palsy
   (a) Progressive spinal muscular atrophy with bulbar palsy
   (b) Infantile and juvenile progressive bulbar palsy (Gomez *et al.* (1962). *Arch. Neurol.*, **6**, 317; Markand & Daly (1971), *Neurology (Minneap.)*, **21**, 753)
   (c) Recessive X-linked bulbar palsy (Tsukagoshi *et al.* (1965). *Arch. Neurol.*, **12**, 597; Kennedy *et al.* (1968). *Neurology (Minneap.)*, **18**, 671)
5. Amyotrophy in the parkinsonism–dementia complex
   Juvenile amyotrophic lateral sclerosis–dementia complex (Staal and Went (1968). *Neurology (Minneap.)*, **18**, 800)
6. Amyotrophy in heredofamilial ataxias
   (a) in Friedreich's ataxia
   (b) in hereditary spastic paraplegia
   (c) ?in Holmes-type cerebellar ataxia
   (d) in recessive X-chromosomal ataxia (Turner and Roberts)
   (e) in dyssynergia cerebellaris myoclonica (Ramsay Hunt)
7. Amyotrophy in Huntington's chorea
8. Amyotrophy in Marinesco-Sjögren syndrome (Alter and Kennedy (1968). *Minn. Med.*, **51**, 901)
9. Amyotrophy in infantile neuraxonal dystrophy (Huttenlocher and Gilles (1967). *Neurology (Minneap.)*, **17**, 1174)

B. *Congenital* (developmental abnormalities)

1. Möbius' syndrome (agenesis of cranial nerve nuclei)
   Möbius' syndrome with peripheral neuropathy and hypogonadotrophic hypogonadism (Abid *et al.* (1978). *J. Neurol. Sci.*, **35**, 309)
   Möbius' syndrome with absence of pectoral muscle

★There is now some evidence to suggest that Guam motor neurone disease may be infective and not genetically determined, but this is not yet proven.

2. Congenital absence of muscles (pectorals, abdominals, etc.) (?possibly better classified under disorders of muscle but it is not known whether the appropriate anterior horn cells are absent)
    (a) congenital absence of pectoral muscle with syndactyly (David (1972). *New Engl. J. Med.*, **287**, 487)
3. Hydromyelia with amyotrophy
4. Spinal dysraphism with amyotrophy
5. Meningomyelocele with amyotrophy
6. Aplasia of spinal cord (amyelia)
7. Syringomyelia or syringobulbia with amyotrophy (note close relationship with Chiari malformation)
8. Anterior horn cell disease with pontocerebellar hypoplasia (Goutières *et al.* (1977), *J. Neurol. Neurosurg. Psychiat.*, **40**, 370)
9. Arthrogryposis multiplex congenita of non-neural and non-myopathic origin

C. Traumatic

C-I. Physical (Amyotrophy due to destruction or compression of anterior horn cells)
1. Birth injury to spinal cord
2. Spinal tumours
3. Haematomyelia
4. Infective masses, e.g.
    (a) tuberculoma
    (b) gumma
    (c) parasitic cyst
5. Other causes of spinal cord compression
6. Ischaemic
    (a) occlusion or stenosis of anterior spinal artery
    (b) progressive vascular myelopathy (Jellinger and Neumayer (1962). *Acta Neurol. Psychiat. Belg.*, **62**, 944)
7. Amyotrophy in multiple sclerosis and neuromyelitis optica
8. Amyotrophy in transverse myelitis
9. Amyotrophy following electrical injury (Farrell and Starr (1968). *Neurology (Minneap.)*, **18**, 601)

C-II. Toxic (Toxins acting on the motor neurone)
1. Tetanus toxin

2. Strychnine
3. Botulinus toxin
4. Lead (Campbell *et al.* (1970). *J. Neurol. Neurosurg. Psychiat.*, **33**, 877; Boothby *et al.* (1974). *Arch. Neurol.*, **31**, 18)
5. Saxitoxin

D. Infective amyotrophy

1. Paralytic acute anterior poliomyelitis
    (a) due to poliomyelitis virus
    (b) due to other enteroviruses (including Coxsackie viruses)
2. Russian spring-summer encephalitis with amyotrophy
3. Herpes zoster (including Ramsay Hunt syndrome—so-called geniculate herpes) (Thomas and Howard (1972). *Neurology (Minneap.)*, **22**, 459)
4. Amyotrophy in Creutzfeldt-Jakob disease (Allen *et al.* (1971). *Brain*, **94**, 715)

E. Amyotrophy of unknown aetiology

1. Motor neurone disease
    (a) progressive bulbar palsy
    (b) progressive muscular atrophy
    (c) amyotrophic lateral sclerosis
2. Juvenile motor neurone disease (van Bogaert (1925). *Rev. neurol.*, **1**, 180; Nelson and Prensky (1972). *Arch. Neurol.*, **27**, 300)
3. ?Progressive amyotrophy following old poliomyelitis (Mulder *et al.* (1972). *Mayo Clinic Proc.*, **47**, 756)
4. Progressive amyotrophy following encephalitis lethargica (Greenfield and Matthews (1954). *J. Neurol. Neurosurg. Psychiat.*, **17**, 50)
5. Amyotrophy in orthostatic hypotension (the Shy-Drager syndrome of progressive multi-system degeneration)
6. Amyotrophy in Pick's Disease (Minauf and Jellinger (1969). *Arch. Psychiat. Nervenkr.*, **212**, 279)
7. Amyotrophy in ataxia telangiectasia (Goodman *et al.* (1969). *Bull Los Angeles Neurol. Soc.*, **34**, 1)
8. Chronic neurogenic quadriceps amyotrophy (Furukawa *et al.* (1977). *Ann. Neurol.*, **2**, 528)

F. Amyotrophy in malignant disease

1. ?Carcinomatous motor neurone disease (Brain *et al.* (1965). *Brain*, **88**, 479)
2. Spinal muscular atrophy in Waldenstrom's macroglobulinaemia (Peters and Chatanoff (1968). *Neurology (Minneap.)*, **18**, 101)

G. Dysfunction of the motor neurone in the metabolic disorders

1. Tetany in
   (*a*) hypocalcaemia
   (*b*) magnesium deficiency
   (*c*) alkalosis
2. ?Hypoglycaemia (organic hyperinsulinism) with amyotrophy (Tom and Richardson (1951). *J. Neuropath. exp. Neurol.*, **10**, 57)

*H. Myokymia, cramps, benign fasciculation**

II. DISORDERS OF MOTOR NERVE ROOTS

A. Congenital

1. Associated with meningomyelocele and other anomalies
2. Arthrogryposis multiplex congenita (radicular type) (Peña *et al.* (1968). *Neurology (Minneap.)*, **18**, 926)

B. Traumatic

B-I. Physical

1. Laceration, contusion, or distraction of roots
2. Compression of roots by:
   (*a*) vertebral osteoarthritis
   (*b*) prolapsed intervertebral disc
   (*c*) Paget's disease
   (*d*) tumour in the spinal canal or intervertebral foramina
   (*e*) vertebral collapse
3. Ischaemia

B-II. Toxic

1. Toxic agents (injected local anaesthetics, phenol, etc.)

*It is not certain that the origin of these disorders lies in dysfunction of the anterior horn cells.
*Only disorders involving motor or mixed nerves are included and those confined to sensory or autonomic nerves have not been included in this classification.

C. Inflammatory

C-I. Infective

1. Radiculopathy in meningitis
2. Syphilis
3. Granulomatous arachnoiditis of other causes
4. Bilharziasis

C-II. Postinfective? allergic

1. Acute postinfective polyradiculoneuropathy (Guillain-Barré syndrome)
2. Polyradiculoneuropathy following inoculation
3. Serum neuropathy
4. 'Neuralgic amyotrophy', including the familial form (Geiger *et al.* (1974). *Brain*, **97**, 87)

D. Neoplastic

1. Neurofibroma
2. Meningioma
3. Metastases
4. Reticulosis
5. Vascular malformations

III. DISORDERS OF PERIPHERAL NERVES*

A. Genetically determined

1. Peroneal muscular atrophy (Charcot-Marie-Tooth disease) (*see* Dyck and Lambert (1968). *Arch. Neurol.*, **18**, 603 and 619 and Behse and Buchthal (1977). *Brain*, 100, 67)
   (*a*) autosomal dominant
   (*b*) autosomal recessive
   (*c*) X-chromosomal type
   (i) Demyelinating type
   (ii) Axonal type
   (iii) Intermediate type (Bradley *et al.* (1977). *J. Neurol. Sci.*, **32**, 123
   (iv) Neuronal type
   (v) Variants (with essential tremor—Salisachs (1976). *J. Neurol. Sci.*, **28**, 17; with heart block—Littler (1970). *Quart. J. Med.*, **39**, 431)

2. Roussy-Levy syndrome (probably a variant of IIIA 1a i)
3. Hereditary hypertrophic interstitial neuropathy (Dejerine and Sottas)
4. Chronic familial infantile polyneuropathy (Kasman *et al.* (1976). *Neurology (Minneap.)*, **26**, 565)
5. Neurofibromatosis (von Recklinghausen)
6. Heredopathia atactica polyneuritiformis (Refsum's syndrome)
7. Familial neuropathy with optic atrophy and nerve deafness (Rosenberg and Chutorian (1967). *Neurology (Minneap.)*, **17**, 827)
8. Familial recurrent polyneuropathy and mononeuropathy (Taylor (1960). *Brain*, **83**, 113; Roos and Thygesen (1972). *Brain*, **95**, 235)
9. Familial recurrent pressure palsies of peripheral nerves (Earl *et al.* (1964). *Quart. J. Med.*, **33**, 481)
10. Hereditary hypertrophic neuropathy with paraproteinaemia (Gibberd and Gavrilescu (1966). *Neurology (Minneap.)*, **16**, 130)
11. Hereditary neuropathy with interstitial nephritis and nerve deafness (Marin and Tyler (1961). *Neurology (Minneap.)*, **11**, 999; Hanson *et al.* (1970). *Neurology (Minneap.)*, **20**, 426)
12. Hereditary 'globular' neuropathy (Dayan *et al.* (1968). *J. Neurol. Neurosurg. Psychiat.*, **31**, 552)
13. Hereditary polyneuropathy with oligophrenia, premature menopause and acromicria (Lundberg (1971). *Europ. Neurol.*, **5**, 84)
14. Hereditary sensory neuropathy with amyotrophy and spinal cord involvement (Khalifeh and Zellweger (1963). *Neurology (Minneap.)*, **13**, 405)
15. Arthrogryposis multiplex congenita (neuropathic form) (Hooshmand *et al.* (1971). *Arch. Neurol.*, **24**, 561)
16. Amyloid neuropathy
    (*a*) Portuguese type (Andrade (1952). *Brain*, **75**, 408)
    (*b*) Indiana type (Rukavina *et al.* (1956). *Medicine (Baltimore)*, **35**, 239)
    (*c*) Iowa type (Van Allen *et al.* (1969). *Neurology (Minneap.)*, **19**, 10)

17. Neuropathy in porphyria
18. A-α-lipoproteinaemic neuropathy (Tangier disease) (Kocen *et al.* (1967). *Lancet*, **1**, 1341; Engel *et al.* (1967). *Arch. Neurol.*, **17**, 1)
19. A-β-lipoproteinaemic neuropathy (Bassen-Kornzweig syndrome) (Schwartz *et al.* (1963). *Arch. Neurol.*, **8**, 438)
20. Neuropathy in leukodystrophy
    (*a*) metachromatic type (sulphatide lipidosis) (Fullerton (1964). *J. Neurol. Neurosurg. Psychiat.*, **27**, 100)
    (*b*) globoid body type (galactosyl ceramide lipidosis) (Hogan *et al.* (1969). *Neurology (Minneap.)*, **19**, 1094)
21. Isoniazid polyneuropathy (genetic predisposition)
22. Neuropathy in Cockayne's syndrome (Moosa and Dubowitz (1970). *Arch. Dis. Child.*, **45**, 674)
23. Neuropathy in the syndrome of Flynn and Aird (1965). *J. neurol. Sci.*, **2**, 161)
24. Fabry's Disease (glycosphingolipid lipidosis) (Bischoff *et al.* (1968). *Klin. Wschr.*, **46**, 666)
25. Peripheral neuropathy in the Riley-Day syndrome (Aguayo *et al.* (1971). *Arch. Neurol.*, **24**, 105)
26. ?Giant axonal neuropathy (probably toxic in many cases—*see* Koch *et al.* (1977). *Ann. Neurol.*, **1**, 438)
27. In primary hyperoxaluria (Moorhead *et al.* (1975). *Brit. Med. J.*, **ii**, 312)

B. Congenital

Hypomyelination neuropathy (Kennedy *et al.* (1977). *Arch. Neurol.*, **34**, 337)

C. Traumatic

C-I. Physical
1. Laceration, contusion, compression or distraction of nerves
2. Birth trauma to brachial plexus
   (*a*) Erb's paralysis
   (*b*) Klumpke's paralysis
3. Entrapment neuropathies
   (*a*) of cranial nerves
      (i) facial nerve compression in the

stylomastoid foramen (Bell's palsy)

(ii) clonic facial spasm (hemifacial spasm)

(iii) Recurrent familial facial palsy (Melkersson's syndrome)

(b) of the upper extremity

(i) thoracic inlet and cervico-axillary canal, including cervical rib

(ii) median nerve in the forearm (pronator syndrome)

(iii) median nerve at the wrist (carpal tunnel syndrome)

(iv) ulnar nerve at the elbow (cubital tunnel syndrome)

(v) ulnar nerve at the wrist or its deep branch in the palm

(vi) radial nerve in the spiral groove

(vii) radial nerve in the forearm

(viii) posterior interosseous nerve in the forearm

(ix) anterior interosseous nerve

(x) suprascapular nerve at the shoulder

(c) of the lower extremity

(i) sciatic nerve at the pelvic exit

(ii) obturator nerve in the obturator canal

(iii) common peroneal nerve around the fibular neck

(iv) deep peroneal nerve (Gutmann (1970). *J. Neurol. Neurosurg. Psychiat.*, **33**, 450)

(v) posterior tibial nerve in the tarsal tunnel

(d) multiple entrapments in mucopolysaccharidosis (Karpati *et al.* (1974). *Arch. Neurol.*, **31**, 418)

4. Electric shock (Farrell and Starr (1968). *Neurology (Minneap.)*, **18**, 601)

5. Burns

6. Radiation injury (Stoll and Andrews (1966). *Brit. Med. J.*, **1**, 834)

7. Ischaemic neuropathy*

(a) giant cell arteritis

(b) mononeuropathy in polyarteritis nodosa

(c) neuropathy in disseminated lupus erythematosus

(d) diabetes mellitus (some cases)

(e) post-irradiation neuropathy

(f) neuropathy in peripheral vascular disease

(g) dysproteinaemic neuropathy

(h) neuropathy in subacute bacterial endocarditis (Jones and Siekert (1968). *Arch. Neurol.*, **19**, 535)

(i) mononeuropathy in amphetamine angiitis (Stafford *et al.* (1975). *Neurology (Minneap.)*, **25**, 570)

(j) neuropathy in rheumatoid arthritis (Dyck *et al.* (1972). *Mayo Clin. Proc.*, **47**, 462)

C-II. Toxic

1. Drugs

barbiturates – clioquinol (subacute myelo-opticoneuropathy) – chloral – chloroquine – cytotoxic agents (especially ethoglyeid, nitrogen mustard and vincristine) – diphenyhydantoin – disulfiram (Bradley and Hewer (1966). *Brit. med. J.*, **2**, 449) – emetine – ethionamide – ? glutethimide – ? hydrallazine – iproniazid – isoniazid – metronidazole (Coxon and Pallis (1976). *J. Neurol. Neurosurg. Psychiat.*, **39**, 403) – nitrofurantoin – perhexiline – phenytoin – sodium cyanate – stilbamidine – streptomycin – sulphanilamide – thalidomide – trichloroethylene – etc.

2. Inorganic substances

(a) heavy metals

antimony – arsenic – bismuth – copper – gold – lead – mercury (Pink disease, Minamata disease) – thallium

(b) other inorganic substances

phosphorus

3. Organic substances (N.B. some of these cause giant axonal neuropathy—*see* Carpenter *et al.* (1974). *Arch. Neurol.*, **31**, 312)

acrylamide – alcohol – aniline – bush tea – carbon disulphide – carbon monoxide* –

---

*Peripheral nerve lesions occurring in these disorders are believed to be ischaemic but other pathological processes may well be involved.

*It is possible that neuropathies arising in patients suffering from carbon monoxide poisoning are toxic, but many are probably pressure palsies arising in the unconscious patient.

carbon tetrachloride – dinitrobenzol – dinitrophenol – hexachlorophene – n-hexane (Herskowitz *et al.* (1971). *New Engl. J. Med.*, **285**, 82) – methyl butyl ketone – pentachlorophenol and DDT (woodworm insecticide) – tetrachlorethane – trichlorethylene – other organic chlorine derivatives – triorthocresylphosphate

4. Toxins derived from bacteria
   (*a*) botulism
   (*b*) diphtheria
   (*c*) dysentery
   (*d*) tetanus
5. Toxins derived from other organisms saxitoxin
6. Buckthorn neuropathy (Mitchell *et al.* (1978). *Neuropath. appl. Neurobiol.*, **4**, 85)

C-III. Of uncertain aetiology (? toxic, ? nutritional)
1. Neuropathy and amyotrophy in
   (*a*) Jamaican and other tropical neuropathy
   (*b*) South Indian paraplegia
   (*c*) neuropathy in tropical ataxia (Nigeria) Williams and Osuntokun (1969). *Arch. Neurol.*, **21**, 475) (probably due to cyanide in cassava root)

D. Inflammatory

D-I. Infective
1. Direct infection of nerves
   (*a*) Leprosy
   (*b*) Syphilis
   (*c*) Brucellosis
   (*d*) Leptospirosis
2. Neuropathies occurring in other infections
   (*a*) Gonorrhoea
   (*b*) Malaria
   (*c*) Meningitis
   (*d*) Mumps
   (*e*) Paratyphoid
   (*f*) Puerperal sepsis
   (*g*) Septicaemia
   (*h*) Smallpox
   (*i*) Tuberculosis
   (*j*) Typhoid
   (*k*) Typhus
   (*l*) In acrodermatitis chronica atrophicans (Hopf (1975). *J. Neurol. Neurosurg. Psychiat.*, **38**, 452)

D-II. Postinfective (allergic)
1. Postinfective neuropathies (?allergic)
   (*a*) Chicken pox
   (*b*) Infectious hepatitis
   (*c*) Measles
   (*d*) Upper respiratory tract infections
   (*e*) Infectious mononucleosis
   (*f*) Influenza
   (*g*) Vaccinia
2. Polyneuropathy of unknown aetiology (?postinfective)
   (*a*) Acute postinfective polyradiculoneuropathy (Guillain-Barré syndrome)
   (*b*) Chronic progressive polyneuropathy
   (*c*) Recurrent polyneuropathy (Austin (1958), *Brain*, **81**, 157)
3. Neuropathy in connective tissue disorders
   (*a*) Systemic lupus erythematosus
   (*b*) Polyarteritis nodosa
   (*c*) Rheumatoid arthritis
   (*d*) Scleroderma (systemic sclerosis)
   (*e*) Thrombotic thrombocytopenic purpura (thrombotic microangiopathy)
   (*f*) Giant cell arteritis
4. Neuropathy in sarcoidosis

E. Metabolic neuropathy

1. Nutritional
   (*a*) specific deficiencies
      i) cyanocobalamin deficiency
      (ii) folic acid deficiency
   (*b*) of uncertain aetiology (probably B_1, B_2 and B_6 vitamin deficiency)
      (i) in chronic alcoholism
      (ii) beri-beri
      (iii) burning feet syndrome
      (iv) famine oedema and kwashiorkor
      (v) in hyperemesis gravidarum
      (vi) in pregnancy
      (vii) pellagra
      (viii) in gluten-sensitive enteropathy (Cooke and Smith (1966). *Brain*, **89**, 683)
2. Neuropathies associated with endocrine disorders
   (*a*) diabetes
      (i) polyneuropathy
      (ii) mononeuropathy (including diabetic amyotrophy)

(b) thyroid disorders

  (i) hyperthyroidism (Feibel and Campa (1976). *J. Neurol. Neurosurg. Psychiat.*, **39**, 491)

  (ii) hypothyroidism (Dyck and Lambert (1970). *J. Neuropath. Exper. Neurol.*, **29**, 631)

  (iii) in thyrotropin deficiency (Grabow and Chou (1968). *Arch. Neurol.*, **19**, 284)

(c) neuropathy in organic hyperinsulinism (Mulder *et al.* (1956). *Neurology (Minneap.)*, **6**, 627)

(d) in acromegaly (Stewart (1966). *Arch. Neurol.*, **14**, 107)

3. Neuropathy in blood dyscrasias

(a) polycythaemia vera

(b) leukaemia

(c) bleeding disorders—haemorrhage into nerves

(d) in sickle cell disease

4. Neuropathy in renal failure

(a) uraemic polyneuropathy (Asbury *et al.* (1963). *Arch. Neurol.*, **8**, 413)

(b) mononeuritis multiplex following dialysis (Meyrier *et al.* (1972). *Brit. med. J.*, **2**, 252)

5. Neuropathy in liver disease including primary biliary cirrhosis (Dayan and Williams (1967). *Lancet*, **2**, 133; Thomas and Walker (1965). *Brain*, **88**, 1079)

6. Neuropathy in porphyria

(a) genetically determined

  (i) acute intermittent porphyria (Swedish type)

  (ii) variegated porphyria (South African type)

  (iii) porphyria cutanea tarda

(b) acquired

  (i) hexachlorobenzene poisoning

7. Dysglobulinaemic neuropathy

(a) macroglobulinaemia

(b) cryoglobulinaemia

(c) with benign IgG paraproteinaemia (Read *et al.* (1978). *J. Neurol. Neurosurg. Psychiat.*, **41**, 215)

F. Neuropathy in malignant disease

1. Carcinomatous neuropathy

2. Neuropathy in reticulosis

3. Neuropathy in myelomatosis

G. Tumours of nerves

1. Arising from supporting structures and/or axons

(a) plexiform neuroma

(b) traumatic neuroma

(c) myelinic neuroma

2. Arising from supporting structures

(a) neurinoma (neurofibroma), including acoustic neuroma

(b) perineural fibroblastoma

(c) neurogenic sarcoma

(d) haemangioma

H. Functional disorders of peripheral nerves*

1. Stiff-man syndrome (Moersch and Woltman (1956). *Proc. Mayo Clin.*, **31**, 421)

2. Myokymia – hyperhidrosis – impaired muscle relaxation (Gamstorp and Wohlfart (1959). *Acta Psychiat. Scand.*, **34**, 181)

3. ?Recurrent muscle spasms of central origin (Satayoshi and Yamada (1967). *Arch. Neurol.*, **16**, 254)

4. ?'Painful legs and moving toes' (Spillane *et al.* (1971). *Brain*, **94**, 541)

5. ?Ekbom's syndrome ('restless legs') (Harriman *et al.* (1970). *Brain*, **93**, 393)

IV. DISORDERS OF NEUROMUSCULAR TRANSMISSION

A. Genetically determined

1. Hereditary myasthenia

(a) congenital and juvenile (Bowman (1948). *Pediatrics*, **1**, 472; *see* Bundey (1972). *J. Neurol. Neurosurg. Psychiat.*, **35**, 41)

(b) myasthenia with myopathy (McQuillen (1966). *Brain*, **89**, 121)

2. Pseudocholinesterase deficiency (suxamethonium paralysis)

B. Toxic

1. Botulism

2. Tick paralysis

*The cause of these disorders is uncertain; they may be due to spinal cord or central neuronal dysfunction.

3. Puff-fish paralysis (tetrodotoxin)
4. Magnesium intoxication
5. Kanamycin and other antibiotics (McQuillen *et al.* (1968). *Arch. Neurol.*, **18**, 402)
6. Penicillamine-induced myasthenia
7. Other drugs (*see* Ch. 25)

C. Autoimmune

1. Myasthenia gravis and its variants
   (*a*) transient neonatal myasthenia (Namba *et al.* (1970). *Pediatrics*, **45**, 488)
   (*b*) ocular myasthenia
      (i) with peripheral neuropathy and spastic paraparesis (Brust *et al.* (1974). *Neurology (Minneap.)*, **24**, 755)
   (*c*) generalised myasthenia
      (i) severe, especially in young women, correlated with HL-A8 antigen
      (ii) in older patients, often with thymoma and with HL-A2 or A3 antigen
   (*d*) myasthenia with thyrotoxicosis
   (*e*) myasthenia with hypothyroidism (Takamori *et al.* (1972). *Arch. Neurol.*, **26**, 326)
   (*f*) myasthenia with other autoimmune diseases
   (*g*) myasthenia with features of the myasthenic–myopathic syndrome (Schwartz and Stalberg (1975). *Neurology (Minneap.)*, **25**, 80)

D. Other myasthenic syndromes

1. Myasthenic–myopathic syndrome (Eaton-Lambert)
   (*a*) with malignant disease
   (*b*) without malignant disease
2. Myasthenic syndrome with end-plate acetylcholinesterase deficiency and reduced acetylcholine release (Engel *et al.* (1977). *Ann. neurol.*, **1**, 315)
3. Symptomatic myasthenia
   (*a*) in polymyositis and systemic lupus
   (*b*) in motor neurone disease
   (*c*) in chronic polyneuropathy

E. Cholinergic paralysis

1. Poisoning with anticholinesterase compounds (e.g. nerve gases)
2. Depolarising drugs
3. Black Widow spider venom

V. DISORDERS OF MUSCLE

A. Genetically determined myopathies

1. The muscular dystrophies
   (*a*) X-linked ('pseudohypertrophic') types
      (i) sex-linked recessive (severe) (Duchenne)
      (ii) sex-linked recessive (mild) (Becker)
   (*b*) facioscapulohumeral (Landouzy and Dejerine)
      (i) autosomal dominant involving face, scapulohumeral and anterior tibial muscles
      (ii) with inflammatory changes in muscle (Munsat *et al.* (1972). *Neurology (Minneap.)*, **22**, 335)
      (iii) with Möbius' syndrome (Hanson and Rowland (1971). *Arch. Neurol.*, **24**, 31)
   (*c*) scapuloperoneal muscular atrophy
      (i) autosomal dominant (Thomas *et al.* (1975). *J. Neurol. Neurosurg. Psychiat.*, **38**, 1008)
      (ii) X-linked (Thomas *et al.* (1972). *J. Neurol. Neurosurg. Psychiat.*, **35**, 208)
      (iii) with inflammatory changes and cardiopathy (Jennekens *et al.* (1975). *Brain*, **98**, 709)
   (*d*) limb-girdle
      (i) autosomal recessive or sporadic (Erb; Leyden and Möbius)
      (ii) myopathy limited to quadriceps
      (iii) autosomal recessive muscular dystrophy in childhood
      (iv) autosomal dominant, of late onset (Coster *et al.* (1974). *Europ. Neurol.*, **12**, 159; Bethlem and van Wijngaarden (1976). *Brain*, **99**, 91)
   (*e*) distal myopathy
      (i) autosomal dominant variety of late onset (Welander)
      (ii) ?ascending distal variety (Barnes)
      (iii) ?juvenile distal type

(*f*) ocular myopathy (progressive external ophthalmoplegia)★
   (i) isolated (dominant)
   (ii) with pigmentary retinal degeneration (dominant or sporadic)
   (iii) with retinal degeneration, short stature, heart block, ataxia, etc. (Kearns and Sayre)
(*g*) oculopharyngeal muscular dystrophy
(*h*) congenital ophthalmoplegia in the Goldenhar-Gorlin syndrome (Aleksic *et al.* (1976). *Neurology (Minneap.)*, **26**, 638)
(*i*) neonatal ophthalmoplegia with microfibres (Hanson *et al.* (1977). *Neurology (Minneap.)*, **27**, 974)

2. Obscure congenital myopathies of unknown aetiology
(*a*) congenital muscular dystrophy (including some cases of arthrogryposis multiplex congenita)
(*b*) benign congenital myopathy without specific features (Turner (1940). *Brain*, **63**, 163)
(*c*) ?congenital universal muscular hypoplasia† (Krabbe (1947). *Nord. Med.*, **35**, 1756)
(*d*) benign congenital or infantile hypotonia (Walton), amyotonia congenita (Oppenheim)‡
(*e*) central core disease
(*f*) nemaline, or rod-body, myopathy
(*g*) the mitochondrial myopathies (no exact classification of these disorders is possible at the present time) (see Chapters 17 and 18)
   (i) hypermetabolic (Luft *et al.* (1962). *J. Clin. Invest.*, **41**, 1776)
   (ii) pleoconial with salt craving and periodic weakness (Shy *et al.* (1966). *Brain*, **89**, 133)
   (iii) megaconial (Shy *et al.* ibid)
   (iv) with fatiguability and mitochondrial

inclusions (Price *et al.* (1967). *J. Neuropath. Exper. Neurol.*, **26**, 475)
   (v) with growth failure and seizures (d'Agostino *et al.* (1968). *Arch. Neurol.*, **18**, 388)
   (vi) with diabetes and distal myopathy (Salmon *et al.* (1971). *Lancet*, **2**, 290)
   (vii) with facioscapulohumeral syndrome (Hudgson *et al.* (1972). *J. Neurol. Sci.*, **16**, 343)
   (viii) with ophthalmoplegia and glycogen storage (DiMauro *et al.* (1973). *Arch. Neurol.*, **29**, 170)
   (ix) with cytochrome b deficiency (Spiro *et al.* (1970). *Arch. Neurol.*, **23**, 103; Morgan-Hughes *et al.* (1977). *Brain*, **100**, 617)
(*h*) myotubular or centronuclear myopathy
   (i) Spiro *et al.* (1966). *Arch. Neurol.*, **14**, 1
   (ii) X-linked variety (Wijngaarden *et al.* (1969). *Neurology (Minneap.)*, **19**, 901)
   (iii) with type I fibre atrophy (Bethlem *et al.* (1970). *Arch Neurol.*, **23**, 70)
(*i*) familial myosclerosis (myodysplasia fibrosa multiplex)
(*j*) myopathy in Marfan's syndrome (Goebel *et al.* (1973). *Neurology (Minneap.)*, **23**, 1257)
(*k*) familial congenital myopathy with cataract and gonadal dysgenesis (Bassöe (1956). *J. Clin. Endocrinol.*, **16**, 1614)
(*l*) myopathies with characteristic histochemical abnormalities
   (i) type I fibre hypotrophy (Engel, W. K. *et al.* (1968). *Arch. Neurol.*, **18**, 435)
   (ii) reducing body myopathy (Brooke and Neville (1971). *Neurology (Minneap.)*, **21**, 412)
(*m*) myopathy with defect in relaxing factor (Brody (1969). *New Engl. J. Med.*, **281**, 187)
(*n*) cardioskeletal myopathy with polysaccharide accumulation (Karpati *et al.* (1969). *Neurology (Minneap.)*, **19**, 553)
(*o*) myopathies with disordered lipid metabolism

★The primary myopathic nature of many of these cases is unproven.
†It is now doubtful whether this disorder is a specific entity as some such cases previously described have been found on further investigation to be suffering from nemaline myopathy.
‡This is probably not a single entity and many such cases are probably not myopathic in origin.

(i) carnitine deficiency and lipid storage

(ii) with cramps and myoglobinuria (Engel, W. K. *et al.* (1970). *New Engl. J. Med.*, **282**, 697)

(iii) carnitine palimityl transferase deficiency

(*p*) myopathies with cytoplasmic inclusions

(i) Nakashima *et al.* (1970). *Arch. Neurol.*, **22**, 270

(ii) with 'finger-print' inclusions (Engel, A. G. *et al.* (1972). *Proc. Mayo Clinic*, **47**, 377)

(*q*) 'multicore disease' (Engel, A. G. and Groover (1971). *Neurology (Minneap.)*, **21**, 413)

(*r*) sarcotubular myopathy (Jerusalem *et al.* (1973). *Neurology (Minneap.)*, **23**, 897)

(*s*) myopathy with tubular aggregates (Morgan-Hughes *et al.* (1970). *Brain*, **93**, 873)

(*t*) myopathy with crystalline intranuclear inclusions (Jenis *et al.* (1969). *Arch. Neurol.*, **20**, 281)

(*u*) autosomal dominant 'spheroid body' myopathy (Goebel *et al.* (1978). *Muscle and Nerve*, **1**, 14)

(*v*) hypertrophic branchial myopathy (Mancall *et al.* (1974). *Neurology (Minneap.)*, **24**, 1166)

(*w*) monomelic hypertrophic myopathy (Celesia *et al.* (1967). *Arch. Neurol.*, **17**, 69)

(*x*) cytoplasmic body neuromyopathy with respiratory failure and weight loss (Jerusalem *et al.* (1979). *J. Neurol. Sci.*, **41**, 1)

3. Myotonic disorders

(*a*) dystrophia myotonica (myotonia atrophica)

(i) adult form

(ii) infantile hypotonic form

(*b*) myotonia congenita (autosomal dominant form, Thomsen)

(*c*) myotonia congenita (autosomal recessive form)

(*d*) myotonia, dwarfism, diffuse bone disease and unusual eye and face abnormality (chrondrodystrophic myotonia—the Schwartz-Jampel syndrome)

(*e*) paramyotonia congenita (Eulenburg)

(*f*) paramyotonia without paralysis on exposure to cold (de Jong)

4. Glycogen-storage diseases

(*a*) glucose-6-phosphatase deficiency (von Gierke) (gives hypotonia without direct muscular involvement)

(*b*) amylo-1,6 glucosidase deficiency (Forbes)

(*c*) amylo-1,4 glucosidase (acid maltase) deficiency (Pompe)

(i) acute infantile form

(ii) adult or late onset variety

(*d*) muscle phosphorylase deficiency (McArdle)

(*e*) hereditary metabolic myopathy with myoglobinuria and abnormal glycolysis

(*f*) ?phosphoglucomutase deficiency

(*g*) myopathy with abnormal glycolytic breakdown at phosphohexoisomerase level

(*h*) phosphofructokinase deficiency

(*i*) multiple enzyme deficiency

5. Familial periodic paralysis and related syndromes

(*a*) familial hypokalaemic periodic paralysis

(*b*) adynamia episodica hereditaria (hyperkalaemic)

(*c*) ?normokalaemic periodic paralysis (Poskanzer and Kerr (1961). *Amer. J. Med.*, **31**, 328)

(*d*) myotonic periodic paralysis

(*e*) thyrotoxic periodic paralysis

6. Generalised myositis ossificans

7. Dysproteinaemic ataxias with myopathy

(*a*) ?ataxia telangiectasia (?secondary to neurogenic atrophy)

(*b*) ?A-β-lipoproteinaemia (acanthocytosis)

8. Myopathy in xanthinuria (Chalmers *et al.* (1969). *J. Path.*, **99**, 45)

9. Familial myoglobinuria of unknown cause

10. Myopathy in malignant hyperpyrexia (Isaacs and Barlow (1970). *Brit. med. J.*, **1**, 275)

11. Progressive muscle spasm, alopecia, diarrhoea and malabsorption (Satoyoshi (1978). *Neurology (Minneap.)*, **28**, 458)

B. Trauma to muscle by external agents

B-I. Physical

1. Crush syndrome

2. Ischaemic infarction or atrophy
   (a) in peripheral vascular disease (Engel and Hawley (1977). *J. Neurol.*, **215**, 161)
   (b) in polyarteritis nodosa and other vasculitides
   (c) in diabetes mellitus (Banker and Chester (1973). *Neurology* (*Minneap.*), **23**, 667)
3. Volkmann's contracture
4. Anterior tibial syndrome
5. Posterior compartment (tibial) syndrome (*Brit. med. J.* (1975), **3**, 193)
6. Congenital torticollis

B-II. Toxic
1. Haff disease
2. Snake-bite by *Enhydrina schistosa* (Malayan sea snake)
3. Saxitoxin poisoning
4. Rhabdomyolysis caused by hornet venom (Shilkin *et al.* (1972). *Brit. med. J.*, **1**, 156)

B-III. Drugs
1. Steroid myopathy
2. Chloroquine myopathy
3. ?Bretylium tosylate myopathy (Campbell and Montuschi (1960). *Lancet*, **2**, 789)
4. Emetine
5. Vincristine
6. Diazocholesterol
7. Clofibrate
8. Carbenoxolone (Mohamed *et al.* (1966). *Brit. med. J.*, **1**, 1581)
9. Amphotericin B (K$^+$ depletion)
10. Anodiaquine
11. Colchicine
12. Meperidine (Aberfeld *et al.* (1968). *Arch. Neurol.*, **19**, 384)
13. Pethidine (Mastaglia *et al.* (1971). *Brit. med. J.*, **iv**, 532)
14. Pentazocine (Steiner *et al.* (1973). *Arch. Neurol.*, **28**, 408)
15. Polymyxin E (Vanhaeverbeck *et al.* (1974). *J. Neurol. Neurosurg. Psychiat.*, **37**, 1343)
16. Triorthocresylphosphate (Prineas (1969). *Arch. Neurol.*, **21**, 150)

C. Inflammatory

C-I. Infections of muscle
1. Viral (presumed)
   (a) Bornholm disease
   (b) Epidemic torticollis
   (c) Following influenza (Middleton *et al.* (1970). *Lancet*, **2**, 533)
   (d) In herpes zoster (Norris *et al.* (1969). *Arch. Neurol.*, **21**, 25)
2. Bacterial
   (a) Gas gangrene (*Cl. welchii*)
   (b) Tetanus (*Cl. tetani*)
   (c) Staphylococci and other pyogenic agents (septic myositis)
   (d) Leprous myositis
   (e) Tropical myositis (usually pyogenic)
3. Nematode
   (a) *Trichinella spiralis* (Trichinosis)
4. Cestode
   (a) Cysticercosis with muscle hypertrophy (Jacob and Mathew (1968). *Neurology* (*Minneap.*), **18**, 767)
   (b) Cysticercosis (asymptomatic)
5. Trypanosomiasis cruzi
6. Toxoplasmosis (Rowland and Greer (1961). *Neurology* (*Minneap.*), **11**, 367)

C-II. Other inflammatory disorders of muscle
1. Polymyositis (Group I of Walton and Adams) (possibly an organ-specific auto-immune disease)
   (a) Acute polymyositis with myoglobinuria
   (b) Subacute polymyositis
   (c) Chronic polymyositis (including chronic myositis fibrosa)
2. Polymyositis or dermatomyositis (Groups II and III of Walton and Adams) when occurring as one feature of what may prove to be a non-organ-specific autoimmune disease
   (a) Dermatomyositis
   (b) Polymyositis in disseminated lupus erythematosus
   (c) Polymyositis in rheumatic fever
   (d) Polymyositis in rheumatoid arthritis
   (e) Polymositis in scleroderma and/or systemic sclerosis
   (f) Scleroderma (morphoea) with myopathy

(g) Ocular myositis (pseudotumour of the orbit)

(h) Muscle infarction and/or polymyositis in polyarteritis nodosa

(i) Polymyopathy in Sjögren's disease (Denka and Old (1969). *Amer. J. Clin. Path.*, **151**, 631)

(j) ?Polymyopathy in Werner's disease (Nature of muscle atrophy uncertain—*see* Epstein *et al.* (1966). *Medicine (Baltimore)*, **45**, 177)

(k) Localised nodular myositis (see Ch. 15)

3. Polymyositis or dermatomyositis (Group IV of Walton and Adams) occurring possibly as a conditioned autoimmune response in malignant disease

4. Polymyositis with associated virus particles (Chou (1967). *Science*, **158**, 1453; Carpenter *et al.* (1970). *Neurology (Minneap.)*, **20**, 889)

C-III. Inflammatory disorders of muscle of unknown aetiology

1. Sarcoidosis with myopathy
2. Granulomatous polymyositis (Lynch and Bansal (1973). *J. Neurol. Sci.*, **18**, 1) and giant cell myositis (Namba *et al.* (1974). *Arch. Neurol.*, **31**, 27)
3. Polymyalgia rheumatica
4. Localised myositis ossificans
5. Fibrositis and nodular fasciitis
6. ? Myopathy in relapsing panniculitis (Weber-Christian syndrome)
7. Myositis with necrotising fasciitis (Carruthers *et al.* (1975). *Brit. med. J.*, **iii**, 355)
8. ? Myopathy in psoriasis (Mormun *et. al.* (1970). *Dermatologia (Basel)*, **140**, 214)
9. Polymyositis in the hypereosinophilic syndrome (Tayzer *et al.* (1977). *Ann. Neurol.*, **1**, 65)
10. Myopathy in Reye's syndrome (Hanson and Urizar (1977). *Ann. Neurol.*, **1**, 431)

D. Muscle disorder associated with endocrine or metabolic disease

1. Thyrotoxicosis
   (a) myopathy
   (b) myasthenia gravis
   (c) periodic paralysis

2. Myxoedema
   (a) girdle myopathy
   (b) Debré-Semelaigne syndrome (cretins) (Debré and Semelaigne (1935). *Amer. J. Dis. Child.*, **50**, 1351)
   (c) Hoffmann syndrome (adults) (Hoffmann (1897). *Deutsch. Z. Nervenheilk*, **9**, 278)
   (d) pseudomyotonia
   (e) ?neuromyopathy following ^{131}I therapy

3. Hypopituitarism with myopathy

4. Acromegaly with muscle hypertrophy (and/or muscular atrophy) (Mastaglia *et al.* (1970). *Lancet*, **2**, 907)

5. Exophthalmic ophthalmoplegia (infiltrative ophthalmopathy or ophthalmic Graves' disease)

6. Cushing's disease myopathy (and corticosteroid myopathy)

7. ACTH myopathy (Prineas *et al.* (1968). *Quart. J. Med.*, **37**, 63)

8. Addison's disease with myopathy

9. Primary aldosteronism (with hypokalaemic periodic paralysis)

10. Hyperparathyroidism with myopathy (Cholod *et al.* (1970). *Amer. J. Med.*, **48**, 700)

11. Myopathy in other forms of metabolic bone disease
    (a) osteomalacia due to
        (i) idiopathic steatorrhoea
        (ii) malabsorption after partial gastrectomy (Ekbom *et al.* (1964). *Acta Med. Scand.*, **176**, 493)
        (iii) renal acidosis
        (iv) hypophosphatnemia (Schott and Wills (1975). *J. Neurol. Neurosurg. Psychiat.*, **38**, 297)
        (v) anticonvulsants (Marsden *et al.* (1973). *Brit. med. J.*, **4**, 526)

12. Myopathy with calcitonin-secreting medullary carcinoma of the thyroid (Cunliffe *et al.* (1970). *Amer. J. Med.*, **48**, 120)

13. Alcoholic myopathy
    (a) acute, with rhabdomyolysis and myoglobinuria
    (b) subacute proximal
    (c) hypokalaemic (Rubinstein and Wainapel (1977). *Arch. Neurol.*, **34**, 553)

14. Nutritional myopathy

(a) Protein deficiency

(b) ?vitamin E deficiency

15. Myopathy in chronic renal failure (Floyd et al. (1974). Quart. J. Med., **43**, 509)

16. Myopathy in lysine-cystinuria (Clara and Lowenthal (1966). J. neurol. Sci., **3**, 433)

17. Myopathy in xanthinuria (Chalmers et al. (1969). Quart. J. Med., **38**, 493)

18. Myopathy in Lafora disease (Coleman et al. (1974). Arch. Neurol., **31**, 396)

E. Myopathy associated with malignant disease

1. Carcinomatous myopathy (other than polymyositis)

2. Myasthenic-myopathic syndrome

3. Carcinomatous embolic myopathy (Heffner (1971). Neurology (Minneap.), **21**, 841)

4. Myopathy in the carcinoid syndrome (Swash et al. (1975). Arch. Neurol., **32**, 572)

F. Myopathy associated with myasthenia gravis

G. Myopathy in thalassaemia

(Logothetis et al. (1972). Neurology (Minneap.), **22**, 294)

H. Other disorders of muscle of unknown aetiology

1. Acute muscle necrosis
   (a) of unknown cause
   (b) in chronic alcoholism
   (c) in carcinoma (Urich and Wilkinson (1970). J. Neurol. Neurosurg. Psychiat., **33**, 398)

2. Paroxysmal myoglobinuria or rhabdomyolysis (Meyer-Betz (1910), see Korein et al. (1959). Neurology, **9**, 767)
   (a) exertional
       (i) in McArdle's disease
       (ii) in other metabolic myopathies (e.g. Kontos et al. (1963). Amer. J. Med., **35**, 283)
   (b) non-exertional (e.g. Bowden et al. (1956). Medicine (Baltimore), **35**, 335; Favara et al. (1967). Amer. J. Med., **42**, 196)
   (c) rhabdomyolysis due to ingestion of quail (Bateman (1977), U.S. Office Naval Research)

3. Amyloid myopathy
   (a) primary familial

(b) primary sporadic

(c) in myelomatosis

(d) with angiopathy (Bruni et al. (1977). Canad. J. Neurol. Sci., **2**, 77)

4. Conditions demonstrating muscular hypertrophy
   (a) ?muscular hypertrophy, extrapyramidal disorders and mental deficiency (de Lange (1934). Amer. J. Dis. Child., **48**, 243)⋆
   (b) hypertrophia musculorum vera
   (c) bilateral hypertrophy of masseters (see VA2(v))

5. Disuse atrophy

6. Muscle cachexia (in wasting diseases and in the elderly)

7. Muscle wasting in contralateral cerebral lesions (particularly of parietal lobe)

I. Tumours of muscle

1. Rhabdomyoma

2. Rhabdomyosarcoma
   (a) adult pleomorphic type
   (b) embryonal botryoid type
   (c) embryonal alveolar type

3. Desmoid fibroma

4. Alveolar sarcoma

5. Angioma

6. Other connective tissue tumours occasionally occurring in muscle

VI. SOME DISORDERS OF SUPRASPINAL TONAL REGULATION WHICH MAY MIMIC NEUROMUSCULAR DISORDERS

1. Muscular hypertrophy, extrapyramidal disorders and mental deficiency (de Lange—see VH 4(a))

2. Prader-Willi syndrome

3. Hypotonia in mental defect

4. Hypotonia in metabolic disorders

5. Hypotonia in cerebral palsy (atonic diplegia)

6. Hypotonia in cerebellar diplegia and other cerebellar ataxias

7. Hypotonia in rheumatic chorea

8. Hypotonia in acrodynia (Pink disease)

9. Hypotonia in the cerebrohepatorenal syndrome (Bowen et al. (1964). Johns Hopkins Med. J., **114**, 402)

⋆This disorder may be identical with congenital hypothyroidism (Debré and Semelaigne, V, D2(b)).

REFERENCES

Adrian, R.H. & Marshall, M.W. (1976) Action potentials reconstructed in normal and mystome muscle fibres. *Journal of Physiology*, **258**, 125.

André-Thomas, Chesni, Y. & Dargassies, S.S.-A. (1960) *The Neurological Examination of the Infant*, Eds R.C. MacKeith, P.E. Polani and E. Clayton-Jones, *Little Club Clinics in Developmental Medicine*, No. 1 (National Spastics Society: London).

Bickerstaff, E.R. (1980) *Neurological Examination in Clinical Practice*. 14th Edn. (Blackwell: Oxford).

Bradley, W.G. (1974) *Disorders of Peripheral Nerves* (Blackwell: Oxford).

Cogan, D.G. (1956) *Neurology of the Ocular Muscles*, 2nd Edn. (Thomas: Springfield, Illinois).

Daniels, L., Williams, M. & Worthingham, C. (1956) *Muscle Testing: Techniques of Manual Examination*, 2nd Edn. (W. B. Saunders: Philadelphia).

Denny-Brown, D. & Nevin, S. (1941) The phenomenon of myotonia. *Brain*, **64**, 1.

Denny-Brown, D. & Pennybacker, J.B. (1938) Fibrillation and fasciculation in voluntary muscle. *Brain*, **61**, 311.

Dubowitz, V. (1978) *Muscle Disorders in Childhood* (Saunders: London, Philadelphia, Toronto).

Edwards, R.H.T. & McDonnell, M. (1974) Hand-held dynamometer for evaluating voluntary muscle function. *Lancet*, **2**, 757.

Gamstorp, I. (1970) *Pediatric Neurology* (Appleton-Century-Crofts: New York).

Gamstorp, I. & Wohlfart, G. (1959) A syndrome characterised by myokymia, myotonia, muscular wasting and increased perspiration. *Acta Psychiatrica Scandinavica*, **34**, 181

Gardner-Medwin, D. & Walton, J.N. (1969) Myokymia with impaired muscular relaxation. *Lancet*, **1**, 127.

Gardner-Medwin, D., Hudgson, P. & Walton, J.N. (1967) Benign spinal muscular atrophy arising in childhood and adolescence. *Journal of the Neurological Sciences*, **5**, 121.

Gray's Anatomy (1967) 34th Edn. Eds D.V. Davies and R.E. Coupland (Longmans: London).

Isaacs, H. (1961) A syndrome of continuous muscle fibre activity. *Journal of Neurology, Neurosurgery and Psychiatry*, **24**, 319.

Jennekens, F.G.I., Tomlinson, B.E. & Walton, J.N. (1971) Histochemical aspects of five limb muscles in old age: an autopsy study. *Journal of the Neurological Sciences*, **14**, 259.

de Jong, R.N. (1979) *The Neurologic Examination*, 4th Edn. (Harper and Row: New York).

de Lange, C. (1934) Congenital hypertrophy of muscles, extrapyramidal motor disturbances and mental deficiency. *American Journal of Diseases of Childhood*, **48**, 243.

Lehoczky, T., Halasy, M., Simon, G. & Harmos, G. (1965) Glycogenic myopathy: a case of skeletal muscle-glycogenosis in twins. *Journal of the Neurological Sciences*, **2**, 366.

Leyburn, P. & Walton, J.N. (1959) The treatment of myotonia: a controlled trial. *Brain*, **82**, 81.

Matthews, W.B. (1966) Facial myokymia. *Journal of Neurology, Neurosurgery and Psychiatry*, **29**, 35.

Medical Research Council (1976) *Aids to the Examination of the Peripheral Nervous System*. Memorandum no. 45 (H.M.S.O.: London).

Mertens, H.-G. & Zschocke, S. (1965) Neuromyotonie. *Klinische Wochenschrift*, **43**, 917.

O'Doherty, D.S., Schellinger, D. & Raptopoulos, V. (1977) Computed tomographic patterns of pseudohypertrophic muscular dystrophy: preliminary results. *Journal of Computer Assisted Tomography*, **1**, 482.

Paine, R.S. & Oppé, T.E. (1966) *Neurological Examination of Children* (Spastics Society and Heinemann: London).

Perkoff, G.T., Hardy, P. & Velez-Garcia, E. (1966) Reversible acute muscular syndrome in chronic alcoholism. *New England Journal of Medicine*, **274**, 1277.

Prineas, J., Hall, R., Barwick, D.D. & Watson, A.J. (1968) Myopathy associated with pigmentation following adrenalectomy for Cushing's syndrome. *Quarterly Journal of Medicine*, **37**, 63.

Salick, A.I. & Pearson, C.M. (1967) Electrical silence of myoidema. *Neurology (Minneapolis)*, **17**, 899.

Satayoshi, E. & Kowa, H. (1967) A myopathy due to glycolytic abnormality. *Archives of Neurology*, **17**, 248.

Vignos, P.J. & Archibald, K.C. (1960) Maintenance of ambulation in childhood muscular dystrophy. *Journal of Chronic Diseases*, **12**, 273.

Wallis, W.E., Poznak, A.V. & Plum, F. (1970) Generalized muscular stiffness, fasciculations, and myokymia of peripheral nerve origin. *Archives of Neurology*, **22**, 430.

Walsh, F.B. & Hoyt, W.F. (1969) *Clinical Neuro-ophthalmology*. 3rd Edn. (Williams and Wilkins: Baltimore).

Welch, L.K., Appenzeller, O. & Bicknell, J.M. (1972) Peripheral neuropathy with myokymia, sustained muscular contraction, and continuous motor unit activity. *Neurology (Minneapolis)*, **22**, 161

Williamson, E. & Brooke, M.H. (1972) Myokymia and the motor unit: a histochemical study. *Archives of Neurology*, **26**, 11.

Wilson, J. & Walton, J.N. (1959) Some muscular manifestations of hypothyroidism. *Journal of Neurology, Neurosurgery and Psychiatry*, **22**, 320.

World Federation of Neurology: Research Group on Neuromuscular Diseases (1968) Classification of the neuromuscular disorders. *Journal of the Neurological Sciences*, **6**, 165.

Progressive muscular dystrophy and the myotonic disorders

INTRODUCTION

The study of the progressive degenerative disorders of muscle began in the mid-nineteenth century, especially in France and Germany. Aran (1850) and Wachsmuth (1855) reviewed the subject with little attempt at classification of disease states or the distinction of neurogenic from myopathic disease. Meryon (1852) gave the first clear account of progressive muscular paralysis in young boys and demonstrated that it was due to 'granular degeneration' of the muscles without changes in the anterior horns of the spinal cord or in the motor roots. Later, Duchenne (1868) gave a vivid description of this disorder, now given his name, and Gowers' (1879) was the first comprehensive account in English and is still one of the finest. Both Duchenne and Gowers emphasised the 'pseudohypertrophic' enlargement of certain muscles. Leyden (1876) and Möbius (1879) de-

scribed a familial form of degeneration affecting the muscles of the pelvic girdle. In 1884 Erb described a juvenile or scapulohumeral form of the disorder, and stressed that this disease was due to a primary degeneration of the muscles which he named muscular dystrophy. The classical description of the facioscapulohumeral form was published by Landouzy and Dejerine (1884), and muscular dystrophy in the external ocular muscles was reported by Hutchinson (1879) and by Fuchs (1890). Shortly afterwards, Batten (1909) suggested that some cases of amyotonia congenita (Oppenheim, 1900) were the result of a simple atrophic variety of congenital muscular dystrophy. Gowers (1902) also described a distal form of the disease. There is now some doubt about the true nature of his cases, but Welander (1951) gave a full account of a distal muscular dystrophy occurring in Sweden. The benign form of sex-linked muscular dystrophy was distinguished from the Duchenne type by Becker and Keiner (1955). Victor, Hayes and Adams (1962) delineated oculopharyngeal muscular dystrophy, distinguishing it from the other ocular myopathies. A scapuloperoneal distribution of muscular weakness is seen in certain cases of spinal muscular atrophy, of which it seems to form a distinct subtype. In some kindreds a similar disorder of myopathic origin constitutes, in effect, another form of muscular dystrophy (Seitz, 1957). It is now apparent that both X-linked and autosomal dominant varieties of scapuloperoneal myopathy exist.

Before the clinical aspects of these disorders are described, the dual problem of the definition of muscular dystrophy and the proper classification of the diseases which have been given this name must be discussed.

The problem of definition

In the nineteenth century, while the clinical syndromes were being delineated, much attention was paid to the distinction between muscular atrophy resulting from pathological changes in the nervous system and those disorders, or myopathies, in which the primary pathological change was in the muscle. The term 'myopathy' has come to apply to any disorder which can be attributed to pathological, biochemical or electrical changes occurring in the muscle fibres or in the interstitial tissues of the voluntary musculature, and in which there is no evidence that such changes are in any way secondary to disordered function in the central or peripheral nervous system; such disorders include many which are inflammatory, metabolic or endocrine in nature. Myopathy, at first identifiable only at autopsy, was correlated gradually with clinical syndromes, while Duchenne defined characteristic responses of muscle to electrical stimulation and Erb, among others, defined typical histological appearances of muscle which could later be used to characterise myopathies in living patients. In particular Erb (1891) described the characteristic histological appearances by which he defined 'muscular dystrophy' (see Ch. 5). His description has not been bettered, although the occurrence of active muscle fibre regeneration has been added to his definition. The investigative techniques of clinical enzymology and electromyography have improved our ability to diagnose muscular dystrophy, but as an operational definition for use in the diagnosis of individual cases we are still dependent upon: (1) the recognition of a specific clinical syndrome; and (2) the recognition of the specific, or at least compatible, histological features in muscle biopsy material. Yet a wider conceptual definition is plainly needed and Walton (1961) suggested that the term 'muscular dystrophy' should be reserved for cases of *progressive, genetically determined, primary, degenerative myopathy.*

As our understanding of the essential lesions underlying each type of muscular dystrophy advances, this definition may become difficult to sustain and will be replaced by more accurate ones. Already some congenital muscular dystrophies are known to be virtually non-progressive and the evidence that they are always genetically determined is inconclusive; furthermore the concept of primary degenerative disorders in general is being eroded by the discovery of underlying specific metabolic disorders in many instances. Some examples of the ocular and oculopharyngeal 'muscular dystrophies' and of the facioscapulohumeral syndrome are now generally considered to be mitochondrial disorders. Some of the 'congenital myopathies', such as nemaline myopathy, are often slowly progressive, thus falling within our definition, yet because of their different but characteristic histology they are not called muscular dystrophies. Finally, the very concept that the muscular dystrophies are primarily myopathic was challenged by Dubowitz (1969), McComas, Sica and Currie (1970) and others, who suggested that a disorder in the nervous system might, after all, determine the development of dystrophic changes in muscle.

Interest in the relationship between muscular dystrophy and neurogenic atrophy was reawakened by Kugelberg and Welander (1956) who described 12 patients with spinal muscular atrophy closely resembling muscular dystrophy. This disorder proved to be a common cause of confusion and its existence necessitated careful clinical, electromyographic and histological examination in every patient to avoid errors in diagnosis. Then followed the discovery that, not only in spinal muscular atrophy but also in other chronic denervating disorders, 'secondary myopathic changes' may occur in muscle (Tyrer and Sutherland, 1961; Drachman, Murphy, Nigam and Hills, 1967) so that, in advanced cases, anterior horn cell disease and primary myopathy may be indistinguishable by any criteria short of autopsy. This has made it necessary to reconsider the pathogenesis of many of the rarer chronic 'myopathies', including the less well-established muscular dystrophies, and this reassessment is still incomplete. A further twist to this already complex situation was added when Dubowitz (1969) suggested that the development of 'dystrophic' changes in muscle might be under a neural influence. This was partly based on re-innervation experiments in animals and partly on the peculiarly selective degeneration of specific muscle groups in each type of dystrophy and the occurrence of mental retardation in Duchenne dystrophy. Subsequent electrophysiological evidence favouring an apparent disorder of anterior horn cell function even in Duchenne muscular dystrophy (McComas, Sica and Currie, 1971) led to a 'neurogenic theory' of the aetiology of the disease which, after a considerable period of popularity in the early 1970s, has now fallen out of favour because of the lack of confirmatory evidence. Those muscular dystrophies which are more difficult to define by strict criteria than the Duchenne type, however, provide a continual source of confusion: cases of limb-girdle, scapuloperoneal and facioscapulohumeral 'syndromes' in which investigation indicates myopathic or neurogenic features, or both, are commonplace in the literature and in clinical practice. It is clear that at this stage no more adequate definition of muscular dystrophy is possible.

The problem of classification

The hereditary nature of the muscular dystrophies was recognised early, but attempts to apply the principles of genetics to certain categories led to much confusion which is not yet fully resolved. Thus, in studying the traditional categories of pseudohypertrophic, pelvic girdle atrophic, facioscapulohumeral and juvenile scapulohumeral forms, Bell (1943) and others found examples of autosomal recessive, dominant and sex-linked recessive inheritance in each of the clinical varieties of the diseases. It was, therefore, apparent that classification according to classical criteria was not satisfactory as a guide either to prognosis or to inheritance.

This confusion has led to many attempts to produce a revised classification, taking into account both clinical and genetic criteria. Notable contributions have been made by Tyler and Wintrobe (1950), Levison (1951), Stevenson (1953), Becker (1953, 1964), Lamy and de Grouchy (1954), Walton and Nattrass (1954), Morton and Chung (1959) and Emery and Walton (1967). Several of these revised classifications have been reviewed in previous editions of this book.

In the absence of any absolute definition of muscular dystrophy or of a known biochemical basis for any of the types, classification consists of listing those disorders which seem to be separate entities on genetic, clinical and pathological grounds and which conform to the operational definition. The sporadic case, in which no genetic evidence is available, presents particular difficulties in diagnosis and classification. In the present state of knowledge, the X-linked and dominant disorders are therefore often better characterised than those of autosomal recessive inheritance. These nosological difficulties are discussed in relation to individual disorders in the sections which follow.

In this Chapter the myotonic disorders are treated separately, and myotonic dystrophy (which differs in so many ways from the 'pure' muscular dystrophies) is therefore excluded from the following working classification. Some of the less well-established clinical types are qualified with question marks.

The pure muscular dystrophies
(a) *X-linked muscular dystrophies*
  Severe (Duchenne)
  Benign (Becker)
  ? Benign with early contractures (Dreifuss)
  Scapuloperoneal
  ? Hereditary myopathy confined to females
(b) *Autosomal recessive muscular dystrophies*
  Scapulohumeral ('limb-girdle')
  ? 'Quadriceps myopathy'
  Autosomal recessive muscular dystrophy in childhood
  Congenital muscular dystrophies
(c) *Autosomal dominant muscular dystrophies*
  Facioscapulohumeral
  Scapuloperoneal
  Late-onset proximal
  Distal (adult-onset)
  Distal (infantile-onset)
  Ocular
  Oculopharyngeal

General principles of diagnosis and management

An unqualified diagnosis of 'muscular dystrophy' is never justifiable. Every case must be allotted firmly to one of the categories listed above; any which seem not to be typical of any specific type should be regarded with great suspicion and should be thoroughly investigated, a point of great importance because several of the other myopathic disorders are treatable. In the early stages, or in any doubtful case, a firm diagnosis should be made only after investigation including estimation of serum enzymes, especially of creatine kinase activity, electromyography (EMG) and muscle biopsy. Nevertheless, the clinical diagnosis of established cases is rarely difficult, especially in the facioscapulohumeral, ocular and oculopharyngeal types and in the myotonic disorders. It is based upon a clear history of the onset and progression of the symptoms, the pattern of inheritance and a detailed examination of the muscles, which will reveal the pattern of selective muscular wasting and weakness that is characteristic of each type of muscular dystrophy. In practice, often the greatest difficulty is in distinguishing between muscular dystrophy and various disorders discussed in the following paragraphs.

When a waddling gait is caused by *disease of the hip joints* there will be no wasting, weakness, hypotonia or reflex change and, in this situation, the hips should always be X-rayed even if passive movements of the joints are full.

Spinal muscular atrophy is an important imitator of muscular dystrophy in childhood and early adult life (Kugelberg and Welander, 1956). There may have been a previously affected sib in the family, sometimes with a more severe infantile form. The weakness may have developed gradually or may apparently have been precipitated by an acute infection, an injury or a prophylactic immunisation. Often the course is variable with periods of improvement. The muscle weakness is chiefly proximal and often selective with corresponding atrophy, and hypertrophy may occur, all points which cause confusion with muscular dystrophy. Unfortunately the selective muscular weakness in spinal muscular atrophy, unlike that of the muscular dystrophies, has no consistent or recognisable pattern: indeed, the recognition that the pattern is slightly 'wrong' for any muscular dystrophy is often the first clue to the diagnosis. Another helpful but inconstant clue is fasciculation of the tongue, which should be sought in all such cases; less often there is fasciculation elsewhere. Such features as tremor, talipes, distal, asymmetrical or even focal muscle weakness and

the loss of tendon reflexes in relatively well-preserved muscles are not constant characteristics of spinal muscular atrophy, but they occur in this disorder more frequently than in the other conditions mentioned here and are helpful clues to the diagnosis when they are found. The serum creatine kinase activity may be normal, but it is often raised. Electromyography and muscle biopsy are the only reliable ways of distinguishing this disorder.

In a small proportion of cases of *motor neurone disease* the weakness is chiefly proximal, but fasciculation and signs of corticospinal tract involvement in the form of brisk reflexes or extensor plantar responses are almost invariable, and clearly distinguish the disorder from muscular dystrophy.

In *polymyositis* the progression of the disease is usually more rapid than in muscular dystrophy, and spontaneous remissions may occur. The generalised proximal (and sometimes also distal) weakness contrasts with the selective weakness in muscular dystrophy and, in particular, often affects the posterior neck muscles. Dysphagia is common in polymyositis and rare in muscular dystrophy, except in the myotonic and oculopharyngeal types. Except in very chronic cases the degree of muscular atrophy in polymyositis is less severe than in dystrophic muscles with an equal degree of weakness; muscle hypertrophy is rare. The tendon reflexes tend to be spared in polymyositis, except in advanced cases, whereas they are lost as soon as there is significant weakness of the relevant muscle in muscular dystrophy. In dermatomyositis the skin changes are often diagnostic.

When all these points are considered, there is rarely doubt as to whether a child has polymyositis or muscular dystrophy. Nevertheless, the diagnosis is so important that a muscle biopsy should always be performed. The same criteria apply to adult cases, but some indolent cases of polymyositis in middle age may be mistaken for 'limb-girdle' dystrophy of late onset. Here the diagnosis is essentially a pathological one, but controversy may persist even after autopsy.

The various *benign congenital myopathies* often present as hypotonia in infancy, but may also cause gait disturbances in later childhood. In occasional cases, clinical diagnosis is possible, for example when a child has the skeletal dysmorphism of nemaline myopathy; however, the diagnosis in this group is essentially pathological, which further underlines the importance of full investigation, including histochemical and electron-microscopic studies of muscle biopsies, in all cases of unusual muscle disease.

The presence of bone pain should raise the possibility of a *myopathy associated with metabolic bone disease*. The absence of muscle wasting and the brisk tendon reflexes are useful clinical points in such cases (Smith and Stern, 1967).

The myopathy sometimes associated with *thyrotoxicosis* can imitate 'limb-girdle' muscular dystrophy, especially when the hyperthyroidism is not clinically obvious. The condition should be excluded by laboratory tests whenever there is proximal weakness and wasting, especially in the upper limbs, with a rather short history or with an unusual pattern of selective muscle involvement.

The differentiation of the many varieties of muscular dystrophy should be made, ideally, on both clinical and genetic grounds. Unfortunately this is rarely possible; many cases have no family history at all and furthermore, the different genetic varieties of the disease cannot always be distinguished clinically. This problem is most acute in cases of the Duchenne and autosomal childhood types and the Becker and 'limb-girdle' types, when the latter is pelvifemoral in onset. Nevertheless, the differentiation of the X-linked disorders from the similar autosomal recessive types is of great importance for genetic counselling. For example, the daughters of a man with Becker dystrophy are all obligate carriers and may transmit the disease to half of their sons, whereas the daughters of a man with 'limb-girdle' dystrophy carry a very small risk of having affected children. On the other hand, the Duchenne, limb-girdle and facioscapulohumeral types can generally be differentiated from each other, even in their early stages, on the basis of the age of onset, the rate of progression and the pattern of selective muscle involvement. Further points in differential diagnosis are discussed in relation to the individual types of muscular dystrophy.

The general principles of management of muscular dystrophy can be summarised as follows:

(1) The first stage of management is diagnosis. Precision in diagnosis is important, not only to exclude treatable disorders but to provide an accurate basis for prognosis and genetic counselling. Furthermore, diagnosis in any disabled patient involves not only identification of the nature of the disease, but also assessment of the degree of handicap, so that appropriate remedial therapy and services can be provided.

(2) Telling the patient, or the parents, the diagnosis and prognosis is a vital stage in management, which will often determine their whole subsequent attitude and approach to the disease. It must be done with sensitivity by a physician who knows the patient personally and has a sound understanding of the disease and its implications. We believe that, in general, adult patients or the parents of affected children should be given a full and accurate account in order to allow them to make constructive plans for the future. It is valuable to balance the bad news with an offer of a programme of management and of continuing practical help and support. Most patients also find some comfort in knowing about the extensive worldwide research into the pathogenesis and potential treatment of the muscular dystrophies.

(3) Genetic advice must be offered at the earliest opportunity, not only to the immediate family but, in the X-linked and dominant disorders, to other relatives at risk of having affected children.

(4) Useful mobility should be maintained as a major priority. Exercise promotes physical fitness and muscle strength, and we believe that regular exercise should become a lifelong habit for all patients. Obesity should be avoided. Contractures can be at least partly controlled by regular stretching. Surgery should be undertaken only with great circumspection, should be as simple and brief as possible and must, above all, be done only in conjunction with well-organised programmes for rapid post-operative mobilisation. In general, surgical procedures should be done only when they are likely to provide an important functional benefit which can be obtained in no other way. Anaesthesia should be avoided, or undertaken only with special precautions to avoid respiratory or cardiac complications. Regular breathing exercises and, where appropriate, postural drainage help to delay the onset of respiratory failure.

(5) A bewildering variety of practical aids and equipment for the disabled has become available in recent years. Many are invaluable, but careful assessment and trial may be necessary to solve specific problems for individual patients. Wheelchairs and lifting equipment, in particular, must be selected with professional skill. Occasional but regular consultation with an occupational therapist, sometimes linked with visits to one of the many 'Aids Centres' now established in Britain, may greatly reduce the disabling effects of the disease. It is of the greatest psychological importance that patients and their families should know in advance of such potential solutions to problems, so that they may live expecting to remain reasonably independent and successful. Professional help should also be provided in planning for ideal access and convenience in the home, school or place of work.

(6) Innumerable practical and emotional problems, large and small, occur during the life of severely handicapped persons, and these commonly affect other members of the family. It is an important part of the management to make sure that an appropriate professional person is available on a continuing basis to suggest solutions and to provide support. A medical social worker with experience of the disease can often fill this role and may be able to foresee and prevent many difficulties. She can also advise on the many grants and special services available for these patients. We have found that psychiatric help is very rarely needed when emotional support and practical help are provided in this way.

(7) Employment, marriage and child-bearing are feasible, and often very successful, in patients with muscular dystrophy in whom the onset is in adolescence or later. Employment and marriage are very rare in the Duchenne type, although sheltered employment is possible for a short period in some cases. It is an important responsibility of the doctor at the time of diagnosis of the late-onset muscular dystrophies to advise about the aspects of the prognosis affecting employment, so that appropriate training and careers may be planned in advance.

Additional points in the management of specific types of muscular dystrophy are discussed in subsequent sections of this Chapter.

THE PURE MUSCULAR DYSTROPHIES

Severe X-linked (Duchenne) muscular dystrophy

This, the commonest muscular dystrophy, is X-linked recessive in inheritance and thus, in its typical form, affects only males and, very rarely, females with Turner's syndrome. Minor or abortive forms may occur in occasional female carriers of the gene, but never in males. It is characterised by: (a) onset usually before the fourth year, rarely as late as the seventh; (b) symmetrical and at first selective involvement of the muscles of the pelvic and pectoral girdles; (c) hypertrophy of the calves and certain other muscles at some stage of the disease in almost every case; (d) relentlessly progressive weakness in every case, leading to inability to walk within 10 years of the onset and later to contractures and thoracic deformity; (e) invariable cardiac involvement; (f) frequent, but not invariable, intellectual impairment; (g) death by the second or third decade, rarely later, caused by respiratory or, less frequently, cardiac failure, often associated with inanition and respiratory infection; (h) very high activity of certain muscle enzymes, notably creatine kinase, in serum in the early stages of the disease; and (i) certain characteristic histological features in muscle.

Incidence. Estimates of the incidence of Duchenne muscular dystrophy range from 13 to 33 per 100 000 liveborn males, and of its prevalence in the population as a whole from 1.9 to 3.4 per 100 000. One-third of cases are new mutants, one-third have a previous family history and one-third are born to unwitting and often mutant carriers (Gardner-Medwin, 1970; Brooks and Emery, 1977; Danieli, Mostacciuolo, Bonfante and Angelini, 1977).

Cases of true Duchenne muscular dystrophy in girls occur only in Turner's syndrome (XO genotype) and are very rare (Walton, 1956a; Ferrier, Bamatter and Klein, 1965; Jalbert, Mouriquand, Beaudoing and Jaillard, 1966). Theoretically, a girl homozygous for the gene might result from the union of a female carrier with a man in whom a gonadal mutation of the Duchenne gene had occurred, but this has never been reported. Occasionally, female heterozygotes show moderately severe manifestations, but these are always less severe than in affected boys. Extreme examples were reported by Gomez, Engel, De wald and Peterson (1977) and Verellen, Freund, de Meyer, Laterre, Ferrière, Scholberg and Frédéric (1978). In the latter case there was a reciprocal translocation of parts of the short arms of chromosomes X and 21 and the authors suggested that this might have affected the random inactivation of the X chromosomes. We have seen a similar case.

Symptoms. The earliest symptom is usually clumsiness in walking, with a tendency to fall. In many cases, the first attempts to walk are delayed and are awkward from the beginning. About half are still unable to walk at the age of 18 months. General developmental delay, especially involving speech, is not uncommon and may divert the clinician's attention from the neuromuscular problem. In other cases, progress may be apparently normal until the third year and very occasionally parents do not report anything abnormal until the sixth or seventh year. Then the child's walking begins to lack briskness and freedom of movement; often this is erroneously attributed to 'laziness' or flat feet, or some other comparatively trivial complaint. It is common to find that parents who have had a dystrophic child can detect the earliest signs of the disease in a second son, at a time when no abnormal signs can be identified by an experienced clinician. Inability to run is often a useful early guide. Soon the boy has increasing difficulty in climbing stairs and in rising from the floor (Fig. 14.1). The method of climbing up the legs to reach a standing position is characteristic (Gowers, 1879). He walks with a waddle and protrudes his abdomen, later rising on to his toes with feet wide apart and shoulders and chin drawn back. Weakness of the upper limbs is often not reported until up to five years after the onset, but it can be found on examination long before this.

Course. At the age of four or five years the boy's growth may outstrip the progress of the disease, giving a false impression of improvement, otherwise deterioration is continuous and most patients become unable to walk between the ages of seven and 11 years. A rapid increase in weakness may

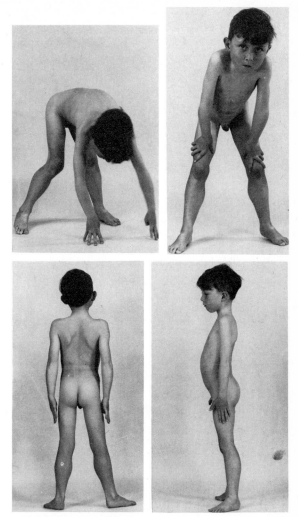

Fig. 14.1   The Duchenne type of muscular dystrophy: note the hypertrophy of the calves and the characteristic method of rising from the floor (Walton, 1962, in Bourne and Golarz *Muscular Dystrophy in Man and Animals*. Basle and New York: Karger)

follow bed rest, but the childhood exanthems rarely affect the condition if the child is kept active. Surgical procedures designed to lengthen Achilles tendons are particularly dangerous in this respect. Archibald and Vignos (1959) stress the importance of early contractures of the hip flexors in accentuating postural difficulties and leading to early confinement to a wheelchair. Once the wheelchair stage is reached, other contractures develop rapidly, especially in the hamstrings and biceps, and weakness of spinal muscles almost invariably leads to increasing scoliosis. Eventually the deformity may make even a wheelchair existence impossible and the patient is confined to bed, able to speak, swallow and breathe, but otherwise retaining feeble power only in the movements of the face, in the grip and in plantar flexion of the feet and toes. Only a quarter of cases survive beyond the age of 21 years and survival beyond 25 years is rare. Death usually results from chest infection with respiratory and sometimes cardiac failure.

Physical examination. Weakness and wasting usually begin in the iliopsoas, quadriceps and gluteus muscles and soon spread to involve the anterior tibial group. In the upper limbs, the costal origin of pectoralis major, the latissimus dorsi, the biceps, triceps and brachioradialis muscles are the first involved. Scapular winging occurs, but is not prominent in the early stages. Hypotonia at the shoulders when the child is lifted is a useful early sign. Later, power is better retained in the wrist flexors than extensors, in the hamstrings than in quadriceps, in the invertors of the foot than in the evertors and in neck extension than in flexion. The calf muscles may remain remarkably strong for several years. Slight facial weakness, especially of movements of the mouth, is usual in the later stages. Late in the course, the intercostal muscles become weak, but diaphragmatic movement is relatively normal. Progressive deterioration of respiratory function occurs, sometimes with severe terminal carbon dioxide retention (Burke, Grove, Houser and Johnson, 1971; Inkley, Oldenburg and Vignos, 1974).

Muscular hypertrophy, later followed by the pseudohypertrophic phase of fatty replacement of muscle, is commonly seen in the calves (Fig. 14.1) and muscles of mastication, less often in the deltoids, wrist extensors and quadriceps and occasionally in other muscles. Denervation of muscle (as in poliomyelitis) may abolish it, and it usually disappears spontaneously as the disease progresses. It is rare for cases of otherwise typical Duchenne muscular dystrophy to show no muscular enlargement at any stage of the disease. Macroglossia is not uncommon.

The tendon reflexes are diminished in the upper limbs early in the disease and the knee jerks also disappear soon. The ankle jerks, however, remain brisk until a comparatively late stage. Contractures generally develop first in the calf muscles and hip flexors and give rise to progressive plantar flexion and inversion of the feet, and to hip contractures with compensatory lumbar lordosis; they are seen later in the hamstrings and biceps brachii.

Some of these children become generally wasted as the disease progresses, but many become very obese, presumably because of a combination of excessive feeding and immobility. Studies of endocrine function have failed to reveal why some are thin and others obese. Sexual development is usually normal, but puberty may be delayed.

Intellectual changes. Intellectual retardation is common in Duchenne muscular dystrophy (Allen and Rodgin, 1960; Worden and Vignos, 1962). Indeed, it occurred in Duchenne's earliest cases and led him to believe at first that the disorder was of cerebral origin. About one-third of cases have an intelligence quotient (IQ) below 75 and a significant minority are below 50; about a tenth are above average. Mean IQ levels in different series vary between about 70 and 85 (Dubowitz, 1965; Zellweger and Hanson, 1967a; Cohen, Molnar and Taft, 1968; Prosser, Murphy and Thompson, 1969; Kozicka, Prot and Wasilewski, 1971; Marsh and Munsat, 1974; Kohno, 1978). However, the most thorough population surveys (Cohen *et al.*, 1968; Kohno, 1978) gave the highest figures for mean IQ. Verbal ability is usually most severely affected. There is no evidence of progressive intellectual deterioration and, except in the series described by Rosman (1970), the severity of the muscular and intellectual involvement are not correlated. The intelligence levels of affected siblings are often similar, but no abnormality has been found in carriers, and the sons of known carriers are no more severely affected than are sporadic cases (Prosser *et al.*, 1969). Kozicka *et al.* (1971) found that the electroencephalogram (EEG) was abnormal more often in retarded cases, but the study by Barwick, Osselton and Walton (1965) revealed no abnormality in the EEG in Duchenne dystrophy. Rosman and Kakulas (1966) found cerebral-neuronal heterotopias at autopsy in three retarded boys with Duchenne dystrophy, but not in four patients with normal intelligence. Their cases were somewhat atypical, however, and Dubowitz and Crome (1969) found no significant abnormality in the brain in 21 autopsied patients, in five of whom the IQ had been below 60.

Skeletal changes. The pattern of skeletal deformity occurring in patients with the Duchenne type muscular dystrophy was reviewed in detail by Walton and Warrick (1954). The changes include narrowing of the shafts and rarefaction of the ends of the long bones (Fig. 14.2), impaired development of flat bones and coxa valga. At a later stage there is almost invariably severe spinal curvature, widespread decalcification and eventually gross distortion and disorganisation of the skeletal system. These changes render the affected bones liable to fracture as a result of minimal trauma, and a child may fracture a femur on falling from a wheelchair. Although it has been suggested that the bony abnormality in some of these cases is an associated inherited dystrophy of bone, Walton and Warrick (1954) gave reasons for concluding that the bone changes are the result of disuse and of

the absence of normal muscular stresses and strains, as well as of the abnormal posture of the body and extremities which results from the muscle disease. A minority of cases develop a long thoracolumbar lordosis instead of the more usual kyphoscoliosis (Wilkins and Gibson, 1976).

Cardiac involvement. This is probably invariable in the true Duchenne form of the disease, although it may not be detectable in the early stages (Zatuchni, Aegerter, Molthan and Shuman, 1951; Walton and Nattrass, 1954; Manning and Cropp, 1958; Perloff, de Leon and O'Doherty, 1966; Slucka, 1968). Persistent tachycardia is common and sudden death from myocardial failure may occur (Berenbaum and Horowitz, 1956) but chronic cardiac failure is rare. Of particular importance is the characteristic electrocardiogram which shows tall R waves in the right precordial leads and deep Q waves in the limb leads and the left precordial leads (Fig. 14.3). Schott, Jacobi and Wald (1955), Skyring and McKusick (1961), Perloff et al. (1966) and Emery (1972) have claimed that this ECG pattern is of diagnostic value in distinguishing between the juvenile forms of muscular dystrophy. Perloff, Roberts, de Leon and O'Doherty (1967) have shown that the pathological basis for this distinctive ECG in two cases was interstitial and

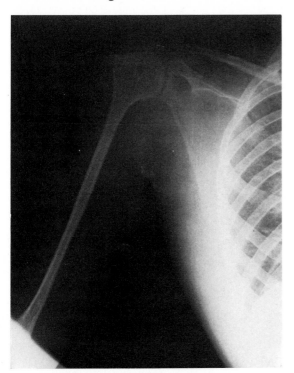

Fig. 14.2 Atrophy of the humerus in an advanced case of Duchenne muscular dystrophy (Walton, 1962)

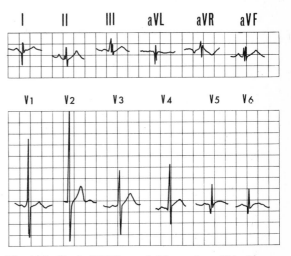

Fig. 14.3 Typical ECG recorded from a boy of 14 with Duchenne muscular dystrophy. There are narrow but deep Q waves in leads I, AVL, V_5 and V_6, and RSR$_1$ pattern in AVR and dominant R waves in V_1 and V_2

replacement fibrosis of the basal part of the left ventricular free wall. Echocardiography has recently indicated relatively good preservation of myocardial function in Duchenne dystrophy, despite the ECG changes. There is, however, some reduction in the rate of diastolic relaxation (Kovick, Fogelman, Abbasi, Peter and Pearce, 1975; Ahmad, Sanderson, Dubowitz and Hallidie-Smith, 1978; Lane, Gardner-Medwin and Roses, 1980). A variety of disturbances of rhythm, including labile tachycardia, may occur. Disease of the nodal arteries may account for some of these (James, 1962; Perloff *et al.*, 1967).

Pathogenesis. This is unknown. Hypotheses in the recent past have suggested a defect in muscle fibre regeneration which interfered with the repair of the normal wear and tear of muscle (Hudgson, Pearce and Walton, 1967); the occurrence of multiple microscopic infarcts of muscle due to a hypothetical vascular lesion in intramuscular arterioles (Mendell, Engel and Derrer, 1971) and a functional defect in spinal anterior horn cells in some way inducing a trophic degenerative lesion in muscle (McComas *et al.*, 1971). None of these hypotheses has stood up to critical investigation, although each is supported by certain items of experimental evidence. At present a hypothesis, rather more promising than the previous ones, postulates a defect in the sarcolemmal membrane which allows a substance or substances, as yet unknown but which could possibly be calcium, to enter the muscle fibre too freely, and there to activate neutral proteases which, in turn, maintain an excessive degree of muscle catabolism and lead to muscle fibre necrosis (Mokri and Engel, 1975; Rowland, 1976; Ebashi and Sugita, 1978; *see also* Ch. 5, 9 and 12).

Diagnosis. The typical distribution of muscular weakness, wasting and hypertrophy, the characteristic gait, best seen when the child attempts to run or to climb stairs, the characteristic very high levels of serum creatine kinase (CK) activity and the rather typical histological appearances in muscle biopsy sections (*see below*) all make the diagnosis, once suspected, relatively easy to confirm.

The conditions most likely to resemble Duch-enne muscular dystrophy in clinical practice are spinal muscular atrophy, polymyositis, the myopathy associated with osteomalacia or renal failure, and certain congenital and metabolic myopathies including central core disease, juvenile acid maltase deficiency and carnitine deficiency. Detailed clinical examination and investigation including electromyography will rarely leave the matter in doubt. The differential diagnosis from autosomal recessive muscular dystrophy in a young boy is discussed in the section on that disorder.

Between the ages of 1 and 5 years, serum CK activity in Duchenne muscular dystrophy is 100–300 times the upper limit of the normal range and other muscle enzymes (aldolase, SGOT, pyruvate kinase, lactic dehydrogenase and others) are also grossly elevated (*see* Ch. 12). No other gradually progressive myopathy gives such high serum enzyme levels. The diagnosis may be made at birth (Heyck, Laudahn and Carsten, 1966). In the neonatal period the normal range of serum CK is higher (Gilboa and Swanson, 1976) but in a large-scale screening survey the activities in newborn cases of Duchenne muscular dystrophy were at least 2.5 times the highest normal figures and 20–50 times the normal mean (Dellamonica, 1978). After birth the CK levels rise over the first year or so and then fall gradually from the age of 2–3 years so that, in very advanced cases, they are only 1–5 times the upper normal limit.

The muscle biopsy in the first few weeks of life may show only a small excess of endomysial connective tissue and the presence of many large hyaline muscle fibres. As the activity of the disease reaches its peak, the muscle fascicles become 'fossilised' by a mesh of perimysial and endomysial connective tissue, the scattered hyaline fibres remain prominent, and active muscle necrosis, phagocytosis and regeneration are conspicuous. Gradually the muscle fibres, which are rounded, often showing splitting and central nuclei, and which vary greatly in size, are replaced by increasing quantities of fat. In the late stages of the disease so little muscle may be left in the mass of fat and fibrous tissue that the biopsy is no longer diagnostic. It is our view that the diagnosis of a new case of muscular dystrophy is so important to the patient and his family that muscle biopsy should always be performed to confirm it.

The confirmation of the diagnosis is usually easy. The difficulty lies in early clinical recognition of the disease. The mean age at diagnosis in the UK is about 5.8 years (Gardner-Medwin, Bundey and Green, 1978). This delay may result in the conception of further preventable cases in the family. The development of a micro-method of CK analysis which can be performed on a dried blood spot (Zellweger and Antonik, 1975) has enabled large-scale neonatal screening projects to be set up in several parts of the world (Zellweger and Antonik, 1975; Beckmann and Scheuer-brandt, 1976; Dellamonica, 1978; Dellamonica, Robert, Cotte, Collombel and Dorche, 1978; Drummond and Veale, 1978). Altogether about 56 000 male neonates have been screened and the incidence of Duchenne muscular dystrophy among them has been 1 in 3500 males. At best, neonatal screening can theoretically prevent 12–15 per cent of cases and is likely to have an unpredict-able and psychologically hazardous effect upon the parents' relationship with their newborn son in all of the families identified. Screening boys with psychomotor developmental delay at the ages of 18 months to 3 years would be less effective but would still be valuable and would probably have less harmful emotional consequences (Gardner-Medwin et al., 1978; Gardner-Medwin, 1979).

The possibility of prenatal diagnosis of Duch-enne muscular dystrophy has been considered since the development of micro-methods of CK estimation and the technique of fetal (placental) blood sampling under direct endoscopic control. Mahoney, Haseltine, Hobbins, Banker, Caskey and Golbus (1977) found an apparently raised CK level in the male fetus of a suspected carrier, terminated the pregnancy and found some evid-ence, in the fetal muscle, of necrosis which they interpreted as confirming the diagnosis. Several males at risk, with 'normal' fetal blood CK levels have subsequently been confirmed as normal at term, but the report of a 'false negative' case by Ionasescu, Zellweger and Cancilla (1978) raises serious doubts about this technique, which would be valuable only if it were capable of distinguish-ing affected from normal male fetuses with a high degree of reliability.

Prevention and carrier detection. About one-third of cases of Duchenne muscular dys-trophy in a population not subjected to genetic counselling are theoretically preventable. The contribution which early diagnosis can make to prevention has already been discussed. Con-siderably more cases could be prevented by the active tracing, investigation and counselling of potential female carriers. The clinician who makes the diagnosis of Duchenne muscular dystrophy thereby acquires the responsibility of making genetic advice available to his patient's female relatives.

The most important achievements of recent muscular dystrophy research have been in carrier detection. For a woman known to be a carrier of the gene for one of the X-linked dystrophies there is a 1 in 4 chance that any pregnancy will result in an affected son. When a woman at risk seeks genetic advice, examination of the family history will allow her to be assigned to one of the following categories (Pearce, Pennington and Walton, 1964; Thompson, Murphy and McAlpine, 1967). *De-finite carriers* are those mothers of an affected son who have also an affected brother, maternal uncle, sister's son or other male relative in the female line of inheritance; also mothers of affected sons by different, non-consanguineous fathers. *Probable carriers* are the mothers of two or more affected sons, who have no other affected relatives. In practice they should be counselled as known carriers. *Possible carriers* are the mothers of isolated cases and the sisters and other female relatives of affected males. The possible carriers may have a high risk of heterozygosity (as in the daughter of a definite carrier where the risk is 1 in 2), or a low risk (as in a distant female cousin with many unaffected males in intervening gen-erations). But in all of them the probability may be calculated after examination of the pedigree (Wiesmann, Moser, Richterich and Rossi, 1965; Emery and Morton, 1968).

The next stage in carrier identification depends upon the fact that many, and perhaps all, true carriers have a slight degree of myopathy which can usually be detected by investigation. Oc-casionally this gives rise to definite muscular hypertrophy (Emery, 1963) or weakness (Chung, Morton and Peters, 1960; Moser, Wiesmann,

Richterich and Rossi, 1964) but in the great majority it is subclinical. There is some evidence that the tendency for carriers to 'manifest' in this way runs in certain families (Moser and Emery, 1974) but Gomez *et al.* (1977) reported extreme discordance of the degree of manifestation in identical twin girls. The most successful method of detecting the myopathy is the estimation of certain serum enzyme levels, of which aldolase and especially CK are the most valuable (Schapira, Dreyfus, Schapira and Demos, 1960). The experience of a number of investigators who have used serum CK estimations was reviewed in previous editions of this chapter and in Gardner-Medwin, Pennington and Walton (1971). Major series have been reported by Hughes (1963), Sugita and Tyler (1963), Milhorat and Goldstone (1965), Wilson, Evans and Carter (1965), Dreyfus, Schapira, Demos, Rosa and Schapira (1966), Emery and Walton (1967), Thompson *et al.* (1967) and Hausmanowa-Petrusewicz, Prot, Niebroj-Dobosz, Hetnarska, Emeryk, Wasowicz, Askanas and Slucka (1968). About 70–75 per cent of definite carriers can be detected in this way. However, in some of these series the normal range of CK levels was rather strictly interpreted and the proportion of carriers with levels above the 97 per cent and 99 per cent confidence limits of the normal range was considerably less than 70 per cent. It is therefore important in interpreting the significance of serum CK levels in potential carriers to know the relative probability of a given CK level being found in a carrier compared with a normal person. This relative probability may then be combined with the prior probability obtained from the pedigree, on Bayesian principles, to obtain the overall risk for the individual (Emery and Morton, 1968; Dennis, Evans, Clayton and Carter, 1976). Spurious elevation of serum CK activity may occur after exercise and falsely low levels have been reported in early pregnancy (Blyth and Hughes, 1971; Emery and King, 1971). Recent reports have also stressed the potential effect of age upon CK levels in carriers and in normal females, in both of whom a decline has been reported in the second and third decades. There is some evidence that carriers may be more readily identified in childhood, but more comparisons with series of normal children are needed before early diagnosis of carriers can be relied upon (Nicholson, Gardner-Medwin, Pennington and Walton, 1979).

Electromyography may also be helpful. The most useful methods have been EMG sampling of multiple muscles as a preliminary to muscle biopsy (Smith, Amick and Johnson, 1966), measurement of the absolute refractory period of muscle fibres (Caruso and Buchthal, 1965), measurement of the duration and number of phases of the motor unit action potentials (van den Bosch, 1963; Hausmanowa-Petrusewicz *et al.*, 1968; Gardner-Medwin, 1968) and analysis of the interference pattern by the use of an automatic spike counter and computer (Willison, 1967; Moosa, Brown and Dubowitz, 1972). However, only 50–70 per cent of definite carriers can, at present, be identified in this way and the most careful comparison with normal control subjects is essential.

The histology of muscle biopsy material is abnormal in some carriers (Dubowitz, 1963; Emery, 1965; Milhorat, Shafiq and Goldstone, 1966; Pearce, Pearce and Walton, 1966; Roy and Dubowitz, 1970) but the difficulty of obtaining a large enough sample means that negative or uncertain results are frequent. Other methods which have been tried, and which may prove to be of value, are muscle electron microscopy (Afifi, Bergman and Zellweger, 1973), studies of the isoenzyme pattern of lactate dehydrogenase in muscle biopsy specimens (Emery, 1964, 1965) and possibly in the serum of some carriers (Hooshmand, Dove and Suter, 1969), electrocardiography (Mann, de Leon, Perloff, Simanis and Horrigan, 1968; Emery, 1969), the measurement *in vitro* of protein synthesis by polyribosomes in biopsied muscle (Ionasescu, Zellweger and Burmeister, 1976), the detection of myoglobinaemia (Adornato, Kagen and Engel, 1978) and the frequency of the 'capping' phenomenon in lymphocytes (Pickard, Gruemer, Verrill, Isaacs, Robinow, Nance, Myers and Goldsmith, 1978). The highest detection rates have so far been obtained by the use of a combination of several methods in each potential carrier (Hausmanowa-Petrusewicz *et al.*, 1968; Radu, Migea, Torok, Bordeianu and Radu, 1968; Gardner-Medwin *et al.*, 1971). However, great caution must be used in interpreting minor deviations from normal in one or more items in a battery of tests, because confidence limits for the normal range for the battery as a whole are not usually available.

Definitely abnormal results from any of these investigations make it highly probable that a woman is indeed a carrier. It is when the results are all normal that difficulties in advising her will arise, because none of the tests is invariably positive in known carriers. In these circumstances, advice can still be given in terms of the probability that she is a carrier, estimated from the precise level of her serum CK within the normal range, together with the application of Bayes' theorem to her pedigree (Emery and Morton, 1968; Emery and Holloway, 1977).

The effectiveness of systematic carrier tracing and counselling has been demonstrated in Ontario, Western Australia and Northern England (Hutton and Thompson, 1976; Kakulas and Hurse, 1978; Gardner-Medwin, 1978).

Management. No treatment is at present known which has any definite influence upon muscular dystrophy. A great many remedies, too numerous to mention, have been tried in the past. Among those given and found wanting have been glycine, vitamin E, corticosteroids, multiple amino acid and vitamin therapy, isoniazid, adenosine triphosphate, high-energy anabolic steroids, 'Laevodosin' and penicillamine. Claims have been made, without adequate evidence and with no independent confirmation, for the efficacy of butylsympathol (Demos, 1963) and allopurinol (Thomson and Smith, 1978). In our view there is no justification for using these, or any other potentially harmful drugs, in this disease except in the context of a properly constituted, controlled, clinical trial.

The absence of specific treatment for muscular dystrophy makes it all the more important to prevent its physical, emotional, social and educational complications and to provide active support for the family throughout the course of the disease. The clinician's first responsibility is to provide an unequivocal diagnosis and enough information and constructive suggestions to enable the family to formulate practical plans for the future. These must be given in relaxed sessions after the initial shock has passed. Females potentially at risk of being carriers should be actively traced and offered genetic advice at this time. In the early stages, the most useful activities for the parents are encouraging regular physical exercise, developing appropriate eating habits to prevent obesity and the stimulation of social activities, sporting and cultural interests, hobbies and education to provide a basis for interests in the later stages of the disease. Vignos and Watkins (1966) showed that organised programmes of maximum resistance exercise may increase muscular strength in the adult forms of muscular dystrophy. Such programmes are more difficult in childhood but it is the common experience that Duchenne boys benefit from active exercise and, conversely, that rest is detrimental. Bed rest for minor illness or trauma should be avoided whenever possible and regular exercise in the form of walking, swimming and games, a little more than the boy really wants to do, should be encouraged. Older boys can do more formal and deliberate exercises and, in the late stages, these should be continued with emphasis on the upper limbs and on breathing exercises. Wheelchair sports provide both exercise and a boost for morale.

Unlike the muscular weakness, contractures are to some extent preventable and reversible. Hip flexion and equinus contractures may significantly alter the stance and interfere with walking at a stage when muscular weakness itself is not severe enough to prevent ambulation. Passive stretching of the hip flexors and iliotibial bands and of soleus and gastrocnemius may therefore be an important part of management. Prone lying to prevent hip flexion contracture is useful. Vignos, Spencer and Archibald (1963) recommend passive stretching for at least 5 seconds repeated 10 times, twice a day. Others suggest more prolonged continuous stretching (Kottke, Pauley and Ptak, 1966) but, in the face of relatively weak antagonist muscles, no regime of stretching will be entirely successful. The dangers of anaesthesia and the increased weakness which follows immobility contraindicate major orthopaedic procedures in these cases, and minor surgery must be undertaken only if immediate postoperative mobilisation is prepared for in advance. Spencer and Vignos (1962) and Vignos et al. (1963) pioneered the active management of the combined weakness and contractures in Duchenne muscular dystrophy, recommending a combination of subcutaneous tenotomy (with brief anaesthesia) and subsequent vigorous physiotherapy and bracing. They enabled some of their patients to walk two or more years longer than usual. Siegel, Miller and Ray (1968), Roy and Gibson (1970) and Dubowitz (1978) recommended similar measures. If tenotomies are to be performed, rapid mobilisation and the maintenance of the corrected position with light alloy calipers are essential. From our own experience we can confirm that it is feasible to prolong ambulation in this way, but one must set against the advantages of this, the sense of relief which patients often feel on accepting a wheelchair existence after a period of exhaustingly difficult walking with frequent falls, and also the time taken up by physiotherapy and the application of complex braces, often at the expense of schooling, and often for the sake of less useful mobility than is possible in a wheelchair (Gardner-Medwin, 1977a). The wheelchair should at first be hand-propelled to provide exercise, but should be replaced with an electrically propelled chair as soon as it no longer provides independent mobility. It is essential, not only to select the right chair for the individual's needs, but to adapt the house and, if necessary, the school, to provide full access for the wheelchair. We often recommend subcutaneous Achilles tenotomy in the early wheelchair state of Duchenne dystrophy with subsequent use of below-knee calipers to prevent the unsightly equinovarus contractures which otherwise occur, simply to allow these boys to wear normal footwear. Contractures at the hips, knees, elbows and wrists occur in the late stages in almost all cases, but these require surgical management only in rare instances where they are persistently painful. Elbow and wrist contractures respond, at least partly, to regular stretching.

Progressive scoliosis usually begins soon after patients become unable to walk (Robin and Brief, 1971) and the prevention of scoliosis is one practical reason for the artificial maintenance of ambulation in appropriate cases. Once it has become established and fixed, it is very difficult to correct or even control and it may go on to cause severe thoracic distortion, respiratory impairment, and a major threat to life. Prevention is often possible, however, in the early stages by careful control of the sitting posture including the position of the legs, with use of leg braces if necessary, and by the use of light spinal braces (Vignos et al., 1963; Dubowitz, 1964; Tunbridge and Diamond, 1966). Respiratory embarrassment must be avoided. Wilkins and Gibson (1976) suggested that the artificial maintenance of a lumbar lordosis in the sitting position might prevent rotation or lateral curvature. They use inserts in specially designed wheelchairs to achieve this and are prepared to undertake spinal fusion if this fails (Gibson, Koreska, Robertson, Kahn and Albisser, 1978). It seems to be possible to induce lumbar lordosis with lightweight moulded polypropylene braces, which allow more active trunk movement than wheelchair inserts. There is no doubt, however, that the management of scoliosis is particularly difficult in this disease and that there is a need for improvement in techniques.

Many aids such as hoists, bath aids and specially adapted clothing are available; these and adaptations to homes and schools can be provided, after their effectiveness and acceptability for each family have been assessed. An occupational therapist may play a dominant part in management when these measures are required. The practical help, advice and emotional support of a social worker are also important. The long inexorable deterioration of the disease is punctuated by crises occurring, for example, at the time of diagnosis, of inability to walk, of changing or leaving school and of illness. Fears of fatal illness, of another child being affected, of pregnancies either in the mother or in her carrier daughters, may be added to the frequent misguided sense of marital guilt on the part of carriers and to the prolonged maintenance of family facades to avoid sharing knowledge, fears and often myths about the disorder. Social isolation is common. Boys may become overprotected, frightened, petulant, resentful, aggressive and lonely. Reactive depression is far commoner in parents than in boys. Many of these problems can be prevented or alleviated by a medical social worker familiar with both the disease and the family.

The combined physical and intellectual handicap presents formidable educational problems. Psychological assessment of aptitudes as well as limitations can assist in planning both education and hobbies. Many boys with poor verbal skills show special competence in design and modelling. The social isolation of home education should be avoided wherever possible and education should be dovetailed with the limited opportunities that are likely to be available when the boy leaves school.

Complications include obesity in the wheelchair stage: this is easier to prevent than to treat. The calorie requirements of some immobile boys are very low and expert dietary advice may be required to maintain a balanced diet. Fractures, especially of the lower end of the femur, often occur in the more adventurous wheelchair users. The atrophic bones mend remarkably well and only very limited splinting is needed, especially in the lower limbs. No attempt should be made to correct contractures at the same time. Anaesthesia may be hazardous (Cobham and Davis, 1964; Boba, 1970; Genever, 1971; Yamashita, Matsuki and Oyama, 1976) and should be administered by an experienced anaesthetist in hospital, even for minor dental and other procedures. Dependent oedema and bedsores are surprisingly rare complications in Duchenne dystrophy.

Respiratory insufficiency gradually increases during the wheelchair stage of the disease (Inkley et al., 1974). This rarely gives rise to symptoms until sudden decompensation occurs during respiratory infections or other sudden stresses. Death may then occur very suddenly in acute respiratory failure, occasionally with terminal heart failure. Cardiac arrhythmias, although often postulated as a cause of sudden death, are rarely observed and delaying respiratory failure seems to be the only useful approach to prophylaxis. Regular breathing exercises and the prevention of scoliosis are important and all parents should be taught to use postural drainage during respiratory infections, together with appropriate antibiotic therapy. Artificial ventilation during acute infections may be appropriate (and effective) in some circumstances, but tracheostomy or long-term ventilation, even on an intermittent nocturnal basis, are rarely justifiable. Sudden fluctuations in serum potassium, perhaps related to the limited total body (muscle) potassium pool, may cause difficulties in the management of acute illness or in postoperative care.

Recent reviews of the management of Duchenne muscular dystrophy include those of Siegel (1977), Robin and Falewski de Leon (1977), Dubowitz (1978) and Bossingham, Williams and Nichols (1979).

Benign X-linked (Becker) muscular dystrophy

The existence of a distinct benign X-linked recessive form of muscular dystrophy was suggested by Becker and Keiner (1955) who described a family and quoted earlier reports of similar pedigrees. Levison (1951), Lamy and de Grouchy (1954), Walton (1955 and 1956a) and Blyth and Pugh (1959) included examples of this form in their series but did not separate them clearly from other categories. In one family, subsequently recognised as being affected with Becker rather than with Duchenne dystrophy, linkage with colour blindness was noted (Philip, Walton and Smith, 1956). Subsequent reports by Becker (1957 and 1962), Dreifuss and Hogan (1961), Moser et al. (1964), Mabry, Roeckel, Munich and Robertson (1965), Rotthauwe and Kowalewski (1965a), Emery and Dreifuss (1966), Markand, North, D'Agostino and Daly (1969), Emery and Skinner (1976), Ringel, Carroll and Schold (1977), Bradley, Jones, Mussini and Fawcett (1978) and others make it clear that the benign cases are distinct and are not simply part of a spectrum of severity. Indeed, the Becker type of muscular dystrophy is now more clearly characterised than some of the traditional categories. Families are occasionally found in which cases of the Becker and Duchenne types seem to coexist (Furukawa and Peter, 1977), but these probably simply reflect the extremes of variation in severity of the two disorders. Genetic linkage data suggest that the Duchenne and Becker genes occupy widely separated loci on the X-chromosome and are not allelic (Skinner, Smith and Emery, 1974; Zatz, Itskan, Sanger, Frota-Pessoa and Saldanha, 1974). The report by Henson, Muller and De Myer (1967), of a hereditary myopathy confined to females, is interesting in this connection. The pedigree suggests an X-linked dominant gene lethal in affected males and may thus represent a yet more severe example of this group of X-linked myopathies.

It may be that even the benign X-linked type of muscular dystrophy should be subdivided. The family reported by Dreifuss and Hogan (1961) and Emery and Dreifuss (1966) differed from typical Becker dystrophy in that the onset was early (age 4–5 years) but the course was benign, contractures were prominent in the early stages, pseudohypertrophy was absent and the myocardium was involved.

Incidence. Perhaps because of the difficulty of identifying sporadic cases, no reliable figures for incidence or prevalence are available. It is our impression that the incidence is of the order of one-tenth to one-fifth and the prevalence of the order of one-third to one-half that of the Duchenne type (Gardner-Medwin, 1970). Emery and Skinner (1976) found the fertility of affected males to be 67 per cent that of their unaffected brothers. These figures imply an incidence of about 3–6 per 100 000 male births, a prevalence of about 1 per 100 000 of the whole population and a mutation rate of about $0.3–0.6 \times 10^{-5}$ per gene per generation, but these figures are very tentative.

Clinical features. The selective muscle involvement is virtually identical to that in Duchenne muscular dystrophy. Symptoms are noticed in the lower limbs 5–10 years before the upper limbs, but examination will usually reveal the typically affected shoulder muscles in any patient with symptoms. There is selective bilateral and symmetrical wasting and weakness of the costal origin of pectoralis major, latissimus dorsi, brachioradialis, hip flexors and extensors and medial vastus of quadriceps. Later the supinator, biceps, triceps, serratus anterior and neck flexors become weak, and the adductors and abductors of the thigh and anterior tibial muscles are involved. Deltoids, the flexors and extensors of the wrists and fingers, small hand muscles, hamstrings and calf muscles are relatively preserved. The face is virtually completely spared, even in the late stages. The tendon reflexes are impaired and later absent in affected muscles. Hypertrophy of the calves is a prominent and almost constant feature, and the deltoids, extensor muscles in the forearm, lateral vasti of the quadriceps and anterior tibial muscles are commonly hypertrophic at some stage of the disease. The calf enlargement affects both the gastrocnemii and soleus muscles and may precede all other symptoms by several years. Muscle cramp in the early stages is more frequent than in any other type of muscular dystrophy except myotonic dystrophy. The first symptoms otherwise are usually difficulty in running or in hurrying up stairs and, later, in doing heavy work with the arms. The lordotic standing posture and waddling gait are very similar to those seen in Duchenne muscular dystrophy. Contractures are not a feature in typical Becker dystrophy until the patient is confined to a wheelchair, but pes cavus is reported in between 15 per cent (Bradley et al., 1978) and 70 per cent (Ringel et al., 1977) of cases. Scoliosis, although emphasised by Ringel et al., is usually not severe and thoracic distortion is very uncommon. No careful studies of respiratory function have been reported but respiratory failure seems to be rare.

Early cardiac involvement is not a feature in typical Becker dystrophy. In the late stages a minority of cases have significant electrocardiographic abnormalities including, in different individuals, bundle-branch block, Q waves, increased R/S ratios and T-wave changes. A few develop clinical cardiac failure and this is sometimes the cause of death (Mabry et al., 1965; Markand et al., 1969; Emery and Skinner, 1976; Bradley et al., 1978) Myocardial involvement seems to be more prominent in a few families (Wadia, Wadgaonkar, Amin and Sardesai, 1976).

Although the great majority of patients with Becker muscular dystrophy are of normal intelligence, and some are of superior intelligence, there does seem to be a significant minority with mental retardation (Zellweger and Hanson, 1967b; Emery and Skinner, 1976; Ringel et al., 1977; Bradley et al., 1978). As in patients with Duchenne dystrophy, this retardation appears to be non-progressive and, in our experience, may be the presenting problem with later recognition of muscle weakness.

Hallen (1970) reported a high incidence of hypogonadism in 'pelvic-girdle' types of muscular dystrophy including the Becker type. We have not encountered this or any other systemic manifestation of this disease, and the fertility of cases reported by Emery and Skinner (1976) and mentioned above is not consistent with hypogonadism.

Course of the disease. This is the principal point of distinction from the Duchenne type. In Becker cases, symptoms may occur as early as one and as late as 45 years of age, but in the great majority the onset is between the ages of five and 15 years. It seems likely that, in cases reporting a very late onset, clinical examination would have revealed signs of involvement earlier. Few patients are able to run after the second decade. Emery and Skinner (1976) reported the following mean ages and ranges for the 'milestones' of the disease: onset 11.1 years (range 2.5–21); inability to walk 27.1 years (range 12–38) (some cases continued to walk up to the age of 63); death 42.2 years (range 23–63). Shaw and Dreifuss (1969) and Bradley et al. (1978) reported very similar figures, but in the experience of Becker (1964) the age at onset extends from five to 30 years and only 10 per cent became unable to walk before the age of 40 years. Emery and Skinner (1976) gave figures for Duchenne cases for comparison as follows: onset 2.8 years (range 0–6); inability to walk 8.5 years (range 6–12); death 16.0 years (range 8–22). They found that in 90 per cent of Becker cases the onset was after 4.7 years and that in 90 per cent of Duchenne cases it was before this age; that 97 per cent of cases became unable to walk after and before 11.2 years respectively, and that 94 per cent died after and before the age of 20.3 years respectively. These figures are of great value in the differential diagnosis. There is no evidence that the course in Becker dystrophy is intermittently progressive or that the disease arrests at any stage, although it may be almost imperceptibly slow for long periods.

Diagnosis. The Becker type of muscular dystrophy is distinguished from the Duchenne type on the basis of severity and rate of progression, and from the scapuloperoneal and limb-girdle forms on the basis of the selective muscle involvement. Detailed muscle examination will usually distinguish cases of spinal muscular atrophy, but cases of the latter with similar selective weakness, muscle hypertrophy and X-linked inheritance have been described (Pearn and Hudgson, 1978).

Investigation will usually leave little doubt about the diagnosis. The serum CK activity is extremely high in the preclinical and early stages of the disease and falls steeply with age (Rotthauwe and Kowalewski, 1965a; Emery and Skinner, 1976; Bradley et al., 1978). In the first 10 years of life the serum CK levels are comparable with those seen in Duchenne cases at the same age (25–200 times normal) and one case has been identified by neonatal screening (Drummond and Veale, 1978). After the age of 20 the serum CK levels are lower, 1–10 times normal in the Emery and Skinner (1976) series and usually 2–60 times normal in the Newcastle series (Bradley et al., 1978). It seems likely, but is not yet certain, that the disease can be ruled out by a normal serum CK level in the preclinical age group.

The EMG usually demonstrates a pattern of short-duration low-amplitude polyphasic potentials with some fibrillation potentials and positive waves (Zellweger and Hanson, 1967b; Markand et al., 1969; Bradley et al., 1978). Bradley et al. reported that the findings in some cases suggested neurogenic atrophy, but giant motor units and grossly reduced interference patterns are not seen in Becker muscular dystrophy. As in Duchenne muscular dystrophy, high-frequency and myotonic discharges are occasionally seen.

The histological findings in Becker muscular dystrophy have been reviewed by Dubowitz and Brooke (1973), Ringel et al. (1977) and Bradley et al. (1978). Random variation in fibre size (both atrophy and hypertrophy), fibre splitting, central nuclei and fibrosis are the major features. Active necrosis and regeneration are more prominent in young patients. Bradley et al. (1978) discuss the difficulty of differentiating the findings from those of neurogenic atrophy in some cases.

Carrier detection and prevention. Carrier detection in Becker muscular dystrophy is even less satisfactory than in the Duchenne type. Carriers only occasionally have detectable muscle weakness (Aguilar, Lisker and Ramos, 1978). Rotthauwe and Kowalewski (1965b) and Wilson et al. (1965) showed that some carriers can be identified by serum CK estimation and a few have abnormal EMGs (Gardner-Medwin, 1968). The largest study was that of Skinner, Emery, Anderson and Foxall (1975) who found that about 60 per cent of definite carriers have serum CK activities above their normal 95 per cent confidence limits (and about 40 per cent above the 99 per cent limit). They found a distinct fall in CK levels with age throughout the first to eighth decades indicating the great importance of early testing for genetic counselling in this disease. Accurate estimates of the risks for potential Becker carriers can be made only in laboratories with extensive experience of the disease.

The principles of counselling in Becker and Duchenne families are the same. All the daughters of affected males are definite carriers of the gene.

X-linked scapuloperoneal myopathy

Cases of a progressive scapuloperoneal syndrome of myopathic origin and with X-linked inheritance were described by Rotthauwe, Mortier and Beyer (1972) and Thomas, Calne and Elliott (1972). The symptoms began in early childhood and progressed over four to six decades. There was wasting and weakness in scapuloperoneal distribution without facial weakness. Muscle hypertrophy was absent. Contractures at the elbows and of the posterior neck muscles and calf muscles were prominent and there was pes cavus. Cardiomyopathy was present in three of the cases of Thomas et al. (1972) and atrioventricular block in some cases described by Rotthauwe et al. (1972), and heart disease was the usual cause of death. The serum CK activity was raised two- to twenty-fold in the first 25 years of life but was normal in older cases. Female carriers had normal serum CK levels (Rotthauwe et al., 1972). The EMG and muscle histology suggested myopathy, without specific diagnostic features. In the family described by Thomas et al. (1972) the disorder was closely linked with deutan colour blindness.

The scapuloperoneal syndrome is much more frequently neurogenic than myopathic in origin (Kaeser, 1965; Emery, Fenichel and Eng, 1968; see also Ch. 20) but some other cases of myopathic origin have been described (see Thomas et al. (1972) for early references; Feigenbaum and Munsat, 1970). Those cases in which autosomal dominant inheritance is recorded and which are

neither neurogenic in origin, nor abortive or incompletely expressed examples of facioscapulohumeral muscular dystrophy (Ricker and Mertens, 1968; Kazakov, Bogorodinsky and Skorometz, 1976), are discussed later in this chapter. The remarkably similar X-linked scapuloperoneal spinal muscular atrophy described by Mawatari and Katayama (1973) and the cases of Waters, Nutter, Hopkins and Dorney (1975) in which both myopathic and neurogenic features occurred, raise the question of whether the myopathic cases described here might have had spinal muscular atrophy with secondary myopathic changes. The balance of evidence makes this unlikely, but it is unfortunate that in the only autopsied case (Thomas et al., 1972) the spinal cord was not examined.

The limb-girdle muscular dystrophies

The term limb-girdle muscular dystrophy was introduced by Walton and Nattrass (1954) to describe cases of both sexes, usually autosomal recessive in inheritance, in which the facial muscles were not involved, and the symptoms of proximal muscle weakness began in the second or third decade and progressed slowly to a stage of severe disability about 20 years after the onset, with some shortening of life expectancy. This definition encompassed the classical pelvic girdle atrophic and juvenile scapulohumeral forms. Since that time, the Becker type of muscular dystrophy, the Kugelberg-Welander 'pseudomyopathic' type of spinal muscular atrophy, the scapuloperoneal syndrome, a variety of 'congenital myopathies' which may sometimes cause symptoms only in the second and third decade and a wide variety of acquired metabolic and other myopathies have been described and characterised. It has also been realised that female carriers of the Duchenne gene may manifest a significant degree of muscle weakness. Undoubtedly, some cases diagnosed as limb-girdle muscular dystrophy in the past have, in fact, suffered from one or other of these disorders. Furthermore, the limb-girdle type of muscular dystrophy has not shared in the rapid increase in research and medical writing about the muscular dystrophies in the last 20 years. A high proportion of cases has always been found to be sporadic (Morton and Chung, 1959) which adds to the difficulty of delineating familial entities. It seems probable that a number of different autosomal recessive entities exist and, in addition, there are reports of families with autosomal dominant inheritance and a 'limb-girdle' syndrome. The following very tentative subdivision of the types of cases which may be seen is therefore proposed.

Cases with scapulohumeral muscular weakness (Erb, 1884). These are the cases for which the term 'limb-girdle dystrophy' remains most useful (Fig. 14.4). They are uncommon. Becker (1964) did not include any in his comprehensive review of myopathies in Baden. The weakness is at first most prominent in the biceps, triceps, trapezius, rhomboid and serratus anterior muscles, and scapular winging is a major feature.

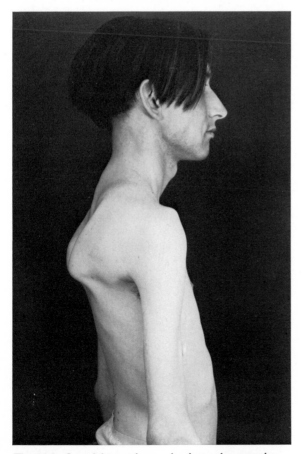

Fig. 14.4 Scapulohumeral muscular dystrophy: note the atrophy of upper limb muscles and the winged scapulae

The deltoid is relatively preserved. The proximal muscles of the lower limbs are affected later, especially the hip flexors and quadriceps with relative preservation of the hamstrings and muscles below the knees. The forearm and hand muscles are also strikingly preserved until the later stages. The condition is usually very slowly but continuously progressive. Ten or even 20 years may elapse before the weakness spreads from the upper to the lower limbs. Moser, Wiesmann, Richterich and Rossi (1966) reported 15 cases of this type from Switzerland where the limb-girdle dystrophies appear to be relatively common. The sexes were equally affected. The age at onset in their cases varied from nine to 31 years but was usually 14–23 years. Hypertrophy of muscles was absent except in one doubtful case, and appears to be rare in this disorder. The serum CK activity was 22 times the normal in the youngest case (aged 14) and normal or only slightly raised (1–5 times normal) in cases over 20 years of age. Our experience is similar.

Contractures often develop in relation to joints in which the active range of movement is limited, but such contractures are not an early feature. The heart is not involved, and intelligence is normal.

The differential diagnosis of this clinical syndrome includes, above all, spinal muscular atrophy. Any patient showing intermittent progression or asymmetry of muscle weakness is particularly likely to have the latter disorder. Nemaline myopathy and thyrotoxic myopathy may present similar features. Diagnosis depends on the clinical and biochemical findings, on the EMG which shows myopathic changes without specific features, and on muscle biopsy to exclude features of the congenital myopathies or denervation. The myopathic features in biopsies of these cases are not specific and are relatively indolent (Dubowitz and Brooke, 1973; Ch. 5).

One of the major disabilities in these patients is in raising the arms. The deltoids may be quite strong, but scapular fixation is very poor. Fixing the scapulae by bracing is not easy and contracture at the shoulder joint may limit the benefit of attempting this. Surgical fixation in carefully selected cases may be valuable (Copeland and Howard, 1978), but the contractures must be overcome first.

Cases with predominant lower-limb weakness. It is this group which has been most severely depleted by the delineation of the spinal muscular atrophies, Becker muscular dystrophy, central core disease, carnitine deficiency, acid maltase deficiency and other genetic myopathies with this pattern of presentation. Acquired myopathies due to polymyositis, sarcoidosis and metabolic bone disease may also present in a similar way. Undoubtedly a pelvifemoral type of autosomal recessive muscular dystrophy exists which presents in childhood or early adult life and which is described in the next section. It is very doubtful whether any separate autosomal recessive lower limb-girdle muscular dystrophy of adult onset exists.

Isolated males presenting in the first three decades of life with pelvifemoral muscular dystrophy associated with muscle hypertrophy are almost all of the Becker type. They should be examined in detail to ascertain whether the precise distribution of muscle weakness conforms to the Becker pattern and, if it does and the investigations are compatible, genetic advice should be given on the basis of X-linked inheritance.

Moser and Emery (1974) have pointed out that the frequency of clinically manifesting female carriers of the Duchenne gene in the population approaches the incidence of undifferentiated limb-girdle muscular dystrophy (20×10^{-6}, Morton and Chung, 1959). While these figures are open to question, it is clear that some apparently isolated female cases of mild to moderately severe muscular dystrophy may well be Duchenne carriers. If a mother or sister were affected, autosomal inheritance might be suspected. Such carriers have weakness in the same distribution as in Duchenne males but it is much less severe, the gait is sometimes waddling with lumbar lordosis, muscle hypertrophy is usually present (sometimes asymmetrically) and the serum CK activity is usually raised several-fold.

'Myopathy confined to the quadriceps' (Bramwell, 1922) should be discussed here. The muscle weakness of adult onset (20–50 years) rarely remains confined to the quadriceps if cases are re-examined after many years (Walton, 1956b; Turner and Heathfield, 1961). Van Wijngaarden, Hagen, Bethlem and Meijer (1968) described two brothers with widespread myopathic changes in the EMG although the clinical involvement was limited to the quadriceps. All other cases have been sporadic. Recent reviews suggest that the condition is heterogeneous, some cases having neurogenic atrophy with secondary myopathic change (Boddie and Stewart-Wynne, 1974; and possibly the cases of Espir and Matthews, 1973), and others a very indolent limb-girdle myopathy. Some may be sporadic cases of the dominant late-onset limb-girdle dystrophy of Bacon and Smith (1971) described in a later section. The serum CK activity may be raised by up to 10-fold.

Childhood muscular dystrophy with autosomal recessive inheritance

This is one of the most difficult categories of muscular dystrophy to characterise. Proof of autosomal recessive inheritance in any given family is rarely possible and therefore the arguments for the existence of this type of the disorder have depended upon the occasional occurrence of muscular dystrophy in girls and in a few families in which consanguinity of the parents has made autosomal recessive inheritance likely. Stevenson (1953) reviewed the early case reports of muscular dystrophy in girls. Lamy and de Grouchy (1954) in their genetic assessment of 102 families with muscular dystrophy with a 'pelvifemoral onset' concluded that in about 90 per cent the inheritance was X-linked and, in about 10 per cent, autosomal recessive. However, in these reports the paucity of clinical information and in particular the lack of EMG or histological evidence make it impossible to be sure that many of the cases described were not, in fact, examples of benign spinal muscular atrophy (Kugelberg and Welander, 1956). The same reservations must be advanced in the assessment of more recent case reports (Stevenson, 1955, Case D58; Blyth and Pugh, 1959; Johnston, 1964) although many of these cases must surely have been examples of muscular dystrophy. Cases which can be fairly confidently accepted as examples of autosomal recessive childhood dystrophy were those of Kloepfer and Talley (1958, Pedigree I), Jackson and Carey (1961), Jackson and Strehler (1968), Ionasescu and Zellweger (1974), Kakulas, Cullity and Maguire (1975),

Shokeir and Kobrinsky (1976) and Dubowitz (1978). Moser *et al.* (1966), in their review of limb-girdle dystrophy in Switzerland, included 14 cases without facial involvement in whom the lower limb muscles were first affected. In nine, the symptoms began between three and nine years of age and in the rest at 15–27 years. It is interesting that the cases of Jackson and Carey (1961) and Shokeir and Kobrinsky (1976) were of Swiss descent. The latter cases had some involvement of facial muscles, and Moser *et al.* (1966) also distinguished a separate autosomal recessive group of seven cases, with onset from the age of 3–17 years, in which the facial muscles were affected. Whether these represent yet another entity within the autosomal recessive muscular dystrophies is not clear. In our experience, slight facial involvement does seem to be a feature in cases with autosomal recessive inheritance. The pure lower limb-girdle group of Moser *et al.* (1966) showed no calf enlargement and their serum CK activities were normal or raised up to 10-fold. The experience of Becker (1964) was different. In south Germany he found that autosomal recessive pelvifemoral dystrophy closely resembled his benign X-linked cases, often showing calf hypertrophy. His recessive cases showed high rates of parental consanguinity and tended to come from small country villages. Our conclusion is that this type of muscular dystrophy is rare, tends to vary in frequency and perhaps in its clinical pattern in different populations and is, in general, much more benign than the Duchenne type from which it is usually easy to distinguish. Penn, Lisak and Rowland (1970) reviewed this subject very thoroughly and concluded that no convincing case of true Duchenne dystrophy had been recorded in a female of normal karyotype and that girls with muscular dystrophy have a separate disorder, generally distinguishable on clinical grounds.

In general, therefore, it seems that this form of the disease is similar to the Duchenne type but rather more benign. The onset may be in the second year or as late as the fourteenth, but is most usual in the second half of the first decade. Progression is comparatively slow and patients usually become unable to walk in their early twenties, sometimes as early as 12 years or as late as 44 years, and many survive to the fifth decade or later (Jackson and Strehler, 1968). The weakness is chiefly proximal and does not appear to have been differentiated clearly in its distribution from that of Duchenne dystrophy, although in some families the facial muscles are spared and in others much more severely affected. Hypertrophy is present in some affected families. ECGs are normal in most cases but this is not a reliable guide because several of the cases described by Jackson and Carey (1961) had QRS changes resembling the typical Duchenne pattern. The serum CK activity is usually only moderately raised (up to 10 times the normal limit); this, perhaps, may not be so in the early stages of the disease, and Jackson and Strehler's cases had much higher levels, some of them in the preclinical stages. In one of the families reported by Kakulas *et al.* (1975) the serum CK approached 100 times the normal level, but the clinical and histological features were less severe than in Duchenne muscular dystrophy. An interesting and very unusual example of severe manifestation of the true X-linked Duchenne gene in one of identical twin girl carriers has been reported by Gomez *et al.* (1977); very rarely, similar isolated cases might masquerade as autosomal recessive muscular dystrophy.

Dubowitz (1978) described some cases of a limb-girdle myopathy associated with cramps and myoglobinuria, in which glycogen- and lipid-storage diseases appeared to have been ruled out. Their significance is not clear.

The principles of management of autosomal recessive childhood muscular dystrophy are the same as for the Duchenne type, taking into account the better prognosis.

Congenital muscular dystrophy

Some of the conditions included in the wider category of the congenital myopathies are discussed in Chapters 17 and 18. The benign congenital myopathy classically described by Batten (1903 and 1909), Turner (1940) and Turner and Lees (1962) differs from the muscular dystrophies in its non-progressive course and in the absence of specific histological features. However, Banker, Victor and Adams (1957), Greenfield, Cornman and Shy (1958), O'Brien (1962), Pearson and

Fowler (1963), Gubbay, Walton and Pearce (1966) and Zellweger, Afifi, McCormick and Mergner (1967) described cases with congenital hypotonia and severe but relatively non-progressive muscular weakness, in which the muscle histology was typical of muscular dystrophy. In several children there was associated arthrogryposis multiplex. The nosological status of these non-progressive congenital muscle disorders remains uncertain and some may even represent non-genetic myopathies acquired *in utero*. Others are undoubtedly autosomal recessive in inheritance (Lebenthal, Shochet, Adam, Seelenfreund, Fried, Najenson, Sandbank and Matoth, 1970).

A few cases of a 'rapidly progressive' type of congenital muscular dystrophy have been reported (de Lange, 1937; Lewis and Besant, 1962; Short, 1963; Wharton, 1965). Of these only Wharton's two cases survived beyond the age of 6 months. The clinical features in these cases varied considerably and the pathological evidence was in general inconclusive. The cases of Short (1963) bear a close resemblance to the X-linked type of centronuclear myopathy (*see* Ch. 17). Further evidence is needed before the existence of a rapidly progressive form of congenital muscular dystrophy can be accepted. In a series of cases from Finland, described by Donner, Rapola and Somer (1975), the symptoms progressed slightly in the first few years of life and thereafter remained static.

The essential features of this disorder are severe hypotonia present from birth, with subsequent development of more or less progressive muscular wasting and weakness. Fetal movements are often impaired. Contractures at birth are common but not invariable, and they may develop later. Some children have difficulty in sucking and breathing in the neonatal period. There is often facial weakness and Donner *et al.* (1975) emphasised severe head lag. The diagnosis can be made with confidence only by examination of the muscle histology. The 'dystrophic' appearances are often severe to a degree that seems out of proportion to the clinical disability, although in some mild cases there are simply non-specific myopathic changes without specific features. Afifi, Zellweger, McCormick and Mergner (1969) emphasised the excessive collagen proliferation and paucity of muscle fibre regeneration. The serum aldolase and CK activities are often normal or only a little raised. Donner *et al.* (1975) reported figures up to 30 times normal in the first three years, falling to 1–5 times normal by the age of five years. Sibs are often affected, but definite evidence of autosomal recessive inheritance is lacking. It is uncommon for cases of Duchenne dystrophy to be hypotonic at birth but, more often, patients with the 'autosomal recessive childhood dystrophy' have been noted to show this sign. For the present, no definite borderline can therefore be drawn between cases of congenital dystrophy and autosomal recessive childhood dystrophy with onset later in life.

In Japan, a separate type of congenital muscular dystrophy is associated with malformation of the central nervous system and severe mental retardation (Kamoshita, Konishi, Segawa and Fukuyama, 1976).

Facioscapulohumeral muscular dystrophy

This variety of muscular dystrophy is characterised by (a) expression in either sex; (b) transmission usually as an autosomal dominant trait, occasionally with apparent sex-limitation in some families; (c) onset at any age from childhood until adult life; (d) the frequent occurrence of abortive or mildly affected cases; (e) initial involvement of the face and shoulder-girdle muscles with subsequent spread to the muscles of the lower limbs; (f) the rarity of muscular hypertrophy; (g) the infrequent occurrence of muscular contractures and skeletal deformity; (h) insidious progress of the disease with prolonged periods of apparent arrest. Although cases occur occasionally in which the disease progresses unusually rapidly, most patients survive and remain active to a normal age.

This type of muscular dystrophy is one of the more clearly defined forms but some cases may cause confusion. Apparently X-linked dominant inheritance may be found in families with no facial weakness (Hertrich, 1957) and, more frequently, apparently isolated or recessive cases of facioscapulohumeral muscular dystrophy may occur (Moser *et al.*, 1966). There is little published evidence as to whether the pattern of muscle involvement is precisely the same in dominant and recessive cases. Cases with minimal facial involvement must be distinguished from examples of the 'scapuloperoneal syndrome' which may be myopathic (Ricker and Mertens, 1968; Thomas, Schott and Morgan-Hughes, 1975) or neurogenic in origin (Kaeser, 1965; Ricker, Mertens and Schimrigk, 1968). Indeed, cases of spinal muscular atrophy may closely resemble facioscapulohumeral muscular dystrophy, even showing dominant inheritance (Fenichel, Emery and Hunt, 1967) but they are more often sporadic. A review of cases with muscular atrophy in facioscapulohumeral distribution undertaken in Newcastle (Bradley, unpublished work) revealed almost equal numbers with 'myopathic' and 'neurogenic' histological findings on muscle biopsy, and a single family with a mitochondrial myopathy (Hudgson, Bradley and Jenkison, 1972; Bradley, Tomlinson and Hardy, 1978). A further diagnostic difficulty was reported by Munsat and Piper (1971), who found inflammatory changes resembling polymyositis in muscle in the early stages of the disease in two families, while true polymyositis with full resolution after therapy may show a similar clinical picture (Rothstein, Carlson and Sumi, 1971). Kazakov, Bogorodinsky, Znoyko and Skorometz (1974), in a study of 200 cases, divided facioscapulohumeral muscular dystrophy into two groups; in the larger, the late lower-limb involvement primarily affected the anterior tibial and peroneal muscles while, in a smaller number, the proximal pelvic girdle muscles were more severely affected. These groups of patients appeared to be genetically distinct. The investigations did not rigorously exclude neurogenic atrophy so some doubts remain about the atypical 'proximal' group.

One of the most striking features of this variety, as previously described by Tyler and Wintrobe (1950) and Walton (1955, 1956a), is the occurrence of partly affected or abortive cases. Many of these patients are unaware that they are suffering from the disease in a mild form and it is therefore very important that, in any study of inheritance, all available family members should be examined. In these abortive cases the disease may remain confined to one or two muscle groups indefinitely.

Incidence. This is quoted as 0.4–5.0 per 100 000 (Morton and Chung, 1959; Becker, 1964). Morton and Chung quoted a prevalence of 0.2 per 100 000. However, the frequency of this type of muscular dystrophy varies considerably in different populations.

Symptoms. The first symptoms of this form of muscular dystrophy are usually seen in the second decade, but there are some patients in whom it begins in the first, while occasionally the onset is apparently delayed until much later in life. Rarely, facial weakness is present at birth or early infancy (Hanson and Rowland, 1971; Brooke, 1977). The symptomatology is virtually identical to that of scapulohumeral muscular dystrophy in that the weakness begins, in most cases, in the shoulder girdles and in the same muscles which are involved in that type. The pelvic girdle muscles are affected much later, but early involvement of the anterior tibial muscles is typical. The additional feature which characterises this form is the facial weakness. Many patients are aware of the progressive change in their facial appearance and realise that they are unable to close their eyes properly and that they cannot whistle. When weakness is advanced they cannot pronounce labials and the speech becomes characteristically indistinct. Scoliosis may occur, but much more often an extensive and severe lumbar lordosis develops. The consequent pelvic tilt, combined with foot-drop and, in some cases, hyperextension of the knees, gives a characteristic gait disability, different from that seen in the other muscular dystrophies.

Course of the disease. This form of muscular dystrophy is very benign in many cases, and there are some who have had the disease since adolescence and who remain active, although with increasing disability, in late life. Even within the same family there may, however, be considerable variation in severity between individuals. There are some in whom the rate of progression is rapid, and walking becomes impossible in middle life, or even in the second or third decade, but this is unusual and in many there are long periods, often of several years, when there is no apparent progression.

The life expectancy in most patients with this form of the disease is therefore normal, but in the more rapidly progressive cases, death from respiratory infection can occur in middle life.

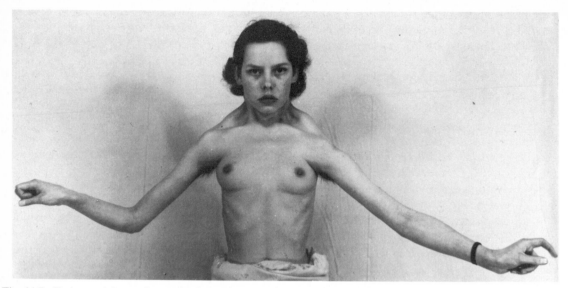

Fig. 14.5   Facioscapulohumeral muscular dystrophy: note the typical facial appearance and bilateral elevation of the scapulae (Walton, 1962)

Physical examination. Muscular hypertrophy is rare in this form, but occasionally occurs in the calves and deltoid muscles.

The facial appearance is characteristic; the face is unlined and wrinkles are often missing from the forehead and around the eyes. There is a typical pouting appearance of the lips and a transverse smile. Affected individuals usually cannot close their eyes or bury their eye-lashes on command, while few can retain air under pressure within the mouth. Occasionally, the facial weakness is so slight as to be difficult to elicit.

The pattern of muscular involvement in the upper and lower limbs is similar to that described above in scapulohumeral dystrophy, but elevation of the scapulae on abduction of the arms (Fig. 14.5) is rather characteristic of the facioscapulohumeral disorder. The neck flexors, serrati, pectorals, biceps, triceps and extensors of the wrists are selectively involved, with relative sparing of the deltoids and wrist flexors. Some asymmetry of muscular weakness and wasting is again seen in a proportion of cases. One helpful distinction is involvement of the anterior tibial muscles, which is often found in the facioscapulohumeral type but is rare in the early stage of scapulohumeral dystrophy. Muscular contractures and skeletal distortion occur late, if at all;

cardiac involvement is rare and the range of intelligence is normal.

Diagnosis and management. Myotonic dystrophy, myotubular, nemaline and mitochondrial myopathies, the Möbius syndrome and myasthenia gravis may all present with various combinations of facial and limb muscle weakness. None of these conforms to the precise pattern of muscle involvement seen in facioscapulohumeral (FSH) muscular dystrophy but, once myasthenia and myotonia have been excluded, muscle biopsy is usually essential to make an accurate diagnosis. The FSH form of spinal muscular atrophy may be suspected because of slightly atypical or asymmetrical muscle weakness or the rapid development of weakness in certain muscles. The EMG and biopsy are diagnostic. In FSH muscular dystrophy, as in spinal muscular atrophy, the serum CK activity is often normal or only slightly raised (up to five times normal, rarely more). The muscle biopsy often shows only minimal myopathic changes. Fibre hypertrophy, scattered very atrophic fibres and occasional 'moth-eaten' fibres are seen (Dubowitz and Brooke, 1973). Preclinical cases do not have raised serum enzyme levels and there is no reliable method of preclinical diagnosis. In few, if any, patients aged over 25 years are there no signs at all of the disease, but very careful examination may be required to detect signs in slightly affected individuals, even in their 50s and 60s.

The inflammatory changes frequently seen in muscle biopsies are often unassociated with symptoms and then require no treatment, but significant muscular aching does occur quite often in this disease and sometimes responds to a short course of steroids. There is no indication for prolonged steroid therapy for this disease, nor is any other effective treatment known. A few patients require operations for scapular fixation or spinal fusion (Copeland and Howard, 1978) but for most, regular active muscle exercise is the only physical treatment necessary.

Autosomal dominant scapuloperoneal myopathy

Cases of sporadic or dominantly inherited scapuloperoneal myopathy have been described by Ricker and Mertens (1968), Thomas et al. (1975) and others. They differ from the X-linked cases in having a later onset in the second to the fifth decade, often with initial foot-drop. The progression is very slow and most patients continue to walk throughout their lives. The serum CK activity is usually only slightly raised but occasionally is very high (Thomas et al., 1975). The condition must be distinguished from the more frequent neurogenic scapuloperoneal syndrome, which may be difficult in the presence of secondary myopathic change in the latter (Feigenbaum and Munsat, 1970). Indeed proof, from examination of the spinal cord at autopsy, of the existence of an autosomal myopathic form has not yet been reported. The possibility that some recorded cases have 'incomplete' or abortive forms of facioscapulohumeral muscular dystrophy is suggested by the large kindred reported by Kazakov et al. (1976) in which facial weakness was a late and mild feature in many cases.

Limb-girdle myopathies of late onset and dominant inheritance

Sporadic cases of 'menopausal' myopathy have been described for many years (Nevin, 1936;

Walton and Adams, 1958; Corsi, Gentili and Todesco, 1965). They may well be heterogeneous and their genetic status is obscure. Large pedigrees with autosomal dominant inheritance have been described by Schneiderman, Sampson, Schoene and Haydon (1969) and Bacon and Smith (1971). Proximal lower-limb weakness predominated, but affected the quadriceps particularly in the cases of Bacon and Smith (1971) and relatively mildly in those of Schneiderman et al. (1969). The myopathic changes on muscle biopsy were non-specific and deteriorated with increasing age (Bacon and Smith, 1971). Serum enzyme activities were normal in the only example recorded. The onset of symptoms was in the late teens or in the third decade and weakness progressed very slowly, walking being maintained until after the seventh decade in some cases. Early diagnosis for genetic counselling appears to depend wholly on careful clinical examination. In the kindred described by Schneiderman et al. (1969) there was close genetic linkage with the Pelger-Huet anomaly of polymorphonuclear leucocyte nuclei. The 'Barnes type of muscular dystrophy' (Barnes, 1932), a dominantly inherited condition of late onset with initial striking muscle hypertrophy, has recently been shown to be of neurogenic origin (Riddoch, D., 1974, personal communication).

Distal myopathy

Distal myopathy was first described by Gowers in 1902; however, many observers now feel that the patient he described may have been suffering from myotonic dystrophy. In 1907 Spiller pointed out that the condition was different from peroneal muscular atrophy (Charcot-Marie-Tooth disease). In the latter condition, muscular atrophy is due to a motor neuropathy, although in some such cases (Greenfield, Shy, Alvord and Berg, 1957; Tyrer and Sutherland, 1961) there are changes suggestive of myopathy in muscle biopsy specimens. Welander (1951, 1957) has had a wide experience of the distal form of muscular dystrophy, which in Sweden is inherited as a dom-character, begins usually between the age of 40 and 60 years, and affects both sexes, although it is commoner in men than in women. The condition usually begins in the small muscles of the hands and slowly spreads proximally; in the legs the anterior tibial muscles and the calves are affected first. The condition is comparatively benign, but proximal weakness occurs in a few more severe cases which are probably homozygous for the dominant gene (Welander, 1957).

Welander's experience of over 250 cases is unique. In Great Britain and in the United States this form of the disease is rare; in Newcastle upon Tyne we have observed a few cases, all of which appeared to be sporadic. Although in these patients the rate of progress of the disease was somewhat more rapid than in the Swedish cases, and although most of them were severely disabled within 10–15 years of the onset, the pattern of muscular involvement was similar to that which she described. The serum CK activity may be as high as 20–100 times normal in cases with symptoms in the third decade (Markesbery, Griggs and Herr, 1977) but is normal or only slightly raised in cases where the onset is much later. Cases with confirmation at autopsy were reported by Tomlinson, Walton and Irving (1974) and the muscle pathology was reviewed by Markesbery et al. (1977).

Biemond (1955) described a juvenile form of distal myopathy which was subsequently found to be neurogenic in origin. Others (Ciani and Gherardi, 1963; Magee and de Jong, 1965; van der Does de Willebois, Bethlem, Meijer and Simons, 1968; Bautista, Rafel, Castilla and Alberca, 1978) have described similar families where the disease seemed more clearly myopathic, although some doubts remain. Like the late form, these early-onset cases are dominant in inheritance. Symptoms begin by the age of two years and progress slowly with eventual arrest. The serum CK activity is up to 20 times normal in some early cases but is normal in later life. Van der Does de Willebois et al. (1968) published histochemical studies in which atrophy of the type I muscle fibres appeared to be a prominent feature.

Initial involvement of peripheral limb muscles serves to distinguish these conditions from the scapulohumeral and scapuloperoneal muscular dystrophies, which they otherwise resemble; in the early stages the appearances in the limbs are similar to those of peroneal muscular atrophy, but

in the latter condition there is usually impairment of vibration sense in the extremities, and impaired nerve conduction. Some cases of mitochondrial myopathy with distal muscle weakness may resemble the juvenile form (Salmon, Esiri and Ruderman, 1971; Lapresle, Fardeau and Godet-Guillain, 1972) and electron microscopy of muscle may be required to distinguish them (Bautista et al., 1978). The difficulty in distinguishing distal myopathy from distal chronic spinal muscular atrophy should not be underestimated (Sumner, Crawfurd and Harriman, 1971).

Ocular myopathy or progressive external ophthalmoplegia

Involvement of the external ocular muscles is extremely unusual in any of the preceding types of muscular dystrophy, but may occur in myotonic dystrophy. Patients who have developed ptosis followed by progressive limitation of ocular movements without significant diplopia were described by Hutchinson (1879) and Fuchs (1890) and were reviewed by Kiloh and Nevin (1951). The symptoms may begin at any time from early childhood to old age. Some upper facial weakness is often associated and about half of the cases have skeletal muscular weakness involving the neck, trunk and limbs, especially the arms (Danta, Hilton and Lynch, 1975). This weakness may be distal. Myasthenia is absent. Fuchs (1890), Sandifer (1946) and Kiloh and Nevin (1951) obtained eyelid muscle during corrective operations and interpreted the histology as showing myopathy. Kiloh and Nevin reviewed the literature on autopsied cases and were unconvinced by descriptions of mild changes in the oculomotor nuclei; they therefore concluded that progressive external ophthalmoplegia is a form of muscular dystrophy. Authors writing more recently agree that it is impossible to make a firm diagnosis of primary myopathy on the basis of external ocular muscle histology alone. Full autopsies showing normal brain stem nuclei and 'dystrophic' changes in ocular and limb muscles were reported by Schwartz and Liu (1954), Cogan, Kuwabara and Richardson (1962) and Ross (1963). Dominant inheritance has been described in a number of families. Ross (1963, 1964) found that some such patients are peculiarly sensitive to curare but they do not improve on anticholinesterase drugs. Surgical correction of ptosis often relieves the only symptom.

The situation, however, is complicated by the frequent occurrence of apparently similar progressive external ophthalmoplegia associated with clinical features of central nervous system involvement and retinal pigmentation (Erdbrink, 1957; Walsh, 1957; Kearns and Sayre, 1958; Drachman, 1968; Rosenberg, Schotland, Lovelace and Rowland, 1968). Some cases have associated spinal muscular atrophy (Rosenberg *et al.*, 1968; Aberfeld and Namba, 1969) or peripheral neuropathy (Stephens, Hoover and Denst, 1958; Drachman, 1968). However, the most frequent association is with a constellation of features occurring in various combinations with ophthalmoplegia which usually begins in childhood (Fig. 14.6). These are pigmentary retinal degeneration (pigment clumps at some distance from the optic disc differing from retinitis pigmentosa), impaired vision, progressive growth failure, delayed menstruation or secondary amenorrhoea in the female, progressive heart block sometimes requiring an artificial pacemaker, skeletal muscle weakness, progressive cerebellar ataxia and neural deafness, increased cerebrospinal fluid protein and (less often) spasticity or dementia (Kearns and Sayre, 1958; Drachman, 1968). Heart block may lead to early death. Most cases with several features of the syndrome have been sporadic, but dominant inheritance of progressive external ophthalmoplegia with retinal pigmentation may be seen (Erdbrink, 1957). The differential diagnosis includes Refsum's syndrome and the Bassen-Kornzweig syndrome (a-β-lipoproteinaemia), in both of which a known biochemical anomaly exists. With so much evidence of involvement of the central nervous system it might reasonably be assumed that the ophthalmoplegia in such cases is nuclear in origin. In a case with spinal muscular atrophy, Aberfeld and Namba (1969) found this to be so. However, Kearns and Sayre (1958) found normal brain stem nuclei at autopsy in one case, although an unexplained vacuolar change involved the central white matter and lenticular nuclei. Daroff, Solitaire, Pincus and Glaser (1966), in a case complicated by terminal features suggesting

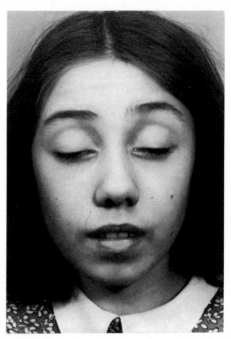

Fig. 14.6   Ocular myopathy in a young girl who had signs of cerebellar degeneration and pigmentary degeneration of the retina (Walton, 1962)

lymphocytic meningitis, found a spongiform encephalopathy which involved the brain stem. This confusing relationship between myopathic and central nervous system pathology in the 'Kearns–Sayre syndrome' has been clarified by the discovery of widespread mitochondrial pathology in these cases. Olson, Engel, Walsh and Einaugler (1972) described seven patients with certain features of this syndrome who had apparently characteristic skeletal muscle biopsy findings, including clusters of normal and abnormal mitochondria (also described by Zintz and Villiger, 1967), and excessive lipid droplets ('ragged-red fibres'). Soon afterwards, Schneck, Adachi, Briet, Wolintz and Volk (1973), in a typical case of the Kearns–Sayre syndrome, found identical mitochondrial changes in skeletal muscle and in a biopsy of the cerebellum. This, and other mitochondrial disorders of the muscle and brain, are discussed further in Chapter 17. It is now clear that a mitochondrial myopathy is also responsible for some, but not all, cases of uncomplicated progressive external ophthalmoplegia (Morgan-Hughes and Mair, 1973; Danta *et al.*, 1975). In this rapidly changing field the term 'ocular muscular dystrophy' is becoming increasingly unfashionable, but it remains the most accurate available description for some otherwise un-explained hereditary ocular myopathies.

Oculopharyngeal myopathy

Victor *et al.* (1962) separated those cases of ocular myopathy with dysphagia as a group, to which they gave the name oculopharyngeal myopathy. Bray, Kaarsoo and Ross (1965) supported this subdivision and defined the other distinguishing features, of which the most valuable was the age of onset (mean 23 years for the ocular cases and 40 for the oculopharyngeal). Many of the reported cases have been of French-Canadian stock (Taylor, 1915; Hayes, London, Seidman and Embree, 1963; Peterman, Lillington and Jamplis, 1964; Barbeau, 1966; Murphy and Drachman, 1968) but occasional cases, often sporadic, have occurred elsewhere. The inheritance in familial cases is dominant. Rebeiz, Caulfield and Adams (1969) confirmed the primary myopathic nature of a case at autopsy. In this type of muscular dystrophy, as in ocular myopathy, muscle biopsy may reveal evidence of a mitochondrial myopathy (Morgan-Hughes and Mair, 1973; Julien, Vital, Vallat, Vallat and le Blanc, 1974).

This disorder bears some resemblance to dystrophia myotonica, not only in some of the clinical and genetic features, but in the probable involvement of smooth muscle (Lewis, 1966) and reports of gonadal atrophy (Lundberg, 1962) and abnormalities of immunoglobulins (Russe, Busey and Barbeau, 1967) in some families.

A very closely similar syndrome with autosomal recessive inheritance and an earlier onset has been described by Fried, Arlozorov and Spira (1975).

MYOTONIC DISORDERS

Introduction

Myotonia, which occurs not only in man but also in certain goats (Brown and Harvey, 1939), is the continued active contraction of a muscle which persists after the cessation of voluntary effort or stimulation; an electrical after-discharge in the EMG can be seen to accompany the phenomenon.

Clinically it is best demonstrated as a slowness in relaxation of the grip, or by a persistent dimpling after a sharp blow on a muscle belly (e.g. in the thenar eminence or tongue). It appears to be caused by an abnormality of the muscle fibre itself, for it persists after section or blocking of the motor nerve and after curarisation (Denny-Brown and Nevin, 1941). Three hereditary myotonic syndromes, all with autosomal dominant inheritance, were classically described. In some individuals (Thomsen, 1876) it affected all the skeletal muscles from birth and the condition was called myotonia congenita (Thomsen's disease). In 1886 Eulenburg described a similar condition, 'paramyotonia', in which, however, the myotonia occurred only on exposure to cold; these patients also suffered from attacks of disabling muscle weakness. Much more common was yet another condition in which there was a progressive atrophy and weakness of the distal muscles of the limbs and of the facial muscles, and in which myotonia was often less striking and localised in a few muscles; this was called myotonia atrophica or dystrophia myotonica (Batten and Gibb, 1909; Steinert, 1909). The clinical features of each may vary considerably, a fact which led to controversy over whether the syndromes are merely different manifestations of the same condition, a view put forward by Maas and Paterson (1939; 1950). The great difference between the course and prognosis of typical cases, and the fact that in the majority of families the conditions breed true, make it clear that they are different diseases (Caughey and Myrianthopoulos, 1963). Further nosological problems arise over the close relationship of paramyotonia to the periodic paralyses. It seems clear that all of these disorders are more closely related to each other than they are to the 'pure' muscular dystrophies.

Recently, Becker (1961; 1971) has confirmed the occurrence of a distinct autosomal recessive form of myotonia congenita and several reports have appeared of a rare disorder, perhaps best called chondrodystrophic myotonia.

Myotonia may also be acquired as a complication of treatment with diazacholesterol (Somers and Winer, 1966). It has been described in association with carcinoma of the lung (Humphrey, Hill and Gordon, 1976).

Various other phenomena may resemble myotonia. In a rare and little-understood syndrome a clinically similar, but probably distinct, phenomenon is associated with myokymia, cramps, hyperhidrosis and sometimes muscle wasting (Gamstorp and Wohlfart, 1959; Greenhouse, Bicknell, Pesch and Seelinger, 1967). The cases of continuous muscle fibre activity described by Isaacs (1961) and Mertens and Zschocke (1965) seem to be similar. Although the failure of relaxation in these cases is similar to that in myotonia, no dimple is induced by percussion. Electromyography shows that the after-discharge is different in form. Brody (1969) described a case with slow relaxation of the muscles after contraction, without myotonia or other abnormal electrical activity, which he attributed to impaired uptake of calcium by the sarcoplasmic reticulum. Another EMG phenomenon superficially resembling myotonia but distinct from it and called pseudomyotonia (Buchthal and Rosenfalck, 1962) but more often nowadays referred to as 'bizarre, high-frequency discharges', is a common finding in polymyositis and muscle glycogenosis, and occurs less often in spinal muscular atrophy, muscular dystrophy and other disorders. Associated *symptomatic* myotonia appears to be very rare but it has been reported in polyneuropathy (Worster-Drought and Sargent, 1952) and polymyositis (Klink and Wachs, 1963). The name pseudomyotonia has also been given to the abnormally slow contraction and relaxation of voluntary muscle that is found in occasional cases of hypothyroidism (Hoffmann, 1897; Wilson and Walton, 1959; Norris and Panner, 1966). This may be distinguished by its failure to improve with exercise and by the absence of myotonic discharges on electromyography. 'Hypertrophia musculorum vera' (Friedreich, 1863; Spiller, 1913) may be identical to Hoffmann's syndrome. Sometimes, most often in paramyotonia congenita, myotonia increases during exertion (myotonia paradoxa) when it must be distinguished from the cramping stiffness of McArdle's disease.

The true myotonias may therefore be classified as follows:

A. Genetically determined
(a) Autosomal dominant myotonia congenita (Thomsen's disease)

(b) Autosomal recessive myotonia congenita (Becker)

(c) Paramyotonia congenita

(d) Dystrophia myotonica

(e) Chondrodystrophic myotonia

B. Acquired
Drug-induced

Myotonia congenita

Thomsen's disease or myotonia congenita (Thomsen, 1876; Nissen, 1923; Thomasen, 1948) usually begins at birth, but symptoms may be delayed to the end of the first or even into the second decade. The myotonia is more widespread than in dystrophia myotonica and may affect the grip and the ocular movements, but most characteristically causes a generalised painless stiffness which is accentuated by rest and cold, and gradually relieved by exercise. Sudden movements may induce widespread 'intention myotonia' and cause falls. There is typically diffuse hypertrophy of muscles which usually persists throughout life, although the myotonia tends to diminish gradually. Affected infants may have a curiously 'strangled' cry and some difficulty in feeding.

Becker (1961; 1971) identified a separate variety of myotonia with autosomal recessive inheritance. In Germany it is commoner than the dominant Thomsen's disease and differs in its later onset (1–12 years or even later), rather greater severity, initial involvement of the legs with later spread to the arms and facial muscles, and in the associated mild distal muscular weakness and atrophy. Some cases can 'work off' both myotonia and weakness by repeated muscle contraction, but the EMG shows a decremental response of muscle evoked potentials on repetitive stimulation of the nerves (Becker, 1971; Harper and Johnston, 1972).

Another possibly distinct type of familial myotonia inherited as an autosomal dominant trait has been described by Becker (1971) and Sanders (1976). Symptoms were first noted in adolescence and painful cramp was much more prominent than in typical Thomsen's disease.

Treatment with quinine, procaine amide or phenytoin alleviates myotonia but many patients prefer to manage without therapy.

Paramyotonia congenita

This condition was first described by Eulenburg (1886). In the families he reported, the affected individuals suffered from myotonia which was apparent only on exposure to cold and, in addition, they experienced attacks of unexplained generalised muscular weakness. Myotonia in all its forms is always made worse by cold, and this criterion is insufficient to distinguish paramyotonia from myotonia congenita. However, the attacks of muscular weakness serve to distinguish this condition, and it is now well recognised that these attacks are similar to those of familial periodic paralysis. The work of Drager, Hammill and Shy (1958) indicated that such attacks are often accompanied by a rise in serum potassium similar to that which occurs in adynamia episodica hereditaria and these authors suggested that paramyotonia congenita and adynamia episodica hereditaria might be identical. However, Walton (1961) and Resnick and Engel (1967) described patients with myotonia who also suffered from attacks of periodic paralysis of the hypokalaemic variety. Magee (1963; 1966), Thrush, Morris and Salmon (1972) and others have reported cases in which repeated muscular contraction induced paradoxical myotonia, and later paralysis, but did so much more readily in the cold; there was no associated change in the serum potassium. At the other end of the spectrum are cases with relatively mild myotonia but with severe attacks of episodic weakness, perhaps best described as myotonic periodic paralysis (van't Hoff, 1962; Saunders, Ashworth, Emery and Benedikz, 1968). Riggs, Griggs and Moxley (1977) found that, in paramyotonia, the myotonia could be abolished by administration of acetazolamide or by induction of hypokalaemia, but that this worsened the weakness, while hyperkalaemia had the opposite effect. Thus, although the nosological status of paramyotonia congenita is confused, it remains a useful diagnostic category for all patients in whom myotonia and weakness are induced by cold, as long as it is recognised that the particular precipitants and any associated electrolyte changes in each family must be worked out if useful advice and treatment are to be given. Generalised muscular hypertrophy and, in longstanding cases, permanent weakness, may occur. The inheritance is autosomal dominant.

Myotonic muscular dystrophy

Dystrophia myotonica (myotonia atrophica) was described by Steinert (1909) and Batten and Gibb (1909) and has been reviewed by Thomasen (1948), Caughey and Myrianthopoulos (1963) and Harper (1979). It is a diffuse systemic disorder in which myotonia and muscular atrophy may be accompanied by cataracts, frontal baldness (in the male), gonadal atrophy, heart disease, impaired pulmonary ventilation, mild endocrine anomalies, bone changes, mental defect or dementia and abnormalities of the serum immunoglobulins. It is inherited as an autosomal dominant trait and affected families tend to show progressive social decline in successive generations, diminished fertility, an increased infant mortality rate and a high incidence of mental backwardness. Characteristically, the pattern of manifestation and the severity of the disease show great variation within families. The impression is often gained that the disease increases in severity and becomes earlier in onset in successive generations. Penrose (1947) argued cogently that this is an illusion attributable largely to the variable age of onset and severity of symptoms.

Incidence. Even the highest published figures for prevalence, of 4.9–5.5 per 100 000 (Klein, 1958; Grimm, 1975) may be underestimates. The incidence at birth is calculated as 13.5 per 100 000 (Todorov, Jéquier, Klein and Morton, 1970). Harper (1979) estimated the mutation rate as 0.625 $\times$ 10^{-5} per gene per generation; this was based on several assumptions and he emphasises that reliable examples of new mutation are rarely found.

Symptoms. These are usually vague. The combination of apathy and lack of insight into their disability, which is typical of patients with dystrophia myotonica, often means that by the time they seek medical attention the characteristic signs of the disease are well advanced. The presenting symptom is usually weakness of the hands, difficulty in walking or a tendency to fall, but questioning will often reveal that myotonia of grip or muscular stiffness has been present for many years. Myotonia is the presenting symptom in about one-third of all cases. It is rarely as severe as in myotonia congenita and may be absent. Patients occasionally present with syncope or cardiac dysrhythmias (Wolintz, Sonnenblick and Engel, 1966). Poor vision, ptosis, impotence or loss of libido and increased sweating are common complaints. The age at the onset of symptoms is commonly between 20 and 50 years but the onset of detectable disease is probably usually in the second decade and many cases are clearly apparent in childhood. A distinctive congenital form presents with severe hypotonia and, in general, the earlier the onset the greater is the severity of the disease. A significant proportion of those who carry the gene never develop symptoms and occasionally it may be difficult to find evidence of the disease, even on careful investigation.

Clinical features and course. The facial appearance is characteristic (Fig. 14.7). Ptosis is very frequent and there may be symmetrical impairment of ocular movements. There is a lack of facial expression with difficulty in closing the eyes, in retracting the corners of the mouth and in pursing the lips; often the lower lip droops. Wasting of the masseters, temporal muscles and sternomastoids gives a characteristic haggard appearance, while the jaw sags and the head hangs forward because of muscular weakness. Dysarthria due to weakness of the facial muscles or to myotonia of the tongue is common. Weakness and

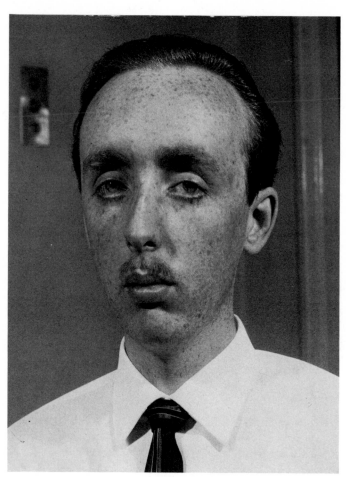

Fig. 14.7 Dystrophia myotonica: note the frontal baldness, the bilateral ptosis and the typical facial appearance

wasting in the limbs affects mainly the muscles of the forearms, the anterior tibial group (leading to early foot-drop) and the calves and peronei. This is quite distinct from the proximal weakness of the other common muscular dystrophies. Abdominal muscular weakness is common. Later, more proximal and more distal limb muscles are involved. Myotonia is often limited to the tongue, forearm and hand but it may be generalised; it tends to become less apparent as the disease progresses in middle life but is absent in early infancy. The tendon reflexes are reduced in the affected muscles and contractures may occur in the later stages.

Slit-lamp examination of the eyes reveals cataracts in about 90 per cent of cases, typically consisting of scintillating white and greenish-coloured posterior subcapsular particles. Later, these develop into stellate cataracts, which may require extraction (Vogt, 1921; Klein, 1958). Ocular hypotension and impaired retinal function are frequent but of less clinical importance (Burian and Burns, 1967).

Cardiac involvement is common; about 65 per cent of patients have ECG abnormalities, usually conduction defects (DeWind and Jones, 1950; Fisch, 1951; Cannon, 1962; Church, 1967; Thomson, 1968). Cardiac failure is a late feature but hypotension and syncope are not infrequent (Lee and Hughes, 1964). The use of propranolol for angina may exacerbate the myotonia (Blessing and Walsh, 1977) and, conversely, the use of procaine amide for myotonia may exacerbate conduction defects (Griggs, Davis, Anderson and Dove, 1975). The pulmonary vital capacity and especially the maximum breathing capacity are often impaired (Kilburn, Eagan, Sieker and Heyman, 1959; Lee and Hughes, 1964; Gillam, Heaf, Kaufman and Lucas, 1964) and the consequent alveolar hypoventilation may contribute to apathy and somnolence but is not the whole explanation for these symptoms (Coccagna, Mantovani, Parchi, Mironi and Lugaresi, 1975). Elevation of part of the diaphragm may be seen in a chest radiograph, and diaphragmatic hypoplasia sometimes contributes to respiratory problems in congenital cases (Aicardi, Conti and Goutières, 1974). Disordered oesophageal contraction may be shown by contrast radiography (Gleeson, Swann,

Hughes and Lee, 1967) or manometry (Siegel, Hendrix and Harvey, 1966) and has been held responsible for dysphagia (Ludman, 1962; Welsh, Haase and Bynum, 1964) and for pulmonary aspiration and bronchiectasis (Pruzanski, 1962). The smooth muscle of the colon may be affected, particularly in congenital cases (Lenard, Goebel and Weigel, 1977). Uterine myopathy sometimes results in prolonged labour (Sciarra and Steer, 1961; Shore, 1975). The testes are usually small, with hyaline change in the seminiferous tubules and this is associated with evidence of unresponsiveness to follicle-stimulating hormone (Harper, Penny, Foley, Migeon and Blizzard, 1972; Sagel, Distiller, Morley, Isaacs, Kay and van der Walt, 1975). Pituitary function is usually normal, but there is often a selective failure of adrenal androgenic function and, occasionally, thyroid activity is impaired (Marshall, 1959; Caughey and Myrianthopoulos, 1963; Lee and Hughes, 1964). Diabetes mellitus occurs in about 5 per cent of cases but in many, although not all, inappropriate hypersecretion of insulin occurs in response to a glucose load and certain other stimuli (Huff, Horton and Lebovitz, 1967; Gorden, Griggs, Nissley, Roth and Engel, 1969; Barbosa, Nuttall, Kennedy and Goetz, 1974; Moxley, Griggs, van Gelder and Thiel, 1978). Hyperostosis of the skull vault, localised or diffuse, and a small sella turcica are frequent radiological findings (Jéquier, 1950; Caughey, 1952; Walton and Warrick, 1954). Both mental defect and progressive dementia occur. Only 24 of Thomasen's 101 cases were of normal intelligence. Rosman and Kakulas (1966) described neuronal heterotopias at autopsy in four cases, of whom three were mentally defective, and investigation in life may reveal EEG abnormalities (Barwick, Osselton and Walton, 1965) or cerebral ventricular enlargement (Refsum, Engeset and Lönnum, 1959; Refsum, Lönnum, Sjaastad and Engeset, 1967). Excessive catabolism of immunoglobulin G has been demonstrated in this disorder by Wochner, Drews, Strober and Waldmann (1966) and low serum concentrations of IgG may be found even in preclinical cases (Roberts and Bradley, 1977).

The course is one of steady deterioration. Most patients who present with muscular symptoms are severely disabled and unable to walk within 15 to

20 years of their onset. However, other patients may continue to walk with little disability throughout their lives. Death occurs before the normal age, usually from chest infections or cardiac failure. Sudden death, attributed to cardiac arrhythmia, has been reported. These patients appear to be particularly at risk during anaesthesia, perhaps partly because of an increased sensitivity to thiopentone (Caughey and Myrianthopoulos, 1963; Gillam *et al.*, 1964).

Congenital myotonic dystrophy. In a small proportion of cases, myotonic dystrophy presents in the newborn period with hypotonia, facial diplegia and feeding difficulties (Vanier, 1960; Harper, 1975). Respiratory difficulties, sometimes fatal, occur in about half of these cases, and talipes and a history of reduced fetal movement or of hydramnios are frequent. Muscular wasting is inconspicuous; cataracts and clinical myotonia are absent. Some patients have associated anomalies of the ribs and diaphragm (Pruzanski, 1966; Aicardi *et al.*, 1974). The affected parent is, in virtually every case, the mother, whose clinical involvement often has not been noticed previously. Diagnosis depends upon the clinical findings in the baby and careful examination of other family members. Muscle biopsy may show atrophy of histochemical type I fibres but is usually unnecessary for diagnosis; myotonia may be found by the persistent electromyographer in some neonatal cases, but is usually apparent in the mother. If the child survives the neonatal period, the condition tends to improve slightly or remain static in childhood, only to deteriorate, as in the adult-onset cases, later in life. Almost all develop clinical myotonia by the age of 10 years. Mental retardation occurs in about 60–70 per cent of cases but is rarely severe (Calderon, 1966; Harper, 1975). Motor and speech development are delayed but even the floppiest babies eventually learn to walk. Dysarthria may necessitate speech therapy and occasional children have persistent dysphagia (Pruzanski, 1966). Harper and Dyken (1972) suggested that a maternal circulating factor may act upon the heterozygous fetus, impairing *in utero* muscle function and development. This might result from involvement both of the fetal and of the maternal components of placental membranes (Gardner-Medwin, 1977b). Subsequently affected siblings usually also suffer from the congenital form, but perhaps not quite invariably so (Harper, 1975).

Diagnosis and prevention. Prevention depends upon early diagnosis and genetic advice, but the latter is rarely sought by patients with this disease. Early case detection is best achieved by combining careful clinical examination with electromyography and slit-lamp examination for cataract (Bundey, Carter and Soothill, 1970; Polgar, Bradley, Upton, Anderson, Howat, Petito, Roberts and Scopa, 1972). Abnormal insulin secretion may also be helpful (Walsh, Turtle, Miller and McLeod, 1970). The results of muscle biopsy, although abnormal and sometimes diagnostic in the clinical stage (Ch. 5), makes disappointingly little contribution to preclinical diagnosis or practical management. Harper (1979) points out that, apart from the problems of early diagnosis, the disorder is easily recognised once it has been considered. Errors and delay in diagnosis result mainly from failure to consider myotonic dystrophy when a patient presents with nonmuscular problems such as cataract, cardiac arrhythmia, dysphagia, constipation, somnolence or obstetric difficulties. In these circumstances, examination of other members of the family is helpful. The discoveries of close genetic linkage between myotonic dystrophy, the ABH secretor status and the Lutheran blood group (Renwick, Bundey, Ferguson-Smith and Izatt, 1970; Harper, Rivas, Bias, Hutchinson, Dyken and McKusick, 1972) and of the feasibility of detecting the ABH secretor status of the fetus by amniocentesis (Harper, Bias, Hutchinson and McKusick, 1971) made it possible, in theory, to diagnose the disease antenatally and to perform selective termination of pregnancy in certain families where the secretor status is appropriately informative. This has, in fact, been achieved (Insley, Bird, Harper and Pearce, 1976).

Pathogenesis. This remains conjectural. Myotonia appears to be a dysfunction of sarcolemmal membrane, possibly related to impaired chloride conductance (Barchi, 1975) (*see* Ch. 30). A widespread dysfunction of cell membranes might well account for the subcapsular cataracts, end-organ resistance to certain hormones (attributable perhaps to lack of receptor sites), rapid catabolism of immunoglobulin G (by the same mechanism) as well as the muscular disorder. Abnormalities of red blood cell membranes have been found which support this hypothesis (Appel and Roses, 1977).

Management. There is no effective treatment for the disease. Myotonia is rarely very troublesome, but if stiffness of the hands or muscular pains are prominent, procaine amide or phenytoin may relieve them (Geschwind and Simpson, 1955; Leyburn and Walton, 1959; Munsat, 1967). Procaine amide seems to be slightly more effective, but Griggs *et al.* (1975) point out that it may exacerbate cardiac conduction defects: for this reason it should probably be used only in young patients with normal ECGs.

Active exercise and avoiding obesity are important here, as in other types of muscular dystrophy. The cardiac, respiratory, endocrine and ocular complications are often asymptomatic or neglected for long periods. They are difficult or impossible to prevent, but can be partially alleviated as they arise. Active medical surveillance, like genetic counselling in this disease, is often unwillingly received and thus provides some ethical problems.

Obstetric supervision is very important because of the special risk of complications, including deterioration of the disorder itself (Hopkins and Wray, 1967), threatened abortion, stillbirth, polyhydramnios and prolonged labour (Shore, 1975). Sarnat, O'Connor and Byrne, 1976). Intensive treatment of respiratory failure in congenital cases may be lifesaving, and tube feeding is often necessary for a few days or sometimes weeks.

Anaesthesia carries special risks of cardiac arrhythmia, or respiratory failure in the postoperative phase, and of aspiration pneumonia (Kaufman, 1960; Gillam *et al.*, 1964). Drugs likely to suppress respiration should be avoided whenever possible: this is particularly important during labour because of their potential effect on the baby.

Chondrodystrophic myotonia (Schwartz-Jampel syndrome)

This syndrome, first described in full by Aberfeld,

Hinterbuchner and Schneider (1965), comprises myotonia, skeletal deformities and short stature. More than 20 cases of both sexes have now been reported and it is clear that the condition is inherited as an autosomal recessive trait (Catel, 1951, quoted by Aberfeld, Namba, Vye and Grob, 1970; Schwartz and Jampel, 1962; Huttenlocher, Landwirth, Hanson, Gallacher and Bensch, 1969; Fowler, Layzer, Taylor, Eberle, Sims, Munsat, Philippart and Wilson, 1974; Pavone, Mollica, Grasso, Cao and Gullotta, 1978, and others). Often choking on cold drinks and hip contractures or dislocations are noticed in infancy, followed by progressive hip deformities, other joint contractures and in some cases pectus carinatus and basilar impression; X-rays of the epiphyses are abnormal. Later, growth fails progressively and the muscles become stiff and sometimes hypertrophied. Tense puckering of the mouth and blepharospasm with small palpebral fissures and irregular eyelashes are evident by the second or third year. Myotonia is present and, in older children, muscular atrophy may occur. Intelligence has usually been normal. A congenital severe variant was described by Cao, Cianchetti, Calisti, de Virgiliis, Ferreli and Tangheroni (1978). Electromyography usually shows true myotonia, but in some cases there is continuous muscle-fibre activity (Fowler *et al.*, 1974; Cao *et al.*, 1978). Minimal EMG changes, including myotonia, are reported in some unaffected close relatives. Electron microscopy of the muscle biopsy reveals minor changes in the T system and dilatation of the sarcoplasmic reticulum in some cases (Fowler *et al.*, 1974; Pavone *et al.*, 1978). A case with recurrent pneumonia and absence of immunoglobulin A in serum was described by Kirschner and Pachman (1976) but the cases of Pavone *et al.* had normal immunoglobulins. Procaine amide therapy has improved the gait and facies in some cases (Huttenlocher *et al.*, 1969).

ACKNOWLEDGEMENTS

Some of the work referred to in this chapter was aided by grants from the Medical Research Council, the Muscular Dystrophy Group of Great Britain and the Muscular Dystrophy Association of America, Inc.

REFERENCES

Aberfeld, D.C., Hinterbuchner, L.P. & Schneider, M. (1965) Myotonia, dwarfism, diffuse bone disease and unusual ocular and facial abnormalities (a new syndrome). *Brain*, **88**, 313.

Aberfeld, D.C. & Namba, T. (1969) Progressive ophthalmoplegia in Kugelberg-Welander disease: report of a case. *Archives of Neurology*, **20**, 253.

Aberfeld, D.C., Namba, T., Vye, M.V. & Grob, D. (1970) Chondrodystrophic myotonia: report of two cases. *Archives of Neurology*, **22**, 455.

Adornato, B.T., Kagen, L.J. & Engel, W.K. (1978) Myoglobinemia in Duchenne muscular dystrophy patients and carriers: a new adjunct to carrier detection. *Lancet*, **2**, 499.

Afifi, A.K., Bergman, R.A. & Zellweger, H. (1973) A possible role for electron microscopy in detection of carriers of Duchenne type muscular dystrophy. *Journal of Neurology, Neurosurgery and Psychiatry*, **36**, 643.

Afifi, A.K., Zellweger, H., McCormick, W.F. & Mergner, W. (1969) Congenital muscular dystrophy: light and electron microscopic observations. *Journal of Neurology, Neurosurgery and Psychiatry*, **32**, 273.

Aguilar, L., Lisker, R. & Ramos, G.G. (1978) Unusual inheritance of Becker type muscular dystrophy. *Journal of Medical Genetics*, **15**, 116.

Ahmad, M., Sanderson, J.E., Dubowitz, V. & Hallidie-Smith, K.A. (1978) Echocardiographic assessment of left ventricular function in Duchenne's muscular dystrophy. *British Heart Journal*, **40**, 734.

Aicardi, J., Conti, D. & Goutières, F. (1974) Les formes néonatales de la dystrophie myotonique de Steinert. *Journal of the Neurological Sciences*, **22**, 149.

Allen, J.E. & Rodgin, D.W. (1960) Mental retardation in association with progressive muscular dystrophy. *American Journal of Diseases of Childhood*, **100**, 208.

Appel, S.H. & Roses, A.D. (1977) Membranes and myotonia. In *Pathogenesis of Human Muscular Dystrophies*, Ed. L.P. Rowland, p. 747 (Excerpta Medica: Amsterdam).

Aran, F.A. (1850) Recherches sur une maladie non encore décrite du système musculaire (atrophie musculaire progressive). *Archives générales de médicine*, **24**, 5.

Archibald, K.C. & Vignos, P.J. (1959) A study of contractures in muscular dystrophy. *Archives of Physical Medicine*, **40**, 150.

Bacon, P.A. & Smith, B. (1971) Familial muscular dystrophy of late onset. *Journal of Neurology, Neurosurgery and Psychiatry*, **34**, 93.

Banker, B.Q., Victor, M. & Adams, R.D. (1957) Arthrogryposis multiplex due to congenital muscular dystrophy. *Brain*, **80**, 319.

Barbeau, A. (1966) The syndrome of hereditary late onset ptosis and dysphagia in French Canada. In *Progressive Muskeldystrophie, Myotonie, Myasthenie*, Ed. E. Kuhn (Springer-Verlag: New York).

Barbosa, J., Nuttall, F.Q., Kennedy, W. & Goetz, F. (1974) Plasma insulin in patients with myotonic dystrophy and their relatives. *Medicine (Baltimore)*, **53**, 307.

Barchi, R.L. (1975) Myotonia: an evulation of the chloride hypothesis. *Archives of Neurology*, **32**, 175.

Barnes, S. (1932) Report of a myopathic family with hypertrophic, pseudohypertrophic, atrophic and terminal (distal in the upper extremities) stages. *Brain*, **55**, 1.

Barwick, D.D., Osselton, J.W. & Walton, J.N. (1965) Electroencephalographic studies in hereditary myopathy. *Journal of Neurology, Neurosurgery and Psychiatry*, **28**, 109.

Batten, F.E. (1903) Three cases of myopathy, infantile type. *Brain*, **26**, 147.

Batten, F.E. (1909) The myopathies or muscular dystrophies; critical review. *Quarterly Journal of Medicine*, **3**, 313.

Batten, F.E. & Gibb, H.P. (1909) Myotonia atrophica. *Brain*, **32**, 187.

Bautista, J., Rafel, E., Castilla, J.M. & Alberca, R. (1978) Hereditary distal myopathy with onset in early infancy. *Journal of the Neurological Sciences*, **37**, 149.

Becker, P.E. (1953) *Dystrophia Musculorum Progressiva* (Georg Thieme: Stuttgart).

Becker, P.E. (1957) Neue Ergebnisse der Genetik der Muskel dystrophien. *Acta Geneticae medicae et gemellologiae (Roma)*, **7**, 303.

Becker, P.E. (1961) Die Heterogenei der Myotonien. In *Proceedings of the 2nd International Congress on Human Genetics*. Vol. 3, p. 1547 (Excerpta Medica: Amsterdam).

Becker, P.E. (1962) Two new families of benign sex-linked recessive muscular dystrophy. *Revue Canadienne de Biologie*, **21**, 551.

Becker, P.E. (1964) Myopathien. In *Humangenetik: Ein kurzes Handbuch in fünf Bänden*, Band III/I, Ed. P.E. Becker, p. 411 (Georg Thieme: Stuttgart).

Becker, P.E. (1971) Genetic approaches to the nosology of muscle disease: myotonias and similar diseases. In *The Clinical Delineation of Birth Defects—Part VII, Muscle*, Ed. D. Bergsma, p. 52 (Williams and Wilkins: Baltimore).

Becker, P.E. & Keiner, F. (1955) Eine neue x-chromosomale Muskeldystrophie. *Archiv für Psychiatrie und Nervenkrankheiten*, **193**, 427.

Beckmann, R. & Scheuerbrandt, G. (1976) Screening auf erhöhte CK-Aktivitäten. *Kinderarzt*, **7**, 1267.

Bell, J. (1943) On pseudohypertrophic and allied types of progressive muscular dystrophy. In *Treasury of Human Inheritance*, Vol. IV, Part IV (Cambridge University Press: London).

Berenbaum, A.A. & Horowitz, W. (1956) Heart involvement in progressive muscular dystrophy. Report of a case with sudden death. *American Heart Journal*, **51**, 622.

Biemond, A. (1955) Myopathia distalis juvenilis hereditaria. *Acta Psychiatrica et Neurologica Scandinavia*, **30**, 25.

Blessing, W. & Walsh, J.C. (1977) Myotonia precipitated by propranolol therapy. *Lancet*, **1**, 73.

Blyth, H. & Hughes, B.P. (1971) Pregnancy and serum-C.P.K. levels in potential carriers of 'severe' X-linked muscular dystrophy. *Lancet*, **1**, 855.

Blyth, H. & Pugh, R.J. (1959) Muscular dystrophy in childhood. The genetic aspect. A field study in the Leeds region of clinical types and their inheritance. *Annals of Human Genetics*, **33**, 127.

Boba, A. (1970) Fatal postanesthetic complications in two muscular dystrophic patients. *Journal of Pediatric Surgery*, **5**, 71.

Boddie, H.G. & Stewart-Wynne, E.G. (1974) Quadriceps myopathy—entity or syndrome? *Archives of Neurology*, **31**, 60.

Bossingham, D.H., Williams, E. & Nichols, P.J.R. (1979) *Severe Childhood Neuromuscular Disease: The Management of Duchenne Muscular Dystrophy and Spinal Muscular Atrophy* (Muscular Dystrophy Group of Great Britain: London).

Bradley, W.G., Tomlinson, B.E. & Hardy, M. (1978) Further studies of mitochondrial and lipid storage myopathies. *Journal of the Neurological Sciences*, **35**, 201.

Bradley, W.G., Jones, M.Z., Mussini, J.-M. & Fawcett, P.R.W. (1978) Becker-type muscular dystrophy. *Muscle & Nerve*, **1**, 111.

Bramwell, E. (1922) Observations on myopathy. *Proceedings of the Royal Society of Medicine*, **16**, 1.

Bray, G.M., Kaarsoo, M. & Ross, R.T. (1965) Ocular myopathy with dysphagia. *Neurology (Minneapolis)*, **15**, 678.

Brody, I.A. (1969) Muscle contracture induced by exercise: a syndrome attributable to decreased relaxing factor. *New England Journal of Medicine*, **281**, 187.

Brooke, M.H. (1977) *A Clinician's View of Neuromuscular Diseases* (Williams and Wilkins: Baltimore).

Brooks, A.P. & Emery, A.E.H. (1977) The incidence of Duchenne muscular dystrophy in the south east of Scotland. *Clinical Genetics*, **11**, 290.

Brown, G.L. & Harvey, A.M. (1939) Congenital myotonia in the goat. *Brain*, **62**, 341.

Buchthal, F. & Rosenfalck, P. (1962) Electrophysiological aspects of myopathy with particular reference to progressive muscular dystrophy. In *Muscular Dystrophy in Man and Animals*, Eds G.H. Bourne & N. Golarz (Basel and New York: Karger).

Bundey, S., Carter, C.O. & Soothill, J.F. (1970) Early recognition of heterozygotes for the gene for dystrophia myotonica. *Journal of Neurology, Neurosurgery and Psychiatry*, **33**, 279.

Burian, H.M. & Burns, C.A. (1967) Ocular changes in myotonic dystrophy. *American Journal of Ophthalmology*, **63**, 22.

Burke, S.S., Grove, N.M., Houser, C.R. & Johnson, D.M. (1971) Respiratory aspects of pseudohypertrophic muscular dystrophy. *American Journal of Diseases of Children*, **121**, 230.

Calderon, R. (1966) Myotonic dystrophy: a neglected cause of mental retardation. *Journal of Pediatrics*, **68**, 423.

Cannon, P.J. (1962) The heart and lungs in myotonic muscular dystrophy. *American Journal of Medicine*, **32**, 765.

Cao, A., Cianchetti, C., Calisti, L., de Virgiliis, S., Ferreli, A. & Tangheroni, W. (1978) Schwartz-Jampel syndrome: clinical, electrophysiological and histopathological study of a severe variant. *Journal of the Neurological Sciences*, **35**, 175.

Caruso, G. & Buchthal, F. (1965) Refractory period of muscle and electromyographic findings in relatives of patients with muscular dystrophy. *Brain*, **88**, 29.

Caughey, J.E. (1952) Radiological changes in the skull in dystrophia myotonica. *Journal of Bone and Joint Surgery*, **34B**, 343.

Caughey, J.E. & Myrianthopoulos, N.C. (1963) *Dystrophia Myotonica and Related Disorders* (Thomas: Springfield, Illinois).

Chung, C.S., Morton, N.E. & Peters, H.A. (1960) Serum enzymes and genetic carriers in muscular dystrophy. *American Journal of Human Genetics*, **12**, 52.

Church, C.S. (1967) The heart in myotonia atrophica. *Archives of Internal Medicine*, **119**, 176.

Ciani, N. & Gherardi, D. (1963) Due casi di myopathia distalis juvenilis hereditaria. *Rivista di Neurologia*, **33**, 731.

Cobham, I.G. & Davis, H.S. (1964) Anesthesia for muscular dystrophy patients. *Anesthesia and Analgesia—Current Researches*, **43**, 22.

Coccagna, C., Mantovani, M., Parchi, C., Mironi, F. & Lugaresi, E. (1975) Alveolar hypoventilation and hypersomnia in myotonic dystrophy. *Journal of Neurology, Neurosurgery and Psychiatry*, **38**, 977.

Cogan, D.G., Kuwabara, T. & Richardson, E.P. (1962) Pathology of abiotrophic ophthalmoplegia externa. *Bulletin of the Johns Hopkins Hospital*, **111**, 42.

Cohen, H.J., Molnar, G.E. & Taft, L.T. (1968) The genetic relationship of progressive muscular dystrophy (Duchenne type) and mental retardation. *Developmental Medicine and Child Neurology*, **10**, 754.

Copeland, S.A. & Howard, R.C. (1978) Thoracoscapular fusion for facioscapulohumeral dystrophy. *Journal of Bone and Joint Surgery*, **60B**, 547.

Corsi, A., Gentili, C. & Todesco, C.V. (1965) The relationship of menopausal muscular dystrophy to other diseases of muscle. A study of 17 cases. *Journal of the Neurological Sciences*, **2**, 397.

Danieli, G.A., Mostacciuolo, M.L., Bonfante, A. & Angelini, C. (1977) Duchenne muscular dystrophy: a population study. *Human Genetics*, **35**, 225.

Danta, G., Hilton, R.C. & Lynch, P.G. (1975) Chronic progressive ophthalmoplegia. *Brain*, **98**, 473.

Daroff, R.B., Solitaire, G.B., Pincus, J.H. & Glaser, G.H. (1966) Spongiform encephalopathy with chronic progressive external ophthalmoplegia. *Neurology (Minneapolis)*, **16**, 161.

Dellamonica, C. (1978) *Etude de la reaction couplée, creatine-kinase/luciferine-luciferase. Application au depistage systematique neonatal de la myopathie de Duchenne de Boulogne.* Thesis for the Université Claude Bernard, Lyon.

Dellamonica, C., Robert, J.M., Cotte, J., Collombel, C. & Dorche, C. (1978) Systematic neonatal screening for Duchenne muscular dystrophy. *Lancet*, **2**, 1100 (letter).

Demos, J. (1963) Essai d'appreciation d'une action thérapeutique éventuelle au cours de la myopathie: étude critique de l'action du p-hydroxy-phényl-butyl-amino-éthanol. *Semaine des Hôpitaux de Paris*, **39**, 572.

Dennis, N.R., Evans, K., Clayton, B. & Carter, C.O. (1976) Use of creatine kinase for detecting severe X-linked muscular dystrophy carriers. *British Medical Journal*, **2**, 577.

Denny–Brown, D. & Nevin, S. (1941) The phenomenon of myotonia. *Brain*, **64**, 1.

DeWind, L.T. & Jones, R.J. (1950) Cardiovascular observations in dystrophia myotonica. *Journal of the American Medical Association*, **144**, 299.

Donner, M., Rapola, J. & Somer, H. (1975) Congenital muscular dystrophy: a clinicopathological and follow-up study of 15 patients. *Neuropädiatrie*, **6**, 239.

Drachman, D.A. (1968) Ophthalmoplegia plus; the neurodegenerative disorders associated with progressive external ophthalmoplegia. *Archives of Neurology*, **18**, 654.

Drachman, D.B., Murphy, S.R., Nigam, M.P. & Hills, J.R. (1967) 'Myopathic' changes in chronically denervated muscle. *Archives of Neurology*, **16**, 14.

Drager, G.A., Hammill, J.F. & Shy, G.M. (1958) Paramyotonia congenita. *Archives of Neurology*, **80**, 1.

Dreifuss, F.E. & Hogan, G.R. (1961) Survival in x-chromosomal muscular dystrophy. *Neurology (Minneapolis)*, **11**, 734.

Dreyfus, J.C., Schapira, F., Demos, J., Rosa, R. & Schapira, G. (1966) The value of serum enzyme determinations in the identification of dystrophic carriers. *Annals of the New York Academy of Sciences*, **138**, 304.

Drummond, L.M. & Veale, A.M.O. (1978) Muscular dystrophy screening. *Lancet*, **1**, 1258 (letter).

Dubowitz, V. (1963) Myopathic changes in a muscular dystrophy carrier. *Journal of Neurology, Neurosurgery and Psychiatry*, **26**, 322.

Dubowitz, V. (1964) Progressive muscular dystrophy: prevention of deformities. *Clinical Pediatrics*, **3**, 323.

Dubowitz, V. (1965) Intellectual impairment in muscular dystrophy. *Archives of Disease in Childhood*, **40**, 296.

Dubowitz, V. (1969) Chemical and structural changes in muscle: the importance of the nervous system. In *Some Inherited Disorders of Brain and Muscle*, Eds J.D. Allan, & D.N. Raine (Livingstone: Edinburgh).

Dubowitz, V. (1978) *Muscle Disorders in Childhood* (Saunders: London).

Dubowitz, V. & Brooke, M.H. (1973) *Muscle Biopsy: A Modern Approach* (Saunders: London).

Dubowitz, V. & Crome, L. (1969) The central nervous system in Duchenne muscular dystrophy. *Brain*, **92**, 805.

Duchenne, G.B. (1868) Recherches sur la paralysie musculaire pseudo-hypertrophique ou paralysie myosclérosique. *Archives générals de médicine*, **11**, 5, 178, 305, 421, 552.

Ebashi, S. & Sugita, H. (1978) The role of calcium in physiological and pathological processes of skeletal muscle. In *Abstracts of the IVth International Congress on Neuromuscular Diseases*, Montreal.

Emery, A.E.H. (1963) Clinical manifestations in two carriers of Duchenne muscular dystrophy. *Lancet*, **1**, 1126.

Emery, A.E.H. (1964) Electrophoretic pattern of lactic dehydrogenase in carriers and patients with Duchenne muscular dystrophy. *Nature*, **201**, 1044.

Emery, A.E.H. (1965) Muscle histology in carriers of Duchenne muscular dystrophy. *Journal of Medical Genetics*, **2**, 1.

Emery, A.E.H. (1969) Abnormalities of the electrocardiogram in female carriers of Duchenne muscular dystrophy. *British Medical Journal*, **2**, 418.

Emery, A.E.H. (1972) Abnormalities of the electrocardiogram in hereditary myopathies. *Journal of Medical Genetics*, **9**, 8.

Emery, A.E.H. & Dreifuss, F.E. (1966) Unusual type of benign X-linked muscular dystrophy. *Journal of Neurology, Neurosurgery and Psychiatry*, **29**, 338.

Emery, A.E.H. & Holloway, S. (1977) Use of normal daughters' and sisters' creatine kinase levels in estimating heterozygosity in Duchenne muscular dystrophy. *Human Heredity*, **27**, 118.

Emery, A.E.H. & King, B. (1971) Pregnancy and serum-creatine-kinase levels in potential carriers of Duchenne X-linked muscular dystrophy. *Lancet*, **1**, 1013.

Emery, A.E.H. & Morton, R. (1968) Genetic counselling in lethal X-linked disorders. *Genetica et Statistica Medica (Basel)*, **18**, 534.

Emery, A.E.H. & Skinner, R. (1976) Clinical studies in benign (Becker type) X-linked muscular dystrophy. *Clinical Genetics*, **10**, 189.

Emery, A.E.H. & Walton, J.N. (1967) The genetics of muscular dystrophy. In *Progress in Medical Genetics*, Eds A.G. Steinberg & A.G. Bearn, Vol. V (Grune & Stratton: New York).

Emery, E.S., Fenichel, G.M. & Eng, G. (1968) A spinal muscular atrophy with scapuloperoneal distribution. *Archives of Neurology*, **18**, 129.

Erb, W.H. (1884) Uber die 'juvenile form' der progressiven muskelatrophie ihre beziehungen zur sogennanten pseudohypertrophie der muskeln. *Deutsches Archiv für klinische Medizin*, **34**, 467.

Erb, W.H. (1891) Dystrophia muscularis progressiva: Klinische und pathologischanatomische Studien. *Deutsche Zeitschrift für Nervenheilkunde*, **1**, 13.

Erdbrink, W.L. (1957) Ocular myopathy associated with retinitis pigmentosa. *Archives of Ophthalmology*, **57**, 335.

Espir, M.L.E. & Matthews, W.B. (1973) Hereditary quadriceps myopathy. *Journal of Neurology, Neurosurgery and Psychiatry*, **36**, 1041.

Eulenburg, A. (1886) Ueber eine familiare, durch 6 generationen verfolgbare form congenitaler paramyotonie. *Neurologisches Zentralblatt*, **5**, 265.

Feigenbaum, J.A. & Munsat, T.L. (1970) A neuromuscular syndrome of scapuloperoneal distribution. *Bulletin of the Los Angeles Neurological Societies*, **35**, 47.

Fenichel, G.M., Emery, E.S. & Hunt, P. (1967). Neurogenic atrophy simulating facioscapulohumeral dystrophy: a dominant form. *Archives of Neurology*, **17**, 257.

Ferrier, P., Bamatter, F. & Klein, D. (1965) Muscular dystrophy (Duchenne) in a girl with Turner's syndrome. *Journal of Medical Genetics*, **2**, 38.

Fisch, C. (1951) The heart in dystrophia myotonica. *American Heart Journal*, **41**, 525.

Fowler, W.M., Layzer, R.B., Taylor, R.G., Eberle, E.D., Sims, G.E., Munsat, T.L., Philippart, M. & Wilson, B.W. (1974) The Schwartz-Jampel syndrome: Its clinical, physiological and histological expressions. *Journal of the Neurological Sciences*, **22**, 127.

Fried, K., Arlozorov, A. & Spira, R. (1975) Autosomal recessive oculopharyngeal muscular dystrophy. *Journal of Medical Genetics*, **12**, 416.

Friedreich, N. (1863) Ueber congenitale halbseitige kopfhypertrophie. *Virchows Archiv für pathologische Anatomie*, **28**, 474.

Fuchs, E. (1890) Ueber isolieren doppelseitige ptosis. *Archiv für Ophthalmologie*, **36**, 234.

Furukawa, T. & Peter, J.B. (1977) X-linked muscular dystrophy. *Annals of Neurology*, **2**, 414.

Gamstorp, I. & Wohlfart, G. (1959) A syndrome characterised by myokymia, myotonia, muscular wasting and increased perspiration. *Acta psychiatrica scandinavica*, **34**, 181.

Gardner-Medwin, D. (1968) Studies of the carrier state in the Duchenne type of muscular dystrophy. 2. Quantitative electromyography as a method of carrier detection. *Journal of Neurology, Neurosurgery and Psychiatry*, **31**, 124.

Gardner-Medwin, D. (1970) Mutation rate in Duchenne type of muscular dystrophy. *Journal of Medical Genetics*, **7**, 334.

Gardner-Medwin, D. (1977a) Objectives in the management of Duchenne muscular dystrophy. *Israel Journal of Medical Sciences*, **13**, 229.

Gardner-Medwin, D. (1977b) Children with genetic muscular disorders. *British Journal of Hospital Medicine*, **17**, 314.

Gardner-Medwin, D. (1978) Strategie per la prevenzione della distrofia muscolare di Duchenne, in *Distrofia Muscolare: alla ricerca di nuove frontiere*, published by the Mario Negri Institute for Pharmacological Research and the Carlo Besta Neurological Institute, Milan. pp. 4–9.

Gardner-Medwin, D. (1979) Controversies about Duchenne

muscular dystrophy; (1) Neonatal screening. *Developmental Medicine and Child Neurology*, **21**, 390.

Gardner-Medwin, D., Bundey, S. & Green, S. (1978) Early diagnosis of Duchenne muscular dystrophy. *Lancet*, **1**, 1102 (letter).

Gardner-Medwin, D., Pennington, R.J. and Walton, J.N. (1971) The detection of carriers of X-linked muscular dystrophy genes: A review of some methods studied in Newcastle upon Tyne. *Journal of the Neurological Sciences*, **13**, 459.

Genever, E.E. (1971) Suxamethonium-induced cardiac arrest in unsuspected pseudohypertrophic muscular dystrophy. *British Journal of Anaesthesia*, **43**, 984.

Geschwind, N.A. & Simpson, J.A. (1955) Procaine amide in the treatment of myotonia. *Brain*, **78**, 81.

Gibson, D.A., Koreska, J., Robertson, D., Kahn, A. & Albisser, A.M. (1978) The management of spinal deformity in Duchenne's muscular dystrophy. *Orthopedic Clinics of North America*, **9**, 437.

Gilboa, N. & Swanson, J.R. (1976) Serum creatine phosphokinase in normal newborns. *Archives of Disease in Childhood*, **51**, 283.

Gillam, P.M.S., Heaf, P.J.D., Kaufman, L. & Lucas, B.G.B. (1964) Respiration in dystrophia myotonica. *Thorax*, **19**, 112.

Glesson, J.A., Swann, J.C., Hughes, D.T.D. & Lee, F.I. (1967) Dystrophia myotonica—a radiological survey. *British Journal of Radiology*, **40**, 96.

Gomez, M.R., Engel, A.G., Dewald, G. & Peterson, H.A. (1977) Failure of inactivation of Duchenne dystrophy X-chromosome in one of female identical twins. *Neurology (Minneapolis)*, **27**, 537.

Gorden, P., Griggs, R.C., Nissley, S.P., Roth, J. & Engel, W.K. (1969) Studies of plasma insulin in myotonic dystrophy. *Journal of Clinical Endocrinology*, **29**, 684.

Gowers, W.R. (1879) *Pseudohypertrophic Muscular Paralysis* (Churchill: London).

Gowers, W.R. (1902) A lecture on myopathy and a distal form. *British Medical Journal*, **2**, 89.

Greenfield, J.G., Cornman, T. & Shy, G.M. (1958) The prognostic value of the muscle biopsy in the 'floppy infant'. *Brain*, **81**, 461.

Greenfield, J.G., Shy, G.M., Alvord, E.C. & Berg, L. (1957) An Atlas of Muscle Pathology in Neuromuscular Diseases (Livingstone: Edinburgh).

Greenhouse, A.H., Bicknell, J.M., Pesch, R.N. & Seelinger, D.F. (1967) Myotonia, myokymia, hyperhidrosis and wasting of muscle. *Neurology (Minneapolis)*, **17**, 263.

Griggs, R.C., Davis, R.J., Anderson, D.C. & Dove, J.T. (1975) Cardiac conduction in myotonic dystrophy. *American Journal of Medicine*, **59**, 37.

Grimm, T. (1975) The ages at onset and at death in dystrophia myotonica. *Journale de Génétique Humaine*, **23** (suppl.), 172.

Gubbay, S.S., Walton, J.N. & Pearce, G.W. (1966) Clinical and pathological study of a case of congenital muscular dystrophy. *Journal of Neurology, Neurosurgery and Psychiatry*, **29**, 500.

Hallen, O. (1970) Zur Frage der Kombination endokriner Symptome und Syndrome mit der Dystrophia musculorum progressiva. *Deutsche Zeitschrift für Nervenheilkunde*, **197**, 101.

Hanson, P.A. & Rowland, L.P. (1971) Möbius syndrome and facioscapulohumeral muscular dystrophy. *Archives of Neurology*, **24**, 31.

Harper, P.S. (1975) Congenital myotonic dystrophy in Britain. I. Clinical aspects *and* II. Genetic basis. *Archives of Disease in Childhood*, **50**, 505 & 514.

Harper, P.S. (1979) *Myotonic Dystrophy* (Saunders: Philadelphia, London & Toronto).

Harper, P.S. & Dyken, P.R. (1972) Early-onset dystrophia myotonica: evidence supporting a maternal environmental factor. *Lancet*, **2**, 53.

Harper, P.S. & Johnston, D.M. (1972) Recessively inherited myotonia congenita. *Journal of Medical Genetics*, **9**, 213.

Harper, P.S., Bias, W.B., Hutchinson, J.R. & McKusick, V.A. (1971) ABH secretor status in the fetus: a genetic marker identifiable by amniocentesis. *Journal of Medical Genetics*, **8**, 438.

Harper, P.S., Penny, R., Foley, T.P., Migeon, C.J. & Blizzard, R.M. (1972) Gonadal function in males with myotonic dystrophy. *Journal of Clinical Endocrinology and Metabolism*, **35**, 852.

Harper, P.S., Rivas, M.L., Bias, W.B., Hutchinson, J.R., Dyken, P.R. & McKusick, V.A. (1972) Genetic linkage confirmed between the locus for myotonic dystrophy and the ABH-secretion and Lutheran blood group loci. *American Journal of Human Genetics*, **24**, 310.

Hausmanowa-Petrusewicz, I., Prot, J., Niebroj-Dobosz, I., Hetnarska, L., Emeryk, B., Wasowicz, B., Askanas, W. & Slucka, C. (1968) Studies of healthy relatives of patients with Duchenne muscular dystrophy. *Journal of the Neurological Sciences*, **7**, 465.

Hayes, R., London, W., Seidman, J. & Embree, L. (1963) Oculopharyngeal muscular dystrophy. *New England Journal of Medicine*, **268**, 163.

Henson, T.E., Muller, J. & De Myer, W.E. (1967) Hereditary myopathy limited to females. *Archives of Neurology*, **17**, 238.

Hertrich, O. (1957) Kasuistiche Mitteilung über eine Sippe mit dominant vererblicher, wahrscheinlich weiblich geschlechtsbebundener progressiver Muskeldystrophie des Schultergürteltyps. *Nervenarzt*, **28**, 325.

Heyck, H., Laudahn, G. & Carsten, P.M. (1966) Enzymaktivatätsbestimmungen bei Dystrophia musculorum progressiva. IV Mitteilung, *Klinische Wochenschrift*, **44**, 695.

Hoffman, J. (1897) Ein fall von Thomsen'scher Krankheit, complicert durch Neuritis multiplex. *Deutsche Zeitschrift für Nervenheilkunde*, **9**, 272.

Hooshmand, H., Dove, J. & Suter, C. (1969) The use of serum lactate dehydrogenase isoenzymes in the diagnosis of muscle diseases. *Neurology (Minneapolis)*, **19**, 26.

Hopkins, A. & Wray, S. (1967) The effect of pregnancy on dystrophia myotonica. *Neurology (Minneapolis)*, **17**, 166.

Hudgson, P., Bradley, W.G. & Jenkison, M. (1972) Familial 'mitochondrial' myopathy: a myopathy associated with disordered oxidative metabolism in muscle fibres. Part I. Clinical, electrophysiological and pathological findings. *Journal of the Neurological Sciences*, **16**, 343.

Hudgson, P., Pearce, G.W. & Walton, J.N. (1967) Preclinical muscular dystrophy: histopathological changes observed on muscle biopsy. *Brain*, **90**, 565.

Huff, T.A., Horton, E.S. & Lebovitz, H.E. (1967) Abnormal insulin secretion in myotonic dystrophy. *New England Journal of Medicine*, **277**, 837.

Hughes, B.P. (1963) Serum enzyme studies with special reference to the Duchenne type dystrophy. In *Research in Muscular Dystrophy. Proceedings of the 2nd Symposium on Current Research in Muscular Dystrophy*, p. 167 (Pitman: London).

Humphrey, J.G., Hill, M.E. & Gordon, A.S. (1976) Myotonia associated with small cell carcinoma of the lung. *Archives of Neurology*, **33**, 375.

Hutchinson, (1879) An ophthalmoplegia externa or symmetrical immobility (partial) of the eye with ptosis. *Transactions of the Medico-Chirurgical Society of Edinburgh*, **62**, 307.

Huttenlocher, P.R., Landwirth, J., Hanson, V., Gallacher, B.B. & Bensch, K. (1969) Osteochondro-muscular dystrophy: a disorder manifested by multiple skeletal deformities, myotonia and dystrophic changes in muscle. *Pediatrics*, **44**, 945.

Hutton, E.M. & Thompson, M.W. (1976) Carrier detection and genetic counselling in Duchenne muscular dystrophy: a follow-up study. *Journal of the Canadian Medical Association*, **115**, 749.

Inkley, S.R., Oldenburg, F.C. & Vignos, P.J. (1974) Pulmonary function in Duchenne muscular dystrophy related to stage of disease. *The American Journal of Medicine*, **56**, 297.

Insley, J., Bird, G.W.G., Harper, P.S. & Pearce, G.W. (1976) Prenatal prediction of myotonic dystrophy. *Lancet*, **1**, 806.

Ionasescu, V. & Zellweger, H. (1974) Duchenne muscular dystrophy in young girls? *Acta Neurologica Scandinavica*, **50**, 619.

Ionasescu, V., Zellweger, H. & Burmeister, L. (1976) Detection of carriers and genetic counseling in Duchenne muscular dystrophy by ribosomal protein synthesis. *Acta Neurologica Scandinavica*, **54**, 442.

Ionasescu, V., Zellweger, H. & Cancilla, P. (1978) Fetal serum-creatine-phosphokinase not a valid predictor of Duchenne muscular dystrophy. *Lancet*, **2**, 1251.

Isaacs, H. (1961) A syndrome of continuous muscle fibre activity. *Journal of Neurology, Neurosurgery and Psychiatry*, **24**, 319.

Jackson, C.E. & Carey, J.H. (1961) Progressive muscular dystrophy: autosomal recessive type. *Pediatrics*, **28**, 77.

Jackson, C.E. & Strehler, D.A. (1968) Limb girdle muscular dystrophy: clinical manifestations and detection of preclinical disease. *Pediatrics*, **41**, 495.

Jalbert, P., Mouriquand, C., Beaudoing, A. & Jaillard, M. (1966) Myopathie progressive de type Duchenne et mosaique XO/XX/XXX: Considerations sur la genèse de la fibre musculaire striée. *Annales Génétiques*, **9**, 104.

James, T.N. (1962) Observations on the cardiovascular involvement, including the cardiac conduction system, in progressive muscular dystrophy. *American Heart Journal*, **63**, 48.

Jéquier, M. (1950) Dystrophie myotonique et hyperostose cranienne. *Schweizerische medizinische Wochenschrift*, **80**, 593.

Johnston, H.A. (1964) Severe muscular dystrophy in girls. *Journal of Medical Genetics*, **1**, 79.

Julien, J., Vital, C., Vallat, J.M., Vallat, M. & le Blanc, M. (1974) Oculopharyngeal muscular dystrophy: A case with abnormal mitochondria and 'fingerprint' inclusions. *Journal of the Neurological Sciences*, **21**, 165.

Kaeser, H.E. (1965) Scapuloperoneal muscular atrophy. *Brain*, **88**, 407.

Kakulas, B.A. & Hurse, P.V. (1978) Twelve years of genetic counselling in muscular dystrophy in Western Australia. In *Abstracts of the IVth International Congress of Neuromuscular Diseases*, Montreal.

Kakulas, B.A., Gullity, P.E. & Maguire, P. (1975) Muscular dystrophy in young girls. *Proceedings of the Australian Association of Neurologists*, **12**, 75.

Kamoshita, S., Konishi, Y., Segawa, M. & Fukuyama, Y. (1976) Congenital muscular dystrophy as a disease of the central nervous system. *Archives of Neurology*, **33**, 513.

Kaufman, L. (1960) Anaesthesia in dystrophia myotonica: A review of the hazards of anaesthesia. *Proceedings of the Royal Society of Medicine*, **53**, 183.

Kazakov, V.M., Bogorodinsky, D.K. & Skorometz, A.A. (1976) The myogenic scapulo-peroneal syndrome. Muscular dystrophy in the K. kindred: Clinical study and genetics. *Clinical Genetics*, **10**, 41.

Kazakov, V.M., Bogorodinsky, D.K., Znoyko, Z.V. & Skorometz, A.A. (1974) The facio-scapulo-limb (or the facioscapulohumeral) type of muscular dystrophy: clinical and genetic study of 200 cases. *European Neurology*, **11**, 236.

Kearns, T.P. & Sayre, G.P. (1958) Retinitis pigmentosa, external ophthalmoplegia and complete heart block. *Archives of Ophthalmology*, **60**, 280.

Kilburn, K.H., Eagan, J.T., Sieker, H.O. & Heyman, A. (1959) Cardiopulmonary insufficiency in myotonic and progressive muscular dystrophy. *New England Journal of Medicine*, **261**, 1089.

Kiloh, L.G. & Nevin, S. (1951) Progressive dystrophy of external ocular muscles (ocular myopathy). *Brain*, **74**, 115.

Kirschner, B.S. & Pachman, L.M. (1976) IgA deficiency and recurrent pneumonia in the Schwartz-Jampel syndrome. *Journal of Pediatrics*, **88**, 1060.

Klein, D. (1958) La dystrophie myotonique (Steinert) et la myotonie congénitale (Thomsen) en Suisse. Étude clinique genetique et demographique. *Journale Génétique Humaine*, suppl. **7**, 1.

Klink, D.D. & Wachs, H. (1963) Polymyositis associated with thyroid carcinoma; report of a case. *Neurology (Minneapolis)*, **13**, 160.

Kloepfer, H.W. & Talley, C. (1958) Autosomal recessive inheritance of Duchenne type muscular dystrophy. *Annals of Human Genetics*, **22**, 138.

Kohno, K. (1978) Mental retardation in Duchenne muscular dystrophy. In *Abstracts of the IVth International Congress on Neuromuscular Diseases*, Montreal.

Kottke, F.J., Pauley, D.L. & Ptak, R.A. (1966) The rationale for prolonged stretching for correction of shortening of connective tissue. *Archives of Physical Medicine*, **47**, 345.

Kovick, R.B., Fogelman, A.M., Abbasi, A.S., Peter, J.P. & Pearce, M.L. (1975) Echocardiographic evaluation of posterior left ventricular wall motion in muscular dystrophy. *Circulation*, **52**, 447.

Kozicka, A., Prot, J. & Wasilewski, R. (1971) Mental retardation in patients with Duchenne progressive muscular dystrophy. *Journal of the Neurological Sciences*, **14**, 209.

Kugelberg, E. & Welander, L. (1956) Heredofamilial juvenile muscular atrophy simulating muscular dystrophy. *Archives of Neurology and Psychiatry*, **75**, 500.

Lamy, M. & de Grouchy, J. (1954) L'hérédité de la myopathie (formes basses). *Journale Génétique Humaine*, **3**, 219.

Landouzy, L. & Dejerine, J. (1884) De la myopathie atrophique progressive (myopathie hereditaire), débutant, dans l'enfance, par le face, sans alteration du système nerveux. *Comptes rendus hebdomadaires des séances de l'Academie des sciences*, **98**, 53.

Lane, R.J.M., Gardner-Medwin, D. & Roses, A.D. (1980) Electrocardiographic abnormalities in carriers of Duchenne muscular dystrophy. *Neurology (Minneapolis)*, **30**, 497.

de Lange, C. (1937) Studien über angeborene Lähmugen bzw. angeborene Hypotonie. *Acta paediatrica*, **20**, Suppl III, 33.

Lapresle, J.M., Fardeau, M. & Godet-Guillain, J. (1972) Myopathie distal congénitale avec hypertrophie des mollets—Présence d'anomalies mitochondriales à la biopsie musculaire. *Journal of the Neurological Sciences*, **17**, 87.

Lebenthal, E., Shochet, S.B., Adam, A., Seelenfreund, M., Fried, A., Najenson, T., Sandbank, U. & Matoth, Y. (1970) Arthrogryposis multiplex congenita: Twenty-three cases in an Arab kindred. *Paediatrics*, **46**, 891.

Lee, F.I. & Hughes, D.T.D. (1964) Systemic effects in dystrophia myotonica. *Brain*, **87**, 521.

Lenard, H.-G., Goebel, H.H. & Weigel, W. (1977) Smooth muscle involvement in congenital myotonic dystrophy. *Neuropadiätrie*, **8**, 42.

Levison, H. (1951) *Dystrophia musculorum progressiva* (Ejnar Munksgaards Forlag: Copenhagen).

Lewis, A.J. & Besant, D.F. (1962) Muscular dystrophy in infancy: Report of 2 cases in siblings with diaphragmatic weakness. *Journal of Paediatrics*, **60**, 376.

Lewis, I. (1966) Late-onset muscular dystrophy: oculopharyngoesophageal variety. *Canadian Medical Association Journal*, **95**, 146.

Leyburn, P. & Walton, J.N. (1959) The treatment of myotonia: a controlled trial. *Brain*, **82**, 81.

Leyden, E. (1876) *Klinik der Rückenmarks-Krankheiten*, Vol. 2, p. 531 (Hirchwald: Berlin).

Ludman, H. (1962) Dysphagia in dystrophia myotonica. *Journal of Laryngology*, **76**, 234.

Lundberg, P.O. (1962) Ocular myopathy with hypogonadism. *Acta Neurologica Scandinavica*, **38**, 142.

Maas, O. & Paterson, A.S. (1939) The identity of myotonia congenita (Thomsen's disease), dystrophia myotonica (myotonia atrophica) and paramyotonia. *Brain*, **62**, 198.

Maas, O. & Paterson, A.S. (1950) The identity of myotonia congenita, dystrophia myotonica and paramyotonia. *Brain*, **73**, 318.

Mabry, C.C., Roeckel, I.E., Munich, R.L. & Robertson, D. (1965) X-linked pseudohypertrophic muscular dystrophy with a late onset and slow progression. *New England Journal of Medicine*, **273**, 1062.

Magee, K.R. (1963) A study of paramyotonia congenita. *Archives of Neurology*, **8**, 461.

Magee, K.R. (1966) Paramyotonia congenita: association with cutaneous cold sensitivity and description of peculiar sustained postures after muscle contraction. *Archives of Neurology*, **14**, 590.

Magee, K.R. & de Jong, R.N. (1965) Hereditary distal myopathy with onset in infancy. *Archives of Neurology*, **13**, 387.

Mahoney, M.J., Haseltine, F.P., Hobbins, J.C., Banker, B.Q., Caskey, C.T. & Golbus, M.S. (1977) Prenatal diagnosis of Duchenne's muscular dystrophy. *New England Journal of Medicine*, **297**, 968.

Mann, O., de Leon, A.C., Perloff, J.K., Simanis, J. & Horrigan, F.D. (1968) Duchenne's muscular dystrophy: the electrocardiogram in female relatives. *American Journal of Medical Science*, **255**, 376.

Manning, G.W. & Cropp, G.J. (1958) The electrocardiogram in progressive muscular dystrophy. *British Heart Journal*, **20**, 410.

Markand, D.N., North, R.R., D'Agostino, A.N. & Daly, D.D. (1969) Benign sex-linked muscular dystrophy. Clinical and pathological features. *Neurology (Minneapolis)*, **19**, 612.

Markesbery, W.R., Griggs, R.C. & Herr, B. (1977) Distal myopathy: electron microscopic and histochemical studies. *Neurology (Minneapolis)*, **27**, 727.

Markesbery, W.R., Griggs, R.C., Leach, R.P. & Lapham, L.W. (1974) Late onset hereditary distal myopathy. *Neurology (Minneapolis)*, **23**, 127.

Marsh, G.G. & Munsat, T.L. (1974) Evidence for early impairment of verbal intelligence in Duchenne muscular dystrophy. *Archives of Disease in Childhood*, **49**, 118.

Marshall, J. (1959) Observations on endocrine function in dystrophia myotonica. *Brain*, **82**, 221.

Mawatari, S. & Katayama, K. (1973) Scapulohumeral muscular atrophy with cardiomyopathy: an X-linked recessive trait. *Archives of Neurology*, **28**, 55.

McComas, A.J., Sica, R.E.P. & Currie, S. (1970) Muscular dystrophy: evidence for a neural factor. *Nature*, **226**, 1263.

McComas, A.J., Sica, R.E.P. & Currie, S. (1971) An electrophysiological study of Duchenne dystrophy. *Journal of Neurology, Neurosurgery and Psychiatry*, **34**, 461.

Mendell, J.R., Engel, W.K. & Derrer, E.C. (1971) Duchenne muscular dystrophy: functional ischaemia reproduces its characteristic lesions. *Science*, **172**, 1143.

Mertens, H.-G. & Zschocke, S. (1965) Neuromyotonie. *Klinische Wochenschrift*, **43**, 917.

Meryon, E. (1852) On granular and fatty degeneration of the voluntary muscles. *Medico-Chirurgical Transactions (London)*, **35**, 73.

Milhorat, A.T. & Goldstone, L. (1965) The carrier state in muscular dystrophy of the Duchenne type: identification by serum creatine kinase level. *Journal of the American Medical Association*, **194**, 130.

Milhorat, A.T., Shafiq, S.A. & Goldstone, L. (1966) Changes in muscle structure in dystrophic patients, carriers and normal siblings seen by electron microscopy, correlation with levels of serum creatine phosphokinase (CPK). *Annals of the New York Academy of Sciences*, **138**, 246.

Möbius, P.J. (1879) Ueber die hereditaren nervenkrankheiten. *Sammlung klinischer Vortäge*, **171**, 1505.

Mokri, B. & Engel, A.G. (1975) Duchenne dystrophy: electron microscopic findings pointing to a basic or early abnormality in the plasma membrane of the muscle fibre. *Neurology (Minneapolis)*, **25**, 1111.

Moosa, A., Brown, B.H. & Dubowitz, V. (1972) Quantitative electromyography: carrier detection in Duchenne type muscular dystrophy using a new automatic technique. *Journal of Neurology, Neurosurgery and Psychiatry*, **35**, 841.

Morgan-Hughes, J.A. & Mair, W.G.P. (1973) Atypical muscle mitochondria in oculoskeletal myopathy. *Brain*, **96**, 215.

Morton, N.E. & Chung, C.S. (1959) Formal genetics of muscular dystrophy. *American Journal of Human Genetics*, **11**, 360.

Moser, H. & Emery, A.E.H. (1974) The manifesting carrier in Duchenne muscular dystrophy. *Clinical Genetics*, **5**, 271.

Moser, von H., Wiesmann, U., Richterich, R. & Rossi, E. (1964) Progressive Muskeldystrophie. VI. Häufigkeit, Klinik und Genetik der Duchenne form. *Schweizerische Medizinische Wochenschrift*, **94**, 1610.

Moser, von H., Wiesmann, U., Richterich, R. & Rossi, E. (1966) Progressive Muskeldystrophie. VIII. Häufigkeit, Klinik und Genetik der Typen I und III. *Schweizerische Medizinische Wochenschrift*, **96**, 169.

Moxley, R.T., Griggs, R.C., van Gelder, V. & Thiel, R. (1978) Insulin insensitivity in myotonic dystrophy: abnormal alanine regulation. *Abstracts of the IVth International Congress on Neuromuscular Diseases*, Montreal.

Munsat, T.L. (1967) Therapy of myotonia: a double-blind evaluation of diphenylhydantoin, procainamide, and placebo. *Neurology (Minneapolis)*, **17**, 359.

Munsat, T.L. & Piper, D. (1971) Genetically determined inflammatory myopathy with facioscapulohumeral distribution. *Neurology (Minneapolis)*, **21**, 440.

Murphy, S.F. & Drachman, D.B. (1968) The oculopharyngeal syndrome. *Journal of the American Medical Association*, **203**, 1003.

Nevin, S. (1936) Two cases of muscular degeneration occurring in late adult life, with a review of the recorded cases of late progressive muscular dystrophy (late progressive myopathy). *Quarterly Journal of Medicine*, **5**, 51.

Nicholson, G.A., Gardner-Medwin, D., Pennington, R.J.T. & Walton, J.N. (1979) Carrier detection in Duchenne muscular dystrophy: assessment of the effect of age on detection-rate with serum-creatine-kinase-activity. *Lancet*, **1**, 692.

Nissen, K. (1923) Beiträge zur kenntnis der Thomsen'schen krankheit (myotonia congenita) mit besonderer berücksichtigung des hereditären momentes und semen beziehungen zu den Mendelschen bererbungsregeln. *Zeitschrift fur klinische Medizin*, **97**, 58.

Norris, F.H. & Panner, B.J. (1966) Hypothyroid myopathy: clinical, electromyographical and ultrastructural observations. *Archives of Neurology*, **14**, 574.

O'Brien, M.D. (1962) An infantile muscular dystrophy: report of a case with autopsy findings. *Guy's Hospital Reports*, **111**, 98.

Olson, W., Engel, W.K., Walsh, G.O. & Einaugler, R. (1972) Oculocraniosomatic neuromuscular disease with 'ragged-red' fibers: histochemical and ultrastructural changes in limb muscles of a group of patients with idiopathic progressive external ophthalmoplegia. *Archives of Neurology*, **26**, 193.

Oppenheim, H. (1900) Ueber allgemeine und localisierte atonie der muskulatur (myatonie) im frühen kindesalter. *Monatsschrift für Psychiatrie und Neurologie*, **8**, 232.

Pavone, L., Mollica, F., Grasso, A., Cao, A. & Gullotta, F. (1978) Schwartz-Jampel syndrome in two daughters of first cousins. *Journal of Neurology, Neurosurgery and Psychiatry*, **41**, 161.

Pearce, G.W., Pearce, J.M.S. & Walton, J.N. (1966) The Duchenne type muscular dystrophy: histopathological studies of the carrier state. *Brain*, **89**, 109.

Pearce, J.M.S., Pennington, R.J.T. & Walton, J.N. (1964) Serum enzyme studies in muscle disease. III. Serum creatine kinase activity in relatives of patients with the Duchenne type of muscular dystrophy. *Journal of Neurology, Neurosurgery and Psychiatry*, **27**, 181.

Pearn, J.H. & Hudgson, P. (1978) A new syndrome—spinal muscular atrophy with adolescent onset and hypertrophied calves, simulating Becker dystrophy. *Lancet*, **1**, 1059.

Pearson, C.M. & Fowler, W.G. (1963) Hereditary non-progressive muscular dystrophy inducing arthrogryposis syndrome. *Brain*, **86**, 75.

Penn, A.S., Lisak, R.P. & Rowland, L.P. (1970) Muscular dystrophy in young girls. *Neurology (Minneapolis)*, **20**, 147.

Penrose, L.S. (1947) The problem of anticipation in pedigrees of dystrophia myotonica. *Annals of Eugenics (London)*, **14**, 125.

Perloff, J.K., de Leon, A.C. & O'Doherty, D. (1966) The cardiomyopathy of progressive muscular dystrophy. *Circulation*, **33**, 625.

Perloff, J.K., Roberts, W.C., de Leon, A.C. & O'Doherty, D. (1967) The distinctive electrocardiogram of Duchenne's progressive muscular dystrophy. *American Journal of Medicine*, **42**, 179.

Peterman, A.F., Lillington, G.A. & Jamplis, R.W. (1964) Progressive muscular dystrophy with ptosis and dysphagia. *Archives of Neurology*, **10**, 38.

Philip, U., Walton, J.N. & Smith, C.A.B. (1956) Colour-blindness and the Duchenne-type muscular dystrophy. *Annals of Human Genetics*, **21**, 155.

Pickard, N.A., Gruemer, H.-D., Verrill, H.L., Isaacs, E.R., Robinow, M., Nance, W.E., Myers, E.C. & Goldsmith, B. (1978) Systemic membrane defect in the proximal muscular dystrophies. *New England Journal of Medicine*, **299**, 841.

Polgar, J.G., Bradley, W.G., Upton, A.R.M., Anderson, J., Howat, J.M.L., Petito, F., Roberts, D.F. & Scopa, J. (1972) The early detection of dystrophia myotonica. *Brain*, **95**, 761.

Prosser, E.J., Murphy, E.J. & Thompson, M.W. (1969) Intelligence and the gene for Duchenne muscular dystrophy. *Archives of Disease in Childhood*, **44**, 221.

Pruzanski, W. (1962) Respiratory tract infections and silent aspiration in myotonic dystrophy. *Diseases of the Chest*, **42**, 608.

Pruzanski, W. (1966) Variants of myotonic dystrophy in pre-adolescent life (the syndrome of myotonic dysembryoplasia). *Brain*, **89**, 563.

Radu, H., Migea, S., Torok, Z., Bordeianu, L. & Radu, A. (1968) Carrier detection in X-linked Duchenne type muscular dystrophy: a pluridimensional investigation. *Journal of the Neurological Sciences*, **6**, 289.

Rebeiz, J.J., Caulfield, J.B. & Adams, R.D. (1969) Oculopharyngeal dystrophy—a presenescent myopathy: a clinico-pathologic study. In *Progress in Neuro-ophthalmology* (Excerpta Medica International Congress Series No. 176), p. 12 (Excerpta Medica: Amsterdam).

Refsum, S., Engeset, A. & Lönnum, A. (1959) Pneumoencephalographic changes in dystrophia myotonica. *Acta Psychiatrica et Neurologica Scandinavica* (Suppl. 137), **34**, 98.

Refsum, S., Lönnum, A., Sjaastad, O. & Engeset, A. (1967) Dystrophia myotonica: repeated pneumoencephalographic studies in ten patients. *Neurology (Minneapolis)*, **17**, 345.

Renwick, J.H., Bundey, S.E., Ferguson-Smith, M.A. & Izatt, M.M. (1970) Confirmation of linkage of the loci for myotonic dystrophy and ABH secretion. *Journal of Medical Genetics*, **8**, 407.

Resnick, J.S. & Engel, W.K. (1967) Myotonic lid lag in hypokalaemic periodic paralysis. *Journal of Neurology, Neurosurgery and Psychiatry*, **30**, 47.

Ricker, K. & Mertens, H.-G. (1968) The differential diagnosis of the myogenic (facio)-scapulo-peroneal syndrome. *European Neurology*, **1**, 275.

Ricker, K., Mertens, H.-G. & Schimrigk, K. (1968) The

neurogenic scapuloperoneal syndrome. *European Neurology*, **1**, 257.

Riggs, J.E., Griggs, R.C. & Moxley, R.T. (1977) Acetazolamide-induced weakness in paramyotonia congenita. *Annals of Internal Medicine*, **86**, 169.

Ringel, S.P., Carroll, J.E. & Schold, C. (1977) The spectrum of mild X-linked recessive muscular dystrophy. *Archives of Neurology*, **34**, 408.

Roberts, D.F. & Bradley, W.G. (1977) Immunoglobulin levels in dystrophia myotonica. *Journal of Medical Genetics*, **14**, 16.

Robin, G.C. & Brief, L.P. (1971) Scoliosis in childhood muscular dystrophy. *Journal of Bone and Joint Surgery*, **53A**, 466.

Robin, G.C. & Falewski de Leon, G. (1977) (editors) Symposium on muscular dystrophy. *Israel Journal of Medical Sciences*, **13**, 85–236.

Rosenberg, R.N., Schotland, D.L., Lovelace, R.E. & Rowland, L.P. (1968) Progressive ophthalmoplegia: report of cases. *Archives of Neurology*, **19**, 362.

Rosman, N.P. (1970) The cerebral defect and myopathy in Duchenne muscular dystrophy: a comparative clinico-pathological study. *Neurology (Minneapolis)*, **20**, 329.

Rosman, N.P. & Kakulas, B.A. (1966) Mental deficiency associated with muscular dystrophy. A neuropathological study. *Brain*, **89**, 769.

Ross, R.T. (1963) Ocular myopathy sensitive to curare. *Brain*, **86**, 67.

Ross, R.T. (1964) The effect of decamethonium on curare sensitive ocular myopathy. *Neurology (Minneapolis)*, **14**, 684.

Rothstein, T.L., Carlson, C.B. & Sumi, S.M. (1971) Polymyositis with facioscapulohumeral distribution. *Archives of Neurology*, **25**, 313.

Rotthauwe, H.-W. & Kowalewski, S. (1965a) Klinische und biochemische Untersuchungen bei Myopathien. III. Mitteilung. Recessive x-chromasomale Muskeldystrophie mit relativ gutartigem Verlauf. *Klinische Wochenschrift*, **43**, 158.

Rotthauwe, H.-W. & Kowalewski, S. (1965b) Klinische und biochemische Untersuchungen bei Myopathien. II Mitteilung. Die Bedeutung der Serum-Kreatin-Phosphokinase und derse Serum-Aldolase für die Idendifizierung von Heterozygoten der recessiv x-chromosomalen Formen der progressiven Muskel-dystrophie (Typ III a und b). *Klinische Wochenschrift*, **43**, 150.

Rotthauwe, H.-W., Mortier, W. & Beyer, H. (1972) Neuer Typ einer recessiv X-chromosomal vererbten Muskeldystrophie: Scapulo-numero-distale Muskeldystrophie mit frühzeitigen Kontrakturen und Herzrhythmusstörungen. *Humangenetik*, **16**, 181.

Rowland, L.P. (1976) Pathogenesis of muscular dystrophies. *Archives of Neurology*, **33**, 315.

Roy, L. & Gibson, D.A. (1970) Pseudohypertrophic muscular dystrophy and its surgical management: review of 30 patients. *Canadian Journal of Surgery*, **13**, 13.

Roy, S. & Dubowitz, V. (1970) Carrier detection in Duchenne muscular dystrophy: a comparative study of electron microscopy, light microscopy and serum enzymes. *Journal of the Neurological Sciences*, **11**, 65.

Russe, H., Busey, H. & Barbeau, A. (1967) Immunoglobulin changes in oculopharyngeal muscular dystrophy. *Proceedings of the 2nd International Congress of Neurogenetics*, Montreal.

Sagel, J., Distiller, L.A., Morley, J.E., Isaacs, H., Kay, G. & van der Walt, A. (1975) Myotonia dystrophica: studies on gonadal function using luteinising-hormone-releasing-hormone (LRH). *Journal of Clinical Endocrinology and Metabolism*, **40**, 1110.

Salmon, M.A., Esiri, M.M. & Ruderman, N.B. (1971) Myopathic disorder associated with mitochondrial abnormalities, hyperglycaemia and hyperketonaemia. *Lancet*, **2**, 290.

Sanders, D.B. (1976) Myotonia congenita with painful muscle contractions. *Archives of Neurology*, **33**, 580.

Sandifer, P.H. (1946) Chronic progressive ophthalmoplegia of myopathic origin. *Journal of Neurology, Neurosurgery and Psychiatry*, **9**, 81.

Sarnat, H.B., O'Connor, T. & Byrne, P.A. (1976) Clinical effects of myotonic dystrophy on pregnancy and the neonate. *Archives of Neurology*, **33**, 459.

Saunders, M., Ashworth, B., Emery, A.E.H. & Benedikz, J.E.G. (1968) Familial myotonic periodic paralysis with muscle wasting. *Brain*, **91**, 295.

Schapira, F., Dreyfus, J.-C., Schapira, G. & Demos, J. (1960) Etudes de l'aldolase et de la créatine kinase du sérum chez les mères de myopathes. *Revue Française d'Études Cliniques et Biologiques*, **5**, 990.

Schneck, L., Adachi, M., Briet, P., Wolintz, A. & Volk, B.W. (1973) Ophthalmoplegia plus with morphological and chemical studies of cerebellar and muscle tissue. *Journal of the Neurological Sciences*, **19**, 37.

Schneiderman, L.J., Sampson, W.I., Schoene, W.C. & Haydon, G.B. (1969) Genetic studies of a family with two unusual autosomal dominant conditions: muscular dystrophy and Pelger-Huet anomaly. *American Journal of Medicine*, **46**, 380.

Schott, J., Jacobi, M. & Wald, M.A. (1955) Electrocardiographic patterns in the differential diagnosis of progressive muscular dystrophy. *American Journal of Medical Science*, **229**, 517.

Schwartz, G.A. & Liu, C.-N. (1954) Chronic progressive external ophthalmoplegia: a clinical and neuropathologic report. *Archives of Neurology and Psychiatry*, **71**, 31.

Schwartz, O. & Jampel, R.S. (1962) Congenital blepharophimosis associated with a unique generalised myopathy. *Archives of Ophthalmology*, **68**, 52.

Sciarra, J.J. & Steer, C.M. (1961) Uterine contractions during labor in myotonic muscular dystrophy. *American Journal of Obstetrics and Gynecology*, **82**, 612.

Seitz, D. (1957) Zur nosologischen Stellung des sogenannten scapulo-peronealen Syndroms. *Deutsche Zeitschrift für Nervenheilkunde*, **175**, 547.

Shaw, R.F. & Dreifuss, F.E. (1969) Mild and severe forms of X-linked muscular dystrophy. *Archives of Neurology*, **20**, 451.

Shokeir, M.H.K. & Kobrinsky, N.L. (1976) Autosomal recessive muscular dystrophy in Manitoba Hutterites. *Clinical Genetics*, **9**, 197.

Shore, R.N. (1975) Myotonic dystrophy: hazards of pregnancy and infancy. *Developmental Medicine and Child Neurology*, **17**, 356.

Short, J.K. (1963) Congenital muscular dystrophy: a case report with autopsy findings. *Neurology (Minneapolis)*, **13**, 526.

Siegel, C.I., Hendrix, T.R. & Harvey, J.C. (1966) The swallowing disorder in myotonia dystrophica. *Gastroenterology*, **50**, 541.

Siegel, I.M. (1977) *The Clinical Management of Muscle Disease* (Heinemann: London).

Siegel, I.M., Miller, J.E. & Ray, R.D. (1968) Subcutaneous lower limb tenotomy in the treatment of pseudohypertrophic muscular dystrophy. *Journal of Bone and Joint Surgery*, **50A**, 1437.

Skinner, R., Smith, C. & Emery, A.E.H. (1974) Linkage between the loci for benign (Becker type) X-borne muscular dystrophy and deutan colour blindness. *Journal of Medical Genetics*, **11**, 317.

Skinner, R., Emery, A.E.H., Anderson, A.J.B. & Foxall, C. (1975) The detection of carriers of benign (Becker-type) X-linked muscular dystrophy. *Journal of Medical Genetics*, **12**, 131.

Skyring, A. & McKusick, V.A. (1961) Clinical, genetic and electrocardiographic studies in childhood muscular dystrophy. *American Journal of Medical Science*, **242**, 534.

Slucka, C. (1968) The electrocardiogram in Duchenne progressive muscular dystrophy. *Circulation*, **38**, 933.

Smith, H.L., Amick, L.D. & Johnson, W.W. (1966) Detection of subclinical and carrier states in Duchenne muscular dystrophy. *Journal of Pediatrics*, **69**, 67.

Smith, R. & Stern, G. (1967) Myopathy, osteomalacia and hyperparathyroidism. *Brain*, **90**, 593.

Somers, J.E. & Winer, N. (1966) Reversible myopathy and myotonia following administration of a hypocholesterolemic agent. *Neurology (Minneapolis)*, **16**, 761.

Spencer, G.E. & Vignos, P.J. (1962) Bracing for ambulation in childhood progressive muscular dystrophy. *Journal of Bone and Joint Surgery*, **44A**, 234.

Spiller, W.G. (1907) Myopathy of the distal type and its relation to the neural form of muscular atrophy (Charcot-Marie-Tooth type). *Journal of Nervous and Mental Disease*, **34**, 14.

Spiller, W.G. (1913) The relation of the myopathies. *Brain*, **36**, 913.

Steinert, H. (1909) Myopathologische beiträge: I. Ueber das klinische und anatomische bild des muskelschwunds der myotoniker. *Deutsche Zeitschrift für Nervenheilkunde*, **37**, 58.

Stephens, J., Hoover, M.L. & Denst, J. (1958) On familial ataxia, neural amyotrophy and their association with progressive extreme ophthalmoplegia. *Brain*, **81**, 556.

Stevenson, A.C. (1953) Muscular dystrophy in Northern Ireland. *Annals of Eugenics*, **18**, 50.

Stevenson, A.C. (1955) Muscular dystrophy in Northern Ireland. An account of nine additional families. *Annals of Human Genetics*, **19**, 159.

Sugita, H. & Tyler, F.H. (1963) Pathogenesis of muscular dystrophy. *Transactions of the Association of American Physicians*, **76**, 231.

Sumner, D., Crawfurd, M.d'A. & Harriman, D.G.F. (1971) Distal muscular dystrophy in an English family. *Brain*, **94**, 51.

Taylor, E.W. (1915) Progressive vagus-glossopharyngeal paralysis with ptosis. A contribution to the group of family diseases. *Journal of Nervous and Mental Disease*, **42**, 129.

Thomas, P.K., Calne, D.B. & Elliott, C.F. (1972) X-linked scapuloperoneal syndrome. *Journal of Neurology, Neurosurgery and Psychiatry*, **35**, 208.

Thomas, P.K., Schott, G.D. & Morgan-Hughes, J.A. (1975) Adult onset scapuloperoneal myopathy. *Journal of Neurology, Neurosurgery and Psychiatry*, **38**, 1008.

Thomasen, E. (1948) *Thomsen's Disease, Paramyotonia, Dystrophia Myotonica* (Universitetsforlaget: Aarhus).

Thompson, M.W., Murphy, E.G. & McAlpine, P.J. (1967) An assessment of the creatine kinase test in the detection of carriers of Duchenne muscular dystrophy. *Journal of Pediatrics*, **71**, 82.

Thomsen, J. (1876) Tonische krämpfe in willkürlich beweglichen muskeln in folge von ererbterpsychischer disposition (ataxia muscularis?). *Archiv für Psychiatrie und Nervenkrankheiten*, **6**, 706.

Thomson, A.M.P. (1968) Dystrophia cordis myotonica studied by serial histology of the pacemaker and conducting system. *Journal of Pathology and Bacteriology*, **96**, 285.

Thomson, W.H.S. & Smith, I. (1978) X-linked recessive (Duchenne) muscular dystrophy and purine metabolism: effects of oral allopurinol and adenylate. *Metabolism*, **27**, 151.

Thrush, D.C., Morris, C.J. & Salmon, M.V. (1972) Paramyotonia congenita: a clinical, histochemical and pathological study. *Brain*, **95**, 537.

Todorov, A., Jéquier, M., Klein, D. & Morton, N.E. (1970) Analyse de la ségrégation dans la dystrophie myotonique. *Journale de Genetique Humaine*, **18**, 387.

Tomlinson, B.E., Walton, J.N. & Irving, D. (1974) Spinal cord limb motor neurones in muscular dystrophy. *Journal of the Neurological Sciences*, **22**, 305.

Tunbridge, P.B. & Diamond, C. (1966) Recent treatment of progressive muscular dystrophy. *Medical Journal of Australia*, **1**, 962.

Turner, J.W.A. (1940) The relationship between amyotonia congenita and congenital myopathy. *Brain*, **63**, 163.

Turner, J.W.A. & Heathfield, K.W.G. (1961) Quadriceps myopathy occurring in middle age. *Journal of Neurology, Neurosurgery and Psychiatry*, **24**, 18.

Turner, J.W.A. & Lees, F. (1962) Congenital myopathy—a fifty year follow up. *Brain*, **85**, 733.

Tyler, F.H. & Wintrobe, M.M. (1950) Studies in disorders of muscle. I. The problem of progressive muscular dystrophy. *Annals of Internal Medicine*, **32**, 72.

Tyrer, J.H. & Sutherland, J.M. (1961) The primary spino-cerebellar atrophies and their associated defects, with a study of the foot deformity. *Brain*, **84**, 289.

van den Bosch, J. (1963) Investigations of the carrier state in the Duchenne type dystrophy. *Proceedings of the 2nd Symposium on Research in Muscular Dystrophy*, p. 23 (Pitman: London).

van der Does de Willebois, A.E.M., Bethlem, J., Meijer, A.E.F.H. & Simons, A.J.R. (1968) Distal myopathy with onset in early infancy. *Neurology (Minneapolis)*, **18**, 383.

Vanier, T.M. (1960) Dystrophia myotonica in childhood. *British Medical Journal*, **2**, 1284.

van't Hoff, W. (1962) Familial myotonic periodic paralysis. *Quarterly Journal of Medicine*, **31**, 385.

van Wijngaarden, G.K., Hagen, C.J., Bethlem, J. & Meijer, A.E.F.H. (1968) Myopathy of the quadriceps muscles. *Journal of the Neurological Sciences*, **7**, 201.

Verellen, C., Freund, M., de Meyer, R., Laterre, C., Ferrière, G., Scholberg, B. & Frédéric, J. (1978) Progressive muscular dystrophy of the Duchenne type in a young girl associated with an aberration of chromosome X. In *Abstracts of the IVth International Congress on Neuromuscular Diseases*, Montreal.

Victor, M., Hayes, R. & Adams, R.D. (1962) Oculopharyngeal muscular dystrophy. A familial disease of late life characterised by dysphagia and progressive ptosis of the eyelids. *New England Journal of Medicine*, **267**, 1267.

Vignos, P.J. & Watkins, M.P. (1966) The effect of exercise in muscular dystrophy. *Journal of the American Medical Association*, **197**, 843.

Vignos, P.J., Spencer, G.E. & Archibald, K.C. (1963) Management of progressive muscular dystrophy of childhood. *Journal of the American Medical Association*, **184**, 89.

Vogt, A. (1921) Die Cataract bei myotonischer Dystrophie. *Schweizerische Medizinische Wochenschrift*, **2**, 669.

Wachsmuth, A. (1855) Ueber progressive Muskelatrophie. Zeitschrift für rationell Medizin, **7**, 1.

Wadia, R.S., Wadgaonkar, S.U., Amin, R.B. & Sardesai, H.V. (1976) An unusual family of benign 'X' linked muscular dystrophy with cardiac involvement. *Journal of Medical Genetics*, **13**, 352.

Walsh, F.B. (1957) *Clinical Neuro-ophthalmology*, 2nd Edn. (Bailliere, Tindall & Cox: London).

Walsh, J.C., Turtle, J.R., Miller, S. & McLeod, J.G. (1970) Abnormalities of insulin secretion in dystrophia myotonica. *Brain*, **93**, 731.

Walton, J.N. (1955) On the inheritance of muscular dystrophy. *Annals of Human Genetics*, **20**, 1.

Walton, J.N. (1956a) The inheritance of muscular dystrophy: further observations. *Annals of Human Genetics*, **21**, 40.

Walton, J.N. (1956b) Two cases of myopathy limited to the quadriceps. *Journal of Neurology and Psychiatry*, **19**, 160.

Walton, J.N. (1961) Muscular dystrophy and its relation to the other myopathies. *Research Publications of the Association of Nervous and Mental Diseases*, **38**, 378.

Walton, J.N. & Adams, R.D. (1958) *Polymyositis* (Livingstone: Edinburgh).

Walton, J.N. & Nattrass, F.J. (1954) On the classification, natural history and treatment of the myopathies. *Brain*, **77**, 169.

Walton, J.N. & Warrick, C.K. (1954) Osseous changes in myopathy. *British Journal of Radiology*, **27**, 1.

Waters, D.D., Nutter, D.O., Hopkins, L.C. & Dorney, E.R. (1975) Cardiac features of an unusual X-linked humeroperoneal neuromuscular disease. *New England Journal of Medicine*, **293**, 1017.

Welander, L. (1951) Myopathia distalis tarda hereditaria. *Acta Medica Scandinavica*, Suppl. **264**, 1.

Welander, L. (1957) Homozygous appearance of distal myopathy. *Acta Geneticae Medicae et Gemellologiae*, **7**, 321.

Welsh, J.D., Haase, G.R. & Bynum, T.E. (1964) Myotonic muscular dystrophy: systemic manifestations. *Archives of Internal Medicine*, **114**, 669.

Wharton, B.A. (1965) An unusual variety of muscular dystrophy. *Lancet*, **1**, 603.

Wiesmann, U., Moser, H., Richterich, R. & Rossi, E. (1965) Progressive Muskeldystrophie. VII. Die Erfassung von Heterozygoten der Duchenne-Muskeldystrophie durch Messung der Serum-Kreatin-Kinase unter lokalisierter Arbeitsbelastung in Anoxie. *Klinische Wochenschrift*, **43**, 1015.

Wilkins, K.E. & Gibson, D.A. (1976) The patterns of spinal deformity in Duchenne muscular dystrophy. *Journal of Bone and Joint Surgery*, **58A**, 24.

Willison, R.G. (1967) Quantitative electromyography: the detection of carriers of Duchenne dystrophy. *Proceedings of the 2nd International Congress of Neurogenetics*, Montreal.

Wilson, J. & Walton, J.N. (1959) The muscular manifestations of hypothyroidism. *Journal of Neurology and Psychiatry*, **22**, 320.

Wilson, K.M., Evans, K.A. & Carter, C.O. (1965) Creatine kinase levels in women who carry genes for three types of muscular dystrophy. *British Medical Journal*, **1**, 750.

Wochner, R.D., Drews, G., Strober, W. & Waldmann, T.A. (1966) Accelerated breakdown of immunoglobulin G (IgG) in myotonic dystrophy: a hereditary error of immunoglobulin catabolism. *Journal of Clinical Investigation*, **45**, 321.

Wolintz, A.H., Sonnenblick, E.H. & Engel, W.K. (1966) Stokes-Adams syndrome and atrial arrythmias as the presenting symptoms of myotonic dystrophy, with response to electro-cardioversion. *Annals of Internal Medicine*, **65**, 1260.

Worden, D.K. & Vignos, P.J. (1962) Intellectual function in childhood progressive muscular dystrophy. *Pediatrics*, **29**, 968.

Worster-Drought, C. & Sargent, F. (1952) Muscular fasciculation and reactive myotonia in polyneuritis. *Brain*, **75**, 595.

Yamashita, M., Matsuki, A. & Oyama, T. (1976) General anaesthesia for a patient with progressive muscular dystrophy. *Anaesthetist*, **25**, 76.

Zatuchni, J., Aegerter, E.E., Molthan, L. & Shuman, C.R. (1951) The heart in progressive muscular dystrophy. *Circulation*, **3**, 846.

Zatz, M., Itskan, S.B., Sanger, R., Frota-Pessoa, O. & Saldanha, P.H. (1974) New linkage data for the X-linked types of muscular dystrophy and G6PD variants, colour blindness and Xg blood groups. *Journal of Medical Genetics*, **11**, 321.

Zellweger, H. & Antonik, A. (1975) Newborn screening for Duchenne muscular dystrophy. *Pediatrics*, **55**, 30.

Zellweger, H. & Hanson, J.W. (1967a) Psychometric studies in muscular dystrophy type IIIa (Duchenne). *Developmental Medicine and Child Neurology*, **9**, 576.

Zellweger, H. & Hanson, J.W. (1967b) Slowly progressive X-linked recessive muscular dystrophy (type IIIb). *Archives of Internal Medicine*, **120**, 525.

Zellweger, H., Afifi, A., McCormick, W.F. & Mergner, W. (1967) Severe congenital muscular dystrophy. *American Journal of Diseases of Childhood*, **114**, 591.

Zintz, von R. & Villiger, W. (1967). Elektronenmikroskopische Befunde bei 3 Fällen von chronisch progressiver okulärer Muskeldystrophie. *Ophthalmologica*, **153**, 439.

Inflammatory myopathies

PART I

POLYMYOSITIS AND RELATED DISORDERS

S. Currie

INTRODUCTION: THE INFLAMMATORY MYOPATHIES

The term myositis can be used for any disorder in which inflammation affects muscle. The inflammation may be confined to a single muscle or involve many. At the microscopic level it may be focal or confluent; in location it is interstitial or perivascular or both. Necrobiotic or degenerative changes in muscle fibre cells accompany the inflammation. This Chapter is concerned mainly with the idiopathic myositides of which polymyositis is the most important. However, the remaining inflammatory myopathies are also discussed. Some of the latter are considered more fully in other chapters and cross-references are made where appropriate. They are mentioned in this chapter for the sake of completeness and because they may be of relevance to the aetiology of the idiopathic disorders. For example, chronic viral myositis and polymyositis have clinical and pathological features in common and a case can be made for calling viral myositis a 'related disorder'.

Table 15.1 Inflammatory myopathies

Idiopathic
  Polymyositis (PM)
    Simple polymyositis
    Dermatomyositis (DM)
    PM–DM with malignancy
    Childhood DM with vasculitis
    PM with connective-tissue (C–T) disorders
      Rheumatoid arthritis (RA)
      Sjögren's syndrome
      Progressive systemic sclerosis (PSS)
      Systemic lupus erythematosus (SLE)
    Localised nodular myositis
  Myasthenia gravis
  Granulomatous myositis
    Sarcoidosis
    Granulomatous myopathy
    'Giant-cell' myositis with thymoma
  Inclusion body myositis

Infective
  Viral
    Coxsackie myositis
    Influenzal myositis
    Bornholm disease
    Benign myalgic encephalomyelitis
  Bacterial
    Pyomyositis—'Tropical' myositis
  Parasitic
    Toxoplasmosis
    Cysticercosis
    Trichinosis

Table 15.1 lists the inflammatory myopathies. This is not an exhaustive list; it serves to place the idiopathic myositides in perspective. Inflammatory conditions which are attributable to infectious agents include tropical myositis with suppuration due to pyogenic organisms; this is a common disorder in the tropics. Viral infections may produce acute or chronic myositis: in man, viral myositides remain ill-defined partly because of the scarcity of pathological studies. The role of viruses in inflammatory myopathy is a complex one because they can cause not only viral myositis directly but also idiopathic myositis indirectly through triggering immune processes. Protozoal and parasitic infections of muscle can result in myositis; these are described by Drs Pallis and Lewis in Part II of this Chapter. Granulomatous myositis occurs in some of these infections, such as toxoplasmosis. Granulomata in muscle are also a feature of sarcoidosis and other granulomatous disorders, sometimes resulting in clinical myopathy. In the literature, the terms granulomatous myositis and giant-cell myositis are used indiscriminately.

Polymyositis is the most notable of the idiopathic myositides in that the myositis is the major feature of the disorder. Myositis is a component of several human disorders of obscure origin. It occurs in the connective-tissue (C–T) disorders, with which polymyositis itself is usually grouped. In these it may be symptomatic, with muscle weakness and pain, or asymptomatic, demonstrable only by muscle biopsy. In one C–T disorder, polymyalgia rheumatica (PMR), muscle pain is common yet the histological changes are slight and not similar to those of myositis. Myositis also occurs in myasthenia gravis; it plays no part in the muscle fatigability, even though its occurrence may have a bearing on the aetiology of the condition.

As myositis localised to a single muscle is rare, there is little need for the term 'polymyositis' to be used as a generic term to cover any disorder in which inflammatory changes affect several muscles. It is better for 'myositis' to be the generic term, with 'polymyositis' reserved for the idiopathic inflammatory necrobiotic myopathies. This point is more than a semantic one, because the indiscriminate use of the term 'polymyositis' has led to many a nosological tangle and also clouds our understanding of the aetiology of these disorders.

POLYMYOSITIS–DERMATOMYOSITIS (PM–DM)

Introduction

The term polymyositis is used for a nonhereditary myopathy in which degenerative changes occur in voluntary muscle, often with inflammation. Typically, there is symmetrical proximal weakness in the limbs, with dysphagia, neck flexor and respiratory muscle involvement in some cases. The presence of an erythematous skin rash in one-third of cases makes the term 'dermatomyositis' appropriate. Most authorities regard polymyositis (PM) and dermatomyositis (DM) as variants of the same disorder. This may be referred to as the polymyositis–dermatomyositis complex; in this chapter the term polymyositis–dermatomyositis is used, abbreviated to PM–DM. Wherever possible, in referring to individual case reports the correct appellation, PM or DM, is given. Arthralgia occurs in about one-third of patients. In a small minority of cases the condition appears to be precipitated by external factors: these include neoplasia, viral infections and the use of certain drugs. Other associations are agammaglobulinaemia and the connective-tissue (C–T) disorders, including rheumatoid arthritis (RA), progressive systemic sclerosis (PSS), Sjögren's syndrome and systemic lupus erythematosus (SLE). PM–DM has traditionally been classified according to such associations as dermatitis, neoplasia and other C–T disorder. The three cardinal investigations in PM–DM are muscle biopsy, electromyography (EMG) and serum creatine kinase estimation. The typical histological changes on muscle biopsy are segmental muscle fibre necrosis with phagocytosis, regeneration with basophilia, perifascicular atrophy and interstitial and perivascular infiltrates, mainly of small lymphocytes. The EMG often shows increased spontaneous activity, small, short polyphasic units on volition and high-frequency discharges. Serum creatine kinase activity is usually raised in active disease. The aetiology of PM–DM remains obscure. A derangement of immune processes may be important. Clinical features which point towards this include the precipitating factors, the associations with agammaglobulinaemia and C–T disorders, the pathological change of muscle-cell necrosis with lymphocytic infiltration, and the efficacy of steroid and immunosuppressive therapy. Experimental studies give further support. The use of immunofluorescent techniques in the examination of muscle biopsy specimens has shown that immune complexes may be a factor. Tests *in vitro* have demonstrated that peripheral blood lymphocytes from patients with PM–DM have undergone sensitisation to some component of muscle. These tests have included transformation, measured by thymidine uptake, and cytotoxicity for cultured muscle cells. The occurrence of this cytotoxicity *in vitro* does not necessarily indicate that a parallel process of damage to muscle cells by lymphocytes has occurred *in vivo*. The animal model experimental autoallergic myositis (EAM) is described in Chapter 11 by Professor Kakulas; it is not a close analogue of any human myositis. The treatment of polymyositis by corticosteroid drugs is well established: high dosage given early in the disorder is usually followed by remission. Other immunosuppressive drugs have been used to treat the condition during the past decade.

Historical

PM was first described by Wagner as long ago as 1863. The more dramatic and clinically apparent subgroup DM was reported by Unverricht (1887) and also by Wagner (1887). Among the series of cases which have been reported are those of Eaton (1954), Walton and Adams (1958), Pearson (1963), Winkelmann, Mulder, Lambert, Howard and Diessner (1968), De Vere and Bradley (1975) and Bohan, Peter, Bowman and Pearson (1977). These authors stressed the need for early diagnosis and treatment with steroid therapy in high dosage. The childhood subgroup, DM with gastrointestinal vascular complications, was delineated by Banker and Victor (1966). Dawkins and Kakulas of Western Australia were pioneers in bringing immunological techniques to bear on the study of both the human and the experimental disorders (Dawkins, 1965; Kakulas, 1966; Dawkins, 1975).

Clinical features

Precipitating factors. Clear-cut precipitating factors can be identified in only a minority of cases

Table 15.2 PM–DM: precipitants and associated disorders

Cause	Incidence
Connective-tissue disorders	20–30% of all cases
Neoplasia	20–30%
Drugs	rare
Viral exanthemata	rare
Gamma-globulin deficiency	rare

(Table 15.2). A time relationship between a possible precipitant, such as a febrile illness or drug therapy, does not, of course, necessarily mean a causal relationship. Nevertheless, the existence of both precipitating factors and associated disorders is of aetiological significance, a point which will be considered in the section on aetiology.

Connective-tissue (C–T) disorders. Semantically, these are associated disorders rather than precipitants of PM–DM and are dealt with more fully in the appropriate section. Use of the term PM is warranted when an inflammatory myopathy with proximal muscular weakness complicates a C–T disorder. In certain of the disorders, such as PSS and Sjögren's syndrome, the myopathy may be the presenting feature and be prominent. In some, including RA, it is usually of less importance both in frequency and severity. In others, such as polyarteritis nodosa (PAN), it is doubtful if true PM ever occurs. The converse of PM complicating other C–T disorders is the presence, in patients with PM, of features suggestive of these disorders. This occurs in between 20–30 per cent of all cases of PM. They include rheumatic symptoms, such as arthralgia or actual arthritis with effusions, and acrosclerosis with long-standing Raynaud's phenomenon and with shiny, atrophic skin in the extremities.

Neoplasia. There is no definite proof of an association between PM–DM and neoplasia. However, the incidence of neoplasia in patients with PM appears to be five times that for the normal population. The association is strongest for DM in elderly men. The neoplasm is most commonly bronchial carcinoma, as in the general population. The possible association is further considered in the section on associated disorders.

Other precipitants. Numerically these are unimportant. Febrile illness, such as viral upper respiratory or gastrointestinal disease, may precede the onset of PM–DM as it may those of RA and acute polyneuritis (Landry-Guillain-Barré-Strohl syndrome). Precise documentation of this is not available. The viral exanthemata and toxoplasmosis (Kagen, 1971) have been reported as triggering factors. Landry and Winkelmann (1972) described a case of rubella followed by DM; this prompted ultramicroscopic study of skin biopsy material in DM, cytoplasmic tubular inclusions being found, as in SLE and other conditions (Hashimoto, Robinson, Velayos and Niizuma, 1971). Hanissian, Martinez, Jabbour and Duenas (1973) described DM after vaccination with live rubella vaccine, the myopathy being accompanied by evidence of myeloradiculoneuritis. Clearly, problems in both diagnosis and semantics may arise when external agents can not only precipitate PM–DM but can themselves cause myositis. Landry and Winkelmann's conclusion seems a reasonable one that 'virus was the initiating factor in the development of inflammatory myositis'. Drugs which have been alleged to precipitate the condition include sulphonamide (Sheard, 1951) and penicillamine (Schraeder, Peters and Dahl, 1972). Pencillamine may also induce three other conditions, *viz.* SLE, myasthenia gravis and pemphigus. An immunopathogenetic mechanism seems possible; thus immune-complex formation was suggested by Cucher and Goldman (1976). Their case was one of PM occurring after the use of D-penicillamine for RA. There was hypocomplementaemia of the C3 and C4 components. In DM, photosensitisation may occur with initiation or exacerbation of erythema by sunlight (Sheard, 1951); this phenomenon may be enhanced by sulphonamide therapy. Lastly, selective or multiple deficiencies in γ-globulins have been reported in isolated cases of PM–DM; this association is considered later.

Initial presentation. Table 15.3 lists the presenting symptoms. The frequency of these varies in the different series of cases which have been reported.

Muscular weakness. Weakness affecting proximal muscles is the commonest presenting symp-

Table 15.3 PM–DM: initial symptoms

Symptoms	Incidence
Muscular weakness	
Legs	30–50%
Arms	25–35%
Skin rash	25%
Joint or muscle pains	25–75%

Table 15.4 Symptoms and signs in PM–DM

Symptom	Incidence
Muscular	
Weakness	
Proximal muscles	
Shoulder girdle	75–100%
Pelvic girdle	75–100%
Distal muscles	30%
Neck flexors	65%
Dysphagia	50%
Facial muscles	rare
Respiratory muscles	rare
Pain or tenderness	50–75%
Contractures	<25%
Atrophy	50%
Skin	
Classical dermatomyositis	30%
Atypical skin changes	25%
Other	
Raynaud's	20–30%
Arthralgia or arthritis	30–50%
Gastrointestinal	rare
Pulmonary	rare
Cardiac	rare (symptomatic)
Peripheral nerve	rare

tom. Weakness may show first in the legs or in the arms. Presentation with dysphagia is exceptional.

Skin rash. This is noticed before muscle weakness in the majority of patients with DM. De Vere and Bradley (1975) found that skin involvement was frequent at presentation. Raynaud's phenomenon is a rare presenting feature, except in myositis with PSS.

Joint and muscular pains. In general, these present in only a minority of cases. However, muscle pains around the shoulder girdles occurred from the outset in three-quarters of De Vere and Bradley's cases.

Clinical pattern. Progression in PM–DM is usually of the order of weeks to months rather than years. In occasional cases the course is spontaneously relapsing and remitting. A rapid onset is often seen in DM, with dysphagia and limb weakness developing over two to three weeks. The myositis in DM is thus frequently 'aggressive' (Bohan and Peter, 1975). The extremes of the spectrum are marked by acute PM or DM, with rapid, generalised weakness and severe constitutional upset, to painless weakness of limb-girdle muscles so indolent in its development that muscular dystrophy is mimicked. In hyperacute PM–DM, actual oedema of muscles may occur. In Table 15.4 the clinical symptoms and signs are listed with a rough guide to their frequency during the course of the disorder.

Muscular manifestations. Weakness occurs during the course of every case. In its absence the clinical diagnosis cannot be made with assurance. When the onset is gradual, weakness affecting the pelvic girdle musculature is noticed, with difficulty in climbing stairs and in standing up from a lying or low sitting position. Loss of strength in the shoulder-girdle muscles is symptomatic in tasks which involve elevation of the arms above shoulder level. Thus, lifting objects to and from high shelves, hanging out clothing and brushing the hair are difficult. Increasing weakness may make lifting the arms barely possible (Fig. 15.1). Weakness of the anterior or flexor muscles of the neck may cause difficulty in raising the head from the pillow while in bed, a symptom which is not often mentioned spontaneously. Involvement of the posterior pharyngeal muscles gives a picture of partial bulbar palsy with dysphagia and dysphonia with a nasal voice. In severe or advanced cases the weakness may be extreme, with the patient confined to chair or bed. Respiratory muscle involvement is unusual and progresses to a fatal outcome only exceptionally.

An atypical distribution of muscle involvement is occasionally found. Generalised weakness may affect the facial and distal as well as the proximal limb muscles (Rothstein, Carlson and Sumi, 1971; Bates, Stevens and Hudgson, 1973). Exceptionally, weakness is predominantly distal (Hollinrake, 1969). The syndrome of isolated quadriceps myopathy is sometimes due to PM, with selective though not exclusive weakness of the quadriceps muscles (Mohr and Knowlson, 1977). The correct

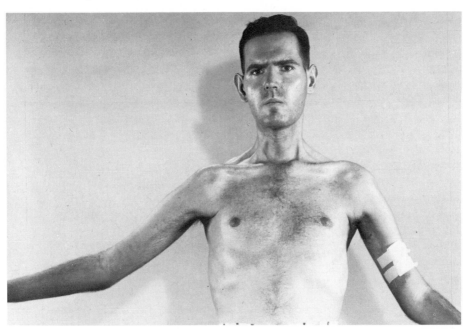

Fig. 15.1 Polymyositis with proximal muscle wasting and weakness and sclerotic skin changes (by courtesy of Dr C.M. Pearson)

diagnosis in these variants depends on the usual clinical investigations and is important because of the implications for therapy. Localised nodular myositis is an even more distinctive variant of PM–DM. Painful nodules recur in various muscles (Cumming, Weiser, Teoh, Hudgson and Walton, 1977b). Pain and stiffness, rather than weakness, give difficulty in using the limbs. Pathologically there are circumscribed areas of inflammatory cell infiltration with adjacent profuse regeneration. These areas are reminiscent of muscle infarction. The disorder may evolve into diffuse PM if left untreated, sometimes with facioscapulohumeral distribution. The condition is distinct from the asymptomatic focal nodular myositis of the C–T disorders. It is probably distinct also from the relapsing myositis of McLetchie and Aikens (1952) in which giant cells occurred in necrotic foci.

True fatigability like that found in myasthenia gravis is not a recognised feature of PM–DM. However, Johns, Crowley, Miller and Campa (1971) described a series of patients with clinical, electrical and pharmacological features of myasthenia gravis and clinical and pathological features of PM. This point is further considered in the section on 'differential diagnosis'.

Contractures or shortening of muscles rarely occur early. They are a feature of advanced or long-standing disease. The muscles which are usually affected are the biceps, with contractures at the elbows, the wrist flexors, preventing full extension of the wrists without flexion of the fingers, and the hamstrings. Contractures may develop early in a variant of PM in which marked fibrosis occurs (Bradley, Hudgson, Gardner-Medwin and Walton, 1973). Atrophy of muscles is also a late event and is rarely marked; thus the degree of weakness is usually disproportionate to that of wasting. This is one of the points of differentiation from advanced muscular dystrophy, in which atrophy is often extensive. Calcinosis of muscles may follow a severe episode of acute myositis and occurs most often in childhood DM.

Skin manifestations. The erythematous skin rash of DM is seen in about a third of cases (Table 15.4), occurring in 15 to 40 per cent of the patients

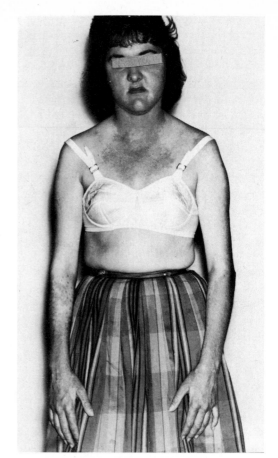

Fig. 15.2 Dermatomyositis with erythematous rash on face, neck and lower arms (by courtesy of Dr C.M. Pearson)

in the reported series. The typical rash (Fig. 15.2) affects the face as a violaceous eruption in butterfly distribution, involving the peri-orbital areas too and spreading to the neck and upper chest. The arms are also involved, both proximally and distally. This component of the rash is an erythema; it may be mottled or diffuse and red or cyanotic in colour. Sometimes the upper eyelids show a dark lilac or heliotrope suffusion, a sign which is thought to be typical of DM. In conjunction with the facial erythema, a thicker, more indurated and scaly rash of dermatitis occurs on the extensor surfaces of the limbs. These dusky red, elevated patches are found over the elbows, the knuckles and, to a lesser extent, over the knees and the medial malleoli. In addition, there is hyperaemia at the base of the fingernails with shiny, red, atrophic skin at the ends of the fingers.

This dermatitis often shows activity *pari passu* with the myositis, the areas or plaques becoming tender and elevated and even ulcerating on occasion. In very acute cases, intradermal and subcutaneous oedema occurs. In quiescent periods the plaques become smaller and paler. Rarely, the typical skin changes of DM occur without clinical or investigatory evidence of myositis. The skin and muscle changes may follow a separate course, in the opinion of Dawkins and Mastaglia (1973), though Banker (1975) felt that 'the muscular weakness and erythematous rash are always conjoined'.

A further one-quarter of patients with PM have some abnormality of the skin. Sclerodermatous changes vary from the shiny, red, atrophic skin of the digits, 'acrosclerosis', to the full-blown widespread skin tethering, with apparent thickening, of PSS. Widespread dermal atrophy (poikiloderma) may be present. Transient erythema or a scaling eruption resembling eczema may occur. Diffuse or focal hyperpigmentation or vitiligo and telangiectasia of the face, anterior chest and shoulders have been described.

Raynaud's phenomenon. The phenomenon of cyanosis or actual blanching of the fingers in response to cold weather or local cooling occurs in less than a third of all patients with PM–DM. It is usually mild in degree, unless the myositis is part of PSS. Indeed, it is unusual to find Raynaud's phenomenon at all, other than in PM with C–T disorder (Bohan and Peter, 1975).

Rheumatic manifestations. Evidence of joint involvement occurs in about one-quarter of patients with PM–DM. As many as one-half of all patients will have arthralgia at some stage (Pearson, 1959). Occasionally the disorder starts with a syndrome which is indistinguishable from early RA with pain and effusions typically in wrists, finger joints and knees. These respond to steroid therapy together with the myositis. Conversely, PM can complicate longstanding RA with proximal myopathy and myositis on biopsy (Pitkeathley and Coomes, 1966; Haslock, Wright and Harriman, 1970). Rarely, signs of RA appear late in the course of PM. Myositis may also occur in Sjögren's syndrome (Silberberg and Drachman, 1962), the variant of RA in which keratoconjunctivitis sicca and xerostomia are found.

Peripheral nerve involvement. This is exceptional and the term 'neuromyositis' can rarely be invoked (Harriman and Currie, 1974). It depends first on clinical evidence, such as sensory symptoms and signs and loss of deep tendon reflexes such as the ankle reflexes, and secondly on confirmation by neurophysiological tests and motor-point muscle and nerve biopsies. The deep tendon reflexes in PM–DM are normal or depressed in parallel with the weakness of the muscles concerned, as in any myopathy. Depression of the reflexes is less likely than it is in muscular dystrophy.

Visceral involvement in PM–DM is also rare, but has been described as affecting many different organs. Involvement of cardiac, respiratory and gastrointestinal systems may be due to associated C–T disorder, such as SLE or PSS, rather than being an integral part of the PM (Bohan and Peter, 1975).

Cardiac involvement. The frequency of cardiac involvement is hard to assess. Diessner, Howard, Winkelmann, Lambert and Mulder (1966) reported a high frequency of abnormality on electrocardiography (ECG). Sharratt, Danta and Carson (1977) found a conduction defect in several patients on ECG and other tests. They felt that such abnormalities fluctuated with the state of the skeletal myopathy. Gottdiener, Sherber, Hawley and Engel (1978) examined 21 patients with PM–DM by echocardiography, phonocardiography and ECG. They noted a relative infrequency of symptomatic involvement. As many as 75 per cent showed abnormality, yet none had cardiac failure. Abnormalities on ECG were found in 52 per cent, including arrhythmias and disturbances in conduction. Myocardial myositis is not a common feature at autopsy. In some of the single case reports with prominent cardiac abnormality the diagnosis of PM–DM has been open to question; an example is that of Schaumburg, Nielsen and Yurchak (1971). The case of Yang, Garner and Beetham (1978) was one of chronic DM in association with carcinoid tumour. The heart was enlarged on chest x-ray and there was a sinus tachycardia. The pathological changes in skin and skeletal muscle were definite and the myocardium showed fibre atrophy and interstitial lymphocytic infiltrates. It should be noted that the condition of granulomatous or giant-cell myocarditis and myositis in association with thymoma is more closely related to myasthenia gravis than to PM–DM (*see* separate section). There are antigenic differences, not only between skeletal and cardiac muscle, but also between myocardium and conducting fibres (Fairfax, 1977). Fairfax envisages selective damage to Purkinje tissue by various immune processes in different diseases.

Parenchymal lung involvement. This has been described, comprising fibrosing alveolitis with a diffusion defect (Camp, Lane and Mowat, 1972). Plowman and Stableforth (1977) described a case of DM with both fibrosing alveolitis and digital vasculitis. The antinuclear antibody test was negative. Clq binding was raised, suggesting the presence of circulating immune complexes. As is often the case, the lung condition was not steroid-responsive and their patient was treated with cyclophosphamide and D-penicillamine in addition. They noted that fibrosing alveolitis might be found in as many as five per cent of cases of PM–DM (Frazier and Miller, 1974).

Gastrointestinal involvement. Oesophageal involvement may include atonicity of the main, smooth muscle, component (Donoghue, Winkelmann and Moersch, 1960); reduced motility was also shown by Diessner *et al.* (1966) using radiological and physiological tests. Both this and a small intestinal disorder may occur when there is acrosclerosis and therefore some evidence of PSS. Such cases illustrate the axiom that multisystem involvement is more likely in PM with C–T disorders. In childhood DM, vasculitis affecting blood vessels in the stomach and upper small bowel may lead to serious abdominal complications, such as gastrointestinal haemorrhage (Banker and Victor, 1966).

Age and sex distribution

Age. PM–DM can occur at any age. However, it is commonest in childhood and in late middle age. It thus shows a bimodal age distribution as was pointed out by Medsger, Dawson and Masi (1970) who suggested that this might mean different immediate precipitants or pathogenesis in childhood and adult PM–DM. In one-fifth of all cases of PM–DM the disease starts when the patient is less than 15 years old. In the series of De Vere and Bradley (1975), two-thirds of the patients were over 40 years of age when the disorder began.

Sex. The condition is twice as common in men as in women. De Vere and Bradley found three women to one man, although there was a preponderance of men in PM–DM with malignancy. The sex ratio also holds for childhood PM–DM.

Incidence. An age-adjusted incidence rate of five per million per year was given by Medsger *et al.* (1970). This figure was very similar to that which Rose and Walton (1966) had estimated for the United Kingdom. It was also in line that that of Pearson (1963) for his own practice in California. Medsger *et al.* (1970) found a significantly higher incidence in black females than in white females. This was also true for PSS and SLE, and the authors speculated that the finding of increased γ-globulins in the serum of normal blacks might be a relevant factor. In contrast, PMR is a disorder occurring almost exclusively in whites, both in South Africa (Bruk, 1967) and the USA (Miller and Stevens, 1978). The incidence of PM–DM in general was half that of SLE.

Genetic aspects. PM–DM is not a hereditary disorder, familial cases being exceptional. Despite this, there are genetic aspects to the condition. Besides the familial occurrence, these comprise racial differences, associations with histocompatibility antigens and lastly the association of DM with hereditary X-linked agammaglobulinaemia.

Familial incidence. The rare instances of familial occurrence of PM–DM include the following cases. Cook, Rosen and Banker (1963) in a series of cases of childhood DM mention the occurrence of DM in identical twins, the disorder developing a year apart. Howard and Thomas (1960) in their series mention that two of their patients each had an affected relative. Lambie and Duff (1963) described DM in first cousins. They found raised serum γ-globulin levels in asymptomatic relatives of these patients. Lewkonia and Buxton (1973) described DM in the daughter of a man with PM; he was of mixed extraction (white and black) which the authors felt might have predisposed him to a disturbance in immunity. As Lambie and Duff suggested, there is the possibility of an underlying, subclinical disturbance in immune processes in the families of patients both with PM–DM and with other C–T disorders.

Racial differences. The higher incidence in black females has already been noted. The most striking example of a racial susceptibility is the apparently high incidence of DM among the Bantu tribe in Transvaal, South Africa (Findlay, Whiting and Simson, 1969). Further evidence is needed about the underlying factors; induction by viruses in a context of inherited predisposition is one possibility.

Histocompatibility studies. Genetic predisposition to PM–DM may also be shown by an association with specific antigens of the histocompatibility complex, the HLA system. The finding of such an association not only indicates a degree of susceptibility to PM–DM, it also implies associations in turn between PM–DM and other disorders in which a particular gene is found to be common. HLA studies have shown an increased incidence of the immune gene HLA–B8 in childhood DM (Pachman, Jonasson, Cannon and Friedman, 1977) and adult PM (Behan, Behan and Dick, 1978). HLA–B8 has also been found in association with myasthenia gravis and PMR. One group of workers has found an increased incidence of HLA–B14 in adult PM (Cumming, Hudgson, Lattimer, Sussman and Wilcox, 1977a). All these findings must be considered as preliminary.

Hereditary X-linked agammaglobulinaemia. This condition may be associated with C–T disorders, including PM–DM. It is considered as an 'associated disorder' in the appropriate section of this Chapter. There is an increasing number of reports of a DM-like syndrome with cerebral vasculitis in boys with hereditary X-linked agammaglobulinaemia (Janeway, Gitlin, Craig and Grice, 1956; Page, Hansen and Good, 1963;

Gotoff, Smith and Sugar, 1972; Rosen, 1974). There is evidence that the immune deficiency has led to viral infection. Echovirus was found in the case of familial hypogammaglobulinaemia associated with DM and encephalitis which was reported by Webster, Tripp, Hayward, Dayan, Doshi, Macintyre and Tyrell (1978). There was improvement in the myopathy when plasma containing antibody to the virus was given. The arthritis which occurs in boys with agammaglobulinaemia is also treatable by γ-globulin therapy. Neither myopathy nor cerebral vasculitis is responsive to steroid or other IS agents. Although there are similarities between the cases of DM and cerebral vasculitis, like that of Gotoff *et al.* (1972) and those of DM and encephalitis, such as that of Webster *et al.* (1978), the cerebral conditions are clearly different.

In addition to X-linked agammaglobulinaemia, hereditary complement deficiency has been reported in a case of DM (Leddy, Griggs, Klemperer and Franks, 1975). They described an elderly man in whom there was a total absence in the serum of the second component of complement (haemolytic complement) activity. Family studies showed an autosomal recessive pattern of inheritance for the abnormality.

Associated disorders

Connective-tissue (C–T) disorders. PM is generally grouped with the C–T disorders. DM has a closer relationship to them than does simple PM, if one accepts that skin involvement is due to systemic vasculitis comparable to that of the C–T disorders. In PM–DM, vasculitis in muscles is uncommon except in childhood DM (Banker, 1975). Myositis, when it occurs in association with other C–T disorders, tends to have a worse prognosis. The disorders overlap in their symptomatology, affecting many systems. Generalised secondary amyloidosis may supervene in these disorders, including DM (Gelderman, Levine and Arndt, 1962). Voluntary muscle may be affected by atrophy from disuse, denervation from motor neuropathy, steroid myopathy and focal infarction from vasculitis, in addition to myositis (Haslock *et al.*, 1970). A short section on myopathy in C–T disorders is included later in this chapter.

Table 15.5 lists the C–T disorders in which polymyositis is known to occur. In SLE, myositis was found in 3 per cent in one series (Estes and Christian, 1971) with proximal muscle weakness, biopsy changes and improvement following steroid therapy. PM in RA may precede or follow the arthritis. It may go unnoticed if there is also difficulty in movement because of the arthritis. Pitkeathley and Coomes (1966) described three cases of PM in association with undoubted erosive RA. In Sjögren's syndrome, myositis is uncommon (Silberberg and Drachman, 1962) even if vasculitis is sometimes found on random muscle biopsy (Bunim, 1961). The inflammatory cell infiltrate in Sjögren's myositis can include many plasma cells. In PSS, clinical myopathy is uncommon (Thompson, Bluestone, Bywaters, Dorling and Johnson, 1969) but myositis does occur. Transitional cases are seen with features of both PSS and of DM (Currie, Saunders and Knowles, 1971a). The typical muscle lesions in polyarteritis nodosa (PAN) and in Wegener's granulomatosis are due to infarction. The significance of any changes in muscle histology in PMR is debatable but it is unlikely that a true myositis ever occurs.

The focal nodular myositis which is found in the C–T disorders is asymptomatic. It has no obvious relationship to the clinical or pathological entity PM–DM.

Table 15.5 PM in connective-tissue disorders

Systemic lupus erythematosus	(SLE)
Rheumatoid arthritis	(RA)
Sjögren's syndrome	
Progressive systemic sclerosis	(PSS)

Neoplasia. PM–DM forms one of the non-metastatic neurological syndromes of neoplasia. Others affecting muscle are necrotising myopathy (Smith, 1969; Urich and Wilkinson, 1970) and 'neuromyopathy' (Croft and Wilkinson, 1965; Campbell and Paty, 1974). These latter conditions are considered in detail by Dr Henson in Chapter 19. The association has been recognised for a long time (Schuermann, 1951; Dowling, 1955) but without firm proof as yet. In the different series, tumour has been found in 5–25 per cent of all cases. The percentage is higher in older men with DM. De Vere and Bradley (1975) reported an incidence of 66 per cent in males over 40 years with DM. It is notable that childhood PM–DM is not associated with malignancy. In general, the incidence appears to be five times that for the normal population (Dowling, 1955) but no firm statistics are available (Barnes, 1976). Barnes felt that the published figures in the literature as a whole did not bear out the higher rate for men. She noted that there was no long-term follow-up study of DM to detect any increased risk of malignancy. The neoplasms which have been reported in association with PM–DM have been various, with bronchial carcinoma the commonest, as in the general population. As well as carcinoma they include reticuloses, such as Hodgkin's disease (Deep, Fraumeni, Tashima and McDivitt, 1964) and lymphosarcoma (Arapakis and Jordanoglou, 1964). Thymoma has occurred concurrently with PM (Klein, Gottlieb, Mones, Appel and Osserman, 1964). The PM–DM which occurs in association with neoplasia is generally stated to be less responsive to steroid therapy than is the condition at large. This belief has not been validated statistically. Cases occasionally run a course which suggests a causal relationship; for example, in the last edition of this book, a case of renal carcinoma with PM was recorded in which improvement occurred only after nephrectomy. However, the situation is a complex one, often made more so by the use of therapy which may affect both disorders.

Myasthenia gravis. The pathological changes in skeletal muscle in myasthenia gravis comprise a form of myositis; and this disorder and PM–DM have some features in common including steroid-responsiveness. This is a point which is mentioned in the sections on differential diagnosis and on aetiology. There are reports of an association between the conditions (Johns et al., 1971; Namba, Brunner and Grob, 1973). Johns et al. found PM appearing during the course of myasthenia gravis; they felt that it was not just an interstitial myositis. Myasthenia gravis and PM were also seen concurrently, but they had no cases of PM followed by myasthenia. There is an increased incidence of the immune gene HLA-B8 in PM–DM as well as in myasthenia gravis, a fact already mentioned in the section on genetics.

Agammaglobulinaemia. The association of hereditary X-linked agammaglobulinaemia and DM has been described already. The peripheral blood in this condition contains normal numbers of T cells but a lack of B cells (Rosen, 1974). Viral infection is more liable in the immunocompromised host. In at least one of these rare cases such infection has been clearly implicated (Webster *et al.*, 1978). In primary acquired agammaglobulinaemia as well as in the hereditary form there is an increased incidence of C–T disorders (Rosen, 1974). The case of DM and encephalitis due to echovirus which was reported by Bardelas, Winkelstein, Seto, Tsai and Rogol (1977) appeared to be a sporadic one of hypogammaglobulinaemia. Treatment with maternal antibody specifically neutralising the echovirus produced temporary improvement. A case of hereditary complement deficiency with DM (Leddy *et al.*, 1975) has been cited in the section on genetic aspects. In two sporadic cases of PM in childhood, Carroll, Silverman, Isobe, Brown, Kelts and Brooke (1976) found IgA deficiency. There was facial muscle involvement, as well as weakness of proximal limb musculature. Intestinal malabsorption with villous atrophy was also present. In each case, muscle strength improved with prednisone. This was notable because the DM which occurs with agammaglobulinaemia is usually unresponsive to steroid therapy. It should be noted that there is no hypogammaglobulinaemia in PM–DM in general (Lisak and Zweiman, 1976).

Classification

Classification traditionally is along the lines which were agreed upon by the World Federation of Neurology Research Group on Neuromuscular Disorders (1968) with three classes: Group I, simple or 'uncomplicated' PM; Group II, dermatomyositis and myositis with C–T disorders, bracketed together; and Group III, PM–DM with malignancy. Classification can be into fewer groupings; thus, PM–DM with malignancy need not be separately classified; or into more, thus DM can be separated from PM with C–T disorder, and childhood DM can be set apart. Such distinctions are important only if making them increases our understanding of the aetiology and management of the disorder.

Group I: simple PM. Simple or uncomplicated PM includes both acute and indolent cases. It has the best prognosis. It is seen in children and adults. Acute rhabdomyolysis is sometimes included, although it may not be a variant of PM at all; the nosological position of this entity is considered in the sections on differential diagnosis and on aetiology.

Group II: DM and myositis with C–T disorders. These can be grouped together in that vasculitis is common to both. Childhood DM, with symptomatic vasculitis affecting the gastrointestinal tract, is perhaps distinctive, with clinical and pathological features which set it apart (Banker, 1975). These are enough to warrant separate classification in the opinion of Bohan and Peter (1975) though not in that of De Vere and Bradley (1975). Soft-tissue contractures, subcutaneous calcification and muscular atrophy are more common in childhood DM. Bohan and Peter (1975) separated DM from myositis with C–T disorders, using for the latter the term 'overlap syndrome'; arthralgia, myalgia and Raynaud's phenomenon were commoner in this sub-group of theirs than in DM or simple PM. The myositis of C–T disorders may have a worse prognosis than has simple PM, although Bohan *et al.* (1977) did not find that this was so. When skin changes are slight, and atypical for DM, placement with Group I (simple PM), rather than with Group II, may be more appropriate. Walton and Adams (1958) put such cases in a separate intermediate group. Most cases of PM fall into this 'transitional' group. While aetiological concepts are still fluid, the issue is not an important one.

Group III: PM–DM with malignancy. The logic in classifying separately PM–DM in association with neoplasia is uncertain. Neoplasia is, after all, only one of the more widely known precipitants of the disorder. The myositis is often said to have a worse natural history and to be refractory to therapy; there is no prospective study of this. The finding of neoplasm in a case of myositis means a fortuitous switching to the separate sub-group. Rowland and Schotland (1965) did not support this separation of myositis with malignancy. Setting apart DM when it occurs with malignancy casts doubt on the correctness of its classification in Group II with the myositis of C–T disorders. This is because the latter have no association with malignancy other than that of neoplasms developing late in their course, as in Sjögren's syndrome. Myolysis in malignancy is of uncertain status, like rhabdomyolysis in general.

Mayo Clinic workers have produced a three-dimensional classification, according to the precipitating factors, the associations and the course (Winkelmann *et al.*, 1968). However, a straightforward list along the lines of the 1968 World Federation of Neurology Research Group seems easier and begs fewer questions (Table 15.6).

Table 15.6 Classification of PM–DM (modified from World Federation of Neurology Research Group on Neuromuscular Disorders, 1968)

Group I	Polymyositis simple
	? Polymyositis with mild skin changes
Group II	Dermatomyositis adult
	Dermatomyositis childhood
	Polymyositis with: RA
	Sjögren's syndrome
	PSS
	SLE
	(? plus 'overlap syndrome' –mixed C–T disorder)
Group III	PM–DM with malignancy

Clinical investigations

Muscle biopsy is the most important single clinical investigation and is considered separately under the section on pathology. The two other cardinal investigations are the EMG and estimation of the serum activity of the enzyme creatine kinase (CK). Other tests do not hold the same value as this triad because they are less specific or reliable. Table 15.7 lists all the investigations, major and minor.

Serum enzyme estimation. The activities of several serum enzymes may be raised, particularly in acute PM–DM; that of the serum CK is the most sensitive and also the most specific for muscle cell damage. High CK activity is usually found in active disease and falls with remission, often some

Table 15.7 Investigations in PM–DM

Major	Serum creatine kinase estimation
	Electromyography
	Muscle biopsy
Minor	Erythrocyte sedimentation rate
	Blood count
	Estimation of other serum enzymes
	Aldolase
	Transaminase
	Lactate dehydrogenase
	Serum myoglobin estimation
	Urinary myoglobin estimation
	Tests for C–T disorders
	LE cell
	Rheumatoid factor
	False positive serological tests
	Positive direct Coombs' test
	Antibodies to cell constituents

weeks before improvement is evident clinically. The level may rise again if the steroid dose is reduced too quickly or when a relapse is impending. Other serum enzymes such as aldolase, transaminase and lactate dehydrogenase are less consistently raised so the serum CK is the best guide to activity (Vignos and Goldwyn, 1972). In chronic PM with slow progression and much muscle fibrosis, the CK activity may not be raised at all. Even at the time of presentation the disease may not be active enough to produce abnormal levels in some cases; thus the serum CK was raised initially in only two-thirds of the cases in the series of De Vere and Bradley (1975).

Electromyography. A triad of EMG findings is characteristic of PM–DM. These findings comprise: (a) spontaneous activity, with fibrillation, positive potentials and increased insertional activity; (b) polyphasic potentials on volitional activity which are of small amplitude and short duration; (c) repetitive high frequency 'pseudomyotonic' discharges which are evoked by mechanical stimulation of the muscle or movement of the electrode. Demonstration of these features may require multiple sampling of several muscles. The spontaneous activity is very like that of denervation and may indeed be due to this, resulting from segmental necrosis of muscle fibres and damage to end-plates and subterminal nerve endings. Such activity may also be seen in other primary myopathies as in the myopathy of periodic paralysis. The small, short polyphasic motor units are typical of myopathy, with loss of muscle fibres from individual motor units. The 'pseudo-myotonic' discharges may be due to abnormal irritability of damaged muscle fibres. In the series of Bohan *et al.* (1977), the EMG showed short, small polyphasic units in 90 per cent of cases, irritability, fibrillation and positive waves in 75 per cent and pseudomyotonic discharges in 40 per cent. Mechler (1974) carried out serial EMG studies in cases of PM over an average period of 2.5 years. He found that the amount of spontaneous activity decreased with chronicity while large, polyphasic potentials of long duration appeared. Possible interpretations of these findings included fibrosis affecting terminal nerve fibres, collateral sprouting and subclinical neuropathy.

The EMG can also help in indicating which muscle to biopsy. A muscle may retain normal power but show marked electrical abnormality. Biopsy can then be of the corresponding muscle on the other side or of vastus internus after sampling of vastus externus. Biopsy at the site of previous EMG needling is best avoided because the needling can cause focal inflammatory changes.

Nerve conduction studies. These rarely show an increase in distal latencies or slowing of motor nerve conduction. There was some evidence of such slowing in the case described by Bauwens (1956) who used the term 'neuromyositis'. Harriman and Currie (1974) reported abnormalities of sensory and motor conduction in two of 31 cases, with histological evidence of denervation.

Pathology: muscle biopsy

Muscle biopsy is of paramount importance in making or confirming the diagnosis of PM (Walton and Adams, 1958). In many cases biopsy may seem superfluous, given a clear-cut clinical picture, with dermal involvement, arthralgia, raised serum enzymes and a positive EMG. Nevertheless, biopsy is a minor surgical procedure with little upset to the patient. It should be carried out without delay to allow an early start with high-dose steroid therapy. Muscle biopsy is thus an integral part of management rather than a means of furnishing data for clinical academic studies. The muscle for biopsy should be carefully chosen,

being one which is neither profoundly weak or atrophic nor of normal strength. A proximal muscle such as deltoid or quadriceps is preferable. Despite forethought in the selection of the muscle for biopsy, abnormalities may be only minimal or atypical, often due to the vagaries of sampling when changes are patchy. Such an experience by no means invalidates the advisability of biopsy. One or more of the three main tests, enzyme studies, EMG and biopsy, can give negative results and diagnosis is based on the clinical and investigatory picture as a whole. A firm and early diagnosis is desirable before a patient is committed to drug therapy, possibly for life. Perhaps the technique of needle biopsy will allow easy sampling of several sites but the specimens obtained may not clearly show changes such as perifascicular atrophy, at low magnification.

The term myositis itself implies that inflammation may be found in muscles, and, indeed, lymphocytic infiltration with muscle-cell damage is the hallmark of the condition. Nevertheless, such infiltration may not be seen on biopsy or even on exhaustive autopsy studies. There are other features characteristic of PM–DM even though none are pathognomonic; these include perifascicular atrophy and changes in the endothelium of blood vessels. Some of the remaining changes are late and non-specific, such as interstitial fibrosis and variation in fibre size.

Muscle: light microscopic changes. The light microscopic changes are obviously the best known and those used for diagnostic purposes. Table 15.8 lists the chief pathological findings.

Table 15.8 PM–DM: pathological changes in muscle on light microscopy

Muscle fibre: segmental necrosis
　　　　　　　degeneration
Regenerating fibres
Infiltrates of inflammatory cells
　　　　　　　epimysial
　　　　　　　interstitial
　　　　　　　perivascular
Phagocytosis of necrotic fibres
Vascular endothelial changes
Interstitial fibrosis
Variation in fibre size
Perifascicular atrophy
Motor nerve and end-plate changes

Degenerative–necrobiotic changes. These are of several kinds and occur in varying proportions. An early change is an alteration of the sarcoplasm, which becomes refractile and highly eosinophilic and shows partial or complete loss of cross-striations. Hyalinisation or granular degeneration may follow. These changes typically affect segments of fibres, often near each other, in a patchy manner (Fig. 15.3). Sometimes large, confluent areas are affected. The periphery of a fascicle is the most liable to damage (Figs 15.4 and 15.5); however, perifascicular atrophy is by no means invariable. Grouping of atrophic fibres may also be seen; it is suggestive of denervation. Vacuolar degeneration sometimes affects muscle fibres, extending over several segments. It was once thought to be characteristic of PM in SLE (Pearson and Yamazaki, 1958).

Regeneration is a common finding in PM–DM. It can be recognised by the lilac-coloured basophilia of the fibres in haematoxylin and eosin stains, the increased number of plump centrally located nuclei, which often appear in rows, and the narrow transverse diameter of the fibres (Fig. 15.6). Such fibres occur singly or in small groups. Actual repair of damaged segments of fibres may be seen (Fig. 15.3). Appropriate staining will show ribonucleic acid in regenerating fibres. The regeneration is orderly and effective (Mastaglia and Kakulas, 1970), unlike that seen in muscular dystrophy.

Inflammatory cell infiltration. The degree of inflammatory cell infiltration varies considerably; it does not closely parallel the necrobiotic changes. With biopsy material the vagaries of sampling are clearly a factor when the changes are patchy; nevertheless, they are only partly explanatory. Typically, multiple foci of inflammatory cells are scattered throughout the muscle specimen. Most of these are adjacent to, or surround, small blood vessels but foci are also endomysial, enclosing groups of muscle fibres, some of which are

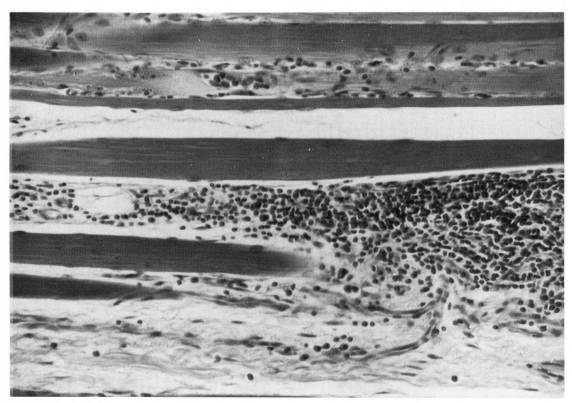

Fig. 15.3   Polymyositis: longitudinal section of muscle. Muscle fibre near top shows necrosis on the right, regeneration on the left. Interstitial lymphocytic infiltration fills the lower field on the right. H & E, ×53 (courtesy of Dr D.G.F. Harriman)

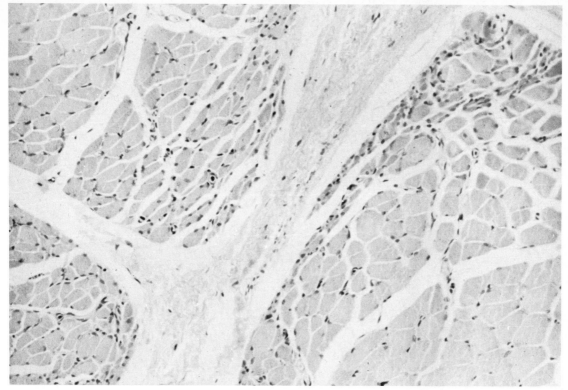

Fig. 15.4 Dermatomyositis; transverse section of muscle. Perifascicular fibre atrophy is seen on either side of the central strand of perimysial connective tissue. H & E, × 22.5 (courtesy of Dr D.G.F. Harriman)

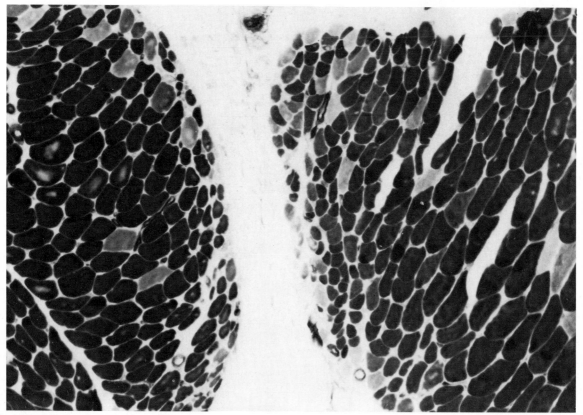

Fig. 15.5 Dermatomyositis; transverse section of muscle. Perifascicular atrophy affecting type I and type II fibres. The predominance of type I fibres is a non-specific feature of myopathy. ATPase, pH 4.3, × 25 (courtesy of Dr D.G.F. Harriman)

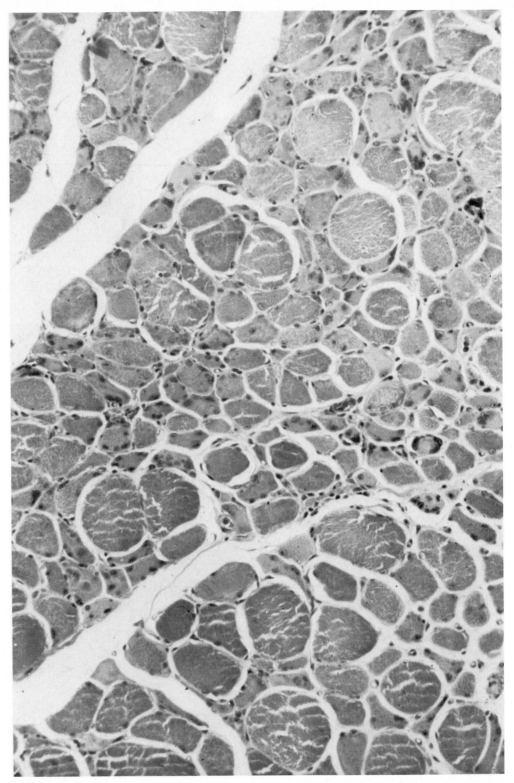

Fig. 15.6 Polymyositis: transverse section of muscle. There is variation in fibre size. In the centre is a cluster of darkly staining cells with large nuclei: these are regenerating fibres. H & E, ×40 (courtesy of Dr D.G.F. Harriman)

degenerating. Inflammatory cells are sometimes sparse rather than collected in foci. The majority of the cells in the infiltrates are small mononuclear cells, lymphocytes, mixed with macrophages and a few plasma cells (Fig. 15.3). Polymorphonuclear leucocytes are scarce. Plasma cells can predominate in the infiltrates in Sjögren's syndrome and are a feature in the myositis of RA in general (Haslock et al., 1970). When inflammatory infiltrates are absent this is not always a matter of sampling. There are well-documented cases in which multiple biopsies or autopsy studies have shown no inflammation. The pathological changes in these cases have otherwise been characteristic (Munsat and Cancilla, 1974; De Vere and Bradley, 1975). Some authorities consider features such as perifascicular atrophy more typical of PM–DM than mononuclear cell infiltration, given that the latter may be found even in hereditary neuropathies and myopathies (Munsat, Piper, Cancilla and Mednick, 1972; Jennekens, Busch, van Hemel and Hoogland, 1975; Hudgson and Fulthorpe, 1975). Inflammatory changes were found in 75 per cent of the cases of PM–DM in the series of Bohan et al. (1977).

Vascular endothelial changes. It is notably in childhood DM that vasculitis is early and prominent in muscle biopsy specimens (Boylan and Sokoloff, 1960; Banker and Victor, 1966; Banker, 1975). Blood vessels in tissues besides muscle are affected, such as those of the connective tissue, gastrointestinal tract, fat and small nerves. Capillaries, arterioles and venules are all involved. Usually there are perivascular inflammatory cells as an early finding, although such infiltrates may be missing (Banker, 1975; Carpenter, Karpati, Rothman and Watters, 1976). Endothelial hyperplasia and necrosis follow, with occlusion by fibrin thrombi. These lead to micro-infarcts of groups of muscle fibres, as opposed to single-fibre necrosis. Type I and type II fibres are affected indiscriminately. This zonal type of necrosis involves one or more fasciculi; all fibres are at the same stage of degeneration. The resulting atrophy is markedly perifascicular; this is paralleled by a reduced number of capillaries at the periphery of fasciculi (Carpenter et al., 1976). These capillaries have narrowed lumina. In the necrotic zones,

regeneration is not a conspicuous feature.

Interstitial fibrosis. An increase in interstitial connective tissue is seen in most specimens. Rarely this is extreme, particularly perimysial, and results clinically in contractures which may be more of a factor than muscle weakness in limiting movement. For these unusual cases the term 'fibrosing myositis' is appropriate (Bradley et al., 1973).

Motor nerve and end-plate changes. Motor point muscle biopsy in PM–DM shows abnormalities in the region of the end-plate in most cases of PM–DM (Harriman and Currie, 1974). In a third of cases there is true collateral reinnervation. Evidence of denervation such as grouped atrophy and type grouping is rare; it occurred in only four of the 31 cases of PM reported by Harriman and Currie. These did not include any cases with an associated C–T disorder, neoplasm or unrelated condition in which neuropathy might occur, such as diabetes. In two of these cases there was sufficient clinical and neurophysiological as well as pathological evidence for the appellation 'neuro-myositis' to be given. In the remainder the changes in the terminal nerves were of no clinical significance and were presumably secondary to muscle cell damage.

Skin: light microscopy changes. In DM the main pathological findings in affected skin are poikiloderma and deposits of mucin. Sometimes there is lymphocytic infiltration as well. Positive findings on biopsy are more likely if this is taken from a clinically affected area of skin rather than from skin at the site of muscle biopsy. Janis and Winkelmann (1968) felt that the poikiloderma, a non-inflammatory oedematous type, was distinctive; taken in conjunction with the mucin deposits, it was an abnormality very suggestive of DM. Sometimes the changes were more like those found in the skin in SLE. Maricq, Spencer-Green and Le Roy (1976) looked at biopsies of digital skin in cases of DM and PSS, with particular attention to the small vessels. They described an abnormal microvascular pattern with dilated and distorted capillary loops alternating with avascular areas. These abnormalities were sometimes seen even in the absence of clinically overt skin disease.

Pathology: ultra-microscopy of muscle.
The abnormalities in muscle which have been demonstrated on ultra-microscopy fall into four categories: these are listed in Table 15.9. The changes are: (1) those affecting the muscle fibres themselves, reflecting the degeneration and regeneration seen on light microscopy; (2) the infiltrates, with ultra-microscopy showing the relationship of individual mononuclear cells to muscle and vascular endothelial cells; (3) alterations in the endothelial cells of small vessels, an early finding in childhood DM; and (4) the demonstration of intranuclear and sarcoplasmic aggregates resembling assorted viruses in several cases of PM–DM. Thus ultra-microscopy adds little in diagnostic information beyond light microscopy but does give findings of aetiological significance.

Table 15.9 PM–DM ultrastructural changes in muscle

Degenerative and regenerative changes
   Shredding, contraction and coagulation of myofibrils
   Focal 'targetoid' areas
   Segmental Z band coagulation
   Vacuolar degeneration
   Sarcomere disruption
   Hyaline degeneration—necrosis
   Myoblast 'embryonal' regeneration

Inflammatory cells
   Lymphocytes
     small
     activated
     perivascular
     juxta-sarcolemmal
   Macrophages

Vascular changes
   Endothelial thickening
   Basement membrane thickening

Virus-like particles
   Coxsackie virus
   Myxovirus
   Papovavirus

Degenerative and regenerative changes. The degenerative changes range from focal alteration to patches of necrosis (Hughes and Esiri, 1975). There is focal shredding of myofilaments (Shafiq, Milhorat and Gorycki, 1967) with central 'targetoid' areas. The segmental muscle fibre necrosis which is seen on light microscopy is found to be hyaline degeneration. This begins as a myofibrillar contracture leading to coagulative necrosis (Mastaglia and Walton, 1971). The sequence is not specific to PM–DM because it occurs in other necrobiotic myopathies such as Duchenne muscular dystrophy. The sarcolemma may form redundant folds. The band structure of fibres may be altered with Z band 'streaming', and the tubular system may be dilated.

The regenerative changes comprise the appearance of myoblastic cells at the edge of necrotic fibres ('embryonal regeneration'); these arise from muscle satellite cells. Thin actin filaments develop in the myoblasts. There is nothing specific about the regeneration in PM–DM as seen at the ultrastructural level.

Inflammatory cells. The infiltration of muscle by inflammatory cells can be studied ultramicroscopically with attention to the relationship of individual mononuclear and muscle cells to each other and to vessels (Mastaglia and Currie, 1971; Hughes and Esiri, 1975). The typical cells are both small and large activated lymphocytes and macrophages. The lymphocytes are found in association with capillaries and closely applied to the sarcolemmal sheaths of muscle fibres. Lymphocytes may also be seen traversing the walls of either capillaries or of venules. Sometimes segmental degenerative changes may be adjacent to activated lymphocytes but this is not a constant relationship. Mastaglia and Currie found cells resembling lymphoid cells within muscle fibres. Macrophages occur near vessels and inside degenerating fibres, showing phagocytosis.

Vascular changes. These comprise endothelial thickening in venules and capillaries with basement-membrane reduplication (Shafiq *et al.*, 1967). The thickening is due to increased cytoplasm with numerous organelles (Gonzalez-Angulo, Fraga, Mintz and Zavala, 1968). In childhood DM, the changes in endothelial cells are conspicuous very early; they show a pattern of degeneration, regeneration, and reduplication which seems to Banker (1975) to be suggestive of a primary abnormality. Tubular inclusions have been described in the endothelial cells in DM by Hashimoto *et al.* (1971) and by others; these may be a non-specific finding.

Virus-like particles. In an increasing number of reports, usually of single cases of PM–DM, virus-like particles have been described in ultramicroscopic studies of muscle. The particles have resembled two groups of virus, picornavirus and myxovirus. The picornavirus has been thought to be Coxsackie virus. Zweymüller demonstrated Coxsackie virus-like particles in PM muscle cells as far back as 1953 (Pearson, 1975) and they have since been shown by Chou and Gutmann (1970), Mastaglia and Walton (1970) and Ben-Bassat and Machtey (1972). They have also been reported as an incidental finding in normal muscle (Caulfield, Rebeiz and Adams, 1968). In the two cases of DM described by Chou and Gutmann, the course was subacute and fatal over months. Chou (1968) found myxovirus-like structures in three separate biopsies from a case of PM during the course of 18 months, suggesting chronic viral replication. A further description was given by Sato, Walker, Peters, Reese and Chou (1971) who went as far as to call chronic PM a 'slow virus' infection. The microtubular inclusions which they found were confined to nuclei in intact muscle cells, but were intrasarcoplasmic as well in damaged cells. Chou and Gutmann postulated that the type of virus might influence the course of the myopathy, picornavirus being associated with subacute PM and myxovirus with chronic PM. Banker (1975) found particles which resembled papovavirus in biopsy material from childhood DM. The particles were intranuclear, but she was not convinced that the structures were more than nucleolar debris. The tubular inclusions in endothelial cells have already been mentioned (Hashimoto et al., 1971).

In no case of PM–DM has the identification of virus been made on stronger grounds than those of morphological appearances. Thus virus must be confirmed by other methods, such as isolation, immunofluorescence and repeated passage (Banker, 1975). The nosological status of 'viral myositis' is discussed in the section on differential diagnosis. The case described by Tang, Sedmak, Siegesmund and McCreadie (1975) was one of chronic myopathy attributable to Coxsackie virus; ultramicroscopy showed foci of myofilament degeneration with a lattice-work of viral particles. The case described by De Reuck, de Coster and Inderadjaja (1977) was similar although lymphocytic infiltrates were present in addition. In the cases of Echovirus infection which were responsible for DM with encephalitis (Bardelas et al., 1977; Webster et al., 1978) the virus was not found in muscle tissue on ultramicroscopy; the muscle fibre necrosis with perivascular and interstitial inflammation were the changes of PM–DM. Clearly, there are similarities to the case of Ben-Bassat and Machtey (1972), which was more obviously one of DM, yet with a fatal outcome and also accompanied by encephalitis; Coxsackie virus-like particles were found in muscle but not isolated. These cases exemplify the problem of what should be classed with the PM–DM complex and what should be excluded.

Minor clinical investigations

Erythrocyte sedimentation rate. This is raised in 50 per cent or more of acute cases; it is increased particularly when there is a marked systemic reaction. Diessner et al. (1966) found an increase in two-thirds of their cases, typically at the height of the disease process; the test held no predictive value. De Vere and Bradley (1975) found that it was raised in only 45 per cent of all their patients, with no correlation with the severity of the disorder. Bohan et al. (1977) concurred with this finding. The blood count is of even less importance. A neutrophil leucocytosis may occur when PM–DM is part of an acute systemic disorder. Anaemia is rare.

Serum enzymes. The serum aldolase and the serum glutamic oxaloacetic transaminase levels are increased when acute muscle cell necrosis occurs; they are used less than the serum CK level which is the most sensitive indicator of activity, according to Pearson and Bohan (1977). These authors did say that estimation of the levels of several enzymes at intervals would almost always demonstrate abnormality at some stage of the clinical course.

Myoglobinaemia. This is considered in the section on special investigations because its assay is not a routine laboratory procedure at present. Like raised serum enzymes, the occurrence of myoglobinaemia reflects muscle-cell necrosis.

Tests for C–T disorders. For obvious reasons these are most likely to show abnormality in PM–DM associated with these disorders. Antinuclear factor is rarely positive in simple PM or DM; it is found in about 10 per cent of cases of PM with C–T disorder (Bohan *et al.*, 1977). The titres of antinuclear antibody may be very high in myositis with SLE. Bohan *et al.* (1977) found that the latex fixation titre for rheumatoid factor was positive (greater than 1:40) in 20 per cent of cases tested. Other tests such as lupus erythematosus (LE) cell preparations, anti-DNA titres and extractable nuclear antigen (ENA) titres gave inconsistent results. Abnormal findings such as cryoglobulins and a positive Coombs test for haemolysis are exceptional.

Special investigations

In the past decade, special techniques have been brought to bear on the study of PM–DM, some purely diagnostic but most in a search for its cause. Many of the studies have involved immunological methods, either for sensitive assay or for the detection of immune disturbance in the condition. The techniques have been an extension of more standard methods of study, such as histopathological and biochemical. Indeed, they are described in a section separate from that on clinical investigations solely because they remain at the research stage without general application to clinical diagnosis and management. The findings of these studies have implications which will be discussed in the section on aetiology and only brief mention of their significance will be given now. The tests are listed in Table 15.10 (not in order of importance).

Humoral immune responses

Skin reactivity and antibodies to tumour extracts. Isolated studies in patients with DM in association with neoplasm are of historical importance as the earliest attempts to look for humoral factors (Grace and Dao, 1959; Curtis, Heckaman and Wheeler, 1961; Alexander and Foreman, 1968). Extracts of tumour tissue from these patients were injected into them. This induced both the formation of serum antibodies against the tumour

Table 15.10 Special investigations in PM–DM

Humoral immune responses
       Skin reactivity
       Antibodies to tumour extracts
       Antibodies to components of muscle
       Specific antinuclear antibody
       Serum immunoglobulin levels
       Serum complement levels
       Immunofluorescence studies

Cellular immune responses
       Transformation with muscle extracts
       Macrophage-migration inhibition with
         muscle antigen
       Cytotoxicity for muscle cells *in vitro*
       Lymphotoxin production *in vitro*

Viral studies

Myoglobin assay Myoglobinaemia
                Myoglobinuria

Radioisotope scanning of muscle

(Experimental myositis)

tissue and skin reactivity to the tissue of humoral type. This reactivity could be passively transferred. Such phenomena have been hailed as evidence of a causative link between neoplasia and DM, with relevance to the aetiology of myositis in general (Pearson and Bohan, 1977). However, similar responses have been shown in patients who have neoplasia but no evidence of myositis (Hellström, Hellström and Pierce, 1969). The phenomenon is probably secondary to tissue damage and of no aetiological significance.

Antibodies to components of muscle. Caspary, Gubbay and Stern (1964) examined the sera of patients with PM–DM for the presence of antibody against myosin, as well as for antinuclear factor. There were positive findings in half the patients but this was also the case for groups of patients with muscular dystrophy and neurogenic muscular atrophy. The results were therefore inconclusive and it appeared that a secondary phenomenon was being detected through a sensitive assay. Similar negative results were subsequently obtained when serum antibodies against extracts of muscle and nuclei were looked for (Stern, Rose and Jacobs, 1967). Fairfax and Gröschel-Stewart (1977) note that, in general, antibodies to myosin are found in the serum only exceptionally. There are two distinct antibodies to smooth muscle, one of which cross-reacts with skeletal, cardiac and other tissue (cytoplasmic) myosin.

Specific antinuclear antibody for polymyositis. An antinuclear antibody specific for a particular C–T disorder can be both diagnostically important and aetiologically significant. The most obvious example is the IgG rheumatoid factor in RA. Studying PM–DM, Reichlin and Mattioli (1976) employed an indirect test on sera from patients. 'Fab' units (fragments antigen binding) were obtained by previous digestion of serum with papain. They were then tested for their capacity to produce significant inhibition of complement fixation by a reference serum reacting with material derived from thymic antigens. In this study about two-thirds of the PM–DM sera and 5 per cent of 'control' sera produced inhibition. The 'control' sera included those from cases of other C–T disorders. Despite the weakness of the precipitin line, Wolfe, Adelstein and Sharp (1977) managed to demonstrate directly a precipitin reaction in their immunodiffusion studies using thymic antigen. A positive reaction was found in two-thirds of the sera from patients with PM. It was present continuously throughout the course of the disorder. It was not found in the sera of patients with other C–T disorders, SLE, PSS, RA and mixed disorders; the results for these were 'uniformly negative', indeed, remarkably so. The authors considered that the factor was an antinuclear antibody which might be a specific serological marker for PM–DM. They felt that they were probably studying the same phenomenon as had Reichlin and Mattioli (1976), using a different method. They thought that the striking demarcation between PM–DM and other C–T disorders might be quantitative rather than qualitative in origin, with a relatively insensitive test giving positive results only when there was clearcut myopathy with sufficient muscle damage. This seems the only reasonable interpretation, given that myositis is common to most of the other C–T disorders.

Serum immunoglobulin levels. Conflicting results have been obtained on measuring immunoglo-bulin levels in PM–DM. Even within individual studies there are inconsistent findings. Dawkins (1975) considers that there is enough evidence of depression of immunoglobulin levels and of humoral competence to fit his concept of PM–DM as a humoral immunodeficiency disorder. Thus IgG concentrations were depressed in the sera of 50 per cent of his cases, and there was a poor antibody response to tetanus toxoid immunisation in a similar percentage. However, Lisak and Zweiman (1976) found that the mean levels of IgG were elevated in PM–DM, and incidentally in myasthenia gravis as well; there was no consistent depression of serum IgA, IgG or IgM to suggest humoral deficiency. In isolated cases of immune deficiency in association with myositis, selective immunoglobulin deficiency may be present. Thus, IgA deficiency was present in a case of childhood myositis (Carroll *et al.*, 1976). Hereditary complement (C2) deficiency in association with DM was reported by Leddy *et al.* (1975), a finding which meant that PM–DM could occur even when the classical complement pathway could not be activated.

Serum complement levels. As with immunoglo-bulins, there are conflicting results in PM–DM which are interpreted differently by those who postulate humoral immune deficiency and those who suggest a role for humoral processes. Dawkins (1975) states from his own studies that hypo-complementaemia was a rare finding. Behan and Behan (1977), on the other hand, found evidence of complement activation in 40 per cent of cases of PM–DM. The components of complement were estimated and serum anticomplementary assays carried out. The cases included ones of uncomplicated PM (Group I). In those cases with hypocomplementaemia, the plasma concentration of the C4 component was low, with positive serum anticomplementary activity; the concentration of the other component of the classical pathway (Clq) was not significantly reduced. The authors felt that, taken together, these findings suggested that circulating soluble immune complexes were present, probably in considerable numbers. Bohan *et al.* (1977) found the B–1–C to be low in 14 of 21 patients; these included patients with uncomplicated PM–DM as well as PM with C–T disorder. However, the total haemolytic complement was decreased in only one patient.

Immunopathological studies (immunofluorescence). The studies of the pathology of muscle by Whitaker and Engel (1972) were directed particularly towards abnormalities of small vessels. Their work included the use of immunofluorescence to demonstrate complement and immunoglobulins in vessel walls. The authors found such deposits, particularly in perimysial veins, in 17 of 39 biopsies. Typically, deposits were in the intima. They were most likely to be present in muscle from cases of childhood DM, and it was in this variant that the greatest number of involved vessels per muscle section were found. The immunoglobulins comprised immunoglobulin G (IgG), IgM and B1C/1A (C3) complement. Fluorescent staining gave a granular or nodular pattern, suggestive of deposition of immune complexes. The vessels which contained deposits were not necessarily abnormal, changes when present comprising endothelial cell proliferation with or without luminal occlusion. Mononuclear cell reaction was not found in association with deposits. Control cases included myasthenia gravis, RA, systemic vasculitides and PSS, none with overt myopathy; cases of muscular dystrophy were also examined. In none of these conditions were granular deposits found in vessels, although deposits occurred in damaged muscle fibres in many conditions. The authors felt that the vascular deposits were unlikely to be secondary to muscle damage and might represent immune complexes. Behan, McQueen and Behan (1980) have recently confirmed these findings. The case of DM with C2 complement deficiency which was reported by Leddy *et al.* (1975) is remarkable in this context, because immunofluorescence studies of vessel walls showed neither immunoglobulins nor C3. There was, in this case, no evidence that there had been activation of the alternative (C3) complement pathway involving the properdin system, a participant in tissue injury mediated by immune complexes.

Cellular immune responses

Lymphocyte transformation with muscle extracts. Peripheral blood lymphocytes from cases of PM–DM were shown to have an increased rate of transformation when cultured with a xenogeneic muscle homogenate (Saunders, Knowles and Currie, 1969; Currie, Saunders, Knowles and Brown, 1971b). The degree of stimulation of these lymphocytes was assessed by measuring their uptake of tritiated thymidine. Lymphocytes from patients with PM–DM showed a significantly higher response to muscle than did lymphocytes from patients with other diseases with and without muscle wasting. Even so, the proliferative response which was obtained with PM–DM lymphocytes was a small one, in absolute terms. The absence of an increased rate in patients with other muscle-wasting disorders was taken to be significant. However, with the much more sensitive technique of cytospherometry, a degree of lymphocyte sensitisation to muscle antigens was subsequently shown by Caspary, Currie and Field (1971). In PM the index of response showed some correlation with the clinical activity of the disorder. Lymphocytes from none of the groups of patients responded to other antigens (collagen, encephalitogenic factor, liver and kidney homogenates). The disorders in the 'control' patients with other diseases were not ones in which immunological mechanisms might be of importance. Esiri, MacLennan and Hazleman (1973) confirmed the finding of PM–DM lymphocyte transformation in the presence of skeletal muscle extract. They studied lymphocytes from patients with other C–T disorders and found an increased rate in PMR but not in RA. De Vere and Bradley (1975) were unable to confirm the findings in PM–DM.

Macrophage migration inhibition. Peripheral blood lymphocytes from patients with PM–DM were studied by Goust, Castaigne and Moulias (1974), using the method of inhibition of macrophage migration in the presence of putative muscle antigen. As in the work of Currie *et al*, (1971b) a xenogeneic muscle extract was used as the antigen with which lymphocytes were cultured. Sensitised lymphocytes were found in almost every case of PM–DM and in the majority of cases of myasthenia gravis, both to muscle and thymus crude antigen.

Lymphocyte cytotoxicity for muscle cells in vitro. Peripheral blood lymphocytes from patients with PM–DM were shown by Currie (1970) to be cytotoxic to human and animal fetal muscle cells in tissue culture. Lymphocytes were added to muscle cultures in Maximow chambers. Those from cases of PM–DM showed agglutination to each other and to muscle cells within hours, and the latter underwent destruction, which was usually marked by 36 hours. Cultures of fibroblasts were destroyed in the presence of lymphocytes from patients with myositis and PSS. Serum from the patients with PM and lymphocytes from those with other muscle-wasting disorders were not cytotoxic to cultures of muscle and other tissues. This work was extended by Currie *et al.* (1971b). They confirmed cytotoxicity for various tissue explants of lymphocytes from patients with PM in association with C–T disorders. However, the presence of clinical features such as skin erythema, Raynaud's phenomenon and arthralgia was not always paralleled by cytotoxicity for cultures other than those of muscle. Antilymphocytic antiserum appeared to prevent cytotoxic action by lymphocytes. The cytotoxicity of PM lymphocytes for muscle cultures was confirmed by Kakulas, Shute and Leclere (1971), using CK release by cultures as a measure of damage, and by Dawkins and Mastaglia (1973) who used the release of radioactive chromium. Cytotoxicity was more likely to occur if the myositis was in an active phase and not already treated by steroid therapy. The cytotoxicity was thought to represent a direct T-cell killing of muscle target cells (Dawkins, 1975). Haas and Arnason (1974) showed cytotoxicity by lymphocytes to muscle cell cultures in Maximow chambers; they also used muscle cultures in Petri dishes and measured the release of CK. Their controls included lymphocytes from patients with other disorders in which immune disturbances are recognised, such as myasthenia gravis, idiopathic polyneuritis and SLE. Unlike Dawkins and Mastaglia (1973), they found destruction of muscle cultures by PM–DM lymphocytes irrespective of the clinical status: *i.e.* in cases of active, quiescent, treated or untreated myopathy. De Vere and Bradley (1975) did not confirm cytotoxicity of PM lymphocytes for muscle cultures.

Lymphotoxin production in vitro. The studies of Johnson, Fink and Ziff (1972) were an extension of the cytotoxicity work. They found that, on incubation with autologous muscle, lymphocytes from patients with PM–DM produced a lymphotoxin which was cytotoxic to muscle cells in culture. Among the control disorders were one case of PAN with muscle lesions and one of muscular dystrophy. Supernatants were obtained after 48–72 h culture of lymphocytes with muscle and applied to monolayers of fetal muscle for 48 h. Cytotoxicity was measured by the reduction in radioactive carbon uptake by the monolayers. There was some evidence that foci of lymphoid cells within muscle explants could release lymphotoxin on appropriate stimulation. The cytotoxic effect was prevented by prednisone. The findings allowed an explanation for muscle cell damage *in vivo* without adjacent lymphocytic infiltration. The possibility of contactual lysis through immunoglobulin was not excluded by the finding of lymphotoxin cytotoxicity.

Viral studies. In the main these comprise the demonstration by ultramicroscopy of virus-like particles, picorna (Coxsackie), myxovirus and papova virus, within muscle cells in biopsy material from cases of PM–DM. These have been described in the section entitled 'Pathology: ultramicroscopy'. In only some of the cases was identification of the viruses attempted by other means such as immunofluorescence and cytopathic effect in culture, and in these instances the results were uniformly negative. Chou and Gutmann (1970) suggested that the virus might comprise defective particles of low infectivity and would therefore be impossible to isolate. Only in cases of myositis which could not be placed firmly within the PM–DM complex have viruses been identified (Echovirus, Coxsackie virus). These cases are referred to in the section on differential diagnosis as examples of viral myositis.

Myoglobin assay. The measurement of myoglobin in blood and urine provides an index of the degree of muscle cell necrosis. However, the amounts of myoglobin are usually small and a sensitive immunological assay is required (Kagen, 1971). In clinical practice, therefore, the estimation of the serum CK level is still the best guide to activity of the disorder. The immuno-assay of myoglobin remains a specialised investigation. Kagen (1977) found myoglobinaemia in 75 per cent of clinically active cases but in only 10 per cent of quiescent cases. The techniques involved immunodiffusion and complement fixation. Myoglobinaemia was present in two-thirds of DM cases, in half the PM cases and in less than half of those of 'overlap' myositis. The concentrations in DM ranged from 10 to 108 μg/ml. There was some correlation with serum CK elevation, but myoglobinaemia was found in a third of the patients in whom the CK activities were normal. Myoglobinaemia disappeared by the second week of prednisone therapy, concomitantly with the fall in serum enzymes.

Radioisotope scanning of muscle. Brown, Swift and Spies (1976) carried out whole-body scanning of muscles. Their work grew out of the use of scanning in the search for occult neoplasm. In PM–DM they found evidence of increased muscle labelling using technetium 99M-polyphosphate with whole-body rectilinear bone scans. There was a correlation with activity; uptake decreased after steroid therapy. The technique gave no help in the localisation of abnormality to particular muscles nor, of course, was it designed to pick up foci of necrosis and inflammation within individual muscles.

Experimental myositis. Experimental auto-allergic myositis is induced in animals by injections of muscle in adjuvant. It is described fully by Professor Kakulas in Chapter 11. Although sometimes referred to as 'animal polymyositis', it is not a close analogue for PM–DM or any other human inflammatory myopathy, such as the myositis of myasthenia gravis (Currie, 1971; Dawkins, 1975). It is a model of a process, not a disorder (Dawkins, 1975). The myositis is monophasic, short-lived and does not produce signs. The pathology comprises focal segmental fibre necrosis and interstitial mononuclear cell infiltration. The condition appears to be due to cell-mediated hypersensitivity and has been passively transferred by lymphoid cells.

Differential diagnosis

The differential diagnosis of PM–DM conventionally is concerned with the criteria for the diagnosis of the condition and with those of the disorders from which this must be differentiated. In addition to this practical aspect, there is the more theoretical question of which disorders should or should not be included under the term 'polymyositis'. Conditions are sometimes classed alongside PM–DM because of clinical or pathological resemblances to it. The UCLA school (Bohan and Peter, 1975; Bohan et al., 1977) are clearly concerned with the criteria for diagnosis in order that a homogeneous group of patients may be studied. Bohan and Peter considered that there were no generally accepted criteria for the diagnosis of PM–DM, as there were, for instance, for SLE and RA. They listed five major criteria. The first is symmetrical weakness of limb-girdle muscles and anterior neck flexors, with progression over weeks to months. The second is muscle biopsy evidence of type I and type II fibre necrosis, phagocytosis, regeneration, atrophy in a perifascicular distribution with an inflammatory exudate, often perivascular. The third is elevation in serum skeletal-muscle enzymes. The fourth is the EMG triad of small polyphasic motor units, fibrillation and repetitive discharges. The fifth is the skin rash of DM, an erythematous dermatitis over extensor surfaces of limbs, and also the face and neck. They regarded four criteria as necessary for a definite diagnosis of PM, three (plus the rash) for DM; a diagnosis of 'possible' PM or DM was justified with fewer criteria. They felt that steroid-responsiveness should not be used as a criterion. The course of other myopathies was sometimes influenced by steroid therapy and some PM–DM cases might be steroid-resistant yet responsive to other IS drugs. De Vere and Bradley (1975) felt that some genuine cases of PM would be left out of any series if there were insistence on positive findings on enzyme estimation, EMG and muscle biopsy. In particular, muscle biopsy in their own series gave the classical pathological changes in only 46 per cent, and in six per cent a single biopsy appeared to be entirely normal.

The main conditions to be taken into account in the differential diagnosis are listed in Table 15.11.

Table 15.11 Differential diagnosis of PM–DM

Hereditary disorders
    Muscular dystrophy
    Chronic spinal muscular atrophy
    Metabolic myopathies

Inflammatory myopathies .
    Granulomatous and giant-cell myopathy
    Sarcoid myopathy
    Viral myositis
    Tropical myositis
    Parasitic myositis
    Myasthenia gravis
    Polymyalgia rheumatica
    Myopathy in Löffler's syndrome
    Inclusion body myositis

Motor neurone disease

Rhabdomyolysis

Acquired metabolic myopathies

Some, like the granulomatous myopathies, are traditionally grouped alongside PM–DM and are included in this Chapter, though they are not clearly related to this. Also considered in separate sections are viral myositis, tropical myositis, parasitic myositis and C–T disorders including PMR.

Hereditary neuromuscular disorders

Muscular dystrophy. Muscular dystrophy, particularly the limb-girdle and facioscapulohumeral types, may be hard to distinguish from chronic PM. Calf enlargement is exceptional in PM although it has been reported in childhood DM (Thompson, 1968). The fact that another member of the family may have the disorder does not in itself rule out PM, even if familial PM is rare. In facioscapulohumeral (FSH) dystrophy (or 'myopathy'), inflammatory infiltrates may occur. Munsat *et al.* (1972) described a variant of FSH dystrophy with autosomal dominant inheritance at a stage of which infiltrates occurred in muscle and steroid therapy resulted in temporary improvement. The condition of FSH myopathy is a heterogeneous one and not a nosological entity. The disorder in their cases differed from PM in the lack of evidence of C–T disorder, in the family history and also in the age of onset, facial involvement and prominent atrophy. An FSH distribution is exceptional in

PM–DM (Bates *et al.*, 1973). They noted that inflammatory changes had been reported to occur at some stage in all the muscular dystrophies. Jennekens *et al.* (1975) described an autosomal dominant disorder with features of both limb-girdle dystrophy and of the scapuloperoneal syndrome. The EMG suggested a neurogenic disorder. However, biopsy showed not only neurogenic atrophy but also myopathic changes including interstitial and perivascular inflammation and vacuolisation of muscle fibres. These disorders could hardly be mistaken for PM, but the occurrence of myositis as part of hereditary myopathy is noteworthy.

Benign chronic spinal muscular atrophy. This usually has a slower tempo and a different distribution from PM; the EMG findings should be clear-cut except that spontaneous activity occurs in both conditions. It should be noted that secondary myopathic change can lead in this condition to very marked increases in CK activity.

Hereditary metabolic myopathies. These, such as McArdle's disease, with muscle pain and weakness, may resemble PM and have been mistakenly treated as such (Mastaglia, McCollum and Larson, 1970). Some lipid storage myopathies may improve with steroid therapy (Engel and Siekert, 1972; Johnson, Fulthorpe and Hudgson, 1973). Carnitine deficiency can present with myalgia and muscle weakness (Johnson *et al.*, 1973; Cumming, Hardy, Hudgson and Walls, 1976). The number of cases of acute childhood PM in some series of PM may have been increased by the erroneous inclusion of cases of metabolic myopathy. Clearly, only full assessment with all the modern techniques will allow differentiation in some patients with myopathy.

Inflammatory myopathies

Granulomatous myopathy. Chronic PM and granulomatous myopathy may be separable only by muscle biopsy: necrobiotic changes and infiltration outside the granulomata will not occur in the latter (Hewlett and Brownell, 1975).

Sarcoidosis. Granulomatous myopathy in sarcoidosis only rarely produces symptoms, such a proximal muscle weakness. Myopathy is typically seen in middle-aged women (Gardner-Thorpe, 1972). It resembles granulomatous myopathy except for the multi-system involvement.

Giant-cell myositis with thymoma. Clinically, this does not present like DM–PM but rather as myasthenia gravis in association with thymoma. The myocardium is involved, as well as skeletal muscle.

Viral myositis. Some muscle disorders which are directly due to viruses are considered by Dr Foster in Chapter 23, and briefly at the end of the present Chapter. Acute viral involvement of muscle such as that seen in pleurodynia and benign myalgic encephalomyelitis may have features in common with PM of acute onset, but differentiation should not be difficult. A greater problem with regard to viral myositis is that of its classification. A DM-like syndrome may occur in immunodeficient individuals, caused either by direct viral action or by virus-induced immune-complex vasculitis. The borderline between PM–DM and viral myositis is blurred in these cases, which are mentioned in the section 'Pathology: ultramicroscopy'. They should be separated from those cases of PM–DM in which virus-like structures are found in muscle biopsy material. Other cases are more easily distinguished from PM–DM. These include the chronic Coxsackie-virus myositis of Tang *et al.*, (1975). This was the case of a child with acute-on-chronic myopathy, affecting the respiratory muscles in particular. Light microscopy showed degenerative changes without inflammation. Deposits of viral particles were seen on ultramicroscopy; these were confirmed as Coxsackie virus. The particles were very like those seen on ultramicroscopy in some cases of PM–DM (Chou and Gutmann, 1970; Mastaglia and Walton, 1971) but identification as virus in the latter cases was not achieved.

Tropical myositis. This is considered in a separate section. It may well be a viral or bacterial myositis. It rarely occurs except in the tropics or in those people who have visited those areas within the preceding year. In this condition fever, arthralgia and focal muscle pains occur. Abscess formation may follow. Its differentiation from PM–DM should not be difficult. It is possible that a form of tropical myositis is responsible for the high incidence of DM which has been reported in the Bantu tribe (Findlay *et al.*, 1969).

Parasitic myositis. Myopathies due to parasites include those occurring in toxoplasmosis and trichinosis. These disorders are considered in the section by Drs Pallis and Lewis in Part II of this Chapter. However, they are mentioned here as they may give problems, both diagnostic and nosological. The case described by Rowland and Greer (1961) was not strictly one of PM, and thus would not have been included in any series of Bohan and Peter (1975), yet the authors called the condition 'toxoplasmic polymyositis', stating that 'polymyositis seems a reasonable appellation'. The presentation was subacute, with pyrexia, muscle aches and tenderness. Serum enzyme activity was raised and the EMG suggested myositis; sternomastoid muscle biopsy was normal. The diagnosis of toxoplasmosis rested on serological tests. Kagen, Kimball and Christian (1974) have claimed serological evidence of toxoplasmosis among patients with PM–DM. Although their results were not convincing, it is possible that Toxoplasma in muscle, like viruses, may trigger off 'idiopathic' myositis.

Myasthenia gravis. This should be separable from PM–DM by the clinical picture, including the distribution of muscular weakness, such as oculomotor and shoulder girdle with sparing of lower limb musculature, and the fatigable nature of the muscle weakness. The response to cholinergic drugs, the sensitivity to D-tubocurarine and the decremental response to nerve stimulation are further features which allow differentiation. However, the two disorders do have several points in common, including some pathological changes and steroid-responsiveness. They have been described in association (Johns *et al.*, 1971; Namba *et al.*, 1973) although this overlap syndrome is not accepted by all (Rowland, Lisak, Schotland and Berg, 1973).

Polymyalgia rheumatica. This C–T disorder is distinguished from PM–DM by the absence of muscle weakness, since incapacity results largely from pain and stiffness. The patients are usually elderly. The ESR is almost always markedly elevated but tests for myopathy give negative results. In some of the C–T disorders, such as RA, difficulty may arise in distinguishing from PM the results of limitation in movement due to pain or to myopathy secondary to steroid therapy. Full investigation including biopsy may be necessary (Haslock *et al.*, 1970).

Myopathy in Löffler's syndrome. Eosinophilic infiltration of muscles has been reported in the hypereosinophilic syndrome of Löffler by Layzer, Shearn and Satya-Murti (1977). Their term 'eosinophilic polymyositis' implies that the condition is a variant of PM–DM, which it is not.

Inclusion body myositis. This is a variety of idiopathic inflammatory myopathy which is distinct from PM–DM in its clinical picture, pathology and the lack of response to immunosuppression (Carpenter, Karpati, Heller and Eisen, 1978); the name was given to the condition by Yunis and Samaha (1971). Men are affected more than women. There are no stigmata of C–T disorder. Distal muscles are involved as well as proximal; weakness is slowly progressive and painless. Serum CK activity is normal or only slightly raised. Electromyography shows marked fibrillation as well as short-duration polyphasic units. The pathological changes in muscle comprise vacuoles, best seen in cryostat sections, cellular infiltration, necrosis and regeneration and capillary proliferation. Ultramicroscopy shows cytoplasmic inclusions comprising masses of filaments and also subsarcolemmal whorls of cytomembranes. Carpenter *et al.* (1978) regard these changes as distinct from those of childhood DM and adult PM–DM. The filaments are not definitely viral in origin. The condition may be commoner than the literature suggests, in view of the techniques required to diagnose it.

Motor neurone disease. Progressive muscular atrophy occasionally gives diagnostic problems. Usually, the distribution of muscular weakness and visible fasciculation of muscles will allow the correct diagnosis. However, proximal limb weakness, EMG changes suggestive of myositis and raised CK activity resulting from secondary myopathy may mean that only muscle biopsy will differentiate successfully. Motor neurone disease with upper as well as lower motor neurone signs presents less difficulty.

Rhabdomyolysis. There is usually an obvious precipitating disorder in rhabdomyolysis with overt myoglobinuria. The conditions range from crush injury, electrocution and heat stroke to infections, notably viral, and convulsions. Bohan and Peter (1975) felt that rhabdomyolysis should not be included as part of the PM–DM spectrum. The condition can occur without any clear precipitant; it may be recurrent. It is commoner in children than in adults. In some of these cases there is an underlying hereditary metabolic myopathy, such as McArdle's phosphorylase deficiency or carnitine palmityl transferase deficiency. A family history may be obtained. PM–DM is rarely so acute that it produces overt myoglobinuria, despite the assertion of Sloan, Franks, Exley and Davison (1978). Neither acute rhabdomyolysis nor the necrotising myopathy of neoplasia (Smith, 1969) can be fitted easily into the PM–DM complex; they are certainly not inflammatory myopathies.

Metabolic myopathies (acquired). Endocrine myopathies, such as those in association with thyroid, parathyroid or adrenal dysfunction and rarely with diabetes mellitus should be easily recognisable. As has been mentioned, sometimes steroid-induced lipid myopathy must be differentiated from symptomatic myositis in a C–T disorder when steroids have been given and proximal muscle weakness has developed. In this regard the needle technique for muscle biopsy could prove useful; lipid changes and atrophy of type II fibres are suggestive of steroid myopathy.

Aetiology

The genesis of the PM–DM complex may lie in a derangement of immune processes. Such a thesis is at once bold, because the evidence for it is both circumstantial and conflicting, and bland, in its very vagueness. The presentation of the clinical features of the condition has provided many items of possible aetiological significance. These have included the precipitants of the disorder, the associated disorders and the investigatory findings both on standard histological examination and on more specialised studies, serological, immunological and pathological. All the evidence must be weighed in the formulation of any aetiological concept. Although it may not be possible to reconcile the conflicting results of different studies or the diametrically opposed views which these results have engendered, the attempt must be made. Thus, the discovery of viral particles on ultramicroscopy of muscle biopsy material in a few cases does not necessarily mean that the myositis in these or other cases is the result of direct viral action. The finding of early abnormalities in blood vessels and of perifascicular atrophy may indicate a vascular factor in the damage to muscle, but PM may be called an ischaemic myopathy only in the narrowest sense. The demonstration of hypo-complementaemia and of immune complexes on immunopathological studies of muscle may be taken to imply that the upset of immune processes consists of humoral overaction with depression of cellular immunity. However, morphological observation of mononuclear cells on muscle histology, the *in vitro* studies of lymphocytes in PM–DM and the existence of the animal model experimental myositis could all be taken to indicate the opposite. In this section on aetiology the main pieces of evidence are considered under individual headings, followed by a conclusion. In Table 15.12, the evidence is given as a list.

Genetic factors

Familial cases. Even if familial cases of PM–DM are exceptional, their occurrence implies an inherited susceptibility, as in the commoner C–T disorders such as RA, and holds aetiological significance for the condition in general. The elevation of serum γ-globulins in a symptomatic relative may be an indication of familial susceptibility.

Histocompatibility studies. The finding of an increased incidence of the immune gene HLA–B8 in both childhood DM and adult PM–DM is of

Table 15.12   PM–DN: aetiological factors

Genetic factors	familial cases histocompatibility antigen studies agammaglobulinaemia
Precipitating factors	viral infection drugs
Associated disorders	connective-tissue disorders neoplasia myasthenia gravis
Pathological findings	mononuclear cell infiltration vasculitis perifascicular atrophy immunoglobulin–complement deposits viral particles
Therapy	steroid therapy other immunosuppressive therapy thymectomy
Humoral immune responses	hypocomplementaemia circulating antibodies skin sensitivity to tumour
Cellular immune responses	*in vitro* lymphocyte studies
Experimental autoallergic myositis	

importance as HLA–B8 is found in association with several disorders thought to have an immunopathogenesis (Oliver, 1977), myasthenia gravis in particular. There is also the implication that there is a common aetiology in childhood DM and adult PM–DM. The increased incidence of HLA–B14 which has also been reported may have been due to serological cross-reactivity.

Genetic immune deficiency. This is a rare concomitant of PM–DM but may be an extreme form of a commoner, less specific deficiency. Genetic predisposition appears to be of more significance in other C–T disorders, such as SLE, with a volume of published work suggesting genetically determined defects in immune responses. Familial or sporadic deficiency in γ-globulins may lead to PM–DM through upset in the regulation of humoral immune processes. The absence of the second component of complement in the case described by Leddy *et al.* (1975), with no immunoglobulins or C3 on immunofluorescence studies of muscle, means that muscle damage in that case must have been mediated through an alternative pathway, if humoral in origin. The same is true for the case described by Gotoff *et al.* (1972) in which DM and cerebral vasculitis occurred, suggestive of immune complex formation despite, or in association with, X-linked agammaglobulinaemia. An alternative, to be elaborated in the next section, on viruses, is that viral action is allowed by immune deficiency, familial hypogammaglobulinaemia in the case described by Webster *et al.* (1978), sporadic in that described by Bardelas *et al.* (1977). Even in these cases, the question remains whether the myositis was directly or indirectly due to the virus. Rosen (1974) discussed the possibility of slow virus infection causing the cerebral component of the DM–cerebral vasculitis syndrome of X-linked agammaglobulinaemia. He also noted that there was an increase in C–T disorders in acquired agammaglobulinaemia. Inherited defects in classical pathway complement result in a diminished capacity to eliminate pathogenic viruses so that circulating immune complexes may be present continuously. Carroll *et al.* (1976) suggested that, in their sporadic cases of IgA deficiency with PM and villous atrophy, a defect in tissue IgA in the intestinal mucosa might allow the absorption of antigens; these could set off immunopathological reactions resulting in tissue damage.

Precipitating factors

Viruses. Febrile illness of presumed viral origin may be a precipitant of PM–DM, although the association is not as clear-cut or as well-documented as, for instance, in acute polyneuritis. The occurrence of PM–DM after viral exanthemata is rare but has long been recognised. Viruses could precipitate the condition by several mechanisms. Some constituent of muscle could be altered, rendering it antigenic and subject to attack by immune processes. Precipitating viruses could activate latent virus or allow secondary invasion by other viruses.

Drugs. Penicillamine is the drug of most interest among those which have been reported as possible precipitants of PM–DM. The PM in the case of Schraeder *et al.* (1972) was part of a mixed C–T disorder resembling SLE; the authors postulated that the damage to muscle and other tissues might be due to immune complex formation between the

drug and tissue components. Cucher and Goldman (1976) concurred with this view. Dawkins (1975), on the other hand, felt that the depression of humoral responses which was known to occur with the drug was in keeping with his concept of PM–DM as a disorder due to imbalance of immune processes, with depressed humoral responses. It is notable that selective IgA deficiency can follow penicillamine therapy.

Associated disorders

Connective-tissue (C–T) disorders. The association of PM–DM with other C–T disorders is of aetiological significance, given the weight of presumptive evidence that these disorders arise from deranged immune processes. The relationship of the asymptomatic focal myositis of the C–T disorders to overt PM–DM is uncertain but there is no doubt that true PM can occur in most of the disorders. Childhood DM, in which systemic vasculitis is frequent, bears the closest resemblance to the C–T disorders, the hallmarks of which are the pathological changes, including vasculitis. On other grounds, childhood DM stands apart from PM and thus does not occur as a component of 'overlap' C–T disorder (*see* 'Classification'). The development of secondary amyloidosis in longstanding PM has implications for the pathogenesis of the disorder.

Neoplasia. The association of neoplasia with PM–DM has not been proved and is of uncertain immunological significance. Possibly a tumour catabolite provokes cross-sensitisation to a component of muscle or forms a complex allergen with one. The frequency is similar to that of thymoma in myasthenia gravis; however, the relationship is less specific and is without the parallel between thymic hyperplasia and neoplasia. PM–DM and the other neuromuscular syndromes of neoplasia are not related. Thus necrotising myopathy and 'carcinomatous neuromyopathy' are separate conditions. Skin tests in patients with carcinoma and DM may be of no aetiological significance, a point discussed later. Dawkins (1975) suggested that both neoplasia and myositis might be secondary to a more fundamental deficiency in immunity. The neoplasms which have been described in association with PM–DM have included reticuloses in which depression of cell-mediated immunity is sometimes marked.

Myasthenia gravis. The overlap between PM–DM and myasthenia gravis, the frequent reports of concurrence and the similarities on muscle histology make the pathogenesis of one disorder relevant to that of the other. Myasthenia gravis is also linked to other C–T disorders. At present, it appears that both T-cell dysfunction and humoral antibodies may be involved and the immunopathology of myasthenia gravis is no clearer than that of PM–DM.

Pathological findings

Mononuclear cell infiltration. The combination of muscle cell damage with interstitial and peri-vascular lymphocytic infiltration is comparable to that of the cellular or delayed hypersensitivity lesion which is induced by the injection of antigen in adjuvant. The approximation of mononuclear and muscle cells in biopsy specimens of PM–DM (Mastaglia and Currie, 1971) was similar to the *in vitro* interaction of sensitised cells and target cells. The enlarged lymphocytes which were found traversing vessel walls were like those seen in experimental allergic neuritis (Astrom, Webster and Arnason, 1968). Lymphocyte-mediated muscle damage could still occur in the absence of infiltrates if lymphotoxins with a remote effect were produced *in vivo* as well as *in vitro* (Johnson *et al.*, 1972). It should also be noted that mononuclear cell infiltration can occur secondarily at the sites of antigen–antibody reaction (Oldstone and Dixon, 1970). The occurrence of an inflammatory phase in several hereditary myopathies is of note. There is not only mononuclear cell infiltration on histological studies but also steroid-responsiveness as if a true myositis had supervened in the context of muscle cell damage due to the primary disorder. Clearly, such a sequence is of relevance to the pathogenesis of PM–DM.

Vasculitis and perifascicular atrophy. The angiopathy of childhood DM and the perifascicular atrophy which is seen commonly in this, and to a lesser extent in adult PM–DM, are suggestive of an ischaemic component in the damage to muscle. Whitaker and Engel (1972) stated that muscular damage was 'more a result of angiopathy than a direct attack on the muscle fibres themselves'. This leaves unanswered the actual mechanism of muscle-cell damage. There is no relationship between damaged fibres and vascular deposits (Bohan and Peter, 1975) and, of course, PM–DM is a feature of agammaglobulinaemia. A vascular factor could precede or coexist with other mechanisms; thus 'it is possible that several mechanisms are operative in leading to the various types of muscle damage' (Whitaker and Engel, 1972). These authors felt that infiltrates were more likely in adult PM, and perifascicular atrophy in childhood DM. At the ultramicroscopic level, experimental ischaemic myopathy, with prominent Z-disc streaming, resembles childhood DM (Karpati, Carpenter, Melmed and Eisen, 1974). In this condition, capillary endothelial changes and other features of childhood DM occur (Munsat, Hudgson and Johnson, 1977).

Immunoglobulin–complement deposits. The finding in both childhood DM and adult PM–DM of vascular deposits of immunoglobulins and complement may represent immune-complex formation with vasculitis and a secondary ischaemic effect on muscles.

Viral-like particles. The significance of the occasional finding of viral-like structures in muscle cells from biopsies in PM remains uncertain. The fact that several different viruses have been demonstrated is, perhaps, evidence against their causing a direct viral myositis, acute or chronic, as also is their occurrence in muscle as an incidental finding. However, many viruses can cause acute myositis, notably Coxsackie virus, the virus which has most often been identified morphologically in PM. Many of the cases of proven viral myositis in man have not resembled the PM–DM complex clinically and pathologically, *e.g.* the case of myositis reported by Tang *et al.* (1975). The curious DM-like syndrome which appears to be due to Echovirus in the immunocompromised host is less easily dismissed as having no relationship to the PM–DM complex. In this condition the viral infection appears to be generalised. In the case described by Webster *et al.* (1978) peripheral blood lymphocytes did not show an increased rate of transformation on incubation with muscle extract, the serum CK activity was normal, the 'dermatitis' element was represented only by transient erythema over the biceps muscles and the muscle disorder improved dramatically with the use of specific antisera. Clearly, there were several respects in which the condition differed from classical PM–DM. However, the histological changes in muscle were those of PM–DM. The case described by Ben-Bassat and Machtey (1972) provides a link between PM–DM and the DM-like syndrome of agamma-globulinaemia. Clinically, it was one of typical acute DM with a heliotrope rash. The DM was accompanied by encephalitis; neither was steroid-responsive and the patient died within three months. Virus-like particles of Coxsackie type were found in muscle cells, although isolation and culture were not undertaken. It should be noted that Dawkins (1975) regarded the finding of viruses persisting in muscle cells in PM–DM as a further reflection of the deficiency in humoral immune processes which he believed to underlie the disorder.

Therapy

Steroid drugs. The apparent efficacy of steroid therapy in PM–DM may be attributable to its anti-inflammatory properties, although it is a potent immunosuppressive agent as well.

Immunosuppressive drugs. All the drugs used, prednisone, methotrexate, azathioprine, cyclophosphamide and chlorambucil, are general immuno-suppressants, and thus do not selectively depress humoral or cell-mediated immune function (Pirofsky and Bardana, 1977). Anti-lymphocytic serum has not yet had a full trial in the treatment of the condition. For this reason no conclusions about the nature of the immune imbalance in PM–DM can be drawn from the efficacy of IS therapy.

Thymectomy has rarely been carried out in PM–DM though its effect appears to be dramatic (Behan and Currie, 1978). The reasons for this are

uncertain, just as they are for remission of myasthenia gravis after thymectomy. Disordered thymic function is implicated in PM–DM.

Humoral immune responses

Hypocomplementaemia. Complement abnormality in active PM–DM with evidence of complement activation made Behan and Behan (1977) feel that circulating soluble immune complexes might have a primary role in the pathogenesis of the disease. Dawkins and Mastaglia (1973) felt that immune complexes were involved in the pathogenesis of the vasculitis rather than that of the myositis itself. This view differs from that of Whitaker and Engel (1972). Banker (1975) thought that the evidence meant that there was more than one type of PM–DM.

Circulating antibodies. Humoral antibodies to components of muscle have been found inconsistently; they are probably not of aetiological importance. The antinuclear antibody specific for PM–DM which was reported by Wolfe *et al.* (1977) places PM–DM alongside other C–T disorders, such as SLE and RA, in which specific IgG autoantibodies occur. It is possible that the antibody is not just a specific serological marker for PM–DM but is a component in immune-complex formation and subsequent vascular damage. It should be noted that there are several muscle-specific antigens, all present within the cytoplasm, not on the cell surface (Dawkins, 1975).

Skin sensitivity to tumour extracts in patients with DM and carcinoma and its passive transfer by serum are of doubtful significance. Their occurrence in patients without myopathy or skin disorder makes it unlikely that such sensitivity reflects a primary role in pathogenesis.

Cellular immune responses. The demonstration of cellular hypersensitivity to muscle antigens measured *in vitro* is an indication of previous sensitisation *in vivo*. Transformation, cytotoxicity and macrophage migration studies leave no doubt that sensitisation of lymphocytes does occur in PM–DM. However, the *in vitro* proliferative response was small and the occurrence of lymphocyte toxicity to muscle cells *in vitro* does not necessarily indicate that a parallel process occurs *in vivo*. Sensitisation could be a phenomenon secondary to muscle damage. The production of lymphotoxin may also be non-specific.

Experimental myositis. Evidence on the pathogenesis of the experimental condition cannot be brought forward in support of a role for cell-mediated immune processes in PM–DM. Experimental myositis is not a true model for PM–DM and its relevance to the occurrence of muscle damage in the inflammatory myopathies is uncertain.

Conclusions. PM–DM cannot be taken as a direct viral myositis, although viruses may be important in its precipitation and perpetuation in some cases. A derangement of immune processes occurs but it is not a simple matter of humoral overaction with cellular immune deficiency, or *vice versa*. Immune complex formation may cause vascular lesions with secondary ischaemic damage to muscle. Immune complexes could also cause damage to muscle cells directly. Thymic auto-regulation may be defective with autoantibody production. Disordered T-cell function may also occur, and possibly T cells destroy muscle cells *in vivo*; the benefits of thymectomy, steroid and other immunosuppressive therapy may be due to depletion of T cells. It appears, therefore, that both humoral and cell-mediated factors are involved in the pathogenesis of PM–DM, perhaps in a phasic manner with a shifting imbalance between the different immune processes. There is an overall uniformity of clinical and pathological features in PM–DM. However, there is no reason why, even in a relatively homogeneous disorder like PM–DM, any immune disturbances should always occur in the same sequence and the same proportions. Some possible factors in the causation of PM–DM are given in Fig. 15.7.

Treatment

There are three recognised forms of therapy for PM–DM: steroid therapy, other immunosuppressive (IS) drugs and thymectomy. The first,

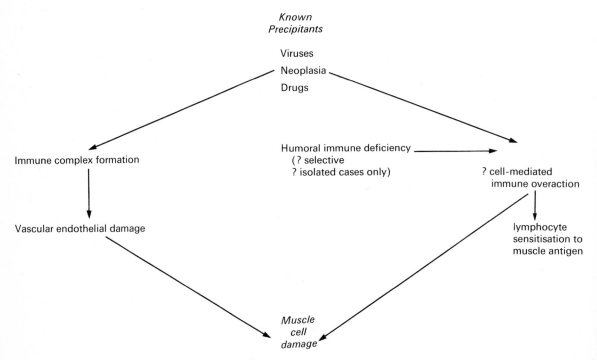

Fig. 15.7   PM–DM: possible factors in muscle cell damage

steroid therapy, is well established even if statistically not fully validated. The second, IS therapy, has been used in few patients, usually after there have been problems with steroid therapy. Thymectomy has been used rarely and is therefore at the experimental stage only. It should be noted that separation of steroid from IS drugs is artificial because steroid drugs themselves are immunosuppressants (Pirofsky and Bardana, 1977).

Steroid therapy. Corticosteroid therapy appears to result in improvement in PM–DM with both a reduction in muscle weakness and other symptoms in the short term, and an improvement in the prognosis in the long term. However, the natural course of the condition varies and is not clearly defined, as cases show differing severity and manner of progression. Thus, comparison of the prognosis in a group of cases from the days before steroid therapy (O'Leary and Waisman, 1940) with that in groups of patients who have received steroids cannot lead to valid conclusions about the efficacy of steroid therapy in the condition. Winkelmann et al. (1968) attempted to compare treated and untreated groups and concluded that the figures for remission and mortality were little different in the two groups. However, the data on which their conclusions were based may have been inadequate (Bohan and Peter, 1975). There has been no controlled trial of steroid therapy in PM–DM and one is unlikely to be carried out, because the role of steroids is so widely accepted that a trial seems unethical (De Vere and Bradley, 1975).

Despite the lack of statistically valid evidence in favour of steroid therapy, its use is to be recommended. Prednisone is preferred to fluorinated steroids, which are more liable to cause steroid myopathy. The initial dose should be 60–80 mg prednisone per day in divided doses; this is maintained over several weeks and then gradually reduced according to the clinical status of the patient and, in acute cases, serial estimations of the serum CK activity. A return of the serum CK activity towards normal usually precedes clinical improvement by two to three weeks; occasionally it heralds a remission despite increasing weakness. Once recovery begins, the prednisone dosage can be slowly reduced, with monitoring of enzyme activity. Rapid lowering of the dosage or attempts to discontinue therapy may be followed by a rise in CK level and the subsequent reappearance of weakness weeks later. Pearson and Bohan (1977) give as guidelines an initial schedule for reducing the dosage, by a 5 mg reduction every two to three weeks, followed by a more gradual lowering. The maintenance dose usually lies between 5–15 mg prednisone per day. This level of dosage can rarely be achieved before six months or so after the first reduction below the initial dosage. In most cases, steroid therapy has to be maintained indefinitely, albeit at low levels. At least five years should elapse before complete withdrawal is contemplated. In this respect PM–DM differs from many disorders for which steroid therapy is used, including other C–T disorders such as PMR. The implication is that treatment with steroid therapy is not curative but merely suppresses the underlying process (Pearson and Bohan, 1977). Both inadequate initial dosage and late commencement of therapy adversely affect the prognosis. In the uncontrolled trial carried out by Winkelmann et al. (1968), inadequate initial dosage may have been one factor responsible for the unimpressive results of steroid therapy. Pearson (1963) stated that steroid therapy should be started within two months of the onset of the disorder if a satisfactory outcome was to be achieved. Late instigation of adequate therapy may explain poor results in some series, such as that of Riddoch and Morgan-Hughes (1975), in which the average time before therapy was over two years, due to factors outside the control of the authors. De Vere and Bradley (1975) reported a much better prognosis, with two-thirds of the surviving patients in their series having no disability, three or more years after the beginning of therapy. They considered that treatment had been adequate in as many as 88 per cent of their cases. The degree of improvement was less marked in those patients who had received inadequate treatment than in those who had been given prednisone therapy early and in high dosage. The use of alternate-day steroid therapy, once considered useful in reducing side effects including adrenal suppression and growth retardation in children, appears to be less fashionable now but could still be considered for childhood DM. Potassium supplements are desirable in many patients who are receiving steroid therapy. Non-specific measures include bed-rest, necessary only during the early stages of acute PM–DM. Physiotherapy, when appropriate, comprises carrying out passive movements initially, followed by gentle exercises. With early, adequate steroid therapy, most patients with acute or subacute PM–DM will show a prompt return of strength and a decline in serum enzyme levels. Improvement almost approaching a return to normal function will be achieved in most cases. In chronic PM–DM with a duration of months or years, definite improvement occurs, with enzyme levels reverting towards normal. Improvement over the pretreatment status averages 50–70 per cent. Moreover, it is maintained, with progressive deterioration halted. In PM–DM with malignancy and with C–T disorders, improvement with steroid therapy is much less predictable and may be short-lived even when it does occur. Serious complications of steroid therapy are rare, in the opinion of Pearson and Bohan (1977).

Immunosuppressive therapy. The drugs used have included methotrexate, azathioprine, cyclophosphamide and chlorambucil. Methotrexate was used over a decade ago by Malaviya, Many and Schwartz (1968). The UCLA group (Metzger, Bohan, Goldberg, Bluestone and Pearson, 1974; Pearson and Bohan, 1977) prefer it used in conjunction with steroid therapy. They have employed the drug usually when there has been an inadequate response to prednisone or to allow a reduction in the dose of prednisone. Over two-thirds of patients have shown a significant improvement in muscle strength and, in about half the patients, worthwhile steroid-sparing has been achieved. Steroid therapy is supplemented by weekly intravenous injections of 25–50 mg methotrexate. The effect of methotrexate as an immunosuppressant is rapid, making it more appropriate for initial use than for maintenance therapy (Pirofsky and Bardana, 1977). Azathioprine is effective, in doses of 2–2.5 mg/kg/day. Pirofsky and Bardana regard this drug as easier to handle than methotrexate. Cyclophosphamide was used alone in the trial conducted by Fries, Sharp, McDevitt and Holman (1973) who compared its efficacy with that of steroids alone and found it

disappointing. The drug appeared to be slow in acting and probably needed to be given for several months to be effective. Their findings did not rule out the possibility of the drug being of benefit as an additive to steroid therapy. Haas (1973) felt that any IS drug had to be given for a minimum of three months for an adequate trial. The pattern for the future may be the use of one of these three drugs for long-term maintenance therapy, with prednisone or parenteral methotrexate for the initial rapid therapy and for relapses. Pirofsky and Bardana made a case for initial therapy with prednisone in doses of about 15 mg daily, with another IS drug, the prednisone being gradually reduced after remission had been achieved, with the IS drug for maintenance. Intermittent parenteral methotrexate would be an alternative to prednisone. The simultaneous use of more than one IS drug in addition to prednisone should be necessary only rarely. Side effects with IS drugs are usually less of a problem than with steroids, the latter being more liable to produce infection. Chlorambucil is the least toxic of the three IS drugs for maintenance treatment. Bone marrow depression is a danger which should not be exaggerated; nevertheless, routine blood counts must be done. The risk of malignancy has been overstated; in the C–T disorders, disturbances of cell-mediated immunity may themselves predispose to the development of malignancy. The amounts of IS drugs are smaller than those used in transplantation work. Antilymphocytic antiserum has been used only occasionally, although with benefit (Pirofsky and Bardana, 1977).

Thymectomy has rarely been used in PM although this is a logical extension of its use in myasthenia gravis and its effect has been described as dramatic (Behan and Currie, 1978).

Prognosis

The natural history of PM–DM has probably been altered by the advent of steroid therapy. In general, prolonged remission occurs in over 50 per cent of cases. In children with concomitant vasculitis resulting in gastrointestinal problems, in patients with other C–T disorders, in those with malignancy and lastly, in the elderly, the prognosis is not as good. De Vere and Bradley (1975) reported a relatively good prognosis in their series of patients, the great majority of whom had been given early steroid therapy in adequate amounts. Relapses occurred in a quarter of their cases, usually within two years of onset. There was a 28 per cent mortality rate, death being more likely when the myositis occurred in association with RA and PSS. Two-thirds of the surviving patients had little disability at four years. There were no cases of childhood DM with vasculitis among their patients. Riddoch and Morgan-Hughes (1975) found a worse prognosis, possibly because diagnosis was made and treatment begun when the disorder was, on average, of more than two years' duration. The prognosis is worse in the older age groups, partly because of the higher percentage of cases with malignancy but also due to coincidental cardiorespiratory disorders. The importance of early therapy (steroid drugs with or without an IS drug) in adequate amounts must be stressed. Delays in considering the diagnosis and in getting a muscle biopsy as well as short low-dosage courses of therapy will mean an increase in the amount of irreparable damage to muscle. The report of Bohan et al. (1977) was one of the first to describe a relatively large group of patients, in one-third of whom IS drugs besides prednisone had been used. Follow-up was short in some of the patients. The mortality rate was 14 per cent. The poorest prognosis was in PM–DM with malignancy where the risks were those of the neoplasm and the myopathy refractory to treatment. In contrast, their patients with other C–T disorders responded well to treatment, unlike those of De Vere and Bradley.

MYOSITIS IN C–T DISORDERS

PM–DM is classed with the C–T disorders and PM can accompany or follow many of them, notably PSS, RA and SLE. This fact has already been acknowledged in several of the sections on PM–DM, including those on associated disorders, classification and aetiology. The frequency with which PM occurs in these disorders has been documented. The majority of patients with PSS have clinical and biochemical evidence of myopathy according to Medsger, Rodnan, Moossy and Vester (1968). They found changes of myositis in 40 per cent of those in whom biopsy was undertaken. Occasionally there was an overlap sufficient to warrant the term 'sclerodermatomyositis'. Despite these findings, much of the muscle-wasting seen in PSS is not caused by myositis. In SLE, myositis, with proximal muscle weakness, biopsy changes and steroid-responsiveness was found in 3 per cent of cases in one series (Estes and Christian, 1971). Vacuolation of segments of muscle fibres has been described in SLE (Pearson and Yamazaki, 1958). It is not specific to SLE. The heterogeneous group of patients with RA who underwent motor-point muscle biopsy by Harriman (Haslock et al., 1970) were pre-selected; muscle-wasting was the commonest reason for biopsy. Their findings therefore did not give an incidence of myositis in RA in general. The abnormalities included myositis, PM and/or focal nodular changes, a chronic myopathy like end-stage dystrophy, changes of denervation and lastly steroid myopathy. They felt that muscle atrophy was due to some effect on muscle-cell metabolism which was not simple disuse. It is clear that, in addition to actual PM, other forms of myopathy occur in these disorders. In PAN, muscle infarction rather than myositis is the principal pathological abnormality. In PMR the changes in muscle are scanty or absent and myositis has not been reported.

Focal nodular myositis

Foci of inflammatory cells are found in the connective tissue of muscles in RA, SLE, PSS and rheumatic fever as well as in PM–DM. Endomysial foci are compact while perimysial collections are larger and more diffuse. Foci are usually near small blood vessels even though the walls of these are unaffected. The cells are mostly small lymphocytes. Adjacent muscle cells are usually intact but may show degenerative changes (Fig. 15.8). Focal nodular myositis is 'a pathological entity without specific clinical connotations' (Cumming et al., 1977b).

Polyarteritis nodosa (PAN)

Symptoms resulting from infarction of muscle are exceptional in this condition, in which renal

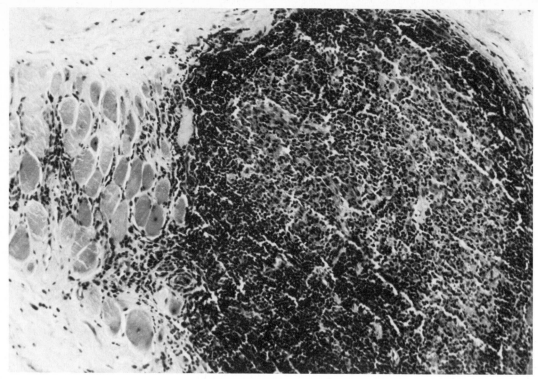

Fig. 15.8 'Focal nodular myositis' in rheumatoid arthritis. A lymphoid follicle with minor myopathic changes in adjacent muscle fibres, thus central nuclei, H & E, ×36 (courtesy of Dr D.G.F. Harriman)

lesions and peripheral nerve damage are the chief effects of vasculitis. Necrotising arteritis in muscle may involve adjacent muscle cells in inflammation. Areas of infarction in muscle occur because of arterial occlusion. Neurogenic muscular atrophy can follow damage to peripheral motor nerves or spinal roots. 'Blind' biopsy of muscle will fail to substantiate a diagnosis of PAN in the majority of patients with the disorder (Wallace, Lattes and Ragan, 1958). Clearly, if a tender spot in a muscle is biopsied, the chances of finding abnormalities are higher. Rarely, multiple tender areas in several muscles occur, with the appearance of a painful proximal myopathy rather like acute PM. Steroid therapy in high dosage may give relief.

Polymyalgia rheumatica (PMR)

This C–T disorder is characterised by aching and stiffness in the proximal musculature, typically of the shoulder girdle. It affects subjects over 55 years old, producing mild anaemia and an elevated ESR (usually much higher than 50 mm/h by the Westergren method). Anorexia, weight loss and malaise occur. Despite its name and similarities to PM–DM, PMR is not a myopathy in that the muscles are not primarily involved. The gross elevation of the ESR and the systemic upset suggest that there is inflammation of major degree yet this does not affect voluntary muscle. The condition is more closely related to RA and to cranial arteritis than to PM–DM; indeed it is among those C–T disorders in which myositis does not occur. Difficulties in use of the limbs result from pain and stiffness and not from muscle weakness. Serum enzyme estimation and EMG give normal findings. Myopathy due to disuse shows on histological study as atrophy of type IIB muscle fibres, with a moth-eaten and whorled appearance, as in RA (Brooke and Kaplan, 1972). PMR is unique among C–T disorders in that it responds rapidly to small doses of steroid drugs; thus less than 10 mg prednisone/day will relieve symptoms within four days. Larger initial doses are generally used as cranial (temporal) arteritis with a risk of visual disturbance may accompany PMR. Large doses are probably unnecessary and should be replaced by careful follow-up (Spiera and Davison, 1978). Unlike other C–T disorders, including PM–DM, PMR is often self-limiting and, in some cases, complete withdrawal of steroid therapy is possible within 2–3 years or less. PMR may be associated with the immune gene HLA–B8, as may PM–DM, as well as with HLA–A10 (Hazleman, Goldstone and Voak, 1977).

Myopathy with glomerulonephritis

The nosological position of this further entity is not clear; however, it has features of the C–T disorders. Judge, McGlynn, Abt, Luderer and Ward (1977) used the term 'immunologic myopathy' for a unique syndrome which possessed some features of Goodpasture's syndrome and of the C–T disorders Wegener's granulomatosis, PAN and PM–DM. The patient had a history of severe generalised muscle weakness and soreness for a long period of nine years. Raynaud's phenomenon had also occurred. Serum enzymes were normal and the EMG did not show myositic changes. Serum C3 activity and total complement values were normal. Muscle biopsy showed type II muscle fibre atrophy with type I hypertrophy. This could have been a non-specific change, resulting from disuse, and there was neither inflammation nor vasculitis. However, direct immunofluorescence showed linear staining for IgG around muscle fibres, with thickening of basement membranes. Terminally, the patient developed renal failure and haemoptysis. Autopsy showed glomerulonephritis and vasculitis affecting skin, lungs and spleen though not involving the central nervous system. In view of the fact that linear staining for IgG on glomerular basement membrane was well recognised in glomerulonephritis, the authors postulated an antigen common to muscle and kidney cells. This curious case has left more questions unanswered than answered.

GRANULOMATOUS OR GIANT-CELL MYOSITIS

Granulomatous myositis occurs in sarcoidosis, giant-cell myositis with thymoma, Wegener's granulomatosis and also as an isolated disorder. In addition, a single case of granulomatous myopathy in Crohn's disease has been described (Ménard, Haddad, Blain, Baudry, Devroede and Massé, 1976).

Sarcoidosis

In this generalised disorder, symptomatic proximal myopathy is unusual; indeed, even asymptomatic involvement yields a positive biopsy rate of less than a third. When myopathy occurs it is typically in middle-aged women (Gardner–Thorpe, 1972) but it does occur in males, particularly of Negro origin. Clinical myopathy results in painless, slowly progressive weakness and wasting of limb-girdle musculature. It may respond to treatment with steroids but inconsistently.

Giant-cell myositis and myocarditis with thymoma

Rundle and Sparks (1963) described thymoma in association with DM but the myopathy resembled DM neither clinically nor pathologically. Painful red lumps occurred in the skin. No proximal myopathy occurred. Myocarditis resulted in heart failure. Giant-cell myositis and myocarditis were found at autopsy. Burke, Medline and Katz (1969) reported a case of myasthenia gravis with malignant thymoma. At autopsy both skeletal muscle (deltoid) and myocardial muscle showed foci of lymphocytes with muscle cell necrosis. There were giant cells in the areas of inflammation. The cells were of Langhans foreign body type, not regenerative multinucleated muscle cells. The authors noted that a third of the reported cases of giant-cell myositis were associated with thymoma.

Wegener's granulomatosis

This condition is related both to other granulomatous conditions and to PAN in that giant-cell granulomata, inflammatory cell infiltrates and a necrotising panarteritis are all present. It also resembles malignant lymphoma of histiocytic type. Wegener's disease affects many systems, notably the kidneys, lungs and skin and should be distinguished from Stewart's midline granuloma affecting the upper respiratory tract. Rarely, skeletal muscle is involved to a degree which produces a painful myopathy. The condition responds to many immunosuppressive drugs including cyclophosphamide (Pirofsky and Bardana, 1977).

Isolated granulomatous myositis

Several authors have reported granulomatous lesions discovered on muscle biopsy in cases of myopathy, which was not clearly a manifestation of generalised sarcoidosis (Lynch and Bansal, 1973; Hewlett and Brownell, 1975). In one of the cases described by Hewlett and Brownell there was widespread muscle cell degeneration and regeneration with raised serum CK activity in addition to well-defined granulomata. There was no inflammatory cell infiltrate apart from lymphocytes in the granulomata, and intramuscular blood vessels were normal. Nevertheless there were grounds for labelling this case as one of 'polymyositis'. In their other cases, and that of

Lynch and Bansal, destruction of muscle cells by granulomata did not lead to raised serum CK activity. Hewlett and Brownell concluded that, exceptionally, a granulomatous process complicates PM, differing from granulomatous myopathy, whether isolated or occurring in sarcoidosis (Fig. 15.9). Both conditions appear to be steroid-responsive, although chronic sarcoid myopathy is less so. The pathology in the case of relapsing myositis described by McLetchie and Aikens (1952) differed from both granulomatous myopathy and PM. Clinically, there were recurrent tender muscle swellings with fever. Biopsy showed necrotic areas of muscle containing giant cells, which appeared to distinguish the condition from the localised nodular myositis of Cumming et al. (1977b).

VIRAL MYOSITIS

Viruses can cause myositis directly, as well as precipitating PM–DM. Some of the reported cases

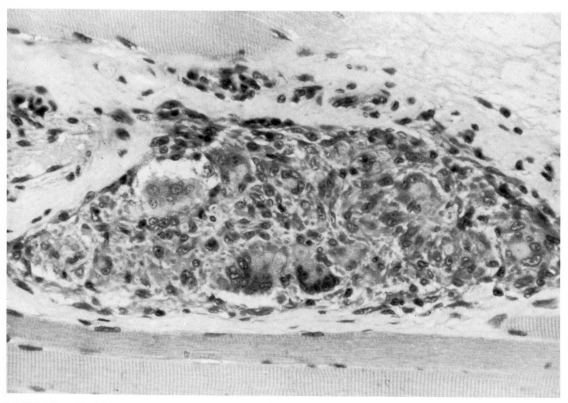

Fig. 15.9 Sarcoidosis: large interstitial granuloma with giant cells and epithelioid cells. The adjacent muscle fibres are intact. H & E, × 19 (courtesy of Dr D. G. F. Harriman)

of viral myositis have been mentioned in the section on differential diagnosis. Myalgia is a component of several acute viral infections in man. They include those due to picornavirus, such as Coxsackie, poliovirus and echovirus, and influenza virus. Two conditions in which myalgia is prominent are pleurodynia, or Bornholm disease, and benign myalgic encephalomyelitis; both are described by Dr Foster in Chapter 23. In pleurodynia, the diaphragm and chest wall muscles are preferentially involved. It is caused by a Coxsackie Type B virus; this can be identified by the inoculation of infected material into suckling mice with the development of florid myositis. In experimental viral myositis the main pathological change is necrotising myopathy, with or without inflammation. In man, the myositis which presumably underlies the myalgia has seldom been demonstrated by pathological studies. An example of this lack of documentation is the myalgic syndrome due to influenza B virus, which was described by Middleton, Alexander and Szymanski (1970). It affects children, producing short-lived myalgia and tenderness in the lower limbs with raised serum CK activity. The acute-on-chronic Coxsackie myositis of Tang et al. (1975) was studied by muscle biopsy late in the course of the disorder, as well as at autopsy. The case was that of a child with life-long muscular weakness gradually spreading to all limb muscles and leading to death from respiratory muscle involvement. Terminally, serum enzymes were raised. At autopsy, the diaphragm was found to be severely affected; there were viral deposits associated with degenerative foci in muscle fibres. Coxsackie Type A9 was shown by fluorescence studies of muscle and was isolated in culture. The light-microscopic appearances were felt to be of an atrophic end-stage of chronic myopathy. There were no infiltrates of inflammatory cells. The relationship of the myopathy in this case to PM–DM is uncertain, even if particles resembling picornarvirus have been found in muscle specimens from cases of PM–DM. Tang et al. referred to the case of congenital Coxsackie myositis in an infant, which was reported by Freudenberg, Roulet and Nicole (1952) and which was alleged to have evolved into 'chronic myositis' subsequently. Acute fulminant myositis with picorna-like crystals was reported by

Fukuyama, Tsunesaburo and Yokota (1977). De Reuck et al. (1977) described a similar case; there was preferential involvement of the diaphragm, as in other examples of Coxsackie myositis. None of these cases were of PM–DM as defined in this chapter. Norris, Dramov, Calder and Johnson (1969) reported virus-like particles in muscle from two cases of myopathy which accompanied recurrent herpes zoster infection. The close temporal relationship between viral infection and myositis resembled that in the case of myositis following live rubella vaccination, which was reported by Hanissian et al. (1973). However, the features of that case were more suggestive of an indirect myositis initiated by virus and classifiable as DM. An intermediate position is held by the DM-like syndrome with echovirus infection which occurs in agammaglobulinaemia (Bardelas et al., 1977; Webster et al., 1978). The myopathy is responsive to plasma containing antibody to echovirus, rather than to steroid therapy. Nevertheless, the histological changes in muscle are those of PM–DM. Thus, viruses can cause acute and chronic myositis both by direct involvement and by the indirect initiation of PM–DM. They may also persist in muscle fibres without any adverse effect on these. Viral myositis and PM–DM can usually be differentiated clinically; thus diagnostic problems are uncommon. However, the nosological status of occasional cases is uncertain and their existence has a bearing on the pathogenesis of the idiopathic condition PM–DM.

TROPICAL MYOSITIS

This condition is known as 'tropical' because it is common in the tropics (Levin, Gardner and Waldvogel, 1971). When it does occur in a temperate zone, the subject has often been resident recently in a tropical region. The disorder may be responsible for as many as 2 per cent of admissions in tropical areas. The condition is sometimes referred to by the name 'pyomyositis' but the suppuration is probably secondary to an unknown primary infection, presumed to be viral. Taylor, Fluck and Fluck (1976) felt that, on epidemiological grounds, viral infection was likely, perhaps by an arenavirus. They carried out ultrastructural studies showing intracellular vesicles resembling viral particles. They could often distinguish an initial illness with fever, arthralgia and muscle pain which might or might not be followed by suppuration. The light-microscopic changes at this stage were slight, comprising patchy cell lysis with lymphocytic infiltration, a 'myositis' of a kind. Eosinophilia, when present, is probably related to coincidental parasitic infection. In general the onset is subacute, with pain in one or more muscles and fever developing in days to weeks. There is local tenderness. Abscesses form deep in large muscles; they are confined by the overlying fascia so that superficial pain, heat and erythema of the skin are absent. The muscles which are typically involved are the biceps, pectoral, gluteal and quadriceps muscles. Children and young adults are those usually affected. The bacterial infection is by *Staphylococcus aureus* in 98 per cent of cases. Spread to several muscles may be haematogenous, but blood cultures are usually negative. Damage to the muscles which contain abscesses is slight, with normal serum enzymes and only rarely residual muscle wasting. This reflects the fact that skeletal muscle is usually resistant to staphylococcal infection. Treatment is by parenteral antibiotics with local incision for drainage.

REFERENCES

Alexander, S. & Foreman, L. (1968) Dermatomyositis and carcinoma. A case report and immunological investigations. *British Journal of Dermatology*, **80**, 86.

Arapakis, G. & Jordanoglou, J. (1964) A case of lymphosarcoma associated with myopathy. *British Medical Journal*, **2**, 32.

Astrom, K.E., Webster, H. de F. & Arnason, B.G. (1968) The initial lesion in experimental allergic neuritis. A phase and electron microscopic study. *Journal of Experimental Medicine*, **128**, 469.

Banker, B.Q. (1975) Dermatomyositis of childhood. Ultrastructural alterations of muscle and intramuscular blood vessels. *Journal of Neuropathology and Experimental Neurology*, **34**, 46.

Banker, B.Q. & Victor, M. (1966) Dermatomyositis (systemic angiopathy) of childhood. *Medicine*, **45**, 261.

Bardelas, J.A., Winkelstein, J.A., Seto, D.S.Y., Tsai, T. & Rogol, A.D. (1977) Fatal Echo 24 infection in a patient with hypogammaglobulinaemia: Relationship to dermatomyositis-like syndrome. *Journal of Pediatrics*, **90**, 396.

Barnes, B.E. (1976) Dermatomyositis and malignancy. A review of the literature. *Annals of Internal Medicine*, **84**, 68.

Bates, D., Stevens, J.C. & Hudgson, P. (1973) 'Polymyositis' with involvement of facial and distal musculature. *Journal of the Neurological Sciences*, **19**, 105.

Bauwens, P. (1956) Variations of the motor unit. *Proceedings of the Royal Society of Medicine*, **49**, 110.

Behan, P.O. & Currie, S. (1978) In *Clinical Neuroimmunology*. Ch. 11, p. 155 (Saunders: London).

Behan, W.M.H. & Behan, P.O. (1977) Complement abnormalities in polymyositis. *Journal of the Neurological Sciences*, **34**, 241.

Behan, W.M.H., Behan, P.O. & Dick, H. (1978) HLA–B8 in polymyositis. *New England Journal of Medicine*, **298**, 1260.

Behan, W.M.H., Mcqueen, A. & Behan, P.O. (1980) Immunogenetic findings in polymyositis (In preparation).

Ben-Bassat, M. & Machtey, I. (1972) Picorna virus-like structures in acute dermatomyositis. *American Journal of Clinical Pathology*, **58**, 245.

Bohan, A. and Peter, J.B. (1975) Polymyositis and dermatomyositis. *New England Journal of Medicine*, **292**, 344 and 403.

Bohan, A., Peter, J.B., Bowman, R.L. & Pearson, C.M. (1977) A computer-assisted analysis of 153 patients with polymyositis and dermatomyositis. *Medicine*, **56**, 255.

Boylan, R.C. & Sokoloff, L. (1960) Vascular lesions in dermatomyositis. *Arthritis and Rheumatism*, **3**, 379.

Bradley, W.G., Hudgson, P., Gardner-Medwin, D. & Walton, J.N. (1973). The syndrome of myosclerosis. *Journal of Neurology, Neurosurgery and Psychiatry*, **36**, 651.

Brooke, M.H. & Kaplan, H. (1972). Muscle pathology in rheumatoid arthritis, polymyalgia rheumatica and polymyositis. A histochemical study. *Archives of Pathology*, **94**, 101.

Brown, M., Swift, T.R. & Spies, S.M. (1976) Radioisotope scanning in inflammatory muscle disease. *Neurology (Minneapolis)*, **26**, 517.

Bruk, M.I. (1967) Articular and vascular manifestations of polymalgia rheumatica. *Annals of Rheumatic Diseases*, **26**, 103.

Bunim, J.J. (1961) A broader spectrum of Sjögren's syndrome and its pathogenetic implications. *Annals of Rheumatic Diseases*, **20**, 1.

Burke, J.S., Medline, N.M. & Katz, A. (1969) Giant cell myocarditis and myositis associated with thymoma and myasthenia gravis. *Archives of Pathology*, **88**, 359.

Camp, A.V., Lane D.J. & Mowat, A.G. (1972) Dermatomyositis with parenchymal lung involvement. *British Medical Journal*, **1**, 155.

Campbell, M.J. & Paty, D.W. (1974) Carcinomatous neuromyopathy: 1. Electrophysiological studies. An electrophysiological and immunological study of patients with carcinoma of the lung. *Journal of Neurology, Neurosurgery and Psychiatry*, **37**, 131.

Carpenter, S., Karpati, G., Heller, I. & Eisen, A. (1978) Inclusion body myositis: a distinct variety of idiopathic inflammatory myopathy. *Neurology (Minneapolis)*, **28**, 8.

Carpenter, S., Karpati, G., Rothman, S. & Watters, G. (1976) The childhood type of dermatomyositis. *Neurology (Minneapolis)*, **26**, 952.

Carroll, J.E., Silverman, A., Isobe, Y., Brown, W.R., Kelts, K.A. & Brooke, M.H. (1976) Inflammatory myopathy, IgA deficiency and intestinal malabsorption. *Journal of Pediatrics*, **89**, 216.

Caspary, E.A., Currie, S. & Field, E.J. (1971) Sensitised lymphocytes in muscular dystrophy: evidence for a neural factor in pathogenesis. *Journal of Neurology, Neurosurgery and Psychiatry*, **34**, 353.

Caspary, E.A., Gubbay, S.S. & Stern, G.M. (1964) Circulating antibodies in polymyositis and other muscle-wasting disorders. *Lancet*, **2**, 941.

Caulfield, J.B., Rebeiz, J. & Adams, R.D. (1968) Viral involvement of human muscle. *Journal of Pathology and Bacteriology*, **96**, 232.

Chou, S.M. (1968) Myxovirus-like structures and accompanying nuclear changes in chronic polymyositis. *Archives of Pathology*, **86**, 649.

Chou, S.M. & Gutmann, L. (1970) Picorna virus-like crystals in subacute polymyositis. *Neurology (Minneapolis)*, **20**, 205.

Cook, C.D., Rosen, F.S. & Banker, B.Q. (1963) Dermatomyositis and focal scleroderma. *Pediatric Clinics of North America*, **10**, 976.

Croft, P.B. & Wilkinson, M. (1965). The incidence of carcinomatous neuromyopathy in patients with various types of carcinoma. *Brain*, **88**, 427.

Cucher, B.G. & Goldman, A.L. (1976) D-penicillamine-induced polymyositis in rheumatoid arthritis. *Annals of Internal Medicine*, **85**, 615.

Cumming, W.J.K., Hardy, M., Hudgson, P. & Walls, J. (1976) Carnitine-palmityl-transferase deficiency. *Journal of the Neurological Sciences*, **30**, 247.

Cumming, W.J.K., Hudgson, P., Lattimer, D., Sussman, M. & Wilcox, C.B., (1977a) HLA and serum complement in polymyositis. *Lancet*, **2**, 978.

Cumming, W.J.K., Weiser, R., Teoh, R., Hudgson, P. & Walton, J.N. (1977b) Localised nodular myositis: a clinical and pathological variant of polymyositis. *Quarterly Journal of Medicine*, **46**, 531.

Currie, S. (1970) Destruction of muscle cultures by lymphocytes from cases of polymyositis. *Acta Neuropathologica (Berlin)*, **15**, 11.

Currie, S. (1971) Experimental myositis. The in-vivo and in-vitro activity of lymph-node cells. *Journal of Pathology*, **105**, 169.

Currie, S., Saunders, M. & Knowles, M. (1971a) Immunological aspects of systemic sclerosis: in vitro activity of lymphocytes from patients with the disorder. *British Journal of Dermatology*, **84**, 400.

Currie, S., Saunders, M., Knowles, M. & Brown, A.E. (1971b) The in-vitro activity of lymphocytes on incubation with muscle antigen and with muscle cultures. *Quarterly Journal of Medicine*, **40**, 63.

Curtis, A.C., Heckaman, J.H. & Wheeler, A.H. (1961) Study of the auto-immune reaction in dermatomyositis. *Journal of the American Medical Association*, **178**, 571.

Dawkins, R.L. (1965) Experimental myositis associated with hypersensitivity to muscle. *Journal of Pathology and Bacteriology*, **90**, 619.

Dawkins, R.L. (1975) Review. Experimental autoallergic myositis, polymyositis and myasthenia gravis. *Clinical and Experimental Immunology*, **21**, 185.

Dawkins, R.L. & Mastaglia, F.L. (1973) Cell-mediated cytotoxicity to muscle in polymyositis: effect of immunosuppression. *New England Journal of Medicine*, **228**, 434.

Deep, W.D., Fraumeni, J.F., Tashima, C.K. & McDivitt, R. (1964) Leukoencephalopathy and dermatomyositis in Hodgkin's disease. *Archives of Internal Medicine*, **113**, 635.

De Reuck, J., de Coster, W. & Inderadjaja, N. (1977) Acute viral polymyositis with predominant diaphragm involvement. *Journal of the Neurological Sciences*, **33**, 453.

De Vere, R. & Bradley, W.G. (1975) Polymyositis: its presentation, morbidity and mortality. *Brain*, **98**, 637.

Diessner, G.R., Howard, F.M., Winkelmann, R.K., Lambert, E.H. & Mulder, D.W. (1966) Laboratory tests in polymositis. *Archives of Internal Medicine*, **117**, 757.

Donoghue, F.D., Winkelmann, R.K. & Moersch, J.H. (1960) Esophageal defects in dermatomyositis. *Annals of Otology*, **69**, 1139.

Dowling. G.B. (1955) Sclerodoma and dermatomyositis. *British Journal of Dermatology*, **67**, 275.

Eaton, L.M. (1954) The perspective of neurology in regard to polymyositis: study of 41 cases. *Neurology (Minneapolis)*, **4**, 245.

Engel, A.G. & Siekert, R.G. (1972) Lipid storage myopathy responsive to prednisone. *Archives of Neurology*, **27**, 174.

Esiri, M., MacLennan, I.C.M. & Hazleman, B.L. (1973) Lymphocyte sensitivity to skeletal muscle in patients with polymyositis and other disorders. *Clinical and Experimental Immunology*, **14**, 25.

Estes, D. & Christian, C.L. (1971) The natural history of systemic lupus erythematosus by prospective analysis. *Medicine*, **50**, 85.

Fairfax, A.J. (1977) Immunological aspects of chronic heart block: A review. *Proceedings of the Royal Society of Medicine*, **70**, 327.

Fairfax, A.J. and Gröschel-Stewart, V. (1977) Myosin auto-antibodies detected by immunofluorescence. *Clinical and Experimental Immunology*, **28**, 27.

Findlay, G.H., Whiting, D.A. & Simson, I.W. (1969) Dermatomyositis in the Transvaal and its occurrence in the Bantu. *South African Medical Journal*, **43**, 694.

Frazier, A.R. & Miller, R.D. (1974) Interstitial pneumonitis in association with polymyositis and dermatomyositis. *Chest*, **65**, 403.

Freudenberg, V.E., Roulet, F. & Nicole, R. (1952) Kongenital Infektion mit Coxsackie-virus. *Annals of Paediatrics*, **178**, 150.

Fries, J.F., Sharp, G.C., McDevitt, H.O. & Holman, H.R. (1973) Cyclophosphamide therapy in systemic lupus erythematosus and polymyositis. *Arthritis and Rheumatism*, **16**, 154.

Fukuyama, Y., Tsunesaburo, A. & Yokota, J. (1977) Acute fulminant myoglobulinuric polymyositis with picorna-like crystals. *Journal of Neurology, Neurosurgery and Psychiatry*. **40**, 775.

Gardner-Thorpe, C. (1972) Muscle weakness due to sarcoid myopathy. Six case reports and an evaluation of steroid therapy. *Neurology (Minneapolis)*, **22**, 917.

Gelderman, A.H., Levine, R.A. & Arndt, K.A. (1962) Dermatomyositis complicated by generalised amyloidosis. *New England Journal of Medicine*, **267**, 858.

Gonzalez-Angulo, A., Fraga, A., Mintz, G. & Zavala, B.J. (1968) Submicroscopic alterations in capillaries of skeletal muscles in polymyositis. *American Journal of Medicine*, **45**, 873.

Gotoff, S.P., Smith, R.D. & Sugar, O. (1972) Dermatomyositis with cerebral vasculitis in a patient with agammaglobulinaemia. *American Journal of Diseases of Children*, **123**, 53.

Gottdiener, J.S., Sherber, H.S., Hawley, R.J. & Engel, W.K. (1978) Cardiac manifestations in polymyositis. *American Journal of Cardiology*, **41**, 1141.

Goust, J.M., Castaigne, A. & Moulias, R. (1974) Delayed hypersensitivity to muscle and thymus in myasthenia gravis and polymyositis. *Clinical and Experimental Immunology*, **18**, 39.

Grace, J.T. & Dao, T.L., (1959) Dermatomyositis in cancer: possible etiological mechanism. *Cancer*, **12**, 648.

Haas, D.C. (1973) Treatment of polymyositis with immunosuppressive drugs. *Neurology (Minneapolis)*, **23**, 55.

Haas, D.C. & Arnason, B.G.W. (1974) Cell-mediated immunity in polymyositis. Creatine phosphokinase release from muscle cultures. *Archives of Neurology*, **31**, 192.

Hanissian, A.S., Martinez, A.J., Jabbour, J.T. & Duenas, D.A. (1973) Vasculitis and myositis secondary to rubella vaccination. *Archives of Neurology*, **28**, 202.

Harriman, D.G.F. & Currie, S. (1974) A propos des neuromyosites. In *Troisièmes Journées Internationales de Pathologie Neuromusculaire*, Eds G. Serratrice, H. Roux & A.M. Recordier, p. 138 (Masson et Cie: Paris).

Hashimoto, K., Robinson, L., Velayos, E. & Niizuma, K. (1971) Electron-microscopic, immunologic and tissue culture studies of paramyxovirus-like inclusions. *Archives of Dermatology*, **103**, 120.

Haslock, D.I., Wright, V. & Harriman, D.G.F. (1970) Neuromuscular disorders in rheumatoid arthritis. A motorpoint muscle biopsy study. *Quarterly Journal of Medicine*, **39**, 335.

Hazleman, B., Goldstone, A. & Voak, D. (1977) Association of polymyalgia rheumatica and giant-cell arteritis with HLA-B8. *British Medical Journal*, **4**, 989.

Hellström, I.E., Hellström, K.E. & Pierce, G.E. (1969) Demonstration of cell-bound and humoral immunity against neuroblastoma cells. *Proceedings of the National Academy of Sciences*, **60**, 1231.

Hewlett, R.H. & Brownell, B. (1975) Granulomatous myopathy: Its relationship to sarcoidosis and polymyositis. *Journal of Neurology, Neurosurgery and Psychiatry*, **30**, 1090.

Hollinrake, K. (1969) Polymyositis presenting as distal muscle weakness. A case report. *Journal of the Neurological Sciences*, **8**, 479.

Howard, F.M. & Thomas, J.E. (1960) Polymyositis and dermatomyositis. *Medical Clinics of North America*, **44**, 1001.

Hudgson, P. & Fulthorpe, J.J. (1975) The pathology of Type II skeletal muscle glycogenosis. A light and electronmicroscopic study. *Journal of Pathology*, **116**, 139.

Hughes, J.T. & Esiri, M.M. (1975) Ultrastructural studies in human polymyositis. *Journal of the Neurological Sciences*, **25**, 347.

Janeway, C.A., Gitlin, D., Craig, J.M. & Grice, D.S. (1956) Collagen disease in patients with congenital agammaglobulinaemia. *Transactions of the Association of American Physicians*, **69**, 93.

Janis, W.F. & Winkelmann, R.K. (1968) Histopathology of the skin in dermatomyositis, a histopathologic study of 55 cases. *Archives of Dermatology*, **97**, 640.

Jennekens, F.G.I., Busch, H.F.M., van Hemel, N.M. & Hoogland, R.A. (1975) Inflammatory myopathy in scapulo-ilio-peroneal atrophy with cardiopathy. *Brain*, **98**, 709.

Johns, T.R., Crowley, W.J., Miller, J.Q. & Campa, J.F.

(1971) The syndrome of myasthenia and polymyositis with comments on therapy. *Annals of the New York Academy of Sciences*, **183**, 64.

Johnson, M.A., Fulthorpe, J.J. & Hudgson, P. (1973) Lipid storage myopathy. A recognisable clinicopathological entity. *Acta Neuropathologica (Berlin)*, **24**, 97.

Johnson, R.L., Fink, C.W. & Ziff, M. (1972) Lymphotoxin formation by lymphocytes and muscle in polymyositis. *Journal of Clinical Investigation*, **51**, 2435.

Judge, D.M., McGlynn, T.J., Abt., A.B., Luderer, J.R. & Ward, S.P. (1977) Immunologic myopathy: Linear IgG deposition and fulminant terminal episode. *Archives of Pathology*, **101**, 362.

Kagen, L.J. (1971) Myoglobinemia and myoglobinuria in patients with myositis. *Arthritis and Rheumatism*, **14**, 457.

Kagen, L.J. (1977) Myoglobinemia in inflammatory myopathies. *Journal of the American Medical Association*, **237**, 1448.

Kagen, L.M., Kimball, A.C. & Christian, C.L. (1974) Serologic evidence of toxoplasmosis among patients with polymyositis. *American Journal of Medicine*, **56**, 186.

Kakulas, B.A. (1966) Destruction of differentiated muscle cultures by sensitized cells. *Journal of Pathology and Bacteriology*, **91**, 495.

Kakulas, B.A., Shute, G.H. & Leclere, A.L.F. (1971) In vitro destruction of human foetal muscle cultures by peripheral blood lymphocytes from patients with polymyositis and lupus erythematosus. *Proceedings of the Australian Association of Neurologists*, **8**, 85.

Karpati, G., Carpenter, S., Melmed, C. & Eisen, A.A. (1974) Experimental ischaemic myopathy. *Journal of the Neurological Sciences*, **23**, 129.

Klein, J.J., Gottleib, A.J., Mones, R.J. Appel, S.H. & Osserman, K.E. (1964) Thymoma and polymyositis. *Archives of Internal Medicine*, **113**, 142.

Lambie, J.A. & Duff, I.F. (1963) Familial occurrence of dermatomyositis. Case reports and a family survey. *Annals of Internal Medicine*, **59**, 839.

Landry, M. & Winkelmann, R.K. (1972) Tubular cytoplasmic inclusion in dermatomyositis. *Mayo Clinic Proceedings*, **47**, 479.

Layzer, R.B., Shearn, M.A. & Satya-Murti, S. (1977) Eosinophilic polymyositis. *Annals of Neurology*, **1**, 65.

Leddy, J.P., Griggs, R.C., Klemperer, M.R. & Franks, M.M. (1975) Hereditary complement (C_2) deficiency with dermatomyositis. *American Journal of Medicine*, **58**, 83.

Levin, M.J., Gardner, P. & Waldvogel, F.A. (1971) Tropical pyomyositis: an unusual infection due to Staphylococcus aureus. *New England Journal of Medicine*, **284**, 196.

Lewkonia, R.M. & Buxton, P.H. (1973) Myositis in father and daughter. *Journal of Neurology, Neurosurgery and Psychiatry*, **36**, 820.

Lisak, R.P. & Zweiman, B. (1976) Serum immunoglobulin levels in myasthenia gravis, polymyositis and dermatomyositis. *Journal of Neurology, Neurosurgery and Psychiatry*, **39**, 34.

Lynch, P.G. & Bansal, D.V. (1973) Granulomatous polymyositis. *Journal of the Neurological Sciences*, **18**, 1.

Malaviya, A.N., Many, A. & Schwartz, R.S. (1968) Treatment of dermatomyositis with methotrexate. *Lancet*, **2**, 485.

Maricq, H.R., Spencer-Green, G. & Le Roy, E.C. (1976) Skin capillary abnormalities as indicators of organ involvement in scleroderma (systemic sclerosis), Raynaud's syndrome and dermatomyositis. *American Journal of*

Medicine, **61**, 862.

Mastaglia, F.L. & Currie, S. (1971) Immunological and ultrastructural observations on the role of lymphoid cells in the pathogenesis of polymyositis. *Acta Neuropathologica (Berlin)*, **18**, 1.

Mastaglia, F.L. & Kakulas, B.A. (1970) A histological and histochemical study of skeletal muscle regeneration in polymyositis. *Journal of the Neurological Sciences*, **10**, 471.

Mastaglia, F.L. & Walton, J.N. (1970) Coxsackie virus-like particles in skeletal muscle in polymyositis. *Journal of the Neurological Sciences*, **11**, 593.

Mastaglia, F.L. & Walton, J.N. (1971) An ultrastructural study of skeletal muscle in polymyositis. *Journal of the Neurological Sciences*, **12**, 473.

Mastaglia, F.L., McCollum, J.P.K. & Larson, P.F. (1970) Steroid myopathy complicating McArdle's disease. *Journal of Neurology, Neurosurgery and Psychiatry*, **33**, 111.

McLetchie, N.G.B. & Aikens, R.L. (1952) Relapsing myositis. *Archives of Pathology*, **53**, 497.

Mechler, F. (1974) Changing electromyographic findings during chronic course of polymyositis. *Journal of the Neurological Sciences*, **23**, 237.

Medsger, T.A., Dawson, W.N. & Masi, A.T. (1970) The epidemiology of polymyositis. *American Journal of Medicine*, **48**, 715.

Medsger, T.A., Rodnan, G.P., Moossy, J. & Vester, J.W. (1968) Skeletal muscle involvement in progressive systemic sclerosis (scleroderma). *Arthritis and Rheumatism*, **11**, 554.

Ménard, D.B., Haddad, H., Blain, J.G., Baudry, R., Devroede, G. & Massé, S. (1976) Granulomatous myositis and myopathy associated with Crohn's disease. *New England Journal of Medicine*, **295**, 818.

Metzger, A.L., Bohan, A., Goldberg, L.S., Bluestone, R. & Pearson, C.M. (1974) Polymyositis and dermatomyositis: combined methotrexate and corticosteroid therapy. *Annals of Internal Medicine*, **81**, 182.

Middleton, P.J., Alexander, R.M. & Szymanski, M.T. (1970) Severe myositis during recovery from influenza. *Lancet*, **2**, 532.

Miller, L.D. & Stevens, M.B. (1978) Skeletal manifestations of polymyalgia rheumatica. *Journal of the American Medical Association*, **240**, 27.

Mohr, P.D. & Knowlson, T.G. (1977) Quadriceps myositis: an appraisal of the diagnostic criteria of quadriceps myopathy. *Postgraduate Medical Journal*, **53**, 757.

Munsat, T. & Cancilla, P. (1974) Polymyositis without inflammation. *Bulletin of the Los Angeles Neurological Society*, **39**, 113.

Munsat, T.L., Hudgson, P. & Johnson, M.A. (1977) Experimental serotonin myopathy. *Neurology (Minneapolis)*, **27**, 772.

Munsat, T., Piper, D., Cancilla, P. & Mednick, J. (1972) Inflammatory myopathy with facioscapulohumeral distribution. *Neurology (Minneapolis)*, **22**, 335.

Namba, T., Brunner, N.G. & Grob, D. (1973) Association of myasthenia gravis with pemphigus vulgaris, Candida albicans infection, polymyositis and myocarditis. *Journal of the Neurological Sciences*, **20**, 231.

Norris, F.H., Dramov, B., Calder, C.D. & Johnson, S.G. (1969) Virus-like particles in myositis accompanying herpes zoster. *Archives of Neurology*, **21**, 25.

Oldstone, M.B.A. & Dixon, F.J. (1970) Pathogenesis of chronic disease associated with persistent lymphocytic choriomeningitis viral infection. *Journal of Experimental Medicine*, **131**, 1.

O'Leary, P.A. & Waisman, M. (1940) Dermatomyositis: A study of forty cases. *Archives of Dermatology and Syphilis*, **41**, 1001.

Oliver, R.T.D. (1977) Histocompatibility antigens and human disease. *British Journal of Hospital Medicine*, **18**, 449.

Pachman, L.M., Jonasson, O., Cannon, R.A. & Friedman, J.M. (1977) HLS–B8 in juvenile dermatomyositis. *Lancet*, **2**, 567.

Page, A.R. Hansen, A.E. & Good, R.A. (1963) Occurrence of leukaemia and lymphoma in patients with agammaglobulinaemia. *Blood*, **21**, 197.

Pearson, C.M. (1959) Rheumatic manifestations of polymyositis and dermatomyositis. *Arthritis and Rheumatism*, **2**, 127.

Pearson, C.M. (1963) Patterns of polymyositis and their response to treatment. *Annals of Internal Medicine*, **59**, 827.

Pearson, C.M. (1975) Myopathy with viral-like structures. *New England Journal of Medicine*, **292**, 641.

Pearson, C.M. & Bohan, A. (1977) The spectrum of polymyositis and dermatomyositis. *Medical Clinics of North America*, **61**, 439.

Pearson, C.M. & Yamazaki, J.N. (1958) Vacuolar myopathy in systemic lupus erythematosus. *American Journal of Clinical Pathology*, **29**, 455.

Pirofsky, B. & Bardana, E.J. (1977) Immunosuppressive therapy in rheumatic disease. *Medical Clinics of North America*, **61**, 419.

Pitkeathley, D.A. & Coomes, E.N. (1966) Polymyositis in rheumatoid arthritis. *Annals of Rheumatic Diseases*, **25**, 127.

Plowman, P.N. & Stableforth, D.E. (1977) Dermatomyositis with fibrosing alveolitis: response to treatment with cyclophosphamide. *Proceedings of the Royal Society of Medicine*, **70**, 738.

Reichlin, M. & Mattioli, M. (1976) Description of a serological reaction characteristic of polymyositis. *Clinical Immunology and Immunopathology*, **5**, 12.

Riddoch, D. & Morgan-Hughes, J.A. (1975) Prognosis in adult polymyositis. *Journal of the Neurological Sciences*, **26**, 71.

Rose, A.L. & Walton, J.N. (1966) Polymyositis: A survey of 89 cases with particular reference to treatment and prognosis. *Brain*, **89**, 747.

Rosen, F.S. (1974) Primary immunodeficiency. *Pediatric Clinics of North America*, **21**. 533.

Rothstein, T.L., Carlson, C.B. & Sumi, S.M. (1971) Polymyositis with facioscapulohumeral distribution. *Archives of Neurology*, **25**, 313.

Rowland, L.P. & Greer, M. (1961) Toxoplasmic polymyositis. *Neurology (Minneapolis)*, **11**, 367.

Rowland, L.P. & Schotland, D.L. (1965) Neoplasms and muscle disease. In *The Remote Effects of Cancer of the Nervous System*, Eds Lord Brain & F.H. Norris, Vol. 1, p. 83 (Grune & Stratton: New York).

Rowland, L.P., Lisak, R.P., Schotland, D.L. & Berg, P. (1973) Myasthenic myopathy and thymoma. *Neurology (Minneapolis)*, **23**, 282.

Rundle, L.G. & Sparks, F.f. (1963) Thymoma and dermatomyositis. *Archives of Pathology*, **75**, 276.

Sato, T., Walker, D.L., Peters, H.A., Reese, H.H. & Chou, S.M. (1971) Chronic polymyositis and myxovirus-like inclusions. *Archives of Neurology*, **24**, 409.

Saunders, M., Knowles, M. & Currie, S. (1969) Lymphocyte stimulation with muscle homogenate in polymyositis and other muscle-wasting disorders. *Journal of Neurology, Neurosurgery and Psychiatry*, **32**, 569.

Schaumburg, H.H., Nielsen, S.L. & Yurchak, P.M. (1971) Heart block in polymyositis. *New England Journal of Medicine*, **284**, 480.

Schraeder, P.L., Peters, H.A. & Dahl, D.S. (1972) Polymyositis and penicillamine. *Archives of Neurology*, **27**, 456.

Schuermann, H. (1951) Maligne Tumoren bei Dermatomyositis und progressiver Sklerodermie. *Archiv für Dermatologie und Syphilis*, **192**, 575.

Shafiq, S.A., Milhorat, A.T. & Gorycki, M.A. (1967) An electron microscope study of muscle degeneration and vascular changes in polymyositis. *Journal of Pathology and Bacteriology*, **94**, 139.

Sharratt, G.P., Danta, G. & Carson, P.H.M. (1977) Cardiac abnormality in polymyositis. *Annals of the Rheumatic Diseases*, **36**, 575.

Sheard, C. (1951) Dermatomyositis. *Archives of Internal Medicine*, **88**, 640.

Silberberg, D.H. & Drachman, D.A. (1962). Late-life myopathy occurring with Sjogren's syndrome. *Archives of Neurology*, **6**, 428.

Sloan, M.F., Franks, A.J., Exley, K.E. & Davison, A.M. (1978) Acute renal failure due to polymyositis. *British Medical Journal*, **1**, 1457.

Smith, B. (1969) Skeletal muscle necrosis associated with carcinoma. *Journal of Pathology*, **97**, 207.

Spiera, H. & Davison, S. (1978) Long-term follow-up of polymyalgia rheumatica. *Mount Sinai Journal of Medicine*, **45**, 225.

Stern, G.M., Rose, A.L. & Jacobs, K. (1967) Circulating antibodies in polymyositis. *Journal of the Neurological Sciences*, **5**, 181.

Tang, T.T., Sedmak, G.V., Siegesmund, K.A. & McCreadie, S.R. (1975) Chronic myopathy associated with Coxsackie virus Type A9. A combined electron microscopical and viral isolation study. *New England Journal of Medicine*, **292**, 608.

Taylor, J.F., Fluck, D. & Fluck, D. (1976) Tropical myositis: ultrastructural studies. *Journal of Clinical Pathology*, **29**, 1081.

Thompson, C.E. (1968) Polymyositis in children. *Clinical Pediatrics*, **7**, 24.

Thompson, J.M., Bluestone, R., Bywaters, E.G.L., Dorling,

J. & Johnson, M. (1969) Skeletal muscle involvement in systemic sclerosis. *Annals of the Rheumatic Diseases*, **28**, 281.

Unverricht, H. (1887) Polymyositis acuta progressiva. *Zeitschrift für Klinische Medizin*, **12**, 533.

Urich, H. & Wilkinson, M. (1970) Necrosis of muscle with carcinoma: myositis or myopathy? *Journal of Neurology, Neurosurgery and Psychiatry*, **33**, 398.

Vignos, P.J. & Goldwyn, J. (1972) Evaluation of laboratory tests in diagnosis and management of polymyositis. *American Journal of Medical Sciences*, **263**, 291.

Wagner, E. (1863) Fall einer seltnen Muskelkrankheit *Archiv der Heilkünde*, **4**, 282.

Wagner, E. (1887) Ein Fall von akuter Polymyositis. *Deutsches Archiv für Klinische Medicin*, **40**, 241.

Wallace, S.L., Lattes, R. & Ragan, C. (1958) Diagnostic significance of the muscle biopsy. *American Journal of Medicine*, **25**, 600.

Walton, J.N. & Adams, R.D. (1958) *Polymyositis* (Livingstone: Edinburgh).

Webster, A.D.B., Tripp, J.H., Hayward, A.R., Dayan, A.D., Doshi, R., Macintyre, E.H. & Tyrell, D.A.J. (1978) Echovirus encephalitis and myositis in primary immunoglobulin deficiency. *Archives of Disease in Childhood*, **53**, 33.

Whitaker, J.N. & Engel, W.K. (1972) Vascular deposits of immunoglobulin and complement in idiopathic inflammatory myopathy. *New England Journal of Medicine*, **286**, 333.

Winkelmann, R.K., Mulder, D.W., Lambert, E.H., Howard, F.M. & Diessner, G.R. (1968) Course of dermatomyositis-polymyositis. Comparison of untreated and cortisone treated patients. *Proceedings of the Mayo Clinic*, **43**, 545.

Wolfe, J.F., Adelstein, E. & Sharp, G.C. (1977) Antinuclear antibody with distinct specificity for polymyositis. *Journal of Clinical Investigation*, **59**, 176.

World Federation of Neurology Research Group on Neuromuscular Disorders (1968) *Journal of the Neurological Sciences*, **6**, 165.

Yang, D., Gardner, R. & Beetham, W.P. (1978) Dermatomyositis, myocardial involvement, and carcinoid syndrome. *Journal of the American Medical Association*, **239**, 1067.

Yunis, E.J. & Samaha, F.J. (1971) Inclusion body myositis. *Laboratory Investigation*, **25**, 240.

PART II

INVOLVEMENT OF HUMAN MUSCLE BY PARASITES

C.A. Pallis and P.D. Lewis

INTRODUCTION

A patchwork of data—dense in parts and diaphanous in others–concerning parasitic involvement of human muscle is available to workers in tropical medicine and related fields. In the limited space at our disposal we have attempted to present this information, emphasising features—both clinical and pathological—which may not be generally known to practising neurologists. Existing textbook contributions on muscle involvement in parasitic disease (Garnham, 1973; Adams, 1975) deal primarily with veterinary aspects or—when dealing with clinical matters—tend to be selective rather than comprehensive.

Muscle lesions (of varying severity and clinical relevance) are encountered in at least four protozoal diseases of man (toxoplasmosis, sarcosporidiosis, African and American trypanosomiasis). The larval stages of the life cycle of at least five cestodes (tapeworms) may develop in human muscle and result in conditions known as cysticercosis, coenurosis, unilocular and alveolar hydatidosis, and sparganosis. Finally the larvae of various nematodes may be found in muscle, causing diseases such as trichinosis and toxocariasis. In the following short accounts of these conditions the parasitological and epidemiologic data are kept to a minimum, and the clinical accounts are somewhat one-sidedly centred on muscle involvement. The parasitic disorders which may affect muscle are summarised in Table 15.13.

PROTOZOAL DISORDERS

Sarcosporidiosis and toxoplasmosis

Protozoal parasites of the class Sporozoasida may be found in the striated muscle of many mammals and some birds. They have occasionally been reported in man. They are given the generic name *Sarcocystis*. The muscle lesions are known as sarcocysts. Sarcocystis and certain species of *Isospora* are probably different stages in the life cycle of the same parasite.

Carnivorism is important in the transmission of this infection. It is believed that the life cycle involves two vertebrate hosts: a 'prey' (ungulates, rodents, birds, etc.) and a 'predator' (dog, cat, cheetah, etc.). The prey is infected by eating sporocysts passed in the faeces of the predator. Asexual multiplication takes place in the lymphoreticular cells of the prey. When predator eats prey, sexual reproduction of the parasite takes place in the intestinal submucosa of the predator and free sporocysts are discharged into the lumen of the gut. There is thus a biologically intriguing alternation of generations in two different vertebrate hosts. Man's fate is sometimes to act as an *Isospora*-passing predator, sometimes as a sarcocyst-ridden prey. The sporocysts most readily available to modern man for ingestion are probably those in his own faeces.

Sarcocysts are cylindrical bodies, usually 400–1000 μm in length and about 100 μm in diameter. They are sometimes much longer and may then be visible to the naked eye as minute white threads. *Sarcocystis lindemanii* (the species found in man) may produce cysts 5 cm long. These cylindrical structures (sometimes referred to as Miescher's tubes) have a hyaline, radially striated limiting membrane, from which septa arise. These divide the tube into compartments containing round, oval or sickle-shaped bodies, 12–16 μm long and 4–10 μm wide, called sporozoites or 'Rainey's corpuscles'.

The only other parasite forming morphologically similar structures in human muscle is *Toxoplasma gondii*. Differentiation is based on the length and diameter of the cysts (smaller in toxoplasmosis), on the thickness and striations of the capsule, on the division of the cyst by septa, and on the size of the sporozoites (more than twice

Table 15.13 Some clinical and pathological features of parasitic involvement of human muscle[1]

Parasite	Refs.[2]	Disease	Weakness	Wasting	Pain	Tenderness	Nodules	Local mass	Diffuse enlargement	Cardiac muscle involvement	Systemic illness	Calcification in muscle	Parasites in muscle fibres	Parasites between fibres	Diffuse inflammatory change	Abscesses	Inflammatory cell aggregates without parasites	'Tracks' in muscle	Involvement of central nervous system	Comments
1. Protozoa																				
Toxoplasma gondii	1–5	Toxoplasmosis	o	o	o	o	o	o	o	+	+	o	+	o	+	o	+	o	+	Possible relation to polymyositis
Sarcocystis lindemanni	6–11	Sarcosporidiosis	[±]	[±]	[±]	[±]	o	o	o	+	o	o	+	o	+	o	+	o	o	Sarcocysts. Possible relation to polymyositis
Trypanosoma gambiense *Trypanosoma rhodesiense*	12–16	African trypanosomiasis	+	+	o	o	o	o	o	+	+	o	o	o	+	o	+	o	+	Not known in what proportions terminal weakness and wasting are 'myopathic', 'neuropathic' or 'cachectic'
Trypanosoma cruzi	17–18	American trypanosomiasis (Chagas' disease)	o	o	o	o	o	o	o	+	+	o	o	o	+	o	+	o	+	Leishmanial phase in muscle 'pseudocysts'
2. Cestodes																				
Taenia solium	19–25	Cysticercosis	[±]	o	[±]	[±]	+	o	[±]	+	[±]	+	o	+	[±]	o	±	o	+	Occasional weakness, pain and tenderness (in pseudo-hypertrophic type only)
Multiceps braumi	26–30	Coenurosis of muscle	o	o	o	o	o	+	o	o	o	o	o	+	[±]	o	[+]	o	o	Cerebral coenurosis is due to a different species (*M. multiceps*)
Echinococcus granulosus	31–37	Unilocular hydatidosis	o	o	[+]	o	o	+	o	+	+	+	+	+	o	o	[±]	o	+	Rupture may cause severe pain and oedema
Echinococcus multilocularis	38–40	Alveolar hydatidosis	o	o	[+]	[+]	o	[+]	o	–	[+]	o	–	+	+	[+]	–	o	+	No capsule. Locally invasive. May metastasise. Local mass may be mobile
S…	41–46	Sparganosis																		

		Calcification, visible microscopically, *not* visible radiologically	Possible relation to 'eosinophilic myositis'	Doubtful involvement of nervous system (? coincidental toxocariasis)
Toxocara canis *Toxocara cati*	[56-58] Toxocariasis (visceral larva migrans)	+	+	+
Ascaris lumbricoides *A. sui, A. devosi, A. columnaris* *Neoascaris vitulorum* *Parascaris equorum* *Toxascaris leonina* *T. transfuga*	[59-60] ? Visceral larva migrans	[+]	+	o

(...cellular parasite 'denervates' part of muscle fibre).

[1]Decreasing degrees of severity are indicated on a scale ranging from ++ to ±. Absence of a feature is shown by o. Parentheses indicate that a particular feature has occasionally been reported. The absence of a symbol implies that information was not available to us.

[2]*References* (Key references are italicised).
[1]Faust *et al*, 1975. [2]Frenkel, 1973. [3]Kagan *et al*, 1974. [4]Rabinowicz, 1971. [5]Samuels & Rietschel, 1976. [6]Dastur & Iyer, 1955. [7]Kean & Breslau, 1964. [8]*Jeffery, 1974.* [9]Liu & Roberts, 1965. [10]Markus *et al*, 1974. [11]McGill & Goodbody, 1957. [12]Goodwin, 1970. [13]Janssen *et al*, 1956. [14]Koten & de Raadt, 1969. [15]Losos & Idede, 1972. [16]Poltera *et al*, 1977. [17]Faust *et al*, 1970. [18]*Köberle, 1968.* [19]Dixon & Lipscomb, 1961. [20]Jacob & Mathew, 1968. [21]Jolly & Pallis, 1971. [22]*MacArthur, 1950.* [23]McGill, 1948. [24]Sawhney *et al*, 1976. [25]Slais, 1970. [26]Fain, 1956. [27]Orihel *et al*, 1970. [28]Raper & Dockeray, 1956. [29]*Templeton, 1968.* [30]Wilson *et al*, 1972. [31]Arana-Iñiguez, 1978. [32]Blanco *et al*, 1949. [33]Devé, 1936. [34]*Devé, 1949.* [35]*Devé, 1951.* [36]Lorenzetti, 1962. [37]Pearson & Rose, 1960. [38]*Abuladze, 1964.* [39]Hunter *et al*, 1976. [40]Schimrigk & Emser, 1978. [41]Ali-Khan *et al*, 1973. [42]Cho & Patel, 1978. [43]Mueller, 1938. [44]Mueller *et al*, 1963. [45]Muller, 1975. [46]*Wirth & Farrow, 1961.* [47]Brashear *et al*, 1971. [48]Davis *et al*, 1976. [49]Despommier *et al*, 1975. [50]Drachman & Tuncbay, 1965. [51]Gould, 1954. [52]*Gould, 1970.* [53]Gross & Ochoa, 1979. [54]Marcus & Miller, 1955. [55]Stoll, 1947. [56]Beaver *et al*, 1952. [57]*Dent et al, 1956.* [58]Woodruff, 1970. [59]Nichols, 1956. [60]Sprent, 1965.

as large in sarcosporidiosis) (see also p. 550).

Patients have occasionally presented with features conceivably related to the presence of parasites in muscle. Thus Liu and Roberts (1965) described a patient with a chronic, painful, indurated area of the chest wall. This was excised and showed sarcocysts, surrounded by areas of lymphocytic and eosinophilic cellular infiltration, giant cells and interstitial fibrosis. Jeffery (1974) reviewed the whole subject of human sarcosporidiosis in some detail. His report included the description of a 21-year-old Gurkha soldier presenting with a painful lump in the thigh. Necrotic muscle tissue was evacuated and sarcocysts were found in an area of relatively unaffected muscle taken from the periphery of the lesion.

Rarely there may be more widespread symptoms, although here again the question of their relationship to sarcosporidiosis is debatable. McGill and Goodbody (1957) described an interesting case of polyarteritis nodosa in which sarcocysts were discovered at necropsy. The authors speculate on a possible relationship between the two conditions, on the basis of 'hypersensitivity'. They suggest that the hyaline capsule of the sarcocysts may be impervious to the passage of antigenic protein, but that cyst rupture may trigger a massive immune response, manifested as polyarteritis.

African trypanosomiasis

African trypanosomiasis is transmitted by the 'bite' of tsetse flies of the genus *Glossina*. These act as biological vectors: part of the life cycle of the parasite takes place in their tissues.

The trypanosomes (*T. rhodesiense* and *T. gambiense*) multiply in the gut of the fly, but do not involve cells. Crithidial forms metamorphose into metacyclic (infective) trypanosomes. It is this form which is 'injected' when man is 'bitten'.

Myositis is a feature of trypanosomal infections in rats (Losos and Idede, 1972). Patients with African trypanosomiasis may show gross muscle wasting, but it remains uncertain to what extent this is 'cachectic' in origin (many patients dying of this disease have concomitant illnesses such as tuberculosis). It is possible however that the wasting may be due, at times, to primary changes in muscle (perhaps immunologically induced). Occasionally it may be of neurogenic origin. Examination of skeletal muscle has very seldom been carried out. Lesions of the spinal roots have been reported (Janssen, van Bogaert and Haymaker, 1956; Poltera, Owor and Cox, 1977). In the otherwise very detailed study of the last-named group of workers, systematic investigation of skeletal muscle was undertaken in only one instance, samples being obtained from the upper and lower limbs, the recti abdominis and the diaphragm. The striated muscles showed atrophic fibres, sometimes accompanied by a patchy chronic cellular infiltration. There were eosinophilic degenerative changes of variagle severity. The changes were most marked in the deaphragm. The illustrated appearande was not that of neural atrophy. Further studies are clearly needed in this field.

American trypanosomiasis

American trypanosomiasis (caused by *Trypanosoma cruzi*) is transmitted through the infected faeces, deposited on human skin, of several species of reduviid or triatomine bugs which 'bite' and defaecate after feeding. Opossums, armadillos, wood and water rats and raccoons act as natural reservoirs. The spread of the disease to man is related to the adaptation of the vector bugs to living and breeding in and around primitive rural habitations. Man himself then becomes an important reservoir host.

Many infections are clinically silent. Swelling is an early local response to the inoculation of infective material and may characteristically involve one eye and one side of the face. There may be generalised lymphadenopathy, fever and malaise. Trypanosomal forms of the parasite are present in the blood during this stage.

The parasites show a predilection for cells of neuroectodermal or mesenchymal origin (cardiac and skeletal muscle, and lympho-reticular cells). There may be early myocarditis or meningoencephalitis. In infected cells the organism goes into a leishmanial phase (unlike what happens in African trypanosomiasis). The Leishmania multiply by binary fission, distend the cell, and produce a leishmanial pseudocyst. Cyst rupture releases crithidial and further trypanosomal forms which re-enter the circulation causing febrile relapses. Death of intracellular Leishmania produces an inflammatory reaction, which may be servere in non-immune individuals.

Skeletal muscle involvement may be florid although it is usually asymptomatic. Chronic myocarditis is common. Chronic Chagas' disease is a late complication of American trypanosomiasis. It is characterised by megacolon and megaoesophagus, brought about by lesions of the intrinsic autonomic innervation of the gastrointestinal tract. Exact pathogenetic mechanisms are still poorly understood.

CESTODES

Cysticercosis

Man is the only definitive host of the cestodes *Taenia solium* and *Taenia saginata*. Ripe proglottids are shed in human faeces. The released ova are consumed by an intermediate host. The pig (occasionally sheep, bears, cats, dogs and monkeys) has this role in the *T. solium* cycle. Various bovidae are involved in the life cycle of *T. saginata*.

The embryos, freed in the gut of the intermediate host, burrow through the intestinal mucosa and are widely distributed through mesenteric venules and lymphatic channels, to skeletal and cardiac muscle, the nervous system and other tissues where, within two to three months, they develop into infective bladder worms or cysticerci. The larval forms of *T. solium* and *T. saginata* are known respectively as *Cysticercus cellulosae* and *Cysticercus bovis*. These forms were recognised and named before their relationship to their parent worms was recognised. The pseudo-generic names have no taxonomic significance.

When parasitised undercooked pork or beef is eaten by man, the scolex (head) of the cysticercus evaginates like the finger of a glove and becomes attached to the gut wall. The human host then develops an adult tapeworm, *not* cysticercosis. The point needs emphasising as it is still widely misunderstood.

Probably the only way in which man can contract *cysticercosis* is by doing what the pig normally does, i.e. by eating *T. solium* ova (his own

or someone else's—usually the latter). It should be noted that, for reasons that are poorly understood, the ingestion by man of the ova of *T. saginata* hardly ever produces cysticercosis.

T. solium taeniasis has virtually disappeared from Europe. The same has happened in many other places. In the Middle East, Muslim Africa, and Indonesia it was always a very rare or non-existent condition because of religious practices which forbid the consumption of pork. Human cysticercosis continues to occur however in India, Mongolia, Korea, China, Central and South America and South Africa (Slais, 1970).

Muscle involvement. Involvement of the central nervous system in cysticercosis is very common and will not be further discussed. Involvement of skeletal muscle has been known since the condition was first recognised. In early accounts it was thought to be rare, but it is now known to be common. There was positive evidence of such invasion in 429 of the 450 cases of cysticercosis surveyed by Dixon and Lipscomb (1961). The morbid anatomy of the condition is well described in standard textbooks and articles (MacArthur, 1950; Trelles and Trelles, 1978) and will not be recapitulated here. Recent developments are reviewed in detail by Slais (1970).

Pseudohypertrophic myopathy. Although it had been described earlier, pseudohypertrophic myopathy in cysticercosis was first drawn to the attention of neurologists by Jacob and Mathew in 1968. In 1971 Jolly and Pallis reviewed seven of the previously reported cases and described two of their own. Since then, further cases have been reported, and it is now possible to describe the clinical and pathological features of this interesting condition in more detail.

All but one of the 16 cases of muscular pseudohypertrophy shown by biopsy to be due to cysticercosis have been reported from India. The main features are summarised in Table 15.14. Eleven males and five females have been affected, their ages ranging from 10 to 45 years.

The thighs, calves, glutei and shoulder girdles are, as a rule, massively enlarged, the patients often being described as having developed a 'Herculean' appearance (Fig. 15.10). The nuchal musculature,

Table 15.14 Summary of clinical and laboratory findings in reported cases of pseudohypertrophic myopathy due to cysticercosis

Authors	Year	Cases reported	Sex	Age	Identifiable initial illness	Weakness	Pain	Tenderness	Subcutaneous nodules	Tongue involvement	Eye involvement	Heart involvement	CNS involvement	Calcified muscle cysts	Ova in stool or history of taeniasis	EMG	CPK	Eosinophila
Priest	1926	1	M	24	+	+	+I	+	+	o	+	+	+	NI	o	o	o	+
McRobert	1944	1	M	25	o	o	o	o	+	o	o	NI	+	o	o	o	o	+
McGill	1947, 1948*	2	M	25	+	++		o	+	+	o	NI	+	? scolices only	o	o	o	+
			M	20	+	++ (calves)	I	o	+	+	o	NI	o	? scolices only	o	o	o	o
Singh and Jolly	1957	1	F	22	o	o	o	±	++	o	papillitis	NI	+	o	o	o	o	++
Prakash and Kumar	1965	1	M	14	o	o	o	+	+	+	o	Abnormal ECG	+	? scolices only	+	o	o	+
Jacob and Mathew	1968	1	M	30	o	±	o	±	+	+	+	Cardiac failure	+	o	o	NI	NI	+
Armbrust-Figueiredo et al	1970	1	F	35	+	+	I	o	o	o	o	Abnormal ECG	+	o	+	NI	NI	o
Jolly and Pallis	1971	2**	M	22	o	o	o	o	o	+	+	o	+	o	o	o	o	NI
			M	25														
Rao et al	1972	1	M	10	o	o	o	o	+	+	o	o	+	o	o	o	o	NI
Salgoakar and Watcha	1974	1	M	11	+	±	o	o	+	+	proptosis; swollen disc	o	+	o	o	NI	N	+
Vigg and Rai	1975	2	F	45	o	+	±	NI	+	+	o	o	+	o	o	o	o	+
			F	35	+	±	±	o	+	o	o	o	+	o	o	o	o	+
Sawhney et al	1976	1	F	24	o	+	+	o	+	o	+	Non-specific T wave changes	+	NI	NI	Abnormal	N	+
Vijayan et al	1977	1	M	17	o	+	o	o	+	+	+	NI	+	o	o	o	o	NI

* Same cases described in two communications
** Cases 3 and 4

I = Initial muscle pain
NI = No information

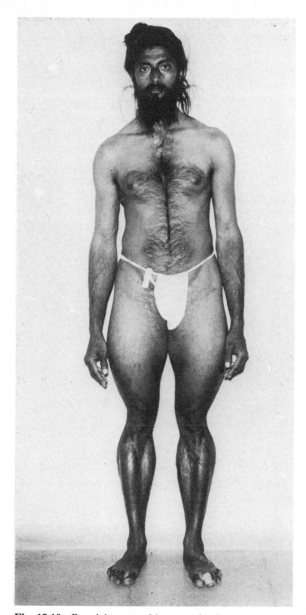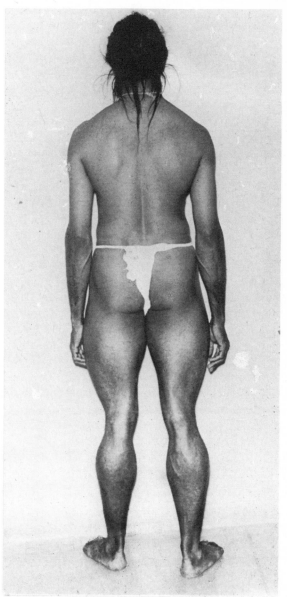

Fig. 15.10   Pseudohypertrophic myopathy due to cysticercosis (reproduced from Jolly and Pallis (1971) with kind permission of the authors, editor and publisher)

erector spinae, masseters and forearm muscles may be notably involved. The pseudohypertrophy is invariably bilateral and symmetrical.

The enlarged muscles are usually firm. There may be slight overlying oedema. No individual nodules can usually be felt, probably because the muscles are so tightly packed with cysticerci. The nodules may occasionally be felt on contraction.

In six instances there was no detectable weak-

ness in the enlarged muscles. In seven cases there was mild to moderate, predominantly proximal paresis, and in one case paresis seems to have been confined to the calf musculature. Two patients were described as very weak. In no case was power increased in a manner commensurate with muscle bulk.

Muscle pain was experienced before the onset of the pseudohypertrophy in several instances, but at the time of presentation was seldom a prominent feature. In most patients the muscular enlargement had been entirely painless throughout the whole of its course. Definite muscle tenderness was elicited in two of the 16 cases and in a further two slight tenderness may have been present.

The muscle enlargement had come on insidiously in all cases, over a period varying from a few weeks to 18 months or more. In six instances an initial illness could be identified, often consisting of fever, pain in the limbs and occasionally urticaria or pruritus. In some cases muscular enlargement had been noted within two or three weeks of such an illness.

In 14 of the 16 patients, muscular enlargement had occurred in a context of palpable subcutaneous nodules, i.e. of clinically obvious cysticercosis. Lingual cysticerci were seen in no fewer than 10 instances and ocular cysticerci in two. Two patients had evidence of cardiac failure and a further three had abnormal electrocardiograms. There was evidence of involvement of the nervous system in 14 instances (usually epilepsy, but occasionally mental change or a focal neurological deficit). Calcification of the parasites in muscle was encountered only twice and seemed to be early (i.e. confined to the scolices).

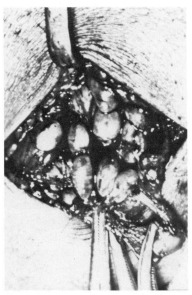

Muscle biopsy will reveal numerous tense cysts, 1 cm or more in length (Fig. 15.11). The muscle fibres are not hypertrophied. Regions in the immediate vicinity of the cysticerci occasionally show variable cellular infiltration with polymorphs, lymphocytes, plasma cells and/or eosinophils, and occasional degenerative changes and areas of focal fibrosis. Sawhney, Chopra, Banerji and Wahi (1976), however, illustrated changes 'not in continuity with the inflammatory reaction seen around the cysts'. These consisted of swollen muscle fibres with loss of cross-striation and central migration of nuclei. Their finding implied, they thought, 'an affection of the muscle fibres *per se* in the disease process'. They did not report, however, on the appearances of sections of muscle from above and below the affected areas. We believe that as likely an explanation for their observations is the phenomenon reported by Drachman and Tuncbay (1965)—in cases of obvious trichinosis—to account for 'extensive myositis without trichinae'.

Electromyography was first used in such cases by Salgaokar and Watcha (1974) who reported normal findings in the proximal muscle groups of their patient. Sawhney *et al.* (1976) reported motor units 'averaging' 300–800 μV and 4–8 ms in duration, 10–15 per cent of which were polyphasic. They interpreted these findings as indicative of myopathy.

We believe muscle enlargement in cysticercosis to be related to larval death, not to the initial dissemination. The cysts found in such cases are invariably very tense and never contain viable parasites. Very little is known of the natural history of the disorder but there is evidence to suggest that it may be a spontaneously reversible condition.

Treatment. Intestinal taeniasis, if present, should be treated. Drug-induced larval death, and the subsequent appearance of further tense cysts, may for a while aggravate the pseudohypertrophy.

Fig. 15.11 Numerous tense cysticerci, presenting at the biopsy site in gastronemius muscle (case of Prakash and Kumar, 1965, reproduced with kind permission of the authors, editor and publisher)

Coenurosis

The word coenurus refers to the polycephalous larval form of certain taeniid worms of the genus *Multiceps*, the adults of which inhabit the intestine of dogs and other canidae. The term is descriptive and has no taxonomic significance.

On farm or field herbivorous mammals may swallow the ova passed by dogs infected by *Multiceps multiceps*. The embryos burrow through the intestinal mucosa and disseminate widely. Affected sheep may develop a neurological disorder known as 'staggers'. Other possible intermediate hosts include rabbits, wild rodents, certain monkeys and—occasionally—man, in whom cerebral symptoms may also be prominent. The cycle is completed when dogs gain access to infected sheep tissue.

In parts of tropical Africa where *M. multiceps* seems to be very rare the taeniid *M. brauni* is found in the gut of the domestic dog, fox and jackal, the usual intermediate hosts being wild rodents or porcupines. Cases of human coenurosis reported from such areas all seem to have shown predominant subcutaneous or muscle involvement.

Coenuri are glistening, globular or ovoid unilocular cysts, each containing several scolices which seem to bud from the inner surface of the cyst wall. The cysts vary in size from that of an almond to that of an apricot. They are usually filled with a milky, gelatinous fluid. They contain neither brood capsules nor daughter cysts. They are surrounded by an adventitious capsule derived from the host, composed of dense collagenous fibrous tissue infiltrated with plasma cells, lymphocytes and occasional histiocytes and eosinophils.

A coenurus is one of the causes of a palpable, occasionally slightly tender, 'tumour' in muscle. The 'tumour' is usually solitary and—in muscle—almost invariably unilocular. The vast majority occur on the trunk. The intercostal and anterior abdominal muscles are favourite sites (Templeton, 1971). Coenuri may also be found in the neck, in relation to the sternomastoid or trapezius muscles.

The pre-operative diagnosis is usually fibroma or lipoma. When the excised 'tumour' is cut across, and the multiple scolices are revealed in the cyst, macroscopic diagnosis should be obvious.

Hydatidosis

The two canid tapeworms (*Echinococcus granulosus* and *Echinococcus multilocularis*) may cause hydatid disease in man. Muscle involvement has been reported with both types of infection.

Ova of *E. granulosus*, discharged in dogs' faeces, are ingested by the intermediate host (usually sheep but occasionally goats, cattle, pigs, wild herbivores or man). After hatching, the embryos penetrate the venules of the intestinal wall and become established in the liver. If they can get beyond the hepatic circulation they lodge in the lungs. A small proportion may reach other tissues such as muscle or bone. The natural cycle is completed when dogs eat ovine offal. In echinococcosis due to *E. multilocularis*, the natural reservoir is in foxes, although dogs and cats may also harbour the parent tapeworm. The usual intermediate hosts are wild rodents. Man may become infected by consuming fruit and vegetables contaminated by the excreta of foxes.

The classic morphological appearance of hydatid cysts due to *E. granulosus* is well described in standard textbooks and will not be recapitulated. Unlike the large single cysts produced by this tapeworm the larval stage of *E. multilocularis* consists of a honeycomb-like aggregate of innumerable small cysts. There is no proper limiting capsule. The lesion may look like the cut surface of a slice of bread. It may have a necrotic centre, resembling an abscess. It behaves locally like an invasive tumour and true metastases may occur.

In sheep-rearing countries, where hydatidosis is common, hydatid disease of muscle is not rare. Muscle is in fact the third most frequent site (after liver and lung) in which cysts may be found. Over 5 per cent of cases of human hydatid disease may show lesions of muscle (Dévé, 1949; Dew, 1951). Goinard and Salasc (1931) reported a personal series of 33 cases.

The initial lesion probably occurs within an individual muscle fibre (Dévé, 1936). Only about a third of muscle hydatids contain viable scolices. They are most commonly encountered in the paravertebral gutters and in the limb-girdle musculature, particularly in the thigh. They are rare distally.

In many parts of the world a hydatid is the

commonest cause of a benign muscle tumour. Physical examination will reveal a deep, slowly growing, poorly mobile, spherical or lobulated mass, of variable size and firm consistency. The exact shape of the tumour will often be influenced by adjacent bone and limiting fascia. Pain is rare, although patients may complain of a dull ache in the relevant muscle after use. A hydatid 'thrill' can seldom be elicited. The lesion may occasionally calcify. Secondary infection of hydatids is not uncommon. The condition may then present as an abscess.

Hydatids in muscle cause neither weakness nor tenderness. The occurrence of myotonia in three out of five members of a family with evidence of muscle involvement due to *E. multilocularis* (Schimrigk and Emser, 1978) was probably fortuitous. The family was thought to be suffering from myotonia congenita.

Sparganosis

Definition. The term sparganosis refers to the extra-intestinal infection of vertebrate hosts by the plerocercoid larvae (or spargana) of pseudo-phyllidean (diphyllobothriid) tapeworms of the genus *Spirometra*. These tapeworms are related to *D. latum* (well known to haematologists and neurologists as an occasional cause of vitamin B_{12} deficiency) but differ in that they cannot complete their life cycle and develop their adult form in man. Two intermediate hosts are needed: the first a copepod crustacean, the second a vertebrate.

The adult worms live in the gut of carnivores. In the Far East '*Spirometra mansoni*' is a common intestinal parasite of dogs and cats. In the United States *Spirometra mansonoides* has been found in bobcats, occasionally in domestic cats and—more rarely—in dogs.

Infected carnivores pass mature proglottids. The ova hatch in ponds or streams, liberating a ciliated coracidium. The coracidia are swallowed by water-fleas of the genus *Cyclops* in whose haemocoele they mature, becoming procercoid larvae. When such larvae are then eaten by frogs, lizards, snakes, birds or small mammals the procercoid larva is liberated in the gut of the vertebrate host, penetrates the intestinal wall and

is distributed to the tissues, where it matures to a migrating, plerocercoid larva.

In the USA, natural paratenic (carrier) hosts include mice, rhesus monkeys, water snakes and the pig, raccoon and opossum. In Korea various species of snake have been incriminated. Unlike *Diphyllobothrium*, the plerocercoids are not found in fish. It is only when the paratenic host is consumed by the definitive (carnivore) host that the life cycle is completed and that an adult tapeworm can again develop.

Man can become infected in one of four ways:

(1) by the accidental ingestion of procercoid-infected copepods (as in drinking unboiled, unfiltered, infected water). The procercoid will then penetrate the human gut and become a plerocercoid;

(2) by eating the infected, uncooked, plerocercoid-containing flesh of frogs, snakes or certain fish, for purposes of nutrition or—more often in parts of South East Asia—as a 'tonic'. The plerocercoid is then transmitted from one paratenic (carrier) host to another. It remains a plerocercoid however, for the adult worm cannot develop in man;

(3) through eating uncooked pork (Becklund, 1962; Corkum, 1966). Spargana are known to develop in pigs allowed to forage in woodland areas, where they may become infected through the ingestion of snakes, frogs or small mammals infected with plerocercoids—or through drinking water from ponds containing infected copepods;

(4) by using the raw flesh of plerocercoid-infected 'split frogs' or snakes as poultices. The practice, long prevalent in Thailand and Vietnam, of dressing ulcers, wounds or infected eyes with such poultices doubtless accounted for many cases of ocular sparganosis.

Clinical features. In ocular sparganosis there is often an intense inflammatory reaction with periorbital oedema. Retrobulbar lesions produce lagophthalmos and the threat of corneal ulceration. The early phases of infection by the gastrointestinal route are usually asymptomatic. In soft tissues the clinical features vary. The usual presentation is as a slightly fluctuant subcutaneous or superficial intramuscular lump, about 5 cm in diameter, often suspected of being a lipoma. Occasionally the lump presents with signs of inflammation. A characteristic although uncommon feature is the tendency of the lumps to move slowly downwards, over several weeks or months—as correctly observed by many patients and repeatedly doubted at first interview by many doctors.

Involved muscles have included the rectus abdominis, thigh muscles, pectoralis major and calf muscles. In many cases, other parts of the body will have been involved, although from the descriptions it is not always clear whether the lesions were entirely subcutaneous or could have extended deeper. In a given lesion there is usually a single, viable larva.

A case in which a live sparganum was extracted from the biceps muscle was reported by Ali-Khan, Irving, Wignall and Bowmer (1973). Cho and Patel (1978) report a case in which the parasite, deep in the right thigh, was surrounded by granulomatous tissue showing a striking histological similarity to the nodules of rheumatoid arthritis. The length of the excised parasite may lead to misdiagnosis of guinea-worm (dracunculiasis).

NEMATODES

Trichinosis

The larvae of *Trichinella spiralis* may be found in the muscles of many facultative or obligatory carnivores. Natural infection is readily transmitted between species—or by cannibalism within a given species.

Trichinosis, among carnivores, is world-wide, its distribution independent of climate. It is encountered from equatorial to arctic regions. The prevalence of human trichinosis, on the other hand, is patchy and deeply influenced by cultural factors.

Human infection takes place through eating parasitised ('measly') pork in the form of raw or undercooked sausage, smoked ham or pickled trotters—or more exotic foods such as boar or bear meat. (Pigs are infected by eating infected rats, or by being fed uncooked swill containing, *inter alia*, the offal of other pigs.)

After ingestion of infected meat, viable larvae are released and pass into the duodenum and jejunum where, after moulting, they very rapidly develop into adult worms. The male dies after copulation but the female (which may reach a size of 4 mm) burrows into the intestinal mucosa and starts producing viviparous larvae within a week of ingestion. During the next two or three weeks each female may produce over a thousand 'second-generation larvae' which enter the systemic circulation (via the lymphatics and the right side of the heart) and seed into many tissues.

In striated muscle the larvae penetrate the sarcolemma and grow until after 16 days they reach a length of 800–1000 μm and a width of 30 μm. They show no preference for any particular fibre type (Ochoa and Pallis, 1980) (Figs. 15.12a, b, c and d). Three weeks after penetration they have increased their length ten-fold, becoming coiled in the process (Fig. 15.13). An ellipsoidal collagenous capsule about 500 μm long and 250 μm wide is formed by the muscle cell around the coiled-up larvae. It takes about three months for this capsule to develop fully. Although widely distributed, the larvae seem to encyst in this manner in striated muscle only. Encysted larvae may remain viable for many years. Calcification may begin within 6–9 months. Following death of the trichinae some cysts may be completely resorbed. The penetration of a striated muscle fibre by a larva results in the destruction both of the penetrated fibre and of some adjacent ones.

The extraocular muscles, masseters, diaphragm, muscles of the tongue, larynx and neck, intercostals and deltoid are most heavily involved. In some epidemics parasitisation predominated in diaphragm, calves and forearm muscles. Sites of attachment to tendons are particularly prone to be affected.

Many infections are asymptomatic, with diaphragm counts of less than 10 larvae per gram. Muscular symptoms probably arise when the larval count reaches 100 per gram. A recently described patient (Davis, Cilo, Plaitakis and Yahr, 1976) survived a deltoid concentration of 4000 larvae per gram. Fatal cases, according to Gould (1970) may carry up to 100 million larvae to the grave with them. A worm's eye view of the human connection could only be depressing for this

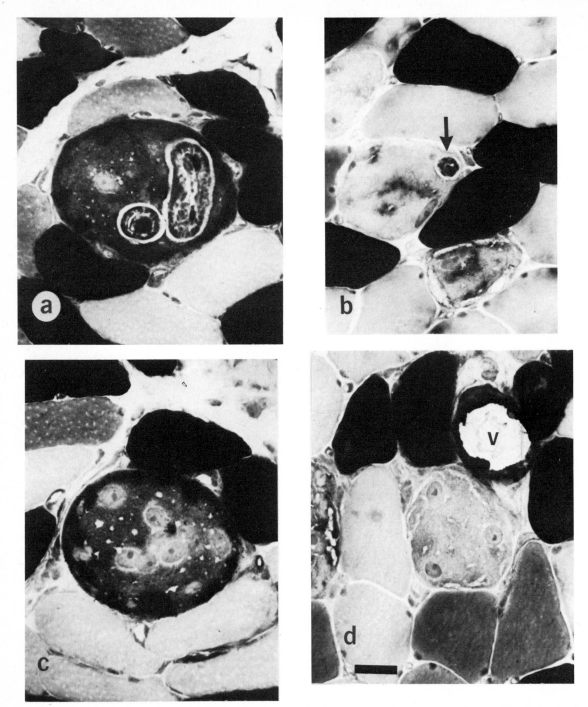

Fig. 15.12   (a) Type I muscle fibre harbouring larva of *Trichinella spiralis*. (b) Type II (A?) fibre cut across parasite (arrowed). (c) Distended type I fibre with reactive nuclei, probably cut close to a parasite. (d) Type II (A?) fibre showing similar changes to those in the fibre in (c)

ATPase pH 4.6: Black = Type I   Common Bar = 25 μm
               White = Type IIA   V = blood vessel
               Intermediate = Type IIB

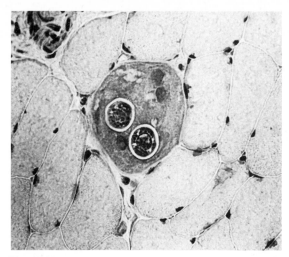

Fig. 15.13   Muscle fibre containing slightly coiled larva of *Trichinella spiralis*, cut across twice

massive parasitisation of man is clearly a demographic dead-end.

Clinical features. The first diagnostically helpful sign is often periorbital oedema. The whole face may be grotesquely bloated. Patients may be misdiagnosed as suffering from angioneurotic oedema or even from renal disease. There may be chemosis, a widespread facial erythema and subconjunctival haemorrhages. Patients may present to ophthalmologists with complaints of conjunctivitis or of pain in one or both eyeballs often related to eye movement. The combination of severe photophobia, fever and headache may lead to misdiagnoses of meningitis. Diagnosis may be very difficult as there may be neck stiffness, probably from myositis of the nuchal musculature. A macular rash, more persistent than that of typhoid, is seen in 10 per cent of cases. Subungual 'splinters' and retinal haemorrhages are not uncommon.

Myalgia is an early and common complaint, although often preceded by fever and by periorbital oedema. Involvement of the ocular muscles, masseters and tongue leave their imprint on the symptomatology. Masticatory difficulties or even trismus may occur. Oedema of the tongue and pharyngeal muscles may cause dysphagia. The calves and forearms are usually painful. Lumbar pains may be excruciating. Myalgia reaches its height during the third week of the illness, seldom extending into the fourth or fifth weeks.

The involved muscles may be patchily tender but the most striking feature is undoubtedly their weakness. In part, this is a genuine paresis. But there is also a considerable reluctance to move, any movement tending to produce 'tension pain' in both agonists and antagonists. Occasionally, the limb muscles may be grossly swollen. An 'oedematous' patient with puffy face, swollen legs and very tender muscles will almost certainly prove to have trichinosis.

The weakness may be extreme, patients rapidly becoming tetraplegic from muscle involvement. There is probably no other disorder of muscle, except periodic paralysis, in which such severe weakness develops in so short a time. The tendon reflexes may be impaired.

Calf pain may result in an early reluctance to stand, of a degree that would not be warranted by paresis or general prostration. Patients may attempt to remain ambulant by walking on their toes. When they take to bed, they tend to remain immobile. Early contractures may ensue.

Involvement of the central nervous system is well documented in the more massive infections. Its manifestations are protean and include stupor, frank meningitis, brain-stem involvement and various combinations of upper motor neurone and radicular signs. These are of variable pathogenesis (haemorrhage, vasculitis, oedema, granulomatous nodules). Larval embolisation into capillaries is encountered but is much less common than vasculitis. The marked response of neurological signs to steroid medication is probably related to these manifestations of hypersensitivity. Confusing symptoms may be encountered. Diplopia is more often than not of myopathic origin. Dyspnoea may be due to asthma, the pain of deep breathing, cardiac failure or ventilatory insufficiency of myopathic type. Misdiagnoses of poliomyelitis, polyneuritis and even myasthenia have been reported.

In severe cases the illness reaches its height in from two to four weeks. Paresis and asthenia may be protracted and convalescence delayed. In various epidemics of human trichinosis, 2–10 per cent of recognised cases have proved fatal. Death usually results from non-specific myocarditis, pneumonia or encephalitis.

Electromyography. Marcus and Miller (1955) described a patient with widespread, severe trichinosis who exhibited 'the most profuse fibrillation of denervation the examiner had ever seen'. There was gross weakness and some wasting. Although the authors attributed the fibrillation, wasting and weakness to 'lower motor neurone changes' we believe a more likely mechanism is the one suggested to account for 'profuse spontaneous fibrillation in all muscles sampled' in the case described by Gross and Ochoa (1979). These authors incriminated 'disconnection of fragments of muscle fibres from their end-plate regions due to focal muscle necrosis'. The implications of such a mechanism are considerable. They might help in the electromyographic differentiation of those parasitic myopathies in which the parasites lie *within* muscle fibres from those in which the parasites lie *between* muscle fibres.

Treatment. The antihelminthic thiabendazole (2-(thiazolyl)-benzimidazole) was introduced into the therapy of human trichinosis in 1964. It also has a profound effect on larvae already in muscle, damaging or killing substantial numbers of them. The suggested intake is 50 mg/kg/day, taken in divided doses. Medication should be continued until symptoms subside or incapacitating side effects appear, but should not be continued for more than 10 days. Side effects include anorexia and various gastrointestinal upsets, slight dizziness, and occasionally, drowsiness.

Treatment of trichinosis with thiabendazole alone may result in a Herxheimer-like reaction. This is probably due to massive dissolution of larvae with abrupt release of protein-breakdown products into the circulation. Corticosteroids are therefore usually prescribed concurrently with— or even a little earlier than—thiabendazole. Such a regime would seem to associate the larvicidal effect of one drug, the immunosuppressive effect of the other and the combined anti-inflammatory effects of both.

Toxocariasis

Toxocara canis is a widely distributed ascarid of dogs, in which species its life cycle resembles that of *Ascaris lumbricoides* in man. Its ova are infective to man. *Toxocara cati* (a common feline ascarid) may also cause human toxocariasis.

Human toxocariasis occurs when ova, present in dog or cat faeces, get into the mouths of children, playing in yards or gardens. The ova hatch in the child's jejunum and the liberated larvae enter mesenteric venules or lymphatics. They are then carried to extraintestinal sites, usually the liver but sometimes to the lungs and even beyond: to brain, eye or muscle. The larvae may remain alive and actively motile in such tissues, boring their way in various directions.

Granulomatous lesions caused by larvae may be few or many, depending on the number of ingested eggs, and on the degree of sensitisation of the invaded host. In the liver they appear as subcapsular white nodules or plaques, 5–10 mm in diameter and easily visible to the naked eye. Lesions in human muscle are less numerous but may nevertheless be detected by the use of a hand lens (Dent, Nichols, Beaver, Carrera and Staggers, 1956). Using a pepsin technique these workers recovered a mean of 5 larvae per gram of skeletal muscle in a child with toxocariasis who had died from a post-transfusion hepatitis. They suggested that the recovery of *Toxocara* larvae by this technique might be applied to muscle and liver biopsy specimens, as a diagnostic procedure in suspected cases. As far as we know, muscle biopsy has seldom been used for this purpose.

Florid disease is rare, the most usual presentation being a chronically ill child with an enlarged liver, pneumonitis and sustained eosinophilia. Muscle pain may occasionally be a feature (Hunter, Swartzwelder and Clyde, 1976).

Diagnostic procedures are reviewed by Woodruff (1970). The morphological differentiation of various larvae capable of causing visceral larva migrans is discussed in detail by Nichols (1956).

REFERENCES

Abuladze, K.I. (1964) Alveococci as parasites in man. In *Taeniata of animals and man and diseases caused by them,* pp. 379–383 (Iztadel'stvo 'Nauka': Moscow. English version: Israel Program for Scientific translations: Jerusalem, 1970).

Adams, R.D. (1975) *Diseases of Muscle: a study in pathology,*

3rd edition (Harper and Row: Hagerstown).

Ali-Khan, Z., Irving, R.T., Wignall, N. & Bowmer, E.J. (1973) Imported sparganosis in Canada. *Canadian Medical Association Journal*, **108**, 590–593.

Arana-Iñiguez, R. (1978) Echinococcus. In *Handbook of Clinical Neurology*, Eds P.J. Vinken & G.W. Bruyn, Vol. 35, pp. 175–208 (North-Holland Publishing Co: Amsterdam).

Armbrust-Figueiredo, J., Speciali, J.G. & Lison, M.P. (1970) Forma miopatica da cisticercose. *Arquivos de Neuro-psiquiatria*, **28**, 385–390.

Beaver, P.C., Snyder, C.H., Carrera, G.M., Dent, J.H. & Lafferty, J.W. (1952) Chronic eosinophilia due to visceral larva migrans. *Pediatrics*, **9**, 7–19.

Becklund, W.W. (1962) Occurrence of a larval trematode (Diplostomatidae) in a larval cestode (Diphyllobothriidae) from Sus scrofa in Florida. *Journal of Parasitology*, **48**, 286.

Blanco, A.E., Mozador, J.L. & Minetti, R. (1949) Los quistes hidatidicos musculares. *Archivos internacionales de la Hidatidosis*, **9**, 221–253.

Brashear, R.E., Martin, R.R. & Glover, J.L. (1971) Trichinosis and respiratory failure. *American Review of Respiratory Diseases*, **104**, 245–249.

Cho, C. & Patel, S.P. (1978) Human sparganosis in Northern United States. *New York State Journal of Medicine*, **78**, 1456–1458.

Corkum, K.C. (1966) Sparganosis in some vertebrates in Louisiana and observations of a human infection. *Journal of Parasitology*, **55**, 444–448.

Dastur, D.K. & Iyer, C.G.S. (1955) Sarcocystis of human muscle. *Bulletin of the Neurological Society of India*, **2**, 25–27.

Davis, M.J., Cilo, M., Plaitakis, A. & Yahr, M.D. (1976) Trichinosis: a severe myopathic involvement with recovery. *Neurology (Minneapolis)*, **26**, 37–40.

Dent, J.H., Nichols, R.L., Beaver, P.C., Carrera, G.M. & Staggers, R.J. (1956) Visceral larva migrans with a case report. *American Journal of Pathology*, **32**, 777–803.

Despommier, D., Aron, L., & Turgeon, L. (1975) Trichinella spiralis: Growth of the intracellular (muscle) larva. *Experimental Parasitology*, **37**, 108–116.

Dévé, F. (1936) Sur le siège initial des kystes hydatiques musculaires. *Comptes rendus de la Société de Biologie*, **123**, 764–765.

Dévé, F, (1949) *L'échinococcose primitive*, p. 79 (Masson: Paris).

Dew, R.H. (1951) Hydated disease. In *British Encyclopaedia of Medical Practice*, 2nd Edn., Ed. Lord Horder. Vol. 6, pp. 587–614 (Butterworth: London).

Dixon, H.B.F. & Lipscomb, F.M. (1961) Cysticercosis: an analysis and follow-up of 450 cases. (Medical Research Council: London), Special Report Series.

Drachman, D.A. & Tuncbay, T.O. (1965) The remote myopathy of trichinosis. *Neurology (Minneapolis)*, **15**, 1127–1135.

Fain, A. (1956) Coenurus of Taenia brauni Setti parasitic in man and animals from the Belgian Congo and Ruanda-Urundi. *Nature*, **178**, 1353.

Faust, E.C., Beaver, P.C. & Jung, R.C. (1975) *Animal Agents and Vectors of Human Disease*. 4th edition, pp. 92–96 (Lea & Febiger: Philadelphia).

Faust, E.C., Russell, P.F. & Jung, R.C. (1970) *Craig and Faust's Clinical Parasitology*, 8th edition (Lea & Febiger: Philadelphia).

Frenkel, J.K. (1973) Toxoplasmosis: parasite life cycle, pathology and immunology of toxoplasmosis. In *The Coccidia : Eimeria, Toxoplasma, Isospora and Related Genera*, Eds D.M. Hammond & P. Long, pp. 343–410 (University Park Press: Baltimore).

Garnham, P.C.C. (1973) Parasitic infections. In *The Structure and Function of Muscle*, 2nd edition, Ed. G.H. Bourne, Vol. 4, pp. 249–288 (Academic Press: New York).

Goinard, P. & Salasc, J. (1931) Sur les kystes hydatiques des muscles volontaires. *Journal de chirurgie*, **54**, 320–331.

Goodwin, L.G. (1970) The pathology of African trypanosomiasis. *Transactions of the Royal Society of Tropical Medicine and Hygiene*, **64**, 797–812.

Gould, S.E. (1954) Eye and orbit in trichinosis. *Bulletin of New York Academy of Medicine*, **30**, 726–729.

Gould, S.E. (1970) *Trichinosis in man and animals*, Ed. S.E. Gould, pp. 147–189 (Thomas: Springfield, Ill.).

Gross, B. & Ochoa, J. (1979) Trichinosis: a clinical report and histochemistry of muscle. *Muscle and Nerve*, **2**, 394–398

Hunter, G.W., Swatzwelder, J.C. & Clyde, D.E. (1976) *Tropical Medicine*. 5th edition (Saunders: Philadelphia).

Jacob, J.C. & Mathew, N.T. (1968) Pseudohypertrophic myopathy in cysticercosis. *Neurology (Minneapolis)* **18**, 767–771.

Janssen, P., van Bogaert, L. & Haymaker, W. (1956) Pathology of the peripheral nervous system in African trypanosomiasis. Study of 7 cases. *Journal of Neuropathology and experimental Neurology*, **15**, 269–287.

Jeffery, H.C. (1974) Sarcosporidiosis in man. *Transactions of the Royal Society of Tropical Medicine and Hygiene*, **68**, 17–29.

Jolly, S.S. & Pallis, C. (1971) Muscular pseudohypertrophy due to cysticercosis. *Journal of the Neurological Sciences*, **12**, 155–162.

Kagan, L.J., Kimball, A.C. & Christian, C.L. (1974) Serologic evidence of toxoplasmosis among patients with polymyositis. *American Journal of Medicine*, **56**, 186–191.

Kean, B.H., & Breslau, R.C. (1964) Cardiac sarcosporidiosis. In *Parasites of the Human Heart*, pp. 74–83 (Grune & Stratton: New York).

Köberle, F. (1968) Chagas' disease and Chagas' syndromes: the pathology of American trypanosomiasis. *Advances in Parasitology*, **6**, 63–116.

Koten, J.W. & de Raadt (1969) Myocarditis in Trypanosoma rhodesiense infections. *Transactions of the Royal Society of Tropical Medicine and Hygiene*, **63**, 485–489.

Liu, C.T. & Roberts, LM. (1965) Sarcosporidiosis in a Bantu woman. *American Journal of Clinical Pathology*, **44**, 639–641.

Lorenzetti, L. (1962) Contributo alla conoscenza dell'echinococcosi primitiva dei muscoli. *Gazzetta internazionale di medicina e chirurgia*, **67**, 2775–2795.

Losos, G.J. & Idede, B.O. (1972) Review of pathology of diseases in domestic and laboratory animals caused by Trypanosoma congolense, T. vivax, T. brucei, T. rhodesiense and T. gambiense. *Veterinary Pathology* (Supplement), **9**, 1–56.

MacArthur, W.P. (1950) *British Encyclopaedia of Medical Practice*, 2nd Edn, Ed. Lord Horder. Vol. 4, p. 111 (Butterworth: London).

McGill, R.J. (1947) Cysticercosis resembling a myopathy. *Indian Journal of Medical Sciences*, **1**, 109–114.

McGill, R.J. (1948) Cysticercosis resembling myopathy. *Lancet*, **2**, 728–730.

McGill, R.J. & Goodbody, R.A. (1957) Sarcosporidiosis in

man with periarteritis nodosa. *British Medical Journal*, **2**, 333–334.

McRobert, G.R. (1944) Somatic taeniasis (solium cysticerosis) *Indian Medical Gazette*, **79**, 399–400.

Marcus, S., & Miller, R.V. (1955) An atypical case of trichinosis with report of electromyographic findings. *Annals of Internal Medicine*, **43**, 615–622.

Markus, M.B., Killick-Kendrick, R. & Garnham, P.C. (1974) The coccidial nature and life-cycle of Sarcocystis. *Journal of Tropical Medicine and Hygiene*, **77**, 248–259.

Mueller, J.F. (1938) Studies on Sparganum mansonoides and Sparganum proliferum. *American Journal of Tropical Medicine*, **18**, 303–328.

Mueller, J.F., Hart, E.P. & Walsh, W.P. (1963) Human sparganosis in the United States. *Journal of Parasitology*, **49**, 294–296.

Muller, R. (1975) *Worms and Disease* (Heinemann: London).

Nichols, R.L. (1956) The etiology of visceral larva migrans. II. Comparative larval morphology of Ascaris lumbricoides, Necator americanus, Strongyloides stercoralis and Ancylostoma caninum. *Journal of Parasitology*, **42**, 363–399.

Ochoa, J. & Pallis, C. (1980) Trichinella thrives in both oxidative and glycoltic human muscle fibres. *Journal of Neurology, Neurosurgery and Psychiatry*, **43**, 281–282.

Orihel, T.C., Gonzales, F. & Beaver, P.C. (1970) Coenurus from neck of Texas woman. *American Journal of Tropical Medicine and Hygiene*, **19**, 255–257.

Pearson, C.M. & Rose, A.S. (1960) The inflammatory disorders of muscle. In *Neuromuscular Disorders (The Motor Unit and its Disorders)*, Eds R.D. Adams, L.M. Eaton & G.M. Shy, Vol. 38, p. 433 (Williams & Wilkins: Baltimore).

Poltera, A.A., Owor, R. & Cox, J.N. (1977) Pathological aspects of human African trypanosomiasis (HAT) in Uganda. A post-mortem survey of 14 cases. *Virchows Archiv A. Pathological Anatomy and Histology*, **373**, 249–265.

Prakash, C. & Kumar, A. (1965) Cysticercosis with taeniasis in a vegetarian. *Journal of Tropical Medicine and Hygiene*, **68**, 100–103.

Priest, R. (1926) A case of extensive somatic dissemination of cysticercus cellulosae in man. *British Medical Journal*, **2**, 471–472.

Rabinowicz, J. (1971) A case of acquired toxoplasmosis in the adult. In *Toxoplasmosis*, Ed. D. Hentsch, pp. 197–219 (Huber: Berne).

Rao, C.M., Sattar, S.A., Gopal, P.S., Reddy, C.C.M. & Sadasivudu, B. (1972) Cysticercosis resembling myopathy. Report of a case. *Indian Journal of Medical Sciences*, **26**, 841–843.

Raper, A.B. & Dockeray, G.D. (1956) Coenurus cysts in man: five cases from East Africa. *Annals of Tropical Medicine and Parasitology*, **50**, 121–128.

Salgaokar, S.V. & Watcha, M.F. (1974) Muscular hypertrophy in cysticercosis: a case report. *Journal of Postgraduate Medicine*, **20**, 148–152.

Samuels, B.S. & Rietschel, R.L. (1976) Polymyositis and toxoplasmosis. *Journal of the American Medical Association*, **235**, 60–61.

Sawhney, B.B., Chopra, J.S., Banerji, A.K. & Wahi, P.L. (1976) Pseudohypertrophic myopathy in cysticercosis. *Neurology (Minneapolis)*, **26**, 270–272.

Schimrigk, K. & Emser, W. (1978) Parasitic myositis by Echinococcus alveolaris. *European Neurology*, **17**, 1–7.

Singh, A. & Jolly, S.S. (1957) Cysticercosis: case report. *Indian Journal of Medical Sciences*, **11**, 98–100.

Slais, J. (1970) The morphology and pathogenicity of bladder worms: Cysticercus cellulosae and Cysticercus bovis (Academia: Prague).

Sprent, J.F.A. (1965) Ascaridoid larva migrans: differentiation of larvae in tissues. *Transactions of the Royal Society of Tropical Medicine and Hygiene*, **59**, 365–366.

Stoll, N.R. (1947) This wormy world. *Journal of Parasitology*, **33**, 1–18.

Templeton, A.C. (1968) Human coenurus infection. A report of 14 cases from Uganda. *Transactions of the Royal Society of Tropical Medicine and Hygiene*, **62**, 251–255.

Templeton, A.C. (1971) Anatomical and geographical location of human coenurus infection. *Tropical and Geographical Medicine*, **23**, 105–108.

Trelles, J.O. & Trelles, L. (1978) In *Handbook of Clinical Neurology*. Eds P.J. Vinken & G.W. Bruyn. Volume 35, pp. 291–320 (North Holland: Amsterdam).

Vigg, B. & Rai, V. (1975) Muscular involvement in cysticercosis with pseudo-hypertrophy of muscles. *Journal of the Association of Physicians of India*, **23**, 593–595.

Vijayan, G.P., Venkataraman, S., Suri, M.L., Seth, H.M. & Hoon, R.S. (1977) Neurological and related manifestations of cysticercosis. *Tropical and Geographical Medicine*, **29**, 271–278.

Wilson, C.V.L.C., Wayte, D.M. & Addae, R.O. (1972) Human coenurosis: the first reported case from Ghana. *Transactions of the Royal Society of Tropical Medicine and Hygiene*, **66**, 611–623.

Wirth, W.A. & Farrow, C.C. (1961) Human sparganosis. Case report and review of the subject. *Journal of the American Medical Association*, **177**, 6–9.

Woodruff, A.W. (1970) Toxocariasis. *British Medical Journal*, **3**, 663–669.

Myasthenia gravis and myasthenic syndromes

HISTORICAL INTRODUCTION

Myasthenia gravis is a specific muscular disease characterised by the development of an abnormal amount of muscular weakness in voluntary muscles following repetitive activation or prolonged tension, with a marked tendency to recovery of motor power after a period of inactivity or lessened muscular tension (Viets, 1958). Some authorities consider that the positive response to anticholinesterase drugs should also be included in the definition. It is important to agree on a definition because the literature contains many reports of cases of doubtful provenance. In particular, the term myasthenia has a less restricted meaning in the French language.

A case described by Thomas Willis (1672) is generally accepted as the first description of the disease. Later landmarks are the papers by Erb, Goldflam and Jolly in the 19th century (see Viets, 1953; Keynes, 1961). The clinical picture was established by the review of Campbell and Bramwell (1900). Laquer and Weigert (1901) first noted a relationship with the thymus gland. Attention was concentrated on the concept of neuromuscular block by the demonstration by Walker (1934) of the beneficial effect of physostigmine. Twenty-five years of electrical and pharmacological studies ignored the pathogenesis until Simpson (1960) suggested that the link between thymus and muscle was immunological, with production of antibody against acetylcholine receptors at the end-plates. The chance finding of Patrick and Lindstrom (1973) that animals used to raise antibody against acetylcholine receptor protein, purified from the electroplaques of the electric eel, became weak with an illness like myasthenia gravis, confirmed the feasibility of the mechanism. Since then this autoimmune hypothesis has been accepted and has become the rationale for modern treatment.

NATURAL HISTORY

Myasthenia gravis affects all races. Estimates of prevalence range from 1 in 50 000 to 1 in 10 000 of the population. Females are affected twice as often as males, the disproportion being 4.5:1 in the first decade, but reversing in later life (Fig. 16.1). The modal age of onset is about 20 years for each sex

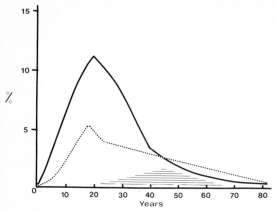

Fig. 16.1   Distribution of age at first myasthenic symptom:

female, no thymoma
male, no thymoma
thymoma, both sexes

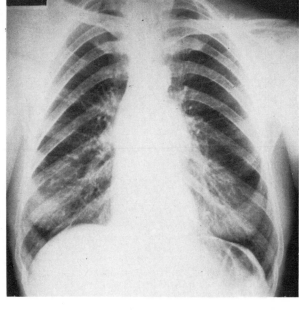

Fig. 16.2   Radiograph of chest showing a thymoma

but because of the different distribution curves the mean age is a little lower for women (26 years) than men (31 years) (Simpson, 1958, 1960). These ages refer to patients without a thymoma. A thymic tumour (Fig. 16.2) is found in 10–15 per cent of cases, about 60 per cent of whom are male (Schwab and Leland, 1953; Simpson, 1958). Myasthenia associated with thymic tumour (benign or malignant) tends to appear at a later age and is rare under the age of 30 years. Muscular weakness is usually severe and difficult to control with any form of treatment, including thymectomy.

If the thymus is not removed the prognosis is worse for women, according to Simpson (1958). The opposite findings, noted by Grob (1958) may have been due to the higher incidence, in females, of the ocular type of myasthenia in his series.

Onset of symptoms is usually insidious but it may be sudden, apparently precipitated by an emotional upset or a febrile illness and less commonly by physical exertion. Symptoms may first appear during pregnancy or in the puerperium. If myasthenia is already present before pregnancy it tends to remit at the end of the first trimester and to relapse soon after childbirth, but this is not invariable. An abnormal response to a relaxant drug used during anaesthesia may be the first indication of myasthenia gravis or of one of the symptomatic myasthenias.

The initial symptom, especially if it is ptosis or diplopia, may subside for months or years, and later remissions may follow relapses. Remissions of more than a month occur in fewer than half of the cases, and usually only in the early years of the illness in patients treated without thymectomy or steroids, becoming less frequent and prolonged as time goes on. More than one long remission is uncommon, and if myasthenic symptoms return after an absence of a year or more and if muscles other than the extraocular are involved, the disease is usually progressive. Relapses are precipitated by the same factors as initial attacks, but additional causes are menstruation, extremes of cold or heat (especially a hot bath or a stuffy atmosphere), inoculation or vaccination and, occasionally, allergy. Bright sunlight may precipitate ptosis and blurred vision, and a few patients declare that it causes generalised weakness.

It is useful to divide the clinical course into three stages (Simpson, 1969a). The clinical state is most labile during the first 5–7 years (Stage 1). Although the most significant remissions occur in Stage 1, most of the deaths directly attributable to the disease occur in this period, particularly during the first year, with a second danger period at 4–7 years, in progressive cases (Simpson, 1958).

To be effective, thymectomy must be carried out in Stage 1 (Simpson, 1958, 1960; Papatestas, Genkins, Horowitz and Kornfeld, 1976). After 10 years (Stage 2) death from myasthenia *per se* rarely occurs, though the patient may be constantly at risk of asphyxiation from inhaled foreign bodies because of the diminished respiratory reserve. Although further progression is unlikely, there is little or no response to thymectomy. Relatively high titres of antireceptor antibody may persist and temporary improvement may be obtained from immunosuppressive treatment or plasma exchange, but the role of the thymus appears to be diminished. After 15 years or more, some cases enter Stage 3, with persisting weakness, higher incidence of muscular atrophy, and a reduced response to anti-cholinesterase drugs. Steroids may still be beneficial in this 'burned out' stage, but thymectomy is of no value and other immunosuppressive regimes have not been assessed. Presumably, permanent morphological changes have occurred at the neuromuscular junctions.

Clinical staging, based on analysis of many cases, is of some value in selecting treatment but it remains difficult to prognosticate for the individual. Grading by 'severity' is less useful. The classification most commonly used (Osserman, 1958) is as follows:

I Ocular myasthenia.

IIA Mild generalised myasthenia with slow progression; no crises; drug-responsive.

IIB Moderate generalised myasthenia; severe skeletal and bulbar involvement, but no crises; drug response is less satisfactory.

III Acute fulminating myasthenia; rapid progression of severe symptoms with respiratory crises and poor drug response; high incidence of thymoma; high mortality.

IV Late severe myasthenia; same as III, but takes 2 years to progress from Classes I or II; crises; high mortality.

These grades, reputed to be a progressive series from I, with good prognosis, to II and IV with poor prognosis, do not represent either discrete types or stages in a progression. It is a tautology to say that purely ocular myasthenia is 'safe' whereas weakness of respiratory muscles in a rapidly deteriorating disorder is dangerous to life. The future course cannot be predicted, although it is widely accepted that it is likely to be benign if signs remain confined to the extraocular muscles for two years. Grob (1953) and Ferguson, Hutchinson and Liversedge (1955) report this type of history in 20–30 per cent of cases, but it has been rare in my experience, except in males. Conversely, the prognosis is worse (with early death) if a thymoma is present, despite initial benefit from thymectomy.

SYMPTOMS AND SIGNS

The characteristic feature of myasthenia gravis is the variability in the strength of the affected muscles, rather than a generalised tiredness. It varies from day to day and even from hour to hour, classically increasing towards the evening. Surprisingly, few patients comment on this until questioned about it. It is not invariable: many patients are weakest on first rising. Short-term weakness is often due to physical exertion but the emotional state is an important determinant. Affected muscles lose further strength if contraction is maintained or repeated (so-called 'pathological fatiguability'). The contracting muscle may lengthen gradually if it is supporting a load, or a coarse tremor develops with increasing 'rest periods' until the attempt to sustain the contraction ceases. In the eye muscles this may cause a pseudonystagmus. Gradual 'fatigue' is not always seen and failure of contraction may be sudden, suggesting a neurotic weakness to the inexperienced. Recovery after rest is often incomplete, even with optimal dosage of anticholinesterases, especially in Stage 2. In Stage 3, there may be weakness which cannot be reversed with anticholinesterase drugs, and muscular atrophy is not uncommon, especially in males (Simpson, 1958). The most commonly affected muscles are the extraocular muscles, triceps brachii, quadriceps femoris, and the tongue. Atrophy of the tongue is curiously selective, giving rise to a triple longitudinal furrowing (Fig. 16.3) which, though rare, is very characteristic of myasthenia gravis (Wilson, 1954). It appears to have been described first by Buzzard in 1905.

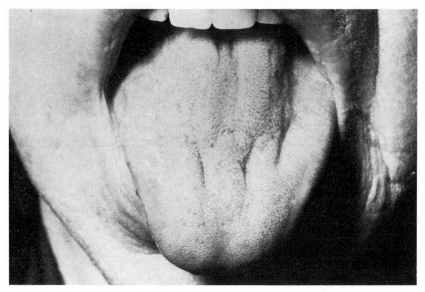

Fig. 16.3   The triple furrowed tongue (there may be four furrows)

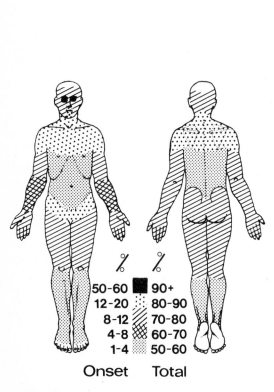

Fig. 16.4   Percentage of cases in which various muscle groups are affected at the onset (left of key) and at some time during the illness (right of key)

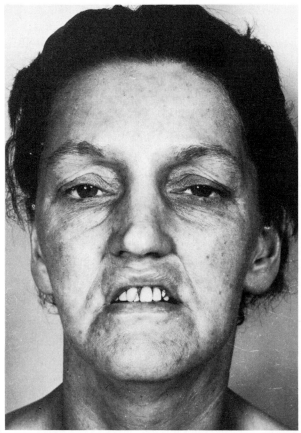

Fig. 16.5   The myasthenic 'snarl' and ptosis

The symptoms associated with weakness of ocular, facial, and other muscles are readily appreciated. The distribution of clinically weak muscles in a large series of cases is shown in Figure 16.4, which also shows that the probability of weakness starting in a muscle group matches its overall probability. Without going into all possible symptoms and signs, attention is drawn to the early and frequent involvement of the extraocular muscles and levatores palpebrarum (more than 90 per cent of cases), usually associated with weakness of orbiculares oculorum, an almost diagnostic combination. The facies is characteristic (Fig. 16.5). Speech and chewing weakness, difficulty in holding up the head, and proximal limb weakness (more in the upper than the lower limbs) are typical. Fortunately, the chest muscles and diaphragm are not involved until later. Nevertheless, any muscle or part of a muscle may be affected and the distribution is commonly asymmetrical. When the history or physical examination suggests the possibility of myasthenia gravis, the most commonly affected muscles should be subjected to a fatigue test and the response to edrophonium assessed. Some appropriate tests for use in doubtful cases are described below, but in most instances an appropriate performance test is readily improvised during the consultation.

Tendon reflexes are surprisingly brisk and clonus may be present (but with a flexor plantar response). If a reflex is elicited repetitively, the jerk may decrease progressively until it disappears. Persistent absence of many tendon reflexes should suggest that weakness is due to carcinomatous myasthenia rather than to myasthenia gravis, but localised absence may be due to muscular atrophy. The differential diagnosis from the carcinomatous syndrome may be difficult because, in Stage 3, responsiveness to anticholinesterases is lost and some patients (usually men) find that muscular power is increased by exercise. Their muscles may show an incrementing response to tetanisation (Simpson, 1966a; Schwartz and Stålberg, 1975a and b).

Abnormalities of sensation

Normal sensation is the rule, though cases of myasthenia gravis have been reported with un-explained sensory loss, especially transitory trigeminal anaesthesia. Paraesthesiae of hands, thighs or face (Harvey, 1948; Simpson, 1960) and the common sensation of 'stiffness' probably have a mechanical explanation. Patients may complain of pain in weak muscles, especially in the neck, the back, and around the eyes. This is normally attributable to the extra effort required to maintain posture, but sometimes there appears to be a true myositis. Sudden substernal ache at the onset of the disease is an occasional and unexplained symptom.

Disorders of other organs

Disorders of the thyroid gland (including subclinical disease indicated by serum antibody studies) are more frequent in a myasthenic population but only a minority have abnormal thyroid function tests, and these patients are as commonly hypothyroid as hyperthyroid (Simpson, 1966b). Millikan and Haines (1953) have found that the incidence of hyperthyroidism before, during, or after detectable myasthenia gravis is about 5 per cent. If all thyroid disorders are added, the incidence may be as high as 9 per cent in males and 18 per cent in females (Simpson, 1958; Downes, Greenwood and Wray, 1966). Many of these patients have thyrotoxic symptoms or signs for only a few months and these may precede myasthenic symptoms by many years. Thyrotoxic symptoms may be subsiding when myasthenia appears and *vice versa*. In a limited period of observation this may lead to the conclusion that the disorders have a 'see-saw' relationship to each other (McEachern and Parnell, 1948).

It was clearly shown by Engel (1961) that myasthenia could not be caused by hyperthyroidism. The linkage between them is probably genetic and immunological rather than hormonal, and involves all non-tumour diseases of the thyroid including non-toxic goitre (Rowland, Hoefer, Aranow and Merritt, 1956; Simpson, 1958, 1968; Bundey, Doniach and Soothill, 1972), spontaneous myxoedema (Feinberg, Underdahl and Eaton, 1957; Sahay, Blendis and Greene, 1965), and Hashimoto's disease (Simpson, 1960, 1964, 1966c; Becker, Titus, McConahey and Woolner, 1964). Many myasthenics resemble thyrotoxic patients in other ways. Slight exophthalmos and thickening of the upper eyelids are common (Simpson, 1960). The 'lid twitch sign' (transient upward overshoot of the upper eyelid on abruptly looking upwards, followed by a slower return to ptosis) described by Cogan (1965) is readily distinguished from thyrotoxic lid-lag. Many patients complain of excessive sweating, even without taking anticholinesterase drugs (Simpson, 1960; Pirskanen, 1976). There may also be a genetic as well as an immunological linkage between myasthenia gravis and other diseases. Primary adrenal insufficiency of autoimmune type is rare (Bosch, Reith and Granner, 1978). An arthropathy resembling rheumatoid arthritis or ankylosing spondylitis is not uncommon in myasthenics or their relatives (Simpson, 1960, 1966c; Oosterhuis, 1964; Namba and Grob, 1970).

Aplastic anaemia associated with a thymic tumour is rare in myasthenic patients (Green, 1958; Simpson, 1960). A more common association is pernicious anaemia (Simpson, 1960, 1964, 1966c) which has a genetic linkage to myasthenia gravis (Simpson, 1976). Other immunological disorders occasionally associated (individually and familially) with myasthenia are systemic lupus erythematosus (Harvey, Shulman, Tumulty, Cowley, and Schoenrich, 1954; Simpson, 1960; Alarcón-Segovia, Galbraith, Maldonado and Howard, 1963; Wolf and Barrows, 1966), pemphigus vulgaris (Wolf, Rowland, Schotland, McKinney, Hoefer and Aranow, 1966; Beutner, Chorzelski, Hale and Hausmanowa-Petrusewicz, 1968; Hausmanowa-Petrusewicz, Chorzelski and Strugalska, 1969; Vetters, Saikia, Wood and Simpson, 1973), ulcerative colitis (Osserman, 1958; Alarcón-Segovia et al., 1963), sarcoidosis (Simpson, 1960; Downes et al., 1966), Sjogren's disease (Downes et al., 1966; Simpson, 1966c; Wolf et al., 1966), and hepatitis (Simpson, 1960; Whitingham, Mackay and Kiss, 1970).

Associated disorders which probably have an immunological basis or cause immunodeficiency are acrocyanosis, haemolytic anaemia, nephritis (Simpson, 1960; Oosterhuis, 1964), reticuloses (Alter and Osnato, 1930; Symmers, 1932; Simpson, 1960; Cohen and Waxman, 1967), diabetes mellitus (Simpson, 1960), and herpes zoster (Simpson, unpublished).

Associated disorders which are relatively more common in myasthenics than those listed above, but in which no immunological pathology has yet been identified, are epilepsy (Hoefer, Aranow and Rowland, 1958; Simpson, 1960) and psychosis (Hayman, 1941; Simpson, 1960; Storm-Mathisen, 1961). Emotional disturbances are common (Brolley and Hollender, 1955; Meyer, 1966). A possible predisposition to cancer is discussed on p. 616.

Neonatal myasthenia

About one in seven live-born children of myasthenic mothers shows evidence of myasthenia at birth and, if the affected child survives, there is complete recovery in 1–12 weeks (mean 18 days) without later relapse. The literature has been reviewed by Namba, Brown and Grob (1970). There is no correlation between the severity of the infant's symptoms and the duration of the mother's illness or the severity of the mother's myasthenia during pregnancy. It is extremely rare for a myasthenic mother to have more than one affected child. Previous thymectomy does not remove the possibility that the baby will be myasthenic, but the transient nature of neonatal myasthenia suggests that the child is affected by a factor transmitted from the mother. The hypothesis that this is an anti-ACh receptor antibody (Simpson, 1960) has been confirmed (Lindstrom, Seybold, Lennon, Whittingham and Duane, 1976b).

Congenital myasthenia

A myasthenic syndrome may be apparent in the new-born child of a mother without myasthenia, and may then persist throughout life (Levin, 1949; Millichap and Dodge, 1960). It is commonly familial and is reported to have a male predominance (Namba, Brunner, Brown, Mugurama and Grob, 1971a; Bundey, 1972), although this has not been my experience. Unlike neonatal myasthenia, in this syndrome the fetal movements are weak and there is striking symmetry of the muscles involved. On these grounds, plus the absence of remissions and a tendency to improve slowly after the age of 6–10 years, Levin (1949) concluded that congenital myasthenia begins prenatally and differs from neonatal myasthenia. It may be a maturation failure, causing persistence of the low safety factor for neuromuscular transmission which is found in normal infants (Churchill-Davidson and Wise, 1963). Response to anticholinesterase drugs is usually described as 'disappointing' and thymectomy rarely causes improvement (Seybold, Howard, Duane, Payne and Harrison, 1971; Whiteley, Schwartz, Sachs and Swash, 1976). It is difficult to decide whether it arrests the disease, because the natural history is benign. Thymic histology is normal (McLean and McKone, 1973; Vetters and Simpson, 1974; Whiteley et al., 1976). Newsom Davis, Pinching, Vincent and Wilson (1978) found no rise in anti-AChR antibody titre in a 25-year-old patient with congenital myasthenia, who previously had been shown to have no clinical improvement with plasmapheresis (Pinching, Peters and Newsom Davis, 1976). This has also been my experience.

Children with congenital myasthenia commonly have low blood levels of IgA (Bundey et al., 1972; Behan, Simpson and Behan, 1976). Two sisters with congenital myasthenia reported by Dick, Behan, Simpson and Durward (1974) had HLA–B8 haplotypes, as in most cases of later-onset myasthenia gravis, but two affected male siblings reported by Whiteley et al. (1976) had different haplotypes, neither being HLA–A1–B8–DW3. Clearly, there is justification for the growing belief that 'congenital myasthenia' is a different disease.

GENETIC FACTORS

Disregarding the debatable status of congenital myasthenia, there is now clear evidence for a genetic factor in myasthenia gravis. Although a genetic study by Jacob, Clack and Emery (1968) showed no secondary cases of myasthenia gravis in 448 relatives of 70 myasthenic patients, and Herrmann (1971) was unable to establish a definite genetic mechanism in his study of families with more than one case of myasthenia gravis, Simpson (1960, 1968) suggested that a genetic factor could have variable expression, accounting for the familial linkage with thyroid disease, arthropathy,

pernicious anaemia and diabetes mellitus (p. 590). Jacob et al. (1968) found no association between myasthenia gravis and the ABO and Rhesus blood groups or with secretor status or the ability to taste phenylthiocarbamide (PTC). Bundey (1972) recognised an early-onset form of childhood myasthenia with autosomal recessive inheritance of the trait. Her study gave limited support to the concept of alternative gene expression.

Linkage with human histocompatibility antigens, reported in the last edition of this book, has been confirmed in many countries (Pirskanen, Tiilikainen and Hokkanen, 1972; Behan, Simpson and Dick, 1973; Fritze, Herrmann, Smith and Walford, 1973; Dick et al., 1974; Feltkamp, van den Berg-Loonen, Nijenhuis, Engelfriet, van Rossum, van Loghem and Oosterhuis, 1974; Pirskanen, 1976). There is a frequent association with HLA–A1–B8–DW3 haplotypes, but it is clear that the association is not a direct one and not obligatory (Dick et al., 1974; Pirskanen, 1976). An increased frequency of HLA–A2 or –A3 in patients with thymoma, reported by Feltkamp et al. (1974) and Fritze, Herrmann, Naeim, Smith and Walford (1974) was not noted by Dick et al. (1974) or by Pirskanen (1976). Another histocompatibility antigen system, such as the LD antigens (Kaakinen, Pirskanen and Tiilikainen, 1975) situated near the SD loci bearing HL–A genes, may exhibit a stronger association with myasthenia gravis and with autoimmune disorders; and both the SD and LD gene loci are close to some loci controlling immunological responsiveness (Ir genes). Genetic factors probably constitute risk factors for autoimmune diseases (Adams (1977) suggests V genes). The relative scarcity of familial cases of myasthenia gravis (3.4 per cent according to Namba et al. 1971a; 7.2 per cent in Finland–Pirskanen, 1977) and involvement of only one of monozygotic twins (Simpson, 1960, 1965; Namba, Shapiro, Brunner and Grob, 1971b) indicate that many aetiological factors may be involved.

CLINICAL CHEMISTRY

There are no consistent changes in blood chemistry in myasthenia gravis. Abnormalities of glucose tolerance (Cohen and King, 1932; Simpson, 1960, 1966b; Frenkel, 1963), adrenocortical hypofunction (Simpson, 1966b; Bosch et al., 1978) and hyper- and hypothyroid function in the absence of clinical endocrinopathies (Simpson, 1966b, 1968) are likely to be due to genetic and/or autoimmune linkage. Diminished pregnanediol excretion (Schrire, 1959) has not been confirmed (Simpson, 1966b).

Hypergammaglobulinaemia occurs in cases associated with other autoimmune diseases (Simpson 1960, 1966b) or with thymoma (Oosterhuis, van der Geld, Feltkamp and Peetoom, 1964) and some of these patients have a raised erythrocyte sedimentation rate (ESR); however, the ESR usually is normal. Isolated instances of monoclonal gammopathy have been described (Rowland, Osserman, Scharfman, Balsam and Ball, 1969). Hypogammaglobulinaemia sometimes occurs (Thévenard and Mende, 1955; Simpson, 1966b) and may be associated with a thymoma (Te Velde, Huber and van der Slikke, 1966; Cohen and Waxman, 1967).

Depressed levels of IgA were found in juvenile-onset myasthenia by Bundey et al. (1972); Simpson, Behan and Dick (1976) found a selective decrease in IgA in 10 of 50 myasthenic patients, which decrease was not influenced by thymectomy. The lowest levels were in three patients with congenital myasthenia who had undergone thymectomy. Bramis, Sloane, Papatestas, Genkins and Aufses (1976) confirmed that serum IgA concentration may be subnormal in myasthenic patients. In their series the lowest concentrations were associated with thymomas or other neoplasms. Decreased IgA concentrations tended to be associated with many or prominent germinal centres in the thymus and levels increased slowly after thymectomy. There were no congenital cases in the series of Lisak and Zweiman (1975) who found normal IgA levels in 19 myasthenic patients. These workers reported a slight but significant depression of the mean IgM level (raised in some subjects, especially with a thymoma). Serum IgG tended to be above normal. There was no consistent pattern and the immuno-globulin levels were not correlated with the clinical state.

Nastuk, Plescia and Osserman (1960) measured serum complement levels serially in myasthenic patients and stated that they were lower during active disease, rising to normal or super-normal levels in remission. Plescia, Segovia and Strampp (1966) found reduced levels of C2 and C4 and inhibitors to these components. Simpson et al. (1976) found no abnormality of Cl_q, C3, C4, C7 and C3 proactivator. They also measured C3 conversion products with C3 activator levels, and CH50 units. All were normal although examined in active and remittent cases. Behan and Behan (1979) re-examined this material when Engel, Lambert and Howard (1977a) demonstrated localisation of IgG and C3 at motor end-plates. Depression of C4 component was found in 34 per cent of myasthenic patients and 29 per cent had circulating immune complexes. The greatest immunological abnormalities were found in patients with mild disease.

Elevated globulin levels in the cerebrospinal fluid (CSF) of 10 patients were recorded by Simpson (1960, 1966b), who reviewed previous isolated reports and concluded that there was associated disease which may be of immunological type: however, recent evidence that anti-ACh receptor antibody may be present in the CSF Lefvert and Pirskanen, 1977) indicates the necessity for re-assessment.

IMMUNOLOGICAL STUDIES

The hypothesis by Simpson (1960) that a thymus-controlled lymphocyte-derived antibody against ACh receptor could be the proximate cause of myasthenia gravis could not be confirmed by the contemporary immunofluorescence techniques (McFarlin, Engel, and Strauss, 1966): however, using high-resolution electron microscopy, Rash, Albuquerque, Hudson, Mayer and Setterfield (1976) found material ('fuzzy coats'), in the region of the receptors in the neuromuscular junction, which resembled IgG in its configuration and dimensions. The presence of IgG and of the C3 component of complement at the postsynaptic membranes of human myasthenic neuromuscular junctions was convincingly demonstrated by Engel et al. (1977a and b) by an immunoperoxidase method. These authors have proposed that subsequent sequential activation of C5–C9 would complete the attack phase of the complement reaction sequence and set the stage for lytic destruction of the postsynaptic membrane. It remains possible that antibody or immune complex may block receptors competitively. The rapid beneficial dffect of plasma exchange (p. 608) might support this concept but not necessarily so, because the regeneration of receptors is probably very rapid (Devreotes and Fambrough, 1975) and there is usually a time lag of two days or more before muscle power is restored (Newsom Davis *et al.*, 1978). Passive transfer of myasthenic immune complexes would help to differentiate between the three main possibilities: i) lysis of postsynaptic membrane, ii) immunopharmacological blockade, and iii) IgG-induced modulation of AChR. Passive transfer of myasthenia from man to mouse by human myasthenic serum has been obtained by Toyka, Drachman, Pestronk and Kao (1975) but not by Rees, Behan, Behan and Simpson (1977). It may be necessary to have previous reduction of the transmission safety factor in order to demonstrate the passive transfer (Stahlberg, Mattson, Uddgard, Heilbronn, Hammarström, Smith, Lefvert, Persson and Matell, 1978) or to use animals of specific H2 haplotype (Fuchs, Nevo, Tarrab-Hazdai and Yaar, 1976). Tissue culture experiments suggest that receptor blockade (Drachman, Kao, Angus and Murphy, 1977) and accelerated degradation of ACh receptors (Anwyl, Appel and Narahashi, 1977; Kao and Drachman, 1977b) may both be involved. Synthesis of AChR appears not to be affected by immunoglobulin from myasthenic patients (Drachman, 1978).

At the time of writing, serum antibody acting directly on acetylcholine receptor sites has not been identified by standard immunological techniques, but its existence is strongly indicated by a number of methods demonstrating the presence in myasthenic serum of an IgG which will prevent access of α-bungarotoxins (α-Bgtx) to nicotinic receptors, indicating high affinity of the immunoglobulin for receptor or closely adjacent material. Early assays, based on measuring the inhibition of binding of α-Bgtx to extrajunctional receptors of denervated rat muscle (Almon, Andrew and Appel, 1974), or to junctional receptors of human muscle (Bender, Ringel, Engel, Daniels and Vogel, 1975), were of low sensitivity. Indirect evidence of an antibody in myasthenic serum

which cross-reacts with AChR from electrogenic tissue of *Torpedo californica* is provided by complement fixation (Aharonov, Tarrab-Hazdai, Abramsky and Fuchs, 1975a).

More sensitive assays are based on the binding of antibody to AChR linked to isotope-labelled α-Bgtx. The antibody-AChR-α-Bgtx complexes are then precipitated, together with carrier immunoglobulin, by adding anti-immunoglobulin and the radioactivity of the resulting pellet is measured (Appel, Almon and Levy, 1975; Lindstrom, 1977). The globulin detected by this method blocks the access of α-Bgtx to the AChR site by binding the receptor complex at a site different from, but in close proximity to, the acetylcholine site which, apparently, is not the target for the antibody. In some reports (Lindstrom *et al.*, 1976b) the titre of antibody measured by this radioimmunoassay correlates reasonably well with the severity of the disease, but only if AChR from human muscle is used. In other reports (Lefvert, Bergström, Matell, Osterman and Pirskanen, 1978; Newsom Davis *et al.*, 1978) the correlation is rather low. No significant titre of this antibody (provisionally termed the receptor antibody) is found in serum from congenital myasthenia (Newsom Davis *et al.*, 1978). The antibody has been detected in sera from infants with neonatal myasthenia, as well as from their mothers (Lindstrom *et al.*, 1976b; Keesey, Lindström, Cokely and Herrman, 1977; Lefvert *et al.*, 1978), but some infants with receptor antibodies have no detectable weakness, possibly because of receptor antigenic difference between mother and child (Simpson, 1960; Keesey *et al.*, 1977). Lefvert *et al.* (1978) have suggested that the IgG antibody detected by radioimmunoassay may not be a primary cause of the disease, because it is sometimes preceded by IgM antibodies in the early stages of myasthenia.

The titre of IgG antibody against AChR is higher in myasthenia gravis associated with thymoma and falls with all the procedures listed later as immunosuppressive (p. 605). It is commonly present in the CSF (Lefvert and Pirskanen, 1977).

Antimyosin antibodies are found in sera from some myasthenics, the titre being highest in those with a thymoma (Strauss, Seegal, Hsu Burkholder, Nastuk and Osserman, 1960; Beutner, Witebsky, Ricken and Adler, 1962; van der Geld,

Feltkamp, and Oosterhuis, 1964; Djanian, Beutner and Witebsky, 1964). Using an immunofluorescence technique, binding of antibody to A-bands of skeletal muscle is seen only with myasthenic sera and is highly correlated with presence of a thymoma (Vetters, 1965). The A-band antibody also reacts with myoid cells in the thymus (Feltkamp-Vroom, 1966). Other antibodies commonly found in sera from myasthenic patients are antinuclear factor, antithyroid and antigastric substances. Rheumatoid factor may also be present in the blood. It does not usually correlate closely with a history of arthritis (Simpson, 1964, 1966b), but may do so (Aarli, Milde and Thunold, 1975). Patients with pemphigus vulgaris have antiepithelial antibody (Noguchi and Nishitani, 1976). Specific antineuronal and antispermatogonia nuclear antibodies in sera of patients with myasthenia gravis have been reported by Martin, Herr, Wanamaker and Kornguth (1974). Clearly, there is a wide spectrum of autoantibodies and they are also more frequent in sera from relatives of myasthenics (Feltkamp et al., 1974), supporting the suggestion of genetic predisposition to autoimmune diseases which may include myasthenia gravis when anti-AChR antibody titre is raised. It is premature to attribute a pathogenetic role to the 'receptor antibody', although changes in titre closely follow the clinical severity of myasthenia and the passive transfer studies described above are impressive.

There is also uncertainty about the significance of cell-mediated immunity. Normal numbers of thymus-dependent (T) cells and thymus-independent (B) lymphocytes are found in peripheral blood of myasthenic patients (Abdou, Lisak, Zweiman, Abramson and Penn, 1974; Sandilands, Gray, Cooney, Anderson, Simpson and Behan, 1975), though lymphocyte subpopulations may differ (Aarli, Heimann, Matre, Thunold and Tönder, 1979). Experiments showing inhibition of leucocyte migration by crude skeletal muscle and myosin-containing fractions, described by a number of workers, were not well controlled and these results could have been caused by differing histocompatibility antigens. Other workers, using different in vitro methods, have shown abnormal lymphocyte proliferation or transformation responses to crude muscle antigen

in myasthenic patients. The extensive literature was reviewed by Behan, Behan and Simpson (1975) who concluded that the cellular reactions demonstrated up to that time are not pathogenic, though impaired T-cell function is present. A mixed leucocyte reaction occurs when thymic cells from patients with myasthenia are cultured in the presence of autologous peripheral blood lymphocytes (Abdou et al., 1974). It must be concluded that abnormalities of numbers, distribution or function of lymphocytes from myasthenic patients are not striking. Ito, Miledi, Vincent and Newsom Davis (1978) point out that lymphocyte transformation in response to fish AChR is not restricted to the cells involved in cell-mediated immunity (antibody-producing cells can also be transformed), and they consider that it would be a mistake to assume that these results necessarily implicate a cellular attack on the end-plate as the cause of the defect in myasthenia gravis. Nevertheless, Abramsky, Aharonov, Webb and Fuchs (1975) and Richman, Patrick and Arnason (1976) have demonstrated in vitro cellular immunity to electroplaque AChR, and there appears to be a definite role for cell-mediated immunity in experimental autoimmune myasthenia gravis.

Experimental autoimmune myasthenia gravis

The affinity of labelled α-Bgtx for acetylcholine receptor provided a method for separating AChR from other proteins of the electric organ of Electrophorus electricus when the toxin was fixed in a chromatography column. To demonstrate that the toxin-binding protein was AChR, Patrick and Lindstrom (1973) raised antibody to it which blocked the response of the electroplaques to carbachol. The AChR, identified and isolated in this way, was injected into rabbits which subsequently became weak and died of a disorder resembling human myasthenia gravis. These findings have been confirmed and extended to other species (Heilbronn, Mattson, Stalberg and Hilton-Brown, 1975; Tarrab-Hazdai, Aharonov, Silman, Fuchs and Abramsky, 1975b). This experimental autoimmune myasthenia gravis (EAMG) is a good model, especially in the monkey (Tarrab-Hazdai et al., 1975b), giving clinical features, including ptosis, which are reversible with edrophonium. Rabbits and monkeys show more severe weakness than guinea pigs and rats, many of which show the electrical and histological changes of EAMG but no clinical weakness. This may be caused by species differences in the safety factor for neuromuscular transmission. As in human myasthenia gravis, strain differences are also important (Fuchs *et al.*, 1976).

The morphological and electrophysiological changes at the neuromuscular junction in the chronic phase of EAMG in the rat closely resemble those of human myasthenia gravis (Engel, Tsujihata, Lindstrom and Lennon, 1976b). Differences which are seen in the acute phase of EAMG but are not observed in the human disease are separation of the postsynaptic region from the muscle fibre, phagocytosis of degenerating postsynaptic folds by macrophages, and an inflammatory reaction confined to those regions of the muscle where the end-plates are located. As the acute phase may be eliminated by omission of pertussis adjuvant from the immunogen (Lindstrom, 1978) it may not be a response to AChR.

The successful production of EAMG depends on there being a certain amount of interspecies cross-reactivity of AChR: at first, the sera of animals immunised with electroplaque AChR have antibodies recognising the electric organ in much higher concentration than that of antibodies recognising the AChR of the animal's muscle. At a later stage of the immune response the absolute amount of antibody against recipient AChR is high (Lindstrom, Engel, Seybold, Lennon and Lambert, 1976a) suggesting true autoimmunity. Passive transfer of EAMG by lymph node cells in the guinea pig (Tarrab-Hazdai, Aharonov, Abramsky, Yaar and Fuchs, 1975a) and rat (Lennon, Lindstrom and Seybold, 1976), and by γ-globulin in the rat (Lindstrom *et al.*, 1976b) supports the theory that the proximate mechanism of myasthenia is autoimmune. But the human disease does not result from inoculation of foreign AChR and present evidence indicates that syngeneic AChR released from damaged muscle does not evoke an antibody response in the human or rat (Lindstrom *et al.*, 1976b). It has been suggested that a source of antibody-stimulating AChR may be the myoid cells of the thymus. Myoid cells have long been

known to cross-react with antimyosin antibody (van der Geld and Strauss, 1966) and they have been shown by Kao and Drachman (1977a) to have surface ACh receptors which may be separate but immunologically related target organs in myasthenia gravis (Aharanov, Tarrab-Hazdai, Abramsky, and Fuchs, 1975b). Goldstein and Whittingham (1966) reported a myasthenic syndrome in guinea pigs inoculated with calf thymus, muscle, or lymph node and attributed this to 'autoimmune thymitis' with liberation from the thymus of a neuromuscular blocking substance. Other workers did not confirm their findings (e.g. Vetters, Simpson and Folkarde, 1969). The conflicting experimental results and conclusions are critically reviewed by Simpson (1978). The Goldstein hypothesis would make it difficult to account for myasthenia originating after thymectomy, or would require *ad hoc* explanations for associated autoimmune disorders if the primary source of autoantigen were the thymic myoid cell.

THYMUS GLAND

There are pathological changes in 70–80 per cent of patients with myasthenia gravis. The most consistent finding is lymphoid hyperplasia of cortex and medulla with T lymphocytes in both parts, not mainly in the cortex as in normal subjects (Aarli *et al.*, 1979). It is commonly associated with numerous germinal centres in the medulla (Castleman and Norris, 1949) (Fig. 16.6). The gland is not involuted, as suggested by earlier observers. Germinal centres are characteristic of a number of autoimmune disorders and not unique to myasthenia gravis. Their significance is uncertain because the prevalence of germinal centres in the thymus bears no clear relationship to the duration or severity of the disease, or to the clinical response to thymectomy (Vetters and Simpson, 1974). Preponderance of B cells in thymic germinal centres (Abdou *et al.*, 1974) has been interpreted as an expression of antibody formation against inappropriate T-cell clones, or excess antibody production attributable to lack of suppressor cells. Papatestas *et al.* (1976) found lower counts of peripheral blood lymphocytes in patients with many germinal centres and have suggested

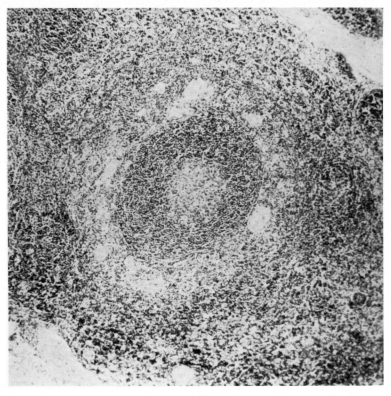

Fig. 16.6   Germinal centre in thymus, H & E, ×42

that the latter may indicate a state of immunosuppression. A. L. Goldstein, Thurman, Cohen and Rossio (1976) have suggested that a thymic hormone, thymosin, influences precursor T cells, possibly via an adenylate cyclase-dependent process, and that genetic factors and/or viral infection may lead to a deficiency of suppressor or regulatory T cells which in turn removes the mechanisms controlling B cell function (including formation of autoantibodies). The source of thymosin is unknown; it would be premature to identify it with the granules described in the thymus by Vetters and MacAdam (1972, 1973). The concept of the role of the thymus in autoimmune disease is more plausible than the alternative that the thymus is itself a target for immunological attack ('thymitis') with consequent release of a neuromuscular blocking substance, as in the theories of Strauss, Smith, Cage, van der Geld, McFarlin and Barlow (1966) and G. Goldstein (Goldstein and Whittingham, 1966). (The 'thymin' of G. Goldstein must not be confused

with the 'thymosin' of A. L. Goldstein). Alternatively, many have considered that myoid cells which can be demonstrated in the thymus may induce B cells which are abnormally reactive to their ACh antigen (*vide infra*).

Whatever the mechanism, there is general agreement that anti-AChR and antimyosin antibody titres are higher in the presence of a thymoma and that this correlates with clinical severity. A thymoma is usually encapsulated and may be cystic and calcified, but it is sometimes malignant. Invasiveness is limited, spread being usually confined to the thorax and occasionally to the lymph nodes of the neck. An account of the histological types described has been given by Iverson (1956). The thymoma which occurs in myasthenia gravis shows a predominance of lymphocytes and epithelial cells which may have an acinar structure. The spindle-celled thymoma has no special association with myasthenia gravis. Indeed, the benign neoplasm may be an associated disorder, the important tissue being the adjacent

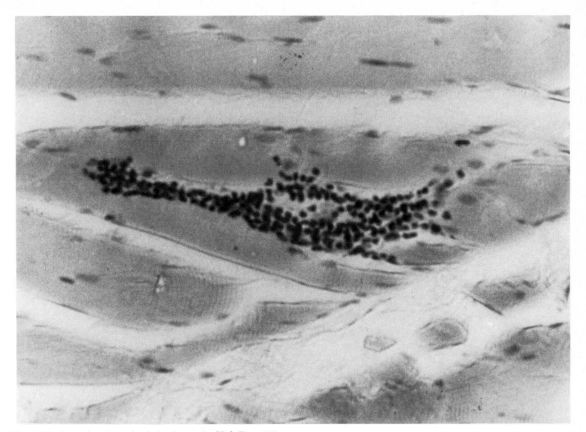

Fig. 16.7   Lymphorrhage in skeletal muscle, H & E, ×189

non-tumour thymus which commonly contains germinal centres (Castleman, 1955).

MUSCLE AND NERVE

Despite frequent statements in the past that myasthenia gravis is a disease without morbid anatomy, the lymphocyte infiltrations of muscle described by Weigert (1901) and termed lymphorrhages (Fig. 16.7) by Buzzard (1905) have been found repeatedly in such cases, but not invariably. According to Oosterhuis and Bethlem (1973) they are seen particularly in patients with a thymoma. On rare occasions they may occur at the end-plates (Wiesendanger and D'Alessandsi, 1963). Buzzard (1905) also reported degenerative changes of muscle fibres which were re-investigated and classified by Russell (1953). These changes were regarded as non-specific. Simpson (1960) sug-

gested that they may indicate cell-mediated immunological damage, a concept supported by Rule and Kornfeld (1971).

In some muscles of a number of patients, denervation atrophy has been reported, the criteria being groups of small muscle fibres with angular cross-sectional contours, and 'target' fibres (Fenichel and Shy, 1963; Brody and Engel, 1964; Oosterhuis and Bethlem, 1973, and others). The histochemical pattern is usually normal but type 2 fibre atrophy is not uncommon (Brooke and Engel, 1969). These changes may not be uniquely associated with denervation due to presynaptic pathology: Coërs and Telerman-Toppet (1976) rarely found the increased terminal innervation ratio which they regard as a sensitive index of denervation with re-innervation.

The peripheral nerve trunks are histologically normal in human myasthenia gravis (Oosterhuis and Bethlem, 1973) and in EAMG (Hill, Lind-

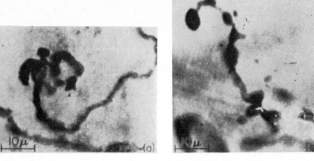

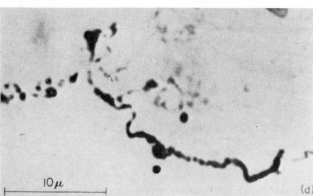

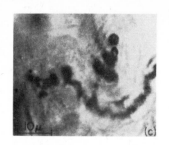

Fig. 16.8 Methylene blue preparations of human motor nerve terminals. (a) Normal end-plate. (b) Elongated end plate from a case of myasthenia gravis. (c) Motor end-plate with shrunken terminal expansions from a case of myasthenia gravis resistant to neostigmine. (d) Axonal sprout with diminutive ending in a case of myasthenia gravis with prominent lymphorrhages—myositic response, previously termed 'dystrophic' (Simpson 1969, by courtesy of the late Dr A.L. Woolf)

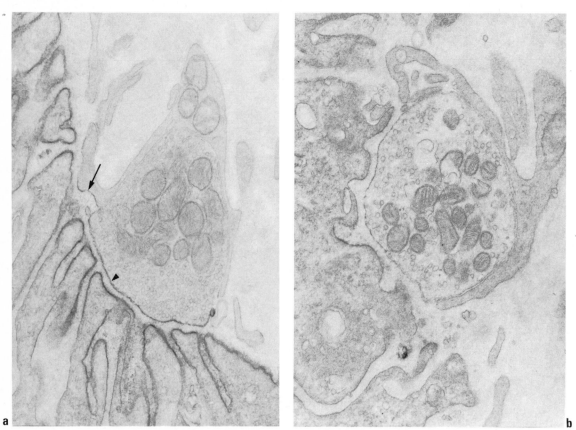

Fig. 16.9 End-plate regions of external intercostal muscles. Acetylcholine receptor sites are stained by α-Bgtx conjugated to horseradish peroxidase, ×22 300 In (a), from a normal subject, AChR is associated with terminal expansions and deeper surfaces of the postsynaptic folds; the presynaptic membrane (arrowhead) stained by leaching, and Schwann's cell membrane (arrow) facing crest of folds are lightly stained. In (b), from a case of moderately severe myasthenia gravis, the postsynaptic regions are simplified, only segments of it react for AChR (Engel, Lindstrom, Lambert and Lennon, 1977b)

strom, Lennon and Dyck, 1977). Collateral sprouting, a hallmark of conventional denervation, is rare in myasthenia gravis and occurs mainly in older patients (Coërs, Telerman-Toppet and Gérard, 1973). By intravital staining with methylene blue, Coërs and Desmedt (1959) demonstrated two types of abnormality of the terminal arborisation of motor nerves (Fig. 16.8), a 'dystrophic' type, considered to be a reaction to muscle fibre degeneration, and a 'dysplastic' type highly characteristic of myasthenia gravis. In the latter there are few terminal knobs and these are arranged serially along a scanty number of terminal branches ending in a remarkably elongated end-plate region, especially in young patients (Coërs and Telerman-Toppet, 1976). Bickerstaff and Woolf (1960) and MacDermot (1960) confirmed these findings and also described prolific ultraterminal sprouting, important evidence of vigorous but aberrant regeneration.

Ultramicroscopic studies of the end-plate region show poor development of junctional folds and of secondary clefts (Zacks, Bauer and Blumberg, 1962; Woolf, 1966; Engel and Santa, 1971; Fardeau, Godet-Guillain and Chevallay, 1974). These changes are accompanied by abnormal reduction of the subneural apparatus (Engel and Santa, 1971) (Fig. 16.9). Bergman, Johns and Afifi (1971) also noted abnormalities of muscle and nerve fibres, damage to Schwann cells, and grossly thickened basement membrane of capillaries but these findings are inconsistent, as are minor changes described in nerve terminals such as dense bodies, myelin figures, mitochondrial abnormalities, and decreased numbers of synaptic vesicles (see review by Engel and Santa, 1971). Fardeau et al. (1974) reported that synaptic vesicles had a normal diameter (about 60 nm) but that the vesicular stacks (at the presumed release sites of ACh) were rarely visible. Nevertheless, they agree with Engel and Santa (1971) that the changes predominate in the subneural apparatus, which is grossly elongated although the mean nerve terminal area is reduced (measured into the folds). It is generally agreed that the postsynaptic membrane disorganisation is not caused by anticholinesterase medication and that it is of functional significance, because the use of labelled α-Bgtx to identify receptor sites has shown reduced

amounts of AChR to a degree which correlates linearly with the decreased miniature end-plate potential amplitude (Engel et al., 1977b). Localisation of the IgG and C3 component of complement to receptors of end-plates obtained only from myasthenic patients has been identified by Engel et al. (1977a) (Fig. 16.10). From morphometric analysis of electron micrographs, these authors found that immune complexes are more abundant in the less severely affected patients than in those with more severe myasthenia gravis (who have less AChR remaining at their end-plates). They interpret this as evidence for a destructive autoimmune reaction involving the postsynaptic membrane. There is functional evidence that anti-AChR antibody increases the degradation of junctional (and extrajunctional) receptors of muscle (Reiness and Weinberg, 1978) and induces modulation of AChR (Heinemann, Merlie and Lindstrom, 1978) without involving complement. Immunopharmacological block, as suggested by Simpson (1960), remains a possibility which is supported by the prompt relapse of myasthenic symptoms noted after retransfusion of homologous cell-free lymph (Matell, Bergström, Franksson, Hammarström, Lefvert, Möller, von Reis and Smith, 1976), and by the indication that serum from myasthenic patients reduces the mepp amplitude of rat endplates, an effect which can be reversed by washing with a control solution (Shibuya, Mori and Nakazawa, 1978).

CAUSATION OF MYASTHENIA GRAVIS

The clinical, pathological, and immunological data now available, with the model provided by EAMG, provide strong support for the Simpson hypothesis of myasthenia gravis as a genetically predisposed autoimmune disorder, the proximate mechanism being destruction of end-plate ACh receptors by a complement-fixing antibody reaction. It is probable, though not proved, that cell-mediated immunity and immunopharmacological blockade of receptors are also important. It is still not known what starts the immunological reaction, although a viral attack on thymus or muscle is an attractive hypothesis. This would account for the occasional finding of IgM antibodies, supplanted

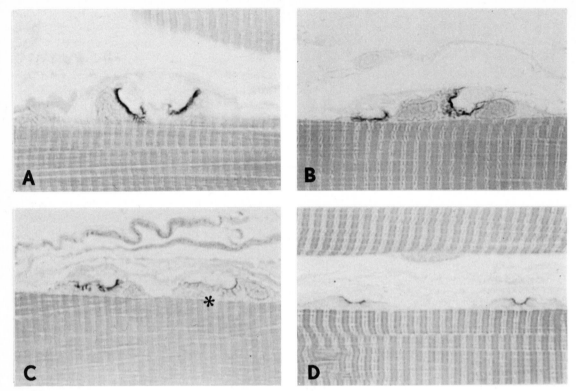

Fig. 16.10   Semi-thin sections of motor end-plates from two cases of myasthenia gravis showing localisation of IgG (A and C) and C3 component of complement (B and D). Reaction at the end-plates is more intense in the case of mild myasthenia gravis (A and B) than in the more severe case (C and D). One of two end-plate regions in C (*) displays only a trace of IgG. Background staining is absent. Unstained sections photographed with a green filter, × 1425 (Engel, Lambert and Howard, 1977a)

by the IgG type in early myasthenia (Lefvert *et al.*, 1978). Tindall, Cloud, Luby and Rosenberg (1978) report elevated titres of complement-fixing antibody to cytomegalovirus (CMV) in myasthenics not treated with thymectomy or steroids. Their suggestion that there is persistent viral antigenic stimulation in the myasthenic thymus, arising from incorporation of viral protein into myoid cell surface membranes with subsequent induction of anti-AChR antibody, would be consistent with the thymitis theory reviewed above; the same criticisms would be valid. Nevertheless, virus-induced breakdown of immune surveillance with lack of recognition of self, a strong possibility in all autoimmune diseases, is more likely to be due to infection of cells of the lymphoid system, as a mutagenic agent, than to infection of target organs. Immunodeficiency is a possible background to myasthenia gravis (Daw-

kins, Robinson and Weatherall, 1975a; Simpson *et al.*, 1976) but also to CMV infection. Some important biological aspects of myasthenia gravis are discussed by Rule and Kornfeld (1971).

NEUROMUSCULAR TRANSMISSION

Performance tests

The abnormal fatigability of skeletal muscles shown by bedside tests (p. 587) may be documented in many ways, providing objective data which may be important in the assessment of the pharmacological tests described below, or in evaluation of treatment. Diaphragmatic movement, or the ability to swallow a mouthful of barium before and after intramuscular injection of edrophonium, may be observed on the fluoroscope; the objective measurement of diplopia, for example with prisms, may be valuable in demonstrating the changing extent of weakness. A recording dynamometer or ergogram (Greene, Rideout and Shaw, 1961) is useful and may be readily improvised. Other techniques for recording the amount of muscular contraction are ocular tonometry (Campbell, Simpson, Crombie and Walton, 1970), nystagmography (Spector and Daroff, 1976) and audio-impedance measurement of the stapedius reflex (Blom and Zakrisson, 1974). These tests may occasionally be useful when muscular weakness is confined to the appropriate sites.

Electrophysiology

In 1895, Jolly showed that the pathological fatigability of myasthenia could be reproduced by faradic stimulation of a motor nerve while the 'fatigued' muscle would still respond to locally applied galvanism. Electromyographic recording shows that the loss of power when the motor nerve is supramaximally and repetitively stimulated is accompanied by a decrement of the evoked action potential of the muscle, while the antidromically conducted nerve action potential is unchanged in amplitude. In view of the recent ultrastructural and immunological data, it is unnecessary to present all the facts of neurophysiological observation relevant to the nature of the functional abnormality. For this purpose the reader is referred to reviews by Slomić, Rosenfalck and Buchthal (1968) and Simpson (1969b). It is now accepted that the essential lesion is degeneration of ACh receptors on the postsynaptic membrane, with or without immunopharmacological blockade, but it is clear from these studies and from computer analysis of evoked motor unit potentials (Ballantyne and Hansen, 1974) that additional, if less important, prejunctional and muscle fibre lesions may co-exist. The essential electrical features are: i) subnormal amplitude of spontaneous miniature end-plate potentials (mepps), ii) transmission failure due to lowered safety factor, and iii) intact prejunctional potentiation mechanisms.

Subnormal amplitudes of mepps, identified by Elmqvist and colleagues, were at first attributed to production of small quanta of ACh following a prejunctional lesion (Elmqvist, 1965), although on theoretical grounds a postjunctional morphological abnormality was at least as probable (Simpson, 1971). The recent evidence for a receptor lesion reconciles the electrophysiological and morphological findings. Decreased amplitude of spontaneous mepps of biopsied intercostal muscle can be used as a diagnostic test because this finding is probably unique to myasthenia gravis, but meticulous technique is necessary for reliable results (Elmqvist and Lambert, 1968). Spontaneous negative discharges recorded with macroelectrodes at the end-plate zone (motor point) of human muscle are considered to be miniature end-plate potentials. Lovelace, Stone and Zablow (1970) reported reduction in frequency of firing and of burst duration, but the amplitude was only slightly reduced. Grob (1971) found no significant difference between these values and those from normal subjects but he had greater difficulty in locating the negative spontaneous discharges in myasthenic subjects. The value of analysis of spontaneous end-plate activity (not to be confused with 'end-plate noise') has not been proved.

Tests of reduced safety factor for transmission

Although space does not permit a full presentation of the electrophysiology of myasthenia, some understanding of the fundamentals is necessary for proper interpretation of diagnostic tests. Demonstration of a lowered safety factor for transmission remains the first approach to diagnosis: myasthenia gravis cannot reasonably be diagnosed in its absence though there are other causes for a reduced safety factor (Simpson, 1966a). There are three methods for demonstrating reduced safety factor, described below.

Decrementing muscular response to repetitive supramaximal stimulation of a motor nerve. This is described in Chapter 26. It is the least sensitive technique: it may be necessary to test a number of muscles or to lower the safety factor still further by preliminary exercise, ischaemia of the limb, or local raising of temperature (Borenstein and Desmedt, 1973; Desmedt and Borenstein, 1977). In some muscles, tetanic and

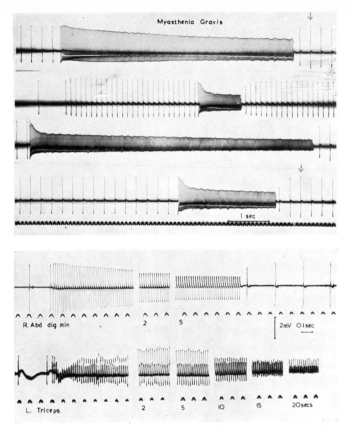

Fig. 16.11 Electromyograms from patients with myasthenia gravis: (a) Ulnar nerve at wrist stimulated with supramaximal shocks repeated 4, 8 and 50 times/s. Action potential recorded from abductor digiti minimi muscle by surface electrodes shows decrement ('fatigue') with fast tetanisation only. Note post-tetanic facilitation at arrows. (b) The classical response from abductor digiti minimi, but the triceps shows a temporary incremental response.

post-tetanic potentiation may be so great that an incrementing response is found, resembling that typical of carcinomatous myasthenia (Fig. 16.11; Simpson, 1966a; Schwartz and Stålberg, 1975a).

Neuromuscular 'jitter' and blocking. End-plate potentials reach the threshold for triggering an action potential of the muscle fibre with random variability, and this results in a little variability of latency between a nerve stimulus and the action potential of the responding muscle fibre. The latencies of responses of fibres belonging to the same motor unit are therefore not quite synchronous; the variability between any fibre(s) and a reference fibre of the same unit is termed the 'jitter'. When the safety factor for transmission is low, the latencies and jitter are increased, there are more response failures ('blockings') and each is

increased by exercising the muscle. This can be detected in human muscles by suitable selective electrodes (single fibre electromyography (EMG)) and the latencies can be studied statistically, usually by a computer, during voluntary contraction (Stålberg, Ekstedt and Broman, 1974) or indirect stimulation (Schwartz and Stålberg, 1975b). The tests are described in Chapter 29.

The 'jitter' phenomena are probably the most sensitive indicators of reduced safety factor, the abnormality being found in all or most muscles, even if clinical myasthenia is confined to the extraocular muscles. The necessity for special electrodes, an experienced physiologist, and computer facilities limit the general usefulness of the method. Increased jitter may have causes other than defective neuromuscular transmission (Stålberg and Ekstedt, 1973) and should be interpreted together with other EMG studies: however, if in a weak muscle, jitter is normal at all end-plates, the diagnosis of myasthenia gravis can be excluded (Stålberg *et al.*, 1974).

Regional curarisation. The lowered safety factor diminishes the amount of curare required to block neuromuscular transmission. The effect may be tested locally by injecting D-tubocurarine intravenously distal to an occlusive cuff and then measuring the decrementing muscular response to supramaximal stimulation (Brown and Charlton, 1975). This test, which is described in Chapter 26, is valuable because it detects reduced safety factor in clinically strong muscles. It is also abnormal in other transmission disorders but not in other, central, diseases which may increase jitter. It is simple and safe for general use in an EMG laboratory, with elementary precautions, but its use is unnecessary if the decrementing response is shown with the provocative techniques listed above.

None of these tests are diagnostic of myasthenia gravis (and if normal they do not exclude it) but that diagnosis is highly probable if a reduced safety factor is demonstrable and if it is promptly raised by injection of edrophonium.

Pharmacological tests

The most widely used tests are those involving a therapeutic response to anticholinesterase drugs, confirming that weakness is of the myasthenic type. Conversely, increased sensitivity to curare and similar drugs may be used to detect latent myasthenia. These tests are dangerous and should not be used where performance or therapeutic tests indicate the diagnosis. They are also inferior to the other tests described here and are largely of historical interest. For these reasons they will not be described in detail, but the interested reader is referred to earlier editions of this book and to original papers. The drugs which have been used are D-tubocurarine (Bennett and Cash, 1943), quinine bisulphate (Eaton, 1943) and deca-methonium (Churchill-Davidson and Richardson, 1952a). The latter is of some importance, as the myasthenic subject shows an abnormal 'dual response' (a brief depolarisation block followed by

a longer, competitive (curare-like) type of block) which should be known to anaesthetists required to paralyse a myasthenic patient.

For diagnostic purposes these tests are inferior to those depending on a temporary therapeutic response to an anticholinerase drug. It will be convenient to describe the additional use of edrophonium to determine the cholinergic status during treatment.

Edrophonium test. The short antimyasthenic effect of edrophonium chloride ('Tensilon') makes it very suitable for a diagnostic test. A syringe is loaded with 1 ml (10 mg) for intravenous injection. Initially 2 mg should be injected to detect sensitivity but if there is no response the remaining 8 mg is injected after 30 s (Osserman and Kaplan, 1953). Within 0.5–1 min there is improvement if weakness is due to myasthenia gravis, but weakness returns in 4–5 min. Some normal subjects experience no obvious effects, while others feel a tight sensation around the eyes and fasciculation may be seen for a few seconds. If weakness is due to cholinergic crisis it is transiently increased and fasciculation may occur. Unfortunately, respiratory weakness may be increased to an extent endangering life.

The positive responses described are valuable and reliable when present, but failure to obtain improvement or fasciculation does not indicate either that weakness is not myasthenic or that it is cholinergic. Negative responses are sometimes found, but false-positive results are very rare provided that only objective criteria are used. Subjective 'improvement' should never be relied on, especially when the test is used to determine the adequacy of treatment. The test is best performed at the time of greatest activity of the therapeutic drug. Where pyridostigmine is being used the test should be performed 2 h after a dose. A second test at 3 h may be necessary when the response is equivocal (Osserman and Kaplan, 1953).

Because of the differing degree of involvement of different muscles, it is very important to test respiratory and bulbar but not ocular muscles when the test is carried out to differentiate between myasthenic and cholinergic weakness. It is possible for these vital muscles to be overdosed while the ocular muscles are still underdosed, and failure to recognise this may lead to fatal overdosage. An equivocal or 'adequate' response should always be taken to mean that further dosage may be dangerous.

Neostigmine test. Though the latency is greater, a favourable response to injection of neostigmine remains the most convincing evidence of myasthenia gravis because its duration is sufficient to permit repeated testing of all muscles (Viets and Schwab, 1935). The duration makes it unsuitable when cholinergic crisis is suspected. Neostigmine methylsulphate is injected intramuscularly (1.5 mg) alone or combined with 0.6 mg of atropine sulphate. Improvement begins in 10–15 min but is most obvious after 30 min. The same preparation may be used intravenously (0.5 mg), when the response is more rapid but the danger of ventricular fibrillation or arrest is greater. The drug should never be given by this route unless accompanied or preceded by atropine. The response to 15 mg of neostigmine bromide orally may be sufficient to make the diagnosis clear. If any of the parenteral tests are equivocal and the diagnosis of myasthenia gravis seems highly probable on clinical grounds, it is worth carrying out a therapeutic trial with oral medication for a week.

Other pharmacological investigations. The abnormal response to decamethonium suggested to Churchill-Davidson and Richardson (1952b) that the motor end-plate was altered in myasthenia gravis and, in view of its similar action, it would be expected that the response to acetylcholine would be altered similarly.

Acetylcholine sensitivity

The response of myasthenic muscle to proximal intra-arterial injection of acetylcholine (ACh) has been a source of much argument and the results reported range from normal to hypersensitive. The conflicting findings were resolved by Engbaek (1951) who showed that most were obtained with unphysiologically large doses of ACh. With suitable dosage it could be demonstrated that myasthenic muscle has a raised threshold to this

drug. Grob, Johns and Harvey (1956) confirmed this conclusion, although the difference from normal was slight. They found abnormalities of the degree and timing of the excitability changes at the end-plate following administration both of ACh and of choline and suggested that an abnormal product of ACh or choline might constitute a 'false transmitter' with competitive blocking activity. This has never been demonstrated, and the abnormal response of the myasthenic muscle can be explained by a postjunctional abnormality (Simpson, 1969a and b, 1971). Elmqvist, Hofmann, Kugelberg, and Quastel (1964) revived the view that excised intercostal muscle of myasthenic patients was normally chemosensitive to bath-applied ACh and other depolarising substances, but in a further series of experiments with intra-arterial injection of graded doses of ACh, using spontaneous end-plate activity as an index, Grob (1971) has confirmed the diminished chemosensitivity of myasthenic muscle.

The Walker effect

Clearly, all of the electrophysiological and pharmacological findings so far described are compatible with the postjunctional lesion demonstrated morphologically. Proponents of the theory of a 'myasthenic toxin' or circulating 'curare-like substance' consider that such a substance produced from the muscles is necessary to account for the claim by Mary Walker (1938) that fatigue of forearm muscles could induce paralysis of extraocular muscles in a myasthenic patient. Many have described ptosis occurring after release of a tourniquet which had occluded venous return from an exercised limb. This test is difficult to evaluate because of the long latency of the response. A modification of the test is to exercise one limb by electrical stimulation distal to a tourniquet and to observe the effect of release of the tourniquet on the indirectly evoked muscle response of the other arm. Johns, Grob and Harvey (1956) found no evidence of release of a blocking substance and my experience is similar, but Tsukiyama, Nakai, Mine and Kitani (1959) reported a decrease of the indirectly evoked muscle response in one arm 1–4 min after release of a cuff from the other arm; the cuff had been inflated during 5 min of supramaximal nerve stimulation at 10/s. This effect was not prevented by previous administration of anticholinesterase. They also reported suppression of the indirectly stimulated muscle response after intra-arterial injection of the myasthenic patient's own serum. Patten (1975) postulated that muscle exercised under hypoxic conditions releases many substances inhibiting muscle function. He has argued that lactic acid, a normal by-product of muscle metabolism, may adversely affect the function of normal and myasthenic muscle and that this would account for the Mary Walker phenomenon (he does not give personal evidence for its existence) and also for the provocative effect of ischaemia in the EMG test described above, possibly by lowering serum calcium levels which might decrease the release of ACh. This interesting hypothesis requires further study.

Until recently there has been no acceptable evidence of a blocking substance in serum (Nastuk, Strauss and Osserman, 1959) but Struppler (1954) claimed to have demonstrated a curare-like effect on frog muscle if the serum is withdrawn after exercise, especially exercise in ischaemic conditions. At present the only evidence for a transmissible blocking substance obtained from resting myasthenic patients is the observation of Matell *et al.* (1976) that if lymph is drained from the thoracic duct of myasthenics the patient improves, but that myasthenia is precipitated by re-transfusion of the cell-free lymph. Passive transfer from human to mouse has been described above. These effects are attributed to an immunoglobulin in serum. There is no convincing evidence for a role of other 'myasthenic toxins' originating in muscle or thymus.

RADIOLOGY OF THYMUS

The thymus gland is not seen in chest radiographs unless there is a thymoma. Small tumours localised to part of the gland may remain invisible, but those seen at surgery before the gland is sectioned can almost always be detected on straight films of the chest (posteroanterior and lateral) (Fig. 16.2) assisted by tomography if necessary. Pneumomediastinography or thymic

venography are unnecessary and not recommended. Isotopic scanning of the mediastinum with selenomethionine-75 (Cowan, Maynard, Witcofski, Janeway and Toole, 1971) or gallium-67 citrate (Swick, Preston and McQuillen, 1976) gives good imaging of thymomas. As the radiopharmaceutical agent accumulates in numerous tissues false-positive studies are reported, but negative studies are considered to be of value in ruling out the presence of a thymoma. Gallium-67 has become the preferred isotope. It may be valuable in detecting recurrences of malignant thymoma after operation.

TREATMENT

There are three facets of treatment: 1) immunosuppression; 2) elevation of the safety factor for neuromuscular transmission; 3) avoidance of factors which lower the safety factor or further embarrass respiration.

Immunosuppressive measures

In principle, the autoimmune disorder may respond to removal or suppression of the thymus, ultrathymic immunosuppression, or removal of antibodies and immuno-aggressive cells.

Thymectomy. For a long time the value of thymectomy was obscured by failure to appreciate that results are different in cases with a thymoma (Keynes, 1955). In cases without a thymoma there is a clear benefit in favour of thymectomy, regardless of age or sex of the patient, provided that the disease is still in Stage 1 (Simpson, 1958). The contrary view of Papatestas, Alpert, Osserman, Osserman and Kark (1971b) was later reversed (Papatestas *et al.*, 1976).

There is no clear indication as to which patients are most likely to benefit, apart from those in whom the disease has been of short duration. Failure of thymectomy to prevent myasthenic death occurs more often in patients requiring a large dose of anticholinesterase drugs, but if they do survive (which is now the rule) the ultimate state is not, apparently, correlated with the preoperative severity. Patients with severe bulbar weakness are most likely to die despite operation. On the other hand, if myasthenia remains confined to the extraocular muscles for two years, the prognosis for life is so good that thymectomy has not been considered justified (Grob, 1953; Ferguson et al., 1955). On the other hand, I believe that it is unusual for weakness to remain so restricted and the operation is now entirely safe, regardless of the surgical method (Fraser, Simpson and Crawford, 1978). The surgical technique (sternal split or transcervical incision) is a matter of choice by the surgeon. Operative morbidity is less with the transcervical approach, but complete removal of the gland is less certain and this is considered desirable if possible. On the other hand, prejudice against the sternal splitting operation is due to the belief that respiratory support by endotracheal intubation is usually necessary. It is generally unnecessary if anticholinesterase medication is not discontinued (Fraser et al., 1978). Undoubtedly, the sites of aberrant thymic tissue are easier to reach with the sternal incision.

Even in Stage 1 (active stage), thymectomy is not a cure for myasthenia gravis. It arrests deterioration, promotes remission and makes the further course more benign. This is increasingly evident with the passage of time (Simpson, 1958; Perlo, Poskanzer, Schwab, Viets, Osserman and Genkins, 1966; Papatestas et al., 1976). It is still controversial whether the pathology of the thymus is important. It is generally agreed that the long-term outlook is much poorer if there is a thymoma, although for 5–10 years the result of thymectomy may be excellent. Indeed, there are many records of myasthenia becoming first clinically apparent months or years after removal of a thymoma (Koch, Regli and Reinle, 1970). There are conflicting reports about the correlation between the presence of germinal centres and the response to surgery. Some reported series are too small for analysis; others have assessed the histology subjectively. Not surprisingly, they disagree with each other. Differing conclusions are: 1) there is no relationship between thymic histology and postoperative response (Castleman and Norris, 1949; Seybold et al., 1971; Reinglass and Brickel, 1973); 2) a favourable response correlates with the presence of numerous germinal centres (MacKay,

Whittingham, Goldstein, Currie and Hare, 1968; Genkins, Papatestas, Horowitz and Kornfeld, 1975; Sambrook, Reid, Mohr and Boddie, 1976); 3) a favourable response is more likely after removal of glands with few germinal centres (Alpert, Papatestas, Kark, Osserman and Osserman, 1971). Vetters and Simpson (1974) used an accurate morphometric technique and also found a tendency for patients with relatively unreactive thymus glands to obtain a better result from thymectomy, but the difference was not statistically significant and others have considered that there is no relationship at all.

The response to thymectomy is unpredictable. It may be immediate or delayed. The more favourable course relative to cases without thymectomy commonly becomes apparent in the second or third year and is most evident with early thymectomy (Simpson, 1958; Genkins et al., 1975). A major relapse is rare but it does occur: a postulated growth of 'aberrant' or incompletely removed thymic tissue has not been confirmed in most cases although it is undoubtedly present in some (Joseph and Johns, 1973). There is often a temporary improvement during the first few days, which may be so rapid that it is obvious as soon as the patient recovers from the anaesthetic, though no neostigmine has been injected throughout the operation. A previous ptosis may be replaced by lid retraction. Unfortunately the dose of anticholinesterase may require progressive increase on the third or fourth day but it is extremely important to recognise the extent of the temporary remission as, during this period, a previously ineffective dose of neostigmine may cause a cholinergic crisis. In the past, many postoperative deaths were caused in this way. To avoid it, many experts stop anticholinesterase medication before operation and resume 2–3 days later, meanwhile supporting breathing by artificial ventilation, commonly by tracheostomy. With careful attention to dosage, neither measure is required (Fraser et al., 1978).

The delayed response to thymectomy, and the inferior response when operation is postponed beyond stage 1, suggest that T cells controlling antibody formation by B cells continue to be active for some time after thymectomy in some extrathymic site, and that it would be rational to follow thymectomy with immunosuppressive drugs aimed at these cells, and not merely in the most seriously affected patients. It might be argued that adequate chemical immunosuppression would remove the need for thymectomy. This should certainly be investigated but the proof will have to be convincing now that thymectomy carries no operative mortality.

Suppression of the thymus. Alternative means of suppressing the thymus have not been shown to be as effective. Carotid sinus denervation, claimed to cause adrenocortical hypertrophy and thymic atrophy, has been abandoned. Radiotherapy as a method of destroying thymic function is less certain than thymectomy and may cause initial deterioration. Preoperative radiotherapy has been advised before removal of a thymoma (Keynes, 1955) and also for non-tumour cases (Schulz and Schwab, 1971). I do not consider that the additional benefit has been proved and I have had no cause to regret abandoning radiotherapy 20 years ago.

Ultrathymic immunosuppression

Cytotoxic drugs. Early reports of improvement of myasthenia after treatment with azathioprine, 6-mercaptopurine, and methotrexate were not impressive, but merit further consideration because of the possibility of response in those cases where the autoimmune process is no longer thymus-dependent. Matell *et al.* (1976) reported gradual improvement, maximal after 6–15 months, with azathioprine, even after apparently unsuccessful thymectomy or steroids. They have shown a decrease in the serum titre of anti-AChR antibody, especially in patients with a thymoma (Lefvert *et al.*, 1978). Further studies are necessary because the duration of illness may be less relevant for ultrathymic immunosuppression than for thymectomy.

Corticosteroids; adrenocorticotrophin. Early reports of 'rebound' remission after initial deterioration of myasthenia treated by ACTH were not followed up because of early fatalities, until the management of crisis situations improved and intensive therapy units became commonplace. It was then possible to use larger doses of ACTH or prednisolone with striking benefit. In the first 7–10 days of treatment there is often clinical deterioration which is associated with a rise of receptor antibody preceding a sustained fall (Lefvert *et al.*, 1978), with marked remission of symptoms. It appears that any corticosteroid or timing regime may be used (Brunner, Berger, Namba and Grob, 1976) at any clinical stage including the most advanced. Serum concentration of anti-AChR antibody decreases and anticholinesterase dosage may be reduced progressively (but not abruptly withdrawn). A recommended regime is prednisone 100 mg daily or on alternate days for a month or more. Results of treatment are impressive, but the side effects and hazards are not negligible (Brunner *et al.*, 1976; Mann, Johns and Campa, 1976). It is not known how long steroid treatment must be continued. In my opinion it is not a treatment of first choice but should be reserved for patients not responding to thymectomy and anticholinesterases and preferably not until three years or more after operation. Some early reports were certainly overenthusiastic and not supported by controlled trial (Howard, Duane, Lambert and Daube, 1976). Indeed it is by no means certain that the benefit from steroids is due to immunosuppression. A direct neuromuscular action is possible, perhaps on regeneration of end-plates.

Antilymphocyte and antithymocyte sera. It is possible that cytotoxic and steroid immunosuppression may act on immunocompetent cells in division, presumably in the reticuloendothelial system, and so the phase of activity may be critical. This limitation may not apply to these sera. Antilymphocyte serum acts to deplete paracortical lymph node areas where recirculation of antigen-sensitive lymphocytes occurs. An additional action may be to coat the receptor sites of the lymphocytes. Antithymocyte serum has been used in myasthenic patients with varying degrees of clinical improvement, especially when used after thymectomy (Pirofsky, Reid, Bardana, and Bayrakci, 1971; Roux, Serratrice and Pollini, 1974). Aureggi, Cirelli, Virno and Nigro (1970) also used antilymphocyte serum. Although of theoretical importance, these antisera appear to be of limited practical value.

Removal of antibodies and immuno-aggressive cells. Drainage of lymph from the thoracic duct, with removal of 0.5–2.0 litres daily, to a total of 4–5 litres, causes improvement of myasthenic weakness within 48 h. Although the lymph volume increases again in a few days, there is maintained improvement for a year or more (Matell et al., 1976). The long-term effect may be due to additional immunosuppressive therapy. In the same series, serum AChR antibody concentration decreased by 10–60 per cent, correlating well with clinical improvement (Lefvert et al., 1978). About 10 per cent of the total blood lymphocytes were removed in these cases but, as the cells reacted normally to mitogenic stimulation, there is no evidence that cell depletion is important. Myasthenic symptoms returned in some cases when homologous cell-free lymph, or an immunoglobulin-containing fraction of lymph, was retransfused.

Plasma exchange (plasmapheresis) is an effective method for reducing serum anti-AChR antibody. Newsom Davis et al. (1978), who first used the treatment, reported progressive improvement in strength, commonly after two days. We have had good results with six exchanges of 4 litres and agree that plasmapheresis followed by immunosuppressive therapy may give long remissions.

Unfortunately relapse at 5–6 months is sometimes severe. Susceptibility to infection is temporarily increased by antibody depletion, the role of which is still being assessed. If it merely removed an immunopharmacological block, antibody depletion would be restricted to the management of myasthenic crises or for preoperative preparation, but it may also permit synthesis of new receptors if followed by long-term immunosuppression (Newsom Davis et al. 1978). The rapid changes in the safety factor for neuromuscular transmission require careful adjustment of anticholinesterase dosage. The efficacy of lymph duct drainage and plasmapheresis depends on the fact that the antireceptor antibody regenerates more slowly than the main pool of immunoglobulin. Nevertheless, increased susceptibility to infection is a hazard, and feedback overproduction of autoantibodies (Bystryn, Schenkein and Uhr, 1971) may be dangerous. A method of inhibiting their production selectively would be ideal.

Induction of anti-idiotypic antibodies. A second-best procedure would be selective destruction of autoantibody. Preliminary experimental induction of anti-idiotypic antibodies by immunisation against AChR-educated lymphocytes has been reported (Schwartz, Novick, Givol and Fuchs, 1978). If confirmed and extended to the human, this would provide a highly effective treatment for myasthenia gravis. Meanwhile, although treatment of the immunological basis of myasthenia gravis must be a prime consideration, it is always necessary to raise the safety factor for neuromuscular transmission. Anticholinesterase medication should be continued in an appropriate dosage throughout all immunosuppressive treatment.

Elevation of the safety factor for transmission

Anticholinesterase drugs. Inhibitors of endplate acetylcholinesterase raise the safety factor for neuromuscular transmission by preventing hydrolysis of ACh and so prolonging the occupancy of receptor sites by ACh. Anticholinesterases do not increase production of ACh and so are effective for as long as the transmitter is released at motor nerve endings and the ACh receptors of the endplates are intact. In stage 3 myasthenia this may not be so, at least in some muscles ('neostigmine resistance'). On the other hand, if inhibition of cholinesterase is carried to excess, so that ACh persists at receptor sites, the end-plate remains depolarised or becomes desensitised ('cholinergic blockade') (see p. 611).

Tertiary amines. Physostigmine (eserine) was the first effective anticholinesterase. An extract of the Calabar bean, it was used as an aboriginal antidote to curare poisoning. It is a carbonate ester no longer used for treatment of myasthenia gravis because it crosses the blood-brain barrier and its action on central cholinergic synapses produces unacceptable symptoms.

Galanthamine hydrobromide (Nivalin) is isolated from the Bulgarian snowdrop. It is used in the USSR and it is said to have a duration of action comparable with neostigmine; unfortunately, it also crosses the blood-brain barrier.

Quaternary ammonium compounds. Drugs of this group have no significant central action in therapeutic dosage. They probably have some action on motor nerve terminals and perhaps directly on the postsynaptic membrane, but it is generally accepted that the anticholinesterase activity is the more important clinically. The drug of choice depends on the required duration of action, peak activity, absence of unwanted effects, margin between dose required for optimum action and that producing cholinergic blockade, and the possibility of cumulative action.

Edrophonium chloride (Tensilon). This hydroxyanilinium salt, administered intravenously (2–10 mg) has a peak action in 2–3 min, which rapidly subsides. Although some effect is still apparent 20–30 min later, this is too brief for therapeutic purposes. It is used to confirm the diagnosis of myasthenia or to differentiate between underdosage and overdosage of anticholinesterases (p. 603).

Neostigmine bromide (Prostigmine). The 15 mg tablet of neostigmine has a cholinergic activity which varies from 2–6 h in different patients. The total and the spacing of doses must be established by individual trial and may vary from 22.5 mg/day in three doses to 45 mg every 2 h (540 mg/day). Exceptional cases requiring even larger doses have been reported, but an average dose is 150 mg daily (Simpson, 1958). After the drug has been given there is a surge of muscular power for 30–60 min, followed by continued activity at a lower level for 2–6 h. Subsequently, strength is rapidly lost, making it difficult to adjust the timing of dosage. Most myasthenics prefer pyridostigmine for this reason. The 'boost' effect of neostigmine is valuable if taken 30 min before a meal or a special physical effort.

Pyridostigmine bromide (Mestinon). Pyridostigmine has less peak effect than neostigmine and its plateau of activity is very little longer but it wanes more slowly, allowing a sustained blood level to be achieved by judiciously timed dosage: this varies from 2–8 h and the frequency must again be established by trial. The 60 mg tablet of pyridostigmine is approximately equivalent to the 15 mg tablet of neostigmine. Each of these drugs should be given by mouth (crushed tablet by oral tube if necessary) in preference to parenteral injection, but in some patients absorption is erratic and it is then necessary to rely on subcutaneous or intramuscular injection of neostigmine methylsulphate (1 mg having an equivalent effect to 15 mg neostigmine or 60 mg pyridostigmine given orally). It should rarely be given intravenously as bradycardia may be dangerous.

Ambenonium chloride (Mysuran, Mytelase). This is a related drug with a slightly longer action than that of 60 mg pyridostigmine, which is approximately equal in potency to 25 mg ambenonium. Muscarinic side effects are less common than with neostigmine or pyridostigmine, but central reactions are more common and the onset of cholinergic crisis may be difficult to detect.

Long-acting neostigmines. Slow-release tablets of neostigmine and pyridostigmine have been claimed to eliminate the need for frequent interruption of sleep, and cumulative side effects have not been prominent. These drugs are little used outside the USA. Bis-neostigmine compounds (e.g. *Hexadistigmin; Ubretid*) have two neostigmine radicals separated by a polymethylene chain of various lengths. This prolongs the activity, but cumulative effects make them unsatisfactory for domiciliary use (Herzfeld, Kraupp, Pateisky and Stumpf, 1957).

Alkyl phosphates. This group of anticholinesterase preparations, which includes diisopropylfluorophosphate (DFP), tetraethylpyrophosphate (TEPP), hexamethyltetraphosphate (HETP), and octamethylpyrophosphoramide (OMPA), had a vogue in the treatment of myasthenia because their long duration of activity was considered desirable. This very property leads to inflexibility of control and they have a greater effect on central synapses than the quaternary ammonium compounds, giving rise to headache, nightmares, and personality disturbance. These drugs have been largely abandoned (Westerberg and Magee, 1955).

Potentiation of ACh release and muscular responsiveness. A number of drugs raise the safety factor for transmission by potentiating release of ACh presynaptically and/or by sensitisation of ACh receptors or muscle contraction. The major action is uncertain and they are inferior to anticholinesterases in treatment of myasthenia gravis.

Guanidine hydrochloride. The antimyasthenic action of guanidine is limited and it is now rarely used for treatment of myasthenia gravis, but it is effective in the management of carcinomatous myasthenia (Lambert, 1966). It is given orally in a dose of 20–50 mg/kg body weight, divided into three doses. It tends to cause circumoral and digital paraesthesiae. It has occasionally caused liver and marrow damage and irreversible nephropathy but in my experience the nephropathy has recovered on withdrawal of guanidine.

4-aminopyridine chloride. By enhancing the influx of calcium ions during the action potential at the nerve terminal, 4-aminopyridine (4-AP) increases the amount of ACh released from motor nerve terminals. This action may restore neuromuscular transmission in myasthenia gravis, carcinomatous myasthenic syndrome and botulism. I have used 4-AP sulphate orally (1.42 mg/kg/day in divided doses) and Lundh, Nilsson and Rosén (1977) also used 4-AP chloride by intravenous injection of 10–20 mg in repeated doses. Circumoral paraesthesiae, photophobia, unsteadiness, and central nervous irritability with a possibility of seizures limit the dose and render the drug less useful than anticholinesterases.

Adrenaline; ephedrine etc. Adrenaline and its amine analogues have exceedingly weak anticholinesterase activity. They are of no practical value for myasthenia gravis but ephedrine may be beneficial by combating the bronchoconstriction caused by anticholinesterases (Ringvist and Ringvist, 1971). The oral dose is 10–25 mg thrice daily.

Veratrum alkaloids; germine esters. Drugs of this group 'amplify' the muscle response by causing repetitive firing of nerve endings and of the stimulated muscle. Potential value is insufficient to compensate for important side effects such as hypotension, cardiac arrhythmias and sensory symptoms, though Flacke, Caviness and Samaha (1966) found these negligible with germine in short-term studies.

Potassium; aldosterone inhibitors. Potassium is used extensively as an adjuvant in myasthenia gravis. The rationale is obscure and the benefit not documented. It may cause nausea and diarrhoea resembling cholinergic crises. Spironolactone, given to conserve potassium (Gottlieb and Laurent, 1961) is of no proven value though it gives a sensation of well-being. Provision of potassium to counteract loss of intracellular potassium during steroid therapy is quite another matter and its use is rational (Critchley, Herman, Harrison, Shields and Liversedge, 1977).

Drugs which may lower the safety factor

Enemas may cause sudden death in myasthenics (Keynes, 1950). The mechanism is unknown, but may involve stretching of a bowel rendered tonic by anticholinesterases. Corticosteroids, adrenocorticotrophin and thyroxin may cause temporary deterioration. Respiratory depressants, including morphine and sedatives, must be used with care, but diazepam is relatively safe. Myasthenic syndromes are very occasionally caused by penicillamine and β-adrenergic blocking drugs (p. 614), but there is no evidence that they aggravate spontaneous myasthenia gravis. A number of substances regularly lower the safety factor for transmission at the neuromuscular junction and should be used (with appropriate adjustment of anticholinesterase dosage) only if the indication is clamant.

Inhibitors of production or release of ACh. A number of aminoglycoside antibiotics have this action, including streptomycin, dihydrostreptomycin, neomycin, kanamycin, gentamycin, viomycin, bacitracin, polymyxin A and B, and colistin, especially with renal insufficiency (Hokkanen, 1964). Low ionised serum calcium may be implicated in a presynaptic action (Wright and McQuillen, 1971).

Blockers of ACh receptors or of muscle response. Any neuromuscular blocking drug must be used with caution in myasthenia gravis. Despite the increased sensitivity to curare (p. 603), D-tubocurarine is the best if relaxation for surgery is required, because its mode of action is unchanged and it is antagonised by neostigmine. The anomalous responses to depolarising drugs (decamethonium, and suxamethonium and others) are dose-dependent and vary in different muscles (Churchill-Davidson and Richardson, 1952a and b).

Membrane stabilisers (hydantoinates, quinine, quinidine, procainamide) are, in principle, harmful but rarely cause significant deterioration in myasthenia gravis.

MYASTHENIC CRISIS

There is little justification for this traditional term, which implies sudden spontaneous exacerbation of activity. Unquestionably, most cases in the past have been unrecognised cholinergic crisis or asphyxia. It is, of course, true that weakness is increased by unusual physical exertion, emotional upset, an infection or childbirth, but it responds to management of the stressful situation. The drugs listed on p. 610, which lower the safety factor for transmission or depress respiration, should be used with caution. Myasthenic crisis is rare in well-managed patients.

The absence of cholinergic signs and the presence of a favourable response to the edrophonium test (p. 603) indicate the cause of the severe weakness. If it is necessary to increase the dose of anticholinesterase medication, the only suitable method in emergency is intramuscular injection of neostigmine. It is necessary to control respiration by endotracheal intubation if pulmonary ventilation is failing, or there is severe dysphagia. Thick, glairy bronchial secretion must be aspirated by bronchoscopic suction. Tracheostomy is not required unless the need for passive ventilation continues for more than one week. Once respiration is safeguarded, treatment can proceed methodically without panic measures, the dose of neostigmine or pyridostigmine being regulated by repeated edrophonium titration (Osserman and Kaplan, 1953). It is possible that plasma exchange may produce rapid improvement but further experience of this mode of treatment is required.

CHOLINERGIC CRISIS

Mild muscarinic effects of anticholinesterase medication (colic, diarrhoea, belching, nausea) are not uncommon in myasthenic patients, although less prominent than in normal subjects taking the same dose. More severe muscarinic signs such as vomiting, sweating, hypersalivation, lachrymation, miosis and pallor are less common and indicate that the dose is nearing a dangerous level. The most valuable indication of impending danger is the size of the pupil. It should not be allowed to contract to less than 2 mm diameter in normal room lighting. Bradycardia is very unusual with oral medication, but may be prominent and lead to cardiac arrest with intravenous medication. Hypotension occurs with severe cholinergic poisoning. In the most severe cases, confusion and coma indicate block of cerebral synapses. The use of an antagonist such as atropine sulphate (0.3–0.6 mg) is obligatory with intravenous dosage, but need not be given if the cholinergic drug is administered orally or by subcutaneous injection, unless colic is intolerable. The disadvantage of suppressing the muscarinic symptoms is that more serious nicotonic signs may be overlooked (Schwab, 1954). There is no evidence that atropine inhibits the nicotinic signs, the earliest of which is fasciculation of muscles. This need not be a serious sign as it will first appear in muscles unaffected by myasthenia. Persistent fasciculation in the leg muscles is consistent with excellent clinical control. Conversely, a depolarisation block may be reached without previous fasciculation, or the latter may be transient and therefore overlooked. A muscle may pass from myasthenic weakness to cholinergic block without passing through a stage of normal strength. Poisoning has reached a dangerous level ('cholinergic crisis') when weakness increases because of depolarisation block. This may be difficult to recognise and undoubtedly accounts for the majority of cases of 'neostigmine resistance' not attributable to atrophy of muscle. It must be emphasised that different muscles will reflect their degree of myasthenic involvement. Thus, some muscles may suffer cholinergic block while others still require further anticholinesterase medication. As the muscles of respiration are often relatively spared by myasthenia, they may be blocked by a dose of neostigmine which is insufficient for the ocular or limb muscles. It is extremely important to measure the effect of a test dose of edrophonium on the respiratory and bulbar muscles as well as on the more easily tested muscles. Even though short-acting, the additional cholinergic effect of edrophonium may be fatal in cholinergic crisis. In these circumstances atropine should be injected first and there should be facilities for immediate assisted respiration. The test is described on page 603.

Cholinergic paralysis requires urgent treatment. A cuffed endotracheal tube should be passed at once and positive-pressure respiration started. Tracheostomy may be necessary if this has to be prolonged. Atropine sulphate should be injected intravenously (2 mg/h) until signs of atropine toxicity develop. Specific antidotes for anticholinesterase poisoning are not satisfactory in clinical practice. Drugs of the oxime group have some effect on overdosage of quaternary ammonium anticholinesterases (Grob and Johns, 1958). Personal experience is limited to pyridine-2-aldoxime (2-PAM) and methane sulphonate (P_2S) but their latency has been found to be too long and their potency and duration of action inadequate for satisfactory treatment. Physiological antagonism can be obtained by the use of D-tubocurarine. I have used this form of treatment of cholinergic crisis, but because it is difficult to judge the dose necessary, this drug is not recommended unless respiration is artificially controlled. In these circumstances there is little need for an antidote other than atropine to protect the cardiovascular system. Controlled respiration and repeated atropine injection pending the recovery of neuromuscular response is the most satisfactory form of treatment available at present. Anticholinesterase medication should not be resumed until there is a clear 'myasthenic type' of response to edrophonium on two successive occasions at intervals of 1 h. On resumption, neostigmine should be given by injection and an adequate dose discovered by trial, guided by edrophonium testing. Only when this has been done should oral medication be resumed, at first with neostigmine and then with longer-acting drugs by cautious substitution and prolongation of dose-interval.

DIFFERENTIAL DIAGNOSIS

Myasthenia gravis has to be differentiated from the symptomatic myasthenias described in the next section. More commonly, the problem is to fail to recognise the existence of a myasthenic disorder; once it is considered the diagnosis is rarely in doubt. Positive EMG tests (p. 601) are confirmatory but negative tests do not invalidate the diagnosis. A properly conducted edrophonium test, with objective response, is very reliable and a raised titre of anti-AChR antibody in the blood is diagnostic of myasthenia gravis.

Myasthenia gravis is commonly mistaken for hysteria because it is so often precipitated by emotional disturbances, and physical signs may be absent if the patient has rested before examination. The intermittent nature of the symptoms and the frequent occurrence of diplopia and dysarthria or other bulbar symptoms may suggest multiple sclerosis. Motor neurone disease, parkinsonism, peripheral neuropathy, and endocrine disorders, particularly thyrotoxicosis, may cause weakness which increases with effort; hypokalaemic states, periodic paralysis, paroxysmal myoglobinuria, craft palsies and other disorders causing transient paralysis may be confused with myasthenia gravis.

The most difficult disorders to differentiate from myasthenia gravis are the condition termed 'pseudoptosis', mitochondrial myopathy and the congenital syndromes with facial and extraocular palsies including congenital ptosis, ocular myopathy and the Von Graefe-Moebius syndrome. None of these conditions responds favourably to anticholinesterase drugs.

OTHER MYASTHENIC SYNDROMES

The syndrome of progressively decreasing muscular power during continuous or repeated contraction, which is relieved by rest, will result from any disorder which lowers the safety factor for neuromuscular transmission, short of complete block. It should be appreciated that many of the types described in the literature are detected only during EMG or pharmacological studies and do not show pathological fatiguability on clinical testing. The lesion may be either pre- or post-junctional. Thus Churchill-Davidson and Wise (1963) examined children under the age of 6 months and found that successive muscle responses to repetitive stimulation of the motor nerve showed a decrement of amplitude, followed by post-tetanic facilitation. Furthermore, such infants were remarkably resistant to high doses of depolarising drugs such as decamethonium. At birth, human motor end-plates are immature, many consisting of terminal clubs, and a terminal arborisation (if present) is simple. Many immature end-plates are seen in children up to the age of 2 yr (Coërs and Woolf, 1959). It is possible that maturation arrest might account for the unusual case of benign congenital myopathy with myasthenic features described by Walton, Geschwind and Simpson (1956) and for the congenital myasthenic syndrome in a 15-year-old boy described by Engel, Lambert and Gomez (1976a). Neither of these patients had a worthwhile response to neostigmine. In the case described by Engel *et al* 1976a) there was acetylcholinesterase deficiency in the subneural apparatus of the motor end-plates and no increase in anti-AChR antibody.

Cholinesterase deficiency

Deficiency of pseudocholinesterase may be genetic or acquired. In normal life there is no muscular weakness, but prolonged apnoea occurs if the affected person is given a depolarising relaxant drug (e.g. succinylcholine) and this disorder must then be distinguished from carcinomatous myasthenia. The genetic variety has a number of phenotypes which may be identified by measuring the inhibitory effect of dibucaine or fluorine (Lehmann and Liddell, 1969). Phenotyping of serum or heparinised blood is available in Britain at the Cholinesterase Research Unit, Department of Chemistry, University of Exeter, Devon (Tel. Exeter 77911).

Acquired deficiency of pseudocholinesterase is caused by liver disease, pregnancy, and use of certain drugs, phenelzine (a monoamine oxidase inhibitor) and echothiophate (an organophosphorus compound used as eye drops for glaucoma) (Pantuck and Pantuck, 1975). The most important and the only necessary treatment for prolonged response to succinylcholine is adequate pulmonary ventilation, continued for several hours if necessary.

Nutritional, metabolic and toxic myasthenia

A disease named kubisagari in Japan was described in the late nineteenth century. This was an outbreak of paralysis with ptosis and bulbar symptoms. Similar epidemics occurred in prisoner-of-war camps in the Far East. Weakness fluctuated in severity and was sometimes worse in the evening. The reports differ regarding the effect of neostigmine but it seems probable that these outbreaks were essentially the same as kubisagari and probably due to nutritional deficiency, though a neurotoxin (such as tick paralysis (Murnaghan, 1960), cannot be excluded. Denny-Brown (1947) reported that parenteral administration of thiamine caused the symptoms to disappear in one week.

In rare cases of peripheral neuropathy a decrementing response to serial stimulation may be seen, as in diabetic neuropathy, Guillain-Barré syndrome and post-zoster motor neuropathy (Simpson and Lenman, 1959; Simpson, 1966a). It is also found in other lower motor neurone diseases including poliomyelitis, syringomyelia and motor neurone disease. This statement refers to the electrophysiological findings: clinical myasthenia is exceedingly rare in disorders of the lower motor neurones. One condition in which it has been described is acute idiopathic porphyria, in which the myasthenic weakness is said to respond to neostigmine (Gillhespy and Smith, 1954).

Muscular weakness of 'myasthenic' type in chewers of tobacco which had fermented as the result of contamination by *Clostridium perfringens* has been described by French authors (Coulonjou and Salaun, 1952). This organism usually causes severe myositis (gas gangrene) and it is possible that minimal muscular damage was responsible for the symptoms described, but it is interesting to consider the possibility of an exotoxin such as that produced by *Cl. botulinum*.

Treatment of patients with a number of β-adrenergic-blocking drugs has resulted in a clinical syndrome described as resembling myasthenia gravis by Herishanu and Rosenberg (1975) who attributed it to a neuromuscular-depressant effect described by previous workers. It should be remembered that serious complications of some β-blockers are immunological in nature (Behan, Behan, Zacharias and Nicholls, 1976).

A number of patients have developed typical myasthenia gravis while taking D-penicillamine for rheumatoid arthritis or Wilson's disease (Bucknall, 1977). Marked falls of serum IgA and other immunoglobulins have been reported with penicillamine treatment for non-immunological diseases (Stephens and Fenton, 1977) and a lupus reaction has been induced (Golding and Walshe, 1977). It therefore seems likely that myasthenia results directly from the drug (and not from association with rheumatoid arthritis) and that it has an immunological pathogenesis. It clears up when D-penicillamine is withdrawn. Nevertheless, as only two cases of myasthenia have occurred during treatment of Wilson's disease (Dawkins, Zilko and Owen, 1975b), existing immunological abnormality or genetic constitution may be important predisposing factors. Three of seven patients with penicillamine-induced myasthenia had HL-A1 HL-A8 haplotypes (Bucknall, 1977).

Polymyositis and related disorders

A myasthenic type of weakness is commonly present at some stage of polymyositis and dermatomyositis (Walton and Adams, 1958). The decrementing neuromuscular response is indistinguishable from myasthenia gravis and there is usually an initial favourable response to edrophonium or neostigmine. Typically, the 'fatigability' is transient or the response to anticholinesterase drugs is not maintained after the first few doses. A similar transient myasthenic syndrome occurs in systemic lupus erythematosus but classical myasthenia gravis also occurs in that disease (Harvey *et al.*, 1954). As interstitial myositis may occur in myasthenia gravis, and the diagnostic status of anticholinesterase responsiveness is debatable, it is clear that the diagnosis will often give rise to disagreement. The most reasonable interpretation is that all are autoimmune diseases which often show clinical and serological overlap and association with thymic tumours. Dermatomyositis is particularly related to carcinoma. The EMG findings have been described by Simpson (1966a) who drew attention to a marked facilitation during rapid stimulation, and occasional slow augmentation of tension and EMG on voluntary contraction (Simpson and Lenman, 1959). These authors and Simpson (1966a) described a number of patients in whom the incrementing response was the major reaction. None of their cases had a malignant tumour or developed one subsequently and some had other EMG or histological characteristics of polymyositis. This intermediate group constitutes an important link between polymyositis and the carcinomatous myasthenic syndrome.

Carcinomatous myasthenic syndrome

The occasional occurrence of a myasthenic type of muscular weakness associated with malignant tumours was first recognised when Anderson, Churchill-Davidson and Richardson (1953) reported prolonged apnoea after administration of succinylcholine to a patient with bronchial neoplasm, and similar patients were reported in the next two years. As the neuromuscular block was reversed by edrophonium, these authors recognised an abnormal end-plate responsiveness resembling that occurring in myasthenia gravis (p. 603). Croft (1958) found abnormal responses to relaxant drugs in patients with carcinomatous neuropathy, not all of whom had symptoms of muscular fatigability, and drew attention to absence of the tendon jerks. The clinical syndrome was first clearly defined by Lambert, Rooke, Eaton and Hodgson (1961), who described EMG characteristics resembling those found by Simpson and Lenman (1959) in non-tumour patients. They found later that the syndrome is related to malignant tumour, either contemporaneously or preceding it by several years, but mainly in men over the age of 40 yr, whereas most women with this syndrome do not develop a recognised neoplasm. The tumour is usually a small-cell or oat-cell carcinoma of bronchus; Greene, Divertie, Brown and Lambert (1968) drew attention to possible histological differences in the tumour cells, suggesting a secretory function. Less commonly the syndrome has occurred with intrathoracic reticulum cell sarcoma (Rooke, Eaton, Lambert and Hodgson, 1960) and with carcinoma of breast, colon, stomach, prostate and other organs (Adams, 1975).

The principal symptoms are weakness and fatigability of proximal muscles of the extremities, particularly of the pelvic girdle and thighs. Careful manual testing often reveals a delay in development of strength at the onset of maximal voluntary contraction, Ptosis may be present, but striking differences from myasthenia gravis are that symptoms of involvement of ocular and bulbar muscular weakness either do not occur, or are mild and transient, and that the tendon reflexes are depressed or absent. Common complaints are aching of the lower limbs, peripheral paraesthesiae, dryness of the mouth, and loss of potency.

The significance of these symptoms is commonly apparent in retrospect after the patient has had prolonged apnoea following administration of a muscle-relaxant drug during surgical procedures. The diagnosis is then readily confirmed by characteristic EMG responses to repetitive supramaximal motor nerve stimulation. The rested muscle shows a pronounced depression of the response to a single stimulus. Low rates of stimulation evoke further decrement: stimulation rates above 10/s evoke markedly incremental responses (Lambert, Okihiro and Rooke, 1965; Lambert, 1966). For further details see Chapter 26. Intracellular recordings from the end-plate region of single muscle fibres reveal normal miniature end-plate potentials but subthreshold end-plate potentials which vary greatly, indicating that a very low number of ACh quanta are released from the nerve ending until it is stimulated repetitively (Elmqvist and Lambert, 1968). The transmission characteristics are similar, but not identical, to those of a normal neuromuscular junction exposed to a high Mg^{+++} concentration. The blood level of Mg^{+++} is normal. The quantum content of the end-plate potential is raised by increasing the external calcium ion concentration and with the addition of guanidine.

Anticholinesterase drugs such as pyridostigmine improve muscular strength, but are much less effective than in myasthenia gravis and tend to become still less effective after 1–2 weeks. Guanidine hydrochloride, though sometimes disappointing in a single test dose, is strikingly effective on prolonged administration. A recommended dosage (Lambert, 1966) is 20–30 mg/kg/day divided into four doses. This will usually restore power to normal and abolish fatigability for many months, sometimes progressively. For dosage and potential adverse effects see page 610. An alternative drug is 4-aminopyridine; Lundh et al. (1977) reported its use in one case. In my experience it has been beneficial, but is greatly inferior to guanidine.

Pathology. The clinical neurophysiology and pharmacology indicate a prejunctional abnormality of ACh release. In light microscopic specimens, stained intravitally with methylene blue, Wise and MacDermot (1962) noted irregularity of calibre and abnormal swelling of axons of intramuscular nerve fibres, increased preterminal branching, and abnormally large and complex end-plates which they regarded as consistent with a mild peripheral neuropathy. Ultramicroscopic studies have not been consistent. Most reports are unable to differentiate the end-plate changes from those of myasthenia gravis (Adams, 1975). Engel and Santa (1971) found no significant abnormality in the mean area of motor nerve terminals, and a normal number of synaptic vesicles, but there was possibly a decrease in the mean diameter of the vesicles and of the mean area of mitochondria in the nerve terminals. They considered that the most significant abnormality was an overdevelopment of the post-junctional region, highly complex secondary clefts and folds, and the sacroplasmic folds contained numerous pinocytotic vesicles. At present it is not understood why the post-junctional region is altered in this way or how it contributes to the functional deficit.

Muscle fibres show minor changes which appear to be similar to those described above in myasthenia gravis. Serum antibody against ACh receptors is not increased (Lindstrom et al., 1976a). There is no report on anti-axonal antibody. Nastuk (in discussion of Lambert et al., 1965) has described A-band fluorescence of muscle reacted with serum globulin from patients with carcinomatous myasthenia, apparently identical to the reaction seen in myasthenia gravis associated with thymoma. This finding has not been reported in detail.

Pathogenesis. Clearly, there are many points of resemblance between this syndrome, true myasthenia gravis, and the myasthenia of polymyositis. About 30 per cent of cases with the Eaton-Lambert syndrome do not have a tumour. An extract of cancer tissue which apparently reduces ACh release is reported by Ishikawa, Engelhardt, Fujisawa, Okamoto and Katjuki (1977). The possibility that a malignant tumour may secret a neurotoxin, in analogy with the well-recognised hormonal secretions, cannot be excluded although it is unlikely in view of the diversity of tumours which may be associated. The myasthenia may precede the tumour by many years and removal of the tumour does not alter the defect of neuromuscular transmission. The relationship is probably indirect, e.g. immunological and associated with a state of immunodeficiency. This would also account for the reported occurrence of the syndrome with Boeck's sarcoid (Adams, 1975). Indeed, it is not impossible that the tumour and the myasthenic syndrome are independent results of a common aetiological factor. Papatestas, Osserman and Kark (1971a) have noted a three-fold increase over the expected incidence of extrathymic neoplasms, in patients with myasthenia gravis who have not had thymectomy while, following thymectomy, the incidence returned to expected levels. As others have suggested that the normal thymus may play a role in immunological defence mechanisms against cancer, Vessey and Doll (1972) examined the hypothesis that thymectomy might increase the risk of cancer and found no evidence that this was so, in agreement with Papatestas et al. (1971a), but the observation of these authors that the thymic disorder associated with myasthenia gravis also predisposes to extrathymic cancer is obviously important with regard to so-called carcinomatous myasthenia. The autoimmune hypothesis of myasthenia gravis has had important repercussions on the concept of autoimmunity and the role of the thymus. It also has important implications for general biology.

ACKNOWLEDGEMENTS

Figure 16.8 is reproduced from the author's chapter on 'The Defect in Myasthenia Gravis' published in 'The Biological Basis of Medicine' edited by Bittar and Bittar (1969), copyright by Academic Press Inc. (London) Ltd. Figures 16.3 and 16.5 are reproduced from 'The motor endplate in myasthenia gravis' by Engel, Lambert and Howard (1977) Proc. Mayo Clin., **52**, 267, with the kind permission of the authors, editor and publishers.

REFERENCES

Aarli, J.A., Milde, E-J. & Thunold, S. (1975) Arthritis in myasthenia gravis. *Journal of Neurology, Neurosurgery and Psychiatry*, **38**, 1048.

Aarli, J.A., Heimann, P., Matre, R., Thunold, S. & Tönder, O. (1979) Lymphocyte subpopulations in thymus and blood from patients with myasthenia gravis. *Journal of Neurology, Neurosurgery and Psychiatry*, **42**, 29.

Abdou, N.I., Lisak, R.P., Zweiman, B., Abramson, I. & Penn, A.S. (1974) The thymus in myasthenia gravis. Evidence for altered cell populations. *New England Journal of Medicine*, **291**, 1271.

Abramsky, O., Aharonov, A., Webb, C. & Fuchs, S. (1975) Cellular immune response to acetylcholine receptor rich fraction in patients with myasthenia gravis. *Clinical and Experimental Immunology*, **19**, 11.

Adams, D.D. (1977) In *Immunology in Medicine*, Eds E.J. Holborow & W.G. Reeves, p. 373 (Academic Press: London).

Adams, R.D. (1975) *Diseases of Muscle. A Study in Pathology*, 3rd edition (Harper and Row: Hagerstown, Maryland).

Aharonov, A., Tarrab-Hazdai, R., Abramsky, O. & Fuchs, S. (1975a) Humoral antibodies to acetylcholine receptor in patients with myasthenia gravis. *Lancet*, **2**, 340.

Aharonov, A., Tarrab-Hazdai, R., Abramsky, O. & Fuchs, S. (1975b) Immunological relationship between acetylcholine receptor and thymus—a possible significance in myasthenia gravis. *Proceedings of the National Academy of Sciences, USA*, **72**, 1456.

Alarcón-Segovia, D., Galbraith, R.F., Maldonado, J.E. &

Howard, F.M. (1963) Systemic lupus erythematosus following thymectomy for myasthenia gravis. *Lancet*, **2**, 662.

Almon, R.R., Andrew, C.G. & Appel, S.H. (1974) Serum globulin in myasthenia gravis: inhibition of α-bungarotoxin binding to acetylcholine receptors. *Science*, **186**, 55.

Alpert, L.I., Papatestas, A., Kark, A., Osserman, R.S. & Osserman, K. (1971) A histologic reappraisal of the thymus in myasthenia gravis. *Archives of Pathology*, **91**, 55.

Alter, N.M. & Osnato, M. (1930) Myasthenia gravis with status lymphaticus and multiple thymic granulomas. *Archives of Neurology and Psychiatry*, **23**, 345.

Anderson, H.J., Churchill-Davidson, H.C. & Richardson, A.T. (1953) Bronchial neoplasm with myasthenia. Prolonged apnoea after administration of succinylcholine. *Lancet*, **2**, 1291.

Anwyl, R., Appel, S.H. & Narahashi, T. (1977) Myasthenia gravis serum reduces acetylcholine sensitivity in cultured rat myotubes. *Nature*, **267**, 262.

Appel, S.H., Almon, R.R. & Levy, N. (1975) Acetylcholine receptor antibodies in myasthenia gravis. *New England Journal of Medicine*, **293**, 760.

Aureggi, A., Cirelli, A., Virno, F. & Nigro, G. (1970) Prime osservazioni sul trattamento della miastenia grave con immunoglobulina antilimfocite ed antitimocite. *Medicina Clinica e Sperimentale*, **20**, 1.

Ballantyne, J.P. & Hansen, S. (1974) Computer method for the analysis of evoked motor unit potentials. 1. Control subjects and patients with myasthenia gravis. *Journal of Neurology, Neurosurgery and Psychiatry*, **37**, 1187.

Becker, K.L., Titus, J.L., McConahey, W.M. & Woolner, L.B. (1964) Morphologic evidence of thyroiditis in myasthenia gravis. *Journal of the American Medical Association*, **187**, 994.

Behan, P.O., Simpson, J.A. & Behan, W.M.H. (1976) Decreased serum IgA in myasthenia gravis. *Lancet*, **2**, 593.

Behan, P.O., Simpson, J.A. & Dick, H. (1973) Immune response genes in myasthenia gravis. *Lancet*, **2**, 1033 & 1220.

Behan, P.O., Behan, W.M.H., Zacharias, F.J. & Nicholls, J.T. (1976). Immunological abnormalities in patients who had the oculomucocutaneous syndrome associated with practolol therapy. *Lancet*, **2**, 984.

Behan, W.M.H. & Behan, P.O. (1979) Immune complexes in myasthenia gravis. *Journal of Neurology, Neurosurgery and Psychiatry*, **42**, 595.

Behan, W.M.H., Behan, P.O. & Simpson, J.A. (1975) Absence of cellular hypersensitivity to muscle and thymic antigens in myasthenia gravis. *Journal of Neurology, Neurosurgery and Psychiatry*, **38**, 1039.

Bender, A.N., Ringel, S.P., Engel, W.K., Daniels, M.P. & Vogel, Z. (1975) Myasthenia gravis: a serum factor blocking acetylcholine receptors of the human neuromuscular junction. *Lancet*, **1**, 607.

Bennett, A.E. & Cash, P.J. (1943) Myasthenia gravis. (Curare sensitivity, a new diagnostic test and approach to causation.) *Archives of Neurology and Psychiatry*, **49**, 537.

Bergman, R.A., Johns, R.J. & Afifi, A.K. (1971) Ultra-structural alterations in muscle from patients with myasthenia gravis and Eaton-Lambert syndrome. *Annals of the New York Academy of Sciences*, **183**, 88.

Beutner, E.H., Chorzelski, T.P., Hale, W.L. & Hausmanowa-Petrusewicz, I. (1968) Autoimmunity in concurrent myasthenia gravis and pemphigus erythematosus. *Journal of the American Medical Association*, **203**, 845.

Beutner, E.H., Witebsky, E., Ricken, D. & Adler, R.H. (1962) Studies on autoantibodies in myasthenia gravis. *Journal of the American Medical Association*, **182**, 46.

Bickerstaff, E.R. & Woolf, A.L. (1960) The intramuscular nerve endings in myasthenia gravis. *Brain*, **83**, 10.

Blom, S. & Zakrisson, J.E. (1974) The stapedius reflex in the diagnosis of myasthenia gravis. *Journal of the Neurological Sciences*, **21**, 71.

Borenstein, S. & Desmedt, J.E. (1973) New diagnostic procedures in myasthenia gravis. In *New Developments in Electromyography and Clinical Neurophysiology*, Ed. J.G. Desmedt, Vol. 1, pp. 350–374 (Karger: Basel).

Bosch, E.P., Reith, P.E. & Granner, D.K. (1978) Myasthenia gravis and Schmidt syndrome. *Neurology (Minneapolis)*, **27**, 1179.

Bramis, J., Sloane, C., Papatestas, A.E., Genkins, G. & Aufses, A.H. (1976) Serum IgA in myasthenia gravis. *Lancet*, **1**, 1243.

Brody, I.A. & Engel, W.K. (1964) Denervation of muscle in myasthenia gravis. *Archives of Neurology*, **11**, 350.

Brolley, N. & Hollender, N.H. (1955) Psychological problems of patients with myasthenia gravis. *Journal of Nervous and Mental Disorders*, **122**, 178.

Brooke, M.H. & Engel, W.K. (1969) The histographic analysis of human muscle biopsies with regard to fiber types. 3. Myotonias, myasthenia gravis, and hypokalemic periodic paralysis. *Neurology (Minneapolis)*, **19**, 469.

Brown, J.C. & Charlton, J.E. (1975) A study of sensitivity to curare in myasthenic disorders using a regional technique. *Journal of Neurology, Neurosurgery and Psychiatry*, **38**, 27.

Brunner, N.G., Berger, C.L., Namba, T. & Grob, D. (1976) Corticotropin and corticosteroids in generalized myasthenia gravis: comparative studies and role in management. *Annals of the New York Academy of Sciences*, **274**, 577.

Bucknall, R.C. (1977) Myasthenia associated with D-penicillamine therapy in rheumatoid arthritis. *Proceedings of the Royal Society of Medicine*, **70** supplement 3, 114.

Bundey, S. (1972) A genetic study of infantile and juvenile myasthenia gravis. *Journal of Neurology, Neurosurgery and Psychiatry*, **35**, 41.

Bundey, S., Doniach, D. & Soothill, J.T. (1972) Immunological studies in patients with juvenile-onset myasthenia gravis and in their relatives. *Clinical and Experimental Immunology*, **11**, 321.

Buzzard, E.F. (1905) The clinical history and post-mortem examination of five cases of myasthenia gravis. *Brain*, **28**, 438.

Bystryn, J-C., Schenkein, I. & Uhr, J.W. (1971) A model for the regulation of antibody synthesis by serum antibody. In *Progress in Immunology*, Ed. B. Amos, pp. 627–636 (Academic Press: New York).

Campbell, H. & Bramwell, E. (1900) Myasthenia gravis. *Brain*, **23**, 277.

Campbell, M.J., Simpson, E., Crombie, A.L. & Walton, J.N. (1970) Ocular myasthenia: evaluation of Tensilon tomography and electromyography as diagnostic tests. *Journal of Neurology, Neurosurgery and Psychiatry*, **33**, 639.

Castleman, B. (1955) Tumors of the thymus gland. In *Atlas of Tumor Pathology*, Section V, fasc. 19, 7–82 (Armed Forces Institute of Pathology: Washington D.C.).

Castleman, B. & Norris, E.H. (1949) The pathology of the thymus in myasthenia gravis. A study of 35 cases. *Medicine (Baltimore)*, **28**, 27.

Churchill-Davidson, H.C. & Richardson, A.T. (1952a) The action of decamethonium iodide (C.10) in myasthenia gravis. *Journal of Neurology, Neurosurgery, and Psychiatry*, **15**, 129.

Churchill-Davidson, H.C. & Richardson, A.T. (1952b) Motor end-plate differences as a determining factor in the mode of action of neuro-muscular blocking substances. *Nature*, **170**, 617.

Churchill-Davidson, H.C. & Wise, R.P. (1963) Neuromuscular transmission in the newborn infant. *Anesthesiology*, **24**, 271.

Coërs, C. & Desmedt, J.E. (1959) Mise en évidence d'une malformation caractéristique de la jonction neuromusculaire dans la myasthénie: correlations histo- et physiopathologique. *Acta Neurologica Belgica*, **59**, 539.

Coërs, C. & Telerman-Toppet, N. (1976) Morphological and histochemical changes of motor units in myasthenia. *Annals of the New York Academy of Sciences*, **274**, 6.

Coërs, C. & Woolf, A.L. (1959) *The Innervation of Muscle. A Biopsy Study* (Blackwell: Oxford).

Coërs, C., Telerman-Toppet, N. & Gérard, J.M. (1973) Terminal innervation ratio in neuromuscular diseases. 1. Methods and controls. 2. Disorders of lower motor neurone, peripheral nerves and muscles. *Archives of Neurology*, **29**, 210 & 215.

Cogan, D.G. (1965) Myasthenia gravis: a review of the disease and a description of lid-twitch as a characteristic sign. *Archives of Ophthalmology*, **74**, 217.

Cohen, S.J. & King, F.H. (1932) Relation between myasthenia gravis and exophthalmic goitre. *Archives of Neurology and Psychiatry*, **28**, 1338.

Cohen, S.M. & Waxman, S. (1967) Myasthenia gravis, chronic lymphocytic leukemia, and autoimmune hemolytic anemia. *Archives of Internal Medicine*, **120**, 717.

Coulonjou, R. & Salaun, A. (1952) Sur un syndrome myasthénique fréquemment rencontré chez des chiqueurs de tabac. *Semaine des Hôpitaux de Paris*, **28**, 3968.

Cowan, R.J., Maynard, C.D., Witcofski, R.L., Janeway, R. & Toole, J.F. (1971) Selenomethionine Se 75 thymus scans in myasthenia gravis. *Journal of the American Medical Association*, **215**, 978.

Critchley, M., Herman, K.J., Harrison, M., Shields, R.A. & Liversedge, L.A. (1977). Value of exchangeable electrolyte measurement in the treatment of myasthenia gravis. *Journal of Neurology, Neurosurgery and Psychiatry*, **40**, 250.

Croft, P.B. (1958) Abnormal responses to muscle relaxants in carcinomatous neuropathy. *British Medical Journal*, **1**, 181.

Dawkins, R.L., Robinson, J. & Wetherall, J.D. (1975a) The significance of immunological disturbances in myasthenia gravis: evidence for two subtypes. In *Recent Advances in Myology*, Eds W.G. Bradley, D. Gardner-Medwin & J.N. Walton, pp. 503–509 (Excerpta Medica: Amsterdam).

Dawkins, R.L., Zilko, P.J. & Owen, E.T. (1975b) Penicillamine therapy, antistriational antibody, and myasthenia gravis. *British Medical Journal*, **4**, 759.

Denny-Brown, D. (1947) Neurological conditions resulting from prolonged and severe dietary restriction. *Medicine (Baltimore)*, **26**, 41.

Desmedt, J.E. & Borenstein, S. (1977) Double-step nerve stimulation test for myasthenic block: sensitization of postactivation exhaustion by ischemia. *Annals of Neurology*, **1**, 55.

Devreotes, P.N. & Fambrough, D.M. (1975) Acetylcholine receptor turnover in membranes of developing muscle fibers. *Journal of Cell Biology*, **65**, 335.

Dick, H.M., Behan, P.O., Simpson, J.A. & Durward, W.F. (1974) The inheritance of HL-A antigens in myasthenia gravis. *Journal of Immunogenetics*, **1**, 401.

Djanian, A.Y., Beutner, E.H. & Witebsky, E. (1964) Tanned-cell haemagglutination test for detection of antibodies in sera of patients with myasthenia gravis. *Journal of Laboratory and Clinical Medicine*, **63**, 60.

Downes, J.M., Greenwood, B.M. & Wray, S.H. (1966) Auto-immune aspects of myasthenia gravis. *Quarterly Journal of Medicine*, **35**, 85.

Drachman, D.B. (1978) Myasthenia gravis. *New England Journal of Medicine*, **298**, 136.

Drachman, D.B., Kao, L., Angus, C.W. & Murphy, A. (1977) Effect of myasthenic immunoglobin on acetylcholine receptors of cultured muscle. *Annals of Neurology*, **1**, 504.

Eaton, L.M. (1943) Diagnostic tests for myasthenia gravis with prostigmin and quinine. *Proceedings of Staff Meetings of the Mayo Clinic*, **18**, 230.

Elmqvist, D. (1965) Neuromuscular transmission with special reference to myasthenia gravis. *Acta Physiologica Scandinavica*, 64 suppl. **249**, 1.

Elmqvist, D. & Lambert, E.H. (1968) Detailed analysis of neuromuscular transmission in a patient with the myasthenic syndrome sometimes associated with bronchogenic carcinoma. *Mayo Clinic Proceedings*, **43**, 689.

Elmqvist, D., Hofmann, W.W., Kugelberg, J. & Quastel, D.M.J. (1964). An electrophysiological investigation of neuromuscular transmission in myasthenia gravis. *Journal of Physiology*, **174**, 417.

Engbaek, L. (1951) Acetylcholine sensitivity in diseases of the motor system with special regard to myasthenia gravis. *Electroencephalography and Clinical Neurophysiology*, **3**, 155.

Engel, A.G. (1961) Thyroid function and myasthenia gravis. *Archives of Neurology*, **4**, 663.

Engel, A.G. & Santa, T. (1971) Histometric analysis of the ultrastructure of the neuromuscular junction in myasthenia gravis and in the myasthenic syndrome. *Annals of the New York Academy of Sciences*, **183**, 46.

Engel, A.G., Lambert, E.H. & Gomez, M.R. (1976a) A new myasthenic syndrome with end-plate acetylcholinesterase (AChE) deficiency, small nerve terminals, and reduced acetylcholine release. *Transactions of the American Neurological Association*, **101**, 11.

Engel, A.G., Lambert, E.H. & Howard, F.M. (1977a) Immune complexes (IgC and C3) at the motor end-plate in myasthenia gravis. Ultrastructural and light microscopic localization and electrophysiologic correlations. *Mayo Clinic Proceedings*, **52**, 267.

Engel, A.G., Lindstrom, J.M., Lambert, E.H. & Lennon, V.A. (1977b) Ultrastructural localisation of the acetylcholine receptor in myasthenia gravis and in its experimental autoimmune model. *Neurology (Minneapolis)*, **27**, 307.

Engel, A.G., Tsujihata, M., Lindstrom, J.M. & Lennon, V.A. (1976b) The motor end plate in myasthenia gravis and in experimental autoimmune myasthenia gravis. *Annals of the New York Academy of Sciences*, **274**, 60.

Fardeau, M., Godet-Guillain, J. & Chevallay, M. (1974) Ultrastructural changes of the motor end-plates in myasthenia gravis and myasthenic syndrome. In *Neurology*, Proceedings of the X International Congress of

Neurology, Barcelona, 1973, Eds A. Subirana & J.M. Espadaler. International Congress Series No. 319, pp. 427–438. (Excerpta Medica: Amsterdam.)

Feinberg, W.D., Underdahl, L.O. & Eaton, L.M. (1957) Myasthenia gravis and myxoedema. *Proceedings of the Staff Meetings of the Mayo Clinic*, **32**, 299.

Feltkamp, T.E.W., van den Berg-Loonen, P.M., Nijenhuis, L.E., Engelfriet, C.P., van Rossum, A.L., van Loghem, J.J. & Oosterhuis, H.J.G.H. (1974) Myasthenia gravis, autoantibodies, and HL-A antigens. *British Medical Journal*, **1**, 131.

Feltkamp-Vroom, T. (1966) Myoid cells in human thymus. *Lancet*, **2**, 1320.

Fenichel, G.M. & Shy, G.M. (1963) Muscle biopsy experience in myasthenia gravis. *Archives of Neurology*, **9**, 237.

Ferguson, F.R., Hutchinson, E.C. & Liversedge, L.A. (1955) Myasthenia gravis. Results of medical management. *Lancet*, **2**, 636.

Flacke, W., Caviness, V.S. & Samaha, F.G. (1966) The action of germine diacetate, a veratrine alkaloid without hypotensive activity, in patients with myasthenia gravis. *New England Journal of Medicine*, **275**, 1207.

Fraser, K., Simpson, J.A. & Crawford, J. (1978) The place of surgery in the treatment of myasthenia gravis. *British Journal of Surgery*, **65**, 301.

Frenkel, M. (1963) The effect of insulin and potassium in myasthenia gravis. *Archives of Neurology*, **9**, 447.

Fritze, D., Herrmann, C., Smith, G.S. & Walford, R.L. (1973) HL-A types in myasthenia gravis. *Lancet*, **2**, 211.

Fritze, D., Herrmann, C., Naeim, F., Smith, G.S. & Walford, R.L. (1974) HL-A antigens in myasthenia gravis. *Lancet*, **1**, 240.

Fuchs, S., Nevo, D., Tarrab-Hazdai, R. & Yaar, I. (1976) Strain differences in the autoimmune response of mice to acetylcholine receptors. *Nature*, **263**, 329.

Geld, H. van der, Feltkamp, T.E.W. & Oosterhuis, H.J.G.H. (1964) Reactivity of myasthenia gravis serum γ-globulin with skeletal muscle and thymus demonstrated by immunofluorescence. *Proceedings of the Society for Experimental Biology and Medicine*, **115**, 782.

Geld, H. van der & Strauss, A.J.L. (1966) Myasthenia gravis. *Lancet*, **1**, 57.

Genkins, G., Papatestas, A.E., Horowitz, S.H. & Kornfeld, P. (1975) Studies on myasthenia gravis: early thymectomy. *American Journal of Medicine*, **58**, 517.

Gillhespy, R.O. & Smith, S.G. (1954) Porphyria treated with neostigmine. *Lancet*, **1**, 908.

Golding, D.N. & Walshe, J.M. (1977) Arthropathy of Wilson's disease. Study of clinical and radiological features in 32 patients. *Annals of Rheumatic Diseases*, **36**, 99.

Goldstein, A.L., Thurman, G.B., Cohen, G.H. & Rossio, J.L. (1976) The endocrine thymus: potential role for thymosin in the treatment of autoimmune disease. *Annals of the New York Academy of Sciences*, **274**, 390.

Goldstein, G. & Whittingham, S. (1966) Experimental autoimmune thymitis. An animal model of human myasthenia gravis. *Lancet*, **2**, 315.

Gottlieb, B. & Laurent, L.P.E. (1961) Spironolactone in the treatment of myasthenia gravis. *Lancet*, **2**, 528.

Green, P. (1958) Aplastic anaemia associated with thymoma. Report of two cases. *Canadian Medical Association Journal*, **78**, 419.

Greene, J.G., Divertie, M.B., Brown, A.L. & Lambert, E.H.

(1968) Small cell carcinoma of lung. Observations on four patients including one with a myasthenic syndrome. *Archives of Internal Medicine*, **122**, 333.

Greene, R., Rideout, D.F. & Shaw, M.L. (1961) Ergometry in the diagnosis of myasthenia gravis. *Lancet*, **2**, 281.

Grob, D. (1953) Course and management of myasthenia gravis. *Journal of the American Medical Association*, **153**, 529.

Grob, D. (1958) Myasthenia gravis. Current status of pathogenesis, clinical manifestations, and management. *Journal of Chronic Diseases*, **8**, 536.

Grob, D. (1971) Spontaneous end-plate activity in normal subjects and in patients with myasthenia gravis. *Annals of the New York Academy of Sciences*, **183**, 248.

Grob, D. & Johns, R.J. (1958) Use of oximes in the treatment of intoxication by anticholinesterase compounds in patients with myasthenia gravis. *American Journal of Medicine*, **24**, 512.

Grob, D., Johns, R.J. & Harvey, A.M. (1956) Studies in neuromuscular function. 3. Stimulating and depressant effects of acetylcholine and choline in normal subjects. *Bulletin of the Johns Hopkins Hospital*, **99**, 136.

Harvey, A.M. (1948) Some preliminary observations on the clinical course of myasthenia gravis before and after thymectomy. *Bulletin of the New York Academy of Medicine*, **24**, 505.

Harvey, A.M., Shulman, L.E., Tumulty, P.A., Cowley, C.L. & Schoenrich, E.H. (1954) Systemic lupus erythematosus. Review of the literature and clinical analysis of 138 cases. *Medicine (Baltimore)*, **33**, 291.

Hausmanowa-Petrusewicz, I., Chorzelski, T. & Strugalska, H. (1969) Three year observation of a myasthenic syndrome concurrent with other autoimmune syndromes in a patient with thymoma. *Journal of the Neurological Sciences*, **9**, 273.

Hayman, M. (1941) Myasthenia gravis and psychosis. Report of a case with observations on its psychosomatic implications. *Psychosomatic Medicine*, **3**, 120.

Heilbronn, E., Mattson, C., Stalberg, E. & Hilton-Brown, P. (1975) Neurophysiological signs of myasthenia in rabbits after receptor antibody development. *Journal of the Neurological Sciences*, **24**, 59.

Heinemann, S., Merlie, J. & Lindstrom, J. (1978) Modulation of acetylcholine receptor in rat diaphragm by anti-receptor sera. *Nature*, **274**, 65.

Herishanu, Y. & Rosenberg, P. (1975) β-Blockers and myasthenia gravis. *Annals of Internal Medicine*, **83**, 834.

Herrmann, C. (1971) The familial occurrence of myasthenia gravis. *Annals of the New York Academy of Sciences*, **183**, 334.

Herzfeld, E., Kraupp, O., Pateisky, K. & Stumpf, C. (1957) Pharmakologische und klinische Wirkungen des Cholinesterasehemnköpers Hexamethylen-bis-(N-methyl-carbaminoyl-1-methyl-3-oxypyridinium-bromid) BC 51. *Wiener klinische Wochenschrift*, **69**, 245.

Hill, P.K., Lindstrom, J.M., Lennon, V.A. & Dyck, P.J. (1977) Experimental autoimmune myasthenia gravis: no morphometric abnormalities of nerve trunks. *Neurology (Minneapolis)*, **27**, 200.

Hoefer, P.F.A., Aranow, H. and Rowland, L.P. (1958) Myasthenia gravis and epilepsy. *Archives of Neurology and Psychiatry*, **80**, 10.

Hokkanen, E. (1964) The aggravating effect of some antibiotics on the neuromuscular blockade in myasthenia gravis. *Acta Neurologica Scandinavica*, **40**, 346.

Howard, F.M., Duane, D.D., Lambert, E.H. & Daube, J.R. (1976) Alternate day prednisone. Preliminary report of a double-blind controlled study. *Annals of the New York Academy of Sciences*, **274**, 596.

Ishikawa, K., Engelhardt, J.K., Fujisawa, T., Okamoto, T. & Katjuki, H. (1977) A neuromuscular transmission block produced by a cancer tissue extract derived from a patient with the myasthenic syndrome. *Neurology (Minneapolis)*, **27**, 140.

Ito, Y., Miledi, R., Vincent, A. & Newsom Davis, J. (1978) Acetylcholine receptors and end-plate electrophysiology in myasthenia gravis. *Brain*, **101**, 345.

Iverson, L. (1956) Thymoma. A review and reclassification. *American Journal of Pathology*, **32**, 695.

Jacob, A., Clack, E.R. & Emery, A.E.H. (1968) Genetic study of sample of 70 patients with myasthenia gravis. *Journal of Medical Genetics*, **5**, 257.

Johns, R.J., Grob, D. & Harvey, A.M. (1956) Studies in neuromuscular function. 2. Effects of nerve stimulation in normal subjects and in patients with myasthenia gravis. *Bulletin of the Johns Hopkins Hospital*, **99**, 125.

Joseph, B.S. & Johns, T.R. (1973) Recurrence of non-neoplastic thymus after thymectomy for myasthenia gravis. *Neurology (Minneapolis)*, **23**, 109.

Kaakinen, A., Pirskanen, R. & Tiilikainen, A. (1975) LD antigens associated with HL-A8 and myasthenia gravis. *Tissue Antigens*, **6**, 175.

Kao, I. & Drachman, D.B. (1977a) Thymic muscle cells bear acetylcholine receptors: possible relation to myasthenia gravis. *Science*, **195**, 74.

Kao, I. & Drachman, D.B. (1977b) Myasthenic immunoglobulin accelerates acetylcholine receptor degradation. *Science*, **196**, 527.

Kessey, J., Lindström, J., Cokely, H. & Herrman, C. (1977) Anti-acetylcholine receptor antibody in neonatal myasthenia gravis. *New England Journal of Medicine*, **296**, 1.

Keynes, G. (1950) Thymectomy for myasthenia gravis. In *Techniques in British Surgery*, Ed. R.H. Maingot, pp. 126–148 (Saunders: Philadelphia).

Keynes, G. (1955) Investigations into thymic disease and tumour formation. *British Journal of Surgery*, **42**, 449.

Keynes, G. (1961) The history of myasthenia gravis. *Medical History*, **5**, 313.

Koch, F., Regli, F. & Reinle, W. (1970) Myasthenia gravis nach Thymektomie. *Schweizerische medizinische Wochenschrift*, **100**, 65.

Laquer, L. & Weigert, C. (1901) Beitrage zur Lehre von der Erb'schen Krankheit ueber die Erb-sche Krankheit (Myasthenia Gravis). *Neurologisches Zentralblatt*, **20**, 594.

Lambert, E.H. (1966) Defects of neuromuscular transmission in syndromes other than myasthenia gravis. *Annals of the New York Academy of Sciences*, **135**, 367.

Lambert, E.H., Okihiro, M. & Rooke, E.D. (1965) Clinical physiology of the neuromuscular junction. In *Muscle*, Eds W.M. Paul, E.E. Daniel, C.M. Kay, & G. Monckton, pp. 487–497 (Pergamon Press: New York).

Lambert, E.H., Rooke, E.D., Eaton, L.M. & Hodgson, C.H. (1961) Myasthenic syndrome occasionally associated with bronchial neoplasm: neurophysiologic studies. In *Myasthenia Gravis*, Ed. H.R. Viets, pp. 362–410 (Thomas: Springfield).

Lefvert, A.K. & Pirskanen, R. (1977) Acetylcholine receptor antibodies in cerebrospinal fluid of patients with myasthenia gravis. *Lancet*, **2**, 351.

Lefvert, A.K., Bergström, K., Matell, G., Osterman, P.O. & Pirskanen, R. (1978) Determination of acetylcholine receptor antibody in myasthenia gravis: clinical usefulness and pathogenetic implications. *Journal of Neurology, Neurosurgery and Psychiatry*, **41**, 394.

Lehmann, H. & Liddell, J. (1969) Human cholinesterase (pseudocholinesterase): genetic variants and their recognition. *British Journal of Anaesthesia*, **41**, 235.

Lennon, V.A., Lindstrom, J.M. & Seybold, M.E. (1976) Experimental autoimmune myasthenia gravis: cellular and humoral immune responses. *Annals of the New York Academy of Sciences*, **274**, 283.

Levin, P.M. (1949) Congenital myasthenia in siblings. *Archives of Neurology and Psychiatry*, **62**, 745.

Lindstrom, J. (1977) An assay for antibodies to human acetylcholine receptor in serum from patients with myasthenia gravis. *Clinical Immunology and Immunopathology*, **7**, 36.

Lindstrom, J. (1978) Pathological mechanisms in myasthenia gravis and its animal model, experimental autoimmune myasthenia gravis. In *The Biochemistry of Myasthenia Gravis and Muscular Dystrophy*, Eds G.G. Lunt & R.M. Marchbanks, pp. 135–156 (Academic Press: London).

Lindstrom, J.M., Engel, A.G., Seybold, M.E., Lennon, V.A. & Lambert, E.H. (1976a) Pathological mechanisms for experimental autoimmune myasthenia gravis. *Journal of Experimental Medicine*, **144**, 739–753.

Lindstrom, J.M., Seybold, M.E., Lennon, V.A., Whittingham, S. & Duane, D.D. (1976b) Antibody to acetylcholine receptor in myasthenia gravis. Prevalence, clinical correlates, and diagnostic value. *Neurology (Minneapolis)*, **26**, 1054.

Lisak, R.P. & Zweiman, B. (1975) Mitogen and muscle extract induced in vitro proliferative responses in myasthenia gravis, dermatomyositis and polymyositis. *Journal of Neurology, Neurosurgery and Psychiatry*, **38**, 521.

Lovelace, R.E., Stone, R. & Zablow, L. (1970) A new test for myasthenia gravis: recording of miniature end-plate potentials in situ. *Neurology (Minneapolis)*, **20**, 385.

Lundh, H., Nilsson, O. & Rosén, I. (1977) 4-Aminopyridine—a new drug tested in the treatment of Eaton-Lambert syndrome. *Journal of Neurology, Neurosurgery and Psychiatry*, **40**, 1109.

MacDermot, V. (1960) The changes in the motor end-plate in myasthenia gravis. *Brain*, **83**, 24.

McEachern, D. & Parnell, J.L. (1948) The relationship of hyperthyroidism to myasthenia gravis. *Journal of Clinical Endocrinology*, **8**, 842.

McFarlin, D.E., Engel, W.K. & Strauss, A.J.L. (1966) Does myasthenic serum bind to the neuromuscular junction? *Annals of the New York Academy of Sciences*, **135**, 656.

MacKay, I.R., Whittingham, S., Goldstein, G., Currie, T.T. & Hare, W.S.C. (1968) Myasthenia gravis: clinical, serological and histological studies in relation to thymectomy. *Australasian Annals of Medicine*, **17**, 1.

McLean, W.T. & McKone, R.C. (1973) Congenital myasthenia gravis in twins. Identical twins with crises in the newborn period. *Archives of Neurology*, **29**, 223.

Mann, J.D., Johns, T.R. & Campa, J.F. (1976) Long-term administration of corticosteroids in myasthenia gravis. *Neurology (Minneapolis)*, **26**, 729.

Martin, L., Herr, J.C., Wanamaker, W. & Kornguth, S.

(1974) Demonstration of specific antineuronal nuclear antibodies in sera of patients with myasthenia gravis. Indirect and direct immunofluorescence. *Neurology (Minneapolis)*, **24**, 680.

Matell, G., Bergström, K., Franksson, C., Hammarström, L., Lefvert, A.K., Möller, E., von Reis, G. & Smith, E. (1976) Effects of some immunosuppressive procedures on myasthenia gravis. *Annals of the New York Academy of Sciences*, **274**, 659.

Meyer, E. (1966) Psychological disturbances in myasthenia gravis: a predictive study. *Annals of the New York Academy of Sciences*, **135**, 417.

Millichap, J.G. & Dodge, P.R. (1960) Diagnosis and treatment of myasthenia gravis in infancy, childhood and adolescence. A study of 51 patients. *Neurology (Minneapolis)*, **10**, 1007.

Millikan, C. & Haines, S.F. (1953) The thyroid gland in relation to neuromuscular disease. In *Metabolic and Toxic Diseases of the Nervous System. Research Publications, Association for Research in Nervous and Mental Disease*, **32**, 61.

Murnaghan, M.F. (1960) Site and mechanism of tick paralysis. *Science*, **131**, 418.

Namba, T. & Grob, D. (1970) Familial concurrence of myasthenia gravis and rheumatoid arthritis. *Archives of Internal Medicine*, **125**, 1056.

Namba, T., Brown, S.B. & Grob, D. (1970) Neonatal myasthenia gravis: report of two cases and review of the literature. *Pediatrics*, **45**, 488.

Namba, T., Brunner, N.G., Brown, S.B., Mugurama, M. & Grob, D. (1971a) Familial myasthenia gravis. Report of 27 patients in 12 families and review of 164 patients in 73 families. *Archives of Neurology*, **25**, 49.

Namba, T., Shapiro, M.S., Brunner, N.G. & Grob, D. (1971b) Myasthenia gravis occurring in twins. *Journal of Neurology, Neurosurgery and Psychiatry*, **34**, 531.

Nastuk, W.L., Plescia, O.J. & Osserman, K.E. (1960) Changes in serum complement activity in patients with myasthenia gravis. *Proceedings of the Society for Experimental Biology and Medicine*, **105**, 177.

Nastuk, W.L., Strauss, A.J.L. & Osserman, K.E. (1959) Search for a neuromuscular blocking agent in the blood of patients with myasthenia gravis. *American Journal of Medicine*, **26**, 394.

Newsom Davis, J., Pinching, A.J., Vincent, A. & Wilson, S.G. (1978) Function of circulating antibody to acetylcholine receptor in myasthenia gravis: investigation by plasma exchange. *Neurology (Minneapolis)*, **28**, 266.

Noguchi, S. & Nishitani, H. (1976) Immunologic studies of a case of myasthenia gravis associated with pemphigus vulgaris after thymectomy. *Neurology (Minneapolis)*, **26**, 1075.

Oosterhuis, H.J.G.H. (1964) Studies in myasthenia gravis. Part I (a clinical study of 180 patients). *Journal of the Neurological Sciences*, **1**, 512.

Oosterhuis, H. & Bethlem, J. (1973) Neurogenic muscle involvement in myasthenia gravis. A clinical and histopathological study. *Journal of Neurology, Neurosurgery and Psychiatry*, **36**, 244.

Oosterhuis, H.J.G.H., van der Geld, H., Feltkamp, T.E.W. & Peetoom, F. (1964) Myasthenia gravis with hypergammaglobulinaemia and antibodies. *Journal of Neurology, Neurosurgery and Psychiatry*, **27**, 345.

Osserman, K.E. (1958) *Myasthenia Gravis* (Grune and Stratton: New York).

Osserman, K.E. & Kaplan, L.I. (1953) Studies in myasthenia gravis: use of edrophonium chloride (Tensilon) in differentiating myasthenia from cholinergic weakness. *Archives of Neurology and Psychiatry (Chicago)*, **70**, 385.

Pantuck, E.J. & Pantuck, C.B. (1975) Cholinesterases and anticholinesterases. In *Muscle Relaxants*, Ed. R. Katz, pp. 143–162 (Excerpta Medica: Amsterdam).

Papatestas, A.E., Osserman, K.E. & Kark, A.E. (1971a) The relationship between thymus and oncogenesis. A study of the incidence of non-thymic malignancy in myasthenia gravis. *British Journal of Cancer*, **25**, 635.

Papatestas, A.E., Genkins, G., Horowitz, S.H. & Kornfeld, P. (1976) Thymectomy in myasthenia gravis: pathologic, clinical and electrophysiologic correlations. *Annals of the New York Academy of Sciences*, **274**, 555.

Papatestas, A.E., Alpert, L.I., Osserman, K.E., Osserman, R.S. & Kark, A.E. (1971b) Studies in myasthenia gravis: effects of thymectomy. *American Journal of Medicine*, **50**, 465.

Patrick, J. & Lindstrom, J. (1973) Autoimmune response to acetylcholine receptor. *Science*, **180**, 871.

Patten, B.M. (1975) A hypothesis to account for the Mary Walker phenomenon. *Annals of Internal Medicine*, **82**, 411.

Perlo, V.P., Poskanzer, D.C., Schwab, R.S., Viets, H.R., Osserman, K.E. & Genkins, G. (1966) Myasthenia gravis: evaluation of treatment in 1,355 patients. *Neurology (Minneapolis)*, **16**, 431.

Pinching, A.J., Peters, D.K. & Newsom Davis, J. (1976) Remission of myasthenia gravis following plasma-exchange. *Lancet*, **2**, 1373.

Pirofsky, B., Reid, R.H., Bardana, E.J. & Bayrakci, C. (1971) Antithymocyte antisera therapy in non surgical immunologic disease. *Transplantation Proceedings*, **111**, 769.

Pirskanen, R. (1976) Genetic associations betwen myasthenia gravis and the HL-A system. *Journal of Neurology, Neurosurgery and Psychiatry*, **39**, 23.

Pirskanen, R. (1977) Genetic aspects of myasthenia gravis. A family study of 264 Finnish patients. *Acta Neurologica Scandinavica*, **56**, 365.

Pirskanen, R., Tiilikainen, A. & Hokkanen, E. (1972) Histocompatibility (HL-A) antigens associated with myasthenia gravis. A preliminary report. *Annals of Clinical Research*, **4**, 304.

Plescia, O.J., Segovia, J.M. & Strampp, A. (1966) An assessment of changes in the complement level of myasthenic sera. *Annals of the New York Academy of Sciences*, **135**, 580.

Rash, J.E., Albuquerque, E.X., Hudson, C.S., Mayer, R.S. & Setterfield, J.R. (1976) Studies of human myasthenia gravis: electrophysiological and ultrastructural evidence compatible with antibody attachment to acetylcholine receptor complex. *Proceedings of the National Academy of Sciences, USA*, **73**, 4584.

Rees, D., Behan, P.O., Behan, W.M.H. & Simpson, J.A. (1977) Myasthenia gravis: passive transfer from man to mouse. In *Symposium on Current Research in Muscular Dystrophy*, abstract 16 (Muscular Dystrophy Group of Gt. Britain: London).

Reiness, C.G. & Weinberg, C.B. (1978) Antibody to acetylcholine receptor increases degradation of junctional and extrajunctional receptors in adult muscle. *Nature*, **274**, 68.

Reinglass, J.L. & Brickel, A.C.J. (1973) The prognostic significance of thymic germinal center proliferation in myasthenia gravis. *Neurology (Minneapolis)*, **23**, 69.

Richman, D.P., Patrick, J. & Arnason, B.G.W. (1976) Cellular immunity in myasthenia gravis. *New England Journal of Medicine*, **294**, 694.

Ringvist, I. & Ringvist, T. (1971) Respiratory mechanics in untreated myasthenia gravis with special reference to the respiratory forces. *Acta Medica Scandinavica*, **190**, 499.

Rooke, E.D., Eaton, L.M., Lambert, E.H. & Hodgson, C.H. (1960) Myasthenia and malignant intrathoracic tumor. *Medical Clinics of North America*, **44**, 977.

Roux, H., Serratrice, G. & Pollini, S. (1974) Antithymic and antilymphocytic globulins in the treatment of some neuromuscular disorders. In *Structure and Function of Normal and Diseased Muscle and Peripheral Nerve*, Eds I. Hausmanowa-Petrusewicz, & H. Jedrzejowska, pp. 265–269 (Polish Medical Publishers: Warsaw).

Rowland, L.P., Hoefer, P.F.A., Aranow, H. & Merritt, H.H. (1956) Fatalities in myasthenia gravis. *Neurology (Minneapolis)*, **6**, 307.

Rowland, L.P., Osserman, E.F., Scharfman, W.B., Balsam, R.F. & Ball, S. (1969) Myasthenia gravis with a myeloma-type, gamma-G (IgG) immunoglobulin abnormality. *American Journal of Medicine*, **46**, 599.

Rule, A.H. & Kornfeld, P. (1971) Studies in myasthenia gravis: biologic aspects. *The Mount Sinai Journal of Medicine*, **38**, 538.

Russell, D.S. (1953) Histological changes in the striped muscles in myasthenia gravis. *Journal of Pathology and Bacteriology*, **65**, 279.

Sahay, B.M., Blendis, L.M. & Greene, R. (1965) Relation between myasthenia gravis and thyroid disease. *British Medical Journal*, **1**, 762.

Sambrook, M.A., Reid, H., Mohr, P.D. & Boddie, H.G. (1976) Myasthenia gravis: clinical and histological features in relation to thymectomy. *Journal of Neurology, Neurosurgery and Psychiatry*, **39**, 38.

Sandilands, G.P., Gray, K., Cooney, A., Anderson, J.R., Simpson, J.A., & Behan, P.O. (1975) Rosette tests following thymectomy. *Lancet*, **1**, 171.

Schrire, I. (1959) Progesterone metabolism in myasthenia gravis. *Quarterly Journal of Medicine*, **28**, 59.

Schulz, M.D. & Schwab, R.S. (1971) Results of thymic (mediastinal) irradiation in patients with myasthenia gravis. *Annals of the New York Academy of Sciences*, **183**, 303.

Schwab, R.S. (1954) Belladonna drugs in cholinergic poisoning during treatment of myasthenia gravis. *Journal of the American Medical Association*, **155**, 1445.

Schwab, R.S. & Leland, C.C. (1953) Sex and age in myasthenia gravis as critical factors in incidence and remissions. *Journal of the American Medical Association*, **153**, 1270.

Schwartz, M., Novick, D., Givol, D. & Fuchs, S. (1978) Induction of anti-idiotypic antibodies by immunisation with syngeneic spleen cells educated with acetylcholine receptor. *Nature*, **273**, 543.

Schwartz, M.S. & Stålberg, E. (1975a) Myasthenia gravis with features of the myasthenic syndrome. An investigation with electrophysiologic methods including single-fiber electromyography. *Neurology (Minneapolis)*, **25**, 80.

Schwartz, M.S. & Stålberg, E. (1975b) Single fibre electromyographic studies in myasthenia gravis with repetitive nerve stimulation. *Journal of Neurology, Neurosurgery and Psychiatry*, **38**, 678.

Seybold, M.E., Howard, F.M., Duane, D.D., Payne, W.S. & Harrison, E.C. (1971) Thymectomy in juvenile myasthenia gravis. *Archives of Neurology*, **25**, 385.

Shibuya, N., Mori, K. & Nakazawa, Y. (1978) Serum factor blocks neuromuscular transmission in myasthenia gravis: electrophysiologic study with intracellular microelectrodes. *Neurology (Minneapolis)*, **28**, 804.

Simpson, J.A. (1958) An evaluation of thymectomy in myasthenia gravis. *Brain*, **81**, 112.

Simpson, J.A. (1960) Myasthenia gravis: a new hypothesis. *Scottish Medical Journal*, **5**, 419.

Simpson, J.A. (1964) Immunological disturbances in myasthenia gravis: with a report of Hashimoto's disease developing after thymectomy. *Journal of Neurology, Neurosurgery and Psychiatry*, **27**, 485.

Simpson, J.A. (1965) Myasthenia gravis. In *Biochemical Aspects of Neurological Disorders*. Second series, Eds J.N. Cumings & M. Kremer, pp. 53–72 (Blackwell: Oxford).

Simpson, J.A. (1966a) Disorders of neuromuscular transmission. *Proceedings of the Royal Society of Medicine*, **59**, 993.

Simpson, J.A. (1966b) The biochemistry of myasthenia gravis. In *Progressive Muskeldystrophie, Myotonie, Myasthenie*, Ed. E. Kuhn, pp. 339–349 (Springer: Berlin).

Simpson, J.A. (1966c) Myasthenia gravis as an autoimmune disease. Clinical aspects. *Annals of the New York Academy of Sciences*, **135**, 506.

Simpson, J.A. (1968) The correlations between myasthenia gravis and disorders of the thyroid gland. In *Research in Muscular Dystrophy. Proceedings of the 4th Symposium*, pp. 31–41 (Pitman: London).

Simpson, J.A. (1969a) Myasthenia gravis. In *Muscle Diseases*, Eds J.N. Walton, N. Canal & G. Scarlato, pp. 14–22 (Excerpta Medica: Amsterdam).

Simpson, J.A. (1969b) The defect in myasthenia gravis. In *The Biological Basis of Medicine—III*, Eds E.E. Bittar & N. Bittar, pp. 345–387 (Academic Press: London).

Simpson, J.A. (1971) A morphological explanation of the transmission defect in myasthenia gravis. *Annals of the New York Academy of Sciences*, **183**, 241.

Simpson, J.A. (1976) Neurological disorders. In *Haematological Aspects of Systemic Disease*, Eds M.C.G. Israels & I.W. Delamore, pp. 440–478 (Saunders: London).

Simpson, J.A. (1978) Myasthenia gravis: a personal view of pathogenesis and mechanism. *Muscle and Nerve*, **1**, 45 & 151.

Simpson, J.A. & Lenman, J.A.R. (1959) The effect of frequency of stimulation in neuromuscular diseases. *Electroencephalography and Clinical Neurophysiology*, **11**, 604.

Simpson, J.A., Behan, P.O. & Dick, H. (1976) Studies on the nature of autoimmunity in myasthenia gravis. Evidence for an immunodeficiency type. *Annals of the New York Academy of Sciences*, **274**, 382.

Slomić, A., Rosenfalck, A. & Buchthal, F. (1968) Electrical and mechanical responses of normal and myasthenic muscle, with particular reference to the staircase phenomenon. *Brain Research*, **10**, 1.

Spector, R.H. & Daroff, R.B. (1976) Edrophonium infrared optokinetic nystagmography in the diagnosis of myasthenia gravis. *Annals of the New York Academy of Sciences*, **274**, 642.

Stahlberg, E., Mattson, C., Uddgard, A., Heilbronn, E.,

Hammarström, L., Smith, E., Lefvert, A.K., Persson, A. & Matell, G. (1978) Increased decremental response in experimental autoimmune myasthenic rabbits following infusion of human myasthenic IgG. In *The Biochemistry of Myasthenia Gravis and Muscular Dystrophy*, Eds G.G. Lunt & R.M. Marchbanks, pp. 179–181 (Academic Press: London).

Stålberg, E. & Ekstedt, J. (1973) Single fibre EMG and microphysiology of the motor unit in normal and diseased human muscle. In *New Developments in Electromyography and Clinical Neurophysiology*, Ed. J.E. Desmedt, Vol. 1, pp. 113–129 (Karger: Basel).

Stålberg, E., Ekstedt, J. & Broman, A. (1974) Neuromuscular transmission in myasthenia gravis studied with single fibre electromyography. *Journal of Neurology, Neurosurgery, and Psychiatry*, 37, 540.

Stephens, A.D. & Fenton, J.C.B. (1977) Serum immunoglobulins in D-penicillamine-treated cystinurics. *Proceedings of the Royal Society of Medicine*, 70, suppl. 3, 31.

Storm-Mathisen, A. (1961) *Myasthenia Gravis* (Aschehoug/Almquist and Wiksell: Oslo/Stockholm).

Strauss, A.J.L., Seegal, B.C., Hsu, K.C., Burkholder, P.M., Nastuk, W.L. & Osserman, K.E. (1960) Immunofluorescence demonstration of a muscle binding, complement-fixing serum globulin fraction in myasthenia gravis. *Proceedings of the Society for Experimental Biology and Medicine*, 105, 184.

Strauss, A.J.L., Smith, C.W., Cage, G.W., van der Geld, H.W.R., McFarlin, D.E. & Barlow, M. (1966) Further studies on the specificity of presumed immune associations of myasthenia gravis and considerations of possible pathogenic implications. *Annals of the New York Academy of Sciences*, 135, 557.

Struppler, A. (1954) Elektromyographische Studien zun Wirkungsmechanismus Endplatten blockierender Stoffe. *Aërztliche Forschung*, 8, 564.

Swick, H.M., Preston, D.F. & McQuillen, M.P. (1976) Gallium scans in myasthenia gravis. *Annals of the New York Academy of Sciences*, 274, 536.

Symmers, D. (1932) Malignant tumours and tumour-like growths of the thymic region. *Annals of Surgery*, 95, 544.

Tarrab-Hazdai, R., Aharanov, A., Abramsky, O., Yaar, I. & Fuchs, S. (1975a) Passive transfer of experimental autoimmune myasthenia by lymph node cells in inbred guinea pigs. *Journal of Experimental Medicine*, 142, 785.

Tarrab-Hazdai, R. Aharanov, A., Silman, I., Fuchs, S. & Abramsky, O. (1975b) Experimental autoimmune myasthenia induced in monkeys by purified acetylcholine receptor. *Nature*, 256, 128.

Te Velde, K., Huber, J. & van der Slikke, L.B. (1966) Primary acquired hypogammaglobulinemia, myasthenia and thymoma. *Annals of Internal Medicine*, 65, 554.

Thévenard, A. & Mende, D. (1955) Etude électrophorétique de protéines sérique par la methode de Tiselius dans la myasthenie d'Erb-Goldflam. *Revue Neurologique (Paris)*, 92, 143.

Tindall, R.S.A., Cloud, R., Luby, J. & Rosenberg, R.N. (1978) Serum antibodies to cytomegalovirus in myasthenia gravis: effects of thymectomy and steroids. *Neurology (Minneapolis)*, 28, 273.

Toyka, K.V., Drachman, D.B., Pestronk, A. & Kao, I. (1975) Myasthenia gravis: passive transfer from man to mouse. *Science*, 190, 397.

Tsukiyama, K., Nakai, A., Mine, R. & Kitani, T. (1959) Studies on a myasthenic substance present in the serum of patient with myasthenia gravis. *Medical Journal of Osaka University*, 10, 159.

Vessey, M.P. & Doll, R. (1972) Thymectomy and cancer—a follow-up study. *British Journal of Cancer*, 26, 53.

Vetters, J.M. (1965) Immunofluorescence staining patterns in skeletal muscle using serum of myasthenic patients and normal controls. *Immunology*, 9, 93.

Vetters, J.M. & MacAdam, R.F. (1972) Hormone production in the human thymus. *Lancet*, 2, 1203.

Vetters, J.M. & MacAdam (1973) Fine structural evidence for hormone secretion by the human thymus. *Journal of Clinical Pathology*, 26, 194.

Vetters, J.M. & Simpson, J.A. (1974) Comparison of thymic histology with response to thymectomy in myasthenia gravis. *Journal of Neurology, Neurosurgery and Psychiatry*, 37, 1139.

Vetters, J.M., Simpson, J.A. & Folkarde, A. (1969) Experimental myasthenia gravis. *Lancet*, 2, 28.

Vetters, J.M., Saikia, N.K., Wood, J. & Simpson, J.A. (1973) Pemphigus vulgaris and myasthenia gravis. *British Journal of Dermatology*, 88, 437.

Viets, H.R. (1953) A historical review of myasthenia gravis from 1672 to 1900. *Journal of the American Medical Association*, 153, 1273.

Viets, H.R. (1958) Discussion on myasthenia gravis. In *Neuromuscular Disorders. Research Publications, Association for Research in Nervous and Mental Disease*, 38, 638.

Viets, H.R. & Schwab, R.S. (1935) Prostigmin in the diagnosis of myasthenia gravis. *New England Journal of Medicine*, 213, 1280.

Walker, M.B. (1934) Treatment of myasthenia gravis with physostigmine. *Lancet*, 1, 1200.

Walker, M.B. (1938) Myasthenia gravis: a case in which fatigue of the forearm muscles could induce paralysis of the extra-ocular muscles. *Proceedings of the Royal Society of Medicine*, 31, 722.

Walton, J.N. & Adams, R.D. (1958) *Polymyositis* (Livingstone: Edinburgh).

Walton, J.N., Geschwind, N. & Simpson, J.A. (1956) Benign congenital myopathy with myasthenic features. *Journal of Neurology, Neurosurgery and Psychiatry*, 19, 224.

Weigert, C. (1901) Pathologisch-anatomischer Beitrag zur Erbach'en Krankheit (Myasthenia Gravis). *Neurologisches Zentralblatt*, 20, 597.

Westerberg, M.R. & Magee, K.R. (1955) Treatment review: myasthenia gravis. *Neurology (Minneapolis)*, 5, 728.

Whiteley, A.M., Schwartz, M.S., Sachs, J.A. & Swash, M. (1976) Congenital myasthenia gravis: clinical and HLA studies in two brothers. *Journal of Neurology, Neurosurgery and Psychiatry*, 39, 1145.

Whittingham, S., Mackay, I.R. & Kiss, Z.S. (1970) An interplay of genetic and environmental factors in familial hepatitis and myasthenia gravis. *Gut*, 11, 811.

Wiesendanger, M. & D'Alessandsi, A. (1963) Myasthenia gravis mit fokaler Infiltration der Endplattenzone. *Acta Neuropathologica*, 2, 246.

Willis, T. (1672) *De Anima Brutorum*, pp. 404–406. Oxford.

Wilson, S.A.K. (1954) *Neurology*, 2nd edition, Ed. A.N. Bruce, p. 1730 (Butterworth: London).

Wise, R.P. & MacDermot, V. (1962) A myasthenic syndrome associated with bronchial carcinoma. *Journal of Neurology, Neurosurgery and Psychiatry*, 25, 31.

Wolf, S.M. & Barrows, H.S. (1966) Myasthenia gravis and

systemic lupus erythematosus. *Archives of Neurology*, **14**, 254.

Wolf, S.M., Rowland, L.P., Schotland, D.L., McKinney, A.S., Hoefer, P.F.A. & Aranow, N. (1966) Myasthenia as an autoimmune disease: clinical aspects. *Annals of the New York Academy of Sciences*, **135**, 517.

Woolf, A.L. (1966) Morphology of the myasthenic neuromuscular junction. *Annals of the New York Academy of Sciences*, **135**, 35.

Wright, E.A. & McQuillen, M.P. (1971) Antibiotic-induced neuromuscular blockade. *Annals of the New York Academy of Sciences*, **183**, 358.

Zacks, S.I., Bauer, W.C. & Blumberg, J.M. (1962) The fine structure of the myasthenic neuromuscular junction. *Journal of Neuropathology*, **21**, 335.

Neuromuscular disorders in infancy and early childhood

INTRODUCTION

In recent years many medical writers have discussed the problem of the floppy baby and in their papers have listed the causes of hypotonia in infancy (*see* review by Dubowitz, 1969). Lists of infantile diseases of which hypotonia is a symptom have intrinsic interest, but they may suggest unreal differential diagnostic situations—unreal partly because, in many of the conditions named, hypotonia is not often the presenting symptom (e.g. mongolism) and partly because the age of the infant may be of critical importance.

There are two main sets of circumstances in which the differential diagnosis of infantile hypotonia arises: these are, first, the rare circum-

stances of relative immobility and limpness at birth or in the first few days and weeks of life; secondly, the common occurrence of delay in the development of control of posture at about 6 months of age and onwards.

We propose to discuss the differential diagnosis of limpness at birth and in later infancy before describing the congenital myopathies and some of the other neuromuscular problems which may be seen in children.

HYPOTONIA AT BIRTH

The normal infant

The normal infant moves its limbs vigorously for about half an hour after birth and, following a period of quiescence, again at about 3–4 hours of age (Desmond, Franklin, Valebona, Hill, Plumb, Arnold and Watts, 1963) and thereafter whenever it is awake and crying—periods of quiet wakefulness in newborn babies being few and brief. Moreover, even when a newborn baby is quiet it exhibits marked flexural tone when lying or suspended, prone or supine, and it is not possible fully to extend the thighs or legs by passive stretching. Passive movements of the limbs give the impression of hypertonia, which should, of course, be equal bilaterally provided that the head is kept in a central position to eliminate the influence of tonic neck reflexes on the limbs. A beat or two of ankle clonus is normal. Even at birth there is some postural control of the head; on being sat up the newborn baby will balance its head for a brief period in the upright position before it flops forward. An anencephalic baby will keep its head upright.

Analysis of muscle tone in the assessment of the neurological status of the newborn has been studied by André-Thomas, Chesni and St.-Anne Dargassies, and an interpretation of the terms used by them is given in the English translation of their book by Mac Keith, Polani and Clayton-Jones (1960). It is clear that the word 'tone' has a somewhat different meaning to French neurologists, because it denotes not only resistance to passive movement but also the power with which active movements are carried out. These authors divide tone into two types, tonus passif and tonus actif. The former is subdivided into extensibilité and passivité. Extensibilité is the capacity of a muscle to be lengthened; as it is measured by the amplitude of slow passive movement of a segment of a limb at a joint, it is presumably also a measure of ligamental laxity. Passivité is the *lack* of resistance to passive movement, as tested for instance by flapping the hand, and may be regarded as the reciprocal of 'tone' as it usually understood by British neurologists. Observation of spontaneous posture and active movements, as well as the power of recoil when a limb is rapidly moved by the examiner from its position of rest, are used in the assessment of tonus actif.

The hypotonic infant

The sight of a newborn infant lying awake and motionless with outstretched limbs is in striking contrast to the appearance of the normal baby. Hypotonia can be confirmed on handling and lifting the infant, when instead of its curling up, the limbs will flop about under the influence of gravity. Resistance to passive movement of the limbs and head will be decreased, 'passivité' will be increased and so will extensibilité, as evinced, for example, by the possibility of wrapping each arm round the neck (the 'scarf' sign) and by flexing the thighs on the trunk with legs extended, when the normal popliteal angle will be obliterated.

Almost all hypotonic infants move less actively than normal babies. Dubowitz (1969; 1978) emphasises the difference between the paralysed floppy baby with neuromuscular disease and the baby with central hypotonia without significant weakness who can withdraw from a painful stimulus or support the limbs briefly against gravity. The distinction is useful but by no means always easy; some disorders of the central nervous system may give rise to severe paralysis.

Causes of hypotonia

Diminished movement and limpness in the newborn baby may be caused by extreme prematurity, by any severe systemic illness, by drugs, and by lesions of the brain, spinal cord, peripheral nerves, myoneural junction, muscles and ligaments. Severe generalised illness (respiratory distress or septicaemia) or intracranial disorders, are by far the commonest causes, but in the absence of obvious illness, and especially when the baby is alert, one must consider the possibility of a number of rare disorders in the differential diagnosis. These include spinal cord injury, spinal muscular atrophy, congenital myotonic dystrophy, the Pompé type of glycogen storage disease which affects the central nervous system as well as heart and muscle, poliomyelitis, myasthenia gravis, various rare forms of congenital myopathy and methaemoglobinaemia with mental defect (Worster-Drought, White and Sargent, 1953). Hypotonia at birth is often a striking feature of Down's syndrome (mongolism), the Prader-Willi syndrome, and of various rarer syndromes associated with severe mental retardation including, for example, the cerebrohepatorenal, Lowe's and Smith-Lemli-Opitz syndromes. An inborn error of metabolism—especially an organic acidaemia—should be suspected in a baby who, well at birth, develops profound hypotonia and respiratory failure within the first few days or even after several months. This is particularly important because some organic acidaemias respond to treatment with biotin or vitamin B_{12} (Keeton and Moosa, 1976; Charles, Hosking, Green, Pollitt, Bartlett and Taitz, 1979). Leigh's disease, which is often associated with lactic acidaemia, also presents with profound hypotonia in a previously normal baby and is often mistaken at first for a neuromuscular disease. The association of hypotonia with hyperventilation is an important clue to the underlying acidosis in these disorders.

Clara and Lowenthal (1966) have described four siblings who had severe generalised hypotonia from birth, with feeding difficulties and respiratory weakness. All showed a persistent selective aminoaciduria, involving ornithine, lysine, cystine and arginine. There was gradual improvement in muscular power, however, and they started to walk at about 3 years. There was no mental defect, but speech defect and dwarfism remained. Hurwitz, Carson, Allen and Chopra (1969) described two floppy babies with limitation of external ocular movements who developed pelvic girdle weakness. Both had persistent aminoaciduria, one having an abnormal clearance of lysine, histidine and glycine and the other of glycine only.

Cerebral causes of hypotonia at birth. The mechanism of higher control of muscle tone in the newborn is not known. Anencephalic and grossly hydranencephalic newborn infants may exhibit normal muscle tone, but whereas *absence* of cerebral hemispheres may not be associated with hyper- or hypotonicity, *damage* to or disease of the hemispheres may.

Muscular hypotonia is characteristic of 'terminal' asphyxia at birth, in which apnoea is associated with pallor, bradycardia and unresponsiveness to physical stimuli. The clinical picture of 'cerebral depression' in the first few days of life, of which absence of vigorous movement and hypotonia are features, may follow severe asphyxia at birth or traumatic labour, or may occur unexpectedly—possibly in the presence of prenatally determined disease or deformity of the brain. Temporary cerebral depression may follow administration of sedative drugs to the mother in labour and hypotonia is a particularly striking feature when diazepam is used in cases of preeclamptic toxaemia. It is characteristic of cerebral depression in the newborn that automatisms, such as the Moro, rooting and sucking reflexes are absent. The nasopalpebral reflex is also frequently absent, and the appearance of a pallid, motionless baby with open eyes is familiar. In fatal cases death is likely to take place within the first 48 hours of life, after increasingly frequent periods of apnoea and cyanosis, and massive intracranial haemorrhage is a common post-mortem finding. In those who survive, however, the hypotonia usually gives place after a day or two either to normal muscle tone and movement or to a clinical state suggesting cerebral irritation, signs of which include hypertonia, hyperactivity, easily elicited automatisms and multifocal fits. Only rarely does the hypotonia caused by an acquired cerebral lesion persist after the first few days of life and in these cases tendon reflexes are usually present, thus differentiating the condition from lower motor neurone or muscular disorders.

Spinal cord injury, tumours and myelodysplasia. Deformity or injury of the spinal cord at birth may result in the classical picture of the floppy infant, but the arms are usually spared. Birth injury to the spinal cord was first accurately described by Crothers (1923). The cord is damaged by stretching or by avulsion of the spinal roots forming the brachial plexus. Most cases follow difficult breech delivery and are occasionally complicated by the rare distal form of brachial plexus palsy (Klumpke) causing paralysis of the small muscles of the hand and the long flexors of the hand and fingers. The minority of spinal cord injuries, namely those complicating difficult vertex delivery, are more commonly associated with brachial plexus palsy of the proximal type (Erb) involving mainly the abductors of the upper arm and flexors and supinators of the forearm (Crothers and Putnam, 1927).

The complete flaccidity and immobility of the lower limbs and trunk in spinal cord injury may result in a mistaken diagnosis of a general neuromuscular disorder, especially if there are also brachial plexus lesions. However, the presence of sphincter and sensory abnormalities will reveal the true diagnosis even if the localised nature of the paralysis is not at first obvious. There is likely to be retention of urine and a patulous anus for several days and pinching the skin of the lower half of the body, although later causing withdrawal, will not result in a cry or grimace. After the first few days, however, normal sphincter action may be regained and sensory loss may be difficult to detect. The cerebrospinal fluid may contain blood. The subject is reviewed by Towbin (1969) and Byers (1975).

Spinal tumours in infancy are uncommon and are easily overlooked at first if there is extensive paralysis involving the intercostal or abdominal muscles as well as the limbs. Tumours extending over many segments of the cord, whether intramedullary (glioma or ependymoma) or extramedullary such as a neuroblastoma, are fairly characteristic at this age. They provide the same pitfalls in diagnosis as extensive cord injury.

Myelodysplasia is usually obvious at birth in the form of meningomyelocele. In cases where the deformity is hidden, however, there are nearly always overlying skin defects (hair, haemangioma, lipoma or congenital dermal sinus) and X-rays will reveal deformity of the vertebral body or cartilaginous spine.

DELAY IN THE DEVELOPMENT OF POSTURAL CONTROL

The normal infant

It is important to realise that the muscle tone of the normal infant diminishes during the first month of life to be regained later. The newborn baby can support his head and may take his weight on his legs more firmly than he will do again until the age of 6–9 months. Control of body posture develops in stages from head to foot (Illingworth, 1972; Touwen, 1976). There is, of course, considerable variability in healthy children. The following is a brief outline of the *average* age at which each accomplishment is acquired.

Head. Some control of the head is evident at birth (*see* above). By about 6 weeks of age a baby can extend its head against gravity to the midline when held prone, by 3 months it can flex against gravity when held supine. By 3 months of age a baby will raise its shoulders and fully extend the head when lying prone; by 5–6 months a baby lying supine will raise its head in anticipation of being picked up.

Arms. By 3 months a baby lying supine will extend its arms towards a proffered object and by 5 months will reach out and grasp the object with one hand.

Trunk and legs. At 6 months most babies will sit with support and even for brief periods without support, propping themselves up by the arms placed between the abducted thighs. Fifty per cent

of normal Newcastle infants are sitting unsupported at 6.4 months, 90 per cent at 8.1 months and 97 per cent at 9.3 months. Fifty per cent are walking unaided at 12.8 months, 90 per cent at 15.8 months and 97 per cent at 18.4 months (Neligan and Prudham, 1969). Note therefore that 3 per cent of normal children will not be walking until after 18.4 months! The percentile figures for Denver infants are a little different, but the Denver Developmental Screening Test is useful and not too difficult to apply by the uninitiated (Frankenburg and Dodds, 1967; Bryant, Davies and Newcombe, 1979).

Hypotonia and developmental delay

There are numerous causes for delay in postural control and a hitherto unexplored problem is the extent to which *all* babies who display retarded motor development give the clinical impression of hypotonia—other, of course, than those with obvious evidence of spasticity. Attempts to measure muscle tone objectively have been made (Rondot, Dalloz and Tardieu, 1958) but not applied in a systematic fashion to this problem. The clinical distinction between ligamentous laxity and muscular hypotonia is not easy, and to base the distinction on the presence or absence of tendon reflexes or muscle weakness is illogical.

Differential diagnosis of hypotonia

As has been hinted above, the differential diagnosis of hypotonia in infancy may embrace all the causes of delay in postural control. Normal variation has been mentioned. It is uncommon for muscular hypotonia and weakness to develop in a previously normal infant so rapidly that they command attention, in themselves, or by causing actual regression in development. Such an event clearly implies a progressive disorder, whether cerebral or neuromuscular in origin. Even these more often result in developmental delay before regression is seen, and timing the 'onset' of the disease, an important point in differential diagnosis, may be a difficult matter, greatly influenced by the parents' experience, powers of observation and memory (Pearn, 1974).

Any chronic debilitating illness in early infancy

and many conditions adversely affecting growth (malnutrition, specific digestive anomalies, malabsorption syndromes, metabolic diseases, congenital heart malformations, congenital defects of the renal tract, chronic pulmonary diseases, etc.) may result in delayed motor control and hypotonia, but can usually be differentiated fairly easily by the history, symptoms and signs. Mental handicap may not be as easily distinguished because the conventional yardsticks of mental development in infancy are so dependent on normal motor abilities; attention must be directed to alertness, awareness, and language development as well as to the specific characteristics of the different conditions underlying mental handicap, for example mongol features or phenylketonuria. It is important not to confuse the absence of facial expression caused by muscle weakness with that of retardation.

It is not uncommon to find delay in postural control and hypotonia, otherwise inexplicable, in infants who have lacked normal mothering in the early weeks and months of life (Buda, Rothney and Rabe, 1972). In such cases the cause may be apparent in simple neglect, frequent change of foster parent or institutional life, but in other cases the lack of normal mothering is by no means always obvious to the clinician—the mother's concern being attributed to the baby's condition, rather than the baby's condition to the mother's endogenous depression and consequent failure to 'identify' with her infant.

If normal variation, chronic disease other than in the nervous system, mental defect and emotional deprivation can be excluded, the causes of hypotonia and delayed development in infancy must lie in disorders of cerebral motor control, spinal cord tracts or anterior horn cells, peripheral nerves or myoneural junction, or of muscles, ligaments and tendons.

Paine's follow-up study (1963) puts the differential diagnostic problem into perspective. The following were the final diagnoses in 111 'floppy' infants: various forms of cerebral palsy, 48; cerebral degenerative disease, 3; brain tumour, 1; mental retardation, 28; spinal cord injury, 1; spinal muscular atrophy, 4; myopathy, 4; benign congenital hypotonia, 18; and disease outside the nervous system, 4. In contrast, no less than 67 of

Walton's (1956) series of 109 cases were eventually diagnosed as spinal muscular atrophy, but there the initial diagnosis in each case was 'amyotonia congenita' and Paine's series of children from 6 months to 20 years of age shows the proportionate causes of hypotonia presenting with delay in postural control.

Cerebral causes of delay in postural control

Static cerebral disorders affecting motor functions (the cerebral palsies) or active degenerative cerebral disease may present in infancy with hypotonia. Persistent atonic cerebral palsy is rare and its pathological basis uncertain. (It is of interest in this context that Woolf (1960) has reported the case of one infant with bilateral cerebral softening secondary to birth asphyxia accompanied by vacuolar degeneration of anterior horn cells.) Flaccidity is, however, often seen in the early months in infants who later prove to be cases of spastic diplegia, athetosis, ataxia or mental defect. The pathological basis for flaccidity in infants with cerebral disorders originating before or at birth may be a delayed maturation of muscle fibres—a fetal or neonatal pattern persisting for longer than usual (Fenichel, 1967). Some cases of 'fibre-type disproportion' seem to fall into this category. In some degenerative diseases of the cerebrum or cerebellum the earliest motor disturbance may take the form of poverty of movement and flaccidity.

The hypotonic stage of spastic diplegia.
The natural history of cerebral spastic diplegia has been described by Ingram (1955), who found that 40 per cent of his cases went through a hypotonic stage in early infancy. After the neonatal period little abnormality may be noticed, but within a few weeks, poverty of movement, especially of the trunk and proximal segments of the limbs, becomes conspicuous. Physical examination shows hypotonia and diminished tendon reflexes, but automatisms such as the Moro reflex and palmar grasp reflexes are too easily elicited at ages when they should have disappeared (about 3 months and 6 months respectively). The hypotonic stage lasts from 6 weeks to 15 months (Ingram, 1955), but the transition to the dystonic stage usually takes place

within 6 months. Paine (1961) emphasised the importance of tonic neck reflexes in the early diagnosis of diplegia, when the characteristic limb posture can be forced on the infant by passive lateral rotation of the head. Hyperadduction of the thighs and plantar flexion of the feet on upright suspension, and an adductor spread of the knee jerk to one or both thighs after the age of 6 months are other signs of an upper motor neurone lesion. Obviously, microcephaly, signs of cerebral sensory defects and intellectual retardation will suggest a cerebral cause for the hypotonia. In the early stages of certain degenerative diseases (especially Tay-Sachs', Niemann-Pick's and Pompé's diseases, generalised gangliosidosis and infantile neuroaxonal dystrophy) the motor disturbance may take the form of flaccidity. In the leucodystrophies and in Tay-Sachs' disease, hypotonia of the neck and trunk muscles may co-exist with spasticity of the limbs. In the Krabbe and metachromatic types of leucodystrophy the associated peripheral neuropathy also causes areflexia in the presence of spasticity.

The hypotonic stage of athetosis. Hypotonia is characteristic of athetosis and choreoathetosis in infancy, but tendon reflexes tend to be brisk in contrast to the diminished muscle tone, and tonic neck reflexes are usually easily elicited. Polani (1959) has studied the natural history of choreoathetosis. About one-third of his patients displayed marked muscular hypotonia from about the second month and this might still be apparent by 1 year of age. Usually opisthotonic attacks begin within the first year; in between attacks the baby is usually floppy.

Ataxic syndromes in infancy. Muscular hypotonia and delay in postural control are often the presenting symptoms of ataxic syndromes of infancy and childhood, whether attributable to static conditions originating before or at the time of birth, or to degenerative processes. An important minority of these cases results from congenital hypothyroidism. Ingram (1962) has described the clinical picture of generalised hypotonia, hyperextensibility of joints, absent automatisms and depressed tendon reflexes, which with a paucity of spontaneous movement and poor postural control is characteristic of both congenital ataxia and congenital ataxic diplegia in early infancy. By the age of 3 or 4 months, however, reflexes are easily elicitable and spasticity may be detected. Intention tremor and incoordination of voluntary movement emerge as the child begins to reach out for objects.

Similarly, degenerative disease producing ataxia may present with delay in acquisition of motor control and hypotonia. Friedreich's ataxia may present thus in infancy and so may ataxia-telangiectasia (Boder and Sedgwick, 1958; Hansen, 1962) in which disease the characteristic combination of athetotic movements with ataxia, the conjunctival telangiectasia and recurrent respiratory infections gradually emerge in the first 10 years of life.

Intermittent ataxia (Blass, Kark and Engel, 1971) whether caused by intoxication, benign paroxysmal vertigo, a IVth ventricular tumour, an aminoacidaemia or lactic acidosis or the syndrome of idiopathic familial intermittent ataxia, may be difficult at first to distinguish from periodic paralysis in very young children.

Mental defect. Delay in postural control in the first year of life is frequently the presenting symptom of mental retardation. Examination at this time may show hypotonia, but later the child proves to have no detectable motor defect, whereas the existence of mental retardation gradually becomes apparent. To what extent muscular hypotonia in infancy is characteristic of all cases of mental retardation is uncertain, but there are two conditions in which it is early and conspicuous. *Down's syndrome* is usually accompanied by flaccidity from birth until about one year of age and the tendon reflexes may be difficult to obtain. In the neonatal period, hypotonia is more frequently found in patients with trisomy 21 than in those with translocations of the 13/21, 15/21 and 21/21 types. Bazelon, Paine, Cowie, Hunt, Houck and Mahanand (1967) have claimed that hypotonia is much improved in mongol children by the oral administration of 5-hydroxytryptophan; this substance is the immediate metabolic precursor of serotonin, the whole-blood level of which is reduced in trisomic mongols (Rosner, Ong, Paine and Mahanand, 1965). It is not known whether the improvement in muscle tone is due to a rise in the serotonin content of the brain or spinal cord (Partington, MacDonald and Tu, 1971). Unfortunately there is no associated improvement in function. *The Prader-Willi syndrome* is an entity characterised by dwarfism, obesity, mental retardation and gonadal hypoplasia (Prader, Labhaft and Willi, 1956; Dubowitz, 1967; Laurence, 1967; Zellweger and Schneider, 1968). Most cases have from birth shown marked generalised hypotonia, areflexia, paucity of movement and feeble sucking. After several months the infants become more active and tendon reflexes are elicitable but the moderate hypotonia may persist. Excessive appetite and obesity develop in the second or third year. Children with the Prader-Willi syndrome have recognisably similar faces (Laurence, 1967).

It is of interest that muscular hypotonia is a feature of several chromosomal defects in addition to Down's syndrome, but peripheral nerve and muscle do not appear to have been studied in these conditions. Benign hypotonia associated with undescended testicles, delayed osseous development and minor facial abnormalities has been reported by Dunn, Ford, Anersperg and Miller (1961) in a child having an additional chromosome in the 21, 22, Y group, who was not a mongol. Muscular hypotonia and multiple malformations have also been reported in trisomy of the 13–15 group (Lubs, Koenig and Brandt, 1961; Taylor, 1968). Hypotonia is characteristic of infants with deletions of the short arm of chromosome No. 4 or No. 5 and in trisomy 18 initial hypotonia is later replaced by hypertonia (Hamerton, 1971). One-third of cases of XXXXY karyotype have been noted to be hypotonic (Smith, 1970). A child presenting at birth with hypotonia and later with seizures and delayed postural control was found to have a 46/47 mosaicism with an extra ring autosome (Atkins, Sceery and Keenan, 1966).

The association of mental retardation with hypotonia by no means rules out serious neuromuscular disease. Both in Duchenne muscular dystrophy and in congenital myotonic dystrophy, mental retardation may be severe and may divert attention from the muscular weakness. Boys with unexplained delay in walking or in speech development should be tested for Duchenne muscular dystrophy by estimation of the serum creatine kinase (CK) activity (*see* Ch. 15).

CONGENITAL MUSCULAR DISORDERS

Most of the neuromuscular disorders which occur in young children are discussed in other chapters of this book. We therefore propose to confine systematic clinical description to the so-called 'congenital myopathies', of which only the genetic and pathological aspects are discussed elsewhere, and to review the others only in the framework of the types of clinical problem which are met with in paediatric practice. The authors' views on many of these disorders are to be found in the previous edition of this book and in Gardner-Medwin (1977); more detailed accounts of neuromuscular disease in childhood include those of Dubowitz (1969; 1978), Brooke (1977), Brooke, Carroll and Ringel (1979) and (for the spinal muscular atrophies) Hausmanowa-Petrusewicz (1978).

The congenital myopathies

Most of the true myopathies present at birth are genetically determined, and in the rest the cause is usually unknown. Some doubt exists as to the genetic basis of some cases of congenital muscular dystrophy. Congenital hypothyroidism may be associated with myopathy (the Debré-Semelaigne syndrome). On the other hand many of the genetic disorders customarily described as *congenital* myopathies do not cause symptoms until later in childhood or even adult life, by which time many acquired myopathies including polymyositis and the metabolic disorders must be considered in the differential diagnosis. It is best therefore to consider these myopathies as 'genetic and idiopathic myopathies' and to classify them more or less in diminishing order of our understanding of their nature as follows. For completeness two final categories of functional disorders of the muscle fibre and disorders of muscle connective tissue are included.

(1)   Genetic myopathies with specific biochemical defects
        Glycogen storage diseases
        Lipid storage diseases

(2) Genetic myopathies with periodic 'metabolic' manifestations
   Periodic paralyses
   Malignant hyperpyrexia
   Familial myoglobinuria and idiopathic rhabdomyolysis
(3) Genetic myopathies with abnormal mitochondria
(4) Genetic myopathies with specific structural changes in fibres
   Central core disease
   Minicore disease
   Nemaline myopathy
   Centronuclear myopathy
   Finger-print myopathy
   Etc.
(5) Genetic myopathies with changes in the histochemical fibre types
(6) Genetic myopathies with progressive degeneration of muscle fibres
   The muscular dystrophies
(7) Genetic myopathies with non-specific changes in fibres
(8) Genetic disorders with abnormal muscle fibre activity
   Myotonic disorders
   Myokymia
   Muscle rigidity
(9) Genetic disorders of muscle connective tissue
   Progressive myositis ossificans
   Myosclerosis

Categories 3–5 and 7 in this list are discussed below. Descriptions of the others will be found in Chapters 14, 18, 20 and 23. We shall concentrate on clinical aspects of the congenital myopathies because their pathological features are described in Chapters 5, 8 and 9.

Genetic myopathies with abnormal muscle mitochondria

Many different types of muscle disease associated with abnormal muscle mitochondria have been described. The mitochondria may be too large or too numerous, are often distorted and may contain paracrystalline or amorphous inclusions. None of these features corresponds with particular clinical features which are equally variable. Mitochondrial myopathy may be suspected on light microscopy when there is an excess of oxidative enzyme activity in the subsarcolemmal regions of type I fibres. Often there is some associated lipid accumulation and in some cases glycogen may accumulate as well (Jerusalem, Angelini, Engel and Groover, 1973). Presumably there is a defect in cellular respiratory function in most of these disorders to which the visible mitochondrial changes are secondary, but some may represent primary disorders of mitochondrial structure. Known metabolic abnormalities include deficiencies of carnitine and carnitine palmityl transferase (see Ch. 18) and disorders of cytochrome function. No rational classification is possible but in this Chapter a simple clinical classification seems appropriate.

Hypermetabolic myopathy. Two cases are known, both with fever, heat intolerance, excessive appetite, polydipsia, weight loss and fatigue starting in childhood with negative family histories (Luft, Ikkos, Palmieri, Ernster and Afzelius, 1962; Haydar, Conn, Afifi, Wakid, Ballas and Fawaz, 1971). Oxidative phosphorylation was uncoupled and thyroid function was normal (DiMauro, Bonilla, Lee, Schotland, Scarpa, Conn and Chance, 1976). Chloramphenicol gave some relief in Haydar's case, presumably by suppressing mitochondrial function.

Progressive muscular weakness and fatigue. Many cases have been described with a slowly progressive myopathy, the symptoms of which usually begin at the age of 5–10 years and in which fatigue is often out of proportion to the degree of muscle weakness but without true myasthenia (Coleman, Nienhuis, Brown, Munsat and Pearson, 1967). Some cases including the original case of 'megaconical myopathy' described by Shy, Gonatas and Perez (1966) have had symptoms from birth. Variations on the theme are reported by van Wijngaarden, Bethlem, Meijer, Hülsmann and Feltkamp (1967) and by Schotland, DiMauro, Bonilla, Scarpa and Lee (1976) who reported a defect in mitochondrial energy supply in a patient aged 37 whose symptoms dated from early childhood.

Hypotonia with salt-craving and periodic muscular weakness. Shy *et al.* (1966) described the case of a child who was hypotonic from birth and who had episodes of severe muscular weakness lasting 10–14 days, associated with salt craving. His otherwise normal brother also craved salt. The muscle contained very numerous mitochondria ('pleoconial myopathy'). The authors recognised the similarity of the symptoms to normokalaemic periodic paralysis but showed that the conditions were different. Spiro, Prineas and Moore (1970) reported a similar case without the periodic exacerbations.

Ophthalmoplegia and the Kearns-Sayre syndrome. This is by far the most frequently encountered clinical pattern in which ptosis, ophthalmoplegia and skeletal muscle weakness are found with various combinations of pigmentary degeneration of the retina, cardiomyopathy, growth failure, nerve deafness, ataxia, dementia and a raised cerebrospinal fluid (CSF) protein level. The syndrome is discussed in Chapter 14 in relation to the ocular form of muscular dystrophy. There is no absolute clinical or histological distinction from other mitochondrial myopathies; for example McLeod, Baker, Shorey and Kerr (1975) reported a mentally retarded patient with many of the features of the Kearns-Sayre syndrome but with normal eye movements.

Distal myopathy with hyperglycaemia. A girl of 5 years described by Salmon, Esiri and Ruderman (1971) had a distal myopathy from the first year of life, fasting hyperglycaemia with ketosis and low insulin levels but a normal insulin response to glucose loading. There were mitochondrial abnormalities and lipid accumulation in the muscle. Male relatives in three generations had raised serum CK activity and hyperglycaemia. Lapresle, Fardeau and Godet-Guillain (1972) reported a family with apparently dominant inheritance of congenital foot drop with facial and sternomastoid weakness and mitochondrial changes in the muscle biopsy.

Facioscapulohumeral syndrome. Hudgson, Bradley and Jenkison (1972) reported a family with at least eight affected members in four generations in which a mitochondrial myopathy gave rise to a facioscapulohumeral syndrome of muscular weakness. The age at onset varied from 6 years to 50 years. The affected child later developed severe lactic acidosis (Bradley, Tomlinson and Hardy, 1978) and has since died of a progressive encephalopathy (Hudgson, personal communication).

Various non-muscular presentations. It is not unusual for cases to be found to have a mitochondrial myopathy in the course of investigation of other symptoms, for example cardiomyopathy and short stature (Rawles and Weller, 1974; Sengers, Stadhouders, Jaspar, Trijbels and Daniels, 1976), progressive ataxia and dementia (Spiro, Moore, Prineas, Strasberg and Rapin, 1970), familial myoclonic epilepsy (Tsairis, Engel and Kark, 1973), Leigh's disease (Crosby and Chou, 1974), Alpers' progressive cortical degeneration of infancy (Sandbank and Lerman, 1972) and Menkes' trichopoliodystrophy (French, Sherard, Lubell, Brotz and Moore, 1972). The cases of Spiro *et al.* (1970) were shown to have a defect in muscle cytochrome b activity.

Mitochondrial myopathy and lactic acidosis. Tarlow, Lake and Lloyd (1973) first drew attention to the association of lassitude and episodic vomiting with lactic and pyruvic acidosis in a child who also had a mitochondrial myopathy, although Van Wijngaarden *et al.* (1967) had found lactic acidosis in one of their cases. Tarlow's case developed symptoms at the age of 4 years and showed some subsequent improvement. Since then, many examples have been reported and it seems likely that many of the syndromes described above may, at times, lead to a critical failure in mitochondrial metabolic function. It is clear, too, that in some cases the mitochondrial disorder is present in many tissues besides muscle, but the extent to which this determines the occurrence of lactic acidosis is not apparent. Certainly, many of the cases to be described have shown an association between acidosis and a subacute and sometimes fatal encephalopathy. In addition, however, to this rather general association between lactic acidosis and mitochondrial disease, a number of more specific syndromes seem to have emerged.

Sengers, ter Haar, Trijbels, Willems, Daniels and Stadhouders (1975) described a syndrome occurring in seven children from three unrelated families in whom cataracts in infancy and effort intolerance were associated with cardiomyopathy, mitochondrial myopathy and lactic acidosis after exercise. No similar cases seem to have been reported but in the brothers described by Rawles and Weller (1974), cardiomyopathy and fatigue (without cataract) occurred with lactic acidosis.

One of the most sinister of the mitochondrial myopathy syndromes is that first described in two papers relating to the same two sisters (D'Agostino, Ziter, Rallison and Bray, 1968; Hackett, Bray, Ziter, Nyhan and Creer, 1973) and later also by Gardner-Medwin, Dale and Parkin (1975), Shapira, Cederbaum, Cancilla, Nielsen and Lippe (1975) and Hart, Chang, Perrin, Neerunjun and Ayyar (1977). The cardinal features in the first decade are the onset of growth failure, headaches, vomiting, fatigue and hirsutism at about the age of 4 years, worsening gradually thereafter. By about 10 years there is marked shortness of stature, the muscles are slim and fatigue easily, but are not very weak, and investigation reveals a degree of nerve deafness, slight pigmentary change in the retinae and lactic acidosis. Episodes of confusion or even coma may follow exertion. Some cases have seizures. There is no ophthalmoplegia, but ptosis and mild facial weakness may occur. Muscle biopsy reveals a mitochondrial myopathy. During the second decade intermittent subacute episodes of encephalopathy occur, associated in our case with patchy 'moth-eaten' areas of low density shown by computerised axial tomography of the brain; these occur mainly in white matter but the clinical effect is patchy loss of cortical function with dysphasia, dyspraxia and agnosia in various combinations. All except one patient (D'Agostino et al., 1968) have died by the age of 16 years. The only detailed autopsies (Shapira et al., 1975) revealed focal cortical neuronal loss with gliosis and vascular proliferation and oedema of the adjacent white matter. No electron microscopy of the central nervous system has yet been reported. Although three pairs of siblings have been reported, the genetic position is not clear because various other relatives suffered similar, less severe symptoms.

Finally, there is now an extensive literature on congenital lactic acidosis of which a number of types with different enzyme defects have been described. These tend to cause severe mental retardation with acidosis. In the case described by van Biervliet, Bruinvis, Ketting, De Bree, Van Der Heider, Wadman, Willems, Brookelman, Van Haelst and Monnens (1977) muscle hypotonia was a dominant feature. They demonstrated a defect in muscle cytochromes aa_3 and b.

Management of mitochondrial myopathy. The diagnosis can often be suspected if one of the clinical syndromes is recognised. The histochemical findings with or without lipid droplets in the muscle fibres are very suggestive, but the diagnosis is generally based on the ultrastructural findings. It is wise to obtain enough muscle at the time of biopsy to rule out carnitine deficiency. Studies of mitochondrial function *in vitro* require several grams of fresh unfrozen muscle tissue and can be performed only in certain laboratories, so that a more specific diagnosis is rarely possible in young children and, indeed, has been achieved in very few adult cases. In the case of Brunette, Delvin, Hazel and Scriver (1972) a specific enzyme defect was found (pyruvate carboxylase). In several cases disorders of cytochrome function have been proved including deficiency of cytochrome b (Spiro, Moore, Prineas, Strasberg and Rapin, 1970; Morgan-Hughes, Darveniza, Kahn, Landon, Sherratt, Land and Clark, 1977) of cytochromes aa_3 and b (van Biervliet et al., 1977) and of cytochrome-c-oxidase (DiMauro, Mendell, Sahenk, Bachman and Scarpa, 1978), or abnormalities of respiration with various substrates (DiMauro, Schotland, Bonilla, Lee, Gambetti and Rowland, 1973).

A few therapeutic manoeuvres may be of limited value. Most important is the recognition of heart block in the Kearns-Sayre syndrome and the provision of a cardiac pacemaker when necessary. Close surveillance is essential because the degree of conduction block can deteriorate rapidly. In cases with lactic acidosis regular bicarbonate therapy may be helpful. Steroids were of temporary benefit in the case described by Shapira et al. (1975) and in the later stages of the disease in the case reported by Gardner-Medwin et al.

(1975). Dubowitz (1978, pp. 99, 102) pointed out that respiratory failure may result partly from a failure in central control of ventilation and he was able to maintain a child's breathing with a home ventilator for a time.

Genetic counselling in the mitochondrial disorders is particularly difficult. Clear evidence of Mendelian inheritance is rarely found but sibs, parents and more distant relatives are quite often affected in various syndromes. Further research into the genetics of the mitochondrial myopathies is clearly needed.

Genetic myopathies with specific structural changes in fibres

Central core disease. Although it was the first of this group of myopathies to be described (Shy and Magee, 1956), central core disease is uncommon. It can be recognised only by histochemical and ultrastructural examination of the muscle. The cores in the muscle fibres may be single or multiple, central or peripheral but they extend for a considerable distance along the fibre. They are seen almost exclusively in type I fibres and are devoid of mitochondria or oxidative enzymes; the myofibril structure in the core may be disrupted or may be intact and the fibres are otherwise normal. Type I fibre predominance is usual and sometimes type II fibres are virtually absent. Morgan-Hughes, Brett, Lake and Tomé (1973) reported a mother with central core disease whose two clinically affected children had muscle with type I predominance but no cores.

Three or more clinical syndromes of central core disease seem to exist, but cores have also been described after experimental tenotomy in association with other types of muscle pathology, so their presence should be interpreted with caution if the clinical situation is unusual.

Most cases present with moderate infantile hypotonia and often with delay in walking until 3 or 4 years of age. Thereafter there is no deterioration, but walking fast and climbing stairs remain difficult. The inheritance is autosomal dominant. Brooke (1977) has pointed out that affected families often recognise and make light of the symptoms and may come under observation only incidentally. The weakness is greater in the legs than in the arms, and muscle wasting is usually slight. The facial muscles are usually, but not always, spared. The tendon reflexes are diminished but present in most cases. A common feature is congenital dislocation of the hips (Armstrong, Koenigsberger, Mellinger and Lovelace, 1971) and in some families talipes is prominent either from birth or later in life while others have flat feet. Kyphoscoliosis may occur.

Dubowitz and Platts (1965) reported an affected brother and sister whose unaffected parents were first cousins, making autosomal recessive inheritance likely. These cases were atypical also in both having focal wasting of the muscles of the right arm from childhood and more generalised weakness in the fourth decade.

The family reported by Bethlem, van Gool, Hülsmann and Meijer (1966) was unique in having only minimal weakness and in having suffered since childhood from severe painless stiffness of the muscles induced by running, climbing stairs or walking on tiptoe, and lasting for several minutes.

In addition, various sporadic and atypical cases have been reported, including one with congenital contractures, who had an unaffected identical twin (Cohen, Duffner and Heffner, 1978), a patient with an extensive family history of malignant hyperpyrexia who was herself susceptible (Denborough, Dennett and Anderson, 1973) and another with late-onset pes cavus with no clinical abnormality of muscle (Telerman-Toppet, Gerard and Coërs, 1973).

The serum CK activity is normal in central core disease. The electromyographic (EMG) abnormalities are often slight and unhelpful. Cruz Martinez, Ferrer, López-Terradas, Pascual-Castroviejo and Mingo (1979) reviewed the EMG findings and reported an increase in the density of muscle fibres belonging to individual motor units, a finding presumably related to the predominance of type I fibres. Isaacs, Heffron and Badenhorst (1975) reported a reduction in calcium uptake by the sarcoplasmic reticulum in two cases. Although both Cruz Martinez et al. and Isaacs et al. interpreted their findings as being evidence of denervation, more direct and definite evidence of a neurogenic basis for central core disease is lacking, its pathogenesis remains obscure and it is probably best to classify it for the present among the congenital myopathies.

Minicore (multicore) disease. Most authors have followed Engel, Gomez and Groover (1971) and Heffner, Cohen, Duffner and Daigler (1976) in calling this condition multicore disease. 'Minicore', proposed by Currie, Noronha and Harriman (1974) distinguishes the typical appearance of the muscle biopsy more precisely from that of central core disease. The minicores extend for only a few sarcomeres, but have the same histochemical and ultrastructural appearance as central cores. Type I fibre predominance is usual but, unlike central cores, minicores occur in both fibre types.

Ten reported cases were reviewed by Taratuto, Sfaello, Rezzonico and Morales (1978), and Dubowitz (1978) recorded three more. With the exception of one case with proximal weakness progressing from the age of 33 years (Bonnette, Roelofs and Olson, 1974) the clinical features have been rather uniform. There is infantile hypotonia, delay in motor development and continuing but non-progressive muscle weakness tending to be proximal in distribution, modest wasting, often some mild asymmetry of involvement, and impairment, rarely absence, of the tendon reflexes. The face is often affected, neck flexion may be weak and one case showed congenital ophthalmoplegia. The serum CK activity is normal and the EMG usually indicates a myopathic disorder.

One of the cases of Engel *et al.* (1971) had a family history of neuromuscular symptoms in three generations; otherwise only sibs or sporadic cases have been affected and the inheritance is therefore probably autosomal recessive.

An unusual case reported by Gadoth, Margalit and Shapira (1978) had muscle biopsy findings perhaps more akin to minicore than central core disease. The patient's non-progressive myopathy was punctuated by exacerbations of weakness during, and for some time after, febrile illnesses.

Nemaline (rod body) myopathy. This condition was first described by Shy, Engel, Somers and Wanko (1963) and by Conen, Murphy and Donohue (1963) and has since become the most frequently reported, best known and most in-

tensively studied of the congenital myopathies. It has been reviewed by Kuitonnen, Rapola, Nopanen and Donner (1972) and Brooke *et al.* (1979).

The characteristic tiny rod bodies (they are not really 'nemaline' or thread-like) are derived from the disorganisation of the material from which the Z bands of the sarcomeres are formed. Their structure is not fully known but appears to include actin (Yamaguchi, Robson, Stromer, Dahl and Oda, 1978). They form clusters or irregular palisades and are often seen near active vesicular nuclei. They may be inconspicuous and are best seen in thick sections stained with toluidine blue or trichrome stains, or under phase contrast when they are usually refractile. Their ultrastructure is also characteristic. As in central core disease, type I fibre predominance is usual and, indeed, rods and cores or minicores may occur together (Afifi, Smith and Zellweger, 1965; Dubowitz, 1978, p. 83). Rods are seen in a variety of clinical and experimental myopathies and are therefore not in themselves specific; nevertheless, the typical clinical features of the congenital myopathy with which they are usually associated have now been so well defined as to leave no doubt that 'nemaline myopathy' is a specific genetic disorder. In addition, however, nemaline rods may be seen in adults with a late-onset progressive myopathy (Heffernan, Rewcastle and Humphrey, 1968) and it is still not clear whether such cases should be considered to be distinct or part of a spectrum of disease severity; the latter seems more likely. The pathogenesis is unknown and, while various pieces of evidence have indicated a neurogenic lesion in some cases, notably the post-mortem evidence of loss of anterior horn cells in a patient with abundant nemaline rods in the muscle fibres (Dahl and Klutzow, 1974), the overall evidence seems still to point to a primary myopathy.

The typical patient is hypotonic in infancy with delayed motor development and with strikingly slender muscles, which are often not as weak as they look. There is usually definite facial weakness and often nasal speech due to palatal weakness. The muscle involvement is indeed universal and the cases of Conen *et al.* (1963) and Hopkins, Lindsey and Ford (1966) were initially diagnosed as having 'Krabbe's universal muscle hypoplasia', a term no longer in use (Krabbe, 1958). The tendon reflexes are reduced or absent. Various skeletal features including a high-arched palate, dental malocclusion, scoliosis and pes cavus, although by no means confined to nemaline myopathy, are common and combine with the facial weakness and muscle hypoplasia to present a striking clinical picture from which the diagnosis may often be suspected. Most cases are moderately severely disabled throughout childhood. The infantile disease may be severe and cause early death (Kolin, 1967; Shafiq, Dubowitz, Peterson and Milhorat, 1967). The disorder is usually considered to be non-progressive, but undoubtedly deterioration can occur. Some relatives may be found to have subclinical involvement, for example, and it is likely that in some cases they will develop symptoms in adult life (Hopkins *et al.*, 1966). Furthermore, progressive respiratory failure is now frequently recognised in the first and second decades (Kuitonnen *et al.*, 1972; Dubowitz, 1978) and often proves fatal. Serial testing of respiratory function may reveal striking abnormalities months or years before serious respiratory symptoms occur, but extensive fatigue and morning headaches are warning symptoms. One of Dubowitz's (1978) cases first presented with acute respiratory failure while hill-walking. One of us (Gardner-Medwin) has found that a negative pressure cuirass ventilator for use at home overnight, together with tracheostomy, has controlled previously severe disabling respiratory failure in a fully ambulant adolescent for a period of over two years.

Many families have now been described with affected parents and children, and autosomal dominant inheritance is very likely. No very extensive pedigrees have been recorded. Sporadic cases with normal biopsies in both parents have been reported. Sex-linked dominant inheritance has been suggested because of an apparent excess of female cases and the predominance of affected mothers (*see* Brooke *et al.*, 1979) but the disorder may apparently be transmitted by a father to his sons (Gonatas, Shy and Godfrey, 1966) so sex-linkage is unlikely.

Centronuclear (myotubular) myopathies. One of the histological characteristics of myopathic disorders in general is the tendency for muscle fibre nuclei to drift away from their normal subsarcolemmal position towards the centre of the fibre. In the centronuclear myopathies, however, central nuclei dominate a histological picture in which abnormal variation in fibre size and often a tendency to type I fibre predominance are the only other major features. Spiro, Shy and Gonatas (1966), who first drew attention to this disorder, described a boy aged 12 years with congenital but progressive muscle weakness and ophthalmoplegia. His muscle fibres contained central nuclei, often vesicular with prominent nuclei, which were surrounded by clear areas devoid of myofibrils and ATPase activity and sometimes lacking oxidative enzyme activity also, but containing mitochondria. They pointed out that these fibres bore a superficial resemblance to the myotubes found in early fetal muscle, postulated that the disorder might represent arrested maturation of muscle fibres, and named it 'myotubular myopathy'. Since then at least 60 cases have been described and the more non-committal name 'centronuclear myopathy' is now generally preferred because the fibres in most of them lack the perinuclear clear areas and in any case differ in several respects from fetal myotubes. Much overlapping clinical, genetic and pathological variation has emerged; for the present purpose a genetic and clinical classification seems to be appropriate.

Early infantile ophthalmoplegic myopathy with autosomal recessive inheritance. Patients in this category closely resemble the case described by Spiro *et al.* (1966) and include those reported by Sher, Rimalovski, Athanassiades and Aronson (1967), Bethlem, Meijer, Schellens and Vroom (1968), Coleman, Thompson, Nienhuis, Munsat and Pearson (1968), Campbell, Rebeiz and Walton (1969), Ortiz de Zarate and Maruffo (1970), Bill, Cole and Proctor (1979). The condition is apparent in the first year of life because of developmental delay, usually without severe hypotonia at first although this may appear later. By the time of diagnosis in the first or second decade there has usually been slight deterioration in gait or some other evidence of gradual progression. Ptosis, strabismus, partial external ophthalmoplegia (for all directions of gaze), facial weakness (not invariable), generalised muscular weakness and wasting, and tendon areflexia are the usual features. Sternomastoid weakness and foot drop are prominent in some cases. Dysarthria is frequent but dysphagia is uncommon. The face may be long and thin and foot deformities and scoliosis may develop. Most cases become unable to walk in the second decade. Intelligence is generally normal but several patients have had convulsions, including the patient of Spiro *et al*. (1966) whose history was complicated by subdural haematomas; it is not yet certain whether the association with convulsions is coincidental. The serum CK activity is normal or, more often, raised two- or three-fold and the EMG shows myopathic abnormalities. The genetic position is puzzling. Both sexes are affected. Most cases are sporadic but affected sibs have been recorded (Sher *et al*., 1967; Bradley, Price and Watanabe, 1970) and in some families subclinical centronuclear myopathy has been found in the mother (Sher *et al*., 1967; Coleman *et al*., 1968). It is, therefore, not yet possible to distinguish autosomal recessive inheritance with manifestation in the heterozygote from autosomal dominant inheritance with variable expressivity. It is possible that the brother and sister reported by Hurwitz *et al*. (1969), with hypotonia and ophthalmoplegia and a family history of aminoaciduria, may have had centronuclear myopathy, as both the clinical and histological features were compatible.

It may be that this category should be defined a little less strictly. In the otherwise typical case of Kinoshita and Cadman (1968) the symptoms developed at the age of 4 years and there was ptosis but no ophthalmoplegia. Similarly, the case of Bethlem, van Wijngaarden, Mumenthaler and Meijer (1970) had no involvement of any cranial musculature; the symptoms developed at 5 years and had progressed only slowly at 35 years. The affected brothers described by Bradley *et al*. (1970) did have ophthalmoplegia but the onset was at 8 and 15 years respectively and they deteriorated and died at the age of 34 years. In contrast, the case of Campbell *et al*. (1969) died at the age of 27 months and occasional cases have had life-threatening hypotonia and respiratory difficulties in the neonatal period (Coleman *et al*., 1967; Bender and Bender, 1977).

Cases with autosomal dominant inheritance and late onset. The family reported by McLeod, Baker, Lethlean and Shorey (1972) is unique in having 16 affected members in five generations. Biopsies were taken from two members. In most, symptoms began in the 3rd decade but in three (including two of the only three children at risk) the disease began in early childhood (in the second year). The myopathy was usually proximal in emphasis but in some cases showed a scapuloperoneal distribution. The eye muscles were spared, but some had slight facial weakness. The symptoms were slowly progressive, but lifespan was normal. The serum CK activity was normal.

There have been other cases with dominant inheritance, mostly with a relatively late onset (Karpati, Carpenter and Nelson, 1970; *see* Brooke *et al*., 1979) and other adult-onset cases have been reported by Vital, Vallat, Martin, LeBlanc and Bergouignan (1970) and Harriman and Haleem (1972).

Severe X-linked centronuclear myopathy. X-linked centronuclear myopathy was reported in two unrelated Dutch families by van Wijngaarden, Fleury, Bethlem and Meijer (1969) and Barth, van Wijngaarden and Bethlem (1975). The males involved were severely affected, often fatally, with hypotonia and respiratory insufficiency at birth, but the survivors tended to improve and two aged 26 and 33 years were not severely disabled. In the cases of van Wijngaarden *et al*. (1969) the clinical features including ophthalmoplegia and facial weakness, as well as the pathology, were remarkably similar to those of the autosomal recessive cases already described.

Earlier, Engel, Gold and Karpati (1968) had reported the case of a severely hypotonic male infant with reduced fetal movements, neonatal apnoea, hypotonia and impairment of sucking and swallowing, who subsequently suffered from recurrent pneumonia and died aged 18 months. The pathology was reported under the title of 'Type I fibre hypotrophy and central nuclei' and for a time this was regarded as a disorder separate from centronuclear myopathy. Then Meyers, Golomb, Hansen and McKusick (1974) studied a second affected brother and obtained a family history of recurrent male stillbirths in the mother's generation, suggesting X-linked inheritance. The second child was apnoeic at birth and profoundly hypotonic, and died at 7 months. These brothers had no facial weakness, and eye movements were normal. The serum CK activities were normal and the EMGs were inconclusive.

A boy with much milder clinical involvement but with at least equally striking 'hypotrophy' of type I fibres was reported by Inokuchi, Umezaki and Santa (1975). He had a mild myopathy at age 14 with areflexia; the eye movements were not mentioned; sucking had been abnormal in infancy. No evidence exists of a mild X-linked type of centronuclear myopathy at present and it is not yet possible to classify this type of case. The nosological situation overlaps here with that of the 'fibre-type disproportions'.

Unusual features associated with centronuclear myopathy. The patient of Harriman and Haleem (1972), a lady of 67 years, had marked hypertrophy of the calves.

Hawkes and Absolon (1975) reported a man of 29 with typical features of the ophthalmoplegic form but, in addition, cataracts and electromyographic myotonia. His father had cataracts and unilateral congenital ptosis. The cataracts were seen only with a slit lamp. Gil-Peralta, Rafel, Bautista and Alberca (1978) described two sibs with clinical myotonia. Myotonic dystrophy seems unlikely in these cases but cannot be ruled out on the evidence.

The association of cardiomyopathy with centronuclear myopathy is recorded by Bethlem, Van Wijngaarden, Meijer and Hülsmann (1969) in a girl of 16 years, and by Verhiest, Brucher, Goddeeris, Lauweryns and de Geest (1976) in two brothers. The boys had earlier sucking difficulties, delayed motor development and generalised myopathy with ptosis, but the eye movements were not mentioned. A boy aged 18 years (case 11) reported by Shafiq, Sande, Carruthers, Killip and Milhorat (1972) had cardiomyopathy and mild myopathy with type I fibre atrophy.

Other congenital myopathies with structural abnormalities in muscle fibres

Finger-print inclusion myopathy. Six cases have been reported by Engel, Angelini and Gomez (1972), Gordon, Rewcastle, Humphrey and Stewart (1974), Fardeau, Tomé and Derambure (1976) and Curless, Payne and Brinner (1978). They include identical twin brothers (Curless *et al.*) half brothers (Fardeau *et al.*) and isolated female cases, of which one had a non-progressive congenital myopathy for 54 years before diagnosis (Gordon *et al.*). Subsarcolemmal inclusions resembling finger-prints were associated with a few small areas of focal loss of myofibrillar structure (not unlike minicores) and, in some cases, type I fibre predominance.

All cases were hypotonic in infancy with delayed motor development (walking at between 2 years and, in Gordon's patient, 12 years) and with no deterioration. The muscles were slim with retained reflexes and mild to moderate weakness. The cranial musculature was normal. Four of the six cases were mildly mentally retarded. Serum CK levels were normal or slightly raised. One patient was thought to show some beneficial response to neostigmine but had no other evidence of myasthenia (Gordon *et al.*, 1974). Finger-print inclusions have also been seen in various other disorders including dermatomyositis, myotonic dystrophy and oculopharyngeal dystrophy (*see* Curless *et al.*, 1978) but the features of the six cases mentioned are sufficiently similar to comprise a clinical entity. The genetic situation is obscure.

Reducing body myopathy. A rather heterogeneous group of six isolated cases has been described by Brooke and Neville (1972), and by Dubowitz and Brooke (1973) (*see also* Dubowitz (1978), Tomé and Fardeau (1975), Sahgal and Sahgal (1977) and Dudley, Dudley, Varakis and Blackburn (1978)). The common factor is the presence of subsarcolemmal inclusion bodies rich in RNA and sulphydryl groups and capable of reducing nitroblue tetrazolium stain. Their ultrastructure is also diagnostic.

The patients of Brooke and Neville were hypotonic in infancy. Their weakness progressed and both died, at 9 months and 2 years of age respectively. The older child had facial weakness and contractures and was of normal intelligence. The serum CK activity was normal. Another infant (Dudley *et al.*, 1978) died at $2\frac{1}{2}$ months of age after a different type of illness consisting of respiratory paralysis due to progressive board-like rigidity of the muscles of the neck, chest and abdomen, and finally of the limbs. His parents were a father and daughter.

Dubowitz's patient developed progressive asymmetrical myopathy at 4 years and died three years later. In addition to reducing bodies, she had histological evidence of a severe degenerative myopathy. Her Coxsackie B virus antibody titre was high and she was treated as having a possible subacute viral polymyositis, responding temporarily to cyclophosphamide but not to steroids.

The patients of Tomé and Fardeau (1975) and of Sahgal and Sahgal (1977) had a non-progressive proximal myopathy and scapuloperoneal myopathy respectively, without facial involvement. The serum CK was normal in both. Intelligence was preserved.

Other congenital myopathies with inclusions. Adams, Kakulas and Samaha (1965) reported a man with lifelong weakness culminating in rapid deterioration for two years. He had a necrotising myopathy and the muscle fibres contained a variety of sarcoplasmic and nuclear inclusions.

Jenis, Lindquist and Lister (1969) described an infant with severe hypotonia and weakness who died, aged 2 months, of respiratory failure. There were numerous crystalline inclusions in muscle fibre nuclei and in the cytoplasm.

Sarcotubular myopathy was reported by Jerusalem, Engel and Gomez (1973) in two brothers with consanguineous parents. There was mild non-progressive myopathy dating from early infancy. The muscle fibres contained vacuoles derived from the sarcoplasmic reticulum and the T system.

'Zebra-body' inclusions were found in the muscle of a boy of 15 years with a vacuolar congenital myopathy (Lake and Wilson, 1975). Their specificity is uncertain.

Other 'structural' congenital myopathies. Ringel, Neville, Duster and Carroll (1978) reported a remarkable child with severe muscular rigidity at birth, and very high serum CK activity (45 times normal) who gradually improved over 10 months. The EMG was electrically silent. Muscle biopsy revealed that the fibres had an unusual trilaminar structure.

Brooke (1977, p. 217) described a lace-like structure of the sarcoplasm of type II fibres on oxidative enzyme staining in two members of a large family of 'toe-walkers'. Electron microscopy gave normal results.

Cancilla, Kalyanaraman, Verity, Munsat and Pearson (1971) reported a brother and sister of 2 and 5 years with infantile hypotonia, delayed motor development and mild weakness without areflexia, whose muscle biopsies showed atrophy of type I fibres and apparent lysis of their myofibrils.

Genetic myopathies with changes in the histochemical fibre types

Details of the techniques of histochemical fibre typing and of the patterns found at various stages of the development of normal muscles in man will be found in Chapter 8.

It has already been made clear that in many of the congenital myopathies, notably central core disease, nemaline myopathy and centronuclear myopathy, an abnormal predominance of type I fibres (those concerned with slow, oxidative, postural activity) is found. Sometimes affected members in families with central core disease may have evidence only of type I fibre predominance on muscle biopsy (Morgan-Hughes et al., 1973). It is not unusual, when investigating a hypotonic child, to find no other pathological change and because such cases tend to improve they are *ipso facto* included in the category 'benign congenital hypotonia'. Indeed, it is not yet clear whether fibre-type predominance is a cause of hypotonia or a result of it. Very similar patterns of fibre-type predominance have been found in muscle biopsies from hypotonic children with primary disorders of the central nervous system (Curless, Nelson and Brimmer, 1978).

However, in addition to inequality of the numbers of type I and II fibres there may be inequality in their size. Usually the small fibres are of type II and this pattern may be found in a wide variety of disorders, especially muscle disuse. Children with small type I fibres have been described as having 'congenital fibre-type disproportion'.

Congenital fibre-type disproportion. Brooke (1973) suggested this name for a group of hypotonic children with no significant pathology other than the small size of their type I fibres. The pattern had emerged from a previous wider analysis of the histochemical patterns found in children's muscle biopsies (Brooke and Engel, 1969). Other cases with the same biopsy findings had been found to have cerebellar disease or myotonic dystrophy, but 22 cases seemed to comprise a clinical entity. There was hypotonia, often quite severe, at or soon after birth, which might deteriorate for up to one year but thereafter remained static. Congenital contractures, often with dislocation of the hips, were frequent and high-arched palates, short stature and later kyphoscoliosis were each seen in about half the cases. The tendon reflexes were usually diminished but present, the serum CK activity was normal or slightly increased and the EMG was normal or mildly 'myopathic'. Walking was delayed beyond 18 months in all but one case and in some beyond 3 years. Brooke emphasised the relatively good prognosis, but has recently modified this because most of his cases have remained significantly disabled (Brooke et al., 1979). One case turned out to have facioscapulohumeral dystrophy. Mild neuromuscular symptoms were present in first degree or more distant relatives of several cases.

Other cases, subsequently described by Fardeau, Harpey, Caille and Lafourcade (1975), Lenard and Goebel (1975), Martin, Clara, Ceuterick and Joris (1976) and Dubowitz (1978) have, on the whole, tended to confirm the existence of this disorder as an entity, although some doubts remain. Martin et al. (1976) found identical biopsy appearances in two cases of globoid cell leucodystrophy and one of Pompe's glycogenosis, and their patient's mother had been alcoholic during her pregnancy. Dubowitz pointed out the importance of making the diagnosis only when the type II muscle fibres were normal or large in size, in order to avoid confusion with congenital myotonic dystrophy. Lenard and Goebel (1975) reported a child with life-threatening hypotonia and respiratory insufficiency in the neonatal period. The occurrence of an apparently dominant mode of transmission in some families was confirmed by Fardeau et al. (1975).

When the clinical and histochemical findings are typical, one is justified in making a provisional diagnosis of congenital fibre-type disproportion, but follow-up assessments for some years are essential. Some cases may be found later to have central hypotonia. Because of the relatively good long-term outlook it is important to prevent and treat spinal deformities enthusiastically to avoid further respiratory insufficiency; the contractures should also be given vigorous attention. There is little doubt that the next few years will bring a clearer understanding of the nature of this disorder and its pathogenesis. Its status as an entity is fragile and as a primary myopathy even more so.

Other abnormalities of size and number of histochemical fibre types. Given two basic fibre types of which either may predominate, or which may be equal in number, and of which either or both may be small or normal (or rarely large) in size, there is wide scope for variation. One may add the presence or absence of central nuclei in the centronuclear myopathies. In practice many of the possible combinations have been reported. Some of these will be found in Chapter 8. From the clinical point of view, little need now be added to the account already given. In congenital myotonic dystrophy there may be relatively small type I fibres, but the type II fibres also are often smaller than normal; however, this situation is not invariable, and Dubowitz and Brooke (1973) emphasise type II fibre hypertrophy in the early stages.

Relatively small type II fibres are unusual in the context of congenital myopathy. Brooke and Engel (1969) and Matsuoka, Gubbay and Kakulas (1974) described children with this finding who had infantile hypotonia, markedly delayed motor development, normal facial and eye movements, preserved reflexes, a non-progressive course and normal intelligence. Dubrovsky, Taratuto and Martino (1978) reported a different clinical pattern associated with type II fibre hypoplasia in a 6-year-old child with non-progressive distal muscle weakness and atrophy, bilateral external ophthalmoplegia and cataracts. The EMG suggested neurogenic atrophy.

Extremely small fibres of both types in a very

hypotonic baby aged 2 weeks reverted to normal at 10 months, together with the hypotonia, but severe congenital ophthalmoplegia and slight facial weakness persisted (Hanson, Mastrianni and Post, 1977).

Congenital myopathies with muscle fibre necrosis

The muscular dystrophies are discussed in detail in Chapter 14. It is only necessary to mention here that both 'congenital muscular dystrophy' and congenital myotonic dystrophy differ sharply from the other muscular dystrophies in being virtually non-progressive. Nevertheless both may cause profound and life-threatening hypotonia and muscular paralysis in the first few days and weeks of life. Both may give rise to congenital contractures which are often widespread in congenital muscular dystrophy, but tend to be restricted to the ankles in myotonic dystrophy.

Genetic myopathies with non-specific changes in fibres

Everyone who investigates children with neuromuscular disorders is familiar with patients who have undoubted muscular weakness without helpful diagnostic features and whose muscle biopsies show equally non-specific changes. When the symptoms date from infancy and the myopathic features include muscle destruction, fatty replacement, fibrosis and marked variation in fibre size, the label used is often 'congenital muscular dystrophy' (q.v., Ch. 14). When the changes are milder, the term 'benign congenital myopathy' or some other non-committal term is applied. Such cases are by no means uncommon but are, naturally, reported in the medical literature only when the author is drawing attention to the problems they pose (Fenichel and Bazelon, 1966) or when they have some unusual feature such as an extensive family history (Turner and Lees, 1962). Undoubtedly, many of the cases diagnosed in the past would have been classified differently had they undergone full histochemical or ultrastructural investigation; in others, no doubt, ill-luck or

ill-judgement in choosing the site for muscle biopsy has led to the failure to reach a more definite conclusion.

In the cases reported by Turner and Lees (1962), six of 13 sibs were affected with hypotonia from birth and had been followed up without evidence of progression of the disorder for 50 years. The pathology was confined to one post-mortem examination of a bedridden patient, but served to confirm the primary myopathic nature of the disorder. Flexion deformities of the fingers occurred in the adult affected members and in an unaffected aunt and a daughter.

Bethlem and van Wijngaarden (1976) described three kindreds in which dominant inheritance of a benign myopathy occurred over four and five generations. Some had congenital torticollis; otherwise the symptoms had started at about 5 years of age and had progressed extremely slowly. Proximal muscles were mainly affected, but flexion contractures of the fingers were a prominent feature. The muscle biopsy findings were non-specific, but lobulated fibres, of the type seen often in the limb-girdle type of muscular dystrophy, were prominent. In this situation the distinction between a 'benign familial myopathy' and a very mild muscular dystrophy is semantic.

Some cases of 'benign congenital myopathy', while clearly not suffering from myasthenia gravis, may show slight and variable responses to anticholinesterase drugs. For example, Rowland and Eskenazi (1956) and Walton, Geschwind and Simpson (1956) reported the cases of two adults, who had first shown symptoms of muscular weakness in early life. There was no marked deterioration, but both cases displayed features of myasthenia and muscular dystrophy; muscle biopsy showed evidence of myopathic changes but there was striking clinical improvement on injection of neostigmine.

Sometimes, non-specific myopathic features in the muscle biopsy may be accompanied by an apparently disproportionate amount of fibrous tissue around and within the fascicles of muscle fibres. The muscles may feel hard and have striking contractures and the electromyographer may encounter a grating sensation as he inserts his needle. Such cases raise the question of whether such a condition as 'primary myosclerosis' exists.

Cases have been reported by Löwenthal (1954) and by Bradley, Hudgson, Gardner-Medwin and Walton (1973) but it must be confessed that considerable doubt remains as to whether they constitute a specific entity. In isolated cases, especially if the pathology is confined to a few muscles, the possibility of fibrosis induced by previous intramuscular drug injection must be considered (*see* Ch. 25). Chronic and benign spinal muscular atrophy sometimes gives a similar picture.

Benign congenital hypotonia

This much-maligned term arose from the work of Walton (1956; 1957) who obtained follow-up information on 109 infants diagnosed as having 'amyotonia congenita' during the period 1930–1954. Oppenheim's concept of 'myatonia', put forward in 1900 for hypotonic children with a favourable prognosis, had become debased and Walton found that, half a century later, the terms 'myatonia' or 'amyotonia congenita' were sometimes used to encompass all of the infantile hypotonias including Werdnig-Hoffmann disease. Seventeen of the 109 cases had hypotonia of unknown cause, but with recovery which was complete in eight and incomplete in nine cases. The term 'benign congenital hypotonia' was 'used as a descriptive title' for these cases whose 'condition appears to have been due to a widespread congenital muscular hypotonia of undetermined aetiology which eventually recovered completely' (Walton, 1956). In the same year, central core disease was first described and, in the period of nearly a quarter of a century which has passed since then, many other disorders giving hypotonia with 'incomplete recovery' have been recognised and are now generally classified as the 'benign congenital myopathies' described earlier in this Chapter. The nature of those cases which show *complete* recovery, and for which Walton now reserves the term 'benign congenital hypotonia', has been less satisfactorily clarified. Brooke and Engel (1969) found that some of them had type I fibre predominance in the muscle biopsy but others have no histological abnormality at all on the evidence of current techniques. No doubt, entities within this group will be identified

in the future; meanwhile 'benign congenital hypotonia' remains, at any particular state of the art, a valuable term for those residual cases for whom, after full investigation, no more accurate label exists. It should be reserved for patients who: (1) are hypotonic at, or soon after, birth, sometimes quite severely; but (2) retain active limb movements and tendon reflexes; and (3) whose motor development is delayed but shows improvement over a period of months or years; and (4) whose serum enzyme activities, EMGs and biopsies are essentially normal. However, it is quite reasonably argued that muscle biopsy is not justified in an apparently benign situation when it can lead to no effective treatment, unless genetic counselling will be influenced by the result. Certainly, biopsy should be performed in this situation only when full histochemical and electron-microscopic studies will be done, for otherwise it is certain to be inconclusive.

The paediatrician with an interest in the development of the child's motor functions tends to look at hypotonia in a different light. For example Lundberg (1979) reviewed 78 children who had delayed development of gross motor functions, such as sitting and walking, but had relatively well-developed manipulative functions and no abnormal neurological signs. She found that only three were diagnosed as having neuromuscular disease. Of 65 children whose walking was delayed beyond 17 months, 71 per cent had been significantly hypotonic in infancy, and 18 per cent had a family history of late walking. Half of them were 'bottom shufflers' and 30 per cent had a family history of bottom-shuffling. A common sign among the late walkers in whom no cause for the delay was found was the 'sitting on air' posture of flexion of the hips and extension of the knees while being suspended under the arms.

Whether one thinks of such children as having 'benign congenital hypotonia' or 'dissociated motor development', the essential need in management is to provide the child with the stimulation and equipment and the family with the understanding of the situation and the support that they need, to allow him to develop without the loss of opportunities which may, in the long run, prove more handicapping than the neuromuscular problem itself.

Skeletal, tendinous and ligamental causes of hypotonia

It may be difficult to make a clinical distinction between ligamental laxity and muscular hypotonia in early infancy. Later in childhood the hyper-extensibility of the joints with relatively normal muscle tone becomes apparent. Certain congenital disorders of connective tissue may be accompanied by delay in postural control and apparent hypotonia due to hyperextensibility of joints. McKusick (1972) records three siblings with extreme ligamentous laxity and multiple joint dislocations whose parents were related. A dominant syndrome of ligamentous laxity and dislocations is perhaps more common (Carter and Sweetnam, 1960). In Marfan's syndrome and especially in a similar 'marfanoid' syndrome (Walker, Beighton and Murdoch, 1969) joint laxity is prominent and in the former some muscular weakness occurs. 'Marfanoid' features have often been mentioned in nemaline myopathy but in fact bear little resemblance to true Marfan's disease. Ehlers-Danlos syndrome must also be considered in the differential diagnosis of the limp child. McKusick (1972) recognises seven varieties of this, of which one (type III) presents with joint laxity as the main feature while, in the others, elastic skin, bruising and other features are more prominent. Osteogenesis imperfecta has been reported as presenting with delay in walking and hypotonia (Tizard, 1949; Dubowitz, 1969).

Disorders of neuromuscular transmission

Myasthenia gravis. It is unusual for myasthenia gravis to present in infancy or childhood. Of 447 cases collected by Millichap and Dodge (1960), 16 showed signs of the disease at, or soon after, birth and 35 presented between the ages of 1 and 16 years. In a series of 217 cases presenting in infancy, childhood or adolescence (Osserman, 1958), 34 had symptoms at, or within a few days of, birth and eight more within the first two years of life.

In most cases of myasthenia gravis presenting at birth, the mother is affected; nevertheless, very few babies born to myasthenic mothers (10 out of 71 in Osserman's series (1958)) have symptoms of the condition, and the severity of the symptoms bears no obvious relation to the severity or duration of the mother's illness. Early diagnosis is important, because, while myasthenia in babies born to myasthenic mothers is a transient illness lasting from a few days to a few weeks, there may be severe generalised weakness which leads to death unless appropriate treatment is given.

Signs may be present at, or within a few hours of, birth and usually consist of generalised hypotonia with respiratory insufficiency—rapid shallow breathing and intermittent cyanosis—or difficulty in sucking and swallowing. The normal newborn baby usually keeps its mouth and eyes shut except when crying or feeding. Reduced mobility of the face, with eyes and mouth open, should suggest the diagnosis, which is supported by the finding of generalised hypotonia.

A test dose of 0.05 mg prostigmine, 0.3 mg pyridostigmine bromide, or 0.1 ml Tensilon (edrophonium chloride 1 mg), by intramuscular injection, will confirm the diagnosis. Maintenance therapy consists of 1–5 mg of prostigmine or 4–20 mg of pyridostigmine bromide orally with feeds. The size and frequency of the dose will have to be adjusted according to the degree and duration of relief of symptoms and must be reduced as spontaneous recovery takes place.

Myasthenia gravis in the newborn infants of non-myasthenic mothers is even rarer. It has the same clinical features and response to treatment but, unlike the condition in babies of myasthenic mothers, is persistent, although usually milder. Bundey (1972) provides evidence for distinguishing cases of myasthenia gravis presenting before and after 2 years of age. The infantile form is probably inherited as an autosomal recessive trait and, while persistent, is mild; however, occasionally severe cases of myasthenia may present in the first six months of life (Oberklaid and Hopkins, 1976). Myasthenia presenting after the age of 2 years resembles the disease in adults.

The muscular weakness of infantile myasthenia is usually widespread, but Ford (1966, p. 1266) reports a family of four affected brothers in whom the extraocular muscles were mainly involved.

Infantile botulism. Two infants, aged 2 and 3 months, who became hypotonic over a period of a few days and had difficulty in sucking and swallowing, were found to have evidence of neuromuscular blockade on electromyography and both botulinus organisms and toxin in the faeces. Both made a spontaneous recovery (Pickett, Berg, Chaplin and Brunstetter-Shafer, 1976). Other cases have been described, all with a similar history (Midura and Arnon, 1976; Turner, Brett, Gilbert, Ghosh and Liebeschuetz, 1978).

Abnormal neuromuscular junction. Examination of the structure of motor nerve endings and motor end-plates has been refined by intravital staining (Coërs, 1952) and electron microscopy (Mair, 1963). Anatomical defects of the neuromuscular junction may account for some otherwise unexplained cases of muscular weakness and hypotonia in infancy. Coërs and Pelc (1954), Woolf and Till (1955) and Woolf (1960) have published examples of non-deteriorating hypotonia in which there were histological defects of axons or end-plates. These findings must be accepted with reserve until more is known of the ultrastructure of neuromuscular junctions in normal subjects (Woolf, 1963).

CLINICAL PROBLEMS IN CHILDREN WITH NEUROMUSCULAR DISORDERS

Arthrogryposis multiplex congenita

The presence of multiple joint contractures at birth is clearly a situation with a wide variety of causes, and individual appraisal of each case is essential if one is to avoid overlooking the relatively unusual cases which have a simple genetic basis, an underlying progressive disease, or important associated anomalies. The great majority of patients show a non-progressive course and most are of normal intelligence.

To qualify as having arthrogryposis multiplex congenita (AMC) a patient must have joint contractures present at birth in at least two different areas of the body (Fisher, Johnstone, Fisher and Goldkamp, 1970). The more limited condition of congenital talipes, however, is analogous in its multifactorial causes which include denervation of the lower limbs (as in spina bifida) and oligohydramnios (perhaps causing restricted movement) and a large group of cases of unknown origin. In a typical case of AMC there is equinovarus deformity of the feet, the hips are abducted and flexed or extended, the knees and elbows incompletely extended, the forearms pronated and the hands flexed with a claw-like apposition of thenar and hypothenar eminences. There may be considerable variation upon this distribution. The muscles acting at the affected joints are typically wasted.

It is currently thought that the condition can result from a number of different pathological processes causing immobilisation of limbs during, or shortly after, the embryonic formation of joints (Dodge, 1960). In support of this view, Jago (1970) described a typical case of arthrogryposis in an infant born to a mother who had had tetanus at the 10th to 12th week of pregnancy and who was treated with d-tubocurarine for 10 days.

The majority of cases are found to have a neurogenic basis for the arthrogryposis (Brandt, 1947; Drachman and Banker, 1963; Besser and Behar, 1967). Typically there is asymmetry of the weakness and joint involvement suggesting patchy loss of anterior horn cells and the spinal cord lesion appears to be non-progressive in almost all cases. Although joint contractures may be found at birth in Werdnig-Hoffmann disease, these are uncommon and never severe, and most of the joint deformity is fully correctable by passive stretching. It seems clear, therefore, that neurogenic arthrogryposis is not a more severe version of Werdnig-Hoffmann disease and, indeed, the two conditions appear to be unrelated entities.

A primary myopathy with features of 'congenital muscular dystrophy' (q.v. Ch. 14) is more rarely the basis of arthrogryposis (Banker, Victor and Adams, 1957; Pearson and Fowler, 1963). The former authors suggested that the posture induced by the contractures was characteristically different in the myopathic disorder, with flexion of the hips and knees and adduction of the legs, as well as kyphoscoliosis, chest deformity and torticollis. It is unlikely that these criteria are reliable for clinical diagnosis. The 'dystrophic' nature of the muscle pathology in myopathic AMC has been questioned by many authors, notably by Dastur, Razzak and Bharucha (1972) who studied the histological and histochemical features of 16 cases of all types. A primary failure of muscle embryogenesis with secondary fibrosis and disorganisation of muscle architecture seems more likely than a degenerative process in these cases. Furukawa and Toyokura (1977) reported another pattern of 'muscular dystrophy' and arthrogryposis in which the proximal muscles of both the upper and lower limbs showed contractures while the distal joints were hyperextensible. The condition was non-progressive.

There is no doubt that both the EMG and the muscle histology may be difficult to interpret in arthrogryposis, presumably because of the chronicity of the lesion, the associated disuse atrophy and the problems of 'secondary myopathic change in denervated muscle'. Nevertheless, investigation will permit most cases to be assigned to a neurogenic or myopathic category (Bharucha, Pandya and Dastur, 1972; Dastur et al., 1972).

Der Kaloustian, Afifi and Mire (1972) report a myopathic form of arthrogryposis in which massive accumulation of glycogen in muscle fibres was found on biopsy.

Neurogenic AMC may be associated with severe malformation of the brain causing severe retardation, microcephaly and optic atrophy (Fowler, 1959; Frischknecht, Bianchi and Pilleri, 1960) and sometimes with more subtle cerebral atrophy and mild educational subnormality (Ek, 1958; Bharucha et al., 1972) but most cases are intellectually normal whether of the neurogenic or myopathic type (Wynne-Davies and Lloyd-Roberts, 1976). Bargeton, Nezelof, Guran and Job (1961) and Peña Miller, Budzilovich and Feigen (1968) described cases of arthrogryposis of autosomal recessive genetic origin, in which the pathology consisted of a peculiar nodular fibrosis of the anterior spinal roots. Congenital familial polyneuropathy may also cause arthrogryposis (confined however to the lower limbs) (Yuill and Lynch, 1974).

Autosomal recessive inheritance occurs in myopathic AMC (Lebenthal, Shocket, Adam, Seelenfreund, Fried, Najenson, Sandbank and Matoth, 1970). Dominant inheritance was reported in a father and two daughters with relatively mild myopathic features (Daentl, Berg, Layzer and Epstein, 1974).

Although the anterior horn cell form of AMC can occur in more than one member of a family (Ek, 1958) it has also been reported in only one of pairs of identical twins; hence the genetic position is uncertain, and the condition may well be heterogenous. In a survey of all the cases of AMC seen in four large centres in Great Britain, Wynne-Davies and Lloyd-Roberts (1976) found none that were familial and concluded that a variety of environmental factors acting *in utero* were responsible, although these could rarely be identified.

Beckerman and Buchino (1978) have reviewed the inherited syndrome complexes in which arthrogryposis may play a part and reported two cases with multiple cervical anomalies including pterygium.

Early and vigorous orthopaedic management of the deformities of arthrogryposis is usually successful in correcting them and because the underlying disorder in the great majority of cases is non-progressive the effort is extremely worthwhile. The treatment has been reviewed by Friedlander, Westin and Wood (1968) and Lloyd-Roberts and Lettin (1970).

Muscle contractures and spinal deformities later in childhood

Congenital contractures, not amounting to arthrogryposis multiplex, occur in several of the congenital myopathies, notably in central core disease, congenital myotonic dystrophy and fibre-type disproportion, and also in nemaline myopathy, some of the congenital polyneuropathies and in some cases of infantile spinal muscular atrophy (SMA). In SMA fixed contractures at birth suggest a degree of chronicity of the lesion that makes it more likely that the case may fall into the slowly progressive or static type II category rather than into the inevitably progressive type I (Werdnig-Hoffmann disease).

Later in childhood, contractures develop especially in the most severe neuromuscular diseases including Duchenne muscular dystrophy and SMA; they may contribute substantially to the child's disability. Regular stretching of the shortened muscles by the parents and the school physiotherapist, while by no means completely successful, makes a major contribution and attention to the sitting posture and sometimes the use of night splints may be valuable. Except at the ankles, where stretching techniques are rarely totally effective, tenotomy is not usually needed when a child has been regularly supervised. The use of tenotomy in the late stages of diseases with a poor prognosis must have a clear purpose, such as improving the child's appearance, posture, or handling, because it will rarely achieve any improvement in function. This is in sharp contrast to its value in arthrogryposis and other congenital contractures with relatively good muscle power. Contractures acquired later, either in the feet or elsewhere, following fractures, immobilisation or neglect, may benefit from the same approach.

Localised contractures in otherwise normal muscles are usually the sequel of earlier intramuscular injections of antibiotics (Norman, Temple and Murphy, 1970: Hoefnagel, Jalbert, Publow and Richtsmeier, 1978).

In some cases of polymyositis in childhood, contractures may develop in a matter of a few days or weeks.

The management of kyphoscoliosis is discussed in relation to Duchenne muscular dystrophy in Chapter 14. The importance of preventive bracing applies *a fortiori* to those disorders with a potentially better prognosis in which thoracic distortion may pose a major threat to life. The chronic childhood spinal muscular atrophies and fibre-type disproportion are particularly important examples. An effective moulded spinal support, fitted to give the maximum comfortable correction of the curvature, should be provided at the first sign of deformity, or preferably just beforehand in patients whose trunk muscles are barely capable of maintaining an off-balance position.

A disorder in which contractures play a major part is the *rigid spine syndrome*, so named by Dubowitz (1973; 1978). Further cases have been described by Goebel, Lenard, Görke and Kunze (1977), Seay, Ziter and Petajan (1977) and Goto, Nagasaka, Nagara and Kuroiwa (1979). The syndrome has been recorded only in males, though Dubowitz (1978) mentions seeing a female case. The patients described had noted the cervical contractures by the age of 6 or 7 years. Some had been normal until that time, others had had earlier muscle weakness and delay in walking. The condition is usually diagnosed late in the second decade, by which time the affected boy has severe contracture of the posterior cervical and paraspinal muscles and slighter elbow and knee contractures. The muscles are generally very thin but only slightly weak. A patient of Professor Sir John Walton's was able to run upstairs but had difficulty in walking down because of severe neck retraction. Neck flexion, however, is very weak and there is no doubt that there is a generalised mild myopathy. Muscle biopsy of the rigid muscles reveals excessive endomysial and perimysial fibrosis, and variation in fibre size. Goebel *et al.* (1977) and Seay *et al.* (1977) found fibre-type disproportion in biceps biopsies in their cases. There are no reports of familial cases at present.

Somewhat similar contractures and muscle weakness are seen in cases of the X-linked type of scapuloperoneal myopathy reported by Thomas, Calne and Elliott (1972) and in the Dreifuss variant of Becker muscular dystrophy (*see* Ch. 15).

Acute muscular weakness in childhood

In the countries which provide immunisation against poliomyelitis it has become a rare event to see a child who has developed severe generalised muscular weakness over a period of hours or a few days.

Poliomyelitis must still be considered, especially in travellers from abroad. ECHO and Coxsackie viruses rarely cause an almost indistinguishable illness. The multifocal distribution of the weakness, the relation to a preceding febrile illness and the development of a purely motor deficit over a few days sometimes accompanied by pain and by fasciculation are all characteristic. Poliomyelitis has been reported as a rare occurrence in newborn babies (Pugh and Dudgeon, 1954; Bates, 1955). It seems clear from the onset of the disease within the first few days of life that the virus can be transmitted via the placenta. In many cases the mother has had the disease in active form shortly before or after the birth of the infant. In other cases, infection through faecal contamination from the mother in the birth process or postanatal infection may have taken place. The infant may have little fever and no diarrhoea. The extent of the paralysis is variable, but in many cases has been widespread with a fatal outcome. Focal myocarditis has been a common post-mortem finding in addition to the typical central nervous system changes.

Some patients who later turn out to have *chronic spinal muscular atrophy* develop symptoms for the first time very suddenly over a few days or even hours in an illness which may resemble poliomyelitis. This often occurs, however, during the course of one of the common childhood fevers or may follow immunisation. Recovery, if any occurs, is very slight after such an episode. Later in the course of the disease, episodes of deterioration are quite often a feature, again with very limited improvement or none at all, so that the disability in these patients tends to deteriorate in a series of steps rather than taking the more continuous downhill course which is seen in the muscular dystrophies, and indeed in many other cases of spinal muscular atrophy.

Other causes of rapidly progressive paralysis which must be considered and which are more fully described in other chapters are acute polyneuritis, the periodic paralyses, myasthenia gravis, acute myositis and acute rhabdomyolysis. Botulism causes bulbar weakness, blurred vision and diplopia followed by generalised flaccid paralysis and areflexia. Poisoning with organophosphorus compounds, curare or an overdose of an anticholinesterase drug may have to be considered in some cases. In young infants, quite acute weakness and hypotonia may occur in Leigh's disease and the organic acidaemias.

Acute postinfectious polyneuritis is uncommon before the age of 4 years and rare before the age of 2 years. The presenting symptoms and course of the illness are similar in childhood and adult life. It is not uncommon to be able to diagnose the preceding viral infection serologically and the Epstein-Barr virus is an important one among many causative agents. The disease as it affects children has been reviewed by Peterman, Daly, Dion and Keith (1959), Paulson (1970) and Eberle, Brinke, Azen and White (1975).

Acute transient viral myositis may cause a rather painful generalised paralysis after a prodromal febrile illness of several days. The serum CK level is 5–50 times normal. Recovery occurs in a few days. McKinlay and Mitchell (1976) described eight patients aged between 5 and 9 years.

Acute weakness may result from *fluctuations in serum potassium levels*. Any condition causing considerable hypokalaemia is likely to be associated with muscular weakness, hypotonia and areflexia. Cushing's disease and primary aldosteronism are rare in young children, but gastrointestinal and renal losses of potassium may occur in a number of infantile diseases, e.g. chronic diarrhoea and vomiting, congenital alkalosis of gastrointestinal origin, renal tubular acidosis and galactosaemia and this produces muscular weakness, hypotonia and depression of tendon reflexes. The hypokalaemic, hyperkalaemic and normokalaemic forms of *periodic paralysis* may all be seen in childhood. Indeed, the hyperkalaemic form almost always begins in the first decade. In their series of 108 cases, Gamstorp, Hauge, Helweg-Larson, Mjönes and Sagild (1957) found that 45 per cent had attacks before the age of 5 years and 90 per cent before the age of 10 years. Their youngest patient was 8 months old at the onset. The symptoms last a few minutes at first but become more prolonged in adolescence. The hypokalaemic form tends to start later but may do so at as early as 3 years (Howes, Price, Pearson and Blumberg, 1966). As the attacks continue, a permanent myopathy may develop and this may be seen even in children (Pearson, 1964; Dyken, Zeman and Rusche, 1969). The normokalaemic form of periodic paralysis also begins before the age of 10 years (Poskanzer and Kerr, 1961) and causes recurrent severe tetraparesis lasting usually for several days or even weeks. A similar clinical pattern of weakness is seen in pleoconial myopathy (Shy *et al.*, 1966).

Acute *focal* muscular weakness of lower motor neurone type may result from birth trauma to the brachial plexus or from poliomyelitis, and two other conditions are of special interest in children. Recurrent attacks of *neuralgic amyotrophy* (brachial neuritis) occur in some families in which the trait is inherited as an autosomal dominant (Geiger, Mancall, Penn and Tucker, 1974; Dunn, Daube and Gomez, 1978). As in the sporadic adult disease, quite severe local pain precedes acute weakness, usually in certain proximal muscles of the upper limb but sometimes in the forearm. There is profound atrophy; recovery takes many months and may be incomplete. Sometimes there is autonomic involvement. Attacks may occur from the first year of life but do so at long intervals, usually of several years. Rarely there is vocal cord paresis. Several authors have noted hypoteleorism in affected members of the families.

Amyotrophy following asthma was first described by Hopkins (1974) in a series of 10 cases. Three more were reported by Danta (1975) and Ilett, Pugh and Smithells (1977). Acute paralysis, preceded in most cases by pain, occurred 4–10 days after an acute asthmatic attack. The weakness resolved slowly and very incompletely. In several of Hopkins' cases the leg was affected, a situation which is very rare in neuralgic amyotrophy if, indeed, it ever occurs. In Hopkins' series, CSF pleocytosis was the rule, often with a raised protein level, but in one of the cases of Ilett *et al.* (1977) the CSF was normal. There seemed to be no consistent relationship to any of the drugs given for the asthma, or to any particular virus infection.

Fluctuating and intermittent muscular weakness in childhood

In addition to the periodic paralyses there are several disorders in which muscular weakness varies from time to time.

Repeated separate episodes of temporary paralysis occur also in pleoconial myopathy (Shy *et al.*, 1966). Recurrent subacute attacks of muscular weakness, especially if they follow physical stress and are associated with nausea or vomiting, should arouse suspicion of carnitine deficiency or mitochondrial myopathy. The discrete episodes of focal neuropathic paralysis in familial brachial neuritis have been mentioned and families have been reported in which recurrent pressure palsies occur against a background of a permanent, subclinical, generalised, peripheral neuropathy. Chronic relapsing polyneuropathy is a sporadic inflammatory disorder in which recurrent episodes of severe demyelinating motor and sensory neuropathy occur and lead to permanent weakness. It is important to recognise this because of the good response to steroids in some cases. The CSF protein is increased. Attacks may start in adolescence. There is an association with certain HLA haplotypes (Thomas, 1979).

The fluctuating weakness and fatigability which occur in myasthenia gravis are not mimicked by any other disorder. A degree of fluctuation over a longer time scale is often seen in the myopathy of carnitine deficiency. A striking sense of fatigue which seems out of proportion to the muscular weakness is a feature of some of the mitochondrial myopathies, but it is not possible to induce true loss of power by repeated muscle contraction in these cases. The degree of weakness in the mitochondrial myopathies may also vary from time to time, but not to a great degree. Rarely one encounters cases of congenital myopathy without specific pathological features in whom fluctuation in symptoms is a prominent feature and some of these cases respond partly to anticholinesterase medication (Rowland and Eskenazi, 1956; Walton *et al.*, 1956).

Progressive muscular weakness

The rate at which muscular weakness develops and progresses is of vital importance both in diagnosis and prognosis. We have attempted, in Table 17.1, to give an indication of the rate of progression of the most important neuromuscular disorders which may be seen for diagnosis at various periods of childhood. This approach has its limitations, however, because the rate of progression may vary from case to case, may change during the course of the illness and in any case may be difficult to gauge in the early stages.

Other valuable clues to diagnosis include the degree of muscle atrophy in relation to the weakness, the broad pattern of distribution of the weakness (whether proximal, distal or generalised), whether the weakness within this broad pattern is highly selective for particular muscles or not, whether the face and other cranial muscles are involved, the presence or absence of fasciculation, fatigability, reflex changes or symptoms and signs of involvement of other tissues, the degree of abnormality in serum CK activity and in other enzymes, and the findings in the EMG and muscle biopsy. Many of these points are discussed in Chapter 13, and here we shall confine discussion of the progressive disorders to a few comments upon some of the most important conditions.

Table 17.1 Progressive muscular weakness

Apparent rate of progression at time of presentation	Onset			
	First 6 months	First 2 years	2–10 years	Adolescence

Progressive over hours or days	Poliomyelitis
	Myasthenia gravis
	Chronic SMA
	Spinal tumour
	Leigh's disease
	Organicacidaemia
	Carnitine deficiency
	Rhabdomyolysis
	Botulism
		Poliomyelitis
		Myasthenia gravis
		Chronic SMA
		Hyperkalaemic P.P.
		Rhabdomyolysis
		(Guillain-Barré)
		Organicacidaemia
		Leigh's disease
			Poliomyelitis
			Guillain-Barré
			  Syndrome
			Hyperkalaemic P.P.
			Hypokalaemic P.P.
			Myasthenia gravis
			Rhabdomyolysis
			Acute myositis
			Pleoconial myopathy
				Poliomyelitis
				
				Guillain-Barré
				  Syndrome
				
				All 3 periodic paralyses
				
				Myasthenia gravis
				Acute myositis

Weeks or months	Werdnig-Hoffmann
	  Disease
	Pompe's Disease
	Congenital M.D.
	Mitochondrial
	  myopathy
	Nemaline myopathy
	
	Centronuclear
	  myopathy
	Reducing body
	  myopathy
	Leigh's disease
	Congenital
	  polyneuropathy
	Metabolic myopathies
		Chronic SMA
		Dermatomyositis
		Myasthenia
		Carnitine deficiency
		Metachromatic
		  leucodystrophy
		
		Reducing body
		  myopathy
		Leigh's disease
		Metabolic myopathies
			Dermatomyositis
			Chronic SMA
			Kearns-Sayre
			  syndrome
			Carnitine deficiency
			Myasthenia
			
			Refsum's disease
			Metabolic myopathies
				Myasthenia
				Polymyositis
				Carnitine deficiency
				MLD Neuropathy
				Dermatomyositis
				Refsum's disease
				Metabolic myopathies

Years	Nemaline myopathy
	Centronuclear
	  myopathy
	Rarely FSH M.D.
	Mitochondrial
	  myopathy
	HMSN type III
	
	Hypothyroidism
		Duchenne M.D.
		Autosomal recessive
		  M.D.
		Rarely polymyositis
		Chronic SMA
		Glycogen storage
		  disease
		
		Kearns-Sayre
		  syndrome
		Carnitine deficiency
		Other mitochondrial
		  myopathies
		Distal M.D. & SMA
		Centronuclear
		  myopathy
			Duchenne M.D.
			Becker M.D.
			Autosomal recessive
			  M.D.
			Chronic SMA
			Polymyositis
			
			Glycogen storage
			  disease
			Carnitine deficiency
			Mitochondrial
			  myopathies
			
			HMSN I and II
			Scapuloperoneal
			M.D.
			Scapuloperoneal
			SMA
				Becker M.D.
				FSH M.D.
				Limb girdle M.D.
				Chronic SMA
				Glycogen storage
				  disease
				
				Carnitine deficiency
				HMSN I and II
				Myotonic M.D.

Static or progressive over decades	Central core disease
	Fibre-type
	  disproportion
	Congenital myotonic
	  M.D.
	Duchenne M.D.
	Congenital M.D.
	Fingerprint
	  myopathy
		Duchenne M.D.
		Autosomal Recessive
		  M.D.
		Fingerprint M.D.
		Central core disease
			Duchenne M.D.
			Autosomal recessive
			  M.D.
			Central core disease
			Myotonic M.D.
			Becker M.D.
				Becker M.D.
				Myotonic M.D.
				FSH M.D.
				Limb girdle M.D.

Duchenne muscular dystrophy. The diagnosis is easy to confirm (Ch. 14). The problem is to remember to consider it when a child presents with the early symptoms. It is not uncommonly overlooked until after another affected child has been born in the family. The earliest sign *in most cases* is delay in walking (50 per cent walk only after the age of 18 months). General psychomotor delay is quite frequent and speech may be immature. At first the gait disturbance is easier to recognise when the patient tries to run or to climb stairs. From an early age, boys with this condition roll on to their faces before standing up from the floor and the full 'Gowers' manoeuvre' of climbing up the legs is not apparent until the age of 4–6 years. A few are hypotonic during the first few months of life. Every child with unexplained developmental delay deserves an estimation of his serum CK activity. Although the very high serum CK levels, present from birth, indicate that active destruction of muscle occurs from the beginning, clinical evidence of progression may not be apparent until the age of 4–7 years.

Spinal muscular atrophy (SMA). After Duchenne muscular dystrophy, SMA is by far the commonest neuromuscular disorder in childhood. We cannot enter here into the complex problems of the nosology of the spinal muscular atrophies. They vary greatly in age at onset, rate of progression and distribution of weakness, but attempts to classify them on these grounds have often proved to be genetically invalid (*see* Chapters 20 and 22), while genetic classifications lead to a state of apparent clinical confusion. The work of Pearn (1971) has done much to clarify the situation and we follow him and Emery (1971) in listing the following categories for a brief discussion of the diagnosis and management. This is in no sense a nosological classification because the criteria for inclusion in the categories are so mixed; but it lists, as clearly as seems possible at present, the apparent genetic entities.

Progressive infantile spinal muscular atrophy ('Acute Werdnig-Hoffmann disease')
Chronic childhood SMA
Adult-onset SMA
Scapuloperoneal SMA

Distal SMA
Facioscapulohumeral SMA
X-linked SMA
Autosomal dominant SMA
Bulbar SMA (Fazio-Londe Disease)

The great majority of cases fall into one of the first two categories, in which the muscular involvement tends to be generalised or predominantly proximal in distribution and in which the inheritance is autosomal recessive. The other rarer types are discussed in Chapter 20.

Progressive infantile SMA may present at any time in the first five months of life and is best distinguished from the chronic cases, not by the age at onset, which may be evident from diminished fetal movement as early as the 35th week of gestation in both acute and chronic cases, but by its relentlessly progressive course. It is therefore prudent to wait for clear evidence of deterioration before offering a prognosis, when the clinical picture of severe paralytic hypotonia, areflexia and fasciculation of the tongue makes the diagnosis of infantile SMA obvious. Muscle biopsy appears not to be of help in distinguishing progressive from non-progressive cases. Other conditions which may present a very similar clinical picture are congenital peripheral neuropathy of the type reported by Lyon (1969), described below, and perhaps infantile botulism.

The term chronic childhood SMA embraces cases of the Kugelberg-Welander syndrome (type III SMA) and of the intermediate or type II variety (Emery, 1971). It covers a wide range of cases in which the onset may be as early as fetal life or as late at least as the end of the first decade and whose severity may vary equally widely. The fact that such variation may occur within a single family suggests that only one genetic entity is involved but undoubtedly the severe infantile case who never learns to sit unsupported and who survives in a helpless condition with major contractures and spinal deformity for anything from a few months to three or more decades presents a very different problem in clinical management from the previously normal 5-year-old who begins to develop a waddling gait. It is also characteristic of chronic SMA that it may progress irregularly, intermittently or not at all, and it is therefore exceptionally difficult to give an accurate prognosis in an individual case, even after a considerable period of observation. A few cases present with the sudden development of weakness over a matter of hours or days, usually in association with an infection or immunisation, and with subsequently a relatively static or chronic course. SMA resembles the muscular dystrophies (and very few other neuromuscular disorders) in causing strikingly selective muscular weakness in many of the later-onset cases. It differs in causing no recognisable pattern of selection and in often being asymmetrical. Fasciculation, so helpful in diagnosis when present, may be absent or inconspicuous in as many as 50 per cent of cases. The feet tend to evert rather than adopting the equinovarus position seen in Duchenne muscular dystrophy. The serum CK may be normal or considerably elevated and even the EMG, so valuable in cooperative adult patients, may be confusing or quite often even normal in children if they are unable to maintain a strong volitional contraction of the needled muscle. It is therefore particularly important to select an appropriate and moderately severely affected muscle for biopsy in trying to reach a definitive diagnosis. It is difficult to assess the power of individual muscles in an uncooperative or obese child; careful palpation of the degree of atrophy will often be helpful in diagnosis and in choosing a muscle for biopsy.

The principles of management of spinal muscular atrophy follow in many respects those laid down for Duchenne muscular dystrophy in Chapter 14. Active orthopaedic measures to deal with contractures and spinal deformity are, however, even more important because of the possibility of prolonged arrest of the progression of the disease and because thoracic distortion due to kyphoscoliosis presents one of the major hazards to life by contributing to respiratory insufficiency. Active spinal bracing as soon as a hypotonic child begins to sit up is therefore usually justified, and spinal fusion during adolescence is often valuable if expertly performed after very careful assessment of respiratory function. Active and intensive postoperative care, including active exercise of limb muscles, is a vital component of this type of management. The provision of light walking-calipers is useful in some cases.

Other progressive myopathies. The other important conditions to consider in a progressive muscular disorder in childhood include dermatomyositis or more uncommonly pure polymyositis, muscle carnitine deficiency, glycogen storage disease (especially acid maltase deficiency and debrancher enzyme deficiency), mitochondrial myopathy, nemaline myopathy, centronuclear myopathy, the Becker, autosomal recessive and facioscapulohumeral types of muscular dystrophy, myotonic dystrophy and the myopathies associated with renal failure, metabolic bone disease, hypothyroidism, Cushing's syndrome (and steroid therapy) and the various peripheral neuropathies. Of these, polymyositis, muscle carnitine deficiency, the juvenile forms of acid maltase and debrancher enzyme deficiency and sometimes the myopathy of metabolic bone disease may mimic muscular dystrophy—a point of great importance because three of these disorders are potentially treatable.

Facial, bulbar and external ocular muscle weakness in infancy

Transient unilateral facial weakness is not uncommon in the newborn and disappears in a few days or weeks. Persistent congenital paralysis is much rarer.

Bell's palsy occurs in young children and may be associated with acute viral infections or occasionally with arterial hypertension. Recurrent attacks, especially if bilateral, raise the possibility of Melkersson's syndrome or very rarely sarcoidosis (Jasper and Denny, 1968). The silent development of facial weakness, first on one side and then on the other, occurs especially in meningeal leukaemia or pontine glioma.

Bilateral facial weakness in the newborn may result from bilateral nuclear agenesis (Möbius' syndrome), usually together with bilateral lateral rectus palsy. Several of the congenital myopathies mentioned earlier may include prominent facial weakness, especially centronuclear myopathy, nemaline myopathy, minicore disease and less often mitochondrial myopathy, central core disease and fibre-type disproportion. Myasthenia gravis must be ruled out. Congenital myotonic dystrophy causes very prominent facial diplegia with a triangular open mouth together with hypotonia and feeding difficulties, and Brooke (1977, p. 114) has pointed out that an infantile form of facioscapulohumeral dystrophy exists in which difficulty in closing the mouth to suck or inability to smile or to close the eyes may be a first symptom. In both of these diseases, examination of the parents gives the essential clue to the diagnosis. Congenital facial weakness, more often unilateral or asymmetrical than otherwise, may be a feature of SMA with the later development of limb muscle weakness. Infantile SMA (Werdnig-Hoffmann disease) certainly affects the face, but rarely profoundly. In Fazio-Londe's disease (Gomez, Clermont and Bernstein, 1962) progressive bulbar paralysis may be accompanied by facial weakness and eventually by paralysis of all the cranial muscles, including those of the eyes. Some cases, but not all, have signs of SMA also. Cranial polyneuritis and meningeal lymphoma or leukaemia must be excluded before this rare disease can justifiably be diagnosed.

Apart from rare cases of congenital or post-infectious lesions of the Xth and XIIth cranial nerves, isolated paralyses are uncommon. A unilateral XIIth nerve lesion may be seen in the Arnold Chiari malformation. Bulbar paralysis may occur in meningeal and medullary neoplasm. Bulbar paralysis in the neonate, in association with more generalised hypotonia or paralysis, suggests myasthenia, Werdnig-Hoffmann disease or congenital myotonic dystrophy, but may also occur in nemaline and centronuclear myopathy, in fibre-type disproportion and in the Prader-Willi syndrome. Later in childhood bulbar paralysis as an important feature of a generalised muscular problem should bring to mind myasthenia or the Guillain-Barré syndrome or, if the pace is slower, polymyositis, myotonic dystrophy, nemaline myopathy or centronuclear myopathy.

External ocular palsies are not uncommon in the newborn period, and must be distinguished from Duane's syndrome and from more extensive external ophthalmoplegia. The congenital neuromuscular disorders most often associated with ophthalmoplegia are myasthenia gravis and centronuclear myopathy, but it may occur in minicore disease. The later development of ophthalmoplegia may result from the same dis-

orders but is also a major feature of the Kearns-Sayre syndrome and rarely of other variants of mitochondrial myopathy and of Fazio-Londe disease. None of these should be diagnosed without considering the possibility of a brain stem lesion or of myasthenia gravis.

Peripheral motor neuropathy in childhood

The distinction between a predominantly motor neuropathy in a child and the very similar distal form of SMA and, even rarer, the distal type of muscular dystrophy, can really be made only on the basis of electrophysiological and histological investigations. Some cases of mitochondrial myopathy also present with distal weakness and, in the facioscapulohumeral and scapuloperoneal syndromes, the distal lower limb involvement may be sufficiently predominant in the early stages to cause confusion.

No attempt will be made here to cover all of the peripheral neuropathies of childhood (see Gamstorp, 1968) and a systematic account will be found in Chapter 21. Diphtheria is now a rare disease and so is acrodynia (Pink disease), since the elimination of mercury from teething powders. Lead poisoning causes an encephalopathy rather than a polyneuropathy in childhood. Certain insecticides and drugs may produce peripheral neuropathy (Watters and Barlow, 1967). In clinical practice the Guillain-Barré syndrome and Charcot-Marie-Tooth disease (hereditary motor and sensory neuropathy type I—HMSN I) are seen far more frequently than other types. The former has been mentioned above in relation to acute muscular weakness.

HMSN I. 'Peroneal muscular atrophy' often begins in childhood and in some cases as early as the first year of life. The foot deformity usually causes more disability than the weakness itself at first, and responds well to orthopaedic treatment. Weakness of the hands may become a serious problem during the school years. Diagnosis is straightforward on the basis of profound slowing of nerve conduction. It is a common experience to find subclinical involvement in one parent and it is important to seek this by clinical and, if necessary, neurophysiological examination for genetic counselling purposes.

HMSN II. The axonal form of 'peroneal muscular atrophy' is also seen but much less frequently in childhood, and both sporadic cases (possibly recessive) and more often dominant inheritance occur. The onset is usually a little later than in HMSN I, but the clinical problems are similar.

HMSN III. Dejerine-Sottas disease is a rare but very disabling disorder, usually producing symptoms in the first two years of life, rarely later. Hypertrophic nerves (also seen in HMSN I), a high CSF protein, and early and severe weakness and deformity are the helpful diagnostic features. Scoliosis is common.

Giant axonal neuropathy. Cases of this rare disorder are described by Asbury, Gale, Cox, Baringer and Berg (1972) and Carpenter, Karpati, Andermann and Gold (1974). A progressive peripheral motor and sensory neuropathy of axonal type begins at the age of 2–3 years and progresses to become severe within a few years. Both children in the above reports were intelligent with abnormal kinky blond hair. Nerve biopsy showed remarkable segmental enlargement of axons, distended with neurofilaments.

Congenital peripheral neuropathies. Charcot-Marie-Tooth disease (HMSN I) may present at birth in rare instances (Vanasse and Dubowitz, 1979). One variant of congenital peripheral neuropathy resembles Werdnig-Hoffmann disease in presenting with severe hypotonia and areflexia in early infancy, but with profound slowing of nerve conduction, a raised CSF protein level and virtually total absence of myelin sheaths in the peripheral nerve and hypertrophic reduplication of the basement membrane (Lyon, 1969; Anderson, Dennett, Hopkins and Shield, 1973; Kasman and Bernstein, 1974; Karch and Urich, 1975; Goebel, Zeman and DeMeyer, 1976; Kennedy, Sung and Berry, 1977). Both parents of one child had slight slowing of nerve conduction (Kennedy *et al.*, 1977). Joosten, Gabreëls, Gabreels-Festen, Vrensen, Korten and Noter-

mans (1974) described two sibs aged 12 and 14 years in whom the symptoms had started in the second or third year of life and had progressed much more in one than the other, but whose nerve pathology was similar to that in the Lyon type. This disorder may be fatal in infancy but most of the cases described have survived at least into their second decade.

A much milder form of congenital peripheral neuropathy was described by Yuill and Lynch (1974) and was inherited as a dominant trait, but there was no information about histology and only one case had nerve conduction studies.

Other genetically determined peripheral neuropathies seen in childhood include Refsum's disease, and several others in which the clinical features of the neuropathy are largely sensory rather than motor (including Friedrich's ataxia, Fabry's disease, Tangier disease, A-β-lipoproteinaemia and the various disorders classified as hereditary sensory neuropathies). A peripheral neuropathy of a clinically significant degree of severity may also occur in some of the progressive degenerative disorders of the central nervous system, particularly in metachromatic leucodystrophy, infantile neuroaxonal dystrophy and Cockayne's syndrome, while a subclinical neuropathy, of no significance to the patient but helpful in diagnosis, may be found by nerve conduction studies in Krabbe's globoid cell leucodystrophy (Moosa, 1971) and in Canavan's disease.

In the commonest infantile form of metachromatic leucodystrophy, deterioration of gait and speech begin at about the age of 1 year and thereafter are progressive over several months to a state of severe retardation with a spastic tetraparesis and optic atrophy. The tendon reflexes are diminished soon after the onset, and severe distal wasting occurs in the late stages. However, in some cases the disorder presents later, usually with cerebral symptoms but occasionally with a progressive demyelinating peripheral neuropathy (Yudell, Gomez, Lambert and Dockerty, 1967). In all forms of the disease the CSF protein level is raised, metachromatic staining may be seen in the nerve biopsy and the underlying deficiency of the enzyme aryl-sulphatase A may be demonstrated in white blood cells.

In infantile neuroaxonal dystrophy, progressive mental retardation and optic atrophy in the first year of life are sometimes associated with severe hypotonia and muscle paralysis resembling that of SMA (Huttenlocher and Gilles, 1967). The diagnosis is difficult without a brain biopsy but can be achieved in at least some cases by the biopsy of peripheral nerve or even by examination of the nerve twigs in a conjunctival biopsy (Arsénio-Nunes and Goutières, 1978).

In Cockayne's dwarfism, progressive growth failure and dementia starting in the first five years of life are associated with a characteristic light-sensitive rash, deep-set eyes and a peripheral neuropathy (Moosa and Dubowitz, 1970). Other features are intracranial calcification and a mild retinal pigmentary degeneration.

Cramps and abnormal muscle contraction

Cramp, although less frequent in childhood than in later life, is no better understood. Limb pains are a common stress symptom in children. Of the overt muscle disorders, patients with the myotonic and, for some reason, the Becker type of muscular dystrophy are most often plagued by cramps. Stiffness on exertion, sometimes amounting to cramp, is a feature of the early stages of McArdle's disease, phosphofructokinase deficiency and carnitine palmityl transferase deficiency. In persistent cases of exertional or post-exertional cramp it is therefore appropriate to do an ischaemic lactate test and to measure the serum CK activity after exercise performed during a fast (see Ch. 18). The urine should also be examined for myoglobin. Painless stiffness of the muscles after exertion may also occur in a variant of central core disease (Bethlem et al., 1966). An unpleasant 'burning, stiffness and aching but not cramping' of the muscle during exertion in two male cousins, one aged 14 years, was traced by Hogan, Lo, Powers and DiMauro (1978) to a deficiency of muscle adenylate deaminase. Both boys had husky voices. Of five other cases of monoadenylate deaminase deficiency reported by Fishbein, Armbrustmacher and Griffin (1978) at least two had symptoms dating from childhood, but the symptoms varied widely from cramps to fatigability, muscle weakness and hypotonia. The muscle biopsies were generally normal on microscopy but the serum CK activity was increased in three of the five cases. Brody (1969) described a single case in which muscle contracture induced by exercise appeared to result from a defect in muscle relaxing factor.

Dystonia and tetany must be considered as possible causes of persistent cramping of muscle during activity. Rigidity, equal in degree to that seen in tetanus, has already been mentioned as one of the presentations of reducing-body myopathy (Dudley et al., 1978) and of a myopathy with trilaminar fibres (Ringel et al., 1978).

The myotonic disorders occurring in childhood are discussed in Chapter 14.

Myokymia with impaired muscular relaxation (also called 'neuromyotonia' and 'continuous muscle fibre activity') is a slowly progressive disorder, which usually begins between the ages of 5–15 years and gives rise to muscular stiffness and cramps (Gardner-Medwin and Walton, 1969). The distal muscles of the feet and hands are mainly affected, but disabling laryngeal spasm occurs in some cases. Claw-like deformities of the feet are common; there may be associated hyperhidrosis and close inspection of the muscles, especially the small hand muscles, reveals irregular undulating contractions which have been likened to a 'bag of worms'. The EMG shows continuous motor unit activity at rest and the activity can be blocked by curare but not by peripheral nerve blockade. Some cases show evidence of a mild peripheral neuropathy; it is not certain whether this is a secondary phenomenon. The condition responds to treatment with carbamazepine or, less certainly, phenytoin. Similar activity occurs in chondrodystrophic myotonia (see Ch. 14).

Myoglobinuria in childhood

Children, like adults, may develop myoglobinuria as a result of crush injury or intoxication (see Ch. 18 and 25).

Paroxysmal myoglobinuria occurring after exertion is a rare phenomenon in childhood. McArdle's disease, though causing stiffness on exertion in some cases during the first decade of life, does not cause myoglobinuria so early. Phosphofructokinase deficiency may do so. Several of the reported cases of carnitine palmityl transferase deficiency have first developed the typical post-exertional cramps and myoglobinuria during childhood. A few cases occur in which these clinical symptoms in childhood are associated with no detectable evidence of glycogen- or lipid-storage myopathy and, no doubt, other comparable metabolic disorders remain to be discovered.

Paroxysmal myoglobinuria occurring without exertion is a much more devastating illness because it results from acute necrosis of muscle (rhabdomyolysis). It tends to follow viral infection in childhood and may happen as early as the first few months of life. Acute muscle weakness and respiratory failure may be complicated by renal failure and may be fatal. Coxsackie virus infections seem to be one of the important precipitants and in some cases evidence may be found of a direct fulminating viral myositis (Fukuyama, Ando and Yokota, 1977). In other cases, attacks may be precipitated by cold (Raifman, Berant and Lenarsky, 1978). Recurrent attacks may affect several sibs in a family (Favara, Vawter, Wagner, Kevy and Porter, 1967; Savage, Forbes and Pearce, 1971). Intensive respiratory care and often renal dialysis are vital in the treatment of this dangerous disorder. Studies of the HLA system would be of interest but do not appear to have been reported yet.

Malignant hyperpyrexia, like acute rhabdomyolysis, may cause sufficient myoglobinuria to induce uraemia in those patients who survive the initial emergency.

Rarely, recurrent myoglobunuria may accompany a progressive myopathy comparable with muscular dystrophy. Meyer-Betz (1910) described this situation in a boy of 13 years and Dubowitz (1978—p. 48) illustrates the case of a boy of 7 years with cramps and myoglobinuria associated with a chronic 'dystrophic' myopathy.

REFERENCES

Adams, R.D., Kakulas, B.A. and Samaha, F.A. (1965). A myopathy with cellular inclusions. *Transactions of the American Neurological Association*, **90**, 213–216.

Afifi, A.K., Smith, J.W. and Zellweger, H. (1965). Congenital non-progressive myopathy: Central core disease and nemaline myopathy in one family. *Neurology (Minneapolis)*, **15**, 371.

Anderson, R.M., Dennett, X., Hopkins, I.J. and Shield, L.K. (1973). Hypertrophic interstitial polyneuropathy in infancy: Clinical and pathologic features in two cases. *Journal of Pediatrics*, **82**, 619–624.

Armstrong, R.M., Koenigsberger, R., Mellinger, J. and Lovelace, R.E. (1971). Central core disease with congenital hip dislocation: study of two families. *Neurology (Minneapolis)*, **21**, 369–376.

Arsénio-Nunes, M.L. and Goutières, F. (1978). Diagnosis of infantile neuroaxonal dystrophy by conjunctival biopsy. *Journal of Neurology, Neurosurgery and Psychiatry*, **41**, 511–515.

Asbury, A.K., Gale, M.K., Cox, S.C., Baringer, J.R. and Berg, B.O. (1972). Giant axonal neuropathy—A unique case with segmental neurofilamentous masses. *Acta Neuropathologica (Berlin)*, **20**, 237–247.

Atkins, L., Sceery, R.T. and Keenan, M.E. (1966). An unstable ring chromosome in a female infant with hypotonia, seizures and retarded development. *Journal of Medical Genetics*, **3**, 134.

Banker, B.Q., Victor, M. and Adams, R.D. (1957). Arthrogryposis multiplex due to congenital muscular dystrophy. *Brain*, **80**, 319–334.

Bargeton, E., Nezelof, C., Guran, P. and Job, J.-C. (1961). Etude anatomique d'un cas d'arthrogrypose multiple congénitale et familiale. *Revue Neurologique*, **104**, 479–489.

Barth, P.G., van Wijngaarden, G.K. and Bethlem, J. (1975). X-linked myotubular myopathy with fatal neonatal asphyxia. *Neurology (Minneapolis)*, **25**, 531–536.

Bates, T. (1955). Poliomyelitis in pregnancy, fetus and newborn. *American Journal of Diseases of Children*, **90**, 189.

Bazelon, M., Paine, R.S., Cowie, V.A., Hunt, P., Houck, J.C. and Mahanand, D. (1967). Reversal of hypotonia in infants with Down's syndrome by administration of 5-hydroxytryptophan. *Lancet*, **1**, 1130.

Beckerman, R.C. and Buchino, J.J. (1978). Arthrogryposis multiplex congenita as part of an inherited symptom complex: two case reports and a review of the literature. *Pediatrics*, **61**, 417–422.

Bender, A.N. and Bender, M.B. (1977). Muscle fiber hypotrophy with intact neuromuscular junctions: A study of a patient with congenital neuromuscular disease and ophthalmoplegia. *Neurology (Minneapolis)*, **27**, 206–212.

Besser, M. and Behar, A. (1967). Arthrogryposis accompanying congenital spinal-type muscular atrophy. *Archives of Disease in Childhood*, **42**, 666.

Bethlem, J. and van Wijngaarden, G.K. (1976). Benign myopathy, with autosomal dominant inheritance: A report on three pedigrees. *Brain*, **99**, 91–100.

Bethlem, J., Meijer, A.E.F.H., Schellens, J.P.M. and Vroom, J.J. (1968). Centronuclear myopathy. *European Neurology*, **1**, 325.

Bethlem, J., van Gool, J., Hülsmann, W.C. and Meijer, A.E.F.H. (1966). Familial non-progressive myopathy with muscle cramps after exercise. A new disease associated with cores in the muscle fibres. *Brain*, **89**, 569.

Bethlem, J., van Wijngaarden, G.K., Meijer, A.E.F.H. and Hülsmann, W.C. (1969). Neuromuscular disease with type I fiber atrophy, central nuclei, and myotube-like structures. *Neurology (Minneapolis)*, **19**, 705.

Bethlem, J., van Wijngaarden, G.K., Mumenthaler, M. and Meijer, A.E.F.H. (1970). Centronuclear myopathy with Type I fiber atrophy and 'myotubes'. *Archives of Neurology*, **23**, 70–73.

Bharucha, E.P., Pandya, S.S. and Dastur, D.K. (1972). Arthrogryposis multiplex congenita. Part I. Clinical and electromyographic aspects. *Journal of Neurology, Neurosurgery and Psychiatry*, **35**, 425–434.

Bill, P.L.A., Cole, G. and Proctor, N.S.F. (1979). Centronuclear myopathy. *Journal of Neurology, Neurosurgery and Psychiatry*, **42**, 548–556.

Blass, J.P., Kark, R.A.P. and Engel, W.K. (1971). Clinical studies of a patient with pyruvate decarboxylase deficiency. *Archives of Neurology*, **25**, 449–460.

Boder, E. and Sedgwick, R.P. (1958). Ataxia telangiectasia. *Pediatrics*, **21**, 526.

Bonnette, H., Roelofs, R. and Olson, W.H. (1974). Multicore disease: report of a case with onset in middle age. *Neurology (Minneapolis)*, **24**, 1039–1044.

Bradley, W.G., Price, D.L. and Watanabe, C.K. (1970). Familial centronuclear myopathy. *Journal of Neurology, Neurosurgery and Psychiatry*, **33**, 687–693.

Bradley, W.G., Tomlinson, B.E. and Hardy, M. (1978). Further studies of mitochondrial and lipid storage myopathies. *Journal of the Neurological Sciences*, **35**, 201–210.

Bradley, W.G., Hudgson, P., Gardner-Medwin, D. and Walton, J.N. (1973). The syndrome of myosclerosis. *Journal of Neurology, Neurosurgery and Psychiatry*, **36**, 651–660.

Brandt, S. (1947). A case of arthrogryposis multiplex congenita. *Acta Paediatrica*, **34**, 365.

Brody, I.A. (1969). Muscle contracture induced by exercise: A syndrome attributable to decreased relaxing factor. *New England Journal of Medicine*, **281**, 187.

Brooke, M.H. (1973). Congenital fiber type disproportion. In *Clinical Studies in Myology*, Ed. B.A. Kakulas, part 2, pp. 147–159 (Excerpta Medica: Amsterdam).

Brooke, M.H. (1977). *A Clinician's View of Neuromuscular Disease* (Williams and Wilkins: Baltimore).

Brooke, M.H. and Engel, W.K. (1969). The histographic analysis of human muscle biopsies with regard to fiber types: 4. Children's biopsies. *Neurology (Minneapolis)*, **19**, 591–605.

Brooke, M.H. and Neville, H.E. (1972). Reducing body myopathy. *Neurology (Minneapolis)*, **22**, 829.

Brooke, M.H., Carroll, J.E. and Ringel, S.P. (1979). Congenital hypotonia revisited. *Muscle & Nerve*, **2**, 84–100.

Brunette, M.G., Delvin, E., Hazel, B. and Scriver, C.R. (1972). Thiamine-responsive lactic acidosis in a patient with deficient low-KM pyruvate carboxylase activity in liver. *Pediatrics*, **50**, 702–711.

Bryant, G.M., Davies, K.J. and Newcombe, R.G. (1979). Standardisation of the Denver developmental screening test for Cardiff children. *Developmental Medicine and Child Neurology*, **21**, 353–364.

Buda, F.B., Rothney, W.B. and Rabe, E.F. (1972). Hypotonia and the maternal-child relationship. *American Journal of Diseases of Children*, **124**, 906.

Bundey, S. (1972). A genetic study of infantile and juvenile myasthenia gravis. *Journal of Neurology, Neurosurgery and Psychiatry*, **35**, 41.

Byers, R.K. (1975). Spinal-cord injuries during birth. *Developmental Medicine and Child Neurology*, **17**, 103–110.

Campbell, M.J., Rebeiz, J.J. and Walton, J.N. (1969). Myotubular, centronuclear or peri-centronuclear myopathy? *Journal of the Neurological Sciences*, **8**, 425–443.

Cancilla, P.A., Kalyanaraman, K., Verity, M.A., Munsat, T. and Pearson, C.M. (1971). Familial myopathy with probable lysis of myofibrils in type I fibers. *Neurology (Minneapolis)*, **21**, 579–585.

Carpenter, S., Karpati, G., Andermann, F. and Gold, R. (1974). Giant axonal neuropathy: A clinically and morphologically distinct neurological disease. *Archives of Neurology*, **31**, 312–316.

Carter, C. and Sweetnam, R. (1960). Recurrent dislocation of the patella and of the shoulder: Their association with familial joint laxity. *Journal of Bone and Joint Surgery*, **42B**, 721–727.

Charles, B.M., Hosking, G., Green, A., Pollitt, R., Bartlett, K. and Taitz, L.S. (1979). Biotin-responsive alopecia and developmental regression. *Lancet*, **2**, 118–120.

Clara, R. and Lowenthal, A. (1966). Familial and congenital lysine-cystinuria with benign myopathy and dwarfism. *Journal of the Neurological Sciences*, **3**, 433.

Coërs, C. (1952). Vital staining of muscle biopsies with methylene blue. *Journal of Neurology, Neurosurgery and Psychiatry*, **15**, 211.

Coërs, C. and Pelc, S. (1954). Un cas d'amyotonie congénitale caractérisé par une anomalie histologique et histochimique de la junction neuromusculaire. *Acta neurologica belgica*, **54**, 166.

Cohen, M.E., Duffner, P.K. and Heffner, R. (1978). Central core disease in one of identical twins. *Journal of Neurology, Neurosurgery and Psychiatry*, **41**, 659–663.

Coleman, R.F., Nienhuis, A.W., Brown, W.J., Munsat, T.L. and Pearson, C.M. (1967). New myopathy with mitochondrial enzyme hyperactivity. *Journal of the American Medical Association*, **199**, 624–630.

Coleman, R.F., Thompson, L.R., Nienhuis, A.W., Munsat, T.L. and Pearson, C.M. (1968). Histochemical investigation of 'myotubular' myopathy. *Archives of Pathology*, **86**, 365–376.

Conen, P.E., Murphy, E.G. and Donohue, W.L. (1963). Light and electron microscopic studies of 'myogranules' in a child with hypotonia and muscle weakness. *Canadian Medical Association Journal*, **89**, 983–986.

Crosby, T.W. and Chou, S.M. (1974). 'Ragged-red' fibers in Leigh's disease. *Neurology (Minneapolis)*, **24**, 49–54.

Crothers, B. (1923). Injury of the spinal cord in breech extractions as an important cause of foetal death and paraplegia in childhood. *American Journal of Medical Science*, **165**, 94.

Crothers, B. and Putnam, M.C. (1927). Obstetrical injuries of the spinal cord. *Medicine (Baltimore)*, **6**, 41.

Cruz Martinez, A., Ferrer, M.T., López-Terradas, J.M., Pascual-Castroviejo, I. and Mingo, P. (1979). Single fibre electromyography in central core disease. *Journal of Neurology, Neurosurgery and Psychiatry*, **42**, 662–667.

Curless, R.G., Nelson, M.B. and Brimmer, F. (1978). Histological patterns of muscle in infants with developmental brain abnormalities. *Developmental Medicine and Child Neurology*, **20**, 159–166.

Curless, R.G., Payne, C.M. and Brinner, F.M. (1978). Fingerprint body myopathy: a report of twins. *Developmental Medicine and Child Neurology*, **20**, 793–798.

Currie, S., Noronha, M. and Harriman, D. (1974). 'Minicore' Disease. In *Abstracts of the IIIrd International Congress on Muscle Diseases*, Ed. W.G. Bradley, p. 12.

(Excerpta Medica: Amsterdam.)

Daentl, D.L., Berg, B.O., Layzer, R.B. and Epstein, C.J. (1974). A new familial arthrogryposis without weakness. *Neurology (Minneapolis)*, **24**, 55–60.

D'Agostino, A.N., Ziter, F.A., Rallison, M.L. and Bray, P.F. (1968). Familial myopathy with abnormal muscle mitochondria. *Archives of Neurology*, **18**, 388–401.

Dahl, D.S. and Klutzow, F.W. (1974). Congenital rod disease: Further evidence of innervational abnormalities as the basis for the clinico-pathologic features. *Journal of the Neurological Sciences*, **23**, 371–385.

Danta, G. (1975). Electrophysiological study of amyotrophy associated with acute asthma (asthmatic amyotrophy). *Journal of Neurology, Neurosurgery and Psychiatry*, **38**, 1016–1021.

Dastur, D.K., Razzak, Z.A. and Bharucha, E.P. (1972). Arthrogryposis multiplex congenita: Part 2: Muscle pathology and pathogenesis. *Journal of Neurology, Neurosurgery and Psychiatry*, **35**, 435–450.

Denborough, M.A., Dennett, X. and Anderson, R.M. (1973). Central-core disease and malignant hyperpyrexia. *British Medical Journal*, **1**, 272–273.

Der Kaloustian, V.M., Afifi, A.K. and Mire, J. (1972). The myopathic variety of arthrogryposis multiplex congenita: A disorder with autosomal recessive inheritance. *Journal of Pediatrics*, **81**, 76.

Desmond, M.M., Franklin, R.R., Valebona, C., Hill, R.M., Plumb, R., Arnold, H. and Watts, J. (1963). The clinical behaviour of the newly born. *Journal of Pediatrics*, **62**, 307.

DiMauro, S., Mendell, R., Sahenk, Z., Bachman, D. and Scarpa, A. (1978). Fatal infantile mitochondrial myopathy due to lack of cytochrome-c-oxidase. In *Abstracts of the IVth International Congress on Neuromuscular Diseases* (Montreal).

DiMauro, S., Schotland, D.L., Bonilla, E., Lee, C.-P., Gambetti, P. and Rowland, L.P. (1973). Progressive ophthalmoplegia, glycogen storage and abnormal mitochondria. *Archives of Neurology*, **29**, 170–179.

DiMauro, S., Bonilla, E., Lee, C.P., Schotland, D.L., Scarpa, A., Conn, H. and Chance, B. (1976). Luft's disease; further biochemical and ultrastructural studies of skeletal muscle in the second case. *Journal of the Neurological Sciences*, **27**, 217–232.

Dodge, P.R. (1960). Neuromuscular disorders. *Research Publications of the Association for Research into Nervous and Mental Disease*, **38**, 497.

Drachman, D.B. and Banker, B.Q. (1963). Arthrogryposis multiplex congenita: Case due to disease of the anterior horn cells. *Archives of Neurology*, **8**, 77–93.

Dubowitz, V. (1967). A syndrome of benign congenital hypotonia, gross obesity, delayed intellectual development, retarded bone age, and unusual facies. *Proceedings of the Royal Society of Medicine*, **60**, 1006.

Dubowitz, V. (1969). *The Floppy Infant* (Spastics International Medical Publications and William Heinemann Medical Books, Ltd.: London).

Dubowitz, V. (1973). Rigid spine syndrome: A muscle syndrome in search of a name. *Proceedings of the Royal Society of Medicine*, **66**, 219–220.

Dubowitz, V. (1978). *Muscle Disorders in Childhood* (Saunders: London).

Dubowitz, V. and Brooke, M.H. (1973). *Muscle Biopsy: A Modern Approach* (Saunders: London).

Dubowitz, V. and Platts, M. (1965). Central core disease of

muscle with focal wasting. *Journal of Neurology, Neurosurgery and Psychiatry*, **28**, 432–437.

Dubrovsky, A.L., Taratuto, A.L. and Martino, R. (1978). Type II hypotrophy and ophthalmoplegia: Another congenital neuromuscular disease? In *Abstracts of the IVth International Congress on Neuromuscular Diseases* (Montreal).

Dudley, A.W., Dudley, M.A., Varakis, J.M. and Blackburn, W.R. (1978). Progressive tetany and reducing bodies in a neonate: A new myopathy. In *Abstracts of the IVth International Congress on Neuromuscular Diseases* (Montreal).

Dunn, H.G., Daube, J.R. and Gomez, M.R. (1978). Heredofamilial brachial plexus neuropathy (hereditary neuralgic amyotrophy with brachial predilection) in childhood. *Developmental Medicine and Child Neurology*, **20**, 28–46.

Dunn, H.G., Ford, J.K., Anersperg, N. and Miller, J.R. (1961). Benign congenital hypotonia with chromosomal anomaly. *Pediatrics*, **28**, 578.

Dyken, M., Zeman, W. and Rusche, T. (1969). Hypokalemic periodic paralysis: Children with permanent myopathic weakness. *Neurology (Minneapolis)*, **19**, 691–699.

Eberle, E., Brinke, J., Azen, S. and White, D. (1975). Early predictors of incomplete recovery in children with Guillain-Barré polyneuritis. *Journal of Pediatrics*, **86**, 356–359.

Ek, J.I. (1958). Cerebral lesions in arthrogryposis multiplex congenita. *Acta Paediatrica Scandinavica*, **47**, 302–316.

Emery, A.E.H. (1971). The nosology of the spinal muscular atrophies. *Journal of Medical Genetics*, **8**, 481–495.

Engel, A.G., Angelini, C. and Gomez, M.R. (1972). Fingerprint body myopathy. *Mayo Clinic Proceedings*, **47**, 377.

Engel, A.G., Gomez, M.R. and Groover, R.V. (1971). Multicore disease: a recently recognised congenital myopathy associated with multifocal degeneration of muscle fibers. *Mayo Clinic Proceedings*, **10**, 666–681.

Engel, W.K., Gold, G.N. and Karpati, G. (1968). Type I fiber hypotrophy and central nuclei. *Archives of Neurology*, **18**, 435–444.

Fardeau, M., Tomé, F.M.S. and Derambure, S. (1976). Familial fingerprint body myopathy. *Archives of Neurology*, **33**, 724–725.

Fardeau, M., Harpey, J.-P., Caille, B. and Lafourcade, J. (1975). Hypotonies neo-natales avec disproportion congenitale des differents types de fibre musculaire, et petitesse relative des fibres de type 1: Demonstration du caractere familial de cette nouvelle entite. *Archives Françaises de Pédiatrie*, **32**, 901–914.

Favara, B.E., Vawter, G.F., Wagner, R., Kevy, S. and Porter, E.G. (1967). Familial paroxysmal rhabdomyolysis in children: A myoglobinuric syndrome. *American Journal of Medicine*, **42**, 196–207.

Fenichel, G.M. (1967). Abnormalities of skeletal muscle maturation in brain damaged children. A histochemical study. *Developmental Medicine and Child Neurology*, **9**, 419.

Fenichel, G.M. and Bazelon, M. (1966). Myopathies in search of a name: Benign congenital forms. *Developmental Medicine and Child Neurology*, **8**, 532–538.

Fishbein, W.N., Armbrustmacher, V.W. and Griffin, J.L. (1978). Monoadenylate deaminase deficiency: A new disease of muscle. *Science*, **200**, 545–548.

Fisher, R.L., Johnstone, W.T., Fisher, W.H. and Goldkamp,

O.G. (1970). Arthrogryposis multiplex congenita: A clinical investigation. *Journal of Pediatrics*, **76**, 255–261.

Ford, F.R. (1966). *Diseases of the Nervous System in Infancy, Childhood and Adolescence*. 5th Edn. (Charles C. Thomas: Springfield, Ill.).

Fowler, M. (1959). A case of arthrogryposis multiplex congenita with lesions in the nervous system. *Archives of Disease in Childhood*, **34**, 505–510.

Frankenburg, W.K. and Dodds, J.B. (1967). The Denver Developmental screening test. *Journal of Pediatrics*, **71**, 181.

French, J.H., Sherard, E.S., Lubell, H., Brotz, M. and Moore, C.L. (1972). Trichopoliodystrophy: 1. Report of a case and biochemical studies. *Archives of Neurology*, **26**, 229–244.

Friedlander, H.L., Westin, G.W. and Wood, W.L. (1968). Arthrogryposis multiplex congenita. A review of 45 cases. *Journal of Bone and Joint Surgery*, **50A**, 89.

Frischknecht, W., Bianchi, L. and Pilleri, G. (1960). Familial arthrogryposis complex congenita. Neuroarthromyodysplasia congenita. *Helvetica Paediatrica Acta*, **15**, 259.

Fukuyama, Y., Ando, T. and Yokota, J. (1977). Acute fulminant myoglobinuric polymyositis with picornavirus-like crystals. *Journal of Neurology, Neurosurgery and Psychiatry*, **40**, 775–781.

Furukawa, T. and Toyokura, Y. (1977). Congenital, hypotonic-sclerotic muscular dystrophy. *Journal of Medical Genetics*, **14**, 426–429.

Gadoth, N., Margalit, D. and Shapira, Y. (1978). Myopathy with multiple central cores: A case with hypersensitivity to pyrexia. *Neuropädiatrie*, **9**, 239–244.

Gamstorp, I. (1968). Polyneuropathy in childhood. *Acta Paediatrica Scandinavica*, **57**, 230.

Gamstorp, I., Hauge, M., Helweg-Larsen, H.F., Mjönes, H. and Sagild, U. (1957). Adynamia episodica hereditaria: A disease clinically resembling familial periodic paralysis but characterised by increasing serum potassium during the paralytic attacks. *American Journal of Medicine*, **23**, 385–390.

Gardner-Medwin, D. (1977). Children with genetic muscular disorders. *British Journal of Hospital Medicine*, **17**, 314–340.

Gardner-Medwin, D. and Walton, J.N. (1969). Myokymia with impaired muscular relaxation. *Lancet*, **1**, 127–130.

Gardner-Medwin, D., Dale, G. and Parkin, J.M. (1975). Lactic acidosis with mitochondrial myopathy and recurrent coma. In *Abstracts of the First International Congress of Child Neurology* (Toronto), p. 47.

Geiger, L.R., Mancall, E.L., Penn, A.S. and Tucker, S.H. (1974). Familial neuralgic amyotrophy: Report of three families with review of the literature. *Brain*, **97**, 97–102.

Gil-Peralta, A., Rafel, E., Bautista, J. and Alberca, R. (1978). Myotonia in centronuclear myopathy. *Journal of Neurology, Neurosurgery and Psychiatry*, **41**, 1102–1108.

Goebel, H.H., Zeman, W. and DeMyer, W. (1976). Peripheral motor and sensory neuropathy of early childhood, simulating Werdnig-Hoffmann disease. *Neuropädiatrie*, **7**, 182–195.

Goebel, H.H., Lenard, H.G., Görke, W. and Kunze, K. (1977). Fibre type disproportion in the rigid spine syndrome. *Neuropädiatrie*, **8**, 467–477.

Gomez, M.R., Clermont, V. and Bernstein, J. (1962). Progressive bulbar paralysis in childhood (Fazio-Londe's disease): Report of a case with pathologic evidence of nuclear atrophy. *Archives of Neurology*, **6**, 317–323.

Gonatas, N.K., Shy, G.M. and Godfrey, E.H. (1966). Nemaline myopathy: The origin of nemaline structures. *New England Journal of Medicine*, **274**, 535–539.

Gordon, A.S., Rewcastle, N.B., Humphrey, J.G. and Stewart, B.M. (1974). Chronic benign congenital myopathy: finger print body type. *Canadian Journal of Neurological Sciences*, **1**, 106–113.

Goto, I., Nagasaka, S., Nagara, H. and Kuroiwa, Y. (1979). Rigid spine syndrome. *Journal of Neurology, Neurosurgery and Psychiatry*, **42**, 276–279.

Hackett, T.N., Bray, P.F., Ziter, F.A., Nyhan, W.L. and Creer, K.M. (1973). A metabolic myopathy associated with chronic lactic acidemia, growth failure and nerve deafness. *Journal of Pediatrics*, **83**, 426–431.

Hamerton, J.L. (1971). In *Human Cytogenetics*, **2**, 278, 356 (Academic Press: New York and London).

Hansen, E. (1962). Ataxia-telangiectasia. *Acta neurologica scandinavica*, **38**, 188.

Hanson, P.A., Mastrianni, A.F. and Post, L. (1977). Neonatal ophthalmoplegia with microfibers: A reversible myopathy? *Neurology (Minneapolis)*, **27**, 974–980.

Harriman, D.G.F. and Haleem, M.A. (1972). Centronuclear myopathy in old age. *Journal of Pathology*, **108**, 237–248.

Hart, Z.H., Chang, C.-H., Perrin, E.V.D., Neerunjun, J.S. and Ayyar, R. (1977). Familial poliodystrophy, mitochondrial myopathy and lactate acidemia. *Archives of Neurology*, **34**, 180–185.

Hausmanowa-Petrusewicz, I. (1978). *Spinal Muscular Atrophy: Infantile and Juvenile Type* (National Science Foundation, Washington, D.C. *and* National Centre for Scientific, Technical and Economic Information, Warsaw, Poland).

Hawkes, C.H. and Absolon, M.J. (1975). Myotubular myopathy associated with cataract and electrical myotonia. *Journal of Neurology, Neurosurgery and Psychiatry*, **38**, 761–764.

Haydar, N.A., Conn, H.L., Afifi, A., Wakid, N., Ballas, S. and Fawaz, K. (1971). Severe hypermetabolism with primary abnormality of skeletal muscle mitochondria: Functional and therapeutic effects of chloramphenicol treatment. *Annals of Internal Medicine*, **74**, 548–558.

Heffernan, L.P., Rewcastle, N.B. and Humphrey, J.G. (1968). The spectrum of rod myopathies. *Archives of Neurology*, **18**, 529–542.

Heffner, R., Cohen, M., Duffner, P. and Daigler, G. (1976). Multicore disease in twins. *Journal of Neurology, Neurosurgery and Psychiatry*, **39**, 602–606.

Hoefnagel, D., Jalberg, E.O., Publow, D.G. and Richtsmeier, A.J. (1978). Progressive fibrosis of the deltoid muscles. *Journal of Pediatrics*, **92**, 79–81.

Hogan, E.L., Lo, H.S., Powers, J.M. and DiMauro, S. (1978). Genetic deficiency of muscle adenylate deaminase. In *Abstracts of the IVth International Congress on Neuromuscular Diseases* (Montreal).

Hopkins, I.J. (1974). A new syndrome: poliomyelitis-like illness associated with acute asthma in childhood. *Australian Paediatric Journal*, **10**, 273–276.

Hopkins, I.J., Lindsey, J.R. and Ford, F.R. (1966). Nemaline myopathy. A long-term clinicopathologic study of affected mother and daughter. *Brain*, **89**, 299.

Howes, E.L., Price, H.M., Pearson, C.M. and Blumberg, J.M. (1966). Hypokalemic periodic paralysis: Electromicroscopic changes in the sarcoplasm. *Neurology (Minneapolis)*, **16**, 242–256.

Hudgson, P., Bradley, W.G. and Jenkison, M. (1972). Familial 'mitochondrial' myopathy: A myopathy associated with disordered oxidative metabolism in muscle fibres. *Journal of the Neurological Sciences*, 16, 343–370.

Hurwitz, L.D., Carson, N.A.J., Allen, I.V. and Chopra, J.S. (1969). Congenital ophthalmoplegia, floppy baby syndrome, myopathy and aminoaciduria. *Journal of Neurology, Neurosurgery and Psychiatry*, 32, 495.

Huttenlocher, P.R. and Gilles, F.H. (1967). Infantile neuroaxonal dystrophy. Clinical, pathologic and histochemical findings in a family with 3 affected siblings. *Neurology (Minneapolis)*, 17, 1174–1184.

Ilett, S.J., Pugh, R.J. and Smithells, R.W. (1977). Poliomyelitis-like illness after acute asthma. *Archives of Disease in Childhood*, 52, 738–740.

Illingworth, R.S. (1972). *The Development of the Infant and Young Child, Normal and Abnormal*, 5th edn. (E. & S. Livingstone: Edinburgh and London).

Ingram, T.T.S. (1955). The early manifestations and course of diplegia in childhood. *Archives of Disease in Childhood*, 30, 244.

Ingram, T.T.S. (1962). Congenital ataxic syndromes in cerebral palsy. *Acta Paediatrica*, 51, 209.

Inokuchi, T., Umezaki, H. and Santa, T. (1975). A case of type I muscle fibre hypotrophy and internal nuclei. *Journal of Neurology, Neurosurgery and Psychiatry*, 38, 475–482.

Isaacs, H., Heffron, J.J.A. and Bandenhorst, M. (1975). Central core disease: A correlated genetic, histochemical, ultramicroscopic and biochemical study. *Journal of Neurology, Neurosurgery and Psychiatry*, 38, 1177–1186.

Jago, R.H. (1970). Arthrogryposis following treatment of maternal tetanus with muscle relaxants. *Archives of Disease in Childhood*, 45, 277–279.

Jasper, P.L. and Denny, F.W. (1968). Sarcoidosis in children: With special emphasis on the natural history and treatment. *Journal of Pediatrics*, 73, 499–512.

Jenis, E.H., Lindquist, R.R. and Lister, R.C. (1969). New congenital myopathy with crystalline intranuclear inclusions. *Archives of Neurology*, 20, 281.

Jerusalem, F., Engel, A.G. and Gomez, M.R. (1973). Sarcotubular myopathy: A newly recognised, benign, congenital familial muscle disease. *Neurology (Minneapolis)*, 23, 897–906.

Jerusalem, F., Angelini, C., Engel, A.G. and Groover, R.V. (1973). Mitochondria-lipid-glycogen (MLG) disease of muscle: A morphologically recessive congenital myopathy. *Archives of Neurology*, 29, 162–169.

Joosten, E., Gabreëls, F., Gabrééls-Festen, A., Vrensen, G., Korten, J. and Notermans, S. (1974). Electron-microscopic heterogeneity of onion-bulb neuropathies of the Déjerine-Sottas type: Two patients in one family with the variant described by Lyon (1969). *Acta Neuropathologica (Berlin)*, 27, 105–118.

Karch, S.B. and Urich, H. (1975). Infantile polyneuropathy with defective myelination: An autopsy study. *Developmental Medicine and Child Neurology*, 17, 504–511.

Karpati, G., Carpenter, S. and Nelson, R.F. (1970). Type I muscle fibre atrophy and central nuclei: A rare familial neuromuscular disease. *Journal of the Neurological Sciences*, 10, 489–500.

Kasman, M. and Bernstein, L. (1974). Chronic progressive polyradiculoneuropathy of infancy. *Neurology (Minneapolis)*, 24, 367.

Keeton, B.R. and Moosa, A. (1976). Organic aciduria: Treatable cause of floppy infant syndrome. *Archives of Disease in Childhood*, 51, 636–638.

Kennedy, W.R., Sung, J.H. and Berry, J.F. (1977). A case of congenital hypomyelination neuropathy: Clinical, morphological and chemical studies. *Archives of Neurology*, 34, 337–345.

Kinoshita, M. and Cadman, T.E. (1968). Myotubular myopathy. *Archives of Neurology*, 18, 265–271.

Kolin, I.S. (1967). Nemaline myopathy. A fatal case. *American Journal of Diseases of Children*, 114, 95.

Krabbe, K.H. (1958). Congenital generalised muscular atrophies. *Acta Psychiatrica*, 33, 94.

Kuitonnen, P., Rapola, J., Noponen, A.L. and Donner, M. (1972). Nemaline myopathy. Report of 4 cases and review of the literature. *Acta Paediatrica Scandinavica*, 61, 353.

Lake, B.D., and Wilson, J. (1975). Zebra body myopathy: Clinical histochemical and ultrastructural studies. *Journal of the Neurological Sciences*, 24, 437–446.

Lapresle, J.M., Fardeau, M. and Godet-Guillain, J. (1972). Myopathie distal congénitale avec hypertrophie des mollets—Présence d'anomalies mitochondriales à la biopsie musculaire. *Journal of the Neurological Sciences*, 17, 87.

Laurence, B.M. (1967). Hypotonia, mental retardation, obesity and cryptorchidism associated with dwarfism and diabetes in children. *Archives of Disease in Childhood*, 42, 126.

Lebenthal, E., Shocket, S.B., Adam, A., Seelenfreund, M., Fried, A., Najenson, T., Sandbank, U. and Matoth, Y. (1970). Arthrogryposis multiplex congenita: Twenty-three cases in an Arab kindred. *Pediatrics*, 46, 891.

Lenard, H.G. and Goebel, H.H. (1975). Congenital fibre type disproportion. *Neuropädiatrie*, 6, 220–231.

Lloyd-Roberts, G.C. and Lettin, A.W.F. (1970). Arthrogryposis multiplex congenita. *Journal of Bone and Joint Surgery*, 52B, 494.

Löwenthal, A. (1954). Un groupe hérédodégénératif nouveau: les myoscléroses hérédofamiliales. *Acta Neurologica et Psychiatrica Belgica*, 54, 155–165.

Lubs, H.A., Koenig, E.U. and Brandt, I.K. (1961). Trisomy 13–15: clinical syndrome. *Lancet*, 2, 1001.

Luft, R., Ikkos, D., Palmieri, G., Ernster, L. and Afzelius, B. (1962). A case of severe hypermetabolism of nonthyroid origin with a defect in the maintenance of mitochondrial respiratory control: a correlated clinical, biochemical and morphological study. *Journal of Clinical Investigation*, 41, 1776–1804.

Lundberg, A. (1979). Dissociated motor development: Developmental patterns, clinical characteristics, causal factors and outcome, with special reference to late walking children. *Neuropädiatrie*, 10, 161–182.

Lyon, G. (1969). Ultrastructural study of a nerve biopsy from a case of early infantile chronic neuropathy. *Acta Neuropathologica (Berlin)*, 13, 131–142.

Mac Keith, R.C., Polani, P.E. and Clayton-Jones, E. (1960). English translation of *The Neurological Examination of the Infant* by André-Thomas, Yves Chesni and S. St. Anne Dargassies (Spastics Society, Heinemann: London).

McKinlay, I.A. and Mitchell, I. (1976). Transient acute myositis in childhood. *Archives of Disease in Childhood*, 51, 135–137.

McKusick, V.A. (1972). *Heritable Disorders of Connective Tissue*, 4th Edn. (C.V. Mosby: St. Louis).

McLeod, J.G., Baker, W. de C., Lethlean, A.K. and Shorey, C.D. (1972). Centronuclear myopathy with autosomal dominant inheritance. *Journal of the Neurological Sciences*, 15, 375–387.

McLeod, J.G., Baker, W. de C., Shorey, C.D. and Kerr, C.B. (1975). Mitochondrial myopathy with multisystem abnormalities and normal ocular movements. *Journal of the Neurological Sciences*, **24**, 39–52.

Mair, W.A.P. (1963). The ultra-structure of muscle in a case of myopathy. In *Research in Muscular Dystrophy*, ed. by members of the Research Committee of the Muscular Dystrophy Group (Pitman Medical: London).

Martin, J.J., Clara, R., Ceuterick, C. and Joris, (1976). Is congenital fibre type disproportion a true myopathy? *Acta Neurologica Belgica*, **76**, 335–344.

Matsuoka, Y., Gubbay, S.S. and Kakulas, B.A. (1974). A new myopathy with type II muscle fibre hypoplasia. *Proceedings of the Australian Association of Neurologists*, **11**, 155–159.

Meyer-Betz, F. (1910). Beobachtungen an einem eigenartigen mit Muskellähmungen verbundenen Fall von Hämoglobinurie. *Deutsches Archiv für klinische Medizin*, **101**, 85.

Meyers, K.R., Golomb, H.M., Hansen, J.L. and McKusick, V.A. (1974). Familial neuromuscular disease with 'myotubes'. *Clinical Genetics*, **5**, 327–337.

Midura, T.F. and Arnon, S.S. (1976). Infant botulism: Identification of Clostridium botulinum and its toxins in faeces. *Lancet*, **2**, 934–936.

Millichap, J.G. and Dodge, P.R. (1960). Diagnosis and treatment of myasthenia gravis in infancy, childhood and adolescence. *Neurology (Minneapolis)*, **10**, 1007.

Moosa, A. (1971). Peripheral neuropathy and ichthyosis in Krabbe's leucodystrophy. *Archives of Disease in Childhood*, **46**, 112.

Moosa, A. and Dubowitz, V. (1970). Peripheral neuropathy in Cockayne's syndrome. *Archives of Disease in Childhood*, **45**, 674–677.

Morgan-Hughes, J.A., Brett, E.M., Lake, B.D. and Tomé, F.M.S. (1973). Central core disease or not? Observations on a family with non-progressive myopathy. *Brain*, **96**, 527–536.

Morgan-Hughes, J.A. Darveniza, P., Kahn, S.N., Landon, D.N., Sherratt, R.M., Land, J.M. and Clark, J.B. (1977). A mitochondrial myopathy characterized by a deficiency in reducible cytochrome b. *Brain*, **100**, 617–640.

Neligan, G. and Prudham, D. (1969). Norms for four standard developmental milestones by sex, social class and place in family. *Developmental Medicine and Child Neurology*, **11**, 413–422.

Norman, M.G., Temple, A.R. and Murphy, J.V. (1970). Infantile quadriceps-femoris contracture resulting from intramuscular injections. *New England Journal of Medicine*, **282**, 964–966.

Oberklaid, F. and Hopkins, I.J. (1976). 'Juvenile' myasthenia gravis in early infancy. *Archives of Disease in Childhood*, **51**, 719–721.

Ortiz de Zarate, J.C. and Maruffo, A. (1970). The descending ocular myopathy of early childhood. Myotubular or centronuclear myopathy. *European Neurology*, **3**, 1.

Osserman, K.E. (1958). *Myasthenia Gravis*. (Grune & Stratton: New York and London.)

Paine, R.S. (1961). The early diagnosis of cerebral palsy. *Rhode Island Medical Journal*, **44**, 522.

Paine, R.S. (1963). The future of the 'floppy infant'. A follow-up study of 133 patients. *Developmental Medicine and Child Neurology*, **5**, 115.

Partington, M.W., MacDonald, M.R.A. and Tu, J.B. (1971). 5-Hydroxytryptophan (5-HTP) in Down's syndrome.

Developmental Medicine and Child Neurology, **13**, 362.

Paulson, G.W. (1970). The Landry-Guillain-Barré syndrome and childhood. *Developmental Medicine and Child Neurology*, **12**, 604.

Pearn, J.H. (1974). The use of motor milestones to determine retrospectively the clinical onset of disease. *Australian Paediatric Journal*, **10**, 147–153.

Pearn, J.H., Bundey, S., Carter, C.O., Wilson, J., Gardner-Medwin, D. and Walton, J.N. (1978). A genetic study of subacute and chronic spinal muscular atrophy in childhood. *Journal of the Neurological Sciences*, **37**, 227–248.

Pearson, C.M. (1964). The periodic paralyses. Differential features and pathology in permanent myopathic weakness. *Brain*, **87**, 341.

Pearson, C.M. and Fowler, W.G. (1963). Hereditary non-progressive muscular dystrophy inducing arthrogryposis syndrome. *Brain*, **86**, 75.

Peña, C.E., Miller, F., Budzilovich, G.B. and Feigen, I. (1968). Arthrogryposis multiplex congenita. *Neurology (Minneapolis)*, **18**, 926.

Peterman, A.F., Daly, D.D., Dion, F.R. and Keith, H.M. (1959). Infectious neuronitis (Guillain-Barré syndrome) in children. *Neurology (Minneapolis)*, **9**, 533–539.

Pickett, J., Berg, B., Chaplin, E. and Brunstetter-Shafer, M.-A. (1976). Syndrome of botulism in infancy: Clinical and electrophysiologic study. *New England Journal of Medicine*, **295**, 770–772.

Polani, P.E. (1959). The natural clinical history of choreoathetoid cerebral palsy. *Guy's Hospital Reports*, **108**, 32.

Poskanzer, D.C. and Kerr, D.N.S. (1961). A third type of periodic paralysis, with normokalemia and favourable response to sodium chloride. *American Journal of Medicine*, **31**, 328–342.

Prader, A., Labhaft, A. and Willi, H. (1956). Ein Syndrome von Adipositas, Kryptorchismus und Oligophrenic nach myatonieartigen Zustand im Neugeborenalter. *Schweizerische medizinische Wochenschrift*, **86**, 1260.

Pugh, R.C.B. and Dudgeon, J.A. (1954). Fatal neonatal poliomyelitis. *Archives of Disease in Childhood*, **29**, 381.

Raifman, M.A., Berant, M. and Lenarsky, C. (1978). Cold weather and rhabdomyolysis. *Journal of Pediatrics*, **93**, 970–971.

Rawles, J.M. and Weller, R.O. (1974). Familial association of metabolic myopathy, lactic acidosis and sideroblastic anemia. *American Journal of Medicine*, **56**, 891–897.

Ringel, S.P., Neville, H.E., Duster, M.C. and Carroll, J.E. (1978). A new congenital neuromuscular disease with trilaminar muscle fibers. *Neurology (Minneapolis)*, **28**, 282–289.

Rondot, P., Dalloz, J.-C. and Tardieu, G. (1958). Mesure de la force des réactions musculaires a l'étirement passif aux cours des raideurs pathologiques par lésions cérébrales. *Revue francaise d'études cliniques et biologiques*, **3**, 585.

Rosner, F., Ong, B.H., Paine, R.S. and Mahanand, D. (1965). Blood-serotonin activity in trisomic and translocation Down's syndrome. *Lancet*, **1**, 1191.

Rowland, L.P. and Eskenazi, A.N. (1956). Myasthenia gravis with features resembling muscular dystrophy. *Neurology (Minneapolis)*, **6**, 667.

Sahgal, V. and Sahgal, S. (1977). A new congenital myopathy: A morphological cytochemical and histochemical study. *Acta Neuropathologica (Berlin)*, **37**, 225–230.

Salmon, M.A., Esiri, M.M. and Ruderman, N.B. (1971). Myopathic disorder associated with mitochondrial abnormalities, hyperglycaemia and hyperketonaemia. *Lancet*, **2**, 290–293.

Sandbank, U. and Lerman, P. (1972). Progressive cerebral poliodystrophy—Alpers' disease: Disorganised giant neuronal mitochondria on electron microscopy. *Journal of Neurology, Neurosurgery and Psychiatry*, **35**, 749–755.

Savage, D.C.L., Forbes, M. and Pearce, G.W. (1971). Idiopathic rhabdomyolysis. *Archives of Disease in Childhood*, **46**, 594–604.

Schotland, D.L., DiMauro, S., Bonilla, E., Scarpa, A. and Lee, C.-P. (1976). Neuromuscular disorder associated with a defect in mitochondrial energy supply. *Archives of Neurology*, **33**, 475–479.

Seay, A.R., Ziter, F.A. and Petajan, J.H. (1977). Rigid spine syndrome: A type 1 fiber myopathy. *Archives of Neurology*, **34**, 119–122.

Sengers, R.C.A., Stadhouders, A.M., Jaspar, H.H.J., Trijbels, J.M.F. and Daniels, O. (1976). Cardiomyopathy and short stature associated with mitochondrial and/or lipid storage myopathy of skeletal muscle. *Neuropädiatrie*, **7**, 196–208.

Sengers, R.C.A., ter Haar, B.G.A., Trijbels, J.M.F., Willems, J.L., Daniels, O. and Stadhouders, A.M. (1975). Congenital cataract and mitochondrial myopathy of skeletal and heart muscle associated with lactic acidosis after exercise. *Journal of Pediatrics*, **86**, 873–880.

Shafiq, S.A., Dubowitz, V., Peterson, H. de C. and Milhorat, A.T. (1967). Nemaline myopathy: Report of a fatal case, with histochemical and electron microscopic studies. *Brain*, **90**, 817–828.

Shafiq, S.A., Sande, M.A., Carruthers, R.R., Killip, T. and Milhorat, A.T. (1972). Skeletal muscle in idiopathic cardiomyopathy. *Journal of the Neurological Sciences*, **15**, 303–320.

Shapira, Y., Cederbaum, S.D., Cancilla, P.A., Nielsen, D. and Lippe, B.M. (1975). Familial poliodystrophy, mitochondrial myopathy and lactate acidemia. *Neurology (Minneapolis)*, **25**, 614–621.

Sher, J.H., Rimalovski, A.B., Athanassiades, T.J. and Aronson, S.M. (1967). Familial myotubular myopathy: a clinical, pathological, histochemical and ultrastructural study. *Journal of Neuropathology and Experimental Neurology*, **26**, 132.

Shy, G.M., Gonatas, N.K. and Perez, M. (1966). Childhood myopathies with abnormal mitochondria. I. Megaconial myopathy. II. Pleoconial myopathy. *Brain*, **89**, 133.

Shy, G.M., Engel, W.K., Somers, J.E. and Wanko, T. (1963). Nemaline myopathy: a new congenital myopathy. *Brain*, **86**, 793.

Shy, G.M. and Magee, K.R. (1956). A new congenital non-progressive myopathy. *Brain*, **79**, 610.

Smith, D.W. (1970). *Recognisable Patterns of Human Malformation*, p. 36 (Saunders: Philadelphia, London, Toronto).

Spiro, A.J., Prineas, J.W. and Moore, C.L. (1970). A new mitochondrial myopathy in a patient with salt craving. *Archives of Neurology*, **22**, 259–269.

Spiro, A.J., Shy, G.M. and Gonatas, N.K. (1966). Myotubular myopathy—persistence of fetal muscle in an adolescent boy. *Archives of Neurology*, **14**, 1–14.

Spiro, A.J., Moore, C.L., Prineas, J.W., Strasberg, P.M. and Rapin I. (1970). A cytochrome-related inherited disorder of the nervous system and muscle. *Archives of Neurology*, **23**, 103–112.

Taratuto, A.L., Sfaello, Z.M., Rezzonico, C. and Morales, R.C. (1978). Multicore disease: Report of a case with lack of fibre type differentiation. *Neuropädiatrie*, **9**, 285–297.

Tarlow, M.J., Lake, B.D. and Lloyd, J.K. (1973). Chronic lactic acidosis in association with myopathy. *Archives of Disease in Childhood*, **48**, 489–492.

Taylor, A.I. (1968). Autosomal trisomy syndromes: a detailed study of 27 cases of Edward's syndrome and 27 cases of Patau's syndrome. *Journal of Medical Genetics*, **5**, 227.

Telerman-Toppet, N., Gerard, J.M. and Coërs, C. (1973). Central core disease: A study of clinically unaffected muscle. *Journal of the Neurological Sciences*, **19**, 207–223.

Thomas, P.K. (1979). Chronic relapsing idiopathic inflammatory polyneuropathy. *Neuropädiatrie*, **10** (Suppl.), 452–453.

Thomas, P.K., Calne, D.B. and Elliott, C.F. (1972). X-linked scapuloperoneal syndrome. *Journal of Neurology, Neurosurgery and Psychiatry*, **35**, 208–215.

Tizard, J.P.M. (1949). Osteogenesis imperfecta presenting with delay in walking. *Proceedings of the Royal Society of Medicine*, **42**, 80.

Tomé, R.M.S. and Fardeau, M. (1975). Congenital myopathy with 'reducing bodies' in muscle fibres. *Acta Neuropathologica (Berlin)*, **31**, 207–217.

Touwen, B. (1976). *Neurological development in infancy* (Heinemann: London).

Towbin, A. (1969). Latent spinal cord and brain stem injury in newborn infants. *Developmental Medicine and Child Neurology*, **11**, 54.

Tsairis, P., Engel, W.K. and Kark, P. (1973). Familial myoclonic epilepsy syndrome associated with skeletal muscle mitochondrial abnormalities. *Neurology (Minneapolis)*, **23**, 408.

Turner, H.D., Brett, E.M., Gilbert, R.J., Ghosh, A.C. and Liebeschuetz, H.J. (1978). Infant botulism in England, *Lancet*, **1**, 1277–1278.

Turner, J.W.A. and Lees, F. (1962). Congenital myopathy—a fifty-year follow-up. *Brain*, **85**, 733–739.

van Biervliet, J.P.G.M., Bruinvis, L., Ketting, D., de Bree, P.K., van der Heiden, C., Wadman, S.K., Willems, J.L., Brookelman, H., van Haelst, U. and Monnens, L.A.H. (1977). Hereditary mitochondrial myopathy with lactic acidemia, a DeToni-Fanconi-Debré syndrome and a defective respiratory chain in voluntary striated muscles. *Paediatric Research*, **11**, 1088–1093.

van Wijngaarden, G.K., Bethlem, J., Meijer, A.E.F.H., Hülsmann, W.C. and Feltkamp, C.A. (1967). Skeletal muscle disease with abnormal mitochondria. *Brain*, **90**, 577.

van Winjgaarden, G.K., Fleury, P., Bethlem, J. and Meijer, A.E.F.H. (1969). Familial 'myotubular' myopathy. *Neurology (Minneapolis)*, **19**, 901.

Vanasse, M. and Dubowitz, V. (1979). Hereditary motor and sensory neuropathy type I in infancy and childhood: A clinical, electro-diagnostic, genetic and muscle biopsy study. *Neuropädiatrie*, **10** (Suppl.), 454–455.

Verhiest, W., Brucher, J.M., Goddeeris, P., Lauweryns, J. and de Geest, H. (1976). Familial centronuclear myopathy associated with 'cardiomyopathy'. *British Heart Journal*, **38**, 504–509.

Vital, C., Vallat, J.-M., Martin, F., LeBlanc, M. and Bergouignan, M. (1970). Étude clinique et ultrastructurale d'un cas de myopathie centronucléaire (myotubular myopathy) de l'adulte. *Revue Neurologique*, **123**, 117–130.

Walker, B.A., Beighton, P.H. and Murdoch, J.L. (1969). The marfanoid hypermobility syndrome. *Annals of Internal Medicine*, **71**, 349–352.

Walton, J.N. (1956). Amyotonia congenita: a follow-up study. *Lancet*, **1**, 1023–1028.

Walton, J.N. (1957). The limp child. *Journal of Neurology, Neurosurgery and Psychiatry*, **20**, 144–154.

Walton, J.N., Geschwind, N. and Simpson, J.A. (1956). Benign congenital myopathy with myasthenic features. *Journal of Neurology, Neurosurgery and Psychiatry*, **19**, 224.

Watters, G.V. and Barlow, C.F. (1967). Acute and subacute neuropathies. *Pediatric Clinics of North America*, **14**, 997.

Woolf, A.L. (1960). Muscle biopsy in the diagnosis of the 'floppy baby': infantile hypotonia. *Cerebral Palsy Bulletin*, **2**, 19.

Woolf, A.L. (1963). Changes in the terminal motor innervation in cases of neuromuscular disease. In *Research in Muscular Dystrophy*, ed. by members of the Research Committee of the Muscular Dystrophy Group (Pitman Medical: London).

Woolf, A.L. and Till, K. (1955). The pathology of the lower motor neuron in the light of new muscle biopsy techniques. *Proceedings of the Royal Society of Medicine*, **48**, 189.

Worster-Drought, C., White, J.C. and Sargent, F. (1953). Familial, idiopathic methaemoglobinaemia associated with mental deficiency and neurological abnormalities. *British Medical Journal*, **2**, 114.

Wynne-Davies, R. and Lloyd-Roberts, G.C. (1976). Arthrogryposis multiplex congenita: Search for prenatal factors in 66 sporadic cases. *Archives of Disease in Childhood*, **51**, 618–623.

Yamaguchi, M., Robson, R.M., Stromer, M.H., Dahl, D.S. and Oda, T. (1978). Actin filaments form the backbone of nemaline myopathy rods. *Nature*, **271**, 265–267.

Yudell, A., Gomez, M.R., Lambert, E.H. and Dockerty, M.B. (1967). The neuropathy of sulfatide lipidosis (metachromatic leukodystrophy). *Neurology (Minneapolis)*, **17**, 103.

Yuill, G.M. and Lynch, P.G. (1974). Congenital non-progressive peripheral neuropathy with arthrogryposis multiplex. *Journal of Neurology, Neurosurgery and Psychiatry*, **37**, 316–323.

Zellweger, H. and Schneider, H.J. (1968). Syndrome of hypotonia—hypomentia—hypogonadism—obesity (HHHO) or Prader-Willi syndrome. *American Journal of Diseases of Children*, **115**, 588.

Metabolic and endocrine myopathies

METABOLIC DISEASES OF MUSCLE

The periodic paralyses

It is convenient to classify the periodic paralyses as primary or secondary and, according to associated changes in the serum K level, as hypokalaemic, normokalaemic or hyperkalaemic. The different types of periodic paralysis share several common features. The paralytic attacks may last from less than one hour to several days. Weakness can be localised or generalised. The deep tendon reflexes are diminished or lost in the course of the attacks. The muscle fibres become unresponsive to either direct or indirect electrical stimulation during the attacks. The generalised attacks usually begin in proximal muscles and then spread to distal ones. Respiratory and cranial muscles tend to be spared but eventually may also become paralysed. Rest after a period of exercise tends to provoke weakness of the muscles that had been exercised, but continued mild exercise may abort the attacks. Exposure to cold may provoke weakness in the primary forms of the disease. Complete recovery usually occurs after initial attacks. Permanent weakness and irreversible pathological changes in muscle can develop after repeated attacks of the primary forms of the disease.

Primary hypokalaemic periodic paralysis. The disease is transmitted by an autosomal dominant gene with reduced penetrance in women. Sporadic cases, especially in men, have also been reported (Talbott, 1941; Sagild, 1959). The attacks typically begin in the first or second decade of life and approximately 60 per cent of the patients are affected before the age of 16 years. Initially the attacks tend to be infrequent, but eventually they may recur daily. Diurnal fluctuations in strength may then appear, so that the patient shows the greatest weakness during the night or in the early hours of the morning and gradually gains strength as the day passes (Allott and McArdle, 1938; Engel, Lambert, Rosevear and Tauxe, 1965). In major attacks the serum potassium level decreases, but not always to below the normal level, and there is urinary retention of sodium, potassium, chloride and water (Biemond and Daniels, 1934; Aitken, Allott, Castelden and Walker, 1937; Allott and McArdle, 1938; Ferrebee, Atchley and Loeb, 1938). Oliguria or anuria develop during such attacks and the patients tend to be constipated. Sinus bradycardia and electrocardiographic signs of hypokalaemia (U waves in leads II, V-2, V-3, and V-4, progressive flattening of T waves and depression of ST segment) appear when the serum potassium falls below normal levels (Van Buchem, 1957; Weisler, 1961). In the fourth and fifth decades of life the attacks become less frequent and may cease altogether. However, the repeated attacks may leave the patient with permanent residual weakness (Bekeny, 1961; Pearson, 1964; Engel *et al.*, 1965; Howes, Price and Blumberg, 1966; Odor, Patel and Pearce, 1967). The metabolic defect of this type of disease can be exacerbated or provoked by a high dietary intake of sodium or carbohydrate and by emotional excitement (Aitken *et al.*, 1937; Ferrebee *et al.*, 1938; Talbott, 1941; McArdle, 1956; Rowley and Kliman, 1960; Shy, Wanko, Rowley and Engel, 1961; Engel *et al.*, 1965).

The diagnosis is supported by a positive family history and a low serum potassium level during major attacks. Depressed serum potassium levels between attacks suggest secondary rather than primary hypokalaemic paralysis. Provocative tests can be done to confirm the diagnosis. The oral administration of glucose, 2 g/kg body weight, combined with 10–20 units of crystalline insulin given subcutaneously may provoke an attack within 2–3 h. If this test fails to induce an attack in adults, it may be repeated after exercise and salt loading (2 g sodium chloride in aqueous solution given orally every hour for a total of four doses). Depression of the serum potassium level during the induced attack and a favourable response to 2.5–7.5 g of potassium chloride given orally must be demonstrated. Negative results do not exclude the diagnosis because patients may, at times, be refractory to such tests (Chen, 1959). Glucose and insulin must never be given to patients already hypokalaemic and potassium must not be given to patients unless they have an adequate renal and adrenal reserve. The intra-arterial epinephrine test is particularly useful in the diagnosis of primary hypokalaemic periodic paralysis (Engel *et al.*, 1965). Two μg/min of epinephrine is infused into the brachial artery for 5 min and the amplitude of the evoked compound muscle action potential is recorded from perfused small hand muscles at intervals before, during and for 30 min after the period of infusion. The test, which is positive when the amplitude of the evoked action potential decreases by more than 30 per cent within 10 min after the infusion, is essentially specific for primary hypokalaemic period paralysis.

Thyrotoxic periodic paralysis. This type resembles the primary hypokalaemic form of the disease in regard to changes in serum and urinary electrolytes during attacks and in its response to glucose, insulin and potassium. However, it is six times more common in males than in females, approximately 75 per cent of the cases occur in Orientals, 85 per cent of the patients first exhibit the attacks between the ages of 20 and 39 years, 95 per cent of the cases are sporadic, and in all cases the attacks cease when the euthyroid state is restored (Engel, 1961). Natural or induced recurrence of the hypermetabolic state causes recurrence of the paralytic attacks (Dunlap and Kepler, 1931; Robertson, 1954; Okihiro and Nordyke, 1966).

Hypokalaemic periodic paralysis secondary to urinary or gastrointestinal potassium wastage. Potassium depletion may be associated with generalised weakness or, less frequently, with periodic paralysis. The latter usually does not occur unless the serum potassium level is less than 3 mmol/l. During the attack the potassium decreases further (Owen and Verner, 1960; River, Kushner, Armstrong, Dubin, Sodki and Cutting, 1960; Staffurth, 1964). The relationship of the attacks to excessive ingestion of carbohydrate or sodium has not been clearly established. The diagnosis of excessive urinary potassium loss may be made if, with an average daily intake of sodium or potassium, the daily urinary potassium excretion exceeds 20 mmol on several consecutive days while the serum potassium remains less than 3 mmol/l at different times of the day (Mahler and Stanbury, 1956; Brooks, McSwiney, Prunty and Wood, 1957). The normal daily faecal potassium excretion is usually small (10 mmol) (Danowsky and Greenman, 1953). Because the serum potassium level is already decreased, provocative tests that may further lower it are contra-indicated.

Various conditions that should be considered in the differential diagnosis are listed in Table 18.1. In addition to periodic or non-periodic weakness, the non-specific effects of chronic potassium depletion may also be present. These include hyposthenuria, polydypsia, and vasopressin-resistant polyuria (Conn, 1955; Dustan, Corcoran and Page, 1956; Milne, Muehrcke and Heard, 1957; Manitius, Levitin, Beck and Epstein, 1960). Chronic pyelonephritis and secondary hypertension leading to secondary aldosteronism and further potassium depletion may develop (Owen and Verner, 1960; Caroll and Davies, 1964). Latent or manifest tetany can occur in several types of potassium depletion (Engel, Martin and

Table 18.1 Differential diagnosis of secondary hypokalaemic periodic paralysis

Paralysis secondary to urinary potassium wastage
Hypertension, alkaline urine, metabolic alkalosis
    Primary hyperaldosteronism (Conn, 1955)
    Liquorice intoxication (Salassa, Mattox and Rosevear, 1962)
    Excessive thiazide therapy for hypertension (Cohen, 1959)
    Excessive mineralocorticoid therapy of Addison's disease
Normotension, alkaline urine, metabolic alkalosis
    Hyperplasia of juxtaglomerular apparatus with hyperaldosteronism (Bryan, MacCardle and Bartter, 1966)
Alkaline urine, metabolic acidosis
    Primary renal tubular acidosis (Owen and Verner, 1960)
    Fanconi's syndrome (Milne, Stanbury and Thomson, 1952)
Acid urine, metabolic acidosis
    Chronic ammonium chloride ingestion (Goulon, Rapin, Lissac, Pocidolo and Mantel, 1962)
    Recovery phase of diabetic coma (Nabarro, Spencer and Stowers, 1952)
    Bilateral ureterocolostomy (Sataline and Simonelli, 1961)
    Recovery phase of acute renal tubular necrosis (Bull, Joekes and Lowe, 1950)

Paralysis secondary to gastrointestinal potassium wastage

Nontropical sprue
Laxative abuse (Schwartz and Relman, 1953)
Pancreatic gastrin-secreting adenoma with severe diarrhoea (Verner and Morrison, 1958)
Villous adenoma of the rectum (Keyloun and Grace, 1967)
Severe or chronic diarrhoea (Keye, 1952)
Draining gastrointestinal fistula
Prolonged gastrointestinal intubation or vomiting
Barium carbonate poisoning (Lewi and Bar-Khayim, 1964)

Taylor, 1949; Fourman, 1954; Conn, 1955; Owen and Verner, 1960; Caroll and Davies, 1964). Growth retardation and proportional dwarfism occur in patients whose potassium has been depleted since infancy (Van Buchem, Doorenbos and Elings, 1956; Caroll and Davies, 1964; Bryan, MacCardle and Bartter, 1966).

Primary hyperkalaemic periodic paralysis. The disease is transmitted by an autosomal dominant gene with high penetrance in both sexes (Helweg-Larsen, Hauge and Sagild, 1955; Gamstorp, 1956; McArdle, 1962; Layzer, Lovelace and Rowland, 1967). Rare sporadic cases have been reported (Dyken and Timmons, 1963). Attacks usually commence in childhood and may be brief or last several days (Layzer *et al.*, 1967). Myalgias

(McArdle, 1962), release of enzymes from muscle into serum and creatinuria (Mertens, Schimrigk, Volkwein and Voigt, 1964; Hudson, Strickland and Wilensky, 1967) can occur during or after paralysis and a permanent myopathy may develop after repeated attacks (French and Kilpatrick, 1957; Hudson, 1963; MacDonald, Rewcastle and Humphrey, 1968). During the attacks the serum potassium increases (French and Kilpatrick, 1957; Egan and Klein, 1959; Van Der Meulen, Gilbert and Kane, 1961; McArdle, 1962; Gamstorp, 1956; Samaha, 1965; Hudson *et al.*, 1967; Layzer, Lovelace and Rowland, 1967) but may not exceed the normal range, and precordial T waves in the electrocardiogram increase in amplitude (French and Kilpatrick, 1957; Egan and Klein, 1959). Potassium, water and possibly sodium diuresis occurs during major attacks and the patient may complain of urinary urgency (Gamstorp, 1956; Egan and Klein, 1959; Klein, Egan and Usher, 1960; Carson and Pearson, 1964; Mertens *et al.*, 1964). Hypocalcaemia during the paralysed state was found in three patients but their urinary calcium excretion was not studied (Dyken and Timmons, 1963; Layzer, Lovelace and Rowland, 1967). The metabolic defect is worsened by exposure to cold, fasting, pregnancy or by potassium administration (Gamstorp, 1956; Drager, Hammill and Shy, 1958; McArdle, 1962; Van't Hoff, 1962; Herman and McDowell, 1963; Hudson, 1963; Layzer, Lovelace and Rowland, 1967).

Myotonic phenomena have been demonstrated in some patients and are especially prone to be present in levator palpebrae and other external ocular muscles and in facial, lingual, thenar and finger extensor muscles (French and Kilpatrick, 1957; Drager *et al.*, 1958; McArdle, 1962; Van't Hoff, 1962; Hudson, 1963; Carson and Pearson, 1964; Layzer, Lovelace and Rowland, 1967). However, no myotonia was found in some patients who had all other typical features of primary hyperkalaemic periodic paralysis (Gamstorp, 1956, 1963), although there was abnormal electrical irritability of the muscle fibres (Buchthal, Engbaek and Gamstorp, 1958). A positive Chvostek sign is frequently observed in attacks (Gamstorp, 1956).

Myotonic hyperkalaemic periodic paralysis and paramyotonia congenita appear to be very similar, if not identical, disorders. The hallmarks of paramyotonia congenita, as described by Eulenburg (1886) and by Rich (1894) were: (1) dominant inheritance with high penetrance; (2) myotonia provoked especially by exposure to cold; (3) predilection of the myotonia for facial, lingual, neck and hand muscles; and (4) attacks of weakness upon exposure to cold and also after exercise. Subsequently, some patients with features of paramyotonia congenita were also found to fulfil the diagnostic criteria of primary hyperkalaemic periodic paralysis, suggesting that the two disorders were, in fact, a single nosologic entity (French and Kilpatrick, 1957; Drager et al., 1958; Van der Meulen, Gilbert and Kane, 1961). However, as mentioned above, even careful electromyographic search disclosed no myotonia in some cases of hyperkalaemic periodic paralysis. Further, in some patients diagnosed as having paramyotonia congenita, potassium loading did not provoke paralytic attacks (Marshall, 1952; Gamstorp, 1963; Garcin, Legrain, Rondot and Fardeau, 1966). Accentuation rather than improvement of the myotonia on repeated muscle contraction ('myotonia paradoxa') has also been cited as a distinguishing feature of paramyotonia (Magee, 1963; Garcin et al., 1966).

The diagnosis of primary hyperkalaemic periodic paralysis is based on the family history, myotonic phenomena (if present) and the provocative effects of orally administered potassium chloride (2–10 g, given in an unsweetened solution just after exercise, in the fasting state). The test is contra-indicated in subjects already hyperkalaemic and unless there is adequate renal and adrenal reserve. An abnormally high serum potassium level between attacks suggests secondary rather than primary hyperkalaemic periodic paralysis.

Secondary hyperkalaemic periodic paralysis. This is associated with renal or adrenal insufficiency and may occur when the serum potassium level exceeds 7 mmol/l. Males tend to be affected more often than females. Rest after exercise provokes weakness in the same manner as it does in other types of periodic paralysis (Bull, Carter and Low, 1953; Marks and Feit, 1953; Richardson and Sibley, 1953; Pollen and Wil-

liams, 1960; Faw and Ewer, 1962; Bell, Hayes and Vosburgh, 1965; Daughaday and Rendleman, 1967). Paraesthesiae in the distal extremities tend to occur when the serum potassium level exceeds 7.5 mmol/l. Electrocardiographic abnormalities (T wave elevation, disappearance of P waves and, eventually, a sinusoidal tracing) evolve as the serum potassium level rises from 7 mmol/l to 9.5 mmol/l (Keith, Osterberg and Burchell, 1942; Finch, Sawyer and Flynn, 1946; Pollen and Williams, 1960). The diagnosis is suggested by the very high serum potassium level during the attack, persistent hyperkalaemia between attacks and by the associated primary disorder.

Normokalaemic, sodium-responsive familial periodic paralysis. A third type of primary periodic paralysis was described by Poskanzer and Kerr (1961). The disease is transmitted by dominant inheritance with high penetrance in both sexes. Paralytic attacks began during the first decade of life and were exacerbated or provoked by rest after exercise, exposure to cold, alcohol in excess and by potassium loading. Large doses of sodium improved the weakness. Glucose administration had no effect on the disease. No consistent changes of serum electrolytes occurred during the attacks but there was increased sodium excretion and potassium retention during the attacks. Another family, described by Meyers, Gilden, Rinaldi and Hansen (1972), suffered from a similar illness but attacks were not provoked by large doses of potassium.

Histopathological alterations in periodic paralysis. The histopathological hallmark of the syndrome is a vacuolar myopathy (Goldflam, 1895). This can be observed in either primary or secondary periodic paralysis, but more commonly in the former than in the latter. The vacuolation is more consistently associated with the permanent myopathy which develops after repeated attacks, than with the acute paralysis (Klein et al., 1960; McArdle, 1963; Samaha, 1965; Resnick and Engel, 1967; Engel, 1977). The vacuoles are typically centrally situated in the fibres and usually one vacuole, but at times multiple vacuoles, appear in a fibre in a single plane of sectioning. Some of the vacuoles are limited by a delicate membrane, some are loculated, and some contain finely granular material which stains positively for glycogen.

Numerous ultrastructural studies in the primary and thyrotoxic periodic paralyses can be summarised as follows. Dilatation and proliferation of sarcoplasmic reticulum (SR) components and abundant networks of transverse tubular (T) system origin have been observed in the muscle fibres (Shy et al., 1961; Howes et al., 1966; Engel, 1966a; Gruner, 1966; Odor et al., 1967; MacDonald et al., 1968; Schutta and Armitage, 1969; Bergman, Afifi, Dunkle and Johns, 1970). The larger and light-microscopically visible vacuoles were thought to arise by coalescence of dilated SR components (Shy et al., 1961; Odor et al., 1967), from fusion of T system networks (Biczyskowa, Fidzianska and Jedrzejowska, 1969), or to be the end-result of focal fibre destruction (MacDonald et al., 1968; Schutta and Armitage, 1969). In view of these divergent results, Engel (1970a) re-examined the morphological sequence of fibre vacuolation in primary hypokalemic periodic paralysis. The steps identified were: (1) evolving vacuole; (2) intermediate-stage vacuole; (3) mature vacuole; and (4) remodelling. Abnormal fibre regions arise containing myriad dilated and at times mineralised SR vesicles, masses of bizarre tubules or osmiophilic lamellae of T system origin, or varied cytoplasmic degradation products (evolving vacuole). The T system proliferates and acts as a membrane source for trapping components of the evolving vacuole. These components are degraded by an autophagic mechanism and a membrane-bound space is formed which contains remnants of the trapped organelles which are now embedded in an amorphous matrix (intermediate-stage vacuole). When all trapped components have undergone lysis, the entire vacuole is filled with matrix (mature vacuole). The intermediate-stage and mature vacuoles communicate with the extracellular space via T tubules and T networks and there is prompt ingress of peroxidase-labelled extracellular fluid into the matrix compartment of the vacuoles. Because these vacuoles are the prevalent ones, most of the vacuolar volume is filled with extracellular fluid. Intermediate-stage and mature vacuoles are remodelled by invaginations of the vacuolar membrane by glycogen-containing sarcoplasm. When the invaginated membrane ruptures, extracellular fluid enters the myofilament space and causes fibre injury. Non-vacuolated fibre regions contain numerous focal dilatations of T tubules, T networks and dilated SR vesicles. Subsequent studies also established that the ultrastructural changes in the different types of periodic paralysis are essentially identical, that electrical inexcitability of a muscle fibre can occur without associated ultrastructural change, and that the morphological changes are reactive and represent delayed consequences of the physiological abnormality (Engel, 1977).

Pathophysiological mechanisms in the periodic paralyses. In primary hypokalaemic periodic paralysis there is a shift of potassium, sodium, chloride and phosphate ions and of water into muscle during generalised attacks. The ionic shifts are reflected by decreased urinary excretion of these ions and by decreased serum potassium levels (Aitken et al., 1937; Ferrebee et al., 1938; Zierler and Andres, 1957; Shy et al., 1961; Engel et al., 1965). The fluid and electrolyte movements must be caused by a muscle membrane abnormality or an increased intracellular demand, or both, and probably occur to maintain osmotic, electrical and Donnan equilibria (Boyle and Conway, 1941).

In thyrotoxic periodic paralysis the fluid and electrolyte shifts are similar to those noted in the primary hypokalaemic form of the disease. In other forms of secondary hypokalaemic periodic paralysis the hypokalaemia and body potassium depletion are more marked and episodic paralysis appears when the exchangeable body potassium has fallen to approximately half-normal levels (Staffurth, 1964). The paroxysmal nature of the attacks is unexplained and it is not known whether the ionic shifts during the attacks are the same as in the primary hypokalaemic form of the disease.

In primary hyperkalaemic periodic paralysis the fluid and electrolyte movements are the opposite of those which occur in the primary hypokalaemic type of disease: the hyperkalaemia is associated with enhanced urinary excretion of potassium, sodium and water suggesting egress of water and electrolytes from muscle (Gamstorp, 1956; Klein et al., 1960; Creutzfeldt, 1961; Carson and

Pearson, 1964). Fluid and electrolyte shifts have not been investigated during paroxysmal attacks of secondary hyperkalaemic periodic paralysis.

Abnormalities of carbohydrate metabolism, such as a block in hexose phosphate utilisation (McArdle, 1956) or in glycogen synthesis (Shy et al., 1961) have been postulated to account for the adverse effects of carbohydrate loading in primary hypokalaemic periodic paralysis. Specific biochemical studies by Engel, Potter and Rosevear (1967) did not confirm these hypotheses. From a different viewpoint, the opposite effects of carbohydrate loading in the primary hypokalaemic and hyperkalaemic syndromes could be related to ionic movements associated with cellular glucose uptake and utilization because potassium movements follow the carbohydrate cycle from muscle to liver and back. Such movements could provoke or correct a defect which is not one of carbohydrate metabolism but which resides in the electrical and biophysical properties of the muscle fibre surface membrane.

Several lines of evidence implicate the muscle fibre surface membrane in the pathogenesis of the paralytic attacks. The resting membrane potential is abnormally low during and even between attacks in both the primary hypokalaemic and primary hyperkalaemic syndromes (Creutzfeldt, Abbott, Fowler and Pearson, 1963; Riecker and Bolte, 1966; McComas, Mrozek and Bradley, 1968; Bradley, 1969; Brooks, 1969; Hofmann and Smith, 1970). The membrane potential alterations cannot be simply secondary to changes in the serum potassium level for, if they were, then the membrane should become hyperpolarised in hypokalaemic periodic paralysis. On the basis of the Goldman constant field equation for the membrane potential (Goldman, 1943), the hypopolarisation in the different types of periodic paralysis can be attributed to increased sodium permeability, decreased chloride permeability, or both. A decrease in the resting membrane potential itself can block the action potential mechanism because sodium activation fails below a resting potential of 60 mV, while potassium activation and membrane repolarisation cannot occur below a resting potential of 40 mV (Jenerick, 1959). Resting membrane potentials lower than 60 mV have, in fact, been recorded during paralytic attacks (Creutzfeldt et al., 1963). A lower than normal membrane input resistance, consistent with increased sodium permeability, has also been observed in the primary hypokalaemic disease by Elmqvist, Engel and Lambert (cited by Engel, 1977) and in the primary hyperkalaemic disease by McComas et al. (1968). There are no reports of membrane potential measurements in the secondary types of periodic paralysis.

The fact that paralysed muscle fibres are unresponsive to either direct or indirect electrical stimulation indicates an abnormality of the extra-junctional ion channels and possibly also of the junctional, acetylcholine-induced ion channels. However, involvement of acetylcholine-induced ion channels is unlikely because an electrical potential was recorded from the end-plate region of paralysed muscle by Grob, Johns and Liljestrand (1957) in the primary hypokalaemic disease. Further, Elmqvist et al. (cited by Engel, 1977) recorded normal or larger than normal end-plate potentials from paralysed muscle fibres in primary hypokalaemic and in primary hyperkalaemic periodic paralysis.

These studies implicated the extrajunctional surface membrane of the muscle fibre in the pathogenesis of the attacks, but did not exclude an abnormality of the contractile mechanism. However, Engel and Lambert (1969) found that direct application of calcium to the myofilament space of electrically inexcitable fibres readily activated the contractile mechanism. Further, the duration of the response to varying doses of calcium was not different from that found in normal fibres. This established that the block in excitation-contraction coupling resided in the membranous components of the fibre (the surface membrane, T system, the SR, or all three) but if the SR was involved, the abnormality was one that affected the release and not the uptake of calcium, for paralysed and control fibres relaxed in comparable manners. It is very possible that both the surface membrane and the T tubules fail to conduct the action potential during attacks, but failure of transverse impulse conduction would be relatively unimportant in the presence of an unresponsive surface membrane.

Treatment of periodic paralyses

Primary hypokalaemic periodic paralysis Acute attacks are treated with 2.0–10.0 g of potassium chloride, given by mouth as an unsweetened 10–25 per cent solution. This dose may be repeated, if necessary, after 3–4 h (Talbott, 1941; McArdle, 1963). Intravenous administration of potassium salts is seldom, if ever, required to terminate an acute attack. Utmost care must be exercised in giving potassium intravenously in order to avoid life-threatening hyperkalaemia, and intravenous fluids must contain no glucose or sodium. The patient's strength and serum potassium must be frequently monitored during treatment of major attacks.

Preventive therapy of the primary hypo-kalaemic form of the disease consists of a relatively low sodium (2.3 g per day) and low carbohydrate (60–80 g per day) diet, avoidance of exposure to cold and overexertion, and supplemental doses of potassium chloride, 2.5–7.5 g, as a 10 per cent aqueous solution taken 2–4 times daily. The dosage must be adjusted according to the frequency and severity of the attacks. Because severely affected patients awaken paralysed in the morning, a dose may have to be taken at 2 a.m. The serum potassium level should not exceed 6 mmol/l during therapy. Acetazolamide (Diamox) is also highly effective in preventing paralytic attacks (Griggs, Engel and Resnick, 1970). Up to 2 g per day of the drug can be used instead of the other preventive measures.

Thyrotoxic periodic paralysis. Treatment consists of antithyroid therapy. Until the patient becomes euthyroid, preventive measures and the treatment of the acute attacks are the same as for the primary hypokalaemic form of the disease. Acetazolamide is ineffective, but propranolol (40 mg q.i.d.) may prevent attacks (Yeung and Tse, 1974).

Other forms of secondary hypokalaemic periodic paralysis. Therapy is directed at the primary disorder and potassium is replaced to compensate for both the static deficits and the dynamic losses. Additional treatment is directed against the metabolic acidosis or alkalosis and other associated electrolyte abnormalities that may be present.

Primary sodium-responsive normokalaemic peri-odic paralysis. In the family studied by Poskanzer and Kerr (1961), therapy with large doses of sodium chloride, or with 0.1 mg 9-α-fluorohydrocortisone and 250 mg acetazolamide per day was effective in preventing paralytic attacks.

Primary hyperkalaemic periodic paralysis. Acute attacks in established cases can be treated with 2g/kg glucose by mouth and 15–20 units of crystalline insulin subcutaneously, but severe attacks may fail to respond to these measures (Gamstorp, 1956; Sagild, 1959). Calcium gluconate, 0.5–2 g administered intravenously, has been reported to terminate attacks in some cases (Gamstorp, 1956; Van der Meulen *et al.*, 1961; Van't Hoff, 1962), but not in others (McArdle, 1962). Preventive therapy consists of frequent meals of high carbohydrate content, avoidance of fasting or of exposure to cold and over-exertion, and use of diuretics promoting kaliuresis, such as acetazolamide or chlorothiazide. The lowest dose of diuretic required to prevent attacks should be used and the amount given should not lower the serum potassium level below 3.7 mmol/l or the serum sodium below 135 mmol/l (McArdle, 1962; Carson and Pearson, 1964; Samaha, 1965).

Secondary hyperkalaemic periodic paralysis. Therapy is again aimed at the primary disorder and should include restriction of dietary potassium intake until the primary cause can be corrected. Intravenous insulin and glucose therapy can temporarily decrease the serum potassium level. In patients with renal failure, severe hyperkalaemia is an indication for haemodialysis.

Disorders of muscle energy metabolism

The glycogen storage diseases

The classification adopted is basically that of Cori (1957), but by now considerable genetic hetero-geneity has been observed in each recognised type of glycogenosis. Skeletal muscle is directly involved in types II (acid maltase deficiency), III (debranching enzyme system deficiency), IV (branching enzyme deficiency), V (myophospho-rylase deficiency) and VII (phosphofructokinase deficiency) and indirectly in type I (glucose-6-phosphatase deficiency). There are also other glycogen or polysaccharide storage syndromes of muscle for which no enzymatic basis has been uncovered to date.

Type I glycogenosis (glucose-6-phosphatase deficiency).

The enzyme normally occurs in liver, kidney and small intestine but not in muscle. Deficiency of the enzyme causes no glycogen excess in muscle but profound hypotonia can occur in affected infants. Transmission is by an autosomal recessive gene. The disease appears to be more highly fatal in some families than others, a finding which suggests genetic heterogeneity. This is further supported by the presence of an immunologically detectable but catalytically inactive enzyme protein in some cases but not in others. The metabolic fault prevents the release from liver of glucose derived from glycogenolysis or gluconeogenesis. The consequences of this are severe fasting hypoglycaemia, lactic acidosis and excessive mobilisation of fat from adipose tissue. Chronic lactic acidosis causes osteoporosis and interferes with the renal excretion of uric acid which results in hyperuricaemia and secondary gout. Fat mobilisation leads to marked hyperlipidaemia, fatty infiltration of liver and xanthoma formation. A haemorrhagic tendency occurs in many patients. All manifestations of the disease tend to improve with age (Moses and Gutman, 1972; Huijing, 1975; Howell, 1978).

Type II glycogenosis (acid maltase deficiency).

Acid maltase, a lysosomal enzyme, hydrolyses both 1,4 and 1,6 α-glycosidic linkages. It is optimally active between pH 4 and 5 and is capable of degrading glycogen completely. The enzyme from human liver can be resolved into several active charge isomers by isoelectric focusing, and into active carbohydrate-containing and carbohydrate-free species by gel chromatography (Murray, Brown and Brown, 1978). Although acid maltase deficiency (AMD) was the first lysosomal disorder to be identified (Hers, 1963), the precise metabolic role of the enzyme is still enigmatic. That massive amounts of glycogen, and at times acid mucopolysaccharides, accumulate in cells lacking the enzyme attest to its biological significance, yet severe deficiency of the enzyme can exist in some cells and tissues without glycogen excess or functional impairment. The disease originally described by Pompe (1932) was a generalised glycogenosis invariably fatal in infancy (Sant'Agnese, 1959). Subsequently, milder forms of AMD, presenting as myopathy, have been observed in children (Hers and van Hoof, 1968) and adults (Engel and Dale, 1968; Hudgson, Gardner-Medwin, Worsfold, Pennington and Walton, 1968; Engel, 1970b). All three forms of the disease are transmitted by autosomal recessive inheritance (Williams, 1966; Nitowsky and Grunfeld, 1967; Engel and Gomez, 1970) and, with one exception (Busch, Koster and van Weerden, 1979), the disease breeds true in each family.

Infantile AMD presents within the first few months of life with generalised and rapidly progressive weakness and hypotonia, and enlargement of the heart, tongue and liver. Respiratory and feeding difficulties are common and death is usually due to cardiorespiratory failure before the age of two years. The electrocardiogram typically shows a short P–R interval, high QRS voltage and left ventricular hypertrophy (Sant'Agnese, 1959; Caddell and Whitemore, 1962; Engel, Gomez, Seybold and Lambert, 1973). Massive amounts of glycogen accumulate in skeletal muscle, heart and liver. Microscopic examination also demonstrates widespread deposition of glycogen in smooth muscle, endothelial and renal tubular cells and in both neural and glial elements of the central nervous system. Most cells of the brain and spinal cord are affected but cerebellar cortical nerve cells are spared. Motor neurones in the brain stem and spinal cord are most severely involved (Mancall, Aponte and Berry, 1965; Hogan, Gutmann, Schmidt and Gilbert, 1969). Glycogen also accumulates in Schwann cells in peripheral nerves (Gambetti, Di Mauro and Baker, 1971). In addition to glycogen, acid mucopolysaccharides also accumulate in skeletal muscle (Martin, de Barsy, Van Hoof and Palladini, 1973; Engel et al., 1973). Acid maltase activity is absent from muscle, liver, heart, leucocytes and cultured fibroblasts (Nitowsky and Grunfeld, 1967; Danzis, Hutzler, Lynfield and Cox, 1969; Brown, Brown and Jeffrey, 1970) but not from kidney (Steinitz and Rutenberg, 1967). However, the renal enzyme is probably different from lysosomal acid maltase (Steinitz and Rutenberg, 1967; Salafsky and Nadler, 1971; Koster, Slee, Van Der Klei-Van Moorsel, Rietra and Lucas, 1976; De Burlet and Sudaka, 1977). A sensitive fluorometric assay, which uses an artificial substrate, reveals that there is no residual enzyme activity in affected tissues in infantile AMD (Mehler and DiMauro, 1977). Catalytically inactive enzyme protein could not be detected by immunological techniques in some patients (de Barsy, Jacquemin, Devos and Hers, 1972; Reuser, Koster, Hoogeveen and Galjaard, 1978; Murray et al., 1978), but such a protein was abundantly present in at least one infant (Beratis, LaBadie and Hirschhorn, 1978). This indicates that even infantile AMD, which appears to be clinically homogeneous, is genetically heterogeneous.

The childhood type of AMD presents clinically in infancy or early childhood as a myopathy. Motor milestones are delayed and weakness is usually greater in proximal than distal limb muscles. Respiratory muscles tend to be selectively severely affected. Calf enlargement may also occur resulting in a clinical picture which simulates muscular dystrophy (Hers and van Hoof, 1968; Swaiman, Kennedy and Sauls, 1968; Engel et al., 1973). The disease progresses relatively slowly and death usually occurs through respiratory failure after repeated bouts of pneumonia. Only few patients survive beyond the second decade. Liver, heart or tongue enlargement occur relatively infrequently. Glycogen excess in muscle is less marked and more variable than in infantile AMD. Autopsy studies reveal little if any increase of glycogen in heart, liver, skin and nervous system (Smith, Amick and Sidbury, 1966; Smith, Zellweger and Afifi, 1967; Engel et al., 1973; Martin, de Barsy, de Schrijver, LeRoy and Palladini, 1976). The enzyme is deficient in muscle, heart and liver (Hers and Van Hoof, 1968; Angelini and Engel, 1972; Mehler and Di Mauro, 1977), cultured fibroblasts (Koster, Slee, Hulsmann and Niermeijer, 1972) and inconsistently in leucocytes (Brown and Zellweger, 1966). Residual acid maltase activity is detected in muscle, liver and heart (Angelini and Engel, 1972; Mehler and Di Mauro, 1977).

The adult form of AMD presents after the age of 20. The symptoms can be those of a slowly progressive myopathy which clinically mimics polymyositis or limb-girdle dystrophy (Engel and Dale, 1968; Hudgson et al., 1968; Engel, 1970b; Carrier, Lebel, Mathieu, Pialat and Devic, 1975; Gullotta, Stefan and Mattern, 1976; Martin, de Barsy and den Tandt, 1976; Karpati, Carpenter, Eisen, Aube and Di Mauro, 1977; Di Mauro, Stern, Mehler, Nagle and Payne, 1978; Bertagnolio, Di Donato, Peluchetti, Rimoldi, Storchi and Cornelio, 1978). However, one-third of the cases present with respiratory failure which may overshadow other manifestations of the disease (Rosenow and Engel, 1978). Respiratory muscle involvement eventually occurs in all cases and respiratory failure is the usual cause of death. Heart and liver enlargement does not occur and cardiac manifestations, if present, are those of cor pulmonale which is secondary to the respiratory failure. Glycogen accumulates in clinically affected muscles but seldom exceeds 5 per cent. In some muscles with histological abnormalities the muscle glycogen content is normal. No glycogen excess is found in tissues other than muscle. Acid mucopolysaccharides, which accumulate in muscle in infants and children with AMD, are sparse or absent from muscle in adults with AMD. Deficiency of acid maltase has been noted in muscle (Engel and Dale, 1968; Hudgson et al., 1968), liver (Engel, 1970b; Engel et al., 1973), heart and central nervous system (Di Mauro et al., 1978) as well as in cultured fibroblasts (Angelini, Engel and Titus, 1972) and cultured muscle cells (Askanas, Engel, Di Mauro, Brooks and Mehler, 1976). A lower than normal leucocyte acid maltase level and a depressed acid/neutral maltase ratio were found by Angelini and Engel (1972) and by Koster, Slee and Hulsmann (1974), but not by Bertagnolio et al. (1968). Residual acid maltase activity is detectable in muscle and other tissues (Engel et al., 1973; Mehler and Di Mauro, 1977).

Serum enzymes of muscle origin (creatine kinase, aspartate aminotransferase) are increased in all three types of AMD, but the increases are usually less than ten-fold over the upper limit of normal. Electromyographic findings indicate a myopathy in all three types of AMD. The abnormalities are more widespread in the infants than in the older patients. In children and adults, some muscles show no electrical abnormalities whereas other muscles have motor unit potentials of abnormally short duration as well as of normal duration. Abnormal insertional activity and myotonic discharges (without clinically detectable myotonia) occur in all patients. Other forms of abnormal electrical activity (fibrillation potentials, positive waves and bizarre repetitive discharges) also occur at rest. In adults, the myotonic discharges are less widely distributed and less intense than in the other patients and appear especially in the paraspinal muscles (Engel *et al.*, 1973).

The common light-microscopic feature in all cases of AMD is a vacuolar myopathy. In infants, virtually all muscle fibres contain large vacuoles. In children, the vacuolation tends to be less marked and some muscle fibres or muscles are spared. In adults, almost all fibres in severely affected muscles display vacuoles. In less severely affected muscles the vacuolation involves 25–75 per cent of the fibres whereas clinically unaffected muscles show few, if any, vacuolated fibres. The vacuoles have a high glycogen content and are strongly reactive for acid phosphatase. Abnormal increases of acid phosphatase activity also occur in muscle fibres with no light-microscopically detectable vacuoles.

Ultrastructural studies show that glycogen accumulates in muscle fibres in four types of spaces: 1) dispersed in the sarcoplasm, displacing, replacing or compressing normal organelles; 2) in sac-like structures, limited by continuous or discontinuous single or double membranes; 3) in ordinary autophagic vacuoles, containing glycogen and miscellaneous cytoplasmic degradation products; 4) in spaces representing transitions between the above. The limiting membranes of the vacuoles are generated by proliferating T-system networks and by the Golgi system. Acid hydrolases are delivered to the vacuoles by vesicles arising from T-system networks (Engel, 1970b; Engel *et al.*, 1973). Because many of the vacuoles are membrane-bound and contain acid hydrolases and cytoplasmic degradation products, they represent secondary lysosomes.

Diagnostic clues in AMD consist of organomegaly in infants and children; the firm consistency of the weak muscles; the selectively severe involvement of respiratory muscles, and also of the hip adductor muscles, in some of the adults; the presence of abnormal electrical irritability, including myotonic discharges without clinical myotonia, in the electromyogram; and a vacuolar myopathy with high glycogen content and acid phosphatase activity of the vacuoles. However, none of the clinical and morphological findings are entirely specific, and confirmatory enzyme studies are essential for the diagnosis. Acid maltase can be readily assayed in muscle, cultured fibroblasts, and also in urine (Salafsky and Nadler, 1973; Mehler and Di Mauro, 1976). Prenatal diagnosis is possible by enzyme assays on cultivated amniotic fluid cells obtained during the 14th and 18th weeks of pregnancy (Galjaard, Mekes, De Josselin de Jong and Niermeijer, 1973).

The marked clinical variability of AMD between infants, children and adults is unexplained. Allelic genes are likely to code for different forms of the disease, but the biochemical mechanisms through which the alleles affect the phenotype are not understood. Angelini and Engel (1972) found that neutral as well as acid maltase was deficient in heart, muscle and liver of infants, but not in liver and muscle of adults, and speculated that this could explain the milder course of the disease in the adults. However, Di Mauro *et al.* (1978) noted that neutral maltase was also deficient in the heart of an adult with AMD. The latter workers postulated that the absolute residual activity of acid maltase determined the severity of tissue involvement. However, this activity was determined with an artificial substrate and the residual enzyme in adult AMD is totally inactive toward glycogen (Di Mauro *et al.*, 1978). There is no explanation for the fact that, in childhood or adult AMD, glycogen content in muscle can vary from normal to moderately high from patient to patient, in different muscles of the same patient, and even in different regions of the same muscle.

Apart from symptomatic management of the cardiac and respiratory insufficiency, there is no satisfactory treatment for AMD. Respiratory support with an oscillating bed during the night, and eventually during the day, may prolong life for a number of years in affected adults. Replacement therapy with fungal or human placental acid maltase has been attempted but delivery of adequate amounts of the enzyme to the tissues without sensitisation of the host, is still impractical (Badhuin, Hers and Loeb, 1964; Hug and Schubert, 1967; De Barsy, Jacquemin, Van Hoof and Hers, 1973). A low-carbohydrate diet combined with epinephrine administration has been tried in a number of adults with AMD (Engel, 1970b; Rosenow and Engel, 1978). Despite transient improvement in the strength of selected limb muscles, the course of the disease was not significantly affected.

Type III glycogenosis (debranching enzyme deficiency). Debranching enzyme is bifunctional: it hydrolyses glycogen branch points (amylo-1,6-glucosidase activity) and transfers those three glucose residues adjacent to the branch points which resist cleavage by phosphorylase (oligo-4→1,/4-glucan transferase activity) (Brown and Illingworth, 1962). The two activities are located at separate catalytic sites on the same enzyme molecule (Gillard and Nelson, 1977). Deficiency of the enzyme leads to the accumulation of glycogen with abnormally short outer chains which resembles phosphorylase limit dextrin (Illingworth and Cori, 1952; Illingworth, Cori and Cori, 1956). The enzyme is normally present in all tissues and can be assayed in leucocytes, erythrocytes, cultured fibroblasts, muscle, liver and heart (Huijing, 1964; Van Hoof, 1967; Justice, Ryan, Hsia and Kromptik, 1970). The disease is transmitted by autosomal recessive inheritance but is genetically heterogeneous. This is evidenced by the existence of subgroups of the disease according to whether the enzyme deficiency involves some or all tissues, the reactivity of the enzyme toward different substrates and the clinical patterns of the disease.

Van Hoof and Hers (1967) determined debranching enzyme activity with four different substrates in tissues of 45 patients. In 34 cases, debranching enzyme activity was very low in muscle, liver and erythrocytes with each method of assay, the glycogen content of the same tissues was high and the outer chains of glycogen were abnormally short. In the remaining 11 cases, enzyme activity was normal or only moderately reduced in one or more tissues with at least one method of assay, and in most of these cases the muscle glycogen content was normal. In another

series investigated by Brown and Brown (1968), seven of 34 patients had normal glycogen content and enzyme activity in muscle. In other cases enzyme activity was absent from liver and muscle but was preserved in leucocytes or erythrocytes (Brandt and De Luca, 1966; Williams and Field, 1968; Deckelbaum, Russell, Shapira, Cohen, Agam and Gutman, 1972).

Two major clinical patterns of the disease have been recognised to date. In the more common form of the disorder, the metabolic disturbance secondary to the hepatic enzyme deficiency dominates the clinical picture. Hepatomegaly, growth retardation and fasting hypoglycaemia, present since infancy, represent the usual findings. In some cases there is also cardiomegaly (Huijing, 1975; Howell, 1978; Moses and Gutman, 1972). The hypoglycaemia causes increased mobilisation and utilisation of fat, hyperlipidaemia and a tendency to develop ketosis (Fernandes and Pikaar, 1969; 1972). Because the outer chains of glycogen can still contribute to blood glucose homeostasis and glucose derived from gluconeogenesis or glycogenolysis can freely leave the liver, the metabolic disturbance is less profound than in type I glycogenosis. The hepatomegaly and fasting hypoglycaemia diminish or disappear after puberty (Brown and Brown, 1968; Cohn, Wang, Hauge, Henningsen, Jensen and Svejgaard, 1975; Howell, 1978). Despite glycogen storage in muscle, the myopathic features in this group are seldom disabling (Levin, Moses, Chayoth, Jagoda and Steinitz, 1967).

In a smaller group of patients there is a clinically significant myopathy (Oliner, Schulman and Larner, 1961; Sidbury, 1965; Brunberg, McCormick and Schochet, 1971; Murase, Ikeda, Muro, Nakao and Sugita, 1973; Di Mauro, Hartwig, Hays, Eastwood, Franco, Olarte, Chang, Roses, Fetell, Schoenfeldt and Stern, 1978). In these there may be a history of protuberant abdomen in childhood which decreased in adolescence, and muscle fatigue or aching on heavy exertion since an early age. Progressive muscle weakness begins in childhood or, more commonly, in adult life and may involve both proximal and distal muscles. Selectively severe involvement of distal forearm muscles occurs in some patients. Persistent hepatomegaly is found in most cases.

The electrocardiogram revealed biventricular hypertrophy in all of five cases studied by Di Mauro, Hartwig *et al.* (1978) and in two of these there was also congestive heart failure. Serum enzymes of muscle origin are increased from twofold to more than ten-fold above the upper limit of normal. The electromyogram shows changes consistent with myopathy. Increased insertional activity, myotonic discharges and fibrillation potentials can also occur (Brunberg *et al.*, 1971; Di Mauro, Hartwig *et al.*, 1978). The muscle glycogen concentration varies between 3–6 per cent and the iodine absorption spectrum of glycogen resembles that of limit dextrin. Histopathological studies reveal a vacuolar myopathy. The abnormal spaces are filled with glycogen which displaces and replaces normal organelles but is not membrane-bound (Neustein, 1969; Brunberg *et al.*, 1971; Murase *et al.*, 1973; Di Mauro, Hartwig *et al.*, 1978). Glycogen excess was also found in erythrocytes in the 5 cases studied by Di Mauro, Hartwig *et al.* (1978).

The diagnostic clues in this myopathy consist of a history of hepatic enlargement, and possibly of hypoglycaemic episodes, during childhood; persistent mild hepatomegaly; cardiomyopathy in some patients; easy fatigability on heavy exertion; a diminished or absent glycaemic response to epinephrine or glucagon; an impaired or absent rise of lactic acid in venous blood flowing from muscles after ischaemic exercise (Brunberg *et al.*, 1971; Di Mauro, Hartwig *et al.*, 1978); abnormal electrical irritability of the muscle fibres in the electromyogram; and a vacuolar myopathy. Confirmatory biochemical studies include glycogen assay and structural analysis and biochemical determination of debranching enzyme activity by more than one method of assay (van Hoof and Hers, 1967; Di Mauro, Hartwig *et al.*, 1978).

There is no effective treatment for the myopathy. Therapy in younger patients consists of prevention of hypoglycaemia by frequent meals of high protein content. After the age of one year, a diet with 45 per cent of the calories from carbohydrate, 20 per cent from fat and the rest from protein is beneficial (Fernandes and Pikaar, 1969). Vigorous exercise, which can provoke arrhythmias in patients with cardiomyopathy, should be avoided.

Type IV glycogenosis (branching enzyme deficiency). The enzyme introduces branch points into glycogen through its α-1,4-glucan : α-1, 4-glucan 6-glycosyl transferase activity. Deficiency of the enzyme was predicted by Illingworth and Cori (1952) on the basis of structural analysis of glycogen isolated from the liver of an affected boy. This glycogen had abnormally long inner and outer chains and fewer than normal branch points, resembling amylopectin. Andersen (1956) described the clinical aspects of this case and the predicted enzyme deficiency was confirmed by Brown and Brown (1966). As the defect is in the synthetic pathway, glycogen storage would not be expected, but in some cases the liver glycogen content is abnormally high. This is probably due to the poor solubility of the abnormal polysaccharide in the cytosol, which may also explain the hepatocellular injury characteristic of the disease. The abnormal glycogen still contains branch points and is heterogeneous in composition (Reed, Dixon, Neustein, Donnell and Landing, 1968; Mercier and Whelan, 1973). Thus, there must be an alternative mechanism for introducing branch points into glycogen: an additional enzyme not detected by the usual assay for branching enzyme (Brown and Brown, 1966), or debranching enzyme acting in reverse (Huijing, Lee, Carter and Whelan, 1970).

The disease is transmitted by autosomal recessive inheritance (Legum and Nitowsky, 1969; Howell, Kaback and Brown, 1971). Abnormal glycogen deposits occur in liver, spleen and lymph nodes and, occasionally, in muscle, kidney, adrenals and the central nervous system (Howell *et al.*, 1971; Schochet, McCormick and Zellweger, 1970). Deficiency of the enzyme has been observed in liver, leucocytes and cultured fibroblasts (Brown and Brown, 1966; Fernandes and Huijing, 1968; Howell *et al.*, 1971) but, thus far, not in muscle. However, the enzyme was not determined in muscle in those cases in which the presence of abnormal glycogen in muscle was documented.

The disorder presents during the first year of life with progressive enlargement of liver and spleen and failure to thrive. The abnormal polysaccharide in liver induces nodular cirrhosis, hepatoparenchymal insufficiency and portal hypertension. Carbohydrate tolerances remain normal. Muscle weakness and atrophy appear in some patients (Sidbury, Mason, Burns and Ruebner, 1962; Levin, Burgess and Mortimer, 1968; Holleman, van der Haar and De Vaan, 1966; Reed *et al.*, 1968; Zellweger, Mueller, Ionasescu, Schochet and McCormick, 1972), but not in others (Brown and Brown, 1966). Death occurs in infancy or early childhood due to hepatic or cardiac failure.

The abnormal polysaccharide stains positively with periodic acid-Schiff (PAS), alcian blue and colloidal iron, gives a brown-blue colour with iodine and resists diastase digestion. It consists of finely filamentous and granular material which intermingles with normal glycogen particles in affected tissues. The presence of normal glycogen particles again suggests that an alternative mechanism for glycogen synthesis is still operative. Deposits in the central nervous system, conspicuous in astroglial cells, resemble Lafora bodies. Different muscles are affected to different extents, but the tongue appears to be especially severely affected (Schochet *et al.*, 1970).

The diagnosis of branching enzyme deficiency is suggested by progressive hepatosplenomegaly and failure to thrive in infancy, muscle weakness (if present), and PAS-positive, diastase-fast deposits in the affected tissues. Enzyme assays and structural analysis of glycogen confirm the diagnosis. Antenatal diagnosis is possible by enzyme assays on fibroblasts cultured from amniotic fluid cells (Howell *et al.*, 1971).

Therapy with fungal α-glucosidase was attempted in two instances (Fernandes and Huijing, 1968; Huijing, Waltuck and Whelan, 1973). Although liver glycogen content was reduced, the course of the disease was not altered.

Type V glycogenosis (myophosphorylase deficiency). McArdle in 1951 described the clinical features of the disease and attributed them to a deficiency of muscle phosphorylase. This prediction was confirmed by Schmid and Mahler (1959) and by Mommaerts, Illingworth, Pearson, Guillory and Seraydarian (1959).

Phosphorylase catalyses the cleavage of 1,4-α-glucosidic linkages, releasing glucose-1-phosphate from non-reducing ends of exposed glycogen chains. Its action comes to a halt when chain length is reduced to four glucose residues which are then removed by the debranching enzyme complex. In resting muscle, phosphorylase is mostly in an inactive *b* form which phosphorylase *b* kinase converts to an active *a* form. Activation of the kinase, and hence of phosphorylase, is mediated by cyclic AMP via activation of adenyl cyclase by epinephrine (in muscle and liver) or glucagon (in liver). Electrical stimulation or exercise activate phosphorylase, probably by calcium released from the sarcoplasmic reticulum (Ozawa, Hosoi and Ebashi, 1967). Phosphorylase *a* is reconverted to phosphorylase *b* by a specific phosphatase which, in turn, is inhibited by cyclic AMP (for reviews *see* Huijing, 1975; Howell, 1978).

Different tissues contain different phosphorylase isoenzymes, and different structural genes code for the isoenzymes present in skeletal muscle, liver and smooth muscle. Cardiac muscle contains isoenzymes found in smooth and skeletal muscle as well as hybrid isoenzymes (Yunis, Fischer and Krebs, 1962; Davis, Schliselfeld, Wolf, Leavitt and Krebs, 1967). Deficiency of muscle phosphorylase occurs independently of other isoenzymes and only skeletal muscle is clinically affected. The syndrome, however, is genetically heterogeneous. This is evinced by subgroups of the disease according to mode of inheritance, clinical patterns, and the presence or absence of catalytically inactive enzyme protein in muscle.

In most instances the disease is transmitted by autosomal recessive inheritance, but there is an unexplained preponderance of males (Huijing, 1975). Possibly, some females remain undiagnosed because they are less likely to engage in the type of exercise which provokes symptoms of the disease. Autosomal dominant transmission of phosphorylase deficiency was reported in one family (Chui and Munsat, 1976).

Symptoms of the disease may date from early childhood, but more typically the capacity for exercise is unimpaired until the second half of the second decade. In contrast to this common pattern, a fatal infantile case, with death due to respiratory insufficiency at the age of 13 weeks, has been reported (Di Mauro and Hartlage, 1978); and 'late-onset' cases have been described in a brother and sister who did not develop symptoms until their fiftieth year (Engel, Eyerman and Williams,

1963) and in a patient who presented with muscle weakness at the age of 74 years (Hewlett and Gardner-Thorpe, 1978).

Catalytically inactive enzyme protein is present in some cases but not in others. The inactive protein has been detected by immunological tests (Dreyfus and Alexandre, 1971) or by SDS poly-acrylamide electrophoresis (Feit and Brooke, 1976; Koster, Slee, Jennekens, Wintzen and Van Berkel, 1979). In one case, the electrophoretic method detected inactive enzyme protein when the immunological method did not (Koster *et al.*, 1979).

The typical symptoms of the disease consist of muscular pain, weakness and stiffness during slight to moderate exertion. Pain on exercise, which is the most prominent feature, can occur in any muscle, even those of the jaw. Rest rapidly relieves the symptoms following moderate exercise, but the more severe or protracted the exercise, the longer the symptoms persist (McArdle, 1951). The pain may disappear with continued exercise if stiffness has not developed. This 'second wind' is related to increased muscle blood flow, and the augmented utilisation by muscle of plasma free fatty acids (Pernow, Havel and Jennings, 1967) and amino acids (Wahren, Felig, Havel, Jorfeldt, Pernow and Saltin, 1973) as energy sources. A frequent and characteristic symptom is inability to extend the fingers fully after sustained gripping movements against resistance; full recovery may take many minutes. After severe exercise, pain, weakness and swelling of muscle may persist for several days. Myoglobinuria after exercise occurs at least once in the course of the disease in half to two-thirds of the cases (Dawson, Spong and Harrington, 1968; Fattah, Rubulis and Faloon, 1970). Muscle weakness and atrophy are detected in about one-third of the cases and are usually mild. Muscles of the pectoral girdle are more likely to be affected than those of the pelvic girdle, and the bulk of the calf muscles may be larger than normal. Moderate exercise provokes the typical muscle symptoms as well as tachycardia, dyspnoea, exhaustion and rarely nausea and vomiting. Ischaemic exercise of the forearm muscles results in rapid fatigue and shortening of the forearm flexors which may persist for some minutes after return of the circulation. It is not a true cramp but a physiological contracture during which the affected muscles remain electrically silent (McArdle, 1951; Rowland, Lovelace, Schotland, Araki and Carmel, 1966). To perform the test, a blood-pressure cuff is placed on the upper arm and is maximally inflated to occlude arterial blood flow. Exercise is by squeezing a rubber bulb against a fixed resistance at a rate of one per second. Normal subjects can readily exercise in this manner for a minute. In occasional patients, weakness develops during the test, which prevents them from exercising to the point of developing a contracture. Because the muscles cannot degrade glycogen to lactic acid during the exercise, there is no rise in lactate in venous blood taken from the forearm muscles after release of the circulation (McArdle, 1951). Normal subjects exhibit a three-fold to five-fold increase of lactate within 5 min of the end of exercise and the lactate level returns to the baseline in about 30 min.

The mechanism of the electrically silent muscle contractures is not understood. One possible explanation would be a deficiency of ATP required for the operation of the sarcoplasmic reticulum (SR) calcium pump. However, Rowland, Araki and Carmel (1965) could not demonstrate a decrease of ATP in muscle during a contracture induced by ischaemic exercise. On the other hand, Gruener, McArdle, Ryman and Weller (1968) found that micro-applications of a calcium-containing solution to skinned muscle fibres elicited prolonged contractures, and Brody, Gerber and Sidbury (1970) noted that isolated SR vesicles accumulated calcium normally in the presence of ATP. The latter two studies are still consistent with the notion that the SR calcium pump fails when ATP becomes unavailable.

The serum levels of muscle enzymes are usually raised at rest. Following exercise, these levels increased markedly within a few hours (Hammett, Bale, Basser and Neale, 1966). Electromyographic studies may show alterations in motor unit potentials indicative of a myopathy and there is electrical silence of muscle fibres during contracture. Repetitive stimulation of motor nerves at 18 Hz was reported to produce an abnormal decrement of the amplitude of the evoked compound muscle action potential (Dyken, Smith and Peake, 1967) but this finding has not been confirmed to date.

Muscle glycogen is usually raised, commonly to between 2–5 per cent, but very occasionally it is normal. Glycogen accumulates subsarcolemmally in blebs and between myofibrils, especially adjacent to I bands (Schotland, Spiro, Rowland and Carmel, 1965). Small pockets of glycogen may also become invaginated into mitochondria (Gruener et al., 1968). Lack of phosphorylase can be demonstrated histochemically in cryostat sections of fresh-frozen muscle. Characteristically, enzyme activity is absent from muscle fibres but is preserved in the smooth muscle cells of the blood vessels. The histochemical demonstration of phosphorylase in muscle depends on the presence of glycogen primer, and the enzyme cannot be demonstrated even in normal muscle depleted of glycogen as, for example, after prolonged storage of a muscle specimen at room temperature, or after death. Biochemical assay of the enzyme is independent of the muscle glycogen content. Although mature skeletal muscle fibres of affected patients lack phosphorylase, regenerating fibres and muscle cells cultured in vitro do show enzyme activity (Roelofs, Engel and Chauvin, 1971). This has been attributed to the synthesis of a fetal isozyme by immature muscle cells (Sato, Imai, Hatayama and Roelofs, 1977; Di Mauro, Arnold, Miranda and Rowland, 1978). Synthesis of the fetal isozyme is repressed by the time of birth.

The diagnosis of myophosphorylase deficiency is suggested by weakness, pain and contractures of muscle on exertion, a history of myoglobinuria, failure to form lactic acid on ischaemic exercise and by histochemical studies of the muscle biopsy specimen. Biochemical assay of the enzyme is required to confirm the diagnosis. In phosphofructokinase deficiency the clinical symptoms can be identical but phosphofructokinase, not phosphorylase, is deficient in muscle, and the isoenzyme characteristic of muscle is also absent from erythrocytes. In debranching enzyme deficiency there is impaired production of lactate on ischaemic exercise, but muscle contractures and myoglobinuria do not occur. The ischaemic exercise test will be negative in other disorders with symptoms that in some respects resemble a glycolytic enzyme deficiency of muscle: carnitine palmityl-transferase deficiency, which can be associated with muscle pain and myoglobinuria on exertion (DiMauro and DiMauro, 1973); the interesting patient described by Slotwiner, Song and Maker (1969) (see below); the painless physiological contractures on exercise associated with a decreased ability of the SR to reaccumulate calcium (Brody, 1969); and the myopathy associated with xanthinuria and with deposition of xanthine and hypoxanthine crystals in muscle (Chalmers, Johnson, Pallis and Watts, 1969; Chalmers, Watts, Bitensky and Chayen, 1969).

The ingestion of glucose or fructose increases exercise tolerance, but their long-term use has proved disappointing. They are awkward to take, predispose to obesity, and fructose may cause colicky pain. A medium-chain triglyceride ketogenic diet has been reported to increase exercise tolerance and to prevent exercise-induced rhabdomyolysis (Brooks, Brumback, Rosenbaum and Engel, 1977). All patients should be advised to keep within the limits of exertion causing significant pain and, as far as possible, to precede vigorous exertion by a period of more gentle activity.

Type VII glycogenosis (muscle phosphofructokinase deficiency). This condition was described by Tarui, Okuno, Ikura, Tanaka, Suda and Nishikawa in 1965. Few additional reports of the disease have been published to date (Layzer, Rowland and Ranney, 1967; Serratrice, Monges, Roux, Aquaron and Gambarelli, 1969; Tobin, Huijing, Porro and Salzman, 1973; Dupond, Robert, Carbillet and Leconte Des Floris, 1977).

The enzyme catalyses the conversion of fructose-6-phosphate to fructose-1,6-diphosphate. The reaction requires ATP and is irreversible. Absence of the enzyme completely inhibits the Embden-Meyerhof pathway and blocks the utilisation of glucose. Glucose-1-phosphate and glucose-6-phosphate levels are increased, and fructose-1,6-diphosphate level is markedly reduced in muscle (Tarui et al., 1965). There is an associated partial enzyme deficiency in erythrocytes which lack the muscle isoenzyme (Tarui et al., 1965; Layzer, Rowland and Ranney, 1967; Tarui, Kono, Nasu and Nishikawa, 1969).

The clinical picture can be similar to that seen with myophosphorylase deficiency and the ischaemic exercise test is positive. In addition, there is a mild haemolytic disease, probably secondary to the partial erythrocyte enzyme defect (Tarui *et al.*, 1969). Autosomal recessive inheritance operates in some families (Tarui *et al.*, 1965; Layzer, Rowland and Ranney, 1967; Dupond *et al.*, 1977) but, in the family reported by Serratrice *et al.* (1969), transmission was probably by autosomal dominant inheritance. In the latter family, the propositus was also atypical in that he had hepatomegaly and suffered from progressive muscle weakness.

The subsarcolemmal glycogen deposits in muscle resemble those seen in myophosphorylase deficiency. Absence of phosphofructokinase can be demonstrated histochemically (Bonilla and Schotland, 1970) but the diagnosis is best established by biochemical assay of the enzyme in muscle.

Other glycogenoses have been reported, some affecting muscle, in which only a single patient or a single family have been described, or in which the enzymic disorder has been insufficiently defined. An example of such a condition affecting muscle is the disorder described by Satoyoshi and Kowa (1967) in two brothers. Both, when 35 years old, developed muscle pain, stiffness and weakness occurring a few hours after moderately heavy exercise. Blood lactate failed to rise after ischaemic exercise except following fructose ingestion. Biopsy studies showed an apparent block at the level of phosphohexoseisomerase, thought to be due to inhibition of the enzyme, associated with a decreased activity of phosphofructokinase. Exercise tolerance improved considerably following fructose, but not glucose, ingestion.

Another example is the 8-year-old boy with pains on exercise, described by Strugalska-Cynowska (1967), who had a very delayed rise in blood lactate following ischaemic exercise. This was attributed, on histochemical grounds, to a disturbance in the activity of phosphorylase-*b*-kinase which converts phosphorylase from the inactive to the active form.

Another glycogenosis was noted in the 4-year-old boy described by Thomson, Maclaurin and Prineas (1963) with a mild myopathy and marked contracture of his calves, having only a slight rise

in blood lactate after ischaemic exercise. His muscles were loaded with glycogen of normal structure. It was thought that there was a partial deficiency of phosphoglucomutase and possibly other glycolytic enzymes.

The case described by Slotwiner *et al.* (1969), with symptoms and many findings resembling phosphorylase deficiency, also poses a difficult problem in classification. The muscle showed the typical subsarcolemmal accumulation of glycogen seen in types V or VII, but biochemically the glycogen was not raised, glycolysis to lactate was normal and thorough investigation failed to reveal any enzymatic defect.

Holmes, Houghton and Woolf (1960) studied a female patient who presented at the age of 21 with symptoms of a myopathy and who died at the age of 31 years. Cardiac and skeletal muscle contained basophilic, PAS-positive, diastase-fast polysaccharide deposits. Similar material was found in hepatocytes and in the lumen of the convoluted tubules. Enzyme assays and structural analysis of the polysaccharide were not performed. A similar disorder was reported by Karpati, Carpenter, Wolfe and Sherwin (1969) in a male patient who died of cardiac failure at the age of 19 years. Post-mortem examination was restricted to muscle and liver. The abnormal polysaccharide had filamentous fine structure and was especially abundant in type II muscle fibres.

Disorders of lipid metabolism

Long-chain fatty acids taken up by skeletal muscle are utilised for energy metabolism or esterified to triglycerides and incorporated into lipid droplets. It is now known that these fatty acids are the major substrate for oxidation by skeletal muscle at rest and during sustained exercise (Andres, Cader and Zierler, 1956; Hagenfeldt and Wahren, 1968; Tancredi, Dagenais and Zierler, 1976; Zierler, 1976). The main steps in the oxidation of long-chain fatty acids, reviewed by Greville and Tubbs (1968) and by Brosnan, Kopec and Fritz (1973), are as follows: (1) fatty acids are esterified with coenzyme (CoA), catalysed by long-chain fatty acyl-CoA synthetase; (2) acyl CoA is converted to acylcarnitine by carnitine palmityltransferase I, located on the outer surface of the inner mitochondrial membrane barrier, permitting passage of acyl carnitine esters through the inner mitochondrial membrane barrier; (3) acyl carnitine esters are reconverted to acyl-CoA by carnitine palmityl-transferase II, located on the inner surface of the inner mitochondrial membrane; (4) intra-mitochondrial β-oxidation of acyl-CoA units; (5) utilisation of acetyl-CoA via the citric acid cycle. Impairment of any step in this scheme may result in triglyceride accumulation within the muscle fibres, or could cause symptoms due to lack of fatty acid substrate for energy metabolism. Lipid storage in muscle, especially in type I muscle fibres, has now been observed in a variety of conditions.

A myopathy associated with triglyceride accumulation in skeletal muscle of a young adult was reported by Bradley, Hudgson, Gardner-Medwin and Walton in 1969. The biochemical basis of the disorder was not defined. In 1970 W.K. Engel, Vick, Glueck and Levy described two patients (identical twins) who had lipid excess in muscle without weakness, cramping pain after exercise, fasting or ingestion of a high-fat, low-carbohydrate diet, and who had previous attacks of myoglobinuria. The twins could form no ketone bodies after fasting or after ingesting long-chain fatty acids, but could produce ketone bodies from short-chain or medium-chain fatty acids. The basic biochemical defect in these patients was not discovered. In 1972, A.G. Engel and Siekert observed a young woman with progressive muscle weakness and lipid excess in muscle, whose symptoms responded favorably to prednisone. In 1973, A.G. Engel and Angelini found that homogenates of this patient's muscle oxidised long-chain fatty acids abnormally slowly, but this could be corrected by the addition of carnitine. They inferred that she suffered from carnitine deficiency and they established this by direct assay of carnitine in five specimens of her muscles. Also in 1973, Di Mauro and Di Mauro described a patient with intermittent myoglobinuria but without lipid excess in muscle, who suffered from muscle carnitine palmityltransferase (CPT) deficiency. In 1975, Chanarin, Patel, Slavin, Wills, Andrews and Stewart reported a further disorder associated with congenital ichthyosis and neutral lipid excess in muscle, liver, gastrointestinal mucosa, leuco-

cytes and cultured fibroblasts. Another patient suffering from a similar illness, but also having steatorrhea and muscle weakness, was reported by Miranda, Di Mauro, Eastwood, Hays, Johnson, Olarte, Whitlock, Mayeaux and Rowland in 1979. The biochemical basis of this disorder remains unsolved. Additional cases of lipid storage myopathies in which the biochemical defect was not established have also been published (Jerusalem, Spiess and Baumgartner, 1975; Mattle, Jerusalem, Nolte and Schollmeyer, 1977). Finally, lipid excess in muscle also occurs in certain mitochondrial myopathies (*see below*). This section considers the two disorders in which distinct defects of lipid metabolism have been discovered to date: carnitine deficiency and CPT deficiency. Clinical and biochemical heterogeneity has been found in both disorders since their description in 1973.

Carnitine deficiency syndromes. Carnitine (γ-trimethylamino-β-hydroxybutyrate) is present in many foods but the daily human requirements are met only by additional biosynthesis. The two main precursors are lysine and methionine. The synthesis involves the formation of ε-N-trimethyllysine, oxidative cleavage of this to glycine and γ-trimethylaminobutyrate followed by β-hydroxylation of the latter compound to carnitine (Haigler and Broquist, 1974; Tanphaichitr and Broquist, 1974; Hulse, Ellis and Henderson, 1978). In man, all the enzymes required for carnitine biosynthesis are found in liver, kidney and brain. Cardiac and skeletal muscle can also participate in biosynthesis but lack the final enzyme, γ-trimethylaminobutyrate hydroxylase (Rebouche and Engel, 1980a). Carnitine formed by liver and kidney is delivered to the other tissues by the circulation. Cardiac and skeletal muscle carnitine levels greatly exceed the serum level, and uptake into these tissues is by an active transport mechanism (Rebouche, 1977; Willner, Ginsburg and Di Mauro, 1978). The possible causes of human carnitine deficiency include impaired biosynthesis, impaired active transport into cells, excessive release from cells, excessive loss from body fluids and excessive catabolism. At present, two main types of carnitine deficiency syndromes have been delineated: a predominantly myopathic form, and a systemic form.

The myopathic form of carnitine deficiency. Including the first patient (Engel and Angelini, 1973; Engel, Angelini and Nelson, 1974), eight cases of the restricted, myopathic type of carnitine deficiency have been reported (Markesbery, McQuillen, Procopis, Harrison and Engel, 1974; VanDyke, Griggs, Markesbery and DiMauro, 1975; Angelini, Lucke and Cantarutti, 1976; Isaacs, Heffron, Badenhorst and Pickering, 1976; Scarlato, Albizzati, Bassi, Cerri and Frattola, 1977; Angelini, Govoni, Bragaglia and Vergani, 1978; Hart, Chang, Di Mauro, Farooki and Ayyar, 1978). Features common with the first case were progressive muscle weakness, lipid excess in muscle and muscle carnitine deficiency. The term of type I lipid storage myopathy has been suggested for this triad of symptoms (Engel *et al.*, 1974). Four of the patients were male and four were female. Muscle weakness was first noted between 18 months and 38 years of age. Serum enzymes of muscle origin were increased in all but one patient. The oldest patient in this group also developed a peripheral neuropathy, and lipid excess was noted in her Schwann cells and leucocytes (Markesbery *et al.*, 1974). Cardiomyopathy was detected in two boys. It was asymptomatic in one (VanDyke *et al.*, 1975) but the other died of congestive heart failure at the age of 3 years (Hart *et al.*, 1978). The serum carnitine level was normal in six patients but decreased in two others (Scarlato *et al.*, 1977; Angelini *et al.*, 1978). Liver carnitine was measured in the first case only and was normal (Engel *et al.*, 1974). Depressed long-chain fatty acid oxidation by muscle homogenates, corrected by carnitine, was demonstrated in the first case. Similar studies were not performed in the other seven patients.

Therapeutic measures used in these patients have included prednisone, carnitine replacement therapy and a low-fat, high-carbohydrate diet. Two of three patients have responded favourably to prednisone and four of five patients responded favourably to carnitine replacement therapy. However, in none of the patients responding to therapy was there an increase in muscle carnitine. Both parents of one patient (Markesbery *et al.*, 1974) and at least one parent of two other patients (Angelini *et al.*, 1976; Hart *et al.*, 1978) had moderately low muscle carnitine levels, a finding which suggests an autosomal recessive inheritance.

The low muscle but normal serum carnitine levels in six patients in this group suggests an impaired active transport of carnitine into muscle cells.

An additional patient, not included in the above series, had severe muscle carnitine deficiency and intermittent episodes of myoglobinuria. Her weakness responded to carnitine therapy but an increase in muscle carnitine was not documented (W.K. Engel, Prockop, Askanas, A.G. Engel, Hutchinson, Galdi, Goldman and Foster, 1980).

Systemic carnitine deficiency. In this syndrome, muscle carnitine deficiency is associated with systemic manifestations. The first case was reported by Karpati, Carpenter, Engel, Watters, Allen, Rothman, Klassen and Mamer (1975). Eight additional cases have been described to date (Boudin, Mikol, Guillard and Engel, 1976; Engel, Banker and Eiben, 1977; Cornelio, DiDonato, Peluchetti, Bizzi, Bertagnolio, D'Angelo and Wiesmann, 1977; Scarlato, Pellegrini, Cerri, Meola and Veicsteinas, 1978; Ware, Burton, McGarry, Marks and Weinberg, 1978; Glasgow, Eng and Engel, 1980). Common features of the syndrome are acute episodes of encephalopathy associated with hepatic dysfunction, progressive muscle weakness, and lipid excess in muscle and other tissues at one stage of illness or at death. Muscle carnitine levels were reduced in all cases. Cardiac carnitine content was decreased in three patients in which it was measured. Serum carnitine, determined in six cases, was reduced in five but higher than normal in one, but the high value was observed at autopsy. Liver carnitine content, measured in six cases, was markedly reduced in four and slightly in two. The kidney carnitine level, measured in two cases, was normal.

The age of onset of the disease ranged from 11 months to 17 years. One or more episodes of encephalopathy preceded the recognition of the muscle weakness in six patients, but in the others the muscle weakness preceded the encephalopathy by several years. The weakness was generally greater proximally than distally, at times also involved facial and cervical muscles, and was associated with decreased muscle bulk. Lipid accumulation was typically more severe in type I than in type II fibres, as in the myopathic form of carnitine deficiency. Seven of the nine patients died in the course of the acute attacks. At autopsy, marked triglyceride excess was found in muscle and liver and, to a lesser extent, in kidney and heart.

The acute attacks are preceded by vomiting which is followed by deepening stupor, confusion and coma. Associated findings include hypoglycaemia, hepatomegaly, hypoprothrombinaemia, hyperammonaemia and an increase in serum enzymes of liver origin. Metabolic acidosis occurs in approximately half of the patients during the acute attacks. In several patients the attacks were provoked by caloric deprivation. The encephalopathic episodes resemble those of Reye's syndrome but, in that disorder, serum and tissue carnitine levels are either normal or only slightly depressed (Glasgow et al., 1980).

Three patients with systemic carnitine deficiency have been treated with carnitine. One improved clinically without change in muscle and liver carnitine (Karpati et al., 1975), one died (Cornelio et al., 1977) and one remained unchanged (Glasgow et al., 1980).

The exact aetiology of the systemic carnitine deficiency is still in doubt. The low serum, muscle and liver carnitine levels suggested a defect in biosynthesis (Karpati et al., 1975). However, this could not account for the fact that replacement therapy did not increase tissue carnitine levels. Recent studies of systemic carnitine deficiency have shown the following: the four hepatic enzymes subserving carnitine biosynthesis were normally active in vitro (Rebouche and Engel, 1980b); there was no block in carnitine biosynthesis from labelled ε-N-trimethyllysine in vivo (Rebouche and Engel, 1980c); the renal plasma threshold for carnitine excretion and the tubular maximum for carnitine reabsorption were lower than normal, but these findings could not entirely account for the decreased muscle carnitine level (Engel, Rebouche, Glasgow and Romshe, 1980). These studies strongly suggest that systemic carnitine deficiency is caused by a generalized defect of carnitine transport.

Carnitine deficiency syndromes probably secondary to other metabolic defects. Lipid excess and low carnitine levels in muscle have been reported in patients where it was presumably secondary to another, but yet unidentified, metabolic lesion. The mechanism and significance of the carnitine deficiency in these cases remains uncertain. An 11-year-old boy described by Smyth, Lake, MacDermot and Wilson (1975) had calcification of basal ganglia, seizures, high-tone hearing loss, increased spinal fluid protein, exertional lactic acidaemia, muscle weakness, frequent vomiting but no acute episodes of encephalopathy. Serum and liver carnitine levels were not assayed. A 51-year-old woman described by Whitaker, Di Mauro, Solomon, Sabesin, Duckworth and Mendell (1977) had progressive muscle weakness, liver dysfunction, and carnitine deficiency in quadriceps but not in biceps muscle. The serum carnitine level was normal. Liver carnitine was not assayed. Prednisone therapy improved the patient's weakness and restored the muscle carnitine content to normal. A young adult woman with progressive weakness and muscle carnitine deficiency had normal serum carnitine levels. Liver carnitine was not assayed. There was impaired oxidation of long-chain fatty acids by muscle homogenates, as in the patient studied by Engel and Angelini (1973), but this could not be corrected by the addition of carnitine. The muscle carnitine deficiency was attributed to a defect of β-oxidation in muscle. The mechanism by which the putative defect might reduce the muscle carnitine level was not explained (Willner, Di Mauro, Eastwood, Hays, Roohi and Lovelace, 1979).

Carnitine deficiency has also been reported in muscles of patients undergoing chronic haemodialysis (Bohmer, Bergrem and Eiklid, 1978), and also in serum and tissues of cachectic, cirrhotic patients (Rudman, Sewell and Ansley, 1977). In addition, decreased muscle carnitine was found in some patients with advanced Duchenne dystrophy (Borum, Broquist and Roelofs, 1977). In another study, the mean muscle carnitine levels were only slightly lower than normal in Duchenne dystrophy (Engel et al., 1977). Borum et al. (1977), suggest that the low carnitine values in dystrophic muscle are a non-specific result of severe muscle damage.

Carnitine palmityltransferase deficiency.
Since the original report of this disorder by Di Mauro and Di Mauro in 1973, a total of 15 cases have been reported in the literature (Bank, Di Mauro, Bonilla, Capuzzi and Rowland, 1975; Cumming, Hardy, Hudgson and Walls, 1976; Herman and Nadler, 1977; Layzer, Havel, Becker and McIlroy, 1977; Carroll, Brooke, DeVivo, Kaiser and Hagberg, 1978; DiDonato, Cornelio, Pacini, Peluchetti, Rimoldi and Spreafico, 1978; Hostetler, Hoppel, Romine, Sipe, Gross and Higginbottom, 1978; Reza, Kar, Pearson and Kark, 1978; Brownell, Severson, Thomson and Fletcher, 1979; Patten, Wood, Harati, Hefferan and Howell, 1979; Scholte, Jennekens and Bouvy, 1979) and four other cases were encountered by the author (A.G.E.). Eighteen of these patients were male and one was female. Transmission is probably by autosomal recessive inheritance with markedly reduced penetrance in women. It is less likely that transmission is by sex-linked recessive inheritance and that female patients represent manifesting heterozygotes. Intermittent symptoms begin during the first or second decade of life. Muscle aching and fatigability occur on sustained exertion. There are recurrent attacks of myoglobinuria, usually, but not invariably, after sustained exertion and especially if exercise is during caloric deprivation or exposure to cold. Severe muscle aching and stiffness precede the myoglobinuria by a few hours and marked muscle weakness can develop in the course of the attack. Renal failure may complicate the myoglobinuria (Bank et al., 1975; DiDonato et al., 1978; Brownell et al., 1979). Serum enzymes of muscle origin increase greatly during the attacks, but may also rise after exercise which does not precipitate overt myoglobinuria. Between attacks, patients are of normal strength and show no electromyographic abnormality. Muscle biopsy at such times shows either no lipid excess (Di Mauro and Di Mauro, 1973; Herman and Nadler, 1977; Carroll et al., 1978) or variable lipid excess, especially in type I muscle fibres (Cumming et al., 1976; Reza et al., 1978). Quantitative electron microscopy in three cases showed that 0.25, 0.74 and 2.8 per cent, respectively, of the muscle fibre volume was occupied by lipid material. In normal muscle the corresponding value is less than 0.2 per cent and,

in carnitine deficiency, values as high as 10 per cent can occur (Engel, Santa, Stonnington, Jerusalem, Tsujihata, Brownell, Sakakibara, Banker, Sahashi and Lambert, 1979). Fasting for 38–72 h is associated with a delayed rise of serum ketone bodies in some patients (Bank et al., 1975; Cumming et al., 1976; Hostetler et al., 1978; Patten et al., 1979), but not in others (Patten et al., 1979; Scholte et al., 1979). The serum creatine phosphokinase level increases abnormally during fasting in some patients, but not in others (Scholte et al., 1979). Increased basal serum triglyceride and cholesterol levels which rose further on fasting were noted in two brothers studied by Bank et al. (1975) but not in other patients.

A partial deficiency of CPT was found in muscles of all patients. CPT I was thought to be decreased in the case reported by Di Mauro and Di Mauro (1973) but Patten et al. (1979) and Scholte et al. (1979) observed a selective decrease of CPT II in their cases. Enzyme deficiency was also found in leucocytes (Layzer et al., 1977; Scholte et al., 1979) and cultured fibroblasts (DiDonato et al., 1978). Impaired oxidation of labelled palmitic acid by muscle homogenates in vitro was detected by Di Mauro and Di Mauro (1973) but not by Layzer et al. (1977). However, the latter workers showed that labelled palmitate was not utilised normally in vivo. Hypothetically, a partial or complete deficiency of CPT I or of CPT II could exist in muscle, or in both liver and muscle. Data on hepatic CPT levels have not been published to date, but it seems likely that those patients not forming ketone bodies normally on fasting have partial deficiency of at least one of the hepatic CPT enzymes. In three cases (Di Mauro and Di Mauro, 1973; Herman and Nadler, 1977; Scholte et al., 1979) there was also an associated deficiency of carnitine acetyltransferase, suggesting a defect in the regulation of short-chain as well as of long-chain acyl transferases. Catalytically inactive but immunologically detectable enzyme protein has not been sought in any of the cases.

It is puzzling that CPT deficiency should be associated with intermittent myoglobinuria, little if any lipid excess in muscle and no permanent weakness, whereas carnitine deficiency causes myoglobinuria infrequently, but is associated with marked lipid excess in muscle and progressive muscle weakness. A possible explanation for the lack of lipid accumulation in muscle in CPT deficiency was offered by Scholte et al. (1979), who found a decreased activity of extrahepatic lipoprotein lipase in their patient.

The diagnosis of the disease is based on the history of exercise intolerance, recurrent myoglobinuria, normal rise of lactate in venous blood flowing from ischaemically exercised muscles and demonstration of CPT deficiency in muscle and possibly other tissues. Treatment consists of a high carbohydrate, low fat diet, frequent feeding and extra carbohydrate intake before and during sustained exertion (Cumming et al., 1976; Reza et al., 1978; Patten et al., 1979).

Mitochondrial myopathies

The term 'mitochondrial myopathies' has been applied previously to muscle diseases in which mitochondria have abnormal structure, function or both. The typical morphological alteration consists of unusually large or excessively abundant mitochondria, often with bizarre cristae and with inclusions of various types. Such organelles usually occur in type I and sometimes in type IIA muscle fibres in which they form subsarcolemmal and intermyofibrillar aggregates. The affected fibres also contain an increased number of small lipid droplets and the mitochondrial aggregates are usually surrounded by glycogen granules. On the basis of their light-microscopic appearance in trichromatically stained sections, the term 'ragged red' has been applied to such fibres (Olson, Engel, Walsh and Einaugler, 1972). A purely morphological definition of mitochondrial myopathies is unsatisfactory, however. In certain disorders with a definite abnormality of mitochondrial metabolism, as in CPT deficiency (Di Mauro and Di Mauro, 1973) or in certain types of exertional lactic acidosis (Sussman, Alfrey, Kirsch, Zweig, Felig and Messner, 1970) there are no structural abnormalities of muscle mitochondria. Conversely, abnormal mitochondria have been found in diseases in which a primary mitochondrial abnormality seems unlikely, as in adult acid maltase deficiency (Engel and Dale, 1968), a few cases of polymyositis (Chou, 1967; Shafiq, Milhorat and Gorycki, 1967) and in certain instances

of denervation atrophy (Gruner, 1963; Shafiq et al., 1967). Finally, similar mitochondrial structural alterations can be associated with divergent abnormalities of mitochondrial function. For these reasons, a biochemical classification of mitochondrial myopathies, even if tentative, is preferable. The classification proposed by Morgan-Hughes, Darveniza, Landon, Land and Clark (1979) will be adopted in this chapter: (1) transport or enzymatic defects of mitochondria causing impaired substrate utilisation; (2) defective mitochondrial energy conservation; (3) specific deficiency of one or more mitochondrial respiratory chain components. The biochemical abnormalities are not necessarily confined to the muscle mitochondria and, in a number of disorders, the myopathy represents but one facet of a multisystem disease. Other features shared by many, but not all, mitochondrial myopathies are: slowly progressive weakness involving proximal and distal muscles since childhood; transiently increased weakness after sustained exertion; and lactic acidaemia after exercise or even at rest.

Mitochondrial disorders associated with transport and enzymatic defects causing impaired substrate utilisation. These syndromes include carnitine deficiency, CPT deficiency and defects of the pyruvate dehydrogenase complex. As CPT and carnitine deficiency were discussed under Disorders of Lipid Metabolism, this section will deal only with defects of the pyruvate dehydrogenase complex. The complex has three components: pyruvate decarboxylase (E_1), dihydrolipoyl transacetylase (E_2) and dihydrolipoyl dehydrogenase (E_3). E_1 exists in an active and inactive form. Formation of the inactive form is catalysed by an ATP-dependent pyruvate dehydrogenase kinase. Inactive E_1 is converted to active E_1 by a calcium- and magnesium-stimulated pyruvate dehydrogenase phosphatase (Robinson and Sherwood, 1975).

Pyruvate decarboxylase deficiency. A patient with this disorder was reported by Blass, Avigan and Uhlendorf (1970). A nine-year-old boy had suffered from attacks of choreoathetosis and ataxia provoked by fever or excitement, since 16 months of age. Blood, urine and cerebrospinal fluid pyruvate levels were abnormally high but lactate levels were rarely abnormal. The enzyme deficiency was demonstrated in cultured fibroblasts and leucocytes. The oxidation of pyruvate was impaired but glutamate, acetate and palmitate were normally oxidised. Muscle specimens revealed an increased number of small lipid droplets, especially in type I fibres, but the patient was not weak (Blass, Kark and Engel, 1971).

Another patient with a deficiency of the pyruvate dehydrogenase complex (in cultured fibroblasts) was a three-year-old girl with microcephaly, hypotonia, spasticity and with persistent pyruvic and lactic acidaemia (Blass, Schulman, Young and Hom, 1972). As the cultured cells showed subnormal oxidation not only of pyruvate but also of citrate and palmitate, the metabolic defect was probably not confined to the pyruvate dehydrogenase complex. No muscle biopsy was taken.

Pyruvate dehydrogenase phosphatase deficiency. This disorder, described by Robinson and Sherwood (1975), caused congenital and chronic lactic acidosis and death in the first year of life. During life, serum lactate, pyruvate, free fatty acid and ketone body levels were increased and there was an associated metabolic acidosis. The enzyme deficiency was demonstrated *post mortem* in muscle, liver and brain. Muscle histopathology was not described.

Dihydrolipoyl dehydrogenase (E_3) deficiency. This was observed by Robinson, Taylor and Sherwood (1978) in a floppy male infant with congenital and chronic lactic, pyruvic, 2-oxoglutaric and branched-chain amino acidaemia. Hypoglycaemia was intermittently present. The enzyme deficiency was demonstrated *post mortem* in all tissues. Muscle histopathology was not described.

Mitochondrial disorders associated with defective energy conservation

Hypermetabolic myopathy. The first case of this disorder was described in detail by Luft, Ikkos, Palmieri, Ernster and Afzelius in 1962. A 35-year-old woman had exhibited profuse perspiration, heat intolerance, polydipsia without polyuria,

hyperphagia and progressive asthenia since early childhood. Her BMR varied between +140 and 210 per cent. Thyroid function studies excluded hyperthyroidism. Morphological studies of muscle revealed a mitochondrial myopathy (the first ultrastructural description) with abundant and large mitochondria harbouring crystalloid and other inclusions. Biochemical studies showed loosely coupled oxidative phosphorylation. Basal ATPase activity was abnormally high and not further stimulated by uncoupling agents. A second case of the same disease was reported by Afifi, Ibrahim, Bergman, Haydar, Mire, Bahuth and Kaylani (1972). Biochemical studies in the second case by Di Mauro, Bonilla, Lee, Schotland, Scarpa, Conn and Chance (1976) confirmed the observations made by Luft *et al.* (1962) and also revealed subnormal accumulation of calcium by the isolated muscle mitochondria. This was attributed to an abnormal release of calcium and it was suggested that the continued recycling of calcium between mitochondria and the cytosol was responsible for the sustained stimulation of respiration and loose coupling.

Mitochondrial myopathies with defective respiratory control without hypermetabolism. The disorders in this group are clinically heterogeneous and it is likely that the loose coupling is secondary to another, but still undefined, abnormality of mitochondrial respiration. Muscle specimens in each instance showed a typical mitochondrial myopathy.

A girl studied by Hülsmann, Bethlem, Meijer, Fleury and Schellens (1967) had severe muscle weakness and atrophy by three years of age. The oxidation of pyruvate-malate and of glutamate was abnormally slow and was not further stimulated by the addition of phosphate acceptor. A boy investigated by Van Wijngaarden, Bethlem, Meijer, Hülsmann and Feltkamp (1967) had shown progressive muscle weakness and mental retardation since the age of 4 years. Lactic acidaemia was present at rest, and increased further on exertion. The basal metabolic rate varied between +5 and 24 per cent. A clinically similar case was reported in a boy with symptoms since the age of 8 years by Schellens and Ossentjuk (1969). Biochemical findings in mitochondria in these cases were similar to those noted by Hülsmann *et al.* (1967). In a kinship investigated by Worsfold, Park and Pennington (1973), four generations were affected with weakness ranging from subclinical to moderately severe in a facioscapulohumeral distribution. Mitochondrial respiration with various substrates showed loose coupling, as in the preceding reports. Another clinical pattern was reported by Spiro, Prineas and Moore (1970). This was the case of a boy who had craved salt since infancy and was noted to have non-progressive weakness since the age of 8 years. He also experienced three episodes of transient, severe generalised weakness lasting several hours, at the age of 13 years. The clinical features resembled those of a child with 'pleoconial myopathy' described by Shy, Gonatas and Perez (1966). However, no biochemical studies were reported by Shy *et al.* (1966).

Another disorder with a defective mitochondrial energy supply was described by Schotland, Di Mauro, Bonilla, Scarpa and Lee (1976). A 37-year-old patient had suffered from non-progressive muscle weakness of limb and torso muscles since early childhood. The electrocardiogram showed biventricular hypertrophy. Mitochondrial respiratory rate and control were markedly reduced with pyruvate-malate, succinate plus rotenone and palmitylcarnitine, but phosphorylative efficiency was normal. The basal, as well as the magnesium-stimulated and 2,4-dinitrophenol-stimulated mitochondrial ATPase activities were also greatly decreased. Thus, the defect involved energy transfer at a level common to all three coupling sites of the respiratory chain, yet, surprisingly, the clinical symptoms were relatively mild.

Defective respiratory control with α-glycerophosphate, but not with other substrates, has been observed in mitochondria isolated from muscles of a patient with oculocraniosomatic muscle weakness (Di Mauro, Schotland, Bonilla, Lee, Gambetti and Rowland, 1973). Muscle glycogen content was also increased but the glycolytic pathway was intact. A similar biochemical abnormality was reported in a 30-year-old man, with slowly progressive muscle weakness since the age of 12 years, who had no ocular or cranial muscle weakness (Black, Judge, Demers

and Gordon, 1975). It is thus clear that this particular biochemical finding is not specific for the oculocraniosomatic myopathy syndrome. Structural mitochondrial abnormalities in limb muscles in this syndrome have been repeatedly observed since Zintz's original observations in 1966. In most patients with mitochondrial myopathies which involve the eye muscles, biochemical studies were not performed. However, in at least one patient, exercise-induced lactic acidaemia was demonstrated (Sulaiman, Doyle, Johnson and Jennett, 1974) which supports the notion of a functional mitochondrial defect.

Defective respiratory control by muscle mitochondria has also been described in some, but not all, patients with Kearns-Sayre syndrome (retinitis pigmentosa, heart block and external ophthalmoplegia) (Kearns and Sayre, 1958; Berenberg, Pellock, Di Mauro, Schotland, Bonilla, Eastwood, Hays, Vicale, Behrens, Chutorian and Rowland, 1977). Lactic and pyruvic acidaemia may also occur in some, but not all, cases (Lou and Reske-Nielsen, 1976). A wider spectrum of the disease includes eighth nerve deficits, ataxia and mental retardation. Structural mitochondrial abnormalities have been reported in this syndrome in muscle and liver (Shy, Silberberg, Appel, Mishkin and Godfrey, 1967), sweat glands (Karpati, Carpenter, Labrisseau and La Fontaine, 1973) and cerebellum (Schneck, Adachi, Brieti, Wolintz and Volk, 1973).

Disorders associated with specific deficiences of one or more mitochondrial respiratory chain components

Deficiency of NADH-Coenzyme Q reductase. This disorder was observed in two sisters who had mild weakness since early childhood. The weakness increased after exertion, fasting or alcohol ingestion and there was lactic acidaemia which became marked after exertion (Morgan-Hughes *et al.*, 1979). Biochemical studies in one sister at the age of 26 years showed that mitochondrial respiratory rates were markedly reduced with NAD-linked, but not other, substrates. The mitochondrial cytochrome components were intact and uncoupling agents did not enhance state 3 respiratory rates in the presence of NAD-linked substrates. The muscle mitochondria were structurally abnormal.

Cytochrome b deficiency. Clinical and morphological features similar to those in the two sisters with NADH-Coenzyme Q reductase deficiency were observed in a 38-year-old man by Morgan-Hughes, Darveniza, Kahn, Landon, Sherratt, Land and Clark (1977). Biochemical studies demonstrated decreased mitochondrial respiratory rates with several substrates either in the presence or absence of phosphate acceptor. Pyruvate dehydrogenase and citrate synthase activities were normal. Spectral analysis of muscle mitochondria revealed a deficiency of reducible cytochrome b.

A deficiency of cytochrome b in muscle mitochondria was also observed by Spiro, Moore, Prineas, Strasberg and Rapin (1970) in a 46-year-old man and his 16-year-old son with progressive muscle weakness, dementia, ataxia, loss of proprioception, hyporeflexia and positive Babinski signs. The son, but not the father, also had bilateral partial external ophthalmoplegia and ptosis. Morphological studies of muscle showed neurogenic as well as myopathic alterations with structurally abnormal mitochondria. The oxidation of glutamate and of succinate plus rotenone by muscle mitochondria was markedly reduced. Spectral analysis revealed a deficiency of cytochrome b as well as of cytochrome a.

Cytochrome c oxidase deficiency with or without cytochrome b deficiency. A distinct clinical syndrome associated with lactic acidosis, features of the DeToni-Fanconi syndrome (hypophosphataemia, hyperphosphaturia, generalised aminoaciduria, glycosuria and polyuria), progressive dementia, muscle weakness and death in infancy is associated with cytochrome c oxidase (cytochrome $a+a_3$) and cytochrome b deficiency (Van Biervliet, Bruinvis, Ketting, De Bree, Van Der Heiden, Wadman, Willems, Bookelman, Van Haelst and Monnens, 1977; Di Mauro, Mendell, Sahenk, Bachman, Scarpa, Scofield and Reiner, 1980). Serum alanine levels were raised. The oxidation of 2-oxoglutarate by muscle mitochondria was reduced because of the primary abnormality of the cytochrome system. Muscle mitochondria were

structurally abnormal. A deficiency of cytochrome oxidase could also be detected in fresh-frozen sections of muscle reacted for this enzyme. No biochemical abnormality was detected in cardiac muscle.

Cytochrome c oxidase deficiency associated with a partial deficiency of the pyruvate dehydrogenase complex was reported by Monnens, Gabreëls and Willems (1975) in an 8-year-old patient with diffuse muscle weakness, nerve deafness, reduced visual acuity and chronic lactic acidaemia. Serum alanine levels were raised. This disorder appears to be clinically and genetically different from that described by Van Biervliet *et al.* (1977).

Cytochrome c oxidase deficiency was also reported in Leigh's disease (subacute necrotising encephalomyelopathy) (Willems, Monnens, Trijbels, Veerkamp, Meyer, Van Dam and Van Haelst, 1977). The patient had recurrent vomiting, hypotonia, motor and mental retardation and ataxia since infancy and died at the age of 6 years of respiratory failure. Serum pyruvate and lactate levels were slightly increased. The enzyme defect was observed in muscle but not in liver. Partial enzyme deficiency was noted in heart. Skeletal muscle mitochondria were structurally abnormal. Defects involving thiamine metabolism, pyruvate carboxylase and pyruvate dehydrogenase had been previously reported in different cases of Leigh's disease (*reviewed* by Willems *et al.* 1977).

A deficiency of terminal mitochondrial respiration due to decreased levels of cytochrome $a+a_3$ in muscle, liver and heart has been reported in trichopoliodystrophy (Menkes' disease) (French, Sherard, Lubell, Brotz and Moore, 1972). This disorder may be related to malabsorption of copper (Danks, Stevens, Campbell, Gillespie, Walker-Smith, Blomfield and Turner, 1972). The clinical features include sparse, coarse, stiff hair with twisted, beaded and fragile shafts, microcephaly, micrognathia, developmental regression and muscle hypotonia.

Structural mitochondrial myopathies of unknown aetiology with lactic acidaemia. Rawles and Weller (1974) observed excessive fatigability, slight generalised weakness, sideroblastic anaemia, congestive heart failure and lactic acidaemia in a 19-year-old man with symptoms persisting since he was 12 years old. The patient's father had asymptomatic lactic acidaemia. Sengers, Ter-Haar, Trijbels, Willems, Daniels and Stadhouders (1975) described congenital cataracts, mitochondrial myopathy, obstructive cardiomyopathy and exercise-induced lactic acidaemia in a 14-year-old boy with symptoms since the age of 8 years.

The triad of poliodystrophy, mitochondrial myopathy and lactic acidaemia has been described by different authors. Schapira, Cederbaum, Cancilla, Nielsen and Lippe (1975) studied a brother and sister whose illness presented around the age of four years and was fatal during the second decade of life. The clinical features included limb weakness, ptosis, possible myocardial involvement, growth retardation, seizures, progressive dementia, macular degeneration, optic atrophy, hirsutism and excessive sweating. Multiple areas of cerebral encephalomalacia with neuronal loss and gliosis, and ferrocalcific deposits in the globus pallidus were found at autopsy. Hart, Chang, Perrin, Neerunjun and Ayyar (1977) described a clinically and pathologically similar disorder in two siblings, but the lactic acidaemia was less marked than in the patients studied by Schapira *et al.* (1975). Markesbery (1979) observed a more benign disorder in a 27-year-old man with muscle weakness, seizures, neurosensory hearing loss, mild peripheral neuropathy, mitochondrial myopathy and calcifications of the basal ganglia. The clinical features resembled those described by Smyth *et al.* (1975) in a patient who also had a low muscle carnitine level. Muscle or serum carnitine was not measured in Markesbery's case.

Lactic and pyruvic acidaemia has also been described in mitochondria-lipid-glycogen myopathy in a 25-month-old girl who had proximal muscle weakness and a tendency to develop ketoacidosis (Di Donato, Cornelio, Balestrini, Bertagnolio and Peluchetti, 1978). The patient had a vacuolar myopathy with lipid and glycogen accumulation and abundant and structurally abnormal mitochondria. The muscle free carnitine level was depressed, but the total muscle carnitine level was normal.

A clinically and biochemically different mitochondria-lipid-glycogen myopathy was reported by Jerusalem, Angelini, Engel and Groover (1973). This was the case of a 7-week-old infant with profound weakness of all but the ocular muscles, hyporeflexia and hepatoglossomegaly. Muscle specimens contained mild glycogen and marked lipid and mitochondrial excess. Glycogen structure was normal and no single glycolytic enzyme defect was identified. Subsequently, the patient improved clinically. At the age of 22 months she no longer had organomegaly, the pathologic changes in muscle were strikingly improved and oxidation of labelled fatty acids and Krebs' cycle intermediates by homogenates of muscle was normal. Muscle free carnitine levels were not depressed

Malignant hyperthermia

Since its recognition (Denborough and Lovell, 1960), this syndrome has aroused great interest among anaesthetists. The current status of the disorder is summarised in reviews by Stephen (1977), Britt (1979), Harriman (1979) and Gronert (1980). In most cases, susceptibility to the disorder is thought to be transmitted by autosomal dominant inheritance with variable penetrance. The reaction is triggered by potent inhalation anaesthetics (halothane, ether, cyclopropane, methoxyflurane, enflurane) or succinylcholine. Premonitory signs include tachycardia, tachypnoea, dysrhythmias, skin mottling, cyanosis, rising body temperature, muscle rigidity, sweating and unstable blood pressure. Failure to obtain muscle relaxation with adequate doses of succinylcholine can also be an early warning sign. The fully developed syndrome is associated with a rapid rise of body temperature (up to 1° C every 5 min); rapidly evolving metabolic acidosis with lactic acidaemia; often, also, respiratory acidosis due to carbon dioxide overproduction; muscle rigidity in 75 per cent of the cases; hyperkalaemia; variable alterations of the serum calcium; very high serum creatine kinase levels; myoglobinaemia and myoglobinuria. Despite wide awareness of the syndrome and symptomatic therapy, the mortality rate remains 60–70 per cent.

The postulated pathophysiological factor is a failure of calcium homeostasis in the muscle fibre. Cytoplasmic calcium concentration may increase because of abnormal calcium release from the sarcoplasmic reticulum or possibly because the muscle fibre plasma membrane is rendered abnormally permeable to calcium by provocative agents. A high intracellular calcium level activates phosphorylase b kinase and myosin ATPase, inhibits troponin and overloads mitochondria with calcium. These events, in turn, cause accelerated glycogenolysis and glycolysis, ATP splitting, uncontrolled muscle contraction, uncoupling of oxidative phosphorylation and excessive production of heat, lactic acid and carbon dioxide. An animal model of the disease has been described and investigated in Landrace or Poland China pigs (Hall, Woolf, Bradley and Jolly, 1966; Gronert, 1980).

Therapy of the acute syndrome consists of termination of anaesthesia, body cooling, intravenous hydration, sodium bicarbonate administration to combat metabolic acidosis, mechanical hyperventilation to decrease the respiratory acidosis, and mannitol or frusemide, as needed, to maintain urine flow. More specific treatment consists of dantrolene, given intravenously, 1–2 mg/kg, which may be repeated each 5–10 min, up to 10 mg/kg (Faust, Gergis and Sokoll, 1979; Gronert, 1980).

Screening of relatives of affected patients for susceptibility to malignant hyperthermia is important. Seventy per cent of the cases at risk have increased serum creatine kinase (CK) activities (Britt, Endrenyi and Peters, 1976). Without this finding, *in vitro* testing of muscle strips for an abnormal contracture response to halothane, caffeine or a combination of both agents can be done. The technique and interpretation of the test are not fully standardised, but the test has been valuable in detecting patients at risk at a number of medical centres (*reviewed by* Gronert, 1980).

An association of malignant hyperthermia with myotonic dystrophy or myotonia congenita (King, Denborough and Zapf, 1972), branchial hypertrophic myopathy (Lambert and Young, 1976) and central core disease (Denborough, Dennett and Anderson, 1973; Eng, Epstein, Engel, McKay and McKay, 1978), has been reported. It is not yet known what proportion of patients with these disorders is, in fact, at risk. The disease can also occur in a congenital myopathy associated with short stature, cryptochordism and skeletal abnormalities which is transmitted by autosomal recessive inheritance (King *et al.*, 1972). Muscle biopsy studies by Harriman (1979) in 105 patients revealed a number of mild and non-specific myopathic changes in two-thirds: increased central nuclei, small angulated fibres, focal decreases in oxidative enzyme activity, focal myofibrillar alterations and, rarely, regenerating fibres. Typical central cores, spanning the entire fibre length, were not observed. No myopathic changes were seen in children under the age of 5 years.

Muscle AMP deaminase deficiency

AMP deaminase converts AMP to IMP with liberation of ammonia. The biological role of the enzyme is not understood; possibly it participates in regulation of ATP levels in muscle. In 1978, Fishbein, Armbrustmacher and Griffin found deficiency of the muscle enzyme in five young men with complaints, often since childhood, of muscle weakness or cramping after exercise. Three patients had mild increases in serum CK and two had abnormal electromyograms. Muscle histology was normal except for mild type I fibre atrophy in one case. Erythrocyte enzyme activity was normal. Ammonia levels failed to rise but lactate values rose normally in venous blood flowing from ischaemically exercised muscles. Subsequently, Schumate, Katnik, Ruiz, Kaiser, Frieden, Brooke and Carroll (1979) observed AMP deaminase deficiency in six patients, four men and two women. In three of these the diagnosis was established after the age of 50 years. One patient suffered from anterior horn cell disease and, in two patients, muscle weakness and pain appeared for the first time after an influenza-like illness. Muscle AMP deaminase deficiency had also been reported in a single case of primary hypokalaemic periodic paralysis (Engel, Potter and Rosevear, 1964). In view of the marked clinical heterogeneity, the significance of muscle AMP deaminase deficiency remains uncertain.

Nutritional and toxic myopathies

Nutritional deficiencies

Although malnutrition is common throughout many parts of the world, its effects on skeletal muscle have not been thoroughly investigated. The negative nitrogen balance and lack of essential nutrients can be expected to cause muscle weakness and wasting, but their relative significance is not clearly understood. Vitamin E deficiency may have a role in causing muscle disease in malabsorption syndromes, as in cystic fibrosis of the pancreas and biliary atresia of childhood (Blanc, Reid and Andersen, 1958) and in a 7-year-old boy with severe malabsorption since birth (Tomasi, 1979). The latter patient presented with progressive external ophthalmoplegia, proximal muscle weakness, peripheral neuropathy and bilateral Babinski signs; the serum CK level was raised and the vitamin E level was low. Replacement therapy with vitamin E decreased the CK level and improved muscle strength. It is also possible that the unusual giant lysosomes observed in muscle fibres of a patient with malabsorption and hypoparathyroidism were related to vitamin E deficiency (Gomez, Engel and Dyck, 1972). The muscle weakness in nutritional osteomalacia has been attributed partly to disuse and partly to malnutrition (Dastur, Gagrat, Wadia, Desai and Bharucha, 1975).

Myopathy in chronic alcoholism

Alcohol may have a direct toxic effect on muscle, or its effects could be mediated by malnutrition and fluid and electrolyte disturbances. Song and Rubin (1972) found that ingestion of ethanol (42 per cent of calories) without malnutrition induced increased CK activity in the serum and non-specific ultrastructural changes in muscle in human volunteers. In ethanol-fed rats, mitochondria show reduced ability to oxidise various substrates, energy production with NAD-dependent substrates, calcium uptake, activity of several enzymes and cytochrome content. These effects may be mediated by acetaldehyde rather than ethanol (Cederbaum and Rubin, 1975).

Two types of clinically distinct myopathy, acute and subacute, have been described in chronic alcoholics. The acute type (Hed, Lundmark, Fahlgren and Orell, 1962) occurs after a bout of acute drinking. In these patients, muscle swelling and tenderness is associated with weakness and myoglobinuria. Hyperkalaemia and renal insufficiency develop in the more severely affected.

A painless variety of acute alcoholic myopathy associated with severe hypokalaemia, marked serum CK elevation, vacuolar myopathy and focal fibre necrosis has been also described (Rubenstein and Wainapel, 1977). The hypokalaemia may be secondary to the combined effects of sweating, vomiting, diarrhoea or renal potassium wastage. The hypokalaemia may be followed by hyperkalaemia as rhabdomyolysis, myoglobinuria and secondary renal failure develop. Histochemical studies in acute alcoholic myopathy reveal focal decreases in oxidative enzyme activity in type I muscle fibres and in necrotic fibres. Ultrastructural changes occur in mitochondria, but some of these changes are secondary to fibre necrosis (Martinez, Hooshmand and Faris, 1973). The subacute alcoholic myopathy described by Ekbom, Hed, Kirstein and Astrom (1964) is associated with symmetrical proximal weakness with little loss of muscle bulk, electromyographic alterations and increased levels of muscle enzymes in serum. In some alcoholics, serum enzyme and electromyographic abnormalities occur without muscle weakness. However, Faris and Reyes (1971) suggest that the sub-clinical group is neuropathic rather than myopathic. Alternatively, a chronic, mild neuropathy exists in alcoholics who also develop a myopathy. The subacute syndrome is reversible within a few months of alcohol withdrawal.

Perkoff, Hardy and Velez-Garcia (1966) drew attention to impaired production of lactate by ischaemically exercised muscles in chronic alcoholics within 48 hours after intoxication. Muscle phosphorylase activity was reduced or low normal in six of seven biopsies. Muscle symptoms, when present, resembled those of phosphorylase deficiency.

Chloroquine myopathy

This quinoline derivative, introduced as an antimalarial drug but useful in the treatment of amoebiasis and certain collagen-vascular diseases, causes undesirable side effects involving the macula, cornea, skeletal muscle and peripheral nerve. The first cases of myopathy were described by Whisnant, Espinosa, Kierland and Lambert (1963). Most of those patients who became weak during chloroquine treatment received 500 mg of the drug per day for a year or longer. Pathologically, it is a vacuolar myopathy mainly affecting type I fibres (Garcin, Rondot and Fardeau, 1964; MacDonald and Engel, 1970; Hughes, Esiri, Oxbury and Whitty, 1971). The vacuoles contain cytoplasmic degradation products and are autophagic in character. In an experimental study, MacDonald and Engel (1970) found that the initial ultrastructural change was a proliferation of the internal membrane system (both T system and SR) and the encirclement of small cytoplasmic areas. Larger vacuoles arose by fusion of smaller ones. The entrapped membranous organelles were degraded to myeloid structures. The limiting membranes of the vacuoles were derived from tubules and labyrinthine networks of T-system origin, and the degraded vacuolar contents reacted strongly for acid phosphatase. Exocytosis of vacuolar contents and frequent fibre splitting occurred after other pathological changes were well established. Chloroquine myopathy is a prototype for those muscle disorders in which an autophagic mechanism becomes excited.

Emetine myopathy
Emetine, an ipecac alkaloid used in the treatment of amoebiasis, inhibits protein synthesis in a variety of cell types (Grollman, 1968). Side effects of the drug include cardiotoxicity and muscle weakness (Klatskin and Friedman, 1948). In experimental animals the drug induces focal decreases in muscle mitochondria, associated with focal myofibrillar degeneration in type I fibres (Duane and Engel, 1970). The lesions in type I fibres closely resemble those observed in multicore disease (Engel, Gomez and Groover, 1971). More advanced pathological changes induced by emetine include muscle fibre necrosis (Bradley, Fewings, Harris and Johnson, 1976).

Diseases associated with myoglobinuria

Myoglobin is a 17 000 dalton protein with a prosthetic haem group and the muscle concentration is about 1 mg/g (Kagen and Christian, 1966). The appearance of myoglobin in the urine is both an indication of severe and acute muscle injury, and a warning that renal damage may result. Any injury to muscle fibres which abnormally increases the permeability or disrupts the integrity of the surface membrane entails leakage of myoglobin into the plasma. The renal threshhold for myoglobin is relatively low (Koskelo, Kekki and Wager, 1967) but still massive and relatively synchronous injury to muscle (rhabdomyolysis) is required before brown discolouration of urine, caused by myoglobin plus metmyoglobin, can be observed. The urinary pigment reacts positively with benzidine. If there is no haemoglobinaemia and no haematuria, the test strongly suggests myoglobinuria. However, microhaematuria can also develop in the course of myoglobinuria. Positive identification of myoglobin requires specific chemical, spectrophotometric or immunological tests. The last are the most sensitive and a recently described immunoprecipitation assay is both quantitative and simple (Markowitz and Wobig, 1977).

Acute attacks of myoglobinuria are characterised by the onset, over a few hours, of muscle weakness, swelling and pain. In addition to myoglobin, phosphate, potassium, creatine, creatinine and muscle enzymes are released into the circulation. The haem pigment in the glomerular filtrate and myoglobin casts in renal tubules may cause proteinuria, haematuria and renal tubular necrosis. Renal failure is more likely if the attack is complicated by hypovolaemia, hypotension or metabolic acidosis. With increasing renal insufficiency, hyperphosphataemia with secondary hypocalcaemia and tetany, and life-threatening hyperkalaemia may develop (Hed, 1955; Bowden, Fraser, Jackson and Walker, 1956; Pearson, Beck and Blahd, 1957; Savage, Forbes and Pearce, 1971; Rowland and Penn, 1972). Death may result from renal or respiratory failure. If the patient survives, the myoglobinuria and proteinuria tend to disappear by the third to fifth day after the onset of the attack; marked hyperenzymaemia, present initially, subsides more gradually; muscle strength returns relatively slowly after major attacks. Electromyographic abnormalities (fibrillation potentials, increased insertional activity and motor unit potential alterations) may persist for several months after severe attacks (Haase and Engel, 1960).

The syndrome has many known causes but in a

substantial proportion of the cases the aetiology remains elusive. The immediate biochemical mechanism which disrupts the plasma membrane remains to be determined. For descriptive purposes, it is convenient to classify the syndrome as metabolic, post-infectious, toxic, ischaemic and/or traumatic, secondary to inflammatory or other myopathies, and idiopathic.

Metabolic. The common denominator is impaired substrate utilisation for energy metabolism, or a critical substrate deficiency in the face of excessive demands for energy. Most diseases in this group were considered earlier in this chapter. Phosphorylase and phosphofructokinase deficiencies block anaerobic glycolysis, and carnitine palmityltransferase deficiency impairs oxidation of long-chain fatty acids. Rare instances of muscle carnitine deficiency may also be associated with myoglobinuria (W.K. Engel *et al.*, (1980). Impaired utilisation of fatty acids probably played a part in the recurrent myoglobinuria of the twin sisters who had a lipid storage myopathy due to an unknown biochemical defect (Engel *et al.* 1970). The syndrome described by Larsson, Linderholm, Müller, Ringqvist and Sörnas (1964) was associated with fatigue, palpitation, dyspnoea, weakness, severe lactic acidaemia and at times myoglobinuria after even moderate exertion. Inheritance appeared to be by an autosomal recessive gene, but in one family the disease was transmitted as a dominant characteristic. Muscle biopsy studies showed that the respiratory functions of mitochondria and glycolytic enzyme activities were normal. The metabolic lesion was not identified.

Critical substrate deficiency in the face of excessive demands for energy probably accounts for the myoglobinuria which occurs in the course of malignant hyperthermia. Substrate deficiency may also be the cause of the myoglobinuria which occurs after unusually severe exercise in untrained but otherwise healthy individuals, as in military recruits (Demos, Gitin and Kagen, 1974) or conga drummers (Furie and Penn, 1974).

Post-infectious. Myoglobinuria has been reported after infections with influenza A, herpes simplex, Epstein-Barr and Coxsackie viruses (Simon, Rovner and Berlin, 1970; DiBona and Morens, 1977; Schlesinger, Gandara and Bensch, 1978). Virus-like structures have been demonstrated by electron microscopy in affected muscle by Fukuyama, Ando and Yokota (1977) and by Gamboa, Eastwood, Hays, Maxwell and Penn (1979). The latter workers were also able to isolate influenza B virus from muscle of a patient who had a fatal attack of myoglobinuria. The muscle biopsy in this individual showed inflammatory changes as well as perifascicular atrophy. The precise mechanism by which viral infections cause rhabdomyolysis is not understood.

Toxic. Myoglobinuria complicating chronic alcoholism was considered above. Almost any other extreme metabolic insult may be associated with myoglobinuria. These include carbon monoxide poisoning, extreme hypoglycaemia, severe hypokalaemia, diabetic acidosis, barbiturate intoxication and uraemic hyperparathyroidism (*reviewed by* Rowland and Penn, 1972). In Haff's disease the eating of fish contaminated by an unidentified toxin induced an epidemic of myoglobinuria along the Baltic coast (Berlin, 1948). In Malayan waters, fisherman bitten by the sea snake *Enhydrina schistosa* develop myalgias, flaccid paralysis, trismus and myoglobinuria (Reid, 1961).

Ischaemic and traumatic. Prolonged massive ischaemia of muscle from whatever cause results in necrosis of muscle fibres and may induce myoglobinuria and renal failure (Bywaters, Delory, Rimington and Smiles, 1941; Bywaters and Stead, 1945). Localised ischaemic necrosis of muscle and occasionally myoglobinuria may occur in severe forms of the anterior tibial syndrome.

Secondary to other myopathies. Myoglobinuria has been described in the course of dermatomyositis (Kessler, Weinberger and Rosenfeld, 1972), and in fulminant polymyositis (Fukuyama *et al.*, 1977; Sloan, Franks, Exley and Davison, 1978; Gamboa *et al.*, 1979). In some of these patients, the myoglobinuria could have been related to a concurrent or underlying viral infection (Fukuyama *et al.*, 1977; Gamboa *et al.*,

1979). Recurrent myoglobinuria was observed by the author in one patient who had classical systemic lupus erythematosus. Finally, anaesthesia-induced myoglobinuria without rigidity or hyperthermia was reported in a patient with Duchenne dystrophy (Miller, Sanders, Rowlinson, Berry, Sussman and Epstein, 1978).

Idiopathic. It is likely that at least some cases initially classified as idiopathic will eventually be shown to have a metabolic or post-infectious aetiology. Thus, the two types of idiopathic myoglobinuria described by Korein, Coddon and Mowrey in 1959 (in young adult males, often with a positive family history; and in children often after an acute infection) may, in fact, have included patients suffering from more recently identified enzyme defects or predisposing viral infections.

ENDOCRINE DISORDERS OF MUSCLE

Muscle disorders associated with hyperthyroidism
Some of these disorders are a direct consequence of the endocrinopathy: others occur more commonly with thyroid dysfunction than predicted by chance and may or may not be affected by the altered endocrine state. Thyrotoxic myopathy, thyrotoxic hypokalaemic periodic paralysis, myasthenia gravis and exophthalmic ophthalmoplegia represent the currently recognised neuromuscular diseases associated with hyperthyroidism. Thyrotoxic hypokalaemic periodic paralysis has been considered in a preceding section.

Thyrotoxic myopathy. Both acute and chronic forms of this condition have been described but it is doubtful that the rare acute type exists as a distinct entity. More likely, it represents instances of acute myasthenia gravis associated with severe thyrotoxicosis (Millikan and Haines, 1953).

Muscle weakness occurs in approximately 80 per cent of untreated cases of hyperthyroidism (Ramsay, 1965). Men are affected more frequently than women and the average duration of muscle symptoms before diagnosis is about six months. Proximal muscle weakness is present in approximately two-thirds, and both proximal and distal muscle weakness in another fifth of the cases. The

thyrotoxicosis is relatively mild and of long duration, or present for only a few weeks before the onset of weakness. The weakness is often out of proportion to visible muscle atrophy, although severe atrophy can occur. The deep tendon reflexes are usually normal or hyperactive, only seldom decreased or absent. The serum CK level is not increased as a rule (in contrast to myxoedema in which it is usually increased, but weakness is uncommon) (Ramsay, 1965, 1968; Fleisher, McConahey and Pankow, 1965). Electromyographic abnormalities are found in about 90 per cent of patients with hyperthyroidism (Havard, Campbell, Ross and Spence, 1963; Ramsay, 1965). These abnormalities consist of a decrease in the mean duration of motor unit potentials and an increase in the incidence of polyphasic potentials. Spontaneous electrical activity (fibrillation potentials, fasciculation, or repetitive discharges) is absent as a rule. After correction of the hyperthyroidism, the electromyographic abnormalities revert to normal.

Light-microscopic studies of muscle may show no abnormality or varying degrees of fatty infiltration and fibre atrophy. Ultrastructural studies have revealed mitochondrial hypertrophy; focal loss of mitochondria from muscle fibres; focal myofibrillar degeneration beginning at the Z disc; focal dilatations of the transverse tubular system; sub-sarcolemmal glycogen deposits; and papillary projections of the surface of the muscle fibres, probably resulting from fibre atrophy (Engel, 1966b; Engel, 1972). None of the ultrastructural changes are specific for thyrotoxic myopathy.

The mechanism of the muscle weakness remains obscure. Physiological investigations have demonstrated shortening of the duration of the active state (Takamori, Gutmann and Shane, 1971) and reduced surface membrane excitability (Gruener, Stern, Payne and Hannapel, 1975). The latter is associated with lower than normal resting membrane potential, and impaired action potential generation on repetitive stimulation secondary to membrane depolarisation and marked afterhyperpolarisation. Biochemical studies have demonstrated a significant decrease in high-energy phosphate compounds in muscle (Satoyoshi, Murakami and Kowa, 1963). The original notion that oxidative phosphorylation was uncoupled by the hyperthyroid state could not be substantiated by Ernster, Ikkos and Luft (1959). Further, Stocker, Samaha and De Groot (1968) found that mitochondria from human thyrotoxic muscle were tightly coupled and had normal respiratory control rates. Other possible causes of the weakness might be related to an abnormally active plasma membrane sodium pump, attributed to an increased number of pump units in the membrane (Philipson and Edelman, 1977), or to an increased number of catecholamine receptor sites in the muscle cell membrane (Williams, Lefkowitz and Watanabe, 1977; Tsai and Chen, 1977). It seems probable that muscle weakness in thyrotoxic myopathy results from a number of different effects rather than from a single action of thyroxine.

Thyroid dysfunction and myasthenia gravis. Incidence of thyroid disorders is much greater in patients with myasthenia gravis than could occur by chance: 5.7 per cent of myasthenic patients are hyperthyroid, 5.3 per cent hypothyroid and 2.1 per cent have non-toxic goiter. Further, about 17 per cent of euthyroid and 40 per cent of thyrotoxic myasthenic patients have circulating antibodies directed against thyroid cell antigens (Osserman, Tsairis and Weiner, 1967). The association of the two diseases is not surprising for both are now recognised to have an autoimmune origin. In myasthenia gravis, circulating antibodies are directed against the nicotinic post-synaptic acetylcholine receptor and induce a deficiency of the receptor (*see* Ch. 16) whereas in Graves' disease thyroid-stimulating autoantibodies bind to components of the thyroid cell membrane and stimulate thyroid growth and hormone release (Solomon and Kleeman, 1976).

The association of Graves' disease with myasthenia gravis, and whether the presence of one disease has a beneficial or adverse affect on the other, has interested neurologists since the turn of the century. Careful case studies (Millikan and Haines, 1953) and the experimental induction of hyperthyroidism in myasthenic patients (Engel, 1961) showed that the hyperthyroidism has an adverse effect on the myasthenia. A plausible explanation for this was obtained by Hofmann and

Denys (1972) who found a decrease in the size of miniature end-plate potentials in hyperthyroid animals.

Few cases of myasthenia gravis associated with spontaneous myxoedema have been reported but it is noteworthy that 19 per cent of myasthenic patients, compared with less than 1 per cent of the general population, have evidence of thyroiditis at autopsy (Becker, Titus, McConahey and Wollner, 1964).

Exophthalmic ophthalmoplegia, Graves' ophthalmopathy. This aspect of Graves' disease may pursue a course independent of the metabolic state. Hyperthyroidism was present in 23 of 50 cases studied by Brain (1959) and in nine there was no history or evidence of thyrotoxicosis. The immediate cause of the exophthalmos is an increase in orbital contents with infiltration of external ocular muscles, lacrimal glands and loose connective tissue. The orbital exudate is composed of lymphocytes, plasma cells, polymorphonuclear leucocytes and a fluid rich in mucoproteins and mucopolysaccharides. The infiltration and subsequent atrophy of ocular muscles results in weakness of ocular movements. The two main symptoms are exophthalmos, usually painful, of one or both eyes and diplopia. Levators and abductors of the globe are most commonly affected, and sometimes ptosis also occurs. The ophthalmoplegia tends to be proportionate to the exophthalmos. This varies in degree and when severe can be associated with chemosis and marked oedema of the eyelids. Corneal ulceration, papilloedema, optic atrophy and blindness may ensue.

The pathogenesis is complex (Havard, 1972). Recent evidence supports the assumption that it involves a delayed hypersensitivity response directed against orbital contents. Thyroglobulin can be detected on normal human orbital muscle. Antibodies directed against this protein may instigate a cell-mediated immune reaction, since patients with Graves' ophthalmopathy consistently demonstrate delayed hypersensitivity to thyroglobulin (Mullin, Levinson, Friedman, Henson, Winand and Kohn, 1977).

The disease is initially sub-acute but tends to be self-limiting. Therapy is mandatory when there is a threat to vision. Prednisone treatment, with or without azathioprine, irradiation of orbital contents behind the lens and surgical decompression of the orbit represent current modes of therapy. Full recovery is rare and some degree of exophthalmos usually remains. Residual diplopia may require operative treatment.

Muscular disorders in hypothyroidism
The main manifestations of the various types of muscle disorder described in hypothyroidism are weakness, cramps, aching or painful muscles, sluggish movements and reflexes, myoidema (i.e. ridging of muscle on percussion) and in some an increase in muscle bulk. The reflex changes are seen in most cases, myoidema and myalgia are less common and weakness occurs in but a few. The serum CK activity is typically elevated even if there are no other clinical symptoms of muscle involvement (Fleischer *et al.*, 1965). Electromyography of the slow contraction and relaxation of the tendon reflex (Lambert, Underdahl, Beckett and Mederos, 1951) and of the myoidema (Salick and Pearson, 1967) would suggest that it is the contractile mechanism of the muscle that is predominantly involved. It seems possible that many enzyme systems are affected, the pattern of involvement determining the clinical type. There is some evidence to suggest impaired glycogenolysis (reduced acid maltase levels in muscle and impaired lactic acid formation on ischaemic exercise) (McDaniel, Pittman, Oh and DiMauro, 1977).

Muscle hypertrophy, with weakness and slowness of movement, constitute the syndrome of Debré-Semelaigne (Debré and Semelaigne, 1935) which occurs predominantly in cretinous children; when accompanied by painful spasms it is given the name of Hoffmann's syndrome and is characteristically seen in myxoedematous adults. However, the two conditions tend to merge into each other and may even occur, though at different times, in the same patient (Wilson and Walton, 1959; Norris and Panner, 1966). Slow relaxation and myoidema are prominent features of Hoffmann's syndrome; superficially, therefore, it resembles myotonia congenita or the very rare cases of true myotonia associated with myxoedema, either iatrogenic or resulting from disease. In the two patients reported by Jarcho and Tyler

(1958) the myxoedema probably abetted a preexisting mild myotonia, because symptomless myotonia was demonstrated in some of the relatives. The occasional association of a girdle myopathy causing mild proximal weakness and atrophy has been described by Åstrom, Kugelberg and Müller (1961). Morphological studies reveal non-specific alterations in hypothyroid myopathy. These include fibre enlargement, increased central nuclei, glycogen and mitochondrial aggregates, dilated SR and proliferating T-system profiles, and focal myofibrillar degeneration (Norris and Panner, 1966; Afifi, Najjar, Mire-Salman and Bergman, 1974; Emser and Schimrigk, 1977). The muscle disorders respond favourably to therapy of the hypothyroid state.

Muscle disorders associated with hyperparathyroidism and with osteomalacia
Parathormone and biologically active forms of vitamin D are important regulators of calcium metabolism and of the serum calcium level. Parathormone mobilises calcium from bone, increases the reabsorption of calcium and excretion of phosphate by the kidney, and stimulates the renal conversion of 25-hydroxy-cholecalciferol to 1,25-dihydroxycholecalciferol, a highly potent form of vitamin D. Biologically active vitamin D promotes intestinal calcium absorption and facilitates mineralisation of osteoid and of newly formed enchondral bone (Habener and Potts, 1978; Haussler and McCain, 1977). Studies in vitamin D-deficient animals also suggest that vitamin D has a direct effect on muscle in augmenting SR and mitochondrial calcium uptake, protein synthesis, ATP stores and force generation (Curry, Basten, Francis and Smith, 1974; Birge and Haddad, 1975; Pleasure, Wyszynski, Sumner, Schotland, Feldmann, Nugent, Hitz and Goodman, 1979).

Muscle weakness can occur in the course of primary and secondary hyperparathyroidism and in osteomalacia. Further, conditions that lead to osteomalacia, such as vitamin D deficiency, renal tubular acidosis or chronic renal failure, are typically also associated with secondary hyperparathyroidism. Vicale in 1949 observed a distinct syndrome in two cases of primary hyperparathyroidism and in one case of renal tubular acidosis. This syndrome is characterised by symmetrical weakness and fatigability which involves especially the proximal muscles, pain on muscular effort, slow, waddling gait, muscle atrophy, creatinuria, weight loss, hyperactive deep tendon reflexes, guarding against passive motion of limbs and tenderness of bone. Electromyography showed no fibrillations or fasciculations. Subsequent reports confirmed the existence of the syndrome in both primary hyperparathyroidism and in osteomalacia (Murphy, ReMine and Burbank, 1960; Bischoff and Esslen, 1965; Prineas, Mason and Henson, 1965; Smith and Stern, 1967; Frame, Heine and Block, 1968; Cholod, Haust, Hudson and Lewis, 1970; Schott and Wills, 1975). The serum alkaline phosphatase level is usually raised; the serum calcium level is typically increased in primary hyperparathyroidism but is low or normal in osteomalacia; the serum phosphate level tends to be low, except in the presence of chronic renal failure.

Muscle biopsy studies have revealed simple atrophy (Bischoff and Esslen, 1965), minimal vacuolar change (Cholod et al., 1970), type II fibre atrophy and changes which might suggest mild denervation atrophy (Patten, Bilezikian, Mallette, Prince, Engel and Aurbach, 1974; Mallette, Patten and Engel, 1975). The latter workers speculate that the muscle involvement in both primary and secondary hyperparathyroidism is neuropathic.

A clearly myopathic and highly malignant syndrome may occur in uraemic hyperparathyroidism. Here, metastatic calcification of vessel walls is associated with intimal proliferation, which causes ischaemia of tissues. This results in gangrenous skin lesions arising on ulcerating areas of livedo reticularis, a necrotising myopathy with hyperenzymaemia and myoglobinuria, and visceral infarcts (Richardson, Herron, Reitz and Layzer, 1969; Goodhue, Davis and Porro, 1972).

Therapy of the various syndromes is directed at removal of the primary cause. When this is not possible, as in chronic renal failure with secondary hyperparathyroidism, long-term treatment with small doses of 1,25-dihydroxycholecalciferol, or its analogue, 1-α-hydroxycholecalciferol, can improve the bone disease and increase muscle strength (Henderson, Ledingham, Oliver, Small,

Russel, Smith, Walton, Preston, Warner and Norman, 1974; Davie, Chalmers, Hunter, Pelc and Kodicek, 1976).

Myopathy associated with hypoparathyroidism
This endocrine disorder is not definitely known to be associated with a myopathy. Increased serum CK activity, but normal muscle histology, has been observed in a few cases by Hower and Struck (1972). Cape (1969) found histochemical deficiency of phosphorylase *a*, but not of phosphorylase *b*, in a case of pseudohypoparathyroidism. A patient studied by Gomez et al. (1972) had a complex disorder involving brain, retina, peripheral nerve and muscle associated with hypoparathyroidism and a malabsorption syndrome. The role of the hypoparathyroidism in the myopathy remains uncertain.

Diseases of the pituitary and suprarenal

Acromegaly and hypopituitarism. Acromegaly in its earlier stages can cause increased muscle bulk and strength, especially if its onset precedes cessation of growth. Later it results in generalised muscle weakness and wasting. Mastaglia, Barwick and Hall (1970) noted mild weakness in six of 11 acromegalics with raised serum CK activity in five. Electromyography demonstrated a decrease in the mean duration of motor unit potentials. Muscle biopsy studies revealed segmental fibre degeneration, foci of small round cell infiltration, thickening of capillary basement membranes, variable hypertrophy and atrophy involving either type I or type II fibres, lipofuscin accumulation, large nuclei with prominent nucleoli and prominent Golgi systems (Mastaglia et al., 1970; Mastaglia, 1973). Pickett, Layzer, Levin, Schneider, Campbell and Sumner (1975) found clinical and electromyographic evidence of myopathy in nine of 17 acromegalics. Carpal tunnel syndrome was a frequent associated finding. They found no abnormalities in muscle biopsies of three patients and none of their patients had increased serum CK activity. The weakness improved slowly after surgical therapy of the acromegaly.

Idiopathic hypopituitarism in children gives rise to dwarfism and poor muscle development.

The reduced mass (when related to age) has been attributed to diminished replication of nuclear DNA (Cheek, Brasel, Elliott and Scott, 1966), a process that can be reversed by giving human growth hormone.

Cushing's syndrome and steroid myopathy. Muscle weakness develops in 50–80 per cent of the patients suffering from Cushing's syndrome (Plotz, Knowlton and Ragan, 1952; Müller and Kugelberg, 1959; Golding, Murray, Pearce and Thompson, 1961) and can also occur as a complication of glucocorticoid hormone treatment (Golding *et al.*, 1961; Perkoff, Silber, Tyler, Cartwright and Wintrobe, 1959; Williams, 1959; Byers, Bergman and Joseph, 1962; Coomes, 1965; Askari, Vignos and Moskowitz, 1976). Fluorinated steroids (dexamethasone, triamcinolone) appear to be more pathogenetic for muscle than non-fluorinated ones (prednisone, cortisone) but the latter also cause myopathy in sufficiently high dosages. The minimal dosage which induces myopathy is not known for any steroid, and considerable individual variation must exist. However, for a given dose of prednisone, women are more susceptible to steroid myopathy than men (Bunch, Worthington, Combs, Ilstrup and Engel, 1980).

The onset of steroid myopathy is usually insidious, but occasionally it can be sudden and accompanied by diffuse myalgias (Askari *et al.*, 1976). Muscles of the pelvic girdle are affected earlier and more severely than those of the pectoral girdle. Proximal muscles are typically weaker than distal ones, but relatively severe weakness of anterior tibial muscles can occur. Normal muscle bulk was found in Cushing's syndrome by Müller and Kugelberg (1959) but muscle atrophy can occur in steroid myopathy (Engel, 1966b). Electromyographic studies have failed to show a consistent pattern (*reviewed by* Askari *et al.*, 1976) but typically there is no spontaneous electrical activity. The serum CK activity is not increased but creatinuria is a constant finding (Askari *et al.*, 1976). The muscle biopsy in Cushing's syndrome shows type II fibre atrophy (Pleasure, Walsh and Engel, 1970). A variety of light-microscopic abnormalities have been described in human steroid myopathy (*reviewed by* Askari *et al.*, 1976)

but earlier reports, based on paraffin sections, included descriptions of artefacts. Type II fibre atrophy, focal increases and decreases in oxidative enzyme activity and focal myofibrillar degeneration were observed by this author (A.G.E.) in human steroid myopathy. Of these, type II fibre atrophy represents the most consistent finding. Ultrastructural studies demonstrate mitochondrial alterations (proliferation, aggregation, degeneration and disappearance), increased numbers of lipid droplets and sub-sarcolemmal glycogen deposits (Engel, 1966b; Afifi, Bergman and Harvey, 1968).

The diagnosis of steroid myopathy poses no problem when the hormones are given for diseases which cause no muscle weakness, such as asthma or psoriasis. However, in polymyositis and in other collagen-vascular diseases treated by steroids, weakness may result from the primary diseases as well as the steroid therapy. In such instances, the following favour the diagnosis of steroid myopathy: a temporal relationship between the exacerbation of the weakness and the appearance of other manifestations of hypercortisonism; increased weakness within a few weeks of the time when steroid dosage was raised; absence of spontaneous electrical activity in the electromyogram; normal serum CK activity but significant creatinuria; and type II fibre atrophy but no inflammation in the muscle biopsy. In practice, the differential diagnosis is difficult because none of the criteria is entirely reliable: high doses of steroids are often started when the primary disease itself becomes more severe, and weakness due to the primary disease and due to steroids can coexist in the same case.

The pathogenesis of steroid myopathy is not fully understood. Morphological studies in experimental animals have shown type II fibre atrophy (Vignos and Greene, 1973), mitochondrial proliferation followed by mitochondrial disappearance and focal myofibrillar degeneration (Tice and Engel, 1967). Electrophysiological studies of rat extensor digitorum longus have revealed decreased resting membrane potentials and reduced membrane excitability which could be prevented by phenytoin treatment (Gruener and Stern, 1972). Biochemical studies in rabbits have demonstrated impaired oxidation of different substrates which correlated with the proportion of type II fibres in the muscle studied (Vignos and Greene, 1973) but mitochondria isolated from rat hind limbs had normal oxidative respiration (Peter, Verhaag and Worsfold, 1970). Impaired calcium uptake and binding by the SR has been noted in steroid myopathy in humans and rabbits (Shoji, Takagi, Sugita and Toyokura, 1976) but not in rats (Peter *et al.*, 1970).

Therapy of steroid myopathy requires withdrawal, if possible, of the offending hormone, or use of the minimum effective dose of a nonfluorinated preparation for control of the primary disease. Muscle strength returns to normal within 1–4 months of cessation of steroid therapy (Askari *et al.*, 1976).

Primary hyperaldosteronism. The periodic paralysis occurring in this condition was discussed earlier in the chapter.

Myopathy and pigmentation after adrenalectomy for Cushing's syndrome. Prineas, Hall, Barwick and Watson (1968) reported a series of patients who developed diffuse pigmentation and severe myopathy accompanied by lipid excess in muscle fibres after adrenalectomy for Cushing's syndrome. The pathogenesis remains obscure.

Addison's disease. Generalised weakness is a characteristic feature of Addison's disease. It is closely related to plasma and muscle water and electrolyte changes and possibly to the associated hypotension. When these are adequately treated, the weakness rapidly disappears. Joint contractures, especially of the knees, have been observed in Addison's disease. They may be caused by a disorder of tendon and fascia rather than by a primary disease of muscle (Thorn, 1949).

REFERENCES

Afifi, A.K., Bergman, R.A. & Harvey, J.C. (1968) Steroid myopathy. Clinical histologic and cytologic observations. *Johns Hopkins Medical Journal*, **123**, 158.

Afifi, A.K., Najjar, S.S., Mire-Salman, J. & Bergman, R.A. (1974) The myopathy of the Kocher-Debré-Semelaigne syndrome. Electromyography, light- and electron-microscopic study. *Journal of the Neurological Sciences*, **22**, 445.

Afifi, A.K., Ibrahim, M.Z.M., Bergman, R.A., Haydar, N.A., Mire, J., Bahuth, N. & Kaylani, F. (1972) Morphologic features of hypermetabolic mitochondrial disease. A light microscopic, histochemical and electron microscopic study. *Journal of the Neurological Sciences*, **15**, 271.

Aitken, R.S., Allott, E.N., Castleden, L.I.M. & Walker, M. (1937) Observations on a case of familial periodic paralysis. *Clinical Science and Molecular Medicine*, **3**, 47.

Allott, E.N. & McArdle, B. (1938) Further observations on familial periodic paralysis. *Clinical Science and Molecular Medicine*, **3**, 229.

Andersen, D.H. (1956) Familial cirrhosis of the liver with storage of abnormal glycogen. *Laboratory Investigation*, **5**, 11.

Andres, R., Cader, G. & Zierler, K.L. (1956) The quantitatively minor role of carbohydrate in oxidative metabolism by skeletal muscle in intact man in the basal state. *Journal of Clinical Investigation*, **35**, 671.

Angelini, C. & Engel, A.G. (1972) Comparative study of acid maltase deficiency. *Archives of Neurology*, **26**, 344.

Angelini, C., Engel, A.G. & Titus, J.L. (1972) Adult acid maltase deficiency. Abnormalities in fibroblasts cultured from patients. *New England Journal of Medicine*, **287**, 948.

Angelini, C., Lucke, S. & Cantarutti, F. (1976) Carnitine deficiency of skeletal muscle: Report of a treated case. *Neurology (Minneapolis)*, **26**, 633.

Angelini, C., Govoni, E., Bragaglia, M.M. & Vergani, L. (1978) Carnitine deficiency: Acute postpartum crisis. *Annals of Neurology*, **4**, 558.

Askanas, V., Engel, W.K., Di Mauro, S., Brooks, D.R. & Mehler, M. (1976) Adult onset acid maltase deficiency. Morphological and biochemical abnormalities reproduced in cultured muscle. *New England Journal of Medicine*, **294**, 573.

Askari, A., Vignos, P.J. & Moskowitz, R.W. (1976) Steroid myopathy in connective tissue disease. *American Journal of Medicine*, **61**, 485.

Åstrom, K.E., Kugelberg, E. & Müller, R. (1961) Hypothyroid myopathy. *Archives of Neurology*, **5**, 472.

Badhin, P., Hers, H.G. & Loeb, H. (1964) An electron microscope and biochemical study of type II glycogenosis. *Laboratory Investigation*, **13**, 1139.

Bank, W.J., Di Mauro, S., Bonilla, E., Capuzzi, D.M. & Rowland, L.P. (1975) A disorder of muscle lipid metabolism and myoglobinuria. Absence of carnitine palmityl transferase. *New England Journal of Medicine*, **292**, 443.

Becker, K.L., Titus, J.H., McConahey, W.M. & Wollner, L.B. (1964) Morphologic evidence of thyroiditis in myasthenia gravis. *Journal of the American Medical Association*, **187**, 994.

Bekeny, G. (1961) Über irreversible Muskelveränderungen, bei der paroxysmalen Lähmung auf grund bioptischer Muskeluntersuchungen. *Deutsche Zeitschrift für Nervenheilkunde*, **182**, 119.

Bell, H., Hayes, W.L. & Vosburgh, J. (1965) Hyperkalemic paralysis due to adrenal insufficiency. *Archives of Internal Medicine*, **115**, 418.

Beratis, N.G., Labadie, G.U. & Hirschhorn, K. (1978) Characterization of the molecular defect in infantile and adult acid α-glucosidase deficiency fibroblasts. *Journal of*

Clinical Investigation, **62**, 1264.

Berenberg, R.A., Pellock, J.M., Di Mauro, S., Schotland, D.L., Bonilla, E., Eastwood, A., Hays, A., Vicale, C.T., Behrens, M., Chutorian, A. & Rowland, L.P. (1977) Lumping or splitting? 'Ophthalmoplegia plus' or Kearns-Sayre syndrome? *Annals of Neurology*, **1**, 37.

Bergman, R.A., Afifi, A.K., Dunkle, L.M. & Johns, R.J. (1970) Muscle pathology in hypokalemic periodic paralysis with hyperthyroidism. *Bulletin of the Johns Hopkins Hospital*, **126**, 100.

Berlin, R. (1948) Haff disease in Sweden. *Acta Medica Scandinavica*, **129**, 560.

Bertagnolio, S., Di Donato, S., Peluchetti, D., Rimoldi, M., Storchi, G. & Cornelio, F. (1978) Acid maltase deficiency in adults. Clinical morphological and biochemical study of three patients. *European Neurology*, **17**, 193.

Biczyskowa, W., Fidzianska, A. & Jedrzejowska, H. (1969) Light and electron microscopic study of the muscles in hypokalemic periodic paralysis. *Acta Neuropathologica*, **12**, 329.

Biemond, A. & Daniels, A.P. (1934) Familial periodic paralysis and its transition into spinal muscular atrophy. *Brain*, **57**, 91.

Birge, S.J. & Haddad, J.G. (1975) 25-Hydroxycholecalciferol stimulation of muscle metabolism. *Journal of Clinical Investigation*, **56**, 1100.

Bischoff, A. & Esslen, E. (1965) Myopathy with primary hyperparathyroidism. *Neurology (Minneapolis)*, **15**, 64.

Black, J.T., Judge, D., Demers, L. & Gordon, S. (1975) Ragged-red fibres. A biochemical and morphological study. *Journal of the Neurological Sciences*, **26**, 479.

Blanc, W.A., Reid, J.D. & Andersen, D.H. (1958) Avitaminosis E in cystic fibrosis of the pancreas. A morphologic study of gastrointestinal and striated muscle. *Pediatrics*, **22**, 494.

Blass, J.P., Avigan, J. & Uhlendorf, B.W. (1970) A defect in pyruvate decarboxylase in a child with an intermittent movement disorder. *Journal of Clinical Investigation*, **49**, 423.

Blass, J.P., Kark, A.P. & Engel, W.K. (1971) Clinical studies of a patient with pyruvate decarboxylase deficiency. *Archives of Neurology*, **25**, 449.

Blass, J.P., Schulman, D., Young D.S. & Hom, E. (1972) An inherited defect affecting the tricarboxylic acid cycle in a patient with congenital lactic acidosis. *Journal of Clinical Investigation*, **51**, 1845.

Bohmer, T., Bergrem, H. & Eiklid, K. (1978) Carnitine deficiency induced during intermittent haemodialysis for renal failure. *Lancet*, **1**, 126.

Bonilla, E. & Schotland, D.L. (1970) Histochemical diagnosis of muscle phosphofructokinase deficiency. *Archives of Neurology*, **22**, 8.

Borum, P.R., Broquist, H.P. & Roelofs, R.I. (1977) Muscle carnitine levels in neuromuscular disease. *Journal of the Neurological Sciences*, **34**, 279.

Boudin, G., Mikol, J., Guillard, A. & Engel, A.G. (1976) Fatal systemic carnitine deficiency with carnitine storage in skeletal muscle, heart, liver and kidney. *Journal of the Neurological Sciences*, **30**, 313.

Bowden, D.H., Fraser, D., Jackson, S.H. & Walker, N.F. (1956) Acute recurrent rhabdomyolysis (paroxysmal myohaemoglobunuria). *Medicine (Baltimore)*, **35**, 335.

Boyle, P.J. & Conway, E.J. (1941) Potassium accumulation in muscle and associated changes. *Journal of Physiology*, **100**, 1.

Bradley, W.G. (1969) Adynamia episodica hereditaria. *Brain*, **92**, 345.

Bradley, W.G., Fewings, J.D., Harris, J.B. & Johnson, M.A. (1976) Emetine myopathy in the rat. *British Journal of Pharmacology*, **57**, 29.

Bradley, W.G., Hudgson, P., Gardner-Medwin, D. & Walton, J.N. (1969) Myopathy associated with abnormal lipid metabolism in skeletal muscle. *Lancet*, **1**, 495.

Brain, W.R. (1959) Pathogenesis and treatment of endocrine exophthalmos. *Lancet*, **1**, 109.

Brandt, I.K. & De Luca, V.A. (1966) Type III glycogenosis: a family with unusual tissue distribution of the enzyme lesion. *American Journal of Medicine*, **40**, 779.

Britt, B.A. (1979) Etiology and pathophysiology of malignant hyperthermia. *Federation Proceedings*, **38**, 44.

Britt, B.A., Endrenyi, L. & Peters, P.L. (1976) Screening of malignant hyperthermia susceptible families by creatine phosphokinase measurement and other clinical investigations. *Canadian Anaesthetists' Society Journal*, **23**, 263.

Brody, I.A. (1969) Muscle contracture induced by exercise. A syndrome attributed to decreased relaxing factor. *New England Journal of Medicine*, **281**, 187.

Brody, I.A., Gerber, C.J. & Sidbury, J.B. (1970) Relaxing factor in McArdle's disease. Calcium uptake by sarcoplasmic reticulum. *Neurology (Mineapolis)*, **20**, 555.

Brooks, B.R., Brumback, R.A., Rosenbaum, R.B. & Engel, W.K. (1977) Triglyceride-mediated prevention of exercise-induced rhabdomyolysis of myophosphorylase deficiency. *Neurology (Minneapolis)*, **27**, 379.

Brooks, J.E. (1969) Hyperkalemic periodic paralysis. *Archives of Neurology*, **20**, 13.

Brooks, R.V., McSwiney, R.R., Prunty, T.F.G. & Wood, F.J.Y. (1957) Potassium deficiency of renal and adrenal origin. *American Journal of Medicine*, **23**, 391.

Brosnan, J.T., Kopec, B. & Fritz, I.B. (1973) The localization of carnitine palmityltransferase in the inner membrane of bovine liver mitochondria. *Journal of Biological Chemistry*, **248**, 4075.

Brown, B.I. & Brown, D.H. (1966) Lack of an α-1,4-glucan: α-1,4-glucan 6-glycosyl transferase in a case of type IV glycogenosis. *Proceedings of the National Academy of Sciences, USA*, **56**, 725.

Brown, B.I. & Brown, D.H. (1968) Glycogen storage diseases: Types I, III, IV, V, VII and unclassified glycogenosis. In *Carbohydrate Metabolism and Its Disorders*, Eds F. Dickens, P.J. Randle & W.J. Whelan, volume 2, p. 123 (Academic Press: New York).

Brown, B.I. & Zellweger, H. (1966) α-1,4-Glucosidase activity in leukocytes from the family of two brothers who lack this enzyme in muscle. *Biochemical Journal*, **101**, 16c.

Brown, B.I., Brown, D.H. & Jeffrey, P.L. (1970) Simultaneous absence of α-1,4-glucosidase and α-1,6-glucosidase activities (pH 4) in tissues of children with type II glycogen storage disease. *Biochemistry*, **9**, 1423.

Brown, D.H. & Illingworth, B. (1962) The properties of an oligo-1,4→1,4 glucantransferase from animal tissues. *Proceedings of the National Academy of Sciences, USA*, **48**, 1783.

Brownell, A.K.W., Severson, D.L., Thomson, C.D. & Fletcher, T. (1979) Cold induced rhabdomyolysis in carnitine palmityltransferase deficiency. *Canadian Journal of Neurological Sciences*, **6**, 367.

Brunberg, J.A., McCormick, W.F. & Schochet, S.S. (1971) Type III glycogenosis. An adult with diffuse weakness and muscle wasting. *Archives of Neurology*, **25**, 171.

Bryan, G.T., MacCardle, R.C. & Bartter, F.C. (1966) Hyperaldosteronism, hyperplasia of the juxtaglomerular complex, normal blood pressure, and dwarfism. *Pediatrics*, **37**, 43.

Buchthal, F., Engbaek, L. & Gamstorp, I. (1958) Paresis and hyperexcitability in adynamia episodica hereditaria. *Neurology (Minneapolis)*, **8**, 347.

Bull, G.M., Carter, A.B. & Lowe, K.G. (1953) Hyperpotassaemic paralysis. *Lancet*, **2**, 60.

Bull, G.M., Joekes, A.M. & Lowe, K.G. (1950) Renal function studies in acute tubular necrosis. *Clinical Science*, **9**, 379.

Bunch, T.W., Worthington, J.W., Combs, J.J., Ilstrup, D.M. & Engel, A.G. (1980) Azathioprine with prednisone for polymyositis. A controlled clinical trial. *Annals of Internal Medicine*, In press.

Busch, H.F.M., Koster, J.F. & Van Weerden, T.W. (1979) Infantile and adult-onset acid maltase deficiency occurring in the same family. *Neurology (Minneapolis)*, **29**, 415.

Byers, R.K., Bergman, A.B. & Joseph, M.C. (1962) Steroid myopathy: report of five cases occurring during treatment of rheumatic fever. *Pediatrics*, **29**, 26.

Bywaters, E.G.L. & Stead, J.K. (1945) Thrombosis of the femoral artery with myoglobinuria and low serum potassium concentration. *Clinical Science*, **5**, 195.

Bywaters, E.G.L., Delory, G.E., Rimington, C. & Smiles, J. (1941) Myohaemoglobin in the urine of the air raid casualties with crushing injury. *Biochemical Journal*, **35**, 1164.

Caddell, J. & Whitemore, R. (1962) Observations on generalised glycogenosis with emphasis on electrocardiographic changes. *Pediatrics*, **29**, 743.

Cape, C.A. (1969) Phosphorylase a deficiency in pseudohypoparathyroidism. *Neurology (Minneapolis)*, **19**, 167.

Caroll, D. & Davies, P. (1964) Renal tubular acidosis presenting with muscle weakness. *Journal of Neurology, Neurosurgery and Psychiatry*, **27**, 5.

Carrier, H., Lebel, M., Mathieu, M., Pialat, J. & Devic, M. (1975) Late familial pseudo-myopathic muscular glycogenosis with α-1,4-glucosidase deficiency. *Pathological Europaea (Bruxelles)*, **10**, 51.

Carroll, J.E., Brooke, M.B., DeVivo, D., Kaiser, K.R. & Hagberg, J.M. (1978) Biochemical and physiological consequences of carnitine palmityltransferase deficiency. *Muscle and Nerve*, **1**, 103.

Carson, M.J. & Pearson, C.M. (1964) Familial hyperkalemic periodic paralysis with myotonia features. *Journal of Pediatrics*, **64**, 853.

Cederbaum, A.I. & Rubin, E. (1975) Molecular injury to mitochondria produced by ethanol and acetaldehyde. *Federation Proceedings*, **34**, 2045.

Chalmers, R.A., Johnson, M., Pallis, C. & Watts, R.W.E. (1969) Xanthinuria with myopathy (with some observations on the renal handling of oxypurines in the disease). *Quarterly Journal of Medicine*, **38**, 493.

Chalmers, R.A., Watts, R.W.E., Bitensky, L. & Chayen, J. (1969) Microscopic studies on crystals in skeletal muscle from two cases of xanthinuria. *Journal of Pathology*, **99**, 45.

Chanarin, I., Patel, A., Slavin, G., Wills, E.J., Andrews, T.M. & Stewart, G. (1975) Neutral lipid storage disease: a new disorder of lipid metabolism. *British Medical Journal*, **1**, 553.

Cheek, D.B., Brasel, J.A., Elliott, D. & Scott, R. (1966) Muscle cell size and number in normal children and in dwarfs (pituitary, cretins and primordial) before and after treatment. *Bulletin of the Johns Hopkins Hospital*, **119**, 46.

Chen, R.F. (1959) Familial periodic paralysis. *Archives of Neurology*, **1**, 475.

Cholod, E.J., Haust, M.D., Hudson, A.J. & Lewis, F.N. (1970) Myopathy in primary familial hyperparathyroidism. Clinical and morphologic studies. *American Journal of Medicine*, **48**, 700.

Chou, S. (1967) Myxovirus-like structures in a case of chronic human polymyositis. *Science*, **158**, 1453.

Chui, L.A. & Munsat, T.L. (1976) Dominant inheritance of McArdle syndrome. *Archives of Neurology*, **33**, 636.

Cohen, T. (1959) Hypokalemic muscle paralysis associated with administration of chlorothiazide. *Journal of the American Medical Association*, **170**, 2083.

Cohn, J., Wang, P., Hauge, M., Henningsen, K., Jensen, B. & Svejgaard, A. (1975) Amylo-1,6-glucosidase deficiency (glycogenosis type III) in the Faroe Islands. *Human Heredity*, **25**, 115.

Conn, J.W. (1955) Presidential address. I. Painting background. II. Primary aldosteronism. *Journal of Laboratory and Clinical Medicine*, **45**, 3.

Coomes, E.N. (1965) Corticosteroid myopathy. *Annals of Rheumatic Diseases*, **24**, 465.

Cori, G.T. (1957) Biochemical aspects of glycogen deposition diseases. *Modern Problems in Paediatrics*, **3**, 344.

Cornelio, F., DiDonato, S., Peluchetti, D., Bizzi, A., Bertagnolio, B., D'Angelo, A. & Wiesmann, U. (1977) Fatal cases of lipid storage myopathy with carnitine deficiency. *Journal of Neurology, Neurosurgery and Psychiatry*, **40**, 170.

Creutzfeldt, O.D. (1961) Die episodiche Adynamie (Adynamia episodica hereditaria Gamstorp), eine familiäre hyperkalämische Lähmung. *Fortschritte der Neurologie, Psychiatrie und Ihre Grenzgebiete*, **29**, 529.

Creutzfeldt, O.D., Abbott, B.C., Fowler, W.M. & Pearson, C.M. (1963) Muscle membrane potentials in episodic adynamia. *Electroencephalograpy and Clinical Neurophysiology*, **5**, 1508.

Cumming, W.J.K., Hardy, M., Hudgson, P. & Walls, J. (1976) Carnitine palmityl-transferase deficiency. *Journal of the Neurological Sciences*, **30**, 247.

Curry, O.B., Basten, J.F., Francis, M.J.O. & Smith, R. (1974) Calcium uptake by sarcoplasmic reticulum of muscle from vitamin D-deficient rabbits, *Nature*, **249**, 83.

Danks, D.M., Stevens, B.J., Campbell, P.E., Gillespie, J.M., Walker-Smith, J., Blomfield, J. & Turner, B. (1972) Menkes' kinky hair syndrome. *Lancet*, **1**, 1100.

Danowski, T.S. & Greenman, L. (1953) Changes in fecal and serum constituents during ingestion of cation and anion exchange. *Annals of the New York Academy of Sciences*, **57**, 273.

Danzis, J., Hutzler, J., Lynfield, J. & Cox, R.P. (1969) Absence of acid maltase in glycogenosis type II (Pompe's disease) in tissue culture. *American Journal of Diseases of Children*, **117**, 108.

Dastur, D.K., Gagrat, B.M., Wadia, N.H., Desai, M.M. & Bharucha, E.P. (1975) Nature of muscular change in osteomalacia: Light and electromicroscope observations. *Journal of Pathology*, **117**, 221.

Daughaday, W.H. & Rendleman, D. (1967) Severe symptomatic hyperkalemia in an adrenalectomized woman due to enhanced mineralocorticoid requirement. *Annals of Internal Medicine*, **66**, 1197.

Davie, M.W.J., Chalmers, T.M., Hunter, J.O., Pelc, B. & Kodicek, E. (1976) l-Alpha-hydroxycholecalciferol in chronic renal failure: studies of the effect of oral doses. *Annals of Internal Medicine*, **84**, 281.

Davis, C.H., Schliselfeld, L.H., Wolf, D.P., Leavitt, C.A. & Krebs, E.G. (1967) Interrelationships among glycogen phosphorylase isoenzymes. *Journal of Biological Chemistry*, **242**, 4824.

Dawson, D.M., Spong, F.Z. & Harrington, J.F. (1968) McArdle's disease: Lack of muscle phosphorylase. *Annals of Internal Medicine*, **69**, 229.

De Barsy, T., Jacquemin, P., Devos, P. & Hers, H.G. (1972) Rodent and human acid α-glucosidase: Purification, assay and inhibition by antibodies. Investigations in type II glycogenosis. *European Journal of Biochemistry*, **31**, 156.

De Barsy, T., Jacquemin, P., Van Hoof, F. & Hers, H.G. (1973) Enzyme replacement in Pompe's disease: An attempt with purified human α-glucosidase. *Birth Defects*, **9**, 184.

Debré, R. & Semelaigne, G. (1935) Syndrome of diffuse muscular hypertrophy in infants causing athletic appearance. Its connection with congenital myxedema. *American Journal of Diseases of Children*, **50**, 1351.

De Burlet, G. & Sudaka, P. (1977) Properties catalitiques de l'α-glucosidase neutre du rein humain. *Biochimie*, **59**, 7.

Deckelbaum, R.J., Russell, A., Shapira, E., Cohen, T., Agam, G. & Gutman, G. (1972) Type III glycogenosis: Atypical enzyme activities in blood cells in two siblings. *Journal of Pediatrics*, **81**, 955.

Demos, M.A., Gitin, E.L. & Kagen, L.J. (1974) Exercise myoglobinemia and acute exertional rhabdomyolysis. *Archives of Internal Medicine*, **134**, 669.

Denborough, M.A. & Lovell, R.R.H. (1960) Anaesthetic deaths in a family. *Lancet*, **2**, 45.

Denborough, M.A., Dennett, X. & Anderson, R.McD. (1973) Central core disease and malignant hyperpyrexia. *British Medical Journal*, **1**, 272.

Di Bona, F.J. & Morens, D.M. (1977) Rhabdomyolysis associated with influenza A. Report of a case with unusual fluid and electrolyte abnormalities. *Journal of Pediatrics*, **91**, 943.

Di Donato, S., Cornelio, F., Balestrini, M.R., Bertagnolio, B. & Peluchetti, D. (1978) Mitochondria-lipid-glycogen myopathy, hyperlactacolisdemia, and carnitine deficiency. *Neurology (Minneapolis)*, **28**, 1110.

Di Donato, S., Cornelio, F., Pacini, I., Peluchetti, D., Rimoldi, M. & Spreafico, S. (1978) Muscle carnitine palmityltransferase deficiency. A case with enzyme deficiency in cultured fibroblasts. *Annals of Neurology*, **4**, 465.

Di Mauro, S. & Di Mauro, P.M.M. (1973) Muscle carnitine palmityltransferase deficiency and myoglobinuria. *Science*, **182**, 929.

Di Mauro, S. & Hartlage, P.L. (1978) Fatal infantile form of muscle phosphorylase deficiency. *Annals of Neurology*, **28**, 1124.

Di Mauro, S., Arnold, S., Miranda, A. & Rowland, L.P. (1978) McArdle disease: The mystery of reappearing phosphorylase activity in muscle culture—a fetal isozyme. *Annals of Neurology*, **3**, 60.

Di Mauro, S., Stern, L.Z., Mehler, M., Nagle, R.B. & Payne, C. (1978) Adult-onset acid maltase deficiency: A postmortem study. *Muscle and Nerve*, **1**, 27.

Di Mauro, S., Schotland, D.L., Bonilla, E., Lee, C.P., Gambetti, P. & Rowland, L.P. (1973) Progressive ophthalmoplegia, glycogen storage and abnormal mitochondria. *Archives of Neurology*, **29**, 170.

Di Mauro, S., Bonilla, E., Lee, C.P., Schotland, D.L., Scarpa, A., Conn, H. and Chance, B. (1976) Luft's disease. Further biochemical and ultrastructural studies of skeletal muscle in the second case. *Journal of the Neurological Sciences*, **27**, 217.

Di Mauro, S., Mendell, J.R., Sahenk, Z., Bachman, D., Scarpa, A., Scofield, R.M. & Reiner, C. (1980) Fatal infantile mitochondrial myopathy and renal dysfunction due to cytochrome-C oxidase deficiency. *Neurology (Minneapolis)*, **30**, 795.

Di Mauro, S., Hartwig, G.B., Hays, A., Eastwood, A.B., Franco, R., Olarte, M., Chang, M., Roses, A.D., Fetell, M., Schoenfeldt, R.S. & Stern, L.Z. (1978) Debrancher enzyme deficiency: Neuromuscular disorder in 5 adults. *Annals of Neurology*, **5**, 422.

Drager, G.A., Hammill, J.F. & Shy, G.M. (1958) Paramyotonia congenita. *Archives of Neurology*, **80**, 1.

Dreyfus, J.C. & Alexandre, Y. (1971) Immunological studies on glycogen storage disease type III and V. Demonstration of the presence of an immunoreactive protein in one case of muscle phosphorylase deficiency. *Biochemical and Biophysical Research Communications*, **44**, 1364.

Duane, D.D. & Engel, A.G. (1970) Emetine myopathy. *Neurology (Minneapolis)*, **20**, 733.

Dunlap, H.F. & Kepler, E.J. (1931) Occurrence of periodic paralysis in the course of exophthalmic goiter. *Proceedings of the Staff Meetings of the Mayo Clinic*, **6**, 272.

Dupond, J.L., Robert, M., Carbillet, J.P. & Leconte Des Floris, R. (1977) Glycogenose musculaire et anémie hémolytique par déficit enzymatique chez aux germains. *La Nouvelle Presse Médicale*, **6**, 2665.

Dustan, H.P., Corcoran, A.C. & Page, I.H. (1956) Renal function in primary aldosteronism. *Journal of Clinical Investigation*, **35**, 1357.

Dyken, M.L., & Timmons, G.D. (1963) Hyperkalemic periodic paralysis with hypocalcemic episode. *Archives of Neurology*, **9**, 508.

Dyken, M.L., Smith, D.M. & Peake, R.L. (1967) An electromyographic diagnostic screening test in McArdle's disease and a case report. *Neurology (Minneapolis)*, **17**, 45.

Egan, T.J. & Klein, R. (1959) Hyperkalemic familial periodic paralysis. *Pediatrics*, **24**, 761.

Ekbom, K., Hed, R., Kirstein, L. & Astrom, K.E. (1964) Muscular affections in chronic alcoholism. *Archives of Neurology*, **10**, 449.

Emser, W. & Schimrigk, K. (1977) Myxedema myopathy: A case report. *European Neurology*, **16**, 286.

Eng, G.D., Epstein, B.S., Engel, W.K., McKay, D.W. & McKay, R. (1978) Malignant hyperthermia and central core disease with congenital dislocating hips. *Archives of Neurology*, **35**, 189.

Engel, A.G. (1961) Thyroid function and periodic paralysis. *American Journal of Medicine*, **30**, 327.

Engel, A.G. (1966a) Electron microscopic observations in primary hypokalemic and thyrotoxic periodic paralysis. *Mayo Clinic Proceedings*, **41**, 797.

Engel, A.G. (1966b) Electron microscopic observations in thyrotoxic and corticosteroid-induced myopathies. *Mayo Clinic Proceedings*, **41**, 785.

Engel, A.G. (1970a) Evolution and content of vacuoles in primary hypokalemic periodic paralysis. *Mayo Clinic Proceedings*, **45**, 774.

Engel, A.G. (1970b) Acid maltase deficiency in adults: Studies in four cases of a syndrome which may mimic muscular dystrophy or other myopathies. *Brain*, **93**, 599.

Engel, A.G. (1972) Neuromuscular manifestations of Graves' disease. *Mayo Clinic Proceedings*, **47**, 919.

Engel, A.G. (1977) Hypokalemic and hyperkalemic periodic paralysis. In *Scientific Approach to Clinical Neurology*, Eds E.S. Goldensohn & S.H. Appel, pp. 1742–1765 (Lea & Febiger: Philadelphia).

Engel, A.G. & Angelini, C. (1973) Carnitine deficiency of skeletal muscle with associated lipid storage myopathy: A new syndrome. *Science*, **173**, 899.

Engel, A.G. & Dale, A.J.D. (1968) Autophagic glycogenesis of late onset with mitochondrial abnormalities: Light and electron microscopic observations. *Mayo Clinic Proceedings*, **43**, 233.

Engel, A.G. & Gomez, M.R. (1970) Acid maltase levels in human heterozygous acid maltase deficiency and in non-weak and neuromuscular disease controls. *Journal of Neurology, Neurosurgery and Psychiatry*, **33**, 801.

Engel, A.G. & Lambert, E.H. (1969) Calcium activation of electrically inexcitable muscle fibers in primary hypokalemic periodic paralysis. *Neurology (Minneapolis)*, **19**, 851.

Engel, A.G. & Siekert, R.G. (1972) Lipid storage myopathy responsive to prednisone. *Archives of Neurology*, **27**, 174.

Engel, A.G., Angelini, C. & Nelson, R.A. (1974) Identification of carnitine deficiency as a cause of human lipid storage myopathy. In *Exploratory Concepts in Muscular Dystrophy II*, Ed. A.T. Milhorat, p. 601 (Excerpta Medica: Amsterdam).

Engel, A.G., Banker, B.Q. & Eiben, R.M. (1977) Carnitine deficiency: Clinical, morphological and biochemical observations in a fatal case. *Journal of Neurology, Neurosurgery and Psychiatry*, **40**, 313.

Engel, A.G., Gomez, M.R. & Groover, R.V. (1971) Multicore disease. A recently recognized congenital myopathy with multifocal degeneration of muscle fibers. *Mayo Clinic Proceedings*, **46**, 666.

Engel, A.G., Potter, C.S. & Rosevear, J.W. (1964) Nucleotides and adenosine monophosphate deaminase activity of muscle in primary hypokalemic periodic paralysis. *Nature*, **292**, 670.

Engel, A.G., Potter, C.S. & Rosevear, J.W. (1967) Studies on carbohydrate metabolism and mitochondrial respiratory activities in primary hypokalemic periodic paralysis. *Neurology (Minneapolis)*, **17**, 329.

Engel, A.G., Gomez, M.R., Seybold, M.E. & Lambert, E.H. (1973) The spectrum and diagnosis of acid maltase deficiency. *Neurology (Minneapolis)*, **23**, 95.

Engel, A.G., Lambert, E.H., Rosevear, J.W. & Tauxe, W.N. (1965) Clinical and electromyographic studies in a patient with primary hypokalemic periodic paralysis. *American Journal of Medicine*, **38**, 626.

Engel, A.G., Rebouche, C.J., Wilson, D.M. & Glasgow, A.M. (1980) Abnormal renal reabsorption of carnitine in systemic carnitine deficiency (SCD). *Neurology (Minneapolis)*, **30**, 368.

Engel, A.G., Santa, T., Stonnington, H.H., Jerusalem, F., Tsujihata, M., Brownell, A.K.W., Sakakibara, H., Banker, B.Q., Sahashi, K. & Lambert, E.H. (1979) Morphometric study of skeletal muscle ultrastructure. *Muscle and Nerve*, **2**, 229.

Engel, F.L., Martin, S.P. & Taylor, H. (1949) On the relation of potassium to the neurological manifestations of hypocalcemic tetany. *Bulletin of the Johns Hopkins Hospital*, **84**, 285.

Engel, W.K., Eyerman, E.L. & Williams, H.E. (1963) Late-onset type of skeletal muscle phosphorylase deficiency. *New England Journal of Medicine*, **268**, 135.

Engel, W.K., Vick, N.A., Glueck, C.J. & Levy, R.I. (1970) A skeletal muscle disorder associated with intermittent symptoms and a possible defect of lipid metabolism. *New England Journal of Medicine*, **282**, 697.

Engel, W.K., Prockop, L.D., Askanas, V., Engel, A.G., Hutchison, R., Galdi, A.P., Williams, J.W., Goldman, A. & Foster, L. (1980) Nearly-fatal lipid-laden myopathy with myoglobinuria and myo-deficiency of carnitine. *Neurology (Minneapolis)*, **30**, 368.

Ernster, L., Ikkos, D. & Luft, R. (1959) Enzymatic activities of human skeletal muscle mitochondria: A tool in clinical metabolic research. *Nature*, **184**, 1851.

Eulenburg, A. (1886) Über eine familiäre durch 6 Generationen verfolgbere form congenitaler Baromyotonie. *Neurologisches Zentralblatt*, **5**, 265.

Faris, A.A. & Reyes, M.G. (1971) Reappraisal of alcoholic myopathy. Clinical and biopsy study on chronic alcoholics without muscle weakness or wasting. *Journal of Neurology, Neurosurgery and Psychiatry*, **34**, 86.

Fattah, S.M., Rubulis, A. & Faloon, W.W. (1970) McArdle's disease: Metabolic studies in a patient and review of the syndrome. *American Journal of Medicine*, **48**, 693.

Faust, D.K., Gergis, S.D. & Sokoll, M.D. (1979) Management of suspected hyperpyrexia in an infant. *Anesthesia and Analgesia*, **58**, 33.

Faw, M.L. & Ewer, R.W. (1962) Intermittent paralysis and chronic adrenal insufficiency. *Annals of Internal Medicine*, **57**, 461.

Feit, H. & Brooke, M.H. (1976) Myophosphorylase deficiency: Two different molecular forms of etiologie. *Neurology (Minneapolis)*, **26**, 963.

Fernandes, J. & Huijing, F. (1968) Branching enzyme deficiency glycogenosis: Studies in therapy. *Archives of Diseases in Childhood*, **43**, 347.

Fernandes, J. & Pikaar, N.A. (1969) Hyperlipidemia in children with liver glycogen disease. *American Journal of Clinical Nutrition*, **22**, 617.

Fernandes, J. & Pikaar, N.A. (1972) Ketosis in hepatic glycogenosis. *Archives of Diseases of Childhood*, **47**, 41.

Ferrebee, J.W., Atchley, D.W. & Loeb, R.F. (1938) A study of the electrolyte physiology in a case of familial periodic paralysis. *Journal of Clinical Investigation*, **17**, 504.

Finch, C.A., Sawyer, C.G. & Flynn, J.M. (1946) Clinical syndrome of potassium intoxication. *American Journal of Medicine*, **1**, 337.

Fishbein, W.N., Armbrustmacher, V.W. & Griffin, J.L. (1978) Myoadenylate deaminase deficiency: A new disease of muscle. *Science*, **200**, 545.

Fleisher, G.A., McConahey, W.M. & Pankow, M. (1965) Serum creatine kinase, lactic dehydrogenase and glutamic-oxaloacetic transaminase in thyroid diseases and pregnancy. *Mayo Clinic Proceedings*, **40**, 300.

Fourman, P. (1954) Experimental observations on the tetany of potassium deficiency. *Lancet*, **2**, 525.

Frame, B., Heine, E.G. & Block, M.A. (1968) Myopathy in primary hyperparathyroidism. Observations in 3 patients.

Annals of Internal Medicine, **68**, 1022.

French, E.B. & Kilpatrick, R. (1957) A variety of paramyotonia congenita. *Journal of Neurology, Neurosurgery and Psychiatry*, **20**, 40.

French, J.H., Sherard, E.S., Lubell, H., Brotz, M. & Moore, C.L. (1972) Trichopoliodystrophy. I. Report of a case and biochemical studies. *Archives of Neurology*, **26**, 229.

Fukuyama, Y., Ando, T. & Yokota, J. (1977) Acute fulminant myoglobinuria polymyositis with picornavirus-like crystals. *Journal of Neurology, Neurosurgery and Psychiatry*, **40**, 775.

Furie, B. & Penn, A.S. (1974) Pigmenturia from conga drumming. *Annals of Internal Medicine*, **80**, 727.

Galjaard, H., Mekes, M., De Josselin de Jong, J.E. & Niermeijer, M.F. (1973) A method for rapid prenatal diagnosis of glycogenosis II (Pompe's disease). *Clinica Chimica Acta* **49**, 361.

Gambetti, P.L., Di Mauro, S. & Baker, L. (1971) Nervous system in Pompe's disease. *Journal of Neuropathology and Experimental Neurology*, **30**, 412.

Gamboa, E.T., Eastwood, A.B., Hays, A.P., Maxwell, J. & Penn, A.S. (1979) Isolation of influenza virus from muscle in myoglobinuric polymyositis. *Neurology (Minneapolis)*, **29**, 1323.

Gamstorp, I. (1956) Adynamia episodica hereditaria. *Acta Paediatrica Scandinavica*, **45**, 1.

Gamstorp, I. (1963) Adynamia episodica hereditaria and myotonia. *Acta Neurologica Scandinavica*, **39**, 41.

Garcin, R., Rondot, P. & Fardeau, M. (1964) Sur les accidents neuromusculaires et en particulier sur une 'myopathie vacuolaire' observés au cours d'un traitement prolongé par la chloroquine. Amélioration rapid apres arrêt due médicament. *Revue Neurologique (Paris)*, **111**, 117.

Garcin, R., Legrain, M., Rondot, P. & Fardeau, M. (1966) Étude clinique et métabolique d'une observation de paramyotonie congénitale d'Eulenberg. Documents ultrastructuraux concernant la biopsie musculaire. *Revue Neurologique*, **115**, 295.

Gillard, B.K. & Nelson, T.E. (1977) Amylo-1,6-glucosidase/4-α-glucano-transferase: Use of reversible substrate model inhibitors to the binding and active sites of rabbit muscle debranching enzyme. *Biochemistry*, **16**, 3978.

Glasgow, A.M., Eng, G. & Engel, A.G. (1980) Systemic carnitine deficiency simulating recurrent Reye's syndrome. *Journal of Pediatrics*, **96**, 889.

Goldflam, S. (1895) Weitere Mittheilung über die paroxysmale, familiäre Lähmung. *Deutsche Zeitschrift fur Nervenheilkunole*, **7**, 1.

Golding, D.N., Murray, S.M., Pearce, G.W. & Thompson, M. (1961) Corticosteroid myopathy. *Annals of Physical Medicine*, **6**, 171.

Goldman, D.E. (1943) Potential, impedance and rectification in membranes. *Journal of General Physiology*, **27**, 37.

Gomez, M.R., Engel, A.G. & Dyck, P.J. (1972) Progressive ataxia, retinal degeneration, neuromyopathy, and mental subnormality in a patient with true hypoparathyroidism, dwarfism, malabsorption and cholelithiasis. *Neurology (Minneapolis)*, **22**, 849.

Goodhue, W.W., Davis, J.N. & Porro, R.S. (1972) Ischemic myopathy in uremic hyperparathyroidism. *Journal of the American Medical Association*, **221**, 911.

Goulon, M., Rapin, M., Lissac, J., Pocidolo, J.J. & Mantel, O. (1962) Quadriplegia with hypokalemia and hypokalemia acidosis secondary to the absorption of ammonium chloride

over a three-year period. *Bulletin de la Societé des Hôpitaux Médicales de Paris*, 113.

Greville, G.G. & Tubbs, P.K. (1968) The catabolism of long chain fatty acids in mammalian tissue. In *Essays in Biochemistry*, Eds P.N. Campbell & G.D. Greville, Vol. 4, p. 155 (Academic Press: London).

Griggs, R.C., Engel, W.K. & Resnick, J.S. (1970) Acetazolamide treatment of hypokalemic periodic paralysis. *Annals of Internal Medicine*, **73**, 39.

Grob, D., Johns, R.J. & Liljestrand, A. (1957) Potassium movement in patients with familial periodic paralysis. *American Journal of Medicine*, **23**, 356.

Grollman, A.P. (1968) Inhibitors of protein biosynthesis. V. Effects of emetine on protein and nucleic acid biosynthesis in HeLa cells. *Journal of Biological Chemistry*, **243**, 4089.

Gronert, G.A. (1980) Malignant hyperthermia. *Anesthesiology*, In press.

Gruener, R., McArdle, B., Ryman, B.E. & Weller, R.O. (1968) Contracture of phosphorylase deficient muscle. *Journal of Neurology, Neurosurgery and Psychiatry*, **31**, 268.

Gruener, R.G. & Stern, L.Z. (1972) Diphenylhydantoin reverses membrane effects in steroid myopathy. *Nature New Biology*, **235**, 41.

Greuner, R.G., Stern, L.Z., Payne, C. & Hannapel, L. (1975) Hyperthyroid myopathy. Intracellular electrophysiological measurements in biopsied human intercostal muscle. *Journal of the Neurological Sciences*, **24**, 339.

Gruner, J.E. (1963) Sur quelques anomalies mitochondriales observées au cours d'affections musculaires variées. *Comptes Rendus des Seances de la Société de Biologie et de ses Filiales*, **157**, 181.

Gruner, J.E. (1966) Anomalies du réticulum sarcoplasmique et prolifération de tubules dans le muscle d'une paralysie périodque familiale. *Comptes Rendus des Seances de la Société de Biologie et de ses Filiales*, **160**, 193.

Gullotta, F., Stefan, H. & Mattern, H. (1976) Pseudodystrophische Muskeglykogenose im Erwachsenenalter (Saure-Maltase-Mangle-Syndrom). *Journal of Neurology*, **213**, 199.

Haase, G.R. & Engel, A.G. (1960) Paroxysmal recurrent rhabdomyolysis. *Archives of Neurology*, **2**, 410.

Habener, J.F. & Potts, J.T. (1978) Parathyroid physiology and primary hyperparathyroidism. In *Metabolic Bone Disease*, Eds L.V. Avioli & S.M. Krane, Vol. 2, p. 1 (Academic Press: New York).

Hagenfeldt, L. & Wahren, J. (1968) Human forearm muscle metabolism during exercise. II Uptake, release and oxidation of individual FFA and glycerol. *Scandinavian Journal of Clinical and Laboratory Investigation*, **21**, 263.

Haigler, H.T. & Broquist, H.P. (1974) Carnitine synthesis in rat tissue slices. *Biochemical and Biophysical Research Communications*, **56**, 676.

Hall, L.W., Woolf, N., Bradley, J.W. & Jolly, D.W. (1966) Unusual reactions to suxamethonium chloride. *British Medical Journal*, **2**, 1305.

Hammett, J.F., Bale, P., Basser, L.S. & Neale, F.C. (1966) McArdle's disease: Three cases in an Australian family. *Proceedings of the Australian Association of Neurologists*, **4**, 21.

Harriman, D.G.F. (1979) Preanesthetic investigation of malignant hyperthermia: Microscopy. *International Anesthesiology Clinics*, **17**, 97.

Hart, Z.W., Chang, C., Di Mauro, S., Farooki, Q. &

Ayyar, R. (1978) Muscle carnitine deficiency and fatal cardiomyopathy. *Neurology (Minneapolis)*, **28**, 147.

Hart, Z.W., Chang, C., Perrin, E.V.D., Neerunjun, J.S. & Ayyar, R. (1977) Familial poliodystrophy, mitochondrial myopathy and lactate acidemia. *Archives of Neurology*, **34**, 180.

Haussler, M.R. & McCain, T.A. (1977) Basic and clinical concepts related to vitamin D metabolism and action. *New England Journal of Medicine*, **297**, 974.

Havard, C.W.H. (1972) Clinical endocrinology: Endocrine exophthalmos. *British Medical Journal*, **1**, 360.

Havard, C.W.H., Campbell, E.D.R., Ross, H.B. & Spence, A.W. (1963) Electromyographic and histological findings in the muscles of patients with thyrotoxicosis. *Quarterly Journal of Medicine*, **32**, 145.

Hed, R. (1955) Myoglobinuria in man, with special reference to familial form. *Acta Medica Scandinavica* (Supplement 303), **151**, 1.

Hed, R., Lundmark, C., Fahlgren, H. & Orell, S. (1962) Acute muscular syndrome in chronic alcoholism. *Acta Medica Scandinavica*, **171**, 585.

Helweg-Larsen, H.F., Hauge, M. & Sagild, U. (1955) Hereditary transient muscular paralysis in Denmark. *Acta Geneticae Medicae et Gemellologiae (Rome)*, **5**, 263.

Henderson, R.G., Ledingham, J.G.G., Oliver, D.O., Small, D.G., Russel, R.G.G., Smith, R., Walton, R.J., Preston, C., Warner, G.T. & Norman, A.W. (1974) Effects of 1,25-dihydroxycholecalciferol on calcium absorption, muscle weakness, and bone disease in chronic renal failure. *Lancet*, **1**, 379.

Herman, J. & Nadler, H.L. (1977) Recurrent myoglobinuria and muscle palmityl-transferase deficiency. *Journal of Pediatrics*, **91**, 247.

Herman, R.G. & McDowell, M.K. (1963) Hyperkalaemic paralysis (adynamia episodica hereditaria). *American Journal of Medicine*, **35**, 749.

Hers, H.G. (1963) α-Glucosidase deficiency in generalized glycogen-storage disease (Pompe's disease). *Biochemical Journal*, **86**, 11.

Hers, H.G. & Van Hoof, F. (1968) Glycogen storage diseases: Type II and type VI glycogenosis. In *Carbohydrate Metabolism and Its Disorders*, Eds F. Dickens, P.J. Randle, W.J. Whelan, Vol. 2, p. 151 (Academic Press: New York).

Hewlett, R.H. & Gardner-Thorpe, C. (1978) McArdle's disease—What limit to the age of onset? *South African Medical Journal*, **53**, 60.

Hofmann, D.D. & Denys, E.H. (1972) Effects of thyroid hormone at the neuromuscular junction. *American Journal of Physiology*, **223**, 283.

Hofmann, W.W. & Smith, R.A. (1970) Hypokalemic periodic paralysis studied in vitro. *Brain*, **93**, 445.

Hogan, G.R., Gutmann, L., Schmidt, R. & Gilbert, E. (1969) Pompe's disease. *Neurology (Minneapolis)*, **19**, 894.

Holleman, L.W.J., Van Der Haar, J.A. & De Vaan, G.A.M. (1966) Type IV glycogenosis. *Laboratory Investigation*, **15**, 357.

Holmes, J.M., Houghton, C.R. & Woolf, A.L. (1960) A myopathy presenting in adult life with features suggestive of glycogen storage disease. *Journal of Neurology, Neurosurgery and Psychiatry*, **23**, 302.

Hostetler, K.Y., Hoppel, C.L., Romine, J.S., Sipe, J.C., Gross, S.R. & Higginbottom, P.A. (1978) Partial deficiency of muscle carnitine palmityl-transferase with normal ketone production. *New England Journal of Medicine*, **298**, 553.

Howell, R.R. (1978) The glycogen storage diseases. In *The Metabolic Basis of Inherited Disease*, 4th Edn. Eds J.B. Stanbury, J.B. Wyngaarden & D.S. Frederickson, p. 137 (McGraw-Hill: New York).

Howell, R.R., Kaback, M.M. & Brown, B.I. (1971) Type IV glycogen storage disease: Branching enzyme deficiency in skin fibroblasts and possible heterozygote detection. *Journal of Pediatrics*, **78**, 638.

Hower, J. & Struck, H. (1972) CPK activity in hypoparathyroidism. (Letter to the editor.) *New England Journal of Medicine*, **287**, 1096.

Howes, E.L., Price, H.M. & Blumberg, J.M. (1966) Hypokalemic periodic paralysis. *Neurology (Minneapolis)*, **16**, 242.

Hudgson, P., Gardner-Medwin, D., Worsfold, M., Pennington, R.J.T. & Walton, J.N. (1968) Adult myopathy from glycogen storage disease due to acid maltase deficiency. *Brain*, **91**, 435.

Hudson, A.J. (1963) Progressive neurological disorder and myotonia congenita associated with paramyotonia. *Brain*, **86**, 811.

Hudson, A.J., Strickland, K.P. & Wilensky, A.J. (1967) Serum enzyme studies in familial hyperkalemic periodic paralysis. *Clinica Chimica Acta*, **17**, 331.

Hug, G. & Schubert, W.K. (1967) Lysosomes in type II glycogenosis: Changes during administration of extract from *Aspergillus niger*. *Journal of Cell Biology*, **35**, C1.

Hughes, J.T., Esiri, M., Oxbury, J.M. & Whitty, C.W.M. (1971) Chloroquine myopathy. *Quarterly Journal of Medicine*, **40**, 85.

Huijing, F. (1964) Amylo-1,6-glucosidase activity in normal leukocytes and in leukocytes of patients with glycogen storage disease. *Clinica Chimica Acta*, **9**, 269.

Huijing, F. (1975) Glycogen metabolism and glycogen storage diseases. *Physiological Reviews*, **55**, 609.

Huijing, F., Waltuck, B.L. & Whelan, W.J. (1973) α-Glucosidase administration: Experiences in two patients with glycogen-storage disease compared with animal experiments. *Birth Defects*, Original Article Series, 9, No. 2, 191.

Huijing, F., Lee, E.Y.C., Carter, J.H. & Whelan, W.J. (1970) Branching action of amylo-1,6-glucosidase/oligo-1,4→1,4-glucantransferase. *FEBS Letters*, **7**, 251.

Hulse, J.D., Ellis, S.R. & Henderson, L.M. (1978) Carnitine biosynthesis. β-Hydroxylation of trimethyllysine by an α-ketoglutarate dependent mitochondrial dioxygenase. *Journal of Biological Chemistry*, **253**, 1654.

Hülsmann, W.C., Bethlem, J., Meijer, A.E.F.H., Fleury, P. & Schellens, J.P.A. (1967) Myopathy with abnormal structure and function of mitochondria. *Journal of Neurology, Neurosurgery and Psychiatry*, **30**, 519.

Illingworth, B. & Cori, G.T. (1952) Structure of glycogen and amylopectins: III. Normal and abnormal human glycogen. *Journal of Biological Chemistry*, **199**, 653.

Illingwoth, B., Cori, G.T. & Cori, C.F. (1956) Amylo-1,6 glucosidase in muscle tissue in generalized glycogen storage disease. *Journal of Biological Chemistry*, **213**, 123.

Isaacs, H., Heffron, J.J.A., Badenhorst, M. & Pickering, A. (1976) Weakness associated with pathological presence of lipid in skeletal muscle: A detailed study of a patient with carnitine deficiency. *Journal of Neurology, Neurosurgery and Psychiatry*, **39**, 1114.

Jarcho, L.W. & Tyler, F.H. (1958) Myxedema, pseudomyotonia and myotonia congenita. *Archives of*

Internal Medicine, **102**, 357.

Jenerick, H. (1959) The control of membrane ionic currents by the membrane potential of muscle. *Journal of General Physiology*, **42**, 923.

Jerusalem, F., Spiess, H. & Baumgartner, G. (1975) Lipid storage myopathy with normal carnitine levels. *Journal of the Neurological Sciences*, **24**, 273.

Jerusalem, F., Angelini, C., Engel, A.G. & Groover, R.V. (1973) Mitochondria-lipid-glycogen (MLG) disease of muscle. A morphologically regressive congenital myopathy. *Archives of Neurology*, **29**, 162.

Justice, P., Ryan, C., Hsia, D.Y. & Kromptik, E. (1970) Amylo-l,6-glucosidase in human fibroblasts: Studies in type III glycogen-storage disease. *Biochemical and Biophysical Research Communications*, **39**, 301.

Kagen, L.J. & Christian, C.L. (1966) Immunologic measurements of myoglobin in human and fetal skeletal muscle. *American Journal of Physiology*, **211**, 656.

Karpati, G., Carpenter, S., Labrisseau, A. & La Fontaine, R. (1973) The Kearns-Shy syndrome. *Journal of the Neurological Sciences*, **19**, 133.

Karpati, G., Carpenter, S., Wolfe, L.S. & Sherwin, A. (1969) A peculiar polysaccharide accumulation in muscle in a case of cardioskeletal myopathy. *Neurology (Minneapolis)*, **19**, 553.

Karpati, G., Carpenter, S., Eisen, A., Aube, M. & Di Mauro, S. (1977) The adult form of acid maltase (α-1,4-glucosidase) deficiency. *Annals of Neurology*, **1**, 276.

Karpati, G., Carpenter, S., Engel, A.G., Watters, G., Allen, J., Rothman, S., Klassen, G. & Mamer, O.A. (1975) The syndrome of systemic carnitine deficiency: Clinical, morphologic, biochemical and pathophysiologic features. *Neurology (Minneapolis)*, **25**, 16.

Kearns, T.P. & Sayre, G.P. (1958) Retinitis pigmentosa, external ophthalmoplegia and complete heart-block. *Archives of Ophthalmology*, **60**, 280.

Keith, N.M., Osterberg, A.E. & Burchell, H.B. (1942) Some effects of potassium salts in man. *Annals of Internal Medicine*, **16**, 879.

Kessler, E., Weinberger, I. & Rosenfeld, J.B. (1972) Myoglobinuric acute renal failure in a case of dermatomyositis. *Israel Journal of Medical Sciences*, **8**, 978.

Keye, J.D. (1952) Death in potassium deficiency. *Circulation*, **5**, 766.

Keyloun, V.E., and Grace, W.J. (1967) Villous adenoma of the rectum associated with severe electrolyte imbalance. *American Journal of Digestive Diseases*, **12**, 104.

King, J.O., Denborough, M.A. & Zapf, P.W. (1972) Inheritance of malignant hyperpyrexia. *Lancet*, **1**, 365.

Klatskin, G. & Friedman, H. (1948) Emetine toxicitiy in man: Studies on the nature of early toxic manifestations, their relationship to the dose level, and their significance in determining safe dosage. *Annals of Internal Medicine*, **28**, 892.

Klein, R., Egan, T. & Usher, P. (1960) Changes in sodium, potassium and water in hyperkalemic familial periodic paralysis. *Metabolism*, **9**, 1005.

Korein, J., Coddon, D.R. & Mowrey, F.H. (1959) The clinical syndrome of paroxysmal myoglobinuria. *Neurology (Minneapolis)*, **9**, 767.

Koskelo, P., Kekki, M. & Wager, O. (1967) Kinetic behavior of ^{131}I-labelled myoglobin in human beings. *Clinica Chimica Acta*, **17**, 339.

Koster, J.F., Slee, R.G. & Hulsmann, W.C. (1974) The use of the leukocytes as an aid in the diagnosis of glycogen storage disease type II (Pompe's disease). *Clinica Chimica Acta*, **51**, 319.

Koster, J.F., Slee, R.G., Hulsmann, W.C. & Niermeijer, M.F. (1972) The electrophoretic pattern and activities of acid and neutral maltase of cultivated fibroblast and amniotic fluid cells from controls and patients with the variant of glycogen storage disease type II (Pompe's disease). *Clinica Chimica Acta*, **40**, 294.

Koster, J.F., Slee, R.G., Jennekens, F.G.I., Wintzen, A.R. & Van Berkel, T.J.C. (1979) McArdle's disease: A study of the molecular basis of two different etiologies of myophosphorylase deficiency. *Clinica Chimica Acta*, **94**, 229.

Koster, J.F., Slee, R.G., Van Der Klei-Van Moorsel, J.M., Rietra, P.J.G.M. & Lucas, C.J. (1976) Physicochemical and immunologic properties of acid α-glucosidase from various human tissues in relation to glycogenosis type II (Pompe's disease). *Clinica Chimica Acta*, **68**, 49.

Lambert, C.D. & Young, J.R.B. (1976) Hypertrophy of branchial muscles. *Journal of Neurology, Neurosurgery and Psychiatry*, **39**, 810.

Lambert, E.H., Underdahl, L.O., Beckett, S. & Mederos, L.O. (1951) A study of the ankle jerk in myxedema. *Journal of Clinical Endocrinology and Metabolism*, **11**, 1186.

Larsson, L.-E., Linderholm, H., Müller, R., Ringqvist, T. & Sörnas, R. (1964) Hereditary metabolic myopathy with paroxysmal myoglobinuria due to abnormal glycolysis. *Journal of Neurology, Neurosurgery and Psychiatry*, **27**, 361.

Layzer, R.B., Lovelace, R.E. & Rowland, L.P. (1967) Hyperkalaemic periodic paralysis. *Archives of Neurology*, **16**, 455.

Layzer, R.B., Rowland, L.P. & Ranney, H.M. (1967) Muscle phosphofructokinase deficiency. *Archives of Neurology*, **17**, 512.

Layzer, R.B., Havel, R.J., Becker, N. & McIlroy, M.B. (1977) Muscle carnitine palmityltransferase deficiency: A case with diabetes and ketonuria. *Neurology (Minneapolis)*, **27**, 379 (abstract).

Legum, C.P. & Nitowsky, H.M. (1969) Studies on leukocyte brancher enzyme activity in a family with type IV glycogenosis. *Journal of Pediatrics*, **74**, 84.

Levin, B., Burgess, E.A. & Mortimer, P.E. (1968) Glycogen-storage disease type IV, amylopectinosis. *Archives of Diseases in Childhood*, **43**, 548.

Levin, S., Moses, S.W., Chayoth, R., Jagoda, N. & Steinitz, K. (1967) Glycogen storage disease in Israel. *Israel Journal of Medical Sciences*, **3**, 397.

Lewi, Z. & Bar-Khayim, Y. (1964) Food poisoning from barium carbonate. *Lancet*, **2**, 342.

Lou, H.C. & Reske-Nielsen, E. (1976) Progressive external ophthalmoplegia: evidence for a disorder in pyruvate-lactate metabolism. *Archives of Neurology*, **33**, 455.

Luft, R., Ikkos, D., Palmieri, G., Ernster, L. & Afzelius, B. (1962) A case of severe hypermetabolism of nonthyroid origin with a defect in the maintenance of mitochondrial respiratory control: a correlated clinical, biochemical, and morphological study. *Journal of Clinical Investigation*, **41**, 1776.

MacDonald, R.D. & Engel, A.G. (1970) Experimental chloroquine myopathy. *Journal of Neuropathology and Experimental Neurology*, **29**, 479.

MacDonald, R.D., Rewcastle, N.B. & Humphrey, J.G. (1968) The myopathy of hyperkalemic periodic paralysis. *Archives of Neurology*, **19**, 274.

McArdle, B. (1951) Myopathy due to a defect in muscle glycogen breakdown. *Clinical Science*, **10**, 13.

McArdle, B. (1956) Familial periodic paralysis. *British Medical Bulletin*, **12**, 226.

McArdle, B. (1962) Adynamia episodica hereditaria and its treatment. *Brain*, **85**, 121.

McArdle, B. (1963) Metabolic myopathies. *American Journal of Medicine*, **35**, 661.

McComas, A.J., Mrozek, K. & Bradley, W.G. (1968) The nature of the electrophysiological disorder in adynamia episodica. *Journal of Neurology, Neurosurgery and Psychiatry*, **31**, 448.

McDaniel, H., Pittman, C.S., Oh, S.J. & Di Mauro, S. (1977) Carbohydrate metabolism in hypothyroid myopathy. *Metabolism*, **26**, 867.

Magee, K.R. (1963) A study of paramyotonia congenita. *Archives of Neurology*, **8**, 461.

Mahler, R.F. & Stanbury, S.W. (1956) Potassium-losing renal disease. *Quarterly Journal of Medicine*, **25**, 21.

Mallette, L.E., Patten, B.M. & Engel, W.K. (1975) Neuromuscular disease in secondary hyperparathyroidism. *Annals of Internal Medicine*, **82**, 474.

Mancall, E.L., Aponte, G.E. & Berry, R.G. (1965) Pompe's disease (diffuse glycogenosis) with neuronal storage. *Journal of Neuropathology and Experimental Neurology*, **24**, 85.

Manitius, A., Levitin, H., Beck, D. & Epstein, F.H. (1960) On the mechanism of impairment of renal concentrating ability in potassium deficiency. *Journal of Clinical Investigation*, **39**, 684.

Markesbery, W.R. (1979) Lactic acidemia, mitochondrial myopathy, and basal ganglia calcification. *Neurology (Minneapolis)*, **29**, 1057.

Markesbery, W.R., McQuillen, M.P., Procopis, P.G., Harrison, A.R. & Engel, A.G. (1974) Muscle carnitine deficiency. Association with lipid myopathy, vacuolar neuropathy and vacuolated leukocytes. *Archives of Neurology*, **31**, 320.

Markowitz, H. & Wobig, G.H. (1977) Quantitative method for estimating myoglobin in urine. *Clinical Chemistry*, **23**, 1689.

Marks, L.J. & Feit, E. (1953) Flaccid quadriplegia, hyperkalemia and Addison's disease. *Archives of Internal Medicine*, **91**, 56.

Marshall, J. (1952) Observations on a case of myotonia paradoxa. *Journal of Neurology, Neurosurgery and Psychiatry*, **15**, 206.

Martin, J.J., De Barsy, T. & Den Tandt, W.R. (1976) Acid maltase deficiency in non-identical adult twins. A morphological and biochemical study. *Journal of Neurology*, **213**, 105.

Martin, J.J., De Barsy, T., Van Hoof, F. & Palladini, G. (1973) Pompe's disease: An inborn lysosomal disorder with storage of glycogen. A study of brain and striated muscle. *Acta Neuropathologica (Berlin)*, **23**, 229.

Martin, J.J., De Barsy, T., De Schrijver, R., LeRoy, J.G. & Palladini, G. (1976) Acid maltase deficiency (type II glycogenosis). Morphological and biochemical studies of a childhood type. *Journal of the Neurological Sciences*, **30**, 155.

Martinez, A.J., Hooshmand, H. & Faris, A.A. (1973) Acute alcoholic myopathy. Enzyme histochemistry and electron microscopic findings. *Journal of the Neurological Sciences*, **20**, 245.

Mastaglia, F.L. (1973) Pathological changes in skeletal muscle in acromegaly. *Acta Neuropathologica (Berlin)*, **24**, 273.

Mastaglia, F.L., Barwick, D.D. & Hall, R. (1970) Myopathy in acromegaly. *Lancet*, **2**, 907.

Mattle, H., Jerusalem, F., Nolte, J. & Schollmeyer, P. (1977) Belastungsinduzierte Muskelschwäche, Myalgien und Kontrakturen. *Schweizerische medizinsiche Wochenschrift*, **107**, 137.

Mehler, M. & Di Mauro, S. (1976) Late-onset acid maltase deficiency. Detection of patients and heterozygotes by urinary enzyme assay. *Archives of Neurology*, **33**, 692.

Mehler, M. & Di Mauro, S. (1977) Residual acid maltase activity in late-onset acid maltase deficiency. *Neurology (Minneapolis)*, **27**, 178.

Mercier, C. & Whelan, W.J. (1973) Further characterization of glycogen from type IV glycogen-storage disease. *European Journal of Biochemistry*, **40**, 22.

Mertens, H.G., Schimrigk, K., Volkwein, U. & Voigt, K.D. (1964) Elektrolyt- und Aldosteronestoffwechsel bei der Adynamia episodica hereditaria, der hyperkaliämschen Form der periodischen Lähmung. *Klinische Wochenschrift*, **42**, 65.

Meyers, K.R., Gilden, D.H., Rinaldi, C.F. & Hansen, J.L. (1972) Periodic muscle weakness, normokalemia, and tubular aggregates. *Neurology (Minneapolis)*, **22**, 269.

Miller, E.D., Sanders, D.B., Rowlinson, J.C., Berry, F.A., Sussman, M.D. & Epstein, R.M. (1978) Anesthesia-induced rhabdomyolysis in a patient with Duchenne's muscular dystrophy. *Anesthesiology*, **48**, 146.

Millikan, C.H. & Haines, S.F. (1953) The thyroid gland in relation to neuromuscular disease. *Archives of Internal Medicine*, **92**, 5.

Milne, M.D., Muehrcke, R.C. & Heard, B.E. (1957) Potassium deficiency and the kidney. *British Medical Bulletin*, **13**, 15.

Milne, M.D., Stanbury, S.W. & Thomson, A.E. (1952) Observations on Fanconi syndrome and renal hyperchloremic acidosis in adults. *Quarterly Journal of Medicine*, **21**, 61.

Miranda, A., Di Mauro, S., Eastwood, A., Hays, A., Johnson, W.G., Olarte, M., Whitlock, R., Mayeaux, R. & Rowland, L.P. (1979) Lipid storage myopathy, ichthyosis and steatorrhea, *Muscle and Nerve*, **2**, 1.

Mommaerts, W.F.H.M., Illingworth, B., Pearson, C.M., Guillory, R.J. & Seraydarian, K. (1959) A functional disorder of muscle associated with the absence of phosphorylase. *Proceedings of the National Academy of Sciences, USA*, **46**, 791.

Monnens, L., Gabreëls, F. & Willems, J.L. (1975) A metabolic myopathy associated with chronic lactic acidosis, growth failure and nerve deafness. *Journal of Pediatrics*, **86**, 983.

Morgan-Hughes, J.A., Darveniza, P., Landon, D.N., Land, J.M. & Clark, J.B. (1979) A mitochondrial myopathy with deficiency of respiratory chain NADH-CoQ reductase activity. *Journal of the Neurological Sciences*, **43**, 27.

Morgan-Hughes, J.A., Darveniza, P., Kahn, S.N., Landon, D.N., Sherratt, R.M., Land, J.M. & Clark, J.B. (1977) A mitochondrial myopathy characterized by a deficiency of reducible cytochrome b. *Brain*, **100**, 617.

Moses, S.W. & Gutman, A. (1972) Inborn error of glycogen metabolism. *Advances in Pediatrics*, **19**, 95.

Müller, R. & Kugelberg, E. (1959) Myopathy in Cushing's syndrome. *Journal of Neurology, Neurosurgery and*

Psychiatry, **22**, 314.

Mullin, B.R., Levinson, R.E., Friedman, A., Henson, D.R., Winand, R.J. & Kohn, L.D. (1977) Delayed hypersensitivity in Graves' disease and exophthalmos. Identification of thyroglobulins in normal human orbital muscle. *Endocrinology*, **100**, 351.

Murase, T., Ikeda, H., Muro, T., Nakao, K. & Sugita, H. (1973) Myopathy associated with type III glycogenosis. *Journal of the Neurological Sciences*, **20**, 287.

Murphy, T.R., ReMine, W.H. & Burbank, M.H. (1960) Hyperparathyroidism: report of a case in which parathyroid adenoma presented primarily with profound muscular weakness. *Proceedings of the Staff Meetings of the Mayo Clinic*, **35**, 629.

Murray, A.K., Brown, B.I. & Brown, D.H. (1978) The molecular heterogeneity of purified liver lysosomal α-glucosidase (acid α-glucosidase). *Archives of Biochemistry and Biophysics*, **185**, 511.

Nabarro, J.D.N., Spencer, A.G. & Stowers, J.M. (1952) Treatment of diabetic ketoacidosis. *Lancet*, **1**, 983.

Neustein, H.B. (1969) Fine structure of skeletal muscle in type III glycogenosis. *Archives of Pathology (Chicago)*, **88**, 130.

Nitowski, H.M. & Grunfeld, A. (1967) Lysosomal α-glucosidase activity in type II glycogenosis: Activity in leukocytes and cell cultures in relation to genotype. *Journal of Laboratory and Clinical Medicine*, **69**, 742.

Norris, F.H. & Panner, B.J. (1966) Hypothyroid myopathy. *Archives of Neurology*, **14**, 574.

Odor, D.L., Patel, A.N. & Pearce, L.A. (1967) Familial hypokalemic periodic paralysis with permanent myopathy. *Journal of Neuropathology and Experimental Neurology*, **26**, 98.

Okihiro, M.M. & Nordyke, R.A. (1966) Hypokalemic periodic paralysis. *Journal of the American Medical Association*, **198**, 949.

Oliner, L., Schulman, M. & Larner, J. (1961) Myopathy associated with glycogen deposition from generalized lack of amylo-1,6-glucosidase. *Clinical Research*, **9**, 243.

Olson, W., Engel, W.K., Walsh, G.O. & Einaugler, R. (1972) Oculocraniosomatic neuromuscular disease with 'ragged-red' fibres. *Archives of Neurology*, **26**, 193.

Osserman, K.E., Tsairis, P. & Weiner, L.B. (1967) Myasthenia gravis and thyroid disease: clinical and immunological correlation. *Mount Sinai Journal of Medicine (New York)*, **34**, 469.

Owen, E.E. & Verner, J.V. (1960) Renal tubular disease with muscle paralysis and hypokalemia. *American Journal of Medicine*, **28**, 8.

Ozawa, E., Hosoi, K. & Ebashi, S. (1967) Reversible stimulation of muscle phosphorylase *b* kinase by low concentrations of calcium ions. *Journal of Biochemistry*, **61**, 531.

Patten, B.M., Wood, J.M., Harati, Y., Hefferan, P. & Howell, R.R. (1979) Familial recurrent rhabdomyolysis due to carnitine palmityltransferase deficiency. *American Journal of Medicine*, **67**, 167.

Patten, B.M., Bilezikian, J.P., Mallette, L.E., Prince, A., Engel, W.K. & Aurbach, G.D. (1974) Neuromuscular disease in primary hyperparathyroidism. *Annals of Internal Medicine*, **80**, 182.

Pearson, C.M. (1964) The periodic paralyses. *Brain*, **87**, 341.

Pearson, C.M., Beck, W.S. & Blahd, W.H. (1957) Idiopathic paroxysmal myoglobinuria. *Archives of Internal Medicine (Chicago)*, **99**, 376.

Perkoff, G.T., Hardy, P. & Velez-Garcia, E. (1966) Reversible acute muscular syndrome in chronic alcoholism. *New England Journal of Medicine*, **274**, 1277.

Perkoff, G.T., Silber, R., Tyler, F.H., Cartwright, G.E. & Wintrobe, M.M. (1959) Studies on disorders of muscle. XII. Myopathy due to the administration of therapeutic amounts of 17-hydroxycorticosteroids. *American Journal of Medicine*, **26**, 891.

Pernow, B.B., Havel, R.J. & Jennings, D.B. (1967) The second-wind phenomenon in McArdle's syndrome. *Acta Medica Scandinavica (Supplement)*, **472**, 294.

Peter, J.B., Verhaag, D.A. & Worsfold, M. (1970) Studies of steroid myopathy. Examination of the possible effect of triamcinolone on mitochondria and sarcotubular vesicles of rat skeletal muscle. *Biochemical Pharmacology*, **19**, 1627.

Philipson, K.D. & Edelman, I.S. (1977) Thyroid hormone control of Na-K-adenosine triphosphatase and K-dependent phosphatase in rat heart. *American Journal of Physiology*, **232**, C 196.

Pickett, J.B.E., Layzer, R.B., Levin, S.R., Schneider, V., Campbell, M.J. & Sumner, A.J. (1975) Neuromuscular complications of acromegaly. *Neurology (Minneapolis)*, **25**, 638.

Pleasure, D.E., Walsh, G.O. & Engel, W.K. (1970) Atrophy of skeletal muscle in patients with Cushing's syndrome. *Archives of Neurology*, **22**, 118.

Pleasure, D., Wyszynski, B., Sumner, D., Schotland, D.L., Feldmann, B., Nugent, N., Hitz, K. & Goodman, D.B.P. (1979) Skeletal muscle calcium metabolism and contractile force in vitamin D-deficient chicks. *Journal of Clinical Investigation*, **64**, 1157.

Plotz, C.M., Knowlton, A.I. & Ragan, C. (1952) The natural history of Cushing's syndrome. *American Journal of Medicine*, **13**, 597.

Pollen, R.H., & Williams, R.H. (1960) Hyperkalemic neuromyopathy in Addison's disease. *New England Journal of Medicine*, **263**, 273.

Pompe, J.C. (1932) Over idiopatsche hypertrophie van het hart. *Nederlands Tijdschrift voor Geneeskunde*, **76**, 304.

Poskanzer, D.C. & Kerr, D.N.S. (1961) A third type of periodic paralysis with normokalemia and favourable response to sodium chloride. *American Journal of Medicine*, **31**, 328.

Prineas, J.W., Hall, R., Barwick, D.D. & Watson, A.J. (1968) Myopathy associated with pigmentation following adrenalectomy for Cushing's syndrome. *Quarterly Journal of Medicine*, **37**, 63.

Prineas, J.W., Mason, A.S. & Henson, R.A. (1965) Myopathy in metabolic bone disease. *British Medical Journal*, **1**, 1034.

Ramsay, I.D. (1965) Electromyography in thyrotoxicosis. *Quarterly Journal of Medicine*, **34**, 255.

Ramsay, I.D. (1968) Thyrotoxic muscle disease. *Postgraduate Medical Journal*, **44**, 385.

Rawles, J.M. & Weller, R.O. (1974) Familial association of metabolic myopathy, lactic acidosis and sideroblastic anemia. *American Journal of Medicine*, **56**, 891.

Rebouche, C.J. (1977) Carnitine movement across muscle cell membranes. Studies in isolated rat muscle. *Biochimica et Biophysica Acta*, **471**, 145.

Rebouche, C.J. & Engel, A.G. (1980a) Tissue distribution of carnitine biosynthetic enzymes in man. *Biochemica et Biophysica Acta*, **630**, 22.

Rebouche, C.J. & Engel, A.G. (1980b) In vitro analysis of hepatic carnitine biosynthesis in human systemic carnitine deficiency. *Clinica Chimica Acta*, In press.

Rebouche, C.J. & Engel, A.G. (1980c) Carnitine biosynthesis in systemic carnitine deficiency (SCD). *Neurology (Minneapolis)*, **30**, 368.

Reed, G.B., Dixon, J.F.P., Neustein, H.B., Donnell, G.N. & Landing, B.H. (1968) Type IV glycogenosis: Patient with absence of a branching enzyme α-1,4-glucan 6-glucosyl transferase. *Laboratory Investigation*, **19**, 546.

Reid, H.A. (1961) Myoglobinuria in sea-snake-bite poisoning. *British Medical Journal*, **1**, 1284.

Resnick, J.S. & Engel, W.K. (1967) Myotonic lid lag in hyperkalaemic periodic paralysis. *Journal of Neurology, Neurosurgery and Psychiatry*, **30**, 478

Reuser, A.J.J., Koster, J.F., Hoogeveen, A. & Galjaard, H. (1978) Biochemical, immunochemical and cell genetic studies in glycogenosis type II. *American Journal of Human Genetics*, **30**, 132.

Reza, J.M., Kar, N.C., Pearson, C.M. & Kark, R.A.P. (1978) Recurrent myoglobinuria due to muscle carnitine palmityltransferase deficiency. *Annals of Internal Medicine*, **88**, 610.

Rich, E.C. (1894) A unique form of motor paralysis due to cold. *Medical News*, **65**, 210.

Richardson, G.O. & Sibley, J.C. (1953) Flaccid quadriplegia associated with hyperpotassemia. *Canadian Medical Association Journal*, **69**, 504.

Richardson, J.A., Herron, G., Reitz, R. & Layzer, R. (1969) Ischemic ulcerations of the skin and necrosis of muscle in azotemic hyperparathyroidism. *Annals of Internal Medicine*, **71**, 129.

Riecker, G. & Bolte, H.D. (1966) Membranpotentiale einzelner Skeletmuskelzellen bei periodischer Muskelparalyse. *Klinische Wochenschrift*, **44**, 894.

River, G.L., Kushner, D.S., Armstrong, S.H., Dubin, A., Sodki, S.J. & Cutting, H.O. (1960) Renal tubular acidosis with hypokalemia and muscular paralysis. *Metabolism*, **9**, 118.

Robertson, E.G. (1954) Thyrotoxic periodic paralysis. *Australian and New Zealand Journal of Medicine*, **3**, 182.

Robinson, B.H. & Sherwood, W.G. (1975) Pyruvate dehydrogenase phosphatase deficiency. A cause of congenital lactic acidosis in infancy. *Pediatric Research*, **9**, 935.

Robinson, B.H., Taylor, J. & Sherwood, W.G. (1978) Deficiency of dihydrolipoyl dehydrogenase (a component of pyruvate and α-ketoglutarate dehydrogenase complexes). A cause of congenital lactic acidosis. *Pediatric Research*, **11**, 1198.

Roelofs, R.I., Engel, W.K. & Chauvin, P. (1971) Demonstration of myophosphorylase activity in muscle grown in tissue culture from patients with muscle phosphorylase deficiency (McArdle's disease). *Journal of Histochemistry and Cytochemistry*, **19**, 715.

Rosenow, E.C. & Engel, A.G. (1978) Acid maltase deficiency in adults presenting as respiratory failure. *American Journal of Medicine*, **64**, 485.

Rowland, L.P. & Penn, A.S. (1972) Myoglobinuria. *Medical Clinics of North America*, **56**, 1233.

Rowland, L.P., Araki, S. & Carmel, P. (1965) Contracture in McArdle's disease. *Archives of Neurology*, **13**, 541.

Rowland, L.P., Lovelace, R.E., Schotland, D.L., Araki, S. & Carmel, P. (1966) The clinical diagnosis of McArdle's disease. Identification of another family with deficiency of muscle phosphorylase. *Neurology (Minneapolis)*, **16**, 93.

Rowley, P.T. & Kliman, B. (1960) The effect of sodium loading and depletion on muscular strength and aldosterone excretion in familial periodic paralysis. *American Journal of Medicine*, **28**, 376.

Rubenstein, A.E. & Wainapel, S.F. (1977) Acute hypokalemic myopathy in alcoholism. A clinical entity. *Archives of Neurology*, **34**, 553.

Rudman, D., Sewell, C.W. & Ansley, J.D. (1977) Deficiency of carnitine in cachectic cirrhotic patients. *Journal of Clinical Investigation*, **60**, 716.

Sagild, U. (1959) *Hereditary Transient Paralysis* (Ejnar Munksgaard: Copenhagen).

Salafsky, I.S. & Nadler, H.L. (1971) Alpha-1,4-glucosidase activity in Pompe's disease. *Journal of Pediatrics*, **79**, 794.

Salafsky, I.S. & Nadler, H.L. (1973) Deficiency of acid alpha-glucosidase in the urine of patients with Pompe's disease. *Journal of Pediatrics*, **82**, 294.

Salassa, R.M., Mattox, V.R. & Rosevear, J.W. (1962) Inhibition of the 'mineralo-corticoid' activity of licorice by spironolactone. *Journal of Clinical Endocrinology and Metabolism*, **22**, 1156.

Salick, A.I. & Pearson, C.M. (1967) Electrical silence of myoedema. *Neurology (Minneapolis)*, **17**, 899.

Samaha, F.J. (1965) Hyperkalemic periodic paralysis. *Archives of Neurology*, **12**, 145.

Sant'agnese, P.A. (1959) Diseases of glycogen storage with special reference to the cardiac type of generalized glycogenosis. *Annals of the New York Academy of Sciences*, **72**, 439.

Sataline, L.R. & Simonelli, J.M. (1961) Potassium paresis following ureterosigmoidostomy. *Journal of Urology*, **85**, 559.

Sato, K., Imai, F., Hatayama, I. & Roelofs, R.I. (1977) Characterization of glycogen phosphorylase isoenzymes present in cultured skeletal muscle from patients with McArdle's disease. *Biochemical and Biophysical Research Communications*, **78**, 663.

Satoyoshi, E. & Kowa, H. (1967) A myopathy due to glycolytic abnormality. *Archives of Neurology*, **71**, 248.

Satoyoshi, E., Murakami, K. & Kowa, H. (1963) Myopathy in thyrotoxocosis: With special emphasis on an effect of potassium ingestion on serum and urinary creatine. *Neurology (Minneapolis)*, **13**, 645.

Savage, D.C.L., Forbes, M. & Pearce, G.W. (1971) Idiopathic rhabdomyolysis. *Archives of Disease in Childhood*, **46**, 594.

Scarlato, G., Albizzati, M.G., Bassi, S., Cerri, C. & Frattola, L. (1977) A case of lipid storage myopathy with carnitine deficiency. Biochemical and electromyographic correlations. *European Neurology*, **16**, 222.

Scarlato, G., Pellegrini, G., Cerri, C., Meola, G. & Veicsteinas, A. (1978) The syndrome of carnitine deficiency: Morphological and metabolic correlations in two cases. *Canadian Journal of Neurological Sciences*, **5**, 205.

Schapira, Y., Cederbaum, S.D., Cancilla, P.A., Nielsen, D. & Lippe, B.M. (1975) Familial poliodystrophy, mitochondrial myopathy and lactate acidemia. *Neurology (Minneapolis)*, **25**, 614.

Schellens, J.P.M. & Ossentjuk, E. (1969) Mitochondrial ultrastructure with crystalloid inclusions in an unusual type of human myopathy. *Virchow Archiv B, Cell Pathology*, **4**, 21.

Schlesinger, J.J., Gandara, D. & Bensch, K.G. (1978)

Myoglobinuria associated with herpes-group viral infection. *Archives of Internal Medicine*, **138**, 422.

Schmid, R. & Mahler, R. (1959) Chronic progressive myopathy with myoglobinuria: Demonstration of a glycogenolytic defect in the muscle. *Journal of Clinical Investigation*, **38**, 1044.

Schneck, L., Adachi, M., Brieti, P., Wolintz, A. & Volk, B.W. (1973) Ophthalmoplegia plus with morphological and clinical studies of cerebellar and muscle tissue. *Journal of the Neurological Sciences*, **19**, 37.

Schochet, S.S., Jr., McCormick, W.F. & Zellweger, H. (1970) Type IV glycogenosis (amylopectinosis). *Archives of Pathology*, **90**, 354.

Scholte, H.R., Jennekens, F.G.I. & Bouvy, J.J.B.J. (1979) Carnitine palmityl-transferase II deficiency with normal carnitine palmityltransferase I in skeletal muscle and leukocytes. *Journal of the Neurological Sciences*, **40**, 39.

Schotland, D.L., Spiro, D., Rowland, L.P. & Carmel, P. (1965) Ultrastructural studies of muscle in McArdle's disease. *Journal of Neuropathology and Experimental Neurology*, **24**, 629.

Schotland, D.L., Di Mauro, S., Bonilla, F., Scarpa, A. & Lee, C.P. (1976) Neuromuscular disorder associated with a defect in mitochondrial energy supply. *Archives of Neurology*, **33**, 475.

Schott, G.D. & Wills, M.R. (1975) Myopathy and hypophosphataemic osteomalacia presenting in adult life. *Journal of Neurology, Neurosurgery and Psychiatry*, **38**, 297.

Schumate, J.B., Katnik, R., Ruiz, M., Kaiser, K., Frieden, C., Brooke, M.H. & Carroll, J.E. (1979) Myoadenylate deaminase deficiency. *Muscle and Nerve*, **2**, 213.

Schutta, H.S. & Armitage, J.L. (1969) Thyrotoxic hypokalemic periodic paralysis. *Journal of Neuropathology and Experimental Neurology*, **28**, 321.

Schwartz, W.B. & Relman, A.S. (1953) Metabolic and renal studies in chronic potassium depletion resulting from overuse of laxatives. *Journal of Clinical Investigation*, **32**, 258.

Sengers, R.C.A., Ter-Haar, B.G.A., Trijbels, J.M.F., Willems, J.L., Daniels, O. & Stadhouders, A.M. (1975) Congenital cataract and mitochondrial myopathy of skeletal and heart muscle associated with lactic acidosis after exercise. *Journal of Pediatrics*, **86**, 873.

Serratrice, G., Monges, A., Roux, H., Aquaron, R. & Gambarelli, D. (1969) Myopathic form of phosphofructokinase deficit. *Revue Neurologique*, **120**, 271.

Shafiq, S.A., Milhorat, A.T. & Gorycki, M.A. (1967) Giant mitochondria in human muscle with inclusions. *Archives of Neurology*, **17**, 666.

Shoji, S., Takagi, A., Sugita, H. & Toyokura, Y. (1976) Dysfunction of sarcoplasmic reticulum in rabbit and human steroid myopathy. *Experimental Neurology*, **51**, 304.

Shy, G.M., Gonatas, N.K. & Perez, M. (1966) Two childhood myopathies with abnormal mitochondria. I. Megaconial myopathy. II. Pleoconial myopathy. *Brain*, **89**, 133.

Shy, G.M., Wanko, T., Rowley, P.T. & Engel, A.G. (1961) Studies in familial periodic paralysis. *Experimental Neurology*, **3**, 53.

Shy, G.M., Silberberg, D.H., Appel, S.H., Mishkin, M.M. & Godfrey, E.H. (1967) A generalised disorder of nervous system, skeletal muscle and heart resembling Refsum's disease and Hurler's syndrome. I. Clinical, pathologic and biochemical characteristics. *American Journal of Medicine*, **42**, 163.

Sidbury, J.B. (1965) The genetics of the glycogen storage diseases. *Progress in Medical Genetics*, **4**, 32.

Sidbury, J.B. Jr., Mason, J., Burns, W.B., Jr & Ruebner, B.H. (1962) Type IV glycogenosis: Report of a case proven by characterization of glycogen and studied at necropsy. *Bulletin of the Johns Hopkins Hospital*, **57**, 157.

Simon, N.M., Rovner, R.N. & Berlin, B.S. (1970) Acute myoglobinuria with type A2 (Hong Kong) influenza. *Journal of the American Medical Association*, **212**, 1704.

Sloan, M.F., Franks, A.J., Exley, K.A. & Davison, A.M. (1978) Acute renal failure due to polymyositis. *British Medical Journal*, **1**, 1457.

Slotwiner, P., Song, S.K. & Maker, H.S. (1969) Myopathy resembling McArdle's syndrome. *Archives of Neurology*, **20**, 586.

Smith, H.L., Amick, L.D. & Sidbury, J.B., Jr. (1966) Type II glycogenosis: Report of a case with four-year survival and absence of acid maltase associated with an abnormal glycogen. *American Journal of Diseases of Children*, **111**, 475.

Smith, J., Zellweger, H. & Afifi, A.K. (1967) Muscular form of glycogenosis, type II (Pompe): Report of a case with unusual features. *Neurology (Minneapolis)*, **17**, 537.

Smith, R. & Stern, G. (1967) Myopathy, osteomalacia and hyperparathyroidism. *Brain*, **90**, 593.

Smyth, D.P.L., Lake, B.D., MacDermot, J. & Wilson, J. (1975) Inborn error of carnitine metabolism ('carnitine deficiency') in man. *Lancet*, **1**, 1198.

Solomon, D.H. & Kleeman, K.E. (1976) Concepts of pathogenesis of Graves' disease. *Advances in Internal Medicine*, **22**, 273.

Song, S.K. & Rubin, E. (1972) Ethanol produces muscle damage in human volunteers. *Science*, **175**, 327.

Spiro, A.J., Prineas, J.W. & Moore, C.L. (1970) A new mitochondrial myopathy in a patient with salt craving. *Archives of Neurology*, **22**, 259.

Spiro, A.J., Moore, C.L., Prineas, J.W., Strasberg, P.M. & Rapin, I. (1970) A cytochrome related inherited disorder of the nervous system and muscle. *Archives of Neurology*, **23**, 103.

Staffurth, J.S. (1964) The total exchangeable potassium in patients with hypokalemia. *Postgraduate Medical Journal*, **40**, 4.

Steinitz, K. & Rutenberg, A. (1967) Tissue α-glucosidase activity and glycogen content in patients with generalized glycogenosis. *Israel Journal of Medical Sciences*, **3**, 411.

Stephen, C.R. (1977) Malignant hyperpyrexia. *Annual Review of Medicine*, **28**, 153.

Stocker, W.W., Samaha, F.J. & De Groot, L.J. (1968) Coupled oxidative phosphorylation in muscle of thyrotoxic patients. *American Journal of Medicine*, **44**, 900.

Strugalska-Cynowska, M. (1967) Disturbances in the activity of phosphorylase-*b*-kinase in a case of McArdle myopathy. *Folia Histochemica et Cytochemica*, **5**, 151.

Sulaiman, W.R., Doyle, D., Johnson, R.H. & Jennett, S. (1974) Myopathy with mitochondrial inclusion bodies. Histologic and metabolic studies. *Journal of Neurology, Neurosurgery and Psychiatry*, **37**, 1236.

Sussman, K.E., Alfrey, A., Kirsch, W.M., Zweig, P., Felig, P. & Messner, F. (1970) Chronic lactic acidosis in an adult. A new syndrome associated with an altered redox state of certain NAD/NADH coupled reactions. *American Journal of Medicine*, **48**, 104.

Swaiman, K.F., Kennedy, W.R. & Sauls, H.S. (1968) Late infantile acid maltase deficiency. *Archives of Neurology*, **18**, 642.

Takamori, M., Gutmann, L. & Shane, S.R. (1971) Contractile properties of human skeletal muscle: Normal and thyroid disease. *Archives of Neurology*, **25**, 535.

Talbott, J.H. (1941) Periodic paralysis. *Medicine (Baltimore)*, **20**, 85.

Tancredi, R.G., Dagenais, G.R. & Zierler, K.L. (1976) Free fatty acid metabolism in the forearm at rest: Muscle uptake and adipose tissue release of free fatty acids. *Johns Hopkins Medical Journal*, **138**, 167.

Tanphaichitr, V. & Broquist, H.P. (1974) Site of carnitine biosynthesis in the rat. *Journal of Nutrition*, **104**, 1669.

Tarui, S., Kono, N., Nasu, T. & Nishikawa, M. (1969) Enzymatic basis for coexistence of myopathy and hemolytic disease in inherited muscle phosphofructokinase deficiency. *Biochemical and Biophysical Research Communications*, **34**, 77.

Tarui, S., Okuno, G., Ikura, Y., Tanaka, T., Suda, M. & Nishikawa, M. (1965) Phosphofructokinase deficiency in skeletal muscle. A new type of glycogenosis. *Biochemical and Biophysical Research Communications*, **19**, 517.

Thomson, W.H.S., MacLaurin, J.C. & Prineas, J.W. (1963) Skeletal muscle glycogenosis: An investigation of two dissimilar cases. *Journal of Neurology, Neurosurgery and Psychiatry*, **26**, 60.

Thorn, G.W. (1949) *The Diagnosis and Treatment of Adrenal Insufficiency*, p. 144 (Thomas: Springfield, Illinois).

Tice, L.W. & Engel, A.G. (1967) The effects of glucocorticoids on red and white muscles in the rat. *American Journal of Pathology*, **50**, 311.

Tobin, W.E., Huijing, F., Porro, R.S. & Salzman, R.T. (1973) A case of muscle phosphofructokinase deficiency. *Archives of Neurology*, **28**, 128.

Tomasi, L.G. (1979) Reversibility of human myopathy caused by vitamin E deficiency. *Neurology (Minneapolis)*, **29**, 1183.

Tsai, J.S. & Chen, A. (1977) L-triiodothyronine increases the level of β-adrenergic receptor in cultured myocardial cells. *Clinical Research*, **25**, 303A.

Van Biervliet, J.P.G.M., Bruinvis, L., Ketting, D., De Bree, P.K., Van Der Heiden, C.K., Wadman, S.K., Willems, J.L., Bookelman, H., Van Haelst, U. & Monnens, L.A.H. (1977) Hereditary mitochondrial myopathy with lactic acidemia, a DeToni-Fanconi-Debré syndrome, and a defective respiratory chain in voluntary striated muscles. *Pediatric Research*, **11**, 1088.

Van Buchem, F.S.P. (1957) The electrocardiogram and potassium metabolism. *American Journal of Medicine*, **23**, 376.

Van Buchem, F.S.P., Doorenbos, H. & Elings, H.S. (1956) Conn's syndrome, caused by adrenocortical hyperplasia. *Acta Endocrinologica*, **23**, 313.

Van Der Meulen, J.P., Gilbert, G.J. & Kane, C.A. (1961) Familial hyperkalemic paralysis with myotonia. *New England Journal of Medicine*, **264**, 1.

Vandyke, D.H., Griggs, R.C., Markesbery, W. & Di Mauro, S. (1975) Hereditary carnitine deficiency of muscle. *Neurology (Minneapolis)*, **25**, 154.

Van Hoof, F. (1967) Amylo-1,6-glucosidase activity and glycogen content of the erythrocytes of normal subjects, patients with glycogen-storage disease and heterozygotes. *European Journal of Biochemistry*, **2**, 271.

Van Hoof, F. & Hers, H.G. (1967) The subgroups of type III glycogenosis. *European Journal of Biochemistry*, **2**, 271.

Van't Hoff, W. (1962) Familial myotonic periodic paralysis. *Quarterly Journal of Medicine*, **31**, 385.

Van Wijngaarden, G.K., Bethlem, J., Meijer, A.E.F.H., Hülsmann, W.C. & Feltkamp, C.A. (1967) Skeletal muscle disease with abnormal mitochondria. *Brain*, **90**, 577.

Verner, J.V. & Morrison, A.B. (1958) Islet cell tumor and a syndrome of refractory watery diarrhea and hypokalemia. *American Journal of Medicine*, **25**, 374.

Vicale, C.T. (1949) The diagnostic features of a muscular syndrome resulting from hyperparathyroidism, osteomalacia owing to renal tubular acidosis and perhaps to related disorders of calcium metabolism. *Transactions of the American Neurological Association*, **74**, 143.

Vignos, P.J. & Greene, R. (1973) Oxidative respiration of skeletal muscle in experimental corticosteroid myopathy. *Journal of Laboratory and Clinical Medicine*, **81**, 365.

Wahren, J., Felig, P., Havel, R.J., Jorfeldt, L., Pernow, B. & Saltin, B. (1973) Amino acid metabolism in McArdle's syndrome. *New England Journal of Medicine*, **288**, 774.

Ware, A.J., Burton, W.C., McGarry, J.D., Marks, J.F. & Weinberg, A.G. (1978) Systemic carnitine deficiency. Report of a fatal case with multisystemic manifestations. *Journal of Pediatrics*, **93**, 959.

Weisler, M.J. (1961) The electrocardiogram in periodic paralysis. *Chest*, **4**, 217.

Whisnant, J.P., Espinosa, R.E., Kierland, R.R. & Lambert, E.H. (1963) Chloroquine neuromyopathy. *Proceedings of the Staff Meetings of the Mayo Clinic*, **38**, 501.

Whitaker, J.N., Di Mauro, S., Solomon, S.S., Sabesin, S., Duckworth, W.C. & Mendell, J.R. (1977) Corticosteroid-responsive skeletal muscle disease associated with partial carnitine deficiency. Studies of liver and metabolic alterations. *American Journal of Medicine*, **63**, 805.

Willems, J.L., Monnens, A.H., Trijbels, J.M.F., Veerkamp, J.H., Meyer, A.E.F.H., Van Dam, K. & Van Haelst, U. (1977) Leigh's encephalomyopathy in a patient with cytochrome c oxidase deficiency of muscle tissue. *Pediatrics*, **60**, 850.

Williams, C. & Field, J.B. (1968) Studies in glycogen-storage disease: Limit dextrinosis, a genetic study. *Journal of Pediatrics*, **72**, 214.

Williams, H.E. (1966) α-Glucosidase activity in human leukocytes. *Biochimica Biophysica Acta*, **124**, 34.

Williams, L.T., Lefkowitz, R.J. & Watanabe, A.M. (1977) Thyroid hormone regulation of β-adrenergic receptor number. *Journal of Biological Chemistry*, **252**, 2787.

Williams, R.S. (1959) Triamcinolone myopathy. *Lancet*, **1**, 698.

Willner, J.H., Ginsburg, S. & Di Mauro, S. (1978) Active transport of carnitine into skeletal muscle. *Neurology (Minneapolis)*, **28**, 721.

Willner, J.H., Di Mauro, S., Eastwood, A., Hays, A., Roohi, F. & Lovelace, R. (1979) Muscle carnitine deficiency: Genetic heterogeneity. *Journal of the Neurological Sciences*, **41**, 235.

Wilson, J. & Walton, J.N. (1959) Some muscular manifestations of hypothyroidism. *Journal of Neurology, Neurosurgery and Psychiatry*, **22**, 320.

Worsfold, M., Park, D. C. & Pennington, R.J. (1973) Familial 'mitochondrial' myopathy. A myopathy associated with disordered oxidative metabolism in muscle fibres. Part 2. Biochemical findings. *Journal of the Neurological Sciences*, **19**, 261.

Yeung, R.T.T. & Tse, T.F. (1974) Thyrotoxic periodic paralysis. Effect of propranolol. *American Journal of Medicine*, **59**, 584.

Yunis, A.A., Fischer, E.H. & Krebs, E.G. (1962) Comparative studies on glycogen phosphorylase. Purification and properties of rabbit heart phosphorylase. *Journal of Biological Chemistry*, **237**, 2809.

Zellweger, H., Mueller, S., Ionasescu, V., Schochet, S.S. & McCormick, W.F. (1972) Glycogenosis IV: A new cause of infantile hypotonia. *Journal of Pediatrics*, **80**, 842.

Zierler, K.L. (1976) Fatty acids as substrates for heart and skeletal muscle. *Circulation Research*, **38**, 459.

Zierler, K.L. & Andres, R. (1957) Movement of potassium into skeletal muscle during spontaneous attack in family periodic paralysis. *Journal of Clinical Investigation*, **28**, 376.

Zintz, R. (1966) Dystrophische Veränderungen in ausseren Augenmuskeln und Schultermuskeln bei der sog. Progressiven Graefeschen Ophthalmoplegie. In *Progressive Muskeldystrophie, Myotonie, Myasthenia*, Ed. E. Kuhn, p. 109 (Springer-Verlag: Berlin).

Neuromuscular disorders associated with malignant disease

INTRODUCTION

The muscular wasting encountered in patients with malignant disease is due to a variety or combination of factors, including cachexia, malnutrition, disuse, infection, toxaemia, arthropathy and old age. It is well known that non-specific pathological abnormalities are found in postmortem specimens of muscle from patients with or without malignant disease, and Pearson (1959) discovered such changes in 54 out of 110 routine autopsies; the lesions are presumably attributable to different or multiple factors, including those mentioned above. Muscular atrophy and weakness deriving from involvement of the lower motor neurones is relatively uncommon and so are the myopathies, such as the myasthenic syndrome and dermatomyositis, described below. In this Chapter, muscular disorders due to metastases affecting nerve or muscle are considered first, followed by a brief mention of nutritional disorders and an extended description of non-metastatic complications of malignant disease as these pertain to the neuromuscular system.

SECONDARY TUMOURS

In spite of the rich blood supply of muscles, the incidence of metastatic tumours in muscle is low. Pearson (1959) found evidence of tumour emboli or actual growths in 6 of 38 cases examined postmortem, a higher incidence than hitherto reported. Nevertheless, it is clear that muscles provide poor soil for the extensive growth of metastases, and biochemical factors are presumably involved in the destruction and regression of tumour emboli which must take place. In Pearson's series there were three cases of metastasis from carcinoma and three from lymphoma, including reticulum cell sarcoma, myeloid leukaemia and giant follicular lymphoma. There were no clinical manifestations of muscular involvement.

Direct invasion of muscles by primary growth is commoner than involvement by metastases; it is seen in both carcinoma and sarcoma. The invasion causes loss of muscle fibres by means of compression atrophy, ischaemia and actual infiltration by tumour cells. A good example of this process is the spread of breast carcinoma into the adjacent pectoral muscles. There is one example of diffuse muscular infiltration with clinically evident weakness in our material; this occurred in a patient with scirrhous carcinoma of the stomach.

METASTATIC INFILTRATION OF NERVE ROOTS AND PERIPHERAL NERVES

Local infiltration

The commonest type of peripheral nerve lesion encountered in malignant disease is compression or infiltration of individual nerves or nerve plexuses by neoplastic tissue deriving from neighbouring growths, either primary or secondary. However, considering the high incidence of carcinoma, sarcoma, and the reticuloses, clinical manifestations of nervous lesions of this type are relatively uncommon. Willis (1952) commented on the way in which nerves escape invasion when enveloped by growth; when invasion does occur, nerve degeneration may not follow. Once infiltration of a nerve takes place there is longitudinal permeation via the perineurium, endoneurium and perineural lymphatics; if nerve damage results there will be muscular wasting and weakness in the distribution of the affected nerve. Familiar examples of this process include lesions of the brachial plexus in Pancoast's tumour, of the lumbar plexus in retroperitoneal lymphosarcoma and of the sacral plexus in pelvic carcinoma.

Diffuse infiltration of peripheral nerves

Diffuse malignant infiltration of peripheral nerves must be extremely rare in any type of carcinoma; indeed, Russell and Rubinstein (1959) knew of no authentic cases in which peripheral nerves or ganglia, other than the trigeminal, were the seat of metastases in carcinoma. However, diffuse infiltration of nerves is seen occasionally in lymphoproliferative disease, myeloma and leukaemia, and in all these complaints the first symptoms may be those of peripheral neuropathy due to this malignant invasion.

Diffuse intraspinal infiltration

Diffuse infiltration of the spinal nerve roots and posterior root ganglia can accompany the peripheral nerve invasion found in the lymphoproliferative disorders and leukaemia, or it may occur independently or in association with intracranial leptomeningeal and cranial nerve involvement. Diagnosis is straightforward when the malignant disease is known to be present; when no signs of the underlying process can be made out the situation may be established by demonstration of neoplastic cells in the spinal fluid. Spinal nerves and ganglia may be the seat of diffuse and nodular infiltration of secondary carcinomatous growth disseminated by the cerebrospinal fluid from a metastasis within the head; such lesions are frequently largest in the lumbar sac, where they involve the cauda equina (Willis, 1952). In these circumstances there is no characteristic clinical syndrome, for symptoms of the major metastasis or intracranial meningeal involvement may predominate. Backache and unilateral or bilateral sciatica may occur with sensory, motor and sphincter symptoms. The course is rather rapidly progressive and the patient soon becomes emaciated. Malignant cells may be found on microscopic examination of the spinal fluid. In other cases spinal carcinomatous meningitis arises in the absence of intracranial metastasis or evidence of cranial nerve involvement (Parsons, 1972). In both cases the sugar content of the cerebrospinal fluid is likely to be decreased and malignant cells may be seen. The common sites of primary growth are bronchus and stomach.

Localised intraspinal metastases

Compression paraplegia due to vertebral and epidural metastases is a well-known feature of carcinoma and the reticuloses. When the lumbar spine is affected, flaccid weakness of the limbs results from compression of lumbosacral nerve roots. Back and root pain are commonly prominent, and sensory loss and sphincter disturbances develop as the condition progresses. Plain X-rays and modern imaging techniques frequently show changes in the affected part of the spine, while lumbar puncture may reveal some degree of spinal block and an increase in the spinal fluid protein. Myelography gives a precise picture of the extent of the lesion. Several nerve roots may be affected by tumour material growing into the spinal canal via the intervertebral foramina from retroperitoneal deposits, but this is rare. Again, pain is usually severe and sensory loss present.

NUTRITIONAL DISORDERS

Pellagra and Wernicke's encephalopathy are known to occur in patients with carcinoma of the alimentary tract, and especially of the stomach.

The relationship of Addisonian anaemia and carcinoma of the stomach is also recognised, but it is not clear whether this association increases the liability to subacute combined degeneration of the spinal cord (Spillane, 1947). Subacute combined degeneration may occur in patients in a cachectic condition due to malignant disease (Brain, 1955). In both pellagra and subacute combined degeneration, muscular weakness may form a part of the neurological syndrome. Diagnosis is simple.

NON-METASTATIC NEUROLOGICAL MANIFESTATIONS OF MALIGNANT DISEASE

Brain introduced the terms carcinomatous neuropathy and neuromyopathy to describe involvement of the central or peripheral nervous system and muscle by non-metastatic processes in patients with cancer. Henson (1970) preferred to use the general diagnosis non-metastatic neurological manifestations of malignant disease, specifying the type of nervous or muscular disorder present. His reasons included the fact that important non-invasive neurological syndromes occur in the reticuloses as well as in carcinoma.

The important neurological disorders associated with malignant disease include encephalomyelitis with carcinoma (Henson, Hoffman and Urich, 1965), cerebellar degeneration, progressive multifocal leucoencephalopathy, peripheral neuropathy and a variety of myopathies. It has proved difficult to determine the incidence of these conditions from the highly selected London Hospital material. Henson (1970) estimated that the combined incidence of symptomatic peripheral neuropathy and encephalomyelitis with carcinoma of the lung was of the order of one or two per cent in an unselected group. Reporting their findings from a prospective longitudinal survey, Wilkinson, Croft and Urich (1967) found that 6.6 per cent of 1465 cases of carcinoma showed clinical evidence of non-metastatic nervous or muscular disorder. The highest incidence was in patients with carcinoma of the lung, ovary and stomach. Fifteen per cent of males with lung cancer were so affected, but this figure falls to approximately 6 per cent if the less

well-defined neuromuscular and muscular syndromes are excluded. Signs of peripheral neuropathy were discovered in 5.3 per cent of 316 patients with lung carcinoma; 2.8 per cent of patients with carcinoma of stomach and 1.2 per cent of those with growths of the breast and large bowel were affected.

Recent electrodiagnostic studies have shown a high yield of abnormalities in patients with lung cancer who made no neurological complaints. These subclinical neuromyopathies were found by Campbell and Paty (1974) in 21 out of 26 patients. The term neuromyopathy is used advisedly here as the abnormalities found reflected disorder in both muscle and nerve in the majority.

Currie, Henson, Morgan and Poole (1970) explored the incidence of non-metastatic neurological syndromes of obscure origin in the reticuloses. There were 11 (1.4 per cent) examples of peripheral neuropathy among 774 patients and 3 (0.4 per cent) of polymyositis. Three additional cases of remarkable cachectic myopathy were also discovered.

The whole subject has been reviewed by Henson (1970), while Currie et al. (1970) and Currie and Henson (1971) have discussed the aetiology of non-metastatic syndromes in the reticuloses.

Neural atrophies

These are attributable to peripheral neuropathy or to anterior horn cell loss in encephalomyelitis with carcinoma. They are distinguished from the myogenic atrophies by the usual criteria, which may include electrodiagnostic tests and muscle biopsy in obscure cases.

Peripheral neuropathy. The clinical features of peripheral neuropathy with carcinoma are commonly those of subacute sensorimotor peripheral neuropathy, but the tempo of the process varies from acute to chronic. In some patients symptoms are limited to distal paraesthesiae and sensory loss, while in others there is profound muscular wasting and weakness and more extensive sensory loss in the limbs (Henson and Urich, 1970). Exceptionally there is acute progressive muscular weakness with little sensory change. The symptoms may precede those of carcinoma and the diagnosis should be remembered in patients with unexplained peripheral neuropathy. Remission can occur. The syndrome is not due to any known nutritional defect and treatment is symptomatic. The associated carcinoma is often bronchial but growths in many other sites have been implicated.

Encephalomyelitis with carcinoma. This condition is usually linked with oat cell bronchial carcinoma, and is characterised pathologically by inflammatory changes with nerve cell destruction in the limbic lobes, brain-stem, spinal cord and posterior root ganglia (Henson, Hoffman and Urich, 1965). The clinical manifestations depend upon the distribution and intensity of lesions and vary from those of limbic encephalitis (Corsellis, Goldberg and Norton, 1968) to an extreme form of sensory neuronopathy (Denny-Brown, 1948). Brain-stem involvement is reflected in ataxia, vertigo, nystagmus, external ophthalmoplegia and bulbar palsy. Disturbances of tone, involuntary movements, increased tendon reflexes and extensor plantar responses may be noted. Spinal cord symptoms are usually limited to muscular wasting and weakness stemming from damage to anterior horn cells; fasciculation may be seen in the affected musculature.

When neuromuscular symptoms are predominant the clinical picture can resemble that of motor neurone disease, but thorough examination in our material has always revealed evidence of brain-stem involvement, such as nystagmus, vertigo and ataxia, or posterior root ganglion lesions. Cord involvement may be patchy or localised; for example, in one patient seen by the author weakness was limited to muscles of the neck and shoulder girdles.

The cerebrospinal fluid protein is often raised in the active stage and there may be a mild lymphocytic pleocytosis. The most important laboratory finding was Wilkinson's discovery of brain-specific complement-fixing antibodies in blood and cerebrospinal fluid in four successive patients (Croft, Henson, Urich and Wilkinson, 1965). However, the significance of this finding has been questioned. Henson and Urich (1979) have reviewed the problem of aetiology.

Encephalomyelitis with carcinoma runs a subacute course from a few months to two years as a rule, duration being largely determined by the growth and extension of the associated cancer. However, the process can be self-limiting and recovery may occur (Henson, 1970).

Motor neurone disease. Brain, Croft and Wilkinson (1965) described a group of patients in whom there was an association between neoplasm and a neurological disorder similar to motor neurone disease. The clinical course was relatively benign compared with that of classical motor neurone disease. There is no evidence of a significant incidence of classical motor neurone disease in patients with carcinoma.

Muscular disorders

Brain and Adams (1965) proposed that the remote muscular effects or complications of carcinoma should be classified under the following heads: (1) polymyopathy, (2) disorders of neuromuscular transmission, (3) dermatomyositis and polymyositis, and (4) endocrine-metabolic myopathies. This classification has the merit of simplicity and will be followed here.

Polymyopathy. There are three conditions to be considered under this head, namely cachectic myopathy, the syndrome of predominantly proximal muscular weakness, and acute muscle necrosis. Problems of terminology arise in dealing with this group because of our ignorance of pathogenesis and our less than full knowledge of the prime sites of disorder. At present the term neuromyopathy appears to be the most appropriate for all three conditions.

Cachectic myopathy (neuromyopathy). In this familiar condition there is great loss of subcutaneous fat. The muscles are diffusely wasted throughout the body. This muscular wasting is associated with widespread, symmetrical weakness, which becomes extreme in the final stages; generally speaking, however, muscular power is remarkably good, considering the degree of atrophy. Myoidema may be present. Depression of tendon reflexes occurs when wasting is extreme. Post-mortem examination reveals thin muscles of a reddish-brown or brown colour. The histological picture is one of variation in the size of muscle fibres, with numbers of unevenly distributed small fibres. In advanced cases fibre necrosis appears, with hyaline, granular and vacuolar degeneration. Ultimately the affected fibres may die, leaving a few sarcolemmal nuclei to mark their disappearance; usually no cellular reaction is seen at these sites of degeneration. There is little correlation between the degree of atrophy and the microscopic changes described. The precise cause of this myopathy is unknown: primary nutritional factors are not necessarily involved, for the patient may be able to take and absorb adequate nourishment. The condition is clinically and pathologically similar to the muscular atrophy which accompanies other chronic debilitating complaints, such as tuberculosis, gastrocolic fistula and steatorrhoea. It must be recalled that some of the pathological changes mentioned above, such as hyaline, granular and vacuolar degeneration and, more rarely, interstitial or perivascular cellular foci, are found in the absence of cachexia or of any clinically discernible muscular disorder on routine examination of muscles at post-mortem examination. Rebeiz (1970) re-explored the subject. Using large blocks of muscle obtained post mortem he noted two types of muscle cell atrophy: (a) randomly distributed atrophic fibres, occurring singly or in groups of two or three; (b) groups of 5–50 closely packed atrophic fibres lying among normal or hypertrophied motor units. These changes were found in patients dying from a variety of carcinomas and from lymphoma. In milder cases the lower limbs only were affected. Rebeiz concluded that the muscular atrophy could not derive from chronic caloric insufficiency. It seemed probable that the two types of atrophy were unrelated and reflected the effect of the neoplastic process on both nervous and muscular systems. The widespread atrophy of motor units or subunits was neurogenic in some cases at least, the primary lesion being in the anterior horn cells of the spinal cord. Engel (1977) wrote that type II fibre atrophy eventually develops in virtually every patient with carcinoma, but it is not necessarily related to disuse or inanition.

A further type of histological change found in chronic cachectic states is granular pigmentary degeneration, and this is also seen in the voluntary muscles and myocardium in aged patients. The contents of muscle cells are transformed into a granular pigment of the lipofuscin group; in extreme examples the cells disappear, leaving an aggregation of degenerate nuclei. Marin and Denny-Brown (1962) found extensive changes of this type in the proximal musculature of patients with carcinoma, so that little remained of the muscle fibres in large areas. The phenomenon was always linked with some degree of cachexia. It appears that this process represents a further type of muscular reaction to carcinoma, presumably of metabolic origin.

Syndrome of proximal muscular weakness (carcinomatous neuromyopathy). The simple clinical observation that patients with malignant disease might present with muscular weakness, which was predominantly, if not entirely, proximal in distribution, was made many years ago (Henson, 1953; Henson, Russell and Wilkinson, 1954). Although the term carcinomatous myopathy was introduced by these workers, they acknowledged that the site and nature of the causal lesion had not been established. Subsequent authors have confirmed the clinical observations made, notably Shy and Silverstein (1965), Campbell and Paty (1974) and Warmolts, Re', Lewis and Engel (1975). Indeed, this is the commonest neurological remote effect of cancer, both in our material and that of others.

Patients with overt or concealed malignant disease complain of weakness affecting the proximal and axial musculature. Myasthenia is not a feature of the condition and clinical evidence of neural lesions is often lacking. The syndrome occurs in patients who are otherwise well preserved. The associated cancer is usually located in the lung, breast, prostate or gastrointestinal tract, but the lung has been implicated most often in our series. It is not unusual for the tumour to be small, and sometimes it is undetectable at initial examination.

Early histopathological studies revealed changes which were disproportionately slight in relation to the degree of weakness. More recently, Warmolts and his colleagues (1975) reported highly predominant type II fibre atrophy and questioned whether the lesion was myopathic or neurogenic. Heffner and Barron (1977) found muscular atrophy, again primarily involving type II fibres, at biopsy; electron microscopic examination showed degenerative changes in intramuscular nerve twigs. Follow-up biopsy demonstrated the changes of denervation. Electromyography may be normal in the early stages or may show mild abnormalities, such as a reduced interference pattern and brief small motor unit potentials, over-abundant on recruitment and polyphasic (Heffner and Barron, 1977). There is, therefore, good evidence of a distal neuropathy in these cases. However, Campbell and Paty (1974) found signs both of myopathy and of neuropathy in their electrodiagnostic studies; clearly, more remains to be learned. The term carcinomatous neuromyopathy seems acceptable in the present state of our knowledge.

The nature of the proximal muscular syndrome remains obscure. It is not necessarily related to weight loss or malnutrition, though Hildebrand and Coërs (1967) regarded these as causal factors, and we do not know whether the condition represents a localised manifestation of the forces at work in malignant cachexia. Pathogenesis may rest on direct or indirect remote effects of the neoplasm.

From the practical point of view, the presence of malignant disease should be suspected in males over the age of 50 with unexplained, acquired weakness of the proximal musculature. The condition is rarer in females. No specific treatment is available but spontaneous remission can occur. Prognosis is determined by the nature of the associated malignant process and its susceptibility to treatment.

Acute necrotising myopathy. Smith (1969) drew attention to the occurrence of necrosis of skeletal muscle in biopsies from three patients with carcinoma of the colon, breast and stomach. Urich and Wilkinson (1970) reported a similar case with full post-mortem examination. A man aged 59 developed a rapidly progressive weakness which involved almost the whole musculature within a few weeks, the patient dying from his muscle disease in about two months. A mucus-producing adenocarcinoma of the stomach was found at necropsy. On histological examination the skeletal muscles showed widespread necrosis with minimal inflammatory reaction. The authors concluded that the process was morphologically, and probably pathogenetically, different from polymyositis. Swash (1974) published a description of a further case, a woman aged 72 with bladder cancer, the patient dying five weeks from the onset. In this patient post-mortem examination showed acute necrotising myopathy and also acute neuropathy. No immune complexes were found in the walls of intramuscular blood vessels.

Brownell and Hughes (1975) described three further cases, all associated with oat cell carcinoma of the lung and all accompanied by degeneration of intramuscular nerve fibres.

It appears that this rare, acute neuromyopathy (a better descriptive term) is usually linked with carcinoma, but no pathogenetic relationship has been established. To date no good evidence of an immunological disorder has been adduced, and toxic and hormonal factors have not been implicated. Treatment with ACTH has been unsuccessful.

Myasthenic syndrome (Eaton-Lambert syndrome). The majority of patients with this complaint prove to be suffering from malignant disease, usually oat cell bronchial carcinoma although other sites have been implicated, notably breast, prostate, stomach and rectum, and there has been a link with reticulum cell sarcoma (Rooke, Eaton, Lambert and Hodgson, 1960; Elmquist and Lambert, 1968). However, the Eaton-Lambert syndrome may occur in the absence of growth, as in four out of six patients described by Brown and Johns (1974). Middle-aged males are often affected. The condition is one of the commoner neuromuscular disorders accompanying carcinoma. Symptoms of neuromuscular disorder commonly precede those of the cancer, sometimes by many months, but they can arise in patients already receiving treatment for malignant disease. Patients with the Eaton-Lambert syndrome have an undue sensitivity to muscle relaxants, so that symptoms are noticed during or after surgical operations in which such agents have been employed. An association of the myasthenic syndrome with myasthenia gravis has been described (Fettel, Shir, Penn, Lovelace and Rowland, 1978), but ordinarily the two conditions are quite distinct.

Clinical features. The clinical picture is characterised by muscular fatigability, a symptom difficult to evaluate because there may be a discrepancy between the severe disability suffered and the relatively slight objective weakness found (Brown and Johns, 1974). Besides the fatigability there are varying degrees of mild wasting and persistent weakness affecting the muscles of the trunk and proximal parts of the limbs. Muscles of the pelvic girdle and thighs are often, but not always, first involved, with consequent difficulty in walking, mounting stairs and rising from a chair; flexion of the hips and extension of the knees are particularly weakened. The arms and shoulder girdles are generally affected sooner or later, but they escape in a few instances. Ptosis oculi, diplopia, dysarthria and dysphagia are rare complaints, but we have seen patients present with drooping lids and double vision, and with myogenic troubles with speech and swallowing. Weakness is often myasthenic, in the sense that it is produced by or follows exertion, and this may be evident on clinical examination. On the other hand, the characteristic facilitation, or temporary increase in power after brief exercise, is not always present (Lambert and Rooke, 1965; Brown and Johns, 1974). Tendon reflexes are diminished or abolished in the affected areas, and sometimes beyond them; the knee jerks are usually depressed first. Fasciculation is not seen. Muscular aching can be a persistent troublesome complaint.

Neurological symptoms may accompany the myopathy, for example, impotence, paraesthesiae in the extremities and dryness of the mouth. We have also noticed unexplained dementia and extensor plantar responses. When the myasthenic syndrome is exceptionally accompanied by another paraneoplastic neurological disorder, such as encephalomyelitis or subacute cortical cerebellar degeneration, there may be initial diagnostic difficulties at the bedside.

The illness is characteristically subacute. The course can be fluctuant, with spontaneous remissions; this usually obtains when neuromuscular symptoms precede local manifestations of the associated growth. However, the degree of improvement is rarely sufficient to enable the patient to return to work. Even in the more favourable cases, socially crippling muscular weakness is the general rule. The whole course of the illness is largely determined by the site and nature of the associated neoplasm. While death is due to the direct effects of the cancer, profound muscular weakness can be a significant contributory factor. Treatment of associated lung cancer cannot be expected to have any beneficial effect on the myasthenic syndrome, but a successful outcome in patients with less malignant forms of tumour may be accompanied by complete recovery (Fontanel, Bethenil, Senechal and Hagneneau, 1973; Metral and Veron, 1975).

Pharmacological responses and electrodiagnostic features. The response of the muscular weakness to an injection of neostigmine or edrophonium hydrochloride is variable; the test is usually negative or equivocal, but occasionally there is measurable relief. There is undue sensitivity to various muscle relaxants as mentioned above, and muscular weakness may be seriously increased if these are used when patients with the syndrome are anaesthetised. Croft (1958) reported five cases of this type after the use of D-tubocurarine, suxamethonium chloride, and gallamine. The results may be fatal and, if recovery occurs, many weeks may elapse before the patient returns to his previous level of muscular power. Wise and MacDermot (1962) reported similar observations. These problems have apparently disappeared with improved anaesthesia in recent years.

Lambert (1968), Rooke (1965) and Elmquist and Lambert (1968) have reviewed the electrodiagnostic features of the syndrome. Briefly, there is no evidence of abnormality of peripheral nerves or muscle fibres to account for the muscular weakness present, but there is a characteristic muscular response to motor nerve stimulation. Rested muscle shows a pronounced depression of the response to a single supramaximal stimulus applied to the motor nerve. At low rates of stimulation, two shocks per second, there may be further transient diminution of the action potential and twitch, but with repetitive stimulation at rates above 10 shocks per second there is a marked increased in the response (Elmquist and Lambert,

1968). Brown and Johns (1974) have claimed that the simplest test is to evoke a muscle action potential before and after voluntary effort; the potential shows a 200- to 1700-fold increase when the test is positive (Lambert, Rooke, Eaton and Hodgson, 1961). Pursuing the defect of neuromuscular transmission, Elmquist and Lambert (1968) studied external intercostal muscle obtained at biopsy from a patient with the syndrome but no evidence of carcinoma. After an elegant series of experiments they concluded that acetylcholine quanta and sensitivity of the muscle endplate receptors to acetylcholine were normal. However, motor nerve stimulation evoked endplate potentials with an amplitude sub-threshold for production of an action potential in most muscle fibres and varying greatly. The quantum content of the end-plate potential increased during repetitive nerve stimulation. It therefore appears that the neuromuscular defect is due to a decrease in the number of acetylcholine quanta released by a nerve impulse. Grob and Namba (1970) observed that the neuromuscular defect was reversed by minute amounts of acetylcholine and also concluded that it was attributable to decreased transmitter release. Guanidine has a beneficial effect (see pp. 610 and 720).

Pathology. Earlier formal histopathological studies showed changes in muscle which were non-specific and disproportionately slight in relation to the clinical disability. However, histochemical studies have shown type II atrophy with target fibres, while electron microscopy has revealed increased development of the subneural apparatus, so that the total post-synaptic membrane area is increased (Castaigne, Rondot, Fardeau, Cathala, Brideau-Dumas and Dudognon, 1977; Lindstrom and Lambert, 1978). The lesions responsible for neurological symptoms have not been displayed, except where there has been an additional coincidental syndrome, such as cerebellar degeneration (Satoyoshi, Kowa and Fukunaga, 1973).

Pathogenesis. As we have seen, Elmquist and Lambert (1968) and Lindstrom and Lambert (1978) have shown that the underlying defect is one of acetylcholine (ACh) release; both ACh and

ACh receptor content are normal, and there is no binding of antibody with the receptors. They suggested that the failure in release might be due to factors produced by oat cell carcinoma, an idea previously given credence by the demonstration by Ishikawa, Engelhardt, Fujisawa, Okamoto and Katsuky (1977) of neuromuscular transmission block, in frog nerve–muscle preparations, by an acetone extract of an oat cell carcinoma removed from a patient with the myasthenic syndrome.

Differential diagnosis. The syndrome must be distinguished from the myopathy of cachexia, myasthenia gravis, polymyositis, other myopathies of late onset, and various neural atrophies.

(i) *Neural atrophies* are easily separated by the usual criteria employed in differentiating neurogenic and myogenic atrophy; nevertheless, the myasthenic syndrome has been confused with motor neurone disease, peripheral neuropathy (which is understandable) and carcinomatous infiltration of nerve roots. Difficulty is most likely to arise when the syndrome is accompanied by other manifestations of paraneoplastic neurological disorder, such as cerebellar dysfunction. (ii) *Myopathy of cachexia.* The muscular wasting and weakness is generalised, and power is well retained considering the degree of wasting. Tendon reflexes are preserved. The electrical responses are normal. (iii) *Myasthenia gravis* occurs predominantly in females, and the age incidence is generally much lower. The distribution of weakness is usually different, for the pelvifemoral muscles are rarely selectively involved first in myasthenia gravis, but this is by no means a safe point of distinction because the external ocular, bulbar or shoulder-girdle musculature may be primarily affected in either complaint. The early onset of wasting and depression or loss of tendon reflexes in the myasthenic syndrome are further differentiating points, as are the various neurological symptoms outlined above. The electrodiagnostic, immunological and histopathological findings in myasthenia are quite different from those described in the myasthenic syndrome (see Ch. 26). (iv) *Polymyositis.* While the clinical features of Eaton-Lambert syndrome resemble those of polymyositis in some ways, there are many points of difference (see Ch. 15). Electrodiagnostic tests and muscle biopsy will resolve any difficulties which may exist. Examination of the thymus in patients dying with the myasthenic syndrome does not reveal histopathological changes of the type seen in myasthenia gravis. (v) *Other myopathies of late onset*. Thyrotoxic myopathy is the most important of these; it is easily diagnosed because signs of thyroid intoxication are found. Muscular dystrophy developing late in life presents no difficulty, for the tempo of this affliction is much slower, the family history may be positive, and there are other dissimilarities evident from the preceding description.

Management and treatment. If no signs of malignant disease are found initially, careful follow-up examinations with serial X-rays of the chest are required. When bronchial carcinoma or another form of malignant disease is demonstrated, treatment is naturally directed towards this.

Guanidine hydrochloride gives the best symptomatic relief of muscle symptoms. This preparation, sometimes used in the treatment of botulism, increases the amount of ACh liberated at the motor end-plate and increases the duration of the action potential. According to Brown and Johns (1974) it is best to give guanidine three-hourly. Most of their patients tolerated 35 mg/kg daily, but side effects were always encountered when the level of 40 mg/kg was exceeded. These unwanted effects are best avoided by introducing guanidine slowly. Early toxic manifestations include vomiting and rashes. With more prolonged medication, renal and haematological complications can follow (Cherington, 1976; Castaigne *et al.*, 1977). Long-term treatment with guanidine must be monitored carefully. Prednisolone may give subjective relief when questions of guanidine toxicity arise. Lundh, Nilsson and Rosen (1977) stated that 4-aminopyridine had a markedly beneficial effect in one patient, but the safety of this drug remains to be assessed.

Myasthenia gravis. Although myasthenia gravis may develop in patients with cancer, there is so far no evidence that the association is significant except in malignant thymoma. Morgan and Dud-ley (1955) reviewed the subject, having examined the records of 44 published cases of malignant thymoma: out of 37 in whom a note on the point was made 26 had myasthenia, four were questionably affected, and seven had no myasthenia. The neuromuscular disorder tended to occur rather late in the course of the cancer. Penn and Hope-Stone (1972) noted that four of their 18 cases of malignant thymoma had symptoms of myasthenia at presentation.

Dermatomyositis and polymyositis. The association of malignant disease and dermatomyositis has been recognised by clinicians for many years. Bohan and Peter (1975) examined the literature and concluded that the association had not been rigorously defined. Overall figures for the coincidence ranged from 15 to 34 per cent. However, Bohan and Peter criticised several previous reviews on the grounds that patient material might have been contaminated by the inclusion of other disease states, such as myopathies, neuropathies and carcinomatous neuromyopathies. Moreover, the diagnosis of one disease facilitates the diagnosis of the other in the hospital setting, 'thereby increasing the discrepancy between inpatients and the general population'. An unpublished personal survey from a neurological department made many years ago gave a figure of five per cent; this series included many patients dying with the acute form of dermatomyositis before the introduction of corticotrophin and corticosteroids in treatment. Bohan and Peter's point on the lack of adequate statistical proof of the association is well made and needs to be met.

Nevertheless, the clinician should undertake a thorough search for malignant disease in patients with dermatomyositis and polymyositis, if only on the basis of anecdotal evidence and past experience. When carcinoma is present it is usually found in the lung, breast, ovary or gastrointestinal tract, but other sites have been implicated, including the thymus.

The clinical and pathological features are similar to those found in dermatomyositis uncomplicated by the presence of malignant disease, and they will not be described here. Sarcoid lesions have been found in muscles, lungs and spleen in dermatomyositis with carcinoma of the lung. The course of the muscular disorder is not modified by the presence of cancer, and remissions occur. Treatment is described in Chapter 15.

Metabolic and endocrine myopathies

Cushing's syndrome and carcinoma. The occurrence of Cushing's syndrome in patients with ACTH-secreting tumours is well recognised. In such cases the myopathy associated with this metabolic disorder may be present, and muscular weakness can form the initial complaint.

Hyponatraemic myopathy. Ross (1963) has shown that muscular weakness may be an important manifestation of hyponatraemia, due to dilution or depletion, in patients with carcinoma of the bronchus. The plasma sodium concentration can be restored, and muscular power improved, by the administration of 9-α-fluorohydrocortisone.

Myopathy in hypercalcaemic states. Muscular weakness and wasting is frequently present in hypercalcaemic states due to benign or malignant tumours of the parathyroid gland. Prineas, Mason and Henson (1965) and Smith and Stern (1967) have shown that the myopathy associated with primary hyperparathyroidism can occur independently of plasma calcium concentration; in such cases osteomalacia is often present, and Prineas *et al.* thought that the muscle disorder might well be linked with deranged vitamin D metabolism. Vitamin D supplements are efficacious in relieving muscle weakness when osteomalacia is present. Hypercalcaemia certainly causes muscular disorder, as evidenced, for example, by the presence of weakness, sometimes profound, in parathyroid carcinoma and malignant disease, with relief as the biochemical situation is restored to normal by surgery or other means (Henson, 1966). The myopathic syndrome is similar whether the cause is hypercalcaemia or metabolic bone disease. In both instances the tendon reflexes are commonly brisk, and this sign constitutes a valuable aid to diagnosis. The commonest cause of hypercalcaemia is malignant disease, but muscular symptoms due to this biochemical disorder are relatively rare. When such symptoms have been encountered in personal experience the associated malignant process has usually been oat cell bronchial carcinoma, breast carcinoma with bony metastases or myeloma.

Carcinoid myopathy. Berry, Maunder and Wilson (1974) and Swash, Fox and Davidson (1975) have reported single examples of myopathy in patients suffering from argentaffin carcinoma with metastases. Swash's patient developed severe proximal weakness, with occasional cramps and muscle tenderness, 10 years after resection of the associated primary tumour in the ileum; secondary deposits had been seen in the liver at operation. In both cases muscle biopsy showed advanced atrophy of type II muscle fibres, scattered necrotic fibres and central nuclei. In Swash's patient, type I fibres were smaller than normal and the diameters of both type I and II fibres were abnormally variable. Electromyography showed a reduced interference pattern with numerous short-duration, low-amplitude, polyphasic potentials.

The serotonin and histamine antagonist, cyproheptadine, improved muscle strength in both cited cases when given in addition to methysergide. The dose of cyproheptadine was 24 mg daily. While muscle weakness in patients with carcinoid syndrome could develop from intestinal malabsorption, hypercalcaemia due to bony metastases, or conceivably due to the release of other active substances by the tumour, the clinical evidence suggests that the cause is circulating serotonin. This view is supported by experimental evidence on serotonin-induced myopathy (Parker and Mendell, 1974; Patten, Oliver and Engel, 1974).

Carcinoid myopathy is a rare condition, but the very fact of its response to treatment renders identification important.

Thyrotoxicosis and malignant disease. Thyrotoxicosis has been recorded as a paraneoplastic complication of oat cell lung cancer and it is conceivable that a patient so afflicted might present with thyrotoxic myopathy.

NEUROMUSCULAR DISORDERS IN THE RETICULOSES

The subjects of cachexia, secondary tumours in muscle, and peripheral neuropathy due to infiltration with neoplastic tissue have been dealt with earlier in this Chapter. Specific nutritional disorders may exceptionally complicate the course of abdominal lymphoproliferative disease through interference with the gastrointestinal tract. The myasthenic syndrome commonly linked with oat cell lung cancer has been reported in reticulum cell sarcoma (Rooke *et al.*, 1960), while dermatomyositis may complicate the course of myeloma, lymphoproliferative disease and leukaemia. Exceptionally, a person with lymphoproliferative disease or myeloma may develop or present with the syndrome of proximal myopathy (p. 716). For example, a recent patient complaining of serious weakness of the limbs and trunk proved to be suffering from otherwise symptomless myeloma; no metabolic abnormality was discovered.

Peripheral neuropathy may occur in myeloma, the lymphoproliferative disorders and leukaemia in the absence of neoplastic infiltration or of a biochemical disorder such as uraemia. Hutchinson, Leonard, Maudsley and Yates (1958) described four cases of this syndrome in patients with Hodgkin's disease, sometimes accompanied by changes in the optic discs and spinal cord. Victor,

Banker and Adams (1958) gave an account of sensorimotor peripheral neuropathy in myeloma. In their patients gross muscular wasting and weakness was a feature, with loss of tendon reflexes and impairment of all forms of sensation. The cerebrospinal fluid protein is usually elevated in such cases, and this may be a mirror of the protein abnormalities in the blood. At post-mortem examination degenerative changes are found in the peripheral nerves, and are more marked distally. Scanty amyloid material may be found. The course of the peripheral neuropathy is unrelated to that of the myeloma; indeed, the presence of myeloma may be discovered only at necropsy, for the neuropathy can be severe enough to cause death on its own account. Myeloma and lymphoproliferative disease should be remembered in the differential diagnosis of obscure cases of peripheral neuropathy.

The cause of peripheral neuropathy in these circumstances is not known. It is not attributable to chemotherapy or to other agents used in the treatment of the primary complaint. Hutchinson *et al.* (1958) felt that there was some evidence of a conditioned vitamin B deficiency in their material. Treatment is symptomatic and supportive for there are no measures which can be relied upon to influence the course of the neuropathy. Spontaneous remission has been observed in patients whose neuropathy has been linked with lymphoproliferative disease.

REFERENCES

Berry, E.M., Maunder, C. & Wilson, M. (1974) Carcinoid myopathy and treatment with cyproheptadine (Periactin). *Gut*, **15**, 34.

Bohan, A. & Peter, J.P. (1975) Polymyositis and dermatomyositis. *New England Journal of Medicine*, **292**, 344. (1st of two parts).

Brain, Lord & Adams, R.D. (1965) In *The Remote Effects of Cancer on the Nervous System*, Eds W.R. Brain & F.H. Norris (Grune & Stratton: New York).

Brain, Lord, Croft, P.B. & Wilkinson, M. (1965). Motor neurone disease as a manifestation of neoplasm. *Brain*, **88**, 479.

Brain, W.R. (1955). *Diseases of the Nervous System*, 5th Edn. (Oxford University Press: London).

Brown, J.C. & Johns, R.J. (1974) Diagnostic difficulties encountered in the myasthenic syndrome sometimes associated with carcinoma. *Journal of Neurology, Neurosurgery and Psychiatry*, **37**, 1214.

Brownell, B. & Hughes, J.T. (1975) Degeneration of muscle in association with carcinoma of the bronchus. *Journal of Neurology, Neurosurgery and Psychiatry*, **38**, 363.

Campbell, M.J. & Paty, D.W. (1974) Carcinomatous neuromyopathy. I. Electrophysiological studies. *Journal of Neurology, Neurosurgery and Psychiatry*, **37**, 131.

Castaigne, P., Rondot, P., Fardeau, M., Cathala, H.P., Brideau-Dumas, J.L. & Dudognon, P. (1977) Syndrome myasthenique de Lambert-Eaton, étude clinique, electrophysiologique, histologique et ultrastructurale. *Revue Neurologique (Paris)*, **133**, 10, 513.

Cherington, M. (1976) Guanidine and germine in Eaton-Lambert syndrome. *Neurology (Minneapolis)*, **26**, 944.

Corsellis, J.A.N., Goldberg, G.J. & Norton, A.R. (1968)

'Limbic encephalitis' and its association with carcinoma. *Brain*, **91**, 481.

Croft, P.B. (1958) Abnormal responses to muscle relaxants in carcinomatous neuropathy. *British Medical Journal*, **1**, 181.

Croft, P.B., Henson, R.A., Urich, H. & Wilkinson, P.C. (1965) Sensory neuropathy with bronchial carcinomas: a study of four cases showing serological abnormalities. *Brain*, **88**, 501.

Currie, S. & Henson, R.A. (1971) Neurological syndromes in the reticuloses. *Brain*, **94**, 307.

Currie, S., Henson, R.A., Morgan, H.G. & Poole, A.J. (1970) The incidence of the non-metastatic neurological syndromes of obscure origin in the reticuloses. *Brain*, **93**, 629.

Denny-Brown, D. (1948) Primary sensory neuropathy with muscular changes associated with carcinoma. *Journal of Neurology, Neurosurgery and Psychiatry*, **11**, 73.

Elmquist, D. & Lambert, E.H. (1968) Detailed analysis of neuromuscular transmission in a patient with the myasthenic syndrome, sometimes associated with bronchial carcinoma. *Proceedings of the Mayo Clinic*, **43**, 689.

Engel, W.K. (1977) Introduction to the myopathies. In *Scientific Approaches to Clinical Neurology*, Eds E.S. Goldensohn & S.H. Appel, vol. 2, pp. 1611–1613 (Lea & Febiger: Philadelphia).

Fettel, M.R., Shir, H.S., Penn, A.S., Lovelace, R.E. & Rowland, L. P. (1978). Combined Eaton-Lambert syndrome and myasthenia gravis. *Neurology (Minneapolis)*, **28**, 398.

Fontanel, J.P., Betheuil, M.J., Senechal, G. & Hagueneau, M. (1973) Un cas de syndrome de Lambert-Eaton secondaire a un epithelioma larynge. *Annales d'OtoLaryngologie et de Chirurgie Cervico-faciale (Paris)*, **90**, 43.

Grob, D. & Namba, T. (1970) Studies on the mechanism of the neuromuscular block in myasthenia gravis and carcinomatous myopathy. In *Muscle Diseases*, Eds J.N. Walton, N. Canal & G. Scarlato, p. 167 (Excerpta Medica: Amsterdam).

Heffner, R.B. & Barron, S.A. (1977) Remote effect of malignancy on intramuscular nerve twigs. *Journal of Neuropathology and Experimental Neurology*. **36**, 605.

Henson, R.A. (1953) Unusual manifestations of bronchial carcinoma. *Proceedings of the Royal Society of Medicine*, **46**, 859.

Henson, R.A. (1966) The neurological aspects of hypercalcaemia: with special reference to primary hyperparathyroidism. *Journal of the Royal College of Physicians (London)*, **1**, 41.

Henson, R.A. (1970). Non-metastatic neurological manifestations of malignant disease. In *Modern Trends in Neurology*, Ed. D. Williams, 5, p. 209 (Butterworth: London).

Henson, R.A. & Urich, H. (1970). Peripheral neuropathy associated with malignant disease. In *Handbook of Clinical Neurology*, Eds P.J. Vinken & G.W. Bruyn, Vol. 8, p. 131 (North-Holland Publishing Co.: Amsterdam).

Henson, R.A. & Urich, H. (1979) Remote effects of malignant disease: certain intracranial disorders. In *Handbook of Clinical Neurology*, Eds P.J. Vinken & G.W. Bruyn, Vol. 38, p. 625 (North-Holland Publishing Co.: Amsterdam).

Henson, R.A., Hoffman, H.L. & Urich, H. (1965) Encephalomyelitis with carcinoma. *Brain*, **88**, 449.

Henson, R.A., Russell, W.R. & Wilkinson, M.I.P. (1954)

Carcinomatous neuropathy and myopathy. *Brain*, **77**, 82.

Hildebrand, J. & Coërs, C. (1967) The neuromuscular function in patients with malignant disease. *Brain*, **90**, 67.

Hutchinson, E.C., Leonard, B.J., Maudsley, C. & Yates, P.O. (1958) Neurological complications of the reticuloses. *Brain*, **81**, 75.

Ishikawa, K., Engelhardt, J.K., Fujisawa, T., Okamoto, T. & Katsuky, H. (1977) A neuromuscular transmission block produced by a cancer tissue extract derived from a patient with the myasthenic syndrome. *Neurology (Minneapolis)*, **27**, 140.

Lambert, E.H. & Rooke, E.D. (1965) Myasthenic state and lung cancer. In *Remote Effects of Cancer on the Nervous System*, Eds W.R. Brain & F.H. Norris, p. 67 (Grune and Stratton: New York & London).

Lambert, E.H., Rooke, E.D., Eaton, L.M. & Hodgson, C.H. (1961) Myasthenic syndrome occasionally associated with bronchial neoplasm: Neurophysiologic studies. In *Second International Symposium on Myasthenia Gravis*, Ed. H.R. Viets (C.C. Thomas: Springfield, Ill.).

Lindstrom, J.M. & Lambert, E.H. (1978) Content of acetycholine receptor and antibodies bound to receptor in myasthenia gravis, experimental autoimmune myasthenia gravis, and Eaton-Lambert syndrome. *Neurology (Minneapolis)*, **28**, 130.

Lundh, H., Nilsson, O. & Rosen, I. (1977) 4-Aminopyridine—a new drug tested in the treatment of Eaton-Lambert syndrome. *Journal of Neurology, Neurosurgery and Psychiatry*, **40**, 1109.

Marin, O. & Denny-Brown, D. (1962) Changes in skeletal muscle associated with cachexia. *American Journal of Pathology*, **41**, 23.

Metral, S. & Veron, J.P. (1975) A propos de trois cas de syndrome de Lambert-Eaton. *Revue d'electro encephalographie et de Neurophysiologie clinique*, **5**, 1.

Morgan, W.L. & Dudley, H.R. (1955) Malignant thymoma and myasthenia gravis. *New England Journal of Medicine*, **253**, 625.

Parker, J.M. & Mendell, J.R. (1974) Proximal myopathy induced by 5 HT-imipramine simulates Duchenne dystrophy. *Nature*, **247**, 103.

Parsons, M. (1972) The spinal form of carcinomatous meningitis. *Quarterly Journal of Medicine*, **41**, 509.

Patten, B.M., Oliver, K.L. & Engel, W.K. (1974) Serotonin-induced muscle weakness. *Archives of Neurology*, **31** 347.

Pearson, C.M. (1959) Incidence and type of pathologic alterations observed in muscle in a routine autopsy survey. *Neurology (Minneapolis)*, **3**, 757.

Penn, C.R.H. & Hope-Stone, H.F. (1972) The role of radiotherapy in the management of malignant thymoma. *British Journal of Surgery*, **59**, 533.

Prineas, J.W., Mason, A.S. & Henson, R.A. (1965) Myopathy in metabolic bone disease. *British Medical Journal*, **1**, 1034.

Rebeiz, J.J. (1970) Amytrophy and cancer. In *Muscle Diseases*, Eds J.N. Walton, N. Canal & G. Scarlato (Excerpta Medica: Amsterdam).

Rooke, E.D., Eaton, L.M., Lambert, E.H. & Hodgson, C.H. (1960) Myasthenia and malignant intrathoracic tumor. *Medical Clinics of North America*, **44**, 977.

Ross, E.J. (1963) Hyponatraemic syndromes associated with carcinoma of the bronchus. *Quarterly Journal of Medicine*, **32**, 297.

Russell, D.S. & Rubinstein, L.J. (1959) *Pathology of Tumours of the Nervous System* (Arnold: London).

Satoyoshi, E., Kowa, H. & Fukunaga, N. (1973) Subacute cerebellar degeneration and Eaton-Lambert syndrome with bronchogenic carcinoma. *Neurology (Minneapolis)*, **23**, 764.

Shy, G.M. & Silverstein, I. (1965) A study of the effects upon the motor unit by remote malignancy. *Brain*, **88**, 515.

Smith, B. (1969) Skeletal muscle necrosis associated with carcinoma. *Journal of Pathology*, **97**, 207.

Smith, R. & Stern, G. (1967) Myopathy, osteomalacia and hyperparathyroidism. *Brain*, **90**, 593.

Spillane, J.D. (1947) *Nutritional Disorders of the Nervous System* (Livingstone: Edinburgh).

Swash, M. (1974) Acute fatal carcinomatous neuromyopathy. *Archives of Neurology*, **30**, 324.

Swash, M., Fox, K.P. & Davidson, A.R. (1975) Carcinoid myopathy. Serotonin-induced muscle weakness in man? *Archives of Neurology*, **32**, 572.

Urich, H. & Wilkinson, M.I.P. (1970) Necrosis of muscle in association with carcinoma of the bronchus. *Journal of Neurology, Neurosurgery and Psychiatry*, **38**, 363.

Victor, M., Banker, B.Q. & Adams, R.D. (1958) The neuropathy of multiple myeloma. *Journal of Neurology, Neurosurgery and Psychiatry*, **21**, 73.

Warmolts, J.R., Re', P.K., Lewis, R.J. & Engel, W.K. (1975) Type II muscle fibre atrophy (II atrophy). An early systemic effect of cancer. *Neurology (Minneapolis)*, **25**, 374.

Wilkinson, M., Croft, P.B. & Urich, H. (1967) The remote effects of cancer on the nervous system. *Proceedings of the Royal Society of Medicine*, **60**, 683.

Willis, R.A. (1952). *The Spread of Tumours in Human Body* (Butterworth: London).

Wise, R.P. & MacDermot, V. (1962) A myasthenic syndrome associated with bronchial carcinoma. *Journal of Neurology, Neurosurgery and Psychiatry*, **25**, 31.

The motor neurone diseases (including the spinal muscular atrophies)

INTRODUCTION

There is a wide range of degenerative disorders of the central nervous system in which involvement of the motor neurones of variable severity occurs, particularly in the spinal cord. Many of these disorders are encompassed by the terms spinocerebellar degeneration or hereditary ataxia. It is also difficult to separate some motor neurone diseases, in which the spinal muscular atrophies may be included, from other forms of hereditary motor neuropathy. Several of the conditions which enter into differential diagnosis will be discussed briefly here but fuller reference will be found elsewhere in this book (*see* Chs 17, 21 and 23). Notably, many disorders involving lower motor neurones (LMN) also affect the primary sensory neurones in the dorsal root ganglia and then present with manifestations of a peripheral neuropathy, with a greater or lesser degree of motor or sensory involvement. These diseases, many of known cause, are dealt with fully in Chapter 21. Finally, in recent years there has been much debate as to whether some forms of muscular dystrophy (*see* Ch. 14) are in fact the result of 'sick' motor neurones or neuronal trophic dysfunction rather than the result of some, as yet unknown, primary disorder of the muscle cell (McComas, Sica and Campbell, 1971). Many workers agree that there is good evidence of neural dysfunction in myotonic dystrophy but the evidence of such dysfunction in Duchenne muscular dystrophy is much less convincing, although, as will be seen, the manifestations of spinal muscular atrophy may closely resemble, both clinically and pathologically, those of many forms of muscular dystrophy, especially the limb-girdle and facioscapulohumeral types.

This chapter will describe those disorders in which the pathological changes are predominantly limited to the lower motor neurones but in some of which upper motor neurones (UMN) are involved as well.

In considering motor neurone diseases we must also clarify certain terms which are commonly employed. Amyotrophy simply means muscle wasting, but is normally used to identify a disorder of the lower motor neurone, although many conditions to which this name has been attached, e.g. diabetic amyotrophy and neuralgic amyotrophy, are probably the result of damage to roots or peripheral nerves and not to the neuronal cell body. Amyotonia is an obsolete term used to indicate hypotonia of muscle due to a central disorder, which may be one of the lower motor neurones, e.g. Werdnig-Hoffmann disease, but may result from cerebral birth trauma and many other processes (*see* Ch. 17). A further source of some confusion lies in the use of the adjective 'spinal', for many of the disorders included in the neurogenic muscular atrophies have signs of brain stem or 'bulbar' involvement; however, the term was originally used to differentiate motor neuronal diseases from those neural atrophies thought to originate in the motor roots or peripheral nerves.

A clinical classification of the motor neurone diseases is given in Table 20.1 and the following discussion will be organised accordingly.

MOTOR NEURONE DISEASE (THE AMYOTROPHIC LATERAL SCLEROSIS COMPLEX)

The descriptive term amyotrophic lateral sclerosis (ALS) was first used by Charcot to describe the pathological findings in a progressive lower and upper motor system disorder, in order to differentiate it from other forms of muscular atrophy. He believed that it was a separate entity from the previously described progressive muscular atrophy (PMA) (Aran, 1850) and from

Table 20.1 Motor neurone diseases

1. Motor neurone disease (the amyotrophic lateral sclerosis complex)
   includes Progressive muscular atrophy
   Progressive bulbar palsy
   Amyotrophic lateral sclerosis
   a) Sporadic forms
   b) Familial forms
   c) Western Pacific types
2. Spinal muscular atrophies
   a) Proximal forms
   b) Distal forms
   c) Scapuloperoneal form
   d) Facioscapulohumeral form
   e) Juvenile progressive bulbar palsy
3. Motor neurone disease associated with other diseases of the central nervous system
   a) Mental disorder
   b) Extrapyramidal disorders
   c) Spinal disease including the hereditary spinocerebellar ataxias
4. Miscellaneous diseases
   a) Infections
   b) Metabolic including hypoglycaemia
   c) Toxicity—heavy metals, organophosphorus compounds
   d) Ischaemic myelopathy including radiation damage
   e) Trauma including electrical injury
   f) Non-metastatic carcinomatous neuromuscular disease

progressive bulbar palsy (PBP) (Duchenne, 1860; Duchenne and Joffroy, 1870), but nowadays these conditions are considered to be clinical variants of the same disease. (For an historical review of the early descriptions and controversies surrounding the delineation of these conditions the reader is referred to Goldblatt, 1969; Bonduelle, 1975; Norris, 1975).

It should be noted that, in Great Britain, the inclusive term commonly used to identify this disease (which embraces the clinical syndromes of progressive muscular atrophy, progressive bulbar palsy and ALS) is motor neurone disease (MND); in the United States, by contrast, motor system disease or, more often, ALS, is occasionally used to cover the whole disease spectrum. In Great Britain ALS refers to that form of MND in which the disease presents at first with prominent signs of UMN dysfunction but comparatively little evidence, at least at first, of muscular weakness, atrophy and fasciculation due to LMN involvement. Nevertheless, UMN signs almost invariably appear ultimately in PMA, and LMN signs in ALS.

Pathology

The clinical and pathological features described by Charcot and Joffroy (1869) and Charcot (1873; 1874) have been modified only in minor detail since that time. The pathological features are those of shrinkage with sclerosis of the antero-lateral pyramidal tracts of the spinal cord, which contrasts with the generally normal appearance of the posterior sensory columns. Progressive degeneration of the large anterior horn neurones, particularly in the cervical cord, occurs with corresponding atrophy of the anterior motor roots and skeletal muscles. Identical lesions are found in the brain stem, particularly involving the motor nuclei of the medulla oblongata. Maximal damage is seen in the nuclei of the Xth, XIth and XIIth cranial nerves and to a lesser extent in the motor nuclei of V and VII but, inexplicably, the oculomotor nuclei are virtually spared. Degeneration is also found in the large Betz cells of the motor cortex; this results in variable degeneration of the pyramidal tracts through the internal capsule, cerebral peduncles and brain stem. Such pyramidal tract degeneration is found even in those clinical cases of pure LMN involvement or progressive muscular atrophy (Friedman and Freedman, 1950). Non-motor neurones and myelinated pathways may occasionally show minor degenerative changes (see Hirano, Malamud, Kurland and Zimmerman, 1969; Castaigne, Lhermitte, Cambier, Escourolle and Le Bigot, 1972). The skeletal muscles show changes of denervation with grouped fibre atrophy; the muscle spindle apparatus is preserved. Smooth muscle is unaffected.

The metabolic abnormality in motor neurones in MND is unknown. Mann and Yates (1974) suggest that the primary defect is one of DNA-directed mRNA synthesis causing inactivation and clumping of nuclear chromatin.

Epidemiology

Motor neurone disease is a progressive fatal disorder which is found world-wide and is responsible for 1 in 1000 adult deaths. It is generally sporadic, with an annual incidence of approximately 1–2 per 100 000 population and a prevalence of 2.5–7 per 100 000 (Bobowick and Brody, 1973; Kurland, Kurtzke, Goldberg and Choi, 1973). Clusters of the disease are found in certain communities of the Western Pacific Islands, notably among the Chamorro Indians on Guam where the prevalence is 400 per 100 000, i.e. almost 100 times the rate in most countries (Brody and Chen, 1969). A high prevalence has also been reported in the Kii peninsula of Japan (see Shiraki and Yase, 1975), New Guinea (Gadjusek, 1963; 1979) and among Filipinos on the Hawaiian islands (Matsumoto, Worth, Kurland and Okazaki, 1972). There is a male preponderance of the sporadic disease which gives a male:female ratio of about 1.6:1 (Kurland, Choi and Sayre, 1969). Between 5 and 10 per cent of cases in most countries are familial with an equal sex distribution and an autosomal dominant pattern of inheritance (Kurland and Mulder, 1955).

Clinical features

The sporadic form of MND may commence at any age in adult life but shows a peak at approximately 55 years of age. A special juvenile type occurs in Madras (Meenakshisundaram, Jagannathan and Ramamurthi, 1970). The disease most commonly presents in the upper limbs (40 per cent of cases), usually with wasting and weakness of the muscles of one hand. The muscles of the thenar eminence are frequently involved and this prevents opposition and adduction of the thumb. The patient complains of loss of fine finger control and difficulty in fastening buttons, picking up small objects and writing. He may be conscious of flickerings beneath the skin, indicating the occurrence of visible fasciculations in scattered muscles. The weakness may be preceded, often by several months, by a history of repeated muscle cramps (Bonduelle, 1975). Cramp is very common in the early stages of the disease and when it occurs repeatedly in forearm or hand muscles it is almost diagnostic of MND; there may also be a history suggesting myotonia of grip. Progressive atrophy of the interossei and lumbrical muscles of the hands allows the unopposed action of the long extensor and flexor muscles causing clawing of the fingers. The atrophy and weakness ascend progressively up the arm to the shoulder girdle muscles and then commonly involve the contralateral hand and upper limb. The next muscles to be involved may be the bulbar muscles or those of the lower extremities. A patchy, asymmetrical progressive muscular atrophy with increasing weight loss is very characteristic of one form of the disease (PMA). However, upper motor neurone (UMN) disease of the legs may predominate causing spastic weakness and reflex spasms especially in bed (ALS). The clinical picture is one of steady progression to disability of all limbs and bulbar muscles. Respiratory muscles are also involved, giving a fall in respiratory muscle strength and maximum breathing capacity, but the vital capacity remains high, approximately 80 per cent of normal, because of the frequent preservation of diaphragmatic function (Braun and Rochester, 1979; Fallat, Jewitt, Bass, Kamm and Norris, 1979; Saunders and Kreitzer, 1979). Dyspnoea is uncommon even when there is severe impairment of respiratory function.

Progressive bulbar palsy. Bulbar palsy running a subacute course may be the presenting feature of the disease, especially in the elderly. Curiously, the overall male preponderance in MND is not evident in this form. Indistinct speech, at first impossible to explain, is often the first manifestation. Visible wasting of the tongue with fasciculations may precede any bulbar symptoms, but then dysarthria may occur from involvement of the palate, tongue and lips. The progressive weakness of the labioglosso-pharyngeal muscles causes difficulty with swallowing and phonation and, later, choking or nasal regurgitation of fluids. Troublesome pooling of saliva often results in drooling from the mouth and a spluttering type of cough. Trigeminal motor neurone involvement causes difficulty in chewing and may even result in subluxation of the jaw, either spontaneously or during yawning. Upper motor neurone involvement is frequent, causing obvious stiffness and slowness in speech, producing a 'strained-strangled voice'. Inappropriate laughter or crying may occur, as in pseudobulbar palsy due to vascular disease, but often the tears are part of an understandable reactive depression or anxiety state.

Speech impairment in motor neurone disease is commonly a 'mixed dysarthria' from a variable involvement of bulbar neurones giving a flaccid weakness and of supranuclear motor pathways causing spasticity. Indirect disturbance may also be caused by a disordered pattern of breathing during speech, arising both through weakness of the intercostal muscles or diaphragm, and through loss of air via the nasal passages (Chevrie-Müller, Dordain and Grémy, 1970). The inability to clear the mouth and throat of food and secretions may cause disturbing gurgling noises or coughing fits during speech. The earliest symptom may be an inability to sing, whistle or speak rapidly, or simply a change in tone or volume (dysphonia). The mixed dysarthria is chiefly characterised by imprecise consonant production, hypernasality, harsh voice quality and slow speaking rate (Darley, Aronson and Brown, 1969). This may be more evident with prolonged speech or fatigue and then compares with myasthenia. Later it may become so severe that speech is unintelligible. Early signs are difficulty with 'blends', e.g. bl or sp, especially during rapid speech.

The consonants affected depend on the locus of weakness. Involvement of the palatopharyngeal sphincter muscles results in difficulty in maintaining intra-oral pressure and affects the articulation of the plosive sounds (p, b, d, g, k and t); thus b and d become m and n (Darley, Aronson and Brown, 1972). An early difficulty commonly arises from wasting and immobility of the tongue, especially of the tip (see Colmant, 1975). An inability to elevate the tip of the tongue affects large numbers of sounds, the linguals (l, r, s, sh and z), the linguadentals (th), the lingua-alveolars (t, d, ch, j and n) and the gutturals or palatal (velar) consonants (g, k and ng). With general weakness of the tongue the vowels (u and o) become difficult to pronounce and finally cannot be articulated at all (Böhme, 1974). Weakness of the facial muscles, including the orbicularis oris and the lips, affects the labial sounds (p, b, m and w) and the labiodentals (f and v) (see Darley et al., 1972).

Physical signs in the bulbar muscles may not be apparent in the early stages of bulbar palsy and may erroneously lead to a diagnosis of hysteria but, later, wasting and fasciculation of the tongue become obvious. Poor voluntary palatal or pharyngeal movement may be associated with a brisk gag reflex or jaw jerk indicating the upper motor neurone involvement. The pattern of breathing may be affected during speech with short, irregular stretches of speech separated by long intervals.

Unusual symptoms. Sensory symptoms of numbness, deadness of paraesthesiae in the extremities are sometimes mentioned. Even allowing for the differing meaning of such symptoms, they occur with such frequency that there may be a minor sensory system involvement. Routine sensory examination is usually normal except in those disabled patients whose clinical pictures are complicated by entrapment or pressure palsies, such as the carpal tunnel syndrome. However, a recent quantitative sensory examination of 10 patients with MND revealed abnormalities of touch-pressure sensibility in 40 per cent (Dyck, Stevens, Mulder and Espinosa, 1975). This would correlate with the minor non-motor and sensory changes which are sometimes found in pathological studies (see Hirano et al., 1969).

Autonomic nervous system involvement is not a feature, even in the terminal stages of the disease.

Constipation may result from the enforced bed-rest and general immobility; hesitancy of micturition or retention of urine may occasionally occur, and may then be secondary to faecal impaction. Libido and sexual function can be retained up to the final weeks of the illness (Jokelainen and Palo, 1976). The normal autonomic function probably accounts at least in part for the absence of skin damage or pressure sores in most patients despite total skeletal muscle paralysis.

Physical findings on examination. The commonest finding is of patchy asymmetrical wasting and weakness of the small hand muscles, especially those of the thenar eminence and the first dorsal interosseus muscle. Other upper limb muscles may also be atrophic and weak. Spontaneous fasciculations are usually seen in the weak muscles, especially in the hands, but often they may be very widespread in the limbs and also in the tongue; they may be more evident in cold weather or after exertion. Muscle tone may be variable depending on the degree of LMN or UMN involvement. Increased tone is commonly found in the lower extremities and corresponds to the finding that tendon reflexes often remain brisk despite the muscular atrophy. Total tendon areflexia is most unusual in MND (less than 5 per cent of cases of PMA) and should raise the question of an alternative, and more favourable, diagnosis such as polyneuropathy. The plantar responses are extensor in about 75 per cent of cases at some stage of the disease, but may disappear later when total paralysis of toe movement occurs. Bulbar symptoms are almost invariably associated with fasciculation and wasting of the tongue, but paresis of the palate and pharynx or spasticity of the lower facial musculature, together with abnormally brisk facial or jaw jerks are also frequently present. Extraocular muscles are unimpaired even at the point of virtually total paralysis of the skeletal musculature of the throat, trunk and limbs.

Investigative findings

There are no specific diagnostic tests for MND, but the single most helpful investigation is an electrophysiological study demonstrating a widespread neurogenic disorder. Needle electro-myography (EMG) demonstrates the presence of scattered spontaneous motor unit discharges (fasciculations), often in all four limbs. These are frequently polyphasic, occurring on average every 4–5 s and accompanied by other features of denervation (Hjorth, Walsh and Willison, 1973). Benign fasciculation in healthy indivuals (see Ch. 13) is distinguished by the absence of other physiological changes of denervation (Trojaborg and Buchthal, 1965). Fasciculations may also occur in a variety of LMN disorders, including cervical spondylosis and lumbar disc disease but, in the latter, they are limited to certain root levels. The most characteristic change in chronic denervation is of a reduced number of motor units being recruited on volition; these are frequently of polyphasic pattern and abnormally large amplitude, and are commonly found throughout the upper and lower extremities, including clinically normal muscles (Lambert, 1969; Brown and Jaatoul, 1974). The typical fibrillation potentials of acute denervation may not be found because of the ready reinnervation by surviving neurones from terminal collateral nerve sprouting (Wohlfart, 1957). This functional compensation may be so efficient that up to 80–90 per cent of motor units may be lost without significant loss of strength (McComas, Upton and Jorgensen, 1975).

The fastest motor and sensory nerve conduction velocities are normal, except in severe denervation when the evoked muscle response is less than 10 per cent of normal (Lambert, 1969). The mild slowing in such cases is probably due to the survival of smaller diameter fibres only, although it could be due to secondary demyelination in degenerating distal motor nerves such as were found in sensory fibres in sural nerve biopsies of MND patients (Dayan, Graveson, Illis and Robinson, 1969). Repetitive nerve stimulation studies show evidence of neuromuscular conduction defects in a high proportion of MND patients and the defect can be partly improved by anti-cholinesterase drugs (Lambert and Mulder, 1957; Mulder, Lambert and Eaton, 1959). Interestingly, similar abnormalities were reported as a late effect of acute anterior poliomyelitis (Buchthal and Honcke, 1944; Hodes, 1948). The neuromuscular fatigue in MND is greatest in patients with florid fasciculation activity (Denys and Norris, 1979) and is thought to be due to variable conduction in the terminal motor nerve twigs, possibly the re-innervative sprouts, causing jitter or intermittent blocking (Stalberg, Schwartz and Trontelj, 1975; Schwartz, Stalberg, Schiller and Thiele, 1976).

Routine blood investigations are generally normal except that the activity, in the serum, of the circulating muscle enzyme, creatine kinase (CK), is mildly to moderately increased in about 40 per cent of cases (Williams and Bruford, 1970). An abnormal response to a glucose load with delayed glucose utilisation and high serum pyruvate levels has been repeatedly demonstrated (Steinke and Tyler, 1964). This was thought to be due to subnormal pancreatic insulin secretion (Gotoh, Kitamura, Koto, Kataska and Arsuyi, 1972) although this finding has not been confirmed by others (Astin, Wilde and Davies-Jones, 1975). Similarly, claims for an abnormality of pancreatic exocrine function (Quick and Greer, 1967) have not been confirmed by other studies (Brown and Kater, 1969; McEwan-Alvarado, Hightower, Carney and Barrier, 1971).

Cerebrospinal fluid studies may show a mild increase in the total protein level and less frequently in the γ-globulins, but all other constituents have been normal (Castaigne, Lhermitte, Schuller and Rouques, 1971).

Radiological investigations are frequently necessary to exclude a local cord lesion in the neck, e.g. extradural compression, tumour or syringomyelia, but usually reveal no significant lesion. Unfortunately, a high proportion of male patients of the age range found in MND have changes of cervical spondylosis and difficulties are sometimes experienced in deciding whether these are relevant (Wilkinson, 1969). Muscular atrophy limited to the hand muscles also requires the exclusion of a cervical rib or apical lung syndrome, although sensory loss in the C8 and T1 dermatome areas is usually clinically evident in the latter conditions.

Course and prognosis

MND in all its clinical variants is a progressive disease which can lead to total paralysis of all limb, trunk, and head and neck muscles with the exception of the extraocular muscles. Diaphrag-matic paralysis is usually incomplete and probably accounts for the absence of dyspnoea until the later stages in most cases. Death usually results from respiratory failure, sometimes complicated by a respiratory infection, but a number of patients have an acute arrhythmia and myocardial ischaemia. It is generally agreed that the mean survival is 3–4 years, but several studies have demonstrated a wide range of survival, including some patients living for over 20 years (Mackay, 1963). Mackay also reported a shorter mean survival for patients with an early onset of bulbar symptoms, and this is the usual experience. Most studies have shown a better prognosis for those patients initially presenting with clinical evidence of spinal neuronal disease (PMA) only (Rosen, 1978), although some of these chronic cases may be examples of the late onset form of spinal muscular atrophy (see below). Mulder and Howard (1976) reported a 20 per cent survival overall at 5 years and a 10 per cent survival at 10 years. Such figures should sound a note of caution in evaluating the apparent benefit of any form of treatment and must point to the necessity of planning proper double-blind trials.

Heredo-familial forms of MND

Europe and the Americas. The familial incidence of MND outside the Western Pacific Islands is generally 5–10 per cent with an autosomal dominant pattern of inheritance showing high penetrance (Kurland and Mulder, 1955; Bobowick and Brody, 1973). The clinical picture is similar to that of sporadic forms except that some patients have shown additional features of dementia or extrapyramidal disease (reviewed by Bonduelle, 1975). The problem of juvenile types of MND is considered here as almost all reports have demonstrated a familial pattern of affliction. Some examples are probably better named familial spastic paraplegia with amyotrophy in view of the predominant upper motor neurone involvement (Refsum and Skillicorn, 1954). Other familial cases of progressive bulbar and proximal muscular atrophy of late onset (Magee, 1960; Kennedy, Alter and Sung, 1968) appear to represent variants of the spinal muscular atrophies (see below).

The mean age of onset in familial MND may be

earlier than in sporadic cases (Kurland and Mulder, 1955) but the usual wide range may be present even among individual families. Equally, there is a wide variation in the clinical course but affected individuals in some pedigrees have had a rapidly fatal disease lasting for months only (Engel, Kurland and Klatzo, 1959; Campbell, 1979).

The pathological changes in familial MND may be identical to those of the sporadic form but Hirano, Kurland and Sayre (1967) reported certain additional pathological features in affected persons in some families. These included clinically silent degeneration in the posterior sensory columns and spinocerebellar tracts with loss of cells in Clarke's column. Hyaline-like cytoplasmic inclusions were present in affected anterior horn cells and sometimes in other neurones. Sometimes the inclusions were dense and rounded, resembling Loewy bodies. However, such inclusions are not confined to familial cases (Schochet, Hardman, Ladewig and Earle, 1969). There have been several reports of major dysfunction of the basal ganglia in addition to that of the motor neurones (Van Bogaert and Radermecker, 1954; Campbell, 1979) and the question of a transitional form between MND and the spinocerebellar ataxias has been discussed by several authors.

Western Pacific Island forms of MND (ALS). Following the occupation by the American Forces of the island of Guam in the Second World War, an abnormally high prevalence of the otherwise typical form of ALS was discovered among the indigenous population of Chamorro Indians (Koerner, 1952). The rate is 50–100 times greater than the rates for MND in most parts of the world and accounts for 13 per cent of all deaths in adult Chamorros. An additional 11 per cent of adult deaths are ascribed to the parkinsonism-dementia complex (P–D), an unusual disease complex with specific pathological findings (Kurland and Brody, 1975). Abnormal clustering of ALS has since been reported from the Kii peninsula of Japan (reviewed by Shiraki and Yase, 1975), remote highland areas of New Guinea (Gajdusek, 1963; 1979) and among Filipinos on Hawaii (Matsumoto et al., 1972).

The pathology of ALS in the Chamorros differs from sporadic ALS in the finding of frequent Alzheimer neurofibrillary bundles and neuro-vacuolar degeneration in neurones (Malamud, Hirano and Kurland, 1961; Hirano et al., 1969). Such changes may be found in the motor neurones commonly affected in ALS, but are more frequently found in cortical neurones in the frontal and temporal lobes and in various basal ganglia. These pathological findings are even more striking in the P–D complex, in which 30 per cent of subjects may show evident muscle wasting. About 10 per cent of Guamanian patients with ALS have terminal evidence of either extrapyramidal or intellectual deficit, although this remains mild (Kurland et al., 1969). Thus it seems probable that the same aetiological factors are responsible for the two diseases. The same pathological changes have been found in other ethnic cases in the Western Pacific and rarely in sporadic cases of ALS elsewhere in the world (Carpenter, 1968; Schochet et al., 1969).

Many attempts to show an environmental factor responsible for MND on Guam have been inconclusive. A possible toxic agent has been the cycad seed, which was a major source of carbohydrate for the local population. Cycad contains a water-soluble hepatotoxic and carcinogenic agent, cyc-asin, but experimental attempts at producing neurological disease have been inconclusive (see Kurland and Brody, 1975). Strong familial clustering, both vertically and horizontally, has been reported from Guam (Mulder and Espinosa, 1969), but despite a high incidence among the immigrant Chamorro population in the USA (Torres, Iriate and Kurland, 1957), a genetic factor remains in doubt (Kurland, Choi and Sayre, 1969). Vertical transmission of an infectious agent rather than Mendelian inheritance is a possible alternative explanation (Bobowick and Brody, 1973). However, transmission studies designed in an attempt to isolate an infectious agent from Guamanian ALS cases have given negative results (Gibbs and Gajdusek, 1972). Recent studies have suggested that host resistance may be abnormal in Guamanian patients with ALS and the P–D complex and may be associated with the genetically determined histocompatibility antigen HLA–BW35 (Hoffman, Robbins, Nolte, Gibbs and Gajdusek, 1978). However, this is a common antigen in Guamanians and its prevalence is not increased in patients with these two chronic degenerative diseases (Hoffman, Robbins, Gibbs, Gajdusek, Garruto and Terasaki, 1977). Diminished cellular immunity in patients in Guam with ALS and P–D was associated with a shorter mean duration of the disease compared with those groups of patients showing normal responses.

Aetiological considerations in MND

The similarity of the pathological and clinical findings in familial and sporadic types of MND suggests a single metabolic defect in motor neurones. This suggestion would have greater validity if we were clearer about the metabolic differences between various neuronal groups. No consistent histochemical abnormality of motor neurones in MND patients compared with the findings in normal spinal cord material has been found in several autopsy studies (Hirsch and Chen, 1969; Engel, 1969).

The superficial similarity to PMA of various motor neuropathies attributable to heavy metal intoxication has led to several studies of such metals in MND patients. No toxic factors have been consistently identified.

Reports of muscle wasting following chronic lead and mercury poisoning (Wilson, 1907; Kantarjian, 1961) have led to several studies of the possible involvement of heavy metals in MND. Currier and Haerer (1968) treated 31 ALS patients, who gave a history of exposure to lead, mercury or arsenic, with various chelating agents but failed to modify the course of the disease, and Engel, Hogenhuis, Collis, Schalch, Barlow, Gold and Dorman (1969) had a similar experience. A similar outcome occurred in seven MND patients who gave a history of exposure to lead, and who were studied by Campbell, Williams and Barltrop (1970). However, a higher incidence of exposure to the heavy metals, lead and mercury, participation in athletics and consumption of large quantities of milk was reported for a group of 25 ALS patients (Felmus, Patten and Swanke, 1976). Conradi, Ronnevi and Vesterberg (1976) found increased levels of lead in the cerebrospinal fluid of patients with ALS, compared with that of control subjects. They also reported increased plasma levels, although the whole blood concentration was not

increased and the plasma concentration in their patients was less than normal control values reported by others (Conradi, Ronnevi and Vesterberg, 1978a). They postulated an uptake of lead by the motor neurones via the motor end-plates but, in a recent study, they failed to show an increase in lead concentration in skeletal muscles (Conradi, Ronnevi and Vesterberg, 1978b). Yase (1972) suggested that the increased incidence of ALS in Japan was related to the high concentration of manganese and calcium in the local soil. Similar speculation about a possible link with selenium was made after the discovery of an apparently high incidence of ALS in a small area of the USA with a high environmental level of this element (Kilness and Hochberg, 1977), but low urinary selenium levels have been found in a separate group of ALS patients (Norris and Sang, 1978). Thus the evidence for a link between MND and heavy metal intoxication is very weak at present.

There have been isolated case reports of the demonstration of virus-like particles in material form, or of isolation of virus from patients with a disease resembling MND, but no consistent pattern has emerged (Johnson, 1976; Johnson, Brooks, Jubelt and Swarz, 1979). A Russian report (Zil'ber, Bajdakova, Gardasjan, Konovalov, Bunina and Barabadze, 1963) of the reproduction of MND in rhesus monkeys by intracerebral inoculation of extracts of brain stem and spinal cords from patients with MND has not been confirmed in extensive studies in the USA under strict quarantine conditions (Gibbs and Gajdusek, 1972); and neuropathological examination of the Russian monkeys by Hirano (1973) did not reveal the changes of ALS. Repeated studies of attempted experimental transmission of MND to primates by the use of post-mortem spinal cord material from sporadic and Guamanian ALS cases have been negative (Gibbs and Gajdusek, 1972) and no cytopathic effects in tissue culture studies have been seen (Cremer, Oshiro, Norris and Lennette, 1973).

Acute poliomyelitis is a cytolytic inflammatory disease of neurones and produces a pathological picture quite unlike that of MND, but several reports have confirmed a higher incidence of previous poliomyelitis infection in patients with MND than could have occurred by chance

(Zilkha, 1962; Poskanzer, Cantor and Kaplan, 1969). Mulder, Rosenbaum and Layton (1972) reviewed the clinical picture in 34 MND patients who had had a previous history of paralytic poliomyelitis 25–40 years earlier. The progressive muscle wasting and weakness commonly began in the same or contralateral limb and generally followed a slow benign course. Electrophysiological studies on patients after acute poliomyelitis showed persistent fasciculation potentials and myasthenic-like neuromuscular fatigue in the surviving motor units (Hodes, 1948). Hence several possible explanations for the late neuronal degeneration after poliomyelitis are possible. The damaged neurones may simply have a shortened life span or may be more susceptible than normal to whatever may be the principal aetiological factor in MND. However, recent studies have renewed the possibility that ALS might represent a chronic infection with poliovirus. A biphasic neuronal disease produced by a similar type C picornavirus, Theiler's virus or murine poliomyelitis, has been re-examined by Lipton and Dal Canto (1976). The late chronic disease excites a mild inflammatory response only. Lipton and Dal Canto were unable to demonstrate the presence of viral antigen, and showed that the immune response to infection was delayed. However, it was during studies of tumour viruses that the most exciting lead arose. Gardner, Henderson, Officer, Rongey, Parker, Oliver, Estes and Huebner (1973), and Gardner, Rasheed, Klement, Rongey, Brown, Dworsky and Henderson (1976), in field studies of tumour viruses, discovered two local colonies of feral mice which developed either a lymphoma or a progressive paralysis of the hind limbs at 12–18 months of age following infection with a type C picornavirus. Transmission of the neurological disease was dose-dependent and was possible only in the neonatal period. High concentration inoculations produced paralysis in 6–12 weeks and the disease was preventable with specific antisera. Cross-breeding produced near-total suppression of virus expression and the development of the disease, which suggests that a genetic factor is involved. Neuropathological studies on the motor neurones (Andrews and Gardner, 1974; Andrews and Andrews, 1976) showed the presence of extracellular and intraneuronal virions and also severe cytomembrane vacuolisation resembling the changes seen in 'Wobbler' mice, a spontaneous neurological mutant, thought to be inherited by an autosomal recessive gene (Duchen and Strich, 1968). Such wobbler mice are abnormally susceptible to the Gardner virus and become ill after a very short incubation period (Andrews and Andrews, 1976) which is further evidence for a genetic factor in the latter disease.

The immune response to foreign antigen was first linked with the major histocompatibility complex in mice by Klein (1975). He suggested that the susceptibility to certain oncogenic viruses was dependent on the H–2 antigenic constitution (equivalent to the HLA system in man) situated on chromosome 17 of the specific mouse strain. This suggestion has been substantiated by several experimental studies in animals, including the variable transmission of scrapie, a non-inflammatory spongiform encephalopathy with neuronal degeneration natural to certain species of sheep (Dickenson and Frazer, 1977). The HLA system in man is located on chromosome 6 with coding for at least four loci, A, B, C and D (Bodmer, 1975). There is evidence to suggest that the major immune response genes are linked with the D locus. Multiple alleles for each locus have been detected and the number is increasing all the time. A strong association of an HLA type with a specific disease indicates that the individual genes coding for the histocompatibility antigen and the disease susceptibility lie close together on the chromosome, e.g. HLA–B27 and ankylosing spondylitis (Dick, Sturrock, Goel, Henderson, Canesi, Rooney, Dick and Buchanan, 1975) and HLA–A3/B7/DW2/DRW2 with multiple sclerosis (Winchester, Ebers, Fu, Espinosa, Zabriskie and Kunkel, 1975). Several studies of HLA typing in series of patients with MND have been reported but no satisfactory study of the important D locus types has yet emerged, mainly because of technical difficulties. No strong link with A or B antigens has been consistently reported. Antel, Arnason, Fuller and Lehrich (1976) reported a significantly increased incidence of A3 antigen in MND patients from Boston and this was supported by a recent study from Israel (Kott, Livni, Zamir and Kuritzky, 1979). The latter authors also found an increased frequency of BW35 but in contrast to their findings in an earlier study (Kott, Livni, Zamir and Kuritzky, 1976) this was not thought to be significant. However, in a study on Guamanian patients with both ALS and P–D (Hoffman *et al.*, 1978), diminished cellular immunity in these two diseases was strongly associated with BW35, although the overall prevalence of this HLA type was not increased in patients with these two chronic degenerative diseases (Hoffman *et al.*, 1977).

Antibody studies to various viruses, including poliovirus, have generally given negative findings in MND (Lehrich, Oger and Arnason, 1974; Jokelainen, Tiilikainen and Lapinleimu, 1977) but in a recent study 68 per cent of ALS patients produced a cell-mediated response to trivalent poliomyelitis antigen whereas no response was obtained in patients with other neurological diseases or in normals. Evidence for immune-complex formation in a number of patients with MND has been reported by Oldstone, Perrin, Wilson and Norris (1976) but the nature of the antigen and antibody have not been determined. Pertschuk and others (Pertschuk, Cook, Gupta, Broome, Vuletin, Kim, Stanek, Brigati, Rainford and Nidzgorski, 1977; Pertschuk, Kim, Prasad, Cook, Gupta and Broome, 1979) have reported the identification of poliovirus antigen in jejunal biopsy material obtained from MND patients with evidence of an immune response locally, but this awaits independent confirmation.

A toxic effect of sera from MND patients upon myelin in experimental tissue culture (Bornstein and Appel, 1965; Field and Hughes, 1969) and on axons from embryonic spinal cord explants (Wolfgram and Myers, 1973; Wolfgram, 1976) has been reported, but such effects could be secondary rather than primary.

Treatment

Not surprisingly, in view of the lack of any clear understanding of the pathogenesis of MND, no form of specific treatment for the disease has yet emerged. Several types of treatment have been tried, based on various putative aetiological factors, all with negative results.

Pancreatic extract and vitamin E preparations have been tried separately or in combination without clear benefit (Brown and Kater, 1969; Dorman, Engel and Fried, 1969). Vitamin B_{12} or hydroxycobalamin injections have been frequently used as placebos, and certainly no beneficial effect has been found from either parenteral or intrathecal administration (Peiper and Fields, 1959). These authors also reported an unsuccessful trial of intrathecal steroid therapy.

In view of the possible relationship to heavy metal intoxication there have been several studies with the chelating agents BAL, Versene (calcium EDTA) and penicillamine, but no persistent benefit has been shown (Engel *et al.*, 1969; Campbell *et al.*, 1970).

The association of ALS with parkinsonism on the island of Guam led to an unsuccessful therapeutic trial of the dopagenic drug levodopa, both in the Guamian and sporadic types of ALS (Mendell, Chase and Engel, 1971). Similarly amantadine, an antiviral drug with dopaminergic properties, failed to produce any significant response (Norris, 1972).

The possibility of viral infection or of indirect involvement of viruses in the aetiology has led to therapeutic trials with several antiviral agents but with negative results. The drugs have included idoxuridine (Liversedge, Swinburn and Yuill, 1970), cytosine arabinoside (Ara–C) (Liversedge, 1973), isoprinosine (Percy, Davis, Johnston and Drachman, 1971), tilorone (Olson, Simons and Halaas, 1978), and polyinosinic-polycytidylic acid (poly-ICLC) (Engel, Cuneo and Levy, 1978). Tilorone and poly-ICLC are both claimed to induce interferon production in animals. Treatment of isolated cases with human fibroblast interferon has also been tried with a report of transient benefit in MND and disappearance of fasciculations (Cook, Pertschuk, Gupta, Nidzgorski, Carter, Horoszewicz, Marcus and Kim, 1979). Norris (1973) and Norris, Calanchini, Fallat, Panchari and Jewett (1974) reported a beneficial effect with guanidine hydrochloride, and an anti-RNA viral agent in some patients with ALS, but this is almost certainly related to its other action in facilitating the release of acetylcholine at the neuromuscular junction (Otsuka and Endo, 1960). Similar symptomatic benefit may also be obtained in some patients with ALS, especially those with bulbar weakness, with the anticholinesterase compound pyridostigmine (Mestinon) in a dose of 60–120 mg taken every 4–6 h. Unfortunately, the improvement is usually short-lived and may be masked by troublesome side effects of increased salivation and muscle cramps. Muscle cramps are more frequent in the early stages of MND and may be diminished in severity and frequency by phenytoin therapy or occasionally by carbamazepine. Treatment with modified snake venom neurotoxin prepared from cobra and Kiart venom (Sanders and Fellowes, 1975; Sanders, Fellowes and Lennox, 1978) has been the subject of considerable controversy but, in a large, double-blind trial, no significant improvement beyond an overall placebo effect was found (Tyler, 1979).

Symptomatic treatment of the bulbar weakness or of the neuromuscular imbalance from the upper motor neurone disorder is often possible. Excessive salivation may respond to anticholinergic drugs, particularly atropine or its synthetic analogues, but occasionally it may be advisable to divide the tympanic plexus and chorda tympani nerves, which reduces salivation by 95 per cent (Zalin and Cooney, 1974; Mullins, Gross and Moore, 1979). The pooling of secretions in the hypopharynx, with the problem of spillage into the larynx and trachea, may also be helped by cricopharyngeal myotomy which lowers the resting intrapharyngeal pressure (Mills, 1973; Lebo, U and Norris, 1976). This operation has been advocated mainly for the management of severe dysphagia and appears to be effective in about a third of patients with pharyngeal paralysis. Tube feeding with a nasogastric polythene tube is frequently required in the end stage of bulbar palsy to alleviate general weakness from inanition. Palliative gastrostomy or oesophagostomy is rarely justified in those patients with restricted severe bulbar weakness and with good limb function. However, tracheostomy with a cuffed tube may be justifiable to prevent the patient from drowning in his own secretions, particularly when bulbar paralysis is severe in a patient who is still mobile.

Other therapeutic provisions may be required to alleviate the physical disability. Physiotherapy and speech therapy are of very limited benefit but are supportive to patients and their relatives. The problem of communication with patients who have severe dysphonia has been aided by the development of small portable electronic communicators (Canon) which provide a 'ticker-tape' print-out. Other electronic aids (e.g. POSSUM, System 7) are available to facilitate simple household tasks, such as operating the door catch, or the controls of radio or television sets, and these provide some measure of independence for the patients. However, considerable fortitude on the part of the patients, relatives and their doctors is required in the face of the relentless progressive paralysis which occurs with preservation of full intellectual faculties.

SPINAL MUSCULAR ATROPHIES

These are heredofamilial disorders of the motor neurones, predominantly affecting those of the spinal cord, but occasionally affecting the motor nuclei in the brain stem, and rarely affecting upper motor neurone pathways. The exact metabolic abnormality is unknown and the various types are distinguished by the age of onset and distribution of weakness. The view that several separate genes are involved has been strengthened in recent years by large studies of intrafamilial cases and sibships (Becker, 1964; Emery, 1971; Pearn, Carter and Wilson, 1973; Pearn, Hudgson and Walton, 1978; Pearn, Bundey, Carter, Wilson, Gardner-Medwin and Walton, 1978).

Acute infantile form (SMA type I)

This disease is characterised by its severe generalised muscle involvement and fatal outcome before 3 years of age (Brandt, 1950; Byers and Banker, 1961). It is thought to be due to a single autosomal recessive gene with a carrier frequency of 1 in 60–80 (Pearn, 1973) and an estimated disease incidence of 1 in 20 000 live births (Pearn, Carter and Wilson, 1973). In at least one-third of cases the disease is manifest before or at birth either by decreased fetal movement or by congenital orthopaedic deformity. In the large study of Pearn and Wilson (1973a) the onset of the disease was before 4 months of age in 95 per cent of cases and all patients showed delayed milestones by 6 months of age. Generalised weakness and hypotonia and feeding difficulties were the commonest symptoms, but breathing difficulties with rapid diaphragmatic movements supersede and are usually responsible for the inevitable fatal outcome. The mean survival is 6 months and 95 per cent of children are dead by 18 months of age.

Fasciculations may be evident in the wasted tongue but are generally invisible elsewhere. Buchthal and Olsen (1970) failed to find any true fasciculation discharges in the EMG in the acute infantile disease but did document a finding, unique to SMA type I, of regularly discharging units occurring with a frequency of 5–15 s in muscles relaxed voluntarily or during sleep. The activity appears to occur in motor units which are still functioning, because the same units can be activated voluntarily. Other EMG features of a central motor neuropathy and chronic denervation are commonly found, particularly in the older age group, but it is possible to have normal EMG findings in small infants.

Pathological studies of the brain and spinal cord show severe loss of motor neurones but some remaining cells are characteristically enlarged with changes resembling those of chromatolysis (Byers and Banker, 1961). The anterior motor roots are very atrophic but sensory roots and tracts are generally normal. However, two recent studies have confirmed older reports of scattered mild abnormalities in the dorsal root ganglia and non-motor pathways (Carpenter, Karpati, Rothman, Watters and Andemann, 1978; Marshall and Duchen, 1978). Histological studies on skeletal muscle show severe denervation changes with scattered small groups or even single hypertrophic fibres.

Chronic infantile form (SMA type II)

There have been many reports since the original papers of Werdnig (1891, 1894) and Hoffmann (1893, 1897, 1900) described a more slowly progressive form of the generalised disease, allowing survival to late childhood or even longer. The identity of this group has been the subject of considerable controversy. Emery (1971) regards it as a separate disease entity, distinct from SMA types I and III. However, two recent large collaborative studies have suggested that a single

autosomal recessive gene accounts for over 90 per cent of the cases which are included in both groups II and III (Bundey and Lovelace, 1975; Pearn, Hudgson and Walton, 1978). Many of the remaining 10 per cent of cases appear to arise by a new dominant mutation which may present at a later stage in childhood and generally causes a milder form of the disease. Zellweger, Simpson, McCormick and Ionasescu (1972) reported a remarkable family of the latter type with 21 cases spanning six generations. The progression was very slow and the disease was more severe in males. The recessive chronic infantile form has a slightly later onset than SMA type I at approximately 6 months of age, and in virtually all cases the disease is manifest before 2 years of age. Clinically, the weakness and wasting is generalised and does not show predominant proximal or distal muscle involvement. Less than 25 per cent of infants are ever able to sit unsupported and none learn to crawl or walk (Pearn and Wilson, 1973b). Fasciculation and atrophy of the tongue is present but fasciculations are not seen in the limbs. However, tremor of the fingers may be evident corresponding to the EMG findings of spontaneous motor unit discharges (Buchthal and Olsen, 1970). The tendon reflexes are diminished and are always absent by 2 years of age. Corticospinal tract involvement does not occur. Life expectancy is very variable, ranging from the 14 months observed in one of Hoffmann's seven patients to more than 30 years in some cases. The clinical progression is slow with occasional sudden deterioration associated with intercurrent infection (Munsat, Woods, Fowler and Pearson, 1969). All children, if untreated (see Ch. 17), develop some degree of scoliosis which can further compromise respiratory ventilation, and gross orthopaedic abnormalities are common in the second decade. Gross chest deformities make management of the inevitable recurrent pneumonia very difficult.

Chronic proximal form (Kugelberg-Welander disease: SMA type III)

Wohlfart, Fex and Eliasson (1955) and Kugelberg and Welander (1956) described a progressive proximal muscular weakness in young adults, which clinically resembled a muscular dystrophy, but showed fasciculations and investigational evidence of a neuropathic disorder. The onset of the weakness was in the quadriceps and hip muscles at 2–17 years of age, but the shoulder girdle muscles became involved within a few years. Fasciculation in limb muscles is seen in at least 50 per cent of cases, but is rarely evident in the tongue; bulbar involvement is rare and, although extensor plantar responses have been reported in a few cases (Gardner-Medwin, Hudgson and Walton, 1967), the tendon reflexes are usually diminished rather than increased. While Emery (1971) regarded this form of SMA as being different from the chronic infantile form, the frequent occurrence within the same sibship of patients with clinical features of both type II and type III suggests that these two clinical categories represent variants of the same disease process, distinct from SMA type I (Pearn et al., 1978).

The usual presentation is with difficulty in walking, especially up stairs, and a waddling gait. Later there is difficulty in lifting the arms and evident winging of the scapulae. The posture is hyperlordotic with a protuberant abdomen. The progression of weakness and disability is slow and distal muscles are seldom severely affected. Patients are usually able to walk for at least 10 years and many are capable of a normal life span. Joint contractures and kyphoscoliosis are common later.

Kugelberg and Welander (1956) found EMG evidence of spontaneous fasciculation and chronic denervation changes with giant residual units. Muscle biopsy in five cases showed fibre type-grouping both of the atrophic and of the hypertrophic muscle fibres, thus indicating the neuropathic nature of the disease. Wohlfart (1942) had previously described two similar clinical cases, also with evident fasciculations, but on noting myopathic changes in a muscle biopsy from one patient had ascribed the disease to a muscular dystrophy. He subsequently reassessed these cases and seven others and confirmed the findings of Kugelberg and Welander (Wohlfart et al., 1955). The 'secondary' myopathic abnormalities often found in muscle sections have been confirmed repeatedly (Kondo, 1969; Mastaglia and Walton 1971) and appear to correlate with the presence of 'myopathic' motor units on EMG studies and also with a frequently increased serum CK activity

(Gath, Sjaastad and Loken, 1969; Mastaglia and Walton, 1971). The few autopsy reports have confirmed the involvement of motor neurones in the spinal cord and have shown no evidence of corticospinal or sensory involvement (Gardner-Medwin et al., 1967; Kohn, 1968).

Juvenile proximal muscular atrophy involves more than one member of a family in about two-thirds of cases (reviewed by Namba, Aberfeld and Grob, 1970). The majority of families have shown an autosomal recessive pattern of inheritance, but both dominant and X-linked recessive forms of the disease have been described (see Emery, 1971). Adult onset of otherwise typical cases showing a benign course was first described by Finkel (1962) and Wiesendanger (1962) and clinically such patients may resemble cases of Becker or limb-girdle muscular dystrophy (Pearn, Hudgson and Walton, 1978). The importance of their recognition lies in distinguishing such cases from MND with its prognosis which is much more grave.

Chronic distal form

Sporadic and familial cases of progressive spinal muscular atrophy of distal distribution have been described. The onset of distal atrophy is usually in the lower limbs and later involves the upper limbs also (Nelson and Amick, 1966; Dyck and Lambert, 1968b; McLeod and Prineas, 1971). However, Meadows and Marsden (1969) described three sibs with an onset of muscle wasting in the hands, in childhood, which spread to the lower legs in later life. Some of these adult distal cases may be indistinguishable from those with the early manifestations of scapuloperoneal atrophy (see below) or the less common neuronal/axonal form of peroneal muscular atrophy (Charcot-Marie-Tooth disease) (see Ch. 21). The latter condition is generally distinguished, however, by the presence of minor sensory abnormalities found either clinically or on electrophysiological studies (Dyck and Lambert, 1968b); the motor conduction velocities in such cases are minimally slowed in contrast to the severe slowing found in the genetically distinct demyelinating form (Dyck and Lambert, 1968a; Thomas and Calne, 1974).

Scapuloperoneal form

The scapuloperoneal syndrome includes a variety of disorders giving rise to proximal weakness around the shoulders and distal weakness in the lower limbs. Some cases appear to be myopathic (*see* Kaeser, 1975), generally with an onset around the shoulder girdle and with features resembling those of facioscapulohumeral muscular dystrophy except that the face is spared (*see below*). Kaeser (1964, 1965) reported the findings in 12 members of a family extending through five generations and with an autosomal dominant pattern of inheritance. The onset was in adult life with symmetrical weakness and wasting of the long extensor muscles of the toes and ankles. After many years the muscles around the shoulder girdle became involved, producing winging of the scapulae and difficulty in raising the arms. The weakness of the legs also spread to involve the calves and quadriceps muscles. In two cases, in the fourth and fifth generations, bulbar muscles became involved, resulting in dysphagia, dysphonia and facial weakness; extraocular weakness was present in one. Tendon reflexes were diminished or absent and sensory examination was normal. EMG studies in three affected members (Kaeser, 1975) revealed abundant fibrillation and fasciculation potentials in some muscles. Severe denervation changes were evident in the legs but a mixed pattern was found in the facial muscles and in muscles around the shoulder girdle. Motor conduction velocities and sensory nerve studies were normal. Muscle biopsies from the lower extremities gave findings which were consistent with chronic denervation but specimens from the deltoid or triceps muscle were thought to be myopathic or pseudomyopathic. An autopsy study of one case showed clear evidence of deterioration of anterior horn cells and bulbar motor nuclei, and a neurogenic type of muscle atrophy including muscles of the upper extremity.

Sporadic cases with a similar distribution of muscle involvement have been described in infancy (Feigenbaum and Munsat, 1970). Zellweger and McCormick (1968) described a single congenital case with talipes equinovarus and progressive inspiratory stridor due to bilateral vocal cord paralysis. A family of three affected sibs with an onset in childhood and a mildly affected mother has been studied in conjunction with Dr B. Berg. The propositus presented with acute bulbar weakness and bilateral vocal cord paralysis requiring tracheostomy. She later developed a scapuloperoneal distribution of muscular atrophy which was evident in two of three brothers and in her mother. The EMG findings in this family, as in the other childhood cases, were of chronic denervation with normal motor conduction velocities.

Dawidenkow (1939) described cases from two families with a scapuloperoneal distribution of weakness, but found a distal sensory loss which caused him to consider the condition to be a variant of Charcot-Marie-Tooth disease. This type has not been reported since then and hence affected patients have not been studied by modern techniques.

Facioscapulohumeral form

Conditions resembling facioscapulohumeral muscular dystrophy in the distribution of muscular atrophy and weakness have been described in a mother and daughter, with onset in adolescence but with pathological evidence of a neuropathy (Fenichel, Emery and Hunt, 1967). Two other sporadic cases with a similar picture were reported by Furukawa, Tsukagoshi, Sugita and Toyokura (1969). There are also some forms of the scapuloperoneal syndrome which could alternatively be included here (Kaeser, 1975).

Progressive juvenile bulbar palsy (Fazio-Londe disease)

The unity of this condition remains in doubt (reviewed by Gomez, 1975). In the only autopsied case, Gomez, Clermont and Bernstein (1962) found a motor neuronal degeneration of the brain stem nuclei including the oculomotor nerves, and to a lesser extent in the cervical and dorsal spinal cord. The child presented at 33 months of age after a generalised convulsion and subsequently had a subacute bulbar palsy together with progressive bilateral facial weakness, ptosis and ophthalmoplegia. Within 6 months she had developed generalised hypotonia and weakness and hyperreflexia with ankle clonus; the plantar responses were flexor. She died at 50 months of age. Apart from the ophthalmoplegia the case resembles a restricted form of SMA type II.

MOTOR NEURONE DISEASE ASSOCIATED WITH OTHER DISEASES OF THE CENTRAL NERVOUS SYSTEM (CNS)

Mental disorders

Certain familial forms of MND may also show features of progressive dementia, as were discussed above, but this discussion will be confined to those mental states where the motor neurone disease is a minor or secondary disorder. Late in the course of many forms of specific dementia, e.g. Alzheimer's or Pick's disease, and Huntington's chorea, progressive muscle wasting and weakness may become apparent and may also be associated with signs of UMN dysfunction. This cachexia cannot be accounted for by inanition and disuse atrophy resulting from being confined to bed, as many of these demented patients have a voracious appetite and remain hyperactive. Histological examination of skeletal muscle from patients with dementia may show identical appearances to those seen in primary neurogenic atrophy (Tomlinson, Walton and Rebeiz, 1969). Such changes have also been seen in elderly, non-demented patients (Jennekens, Tomlinson and Walton, 1971) and hence the muscle changes in dementia may simply represent an accelerated ageing process. Campbell, McComas and Petito (1973), in an electrophysiological study of healthy elderly patients, found evidence of progressive loss of motor units after the age of 60 years, but without significant impairment of nerve conduction or muscle fibre contraction, and concluded that this presumably resulted from neuronal loss in the spinal cord. Tomlinson and Irving (1977) have shown that the total numbers of neurones in the anterior horns of the spinal cord decline with increasing age.

The association of MND and Pick's disease has been known for a long time although few neuropathological studies have been reported (De Morsier, 1967; Minauf and Jellinger, 1969). In addition to the specific changes both of Pick's disease and of MND, degenerative changes in the basal ganglia, including the substantia nigra, have been found. Several sporadic cases of presenile dementia and MND but without the pathological changes of either Pick's or Alzheimer diseases have been reported from Japan (Mitsuyama and Takamiya, 1979). Other cases of dementia with extrapyramidal and motor system disorders are perhaps best described by the term corticostriatospinal atrophy. Several families with such progressive syndromes have been described over the years even before the reports from Guam (Worster-Drought, Hill and McMenemy, 1933; Staal and Went, 1968; Bonduelle, 1975). The European cases have not shown the typical neurofibrillary degenerative changes of the P–D and ALS cases from Guam. There is also considerable overlap with the original descriptions of Jakob-Creutzfeldt disease in which the degeneration also involved the cerebellum and spinal neurones. However, this term is now confined to a subacute multisystem disease due to spongiform encephalopathy with recurrent myoclonus, dementia and a fatal outcome usually within months. Some cases have been reported where the presenting feature was progressive muscular wasting, the so-called amyotrophic form (Allen, Dermott, Connelly and Hurwitz, 1971). Characteristic pathological changes are found on brain biopsy or on autopsy. These consist of widespread neuronal degeneration with intense astrocytic proliferation, and spongiosis of the neuropil, consisting of vacuolated astrocytic processes and neuronal soma. The similarities of these changes in the basal ganglia and cerebellum to those in kuru (Klatzo, Gajdusek and Zigas, 1959) and also to scrapie, a naturally occurring transmissable disease of sheep, led to the successful transmission experiments of Jakob-Creutzfeldt disease to primates (Gibbs, Gajdusek, Asher, Alpers, Beck, Daniel and Matthews, 1968). The exact nature of the very small transmissable agent is still the subject of considerable study.

Extrapyramidal disorders

The association of familial MND with extrapyramidal features was referred to earlier, but isolated cases of Parkinson's disease with the late development of an ALS-like picture have also been described (Bonduelle, 1975). Several of these cases have followed documented encephalitis lethargica (Greenfield and Matthews, 1954; Pallis, 1976). It seems unlikely that the association of these disease states occurs by chance and thus there appears to be a considerable overlap with other degenerative CNS disorders.

Spinal disorders and spinocerebellar ataxias

The problem of differentiation of hereditary spastic paraplegia with amyotrophy, and certain hereditary motor neuropathies including Charcot-Marie-Tooth disease, from other forms of MND has been mentioned earlier. Several other heredo-familial disorders may be associated with progressive muscle wasting, particularly in the distal parts of the limbs, e.g. Friedreich's ataxia. In general, the prominent sensory disturbance and ataxia is a clear distinguishing feature, but the undoubted muscular atrophy is clearly evident, especially in the feet, which show pes cavus. Electrophysiological studies of several forms of spinocerebellar ataxia show evidence of motor unit loss and, in some cases, mild slowing of nerve conduction (Dyck and Lambert, 1968b; McLeod, 1971). Pathological studies have confirmed the degeneration of motor neurones in addition to those of the sensory system (Greenfield, 1954).

MISCELLANEOUS DISEASES

Infections

Acute poliomyelitis is the archetype of a necrotising infection of the large motor neurones of the spinal cord, brain stem and cortex, although in fatal cases there is pathological evidence of involvement of non-motor neurones (Bodian, 1952). Poliovirus is an enterovirus which may exist as a commensal in the bowel but causes a mild systemic upset only, without neurological features in most cases. This may be associated with features of an aseptic meningitis. Paralytic disease occurs in less than 10 per cent of infected individuals and may show a familial clustering even at times of severe epidemics (Aycock, 1942). This suggests a

genetic predisposition to the development of poliomyelitis (Addair and Snyder, 1942; Herndon and Jennings, 1951). An association between HLA–A3 and poliomyelitis has been reported by Pietsch and Morris (1975) but denied by others (Lasch, Joshua, Gazit, El-Nasri, Marcus and Zamie, 1979). The paralytic illness often commences with fasciculation and considerable muscular pain and tenderness. The paralysis may be localised or widespread and of variable severity. Asymmetry or selective involvement of muscles is quite common. Maximum severity is reached within a few days and recovery may commence within a week of the onset of paralysis. Severe cases involve the brain stem vital centres, but respiratory paralysis may also occur from peripheral involvement of the diaphragm and intercostal muscles. Fortunately, only a small proportion of affected muscles become permanently paralysed, but it is uncertain whether this implies that affected neurones are capable of recovery from viral infection and replication. The recovery of muscle power may be the result of sparing of individual motor neurones, but certainly electrophysiological studies demonstrate that reinnervative sprouting in surviving motor units occurs to produce greatly hypertrophied units (McComas, Sica, Campbell and Upton, 1971). It is probable that suboptimal conduction in these reinnervative terminal nerve fibres is responsible for the neuromuscular transmission defects which are demonstrable (Buchthal and Honcke, 1944; Hodes, 1948). Treatment of acute paralytic poliomyelitis is supportive and may require tracheostomy and ventilatory assistance. The mortality appears to vary between five per cent and 30 per cent.

Rarely, polioclastic infections of spinal neurones have been associated with infection with other viruses, notably of the Coxsackie and ECHO groups. The encephalomyelitic picture which very occasionally complicates neoplastic disease, especially lymphomas, may also be attributable to such viruses, although full virological studies have never been fully undertaken (Walton, Tomlinson and Pearce, 1968; Castleman, 1970).

Herpes zoster or shingles is an acute viral infection of sensory ganglion cells and produces a painful vesicular rash but occasionally herpes simplex virus may be responsible. Rarely, the viral infection spreads to adjacent areas of the spinal cord to produce a segmental myelitis (Thomas and Howard, 1972) and sometimes a generalised encephalomyelitis may occur (Gardner-Thorpe, Foster and Barwick, 1976). Segmental myelitis may be associated with local invasion and destruction of motor neurones, resulting in localised muscular atrophy and weakness. Such motor complications appear to occur more commonly with involvement of the lower spinal cord or cauda equina. Recovery from such weakness is possible but usually incomplete. Cranial motor nerve involvement is also known, but may result from local peripheral infection and swelling rather than in the brain stem, e.g. oculomotor paralysis from orbital infection with ophthalmic zoster, or facial nerve paralysis from geniculate ganglion herpes (Ramsay Hunt syndrome).

Metabolic disorders with amyotrophy

Several workers have suggested an association between motor neurone disease and previous gastrectomy, but it seems probable that this is fortuitous (Ask-Upmark, 1950, 1961; Norris, 1975). A progressive muscle wasting disorder has been described in patients having hypoglycaemic symptoms following partial gastrectomy (Silfver-skiold, 1946; Williams, 1955) but the majority of cases of hypoglycaemic amyotrophy have been associated with insulin-secreting tumours (Tom and Richardson, 1951; Mulder, Bastron and Lambert, 1956). Such patients commonly experience paraesthesiae although the sensory involvement has been minimal. Surgical removal of the tumour has led to disappearance of the paraesthesiae and at least stabilisation of the muscle weakness, and in some cases electrophysiological evidence of improvement has been shown (Lambert, Mulder and Bastron, 1960). The evidence that this disease is due to a neuronal disorder rather than a predominantly motor peripheral neuropathy requires further study.

Diabetic amyotrophy is characterised by an asymmetrical proximal wasting and weakness of the legs, often accompanied by severe local pain in the anterior thighs and sometimes in the lumbar region or perineum. Garland and Taverner (1953) pointed out the frequent finding of extensor plantar responses and this, together with the appearance of fasciculations, can cause confusion with classical motor neurone disease. The patients are invariably middle-aged or elderly and the neuromuscular syndrome may be the presenting feature of maturity-onset diabetes. Good metabolic control may be associated with excellent recovery of function (Casey and Harrison, 1972). Garland and Taverner (1953) initially attributed the disorder to a myelopathy but later were non-committal and coined the term diabetic amyotrophy (Garland, 1955). The condition has been attributed to a local femoral neuropathy because of the prolonged latency of the knee jerk (Gilliatt and Willison, 1962) and also a prolonged femoral conduction time (Chopra and Hurwitz, 1968; Lamontagne and Buchthal, 1970) but the frequent involvement of other muscle groups and the absence of sensory loss makes this an incomplete explanation. Pathological involvement of the femoral nerve has been shown in some such cases (Raff, Sangalang and Asbury, 1968).

Chronic renal failure or uraemia is usually associated with a mixed motor and sensory polyneuropathy. However, the motor involvement may predominate and cause a distal weakness of the legs and, to a lesser extent, of the arms, with depressed tendon reflexes. Distal dysaesthesiae are common, although rarely painful and may be associated with muscle cramps and a 'restless legs' syndrome (Asbury, 1975). Electrophysiological studies have shown mild slowing of motor and sensory conduction (Jebsen, Tenckhoff and Honet, 1967). Asbury, Victor and Adams (1963), in an autopsy study of four cases of uraemic polyneuropathy, found a striking loss of nerve fibres in the distal parts of the nerves, with little or no involvement of the proximal portions or nerve roots. They also noted striking myelin breakdown. Central chromatolysis was noted in the spinal motor neurones. They concluded that the changes are those of an axonal degeneration. The demyelinative changes in fresh sural nerve biopsies have been stressed by some workers (Dinn and Crane, 1970), but in an elegant combined electrophysiological and histological study by Dyck, Johnson, Lambert and O'Brien (1971) the demyelination was shown to be non-random and present in nerve fibres undergoing axonal degeneration.

Chronic hepatic failure is commonly associated with muscle wasting and weakness. In many cases a frank polyneuropathy may be present, but until recently this was thought to be usually the result of alcoholism or diabetes which may also be present. Pathological studies on sural nerve biopsies have shown a mild, usually asymptomatic, demyelinating neuropathy in patients with liver disease, and this finding was not restricted to alcoholic cases (Dayan and Williams, 1967). Electrophysiological studies have shown that there is a significant incidence of subclinical polyneuropathy, affecting sensory fibres more than motor, including non-alcoholic cases (Seneviratne and Peiris, 1970; Morgan, Read and Campbell, 1979). The mild degree of slowing of nerve conduction suggests that this is primarily an axonal degenerative disorder similar to that observed in uraemia, but further studies are required to clarify this.

The muscle wasting in hyperthyroidism is generally thought to be a myopathic disorder, but histological studies have shown remarkably little abnormality in the majority of cases. Neither specific myopathic nor denervation changes have been described. McComas, Sica, McNabb, Goldberg and Upton (1973) have described electrophysiological findings of a reversible motor neuropathy in thyrotoxicosis, but this awaits independent confirmation.

Muscle weakness may also be a feature of acromegaly or gigantism caused by a pituitary tumour. In some cases this may be rapidly reversed with treatment of the tumour and lowering of the circulating growth hormone levels. No adequate explanation for this phenomenon has been given. The carpal tunnel syndrome is quite common in acromegaly and a diffuse hypertrophic neuropathy has been described very occasionally since the last century (Marie and Marinesco, 1891). Histological studies have shown an increase of endoneural and perineural connective tissue with loss of myelinated nerve fibres (Stewart, 1966) and recently Dinn (1970) described changes of a primary demyelinating disorder. However, nerve conduction is only mildly slowed in addition to the moderate reduction in nerve action poten-

tials, which suggests a mainly axonal degeneration with non-random demyelination (Low, McLeod, Turtle, Donnelly and Wright, 1974: Pickett, Layzer, Levin, Schneider, Campbell and Sumner, 1975).

Hyperlipoproteinemia has been associated with progressive muscular atrophy, but it is uncertain whether such cases represent an adult onset form of spinal muscular atrophy with an associated genetic abnormality of lipid metabolism (Quarfordt, Devino, Engel, Levy and Fredrickson, 1970).

Toxic motor neuropathies

Early in the course of a toxic polyneuropathy, the impaired function is associated with irritability or hypersensitivity, and paraesthesiae or dysaesthesiae. Motor involvement is associated with weakness and impaired tendon reflexes, progressing to atrophy and areflexia. Endogenous toxic causes have been discussed under the heading of metabolic diseases. Many exogenous toxins have been associated with peripheral neuropathies but few cause a predominantly motor syndrome.

The possible association of lead poisoning and motor neurone disease has been discussed earlier. Lead intoxication may affect the central nervous system or the peripheral nerves. Motor involvement predominates, although paraesthesiae and pain are common. The motor weakness is greatest in muscles receiving the most use; hence the wrist drop in painters intoxicated by lead paints. In children, the CNS involvement predominates, but foot drop may be evident in association with brisk reflexes and extensor plantar responses (Seto and Freeman, 1964). Pathological studies have shown evidence of axonal degeneration and also demyelination, which is dose-dependent to a certain extent (Fullerton, 1966).

Several other heavy metal intoxications have been associated with peripheral neuropathy. In arsenic poisoning, sensory involvement is prominent and causes painful dysaesthesiae in addition to distal weakness. In other metal intoxications the initial sensory disturbance may subside and produce a predominant distal motor weakness, for example in gold therapy (Endtz, 1958), and in chronic mercurial poisoning (Kantarjian, 1961). Mercury intoxication, particularly with organic compounds, e.g. methyl-mercury (Minamata disease) may affect the central nervous system and produce mental and extra-pyramidal disorders (McAlpine and Araki, 1958; Kurland, Faro and Siedler, 1960).

Organophosphorus compounds have been widely used in industry, mainly as pesticides. They are powerful inhibitors of carboxylic esterase enzymes, including cholinesterase. In man, acute intoxication causes inhibition of acetylcholinesterase of the nervous system, resulting in accumulation of acetylcholine at the synapses, and a paralytic cholinergic crisis. If respiratory paralysis is treated and the airway is protected from the excessive secretions, complete recovery occurs within 10 days (Namba, Nolte, Jackrel and Grob, 1971). Bidstrup, Bonnell and Beckett (1953) described three cases of a delayed neuropathy after an acute cholinergic illness in workers manufacturing the compound 'Mipafox'. However, the delayed neuropathy in organophosphorus poisoning generally occurs without an antecedent cholinergic illness. Tri-orthocresyl phosphate (TOCP), a weak insecticide and a high-temperature industrial lubricant, has been responsible for the greatest number of cases of neuropathy in man. The largest outbreak of poisoning occurred in 1930–31 in the United States when alcoholic extracts of ginger and rum were adulterated by TOCP and freely used as an alcoholic drink. An estimated 16 000 cases of polyneuropathy (ginger jake paralysis) occurred at that time (Namba et al., 1971), and several other major outbreaks have resulted from contaminated cooking oil since then. The neuropathy develops after an interval of 7–21 days, beginning with paraesthesiae and swiftly followed by a spreading distal weakness (Hopkins, 1975). The paralysis progresses rapidly over a period of several days. The affected muscles waste. Sensory loss is trivial or absent and the paraesthesiae disappear early in the course of the disease. The tendon reflexes may be lost, but sometimes are increased because of pyramidal tract involvement; spasticity may develop later. Recovery from the neuropathy attributable to organophosphorus poisoning is poor. Pathological studies in man and experimental animals have shown an axonal degeneration present only in the distal ends of the motor nerves, and also changes in the spinal cord (Cavanagh, 1964).

Ischaemic myelopathy

Acute occlusion of arteries supplying the spinal cord causes an initial paraplegia with sensory loss up to the level which is ischaemic, but in certain cases good sensory recovery has occurred, leaving a residual motor neuropathy (Dodson and Landau, 1973). Less acute aortic disease has been associated with selective poliomyelomalacia, particularly of the ventral grey matter of the spinal cord (Herrick and Mills, 1971) and a chronic motor neurone syndrome has been described in relation to arteriosclerosis or hypertension (Jellinger and Neumayer, 1962; Hughes and Brownell, 1966; Jellinger, 1967). The latter is a progressive disease with a picture of weakness and wasting, mainly in the lower limbs, and mild but definite sensory impairment. The pathological changes are confined to the territory of the anterior spinal artery. Ischaemic lacunae are present in the spinal grey matter involving the motor nerve cells, and the lesions may extend laterally into the territory of the spinothalamic tracts or dorsally into the base of the posterior columns. Atherosclerosis does not appear to occur in the anterior spinal artery or its branches, but mesial thickening of the wall has been found, particularly in hypertensive patients. It seems unlikely that this disease state, which is largely restricted to the lower limbs, could be confused with MND. Its restriction to the territory of the anterior spinal artery is probably related to the architectural deficiency of the blood supply to the anterior two-thirds of the spinal cord, and its vulnerability to ischaemia (Jellinger and Neumayer, 1969).

The occasional chronic myelopathy with progressive muscle wasting and weakness which follows radiation therapy to the spinal region including the spinal cord, is thought to be largely due to ischaemia. Prominent abnormalities of small and medium-sized arterioles are found in the damaged areas. Hyalinisation, fibrinoid necrosis and thrombosis of vessels are seen in relation to local necrosis and astrocytosis (Pennybacker and Russell, 1948). Several authors have described a clinical syndrome of muscular atrophy and weakness in the lower extremities, with preserved sensation, which has occurred several months after irradiation (Greenfield and Stark, 1948; Sadowsky, Sachs and Ochoa, 1976).

Trauma, including electrical injury

Cases of motor neurone disease with a previous history of significant trauma have been reported by many authors, but are thought to be chance associations (see Bonduelle, 1975). However, a distinctive syndrome of benign post-traumatic amyotrophy developing several months after major local trauma has been described (Norris, 1972). The wasting was confined to the injured limb and after several months there was complete recovery: this is reminiscent of neuralgic amyotrophy or allergic brachial neuritis. A few cases of apparent post-traumatic MND were subsequently proved to be attributable to cervical arachnoiditis (Puech, Grossiard, Brun and Denis, 1947; Kissel, 1948).

The neurological effects of electrical trauma have been comprehensively reviewed by Panse (1970). Transient sensorimotor paralysis of limbs, persisting for up to two weeks, has been described in survivors of severe electrical trauma involving moderate or high energies (voltages of 1000 V or more and current in the range 25 mA–5 A) and also in those who have been struck by lightning. The site of damage has depended on the path taken by the electrical current through the body. Spinal amyotrophy following lightning accidents has been known for more than a century. It is also well known after passage of electricity from limb to limb, or trunk to limb. The muscular atrophy is commonly unilateral and is roughly confined to the neurological distribution of sensory dermatomes related to the point of contact. Hence, weakness and wasting around the shoulder and upper arm may develop after electrical burns to the thumb and index fingers. Not all victims show electrical burns or scars at the site of contact and roughly only a half have suffered loss of consciousness at the time of injury. Apparently, the weakness may be immediate or delayed by as long as a few months, and the atrophy can be progressive for a few months

before becoming static or showing regression. Loss of the local tendon reflexes is the general rule, but sensory loss is usually slight. Spasticity or other pyramidal signs have been described and indicate more extensive damage to the spinal cord. There have been a few descriptions of typical clinical cases of MND following electrical trauma, but these are generally regarded as being coincidental. There have been no reports of electrophysiological or pathological studies of these cases of localised amyotrophy.

Non-metastatic carcinomatous neuromuscular disease

The various forms of neuromuscular disease occurring in association with cancer are discussed fully in Chapter 19. Reference here will be limited to those cases where a direct involvement of motor neurones is apparent. The question of a viral aetiology of the encephalomyelitic syndromes related to cancer, where there is inflammatory disease of motor and sensory neurones, was referred to in the section on infections. Non-inflammatory degeneration of anterior horn cells and of dorsal ganglion cells has been described in sensorimotor polyneuropathies (Norris, Rudolf and Barney, 1964; Victor, 1965; Henson and Urich, 1970). However, the direct association of cancer with a pure motor neurone disease state remains controversial and in most cases is coincidental (Norris and Engel, 1965; Norris, McMenemey and Barnard, 1969; Brownell, Oppenheimer and Hughes, 1970).

The advent of modern electrophysiological techniques has revealed evidence of subclinical neuropathy in up to 50 per cent of cases with malignancy (McLeod, 1975). These cases correspond to the carcinomatous 'neuromyopathy' of Brain and Henson (1958) and in some cases to the 'mild terminal neuropathy' which complicates known cancer (Croft, Urich and Wilkinson, 1967; Croft and Wilkinson, 1969). This disorder presents with symmetrical, mainly proximal, limb weakness and wasting in association with minor sensory symptoms such as paraesthesiae or mild numbness. The examination findings are of depressed tendon reflexes and, frequently, occasional fasciculations or distal sensory loss, especially to vibration. Electromyography reveals a high incidence of chronic denervation changes together with spontaneous discharge of fibrillation and short-duration fasciculation potentials; active 'myopathic' units may also be found, particularly in proximal muscles (Trojaborg, Frantzen and Andersen, 1969; Campbell and Paty, 1974). Motor conduction velocity frequently may be normal but may be mildly slowed, especially in the terminal nerve segments. Sensory conduction is frequently impaired and sensory action potentials may be absent or markedly reduced. Evidence has been presented to show that the disorder is a progressive neuronal dysfunction but with involvement of motor to a greater extent than of sensory neurones (Campbell and Paty, 1974).

The mechanism by which non-metastatic polyneuropathy and neuronal disease are produced is unknown. The possibility that they are caused by toxic factors released by the tumour has been suggested by many authors (Costa and Holland, 1965). Certainly, the incidence of clinical neurological disease is apparently higher in association with undifferentiated cell tumours of the lung, which may produce a wide range of hormone-like compounds (Lebovitz, 1965; Ross, 1972). The possibility of neuronal damage from viral invasion was discussed earlier and this could be linked with an immune mechanism. Brain and Henson (1958) speculated on a crossed reaction to shared antigenic sites between tumour and nervous tissue proteins. This was supported by the finding of anti-CNS antibodies in the serum of four patients with subacute sensory neuropathy but not in other forms of neuropathy (Wilkinson, 1964). The demonstration of circulating lymphocytes sensitised to peripheral nervous tissue was thought, like the serum antibodies, to be a secondary phenomenon to sequestrated or damaged neural proteins (Paty, Campbell and Hughes, 1974).

REFERENCES

Addair, J. & Snyder, L.H. (1942) Evidence for an autosomal recessive gene for susceptibility to paralytic poliomyelitis. *Journal of Heredity*, **33**, 306–9.

Allen, I.V., Dermott, E., Connelly, J.H. & Hurwitz, L.J. (1971). A study of a patient with the amyotrophic form of Creutzfeld-Jakob disease. *Brain*, **94**, 715.

Andrews, J.M. & Andrews, R.L. (1976) The comparative neuropathology of motor neuron diseases. In *Amyotrophic Lateral Sclerosis. Recent Research Trends*, Eds J.M. Andrews, R.T. Johnson & M. Brazier, pp. 181–216 (Academic Press: New York).

Andrews, J.M. & Gardner, M.B. (1974) Lower motor neuron degeneration associated with type C RNA virus infection in mice. Neuropathological features. *Journal of Neuropathology and Experimental Neurology*, **33**, 285–307.

Antel, J.P., Arnason, B.E.W., Fuller, T.C. & Lehrich, J.R. (1976) Histocompatibility typing in amyotrophic lateral sclerosis. *Archives of Neurology*, **33**, 423–5.

Aran, F.A. (1850) Recherches sur une maladie non encore décrite du système musculaire (atrophie musculaire progressive) *Archives of General Medicine*, **24**, 5–35.

Asbury, A.K. (1975) Uremic Neuropathy. In *Peripheral Neuropathy*, Eds P.J. Dyck, P.K. Thomas & E.H. Lambert, pp. 982–92 (Saunders: New York).

Asbury, A.K., Victor, M., & Adams, R.D. (1963) Uremic polyneuropathy. *Archives of Neurology*, **8**, 413.

Ask-Upmark, E., (1950) Amyotrophic lateral sclerosis observed in 5 persons after gastric resection. *Gastroenterologia (Basel)*, **15**, 257–259.

Ask-Upmark, E. (1961) Precipitating factors in the pathogenesis of amyotrophic lateral sclerosis. *Acta medica scandinavica*, **170**, 717–23.

Astin, K.J., Wilde, C.E. & Davies-Jones, G.A.B. (1975) Glucose metabolism and insulin response in the plasma and cerebrospinal fluid in motor neurone disease. *Journal of the Neurological Sciences*, **25**, 205–10.

Aycock, W.L. (1942) Familial aggregation in poliomyelitis. *American Journal of the Medical Sciences*, **203**, 452–65.

Becker, P.E. (1964) Atrophia musculorum spinalis pseudomyopathica. Hereditare neurogene proximale Amyotrophie von Kugelberg und Welander. *Zeitschrift für Menschliche Vererbungs- und Konstitutionslehre*, **37**, 193.

Bidstrup, P.L., Bonnell, J.A. & Beckett, A.G. (1953) Paralysis following poisoning by a new organic phosphorus insecticide (mipafox). Report on two cases. *British Medical Journal*, **1**, 1068–72.

Bobowick, A.R. & Brody, J.A. (1973) Epidemiology of motor neuron diseases. *New England Journal of Medicine*, **288**, 1047–55.

Bodian, D. (1952) Virus and host factors determining the nature and severity of lesions and of clinical manifestations. Poliomyelitis. *Proceedings of the 2nd International Polio Conference*, pp. 61–87 (Lippincott: Philadelphia).

Bodmer, W.F. (1975) Histocompatibility testing international. *Nature*, **256**, 696–8.

Böhme, G. (1974) *Stimm-, Sprech- und Hörstörungen. Aetiologie, Diagnostik, Therapie* (Fischer Verlag: Stuttgart).

Bonduelle, M. (1975) Amyotrophic lateral sclerosis. In *Handbook of Clinical Neurology*, Eds P.J. Vinken & G.W. Bruyn, Vol. 22, pp. 281–338 (North Holland: Amsterdam).

Bornstein, M.B. & Appel, S.H. (1965) Tissue culture studies of demyelination. *New York Academy of Sciences*, **122**, 280–6.

Brain, W.R. and Henson, R.A. (1958) Neurological

syndromes associated with carcinoma. *Lancet*, **2**, 971.

Brandt, S. (1950) Course and symptoms of progressive infantile muscular atrophy. A follow-up study of 112 cases in Denmark. *Archives of Neurology and Psychiatry*, **63**, 218.

Braun, N.M.T. & Rochester, D.F. (1979) Muscular weakness and respiratory failure. *American Revue of Respiratory Diseases*, **119** (2 part 2), 123–5.

Brody, J.A. & Chen, K.M. (1969) Changing epidemiologic patterns of amyotrophic lateral sclerosis and Parkinsonism-dementia on Guam. In *Motor Neuron Disease*, Eds F.H. Norris & L.T. Kurland, p. 61 (Grune and Stratton: New York).

Brown, J.C. & Kater, R.M.H. (1969) Pancreatic function in patients with amyotrophic lateral sclerosis. *Neurology (Minneapolis)*, **19**, 185–9.

Brown, W.F. & Jaatoul, N. (1974) Amyotrophic lateral sclerosis. Electrophysiological study. (Number of motor units and rate of decay of motor units) *Archives of Neurology*, **30**, 242–8.

Brownell, D.B., Oppenheimer, D.R. & Hughes, J.T. (1970) The central nervous system in motor neurone disease. *Journal of Neurology, Neurosurgery and Psychiatry*, **33**, 338–57.

Buchthal, F. & Honcke, P. (1944) Electromyographical examination of patients suffering from poliomyelitis ant. ac. up to six months after the acute stage of the disease. *Acta. Medica Scandinavica*, **116**, 148–64.

Buchthal, F. & Olsen, P.Z. (1970). Electromyography and muscle biopsy in infantile spinal muscular atrophy. *Brain*, **93**, 15.

Bundey, S. & Lovelace, R.E. (1975) A clinical and genetic study of chronic proximal spinal muscular atrophy. *Brain*, **98**, 455–72.

Byers, R.K. & Banker, B.Q. (1961) Infantile muscular atrophy. *Archives of Neurology*, **5**, 140–164.

Campbell, A.M.G., Williams, E.R. & Barltrop, D. (1970). Motor neurone disease and exposure to lead. *Journal of Neurology, Neurosurgery and Psychiatry*, **33**, 872–85.

Campbell, M.J. (1979) Genetic aspects of motor neurone disease. In *Progress in Neurological Research*, Eds P.O. Behan & F.C. Rose, pp. 135–44 (Pitman: London).

Campbell, M.J. & Paty, D.W. (1974) Carcinomatous neuromyopathy: an electrophysiological and immunological study of patients with carcinoma of the lung. I. Electrophysiological studies. *Journal of Neurology, Neurosurgery and Psychiatry*, **37**, 131–41.

Campbell, M.J., McComas, A.J. & Petito, F. (1973) Physiological changes in ageing muscle. *Journal of Neurology, Neurosurgery and Psychiatry*, **36**, 174–82.

Carpenter, S. (1968) Proximal axonal enlargement in motor neuron disease. *Neurology (Minneapolis)*, **18**, 841–51.

Carpenter, S., Karpati, G., Rothman, S., Watters, G. & Andemann F. (1978) Pathological involvement of primary sensory neurons in Werdnig-Hoffmann disease. *Acta Neuropathologica*, **42**, 91–7.

Casey, E.B. & Harrison, M.J.G. (1972) Diabetic amyotrophy: a follow-up study. *British Medical Journal*, **1**, 656.

Castaigne, P., Lhermitte, F., Schuller, E. & Rouques, C. (1971) Les proteines du liquids cephalo-rachidien au cours de la sclerose laterale amyotrophique. *Revue Neurologique*. **125**, 393–400.

Castaigne, P., Lhermitte, F., Cambier, J., Escourolle, R. & Le Bigot, P. (1972) Etude neuropathologique de 61

observations de sclerose laterale amyotrophique. Discussion nosologique. *Revue Neurologique*, **127**, 401–14.

Castleman, B. (1970). (Ed.) Case records of the Massachusetts General Hospital (case 42–1970). *New England Journal of Medicine*, **283**, 806.

Cavanagh, J.B. (1964) Peripheral nerve changes in orthocresyl phosphate poisoning in the cat. *Journal of Pathology and Bacteriology*, **87**, 365–83.

Charcot, J.M. (1873) *Lecons sur les maladies du systeme nerveaux*. IInd series, collected by Bourneville, Paris, Delahaye (English translation by Sigerson, G., London, New Sydenham Society, 1881).

Charcot, J.M. (1874). De la sclerose laterale amyotrophique. *Progrès Médical (Paris)*, **2**, 325, 341, 453.

Charcot, J.M. & Joffroy, A. (1869) Deux cas d'astrophie musculaire progressive avec lesions de la substance grise et des faisceaux anterolateraux de la moelle epiniere. *Archives of Physiology*, **2**, 354, 629 and 744.

Chevrie-Müller, C., Dordain, N. & Grémy, F. (1970) Etude phoniatrique clinique et instrumentale des dysarthries. II Resultat chez les malades presentant des syndromes bulbaires et pseudo-bulbaires. *Revue Neurologique*, **122**, 123–38.

Chopra, J.S. & Hurwitz, L.J. (1968) Femoral nerve conduction in diabetes and chronic occlusive vascular disease. *Journal of Neurology, Neurosurgery and Psychiatry*, **31**, 28–33.

Colmant, H.J. (1975) Progressive bulbar palsy in adults. In *Handbook of Clinical Neurology*, Eds P.J. Vinken & G.W. Bruyn, Vol. 22, pp. 111–56 (North Holland: Amsterdam).

Conradi, S., Ronnevi, L.-O., & Vesterberg, O. (1976) Abnormal tissue distribution of lead in amyotrophic lateral sclerosis. *Journal of Neurological Sciences*, **29**, 259–65.

Conradi, S., Ronnevi, L.-O., & Vesterberg, O., (1978a) Increased plasma levels of lead in patients with amyotrophic lateral sclerosis compared with control subjects as determined by flameless atomic absorption spectrophotometry. *Journal of Neurology, Neurosurgery and Psychiatry*, **41**, 389–93.

Conradi, S., Ronnevi, L.-O., & Vesterberg, O., (1978b) Lead concentration in skeletal muscle in amyotrophic lateral sclerosis patients and control subjects. *Journal of Neurology, Neurosurgery and Psychiatry*, **41**, 1001–4.

Cook, A.W., Pertschuk, L.P., Gupta, K., Nidzgorski, F., Carter, W., Horoszewicz, J.S., Marcus, E.L. & Kim, D.S. (1979) The effect of antiviral agents on jejunal immunopathology in amyotrophic lateral sclerosis. In *Progress in Neurological Research*, Eds P.O. Behan & F.C. Rose, pp. 62–72 (Pitman: London).

Costa, G. & Holland, J.F. (1965) Systemic effect of tumors with special reference to the nervous system. In *The Remote Effects of Cancer on the Nervous System*, Eds Lord Brain and F.H. Norris Jr., pp. 125–133 (Grune and Stratton: New York).

Cremer, N.E., Oshiro, L.S., Norris, F.H. & Lennette, E.H. (1973) Cultures of tissues from patients with amyotrophic lateral sclerosis. *Archives of Neurology*, **29**, 331–3.

Croft, P.B. & Wilkinson, M. (1969) The course and prognosis in some types of carcinomatous neuromyopathy. *Brain*, **92**, 1–8.

Croft, P.B., Urich, H. & Wilkinson, M. (1967) Peripheral neuropathy of sensorimotor type associated with malignant disease. *Brain*, **90**, 31–66.

Currier, R.D. & Haerer, A.F. (1968) Amyotrophic lateral

sclerosis and metallic toxins. *Archives of Environmental Health*, **17**, 712–9.

Darley, F.L., Aronson, A.E. & Brown, J.R. (1969) Differential diagnostic patterns of dysarthria. *Journal of Speech and Hearing Research*, **12**, 246–69.

Darley, F.L., Aronson, A.E. & Brown, J.R. (1972) *Motor Speech Disorders* (Saunders: Philadelphia).

Dawidenkow, S. (1939) Scapulo-peroneal amyotrophy. *Archives of Neurology and Psychiatry*, **41**, 694.

Dayan, A.D. & Williams, R. (1967) Demyelinating peripheral neuropathy and liver disease. *Lancet*, **2**, 133–34.

Dayan, A.D., Graveson, G.S., Illis, L.S. & Robinson, P.K. (1969) Schwann cell damage in motor neuron disease. *Neurology (Minneapolis)*, **19**, 242–6.

De Morsier, G. (1967) Un cas de maladie de Pick avec sclerose laterale amyotrophique terminale. Contribution a la semeiologie temporale. *Revue Neurologique*, **116**, 373–82.

Denys, E.H. & Norris, F.H. (1979) Amyotrophic lateral sclerosis. Impairment of neuromuscular transmission *Archives of Neurology*, **36**, 202–5.

Dick, H.M., Sturrock, R.D., Goel, G.K., Henderson, N., Canesi, B., Rooney, P.J., Dick, W.C. & Buchanan, W.W., (1975) HL–A antigens, ankylosing spondylitis and sacroilitis. *Tissue Antigens*, **5**, 26–32.

Dickinson, A.G. & Fraser, H. (1977) In *Slow Virus Infections of the Central Nervous System*, Eds ter V. Meulen & M. Katz, Ch. 1 (Springer-Verlag: New York).

Dinn, J.J. (1970) Schwann cell dysfunction in acromegaly. *Journal of Clinical Endocrinology and Metabolism*, **31**, 140.

Dinn, J.J. & Crane, D.L. (1970) Schwann cell dysfunction in uraemia. *Journal of Neurology, Neurosurgery and Psychiatry*, **33**, 605.

Dodson, W.E. & Landau, W.M. (1973) Motor neuron loss due to aortic clamping in repair of coarctation. *Neurology (Minneapolis)*, **23**, 539–42.

Dorman, J.D., Engel, W.K. & Fried, D.M. (1969) Therapeutic trial in amyotrophic lateral sclerosis. *Journal of the American Medical Association*, **209**, 257.

Duchen, L.W. & Strich, S.J. (1968) An hereditary motor neurone disease with progressive denervation of muscle in the mouse: The mutant 'wobbler'. *Journal of Neurology, Neurosurgery and Psychiatry*, **31**, 535–42.

Duchenne, G. (1860) Paralysie musculaire progressive de la langue, du voile du palais et des levres. *Archives Générales de Médecine*, **16**, 283, 431.

Duchenne, G. & Joffroy, A. (1870) De l'atrophie aigue et chronique des cellules nerveuses de la moelle et du bulbe rachidien, a propos d'une observation de paralysie glossolabio-laryngie, *Archives of Physiology*, **3**, 499.

Dyck, P.J. & Lambert, E.H. (1968a) Lower motor and primary sensory neuron diseases with peroneal muscular atrophy. 1. Hereditary polyneuropathies. *Archives of Neurology*, **18**, 603.

Dyck, P.J. & Lambert, E.H. (1968b) *Ibid.* ii. Various neuronal degenerations. *Archives of Neurology*, **18**, 619.

Dyck, P.J., Johnson, W.J., Lambert, E.H. and O'Brien, P.C. (1971) Segmental demyelination secondary to axonal degeneration in uremic neuropathy. *Mayo Clinic Proceedings*, **46**, 400–31.

Dyck, P.J., Stevens, J.C., Mulder, D.W. & Espinosa, R.E. (1975) Frequency of nerve fiber degeneration of peripheral motor and sensory neurons in amyotrophic lateral sclerosis. Morphometry of deep and superficial peroneal nerves. *Neurology (Minneapolis)*, **25**, 781–5.

Emery, A.E.H. (1971) The nosology of the spinal muscular atrophies. *Journal of Medical Genetics*, **8**, 481–95.

Endtz, L.J., (1958) Complications nerveuses du traitement aurique. *Revue Neurologique*, **99**, 395–410.

Engel, W.K. (1969) Motor neuron histochemistry in ALS and infantile spinal muscular atrophy. In *Motor Neuron Diseases*, Eds F.H. Norris & L.T. Kurland, pp. 218–34 (Grune and Stratton: New York).

Engel, W.K., Cuneo, R.A. & Levy, H.B. (1978) Polyinosinicpolycytidylic acid treatment of neuropathy (Letter) *Lancet*, **1**, 503–4.

Engel, W.K., Kurland, L.T. & Klatzo, I. (1959) An inherited disease similar to amyotrophic lateral sclerosis with a pattern of posterior column involvement. An intermediate form? *Brain*, **82**, 203–20.

Engel, W.K., Hogenhuis, L.A.H., Collis, W.J., Schalch, D.S., Barlow, M.H., Gold, E.N. & Dorman, J.D. (1969) Metabolic studies and therapeutic trials in amyotrophic lateral sclerosis. In *Motor Neuron Diseases*, Eds F.H. Norris & L.T. Kurland, pp. 199–208 (Grune and Stratton: New York).

Fallat, R.J., Jewitt, B., Bass, M., Kamm, B. & Norris, F.H. Jr. (1979) Spirometry in amyotrophic lateral sclerosis. *Archives of Neurology*, **36**, 74–80.

Feigenbaum, J.A. & Munsat, T.L. (1970) A neuromuscular syndrome of scapuloperoneal distribution. *Bulletin of the Los Angeles Neurological Society*, **35**, 47–57.

Felmus, M.T., Patten, J.P. & Swanke, D. (1976) Antecedent events in amyotrophic lateral sclerosis. *Neurology (Minneapolis)*, **26**, 167–72.

Fenichel, G.M., Emery, E.S. & Hunt, P. (1967) Neurogenic atrophy simulating facio-scapulo-humeral dystrophy. A dominant form. *Archives of Neurology*, **17**, 257–60.

Field, E.J. & Hughes, D. (1969) Toxicity of serum from motor neuron disease for myelin and glial cells in tissue culture. In *Motor Neuron Diseases*, Eds F.H. Norris & L.T. Kurland, pp. 179–82 (Grune and Stratton: New York).

Finkel, N. (1962) A forma psuedomiopatica tardia da atrophia muscular progressiva heredo-familial. *Archivos de Neuropsiquiatria*, **4**, 307.

Friedman, A.P. & Freedman, D. (1950) Amyotrophic lateral sclerosis. *Journal of Nervous and Mental Disease*, **111**, 1–18.

Fullerton, P.M. (1966) Chronic peripheral neuropathy produced by lead poisoning in guinea-pigs. *Journal of Neuropathology and Experimental Neurology*, **25**, 214.

Furukawa, T., Tsukagoshi, H., Sugita, H. & Toyokura, Y. (1969) Neurogenic muscular atrophy simulating facioscapulohumeral muscular dystrophy. *Journal of the Neurological Sciences*, **9**, 389.

Gajdusek, D.C. (1963) Motor-neuron disease in natives of New Guinea. *New England Journal of Medicine*, **268**, 474–6.

Gajdusek, D.C. (1979) A focus of high incidence amyotrophic lateral sclerosis and Parkinsonism and dementia syndromes in a small population of Auyn and Jakai people of Southern West New Guinea. In *Amyotrophic Lateral Sclerosis*, Eds T. Tsubaki & Y. Toyokura, pp. 287–305 (University of Tokyo Press: Tokyo).

Gardner, M.B., Rasheed, S., Klement, V., Rongey, R.W., Brown, J.C., Dworsky, R. & Henderson, B.E. (1976). Lower motor neuron disease in wild mice caused by indigenous Type C virus and search for a similar etiology in human amyotrophic lateral sclerosis. In *Amyotrophic*

Lateral Sclerosis. Recent Research Trends, Eds J.M. Andrews, R.T. Johnson & M. Brazier, pp. 217–34 (Academic Press: New York).

Gardner, M.B., Henderson, B.E., Officer, J.E., Rongey, R.W., Parker, J.C., Oliver, C., Estes, J.D. & Huebner, R.J. (1973) A spontaneous lower motor neuron disease apparently caused by indigenous Type-C RNA virus in wild mice. Journal of the National Cancer Institute, 51, 1243–54.

Gardner-Medwin, D., Hudgson, P. & Walton, J.N. (1967) Benign spinal muscular atrophy arising in childhood and adolescence. Journal of the Neurological Sciences, 5, 121–58.

Gardner-Thorpe, C., Foster, J.B. & Barwick, D.D. (1976) Unusual manifestations of herpes zoster: A clinical and electrophysiological study. Journal of the Neurological Sciences, 28, 427–47.

Garland, H. (1955) Diabetic amyotrophy. British Medical Journal, 2, 1287.

Garland, H. & Taverner, D. (1953). Diabetic myelopathy. British Medical Journal, 1, 1405.

Gath, I., Sjaastad, O. & Loken, A.C. (1969) Myopathic electromyographic changes correlated with histopathology in Wohlfart-Kugelberg-Welander disease. Neurology (Minneapolis), 19, 344.

Gibbs, C.J. & Gajdusek, D.C. (1972) Amyotrophic lateral sclerosis, Parkinson's disease and the amyotrophic lateral sclerosis-Parkinsonism-dementia complex on Guam: a review and summary of attempts to demonstrate infection as the aetiology. In Host-Virus Reactions with Special Reference to Persistent Agents, Ed. G. Dick, Journal of Clinical Pathology, 25, suppl. 6, 132.

Gibbs, C.J., Jr., Gajdusek, D.C., Asher, D.M., Alpers, M.P., Beck, E., Daniel, P.M. & Matthews, W.B. (1968) Creutzfeldt-Jakob disease (spongiform encephalopathy): Transmission to the chimpanzee. Science, 161, 388.

Gilliatt, R.W. & Willison, R.G. (1962) Peripheral nerve conduction in diabetic neuropathy. Journal of Neurology, Neurosurgery and Psychiatry, 25, 11.

Goldblatt, D. (1969) Motor neuron disease: historical introduction. In Motor Neuron Diseases, Eds F.H. Norris Jr. & L.T. Kurland, pp. 3–11 (Grune and Stratton: New York).

Gomez, M.R. (1975) Progressive bulbar paralysis of childhood (Fazio-Londe disease). In Handbook of Clinical Neurology, Eds P.J. Vinken & G.W. Bruyn, 22, pp. 103–110 (North-Holland: Amsterdam).

Gomez, M.R., Clermont, V. & Bernstein, J. (1962). Progressive bulbar palsy in children (Fazio-Londe's disease). Archives of Neurology and Psychiatry, 6, 317.

Gotoh, F., Kitamura, A., Koto, A., Kataoka, K. & Atsuji, H. (1972) Abnormal insulin secretion in amyotrophic lateral sclerosis. Journal of the Neurological Science, 16, 201.

Greenfield, J.G. (1954). The Spino-cerebellar Degenerations (Blackwell: Oxford).

Greenfield, J.G. & Matthews, W.B. (1954) Post-encephalitic Parkinsonism and amyotrophy. Journal of Neurology and Psychiatry, 17, 50.

Greenfield, J.G. & Stark, F.M. (1948) Post-irradiation neuropathy. American Journal of Roentgenology, Radium Therapy and Nuclear Medicine, 60, 617–22.

Henson, R.A. & Urich, H. (1970) In Handbook of Clinical Neurology, Eds P.J. Vinken & G.W. Bruyn, Vol. 8, pp. 131–148 (North Holland: Amsterdam).

Herndon, C.N. & Jennings, R.G. (1951) A twin-family study of susceptibility to poliomyelitis. American Journal of Human Genetics, 3, 17–46.

Herrick, M.K. & Mills, P.E. (1971) Infarction of the spinal cord. Archives of Neurology, 24, 228.

Hirano, A. (1973) Progress in the pathology of motor neuron diseases. Progress in Neuropathology, 2, 181–215.

Hirano, A., Kurland, L.T. & Sayre, G.P. (1967) Familial amyotrophic lateral sclerosis. Archives of Neurology, 16, 232.

Hirano, A., Malamud, N., Kurland, L.T. & Zimmerman, H.W. (1969) A review of the pathological findings in amyotrophic lateral sclerosis. In Motor Neuron Diseases, Eds F.H. Norris Jr. & L.T. Kurland, pp. 51–60 (Grune and Stratton: New York).

Hirsch, H.E. (1968) Enzyme levels in individual motor neurons in amyotrophic lateral sclerosis. Neurology (Minneapolis), 18, 294.

Hirsch, H.E. & Chen, K.M. (1969) Enzyme activities in individual motor neurons in amyotrophic lateral sclerosis. Journal of Neuropathology and Experimental Neurology, 28, 267–77.

Hjorth, R.J., Walsh, J.C. & Willison, R.G. (1973) The distribution and frequency of spontaneous fasciculations in motor neurone disease. Journal of the Neurological Sciences, 18, 469–74.

Hodes, R. (1948) Electromyographic study of defects of neuromuscular transmission in human poliomyelitis. Archives of Neurology and Psychiatry, 60, 457.

Hoffmann, J. (1893). Uber chronische spinale Muskelatrophie im Kindesalter, auf familiärer Basis. Deutsche Zeitschrift für Nervenheilkunde, 3, 427.

Hoffmann, J. (1897) Weiter Beitrag zur Lehre von der hereditaren progressiven spinalen. Muskelatrophie im Kindesalter. Deutsche Zeitschrift für Nervenheilkunde, 10, 292 (and Ibid 18, 217, 1900).

Hoffman, P.M., Robbins, D.S., Nolte, M.T., Gibbs, C.J. & Gajdusek, D.C. (1978) Cellular immunity in Guamanians with amyotrophic lateral sclerosis and parkinsonism-dementia. New England Journal of Medicine, 299, 680–5.

Hoffman, P.M., Robbins, D.S., Gibbs, C.J., Gajdusek, D.C., Garruto, R.M. & Terasaki, P.I. (1977) Histocompatibility antigens in amyotrophic lateral sclerosis and parkinsonism-dementia on Guam. Lancet, 2, 717.

Hopkins, A. (1975) Toxic neuropathy due to industrial agents. In Peripheral Neuropathy, Eds P.J. Dyck, P.K. Thomas & E.H. Lambert, pp. 1207–26 (Saunders: New York).

Hughes, J.T. & Brownell, D.B. (1966) Spinal cord ischaemia due to arteriosclerosis. Archives of Neurology, 15, 189–202.

Jebson, R.H., Tenckhoff, H. & Honet, J.C. (1967) Natural history of uremic polyneuropathy and effects of dialysis. New England Journal of Medicine, 277, 327.

Jellinger, K. (1967) Arteriosclerosis of the spinal cord and progressive vascular myelopathy. Journal of Neurology, Neurosurgery and Psychiatry, 30, 195–206.

Jellinger, K. & Neumayer, E. (1962) Myelopathie progressive d'origine vasculaire. Revue Neurologique, 106, 666.

Jellinger, K. & Neumayer, E. (1969). Intermittent claudication of the cord and cauda equina. In Handbook of Clinical Neurology, Eds P.J. Vinken & G.W. Bruyn, Vol. 13, p. 507 (North Holland: Amsterdam).

Jennekens, F.G.I., Tomlinson, B.E. & Walton, J.N. (1971) Data on the distribution of fibre types in five human limb muscles. An autopsy study. Journal of the Neurological

Sciences, **14**, 245–57.

Johnson, R.T. (1976) Virological studies of amyotrophic lateral sclerosis: an overview. In *Amyotrophic Lateral Sclerosis. Recent Research Trends,* Eds J.M. Andrews, R.T. Johnson & M. Brazier, pp. 173–80 (Academic Press: New York).

Johnson, R.T., Brooks, B.R., Jubelt, B. and Swarz, J.R. (1979) Viruses and Motor Neurone Diseases. In *Progress in Neurological Research,* Eds P.O. Behan & F.C. Rose, pp. 36–43 (Pitman: London).

Jokelainen, M. & Palo, J. (1976) Letter: Amyotrophic lateral sclerosis and autonomic nervous system. *Lancet,* **1,** 1246.

Jokelainen, M., Tiilikainen, A. & Lapinleimu, K. (1977) Polio antibodies, HLA antigens and amyotrophic lateral sclerosis. *Tissue Antigens,* **10,** 259–66.

Kaeser, H.E. (1964) Die familiare scapulo-peroneale Muskelatrophie. *Deutsche Zeitschrift für Nervenheilkunde,* **186,** 379.

Kaeser, H.E. (1965) Scapuloperoneal muscular atrophy. *Brain,* **88,** 407.

Kaeser, H.E. (1975) Scapulo-peroneal syndrome. In *Handbook of Clinical Neurology,* Eds P.J. Vinken & G.W. Bruyn. Vol. 22, pp. 57–65 (North Holland: Amsterdam).

Kantarjian, A.D. (1961) A syndrome clinically resembling amyotrophic lateral sclerosis following chronic mercurialism. *Neurology (Minneapolis),* **11,** 639.

Kennedy, W.R., Alter, M. & Sung, J.H. (1968) Progressive proximal spinal and bulbar muscular atrophy of late onset: a sex-linked recessive trait. *Neurology (Minneapolis),* **18,** 671.

Kilness, A.W. & Hochberg, F.H. (1977) Amyotrophic lateral sclerosis in high Selenium environment. *Journal of the American Medical Association,* **237,** 2843–4.

Kissel, P. (1948) Syndrome de sclérose latérale amyotrophique avec paralysie labio-glosso-laryngée par arachnoïdite cervicale post-traumatique. Vérification opératoire. *Revue Neurologique,* **80,** 771–3.

Klatzo, L., Gajdusek, D.C. & Zigas, V. (1959). Pathology of Kuru. *Laboratory Investigation,* **8,** 799.

Klein, J. (1975) *Biology of the Mouse Histocompatibility—2 Complex* (Springer Verlag: Berlin and New York).

Koerner, D.R. (1952). Amyotrophic lateral sclerosis on Guam: a clinical study and review of the literature. *Annals of Internal Medicine,* **37,** 1204–20.

Kohn, R. (1968) Postmortem findings in a case of Wohlfart-Kugelberg-Welander disease. *Confinia Neurologica,* **30,** 253.

Kondo, K. (1969) Contribution to the 'pseudo-dystrophic' nature of muscular atrophy in Wohlfart-Kugelberg-Welander's disease. *Acta Neuropathologica (Berlin),* **13,** 29.

Kott, E., Livni, E., Zamir, R. & Kuritzky, A. (1976) Amytrophic lateral sclerosis: Cell-mediated immunity to polio virus and basic myelin protein in patients with high frequency of HLA-BW35. *Neurology (Minneapolis),* **26,** 376–7.

Kott, E., Livni, E., Zamir, R. & Kuritzky, A. (1979) Cell-mediated immunity to polio and HLA antigens in amyotrophic lateral sclerosis. *Neurology (Minneapolis),* **29,** 1040–44.

Kugelberg, E. & Welander, M. (1956) Heredofamilial juvenile muscular atrophy simulating muscular dystrophy. *Archives of Neurology and Psychiatry,* **75,** 500.

Kurland, L.T. & Brody, J.A. (1975) Amyotrophic lateral sclerosis Guam type. In *Handbook of Clinical Neurology,* Eds P.J. Vinken & G.W. Bruyn, Vol. 22, pp. 339–47

(North Holland: Amsterdam).

Kurland, L.T. & Mulder, D.W. (1955) Epidemologic investigations of amyotrophic lateral sclerosis. *Neurology (Minneapolis)* **5,** 182.

Kurland, L.T., Choi, N.W. & Sayre, G.P. (1969) Implications of incidence and geographic patterns on the classification of amyotrophic lateral sclerosis. In *Motor Neuron Diseases,* Eds F.H. Norris & L.T. Kurland, p. 28 (Grune and Stratton: New York).

Kurland, L.T., Faro, S.N. & Siedler, H. (1960) Minamata disease: the outbreak of a neurologic disorder in Minamata, Japan, and its relationship to the ingestion of seafood contaminated by mercuric compounds. *Neurology (Minneapolis),* **1,** 370.

Kurland, L.T., Kurtzke, J.F., Goldberg, I.D. & Choi, N.W. (1973) Amyotrophic lateral sclerosis and other motor neuron diseases. In *Epidemiology of Neurologic and Sense Organ Disorders,* Eds L.T. Kurland, J.F. Kurtzke & I.D. Goldberg, pp. 108–27 (Harvard University Press: Cambridge, Mass.).

Lambert, E.H. (1969) Electromyography in amyotrophic lateral sclerosis. In *Motor Neuron Diseases,* Eds F.H. Norris & L.T. Kurland, p. 135 (Grune and Stratton: New York).

Lambert, E.H. & Mulder, D.W. (1957) Electromyographic studies in amyotrophic lateral sclerosis. *Proceedings of the Staff Meetings of the Mayo Clinic,* **32,** 441–7.

Lambert, E.H., Hulder, D.W. & Bastron, J.A. (1960) Regeneration of peripheral nerves and hyperinsulin neuronopathy. *Neurology (Minneapolis),* **10,** 851–4.

Lamontagne, A. & Buchthal, F. (1970) Electrophysiological studies in diabetic neuropathy. *Journal of Neurology, Neurosurgery and Psychiatry,* **33,** 442.

Lasch, E.E., Joshua, K., Gazit, E., El Nasri, M., Marcus, O. & Zamir, R. (1979). Study of the HLA antigens in Arab children with paralytic poliomyelitis. *Israel Journal of Medical Sciences,* **15,** 12–13.

Lebo, C.P., U., K.S. and Norris, F.H. Jr. (1976) Cricopharyngeal myotomy in amyotrophic lateral sclerosis. *Laryngoscope,* **86,** 862–8.

Lebovitz, H.E. (1965) Endocrine-metabolic syndromes associated with neoplasms. In *The Remote Effects of Cancer on the Nervous System,* Eds Lord Brain and F.H. Norris Jr., pp. 104–11 (Grune and Stratton: New York).

Lehrich, J.R., Oger, J. & Arnason, B.G.W. (1974) Neutralizing antibodies to poliovirus and mumps virus in amyotrophic lateral sclerosis. *Journal of the Neurological Science,* **23,** 537–40.

Lipton, H.L. & Dal Canto, M.C. (1976) Theiler's virus-induced CNS disease in mice. In *Amyotrophic Lateral Sclerosis. Recent Research Trends,* Eds J.M. Andrews, R.T. Johnson & M. Brazier, pp. 263–77 (Academic Press: New York).

Liversedge, L.A. (1973) The use of cytosine arabinoside in the treatment of motor neurone disease. Unpublished observations.

Liversedge, L.A., Swinburn, W.R. & Yuill, G.M. (1970). Idoxuridine and motor neurone disease. *British Medical Journal,* **1,** 755.

Low, P.A., McLeod, J.G., Turtle, J.R., Donnelly, P. & Wright, R.G. (1974) Peripheral neuropathy in acromegaly. *Brain,* **97,** 139–152.

McAlpine, D. & Araki, S. (1958) Minamata disease: an unusual neurological disorder caused by contaminated fish. *Lancet,* **2,** 629.

McComas, A.J., Sica, R.E.P. & Campbell, M.J. (1971) 'Sick' motorneurones. A unifying concept of muscle disease. *Lancet*, **1**, 321–325.

McComas, A.J., Upton, A.R.M. & Jorgensen, P.B. (1975) Patterns of motoneurone dysfunction and recovery. *Candian Journal of Neurological Science*, **2**, 5–15.

McComas, A.J. Sica, R.E.P., Campbell, M.J. & Upton, A.R.M. (1971) Functional compensation in partially denervated muscles. *Journal of Neurology, Neurosurgery and Psychiatry*, **34**, 453–460.

McComas, A.J., Sica, R.E.P., McNabb, A.R., Goldberg, W. & Upton, A.R.M. (1973) Neuropathy in thyrotoxicosis. *New England Journal of Medicine*, **289**, 219–220.

McEwan-Alvarado, G., Hightower, N.C., Carney, L.R. & Barrier, C.W. (1971) Exocrine pancreatic function in patients with amyotrophic lateral sclerosis. *American Journal of Digestive Diseases*, **16**, 107.

Mackay, R.P. (1963) Progressive course in amyotrophic lateral sclerosis. *Archives of Neurology*, **8**, 117–127.

McLeod, J.G. (1971) An electrophysiological and pathological study of peripheral nerves in Friedreich's ataxia. *Journal of the Neurological Sciences*, **12**, 333–349.

McLeod, J.G. (1975) Carcinomatous neuropathy. In *Peripheral Neuropathy*, Eds P.J. Dyck, P.K. Thomas & E.H. Lambert, pp. 1301–1313 (Saunders: New York).

McLeod, J.G. & Prineas, J.W. (1971) Distal type of chronic spinal muscular atrophy: clinical electrophysiological and pathological studies. *Brain*, **94**, 703–14.

Magee, K.R. (1960) Familial progressive bulbar-spinal muscular atrophy. *Neurology (Minneapolis)*, **10**, 275.

Malamud, N., Hirano, A., & Kurland, L.T. (1961) Pathoanatomic changes in amyotrophic lateral sclerosis on Guam. *Archives of Neurology*, **5**, 301.

Mann, D.M.A. & Yates, P.O. (1974) Motor neurone disease: the nature of the pathogenic mechanism. *Journal of Neurology, Neurosurgery and Psychiatry*, **37**, 1036–1046.

Marie, P. & Marinesco, G. (1891) Sur l'anatomie pathologique de l'acromégalie. *Archives de médecine expérimental et d'anatomie Pathologique (Paris)*, **3**, 539.

Marshall, A. & Duchen, L.W. (1978) Sensory system involvement in infantile spinal muscular atrophy. *Journal of the Neurological Sciences*, **26**, 349–59.

Mastaglia, F.L. & Walton, J.N. (1971) Histological and histochemical changes in skeletal muscle from cases of chronic juvenile and early adult spinal muscular atrophy (the Kugelberg-Welander syndrome). *Journal of the Neurological Sciences*, **12**, 15.

Matsumoto, N., Worth, R.M., Kurland, L.T. & Okazaki, H. (1972) Epidemiologic study of amyotrophic lateral sclerosis in Hawaii: Identification of high incidence among Filipino men. *Neurology (Minneapolis)*, **22**, 934.

Meadows, J.C. & Marsden, C.D. (1969) A distal form of chronic spinal muscular atrophy. *Neurology (Minneapolis)*, **19**, 53.

Meenakshisundaram, E., Jagannathan, K. & Ramamurthi, B. (1970) Clinical pattern of motor neuron disease seen in younger aged groups in Madras. *Neurology (India)*, **18**, Suppl. 1, 109–112.

Mendell, J.R., Chase, T.N. & Engel, W.K. (1971) Amyotrophic lateral sclerosis. A study of central monamine metabolism and a therapeutic trial of levodopa. *Archives of Neurology*, **25**, 320.

Mills, C.P. (1973) Dysphagia in pharyngeal paralysis treated by cricopharyngeal sphincterotomy. *Lancet*, **1**, 455–457.

Minauf, M. & Jellinger, K. (1969) Combination of amyotrophic lateral sclerosis with Pick's disease. *Archiv für Psychiatrie und Nervenkrankheiten*, **212**, 279.

Mitsuyama, Y. & Takamiya, S. (1979) Presenile dementia with motor neuron disease in Japan. *Archives of Neurology*, **36**, 592–593.

Morgan, M.H., Read, A.E. & Campbell, M.J. (1979) Clinical and electrophysiological studies of peripheral nerve function in patients with chronic liver disease. *Clinical Science*, **57**, 31–37.

Mulder, D.W. & Espinosa, R.E. (1969) Amyotrophic lateral sclerosis: Comparison of the clinical syndrome in Guam and the United States. In *Motor Neurone Diseases*, Eds F.H. Norris & L.T. Kurland, p. 12 (Grune and Stratton: New York).

Mulder, D.W. & Howard, F.M. (1976) Patient resistance and prognosis in amyotrophic lateral sclerosis. *Mayo Clinic Proceedings*, **51**, 537–541.

Mulder, D.W., Bastron, J.A. & Lambert, E.H. (1956) Hyperinsulin neuronopathy. *Neurology (Minneapolis)*, **6**, 627–635.

Mulder, D.W., Lambert, E.H. & Eaton, L.M. (1959) Myasthenic syndrome in patients with amyotrophic lateral sclerosis. *Neurology (Minneapolis)*, **9**, 627.

Mulder, D.W., Rosenbaum, R.A. & Layton, D.D. (1972) Late progression of poliomyelitis or forme fruste amyotrophic lateral sclerosis? *Mayo Clinic Proceedings*, **47**, 756.

Mullins, W.M., Gross, C.W. & Moore, J.M. (1979) Long-term follow-up of tympanic neurectomy for sialorrhoea. *Laryngoscope*, **89**, 1219–1223.

Munsat, T.L., Woods, R., Fowler, W. & Pearson, C.M. (1969). Neurogenic muscular atrophy of infancy with prolonged survival. *Brain*, **92**, 9–24.

Namba, T., Aberfeld, D.C. & Grob, D. (1970) Chronic proximal spinal muscular atrophy. *Journal of the Neurological Sciences*, **11**, 401.

Namba, T., Nolte, C.T., Jackrel, J. & Grob, D. (1971) Poisoning due to organophosphate insecticides. Acute and chronic manifestations. *American Journal of Medicine*, **50**, 475–492.

Nelson, J.W. & Amick, L.D. (1966) Heredofamilial progressive spinal muscular atrophy. *Neurology (Minneapolis)*, **16**, 306 (Abstract).

Norris, F.H. (1972) Amantadine in Jakob-Creutzfeld disease. *British Medical Journal*, **2**, 349.

Norris, F.H. (1972) Benign post-traumatic amyotrophy. *Archives of Neurology*, **27**, 269–270.

Norris, F.H. (1973) Guanidine in amyotrophic lateral sclerosis. *New England Journal of Medicine*, **288**, 690.

Norris, F.H. & Engel, W.K. (1965) Carcinomatous anyotrophic lateral sclerosis. In *The Remote Effects of Cancer on the Nervous System*, Eds W.R. Brain & F.H. Norris, p. 24 (Grune and Stratton: New York).

Norris, F.H. & Sang, K. (1978) Amyotrophic lateral sclerosis and low urinary selenium levels. (Letter) *Journal of the American Medical Association*, **239**, 404.

Norris, F.H., McMenemey, W.H. & Barnard, R.O. (1969) Anterior horn cell pathology in carcinomatous neuromyopathy compared with other forms of motor neurone disease. In *Motor Neurone Diseases*, Eds F.H. Norris & L.T. Kurland, p. 100 (Grune and Stratton: New York).

Norris, F.H. Jr. (1975) Adult spinal motor neuron disease. In *Handbook of Clinical Neurology*, Eds P.J. Vinken & G.M. Bruyn, Vol. 22, 156 (North Holland: Amsterdam).

Norris, F.H. Jr., Rudolf, J.H. & Barney, M. (1964) Carcinomatous neuropathy. *Neurology (Minneapolis)*, **14**, 202.

Norris, F.H. Jr., Calanchini, P.R., Fallat, R.J., Panchari, R.P.T. & Jewett, B. (1974) The administration of guanidine in amyotrophic lateral sclerosis. *Neurology (Minneapolis)*, **24**, 721–728.

Oldstone, M.B.A., Perrin, L.H., Wilson, C.B. & Norris, F.H. (1976) Evidence for immune-complex formation in patients with 'ALS'. *Lancet*, **2**, 169.

Olson, W.H., Simons, J.A. & Halaas, G.W. (1978) Therapeutic trial of tilorone in ALS. Lack of benefit in a double-blind placebo-controlled study. *Neurology (Minneapolis)*, **28**, 1293–1295.

Otsuka, M. & Endo, M. (1960). The effect of guanidine on neuromuscular transmission. *Journal of Pharmacology and Experimental Therapeutics*, **128**, 273.

Pallis, C. (1976) In *Motor Neurone Disease*, Ed. F.C. Rose (Pitman: London).

Panse, F. (1970) Electrical lesions of the nervous system. In *Handbook of Clinical Neurology*, Eds P.J. Vinken & G.W. Bruyn, Vol. 7, 344–387 (North Holland: Amsterdam).

Paty, D.W., Campbell, M.J. & Hughes, D. (1974). Carcinomatous neuromyopathy; an electrophysiological and immunological study of patients with carcinoma of the lung. II Immunological studies *Journal of Neurology, Neurosurgery and Psychiatry*, **37**, 142–151.

Pearn, J.H. (1973) The gene frequency of acute Werdnig-Hoffmann disease (SMA type I). A total population survey in North-East England. *Journal of Medical Genetics*, **10**, 260–265.

Pearn, J.H. (1978) Autosomal dominant spinal muscular atrophy—A clinical and genetic study. *Journal of the Neurological Sciences*, **38**, 263–275.

Pearn, J.H. & Wilson, J. (1973a) Acute Werdnig-Hoffmann disease. *Archives of Disease in Childhood*, **48**, 425–430.

Pearn, J.H. & Wilson, J. (1973b) Chronic generalised spinal muscular atrophy of infancy and childhood. *Archives of Disease in Childhood*, **48**, 768–774.

Pearn, J.H., Bundey, S., Carter, C.O., Wilson, J., Gardner-Medwin, D. & Walton, J.N., (1978) A genetic study of subacute and chronic spinal muscular atrophy in childhood—A nosological analysis of 124 index patients. *Journal of the Neurological Sciences*, **37**, 227–248.

Peiper, S.J. & Fields, W.S. (1959) Failure of amyotrophic lateral sclerosis to respond to intrathecal steroid and vitamin B12 therapy. *Archives of Neurology*, **9**, 522.

Pennybacker, J. & Russell, D.S. (1948) Necrosis of the brain due to radiation therapy. *Journal of Neurology, Neurosurgery and Psychiatry*, **11**, 183–198.

Percy, A.K., Davis, L.E., Johnston, D.M. & Drachman, D.B. (1971) Failure of isoprinosine in amyotrophic lateral sclerosis. *New England Journal of Medicine*. **285**, 689.

Pertschuk, L.P., Kim, D.S., Prasad, I., Cook, A.W., Gupta, J.K. & Broome, J.D. (1979) Jejunal mucosa in motor neurone disease and other chronic neurological disorders. In *Progress in Neurological Research*, Eds P.O. Behan & F.C. Rose, pp. 44–61 (Pitman: London).

Pertschuk, L.P., Cook, A.W., Gupta, J.K. Broome, J.D., Vuletin, J.C., Kim, D.S., Stanek, A.E., Brigati, D.J., Rainford, E.A. and Nidzgorski, F. (1977) Jejunal immunopathology in amyotrophic lateral sclerosis and multiple sclerosis. Identification of viral antigens by immunofluorescence. *Lancet*, **1**, 1119.

Pickett, J.B.E., Layzer, R.B., Levin, S.R., Schneider, V.,

Campbell, M.J. & Sumner, A.J. (1975) Neuromuscular complications of acromegaly. *Neurology (Minneapolis)*, **25**, 638–645.

Pietsch, M.C. & Morris, P.J. (1975) An association of HLA 3 and HLA 7 with paralytic poliomyelitis. *Tissue Antigens*, **4**, 50.

Poskanzer, D.C., Cantor, H.M. & Kaplan, G.S. (1969) The frequency of preceding poliomyelitis in amyotrophic lateral sclerosis. In *Motor Neuron Diseases*, Eds F.H. Norris & L.T. Kurland, p. 286 (Grune & Stratton: New York).

Puech, P., Grossiard, A., Brun, M. & Denis, J.P. (1947) Tableau clinique de sclérose latérale amyotrophique. Arachnoidite cervicale en virole á l'intervention. *Revue Neurologique*, **79**, 358–359.

Quarfordt, S.H., Devino, D.C., Engel, W.K., Levy, R.I. & Fredrickson, D.S. (1970) Familial adult-onset proximal spinal muscular atrophy. *Archives of Neurology*, **22**, 541–549.

Quick, D.T. & Greer, M. (1967) Pancreatic dysfunction in amyotrophic lateral sclerosis. *Neurology (Minneapolis)*, **17**, 112.

Raff, M.C., Sangalang, V. & Asbury, A.K. (1968) Ischemic mononeuropathy multiplex associated with diabetes mellitus. *Archives of Neurology*, **18**, 487.

Refsum, S. & Skillicorn, S.A. (1954) Amyotrophic familial spastic paraplegia. *Neurology (Minneapolis)*, **4**, 40.

Rosen, A.D. (1978) Amyotrophic lateral sclerosis. Clinical features and prognosis. *Archives of Neurology*, **35**, 638–642.

Ross, E.J. (1972) Endocrine and metabolic manifestations of cancer. *British Medical Journal*, **1**, 735–8.

Sadowsky, C.H., Sachs, E. & Ochoa, J. (1976) Post-radiation motor neuron syndrome. *Archives of Neurology*, **33**, 786–8.

Sanders, M. & Fellowes, J. (1975) Use of detoxified snake neurotoxin as a partial treatment for amyotrophic lateral sclerosis. *Journal of Cancer and Cytology*. **15**, 26–30.

Sanders, M., Fellowes, O.N. & Lennox, A.C. (1978) Refinements of the method to produce modified snake venom neurotoxin and of the methods used in the partial treatment of amyotrophic lateral sclerosis. *Toxicon Supplement*, (1) 481–488.

Saunders, N.A. & Kreitzer, S.M. (1979) Diaphragmatic function in amyotrophic lateral sclerosis. *American Review of Respiratory Diseaseas*, **119**, 127–130.

Schochet, S.S., Hardman, J.M., Ladewig, P.P. and Earle, K.M. (1969) Intraneuronal conglomerates in sporadic motor neuron diseases: a light and electron microscopy study. *Archives of Neurology*, **20**, 548.

Schwartz, M.S., Stalberg, E., Schiller, H.H. & Thiele, B.L. (1976) The reinnervated motor unit in man. A SFEMG multielectrode investigation. *Journal of the Neurological Sciences*, **27**, 303–312.

Seneviratne, K.N. & Peiris, O.A. (1970) Peripheral nerve function in chronic liver disease. *Journal of Neurology, Neurosurgery and Psychiatry*, **33**, 609.

Seto, D.S.Y. & Freeman, J.M. (1964) Lead neuropathy in childhood. *American Journal of Diseases of Children*, **107**, 337.

Shiraki, H. & Yase, Y. (1975) Amyotrophic lateral sclerosis in Japan. In *Handbook of Clinical Neurology*, Eds P.J. Vinken & G.W. Bruyn, Vol. 22, pp. 353–419 (North Holland: Amsterdam).

Silfverskiold, B.P. (1946) Polyneuritic hypoglycaemia. Late peripheral paresis after hypgolycemic attacks in two insulinoma patients. *Acta medica Scandinavica*, **125**, 502–504.

Stalberg, E., Schwartz, M.S. & Trontelj, J.V. (1975) Single fibre electromyography in various processes affecting the anterior horn cell. *Journal of the Neurological Sciences*, **24**, 504–415.

Staal, A. & Went, L.N. (1968) Juvenile ALS-dementia complex in a Dutch family. *Neurology (Minneapolis)*, **18**, 800.

Steinke, J. & Tyler, R.H. (1964) The association of amyotrophic lateral sclerosis (motor neuron disease) and carbohydrate intolerance, a clinical study. *Metabolism*, **13**, 1376.

Stewart, B.M. (1966) The hypertrophic neuropathy of acromegaly: a rare neuropathy associated with acromegaly. *Archives of Neurology*, **14**, 107.

Thomas, J.E. & Howard, F.M. (1972) Segmental zoster paresis: A disease profile. *Neurology (Minneapolis)*, **22**, 459–466.

Thomas, P.K. & Calne, D.B. (1974) Motor nerve conduction velocity in peroneal muscular atrophy: evidence for genetic heterogeneity *Journal of Neurology, Neurosurgery and Psychiatry*, **37**, 68–75.

Tom, M.I. & Richardson, J.C. (1951) Hypoglycaemia from islet cell tumour of pancreas with amyotrophy and cerebrospinal nerve cell changes. *Journal of Neurology, Neurosurgery and Psychiatry.* **10**, 51–66.

Tomlinson, B.E. & Irving, D. (1977) The numbers of limb motor neurons in the human lumbosacral cord throughout life. *Journal of the Neurological Sciences*, **34**, 213.

Tomlinson, B.E., Walton, J.N. & Rebeiz, J.J. (1969) The effects of ageing and of cachexia upon skeletal muscle. A histopathological study. *Journal of the Neurological Sciences*, **9**, 321.

Torres, J., Iriate, L.L.G. & Kurland, L.T. (1957) Amyotrophic lateral sclerosis among Guamanians in California. *California Medicine*, **86**, 385.

Trojaborg, W. & Buchthal, F. (1965) Malignant and benign fasciculations. *Acta psychiatrica et neurologica scandinavica*, **41**, 251–254.

Trojaborg, W., Frantzen, E. & Andersen, I. (1969) Peripheral neuropathy and myopathy associated with carcinoma of the lung. *Brain*, **92**, 71–82.

Tyler, H.R. (1979) Double-blind study of modified neurotoxin in motor neurone disease. *Archives of Neurology*, **29**, 77–81.

Van Bogaert, L. & Radermecker, M.A. (1954) Scleroses laterales amyotrophiques typiques et paralysies agitantes hereditaires, dans une même famille, avec une forme de passage possible entre les deux affections. *Monatsschrift für Psychiatrie und Neurologie*, **127**, 185–203.

Victor, M. (1965) The effects of nutritional deficiency on the nervous system. A comparison with the effects of carcinoma. In *The Remote Effects of Cancer on the Nervous System*, Eds Lord Brain & F.H. Norris Jr., pp. 134–61 (Grune and Stratton: New York).

Walton, J.N., Tomlinson, B.E. & Pearce, G.W. (1968) Subacute 'poliomyelitis' and Hodgkins disease. *Journal of the Neurological Sciences*, **6**, 435–445.

Werdnig, G. (1891) Zwei frühinfantile hereditäre Fälle von progressiver Muskel-atrophie unter dem bilde der Dystrophie, aber auf neurotischer Grundlag. *Archiv Psychiatrie und Nervenkrankheiten*, **22**, 437–480.

Werdnig, G. (1894) Die früh-infantile progressive spinale Amyotrophie. *Archives of Psychiatry*, **26**, 706.

Wiesendanger, M. (1962) Uber die hereditäre, neurogene proximale Amyotrophie (Kugelberg-Welander). *Archiv der Julius Klaus-Stiftung für Vererbungsforschung*, **37**, 147.

Wilkinson, M. (1969) Motor neuron disease and cervical spondylosis. In *Motor Neuron Diseases*, Eds F.H. Norris & L.T. Kurland, pp. 130–134 (Grune and Stratton: New York).

Wilkinson, P.C. (1964) Serological findings in carcinomatous neuropathy. *Lancet*, **1**, 1301–1303.

Williams, C.J. (1955) Amyotrophy due to hypoglycaemia. *British Medical Journal*, **1**, 707–708.

Williams, E.R. & Bruford, A. (1970) Creatine phosphokinase in motor neurone disease. *Clinical Chimica Acta*, **27**, 53.

Wilson, S.A.K. (1907) The amyotrophy of chronic lead poisoning: amyotrophic lateral sclerosis of toxic origin. *Review of Neurology and Psychiatry*, **5**, 441.

Winchester, R.J., Ebers, G., Fu, S.M., Espinosa, L., Zabriskie, J. & Kunkel, H.G. (1975). B-cell alloantigen Ag-7a in multiple sclerosis. *Lancet*, **2**, 814.

Wohlfart, G. (1942) Zwei Fälle von Dystrophia musculorum progressiva mit fibrillären Zuckungen and atypischen Muskelbefund. *Deutsche Zeitschrift für Nervenheilkuncle*, **153**, 189.

Wohlfart, G. (1957) Collateral regeneration from residual motor nerve fibers in amyotrophic lateral sclerosis. *Neurology (Minneapolis)*, **7**, 124–134.

Wohlfart, G., Fex, J. & Eliasson, S. (1955) Hereditary proximal spinal muscle atrophy simulating progressive muscular dystrophy. *Acta psychiatrica et neurologica*, **30**, 395.

Wolfgram, F. (1976) Blind studies on the effect of amyotrophic lateral sclerosis sera on motor neurons in vitro. In *Amyotrophic Lateral Sclerosis. Recent Research Trends*, Eds J.M. Andrews, R.T. Johnson & M. Brazier, pp. 145–9 (Academic Press: New York).

Wolfgram, F. & Myers, L. (1973) Amyotrophic lateral sclerosis: Effect of serum on anterior horn cells in tissue culture. *Science*, **179**, 579–580.

Worster-Drought, C., Hill, T.R. & McMenemey, W.H. (1933) Familial presenile dementia with spastic paralysis. *Journal of Neurology and Psychopathology*, **14**, 27–34.

Yase, Y. (1972) The pathogenesis of amyotrophic lateral sclerosis. *Lancet*, **2**, 292–296.

Zalin, H. & Cooney, T.C. (1974) Chorda tympani neurectomy—a new approach to sub-mandibular salivary obstruction. *British Journal of Surgery*, **61**, 391–4.

Zellweger, H. & McCormick, W.F. (1968). Scapuloperoneal dystrophy and scapuloperoneal atrophy. *Helvetica Paediatrica Acta*, **6**, 643.

Zellweger, H., Simpson, J., McCormick, W.F. & Ionasescu, U. (1972). Spinal muscular atrophy with autosomal dominant inheritance. *Neurology (Minneapolis)*, **22**, 957–63.

Zil'ber, L.A., Bajdakova, Z.L., Gardasjan, A.N., Konovalov, N.V., Bunina, T.L. & Barabadze, E.M. (1963) Study of the etiology of amyotrophic lateral sclerosis. *Bulletin of the World Health Organisation*, **29**, 449.

Zilkha, K.J. (1962) Contribution to discussion on motor neurone disease. *Proceedings of the Royal Society of Medicine*, **55**, 1028.

The neuropathies

INTRODUCTION

A peripheral neuropathy may be defined as a disease causing disordered function and structure of the peripheral nervous system. The latter includes not only the spinal nerves, plexuses, main nerve trunks and terminal ramifications, but also the perikarya (anterior horn cell and dorsal root ganglion neurone), the nerve roots and the presynaptic parts of the neuromuscular junctions. Certain parts of this system in fact lie within the central nervous system, namely the anterior horn cells and the central branch of the primary sensory neurone which runs the entire length of the dorsal columns in the spinal cord. These parts may therefore be damaged by central nervous diseases.

Little discussion can be given to the perikaryon, nerve roots or neuromuscular junction in this chapter. Reference is made to reviews of myelopathies affecting anterior horn cells (Bradley, 1975a), anterior horn cell degenerations (Ch. 20), dorsal root ganglion degenerations, and to diseases of the roots (Bradley, 1975b) and neuromuscular junction (Chapters 7 and 16).

The incidence of peripheral nerve disease is at least as high as that of primary muscle disease, and it is therefore impossible in this chapter to go into as great detail as in the remainder of the book. For a fuller consideration of peripheral nerve disease, the reader is referred to Vinken and Bruyn (1970a, b), Bradley (1974) and Dyck, Thomas and Lambert (1975).

CLINICAL SYMPTOMS AND SIGNS INDICATIVE OF PERIPHERAL NERVE DAMAGE

Sensory symptoms may be divided into negative and positive phenomena, and into those due to damage to the large myelinated or to the small myelinated and non-myelinated fibres. Of the *negative* phenomena, loss of large fibre function, as in tabes dorsalis and some toxic neuropathies, causes loss of joint position and touch sensation. Patients complain of numbness, are unable to recognise objects with their eyes closed, and have a sensory ataxia in the dark. Loss of small myelinated and non-myelinated fibre function causes loss of pain and temperature sensation, which may lead to injury and ulceration because of loss of protective reflexes. Of the *positive* phenomena, pain from peripheral nerve compression is easy to understand, but many of the other positive sensory symptoms are less explicable. They include prickling paraesthesiae, burning sensations and lightning, lancinating pains. Hyperpathia, where light touch and pin-prick have an excessive painful quality often with a raised threshold, may occur both with thalamic and peripheral nerve damage. The explanation of these phenomena may rest on the holistic interpretation of sensory inputs requiring the integration of all modalities, similar to the gate theory of Melzack and Wall (1965).

Sensory signs. The clinical examination of sensation usually employed tests the awareness and subjective quality of a light touch with cotton wool, the perception of movements of the joints, of vibration of a tuning fork with a frequency of 128 Hz or less placed on bony points, and the minimum separation over which it is possible to discriminate two separate points. The presence and the subjective quality of pain sensation are assessed with a pin-prick, and temperature sensation by the ability to recognise objects at 40°C and 30°C as hot and cold respectively. It is usual to find that loss of pain and temperature sensation on the one hand, and loss of joint position sense, vibration and two-point discrimination on the other, tend to be grouped together.

Such a sensory examination is time-consuming particularly in unreliable patients, though it is still relatively crude. Many refinements have been introduced since von Frey introduced graded hairs for pressure quantitation (*see* Dyck, Lambert and Nichols, 1971; Dyck, Schultz and O'Brien, 1972). Unfortunately, even with these sophisticated techniques, the patient still has to make a subjective response.

Motor symptoms. These usually comprise difficulty in performing certain manoeuvres such as opening a bottle, walking upstairs or mounting the kerb. Patients note rapid fatigue, and may be aware of wasting of muscles. With insidious diseases, the patient may unconsciously adopt trick movements, so that severe weakness has appeared before he presents to the doctor.

Motor signs. Wasting is most easily seen where it is asymmetrical. Weakness of individual muscle groups is important to assess, but involves the cooperation of the patient. Care must be taken to recognise weakness due to functional problems and local pain. Power may be graded 0–5 on the Medical Research Council Scale described in Chapter 13. Grade 4 embraces a wide range of

degrees of weakness, and requires subdivision. It is possible to measure the maximum power of most muscle groups with suitable dynamometers, and to compare this with the normal range.

The tendon reflex requires the function of the γ-motor neurone, the muscle spindles, the spindle sensory afferent fibres, the α-motor neurone and the extrafusal muscle fibres. The tendon reflexes will be lost with damage to any of these. In peripheral nerve disease, however, the reflexes are commonly lost while the power and bulk of the muscle are relatively normal. In comparison, the reflexes are lost relatively late in primary muscle diseases, though this rule is not invariable.

Autonomic symptoms. These may be peripheral, such as complaints of coldness of the limbs, or central, such as postural syncope, urinary and faecal incontinence, bouts of precipitate nocturnal watery diarrhoea, and impotence in the male.

Autonomic signs. These include impaired pupillary responses to light and accommodation, trophic changes in the skin and a marked postural fall of blood pressure.

PATTERNS OF NEUROPATHIES

The commonest type of neuropathy is a *mixed sensorimotor distal symmetrical polyneuropathy* producing a glove and stocking loss of one or more modalities of sensation, a predominantly distal weakness including the small muscles of the hands and a foot-drop, and involving all limbs. Some patients have a *pure sensory* or *pure motor distal symmetrical polyneuropathy*. Less common is a *mononeuropathy* where only one nerve is damaged. Where several individual nerves are involved, the term *multiple mononeuropathy* is given. A *proximal motor polyneuropathy* is occasionally seen with little or no sensory loss. A purely *autonomic neuropathy* is rare, and is more commonly intermixed with a sensorimotor polyneuropathy.

The disease may be *chronically progressive* or less commonly *acute* or *subacute*. As a rule of thumb, significant neuropathies developing in less than three weeks may be termed acute, those developing over three weeks to three months may be termed subacute, and where progression occurs for more than three months, the term chronic is given. Rarely, *recurrent* neuropathies occur, with *relapses* and *remissions*.

INVESTIGATIONS INDICATING PERIPHERAL NERVE DAMAGE

Electrophysiology. The most important investigations indicating peripheral nerve damage are motor and sensory nerve conduction studies and electromyography (EMG). The techniques, normal values and changes with disease are discussed in greater detail in Chapters 27 and 28. A demyelinating neuropathy (*see* Ch. 6) produces a marked decrease in nerve conduction velocity, for example from the normal value of more than 45 m/s in the ulnar nerve to as low as 7–30 m/s (Cragg and Thomas, 1964b; Kaeser, 1970). The terminal latency is also increased, and the nerve action potential (sensory or mixed) is decreased in amplitude. Denervation changes in the muscle on electromyography are often minor. In neuropathies with axonal degeneration (*see* Ch. 6), there is either no change or only a minor decrease in nerve conduction velocity right up to the stage of complete nerve failure, though the terminal latency may be disproportionately increased (Cragg and Thomas, 1964; Kaeser, 1970). However, the sensory or mixed nerve action potential is markedly decreased in amplitude, indicating a loss of myelinated fibres. This applies equally, whether the axonal degeneration is due to damage in the nerve trunks, such as by a vascular lesion, or in the perikarya as in motor neurone disease or a hereditary ganglioneuropathy.

It is important to recognise that maximal conduction velocity studies and measurement of the amplitude of the nerve action potential *in vivo* both relate only to the largest myelinated fibres. If the neuropathy causes severe degeneration of the small myelinated and non-myelinated fibres, but spares the large myelinated fibres, these parameters will be normal. It is possible to gain some insight into such a condition by estimating the range of conduction velocities by techniques such as those of Thomas, Sears and Gilliatt (1959) and Hopf (1963), and by the dispersion of the nerve

action potential or evoked motor action potential. Lambert and Dyck (1968) showed that it is possible to overcome this problem by studying the evoked action potentials of nerve biopsies *in vitro*.

EMG changes in peripheral neuropathies (*see* Ch. 28) may be divided into evidence of *denervation*, with fibrillation potentials (which may also be seen in primary conditions of the muscle, including polymyositis and the muscular dystrophies) and loss of motor units with a reduced interference pattern, and evidence of *reinnervation*, the motor action potentials being polyphasic, larger in amplitude and duration than normal, with an increased motor unit territory. All these changes occur equally in diseases of the perikarya or axons. In segmental demyelination there is usually little change in the EMG other than a decrease in the interference pattern.

Lesions of the nerve roots may be recognised by preservation of the sensory nerve action potential and axon flare in an anaesthetic area, and by EMG signs of denervation in the axial muscles (*see* Bradley, 1975b).

Pathology. This is considered in detail in Chapter 6.

Autonomic functions. Abnormalities may be indicated by an excessive postural fall in blood pressure, by the loss of the usual reciprocal relationship between blood pressure and pulse rate, and the loss of the overshoot reaction in the Valsalva manoeuvre. There may be an increased sensitivity (denervation supersensitivity) to an intravenous infusion of noradrenalin. Gastrointestinal studies may show decreased peristalsis. For further details, the reader is referred to Bannister (1971), Thomashefsky, Horwitz and Feingold (1972) and Bradley (1974).

Cerebrospinal fluid (CSF) may be abnormal in peripheral nerve disease if the perikarya or nerve roots are involved, though it may also be abnormal with many other diseases. The protein concentration is raised without a pleocytosis in radiculoneuropathies such as the Guillain-Barré-Strohl syndrome (albumino-cytologic dissociation). Examination of the cerebrospinal fluid and of the subarachnoid space may reveal many processes such as tumours and arachnoiditis damaging the nerve roots and perikarya (Bradley, 1975a, b).

Many other laboratory investigations are required to elucidate the aetiology of peripheral neuropathies, including measurement of the blood sugar, vitamin B_{12} level, porphyrins, phytanic acid and so on.

DIFFERENTIAL DIAGNOSIS OF THE SITE OF NEUROMUSCULAR INVOLVEMENT

In the classical case it is easy to decide upon the site of the disease. In a primary muscle disease there is only weakness and wasting with no sensory loss, and the reflexes are preserved until muscle wasting is relatively advanced. In peripheral nerve disease there is usually loss of sensory and motor function and of reflexes. In an upper motor neurone lesion there is little wasting, and the weakness is in a characteristic distribution with increased tone and reflexes. In myasthenia gravis there are usually ptosis, external ocular movement disorders, dysphagia, proximal weakness, prominent fatiguability, and no sensory loss with relative preservation of reflexes.

However it is not always as easy as this. Minimal disease may cause symptoms with no signs, and it may be difficult to separate the paraesthesiae of multiple sclerosis from those of a sensory neuropathy, or the weakness of a pure motor neuropathy from a primary muscle disease. Electrophysiological and other investigations are often required to define the site of the disease as well as to elucidate its nature. It is important to avoid the diagnostic catch of a disease which is damaging both the muscle and the nerve separately, as seen in many toxic conditions (Bradley, 1970; Bradley, Lassman, Pearce and Walton, 1970).

INCIDENCE AND AETIOLOGY

It is impossible accurately to state the incidence of peripheral nerve diseases. This varies greatly in different parts of the world according to the different indigenous diseases. Vitamin deficiency neuropathies and leprosy are common in tropical countries, and toxic neuropathies are more commonly seen in industrial societies. It is also clear that many diseases cause subclinical damage in a large number of patients, though only a few present with symptoms. Thus the incidence depends upon the type of investigation used in ascertainment. Finally, the incidence is totally dependent upon whether cases are collected by referral to hospital or by a population survey. In a population study in Carlisle (Brewis, Poskanzer, Rolland and Miller, 1966) the incidence of patients with a diagnosis of the carpal tunnel syndrome was $2.3/10^5$/yr, of the Guillain-Barré-Strohl syndrome $0.6/10^5$/yr, and of peroneal muscular atrophy $0.2/10^5$/yr. The incidence of subacute combined degeneration, which often involves a peripheral neuropathy, was $2.3/10^5$/yr. Clinical experience in industrialised civilisations suggests that the total incidence of peripheral neuropathies is perhaps more than 20 times that of the carpal tunnel syndrome, that is at least $50/10^5$/yr.

The three major causes of neuropathy in the world today are leprosy, diabetes and old age. The order of frequency depends upon many factors, including the country under investigation and the age of the population. The fourth major category is 'undiagnosed'. The proportion falling into this group in a general hospital in the United Kingdom is about 40 per cent (Prineas, 1970a), but it is up to 50–70 per cent in specialised units (Elkington, 1952; Matthews, 1952; Rose, 1960; Bradley, 1967), for the more easily diagnosed cases have already been filtered out by this stage. Most such patients have a chronic progressive sensorimotor distal symmetrical polyneuropathy. Dyck (1980) has recently shown that in this group of 'idiopathic polyneuropathies' about half have a familial neuropathy demonstrated by abnormal clinical, electrophysiological or pathological examinations of the peripheral nervous system on other members of the family. A proportion of the remaining 'non-familial idiopathic' cases may have chronic inflammatory polyneuropathy, which may respond to corticosteroid therapy.

INDIVIDUAL DISEASES CAUSING PERIPHERAL NERVE DAMAGE

For clarity, this section deals with peripheral neuropathies in aetiological groups, although for diagnostic purposes the clinical presentation and investigations are of more help (*see* p. 777). It is impossible to consider every cause of peripheral neuropathy, and a brief outline can be given of only a few. The first two conditions discussed are trauma and diphtheritic neuropathy because they are archetypes of axonal degeneration and segmental demyelination respectively, the two main pathological processes occurring in nerve (*see* Ch. 6).

Trauma

The nerves are generally buried deep within a muscle mass and are thereby protected, except against penetrating wounds. There are, however, certain vulnerable sites, such as the radial nerve in the spiral groove where it may be damaged by a fractured humerus, the lateral popliteal nerve at the head of the fibula, and the ulnar nerve behind the medial epicondyle of the humerus. Seddon (1943) defined three grades of injury, and Sunderland (1968) five. The following classification incorporates both:

(1) blockage of nerve conduction without loss of continuity of the axon (*neurapraxia*— Seddon). This is usually transient;

(2) damage to the axon with subsequent Wallerian degeneration, although the connective tissue including the Schwann cell basement membrane remains intact (*axonotmesis*—Seddon). Regeneration occurs at 1–2 mm/day and is usually effective unless the lesion is very proximal;

(3) damage to the axon and connective tissue, but preservation of the perineurium and fascicular architecture of the nerve. Regeneration is less complete than (2), but is still relatively effective;

(4) damage to the axon, connective tissue and perineurium, although the nerve remains macrosopically intact. Regeneration is poorly orientated and less effective;

(5) complete anatomical section of the nerve.

Types (3)–(5) were included in Seddon's term '*neurotmesis*'. In category (5), the best plan is to suture the nerve five days to two weeks after the injury (Ducker, Kempe and Hayes, 1969). A nerve graft may be required to bridge the gap. An autograft is the best for this, although this necessitates producing a lesion of another nerve. Heterografts are only moderately effective, although immunosuppression for the time required for the nerve axons to grow through the graft will produce a better result (Pollard, Guy and McLeod, 1971).

In addition to external trauma, the nerve may be compressed at many sites by anatomical structures within the body producing the so-called *entrapment* or *compressive neuropathies* (Staal, 1970; Kopell and Thompson, 1976). The commonest such condition is compression of the median nerve in the carpal tunnel; this and other common entrapment neuropathies are described in Chapter 23. The pathological changes are described in Chapter 6. In mild cases of the carpal tunnel syndrome, where there is segmental demyelination only, rapid recovery of function can be expected after decompression. However in the more severe cases, where there is axonal degeneration and loss of myelinated nerve fibres, recovery is slower.

Diphtheritic Neuropathy

Diphtheria was once a scourge in many parts of the world, but immunisation in early childhood and the frequent use of antibiotics have now made it a rare disease in developed countries. It was first described by Trousseau and Lassegue (1851). Kinnier Wilson's textbook (1954) gives a full review. The responsible organism is *Corynebacterium diphtherii*, which usually causes an acute pharyngitis characterised by a grey membrane, but which can infect a skin wound. The dangerous complications are delayed and are due to a cardiotoxin and a neurotoxin. In experimental animals, the severity of the disease is proportional to the dose of neurotoxin used. However, the amount of neurotoxin produced by the *Corynebacterium* varies from strain to strain. In human infections it is therefore impossible to relate the severity of the infection to the severity of the delayed complications.

The major nerve damage due to the neurotoxin is usually delayed for 15–40 days after the onset of pharyngitis, though occasionally a precocious paralysis may develop 3–10 days after infection, being limited to the local area, particularly the palate, and relatively benign. The major paralysis often begins in the palate but rapidly spreads to involve all the nerves, both motor and sensory. The patient may require tracheostomy and artificial respiration to prevent death from paralysis of bulbar and respiratory muscles.

Neither the reason for the delay nor the mode of action of the diphtheria toxin is known. The toxin is rapidly fixed in the body; one hour after injection into experimental animals its effect can no longer be neutralised by an injection of massive doses of antitoxin. As discussed in Chapter 6, the toxin causes segmental demyelination by damaging the Schwann cells of the peripheral nerves in a patchy fashion. There is breakdown of the myelin sheaths, but the axons remain intact unless the neuropathy is very severe. This produces a marked slowing of nerve conduction or a complete conduction block and paralysis. However, remyelination occurs quickly and the paralysis disappears in 15–30 days if death from complications does not supervene. In the experimental animal, clinical recovery occurs at a stage when nerve conduction remains slowed (Morgan-Hughes, 1968).

Leprosy

This is certainly the major cause of severe peripheral nerve disease in the world today. The chronic infection insidiously damages the peripheral nervous system over many years. There is a predilection for the cutaneous nerves with severe anaesthesia causing injuries and mutilation. There is loss of digits and facial structures, together with penetrating ulcers, secondary infections and Charcot (neuropathic) joints.

Two major forms of leprosy may be distinguished, *lepromatous* and *tuberculoid*, though *intermediate* forms are common (Rees and Waters, 1971). In the lepromatous type, hypertrophic skin lesions are frequent, and all elements of the nerves are teeming with *Microbacterium leprae* (Boddingius, 1972). The immunological response is humoral, with a marked increase in serum immunoglobulins and enlargement of the lymph nodes, but the lepromin skin test is negative. The neuropathy is generally distal, symmetrical and predominantly sensory in type, although multiple mononeuropathies may be seen (Rosenberg and Lovelace, 1968). It has been suggested that the *Microbacterium* has a predilection for skin areas of lower temperature (Sabin, 1969). In the tuberculoid form of the neuropathy there is atrophy and depigmentation of the skin, and neuropathic phenomena are prominent. It is extremely difficult to find bacilli in the nerve, and the immunological response is cellular with a positive lepromin skin test. The pattern is usually of multiple mononeuropathies with nodular thickening of the nerve and fibrous tethering to underlying structures.

Therapy with DDS and other sulphones has been available for a number of years and is known to be slowly effective in suppressing the disease. Even so, relapses can occur after many years of therapy. The success in growing *Microbacterium leprae* in the mouse foot-pad (Rees and Waters, 1971) has allowed the experimental investigation of the treatment of this difficult disease. Many other drugs have now been screened, and it has been shown that DDS is bacteriostatic, while rifampicin is rapidly bactericidal. When the disease has been suppressed, it is possible to consider palliative procedures such as tendon transplants, and excision of fibrosed segments with heterologous nerve grafts (Antia, Pandya and Dastur, 1970).

Diabetes mellitus

Distal, symmetrical, predominantly sensory polyneuropathy is the commonest neuropathy associated with diabetes mellitus. Patients complain of numbness and paraesthesiae of the toes and feet, and later the fingers, sometimes of a burning quality, with tender calves. Relatively painless perforating ulcers of the feet of diabetics may result from the loss of pain sensation combined with metabolic damage to the tissue, and the poor vascular supply. Loss of touch, pain and vibration sensation extends in a glove and stocking distribution, and the reflexes are depressed distally. The syndrome of *diabetic pseudotabes* results when there is marked impairment of joint position sense together with damage to the iris from attacks of uveitis. Charcot joints may also occur.

The prevalence of the polyneuropathy is difficult to define for it depends on the intensity of the search. Patients complain of symptoms relatively infrequently unless they suffer from 'burning feet' or ulcers. However, an asymptomatic polyneuropathy is more often found on clinical examination, and subclinical damage to nerves is even more frequently revealed by electrophysiological studies. Perhaps about 5 per cent of diabetics have significant symptoms and signs of a distal predominantly sensory polyneuropathy (Bruyn and Garland, 1970). It is generally believed that the neuropathy is less common in children (Hoffman, 1964) although quite a high incidence of asymptomatic electrophysiological abnormalities is found in children (Lawrence and Locke, 1963; Gamstorp, Shelburne, Engleson, Redondo and Traisman, 1966).

There is a tendency for the prevalence and severity of a neuropathy to vary with the age at presentation and the degree of control of the diabetes, though the relationship is not precise (Rundles, 1945). Gregersen (1967, 1968a, b) showed that the average motor and sensory nerve conduction velocities were decreased and the vibration perception threshold raised, in a large group of diabetic patients, whether their illness was recently diagnosed or long-standing. The impairment is greater in those with symptomatic neuropathies, those with diabetes of longer duration, and those with poor control (Gamstorp *et al.*, 1966; Gregersen, 1967, 1968a and b; Ward, Fisher, Barnes, Jessop and Baker, 1971). Greenbaum (1964) showed that the neuropathy tended to begin around the time of diagnosis, or at times of poor control of blood sugar levels. Interestingly in early diabetes there is a widespread sensory abnormality which also involves the threshold for taste and the critical fusion frequencies for sound and light (Chochinov, Ullyot and Moorhouse, 1972).

However, individual patients may vary from this prediction. Particularly in the older group, diabetes may be brought to light only when investigating a patient presenting with a peripheral neuropathy. Similarly, in other patients the neuropathy advances despite adequate control of the blood sugar level and the absence of hypoglycaemic episodes which may themselves damage the peripheral nerves (Danta, 1969; Bruyn and Garland, 1970). The explanation rests upon an understanding of the underlying biochemical defect in diabetes, which probably causes impairment of the transport of glucose into cells long before hyperglycaemia and the classic symptoms of polyuria and polydipsia appear (Reaven, Olefsky and Farquhar, 1972). The nerves may be undergoing damage during the whole of the 'pre-diabetic phase', and the underlying defect is not necessarily corrected by the administration of insulin.

As described in Chapter 6, the neuropathy is predominantly demyelinating, with some axonal degeneration in severe cases. Onion-bulb hypertrophic neuropathy may occur very occasionally. Although lower limb ischaemia may produce segmental demyelination (Chopra and Hurwitz, 1967; Eames and Lange, 1967), and large-vessel arterial disease is common in diabetes, the degree of segmental demyelination in diabetic polyneuropathy is greater than that seen in ischaemic neuropathy. The majority view is, therefore, that the Schwann cell damage is metabolic and not ischaemic in origin (Rundles, 1945; Greenbaum, 1964; Thomas and Lascelles, 1966; Chopra, Hurwitz and Montgomery, 1969), although many authors have taken the opposite view, emphasising the arteriosclerotic changes in the major feeding arteries (Woltman and Wilder, 1929; Martin, 1953), and the thickening of the walls of arterioles and capillaries, with hyaline degeneration, endothelial proliferation and deposition of PAS-positive material (Fagerberg, 1959). The mechanism of the polyneuropathy cannot be regarded as conclusively settled at present.

It is important to remember that the demonstration of an impaired glucose tolerance does not prove that the neuropathy is due to the diabetes. The increased incidence of other diseases of the 'autoimmune' type, such as pernicious anaemia, must be remembered (Khan, Wakefield and Pugh, 1969).

Proximal acute mononeuropathies. Patients with diabetes, especially those with a distal sensory polyneuropathy, frequently have weak and wasted quadriceps femoris muscles (Hirson, Feinmann and Wade, 1953). Goodman (1954) reviewed 17 cases of femoral neuropathy and found that 16 of them were diabetic. This chronic, predominantly motor, femoral neuropathy is perhaps a tenth as common as the chronic, mainly sensory, distal symmetrical polyneuropathy, and is often asymptomatic. The more striking subacute painful proximal neuropathy of diabetes is even less common. Patients suffer severe pain usually in the distribution of one femoral nerve, and soon develop wasting and weakness of the quadriceps muscle with loss of the knee jerk and sometimes a small area of superficial sensory loss on the front of the upper thigh. The pain may last two or three months, then gradually remits. The femoral nerve is the commonest to be involved but others, including the obturator and lateral popliteal nerves, may also be affected. The control of the blood sugar level is often poor at the time of presentation, and, with correction, the condition improves. Casey and Harrison (1972) studied 12 patients 10 months to 12 years after the onset of the condition, and found that 11 had improved, and seven made a good functional recovery.

The history of the condition is interesting. Bruns (1890) first reported a proximal mononeuropathy in diabetes, recognising that the site of the lesion lay in the peripheral nerve. Other reports appearing from time to time thereafter failed to diagnose the site of the lesion correctly (Bruyn and Garland, 1970). Interest in the condition was reawakened by the description by Garland of five further cases (Garland and Taverner, 1953; Garland, 1955). He originally mistook the site of the damage as well, terming the condition 'diabetic myelopathy' because three of the five cases had extensor plantar responses, and four of the five an increased concentration of protein in the CSF. Skanse and Gydell (1956) described a diabetic patient with bilateral femoral neuropathies in whom the quadriceps EMG was neuropathic, and in whom at autopsy there was myelin degeneration in the femoral nerve. Lindén (1962) described severe degeneration in the lumbar plexus with mild retrograde changes in the roots and anterior horn cells. As described in Chapter 6, Raff et al. (1968) have clearly shown the condition to be caused by infarcts of the nerve, only a few of which are related to occluded vasa nervorum. Axonal degeneration results in most

cases, though the femoral nerve motor conduction velocity may occasionally be as low as 44 per cent of normal, suggesting that segmental demyelination may at times be the predominant process (Chopra and Hurwitz, 1968).

Autonomic neuropathy. The autonomic nervous system is frequently damaged in diabetes. Impotence in the male is probably the most frequent symptom, followed by diabetic diarrhoea. There is marked loss of potency in about 50 per cent of diabetic males (Martin, 1953; Ellenberg, 1971). Retrograde ejaculation may also occur (Greene, Kelalis and Weeks, 1963) because of lack of relaxation of the external sphincter during orgasm. The bladder is frequently involved in diabetic autonomic neuropathy, producing an increased residual volume and decreased detrusor muscle activity. This rarely leads to retention with overflow, though it predisposes to urinary infections, and is particularly common in those with impotence (Ellenberg, 1971).

Severe diabetic diarrhoea is relatively uncommon, although investigations demonstrate that gastrointestinal function is quite commonly abnormal (Rundles, 1945; Bruyn and Garland, 1970). The diarrhoea is usually post-prandial or nocturnal, profuse, watery, explosive and distressing (Malins and Mayne, 1969).

Symptomatic postural hypotension is another uncommon autonomic complication of diabetes (Fabré, 1965), though again impaired cardiovascular reflexes are found in 20 per cent of diabetics (Sharpey-Shafer and Taylor, 1960; Moorhouse, Carter and Doupe, 1966). Some patients exhibit peripheral red shiny atrophic skin with decreased sweating, while others have cold, white limbs with hyperhidrosis (Martin, 1953). The latter may be due to postganglionic degeneration with arteriolar denervation supersensitivity (Pickering, 1960).

The pathological basis of the autonomic dysfunction probably rests in degeneration of the neurones of the autonomic ganglia and their processes (Appenzeller and Richardson, 1966; Hensley and Soergel, 1968).

Ageing

Increasing age brings a mixed bag of joys and

sorrows, the latter comprising the many ills to which the ageing body is liable. It is well known that from the seventh decade onwards the vibration sensation, two-point discrimination, taste discrimination, and coordination become impaired, the ankle jerks become depressed, and deafness and cataracts may appear (Pearson, 1928; Critchley, 1931; Howell, 1949). A decrease of the maximum conduction velocity occurs in motor and sensory nerves (see Kaeser, 1970). The decrease is about 10 per cent of the velocity in the third decade, and is more in those with dementia.

Although degeneration of the nerves is prominent from the seventh decade onwards, it probably occurs progressively from early adult life. Dyck et al. (1972) demonstrated a progressive increase of pressure threshold with age from the third decade. Campbell and McComas (1970) found that the estimated number of motor units in the extensor digitorum brevis muscle fell significantly after the age of 60, though their graphs show a trend for the estimate to fall before this time. Jennekens, Tomlinson and Walton (1971) found that the extensor digitorum brevis muscle in fact shows changes of denervation and reinnervation progressively from the first decade. Harriman, Taverner and Woolf (1970) found the complexity of the intramuscular terminal innervation and spherical axonal swellings to be more marked with increasing age. Though the changes are earlier and greater distally, particularly in the lower limb, they also involve more proximal parts of the nervous system (Corbin and Gardner, 1937; Cottrell, 1940; Gardner, 1940).

The nerves of the elderly show degenerative changes of the vasa nervorum, increased fibrosis, and both segmental demyelination and axonal degeneration with regeneration (Cottrell, 1940; Vizoso, 1950; Lascelles and Thomas, 1966; Arnold and Harriman, 1970). The non-myelinated nerve fibres are also involved in the process, showing progressive degeneration; complex plates of Remak cells develop (Ochoa and Mair, 1969a, b).

The problem with all degenerative conditions associated with age is to know whether they are due to ageing itself or to some other disease which is common in old age. This is almost a philosophical point, and it is probably more relevant to ask why

some patients show degenerative changes at 45 years while others show none at the age of 80. This variability makes it very important to choose 'controls' carefully in any study of peripheral nerve function in a certain disease. It is necessary not only to match for age and sex, but also potentially for the degree of 'infirmity'. The neuropathy of old age certainly has many possible origins including ischaemia, entrapments, the cumulative effect of multiple traumata throughout life with a gradual decrease in the regenerative capacity, and the possibility of an underlying neoplasm.

Exogenous toxins

A wide range of chemical agents may cause damage to the peripheral nervous system, including inorganic substances, particularly metals, and organic chemicals. The latter may be derived from plants, animals or the ingenuity of the organic chemist. The short length of this section devoted to toxic neuropathies is no indication of their importance, but is simply due to the large number of such chemicals and the small amount which is known about the action of most of them.

Care is required before accepting all reports of neuropathies due to toxic substances, particularly those recording uncommon reactions to drugs. The neuropathy may in fact be due to the underlying disease for which the drug was first given, or the association may be fortuitous. Moreover, allergic immunological reactions to almost any agent can occur. The agent acts as a hapten, binds to protein, which then becomes an antigen against which the body reacts. Such reactions are usually no more common with one agent than another, the 'allergic predisposition' being more a characteristic of the individual.

Other idiosyncratic reactions may indicate an underlying metabolic abnormality. Isoniazid intoxication occurs particularly in slow inactivators of the drug. In these individuals hepatic acetylation is slow and consequently, blood levels are abnormally high, the major mechanism for drug elimination being urinary excretion (Evans, Manley and McKusick, 1960; Evans, 1963). This tendency is inherited as an autosomal recessive trait, heterozygotes showing intermediate rates of inactivation.

The importance of the understanding of toxic neuropathies is two-fold. First, a diligent search for, and the recognition of, intoxication of a patient with a peripheral neuropathy, will allow the withdrawal of the agent and, potentially, the recovery of the patient. Secondly, investigation of these diseases should allow greater understanding of the basic biochemistry of peripheral nerve disease. Poisons may affect many sites and are rarely entirely specific, though many have a predilection for certain parts of the peripheral nervous system. Botulinum toxin blocks the release of transmitter vesicles at the neuromusclar junctions (Duchen, 1970). Saxitoxin and tetrodotoxin block the depolarisation of axonal and neuronal membranes (Evans, 1969). Diphtheria toxin has a particular effect on the Schwann cells (*see* above and Ch. 6) causing demyelination with relative sparing of the axons. However, in most cases of toxic neuropathies the agent acts mainly on the perikaryon and axon, producing axonal degeneration. In triorthocresyl phosphate (TOCP) (Cavanagh, 1964) and acrylamide neuropathies (Fullerton and Barnes, 1966) this has been particularly well studied. Frequently, the pattern of degeneration is the 'dying-back' type affecting the distal parts of the largest fibres (*see* Ch. 6). The presence of a mild toxic neuropathy may predispose to the development of a second disease of the nerve, such as entrapment (Hopkins and Morgan-Hughes, 1969).

Drugs and other agents are usually screened before release for neurotoxic effects by administration to animals. Unfortunately there are considerable differences in the susceptibility of various species. For instance, the rat is more resistant to lead, vincristine and TOCP than are the guinea pig and many other animals (Smith, Elvove and Frazier, 1930; Fullerton, 1966; Bradley, 1970).

An indication of the types of agents responsible for peripheral nerve damage is given in Table 21.1.

Vitamin deficiencies

Peripheral nerve damage occurs in a number of vitamin deficiencies, the most important clinically being those of beriberi, pernicious anaemia and malabsorption. Leaving aside the deficiency of vitamin B_{12}, deficiencies of other vitamins usually occur in the setting of malnutrition, where multiple deficiencies coexist. In experimental work it has been difficult to prove the requirement of an individual vitamin for peripheral nerve function, with the exception of thiamine (Victor, 1965). For an extensive recent review of this problem the reader is referred to Erbslöh and Abel (1970).

Thiamine-vitamin B_1. The active form of this vitamin is thiamine pyrophosphate which is the co-enzyme for at least three important enzymes of carbohydrate metabolism, pyruvate decarboxylase, α-ketoglutarate decarboxylase and transketolase. Deficiency causes an accumulation

Table 21.1 Some of the causes of toxic neuropathies

Metals :	Lead, arsenic, mercury, thallium, gold.
Industrial Organic Compounds :	*Solvents :* n-hexane, petrol, trichlorethylene, carbon tetrachloride, carbon disulphide, dimethylsulphoxide
	Insecticides and herbicides : dieldrin, aldrin, 2,4-D, DDT
	Others : TOCP, acrylamide, diethylthiocarbamate, p-bromophenylacetylurea
Drugs :	*Anticonvulsants :* phenytoin
	Chemotherapeutic : isoniazid, furans (nitrofurantoin, furaltadone), ethambutol, ethionamide, amphotericin B, sulphonamides, clioquinol, chloroquine
	Antimitotic : nitrogen mustards, ethoglucid, *Vinca* alkaloids (vincristine, vinblastine)
	Sedatives : thalidomide, glutethimide
	Others : Imipramine, monoamine oxidase inhibitors, disulfiram, hydrallazine, stilbamidine, nitrofurazone
Foods :	Cyanogens (cassava, cycasin), alcohol, lathyrogens
Bacterial and Viral :	Diphtheria, [Guillain-Barré-Strohl syndrome]

of pyruvate and lactate, with impairment of energy metabolism in both the neurone and in Schwann cells. Although starvation alone in the presence of vitamin therapy may cause a peripheral neuropathy (Mattson and Lecocq, 1968), the typical setting for thiamine deficiency was such as that occurring in the Japanese prisoner-of-war camps in the Second World War. The diet consisted predominantly of polished rice, which contains carbohydrate but no vitamins because of the removal of the rice husks. The result was damage to the peripheral nerves (dry beriberi) and to the heart with congestive cardiac failure (wet beriberi). The incidence of symptomatic neuropathy depended upon the severity of deprivation. Most of the patients showed signs of a distal, symmetrical polyneuropathy, which in 50 per cent was mixed sensorimotor, in 30 per cent mainly sensory, and 20 per cent mainly motor (Cruickshank, 1952). Treatment with thiamine at a dose of more than 100 mg/day led to a slow recovery which often took more than six months. Those who had suffered prolonged and severe starvation made a lesser degree of recovery, residual dysaesthesiae being particularly common.

In experimental thiamine deficiency in rats, the maximum motor conduction velocity of the sciatic nerve was decreased by 50–60 per cent of normal, suggesting a major degree of segmental demyelination (Erbslöh and Abel, 1970). Earlier reports of the pathological changes in thiamine deficiency suggested the presence of segmental demyelination; Collins, Webster and Victor (1964) showed that the earliest change was an increase in the normal irregularities of the myelin sheaths. Nevertheless, it is clear that axonal degeneration predominates (Collins et al., 1964; Prineas, 1970b), leading to a consequently greater denervation atrophy of the muscle than would be expected with segmental demyelination (Erbslöh and Abel, 1970). This is in keeping with the slow recovery seen in the clinical situation, which suggests axonal degeneration with recovery by axonal regrowth.

Vitamin B$_{12}$ is involved in the metabolism of methyl units, in nucleic acid metabolism, and probably in cell membrane synthesis. Deficiency is most commonly due to loss of intrinsic factor

produced by the gastric mucosa and required for the intestinal absorption of vitamin B$_{12}$. This is usually due to autoimmune damage to the gastric parietal cells by circulating autoantibodies. There is a familial tendency, and the disease usually presents in middle age. More rarely there is congenital absence of intrinsic factor, and the disease presents in the juvenile. Other causes of malabsorption of vitamin B$_{12}$ include the blind loop syndrome, ileal resection, the fish tapeworm, and the dietary fads of vegans. The mechanism of damage of the peripheral nerves in vitamin B$_{12}$ deficiency is not certain. Clinically, the central nervous system changes predominate, particularly those in the spinal cord, with progressive signs of damage to the pyramidal tracts and dorsal columns. In addition, many patients have paraesthesiae in the hands and feet and a mild glove and stocking impairment of the modalities of sensation conveyed by the larger fibres, together with loss of the ankle jerks.

There is slowing of the maximum motor and sensory conduction velocities by 10–20 per cent of normal in the distal parts of the peripheral nerves, with no change in the proximal parts (Mayer, 1965). The response to treatment with intramuscular vitamin B$_{12}$ at a dose of 1000 μg/day is relatively quick, the paraesthesiae disappearing within a few days and the distal reflexes returning within one or two months. Similarly, the distal nerve conduction velocity returns to normal within one month (Mayer, 1965). However, the spinal cord disease is much less responsive to therapy, and the prognosis is entirely dependent upon this. The physiological studies suggest that the neuropathy is a 'dying-back' type of axonal degeneration, and this suggestion is supported by pathological studies in man, there being loss of the larger myelinated fibres in distal sensory nerves with the changes of axonal degeneration in teased single fibres (Greenfield and Carmichael, 1935; McLeod, Walsh and Little, 1969). However, in experimental vitamin B$_{12}$ deficiency in monkeys, segmental demyelination apparently predominates (Torres, Smith and Oxnard, 1971).

Malabsorption and other causes of vitamin deficiencies. A variety of nervous and muscular syndromes have been reported with diseases causing malabsorption, a progressive symmetrical distal mixed polyneuropathy being the commonest, with sensory ataxia, paraesthesiae and spontaneous pains (Cook and Smith, 1966; Cook, Johnson and Woolf, 1966; Erbslöh and Abel, 1970). Malabsorptions of all types may cause deficiencies, particularly of the fat-soluble vitamins and folic acid. However, supplementation with all known vitamins, together with replacement of pancreatic enzymes or the institution of a gluten-free diet as required, will still not correct some of the neuropathies. Pathological changes are axonal and distal; however, more studies are required of this interesting group of conditions (Cook et al., 1966).

Alcoholics. These subjects frequently have a peripheral neuropathy similar in presentation to that of thiamine deficiency, and have been shown to have deficiencies of thiamine, folic acid, pyridoxin, pantothenic acid and riboflavin (Fennelly, Frank, Baker and Leevy, 1964) with evidence of malabsorption of thiamine (Tomasulo, Kater and Iber, 1968). Their high calorie intake in the form of alcohol, with deficiency of thiamine, may be responsible for the nerve damage in many. Some, however, fail to improve with replacement of vitamins of the B group, and the direct toxic effect of alcohol and the possible effect of liver damage must also be considered.

Epileptics may show signs of a peripheral neuropathy with areflexia, slight slowing of maximum motor and sensory conduction velocities, and evidence of denervation on electromyography (Horwitz, Klipstein and Lovelace, 1967). The serum folic acid is often low in these patients but replacement does not always improve the neuropathy. The peripheral nerve damage is probably due to the chronic effects of the anticonvulsants, perhaps exacerbated by recurrent anoxic and traumatic episodes during the epileptic fits.

Pyridoxine (vitamin B_6). Deficiency of pyridoxine, whose active derivative pyridoxal-5-phosphate is a co-enzyme for many decarboxylases and transaminases, experimentally produces a peripheral neuropathy (Follis and Wintrobe, 1945; Vilter, Müller, Glazer, Jarrold, Abraham,

Thompson and Hawkins, 1953). This is predominantly a distal, symmetrical sensory polyneuropathy, though central nervous system changes also occur. In the pig it is probably mainly an axonal degeneration, although single-fibre studies have not been undertaken (Follis and Wintrobe, 1945). Isoniazid produces an essentially identical neuropathy by interfering with pyridoxine metabolism, probably with the formation of the isonicotinyl hydrazone of pyridoxine (Aspinall, 1964). The pathological changes of axonal degeneration in isoniazid neuropathy are well described (Cavanagh, 1967; Hildebrand and Coërs, 1967; Ochoa, 1970).

In pellagra which is due to *nicotinic acid* deficiency, a painful burning distal symmetrical sensory polyneuropathy may occur, although the central nervous system changes predominate (Erbslöh and Abel, 1970). The burning-feet syndrome may at times be due to *riboflavin* deficiency (Lai and Ransome, 1970).

Acute intermittent porphyria

Acute nervous crises, particularly of the acute intermittent type, occur in porphyria. They take the form of severe episodes of abdominal pain, psychiatric disorders, and peripheral neuropathies. The characteristics of the neuropathy were reviewed in 25 patients by Ridley (1969). It is an acute, severe and chiefly motor neuropathy leading to flaccid paralysis and loss of reflexes. There is a *proximal* predominance, the upper limbs being involved more than the lower limbs. The cranial nerves, trunk and respiratory muscles and sphincters are often involved. In about 50 per cent of patients there is some sensory impairment, which may be either proximal or distal and which affects all modalities. The most classic picture is of a proximal muscle weakness with sensory loss in a bathing trunk distribution, and paradoxical preservation of the ankle jerks. Muscle wasting is rapid.

Pathological changes are predominantly of axonal degeneration, which in the motor nerves affects particularly the distal parts of the larger fibres in the intramuscular nerves, and in the sensory fibres affects predominantly the centrally directed axons of the dorsal roots (Cavanagh and

Mellick, 1965). In both instances there is, therefore, a 'dying-back' distribution in individual axons, although the longest fibres are not involved as is usual in the 'dying-back' type of condition. It has been suggested that the effects fall particularly on those fibres with the largest motor units, although this appears unlikely in view of the similar distribution of damage in the sensory fibres. In some cases there may be segmental demyelination (Thomas, 1971).

In severe attacks, respiratory and bulbar paralysis may cause death, and tracheostomy and artificial respiration are often required. A few patients make a rapid recovery (Heirons, 1957), although in most the recovery is relatively slow, as might be expected with axonal regeneration. Sørensen and With (1971) reviewed 95 patients with acute intermittent porphyria, 41 of whom had suffered from paralytic episodes. Of these 41, 17 had died, and 12 of the 24 survivors had residual paralyses after three years which, in most cases, remained permanent thereafter. Recovery was less rapid and complete in males.

Attacks of acute intermittent porphyria occur either spontaneously or are precipitated by drugs, such as alcohol in excess, barbiturates and sulphonamides. The disease has a dominant mode of inheritance with incomplete penetrance (Pratt, 1967). It has been shown that the attacks are associated with the induction of high levels of δ-aminolaevulinic acid synthetase in the liver causing increased excretion of δ-aminolaevulinic acid and porphobilinogen in the urine (Cavanagh and Ridley, 1967; Sweeney, Pathack and Asbury, 1970). The enzyme requires pyridoxal-5-phosphate as its co-enzyme, and it has been suggested that the induction of this enzyme causes a deficiency of pyridoxine, which produces the neuropathy. However, the picture of porphyric neuropathy differs from that of deficiency of pyridoxine, and there is no correlation between the pyridoxal-5-phosphate level and the neuropathy (Hamfelt and Wetterberg, 1968). Meyer, Strand, Doss, Rees and Marver (1972) doubted that δ-aminolaevulinic acid synthetase induction causes the syndrome, and found a decrease of the red cell urobilinogen I-synthetase activity, although the part played by this in the neuropathy is not clear. Treatment with glucose and haematin appears to be effective in aborting an attack of porphyric neuropathy; the haematin probably produces feed-back inhibition of the abnormally increased enzymes of the early parts of the pathway for haem synthesis (Bosch, Pierach, Bossenmaier, Cardinal and Thorson, 1977).

Metabolic neuropathies

Under this heading might be included diabetes mellitus and porphyria, which have already been considered, as well as the neuropathies of hepatic, renal and thyroid disease, and of hypoglycaemia as well as a small group of neuropathies associated with rare metabolic abnormalities. General reviews of this group of conditions have been published by Henson and Urich (1970a) and Bruyn and Garland (1970). All are associated with general medical diseases and, in all, the incidence of symptomatic neuropathies is greatly exceeded by that of asymptomatic damage of the nerve, either producing signs on examination or abnormalities in electrophysiological studies.

Uraemic neuropathy. With the longer survival of patients with uraemia as a result of peritoneal or haemodialysis, many such patients develop a chronic, distal, symmetrical, predominantly sensory polyneuropathy. Several useful reviews of this condition include those of Asbury, Victor and Adams (1963), Tyler (1968), Nielsen (1971), and Thomas, Hollinrake, Lascelles, O'Sullivan, Baillod, Moorhead and McKenzie (1971). It is usually not seen until the blood urea exceeds 250 mg/100 ml, and the creatinine clearance falls below 5 ml/min. However, the severity of the neuropathy is not directly related to the degree of uraemia or electrolyte disturbance (Preswick and Jeremy, 1964). The exact cause of the neuropathy is not clear, although there is some evidence of an inhibitor of transketolase in uraemics, which is removed by dialysis but not overcome by thiamine administration (Sterzel, Semar, Lonergan, Treser and Lange, 1971). Dialysis may prevent the progression of the neuropathy and allow some recovery (Konotey-Ahulu, Baillod, Comty, Heron, Shaldon and Thomas, 1965; Jebsen, Tenckhoff and Honet, 1967). However, the occasional acute appearance or deterioration of the neuropathy following the institution of dialysis therapy in some patients (Tenckhoff, Boen, Jebsen and Spiegler, 1965) suggests that acute changes in osmotically active chemicals and loss of essential substances may play some part in the neuropathy. The neuropathy responds fairly well to renal transplantation.

The symptoms, which are present in about 75 per cent of patients having chronic dialysis, include burning paraesthesiae, restless legs, hyperpathia and numbness spreading upwards from the feet, and only later involving the hands. Motor involvement is milder, although a foot drop may result. There is mild slowing of the maximum motor and sensory nerve conduction velocities by about 5–10 per cent with a decrease of the amplitude of the sensory nerve action potential, the changes being suggestive of an axonal neuropathy (Konotey-Ahulu et al., 1965; Jebsen et al., 1967). It has been suggested that a fall in the maximum nerve conduction velocity is sufficient to indicate that dialysis is inadequate, although it is unlikely to be helpful in an individual case (Kominami, Tyler, Hampers and Merritt, 1971). However, pathological studies have shown definite segmental demyelination as well as signs of axonal degeneration (Asbury et al., 1963; Dayan, Gardner-Thorpe, Down and Gleadle, 1970; Dinn and Crane, 1970; Appenzeller, Kornfeld and McGee, 1971; Thomas et al., 1972), although as emphasised in Chapter 6, segmental demyelination is easier to see than axonal degeneration in teased single-fibre studies. Asbury et al. (1963) showed loss of Schwann cells, and Dyck, Johnson, Lambert and O'Brien (1971) showed that segmental demyelination was restricted to some fibres preferentially (secondary segmental demyelination, see Ch. 6).

Hepatic neuropathy. The central nervous effects of chronic liver failure far outweigh the peripheral ones. Few patients with chronic liver failure have symptoms of the latter, though a fifth have signs of peripheral nerve damage, usually with depression of reflexes distally. There is also slight slowing (by about 10 per cent) (Knill-Jones, Goodwill, Dayan and Williams, 1972) and up to two-thirds of patients have an increased peripheral latency of sensory and motor conduction and a decrease in the sensory nerve action potential

amplitude (Seneviratne and Peiris, 1970). The peripheral nerves of most patients show segmental demyelination with a lesser degree of loss of myelinated nerve fibres, probably indicating some axonal degeneration (Dayan and Williams, 1967; Knill-Jones et al., 1972). In most such series many of the patients had alcoholic cirrhosis, and the effects of the alcohol and vitamin deficiencies in this condition cannot be excluded (see above). However, similar damage can be found in primary biliary cirrhosis. Thomas and Walker (1965) reported three patients with cutaneous xanthomata, who had a mild distal symmetrical sensory polyneuropathy with xanthomatous infiltrations within the peripheral nerve causing loss of myelinated nerve fibres.

Neuropathies associated with thyroid disease. The proximal myopathy associated with myxoedema is described in Chapter 18. In the peripheral nerves, a carpal tunnel syndrome is relatively common due to infiltration of the tissue within the tunnel by myxoid material (Murray and Simpson, 1958), and other entrapments may also occur. About 45 per cent of myxoedematous patients have sensory symptoms, and 10 per cent of these have signs of a mild distal, symmetrical, predominantly sensory, polyneuropathy (Nickel and Frame, 1958). In most there is slowing of the maximum sensory nerve conduction velocity by about 30 per cent and decrease in amplitude of the sensory nerve action potentials; in some there is slowing of the maximum motor nerve conduction velocity (Fincham and Cape, 1968; Grabow and Chou, 1968). Dyck and Lambert (1970) presented physiological and histological evidence of segmental demyelination and remyelination of myelinated nerve fibres, with no change in non-myelinated nerve fibres, in myxoedematous neuropathy. The symptoms and signs of the neuropathy largely recover with thyroid replacement.

In thyrotoxicosis the proximal myopathy is the main neuromuscular disorder (see Ch. 18). However, electromyographic evidence of distal denervation has been reported in this condition, and some patients have mild symptoms and signs of sensory involvement suggesting the presence of a peripheral neuropathy (Ludin, Spiess and Koenig, 1969).

Hypoglycaemic neuropathy. The peripheral nervous system is by no means as sensitive to hypoglycaemia as the central nervous system, but cases of a distal symmetrical mixed polyneuropathy have been reported in patients with insulinomata (Danta, 1969; Bruyn and Garland, 1970). Central nervous system symptoms predominate, but there may be initial sensory symptoms in the limbs and later a rapidly progressive distal motor neuropathy. Cases which have come to autopsy show degeneration of the perikarya within the spinal cord and dorsal root ganglia. The possible rôle of hypoglycaemic episodes in 'fragile' diabetics who develop a neuropathy must be considered.

Neuropathies with other metabolic abnormalities. In a few, relatively rare, diseases of peripheral nerve, a metabolic abnormality has been described which may perhaps be the cause of the neuropathy. Several of these diseases affect the central nervous system more than the peripheral.

Bassen-Kornzweig's disease. This gives neurological damage including ataxia from posterior column and spinocerebellar tract degeneration, pyramidal tract degeneration, atypical retinitis pigmentosa, areflexia and anterior horn cell degeneration. There is also malabsorption, particularly of fat. Beta-lipoproteins are absent from the plasma. The plasma cholesterol is very low. The red-cell membrane is abnormal, leading to the formation of burr cells (acanthocytes) (Farquhar and Ways, 1966). The exact part played by the abetalipoproteinaemia in the neuropathy is not known.

Tangier disease. This consists of the deposition of cholesterol esters throughout the reticuloendothelial system, particularly the tonsils, associated with a very low plasma cholesterol and absent α-lipoproteins in the plasma. A progressive or recurrent sensorimotor neuropathy has been recorded in this disease, with loss both of myelin sheaths and axons (Kocen, Lloyd, Lascelles, Fosbrooke and Williams, 1967; Engel, Dorman, Levy and Fredrickson, 1967). The relationship between the biochemical abnormality and the neuropathy requires clarification.

Fabry's disease. The stigmata of Fabry's disease (angiokeratoma corporis diffusum) include typical skin lesions, corneal opacities, dilated conjunctival capillaries and abnormal deposition of lipids in many tissues. The lipids in blood vessel walls lead to cerebral and myocardial infarction and renal failure. Similar lipid accumulation, mainly of ceramide trihexosides, also occurs in many neurones. Spontaneous pains in the limbs are a frequent feature of the disease, even when clinical signs of neuropathy are slight or absent, and lipid deposits in the perineurium and a moderate loss of myelinated nerve fibres may be found in peripheral nerves (Kocen and Thomas, 1970). Ceramide trihexosidase is deficient in these patients, presumably leading to the formation of abnormal membranes, including myelin.

Metachromatic leucodystrophy. In this disease, although central nervous white matter degeneration predominates, the peripheral nervous system is also involved. This leads to progressive areflexia and sometimes hypotonia superimposed upon the picture of decorticate spasticity. Nerve conduction velocities are greatly slowed, and there is extensive segmental demyelination with accumulation of metachromatic lipids in Schwann and other cells (*see* Ch. 6). These consist of ceramide hexoside sulphates, and result from a deficiency of the enzyme aryl sylphatase A (Dayan, 1967; Yudell, Gomez, Lambert and Docherty, 1967).

The accumulation of phytanic acid in Refsum's syndrome and of ceramide hexosides and ceramide hexoside sulphates in hypertrophic neuropathy of the Dejerine-Sottas variety are described on p. 771 of this chapter. The finding of aminoaciduria or of an abnormal pyruvate tolerance test (Hutchinson, Leonard, Maudsley and Yates, 1958; Hockaday, Hockaday and Rushworth, 1966) occasionally in a patient, suggests the presence of an underlying biochemical defect awaiting discovery.

Hereditary neuropathies

A number of inherited diseases of peripheral nerves have now been characterised, although they make up only a small part of the whole group of peripheral neuropathies. Porphyria has already been mentioned in this context. There is space to consider only a few of these diseases briefly here.

In several diseases where the central nervous system changes predominate, such as Friedreich's ataxia (Hughes, Brownell and Hewer, 1968; McLeod, 1971), metachromatic leucodystrophy, globoid leucodystrophy, the lipidoses, Canavan's disease, and neuroaxonal dystrophy (see Ch. 6), peripheral nerve involvement may be demonstrated clinically, physiologically and pathologically. Sometimes this allows diagnosis of the condition by peripheral nerve biopsy, thereby avoiding brain biopsy (see Ch. 6). The other conditions which will be considered below are amyloidosis, hereditary sensory ganglioneuropathy, peroneal muscular atrophy and Refsum's disease. Pratt (1967) mentions a number of other hereditary neuropathies.

Amyloidosis. Three main types of familial amyloidosis with different clinical patterns have been described. All have a dominant mode of inheritance, and they have been reviewed by Andrade, Araki, Block, Cohen, Jackson, Kuroiwa, McKusick, Nissim, Sohar and Van Allen (1970).

1. *The Andrade type.* This condition is endemic in the part of Northern Portugal around Oporto (Andrade, 1952). It also occurs in Portuguese descendants in other parts of the world, and in those with no Portuguese blood (Araki, Mawatari, Ohta, Nakajima and Kuroiwa, 1968; Andersson, 1970). The disease begins between 25–35 years of age, and leads to death within 7–15 years. It presents with sensory symptoms starting in the lower limbs, including painful dysaesthesiae and spontaneous shooting pains. Pain and temperature sensation and autonomic function are preferentially lost (viz. small myelinated and non-myelinated fibres are particularly involved), leading to trophic ulceration of the feet. There is general debility, and the autonomic involvement produces diarrhoea, sphincter impairment, impotence in the male, decreased gastrointestinal motility, postural hypotension, and disordered cardiac conduction. Death may be due to inanition, or from chronic renal failure due to chronic pyelonephritis or amyloid infiltration of the kidneys.

Amyloid is found not only in the peripheral nerves (see Ch. 6), but also in the kidneys, skin blood vessels, and rectal submucosa. The maximum motor and sensory nerve conduction velocities may be normal or decreased only by about 10 per cent, although there is a progressive fall in the sensory nerve action potential amplitude until total failure of peripheral nerve conduction occurs (Dyck and Lambert, 1969; Araki et al., 1968; Andersson and Blom, 1972). Dyck and Lambert (1969) showed that the loss of C fibre potential in the sural nerve in vitro corresponded to the early and almost specific loss of non-myelinated nerve fibres seen pathologically.

2. *The Rukavina type.* A large kinship of Swiss origin with amyloid polyneuropathy was described from Indiana by Rukavina, Block, Jackson, Falls, Carey and Curtis (1956), and subsequently a further unrelated kinship of German origin has been reported from Maryland (Mahloudji, Teasdall, Adamkiewicz, Hartmann, Lambird and McKusick, 1969). This condition is much more benign than the Andrade type, males, however, being more severely affected than females. It presents usually at about the age of 45 years with a bilateral carpal tunnel syndrome (see above). At this stage surgical decompression can cure the local symptoms and amyloid is found infiltrating the flexor retinaculum, causing the compression (Lambird and Hartmann, 1969).

Later in the disease, a progressive, distal, symmetrical polyneuropathy develops, affecting particularly the large myelinated fibres and the legs more than the arms. This often remains mild, and some patients live to the eighties with little disability. Vitreous opacities are common, requiring surgical evacuation of the vitreous. Autonomic and renal involvement occur only late in this type of amyloidosis. Electrophysiological studies show a minimal decrease of the maximum motor nerve conduction velocity in the nerve trunks, although the terminal motor and sensory latency are increased.

3. *The Van Allen type.* Van Allen, Frohlich and Davis (1969) reported a large kinship in Iowa originating from the British Isles, who presented at about the age of 30–35 years with a painful distal symmetrical sensorimotor polyneuropathy start-

ing in the lower limbs. The carpal tunnel syndrome was not seen, nor was there significant autonomic disturbance. However, a progressive nephropathy and peptic ulceration were prominent features in this family. Progressive renal failure caused death within 15–20 years, by which time there was significant loss of all modalities of sensation distally in the arms and legs, with amyotrophy. The CSF protein concentration was raised in most cases.

The pathological changes in the amyloidosis are described in Chapter 6. Unfortunately only symptomatic therapy is available for these conditions.

Hereditary sensory radicular neuropathy. Denny-Brown (1951) described the pathological changes in this condition reported by many previously without pathological confirmation (see Campbell, 1970). The disease generally has an autosomal dominant mode of inheritance, and usually presents with painless penetrating ulcers of the feet around the age of 20–30 years. This led Thévenard (1942) to give the condition the name 'l'acropathie ulcero-mutilante familiale'. Destructive changes in the fingers also occur. The patients have marked loss of pain and temperature sensation distally, though later other modalities of sensation and the distal motor fibres become involved in the process. The proximal tendon reflexes are usually spared. Lightning-like pains in the limbs may occur. Early in the condition the maximum motor and sensory nerve conduction velocities are normal, although there is a slight decrease in the amplitude of the nerve action potential and an increased terminal latency. The later presence of EMG signs of denervation distally indicates minor degrees of motor neurone degeneration. The condition progresses gradually, and death results from uncontrolled infection or secondary amyloid infiltration of the kidney.

The primary pathological change is shrinkage and loss of the small neurones in the dorsal root ganglia, and of the small myelinated and non-myelinated fibres in the peripheral nerves. It is assumed that the primary site of the disease is in the small dorsal root ganglion neurones. Later there is quite extensive damage to the larger neurones and fibres (Turkington and Stiefel, 1965). Fig. 21.1

shows a sural nerve from such a patient in which no myelinated nerve fibres remain. The finding, by Denny-Brown (1951), of amyloid in the dorsal root ganglion has not been confirmed by others (Wallace, 1970), and may have been due simply to secondary amyloidosis.

A number of other neurological features have been reported in some families with this condition, including nerve deafness, optic atrophy and central nervous involvement. Other diseases which may cause a very similar picture include tabes dorsalis, although the large rather than the small fibre function is especially involved in this condition, diabetic sensory polyneuropathy (see above), alcoholic acrodystrophic neuropathy (Bureau, Barrière, Kerneis and de Ferron, 1957; Mota-Revetllat, 1966), sensory neuropathy of carcinoma (see below), and congenital insensitivity to pain. The characteristic of the latter is the absence of perception of pain over the whole body in the presence of otherwise entirely normal sensation (Jewsbury, 1970). Even in this condition, although Baxter and Olszewski (1960) did not observe any abnormality of dorsal roots, skin nerve endings, spinal cord or brain, Swanson, Buchan and Alvord (1965) found an absence of small neurones and non-myelinated nerve fibres in the dorsal roots. A personally observed case with insensitivity to pain over the whole body, though with signs and pathological evidence (see Fig. 21.1) of a sensory radiculoneuropathy, indicates that the separation of these conditions is not always clear.

Charcot-Marie-Tooth disease and hypertrophic neuropathy. The history of peroneal muscular atrophy goes back to the descriptions by Charcot and Marie (1886) and Tooth (1886) who described families with progressive distal wasting and weakness producing a 'stork-leg' appearance, with motor involvement later spreading to the hands and relatively little involvement of the sensory nerves. That of hypertrophic neuropathy goes back to the original descriptions by Dejerine and Sottas (1893) and Dejerine and André-Thomas (1906) of a brother and sister presenting in their teens with a relatively rapidly progressive distal sensorimotor neuropathy, in whom the peripheral nerves were hypertrophied with 'onion-bulb' formation (see Ch. 6). It is only in

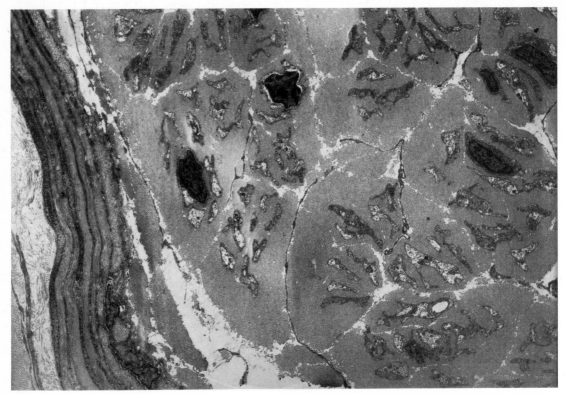

Fig. 21.1 Electron micrograph of transverse section of sural nerve biopsy of a patient with total insensitivity to pain over the whole body, and a peripheral sensory radicular neuropathy of the Denny-Brown type. The perineurium can be seen to the left. The nerve consists entirely of collagen and residual atrophic Schwann cell processes. There is total loss of nerve fibres (buffered formalin fixation)

recent times that the relationship between these diseases and a number of other conditions with a similar clinical and pathological picture has been elucidated. This has largely been the result of the work of Dyck and Lambert (1968a and b) who surveyed a large number of individuals from families with this condition, and proposed the following classification:

1. *Charcot-Marie-Tooth disease of the hypertrophic type with dominant inheritance.* This group includes kinships similar to those described by Charcot and Marie (1886), Tooth (1886) and Roussy and Lévy (1926). The earliest sign is usually pes cavus, and some gait disturbance often appears by the second decade due to progressive atrophy of the anterior and posterior tibial groups of muscles. A progressive foot-drop develops, and later difficulty in manipulating the fingers. Sensory impairment appears late and is less severe

than the motor involvement, affecting especially the large fibre modalities. Some relatives with no symptoms show marked slowing of nerve conduction (Bradley and Aguayo, 1969). The condition is very slowly progressive, and many patients can still walk with aids 30 years after the onset. The maximum motor and sensory nerve conduction velocities are 5–20 m/s, and the nerve shows extensive segmental demyelination and hypertrophy with 'onion-bulb' formation. Signs of spinal cord damage may occasionally be present, perhaps from compression by hypertrophic nerve roots (Symonds and Blackwood, 1962).

2. *Charcot-Marie-Tooth disease of the hypertrophic type, sporadic, dominant with poor expression, or recessive inheritance.* These cases are identical to 1 above, but with a different family pattern.

3. *Hypertrophic neuropathy of the Dejerine-Sottas type.* This group includes kinships similar to those originally described by Dejerine and Sottas. The onset is usually in the first few years of life, with delayed walking. The condition progresses slowly so that the patient becomes wheelchair-bound from 20–30 years of age. There is a progressive symmetrical glove and stocking loss of sensation. The electrophysiological and pathological changes are essentially similar to those described in 1 above, though the surviving myelin sheaths tend to be thinner.

4. *The neuronal sensorimotor type of Charcot-Marie-Tooth disease with dominant inheritance.* The clinical pattern is similar to 1 above, but the onset is in middle age, there is less hand and more leg involvement, and no enlargement of the peripheral nerves. The maximum motor nerve conduction velocity in the ulnar and median nerves is normal, and sensory loss is mild compared with motor impairment. Sensory nerve biopsies show loss of the larger myelinated nerve fibres and no segmental demyelination or hypertrophic change. The site of the lesion may be in the motor axons or anterior horn cells and the dorsal root ganglion neurones.

5. *Progressive spinal muscular atrophy of the Charcot-Marie-Tooth type.* These are sporadic cases with onset in the second and third decades of life. There is distal symmetrical weakness of the lower limbs subsequently spreading to the hands and forearms. Wasting is severe and extends to the mid-thigh and forearm. There is no sensory abnormality, clinically or electrophysiologically. The maximum motor nerve conduction velocity is normal and the nerves are not hypertrophied.

Peroneal muscular atrophy may occur with other diseases in which there is central nervous degeneration.

In Dyck and Lambert's series, type 1 *above* was the most frequent (about 70 per cent), and type 2 was the next most common (about 10 per cent). The remainder were less common. At present there is no knowledge of the aetiology of the conditions, though Dyck, Ellefson, Lais, Smith, Taylor and Van Dyke (1970) found evidence of an abnormal metabolism of ceramide hexosides and ceramide hexoside sulphates in hypertrophic neuropathy of the Dejerine-Sottas type. A more recent survey has suggested the presence of an intermediate group of families falling between the dominant hypertrophic and the dominant neuronal sensorimotor forms of Dyck and Lambert (Madrid, Bradley and Davis, 1977; Bradley, Madrid and Davies, 1977; Davis, Bradley and Madrid, 1979).

Hypertrophic neuropathy may occur in many other conditions including diabetes (*see above*), relapsing polyneuropathy (Austin, 1958; Cazzato, 1965), acromegaly (Stewart, 1966), multifocal enlargement of peripheral nerves (Adams, Asbury and Michelsen, 1965; Simpson and Fowler, 1966), and in Refsum's disease (Cammermeyer, 1956) in which inheritance is probably by an autosomal recessive trait. The latter disease was described by Refsum (1946) under the title of *heredopathia atactica polyneuritiformis.* Symptoms appear in the first and second decades of life, with the development of a chronic progressive symmetrical distal sensorimotor polyneuropathy which may show relapses and remissions. There is cerebellar dysfunction with ataxia and nystagmus, and atypical retinitis pigmentosa which lacks the classical 'bone corpuscle' pigment cells. The cerebrospinal fluid protein concentration is raised, and there are often nerve deafness, ichthyosis, cardiac and pupillary abnormalities. The condition is rare, only about 50 cases having been described in the literature, but is of interest because of a knowledge in part of the underlying biochemistry of the condition and treatment thereof. There is an increased amount of one of the fatty acids, namely phytanic acid (3,7,11,15-tetramethyl-hexadecanoic acid) in the blood and many tissues of the body (Klenk and Kahlke, 1963), due to impaired metabolism of phytols in the diet, the exclusion of which produces a considerable improvement in some patients (Steinberg, Mize, Herndon, Fales, Engel and Vroom, 1970).

Acute inflammatory polyneuropathy (Guillain-Barré-Strohl syndrome)

Landry (1859) described a group of patients with acute ascending paralysis now recognised to embrace both patients with inflammatory poly-neuropathy and transverse myelitis. Guillain, Barré and Strohl (1916) collected a series of patients with polyradiculoneuritis, stressing the albuminocytologic dissociation in the cerebro-spinal fluid. Many such patients have been de-scribed since and much is known about the aetiology of the condition, although the criteria for diagnosis still remain difficult to define. Although it is probable that there is only one single disease entity here, a spectrum of disease is seen ranging from the acute, with a relatively good prognosis, to the subacute and chronic cases where continuing activity of the disease causes a worsening of the prognosis. In order to achieve a group with a relatively homogeneous clinical course and prog-nosis, many require criteria to be satisfied before making the diagnosis. Emphasis is particu-larly given to the duration between the onset and peak of the weakness (Cambier and Brunet, 1970). Osler and Sidell (1960) in a list of 12 criteria, set two weeks as the limit for this interval. Prineas (1970a) allowed three weeks. Ravn (1967) accepted 46 days. Pleasure, Lovelace and Duvoisin (1968) set the limit at two months, while two of the cases of Asbury, Arnason and Adams (1969) worsened over three months. All such cases seemed essen-tially to be of the same disease, which illustrates the difficulty in defining acceptable diagnostic criteria.

The following gives an outline of the *clinical pattern* of the condition drawn from the reviews quoted above. Over 50 per cent of patients give a history of some preceding viral infection 2–4 weeks before the onset of the neuropathy. Over a quarter begin with paraesthesiae in the feet, spreading proximally and then involving the hands. Over a third have moderately severe pains, particularly in the back and limbs, which may cause diagnostic difficulties. Sensory loss is usually slight and may be absent in a third of patients, while motor involvement is the most striking feature. In half of the patients weakness is diffuse from the onset, while in the remainder it spreads up from the lower limbs to involve the upper limbs, the respiratory and then bulbar muscles in the most severe cases. On average the condition progresses for 1–2 weeks and, at its maximum, tracheostomy and artificial respiration are re-quired to support life in about 10–20 per cent of cases. In terms of a peripheral neuropathy, such a progress is *acute*.

The paresis is at its maximum for 1–4 weeks. Thereafter there is gradual recovery, although it may take 3–6 months in some, and about 3–6 per cent of patients have relapses.

The cerebrospinal fluid protein concentration is raised in almost all patients at some time during the illness, particularly after the first seven days. The maximum rise is seen from the 10th–20th days, and the level may rise to 2 g/100 ml. The proportion of gamma-globulin is raised in most cases. Papilloedema, which occurs in 5–10 per cent of cases, may be due to the increased protein concentration causing impairment of the absorp-tion of cerebrospinal fluid (Morley and Re-ynolds, 1966). Although Guillain *et al.* (1916) emphasised the albuminocytologic dissociation, about a quarter of patients have a raised cell count in the CSF, though rarely to more than 40 cells/mm³. As described in Chapter 6, in-flammatory infiltration with lymphocytes and segmental demyelination involve both the roots and the peripheral nerves. Pathologically, involved nerves show a decrease of maximum conduction velocity to 50 per cent of normal, but studies undertaken early in the condition and in those cases where only the nerve roots are involved, may give entirely normal results. Investigation of the late (F and H) waves of the evoked motor action potential may help to demonstrate this root involvement.

The overall prognosis for recovery is good, considering the parlous state of the patients. It might be hoped that no patient would die, even in those requiring intermittent positive pressure respiration, although most series still have a mortality rate of more than 10 per cent. About 18 per cent of patients followed for more than three years have some residual permanent signs and symptoms. In children, this figure surprisingly rises to 26 per cent (Ravn, 1967). Those more severely paralysed have a worse prognosis; of those on a respirator, 17 per cent remain severely disabled and an additional 10 per cent have residual signs but lead a normal life (Hewer, Hilton, Crampton-Smith and Spalding, 1968). No other features of the disease have been found to assist the forecast.

A less common variation of this condition affects predominantly the cranial nerves including the extraocular muscles, ataxia and areflexia usually being the sole indication of peripheral nerve involvement (Fisher, 1956; Elizan, Spire, Andiman, Baughman and Lloyd-Smith, 1971). Autonomic involvement can also occur in the Guillain-Barré-Strohl syndrome (Appenzeller and Marshall, 1963; Birchfield and Shaw, 1964) and may even occur without peripheral nerve involvement (Thomashefsky et al., 1972). Orthostatic hypotension on tipping patients on a respirator is common, but spontaneous episodes of hypotension, hypertension and cardiac dysrrhythmia may also occur (Hewer et al., 1968; Davies and Dingle, 1972). These may result from partial blockage of the cardiovascular reflexes on the afferent and efferent sides, and from the high circulating levels of catecholamines together with denervation supersensitivity of the blood vessels and heart.

Aetiology. Uncertainty still exists concerning the exact aetiology of this condition, although most agree that a preceding viral infection is often important. The condition may, however, occur following other precipitants such as surgical operations (Arnason and Asbury, 1968). Some authors (Melnick and Flewett, 1964) have found an increased incidence of antibodies to a wide range of viruses in the sera of these patients. In many cases of the Guillain-Barré-Strohl syndrome, antibodies to nervous tissue (Melnick, 1963), circulating myelinotoxins (Cook, Dowling, Murray and Whitaker, 1971) and lymphocytes in the peripheral blood sensitive to peripheral nerve antigen (Knowles, Saunders, Currie, Walton and Field, 1969; Cook, Dowling and Whitaker, 1970; Currie and Knowles, 1971; Caspary, Currie, Walton and Field, 1971) may be found. It has been suggested that those with a higher proportion of reactive lymphocytes in the peripheral blood at the onset of the disease have a worse prognosis (Cook et al., 1970). IgM and complement (Luijtens and Baart de la Faille-Kuyper, 1972), and lymphocytes (Haymaker and Kernohan, 1949; Asbury et al., 1969) are found in the peripheral nerves in the Guillain-Barré-Strohl syndrome. The argument

continues about whether the antibodies or the lymphocytes are the primary cause of the syndrome.

An experimental analogue of this condition is available, namely experimental allergic neuritis (EAN) produced by the injection of peripheral nerve protein together with Freund's adjuvant (Waksman and Adams, 1955, 1956), and this might be expected to help in elucidating the problem. Aström, Webster and Arnason (1968) clearly showed that lymphocytic infiltration of the peripheral nerves preceded pathological alterations in the myelin sheaths and signs of the disease. There are opposing views concerning the role of circulating myelinotoxic agents in EAN, but there seems little doubt that the experimental disease is due to a delayed hypersensitivity reaction of the cellular type.

The question remains as to what attracts the lymphocytes and antibodies into the peripheral nerve. One suggestion is that, during the preceding illness, the virus enters the Schwann cell, replicating there. Lymphocytes and antibodies reacting against this are thereby attracted into the nerve, where they damage the infected Schwann cells. This autoimmune mechanism is similar, therefore, to that suggested for post-viral encephalomyelitis. The finding of similar pathological changes in a proved viral disease of chickens (Marek's disease) supports this suggestion (Wight, 1969). However, cases of the Guillain-Barré-Strohl syndrome arising during immunosuppressive therapy (Drachman, Paterson, Berlin and Roguska, 1970) and following other precipitants show that this is not the whole story.

Treatment. If the autoimmune theory were true, treatment with immunosuppressive agents would be sensible. There is, however, argument about the effectiveness of these agents. Some patients show a dramatic response to corticosteroid therapy, but others show an equally dramatic relapse when the dosage is reduced, and some become corticosteroid-dependent (Matthews, Howell and Hughes, 1970). Heller and DeJong (1963) reviewed cases from the literature, and concluded that ACTH or corticosteroid therapy was beneficial. Prineas (1970a) came to a similar conclusion with patients who received the treatment early in their disease. Ravn (1967) disagreed however, and controlled trials of ACTH and prednisone have failed to show benefit (McQuillen, 1971; Hughes, Newsom-Davis, Perkin and Pearce, 1978). Some authors have reported a beneficial effect of cytotoxic immunosuppressive therapy (Yuill, Swinburn and Liversedge, 1970; Heathfield and Dallos, 1970).

The theoretical objection to such treatment is that when symptoms and signs have appeared, the lymphocytes are already in the nerves. The best time to administer immunosuppressive therapy would be *before* this, which is obviously impossible in the clinical situation. Large double-blind controlled trials are required to elucidate the matter. The author's view is that a short trial of about one week of corticosteroid treatment is indicated when the condition is deteriorating or severe. If there is no improvement, cytotoxic immunosuppressive therapy may be added for the second week. If no improvement results, both treatments are gradually withdrawn. The most important treatment is the general support, including tracheostomy and artificial respiration where required.

Carcinomatous neuropathy

That carcinoma can produce degeneration of the nervous system by its remote effects without direct invasion has been known for more than 40 years (Weber and Hill, 1933; Greenfield, 1934), and carcinomatous cachexia has been known since time immemorial. A number of reviews of carcinomatous neuropathy have appeared (Brain and Norris, 1965; Henson and Urich, 1970b). It is now recognised that a neuropathy may be caused by almost any cancer, but that it is especially common with carcinoma of the bronchus, ovary, breast, and stomach, and the reticuloses. Certain tumours tend to produce certain types of neuropathy. The central nervous and peripheral nervous systems as well as the neuromuscular junction and the muscle may be affected (*see* Chapters 15, 16, and 19). Although some doubt the existence of carcinomatous neuropathy (Wilner and Brody, 1968), and others have suggested that it is predominantly the result of malnutrition (Hildebrand and Coërs, 1967), it is generally acknowledged that there is an increased incidence of these syndromes with carcinoma. In fact, Newman and Gugino (1964) followed up eight patients, who were more than 65 years of age and who had an unexplained neuropathy, and found that all developed carcinoma within 18 months. The number was small, and there was no control series, but this report does illustrate that an occult neoplasm is an important cause of chronic progressive polyneuropathy in old age.

The incidence of carcinomatous polyneuropathy is difficult to define because it depends upon the intensity of the search. Croft and Wilkinson (1965) found 'neuromyopathy' in 16 per cent of patients with carcinoma of the lung, although they included those with simple areflexia which might have been due to ageing. Trojaborg, Frantzen and Andersen (1969) found clinical signs of a peripheral neuropathy in only 5 per cent of patients with carcinoma of the lung, and Hildebrand and Coërs (1967) found such signs in only 4 per cent of a group of patients with various carcinomata. Two to 5 per cent of patients with reticuloses have signs of peripheral neuropathy (Hutchinson *et al.*, 1958; Currie and Henson, 1971). Electrophysiological evidence of peripheral nerve damage was present in 32 per cent of Trojaborg's series, and 41 per cent of Hildebrand and Coërs' series showed histological abnormality of the terminal motor innervation. This was particularly common in wasted patients. The commonest electrophysiological abnormalities are signs of denervation in the EMG, with a slight increase in the terminal latency of motor conduction, although there are normal sensory and motor nerve conduction velocities in the main nerve trunks.

The commonest peripheral nerve disease caused by carcinoma is a mixed sensorimotor distal symmetrical polyneuropathy which makes up more than 80 per cent of such cases (Croft, Urich and Wilkinson, 1967). In some this is an insignificant part of their terminal carcinomatous illness, but in others it is a more severe disease, occasionally relapsing and remitting. A pure sensory neuropathy makes up the remainder of the group, the condition originally having been shown by Denny-Brown (1948) to be due to degeneration of the neurones of the dorsal root ganglia, with perivascular lymphocytic infiltration in the ganglia

(Henson and Urich, 1970b). A form of motor neurone disease has also been reported in association with carcinoma (Brain, Croft and Wilkinson, 1965), but it is uncertain whether this is more than a chance association. The critical criterion of cure of the carcinomatous syndrome following total removal of the carcinoma has been shown in very few patients (*see* Chapters 19 and 20).

There is some uncertainty about the underlying pathology in the mixed sensorimotor neuropathies of carcinoma. Croft *et al.* (1967) found changes suggestive of segmental demyelination in 10 cases, confirmed by teasing the single nerve fibres in two patients. Henson and Urich (1970b) found both axonal degeneration and segmental demyelination, the latter predominating. However, Webster, Schröder, Asbury and Adams (1967) in a patient with bronchial carcinoma, and Walsh (1971) in 5 patients with multiple myeloma, found only axonal degeneration. The aetiology of the condition is uncertain. Lymphocytic infiltration in the peripheral nerves of three of the cases of Croft *et al.* (1967) raised the possibility of an autoimmune process. Another possibility is of a virus which is allowed to infiltrate the nerves as a result of the decreased immunological competence due to the carcinomatous process.

Ischaemic neuropathies and collagen-vascular diseases

As outlined in Chapter 6, although the peripheral nerves have an extensive plexus of blood vessels, occlusion of several major feeding vessels or of many smaller vasa nervorum can cause a neuropathy. This is usually asymmetrical, acute, and mixed sensorimotor in type. Large artery disease causes symptoms which are due to the ischaemic muscles (intermittent claudication) or gangrene of the whole limb, but in a survey of 32 patients with symptomatic arterial disease, 63 per cent showed paraesthesiae (Eames and Lange, 1967). Examination revealed sensory abnormalities in up to 87.5 per cent of cases, usually patchy, asymmetrical and distal in the lower limbs. Depressed ankle jerks were found in 41 per cent; 51 per cent had weakness of one or both legs, and 31 per cent had muscle wasting which was often asymmetrical. Pathological examination often showed severe loss

of myelinated fibres with both Wallerian degeneration and segmental demyelination (Eames and Lange, 1967; Chopra and Hurwitz, 1967). An acute asymmetrical mononeuropathy may occur in subacute bacterial endocarditis because of embolisation of the major feeding vessels (Jones and Seikert, 1968). The proximal ischaemic mononeuropathy of diabetes has already been described, and the part played by ischaemia in the distal symmetrical polyneuropathy of diabetes has been discussed. Ischaemia due to amyloid infiltration of the walls of the blood vessels may play a part in amyloid neuropathy.

Most of the collagen-vascular diseases can damage the nerves by ischaemia. A review of this group of conditions was prepared by Glaser (1970). The incidence of peripheral nerve involvement is highest in polyarteritis nodosa in which up to 20–30 per cent of patients have a neuropathy (Lovshin and Kernohan, 1948; Bleehen, Lovelace and Cotton, 1963). The picture usually is of multiple mononeuropathies with acute lesions of several individual nerves, although later it may blend into a progressive distal symmetrical sensorimotor polyneuropathy. Individual infarcts of the nerve are often painful. Pathology is outlined in Chapter 6. The treatment of polyarteritis nodosa with corticosteroids alone is not completely effective, and combination with cytotoxic immunosuppressive agents is often required.

The incidence of involvement of the peripheral nervous system in systemic lupus erythematosus varies from 3–13 per cent (Dubois, 1966; Johnson and Richardson, 1968), central nervous system involvement being considerably more frequent. Again the pattern is usually of multiple mononeuropathies, although in some patients there is a distal symmetrical sensorimotor polyneuropathy. Occasionally a picture resembling an acute inflammatory polyneuropathy may occur. A peripheral neuropathy can occur in giant cell arteritis (Warrell, Godfrey and Olsen, 1968), scleroderma (Richter, 1954; Kibler and Rose, 1960), dermatomyositis (McEntee and Mancall, 1965) and Wegener's granulomatosis (Stern, 1970).

Several types of clinically symptomatic peripheral neuropathy have been described in rheumatoid arthritis. They are best classified into four types (modified from Pallis and Scott, 1965).

1. *Lesions of the major nerves of the upper and lower limbs.* These comprise 37 per cent of this group of conditions. They are mainly caused by compression of the nerve within a fascial sheath or bony canal by an effusion within a joint, swelling of the joint capsule, osteophytes or displacement of a bone. Lesions of the lateral popliteal nerve at the femoral head and of the median nerve in the carpal tunnel are the commonest, with all the features of an entrapment neuropathy (*see above*). Local injection of corticosteroids or surgical decompression may be required to relieve the pressure. Occasionally such lesions of the major nerves may be due to an underlying arteritis.

2. *Distal symmetrical sensory polyneuropathy of the lower limbs* (35 per cent). This condition is insidious in onset, with paraesthesiae, numbness and loss of pain and vibration sense up to the ankles. The ankle jerks may be absent.

3. *Digital neuropathy* (22 per cent). This condition is caused by individual digital arteries producing sensory loss on one side of one finger. The condition is usually not severe.

4. *Distal symmetrical mixed sensorimotor polyneuropathy of upper and lower extremities.* This is the smallest group (6 per cent) but is the most severe and has the poorest prognosis. It often presents initially as multiple mononeuropathies before progressing to a distal symmetrical sensorimotor polyneuropathy. The course is relatively rapid over a few months, and most patients die within two years from a widespread vasculitis.

All forms of neuropathy are commonest in seropositive patients with nodules (Hart, 1966), and this is particularly true of the fourth (severe) type of neuropathy (Chamberlain and Bruckner, 1970). It has been suggested that corticosteroid therapy of rheumatoid arthritis predisposes to the development of a peripheral neuropathy, although the mechanism is not clear (Ferguson and Slocumb, 1961).

Electrophysiological investigations may help to elucidate the condition in patients with rheumatoid arthritis. In the first type, nerve conduction will show a focal delay at the point of compression. Many patients with the second type of neuropathy have maximum sensory conduction velocities reduced to about 50 per cent of normal, that is to the level expected in segmental demyelination. Patients with the fourth type of neuropathy show little or no slowing of nerve conduction, together with severe EMG evidence of denervation, the whole picture suggesting axonal degeneration (Chamberlain and Bruckner, 1970).

Pathological studies have generally shown a diffuse vasculitis with occlusion of the vasa nervorum, more marked in the fourth type of neuropathy than in the second type. The infarcts are particularly in the upper arm and mid-thigh levels, involving the centre of the fasciculi, and these areas may constitute 'watershed territories' in the peripheral nerves (Dyck, Conn and Okazaki, 1972). The nerves may show segmental demyelination, although Wallerian degeneration predominates, particularly in the more severe cases (Haslock, Wright and Harriman, 1970; Weller, Bruckner and Chamberlain, 1970; Dyck *et al.*, 1972). Treatment is extremely difficult. In the second type of sensory polyneuropathy it is best to avoid corticosteroid therapy as far as possible. In the fourth type of neuropathy, cytotoxic immunosuppressive agents are worthy of trial because of the poor prognosis. D-penicillamine may also be of value (Golding, 1971).

Radiation neuropathy

The peripheral nerves are relatively resistant to X-radiation damage, but may be damaged if they are included in the field of deep X-ray therapy (Innes and Carsten, 1961; Stoll and Andrews, 1966). The commonest radiation damage of peripheral nerves is where the brachial plexus is injured as a result of radiotherapy for carcinoma of the breast, although the lumbosacral plexus may also be damaged by treatment of the pelvic areas. A dose of more than 5000 rads is liable to cause a progressive syndrome of paraesthesiae, muscle weakness and atrophy. Occasionally, as in radiation myelopathy, a sudden onset suggests a vascular occlusion secondary to endarteritis. The progressive syndrome probably also has a vascular basis, radiation damage to parenchymatous elements *per se* being less important. An interval of three months to three years following radiotherapy is usual, and no treatment

Table 21.2 An outline clinical approach to the diagnosis of peripheral neuropathies (from Bradley, 1974)

Clinical type	Clinical Features	Electrophysiology Nerve conduction	EMG	Pathology	Causes
I: Acute severe polyneuropathy	Proximal or ascending. Mainly motor. Artificial ventilation often required. Often little sensory loss	Demyelination type	No abnormality	Segmental demyelination — Lymphocytic infiltration roots and nerves. Only macrophages	Acute inflammatory polyneuropathy of Guillain, Barré and Strohl. Diphtheritic neuropathy
		Bathing trunk area sensory loss	Normal	Denervation	Axonal degeneration roots and nerves. Some segmental demyelination.	Acute hepatic porphyria
II: Single or multiple mononeuropathies	One or several nerves. Acute or subacute. Often painful.	Proximal	Axonal or demyelination type	Denervation	Occlusion of vasa nervorum. Mainly axonal degeneration.	Diabetic amyotrophy. Neuralgic amyotrophy.
		Various	Focal slowing	Normal or mild denervation	Segmental demyelination secondary to nerve compression	Entrapment neuropathies
			No conduction or axonal type	Denervation	Mainly axonal degeneration — Occlusion of vasa nervorum. Focal damage	Collagen-vascular disease. Trauma. Leprosy
III: Distal symmetrical sensorimotor polyneuropathy. Subacute or chronic	Distal preponderance. Lower extremity more than upper. Sensory loss often exceeds motor	Hypertrophic nerves	Demyelination type	Normal	Segmental demyelination, 'onion bulbs'	Hypertrophic neuropathies of Dejerine-Sottas and Charcot-Marie-Tooth types. Refsum's disease. Diabetic polyneuropathy
		Normal size nerves	Mixed type	Moderate denervation	Mixed segmental demyelination and axonal degeneration	Familial: axonal type of Charcot-Marie-Tooth, amyloidosis. Metabolic: uraemia, hepatic, hypoglycaemia. Vitamin deficiency: B_1, B_6, B_{12}. Carcinoma. Toxic. Leprosy. Old age
			Axonal type	Denervation	Mainly axonal degeneration. Some segmental demyelination.	
V: Recurrent polyneuropathy	Relapses and varying degrees of remission. Mixed sensorimotor	Steroid-responsive	Demyelination type	Mild denervation	Segmental demyelination. Some 'onion-bulb' hypertrophy.	Recurrent autoimmune polyneuropathy. Steroid-dependent polyneuropathy
		Non-steroid responsive	Axonal type	Denervation	Axonal degeneration	Ischaemic neuropathies. Tangier disease

is of avail once the neuropathy has started. Immediate and late anterior horn cell degeneration following electrocution injuries may also be mentioned in this context (Panse, 1970).

Nerve tumours

These are outside the scope of this book, and the reader is referred to Russell and Rubinstein (1963) and Kramer (1970).

A DIAGNOSTIC SYNOPSIS

A physician confronted by a list of several hundred causes of peripheral nerve disease has difficulty in separating the wood from the trees when attempting to arrive at a clinical and aetiological diagnosis. This Chapter has been designed to try to bring some order into this situation, the diseases being classified into aetiological groups. However, clinical classification is of more use when attempting to arrive at a diagnosis in a patient.

Peripheral neuropathies may be classified in at least five different ways:

(1) *Rate of progress*—acute, subacute, chronic.

(2) *Distribution*—proximal, distal, diffuse.

(3) *Type of fibre involved*—motor, sensory, mixed; large or small fibre.

(4) *Pattern*—polyneuropathy, mononeuropathy, multiple mononeuropathy, radiculopathy.

(5) *Pathological*—axonal degeneration, segmental demyelination, mixed.

A simplified approach to the diagnosis originally suggested by Asbury (1967, personal communication) is to divide all peripheral neuropathies into:

I *Acute severe polyneuropathies;*
II *Mononeuritis or mononeuritis multiplex;*
III *Subacute or chronic distal symmetrical sensorimotor polyneuropathy;*
IV *Recurrent and hypertrophic polyneuropathy.*

The order of this classification is dictated by the diagnostic approach, and not by the frequency of the individual types of presentation. Type III is by far the largest group, and the most difficult in which to diagnose the underlying aetiology. Some further sub-divisions and aetiological factors are shown in Table 21.2, which is intended neither to be complete, nor to be like a diagnostic 'multiple-choice paper', but rather to indicate the lines of thought that are required to diagnose the cause of the disease in a patient presenting with a peripheral neuropathy.

REFERENCES

(N.B. Any references quoted in the text of this Chapter and not found in this bibliography will be found in the reference list which follows Chapter 6).

Adams, R.D., Asbury, A.K. & Michelsen, J.J. (1965) Multifocal pseudohypertrophic neuropathy. *Transactions of the American Neurological Association*, **90**, 30.

Andersson, R. (1970) Hereditary amyloidosis with polyneuropathy. *Acta medica Scandinavica*, **188**, 85–94.

Andersson, R. & Blom, S. (1972) Neurophysiological studies in hereditary amyloidosis with polyneuropathy. *Acta medica Scandinavica*, **191**, 233.

Andrade, C. (1952) A peculiar form of peripheral neuropathy. Familial atypical generalised amyloidosis with special involvement of the peripheral nerves. *Brain*, **75**, 408.

Andrade, C., Araki, S., Block, W.D., Cohen, A.S., Jackson, C.E., Kuroiwa, Y., McKusick, V.A., Nissim, J., Sohar, E. & Van Allen, M.W. (1970) Hereditary amyloidosis. *Arthritis and Rheumatism*, **13**, 902.

Antia, N.H., Pandya, S.S. & Dastur, D.K. (1970) Nerves in the arm in leprosy. I: Clinical, electrodiagnostic and operative aspects. *International Journal of Leprosy*, **38**, 12.

Appenzeller, O. & Marshall, J. (1963) Vasomotor disturbance in Landry-Guillain-Barré syndrome. *Archives of Neurology*, **9**, 368.

Appenzeller, O. & Richardson, E.P. (1966) The sympathetic chain in patients with diabetes and alcoholic polyneuropathy. *Neurology (Minneapolis)*, **16**, 1205.

Appenzeller, O., Kornfield, M. & McGee, J. (1971) Neuropathy in chronic renal disease. A microscopic, ultrastructural and biochemical study of sural nerve biopsy. *Archives of Neurology*, **24**, 449.

Araki, S., Mawatari, S., Ohta, M., Nakajima, A. & Kuroiwa, Y. (1968) Polyneuritic amyloidosis in a Japanese family. *Archives of Neurology*, **18**, 593.

Arnason, B.G. & Asbury, A.K. (1968) Idopathic polyneuritis after surgery. *Archives of Neurology*, **18**, 500.

Arnold, N. & Harriman, D.G.F. (1970) The incidence of abnormality in control human peripheral nerves studied by single axon dissection. *Journal of Neurology, Neurosurgery and Psychiatry*, **33**, 55.

Asbury, A.K., Victor, M. & Adams, R.D. (1963) Uraemic polyneuropathy. *Archives of Neurology*, **8**, 413.

Aspinall, D.L. (1964) Multiple deficiency state associated with isoniazid therapy. *British Medical Journal*, **2**, 1177.

Aström, K.E., Webster, H. de F. & Arnason, B.G. (1968) The initial lesion in experimental allergic neuritis. A phase and electron microscopic study. *Journal of Experimental Medicine*, **128**, 469.

Austin, J.H. (1958) Recurrent polyneuropathies and their corticosteroid treatment. *Brain*, **81**, 157.

Bannister, R. (1971) Degeneration in the autonomic nervous system. *Lancet*, **2**, 175.

Baxter, D.W. & Olszewski, J. (1960) Congenital universal insensitivity to pain. *Brain*, **83**, 381.

Birchfield, R.J. & Shaw, C.M. (1964) Postural hypotension in the Guillain-Barré syndrome. *Archives of Neurology* **10**, 149.

Bleehan, S.S., Lovelace, R.E. & Cotton, R.E. (1963) Mononeuritis multiplex in polyarteritis nodosa. *Quarterly Journal of Medicine*, **32**, 193.

Boddingius, J. (1972) Ultrastructural changes in peripheral nerves in leprosy. *Journal of Anatomy*, **111**, 516.

Bosch, E.P., Pierach, C.A., Bossenmaier, I., Cardinal, R. & Thorson, M. (1977) Effect of hematin in porphyric neuropathy. *Neurology (Minneapolis)*, **27**, 1053.

Bradley, W.G. (1967) Unpublished observations.

Bradley, W.G. (1970) The neuromyopathy of vincristine in the guinea pig. An electrophysiological and pathological study. *Journal of the Neurological Sciences*, **10**, 133.

Bradley, W.G. (1974) *Disorders of Peripheral Nerves* (Blackwell Scientific Publications: Oxford).

Bradley, W.G. (1975a) Myelopathies affecting anterior horn cells. In *Peripheral Neuropathies*, Eds P.J. Dyck, P.K. Thomas & E.H. Lambert, Chap. V. Cl (Saunders: London).

Bradley, W.G. (1975b) Diseases of spinal roots. In *Peripheral Neuropathies*. Eds. P.J. Dyck, P.K. Thomas & E.H. Lambert, Chap. V. C2 (Saunders: London).

Bradley, W.G. & Aguayo, A. (1969) Hereditary chronic neuropathy. Electrophysiological and pathological studies in an affected family. *Journal of the Neurological Sciences*, **9**, 131.

Bradley, W.G., Madrid, R. & Davis, C.J.F. (1977) The peroneal muscular atrophy syndrome. Part 3: Clinical, electrophysiological and pathological correlations. *Journal of the Neurological Sciences*, **32**, 123.

Bradley, W.G., Lassman, L.P., Pearce, G.W. & Walton, J.N. (1970) The neuromyopathy of vincristine in man. Clinical, electrophysiological and pathological studies. *Journal of the Neurological Sciences*, **10**, 107.

Brain, W.R., Croft, P.B. & Wilkinson, M. (1965) Motor neurone disease as a manifestation of neoplasm. *Brain*, **88**, 479.

Brain, Lord & Norris, F.H. Jr. Eds. (1965) *The Remote Effects of Cancer on the Nervous System* (Grune and Stratton: New York).

Brewis, M., Poskanzer, D.C., Rolland, C. & Miller, H. (1966) Neurological disease in an English city. *Acta neurological Scandinavica*, Suppl. **24**, 1.

Bruns, L. (1890) Über neuritische Lähmungen beim Diabetes mellitus. *Berlinen klinische Wochenschrift*, **27**, 509.

Bruyn, G.W. & Garland, H. (1970) Neuropathies of endocrine origin. In *Handbook of Clinical Neurology*, Vol. 8, Eds. P.J. Vinken & G.W. Bruyn, pp. 29–71 (North Holland: Amsterdam).

Bureau, Y., Barrière, H., Kerneis, J.-P. & de Ferron, A. (1957) Acropathies ulcero-mutilantes pseudosyringomyliques non-familiales des membres inférieurs. *Presse médicale*, **65**, 2127.

Cambier, J. & Brunet, P. (1970) *Le syndrome de Guillain et Barré* (Ballière et fils: Paris).

Campbell, A.M.G. (1970) Hereditary sensory neuropathy. In *Handbook of Clinical Neurology*, Vol. 8, Eds. P.J. Vinken & G.W. Bruyn, pp. 180–186 (North Holland: Amsterdam).

Campbell, M.J. & McComas, A.J. (1970) The effects of ageing on muscle function. *5th Symposium on Current Research in Muscular Dystrophy* (Abstract) (Muscular Dystrophy Group: London).

Casey, E.B. & Harrison, M.J.G. (1972) Diabetic amyotrophy: a follow-up study. *British Medical Journal*, **1**, 656.

Cavanagh, J.B. (1967) Pattern of change in peripheral nerves produced by isoniazid intoxication in rats. *Journal of Neurology, Neurosurgery and Psychiatry*, **30**, 26.

Cavanagh, J.B. & Ridley, A.R. (1967) The nature of the neuropathy complicating acute intermittent porphyria. *Lancet*, **2**, 1023.

Cazzato, G. (1965) Rapporti fra 'poliradiculonevrite recidivanti' e 'nevrite interstiziale ipertrofica progressiva sporadica dell'adulto'. *Rivistadi patologia nervosa e mentale*, **86**, 325.

Chamberlain, M.A. & Bruckner, F.E. (1970) Rheumatoid neuropathy. Clinical and electrophysiological features. *American Journal of Rheumatic Diseases*, **29**, 609.

Charcot, J.M. & Marie, P. (1886) Sur une forme particulière d'atrophie musculaire progressive souvent familial débutant par les pieds et les jambes et atteignant plus tard les mains. *Revue de médecine (Paris)*, **6**, 97.

Chochinov, R.H., Ullyot, L.E. & Moorhouse, J.A. (1972) Sensory thresholds in patients with juvenile diabetes and their close relatives. *New England Journal of Medicine*, **286**, 1233.

Chopra, J.S. & Hurwitz, L.J. (1968) Femoral nerve conduction in diabetes and chronic occlusive vascular disease. *Journal of Neurology, Neurosurgery and Psychiatry*, **31**, 28.

Chopra, J.S., Hurwitz, L.J. & Montgomery, D.A.D. (1969) The pathogenesis of sural nerve changes in diabetes mellitus. *Brain*, **92**, 391.

Collins, G.H., Webster, H. de F. & Victor, M. (1964) The ultrastructure of myelin and axonal alterations in sciatic nerves of thiamine deficient and chronically starved rats. *Acta neuropathologica (Berlin)*, **3**, 511.

Cook, S.D., Dowling, P.C. & Whitaker, J.N. (1970) The Guillain-Barré syndrome. Relationship of circulating immunocytes to disease activity. *Archives of Neurology* **22**, 470.

Cook, S.D., Dowling, P.C., Murray, M.R. & Whitaker, J.N. (1971) Circulating demyelinating factors in acute idiopathic polyneuritis. *Archives of Neurology*, **24**, 136.

Cooke, W.T. & Smith, W.T. (1966) Neurological disorders associated with adult coeliac disease. *Brain*, **89**, 683.

Cooke, W.T., Johnson, A.G. & Woolf, A.L. (1966) Vital staining and electron microscopy of the intramuscular nerve endings in the neuropathy of adult coeliac disease. *Brain*, **89**, 663.

Corbin, K.B. & Gardner, E.D. (1937) Decrease in number of myelinated fibres of human spinal roots with age. *Anatomical Record*, **68**, 63.

Cottrell, L. (1940) Histologic variations with age in apparently normal nerve trunks. *Archives of Neurology and Psychiatry*, **43**, 1138.

Cragg, B.G. & Thomas, P.K. (1964) Changes in nerve

conduction in experimental allergic neuritis. *Journal of Neurology, Neurosurgery and Psychiatry*, **27**, 106.

Critchley, M. (1931) The neurology of old age. *Lancet*, **2**, 1119, 1221, 1331.

Croft, P.B. & Wilkinson, M. (1965) The incidence of carinomatous neuromyopathy in patients with various types of carcinoma. *Brain*, **88**, 427.

Croft, P.B., Urich, H. & Wilkinson, M. (1967) Peripheral neuropathy of sensorimotor type associated with malignant disease. *Brain*, **90**, 31.

Cruikshank, E.K. (1952) Dietary neuropathies. *Vitamins and Hormones*, **10**, 1.

Currie, S. & Henson, R.A. (1971) Neurological syndromes in the reticuloses. *Brain*, **94**, 307.

Currie, S. & Knowles, M. (1971) Lymphocyte transformation in the Guillain-Barré syndrome. *Brain*, **94**, 109.

Danta, G. (1969) Hypoglycaemic peripheral neuropathy. *Archives of Neurology*, **21**, 121.

Davies, A.G. & Dingle, H.R. (1972) Observations on cardiovascular and neuroendocrine disturbances in the Guillain-Barré syndrome. *Journal of Neurology, Neurosurgery and Psychiatry*, **35**, 176.

Davis, C.J.F., Bradley, W.G. & Madrid, R. (1979) The peroneal muscular atrophy syndrome. 1: Clinical, genetic, and electrophysiological findings and classification. *Journal de génétique humaine*, **26**, 311.

Dayan, A.D. & Williams, R. (1967) Demyelinating peripheral neuropathy and liver disease. *Lancet*, **2**, 133.

Dayan, A.D., Gardner-Thorpe, C., Down, P.F. & Gleadle, R. (1970) Peripheral neuropathy in uraemia. Pathological studies of peripheral nerves from 6 patients. *Neurology (Minneapolis)*, **20**, 649.

Dejerine, J. & Andre-Thomas (1906) Sur la névrite interstitielle et hypertrophique de l'enfance (Observation suivie d'autopsie). *Nouvelle iconographie de la Salpètriène*, **19**, 477.

Denny-Brown, D. (1948) Primary sensory neuropathy with muscular changes associated with carcinoma. *Journal of Neurology, Neurosurgery and Psychiatry*, **11**, 73.

Denny-Brown, D. (1951) Hereditary sensory radicular neuropathy. *Journal of Neurology, Neurosurgery and Psychiatry*, **14**, 237.

Dinn, J.J. & Crane, D.L. (1970) Schwann cell dysfunction in uraemia. *Journal of Neurology, Neurosurgery and Psychiatry*, **33**, 605.

Drachman, D.A., Paterson, P.Y., Berlin, B. & Roguska, J. (1970) Immunosuppression and the Guillain-Barré syndrome. *Archives of Neurology*, **23**, 385.

Dubois, E.L. Ed. (1966) *Lupus Erythematosus* (McGraw-Hill: New York).

Duchen, L.W. (1970) Changes in motor innervation and cholinesterase localization induced by botulinum toxin and skeletal muscle of the mouse: difference between fast and slow muscles. *Journal of Neurology, Neurosurgery and Psychiatry*, **33**, 40.

Ducker, T.B., Kempe, L.G. & Hayes, G.J. (1969) The metabolic background for peripheral nerve surgery. *Journal of Neurosurgery*, **30**, 270.

Dyck, P.J. (1980) Personal communication.

Dyck, P.J. & Lambert, E.H. (1968a) Lower motor and primary sensory neuron diseases with peroneal muscular atrophy. I: Neurologic, genetic and electrophysiologic findings in hereditary polyneuropathies. *Archives of Neurology*, **18**, 603.

Dyck, P.J. & Lambert, E.H. (1968b) II: Neurologic, genetic and electrophysiologic findings in various neuronal degenerations. *ibid*, **18**, 619.

Dyck, P.J. & Lambert, E.H. (1970) Polyneuropathy associated with hypothyroidism. *Journal of Neuropathology and Experimental Neurology*, **29**, 631.

Dyck, P.J., Lambert, E.H. & Nichols, P.C. (1971) Quantitative measurement of sensation related to compound action potential and number of sizes of myelinated and unmyelinated fibres of sural nerve in health, Friedreich's ataxia, hereditary sensory neuropathy and tabes dorsalis. *Handbook of Electroencephalography and Clinical Neurophysiology*, Vol. 9, pp. 9–83 (North Holland: Amsterdam).

Dyck, P.J., Schultz, P.W. & O'Brien, P.C. (1972) Quantitation of touch-pressure sensation. *Archives of Neurology*, **26**, 465.

Dyck, P.J., Thomas, P.K. & Lambert, E.H. (1975) *Peripheral Neuropathy* (Saunders: London).

Elizan, T.S., Spire, J.P., Andiman, R.M., Baughman, F.A. & Lloyd-Smith, D.L. (1971) Syndrome of acute idiopathic ophthalmoplegia with ataxia and areflexia. *Neurology (Minneapolis)*, **21**, 281.

Elkington, J. St. C. (1952) Recent work on the peripheral neuropathies. *Proceedings of the Royal Society of Medicine*, **45**, 661.

Ellenberg, M. (1971) Impotence in diabetes: the neurologic factor. *Annals of Internal Medicine*, **75**, 213.

Engel, W.K., Dorman, J.D., Levy, R.I. & Fredrickson, D.S. (1967) Neuropathy in Tangier disease. *Archives of Neurology*, **17**, 1.

Erbslöh, F. & Abel, M. (1970) Deficiency neuropathies. In *Handbook of Clinical Neurology*, Vol. 7, Eds P.J. Vinken & G.W. Bruyn, pp. 558–663 (North Holland: Amsterdam).

Evans, D.A.P. (1963) Pharmacogenetics. *American Journal of Medicine*, **34**, 639.

Evans, D.A.P., Manley K.A. & McKusick, V.A. (1960) Genetic control of isoniazid metabolism in man. *British Medical Journal*, **2**, 485.

Evans, M.H. (1969) Mechanism of saxitoxin and tetrodotoxin poisoning. *British Medical Bulletin*, **25**, 263.

Fabré, S. (1965) Les expressions péripheriques de la neuropathie végétative du diabète sucre. *Montpellier médical*, **67**, 104.

Fagerberg, S.-E. (1959) Diabetic neuropathy. A clinical and histological study on the significance of vascular affections. *Acta medica Scandinavica, Supplement*, **343**, 5.

Farquhar, J.W. & Ways, P. (1966) Abetalipoproteinemia. In *Metabolic Basis of Inherited Diseases*, 2nd Edn. Eds J.B. Stanbury, J.B. Wyngaarden & D.S. Fredrickson, pp. 509–522 (McGraw-Hill: New York).

Fennely, J., Frank, O., Baker, H. & Leevy, C.M. (1964) Peripheral neuropathy of the alcoholic. Aetiologic role of aneurin and other B-complex vitamins. *British Medical Journal*, **2**, 1290.

Ferguson, R.H. & Slocumb, C.H. (1961) Peripheral neuropathy in rheumatoid arthritis. *Bulletin on Rheumatic Diseases*, **11**, 251.

Fincham, R.W. & Cape, C.A. (1968) Neuropathy in myxoedema. *Neurology (Minneapolis)*, **19**, 464.

Fisher, C.M. (1956) An unusual variant of acute idiopathic polyneuritis (syndrome of ophthalmoplegia, ataxia and areflexia). *Journal of Medicine*, **255**, 57.

Follis, R.H. Jr. & Wintrobe, M.M. (1945) A comparison of

the effects of pyridoxine and pantothenic acid deficiency on nervous tissue of swine. *Journal of Experimental Medicine*, **81**, 539.

Fullerton, P.M. (1966) Chronic peripheral neuropathy produced by lead poisoning in guinea pigs. *Journal of Neuropathology and Experimental Neurology*, **25**, 214.

Gamstorp, I., Shelburne, S.A. Jr., Engelson, G., Redondo, D. & Traisman, H.S. (1966) Peripheral neuropathy in juvenile diabetes. *Diabetes*, **15**, 411.

Gardner, E.D. (1940) Decrease in human neurones with age. *Anatomical Record*, **77**, 529.

Garland, H. (1955) Diabetic amyotrophy. *British Medical Journal*, **2**, 1287.

Garland, H. & Taverner, D. (1953) Diabetic myelopathy. *British Medical Journal*, **1**, 1405.

Glaser. G.H. (1970) Neuropathies in collagen diseases. In *Handbook of Clinical Neurology*, Vol. 8. Eds P.J. Vinken & G.W. Bruyn, pp. 118–130 (North Holland: Amsterdam).

Golding, D.N. (1971) Rheumatoid neuropathy. *British Medical Journal*, **2**, 169.

Goodman, J.J. (1954) Femoral neuropathy in relation to diabetes mellitus. *Diabetes*, **3**, 266.

Grabow, J.D. & Chou, S.M. (1968) Thyrotropin hormone deficiency with a peripheral neuropathy. *Archives of Neurology*, **19**, 284.

Greenbaum, D. (1964) Observations on the homogeneous nature and pathogenesis of diabetic neuropathy. *Brain*, **87**, 215.

Greene, L.F., Kelalis, P.P. & Weeks, R.E. (1963) Retrograde ejaculation of semen due to diabetic neuropathy. Report of 4 cases. *Fertility and Sterility*, **14**, 617.

Greenfield, J.G. (1934) Subacute spinocerebellar degeneration occurring in elderly patients. *Brain*, **57**, 161.

Gregersen, G. (1967) Diabetic neuropathy: influence of age, sex, metabolic control, and duration of diabetes on motor conduction velocity. *Neurology (Minneapolis)*, **17**, 972.

Gregersen, G. (1968a) Latency time, maximal amplitude and electromyography in diabetic patients. *Acta medica Scandinavica*, **183**, 55.

Gregersen, G. (1968b) Vibratory perception threshold and motor conduction velocity in diabetes and non-diabetics. *ibid.*, **183**, 61.

Guillain, G., Barré, J. & Strohl, H. (1916) Sur un syndrome de radiculonévrite avec hyperalbuminose du liquide céphalo-rachidien sans reaction cellulaire. *Bulletin et mémoires de la Société médicale des hôpitaux de Paris*. 1462.

Hamfelt, A. & Wetterberg, L. (1968) Neuropathy in porphyria. *Lancet*, **1**, 50.

Harriman, D.G.F., Taverner, D. & Woolf, A.L. (1970) Ekbom's syndrome and burning paraesthesiae. A biopsy study by vital staining and electron microscopy of the intramuscular innervation, with a note on the age changes in motor nerve endings in distal muscles. *Brain*, **93**, 393.

Hart, F.D. (1966) Complicated rheumatoid disease. *British Medical Journal*, **2**, 131.

Haslock, D.I., Wright, V. & Harriman, D.G.F. (1970) Neuromuscular disorders in rheumatoid arthritis. A motor-point biopsy study. *Quarterly Journal of Medicine*, **39**, 335.

Haymaker, W. & Kernohan, J.W. (1949) The Landry-Guillain-Barré syndrome. *Medicine (Baltimore)*, **28**, 59.

Heathfield, K. & Dallos, V. (1970) Treatment of polyneuropathy with azathioprine. *Lancet*, **2**, 1030.

Heirons, R. (1957) Changes in the nervous system in acute porphyria. *Brain*, **80**, 176.

Heller, G.L. & DeJong, R.N. (1963) Treatment of the Guillain-Barré syndrome: use of corticotropin and glucocorticoids. *Archives of Neurology*, **8**, 179.

Hensley, G.T. & Soergel, K.H. (1968) Neuropathologic findings in diabetic diarrhoea. *Archives of Pathology*, **85**, 587.

Henson, R.A. & Urich, H. (1970a) Metabolic neuropathies. In *Handbook of Clinical Neurology*, Vol. 8. Eds P.J. Vinken & G.W. Bruyn, pp. 1–28 (North Holland: Amsterdam).

Henson, R.A., & Urich, H. (1970b) Peripheral neuropathy associated with malignant disease. In *Handbook of Clinical Neurology*, Vol. 8. Eds P.J. Vinken & G.W. Bruyn, pp. 131–148 (North Holland: Amsterdam).

Hewer, R.L., Hilton, P.J., Crampton-Smith, A. & Spalding, J.M.K. (1968) Acute polyneuritis requiring artificial respiration. *Quarterly Journal of Medicine*, **37**, 479.

Hildebrand, J. & Coërs, C. (1967) Neuromuscular function in patients with malignant tumours. *Brain*, **90**, 67.

Hirson, C., Feinmann, E.L. & Wade, H.J. (1953) Diabetic neuropathy. *British Medical Journal*, **1**, 1408.

Hockaday, T.D.R., Hockaday, J.M. & Rushworth, G. (1966) Motor neuropathy associated with abnormal pyruvate metabolism unaffected by thiamine. *Journal of Neurology, Neurosurgery and Psychiatry*, **29**, 119.

Hoffmann, J. (1964) Peripheral neuropathy in children with diabetes mellitus. *Acta neurologica Scandinavica, Suppl.*, **8**, 1.

Hopf, H.C. (1963) Electromyographic study on so-called mononeuritis. *Archives of Neurology*, **9**, 307.

Hopkins, A.P. & Morgan-Hughes, J.A. (1969) Effect of local pressure in diphtheritic neuropathy. *Journal of Neurology, Neurosurgery and Psychiatry*, **32**, 614.

Horwitz, S.J., Klipstein, F.A. & Lovelace, R.E. (1967) Folic acid and neuropathy in epilepsy. *Lancet*, **2**, 1305.

Howell, T.H. (1949) Senile deterioration of the central nervous system. A clinical study. *British Medical Journal*, **1**, 56.

Hughes, J.T., Brownell, B. & Hewer, R.L. (1968) The peripheral sensory pathway in Friedreich's ataxia. An examination by light and electron microscopy of posterior nerve roots, posterior root ganglia and peripheral sensory nerves in cases of Friedreich's ataxia. *Brain*, **91**, 803.

Hughes, R.A.C., Newsom Davis, J.M., Perkin, J.D. & Pearce, J.M. (1978) Controlled trial of prednisolone in acute polyneuropathy. *Lancet*, **2**, 750.

Hutchinson, E.C., Leonard, B.J., Maudsley, C. & Yates, P.C. (1958) Neurological complications of reticuloses. *Brain*, **81**, 75.

Innes, J.R.M. & Carsten, A. (1961) Delayed effects of localised x-irradiation on the nervous system of experimental rats and monkeys. *Brookhaven Symposia in Biology*, **14**, 200.

Jebsen, R.H., Tenckhoff, H. & Honet, J.C. (1967) Natural history of uraemic polyneuropathy and effects of dialysis. *New England Medical Journal*, **277**, 327.

Jennekens, F.G.I., Tomlinson, B.E. & Walton, J.N. (1971) Data on the distribution of fibre types in five human limb muscles. An autopsy study. *Journal of the Neurological Sciences*, **14**, 245.

Jewesbury, E.C.O. (1970) Congenital indifference to pain. In *Handbook of Clinical Neurology*, Vol. 8. Eds P.J. Vinken & G.W. Bruyn, pp. 187–204 (North Holland: Amsterdam).

Johnson, R.T. & Richardson, E.P. (1968) The neurological manifestations of systemic lupus erythematosus. *Medicine (Baltimore)*, **47**, 333.

Jones, H.R. & Siekert, R.G. (1968) Embolic mononeuropathy and bacterial endocarditis. *Archives of Neurology*, **19**, 535.

Kaeser, H.E. (1970) Nerve conduction velocity measurements. In *Handbook of Clinical Neurology*, Vol. 7. Eds P.J. Vinken & G.W. Bruyn, p. 116 (North Holland: Amsterdam).

Khan, M.A., Wakefield, G.S. & Pugh, D.W. (1969) Vitamin B_{12} deficiency and diabetic neuropathy. *Lancet*, **2**, 768.

Kibler, R.F. & Rose, F.C. (1960) Peripheral neuropathy in the 'collagen diseases'. A case of scleroderma neuropathy. *British Medical Journal*, **1**, 1781.

Klenk, E. & Kahlke, W. (1963) Über das Vorkommen, der 3, 7, 11, 15-tetra-methyl-Hexadecansaure in den Cholisterniestern und anderen Lipoidfraktionen der Organe bein einem Krankheitsfall unbebannter Genese (Verdacht auf Heredopathia atactica polyneuritiformis (Refsum-Syndrom)). *Hoppe-Seyler's Zeitschrift für physiologische Chemie*, **333**, 133.

Knill-Jones, R.P., Goodwill, C.J., Dayan, A.D. & Williams, R. (1972) Peripheral neuropathy in chronic liver disease: clinical, electrodiagnostic and nerve biopsy findings. *Journal of Neurology, Neurosurgery and Psychiatry*, **35**, 22.

Knowles, M., Saunders, M., Currie, S., Walton, J.N. & Field, E.J. (1969) Lymphocyte transformation in the Guillain-Barré syndrome. *Lancet*, **2**, 1168.

Kocen, R.S., Lloyd, J.K., Lascelles, P.T., Fosbrooke, A.S. & Williams, D. (1967) Familial lipoprotein deficiency (Tangier disease) with neurological abnormalities. *Lancet*, **1**, 1341.

Kocen, R.S. & Thomas, P.K. (1970) Peripheral nerve involvement in Fabry's disease. *Archives of Neurology*, **22**, 81.

Kominami, N., H.R., Hampers, C.L. & Merritt, J.P. (1971) Variations in motor nerve conduction velocity in normal and uraemic patients. *Archives of Internal Medicine*, **128**, 235.

Konotey-Ahulu, F.I.D., Baillod, R., Comty, C.M., Heron, J.R., Shaldon, S. & Thomas, P.K. (1965) Effect of periodic dialysis on the peripheral neuropathy of end-stage renal failure. *British Medical Journal*, **2**, 1212.

Kopell, H.P. & Thompson, W.A.L. (1976) *Peripheral Entrapment Neuropathies*. 2nd Edn. (Williams and Wilkins: Baltimore).

Lai, C.S. & Ransome, G.A. (1970) Burning feet syndrome: a case due to malabsorption and responding to riboflavine. *British Medical Journal*, **2**, 151.

Lambert, E.H. & Dyck, P.J. (1968) Compound action potentials of human sural nerve biopsies. *Electroencephalography and Clinical Neurophysiology*, **25**, 399.

Lambird, P.A. & Hartmann, W.H. (1969) Hereditary amyloidosis, the flexor retinaculum and the carpal tunnel syndrome. *American Journal of Clinical Pathology*, **52**, 714.

Landry, O. (1859) Note sur la paralysie ascendante aigue. *Gazette hebdomadaire de médicine et de Chirugie*, **6**, 472; 486.

Lascelles, R.G. & Thomas, P.K. (1966) Changes due to age in internodal length in sural nerve in man. *Journal of Neurology, Neurosurgery and Psychiatry*, **29**, 40.

Lawrence, D.G. & Locke, S. (1963) Neuropathy in children with diabetes mellitus. *British Medical Journal*, **1**, 784.

Lindén, L. (1962) Amyotrophia diabetica. *Svenska Lakantidningen*, **59**, 3368.

Lovshin, L.L. & Kernohan, J.W. (1948) Peripheral neuritis in periarteritis nodosa. *Archives of Internal Medicine*, **82**, 321.

Ludin, H.P., Spiess, H. & Koenig, M.P. (1969) Neuromuscular dysfunction associated with thyrotoxicosis. *European Neurology*, **2**, 269.

Luijtens, J.A.F.M. & Baart de la Faille-Kuyper, E.H. (1972) The occurrence of IgM and complement factors along myelin sheaths of peripheral nerves. An immunohistochemical study of the Guillain-Barré syndrome. *Journal of the Neurological Sciences*, **15**, 219.

McEntee, W.J. & Mancall, E.L. (1965) Neuromyositis: a reappraisal. *Neurology (Minneapolis)*, **15**, 69.

McLeod, J.G. (1971) An electrophysiological and pathological study of peripheral nerves in Friedreich's ataxia. *Journal of the Neurological Sciences*, **12**, 333.

McLeod, J.G., Walsh, J.C. & Little, J.M. (1969) Sural nerve biopsy. *Medical Journal of Australia*, **ii**, 1092.

McQuillen, M.P. (1971) Idiopathic polyneuritis: several studies of nerve and immune functions. *Journal of Neurology, Neurosurgery and Psychiatry*, **34**, 607.

Madrid, R., Bradley, W.G. & Davis, C.J.F. (1977) The peroneal muscular atrophy syndrome. Part 2: Observations on the pathological changes in sural nerve biopsies. *Journal of the Neurological Sciences*, **32**, 91.

Malins, J.M. & Mayne, N. (1969) Diabetic diarrhea. *Diabetes*, **18**, 858.

Martin, M.M. (1953) Diabetic neuropathy. A clinical study of 150 cases. *Brain*, **76**, 594.

Matthews, W.B. (1952) Cryptogenic polyneuritis. *Proceedings of the Royal Society of Medicine*, **45**, 667.

Matthews, W.B., Howell, D.A. & Hughes, R.C. (1970) Relapsing corticosteroid-dependent polyneuritis. *Journal of Neurology, Neurosurgery and Psychiatry*, **33**, 330.

Mayer, R.F. (1965) Peripheral nerve function in vitamin B_{12} deficiency. *Archives of Neurology*, **13**, 355.

Melnick, S.C. (1963) Thirty-eight cases of the Guillain-Barré syndrome: an immunological study. *British Medical Journal*, **1**, 368.

Melnick, S.C. & Flewett, T.H. (1964) Role of infection in the Guillain-Barré syndrome. *Journal of Neurology, Neurosurgery and Psychiatry*, **27**, 395.

Melzack, R. & Wall, P.D. (1965) Pain mechanisms: a new theory. *Science*, **150**, 971.

Meyer, U.A., Strand, L.J., Doss, M., Rees, A.C. & Marver, H.S. (1972) Acute intermittent porphyria: demonstration of a genetic defect in porphobilinogen metabolism. *New England Journal of Medicine*, **286**, 1277.

Moorhouse, J.A., Carter, S.A. & Doupe, J. (1966) Vascular responses in diabetic peripheral neuropathy. *British Medical Journal*, **1**, 883.

Morley, J.B. & Reynolds, E.H. (1966) Papilloedema and the Landry-Guillain-Barré syndrome. *Brain*, **89**, 205.

Mota-Revetllat, J. (1966) Acropatia ulceromutilante: enfermedad de Thévenard. Forme esporadica. *Medicina Clinica (Barcelona)*, **47**, 322.

Murray, I.P.C. & Simpson, J.A. (1958) Acroparaesthesia in myxoedema: a clinical and electromyographic study. *Lancet*, **1**, 1360.

Newman, M.K. & Gugino, R.J. (1964) Neuropathies and myopathies associated with occult malignancies. *Journal of the American Medical Association*, **190**, 575.

Nickel, S.N. & Frame, B. (1958) Neurologic manifestations of myxedema. *Neurology (Minneapolis)*, **81**, 511.

Nielsen, V.K. (1971) The peripheral nerve function in chronic renal failure. *Acta medica Scandinavica*, **190**, 105.

Ochoa, J. (1970) Isoniazid neuropathy in man. Quantitative electron microscopic study. *Brain*, **93**, 831.

Ochoa, J. & Mair, W.G.P. (1969a) The normal sural nerve in man. I: Ultrastructure and numbers of fibres and cells. *Acta neuropathologica (Berlin)*, **13**, 197.

Ochoa, J. & Mair, W.G.P. (1969b) The normal sural nerve in man. II: Changes in the axons and Schwann cells due to ageing. *ibid*, **13**, 217.

Osler, L.D. & Sidell, A.D. (1960) The Guillain-Barré syndrome. The need for exact diagnostic criteria. *New England Journal of Medicine*, **262**, 964.

Pallis, C.A. & Scott, J.T. (1965) Peripheral neuropathy in rheumatoid arthritis. *British Medical Journal*, **1**, 1141.

Panse, F. (1970) Electrical lesions of the nervous system. In *Handbook of Clinical Neurology*, Vol. 7. Eds P.J. Vinken & G.W. Bruyn, pp. 344–387 (North Holland: Amsterdam).

Pearson, G.H.J. (1928) The effect of age on vibratory sensibility. *Archives of Neurology and Psychiatry*, **20**, 482.

Pickering, G.W. (1960) The anatomical and functional aspects of the neurological lesions of diabetes. *Proceedings of the Royal Society of Medicine*, **53**, 142.

Pleasure, D.E., Lovelace, R.E. & Duvoisin, R.C. (1968) Prognosis of acute polyradiculoneuritis. *Neurology (Minneapolis)*, **18**, 1143.

Pollard, J.D., Guy, R.S. & McLeod, J.G. (1971) Peripheral nerve grafting. *Proceedings of the IInd International Congress on Muscle Diseases*. Perth: Western Australia.

Pratt, R.T.C. (1967) *The Genetics of Neurological Disorders* (Oxford University Press: London).

Preswick, G. & Jeremy, D. (1964) Subclinical polyneuropathy in renal insufficiency. *Lancet*, **2**, 731.

Prineas, J. (1970a) Polyneuropathies of undetermined cause. *Acta neurologica Scandinavica, Suppl.* **44**, 1.

Prineas, J. (1970b) Peripheral nerve changes in thiamine-deficient rats. An electron microscopic study. *Archives of Neurology*, **23**, 541.

Ravn, H. (1967) The Landry-Guillain-Barré syndrome. *Acta neurologica Scandinavica, Supplement* **30**, 1.

Reaven, G.M., Olefsky, J. & Farquhar, J.W. (1972) Does hypoglycaemia or hyperinsulinaemia characterize the patient with chemical diabetes? *Lancet*, **1**, 1247.

Rees, R.J.W. & Waters, M.F.R. (1971) Recent trends in leprosy research. *British Medical Bulletin*, **28**, 16.

Refsum, S. (1946) Heredopathia atactica polyneuritiformis: familial syndrome not hitherto described. *Acta psychiatrica et neurologica Scandinavica 38*.

Richter, R.B. (1954) Peripheral neuropathy and connective tissue disease. *Journal of Neuropathology and Experimental Neurology*, **13**, 168.

Ridley, A. (1969) The neuropathy of acute intermittent porphyria. *Quarterly Journal of Medicine*, **38**, 307.

Rose, F.C. (1960) Peripheral neuropathy. *Proceedings of the Royal Society of Medicine*, **53**, 51.

Rosenberg, R.N. & Lovelace, R.E. (1968) Mononeuritis multiplex in lepromatous leprosy. *Archives of Neurology*, **19**, 310.

Roussy, G. & Lévy, G. (1926) Sept cas d'une maladie familiale particulière: Trouble de la marche, pied bots et aréfléxie tendineuse généralisée, avec accessoirement,

légère maladresse des mains. *Revue Neurologique*, **1**, 427.

Rukavina, J.G., Block, W.D., Jackson, C.E., Falls, H.F., Carey, J.H. & Curtis, A.C. (1956) Primary systemic amyloidosis: a review and an experimental genetic and clinical study of 29 cases with particular emphasis on the familial form. *Medicine (Baltimore)*, **35**, 239.

Rundles, R.W. (1945) Diabetic neuropathy: a general review with a report of 125 cases. *Medicine (Baltimore)*, **24**, 111.

Russell, D.S. & Rubinstein, L.J. (1963) *Pathology of Tumours of the Nervous System*. 2nd Edn. (Arnold: London).

Sabin, T.D. (1969) Temperature-linked sensory loss. A unique pattern in leprosy. *Archives of Neurology*, **20**, 257.

Seddon, H.J. (1943) Three types of nerve injury. *Brain*, **66**, 237.

Seneviratne, K.N. & Peiris, O.A. (1970) Peripheral nerve function in chronic liver disease. *Journal of Neurology, Neurosurgery and Psychiatry*, **33**, 609.

Sharpey-Shafer, E.P. & Taylor, P.J. (1960) Absent circulatory reflexes in diabetic neuritis. *Lancet*, **1**, 559.

Simpson, D.A. & Fowler, M. (1966) Two cases of localised hypertrophic neurofibrosis. *Journal of Neurology, Neurosurgery and Psychiatry*, **29**, 80.

Skanse, B. & Gydell, K. (1956) A rare type of femoral sciatic neuropathy in diabetes mellitus. *Acta medica Scandinavica*, **155**, 463.

Smith, M.I., Elvove, E. & Frazier, W.H. (1930) The pharmacological action of certain phenol esters, with special reference to the aetiology of so-called ginger paralysis. *U.S. Treasury Public Health Reports*, **45**, 2509.

Sørensen, A.W.S. & With, T.K. (1971) Persistent paresis after porphyric attacks. *Acta medica Scandinavica*, **190**, 219.

Staal, A. (1970) The entrapment neuropathies. In *Handbook of Clinical Neurology*, Vol. 7. Eds P.J. Vinken & G.W. Bruyn, pp. 285–325 (North Holland: Amsterdam).

Steinberg, D., Mize, C.E., Herndon, J.H. Jr., Fales, H.M., Engel, W.K. & Vroom, F.Q. (1970) Phytanic acid in patients with Refsum's syndrome and response to dietary treatment. *Archives of Internal Medicine*, **125**, 75.

Stern, G. (1970) The peripheral nerves in Wegener's granulomatosis. In *Handbook of Clinical Neurology*. Eds P.J. Vinken & G.W. Bruyn, pp. 112–117 (North Holland: Amsterdam).

Sterzel, R.B., Semar, M., Lonergan, E.T., Treser, G. & Lange, K. (1971) Relationship of nerve tissue transketolase to neuropathy of chronic uraemia. *Journal of Clinical Investigation*, **50**, 2295.

Stoll, B.A. & Andrews, J.T. (1966) Radiation-induced peripheral neuropathy. *British Medical Journal*, **2**, 834.

Sunderland, S. (1968) *Nerve and Nerve Injuries* (Livingstone: Edinburgh).

Swanson, A.G., Buchan, G.C. & Alvord, E.C. Jr. (1965) Anatomic changes in congenital insensitivity to pain: absence of small primary sensory neurons in ganglia roots and Lissauer's tract. *Archives of Neurology*, **12**, 12.

Sweeney, V.P., Pathak, M.A. & Asbury, A.K. (1970) Acute intermittent porphyria: increased ALA-synthetase activity during an acute attack. *Brain*, **93**, 369.

Tenckhoff, H.A., Boen, F.S.T., Jebsen, R.H. & Spiegler, J.H. (1965) Polyneuropathy in chronic renal insufficiency. *Journal of the American Medical Association*, **192**, 1121.

Thévenard, A. (1942) L'acropathie ulcero-mutilante familiale. *Revue Neurologique*, **74**, 193.

Thomas, P.K. & Lascelles, R.G. (1966) The pathology of diabetic neuropathy. *Quarterly Journal of Medicine*, **35**, 489.

Thomas, P.K., Sears, T.A. & Gilliatt, R.W. (1959) The range of conduction velocity in normal motor nerve fibres to the small muscles of the hand and foot. *Journal of Neurology, Neurosurgery and Psychiatry*, **22**, 175.

Thomashefsky, A.J., Horwitz, S.J. & Feingold, M.H. (1972) Acute autonomic neuropathy. *Neurology (Minneapolis)*, **22**, 251.

Tomasulo, P.A., Kater, R.M.H. & Iber, F.L. (1968) Impairment of thiamine resorption in alcoholism. *American Journal of Clinical Nutrition*, **21**, 1340.

Tooth, H.H. (1886) *The Peroneal Type of Progressive Muscular Atrophy*. Thesis, University of London (H.K. Lewis: London).

Torres, I., Smith, W.T. & Oxnard, C.E. (1971) Peripheral neuropathy associated with vitamin B_{12} deficiency in captive monkeys. *Journal of Pathology*, **105**, 125.

Trojaborg, W., Frantzen, E. & Andersen, I. (1969) Peripheral neuropathy and myopathy associated with carcinoma of the lung. *Brain*, **92**, 71.

Trousseau, A. & Lassegue, G. (1851) Du nassonnement de la paralysie du voile du palais. *L'Union médicale*, **5**, 471.

Turkington, R.W. & Stiefel, J.W. (1965) Sensory radicular neuropathy. *Archives of Neurology*, **12**, 19.

Tyler, H.R. (1968) Neurologic disorders in renal failure. *American Journal of Medicine*, **44**, 734.

Victor, M. (1965) The effects of nutritional deficiency on the nervous system. A comparison of the effects of carcinoma. In *The Remote Effects of Cancer on the Nervous System*. Eds Lord Brain & F.H. Norris, Jr. pp. 134–161 (Grune and Stratton: New York).

Vilter, R.W., Müller, J.F., Glazer, H.S., Jarrold, T., Abraham, J., Thompson, C. & Hawkins, V.R. (1953) The effect of vitamin B_6 deficiency by desoxyptridoxine in human beings. *Journal of Laboratory and Clinical Medicine*, **42**, 335.

Vinken, P.J. & Bruyn, G.W. (Eds) (1970a) Diseases of nerve, Part I, *Handbook of Clinical Neurology*. Vol. 7 (North Holland: Amsterdam).

Vinken, P.J. & Bruyn, G.W. (Eds) (1970b) Diseases of nerve, Part II *Handbook of Clinical Neurology*. Vol. 8 (North Holland: Amsterdam).

Vizoso, A.D. (1950) The relationship between internodal length and growth in human nerves. *Journal of Anatomy*, **84**, 342.

Wallace, D.C. (1970) Hereditary sensory radicular neuropathy. A family study. *Australian Medical Association Mervyn Archdall Medical Monographs*, **8**. (Australian Medical Association: Sydney.)

Walsh, J.C. (1971) The neuropathy of multiple myeloma. An electrophysiological and histological study. *Archives of Neurology*, **25**, 404.

Ward, J.D., Fisher, D.J., Barnes, C.G., Jessop, J.D. & Baker, R.W.R. (1971) Improvement in nerve conduction following treatment in newly diagnosed diabetics. *Lancet*, **1**, 428.

Warrell, D.A., Godrey, S. & Olden, E.G.J. (1968) Giant-cell arteritis with peripheral neuropathy. *Lancet*, **1**, 1010.

Weber, F.P. & Hill, T.R. (1933) Complete degeneration of the posterior columns of the spinal cord with chronic polyneuritis in a case of widespread carcinomatous disease elsewhere. *Journal of Neurology and Psychopathology*, **14**, 57.

Weller, R.O., Bruckner, F.E. & Chamberlain, M.A. (1970) Rheumatoid neuropathy: a histological and electrophysiological study. *Journal of Neurology, Neurosurgery and Psychiatry*, **33**, 592.

Wight, P.A.L. (1969) The ultrastructure of sciatic nerves affected by fowl paralysis (Marek's disease). *Journal of Comparative Pathology and Therapeutics*, **79**, 563.

Williams, P.L. & Landon, D.N. (1963) Paranodal apparatus of peripheral myelinated nerve fibres of mammals. *Nature*, **198**, 670.

Wilner, E.C. & Brody, J.A. (1968) An evaluation of the remote effects of cancer on the nervous system. *Neurology (Minneapolis)*, **18**, 1120.

Wilson, S.K.A. (1954) *Neurology*. 2nd Edn. Ed. A.N. Bruce, p. 738 (Butterworth: London).

Woltman, H.W. & Wilder, R.M. (1929) Diabetes mellitus. Pathologic changes in the spinal cord and peripheral nerves. *Archives of Internal Medicine*, **44**, 476.

Yudell, A., Gomez, M.R., Lambert, E.H. & Docherty, M.B. (1967) Neuropathy of sulfatide lipidosis (metachromatic leucodystrophy). *Neurology (Minneapolis)*, **17**, 103.

Yuill, G.M., Swinburn, W.R. & Liversedge, L.A. (1970) Treatment of polyneuropathy with azathioprine. *Lancet*, **2**, 854.

Genetic aspects of neuromuscular disease

INTRODUCTION

All the disorders to be discussed in this Chapter
are genetic. This means that in each case the basic
defect resides within the genes which are composed of deoxyribonucleic acid (DNA). The latter
consists of two chains of nucleotides arranged in a
double helix. Each nucleotide is composed of a
nitrogenous base, a sugar molecule (deoxyribose)
and a phosphate molecule. The backbone of each
nucleotide chain is formed by sugar–phosphate
molecules, and the two chains are held together by
hydrogen bonds between the nitrogenous bases
which point inward toward the centre of the helix.
There are four bases: adenine, thymine, guanine
and cytosine. The arrangement of bases in each
strand of the DNA molecule is not random but is
in the form of triplet codes, each triplet specifying
a particular amino acid. The latter join together to
form polypeptides and proteins such as enzymes or
structural proteins (e.g. membranes). In genetic
disorders there is a change (called a mutation) in a
particular triplet (or group of triplets) resulting
ultimately in the formation of an abnormal
protein, or a protein with no biological activity or
even no protein at all. Apart from the glycogenoses
and one or two rare myopathies, the basic genetic
defect is not known in any of the hereditary
neuromuscular disorders afflicting man. However,
from the known function and fine structure of
genes as described in micro-organisms, there is
considerable scope for alterations in the genetic
code and, therefore, genetic heterogeneity in a
group of disorders such as the neuromuscular
disorders is to be expected.

At the clinical level it is convenient to consider
genetic disorders as being autosomal dominant,
autosomal recessive or X-linked. For each particular genetic trait an individual possesses two
genes which may be alike, in which case the
individual is said to be homozygous, or they may
be different in which case he is said to be
heterozygous. A trait manifest in the heterozygote
is dominant, whereas one which is manifest only in
the homozygote is recessive. A classical dominant
disorder affects both males and females and is
transmitted from one generation to another. There
is a 1 in 2 chance that any child of an affected parent
will inherit the mutant gene and will therefore be
affected.

Dominant disorders often show considerable
variation in severity, sometimes referred to as
expressivity. Occasionally a trait may not be
manifest in all heterozygotes. In those who appear
to be unaffected the gene is said to be non-
penetrant. For any dominant disorder the proportion of heterozygotes who are affected (even if

only minimally) is referred to as the 'penetrance' of the gene. Thus in epiloia penetrance is reduced to about 80 per cent because in 20 per cent of heterozygotes the trait is apparently not manifest.

Recessive disorders also affect both males and females but in this case only sibs (brothers and sisters) are affected and these disorders are not transmitted from one generation to another. The risk of recurrence after one affected child is 1 in 4. Affected individuals themselves can usually be reassured regarding the risks to their children because their children will be affected only if the affected parent marries a heterozygote which, in the case of an unrelated person, is very unlikely with a rare disorder.

X-linked disorders are caused by mutant genes on the X chromosome. Almost all such disorders are recessive and therefore female heterozygotes (or carriers) are usually normal and only males (who are hemizygous) are affected. In the case of a carrier female there is a 1 in 2 chance that any of her sons will be affected and a 1 in 2 chance that any of her daughters will be carriers. In the case of an affected male, none of his sons will be affected because they inherit their father's Y chromosome, but all his daughters will be carriers because they inherit their father's X chromosome which has the mutant gene.

As there is no effective treatment for any of the inherited neuromuscular disorders the only approach to the problem is prevention. This is possible through genetic counselling and prenatal diagnosis. Genetic counselling involves explaining the nature of the disorder, its prognosis and the chances of recurrence. Important advances in this field in the last few years have been the development of tests for detecting preclinical cases of certain genetic disorders such as myotonic dystrophy, and methods for identifying healthy female carriers of various X-linked disorders such as Duchenne muscular dystrophy. In those disorders where the basic biochemical defect is known (e.g. Pompe's disease) prenatal diagnosis is possible from the biochemical study of cultured amniotic fluid cells obtained by transabdominal amniocentesis carried out at about the 15th week of gestation. If the fetus proves to be affected the parents can be offered therapeutic abortion. In the case of X-linked recessive disorders where the basic

biochemical defect is not yet known (e.g. Duchenne muscular dystrophy) it is possible to sex the fetus in utero and, through selective abortion of any male fetuses, guarantee that a mother who is a carrier will have a daughter who will not be affected.

PROGRESSIVE MUSCULAR DYSTROPHY

Until Walton and Nattrass (1954) attempted a classification based on genetic considerations, studies were handicapped by the use of categories which embraced a conglomeration of genetic entities. Some of the modifications in classification which clarify further the separation of genetic entities include suggestions made by Becker (1953, 1964), Lamy and de Grouchy (1954), Becker and Kiener (1955), Kloepfer and Talley (1958), Chung and Morton (1959), Morton and Chung (1959), Rotthauwe and Kowalewski (1965) and Emery and Walton (1967).

Duchenne and Becker muscular dystrophy

Stevenson (1953, 1958), in his series of 27 families of Duchenne type muscular dystrophy, excluded affected individuals and families in which the gene was not X-linked, the onset was not early, and progression was not rapid. Other investigators have included families with muscular dystrophy in which the gene was X-linked, but in which onset age was later and progression was slower. Becker and Kiener (1955) defined the severe form as having an age of onset before 10 years, inability to walk usually by age 11 years, and death by age 20, while the mild form usually has onset age after 10 years, ability to walk in maturity, and death after age 25. The severe and mild forms of X-linked muscular dystrophy never occur in the same family (Blyth and Pugh, 1959). From the X-linked pedigrees of Walton (1955, 1956) it would seem that about 9 out of 10 pedigrees represent the rapidly progressive Duchenne type.

Clinically severe X-linked recessive Duchenne type of muscular dystrophy. This form of muscular dystrophy is characterised by: (*a*) transmission as an X-linked recessive trait; (b) expression limited to males except occasionally in carrier females (Emery, 1963) and in females with Turner's syndrome (Walton, 1957a; Ferrier, Bamatter and Klein, 1965); (c) onset usually in the first five years of life; (d) symmetrical involvement first of pelvic girdle muscles, later of the shoulder girdle; (e) pseudohypertrophy, particularly of the calf, in about 80 per cent of cases; (f) steady and rapid progression leading usually to inability to walk by 11 years of age and subsequently causing progressive deformity with muscular contractures; (g) occasional facial weakness in terminal stages; (h) serum creatine kinase levels elevated except in terminal stages with high levels even at birth (Heyck, Laudahn and Carsten, 1966); (i) death from inanition or respiratory infection, usually in the second decade.

It has been generally assumed that the gene for Duchenne muscular dystrophy is 100 per cent penetrant in hemizygous (XY) males. However there have been reports which suggest that occasionally males may be hemizygous for the mutant gene and yet do not have clinical symptoms of the disease (Thompson, Ludvigsen and Monckton, 1962; Richterich, Rosin, Aebi and Rossi, 1963). In a proportion of apparently unaffected male sibs and in some fathers of affected boys slight abnormalities in serum creatine kinase levels, electromyography and even muscle histology have been reported (Beckmann and Jerusalem, 1966; Smith, Amick and Johnson, 1966). However, Emery and Spikesman (1970), using carefully matched controls, concluded that slightly elevated serum creatine kinase levels in male relatives were not associated with a subclinical form of X-linked Duchenne muscular dystrophy or with the heterozygous state of autosomal recessive Duchenne muscular dystrophy.

We have recently reviewed the findings in a number of studies of the incidence of Duchenne muscular dystrophy which have been carried out over the last 30 years (Stephens and Tyler, 1951; Walton, 1955; Stevenson, 1958; Blyth and Pugh, 1959; Moser, Weismann, Richterich and Rossi, 1964; Kuroiwa and Miyazaki, 1967; Gardner-Medwin, 1970; Prot, 1971; Lawrence, Brown and Hopkins, 1973; Brooks and Emery, 1977). Out of 1 532 218 male births, 324 were affected, which

gives an overall mean incidence ($\pm$ S.E.) of 21.1 $\pm$ 1.2 $\times$ 10^{-5} or approximately 1 in 4800 male births (Emery, 1977a). Incidences in fact ranged from 1 in 7689 to 1 in 3067, probably because of different degrees of ascertainment in different populations. In our own studies in S.E. Scotland over the period 1953–68 the incidence was 26.5 $\times$ 10^{-5} or approximately 1 in 3774 male births (Brooks and Emery, 1977).

In an X-linked recessive condition in which affected males do not survive to have children, the mutation rate is one-third the birth incidence. Using the overall mean incidence of 21.1 $\times$ 10^{-5} the mutation rate is therefore 70 $\times$ 10^{-6}. This figure is higher than values obtained for other X-linked disorders, one possible explanation being that there is more than one form of severe X-linked Duchenne muscular dystrophy (Emery, Skinner and Holloway, 1979b).

Clinically milder X-linked recessive types of muscular dystrophy. A milder X-linked form of muscular dystrophy was recognised first by Becker (Becker, 1955, 1957, 1962). This is clinically similar to the Duchenne type muscular dystrophy but differs in that the disease usually manifests itself in the teens or early twenties and affected individuals usually survive at least to the third decade. Other investigators have also reported families with X-linked muscular dystrophy in which the onset was later and the progression slower than in the classical Duchenne type of muscular dystrophy (Levison, 1951; Lamy and de Grouchy, 1954; Walton, 1955, 1956; Blyth and Pugh, 1959; Rotthauwe and Kowalewski, 1966a; Zellweger and Hanson, 1967; Markand, North, D'Agostino and Daly, 1969; Radu and Stenzel, 1969a; Conomy, 1970). From a detailed study of 10 extensive families with benign (Becker type) X-linked muscular dystrophy, Emery and Skinner (1976) have defined the clinical features of this disease and the differences from Duchenne muscular dystrophy. Both disorders are characterised by predominantly proximal muscle weakness with pseudohypertrophy of the calf muscles. However, unlike Duchenne muscular dystrophy, in Becker muscular dystrophy there is no evidence of right ventricular preponderance on electrocardiography and cardiac involvement, when present, is a late manifestation. The best criterion for distinguishing between the two disorders is the age of becoming chair-bound: nearly 97 per cent of boys with Duchenne muscular dystrophy become chair-bound *before* the age of 11 whereas 97 per cent of patients with Becker muscular dystrophy become chair-bound *after* the age of 11 (Emery and Skinner, 1976). In both diseases the serum level of creatine kinase is raised, particularly in the early stages, and in this way preclinical cases may be identified.

Mabry, Roeckel, Munich and Robertson (1965) have described a large family with a benign X-linked form of muscular dystrophy which appears to differ from the Becker type in age of onset and the greater degree of disability which it produces. Emery and Dreifuss (1966) have described another benign form of muscular dystrophy in which there was no pseudohypertrophy and muscular contractures were an *early* and prominent feature. Similar families have also been described (Cammann, Vehreschild and Ernst, 1974). To these benign X-linked forms of muscular dystrophy with mainly proximal muscle involvement might also be added the type in which the scapular and peroneal muscles are predominantly affected (Waters, Nutter, Hopkins and Dorney, 1975). The main distinguishing features between the various forms of X-linked muscular dystrophy are summarised in Table 22.1.

The locus for Duchenne muscular dystrophy has been shown not to be within measurable distance of the loci for colour blindness (Emery, 1966; Greig, 1977), glucose-6-phosphate dehydrogenase (G6PD) deficiency (Zatz, Itskan, Sanger, Frota-Pessoa and Saldanha, 1974) or the Xg blood group (Blyth, Carter, Dubowitz, Emery, Gavin, Johnston, McKusick, Race, Sanger and Tippett, 1965). On the other hand, though the loci for Becker muscular dystrophy and the Xg blood group are not close to each other, the former is within measurable distance of both the loci for colour blindness (Emery, Smith and Sanger, 1969; Skinner, Smith and Emery, 1974) and G6PD (Zatz *et al.*, 1974), the latter two loci being very closely linked. Thus the genes for Duchenne and Becker types of muscular dystrophy are not alleles but are located at two different sites on the X-chromosome and therefore presumably have a different biochemical basis.

Autosomal recessive Duchenne type of muscular dystrophy. Stevenson (1953) suggested that the name Duchenne be limited to that type of muscular dystrophy which affects boys and has early onset and rapid progression. However, many investigators have found the Duchenne clinical description useful whether or not affection is limited to males (Becker, 1953). Lamy and de Grouchy (1954) found the Duchenne clinical description applicable to cases inherited as an autosomal recessive trait in about 1 out of 10 pedigrees in their series of 102 families totalling 160 cases. Walton (1955) included two girls among his 56 cases of Duchenne type with the comment that they 'have shown no significant difference in clinical manifestations and course from several of the boys'. Kloepfer and Talley (1958) studied the occurrence of Duchenne type muscular dystrophy (three males and four females) in four related sibships in which all eight parents had a common

Table 22.1 X-linked muscular dystrophies

Type	Onset	Course	Weakness	Pseudo-hypertrophy	Myocardial involvement	Contrac-tures
Duchenne	<5	severe	proximal	+++	+	+ (late)
Becker	3–25	benign	proximal	+++	–	–
Mabry	11–13	benign	proximal	+++	+	–
Emery-Dreifuss	<5	benign	proximal	–	+	+ (early)
Scapuloperoneal	<10	benign	scapuloperoneal	–	+	+ (early)

ancestor. There was no doubt that an autosomal recessive pattern of inheritance was involved. Age of onset ranged from 5 to 13 years. Blyth and Pugh (1959) accepted this category and Dubowitz (1960) presented a pedigree. Jackson and Carey (1961) reported 14 affected individuals (including five girls) distributed in seven related sibships with clinical stigmata typically similar to the Duchenne type which they found to be transmitted as an autosomal recessive trait. Age of onset was from 5 to 13 years. Milhorat (1961) reported the occurrence of 25 females clinically similar to 185 X-linked recessive males of the Duchenne type. Others have also studied and commented upon the occurrence of muscular dystrophy in young girls (Johnston, 1964; Radu and Stenzel, 1969b; Penn, Lisak and Rowland, 1970). However, it is now believed that this is an uncommon condition and that many of the cases reported in the past probably had spinal muscular atrophy and not muscular dystrophy.

Facioscapulohumeral muscular dystrophy

Facioscapulohumeral muscular dystrophy is characterised as follows: (*a*) transmission as an autosomal dominant trait; (*b*) expression in either sex; (*c*) onset usually in adolescence, but possibly at any age from childhood until late adult life; (*d*) occurrence of abortive or mildly affected cases is common; (*e*) initial involvement, sometimes asymmetrical, of facial and scapulohumeral muscles, usually with spread within 20 or 30 years to the pelvic muscles; (*f*) pseudohypertrophy is very rare; (*g*) slow insidious progression with periods of long arrest of the disease; (*h*) rarely severe disability and usually slight skeletal changes; (*i*) high patient survival and ability to remain active to normal age; (*j*) usually normal or slightly raised serum creatine kinase levels.

All studies of this entity including those of Bell (1943), Boyes, Fraser, Lawler and Mackenzie (1949), Tyler and Stephens (1950), Becker (1953), Walton and Nattrass (1954) and Morton, Chung Peters (1963), are in agreement that transmission is as a dominant trait which is completely penetrant (Morton and Chung, 1959) in both sexes. However, expression of the gene may be so mild that the condition goes unrecognised. For example

Walton (1955) emphasised the unreliability of family histories when he said 'The affected girls in generation III were examined on two occasions and each time II.4 was interviewed. It was only at a late stage of the second interview that the author's suspicions of facial involvement in II.4 were aroused and examination subsequently revealed that she was undoubtedly an abortive case. She had insisted previously that all her sibs were well; however, when they, too, agreed to be examined it was discovered that II.9 was another abortive case, and that II.7 was quite severely affected.'

Morton and Chung (1959) found the incidence rate of facioscapulohumeral muscular dystrophy to be 38×10^{-7} when determined from their own Wisconsin data and 92×10^{-7} when based on pooled data. From these same data prevalence rates were 23×10^{-7}, and 56×10^{-7}, respectively. In the studies of Tyler and Stephens (1950), Walton (1955), Race (1955), and Stevenson, Cheeseman and Huth (1955) data were insufficient to establish linkage between the gene for facioscapulohumeral muscular dystrophy and genes for the ability to taste phenylthiocarbamide (PTC), for blood groups, and the secretor factor.

Limb-girdle muscular dystrophy

This form of muscular dystrophy, according to Walton and Nattrass (1954) and Morton, Chung and Peters (1963), is characterised by: (*a*) transmission as an autosomal recessive trait in 59 per cent of the cases, and sporadic occurrence in the remaining 41 per cent; (*b*) expression in either sex; (*c*) onset usually late in the first or in the second or third decades, but occasionally in middle age; (*d*) primary involvement of either the shoulder girdle muscles (usually) or of the pelvic girdle (rarely) with spread to other areas after a variable period; (*e*) only rare occurrence of muscular pseudohypertrophy; (*f*) rare occurrence of abortive cases; (*g*) variable severity and rate of progression, intermediate between the Duchenne and facioscapulohumeral forms; (*h*) in most cases severe disability in middle life and death at a younger than normal age; (*i*) occasional slight facial weakness in late stages; (*j*) usually normal or slightly raised serum creatine kinase levels.

Many investigators, including Bell (1943),

Stevenson (1953), Becker (1953), Walton (1955, 1956), Morton and Chung (1959), and Morton, Chung and Peters (1963), have found limb-girdle muscular dystrophy to be inherited as an autosomal recessive trait which is probably 100 per cent penetrant in both sexes in the homozygous genotype, but not all cases are believed to be autosomal recessive even after misdiagnosed cases of facioscapulohumeral and Duchenne types are eliminated. Morton and Chung (1959) found that 59 per cent of all limb-girdle cases were recessive. Morton, Chung and Peters (1963) believe there is no genetic value to be gained by subdividing this category on the basis of onset and severity (Blyth and Pugh, 1959), scapulohumeral or pelvifemoral onset (Becker, 1953), and the presence or absence of pseudohypertrophy (Bell, 1943), because within families a continuous mixture of these categories occurs.

Autosomal recessive limb-girdle muscular dystrophy. Morton and Chung (1959) found the age of onset to range from 10 to 50 years with a median of 30 years. They found no clinical distinction between recessive and sporadic types. Although they did not estimate incidence and prevalence rates separately for these two genetic types, these values may be obtained readily for the recessive gene by multiplying their combined values by 59 per cent. Using this procedure the incidence rate was 385×10^{-7} from their Wisconsin data and 468×10^{-7} when based on their pooled data. From these same data prevalence rates were 118×10^{-7} and 142×10^{-7}, respectively.

Stevenson et al. (1955) had insufficient data to establish linkage relations between the gene for limb-girdle muscular dystrophy and genes for P.T.C., blood groups, and secretor factor.

Sporadic limb-girdle muscular dystrophy. Morton and Chung (1959) and Morton, Chung and Peters (1963) found 41 per cent of all limb-girdle types of muscular dystrophy to be sporadic after exclusion of isolated cases of autosomal recessive genotypes by segregation analysis. These authors postulated that the most probable explanation for the occurrence of this category is the occasional expression of a recessive

gene in the heterozygous genotype. This means that similar secondary cases would be expected rarely in other members of a family. However, chronic polymyositis (Walton and Adams, 1958; Pearson and Rose, 1960), benign spinal muscular atrophy and some rare forms of metabolic myopathy could account for many cases in this sporadic group.

In a manner similar to that used for the autosomal recessive variety, incidence and prevalence values may be obtained for sporadic limb-girdle muscular dystrophy by multiplying by 41 per cent the combined values found by Morton and Chung (1959). The incidence rate was 268×10^{-7} from their Wisconsin data and 326×10^{-7} when based on pooled data. From these same data prevalence rates were 82×10^{-7} and 99×10^{-7} respectively.

Limb-girdle muscular dystrophy clearly inherited as an autosomal dominant trait has been described but appears to be very rare (Schneiderman, Sampson, Schoene and Haydon, 1969; Bacon and Smith, 1971). In one such family, linkage with the Pelger-Huet anomaly has been reported (Schneiderman et al., 1969).

Manifesting carriers of X-linked muscular dystrophy. It has been estimated that about 8 per cent of all female carriers of X-linked Duchenne muscular dystrophy may have varying degrees of muscle weakness (Moser and Emery, 1974). In its more extreme form this weakness may resemble limb-girdle muscular dystrophy, the incidence of which is roughly the same as the incidence of manifesting carriers of Duchenne muscular dystrophy. The distinction between these two conditions is important because in limb-girdle muscular dystrophy an affected woman (or her unaffected sister) is most unlikely to have affected children, but in the case of a manifesting carrier of X-linked Duchenne muscular dystrophy there is a 1 in 2 chance that any son she has will be affected and her sister may also be at risk of having affected sons. Some distinguishing features between these two conditions are summarised in Table 22.2.

Distal muscular dystrophy

This characteristically benign disease begins in the

Table 22.2 Some distinguishing features between manifesting female carriers of X-linked Duchenne muscular dystrophy and limb-girdle muscular dystrophy

Features	Manifesting carriers	Limb-girdle dystrophy
Pseudohypertrophy	80%	rare
Asymmetrical weakness	60%	rare
ECG abnormalities	5–10%	–
Serum creatine kinase increased	>95% often very high	60% rarely high

small muscles of the hands, feet and legs. From 78 propositi Welander (1951) examined 249 individuals with distal muscular dystrophy who were distributed in 72 pedigrees. The age of onset ranged from 20 to 77 with a mean of 47 years. Transmission was as an autosomal dominant trait which was about 80 per cent penetrant in males and 69 per cent penetrant in females. As prevalence in the population studied was as high as 1 in 55 for individuals who were 65 years or older, it was possible to observe a mating between two affected parents who had 15 offspring, of whom two were severely affected and therefore considered to be homozygous for the dominant gene (Welander, 1957). Walton (1963) studied six cases of distal muscular dystrophy, and though there was no evidence of the disease in any of their relatives they were all severely affected in a way comparable to Welander's patients whom she considered to be homozygotes. Six individuals with distal muscular dystrophy have been described in an English family where the mode of inheritance was consistent with that of an autosomal dominant trait (Sumner, Crawfurd and Harriman, 1971). Affected males had an earlier onset and wider distribution of muscle weakness than affected females and the authors considered this to be a different disease from that described by Welander.

Ocular muscular dystrophy

When extrinsic ocular muscles are affected by ocular muscular dystrophy, the clinical symptoms begin with ptosis or diplopia and progress to complete bilateral ophthalmoplegia. Upper facial muscles are usually weak and atrophy of neck, trunk and limb muscles may also occur. The disease usually begins in early adult life but may be manifest even in infancy.

Though the disease frequently follows an autosomal dominant mode of inheritance, the large number of isolated cases described in various reports and reviewed by Kiloh and Nevin (1951) and by Lees and Liversedge (1962) suggest either that penetrance is often reduced, or the mutation rate is high, or that the condition may be due to more than one gene and that whereas one such gene is clearly an autosomal dominant others may be recessive.

The so-called 'oculopharyngeal' type of muscular dystrophy, in which the onset is in middle age (Bray, Kaarsoo and Ross, 1965) and progressive dysphagia is a prominent feature, is a distinct entity. A large proportion of cases with this type of muscular dystrophy have been of French-Canadian extraction (Taylor, 1915; Victor, Hayes and Adams, 1962; Hayes, London, Seidman and Embree, 1963; Peterman, Lillington and Jamplis, 1964).

Congenital myopathies

The syndrome of generalised muscular hypotonia, feebleness of voluntary movements and depressed or absent tendon reflexes present at birth or manifest during early infancy, has been variously referred to as amyotonia congenita, myatonia congenita or Oppenheim's disease. Batten (1910) was the first to recognise that the syndrome could be myopathic in origin or result from a lesion in the anterior horn cells of the spinal cord (infantile spinal muscular atrophy or Werdnig-Hoffmann's disease). In fact, more recent studies have shown that the syndrome may result from many causes (Brandt, 1950; Walton, 1957b) though Werdnig-Hoffmann's disease and congenital myopathies, of one form or another, account for most cases. The congenital myopathies themselves are a heterogenous group of disorders though they all have in common muscular weakness dating from birth or early infancy. A classification of the congenital myopathies is given in Table 22.3, details of which have been discussed elsewhere (Emery and Walton, 1967). Zellweger (1966) and Dubowitz (1978) have reviewed their differential diagnosis in detail.

An understanding of the pathogenesis of this group of diseases is urgently needed, both for genetic counselling and for determining the prognosis in the individual case. Serum enzyme studies and refinements in histological and histochemical techniques may soon make this possible.

Table 22.3 Classification of the congenital myopathies

1. *Congenital muscular dystrophies proper*
   Muscle histology characteristic of dystrophy
   Serum enzymes usually normal
   Autosomal recessive inheritance probable
   A. Rapidly progressive
      Death in infancy or early childhood.
      (Banker, Victor and Adams, 1957; O'Brien, 1962; Short, 1963; Wharton, 1965).
   B. Slowly progressive
      (Greenfield, Cornman and Shy, 1958; Fukuyama, Kawozura and Haruna, 1960; Pearson and Fowler, 1963).

2. *Exceptional early onset in forms of muscular dystrophy which usually begin in childhood.*
      e.g. Duchenne muscular dystrophy (Walton and Nattrass, 1954)
      Myotonic dystrophy (Vanier, 1960; Dodge, Gamstorp, Byers and Russell, 1965; Sarrouy, Farouz, Robert, Sabatini, Vaillaud and Poncet, 1966)
      Distal muscular dystrophy (Magee and de Jong, 1965)

3. *Congenital 'myopathies'**
      Muscle histology may be normal with conventional staining techniques
      Serum enzymes usually normal

   †A. Benign congenital hypotonia
      (Walton, 1957b; Greenfield, Cornman and Shy, 1958; Gordon, 1966)
   †B. Congenital universal muscular hypoplasia (Krabbe's disease)
      (Schreier and Huperz, 1956; Krabbe, 1958; Ford, 1966)
   C. Central core disease
      ? Autosomal dominant
      (Shy and Magee, 1956; Engel, Foster, Hughes, Huxley and Mahler, 1961; Dubowitz and Platts, 1965; Dubowitz and Roy, 1970)
   D. Nemaline myopathy
      Autosomal recessive
      (Karpati, Carpenter and Andermann, 1971)
      Autosomal dominant
      (Shy, Engel, Somers and Wanko, 1963; Spiro and Kennedy, 1965; Hopkins, Lindsey and Ford, 1966)
   E. Myotubular myopathy (centronuclear myopathy)
      (Spiro, Shy and Gonatas, 1966; Schochet, Zellweger, Ionasescu and McCormick, 1972)
      Autosomal recessive
      (Bradley, Price and Watanabe, 1970)
      Autosomal dominant
      (McLeod, Baker, Lethlean and Shorey, 1972)
      X-linked recessive
      (Meyers, Golomb, Hansen and McKusick, 1974)
   F. Mitochondrial abnormalities
      'megaconial myopathy' (Shy and Gonatas, 1964)
      'pleoconial myopathy' (Shy, Gonatas and Perez, 1966)
      with salt craving (Spiro, Prineas and Moore, 1970)
   G. Myopathy with crystalline intranuclear inclusions:
      possibly a variant of nemaline myopathy (Jenis, Lindquist and Lister, 1969)
   H. Sarcotubular myopathy
      (Jerusalem, Engel and Gomez, 1973)
      Autosomal recessive
   I. Fingerprint body myopathy
      (Engel, Angelini and Gomez, 1972)
   J. Familial type I fibre atrophy
      (Kinoshita, Satoyoshi and Kurmagai, 1975).
      ? Autosomal dominant

4. *Arthrogryposis multiplex congenita*
      (myopathic form)
      ?Autosomal recessive
      (Pearson and Fowler, 1963; Kaloustian, Afifi and Mire, 1972)

5. *Hereditary carnitine deficiency*
      Autosomal recessive
      (Van Dyke, Griggs, Markesbery and DiMauro, 1975)

Carrier detection in muscular dystrophy

From the point of view of genetic counselling, carrier detection is more important in X-linked than in autosomal recessive disorders. With regard to carriers of X-linked Duchenne muscular dystrophy, a small proportion of such women have enlarged calves and some may even have quite marked muscle weakness (Emery, 1963). It has been estimated that about 8 per cent of carriers exhibit some degree of weakness (Moser and Emery, 1974) which may mimic limb-girdle muscular dystrophy (see p. 790). However, the majority of carriers are symptom-free and their detection is important for genetic counselling. The

*May present with muscle weakness in infancy.
†Groups 3A and 3B may rightly belong to 3C or 3D etc.
(see Hopkins, Lindsey and Ford, 1966; Emery and Walton, 1967).

simplest and most reliable test has proved to be estimation of the serum level of creatine kinase first employed by Okinaka, Sugita, Momoi, Toyokura, Kumagai, Ebashi and Fujie in 1959. Results from many centres have shown that about two-thirds of carriers have significantly elevated levels of serum creatine kinase (Emery, 1969a). Attempts have been made to improve the detection rate by studying the effects of controlled exercise on serum enzyme levels (Emery, 1967) or by using other methods but none of these has so far proved superior to the serum level of creatine kinase.

Abnormalities reported in a proportion of carriers include a reduction in peripheral circulation time (Démos, Dreyfus, Schapira and Schapira, 1962) though not in limb blood flow (Emery and Schelling, 1965), electrocardiographic changes (Emery, 1969b; Hausmanowa-Petrusewicz, Prot, Dobosz, Emeryk, Rowinska, Rubach, Kopeć and Kopeć, 1971) and certain electromyographic changes (Caruso and Buchthal, 1965; Gardner-Medwin, Pennington and Walton, 1971; Moosa, Brown and Dubowitz, 1972) though there are no significant changes with simple quantitative electromyography (Emery, Teasdall and Coomes, 1966).

In a proportion of carriers, abnormalities have also been observed in muscle histology by light microscopy (Dubowitz, 1963; Emery, 1963, 1965; Pearson, Fowler and Wright, 1963; Macciotta, Costa, Cao, Sforza and Scano, 1964; Stephens and Lewin, 1965; Kowalewski, Rotthauwe, Mölbert and Mumenthaler, 1966; Pearce, Pearce and Walton, 1966; Smith *et al.*, 1966), by electron microscopy (Roy and Dubowitz, 1970) and by histochemical studies (Morris and Raybould, 1971). Various biochemical abnormalities in muscle tissue from carriers have been reported, including a significant reduction in LDH-5 (Emery, 1964; Mannucci, Idèo, Cao and Macciotta, 1965; Johnston, Wilkinson, Withycombe and Raymond, 1966; Pearson and Kar, 1966), and increased protein synthesis (Ionasescu, 1975). The proportion of echinocytes in peripheral blood may also be increased (Lumb and Emery, 1975). None of these various techniques has, however, replaced the serum level of creatine kinase as being the most practical and sensitive test for the carrier state in Duchenne muscular dystrophy. Carriers of Becker

muscular dystrophy also have elevated levels of serum creatine kinase (Rotthauwe and Kowalewski, 1966b; Emery, Clack, Simon and Taylor, 1967) and a recent study indicates that about 60 per cent have levels which exceed the normal 95th percentile (Skinner, Emery, Anderson and Foxall, 1975). In both Duchenne and Becker types of muscular dystrophy there is therefore the problem of counselling a suspected carrier whose serum creatine kinase level falls within the normal range. Simple statistical techniques have been devised which can be applied in such situations and which take into account enzyme levels, not only in the potential carrier, but also in her sisters and mother, and also include information on normal brothers and sons (Emery, 1976; Emery and Holloway, 1977). In these various calculations we assume that the mutation rates in male and female germ lines are equal, from which it follows, according to classical genetic theory, that one-third of all cases of Duchenne muscular dystrophy are the result of new mutations and their mothers are not therefore carriers. However Roses, Metcalf, Hull, Nicholson, Hartwig and Roe (1977) have challenged this idea and claim to have been able to detect abnormalities indicative of the carrier status in nearly all mothers of affected boys. If true, this would have important implications for genetic counselling because the mother of an isolated case would almost certainly be a carrier. However, Davie and Emery (1978), using a variety of statistical methods, have shown that the proportion of new mutants does not, in fact, differ significantly from the theoretical value of one-third.

In calculating the probability of a woman being a carrier it is necessary to know the distribution of serum creatine kinase levels in known carriers as well as in normal women and this is best determined by each laboratory. We have so far studied the distribution of enzyme levels in 71 known carriers and, for illustrative purposes, the probabilities of a woman, who has an affected son, being a carrier in various family situations, are given in Table 22.4.

The various clinical, histological and biochemical manifestations in carriers of X-linked muscular dystrophy may be explained in terms of the Lyon hypothesis (Lyon, 1961, 1962) concerning gene

Table 22.4 Probabilities of a mother of a sporadic case of Duchenne muscular dystrophy being a carrier in various family situations (normal SCK 95th percentile >85 IU/l)

Serum creatine kinase activity Mother	Grandmother	Number of normal sons	Number of normal brothers	Probability of mother being a carrier (%)
0–50	–	0	0	35
	0–50	0	0	26
	0–50	0	1	23
	0–50	0	2	22
	0–50	1	0	15
	0–50	1	1	14
	0–50	1	2	13
	51–70	0	0	31
	51–70	0	1	26
	51–70	0	2	24
	51–70	1	0	18
	51–70	1	1	15
	51–70	1	2	14
51–70	–	0	0	56
	0–50	0	0	45
	0–50	0	1	42
	0–50	0	2	41
	0–50	1	0	29
	0–50	1	1	27
	0–50	1	2	25
	51–70	0	0	51
	51–70	0	1	46
	51–70	0	2	43
	51–70	1	0	34
	51–70	1	1	30
	51–70	1	2	27

action in the X chromosome of females. It is presumed that in those carriers with clinical manifestations, high serum creatine kinase activity and abnormal muscle histology, the proportion of cells in which the active X chromosome bears the muscular dystrophy gene is greater than in carriers who have no clinical manifestations, normal serum enzymes and normal histology. However, difficulties have been encountered in trying to interpret muscle histology in carriers in terms of the Lyon hypothesis, because two distinct populations of muscle fibres have not been found (Emery, 1965).

Prenatal diagnosis of muscular dystrophy

Until comparatively recently, a woman who considered her risk of having a child who might develop muscular dystrophy to be unacceptably high, had no alternative other than family limitation. However, in the case of X-linked Duchenne muscular dystrophy, with the advent of fetal sexing and selective abortion of male fetuses, such a woman can be guaranteed a daughter who will not be affected but may be a carrier. This is an unsatisfactory solution to the problem because a proportion of aborted male fetuses will be normal. What is required therefore is a reliable prenatal test for affected male fetuses. However, as the basic biochemical defect is unknown, unlike the situation in several inborn errors of metabolism, prenatal diagnosis cannot be achieved from the biochemical study of amniotic fluid cells. Indirect tests, such as the fetal serum creatine kinase level, are therefore being considered. It is known that muscle histology is abnormal in a proportion of at-risk male fetuses, as early as the second trimester of pregnancy (Emery, 1977b). These abnormalities include increased mean fibre diameter, increased variation in fibre size and an increase in the proportion of hyaline fibres. Similar abnormalities have now been reported in muscle obtained at termination from at risk male fetuses in which SCK levels were apparently elevated (Stengel-Rutkowski, Scheuerbrandt, Beckmann and Pongratz, 1977; Mahoney, Haseltine, Hobbins, Banker, Caskey and Golbus, 1977). Disconcerting, however, have been more recent reports of normal fetal SCK levels with the subsequent birth of affected boys (Ionasescu, Zellweger and Cancilla, 1978; Golbus, Stephens, Mahoney, Hobbins, Haseltine, Caskey and Banker, 1979), and we have reported at risk fetuses in which the fetal SCK levels were normal yet the histology of cryostat sections of muscle obtained at termination was abnormal (Emery, Burt, Dubowitz, Rocker, Donnai, Harris and Donnai, 1979a). These results cast doubt on the reliability of fetal SCK in antenatal diagnosis. However, the parameters used to indicate an abnormal fetus (increased mean fibre diameter, increased variation in fibre size and increase in the proportions of hyaline and eosinophilic fibres) have been shown to be reproducible, and there has also been very good agreement between two independent observers concerning the general assessment of fetal muscle histology (Emery et al., 1979a). Thus quantitative studies on unfixed cryostat sections of fetal muscle might well provide a useful means of checking the validity of any future presumptive antenatal diagnostic test.

MYOTONIA

Myotonia is a failure of voluntary muscle to relax immediately following contraction. Morton *et al.* (1963) agree with the conclusions of Bell (1947), Thomasen (1948), Stephens (1953) and de Jong (1955) that myotonia congenita, dystrophia myotonica, and paramyotonia are clinically and genetically distinct.

Myotonia congenita

This condition is usually present at birth and is characterised by stiffness which is accentuated by cold and relieved by exercise. Generalised muscular hypertrophy is common. A dominant gene with high penetrance in both sexes is the typical pattern of inheritance for myotonia congenita (Birt, 1908; Bell, 1947; Thomasen, 1948). Becker (1977), however, has shown that the disease may also be inherited as an autosomal recessive trait. In the dominant form myotonia is less severe and muscle weakness less common than in the recessive form.

Dystrophia myotonica

Dystrophia myotonica (Steinert, 1909; Batten and Gibb, 1909) typically begins in adult life with myotonia localised to the small hand muscles, forearms and tongue. Other manifestations include cataract, frontal baldness in males, gonadal atrophy, mental retardation, facial myopathy, sternomastoid weakness, and progressive myopathy of peripheral distribution in the limbs. All studies, including those of Maas and Paterson (1943), Bell (1947), Thomasen (1948), de Jong (1955) and Lynas (1957), have reported transmission by an autosomal dominant gene which Klein (1961) found to be 100 per cent penetrant in male heterozygotes and 64 per cent penetrant in female heterozygotes. Maas and Paterson (1943) found an incidence of 120×10^{-5} and Lynas (1957) found a prevalence of 24×10^{-6} in

Northern Ireland. Klein (1961) estimated a prevalence of 5×10^{-5} in Switzerland. Mutation rates according to Lynas (1957) and Klein (1961) were 8×10^{-6} and 16×10^{-6} respectively. From observations of 33 affected males and 22 affected females Lynas (1957) observed that the percentage of affected individuals with myotonia was 47.3 per cent; with cataract 41.8 per cent; with baldness 43.6 per cent; with myopathic facies 63.6 per cent; with atrophy of sternomastoids 54.5 per cent; with atrophy of hands 40 per cent; with atrophy of arms 34.5 per cent; with atrophy of legs 29.1 per cent. Klein observed cataract in 97.9 per cent of his cases, testicular atrophy in 70 per cent of the males, and sexual disorders in 47 per cent of the females. A congenital form of myotonic dystrophy, characterised by hypotonia, mental retardation and various congenital abnormalities, has been described in the offspring of mothers with myotonic dystrophy, probably attributable to the combination of a genetic predisposition and as yet unidentified 'humoral' factors (Harper, 1975).

The original claim of an additional small acrocentric chromosome in a proportion of cells in some patients with dystrophia myotonica (Fitzgerald and Caughey, 1962), has been disproved (Jackson, 1965). However, Mutton and Gross (1965) have reported a significantly higher frequency of chromatid and isochromatid breaks in some patients with this disease.

It has been shown that the loci for dystrophia myotonica and ABH secretion are linked with a mean recombination value of 0.07 (Renwick, Bundey, Ferguson-Smith and Izatt, 1971). The detection of preclinical cases of this disease is important in genetic counselling. In this regard, the linkage with secretor status may be helpful in some families, and preclinical detection might also be accomplished by a combination of electromyography and careful slit-lamp examination for cataracts (Bundey, Carter and Soothill, 1970; Pescia and Emery, 1976).

Paramyotonia

Paramyotonia (Eulenburg, 1886) resembles myotonia congenita except that myotonia appears only after exposure to cold and is followed by severe generalised weakness like that of periodic paralysis. The pattern of inheritance is that of an autosomal dominant trait (Stephens, 1953; de Jong, 1955; Hudson, 1963) which is almost 100 per cent penetrant in heterozygotes of both sexes.

PERIODIC PARALYSIS

This condition may be subdivided into three genetic categories primarily because affected individuals within kindreds are typically hypokalaemic, hyperkalaemic or normokalaemic (Pearson, 1964). However, normokalaemic cases are comparatively rare and as this sub-variety seems closely related to the hyperkalaemic type it will not be considered separately here.

Hypokalaemic periodic paralysis

Mitchell, Flexner and Edsall (1902) and Holtzapple (1905) recommended administration of potassium in periodic paralysis on purely empirical grounds, and Biemond and Daniels (1934) demonstrated that serum potassium was decreased during attacks, which could be provoked by the administration of glucose (Aitken, Allott, Castleden and Walker, 1937; Jantz, 1947; McQuarrie and Ziegler, 1952). The age of onset of attacks ranged from age 4 to 40 years with a median of about 15 years, and the frequency of attacks ranged from one to 200 per year (Oliver, McQuarrie and Ziegler, 1944). Duration of attacks varied from one to 96 h with an average of 12 h (Meyers, 1949) and they usually occurred at night (Cerny and Katzonstein-Sutro, 1952). Most family studies (Gaupp, 1940; Meyers, 1949; Sagild and Helweg-Larsen, 1955) show transmission as an autosomal dominant trait which, according to the pedigrees of Helweg-Larsen, Hauge and Sagild (1955), is almost 100 per cent penetrant in males and about 8 per cent penetrant in females. These authors estimated an incidence of 8×10^{-6} in Denmark.

Hyperkalaemic periodic paralysis

From a review of the literature and personal examination of 68 cases (17 in hospital) Gamstorp (1956) found that serum potassium was typically increased during attacks of this type of periodic paralysis which could be provoked by the administration of potassium. She called this condition 'adynamia episodica hereditaria'. The age of onset ranged from one to 31 years with an average of six years and the frequency of attacks was usually once a week with a duration typically about 1 hour. Attacks occurred usually during the day. Transmission was as an autosomal dominant trait which was completely penetrant in both sexes. Incidence in Sweden was 2×10^{-6}. Data were insufficient for Tyler, Stephens, Gunn and Perkoff (1951) to find linkage relations between the gene for this condition and genes for the blood groups or for PTC detection.

OTHER DISEASES OF MUSCLE

Myasthenia gravis

An abnormal degree of fatigability of skeletal muscle, which may be reversed by anticholinesterase drugs, characterises myasthenia gravis. There appear to be at least three forms of this disease. A neonatal form, which occurs in about 1 in 10 newborn babies of myasthenic mothers, is transient and lasts only a few weeks. This is not genetic but is probably the result of some humoral factor which has crossed the placental barrier. Secondly there is an inherited, probably recessive form, beginning usually in childhood (Bundey, 1972) which has a relatively better prognosis than the commonest adult form. Although adult familial cases are rare (Jacob, Clack and Emery, 1968), when they are reported the high frequency of occurrence over two generations rather than one generation and the absence of consanguinity in the parents (Wilson and Stoner, 1944; Stone and Rider, 1949; Foldes and McNell, 1960) is compatible with transmission by an autosomal dominant gene with low penetrance or more likely multifactorial inheritance. In a review of 1873 cases, Namba, Brunner, Brown, Muguruma and Grob (1971) found a family history of secondary cases in 64 (3.4 per cent).

Myosclerosis

Familial information about myosclerosis, characterised by progressive sclerosis of intramuscular connective tissue, is limited to a study by Löwenthal (1954) in which one male and three female sibs were affected in one family and in another family four individuals were affected in three generations. If only one genotype is involved, then a dominant gene with reduced penetrance probably accounts for the occurrence of myosclerosis in these families.

Myoglobinuria

In individuals who have not had a crush injury (Bywaters, Delory, Rimington and Smiles, 1941) or polymyositis (Walton and Adams, 1958), familial myoglobinuria (Meyer-Betz, 1911) is characterised by paroxysmal attacks of generalised muscular pains, often after exercise, accompanied by myoglobinuria which is sometimes associated with permanent muscular wasting. Evidence for the role of genetic factors in this condition is limited to the observation of two affected sibs by Acheson and McAlpine (1953) and of three brothers by Hed (1955). Most reported cases have been sporadic (Reiner, Konikoff, Altschule, Dammin and Merrill, 1956). This information suggests an autosomal recessive pattern of inheritance but the available data is insufficient to rule out other possibilities. There is increasing evidence to suggest that this condition may be due to carnitine palmityl transferase deficiency (see Chapter 18).

Myositis ossificans

Progressive sclerosis of intramuscular connective tissue which is followed by deposition of bone, characterises myositis ossificans (Mair, 1932). Bone is laid down directly without an intermediate stage of calcification. Most cases show congenital anomalies of the great toes and thumbs (van Creveld and Soeters, 1941). Evidence that this condition may be transmitted as a dominant trait with reduced penetrance is suggested by its occurrence in a father and son (Burton-Fanning and Vaughan, 1901) and in a two-generation family (Gaster, 1905). The condition has also been observed in two pairs of monozygotic twins (Vastine, Vastine and Arango, 1948; Eaton, Conkling and Daeschner, 1957). Finally there is a paternal age effect in sporadic cases which also suggests dominant inheritance (Tünte, Becker and Knorre, 1967).

NEUROMUSCULAR DISEASES

Motor neurone disease

Motor neurone disease (MND) may present in one of three forms: progressive bulbar palsy, progressive muscular atrophy and amyotrophic lateral sclerosis. MND may run a rapidly progressive course leading to death within a year or so from the onset. Most cases are non-familial and the cause is obscure. In 10 studies of the familial occurrence of motor neurone disease, 32 secondary cases have been found among 1008 relatives, compared with a prevalence of about 50×10^{-6} in the general population (Pratt, 1967). If the condition is caused by a single autosomal gene then penetrance must be very low. Alternatively, the condition may be due to the operation of several genes (multifactorial). It is also possible that the rare occurrence of the condition in relatives may be due to exposure to a common aetiological agent. Families in which the disease is clearly inherited as an autosomal dominant trait have been described, but are uncommon (Kurland and Mulder, 1955; Engel, Kurland and Klatzo, 1959; Roe, 1964). In 58 consecutive cases studied by Kurland and Mulder (1955) a positive family history was found in only five.

A genetic basis for amyotrophic lateral sclerosis and the parkinsonism–dementia complex, which account for about 1 in 10 adult deaths in the island of Guam, has not yet been proved (Hirano, Malamud, Elizan and Kurland, 1966).

A slowly progressive benign form of motor neurone disease has been described. Many such cases have been sporadic (Pearce and Harriman, 1966) but families have been reported in which the condition appears to be inherited as an autosomal dominant trait (Espinosa, Okihiro, Mulder and Sayre, 1962).

Spinal muscular atrophy

The spinal muscular atrophies (SMA) may be defined as a group of inherited disorders in which the primary defect is degeneration of the anterior horn cells of the spinal cord and often of bulbar motor nuclei but with no evidence of peripheral nerve or long tract involvement. When so defined, motor neurone disease and its variants and the various forms of 'amyotrophy' are excluded as are congenital abnormalities of the spinal cord and traumatic, toxic, infective and neoplastic causes of anterior horn cell degeneration (see Ch. 13).

In an international collaborative study of SMA involving over 500 established cases (Emery, Davie, Holloway and Skinner, 1976a) there was considerable variation in age of onset, though in over three-quarters onset was before 4 years of age and in these cases the prognosis was much worse than where onset was after 4 years of age. A febrile episode, often of viral origin, was occasionally noted at the time of onset which might possibly be of aetiological significance, perhaps by precipitating the disease in a genetically predisposed individual. Proximal limb muscles were predominantly affected and cranial nerves were rarely affected. Almost 10 per cent of cases were reported as being mentally retarded. Muscle fasciculations were present in about half the cases. Electromyography and muscle histology were the most reliable diagnostic criteria, the serum level of creatine kinase being rarely high and in more than half the cases it was normal (Emery et al., 1976a). Most of the cases dealt with in this particular study were of the childhood types of proximal SMA (see below).

Analysis of the genetic data suggested that the majority of these cases were attributable to at least one (but probably several) autosomal recessive genes, very few being inherited as a dominant trait, and in only one out of the 403 families was there any suggestion of X-linked inheritance (Emery, Hausmanowa-Petrusewicz, Davie, Holloway and Skinner, 1976b).

A classification of the spinal muscular atrophies based on clinical and genetic differences has been proposed previously (Emery, 1971, 1973) and will be adopted in the following discussion (Table 22.5).

Table 22.5 A clinicogenetic classification of the spinal muscular atrophies

I *Proximal SMA*
  A. Infantile
    Autosomal recessive
      1. Without arthrogryposis multiplex congenita
      2. With arthrogryposis multiplex congenita
  B. Intermediate
    Autosomal recessive
  C. Juvenile
    1. Autosomal recessive
      a. Usual form (Kugelberg-Welander)
      b. 'Ryukyuan' SMA
      c. With microcephaly and mental subnormality
    2. Autosomal dominant
  D. Adult
    1. Autosomal recessive
    2. Autosomal dominant
    3. X-linked recessive
II *Distal SMA*
    1. Autosomal recessive
    2. Autosomal dominant
III *Juvenile progressive bulbar palsy*
    Autosomal recessive
      1. Usual form (Fazio-Londe)
      2. With nerve deafness (Van Laere)
IV *Scapuloperoneal SMA*
    1. Autosomal dominant
    2. Autosomal recessive
V *Facioscapulohumeral SMA*
    Autosomal dominant

Proximal SMA. The spinal muscular atrophies with predominantly proximal muscle involvement are much commoner than other forms, and can be further subdivided according to age of onset, clinical severity and certain other features (Table 22.6).

Not all investigators agree that proximal SMA can be so subdivided and suggest there is a 'spectrum of clinical variation' ranging from the severe infantile to the more benign forms. If distinct forms exist there should be little variation within a family. We have analysed the clinical and genetic data in 24 published reports involving 201 families of patients with proximal SMA with onset before adulthood (Emery, 1973). The results indicated that there was a high degree of correlation in age of onset and various clinical features within families. Reported families showing considerable clinical variation in different affected members are therefore the exception and are probably highly selective.

Infantile Werdnig-Hoffmann disease. Although mild contractures are frequently found in infants with the infantile (Werdnig, 1891; Hoffmann, 1893) form of proximal SMA, the reported association with arthrogryposis multiplex congenita may well represent a distinct clinical entity. *Both* disorders have been described in several sibs in the same family (Frischknecht, Bianchi and Pilleri, 1960; Bargeton, Nezelof, Guran and Job, 1961).

Table 22.6 Distinguishing features of the various forms of proximal spinal muscular atrophy

Type	Age (Usual) onset	survival	Ability to sit without support*	Fascicula-tions of skeletal muscles	Serum creatine kinase
Infantile	<9 months	<4 years	never	+ / −	normal
Inter-mediate	3–18 months	>4 years	usually	+ / −	usually normal
Juvenile	>2 years	adulthood	always	+ +	often raised
Adult	>30 years	50 years +	always	+ +	often raised

*At some time during the course of the illness.

Intermediate. It has been suggested that an autosomal recessive form of SMA intermediate in severity between the infantile (Werdnig-Hoffmann) and juvenile (Wohlfart-Kugelberg-Welander) forms may exist (Fried and Emery, 1971; Emery, 1971; 1973). Though there is some overlap in age of onset with the infantile form, patients with the intermediate type survive longer, even into the late teens.

Juvenile. Clinical features of the usual autosomal recessive form of juvenile, Wohlfart-Kugelberg-Welander SMA (Wohlfart, Fex and Eliasson, 1955; Kugelberg and Welander, 1956) have been well documented. Possible variants include the autosomal recessive form described in an inbred community in the Ryukyuan islands off Japan, the clinical features of which include pes cavus and scoliosis (Kondo, Tsubaki and Sakamoto, 1970). An autosomal recessive form of juvenile proximal SMA associated with microcephaly and mental subnormality has been described by Spiro, Fogelson and Goldberg (1967) in three brothers. An autosomal dominant form of juvenile proximal SMA has also been described (Kugelberg and Welander, 1956).

Adult. The adult form of proximal SMA may be inherited in different families as an autosomal recessive, autosomal dominant or X-linked recessive trait.

Distal SMA is a relatively benign condition transmitted either as an autosomal recessive or autosomal dominant trait. Onset is usually in early childhood (Meadows and Marsden, 1969). Clinically, the condition resembles peroneal muscular atrophy. However, in the latter condition the legs are typically more severely affected than the arms, peripheral sensory abnormalities can usually be detected if carefully sought, motor nerve conduction velocities are usually reduced and the pathology of peripheral nerves is abnormal, features not found in distal SMA.

Juvenile progressive bulbar palsy (Fazio-Londe's disease) is inherited as an autosomal recessive trait and is characterised by progressive cranial nerve paralyses usually dating from early childhood (Gomez, Clermont and Bernstein, 1962). The association with bilateral perceptive deafness (Van Laere's syndrome) appears to be a different disorder (Boudin, Pepin, Vernant, Gautier and Gouerou, 1971) but is also inherited as an autosomal recessive trait.

Scapuloperoneal muscular atrophy. Most cases of scapuloperoneal SMA are inherited as an autosomal dominant trait but instances of autosomal recessive inheritance have also been described (Feigenbaum and Munsat, 1970; Emery, 1971). The weakness is mainly localised to the pectoral girdle musculature and the peroneal muscles. It may be myopathic or neuropathic (SMA) in origin and the latter group itself is probably heterogeneous as the onset in some cases is in the second or third decade of life, but in others it begins in childhood.

Facioscapulohumeral muscular atrophy. This clinically resembles facioscapulohumeral muscular dystrophy, from which it can be differentiated only on the basis of muscle histology and electromyography. This rare form of SMA can apparently be inherited as an autosomal dominant trait (Fenichel, Emery and Hunt, 1967).

Peroneal muscular atrophy

Slowly progressive weakness and wasting of the peripheral lower limb muscles to give a typical 'champagne bottle' appearance, and wasting of the small muscles of hands and forearm characterise peroneal muscular atrophy (Charcot and Marie, 1886; Tooth, 1886). Although in many studies data have not been sufficient to allow determination of patterns of inheritance, in many cases the disease is clearly inherited as a recessive trait, but studies of several large kindreds (England and Denny-Brown, 1952; Hierons, 1956) clearly demonstrate dominant inheritance. Erwin (1944) presented a pedigree with seven affected males in three generations consistent with an X-linked recessive pattern of inheritance. In a population survey in Norway, Skre (1974) estimated that the relative prevalences of the autosomal recessive, autosomal dominant and X-linked recessive forms of this disease were 1.4, 36 and 3.6 per 100 000 respectively.

Killian and Kloepfer (unpublished) report a kindred with 70 or more heterozygous individuals affected with the classical type of Charcot-Marie-Tooth disease with hypertrophy of peripheral nerves, as described by Dyck, Lambert and Mulder (1963). In this kindred a marriage between two heterozygotes produced a male and a female homozygote with stigmata simulating Dejerine-Sottas syndrome. Dyck and Lambert (1968a, b) have distinguished three main varieties of peroneal muscular atrophy; one is characterised by a hypertrophic neuropathy, is usually of dominant inheritance and is much more benign than Dejerine-Sottas disease. The second, or neuronal variety is also usually dominant but is more severe clinically, while the third and rarest type is probably a form of spinal muscular atrophy, often recessively inherited (distal SMA as defined above). It may well be possible to differentiate the two dominant forms on the basis of nerve conduction studies (Thomas, Calne and Stewart, 1974).

Friedreich's ataxia

Muscular atrophy is seen in some cases of Friedreich's ataxia (Friedreich, 1863) which is characterised by ataxia, spastic paraparesis, sensory tract disorders, nystagmus and pes cavus. The two genetic types of this condition have not been separated clinically.

Autosomal recessive type of Friedreich's ataxia. Bell and Carmichael (1939) reviewed 124 pedigrees of Friedreich's ataxia (351 cases) in which the mode of inheritance was consistent with that of an autosomal recessive trait. Consanguinity between parents was 17.9 per cent. Sjögren (1943) reported seven pedigrees in Sweden in which a similar pattern was observed. McKusick (1978) considers that all cases which legitimately deserve the designation Friedreich's ataxia have recessive inheritance and that cases of dominant inheritance are probably not Friedreich's ataxia.

Autosomal dominant type of Friedreich's ataxia. Bell and Carmichael (1939) reviewed 12 pedigrees (125 cases) in which transmission seemed to be due to an autosomal dominant gene. The rate of consanguinity between parents was not increased. Sjögren (1943) reported seven pedigrees in Sweden in which transmission was as an autosomal dominant trait with complete penetrance in both sexes (see also McKusick, 1978).

Hypertrophic polyneuropathy

A palpable hypertrophy of the sheath of Schwann in peripheral nerve trunks characterises progressive hypertrophic polyneuropathy (Dejerine and Sottas, 1893). In this condition the muscular weakness and wasting is similar to that observed in peroneal muscular atrophy, to which it is closely related (*see above*). Pupillary abnormalities, such as anisocoria, and a slow light reflex, are common (François and Descamps, 1949). From a pedigree presented by Russell and Garland (1930) in which nine individuals were affected in four generations and from that presented by Bedford and James (1956) in which eight were affected in five generations, it may be concluded that this condition is inherited as an autosomal dominant trait with high penetrance in both sexes. Thévenard, van Bogaert, Berdet and Rougerie (1956) found five out of seven sibs affected. When affection is limited to one sibship or to isolated cases and other relatives are not examined, the evidence for reduced penetrance or for inheritance as an autosomal recessive trait may be more apparent than real as subclinical cases may be revealed by clinical examination or nerve conduction velocity measurement.

GENERAL CONCLUSIONS

All neuromuscular disorders have a genetic component to their aetiology though this is relatively less important in some disorders, such as mature onset myasthenia gravis, than in others such as Duchenne muscular dystrophy. The recognition of genetic heterogeneity within what clinically may appear to be a single disorder is important for a number of reasons. Disorders inherited differently presumably have a different biochemical basis, they may have different prognoses and might conceivably respond differently to a particular treatment should such become available. However, the most important reason for understanding the genetic basis of a particular neuromuscular disorder is for reliable genetic counselling. Hereditary disorders, including neuromuscular disorders, are invariably serious, rarely treatable and never curable. The only approach at present is therefore prevention through genetic counselling. This is likely to become increasingly effective in the future when the basic biochemical defects in these disorders are better understood, because this would then lead to reliable tests for detecting carriers and preclinical cases and would probably make prenatal diagnosis possible.

REFERENCES

Acheson, D. & McAlpine, D. (1953) Muscular dystrophy associated with paroxysmal myoglobinuria and excessive excretion of ketosteroids. *Lancet*, **2**, 327.

Aitken, R.S., Allott, E.N., Castleden, L.I.M. & Walker, M. (1937) Observations on a case of familial periodic paralysis. *Clinical Science*, **3**, 47.

Bacon, P.A. & Smith, B. (1971) Familial muscular dystrophy of late onset. *Journal of Neurology, Neurosurgery and Psychiatry*, **34**, 93.

Banker, B.Q., Victor, M. & Adams, R.D. (1957) Arthrogryposis multiplex due to congenital muscular dystrophy. *Brain*, **80**, 319.

Bargeton, E., Nezelof, C., Guran, P. & Job, J.C. (1961) Etude anatomique d'un cas d'arthrogrypose multiple congénitale et familiale. *Revue Neurologique (Paris)*, **104**, 479.

Batten, F.E. (1910) Critical review: the myopathies or muscular dystrophies. *Quarterly Journal of Medicine*, **3**, 313.

Batten, F.E. & Gibb, H.P. (1909) Myotonia atrophica. *Brain*, **32**, 187.

Becker, P.E. (1953) *Dystrophia musculorum progressiva. Eine genetische und klinische Untersuchung der Muskeldystrophien.* (Georg Thieme: Stuttgart.)

Becker, P.E. (1955) Zur Genetik der Myopathien. *Deutsche Zeitschrift für Nervenheilkunde*, **173**, 482.

Becker, P.E. (1957) Neue Ergebnisse der Genetik der Muskeldystrophien. *Acta genetica et statistica medica (Basel)*, **7**, 303.

Becker, P.E. (1962) Two new families of benign sex-linked recessive muscular dystrophy. *Revue canadienne de biologie*, **21**, 551.

Becker, P.E. (1964) Myopathien. In *Humangenetik, Ein Kurzes Handbuch*. Vol. 3. Ed. P.E. Becker (Georg Thieme: Stuttgart).

Becker, P.E. (1977) *Myotonia congenita and syndromes associated with myotonia* (Georg Thieme: Stuttgart).

Becker, P.E. & Kiener, F. (1955) Eine neue X chromosomale Muskeldystrophie. *Zeitschrift für Neurologie*, **193**, 427.

Beckmann, R. & Jerusalem, F. (1966) Male carriers of Duchenne-type muscular dystrophy? *Lancet*, **2**, 1138.

Bedford, P.D. & James, F.E. (1956) A family with progressive hypertrophic polyneuritis of Dejerine and Sottas. *Journal of Neurology and Psychiatry*, **19**, 46.

Bell, J. (1943) Nervous diseases and muscular dystrophies. On pseudohypertrophic and allied types of progressive muscular dystrophy. *Treasury of Human Inheritance*, **4** (Part IV), 283.

Bell, J. (1947) On dystrophia myotonica, myotonia congenita and paramyotonia. *Treasury of Human Inheritance*, **4** (Part V), 343.

Bell, J. & Carmichael, E.A. (1939) On hereditary ataxia and spastic paraplegia. *Treasury of Human Inheritance*, **4** (Part III), 137.

Biemond, A. & Daniels, A.P. (1934) Familial periodic paralysis and its transmission into spinal muscular atrophy. *Brain*, **57**, 91.

Birt, A. (1908) A study of Thomsen's disease (congenital myotonia) by a sufferer from it. *Montreal Medical Journal*, **37**, 771.

Blyth, H. & Pugh, R.J. (1959) Muscular dystrophy in childhood. The genetic aspect. *Annals of Human Genetics*, **23**, 127.

Blyth, H., Carter, C.O., Dubowitz, V., Emery, A.E.H., Gavin, J., Johnston, H.A., McKusick, V.A., Race, R.R., Sanger, R. & Tippett, P. (1965) Duchenne's muscular dystrophy and the Xg blood groups: A search for linkage. *Journal of Medical Genetics*, **2**, 157.

Boudin, G., Pepin, B., Vernant, J.C., Gautier, B. & Gouerou, H. (1971) Cas familial de paralysie bulbo-pontine chronique progressive avec surdité. *Revue Neurologique (Paris)*, **124**, 90.

Boyes, J.W., Fraser, F.C., Lawler, S.D. & Mackenzie, H.J. (1949) A pedigree of progressive muscular dystrophy. *Annals of Eugenics*, **15**, 46.

Bradley, W.G., Price, D.L. & Watanabe, C.K. (1970) Familial centronuclear myopathy. *Journal of Neurology, Neurosurgery and Psychiatry*, **33**, 687.

Brandt, S. (1950) Werdnig-Hoffman's infantile progressive

muscular atrophy. *Opera ex domo biologiae hereditariae humanae Universitatis hafniensis*, Vol. 22.

Bray, G.M., Kaarsoo, M. & Ross, R.T. (1965). Ocular myopathy with dysphagia. *Neurology (Minneapolis)*, **15**, 678.

Brooks, A.P., & Emery, A.E.H. (1977) The incidence of Duchenne muscular dystrophy in the south-east of Scotland. *Clinical Genetics*, **11**, 290.

Bundey, S. (1972) A genetic study of infantile and juvenile myasthenia gravis. *Journal of Neurology, Neurosurgery and Psychiatry*, **35**, 41.

Bundey, S., Carter, C.O. & Soothill, J.F. (1970) Early recognition of heterozygotes for the gene for dystrophia myotonica. *Journal of Neurology, Neurosurgery and Psychiatry*, **33**, 279.

Burton-Fanning, F.W. & Vaughan, A.L. (1901) A case of myositis ossificans. *Lancet*, **2**, 849.

Bywaters, E.G.L., Delory, G.E., Rimington, C. & Smiles, J. (1941) Myohaemoglobin in the urine of air raid casualties with crushing injury. *Biochemical Journal*, **35**, 1164.

Cammann, R., Vehreschild, T. & Ernst, K. (1974) Eine neue Sippe von X-chromosomaler benigner Muskeldystrophie mit Frühkontrakturen (Emery-Dreifuss). *Psychiatrie Neurologie und medizinische Psychologie (Leipzig)*, **26**, 431.

Caruso, G. & Buchthal, F. (1965) Refractory period of muscle and electromyographic findings in relatives of patients with muscular dystrophy. *Brain*, **88**, 29.

Cerny, A. & Katzonstein-Sutro, E. (1952) Die paroxysmale Lähmung. *Schweizer Archiv für Neurologie und Psychiatrie*, **70**, 259.

Charcot, J.M. & Marie, P. (1886) Sur une forme particulière d'atrophie musculaire progressive, souvent familiale, débutant par les pieds et les jambes, et atteignant plus tard les mains. *Revue médicale française*, **6**, 97.

Chung, C.S. & Morton, N.E. (1959) Discrimination of genetic entities in muscular dystrophy. *American Journal of Human Genetics*, **11**, 339.

Conomy, J.P. (1970) Late-onset slowly progressive sex-linked recessive muscular dystrophy. *Military Medicine*, **135**, 471.

Davie, A. & Emery, A.E.H. (1978) Estimation of the proportion of new mutants among cases of Duchenne muscular dystrophy. *Genetics*, **15**, 339.

Dejerine, J. & Sottas, J. (1893) Sur la névrite interstitielle hypertrophique et progressive de l'enfance; affection souvent familiale et a début infantile, caractérisée par une atrophie musculaire des extremités, avec troubles marques de la sensibilité et ataxie des mouvements et rélévant d'une névrite interstitielle hypertrophique à marche ascendante avec lesions medullaires consécutives. *Comptes rendus des séances de la Société de biologie et de ses filiales (Paris)*, **5**, 63.

Démos, J., Dreyfus, J.C., Schapira, F. & Schapira, G. (1962) Anomalies biologiques chez les transmetteurs apparemment sains de la myopathie. *Revue canadienne de biologie*, **21**, 587.

Dodge, P.R., Gamstorp, I., Byers, R.K. & Russell, P. (1965) Myotonic dystrophy in infancy and childhood. *Pediatrics*, **35**, 3.

Dubowitz, V. (1960) Progressive muscular dystrophy of the Duchenne type and its mode of inheritance. *Brain*, **83**, 432.

Dubowitz, V. (1963) Myopathic changes in muscular dystrophy carriers. *Proceedings of the Royal Society of Medicine*, **56**, 810.

Dubowitz, V. (1978) *Muscle Disorders in Childhood* (Saunders: London).

Dubowitz, V. & Platts, M. (1965) Central core disease of muscle with focal wasting. *Journal of Neurology, Neurosurgery and Psychiatry*, **28**, 432.

Dubowitz, V. & Roy, S. (1970) Central core disease of muscle: clinical, histochemical and electron microscopic studies of an affected mother and child. *Brain*, **93**, 133.

Dyck, P.V. & Lambert, E.H. (1968a, b). Lower motor and primary sensory neurone disease with peroneal muscular atrophy. I. Neurologic, genetic and electrophysiologic findings in hereditary polyneuropathies. II. Neurologic, genetic and electrophysiologic findings in various neuronal degenerations. *Archives of Neurology*, **18**, 603, 619.

Dyck, P.J., Lambert, E.H. & Mulder, D.W. (1963) Charcot-Marie-Tooth disease: nerve conduction and clinical studies of a large kindred. *Neurology (Minneapolis)*, **13**, 1.

Eaton, W.L., Conkling, W.S. & Daeschner, C.W. (1957) Early myositis ossificans progressiva occurring in homozygotic twins; a clinical and pathological study. *Journal of Pediatrics*, **50**, 591.

Emery, A.E.H. (1963) Clinical manifestations in two carriers of Duchenne muscular dystrophy. *Lancet*, **1**, 1126.

Emery, A.E.H. (1964) The electrophoretic pattern of lactic dehydrogenase in carriers and patients with Duchenne muscular dystrophy. *Nature*, **201**, 1044.

Emery, A.E.H. (1965) Muscle histology in carriers of Duchenne muscular dystrophy. *Journal of Medical Genetics*, **2**, 1.

Emery, A.E.H. (1966) Genetic linkage between the loci for colour blindness and Duchenne type muscular dystrophy. *Journal of Medical Genetics*, **3**, 92.

Emery, A.E.H. (1967) The use of serum creatine kinase for detecting carriers of Duchenne muscular dystrophy. In *Exploratory concepts in muscular dystrophy and related disorders*. Ed. A.T. Milhorat, p. 90 (Excerpta Medica International Congress ser. 147: Amsterdam).

Emery, A.E.H. (1969a) Genetic counselling in X-linked muscular dystrophy. *Journal of the Neurological Sciences*, **8**, 579.

Emery, A.E.H. (1969b) Abnormalities of the electrocardiogram in female carriers of Duchenne muscular dystrophy. *British Medical Journal*, **2**, 418.

Emery, A.E.H. (1971) The nosology of the spinal muscular atrophies. *Journal of Medical Genetics*, **8**, 481.

Emery, A.E.H. (1973) The nosology of the spinal muscular atrophies. In *Clinical Studies in Myology*. Ed. B.A. Kakulas p. 439 (Excerpta Medica: Amsterdam).

Emery, A.E.H. (1976) *Methodology in Medical Genetics—An Introduction to Statistical Methods* (Churchill Livingstone: Edinburgh, London and New York).

Emery, A.E.H. (1977a) Genetic considerations in the X-linked muscular dystrophies. In *Pathogenesis of Human Muscular Dystrophies*. Ed. L.P. Rowland. p. 42 (Excerpta Medica: Amsterdam).

Emery, A.E.H. (1977b) Muscle histology and creatine kinase levels in the fetus in Duchenne muscular dystrophy. *Nature*, **266**, 472.

Emery, A.E.H. & Dreifuss, F.E. (1966) Unusual type of benign X-linked muscular dystrophy. *Journal of Neurology, Neurosurgery and Psychiatry*, **29**, 338.

Emery, A.E.H. & Holloway, S. (1977) Use of normal daughters' and sisters' creatine kinase levels in estimating heterozygosity in Duchenne muscular dystrophy. *Human Heredity*, **27**, 118.

Emery, A.E.H. & Schelling, J.L. (1965) Limb blood flow in patients and carriers of Duchenne muscular dystrophy.

Acta genetica et statistica medica (Basel), **15**, 337.

Emery, A.E.H. & Skinner, R. (1976) Clinical studies in benign (Becker type) X-linked muscular dystrophy. *Clinical Genetics*, **10**, 189.

Emery, A.E.H. & Spikesman, A. (1970) Evidence against the existence of a subclinical form of X-linked Duchenne muscular dystrophy. *Journal of the Neurological Sciences*, **10**, 523.

Emery, A.E.H. & Walton, J.N. (1967) The genetics of muscular dystrophy. In *Progress in Medical Genetics*. Vol. 5. Eds A.G. Steinberg and A.G. Bearn, p. 116 (Grune and Stratton: New York).

Emery, A.E.H., Skinner, R. & Holloway, S. (1979b) A study of possible heterogeneity in Duchenne muscular dystrophy. *Clinical Genetics*, **15**, 444.

Emery, A.E.H., Smith, C.A.B. & Sanger, R. (1969) The linkage relations of the loci for benign (Becker type) X-borne muscular dystrophy, colour blindness and the Xg blood groups. *Annals of Human Genetics*, **32**, 261.

Emery, A.E.H., Teasdall, R.D. & Coomes, E.N. (1966) Electromyographic studies in carriers of Duchenne muscular dystrophy. *Bulletin of the Johns Hopkins Hospital*, **118**, 439.

Emery, A.E.H., Clack, E.R., Simon, S. & Taylor, J.L. (1967) Detection of carriers of benign X-linked muscular dystrophy. *British Medical Journal*, **4**, 522.

Emery, A.E.H., Davie, A.M., Holloway, S. & Skinner, R. (1976a) International collaborative study of the spinal muscular atrophies Part 2. Analysis of genetic data. *Journal of the Neurological Sciences*, **30**, 375.

Emery, A.E.H., Hausmanowa-Petrusewicz, I., Davie, A.M., Holloway, S. & Skinner, R. (1976b). International collaborative study of the spinal muscular atrophies. Part 1. Analysis of clinical and laboratory data. *Journal of the Neurological Sciences*, **29**, 83.

Emery, A.E.H., Burt, D., Dubowitz, V., Rocker, I., Donnai, D., Harris, R. & Donnai, P. (1979a) Antenatal diagnosis of Duchenne muscular dystrophy. *Lancet*, **1**, 847.

Engel, W.K., Kurland, L.T. & Klatzo, I. (1959) An inherited disease similar to amyotrophic lateral sclerosis with a pattern of posterior column involvement. An intermediate form? *Brain*, **82**, 203.

Engel, W.K., Foster, J.B., Hughes, B.P., Huxley, H.E. & Mahler, R. (1961) Central core disease—An investigation of rare muscle cell abnormality. *Brain*, **84**, 167.

England, A.C. & Denny-Brown, D. (1952) Severe sensory changes and trophic disorder in peroneal muscular atrophy (Charcot-Marie-Tooth type). *Archives of Neurology and Psychiatry*, **67**, 1.

Erwin, W.G. (1944) A pedigree of sex-linked recessive peroneal atrophy. *Journal of Heredity*, **35**, 24.

Espinosa, R.E., Okihiro, M.M., Mulder, D.W. & Sayre, G.P. (1962) Hereditary amyotrophic lateral sclerosis. *Neurology (Minneapolis)*, **12**, 1.

Eulenburg, A. (1886) Ueber eine familiare, durch 6 Generationen verfolgbare form congenitaler Paramiotonie. *Neurologisches Zentralblatt*, **5**, 265.

Feigenbaum, J.A. & Munsat, T.L. (1970) A neuromuscular syndrome of scapuloperoneal distribution. *Bulletin of the Los Angeles Neurological Society*, **35**, 47.

Fenichel, G.M., Emery, E.S. & Hunt, P. (1967) Neurogenic atrophy simulating facioscapulohumeral dystrophy. *Archives of Neurology*, **17**, 257.

Ferrier, P., Bamatter, F. & Klein, D. (1965) Muscular dystrophy (Duchenne) in a girl with Turner's syndrome.

Journal of Medical Genetics, **2**, 38.

Fitzgerald, P.H. & Caughey, J.E. (1962) Chromosome and sex chromatin studies in cases of dystrophia myotonica. *New Zealand Medical Journal*, **61**, 410.

Foldes, F.C. & McNell, P.G. (1960) Unusual occurrence of myasthenia gravis. *Journal of the American Medical Association*, **174**, 418.

Ford, F.R. (1966) *Diseases of the nervous system in infancy, childhood and adolescence*. 5th Edn. (Thomas: Springfield, Illinois).

François, J. & Descamps, L. (1949) Etude neuro-ophthalmologique de deux sources d'amyotrophie neurale hérédo-dégénerative, l'une du type Charcot-Marie-Tooth (famille Joly), l'autre du type névrite hypertrophique de Dejerine-Sottas (famille Molle). *Acta Neurologica et psychiatrica Belgica*, **49**, 648.

Fried, K. & Emery, A.E.H. (1971) Spinal muscular atrophy type II. *Clinical Genetics*, **2**, 203.

Friedreich, N. (1863) Ueber degenerative Atrophie der spinalen Hinterstränge. *Virchows Archiv für pathologische Anatomie und Physiologie und für klinische medizin*, **26**, 391.

Frischknecht, W., Bianchi, L. & Pilleri, G. (1960) Familiare Arthrogryposis multiplex congenita Neuro-arthro-myodysplasia congenita. *Helvetica Paediatrica Acta*, **15**, 259.

Fukuyama, F., Kawozura, M. & Haruna, H. (1960) A peculiar form of congenital muscular dystrophy. Report of 15 cases. *Paediatrics (Tokyo)*, **4**, 5.

Gamstorp, I. (1956) Adynamia episodica hereditaria. *Acta paediatrica (Stockholm)*, Suppl. 108.

Gardner-Medwin, D. (1970) Mutation rate in Duchenne type of muscular dystrophy. *Journal of Medical Genetics*, **7**, 334.

Gardner-Medwin, D., Pennington, R.J. & Walton, J.N. (1971) The detection of carriers of X-linked muscular dystrophy genes. A review of some methods studied in Newcastle upon Tyne. *Journal of the Neurological Sciences*, **13**, 459.

Gaster, D. (1905) A case of myositis ossificans. *West London Medical Journal*, **10**, 37.

Gaupp, R. (1940) Erblichkeitsuntersuchungen beiparoxysmaler Lahmung. *Zeitschrift für die gesamte Neurologie und Psychiatrie*, **170**, 108.

Golbus, M.S., Stephens, J.D., Mahoney, M.J., Hobbins, J.C., Haseltine, F.P., Caskey, C.T. & Banker, B.Q. (1979) Failure of fetal creatine phosphokinase as a diagnostic indicator of Duchenne muscular dystrophy. *New England Journal of Medicine*, **300**, 860.

Gomez, M.R., Clermont, V. & Bernstein, J. (1962) Progressive bulbar paralysis in childhood (Fazio-Londe's disease). *Archives of Neurology*, **6**, 317.

Gordon, N. (1966) Benign congenital hypotonia. A syndrome or a disease? *Developmental Medicine and Child Neurology*, **8**, 330.

Greenfield, J.G., Cornman, T. & Shy, G.M. (1958) The prognostic value of the muscle biopsy in the 'floppy infant'. *Brain*, **81**, 461.

Greig, D.N.H. (1977) Family in which Duchenne's muscular dystrophy and protan colour blindness are segregating. *Journal of Medical Genetics*, **14**, 130.

Harper, P.S. (1975) Congenital myotonic dystrophy in Britain. II. Genetic basis. *Archives of Disease in Childhood*, **50**, 514.

Hausmanowa-Petrusewicz, I., Prot, J., Dobosz, I., Emeryk, B., Rowinska, K., Rubach, K., Ropeć, A & Kopeć, J. (1971) Further studies concerning the detection of carriership in the Duchenne type of dystrophy. *European Neurology*, **5**, 186.

Hayes, R., London, W., Seidman, J. & Embree, L. (1963) Oculopharyngeal muscular dystrophy. *New England Journal of Medicine*, **268**, 163.

Hed, R. (1955) *Myoglobinuria in Man*. (Norstedt: Stockholm.)

Helweg-Larson, H.F., Hauge, M. & Sagild, E. (1955) Periodic paralysis. *Acta genetica et statistica medica (Basel)*, **5**, 263.

Heyck, H., Laudahn, G. & Carsten, P.M. (1966) Enzymaktivitätsbestimmungen bei Dystrophia musculorum progressiva. IV. Die Serumenzymkinetik im präklinischen Stadium des Typus Duchenne während der ersten 2 Lebensjahre. *Klinische Wochenschrift*, **44**, 695.

Hierons, R. (1956) Familial peroneal muscular atrophy and its association with familial ataxias and tremor and longevity. *Journal of Neurology, Neurosurgery and Psychiatry*, **19**, 155.

Hirano, A., Malamud, N., Elizan, T.S. & Kurland, L.T. (1966) Amyotrophic lateral sclerosis and Parkinsonism-dementia complex on Guam. *Archives of Neurology*, **15**, 35.

Hoffmann, J. (1893) Ueber chronische spinale Muskelatrophie im Kindesalter auf familiarer basis. *Deutsche zeitschrift für Nervenheilkunde*, **3**, 427.

Holtzapple, G.E. (1905) Periodic paralysis. *Journal of the American Medical Association*, **45**, 1224.

Hopkins, I.J., Lindsey, J.R. & Ford, F.R. (1966) Nemaline myopathy. A long term clinicopathologic study of affected mother and daughter. *Brain*, **89**, 299.

Hudson, A.J. (1963) Progressive neurological disorder and myotonia congenita associated with paramyotonia. *Brain*, **86**, 811.

Ionasescu, V. (1975) Distinction between Duchenne and other muscular dystrophies by ribosomal protein synthesis. *Journal of Medical Genetics*, **12**, 49.

Ionasescu, V., Zellweger, H. & Cancilla, P. (1978) Fetal serum-creatine-phosphokinase not a valid predictor of Duchenne muscular dystrophy. *Lancet*, **2**, 1251.

Jackson, C.E. & Carey, J.N. (1961) Progressive muscular dystrophy; autosomal recessive type. *Pediatrics*, **28**, 77.

Jackson, J.F. (1965) Chromosomes in dystrophia myotonica. *Lancet*, **1**, 1225.

Jacob, A., Clack, E.R. & Emery, A.E.H. (1968) Genetic study of sample of 70 patients with myasthenia gravis. *Journal of Medical Genetics*, **5**, 257.

Jantz, H. (1947) Stoffwechsel untersuchungen bei paroxysmaler Lähmung. *Nervenarzt*, **18**, 360.

Jenis, E.H., Lindquist, R.R. & Lister, R.C. (1969) New congenital myopathy with crystalline intranuclear inclusions. *Archives of Neurology*, **20**, 281.

Jerusalem, F., Engel, A.G. & Gomez, M.R. (1973) Sarcotubular myopathy. *Neurology (Minneapolis)*, **23**, 897.

Johnston, H.A. (1964) Severe muscular dystrophy in girls. *Journal of Medical Genetics*, **1**, 79.

Johnston, H.A., Wilkinson, J.H., Withycombe, W.A. & Raymond, S. (1966) Alpha-hydroxybutyrate dehydrogenase activity in sex-linked muscular dystrophy. *Journal of Clinical Pathology*, **19**, 250.

de John, J.G.Y. (1955) *Myotonia* (Van Gorcum: Assen).

Kaloustian, V.M., Afifi, A.K. & Mire, J. (1972) The myopathic variety of arthrogryposis multiplex congenita: a disorder with autosomal recessive inheritance. *Journal of Pediatrics*, **81**, 76.

Karpati, G., Carpenter, S. & Andermann, F. (1971) A new

concept of childhood nemaline myopathy. *Archives of Neurology*, **24**, 291.

Kiloh, L.G. & Nevin, S. (1951) Progressive dystrophy of the external ocular muscles. *Brain*, **74**, 115.

Kinoshita, M., Satoyoshi, E. & Kumagai, M. (1975) Familial type I fiber atrophy. *Journal of the Neurological Sciences*, **25**, 11.

Klein, D. (1961) Dystrophia Myotonica and the Clinical and Genetic Aspects of the Problems of Myotonia, *2nd International Conference of Human Genetics*: Rome, p. 81.

Kloepfer, H.W. & Talley, C. (1958) Autosomal recessive inheritance of Duchenne-type muscular dystrophy. *Annals of Human Genetics*, **22**, 138.

Kondo, K., Tsubaki, T. & Sakamoto, F. (1970) The Ryukyuan muscular atrophy. An obscure heritable neuromuscular disease found in the islands of Southern Japan. *Journal of Neurological Sciences*, **11**, 359.

Kowalewski, S., Rotthauwe, H.W., Mölbert, E. & Mumenthaler, M. (1966) Female carriers of muscular dystrophy. *Lancet*, **1**, 1216.

Krabbe, K.H. (1958) Congenital generalized muscular atrophies. *Acta psychiatrica et neurologica*, **33**, 94.

Kugelberg, E. & Welander, L. (1956) Heredofamilial juvenile muscular atrophy simulating muscular dystrophy. *Archives of Neurology and Psychiatry*, **75**, 500.

Kurland, L.T. & Mulder, D.W. (1955) Epidemiologic investigations of amyotrophic lateral sclerosis—familial aggregations indicative of dominant inheritance. *Neurology (Minneapolis)*, **5**, 182.

Kuroiwa, Y. & Miyazaki, T. (1967) Epidemiological study of myopathy in Japan. In *Exploratory Concepts in Muscular Dystrophy*. Ed. A.T. Milhorat. p. 98 (Excerpta Medica: Amsterdam).

Lamy, M. & de Grouchy, J. (1954) L'hérédité de la myopathie (formes basses). *Journal de génétique humaine*, **3**, 219.

Lees, F. & Liversedge, L.A. (1962) Descending ocular myopathy. *Brain*, **85**, 701.

Levison, H. (1951) Dystrophia musculorum progressiva; clinical and diagnostic criteria; inheritance. *Acta psychiatrica et Neurologica*, suppl., **76**, 1.

Löwenthal, A. (1954) Myosclérose familiale. *Études presentées à la 1re réunion neurologique*, p. 62. (Belgo-Suisse: Vevey.)

Lumb, E.M. & Emery, A.E.H. (1975) Erythrocyte deformation in Duchenne muscular dystrophy. *British Medical Journal*, **2**, 467.

Lynas, M. (1957) Dystrophia myotonica with special reference to Northern Ireland. *Annals of Human Genetics*, **21**, 318.

Lyon, M.F. (1961) Gene action in the X-chromosomes of the mouse (*Mus. musculus* L.). *Nature*, **190**, 372.

Lyon, M.F. (1962) Sex chromatin and gene action in the mammalian X-chromosome. *American Journal of Human Genetics*, **14**, 135.

Maas, O. & Paterson, A.S. (1943) Genetic and familial aspects of dystrophia myotonica. *Brain*, **66**, 55.

Mabry, C.C., Roeckel, I.E., Munich, R.L. & Robertson, D. (1965) X-linked pseudohypertrophic muscular dystrophy with a late onset and slow progression. *New England Journal of Medicine*, **273**, 1062.

Macciotta, A., Costa, V., Cao, A., Sforza, F. & Scano, V. (1964) Studio istologico sul tessuto muscolare die genitori di un bambino con Miodistrofia pelvi-femoral tipo Duchenne. *Annali Italiani di Pediatria*, **17**, 1.

Magee, K.R. & de Jong, R.N. (1965) Hereditary distal myopathy with onset in infancy. *Archives of Neurology*, **13**, 387.

Mahoney, M.J., Haseltine, F.P., Hobbins, J.C., Banker, B.Q., Caskey, C.T. & Golbus, M.S. (1977) Prenatal diagnosis of Duchenne's muscular dystrophy. *New England Journal of Medicine*, **297**, 968.

Mair, W.E. (1932) Myositis ossificans progressiva. *Edinburgh Medical Journal*, **29**, 13, 69.

Mannucci, P.M., Idéo, G., Cao, A. & Macciotta, A. (1965) Gli isoenzimi della latticodeidrogenasi (LDH) e della transaminasi glutammico-ossalacetica (TGO) nel muscolo fetale, adulto, e di Sogetti affetti da distrofia muscolare, progressiva tipo Duchenne. *Rassegna medica Sarda*, **68**, 287.

Markand, O.N., North, R.R., D'Agostino, A.M. & Daly, D.D. (1969) Benign sex-linked muscular dystrophy. *Neurology (Minneapolis)*, **19**, 617.

McKusick, V.A. (1978) *Mendelian Inheritance in Man*. 5th edition (Heinemann: London).

McQuarrie, I. & Ziegler, M.R. (1952) Hereditary periodic paralysis; effects of fasting and of various types of diet on occurrence of paralytic attacks. *Metabolism*, **1**, 129.

McLeod, J.G., Baker, W. de C., Lethlean, A.K. & Shorey, C.D. (1972) Centronuclear myopathy with autosomal dominant inheritance. *Journal of the Neurological Sciences*, **15**, 375.

Meadows, J.C. & Marsden, C.D. (1969) A distal form of chronic spinal muscular atrophy. *Neurology (Minneapolis)*, **19**, 53.

Meyer-Betz, F. (1911) Zur vergleichenden Pathologie der paroxysmalen Hemoglobinurie. *Deutsches Archiv für Klinische Medizin*, **103**, 150.

Meyers, K.R., Golomb, H.M., Hansen, J.L. & McKusick, V.A. (1974) Familial neuromuscular disease with 'myotubes'. *Clinical Genetics*, **5**, 327.

Meyers, W.A. (1949) Familial periodic paralysis as traced in one family for five generations. *Pennsylvania Medical Journal*, **52**, 1060.

Milhorat, A.T. (1961) Clinico-genetic Aspects of Muscular Dystrophy. *2nd International Conference of Human Genetics*: Rome, p. 83.

Mitchell, J.K., Flexner, S. & Edsall, D.L. (1902) A brief report of the clinical, physiological and chemical study of three cases of family periodic paralysis. *Brain*, **25**, 109.

Moosa, A., Brown, B.H. & Dubowitz, V. (1972) Quantitative electromyography: carrier detection in Duchenne type muscular dystrophy using a new automatic technique. *Journal of Neurology, Neurosurgery and Psychiatry*, **35**, 841.

Morris, C.J. & Raybould, J.A. (1971) Histochemically demonstrable fibre abnormalities in normal skeletal muscle and in muscle from carriers of Duchenne muscular dystrophy. *Journal of Neurology, Neurosurgery and Psychiatry*, **34**, 348.

Morton, N.E. & Chung, C.S. (1959) Formal genetics of muscular dystrophy. *American Journal of Human Genetics*, **11**, 360.

Morton, N.E., Chung, C.S. & Peters, H.A. (1963) Genetics of muscular dystrophy. In *Muscular Dystrophy in Man and Animals*. Ed. G.H. Bourne & N. Golarz (Karger: Basel).

Moser, H., & Emery, A.E.H. (1974) The manifesting carrier in Duchenne muscular dystrophy. *Clinical Genetics*, **5**, 271.

Moser, H., Wiesmann, U., Richterich, R. & Rossi, E. (1964) Progressive muskeldystrophie VI. Häufigkeit, Klinik und Genetik der Duchenne-Form. *Schweizerische medizinische Wochenschrift*, **94**, 1610.

Mutton, D.E. & Gross, N. (1965) Chromosomes in dystrophia myotonica. *Lancet*, **2**, 289.

Namba, T., Brunner, N.G., Brown, S.B., Muguruma, M. & Grob, D. (1971) Familial myasthenia gravis. *Archives of Neurology*, **25**, 49.

O'Brien, M.D. (1962) An infantile muscular dystrophy. Report of a case with autopsy findings. *Guy's Hospital Reports*, **111**, 98.

Okinaka, S., Sugita, H., Momoi, H., Toyokura, Y., Kumagai, H., Ebashi, S. & Fujie, Y. (1959) Serum creatine phosphokinase and aldolase activity in neuromuscular disorders. *84th annual meeting of the American Neurological Association*: Atlantic City.

Oliver, C.P., McQuarrie, I. & Ziegler, M. (1944) Hereditary periodic paralysis in a family showing varied manifestations. *American Journal of Diseases of Children*, **69**, 308.

Pearce, G.W., Pearce, J.M.S. & Walton, J.N. (1966) The Duchenne type muscular dystrophy: histopathological studies of the carrier state. *Brain*, **89**, 109.

Pearce, J.M.S. & Harriman, D.G.F. (1966) Chronic spinal muscular atrophy. *Journal of Neurology, Neurosurgery and Psychiatry*, **29**, 509.

Pearson, C.M. (1964) The periodic paralyses: differential features and pathological observations in permanent myopathic weakness. *Brain*, **87**, 341.

Pearson, C.M. & Fowler, W.M. (1963) Hereditary non-progressive muscular dystrophy inducing arthrogryposis syndrome. *Brain*, **86**, 75.

Pearson, C.M. & Kar, N.C. (1966) Isoenzymes: general considerations and alterations in human and animal myopathies. *Annals of the New York Academy of Sciences*, **138**, 293.

Pearson, C.M. & Rose, A.S. (1960) The inflammatory disorders of muscle. *Research Publications, Association for Research in Nervous and Mental Disease*, **38**, 422.

Pearson, C.M., Fowler, W.M. & Wright, S.W. (1963) X-chromosome mosaicism in females with muscular dystrophy. *Proceedings of the National Academy of Sciences of the United States of America*, **50**, 24.

Penn, A.S., Lisak, R.P. & Rowland, L.P. (1970) Muscular dystrophy in young girls. *Neurology (Minneapolis)*, **20**, 147.

Pescia, G. & Emery, A.E.H. (1976) Valeur et limites de l'examen biomicroscopique du cristallin dans la detection des heterozygotes pour la dystrophie myotonique. *Journal de Génétique humaine*, **24**, 227.

Peterman, A.F., Lillington, G.A. & Jamplis, R.W. (1964) Progressive muscular dystrophy with ptosis and dysphagia. *Archives of Neurology*, **10**, 38.

Pratt, R.T.C. (1967) *The Genetics of Neurological Disorders*. (Oxford University Press: London.)

Prot, J. (1971) Genetic-epidemiological studies in progressive muscular dystrophy. *Journal of Medical Genetics*, **8**, 90.

Race, R.R. (1955) On the inheritance of muscular dystrophy. A note on the blood groups. *Annals of Human Genetics*, **20**, 13.

Radu, H. & Stenzel, K. (1969a) Beiträge zum Studium der pseudohypertrophischen Muskeldystrophien I. Gutartige pseudohypertrophische Muskeldystrophie. *Deutsche Zeitschrift für Nervenheilkunde*, **196**, 92.

Radu, H. & Stenzel, K. (1969b) Beiträge zum Studium der pseudohypertrophischen Muskeldystrophien II. Pseudohypertrophische Muskeldystrophie bei Mädchen. *Deutsche Zeitschrift für Nervenheilkunde*, **196**, 116.

Reiner, L.R., Konikoff, N., Altschule, M.D., Dammin, G.J. & Merrill, J.P. (1956) Idiopathic paroxysmal myoglobinuria; report of 2 cases and evaluation of syndrome. *Archives of Internal Medicine*, **97**, 537.

Renwick, J.H., Bundey, S.E., Ferguson-Smith, M.A. & Izatt, M. (1971) Confirmation of linkage of the loci for myotonic dystrophy and ABH secretion. *Journal of Medical Genetics*, **8**, 407.

Richterich, R., Rosin, S., Aebi, U. & Rossi, E. (1963) Progressive muscular dystrophy V. The identification of the carrier state in the Duchenne type by serum creatine kinase determination. *American Journal of Human Genetics*, **15**, 133.

Roe, P.F. (1964) Familial motor neurone disease. *Journal of Neurology, Neurosurgery and Psychiatry*, **27**, 140.

Roses, A.D., Roses, M.J., Metcalf, B.S., Hull, K.L., Nicholson, G.A., Hartwig, G.B. & Roe, C.R. (1977) Pedigree testing in Duchenne muscular dystrophy. *Annals of Neurology*, **2**, 271.

Rotthauwe, H.W. & Kowalewski, S. (1965) Klinische und biochemische Untersuchungen bei Myopathien I. Serumenzyme bei progressiver Muskeldystrophie (Typ I, II, IIIa). *Klinische Wochenschrift*, **43**, 144.

Rotthauwe, H.W. & Kowalewski, S. (1966a) Gutartige recessiv X-chromosal vererbte Muskeldystrophie I. Untersuchungen bei Merkmalsträgern. *Humangenetik*, **3**, 17.

Rotthauwe, H.W. & Kowalewski, S. (1966b) Gutartige recessiv X-chromosomal vererbte Muskeldystrophie II. Untersuchungen bei Konduktorinnen. *Humangenetik*, **3**, 30.

Roy, S. & Dubowitz, V. (1970) Carrier detection in Duchenne muscular dystrophy. A comparative study of electron microscopy, light microscopy and serum enzymes. *Journal of the Neurological Sciences*, **11**, 65.

Russell, W.R. & Garland, H.G. (1930) Progressive hypertrophic polyneuritis with case reports. *Brain*, **53**, 376.

Sagild, U. & Helweg-Larsen, H.F. (1955) Clinical picture of hereditary transitory muscular paralysis: periodic adynamia and periodic paralysis. *Nord Medical*, **53**, 981.

Sarrouy, C., Farouz, S., Robert, J.M., Sabatini, R., Vaillaud, J.C. & Poncet, J. (1966) La maladie de Steinert chez l'enfant. *Semaine des hôpitaux de Paris (Annals de pediatrie)*, **42**, 1.

Schneiderman, L.J., Sampson, W.I., Schoene, W.C. & Haydon, G.B. (1969) Genetic studies of a family with two unusual autosomal dominant conditions: muscular dystrophy and Pelger-Huet anomaly. *American Journal of Medicine*, **46**, 380.

Schochet, S.S., Zellweger, H., Ionasescu, V. & McCormick, W.F. (1972) Centronuclear myopathy: disease entity or a syndrome? *Journal of the Neurological Sciences*, **16**, 215.

Schreier, K. & Huperz, R. (1956) Über die hypoplasia musculorum generalisata congenita. *Annals Paediatrici*, **186**, 241.

Short, J.K. (1963) Congenital muscular dystrophy, a case report with autopsy findings. *Neurology (Minneapolis)*, **13**, 526.

Shy, G.M. & Gonatas, N.K. (1964) Human myopathy with giant abnormal mitochondria. *Science*, **145**, 493.

Shy, G.M. & Magee, K.R. (1956) A new congenital non-progressive myopathy. *Brain*, **79**, 610.

Shy, G.M., Gonatas, N.K. & Perez, M. (1966) Two childhood myopathies with abnormal mitochondria. I. Megaconial myopathy. II. Pleoconial myopathy. *Brain*, **89**, 133.

Shy, G.M., Engel, W.K., Somers, J.E. & Wanko, T. (1963) Nemaline myopathy, a new congenital myopathy. *Brain*, **86**, 793.

Sjögren, T. (1943) Klinische und erbbiologische Untersuchungen uber die Heredotaxien. *Acta psychiatrica et neurologica*, Suppl. 27.

Skinner, R., Smith, C. & Emery, A.E.H. (1974) Linkage between the loci for benign (Becker-type) X borne muscular dystrophy and deutan colour blindness. *Journal of Medical Genetics*, **11**, 317.

Skinner, R., Emery, A.E.H., Anderson, A.J.B. & Foxall, C. (1975) The detection of carriers of benign (Becker-type) X-linked muscular dystrophy. *Journal of Medical Genetics*, **12**, 131.

Skre, H. (1974) Genetic and clinical aspects of Charcot-Marie-Tooth's disease. *Clinical Genetics*, **6**, 98.

Smith, H.L., Amick, L.D. & Johnson, W.W. (1966) Detection of subclinical and carrier states in Duchenne muscular dystrophy. *Journal of Pediatrics*, **69**, 67.

Spiro, A.J. & Kennedy, C. (1965) Hereditary occurrence of nemaline myopathy. *Archives of Neurology*, **13**, 155.

Spiro, A.J., Fogelson, M.H. & Goldberg, A.C. (1967) Microcephaly and mental subnormality in chronic progressive spinal muscular atrophy of childhood. *Developmental Medicine and Child Neurology*, **9**, 594.

Spiro, A.J., Prineas, J.W. & Moore, C.L. (1970) A new mitochondrial myopathy in a patient with salt craving. *Archives of Neurology*, **22**, 259.

Spiro, A.J., Shy, G.M. & Gonatas, N.K. (1966) Myotubular myopathy. *Archives of Neurology*, **14**, 1.

Steinert, H. (1909) Myopathologische Seitrage. *Deutsche Zeitschrift für Nervenheilkunde*, **37**, 58.

Stengel-Rutkowski, L., Scheuerbrandt, G., Beckmann, R. & Pongratz, D. (1977) Prenatal diagnosis of Duchenne's muscular dystrophy. *Lancet*, **1**, 1359.

Stephens, F.E. (1953) Inheritance of diseases primary in the muscle. *American Journal of Medicine*, **15**, 558.

Stephens, F.E. & Tyler, F.H. (1951) Studies in disorders of muscle. V. The inheritance of childhood progressive muscular dystrophy in 33 kindreds. *American Journal of Human Genetics*, **3**, 111.

Stephens, J. & Lewin, E. (1965) Serum enzyme variations and histological abnormalities in the carrier state in Duchenne dystrophy. *Journal of Neurology, Neurosurgery and Psychiatry*, **28**, 104.

Stevenson, A.C. (1953) Muscular dystrophy in Northern Ireland. I. An account of 51 families. *Annals of Eugenics (London)*, **18**, 50.

Stevenson, A.C. (1958) Muscular dystrophy in Northern Ireland. IV. Some additional data. *Annals of Human Genetics*, **22**, 231.

Stevenson, A.C., Cheeseman, E.A. & Huth, M.C. (1955) Muscular dystrophy in Northern Ireland. III. Linkage data with particular reference to autosomal limb-girdle muscular dystrophy. *Annals of Human Genetics*, **19**, 165.

Stone, C.T. & Rider, J.A. (1949) Treatment of myasthenia gravis. *Journal of the American Medical Association*, **141**, 107.

Sumner, D., Crawfurd, M.D'A. & Harriman, D.G.F. (1971) Distal muscular dystrophy in an English family. *Brain*, **94**, 51.

Taylor, E.W. (1915) Progressive vagus-glossopharyngeal paralysis with ptosis. A contribution to the group of family diseases. *Journal of Nervous and Mental Disease*, **42**, 129.

Thévenard, A., van Bogaert, L., Berdet, H. & Rougerie, J.

(1956) Progressive hypertrophic polyneuritis. *Revue Neurologique*, **94**, 3.

Thomas, P.K., Calne, D.B. & Stewart, G. (1974) Hereditary motor and sensory polyneuropathy (peroneal muscular atrophy). *Annals of Human Genetics*, **38**, 111.

Thomasen, E. (1948) 'Myotonia', Vol. 17. (Hereditarae Humanae Universitates Hafniensis: Aarhus.)

Thompson, M.W., Ludvigsen, B. & Monckton, G. (1962) Some problems in the genetics of muscular dystrophy. *Revue canadianne de biologie*, **21**, 543.

Tooth, H.H. (1886) *The Peroneal Type of Progressive Muscular Atrophy* (Lewis: London).

Tünte, W., Becker, P.E. & Knorre, G. (1967) Zur Genetik der Myositis ossificans progressiva. *Humangenetik*, **4**, 320.

Tyler, F.H. (1950) Studies in disorders of muscle: pseudohypertrophy of muscle in progressive muscular dystrophy and other neuromuscular diseases. *Archives of Neurology and Psychiatry*, **63**, 425.

Tyler, F.H. & Stephens, F.E. (1950) Studies in disorders of muscle. II. Clinical manifestations and inheritance of facioscapulohumeral dystrophy in a large family. *Annals of Internal Medicine*, **32**, 640.

Tyler, F.H., Stephens, F.E., Gunn, F.D. & Perkoff, G.T. (1951) Studies in disorders of muscle. VII. Clinical manifestations and inheritance of periodic paralysis without hypopotassemia. *Journal of Clinical Investigations*, **30**, 492.

van Creveld, S. & Soeters, J.M. (1941) Progressive myositis ossificans. *American Journal of Diseases of Children*, **62**, 1000.

van Dyke, D.H., Griggs, R.C., Markesbery, W. & DiMauro, S. (1975) Hereditary carnitine deficiency of muscle. *Neurology (Minneapolis)*, **25**, 154.

Vanier, T.M. (1960) Dystrophia myotonica in childhood. *British Medical Journal*, **2**, 1284.

Vastine, J.H., Vastine, M.F. & Arango, O. (1948) Myositis ossificans progressiva in homozygotic twins. *American Journal of Roentgenology*, **59**, 204.

Victor, M., Hayes, R. & Adams, R.D. (1962) Oculopharyngeal muscular dystrophy. A familial disease of late life characterized by dysphagia and progressive ptosis of the eyelids. *New England Journal of Medicine*, **267**, 1267.

Walton, J.N. (1955) On the inheritance of muscular dystrophy. *Annals of Human Genetics*, **20**, 1.

Walton, J.N. (1956) The inheritance of muscular dystrophy: further observations. *Annals of Human Genetics*, **21**, 40.

Walton, J.N. (1957a) The inheritance of muscular dystrophy. *Acta genetica et statistica medica (Basel)*, **7**, 318.

Walton, J.N. (1957b) The limp child. *Journal of Neurology, Neurosurgery and Psychiatry*, **20**, 144.

Walton, J.N. (1963) Clinical aspects of human muscular dystrophy. In *Muscular Dystrophy in Man and Animals*. Eds G.H. Bourne and Ma. Nelly Golarz. p. 263 (Hafner: New York).

Walton, J.N. & Adams, R.D. (1958) *Polymyositis.* (Livingstone: Edinburgh.)

Walton, J.N. & Nattrass, F.J. (1954) On the classification, natural history and treatment of the myopathies. *Brain*, **77**, 169.

Waters, D.D., Nutter, D.O., Hopkins, L.C. & Dorney, E.R. (1975) Cardiac features of an unusual X-linked humeroperoneal neuromuscular disease. *New England Journal of Medicine*, **293**, 1017.

Welander, L. (1951) Myopathia distalis tarda hereditaria; 249 examined cases in 72 pedigrees. *Acta medica scandinavica*, **141**, Suppl. 265, 41.

Welander, L. (1957) Homozygous appearance of distal myopathy. *Acta genetica et statistica medica (Basel)*, **7**, 321.

Werdnig, G. (1891) Zwei fruhinfantile hereditare Falle von progressiver Muskelatrophie unter dem bilde der Dystrophie aber auf neurotischer Grundlage. *Archiv für Psychiatrie und Nervenkrankheiten*, **22**, 437.

Wharton, B.A. (1965) An unusual variety of muscular dystrophy. *Lancet*, **1**, 248.

Wilson, A. & Stoner, H.B. (1944) Myasthenia gravis: a consideration of its causation in a study of 14 cases. *Quarterly Journal of Medicine*, **13**, 1.

Wohlfart, G., Fex, J. & Eliasson, S. (1955) Hereditary proximal spinal muscular atrophy—a clinical entity stimulating progressive muscular dystrophy. *Acta psychiatrica et neurologica*, **30**, 395.

Zatz, M., Itskan, S.B., Sanger, R., Frota-Pessoa, O. & Saldanha, P.H. (1974) New linkage data for the X-linked types of muscular dystrophy and G6PD variants, colour blindness and Xg blood groups. *Journal of Medical Genetics*, **11**, 321.

Zellweger, H. (1966) Congenital myopathies and their differential diagnosis. *Pädologie Fortbildungskurse*, **18**, 105.

Zellweger, H. & Hanson, J.W. (1967) Slowly progressive X-linked recessive muscular dystrophy (Type IIIb). *Archives of Internal Medicine*, **120**, 525.

The clinical features of some miscellaneous neuromuscular disorders

INTRODUCTION

Several disorders of the spinal cord or nerve roots and trunks present no problem of pathogenesis, and yet are important because of their frequency in clinical practice. Although affecting voluntary muscles secondarily, they should be considered in any comprehensive treatise on disorders of muscle. Denervation atrophy is the resulting change in muscle affected by lesions of its motor nerve supply and the histological changes of neurogenic atrophy are non-specific, regardless of the cause. These changes have been considered in detail elsewhere (Ch. 5). Any disorder of the motor neurone may result in this type of change, whether that disorder be of the axons themselves or of their cells of origin, produced either by direct implication in a pathological process or because of ischaemia or compression arising from some extraneuronal lesion.

SPINAL CORD

Any pathological process, whether congenital or acquired, inflammatory, neoplastic or resulting from trauma, may affect the innervation of voluntary muscle by damaging the final common path from the anterior horn. Certain disease processes present a uniform clinical picture of muscle wasting, e.g. the motor neurone diseases, and, therefore, deserve separate consideration. But in others the loss of muscle tissue is often an epiphenomenon.

Craniovertebral anomalies and syringomyelia

Congenital bony anomalies at the craniovertebral junction, including occipitalisation of the atlas, basilar impression, Klippel-Feil deformity, etc., have recognisable clinical and radiological characteristics (Spillane, Pallis and Jones, 1957). The association between syringomyelia and these anomalies is well known, but more recently (Gardner, 1965; Appleby, Foster, Hankinson and Hudgson, 1968) it has been noted that an abnormal dilatation of the central canal may accompany congenital anomalies of the neuraxis at the cervicomedullary junction *viz*. the Chiari group of malformations (Chiari, 1891).

The clinical features of syringomyelia are distinctive and include lower motor neurone wasting of muscles, often most evident in those innervated from the first dorsal segment. Areflexia and the characteristic dissociated anaesthesia which implies central cord cavitation are seen in most cases. Classical syringomyelia with its onset in early life cannot, on clinical grounds, be differentiated from the syringomyelia-like syndromes which accompany the cervicomedullary anomalies and which may present in adult life. In some cases early involvement of posterior column function, i.e. loss of the appreciation of joint position sense in the hands, suggests high cervical cord compression and a history of onset following trauma to the neck is suggestive of a Chiari malformation. Radiology may reveal the underlying bony abnormality, but there are many cases where the lesion is limited to neural tissue and in which supine myelography is necessary to demonstrate the associated Chiari malformation (ectopia of the cerebellar tonsils) or the adhesive arachnoidal thickening which prevents free communication between the fourth ventricle and the cisterna magna. It is thought that this relative impermeability of the cerebrospinal fluid (CSF) pathway at this point causes the dilatation of the central canal (hydromyelia). A breach of the lining ependymal layer is followed by dissection of the neural tissue by CSF and the resulting clinical features of syringomyelia. More complete occlusion may result in an associated hydrocephalus. The muscle wasting, which often begins in small hand muscles, results from direct destruction of anterior horn cells by the expanding central canal or the serpiginous extensive cavitation of the syrinx. However, simple cord compression at a high cervical level may be associated with significant wasting of the small muscles of the hand, the true pathogenesis of which remains conjectural (Symonds and Meadows, 1937) although a vascular mechanism has been postulated. The clinical recognition of these cases and their distinction from classical syringomyelia, if such exists *sui generis*, is of considerable importance since surgical decompression at a high cervical level often results in clinical improvement, especially in cases of short duration (Appleby *et al.*, 1968; Hankinson, 1970; Barnett, Foster and Hudgson, 1973). In both groups, a common presenting feature is weakness and wasting of the small hand muscles.

Although syringomyelia rarely extends to, and does not begin in, the lumbar region, many cases of spinal dysraphism are associated with clinical features suggesting a central cord lesion, e.g. diastematomyelia; often these are associated with a true duplex cord, or the lower-limb wasting can be ascribed to an associated hydromyelic dilatation of the central canal. Again, considerable improvement can follow surgical decompression (James and Lassman, 1962a, 1962b, 1964).

Myelitis

Polioclastic viral invasion of the nervous system can give extensive anterior horn cell destruction as typically seen in acute anterior poliomyelitis, in which, during the second phase of the illness, fever and meningism may be followed by profound or total muscle weakness. In part this is due to the inflammatory change and oedema in the anterior horn so that, even after severe invasion, there may be recovery of some neurones and the initial dismal prognosis may prove to be better for certain muscle groups after the acute phase of the illness is past. However, in the severe case there is massive destruction and necrosis of anterior horn cells with neurophagia. The poliomyelitis virus is not alone in its intense polioclastic properties and, following effective immunisation, other viral myelitides have shown a proportional increase in incidence.

The Coxsackie viruses have been held responsible for a poliomyelitic illness (Chumokov, Voroshilova, Zhevandrova, Mironova, Itzelis and Robinson, 1956). The virus first identified as AB-IV or poliovirus 4 was later recognised to be Coxsackie virus A-7 (Johnsson and Lundmark, 1957; Dalldorf, 1958), and the lesions caused when it invades the nervous system of the monkey may be indistinguishable from those caused by poliovirus (Habel and Loomis, 1957).

The virus of herpes zoster, usually confined to the posterior root ganglia, may invade the substance of the spinal cord and produce various clinical effects, notably anterior horn cell damage with associated focal muscle wasting, more extensive cord damage with an incomplete Brown-Séquard syndrome or rarely a devastating transverse myelitis of poor prognosis. Rarely, the infection is followed by a clinical picture indistinguishable from the other postinfective radiculopathies with ascending motor weakness and sensory impairment (Knox, Levey and Simpson, 1961).

Tetanus

Traumatic inoculation with the bacillus *Clost-*

ridium tetani is followed after a variable incubation period of one, two or more weeks by restlessness leading to stiffness of muscles and the noise-induced spasms of classical clinical tetanus. The exotoxin of the bacillus is fatal to man in a dose of 0.22 mg and although spasm is often maximal in muscles closely related to the point of entry there is general agreement that the toxin reaches the central nervous system by the blood stream, where it possibly acts by blocking the Renshaw cell inhibitory system (Eccles, 1957). There is no consistent or specific neuropathological change in muscle or neural tissue in the fatal cases, even when prolonged spasm has resulted in tonic contracture of skeletal muscle (Adams, Denny-Brown and Pearson, 1962). However, many patients recovering from the illness suffer irritability, fits and myoclonus, sleep disturbances, decreased libido and postural hypotension. These features may be reflected in abnormalities in the electroencephalogram (Illis and Taylor, 1971). Recent clinical interest in the management of cases of tetanus has concerned the establishment of centres for its treatment and more specifically the control of spasms by early tracheostomy, the use of muscle-relaxant drugs and positive pressure respiration.

NERVE ROOT LESIONS

Intervertebral disc disease

Progressive disc degeneration in middle life, more prevalent in the male and related to activity and previous trauma (Irvine, Foster, Newell and Klukvin, 1965) results in structural change in the vertebral column and the stimulation of new bone formation (osteophytosis), distortion of foramina and fibrosis of root sleeves. The clinical pattern of cervical spondylosis is dependent upon the precise levels and extent of pathological change in root foramina and the spinal canal giving root compression in one instance, or cord ischaemic change and myelopathy in another. When root involvement is extensive this is reflected in the appropriate limb, where reflex asymmetry and focal wasting may be apparent, indicative of damage to the motor root or spinal nerve. Pain in the appropriate dermatome is almost always a pre-cursor of the motor change and degenerative spondylosis accounts for most cases of so-called 'brachial neuritis' in middle life. Very rarely cervical root lesions are associated with a pseudomyotonic syndrome or carpal spasm (Frykholm, 1951; Satoyoshi, 1972). The phenomenon occurs as a result of simultaneous contraction of the antagonistic muscles of the extensors and flexors of the forearm and is thought to result from ectopic reinnervation in cervical roots.

In a separate category, and always to be considered as a distinct clinical group, are the patients with or without degenerative spondylosis who suffer acute trauma to the spine, with resultant annular rupture and direct root or cord compression from prolapsed nuclear material. In such cases the onset of pain and weakness is temporally related directly to the trauma. The muscle wasting in the upper and lower limbs may be extensive following acute disc prolapse and can provide one of the indications for surgical treatment. Whereas 'brachial neuritis' does not always imply nuclear herniation, because the associated trauma may be minimal, in the lower limb sciatica of acute onset usually does mean annular rupture and true disc prolapse. Here, as in the upper limb, a clinical assessment of the spinal level of the lesion can be made if particular roots are compressed, as the resulting wasting and weakness of muscle groups innervated from their cord segments is clinically detectable (*see* Ch. 13). However, pain is the predominant feature of any disc lesion, and muscle weakness, especially in the upper limb, may be evident only on examination.

Spinal tumours

The pain of extramedullary, intraspinal neoplasm can closely resemble that of disc herniation or rupture, particularly in the lumbar region, and may be associated with similar focal muscle wasting and weakness. Certain clinical points allow differentiation. Thoracic disc prolapse producing girdle pain is rare. Thoracic or dorsal meningioma in the middle-aged woman is not. The pain of spinal neurofibroma tends to be aggravated by rest and relieved by movement, the pain of disc prolapse the reverse, although the root pain from both is aggravated by coughing and straining. The cutaneus stigmata of neurofibromatosis may be visible when an underlying neurofibroma is the cause. Intrinsic cord tumours, which are often painful, tend to give more widespread muscle wasting and weakness than those which are extramedullary. For example, an ependymoma of the conus, cauda equina or filum usually presents with low back pain and later with marked weakness and wasting of the leg muscles. Clinical examination will reveal the segmental level of the lesion. The clinical presentation may suggest the nature of the lesion but radiography is always necessary, with straight films often providing the clue and myelography the conclusive evidence before surgical exploration. Foraminal erosion with a dense bony rim to the foramen or, in the anteroposterior projection, pedicular erosion, may indicate neurofibroma. Widening of the interpedicular distance at a particular segmental level may indicate the situation of the intraspinal growth. Extradural compression from metastases or myeloma with or without vertebral collapse can similarly present with girdle or sciatic pain, but here radiology usually reveals the destruction associated with metastatic deposits. If plain radiographs are normal, then myelography may again be required.

Neuralgic amyotrophy and serum neuropathy

Following the injection of antitetanus serum, or other sera containing foreign protein, a syndrome of arthralgia, rash and fever may appear and may be associated with extensive weakness and, later, wasting of the muscles of one (or rarely both) shoulder girdle and upper limb. The prognosis of the muscle weakness and of the serum sickness itself is good, but occasional focal pareses persist, e.g. paresis of serratus anterior. Closely allied to serum neuropathy is the syndrome of neuralgic amyotrophy, a shoulder-girdle neuritis in which some 10–14 days after a specific or non-specific illness or sometimes without obvious precipitant, severe pain in the shoulder on one side or both is followed after a few days' interval by weakness and, later, wasting of muscle. The muscles innervated by the fifth and sixth cervical roots are usually affected and there is often some sensory impairment within the distribution of the axillary

nerve, i.e. over the lower belly and insertion of the deltoid. Paralysis of serratus anterior is common and often associated with weakness of the deltoid and spinati. Less commonly groups innervated by the sixth and seventh roots, i.e. in the forearm, may be involved. This disorder affects young adults and was first clearly delineated as an entity during wartime (Parsonage and Turner, 1948). It is curiously common in the United Kingdom and European countries. The prognosis is excellent but recovery of the paralysed muscle may be extremely slow, taking up to 18 months. There appears to be no equivalent disorder involving the lumbosacral roots and plexus and, when such a syndrome of pain and weakness of the lower limbs presents, then some pathological process other than one of a putative allergic monoradiculopathy must be considered.

PERIPHERAL NERVE

Facial palsy

Lower motor neurone paralysis of the muscles innervated by the seventh cranial nerve is one of the most common clinical examples of neurogenic muscle atrophy and yet its pathogenesis remains obscure. From a large group of patients presenting with facial weakness a proportion is found to be suffering from systemic disease, of which the facial weakness is but a part. One such example is the nuclear palsy of poliomyelitis, where the symptoms of the attendant viraemia and its general setting in epidemic situations suggest the diagnosis. Infranuclear palsy in multiple sclerosis, in which pain is frequently absent and taste is spared, or the progressive facial paralysis of cerebellopontine angle tumour, can readily be differentiated. Tumours of the facial canal may rarely cause progressive facial weakness as may pathological conditions of the parotid glands (e.g. sarcoidosis). Facial paralysis may also be a rare presenting symptom of acute leukaemia. In such instances clinical and radiological evidence point to the correct diagnosis. Paralysis following inadvertent puncture of the parotid sheath in dental anaesthesia is readily recognised. Facial palsy due to herpes zoster (the Ramsay Hunt syndrome) is often associated with ipsilateral facial sensory loss, partial deafness and vesicles in the ear or on the soft palate. Occasional cases of postinfective polyradiculopathy present with facial palsy of infranuclear type and when the onset is unilateral the differentiation from simple Bell's palsy may be difficult, but here, as in the other examples quoted, pain is unusual and progressive muscle weakness elsewhere soon indicates a more generalised radiculopathy. The author has seen three cases of post-infective polyradiculopathy in which the presenting feature was facial weakness, unilateral in one, but bilateral in two.

Bell's palsy is well recognised. Frequently following a period of exposure, the patient will first notice his facial weakness on waking or may describe pain in the region of the ear and stylomastoid foramen which precedes the onset of the palsy. Weakness is usually complete in one to three hours. In some patients where the chorda tympani is thought to be involved, there is loss of taste on the affected side, or hyperacusis may be noticed when the nerve to stapedius is involved. The lesion usually lies below the geniculate ganglion (Jepson, 1965; Zilstorff-Pederson, 1965) and in half of these, below the origin of the chorda tympani. Electrodiagnostic techniques reveal that 50 per cent of all patients show no impairment of nerve conduction, with an attendant excellent prognosis (see Ch. 27). Of the remainder, some 40 per cent show changes indicative of partial denervation (Taverner, 1959). In this group such tests may give some indication of ultimate prognosis (Taverner, 1959; Langworth and Taverner, 1963). In a small proportion of cases the nerve is electrically unresponsive due to complete denervation within the first week. Only a small proportion of patients with Bell's palsy fail to recover, and have evident clinical and/or cosmetic disability. With such a good overall tendency to natural recovery, specific treatment is difficult to assess, and although surgical decompression of the facial canal in the early stages has had its advocates, no satisfactory trial has demonstrated the effectiveness of this procedure (Miller, 1967). Personal experience and published observations (Taverner, Fearnley, Kemble, Miles and Peiris, 1966) have suggested that the very early use of corticotrophin may shorten the period of paralysis and perhaps improve the prognosis of that small group of cases in which early denervation implies limited recovery. More recent trials of corticotrophin and steroids suggest that prednisolone is the drug of choice (Taverner, Cohen and Hutchinson, 1971).

Entrapment neuropathies

Focal muscle weakness and wasting in a limb may indicate that the nerve of supply to the afflicted muscle is damaged by entrapment or constriction at a point in its course in the limb. Most such entrapments are the result of the nerve being compressed and/or rendered ischaemic as it passes through a fibro-osseous tunnel or where it alters course over a fibrous or aponeurotic band. When compression at a point is clinically apparent and can be demonstrated either by electrodiagnostic techniques or at operation, the pathogenesis may be evident. Space-occupying lesions such as ganglia, lipoma, local tenosynovitis or rheumatoid disease, with associated joint capsular swelling, have all been implicated but occasionally a post-traumatic fibrous band or more obvious local anatomical aberration, e.g. cervical rib, may be responsible. Where more vascular nerve trunks, for example the median, are compressed, compression first induces paraesthesiae thought to be the result of local arterial insufficiency (Fullerton, 1963; Thomas and Fullerton, 1963). The first symptoms are more commonly motor and again it was thought that the weakness resulted from direct and immediate ischaemia, perhaps due to obliteration of the vasa nervorum (Richards, 1951; British Medical Journal, 1970). Recently, however, (Ochoa, Fowler and Gilliatt, 1972; Gilliatt, 1975) experimental evidence has been produced suggesting that the defective nerve conduction may have a mechanical basis and result from direct applied pressure, where displacement of the node of Ranvier on individual fibres is associated with stretching of paranodal myelin to one side of the node and invagination of the paranodal myelin on the other, resulting in lateral movement of the axon and paranodal myelin relative to the surrounding Schwann cells. Local rupture of the Schwann cell membrane follows. So-called idiopathic cases of nerve compression are often associated with frozen shoulder, tennis elbow, and supraspinatus tendinitis, and this has led to the suggestion that thickening of the fibro-osseous sheaths may be part of a more diffuse abnormality of fibrous tissue (Lam, 1967), analogous to the autoimmune concept of Dupuytren's contracture (Burch, 1966) where the histology of the fibrosis can resemble the changes seen in long-standing cases of carpal tunnel syndrome.

Patients with peripheral entrapment may complain of proximal symptoms; for example, pain in the neck and shoulder may accompany median nerve compression in the carpal tunnel. In patients with a metabolic neuropathy, peripheral nerve entrapment syndromes occur with increased frequency. A theory to explain these and other clinical phenomena in the entrapment syndromes has been propounded (Upton and McComas, 1973). Impairment of axoplasmic flow by a compressive proximal lesion may induce clinical symptoms from an otherwise subclinical distal compressive lesion, while neurones with a defective perikaryon metabolism may fail to maintain a sufficient distal flow of 'trophic messenger substance' when the peripheral axon is compressed as, for example, in some hereditary neuropathies, or in the neuropathy of diabetes and renal failure. This explanation has been termed the 'double crush' phenomenon (McComas, 1977).

The upper limb

Median nerve. Most patients in middle life (especially women) who complain of acroparaesthesiae are suffering from median-nerve compression at the wrist (*the carpal tunnel syndrome*). Typically, the patient complains of tingling, numbness and often pain in median distribution in the hand. The symptoms are often worse after use of the hand and frequently waken the patient from sleep, causing her to hold the hand out of the bed and shake it in an abortive attempt to obtain relief. Often the pain extends up to and even above the elbow, and thus mimics the 'brachial neuralgia' of cervical root compression. In the established case, clinical examination may reveal tenderness over the carpal tunnel, sensory impairment within median nerve distribution in the hand and, eventually, detectable weakness and wasting of the short abductor of the thumb. Nerve conduction studies reveal delay in the nerve as it passes under

the flexor retinaculum. Since the carpal tunnel syndrome was recognised and effective surgical treatment described (Brain, Wright and Wilkinson, 1947) many reviews of its pathogenesis and treatment have appeared (Nissen, 1952; Kremer, Gilliatt, Golding and Wilson, 1953; Garland, Bradshaw and Clark, 1957; Phalen and Kendrick, 1957; Foster, 1960). Undoubtedly, surgical division of the flexor retinaculum produces effective and permanent relief and is the treatment of choice, but when for medical reasons (e.g. in severe rheumatoid arthritis, pregnancy, and associated disorders) surgery is not advised, or where the diagnosis is not certain, hydrocortisone injected into the tunnel may afford relief, albeit temporary.

The carpal tunnel syndrome is not common in men and usually there is a recognisable pathogenic mechanism, e.g. acromegaly, myxoedema, rheumatoid disease at the wrist, ganglion, old fracture of the carpal bones, etc. However, a similar picture presenting in the dominant limb may result from median nerve compression as it enters the forearm. Here, the nerve runs between the two heads of pronator teres and deep to the flexor digitorum profundus (*the pronator syndrome*). There may be an anatomical aberration in the relationship of the nerve to the muscle, an abnormal fascial band, or the nerve may be compressed by a hypertrophied pronator teres muscle. In either case the sensory symptoms are identical to those of carpal tunnel compression but there are no nocturnal exacerbations and there may be, in addition to weakness of the small thumb abductor, detectable weakness of the median-innervated long flexors of the fingers. Electromyography confirms a conduction delay in the forearm and surgical decompression is effective in relieving the symptoms.

Ulnar nerve. Ulnar compression may occur at the wrist, in the palm or at the inner side of the elbow. The commonest cause of compression at the elbow is an entrapment by the fibrous arch or origin of flexor carpi ulnaris (*cubital tunnel syndrome*) (Osborne, 1957), which joins the two heads of the muscle and runs from the medial epicondyle to the olecranon. Decompression at this point, implicit in anterior transposition of the nerve, is a simple and effective surgical treatment (Harrison and Nurick, 1970) and in only a small proportion of cases of 'tardy ulnar palsy' can ganglion, osteoarthritis involving the ulnar groove, old fracture, hypermotility or rheumatoid disease be implicated. An *ulnar tunnel syndrome* results from compression of the nerve trunk as it enters the hand on the volar aspect of the forearm. At this point it is enclosed in a fibro-osseous tunnel beyond which it divides into its superficial (motor and sensory) and deep (motor) branches. A traumatic ganglion (Brooks, 1952) compressing the deep branch will result in wasting and weakness of small hand muscles or, if the undivided trunk is involved, motor weakness of the ulnar-innervated muscles and sensory disturbance in the fifth finger and in the medial aspect of the fourth. Oedema secondary to rheumatoid arthritis or tenosynovitis, the inflammatory swelling of gout, deformity following Colles' fracture and osteoarthritis of the pisiform-triquetral joint have also been implicated. In ulnar compression, both at the elbow and wrist, the hand assumes a typical posture and testing will reveal selective weakness of the ulnar-innervated muscles. Paraesthesiae caused by compression at the wrist do not extend into the palm and electrophysiological tests will confirm that the lesion lies at or beyond the wrist.

Radial nerve. Pain over the lateral aspect of the elbow joint and detectable weakness of the wrist and finger extensors ensue when the posterior interosseous nerve is compressed by lipoma, ganglion, fibroma or post-traumatic fibrosis, or when the nerve is compressed between the two layers of the supinator against the aponeurosis of the extensor carpi radialis brevis. However, radial nerve palsy is more often the result of acute compression in its humeral spiral groove (*Saturday-night palsy*); the motor nerve damage is not accompanied by significant paraesthesiae which could alert the patient to his position and predicament.

Syndromes of the thoracic outlet. These result from anatomical variations in the relations of the lower cord of the brachial plexus causing compression of the neurovascular bundle. The cord may be 'post-fixed' or abnormally 'prefixed' and compressed by a cervical rib or its unossified analogue, or compressed because of abnormal disposition of the scalenus anticus or medius. Hypertrophy of the scalenus medius itself or its abnormal insertion on the first rib may cause angulation of the plexus. In other cases a fibrous band, often considered to be a fibrotic scalenus minimus muscle, may produce the distortion and the painful sequelae. Pain, often of long standing, is aggravated by carrying with the affected arm, distributed along the medial border of the limb, and is associated in some cases with weakness and wasting of the muscles innervated by the first dorsal root. In one-third of patients the wasting is confined to the lateral part of the thenar pad (Gilliatt, Le Quesne, Logue and Sumner, 1970). Various manoeuvres may aid diagnosis; most depend upon compression of the vascular bundle, and pressure in the supraclavicular fossa may induce the pain and the paraesthesiae. Occasionally the pain and wasting are associated with vascular phenomena such as Raynaud's phenomenon or poststenotic dilatation of the subclavian artery and embolus formation. Rarely this results in axillary artery occlusion and ischaemia of the arm, or retrograde embolism in the vertebral artery with brain stem infarction.

With recognition of other forms of entrapment neuropathy in the upper limb and of the frequency with which degenerative cervical spine disease causes brachial pain, fewer cases of thoracic outlet syndrome are diagnosed. However, those fulfilling the above clinical criteria, especially when cervical rib is demonstrated or a fibrous band is found at exploratory operation, are greatly benefited by decompression. Where damage to the subclavian artery has occurred, reconstructive vascular surgery may be required.

Lower limb. Significant muscle involvement following entrapment neuropathy in the lower limb is confined to the major motor nerves, i.e. lateral popliteal and sciatic nerves.

Lateral popliteal (common peroneal) nerve. A frequent cause of drop-foot is damage to the lateral popliteal nerve as it courses round the fibular neck, but this is not necessarily accompanied by entrapment. Pressure applied to the nerve from tight stockings, supports, calipers, plasters, industrial kneeguards, due to the posture adopted in certain occupations (as in roof-layers), or even from the opposite limb or bedcage in a stuporose patient, may be followed by paralysis of the anterior crural muscles. A ganglion in the popliteal fossa, or a popliteal cyst, may also compromise the nerve. Examination reveals weakness of the appropriate muscles, *viz.* the anterior crural group and peroneals, with sparing of the tibialis posterior, a useful diagnostic point in differentiating the drop-foot of peroneal palsy from that caused by a centrally placed fifth lumbar root lesion.

Sciatic nerve. The main motor nerve to the lower limb may be entrapped in the sciatic notch, damaged by a misplaced injection or, rarely, by direct trauma. The gluteal muscles are spared but the hamstrings and anterior and posterior crural groups are weakened according to the anatomical distribution of sciatic nerve fibres.

Restless legs syndrome

Formication, prickling and crawling sensations in the legs, felt particularly between the knee and ankle, often relieved by movement, form the clinical syndrome of restless legs. First described by Thomas Willis in 1685, the clinical features have been reviewed by Beard (1880), Oppenheimer (1923), Norlander (1954), Wittmach (1961) and Gorman, Dyck and Pearson (1965), with a recent definitive review by Ekbom (1960), whose name is now frequently associated with the syndrome.

The symptoms may spread into the thighs and feet and, rarely, the hands and arms may be involved. The symptoms occur most frequently in bed at night and prevent sleep. It was Ekbom's initial belief that the symptoms had a vascular pathogenesis but this has not been substantiated. While in most cases there is no evident pathology, these symptoms which constitute Ekbom's syndrome have been described in association with drug therapy, notably prochlorperazine, with barbiturate withdrawal, prolonged exposure to cold, carcinoma, iron deficiency anaemia and avitaminosis, diabetic neuropathy, prostatitis and uraemic neuropathy (Callaghan, 1966). The syndrome has also been reported in association with chronic pulmonary disease (Spillane, 1970). The

paraesthesiae are more frequent in women, especially in pregnancy, and not accompanied by evidence of polyneuropathy; it has been suggested that the basic pathology lies in the spinal cord (Ask-Upmark, 1954). There is a strikingly high incidence of psychoneurotic symptoms in patients suffering from this syndrome, especially anxiety, tension and depression. Myokymia is present in some affected individuals, but distressing sensory symptoms differentiate 'restless legs' from other disorders where myokymia is a feature; for example the syndrome of continuous muscle fibre activity (Isaacs, 1961), or quantal squander myokymia (McComas, 1977) (*see* below).

When the sensation in the legs is pain, there may be an associated spontaneous movement of the toes (Spillane, Nathan, Kelly and Marsden, 1971). Recent work suggests that in this distinctive disorder the lesion responsible is in the afferent fibres of the posterior nerve roots (Nathan, 1978).

Although there is no recognisable pathogenesis in the spontaneously occurring cases, treatment with phenothiazines or diazepam may be successful. Chlorpromazine 50 mg given last thing at night may alleviate the troublesome nocturnal symptoms. In otherwise refractory cases relief has been obtained by using procaine hydrochloride i.v., in a dose of 500 mg in 0.5 litre of normal saline infused over a period of 30–40 min on three consecutive days.

NEUROMUSCULAR JUNCTION

Botulism

Rapid death from bulbar paralysis results from the injection of the exotoxin of *Clostridium botulinum*. The bacillus is strictly anaerobic and is found in all soils and animal faeces; outbreaks of botulism have usually been associated with improperly prepared canned and bottled foods. The toxin is the most powerful poison recognised, 0.05 mg being fatal to man. It has a specific action in blocking terminal motor nerve filaments (Brooks, 1956). Experimental botulinus paralysis in the rabbit is due to a block of cholinergic fibres (Ambache, 1949) with a specific action in blocking the terminal nerve filaments at the presynaptic level and of interfering with acetylcholine release. The neuromuscular block differs from that due to curare in that, although paralysed muscle will no longer respond to nerve stimulation, it contracts after the intra-arterial injection of acetylcholine. Symptoms appear two to 36 hours after ingestion. At first confined to the bulbar muscles with diplopia, ptosis, irritability, and giddiness, the paralysis spreads to give respiratory failure of both central and peripheral type. Sensation is not affected (Lamanna, 1959).

Repetitive nerve stimulation shows a defect of neuromuscular transmission similar to that seen in myasthenia gravis and the Eaton-Lambert syndrome. Motor nerve conduction velocity and sensory latencies are not affected. Since guanidine has been used with benefit in the Eaton-Lambert syndrome (Lambert and Rooke, 1965), Cherington and Ryan (1969) used the compound successfully in botulism in doses of 35–50 mg/kg body weight. Guanidine acts by enhancing the release of acetylcholine (Otsuka and Endo, 1960) and its salts can inactivate botulinum toxin directly (Stefanye, Iwamasa, Schantz and Spero, 1964). Polyvalent antitoxin and neostigmine are ineffective, and further experience with guanidine in botulism has shown that it is of value.

Myokymia, continuous muscle fibre activity

Three forms of myokymia have been described in clinical practice. One of these takes the form (Harman and Richardson, 1954) of continuous undulating movement in the muscles of the face (facial myokymia) or sometimes in those of the limbs and trunk. Electromyographically in these cases there are stereotyped groups of from two to over 200 motor unit potentials (multiplets) occurring at intervals of about 20 ms. Facial myokymia is occasionally a manifestation of multiple sclerosis (Matthews, 1966) or even of pontine tumour, but the variety which affects the limbs and trunk and which may be particularly prominent in calf muscles is usually benign.

Another form of myokymia, known as 'live flesh', takes the form of a brief series of twitches of the lower eyelid) or of a calf muscle, often related to fatigue and again of no pathological significance.

The third variety, first described by Gamstorp and Wohlfart (1959) and later by Isaacs (1961)

under the title of 'continuous muscle fibre activity and spasm', is characterised by diffuse coarse fasciculation and muscle stiffness and cramps with impaired relaxation after contraction which are transiently improved by repeated contraction. Sometimes there is marked stiffness of gait and movement and some patients develop laryngeal and other localised spasms or occasionally progressive deformity of the feet. Hyperhidrosis is common and some patients go on to develop atrophy of distal limb muscles (Gardner-Medwin and Walton, 1969).

The electromyogram shows continuous spontaneous repetitive discharges of potentials resembling motor unit potentials, but myotonic discharges are usually absent from the EMG and as a rule no fibrillation potentials are seen. Peripheral nerve block has no influence upon the activity but neuromuscular block abolishes it. Ultrastructural studies of motor end-plates have given normal findings (Sigwald, Raverdy, Fardeau, Gremy, Mace de Lepinay, Bouttier and Danic, 1966), although Mertens and Zschocke (1965), who entitled the same disorder 'neuromyotonia', thought that there were minor end-plate abnormalities in methylene blue preparations. Isaacs (1961) suggested that the condition was a functional anomaly of the distal part of the motor nerve fibres and postulated excessive release of acetylcholine at motor end-plates ('quantal squander'). However, other evidence suggests a post-synaptic defect with increasing sensitivity of the muscle fibre membrane to acetylcholine. The condition is almost specifically relieved by phenytoin and by other membrane stabilising drugs (Isaacs and Heffron, 1974), although in the more severe cases the muscular atrophy may prove to be progressive even if the myokymia is relieved.

MUSCLE

Acute muscle compartment compression syndromes

Severe boring pain in the tibialis anterior muscle may occur in male adults, and especially those who undertake unaccustomed exercise (tibialis anticus syndrome). The pain is also recognised in athletes with gross hypertrophy of the anterior crural group of muscles, and is thought to be ischaemic. Exercise of the anterior crural group encased in their osseofibrous sheath results in swelling and increased vascularity. Oedema followed by ischaemic necrosis within the anterior crural compartment may also be due to arterial embolism or thrombosis, direct trauma or even fracture of the tibia and fibula. The resultant damage to the muscle and the anterior tibial nerve results in foot-drop and impaired walking. Most patients with the anterior tibial syndrome are able to obtain complete relief by resting, but occasionally the pain persists and decompression of the anterior crural compartment has been recommended in order to prevent permanent muscle damage (Sirbou, Murphy and White, 1944). The long flexors of the toes lying in the deep posterior compartment of the lower leg are also susceptible to compression necrosis, usually following fracture of the tibia. Such a fracture may damage the posterior tibial or peroneal arteries with subsequent necrosis and fibrosis of the long flexor muscles.

Volkmann's ischaemic contracture

Postischaemic fibrosis of the long flexors of the fingers, first described in 1881 by Volkmann, is specifically associated with supracondylar fractures of the humerus in childhood. The onset is often rapid, accompanied by burning pain in the hand and forearm. Diminution of the radial pulse may be observed, and paralysis of the long flexor muscles develops without sensory loss. After the oedema has settled, the atrophic muscles become fibrosed and essentially useless. Similar post-ischaemic contraction may follow arterial embolism. Thus the syndrome is very similar to that occurring in the anterior and posterior crural compartments, ischaemia being followed by infarction and consequent fibrosis.

Myositis ossificans

In the literature there are reports of some 350 patients, mostly children, often suffering from a congenital anomaly of their great toes or other digits, in whom sclerosis of muscle connective tissue is followed by the deposition of bone—fibrodysplasia ossificans progressiva (McKusick,

1956) or *progressive myositis ossificans*. There is some evidence that this disorder may be transmitted by a dominant gene (Gaster, 1905; Eaton, Conkling and Daeschner, 1957) or be due to autosomal dominant mutations exposed to strong selection pressure, i.e. almost all cases are new mutants (Tünte, Becker and Knorre, 1967), but its pathogenesis is unknown. Chromosome studies show a normal karyotype (Viparelli, 1963). Children or young adults are affected, with the involvement of aponeuroses, tendons and fascia in addition to the connective tissue of the muscle itself. Commonly, the child presents with a swelling or swellings in the neck, mimicking congenital torticollis. These may be fluctuant or hard and tend to vary in size and consistency but ultimately become hardened as the bone is deposited. Although frequently painless, in some cases the swellings are very tender and this picture, together with swelling of joints and fever, may superficially resemble acute rheumatism. Ulceration of the tense, overlying skin may expose the ossified muscle and result in secondary infection. Although almost any voluntary muscle may be involved, in most cases the most severely affected muscles are those of the back, shoulder and pelvic girdles. Ultimately large groups of muscles become ossified and the bone tends to conform to the shape of the muscle involved. Although the diaphragm itself is very rarely affected, the general fixation of the ribs results in a terminal aspiration pneumonia and death from infection and/or asphyxia. Corticotrophin and steroids have been used in treatment and a diphosphonate, disodium etidronate, has been recommended following its use in preventing ectopic calcification in the experimental animal (Russel, Smith, Bishop, Price and Squire, 1972).

Direct and indirect trauma to muscle with resulting rupture, contusion or frank haemorrhage is common in industrial accidents and in various sports. In the large majority of cases, treatment results in complete clinical recovery. In a few, however, the traumatic incident is followed by increasing stiffness in the muscle over the next one to four weeks and the development of a firm, painful calcified mass, palpable at the site of the injury. Similar calcification or ossification, particularly in thigh muscles and in the region of the hip joints, may be seen in cases of paraplegia or paraparesis, as after partial recovery from transverse myelitis. Radiography will indicate calcification of feathery pattern in the swelling (Howard, 1946) where a haematoma has dissected along the fasciculae, or a more common irregular circumscribed area of variable density where a solitary haematoma is calcified. Post-traumatic inflammatory change in connective tissue is replaced by islands of cartilage and eventually by bone in the thickened septa. The clinical disability which results is largely dependent upon the precise situation of the new bone: that close to joints may cause by direct mechanical interference the most severe disability, whereas an area of bone formation in the belly of a muscle at a distance from its origin or insertion may scarcely be discernible to the patient except perhaps for pain and stiffness in the muscle itself.

Less common than this *myositis ossificans circumscripta* is the ossification of specific muscles as a result of their repeated involvement in the trauma of certain exercises or occupations. Riders and infantrymen have suffered from local ossification in the adductors of the thighs (rider's bone) and the deltoid and pectorals (drill bone) respectively. Fencers and athletes throwing a weapon or weight may develop ossification in biceps, brachialis and brachioradialis of the arm involved. *Traumatic ossifying myositis* may not be evident to the victim and may be discovered on routine radiology, but in the majority of cases the new bone is tender and restricts normal movement. Spontaneous reabsorption is reported on cessation of the provocative activity, but most cases come to surgery. The histological appearance of the muscle is similar in both the acute and subacute varieties.

Tumours of muscle

Although direct invasion of muscle tissue by adjacent carcinoma or other malignant neoplasm is relatively common, primary muscle tumours and metastatic tumour spread to muscle tissue are rare. Direct invasion causes muscle atrophy from compression and the histological changes are those of the invasive tumour itself. Despite the extensive vascular supply of skeletal muscle, the autopsy finding of metastatic deposits in muscle is very rare, perhaps because of some local change in pH or metabolism which does not allow implantation and development of tumour emboli. However, Pearson (1959) examined the muscles histologically post mortem in 38 cases of malignancy and found tumour emboli and growths in six. Fourteen muscles were involved out of a total of eight to nine muscles examined in each of the 38 cases. This work suggests that tumour embolisation to muscle is not as rare as was formerly believed. However, in the terminal stages of malignancy it is very unlikely that such small metastatic deposits would be clinically recognisable or would exert an influence to be distinguished from the generalised cachexia of the primary disease. Patients with visceral carcinoma, especially carcinoma of the gastrointestinal tract, may suffer a migrating monomyositis multiplex (Heffner, 1971) caused by systemic emboli from non-bacterial thrombotic endocarditis. The condition mimics polymyositis but is more focal, with severe pains of sudden onset lasting for a few days. The muscles of the lower leg are preferentially affected, and the underlying pathology is embolic infarction of muscle tissue.

A tumour or swelling in the substance of voluntary muscle does not necessarily imply new growth, and abscess formation due either to aerobic or anaerobic organisms is seen in various conditions, notably diabetes mellitus or tropical myositis. Frequently the cardinal signs of acute inflammation are absent and the abscess has to be distinguished from old haematoma or localised nodular myositis (*see* Ch. 15). Of the tumours of supporting tissues, angioma is uncommon, whether of cavernous, capillary or arteriovenous type, but dermoid tumours and benign fibrous growths are more common and particularly involve the anterior abdominal wall. They may be associated with dull, aching pain and are evident on palpation. In the limbs, neurofibromata may cause severe pain aggravated by contraction of the surrounding muscle and often provoked by palpation of the tumour itself. There is frequently a curious wasting of the surrounding muscle, perhaps because of disuse, a wasting which frequently recovers after surgical removal of the lesion. Rupture of a tendon (e.g. of biceps brachii) or a muscle hernia (through the deep fascia) may give an appearance of local swelling which can be misconstrued by the unwary.

Primary tumours of muscle are fortunately uncommon and fall into three distinct histological groups:

Rhabdomyoma. These rare tumours of skeletal muscle may be circumscribed, diffuse, solitary or multiple. A distinctive form is seen as a congenital tumour of cardiac muscle often associated with tuberous sclerosis.

The rhabdomyosarcoma is an extremely malignant tumour estimated by Stout (1946) to be associated with a less than four per cent survival at five years. It tends to occur in the muscles of the extremities, especially the legs and involves patients between the ages of 40 and 60 in particular. The tumour presents as a deep-seated muscle swelling which is relatively immobile and spreads by local invasion. Unfortunately, the tumour is not particularly radiosensitive and only radical surgery can offer a better prognosis—35 per cent survival at five years (Pack and Ariel, 1958).

Mid-line teratomas, wherever their situation, may contain elements of striated muscle and the clinical features here are largely determined by the situation of the lesion. Particularly common are those involving the genital organs where primitive muscle tissue may form a sarcomatous mass (sarcoma botryoides in the female or a malignant rhabdomyoma of the prostate in the male).

The granular cell myoblastoma is an uncommon tumour; 30 per cent appear in the tongue, others in the skin, subcutaneous tissues or breast. Surgical treatment with total extirpation is often feasible.

Stiff-man syndrome

From the Mayo Clinic in 1956 Moersch and Woltman reported 14 patients who had suffered a progressive, fluctuating muscle rigidity and spasm; they used the term stiff-man syndrome to describe these patients. Since then some 26 further reports have appeared in the neurological literature describing patients suffering from similar stiffness and rigidity and, in a critical survey of the literature, Gordon, Janusko and Kaufman (1967) laid down certain criteria for the diagnosis. The disorder is more common in men and tends to affect adults in middle life. The first symptoms are brief episodes of aching and tightness of the axial muscles which, after some weeks, become more persistent and eventually involve the limb girdles and limb muscles producing a symmetrical continuous stiffness of the systemic musculature. The muscles become board-like and rigid and any attempt at passive movement or sudden noise may precipitate excruciatingly painful muscle spasms causing the patient to cry out; they are associated with adrenergic concomitants such as tachycardia and sweating. The spasms may be initiated by talking, chewing, swallowing or attempted voluntary movement. The muscle involvement is unselective in that agonists and antagonists are equally involved, so that the patient becomes rigid in extension. In some patients dysphagia has been described, and in others the facial muscles have been involved by similar rigidity. Patients are described in whom the respiratory muscles have also shown this stiffness with resulting difficulty in breathing. During sleep the muscles relax and, indeed, general anaesthesia will produce complete relaxation (Price and Allott, 1958). In those cases accepted by Gordon and his colleagues as fulfilling these clinical criteria there were no neurological abnormalities, save for the extreme rigidity. Corticospinal signs were absent and there was no sensory impairment. Intellectually, these patients are intact and electromyographic examination of the involved muscles show these to be in persistent tonic contraction, even at rest. The action potentials are normal (Moersch and Woltman, 1956; Howard, 1963; Trethowan, Allsop and Turner, 1960). The spasm can be abolished by spinal anaesthetic (Werk, Sholiton and Monell, 1961) and by procaine infiltration around an appropriate nerve trunk (Gordon, Janusko and Kaufman, 1967). Myoneural blocking agents, for example, curare (Brage, 1959), tubocurarine (Stuart, Henry and Holley, 1960) and succinylcholine (Werk *et al.*, 1961) have all been shown to relieve the spasms. In 1963 Howard described the use of diazepam (Valium) following the demonstration that the drug blocked strychnine convulsions in mice and spinal reflexes in cats. He was able with this drug to induce electromyographic silence when the involved muscles were at rest. More recently the effectiveness of baclofen, clonazepam and diazepam have been assessed, and the ineffectiveness of dipropylacetate has been confirmed (Martinelli, Pazzaglia, Montagna, Coccagna, Rizzuto, Simonati and Lugaresi, 1978).

There has been much conjecture about the pathogenesis of this strange and rare disorder. Gordon and his colleagues (1967) suggested that the persisting α-neurone bombardment of the muscle is probably maintained by abnormal γ-motor system activity, perhaps initiated from higher centres. The pain of the spasms is thought to be due to further intensification of the contraction resulting from exteroceptive and enteroceptive stimuli and emotional factors. In their case the presence of a non-glucose reducing substance in the urine suggested a possible metabolic factor. An association between this disease, nocturnal myoclonus and epilepsy has recently been suggested (Martinelli et al., 1978). However, in our current stage of knowledge the pathogenesis still remains unresolved. One report (Kasperek and Zebrowski, 1971) described a patient whose clinical signs were characteristic and in whom, at autopsy some 11 months after the onset of the stiffness, changes of a subacute encephalomyelitis, presumed to be viral, were found. Most of the pathological abnormalities were in the brain stem and spinal cord. On the basis of pharmacological evidence it has been suggested that the syndrome depends upon an imbalance between the cholinergic systems and the GABA system (Martinelli et al., 1978), giving excessive activity in interneurones in the spinal cord.

Diagnosis from other organic disorders of the nervous system is not usually difficult. Cervical spondylosis with myelopathy may produce severe cortico-spinal rigidity. Extra-pyramidal disease such as torsion dystonia, Wilson's disease and parkinsonism may all produce a somewhat similar clinical picture, but usually give rise to little diagnostic difficulty. Chronic tetanus, McArdle's myopathy, myotonia and dermatomyositis have all mimicked the stiff-man syndrome, and severe generalised arthritis with resulting muscle spasm has also been confused with it. However, in the stiff-man syndrome the pain and stiffness are confined to the muscles and are not periarticular, as they would be in a diffuse arthropathy.

Occasionally the spasms are severe enough to cause spontaneous fractures and gross deformity of the limbs (Asher, 1958) and it is not, therefore, surprising that several biopsy reports have described changes in the muscles. However, occasional degenerative foci, nerve-sprouting and slight fibrosis could all result from the intense spasms themselves, producing, as they must, relative ischaemia of muscle. In most biopsies, however, the muscle fibres, the myomesium and the intramuscular nerve endings show no consistent abnormality.

The absence of objective organic change in these patients has led to the suggestion that many of the spasms may be 'hysterical'. However, the personality of the patient suffering from this syndrome does not conform to that of the true hysteric and the extreme distress, immobility and eventual bed-dependence do not support this suggestion.

Epidemic myalgia, pleurodynia (Bornholm disease)

The first clinical descriptions of this disease are found in the Norwegian literature (Daae, 1872, and Homann, 1872), and in 1934 Sylvest published his classic monograph on the subject from Copenhagen.

It is now recognised that viruses of the Coxsackie Group B are responsible for the clinical picture of headache, fever, and pain in the lower chest and abdomen of sudden onset. The pain is made worse by respiratory movements and frequently pleural friction can be heard, with tenderness and skin hyperaesthesia over the lower chest wall (Curnen, Shaw and Melnick, 1949; Weller, Enders, Buckingham and Finn, 1950; Kilbourne, 1950). B-1 types of virus and also strains of B-3 have been recovered from patients with pleurodynia and the condition has been associated with B-4 infection in South Africa (Patz, Measroch and Gear, 1953; Wilkins, Kotze, Melvin, Gear, Prinsloo and Kirsch, 1955), so that many B strains of virus have been implicated but Group A viruses are not responsible.

Focal inflammatory and necrotic foci similar to those seen in the muscle of infected mice have been seen in the few recorded biopsies from human cases. The disease is short-lived; its main clinical interest lies in its epidemic qualities and, when endemic, in its differentiation from more significant pleural and peritoneal inflammatory disorders.

Epidemic myalgic encephalomyelitis

At the Royal Free Hospital in London in 1955 an outbreak of this disease affected more than 300 people. The disorder tends to occur in the summer months, and affects young people who suffer headache, muscle pains, occasional lymphadenopathy and fever. Neurological signs have been detected, e.g. nystagmus, myoclonus, and weakness of the bulbar muscles together with generalised muscle weakness and hyporeflexia. The majority of the patients complain of peripheral paraesthesiae and peripheral sensory loss is often described. The disease is associated with a feeling of generalised fatigue, and the frequent psychiatric disturbance has suggested to some that the disease is not organically determined. The exact nosology of this disorder is still in doubt, and terms such as neuromyasthenia have been suggested. An organic basis is supported by the abnormal lymphocytes found in the peripheral blood of some patients (Wallis, 1957). During a recent outbreak in London a high incidence of serum anticomplementary activity together with ill-defined aggregates on electron microscopy of acute phase sera were described (Dillon, Marshall, Dudgeon and Steigman, 1974).

REFERENCES

Adams, R.D., Denny-Brown, D. & Pearson, C.M. (1962) *Diseases of Muscle: a Study in Pathology*, 2nd Edn. (Hoeber: New York).

Ambache, N. (1949) The peripheral action of Cl. botulinum toxin. *Journal of Physiology*, **108**, 127.

Appleby, A., Foster, J.B., Hankinson, J. & Hudgson, P. (1968) The diagnosis and management of the Chiari anomalies in adult life. *Brain*, **91**, 131.

Asher, R.A. (1958) A woman with stiff-man syndrome. *British Medical Journal*, **1**, 265.

Ask-Upmark, E. (1954) Contribution to the pathogenesis of the syndrome of restless legs. *Acta medica Scandinavica*, **164**, 231.

Barnett, H.J.M., Foster, J.B. & Hudgson, P. (1973) *Syringomyelia* (Saunders: London).

Beard, G.M. (1880) *A practical treatise in nervous exhaustion*, p. 41 (W. Wood & Co.: New York).

Brage, D. (1959) Stiff-man syndrome. *Revista clinica española*, **72**, 30.

Brain, W.R., Wright, A.D. & Wilkinson, M. (1947) Spontaneous compression of both median nerves in the carpal tunnel. *Lancet*, **1**, 277.

British Medical Journal (1970) Entrapment neuropathies, Leading Article, **1**, 645.

Brooks, D.M. (1952) Nerve compression by simple ganglia. *Journal of Bone and Joint Surgery*, **34B**, 391.

Brooks, V.B. (1956) The action of botulinum toxin on motor-nerve filaments. *Journal of Physiology*, **134**, 264.

Burch, P.R.J. (1966) Dupuytren's contracture: an autoimmune disease? *Journal of Bone and Joint Surgery*, **48B**, 312.

Callaghan, N. (1966) Restless legs syndrome in uraemic neuropathy. *Neurology (Minneapolis)*, **16**, 359.

Cherington, M. & Ryan, D.W. (1969) Botulism and guanidine. *New England Journal of Medicine*, **278**, 931.

Chiari, H. (1891) Über Veränderung des Kleinhirns infolge von Hydrocephalie der Grosshirns, *Deutsche medizinische Wochenschrift*, **17**, 1172.

Chumokov, M.P., Voroshilova, M.K., Zhevandrova, V.I., Mironova, L.L., Itzelis, F.I. & Robinson, I.A. (1956) New methods of detection and identification of poliomyelitis virus. *Problems of Virology*, **1**, 16.

Curnen, E.C., Shaw, E.W. & Melnick, J.L. (1949) Diseases resembling nonparalytic poliomyelitis associated with a virus pathogenic for infant mice. *Journal of the American Medical Association*, **141**, 894.

Daae, A. (1872) Epidemi i drangedal af miskel—reumatisme udbredt ved smitte. *Norsk magzizin fau Laegevidenskaben*, **2**, 409.

Dalldorf, G. (1958) The Coxsackie viruses—1957. In *Poliomyelitis. 4th International Poliomyelitis Conference, Philadelphia* (Lippincott: Philadelphia).

Eaton, W.L., Conkling, W.S. & Daeschner, C.W. (1957) Early myositis ossificans progressiva occurring in homozygotic twins; a clinical and pathological study. *Journal of Pediatrics*, **50**, 591.

Eccles, J.C. (1957) In *The Physiology of Nerve Cells* (Oxford University Press: London).

Ekbom, K.A. (1960) Restless legs syndrome. *Neurology (Minneapolis)*, **10**, 868.

Foster, J.B. (1960) Hydrocortisone and the carpal tunnel syndrome. *Lancet*, **1**, 454.

Frykholm, R. (1951) Cervical nerve root compression resulting from disc degeneration and root fibrosis. *Acta Chirurgica Scandinavica*, **160**, 148 (supp.).

Fullerton, P.M. (1963) The effect of ischaemia on nerve conduction in the carpal tunnel syndrome. *Journal of Neurology, Neurosurgery and Psychiatry*, **26**, 785.

Gamstorp, I. & Wohlfart, G. (1959) A syndrome characterised by myokymia, myotonia, muscular wasting and increased perspiration. *Acta Psychiatrica et Neurologica*, **34**, 181.

Gardner, W.J. (1965) Hydrodynamic mechanism of syringomyelia: its relationship to myelocele. *Journal of Neurology, Neurosurgery and Psychiatry*, **25**, 247.

Gardner-Medwin, D. & Walton, J.N. (1969) Myokymia with

impaired muscular relaxation. *Lancet*, **1**, 127.

Garland, H., Bradshaw, J.P.P. & Clark, J.M.P. (1957) Compression of median nerve in carpal tunnel and its relation to acroparaesthesiae. *British Medical Journal*, **1**, 730.

Gaster, D. (1905) A case of myositis ossificans. *West London Medical Journal*, **10**, 37.

Gilliatt, R.W. (1975) Peripheral nerve compression and entrapment (the Oliver Sharpey Lecture). Proceedings of a Conference held at the Royal College of Physicians of London, February 1975.

Gilliatt, R.W., Le Quesne, P.H., Logue, V. & Sumner, A.J. (1970) Wasting of the hand associated with a cervical rib or band. *Journal of Neurology, Neurosurgery and Psychiatry*, **33**, 615.

Gordon, E.E., Janusko, D.M. & Kaufman, L. (1967) A critical survey of the stiff-man syndrome. *American Journal of Medicine*, **42**, 582.

Gorman, C.A., Dyck, P.J. & Pearson, J.S. (1965) Symptoms of restless legs. *Archives of Internal Medicine*, **155**, 155.

Habel, K. & Loomis, L.N. (1957) Coxsackie A₂ virus and the Russian 'Poliovirus Type 4'. *Proceedings of the Society for Experimental Biology and Medicine*, **95**, 597.

Hankinson, J. (1970) Syringomyelia and the surgeon. In *Modern Trends in Neurology*, Vol. 5, Ed. D. Williams, p. 127 (Butterworths: London).

Harman, J.B. & Richardson, A.T. (1954) Generalised myokymia in thyrotoxicosis: Report of a case. *Lancet*, **2**, 473.

Harrison, M.J.G. & Nurick, S. (1970) Results of anterior transposition of the ulnar nerve for ulnar neuritis. *British Medical Journal*, **1**, 27.

Heffner, R.R. (1971) Myopathy of embolic origin in patients with carcinoma. *Neurology (Minneapolis)*, **21**, 840.

Homann, C. (1872) Om en i Kragerø Laegedistrikt Lerskende Smitsom Febersygdom. *Norsk magazin for laegevidenskaben*, **2**, 542.

Howard, C. (1946) Traumatic ossifying myositis. *United States Naval Medical Bulletin*, **46**, 724.

Howard, F.M. (1963) A new and effective drug in the treatment of stiff-man syndrome. *Proceedings of the Staff of the Mayo Clinic*, **38**, 203.

Illis, L.S. & Taylor, F.M. (1971) Neurological and electroencephalographic sequelae of tetanus. *Lancet*, **1**, 826.

Irvine, D.H., Foster, J.B., Newell, D.J. & Klukvin, B.N. (1965) Prevalence of cervical spondylosis in general practice. *Lancet*, **1**, 1089.

Isaacs, H. (1961) A syndrome of continuous muscle-fibre activity. *Journal of Neurology, Neurosurgery and Psychiatry*, **24**, 319.

Isaacs, H. & Heffron, J.J.A. (1974) The syndrome of 'continuous muscle-fibre activity' cured: further studies. *Journal of Neurology, Neurosurgery and Psychiatry*, **37**, 1231.

James, C.C.M. & Lassman, L.P. (1962a) Spinal dysraphism. The diagnosis and treatment of progressive lesions in spina bifida occulta. *Journal of Bone and Joint Surgery*, **44B**, 828.

James, C.C.M. & Lassman, L.P. (1962b) Spinal dysraphism. Spinal cord lesions associated with spina bifida occulta. *Physiotherapy*, **48**, 154.

James, C.C.M. & Lassman, L.P. (1964) Diastematomyelia. A critical review of 24 cases submitted to laminectomy. *Archives of Disease in Childhood*, **39**, 124.

Jepson, O. (1965) Topognosis (Topographic diagnosis) of facial nerve lesions. *Archives of Otolaryngology*, **81**, 446.

Johnsson, T. & Lundmark, C. (1957) Identification of the 'fourth type' of poliomyelitis virus. *Lancet*, **1**, 1148.

Kasperek, S. & Zebrowski, S. (1971) Stiff-man syndrome and encephalomyelitis. *Archives of Neurology*, **24**, 22.

Kilbourne, E.D. (1950) Diverse manifestations of infection with a strain of Coxsackie virus. *Federation Proceedings*, **9**, 581.

Knox, J.D.E., Levy, R. & Simpson, J.A. (1961) Herpes zoster and the Landry-Guillain-Barré syndrome. *Journal of Neurology, Neurosurgery and Psychiatry*, **24**, 167.

Kremer, M., Gilliatt, R.W., Golding, J.S.B. & Wilson, G.T. (1953) Acroparaesthesiae in the carpal tunnel syndrome. *Lancet*, **2**, 590.

Lam, S.D.S. (1967) Peripheral nerve compression syndromes in the upper limb. *Guy's Hospital Reports*, **116**, 131.

Lamanna, C. (1959) Most poisonous poison. *Science*, **130**, 763.

Lambert, E.H. & Rooke, E.D. (1965) Myasthenic state and lung cancer. In *The remote effects of cancer on the nervous system*. Proc. of symposium. Ed. Lord Brain & F.H. Norris (Grune & Stratton: New York).

Langworth, E.P. & Taverner, D. (1963) The prognosis in facial palsy. *Brain*, **86**, 465.

Martinelli, P., Pazzaglia, P., Montagna, P., Coccagna, G., Rizzuto, N., Simonati, S. & Lugaresi, E. (1978) Stiff-man syndrome associated with nocturnal myoclonus and epilepsy. *Journal of Neurology, Neurosurgery and Psychiatry*, **41**, 458.

Matthews, W.B. (1966) Facial myokymia. *Journal of Neurology, Neurosurgery and Psychiatry*, **29**, 35.

McComas, A.J. (1977) In *Neuromuscular Function and Disorders*, Vol. 22, p. 257 (Butterworths: London).

McKusik, V. (1956) *Heritable disorders of connective tissue*, p. 184 (Mosby: St. Louis).

Mertens, H.-G. & Zschocke, S. (1965) Neuromyotonia. *Klinische Wochenschrift*, **43**, 917.

Miller, H. (1967) Facial paralysis. *British Medical Journal*, **3**, 815.

Moersch, F.P. & Woltman, H.W. (1956) Progressive fluctuating muscular rigidity and spasm (stiff-man syndrome). *Proceedings of the Staff of the Mayo Clinic*, **31**, 421.

Nathan, P.W. (1978) Painful legs and moving toes: evidence on the site of the lesion. *Journal of Neurology, Neurosurgery and Psychiatry*, **41**, 934.

Nissen, K.I. (1952) Aetiology of carpal tunnel compression of the median nerve. *Journal of Bone and Joint Surgery*, **34B**, 514.

Norlander, N.B. (1954) Restless legs. *British Journal of Physical Medicine*, **17**, 160.

Ochoa, J. Fowler, T.J., & Gilliatt, R.W. (1972) Anatomical changes in peripheral nerves compressed by a pneumatic tourniquet. *Journal of Anatomy*, **113**, 433.

Oppenheimer, H. (1923) *Lehrbuch der Nervenkrankheiten*, p. 1774 (S. Karger: Berlin).

Osborne, G.V. (1957) The surgical treatment of tardy ulnar neuritis. *Journal of Bone and Joint Surgery*, **34B**, 782.

Otsuka, M. & Endo, M. (1960) Effect of guanidine on neuromuscular transmission. *Journal of Pharmacology and Experimental Therapeutics*, **128**, 273.

Pack, G.T. & Ariel, I.M. (1958) *Tumours of the soft somatic tissues; a clinical treatise* (Hoeber: New York).

Parsonage, M.J. & Turner, J.W.A. (1948) Neuralgic amyotrophy, the shoulder girdle syndrome. *Lancet*, **1**, 973.

Patz, I.M., Measroch, V. & Gear, J. (1953) Bornholm disease, pleurodynia or epidemic myalgia: outbreak in Transvaal associated with Coxsackie virus infection. *South African Medical Journal*, **27**, 397.

Pearson, C.M. (1959) The incidence and type of pathologic alterations observed in muscles in a routine autopsy survey. *Neurology (Minneapolis)*, **9**, 757.

Phalen, G.S. & Kendrick, J.I. (1957) Compression neuropathy of the median nerve in the carpal tunnel. *Journal of the American Medical Association*, **164**, 525.

Price, T.M.L. & Allott, E.H. (1958) The stiff-man syndrome. *British Medical Journal*, **1**, 682.

Richards, R.C. (1951) Ischaemic lesions of peripheral nerve: a review. *Journal of Neurology, Neurosurgery and Psychiatry*, **14**, 76.

Russel, R.G.G., Smith, R., Bishop, M.C., Price, D.A. & Squire, C.M. (1972) Treatment of myositis ossificans progressiva with a diphosphonate. *Lancet*, **1**, 10–12.

Satoyoshi, E. (1972) Pseudomyotonia in cervical roof lesions with myelopathy. *Archives of Neurology*, **27**, 307.

Sigwald, J., Raverdy, P., Fardeau, M., Gremy, F., Mace de Lepinay, A., Bouttier, D. & Danic, M. (1966) Pseudo-myotonie. Forme particulière d'hypertonie musculaire à prédominance distale. *Revue Neurologique*, **115**, 1003.

Sirbou, A.B., Murphy, M.J. & White, A.S. (1944) Soft tissue complications of fractures of the leg. *California and Western Medicine*, **60**, 63.

Spillane, J.D. (1970) Restless legs in chronic pulmonary disease. *British Medical Journal*, **4**, 796.

Spillane, J.D., Pallis, C. & Jones, A.M. (1957) Developmental abnormalities in the region of the foramen magnum. *Brain*, **80**, 11.

Spillane, J.D., Nathan, P.W., Kelley, R.E. & Marsden, C.D. (1971) Painful legs and moving toes. *Brain*, **94**, 541.

Stefanye, K., Iwamasa, R.T., Schantz, E.J. & Spero, L. (1964) Effect of guanidium salts on toxicity of botulinum toxin. *Biochemica et biophysica acta*, **86**, 412.

Stout, A.P. (1946) Rhabdomyosarcoma of the skeletal muscles. *Annals of Surgery*, **123**, 447.

Stuart, F.S., Henry, M. & Holley, H.L. (1960) The stiff-man syndrome. *Arthritis and Rheumatism*, **3**, 229.

Sylvest, E. (1934) *Epidemic myalgia: Bornholm disease* (Levin and Munksgaard: Copenhagen).

Symonds, C.P. & Meadows, S.P. (1937) Compression of the spinal cord in the neighbourhood of the foramen magnum.

Brain, **60**, 52.

Taverner, D. (1959) The prognosis and treatment of spontaneous facial palsy. *Proceedings of the Royal Society of Medicine.*, **52**, 1077.

Taverner, D., Cohen, S.B. & Hutchinson, B.C. (1971) Comparison of corticotrophin and prednisolone in the treatment of idiopathic facial paralysis (Bell's palsy). *British Medical Journal*, **4**, 20.

Taverner, D., Fearnley, M.E., Kemble, F., Miles, D.W. & Peiris, O.S. (1966) Prevention of denervation in Bell's palsy. *British Medical Journal*, **1**, 391.

Thomas, P.K. & Fullerton, P.M. (1963) Nerve fibre size in the carpal tunnel syndrome. *Journal of Neurology, Neurosurgery and Psychiatry*, **26**, 520.

Trethowan, W.H., Allsop, J.L. & Turner, B. (1960) The stiff-man syndrome. *Archives of Neurology*, **3**, 448.

Tünte, W., Becker, P.E. & Knorre, G.V. (1967) Zur Genetik der Myositis ossificans progressiva. *Humangenetik*, **4**, 320.

Upton, A.R.M. & McComas, A.J. (1973) The double-crush in nerve entrapment syndromes. *Lancet*, **2**, 359.

Viparelli, V. (1963) La miosite ossificante progressiva. *Annali di Neuropsichiatria e Psicoanalisi*, **9**, 297.

Volkmann, R. (1881) Die ischaemischen Muskellähmungen und Kontrakturen. *Zentralblatt für Chirurgie*, **8**, 801.

Wallis, A.L. (1957) M.D. Thesis. Edinburgh University— cited by *British Medical Journal*, leading article (1978), **1**, 1436.

Weller, T.H., Enders, J.F., Buckingham, M. & Finn, J.J. Jr. (1950) The aetiology of epidemic pleurodynia; a study of two viruses isolated from a typical outbreak. *Journal of Immunology*, **65**, 337.

Werk, E.E., Sholiton, L.J. & Monell, R.J. (1961) The stiff-man syndrome and hyperthyroidism. *American Journal of Medicine*, **31**, 647.

Wilkins, A.J.W., Kotze, D.M., Melvin, J., Gear, J., Prinsloo, F.R. & Kirsch, Z. (1955) Meningo-encephalitis due to Coxsackie B virus in Southern Rhodesia. *South African Medical Journal*, **29**, 25.

Willis, T. (1685) *The London Practice of Physic*, p. 404 (Barsett & Cooke: London).

Wittmach, T. (1961) *Pathologie und Therapie der sensibilitat-Neurosen*, p. 459 (E. Shafer: Leipzig).

Zilstorff-Pedersen, K. (1965) Quantitative measurements of the nasolacrimal reflex. *Archives of Otolaryngology*, **81**, 457.

Myopathies in animals

INTRODUCTION

Animals differ from man in that their gestations tend to be shorter, and their rates of fetal growth greater, when these are expressed as a function of maternal body weight (Blaxter, 1964). There is a wide range in litter size; young may be relatively immature and helpless at birth, or well-developed and active. Regardless of the number of offspring or their functional state, lower animals grow more rapidly than man, and reach maturity at an earlier age. These characteristics have been exaggerated by genetic selection in farm animals bred for production. This intensification has led to the unmasking of hitherto unsuspected nutritional deficiencies or limiting factors, as greater growth rates are achieved; this is particularly apparent when the animals are housed, and fed on locally grown crops. Examples of nutritional myopathies so induced are discussed in this Chapter.

When the product is meat, intended to suit modern tastes, selection and husbandry have tended to favour the well-muscled animal, free from excess fat. As a consequence, there seems to have been an inadvertent selection of somewhat doubtful virtues such as 'double muscling' in cattle, and of unwanted characteristics such as susceptibility to the porcine stress syndrome in 'improved' pigs. Livestock may also be subjected to long-distance droving or transportation and may thereby suffer metabolic injuries resulting in 'transport myopathy', while the horse, bred for work, is susceptible to the notorious condition of paralytic myoglobinuria.

Thus, selection and genetic manipulation by man, combined with modern methods of intensive management, have been much concerned with muscle; it is clear, however, that while farm animals depend on man for their breeding programme and their diet, they do not constantly have, as wild animals do, natural selection as a final arbiter.

This Chapter is based on the earlier work of Sir Kenneth Blaxter, who contributed so much to the knowledge of nutritional myopathies of farm animals. In building on his earlier work we have encountered problems; because of the large amount of information now available, we have restricted the topic principally to the primary myopathies of non-primate mammals.

We have not dealt with inflammatory diseases of known aetiology. Although some of these, for example toxoplasmosis, cysticercosis, trichinosis and clostridial myonecrosis, are of considerable economic importance, or are of interest to the epidemiologist, we consider that adequate descriptions are to be found in the texts of Hadlow (1962), Nieberle and Cohrs (1967) and Jubb and Kennedy (1970).

An attempt has been made to introduce a classification of the myopathies; this, however, is not precise. It is very probable that in some instances the primary defect leading to a myopathy develops during gestation, and yet clinical manifestations may not appear until some days or weeks after birth. Because of gaps in knowledge about the genesis of some diseases in this category we have classified them as 'Congenital or neonatal'.

With regard to pathology, in general it is not possible to characterise the different diseases of each species by specific pathological features because, in many instances, these are lacking. Muscle cells suffering acute damage from different causes tend to go through common pathways of degenerative change. The most useful basis for classification at present is aetiology, although this may be unknown or complex. The aetiological factors are hereditary, nutritional, toxic, metabolic and possibly immunological.

In some instances the question of heritability has been a problem. We have classified a myopathy as heritable where it has been established that this aspect of phenotypic variation is due to additive gene effects. Otherwise, where a myopathy has been detected in a small number of animals which had a common parent, or where it affects a single breed, we have classified it as familial provided that the condition does not occur in other animals of the same species, reared in the same environment, at the same time. Such considerations quickly lead to the concept of 'liability' and the acceptance that all diseases have a genetic component.

The physiological specialisation of muscle cell types is similar in farm animals to that of the intensively studied laboratory animals, and fibre-typing is usually based on standard histochemical methods. The alkali-stable myosin ATPase reaction (Guth and Samaha, 1970) is particularly useful, and is the basis for the type I, intermediate, and type II system of classification we have adopted in this Chapter. Table 24.1 shows the corresponding nomenclature in other systems of classification. We accept, however, that the functional state of a muscle cell is dynamic; it can change with age and training, and is dependent on normal innervation. There are species differences, such as the gradation according to body size, from mouse to horse, that occurs in the proportion of fast-twitch, aerobic cells in the diaphragm (Davies and Gunn, 1972). Furthermore, some muscles of pigs have, as a normal feature, intrafascicular groups of type I cells, giving an appearance which deceptively resembles the pathological change known as fibre-type grouping.

There are also differences between species in the histochemical cell types of the masseter muscle, which in the ox and sheep appears to have the histochemical characteristics appropriate to a functional demand for slow, sustained work (Suzuki, 1977). Comprehensive differences between breeds within a species have also been described (Gunn, 1975).

As in man, dystrophic or injured muscle cells are either abnormally permeable, or suffer total structural breakdown. Loss of normal membrane function tends to result in leakage of potassium from, and entry of sodium and calcium ions into,

Table 24.1 The relationship between physiological, biochemical and histochemical parameters and three systems of cell-type nomenclature

Contraction speed	$\begin{bmatrix} ATPase \\ pH\ 10.4 \\ reaction \end{bmatrix}$	Energy method	$\begin{bmatrix} NADH\text{-}TR \\ reaction\ or \\ haemoglobin \\ content \end{bmatrix}$		Type	
Slow	[Low]	Oxidative (aerobic)	[High]	SO	I	β red
Fast	[Intermediate]	Oxidative/ glycolytic (combined)	[Intermediate]	FOG	INT	α red
Fast	[High]	Glycolytic (anaerobic)	[Low]	FG	II	α white

the muscle cells, irrespective of the cause of injury. Wrogemann and Pena (1976) have suggested that the increased net influx of Ca^{++} is the basis of a final common pathogenic mechanism for muscle necrosis in a wide variety of muscle disorders, independent of their aetiology. It is probable that muscle necrosis is due to mitochondrial Ca^{++} overload, leading to energy deficiency, a failure of energy-dependent calcium-pumping mechanisms, and an increase in the concentration of sarcoplasmic calcium. The build-up of sarcoplasmic Ca^{++} induces local sarcomere contraction and rupture of the contractile elements within the cell. These combined changes are seen on histological examination as hyaline, floccular and granular effects.

As a further result of the impairment of membrane function and integrity, enzymes normally present in muscle escape and can be detected in increased amounts in the blood, so providing the basis for a range of diagnostic tests. Of the many enzymes so liberated, creatine kinase (CK, E.C. 2.7.3.2.) is one of the most useful indicators of acute muscle damage. It is present in relatively large amounts in the skeletal and cardiac muscle of cattle (Keller, 1971), horses, pigs and sheep (Boyd, 1976) but also occurs in the brain. Three isoenzymes are present in different proportions in these three tissues (Mercer, 1974).

Such enzymes, however, may be liberated during exercise, have relatively short half-lives in the blood (four hours in cattle; Anderson, Berrett and Patterson (1976)) and are not structural components of the muscle cell. Recent investigations have established that, under physiological conditions, 3-methyl histidine is, in some species, a valid index of muscle protein degradation (Harris, Milne, Lobley and Nicholas, 1977). 3-methyl histidine occurs only in the myosin and actin components of total muscle protein and, when released as a metabolite, it is not re-utilised during protein turnover. During myofibrillar protein catabolism it may be rapidly and quantitatively excreted in the urine. Recent work has shown that urinary excretion of 3-methyl histidine is not a reliable measure of muscle protein degradation in sheep (Harris and Milne, 1977) or pigs (Milne and Harris, 1978), but that it may be a valid index of muscle protein degradation

in cattle (Harris and Milne, 1978). The usefulness of this metabolite as an indicator of myopathy remains to be explored (Ward and Buttery, 1978).

DEVELOPMENTAL DISORDERS OF SKELETAL MUSCLE

Hereditary disorders manifested congenitally or neonatally

Double-muscling is an hereditary, congenital disorder in which the muscles are not duplicated, but are larger than normal. Some or all of the muscles may be hypertrophied; the muscles of the upper hind limb, however, are always involved, and usually also those of the back and shoulders. The clinical appearance is of bulging muscles (Fig. 24.1) which, because there is very little subcutaneous fat, are separated by well-defined grooves. The condition is mainly associated with cattle, but has been reported occasionally in sheep. The subject has been reviewed by Swatland (1974), and Bradley (1978a).

The anatomical basis for the muscular hypertrophy is muscle cell hyperplasia, with a change from the normal proportions of muscle fibre types. There are reduced numbers of type I (β, red; slow, oxidative) and intermediate (α, red; fast, oxidative, glycolytic) cells, and increased numbers of type II (α, white; fast, glycolytic), the last being hypertrophied (Holmes and Ashmore, 1972). Muscles of normal size in affected calves may exhibit muscle cell hyperplasia with hypotrophy; such animals

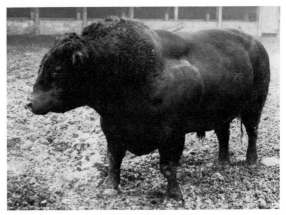

Fig. 24.1   Double muscling. A double muscled Aberdeen Angus bull

may develop the clinical features of double-muscling as they grow older.

Double-muscling has been observed in many breeds of cattle and is of considerable economic importance. It is a cause of dystocia due to relative oversize of the calf, while mature animals are susceptible to stress (*see* Porcine stress syndrome), and may produce a carcass of poor quality. On the other hand, a double-muscled carcass contains little fat and has an advantageous muscle–bone ratio. The condition is inherited as an autosomal recessive trait, and there is a variable expression of the gene in the heterozygous animal.

Limber legs of Jersey cattle. This is a semi-lethal, congenital abnormality of Jersey cattle in which there is abnormal flexion and extension of the limb joints. There is splaying of the limbs as in 'splayleg' of the newborn pig. Under-development of the limb muscles gives the illusion of joint enlargement. Lamb, Arave and Shupe (1976) investigated the pedigrees of 105 cases and concluded that it was inherited as an autosomal recessive trait. The site and nature of the lesion has not been determined; histological lesions were not found in bone or muscle.

Myotonia in some instances hereditary, has been recorded in several species of farm animals; it is discussed more appropriately in a later section (p. 840). Fetal myotonia may, however, be one of the aetiological factors which lead to the development of congenital articular rigidity which is also discussed later.

'Daft lamb' disease of Border Leicester sheep. A hereditary and congenital disease of Border Leicester lambs, clinically indistinguishable from the 'daft' lambs of Innes, Rowlands and Parry (1949), but without cerebellar lesions, was reported by Terlecki, Richardson, Bradley, Buntain, Young and Pampiglione (1978). It was characterised by skeletal fragility and a specific, progressive myopathy. The lambs were clinically affected at birth but histological evidence of myopathy was not detected until the lambs were 3 months old. The lesions, which occurred particularly in the neck muscles, were described in terms of their histopathological and histochemical features by Bradley and Terlecki (1977), and in terms of their fine structure by Bradley (1978b).

Affected muscles showed abnormal variation in cell size (Fig. 24.2), without degenerative or

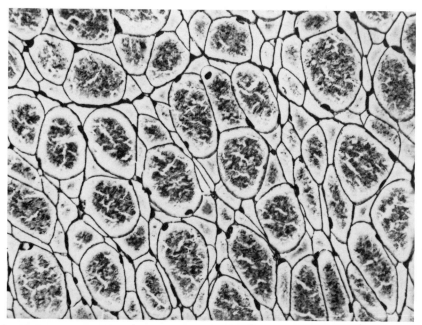

Fig. 24.2 'Daft lamb' disease. *M. splenius* of a 3-month-old 'daft lamb' showing a wide variation in cell size, with large intrafascicular cells. Gomori's reticulin stain, ×275

inflammatory lesions, or change in histochemical profile. The pathognomonic lesion was abnormal enlargement of some of the intrafascicular type I cells, while other type I cells, and the type II cells, were smaller than normal. Light and electron-microscopic studies of intramuscular nerves showed that 28 per cent of such axons contained lamellated dense bodies, and in some axon terminals there were distended mitochondria which themselves contained membranous bodies. These findings suggested that the mechanism of the myopathy might be a defect in neuromuscular transmission, leading to delayed development of some muscle cells. It was not clear, however, whether there was a primary defect in the muscle cells, either alone or together with a neuropathy. The disease is inherited as an autosomal recessive trait.

Mitochondrial myopathy of dogs. Myopathy with a possible recessive X-linked inheritance in a litter of Irish terrier pups was described by Wentink, van der Linde-Sipman, Meijer, Kamphuisen, van Vorstenbosch, Hartman and Hendriks (1972). Clinical signs, which did not appear until the animals were eight weeks old, were stiffness, muscle atrophy and difficulty in swallowing. Serum CK and other muscle enzyme activities were markedly increased. The muscles were pale, with yellowish-white streaks; histological examination showed patchy myodegeneration with phagocytosis and calcification. In severely affected muscles the histochemical distinctions between type I and type II fibres were obscured; phosphorylase, dehydrogenase and oxidase activity were also lost. Electron microscopy showed the presence of abnormal mitochondria and electron-dense bodies.

Later, Wentink, Meijer, van der Linde-Sipman and Hendriks (1974) described the biochemical characteristics of mitochondria isolated from the triceps brachii and quadriceps femoris muscles of an affected dog. The organelles appeared to have normal oxidative phosphorylation but lacked respiratory control (loosely coupled mitochondria).

Muscular dysgenesis of mice. A lethal mutation in the mouse, termed muscular dys-

genesis (mdg) was described by Pai (1965a, b). It occurred in an inbred stock of tailless mice and was transmitted as a single autosomal recessive gene.

The most striking effect in newborn mice homozygous for the mdg mutation is a severe, generalised deficiency of skeletal musculature caused by failure of skeletal muscle cell differentiation. Cardiac and smooth muscle cells appear to be normal. Abnormalities are first apparent at the time when myoblasts differentiate into striated myotubes. Subsequently, degenerative changes occur in the muscle cells. The central and peripheral nervous systems, and the cholinesterase reaction of motor end-plates, appear to be normal.

Skeletal changes also occur, and there is an excessive accumulation of brown fat bodies in affected animals. Pai suggested that these lesions were secondary in nature and resulted from a lowered energy requirement of mutant fetuses.

'Sprawling' defect of mice. A disorder of mice transmitted by a fully penetrant autosomal dominant gene (Swl) results in the 'sprawling' syndrome (Duchen, 1975a). The clinical condition, which particularly affects the hind legs, becomes evident 7–10 days after birth. The hind legs move stiffly and jerkily; when the mouse is lifted by the tail, the hind limbs are abnormally flexed. At rest, in the fully developed syndrome, the hind limbs are stiffly extended forwards under the body.

There is a reduction in the number of muscle spindles, especially in the lumbosacral, axial and hind limb muscles. There is no progressive disease of the nervous system but there is a failure of maturation and myelination of sensory axons.

Congenital muscular dystrophy of mice. Muscular dystrophy occurred as a spontaneous recessive autosomal mutation in the Bar Harbor strain of mouse 129/Re. The early onset of clinical effects prevented normal breeding of affected animals but techniques such as transplantation of dy/dy ovaries, and artificial insemination of dystrophic young females with sperm collected from dystrophic males, have allowed all-dystrophic litters to be produced. Investigations of fetuses so produced revealed prenatal, preclinical effects on skeletal muscle fibres (Meier, West and Hoag, 1965; Platzer, 1971). Only differentiated muscle cells are involved, however, and it seems more appropriate to discuss this condition in a later section (p. 838).

Other disorders of complex or unknown aetiology, manifested congenitally or neonatally

Congenital articular rigidity (CAR). This term is used to indicate a congenital dysfunction of one or more joints. The condition in cattle was reviewed by Done (1976), in pigs by Bradley and Wells (1978) and in farm animals generally, by Swatland (1974).

CAR is one of the more common developmental defects of cattle, and is frequently the cause of dystocia. It is sometimes accompanied by other defects such as hydrocephalus, spinal dysraphism and cleft palate. Myopathic changes usually take the form of reduced muscle size, and atrophy of myofibres without regeneration; in severely affected muscles there may be replacement of myofibres with adipose tissue (Fig. 24.3). Such

changes may be neurogenic because of loss of neurones accompanying abnormal development of the central nervous system, or from aberrations of peripheral nerves.

CAR in cattle. An apparently specific, non-lethal and mild form of CAR affecting the fore and sometimes the hind fetlock and pastern joints of dairy cattle has been observed in Southern England (Bradley, unpublished; Greenough, MacCallum and Weaver, 1972). Affected calves may recover spontaneously in the course of a few weeks.

Congenital articular rigidity may be produced by viral teratogens such as akabane virus (Hartley, Wanner, Della-Porta and Snowdon, 1975; Shimshony, 1978) or by plant teratogens such as *Lupinus sp.* (Shupe, Binns, James and Keeler, 1967), acting at critical stages of pregnancy. A second class of aetiological factor, exemplified by the arthrogryposis–cleft palate syndrome of Charolais cattle (Jackson, 1978), is heredity. Hereditary CAR is almost always attributable to a recessive gene (Swatland, 1974).

The mechanism of CAR has not been estab-

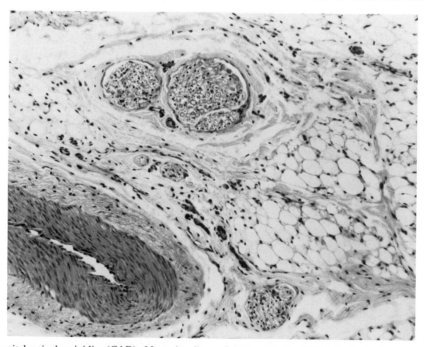

Fig. 24.3 Congenital articular rigidity (CAR). *M. semitendinosus* from a calf with CAR. The fascicular architecture is normal but the cells that compose the fascicles are adipose cells. Some contain single large lipid droplets; others contain variable numbers of smaller lipid droplets. The intramuscular nerves and vasculature appear normal. H & E, ×85

lished. Histological studies reveal little except the terminal results, which are dominated by the non-specific effects of immobilisation (Swatland, 1974). The events leading to the development of CAR may be motor neuronal failure, which would result in defective prenatal muscular movements, myofibre atrophy and possibly prenatal joint immobilisation. Skeletal or connective tissue abnormalities due to teratogenic factors are also possible causes of the condition. A myogenic cause, such as fetal myotonia, is suspected when the central and peripheral nervous systems appear normal. Myotonia has been reported in the calf (Van Niekerk and Járos, 1970), and very probably has been observed in the sheep fetus (Swatland, 1974).

A possible instance in which primary myopathy formed part of the CAR syndrome was reported by Ball (1936). Muscles relating to the rigid joints of a calf appeared to have a normal vascular and nerve supply but the muscle fibres showed degenerative changes and were extensively replaced with adipose cells. There was also evidence of myofibre regeneration.

CAR in horses. The condition also occurs in horses. Rooney (1966) stated that the lesions almost invariably accompany axial skeletal malformation; he was unable to find lesions in the skeletal musculature of such animals. Nevertheless lesions were found by Gunn (1976) in the *M. flexor digitorum profundus* from two Thoroughbred foals with contractions of the distal joints of both fore legs. The foals did not have axial skeletal abnormalities but the limb contractures were sufficient to cause dystocia. The ratio of muscle weight to tendon weight of the humeral head of the deep digital flexor was less in affected than in normal animals. Throughout most of the muscle of affected animals there was an increase in fibrous tissue and a decrease in the area occupied by muscle cells, although the total number of cells was the same as in normal foals. There was no evidence of reinnervation, that is, of muscle cell-type grouping. Gunn concluded that the condition was myogenic rather than neurogenic in origin, and was characterised by muscle cell hypotrophy, normal muscle cell number and an increase in connective tissue.

CAR in sheep. In sheep, CAR may be induced by environmental factors to which the ewe may be exposed at critical stages of pregnancy. Factors which have been incriminated are teratogenic plant toxins such as that from locoweed, viruses such as akabane virus (Parsonson, Della-Porta and Snowdon, 1977; Shimshony, 1978), Wesselsbron and Rift Valley fever viruses (Coetzer and Barnard, 1977), chemical agents such as methyl-5(6)-butyl-2-benzimidazole carbamate (Szabo, Miller and Scott, 1974) and diets deficient in vitamin E or selenium.

Genetically determined primary myopathies causing CAR have been described in Welsh Mountain lambs by Fraser Roberts (1929) and in Merino lambs by Morley (1954). Both types are inherited as autosomal recessive traits. The condition in Welsh Mountain sheep does not involve the central or peripheral nervous systems; in Morley's cases however the brain was decreased in size and the superior frontal gyrus (motor area) was poorly developed. The muscles were replaced with fibrous tissue. Fraser Roberts found that muscles were atrophic and sometimes fused into irregular, fibrous masses in which there was little muscle tissue.

CAR in pigs. In his review of this topic, Swatland (1974) draws attention to hereditary forms of CAR in pigs that may be inherited as simple autosomal recessive traits. As far as we are aware, studies of muscle pathology have not been reported. Environmentally induced CAR in pigs can occur in vitamin A deficiency, in manganese deficiency or after ingestion of toxic plants including *Nicotiana tabacum* (tobacco), *Datura stramonium* (thorn apple), *Conium maculatum* (hemlock) and *Prunus serotina* (black cherry). In these circumstances it is very probable that myopathies, so far inadequately described, are secondary to neural lesions.

Rigid lamb syndrome. A condition which has been termed rigid lamb syndrome has been encountered locally and sporadically in Rhodesia (Rudert, Lawrence, Foggin and Barlow, 1978). Lambs are born with varying degrees of rigidity of the limbs and spine. In the mildest cases there is exaggerated extensor tone of fore and hind limbs.

Histopathological lesions appear to be confined to the neuromuscular system, and consist principally of widespread neuronal degeneration with arrest of myelination, and secondary degenerative changes in the white matter of the central nervous system.

The muscles are underdeveloped but in many cases there is no detectable myopathy. In others, a variable degree of muscle degeneration is present, sometimes being severe and widespread, and appearing macroscopically as pale areas. When seen under the microscope, the myopathic lesions range from very mild changes to necrosis with macrophage infiltration and replacement fibrosis.

The aetiology of the disease is not known but the condition appears to be exacerbated by the application of sulphur to the pasture grazed by pregnant ewes. Rudert et al. (1978) suggested that the syndrome may be nutritional in origin, and may be caused by interference with selenium metabolism by the presence of relatively large quantities of cyanogenic glycosides and sulphur in the herbage. Various feeding trials with pregnant ewes did not lead to experimental induction of the disease; the incidence of the condition was reduced, however, by the administration of vitamin E and selenium to pregnant ewes. Shimshony (1978) has suggested that there is justification for examining the possibility of viral aetiology in the rigid lamb syndrome.

Congenital myopathy of lambs. Nisbet and Renwick (1961) described two congenital abnormalities, in which muscle degeneration occurs, of Suffolk lambs in Scotland. The first defect consists of a flexion of the fetlocks and carpal joints. This leads to abnormality of gait but the lambs invariably recover spontaneously within three months. The second consists of bilateral weakness of the neck muscles associated with inability to raise the head and to reach the teat. Most lambs recover spontaneously within a few months.

Lesions found in lambs with flexed limbs at birth were myodegeneration with calcification and regeneration. In older animals, which failed to recover from the cervical muscle defect, there was fibrosis in the M. longissimus cervicis accompanied by muscle cell atrophy and replacement with fat

cells. There were few signs of active myodegeneration or regeneration. No lesions were found in the central nervous system. Nisbet and Renwick suggested that the lesions may have been caused by deficiency of vitamin E or selenium. For the neck lesions they proposed, in addition, a possible idiopathic primary ischaemia, perhaps due to an hereditary factor, or an ischaemia resulting from prolonged labour.

Splayleg is typically a transient clinical syndrome of the newborn piglet. The syndrome affects the hind and sometimes the fore limbs; it is manifested as a failure of limb adduction that leads to postural collapse. The sequel may be death, usually due to failure to compete successfully with littermates for a teat, or overlaying by the sow. Piglets which survive, recover spontaneously within a week.

The subject has been critically reviewed by Ward (1978) who states that it occurs in 60 000 piglets in Britain each year, with an overall incidence of 0.4 per cent and a mortality rate of the order of 50 per cent.

The aetiology and pathogenesis are not known. It has been attributed to a dominant sex-linked hereditary factor with incomplete penetrance (Lax, 1971); trauma, due to slippery floors (Kohler, Cross and Ferguson, 1969); defective maternal nutrition, caused in particular by a reduced intake of choline and methionine (Cunha, 1968); ingestion, by the pregnant sow, of food contaminated with the fungal toxin fusarium F_2 (Miller, Hacking, Harrison and Gross, 1973); dysmaturity of skeletal musculature (Deutsch and Done, 1971); and to developmental (hypoplastic) and myopathic (dystrophy-like) defects (Bergmann, 1976a, b).

Ward (1978) concludes that there is considerable evidence to indicate that splayleg is most usefully considered as a multifactorial disorder to which the concept of 'liability' may be applied.

The histological and electron-microscopical examination of affected muscles reveals a deficiency of myofibrils—myofibrillar hypoplasia (Thurley, Gilbert and Done, 1967; Deutsch and Done, 1971). The increased sarcoplasmic space is filled with granular material which appears to be a mixture of glycogen and ribosomes (Fig. 24.4).

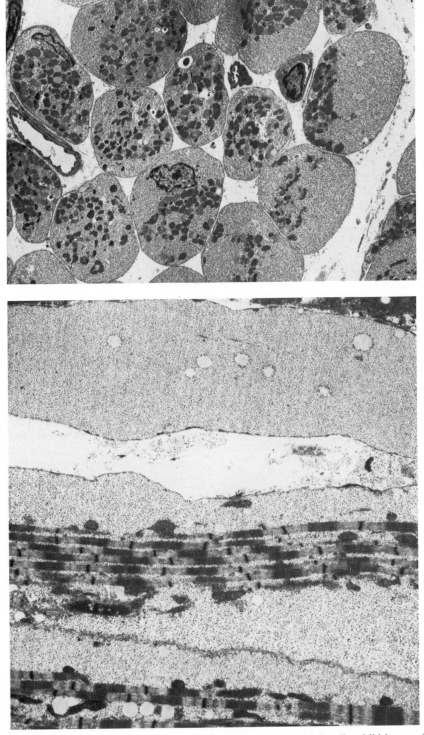

Fig. 24.4   Myofibrillar hypoplasia. A: *M. sartorius* of a newborn piglet, showing muscle cells exhibiting myofibrillar hypoplasia. The areas not occupied by myofibrils contain granular material, ×2000. B: longitudinal section of a similar area. Myofibrils have a normal sarcomere structure, but do not fill the sarcoplasmic space, ×2500

However, pathological definition is not yet possible because there is a continuous gradation in the numbers of myofibrils present in muscle fibres of severely affected and normal piglets. This makes it difficult to appreciate the relevance of the myofibrillar deficiency to the postural defect, and renders morphological diagnosis in the middle of the range impracticable. In short, 'myofibrillar hypoplasia' is not pathognomonic of 'splayleg', which is reliably indicated only by its clinical manifestations. Patterson, Sweasey, Allen, Berrett and Thurley (1969) suggested that alterations in membrane permeability were involved because, in affected animals, there was an increase in serum enzyme activities of muscle origin, and the ratio of intracellular to extracellular potassium was reduced.

Myofibrillar hypoplasia in the calf. Myofibrillar hypoplasia, indistinguishable from that seen in the muscles of some newborn piglets, was observed by Bradley (1979) in the skeletal muscle of a solitary bovine calf. The calf appeared normal at birth but became progressively weaker until it was unable to stand. The animal was killed when aged 6 weeks, at which time no gross lesion other than muscle atrophy was detected. On histological examination the myocardium appeared to be normal; there were, however, diffuse and widespread changes in the skeletal muscle. The fascicles were abnormally small. The cross-sectional areas of muscle cells were reduced, and the cells were incompletely filled with myofibrils. Muscle-cell nuclei were numerous, often of bizarre shape, and some were situated internally in chain formations. Electron-microscopic examination revealed electron-dense inclusions and an absence of Z discs.

Familial or hereditary defects manifested during somatic growth

Weaver syndrome of Brown Swiss cattle. A possibly hereditary, primary myopathy occurring in three Brown Swiss cattle was described by Leipold, Blaugh, Huston, Edgerly and Hibbs (1973). The disease developed when the animals were about 6 months old, and was progressive. The gait of the hind limbs became abnormal and erratic until the animals became permanently recumbent. This occurred when they were aged between 18 and 32 months.

Neurological examination showed normal reflexes. Histological examination of the central and peripheral nervous systems and vasculature did not reveal any abnormality. Lesions were restricted to the skeletal musculature of the loins and hindquarters. The muscles did not appear to be atrophied, but some muscles were greyish-white at the periphery. Some muscle cells were hyaline, while others were vacuolated or split and fragmented. There were no signs of regeneration but there was proliferation of sarcolemmal nuclei. Strands of connective tissue traversed the muscle; a conspicuous feature was the presence of rows of fat cells which were erratically arranged at the periphery of the muscle.

Type II muscle cell deficiency in the dog. A muscle disorder in young Labrador Retrievers was described by Kramer, Hegreberg, Bryan, Meyers and Ott (1976). On clinical examination the animals were found to have poor conformation because of a marked deficiency of muscle, abnormal positioning of the head and neck, and a stiff, hopping gait. These characteristics were aggravated by exercise, cold or excitement, and were associated with an electromyographic (EMG) pattern which indicated a myotonic defect. Histochemical study of muscle biopsies showed a predominance of type I cells and a deficiency of type II muscle cells. Kramer *et al.* (1976) suggested that the condition was possibly inherited as an autosomal recessive trait.

Dystonia musculorum of mice. The clinical and pathological findings in dystonia musculorum of the mouse were described by Duchen, Strich and Falconer (1964). This condition, which is the result of a spontaneous mutation, and is transmitted by a single autosomal recessive gene *(dt)*, is characterised by progressive muscular incoordination without paralysis. Duchen *et al.* (1964) found that the main pathological features occurred in central and peripheral branches of sensory ganglion cells, with degeneration and progressive loss of nerve fibres in sensory peripheral structures. These changes were accompanied by atrophy of neuromuscular spindles.

Other disorders of unknown aetiology manifested during somatic growth

Asymmetric hindquarter syndrome of the pig. Asymmetry of the hindquarters in pigs was first described in Germany by Bickhardt, Ueberschär and Giese (1967). They suggested that the condition, which showed degenerative and atrophic changes of muscle with interstitial and perineural fibrosis, was the result of neurogenic atrophy. Later, a similar case was reported in Belgium by Hoorens and Oyaert (1970) who considered that perivascular fibrosis of the arteriolar system within affected muscles was the cause. The condition has also occurred in England, where it was studied by Done, Allen, Bailey, de Gruchy and Curran (1975).

The asymmetry is usually recognised clinically when the pigs reach about 30 kg live weight (Fig. 24.5). The condition does not cause lameness, but adversely affects carcase composition. One limb is smaller than the other and frequently, within a herd, a majority of the affected pigs have the smaller limb on the same side; thus there are either 'right-handed' or 'left-handed' affected herds. The principal asymmetrical muscles are those of the posterior thigh (Fig. 24.6). There is strong evidence of a familial tendency; test matings, however, provided evidence that the condition is not attributable to a single gene with complete penetrance (Done *et al.*, 1975).

The same authors found a variety of degenerative and dystrophic changes in the muscles of AHQS pigs, but these changes were not confined to 'undersized' muscles. There was evidence of single-fibre degeneration similar to that described by Muir (1970) in many muscles of most of the pigs, and there was considerable interstitial fibrosis. Larger collections of uniformly small fibres suggestive of neurogenic atrophy were occasionally seen, usually in muscles with obvious perineural fibrosis. The dystrophic/atrophic changes tended to be more severe in the smaller muscle of an asymmetrical pair, but myofibre degeneration and interstitial

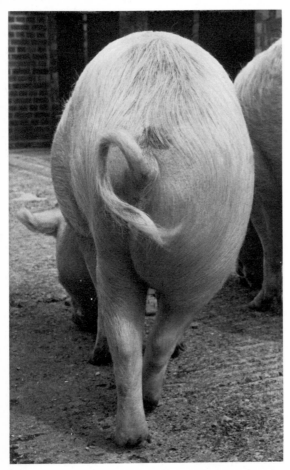

Fig. 24.5 Asymmetric hindquarter syndrome. An affected pig

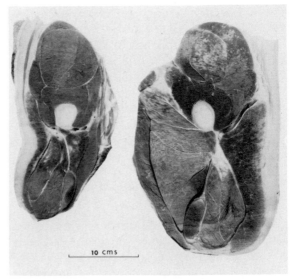

Fig. 24.6 Asymmetric hindquarter syndrome. Transverse section at mid-femur level of the hind limbs of the pig illustrated in Fig. 24.5. The quadriceps muscles (top) are similar in size but the muscle mass of the posterior thigh on the left side is conspicuously reduced

fibrosis were not restricted to such 'undersized' muscles.

There was a gross deficiency of fibres in the 'undersized' muscles, with a degree of compensatory hypertrophy. This may have been caused by aberrations of growth or remodelling processes. The asymmetrical appearance may also be due in part to unequal distribution of subcutaneous fat. Done and his colleagues were unable to resolve the aetiology of the syndrome but concluded that it probably develops postnatally, and that some pigs have a genetic liability to develop the condition. More recently, Bradley and Wells (1978) suggested that another possible cause of the condition might be an asymmetrical distribution of motor neurones in the spinal cord.

FAMILIAL OR HEREDITARY MYOPATHIES AFFECTING DIFFERENTIATED MUSCLE CELLS

Dystrophy-like myopathies

Diaphragm myopathy of Meuse-Rhine-Yssel cattle. This unique disease was first described by Hoebe (1975) and later by Goedegebuure and Hoebe (1976). The associations of parentage suggest a familial origin, because it occurs only in Meuse-Rhine-Yssel cattle from an area of Eastern Holland where this breed forms half the population. The condition is progressive, with clinical signs of digestive disturbances, ruminal tympany due to difficulty in eructation, and dyspnoea which leads finally to asphyxia. The phrenic nerves appear to be histologically normal, and have a normal conduction velocity. The disease seems to be a primary myopathy which always affects the diaphragm; in about 5 per cent of cases the intercostal muscles are also involved.

The gross appearance is of a pale, hard and swollen diaphragm with a normal centrum tendineum. There are white areas which are always fibrous, and which sometimes contain fat.

Under the microscope, dramatic changes can be seen, dominated by pathological alterations which involve both type I and type II muscle cells. The lesions include fibre hypertrophy and splitting, vacuolar change, floccular degeneration and phagocytosis (Fig. 24.7). There are numerous target and targetoid cells, that is, cells with an abnormal appearance caused by zonation of enzyme reactions (Dubowitz and Brooke, 1973). Some cells are angular and atrophic, and there is an increase in muscle-cell nuclei, some of which are internal. There is variable, but usually slight, endomysial fibrosis.

Serum CK and LDH enzyme activities are not increased, but there is reduced CK and LDH 1 isoenzyme activity in affected muscle.

Primary myopathy of Merino sheep. A progressive myopathy of Merino lambs, inherited as an autosomal recessive trait, was described by McGavin and Baynes (1969), and McGavin (1974). Clinically, signs of stiffness are usually detected when the lambs are about 1 month old; when driven, affected lambs develop a 'rocking horse' type of gait because they are unable to extend the stifle and flex the hock joints. The condition is progressive and, under range conditions, results in death from starvation.

Lesions sometimes occur in the *M. triceps brachii*, always in the *M. quadriceps femoris*, and consistently in the *M. vastus intermedius*. Lesions are bilaterally symmetrical and are visible to the naked eye as white areas, or indeed whole white muscles, because of replacement of muscle fibres with fat cells.

The histological lesions are distinctive. In lambs aged 6 weeks, the muscle cells are rounded in cross-section and vary from 15 to 100 μm in diameter. Some have central and peripheral sarcoplasmic masses, while others are vacuolated (Fig. 24.8). There is an increase in muscle-cell nuclei which may be vesicular, and which may occur internally in long chains. There is a slight increase in, or condensation of, endomysial connective tissue. Type I cells are particularly affected; the *M. vastus intermedius* of Merino sheep is composed entirely of this type of cell. As the lambs age there is a reduction in the number of muscle cells. These are progressively replaced with fat cells until, at five years, more than 90 per cent of an affected muscle may be replaced with fat. Significant lesions have not been found in the central or peripheral nervous systems.

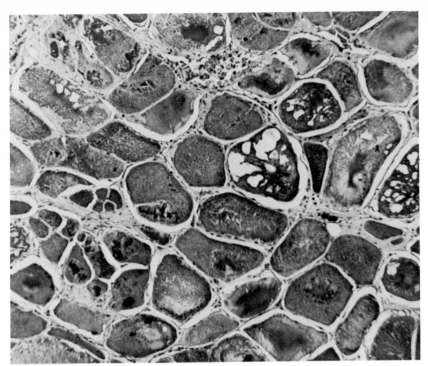

Fig. 24.7 Diaphragm myopathy. Diaphragm muscle of a Meuse-Rhine-Yssel cow affected with diaphragm myopathy. Many muscle cells show vacuolar change, target or targetoid formation and splitting. There is also an increase in endomysial connective tissue. Masson's trichrome, ×85 (section supplied by courtesy of Dr S. A. Goedegebuure)

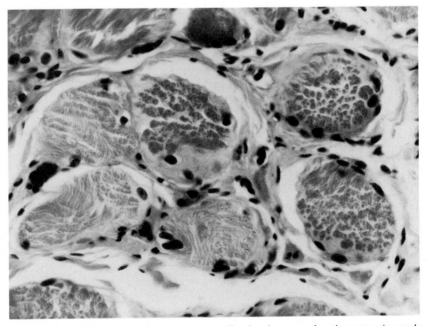

Fig. 24.8 Primary myopathy of Merino sheep. *M. vastus intermedius* showing sarcoplasmic masses, internal nuclei and a slight increase or condensation of endomysial connective tissue. H & E, ×275 (section supplied by courtesy of Dr R. B. Richards)

Pietrain creeper syndrome appears to be an inherited, progressive, primary myopathy in a breed of pigs particularly susceptible to stress. The genetic basis of the condition remains to be clarified. The Pietrain creeper syndrome has been recognised in one pure-bred herd, in which selection for susceptibility to the porcine stress syndrome has been practised for experimental purposes, and in one commercial herd. Usually only two or three pigs in each affected litter show the characteristic clinical features (Bradley and Wells, 1978).

The pigs appear to be normal until they are about three weeks old, when they develop static tremor in fore and hind quarters when standing, and a reluctance to stand for more than a few seconds. The condition is progressive. Although the pigs grow well at first, after four or five weeks recumbency becomes almost continuous, brief periods of standing being accompanied by carpal flexion. By 10 or 12 weeks, carpal extension is restricted and infrequent movement is limited to a creeping type of gait.

Macroscopically, affected muscles appear atrophic. Histological examination shows that all major muscles are affected but the severity of pathological change varies between muscles. The proximal limb muscles are most affected. The main pathological features are a wide variation in muscle-cell diameter (Fig. 24.9), an increase in the number of internal nuclei, and focal myodegeneration and regeneration in excess of that observed in normal Pietrain pig muscle (*see* Focal myopathy). Both type I and type II muscle fibres are involved, and there are marked changes in the normal distribution pattern of muscle fibre types. Target cells do not occur, but there is an abnormal distribution of histochemical enzyme reaction products within the cells.

Significant abnormalities have not been detected in the central or peripheral nervous systems, the motor end-plates or the neuromuscular spindles.

Muscular dystrophy in the dog. Apparently spontaneous, dystrophy-like myopathies with

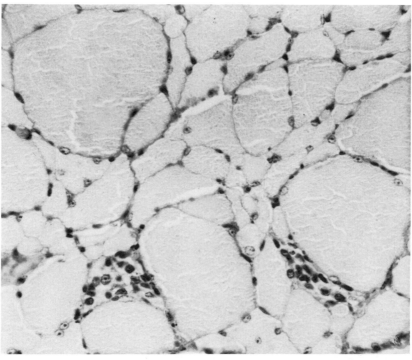

Fig. 24.9 Pietrain creeper syndrome. *M. semitendinosus* of a 12-week-old pig. There is a marked increase in the range of cell size with some focal myodegeneration. A few cells contain internal nuclei. Collagen/elastin, ×275

inconspicuous attempts at regeneration occur, but cases are usually isolated and the aetiology obscure. The diseases are briefly discussed in a later section (p. 858).

Muscular dystrophy of mink is a progressive myopathy of mink in which the histopathological lesions resemble those in amyotonic muscular dystrophy of man. The disorder has a familial pattern, suggesting an autosomal recessive form of inheritance. It has been described by Hegreberg, Camacho and Gorham (1974), Hamilton, Hegreberg and Gorham (1974) and Hegreberg, Hamilton, Comacho and Gorham (1974) with regard to the histopathology, histochemistry and biochemistry respectively.

Clinical signs may appear at 2 months of age and follow a progressive course, resulting in motor dysfunction, dysphagia, muscle weakness and atrophy. The temporal and masseter muscles, and the proximal muscles of the limbs, are particularly affected.

The macroscopic changes consist of pale streaks extending through affected, atrophic muscles. Histopathological changes are confined primarily to skeletal muscles, which are affected to varying degrees and show a wide spectrum of changes. These include variation in muscle fibre diameter, internal nuclei, myodegeneration, increased amounts of endomysial and perimysial connective tissue, and attempts at regeneration. The myonecrotic process appears to involve individual fibres in a random manner. There are neither inflammatory reactions nor calcification. Both type I and type II cells are affected. The perinuclear halos and severe myonecrosis that occur in the myopathy of the Syrian hamster (Homburger, Baker, Nixon, Wilgram and Harrop, 1965) do not occur, neither do the long rows of central nuclei which are a conspicuous feature of muscular dystrophy in the mouse (Pearce and Walton, 1963). Serum levels of enzymes of muscular origin are markedly increased.

Muscular dystrophy of mice. Two muscular dystrophies of the Bar Harbor strain 129 of mouse have been described and studied in detail. The first, more severe (*129/Re*) form, has been used extensively as an experimental model; many of the

findings were summarised by Harman, Tassoni, Curtis and Hollinshead (1963).

The ultrastructural changes occurring in muscle fibres of affected fetal mice were described by Platzer (1971). Banker (1967), and Bray and Banker (1970), reported the ultrastructural findings in mice aged two weeks, and in older mice respectively.

The disease is first recognisable at about 2 weeks of age, when affected mice drag their hind limbs. There is reduced activity and rapidly progressive muscular weakness. Functional control of the hind legs is lost; attempts at movement are made by the atrophied fore limbs. Head nodding, muscular tremors and gasping respiration are also features which occur in some mice. Kyphosis and contractures supervene as late manifestations and the mice die when about four months old.

One of the most striking histological features of the diseased muscle is a wide variation in the diameter of the fibres, with intermingling of hypertrophic and atrophic fibres. Partial and complete segmental coagulation necrosis occurs, with phagocytosis of debris. Regenerative activity occurs from portions of affected fibres but this tends to be abortive, and particularly so when there is also proliferation of connective tissue. Numerous enlarged, internal nuclei occur, often in prominent rows. Endomysial and perimysial fibrosis is usually slight; there is also relatively little replacement of muscle fibres with fat cells.

Opinions about the basic ultrastructural change have centred mainly on the sarcoplasmic reticulum as the site of the fundamental abnormality (Platzer, 1971), although lesions occur in mitochondria, myofibrils and sarcolemma, and there is an increase in lysosomal activity. There is also evidence to suggest that the muscular dystrophy may be attributable to a neuronal abnormality. James and Meek (1975) were, however, unable to find an ultrastructural abnormality in any of the muscle spindles of dystrophic mice. They commented that if the 'neurogenic hypothesis' of muscular dystrophy were true, then changes in these richly innervated structures might be expected.

There is a marked increase in the free fatty acid content of the muscle. Pentose shunt enzymes operating in dystrophic muscle are thought to be important, because increased activity of these enzymes leads to increased production of NADPH$_2$ in the system. The NADPH$_2$ so formed is probably responsible for the increase in fatty-acid synthesis (Susheela, Hudgson and Walton, 1968). These authors also suggested that cellular damage in dystrophic muscle could possibly be a secondary effect of free fatty acid accumulation.

A second hereditary myopathy of the inbred mouse was discovered by Meier and Southard (1970). This also is attributable to an autosomal recessive gene which is an allele at the muscular dystrophy locus (gene symbol dy^{2J}). Clinical signs of the myopathy are progressive in these mutants but the disease is milder than in the dy mutant and the animals can breed successfully. The pathological effects are, however, complicated by gene interactions. In the course of the studies of muscle from dy^{2J} mice, Meier and MacPike (1973) recognised two types of lesions. Some mice (dy^{2J}/dy^{2J}) showed lesions that were similar to, but milder than, those found in the original dy mutation, whereas others had additional qualitative changes, particularly of mitochondria. While the pathological picture in the dy^{2J}/dy^{2J} mice resembled that of the Duchenne type of dystrophy, that of the other genotypes was more suggestive of myotonia dystrophica. They also showed that the action of an 'irrelevant' gene (W) can modify or contribute to the pathological effects of the dy^{2J} gene, thus leading to new or different features. In both the severe $129\ ReJ\ dy/dy$ and the milder dy^{2J}/dy^{2J} forms, prominent amyelination in cranial nerves and spinal roots have been described (Bradley and Jenkison, 1975). These neural abnormalities distinguish the mouse disease from any form of human muscular dystrophy

'Motor end-plate disease' myopathy of mice.

An autosomal recessive gene is responsible for 'motor end-plate disease' of mice. The disease becomes apparent about 10 days after birth and is accompanied by progressive muscle weakness leading to death within the next two weeks. The disease appears to involve a block in neuromuscular transmission and, as the condition progresses, the muscle fibres become severely atrophied. The disorder was first described by Duchen, Searle and Strich (1967), and has been reviewed by Duchen (1975b).

Dystrophy-like myopathy of the Syrian hamster.

Dystrophy-like myopathy in an inbred line (BIO 1.50 (Whitney) strain) of the Syrian hamster was first recognised and described by Homburger, Baker, Nixon and Wilgram (1962). It was quickly determined that this muscle disease was hereditary and transmitted by an autosomal recessive gene (Homburger, Nixon, Harrop, Wilgram and Baker, 1963). The topic has been reviewed by Homburger (1972), and aspects of the pathology reappraised by Caulfield (1972).

Muscular weakness usually becomes apparent clinically when animals are between 60 and 200 days old, but its presence can be quickly unmasked in weanlings by forced swimming. When fatigued by this method, dystrophic animals show weakness of the adductor muscles and the hind legs splay sideways. The muscular weakness is progressive throughout the life of the animals, but the pathological changes do not usually reach the advanced stage seen in dystrophic mice because dystrophic hamsters are short-lived. Congestive heart failure due to myocardial lesions kills most animals about half-way through the normal life span.

The cheek pouch retractor muscle is suitable for biopsy studies; in older animals a very high percentage of such biopsies reveals dystrophic lesions. The histological lesions, which are aggravated by exercise, crowding or defective nutrition, are similar to those found in dystrophic mice. There is loss of muscle fibres through atrophy and fragmentation, great variation in muscle fibre diameter, granular degeneration and coagulation necrosis with phagocytosis of debris (Fig. 24.10).

There is an increase in the number of sarcolemmal nuclei, some of which are internal and occur in long chains. Nucleoli are prominent. Cells containing these forms are probably regenerating by the linear fusion of basophilic myoblasts. The multinucleated myotubes do not repair or replace more than a few of the necrotic fibres. Increases in the amount of connective tissue and fat cells occur, but these are not conspicuous features of the pathology. The dystrophic process affects both type I and type II fibres (Homburger *et al.*, 1965; Homburger, Baker, Wilgram, Caulfield and Nixon, 1966).

Homburger (1972) emphasised the similarity

between these lesions and the changes found in myotonia atrophica and Duchenne's dystrophy in man.

Ultrastructural investigations (Caulfield, 1966, 1972) revealed non-specific lesions similar to those seen in a variety of myopathies. One of the earliest detectable changes was deposition of lipid between the rows of myofilaments. Later, there was degeneration and disintegration of Z and I bands, condensation of the cell, and mineralisation of mitochondria. Early changes in the form of distension of the sarcotubular system have been interpreted in terms of the concept that defective calcium transport, and failure of the relaxing system of the cell, may well be a fundamental lesion. Caulfield (1972), however, pointed out that the appearance of dilated components of the sarcotubular system is a non-specific change; attempts to relate this lesion to defective function of the relaxing system have been unsuccessful.

The serum levels of enzymes of muscular origin are markedly raised in dystrophic animals.

Myotonic syndromes

Myotonia of sheep, goats and dogs is characterised clinically by the involuntary per-sistence of voluntary contraction. The muscles are extremely sensitive to mechanical stimulation; tapping, stretching or the insertion of electrodes cause contraction of the muscle due to long-lasting, irregular tetanus in groups of muscle fibres. As discussed on p. 830 it is possible that fetal myotonia may be a factor leading to the development of congenital articular rigidity. Myotonia has been recognised in a calf (Van Niekerk and Járos, 1970) and in a Thoroughbred filly (Steinberg and Botelho, 1962).

Myotonia in sheep. A myotonia-like syndrome in Shropshire lambs was described by Rings, Hoffsis and Donham (1976). The lambs, when startled, would fall nose-first on to their sides with limbs in rigid extension. There were some deaths due to respiratory failure. The lambs were normal at birth, and were given vitamin E and selenium injections when 1 week old. The condition developed when they were about 3 months old; by this age the lambs appeared 'double muscled', and had a waddling gait. Plasma CK and LDH activities were raised. The EMG pattern was suggestive of diffuse myopathy with possible myotonic discharges. There was enlargement of the heart, diaphragm and skeletal muscles; his-

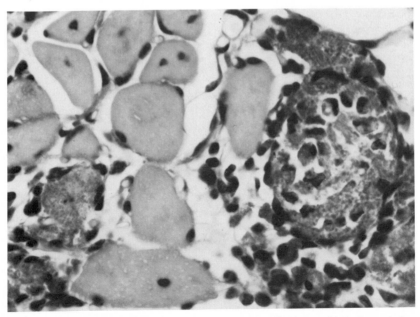

Fig. 24.10   Dystrophy-like myopathy of the Syrian hamster. Some muscle cells are atrophic and contain internal nuclei. Myodegeneration and phagocytosis are prominent. H & E, ×400

tological changes comprised muscle cell hyperplasia and hypertrophy, and possibly some myodegeneration. The fat content of the carcase was lower than usual. It was not possible to establish the hereditary nature of the disease because breeding records were not available.

Myotonia in goats. In goats, the disorder develops within a few weeks of birth, and becomes increasingly severe with age. In pregnant females it tends to disappear at about the time of parturition. It is not accompanied by gross or histopathological lesions. When startled, affected animals become rigid and may be unable to move for several seconds. During such an episode the animal may fall over. The neurotransmitting apparatus is not directly involved; myotonia persists in denervated muscles, and curarisation does not modify the characteristic response of the myotonic muscle to mechanical stimulus; affected muscles are, however, hypersensitive to potassium ions (Brown and Harvey, 1939). The functional defect is not unpropagated contracture but is caused by loss of accommodation to maintained or slowly increasing stimuli, and lowered threshold to any depolarising influence (Bryant, Lipicky and Herzog, 1968). In myotonia of man and goat, the loss of accommodation is apparently caused by a defect in the sarcolemma, which has increased resting membrane resistance due to low chloride conductance (Lipicky, Bryant and Salmon, 1971). Myotonic responses can be produced by drugs such as 20,25-diazocholesterol (Rüdel and Senges, 1972) and other pharmacological agents (Bryant and Morales-Aguilera, 1971) which are known to alter membrane resistance and to reduce chloride conductance. Adrian and Bryant (1974) have suggested that the mechanism of myotonia depends in part on the accumulation of potassium within the transverse tubular system, following a normal propagated action potential. When this occurs in a fibre with low surface conductance, accumulation of potassium within the tubules may initiate the myotonic discharge; in other words, cumulative after-depolarisation can become large enough to initiate a self-maintaining activity.

Myotonia in dogs. Myopathic changes accompany myotonia in dogs. Griffiths and Duncan (1973) reported the clinical findings in four cases of myotonia. Muscle cells were rounded in cross-section on histological examination and very variable in size. There were numerous internal nuclei, many of which were in chains. Muscle-cell splitting, myodegeneration, regeneration and endomysial and perimysial fibrosis occurred (Duncan, Griffiths and McQueen, 1975). The peripheral and central nervous systems were normal. Myotonia may also occur in canine Cushing's syndrome but is thought to have a neurogenic origin (Duncan, Griffiths and Nash, 1977).

MYOPATHY DUE TO TRANSITORY DEFECTS OF CELL METABOLISM

Paralytic myoglobinuria of the adult horse. The typically severe, and frequently fatal, form of paralytic myoglobinuria (also known as azoturia) is an acute myopathy of in-work draught horses which occurs most commonly during the spring (Hadlow, 1962, 1973). A milder form of the disease, known as 'tying-up', or 'set-fast', occurs in Thoroughbreds (Bone, 1963) and in riding horses and ponies. Exercise is the precipitating factor. In draught horses it is usual to find that the disease occurs within an hour of being put to work after a period of 2–5 days' rest, while fed a high-energy diet (Tutt, 1964).

Severely affected horses may collapse between the shafts, showing clinical signs of muscular weakness, spasm, profuse sweating and myoglobinuria. Animals affected in this way usually die from renal failure within a few days. In milder cases there may be complete recovery; some may show residual atrophy of muscle. In riding horses the milder form of the disease is characterised by muscular stiffness, especially of the hind limbs, swelling and hardening of the back and quarter muscles, and profuse sweating. There are no renal complications, and the animals usually recover completely.

The precise cause is uncertain, but it is a widely held view that during the rest period intramuscular glycogen storage reaches maximum levels; the glycogen is rapidly broken down when exercise begins. It is very probable that the cause of muscle fibre necrosis, and consequent liberation

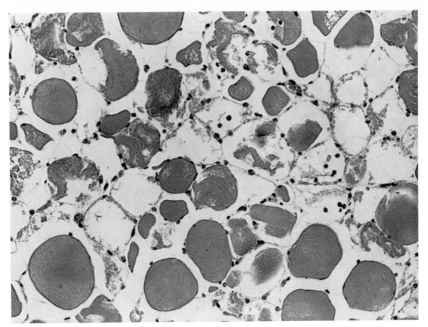

Fig. 24.11 Paralytic myoglobinuria of the horse. *M. longissimus dorsi* showing rounded and hyaline muscle cells, floccular change, empty endomysial tubes and a minimal infiltration of inflammatory cells. H & E, ×125

of myoglobin, is the combination of massive production of lactic acid with tissue hypoxia.

Histological lesions may be widespread in the skeletal musculature, and may occur in the myocardium, but lesions are most evident macroscopically in the lumbar, gluteal and quadriceps muscles. These take the form of greyish-yellow patches and pallor. Sometimes haemorrhages are present. Histological examination shows groups of muscle cells with hyaline or floccular change, empty endomysial tubes, and usually infiltration with inflammatory cells (Fig. 24.11).

In draught oxen, paralytic myoglobinuria is probably attributable to nutritional deficiency of vitamin E and/or selenium, clinical disease being precipitated by a stress factor such as sudden muscular exertion. Although it superficially resembles paralytic myoglobinuria of the horse, it is more probably related to transport myopathy.

Myopathy of cattle due to exercise and environmental factors. During investigations of the interaction between environmental and nutritional factors in the aetiology of nutritional myodegeneration, Anderson, Bradley, Berrett and Patterson (1977) detected two distinct episodes of

myodegeneration, the first of which appeared to be unrelated to the vitamin E and selenium status of the animals. Housed cattle aged 6–16 months were maintained for at least four months on a diet deficient in vitamin E and selenium. They were turned out to pasture during inclement weather in the autumn and spring. At the latter time, five control cattle were included in the group. These had been supplemented with vitamin E and selenium injections five times, at two-week intervals. Following turnout, plasma CK was raised in 80 per cent of the calves whether or not they were deficient in vitamin E and selenium. This episode was accompanied by acute myodegeneration of some of the distal flexor muscles of the fore limb. The plasma CK activity fell to normal within 24–48 h, indicating that the myodegenerative process had stopped. The myodegeneration and rise in CK were assumed to be caused by the sudden increase in exercise induced by grazing.

Subsequently, a second rise in CK activity occurred in 50 per cent of the calves. This was observed only in the nutritionally deficient animals. It was associated with myodegeneration of the *M. biceps femoris* and was considered to be a mild form of the naturally occurring disease induced by nutritional deficiency of vitamin E and selenium, in combination with the effects of increased exercise and inclement weather.

Porcine stress syndrome (PSS). This acute stress syndrome is commonly associated with certain breeds or strains of pig that have been improved by selection for lean carcase composition. It causes sudden death, following stress such as that caused by transport, excitement or exposure to high environmental temperature, and occurs most frequently in heavily muscled pigs at the time of marketing. The syndrome can also be precipitated by exposure to certain anaesthetics, of which halothane is the most notorious. The last-mentioned phenomenon has been studied extensively with the aim of elucidating the mechanism of anaesthetic-induced malignant hyperpyrexia (hyperthermia) of man. Much has been written about PSS. The reader is referred to the review by Swatland (1974) and, for more recent advances, to the Proceedings of the Third International Production Disease Conference, Wageningen, The Netherlands, September, 1976.

Affected animals appear distressed; blood pO_2 is greatly reduced, the lactate content of blood and muscle is markedly increased and, after death, the muscle appears pale, soft and exudative. Thus, in addition to losses during transport, PSS is frequently associated with economic loss due to the production of pale, soft, exudative pork caused by pathological changes occurring immediately before, or during slaughter.

Morphological examination of the muscles of stress-susceptible pigs, before the pathological syndrome has been triggered, do not reveal any abnormal features except the presence of small foci of myodegeneration and regeneration, which Muir (1970) interpreted as indications of a continuous dynamic process. Histochemical methods show that, in affected muscles of stress-susceptible pigs, the proportion of type II (glycolytic and oxidative/glycolytic) cells is increased at the expense of type I (oxidative) cells. There is also a tendency for type II cells to be larger than type I cells. The results of numerous studies of this kind can be integrated into a consistent thesis (Swatland, 1974) namely, that stress susceptibility is related to an increase in the mass of muscles which

in turn is caused by an increase in the proportion of myofibres with strong histochemical reactions for both alkali-stable myosin ATPase and for phosphorylase. In this respect, stress susceptibility in pigs differs markedly from malignant hyperpyrexia in man. Swatland and Cassens (1972) compared the muscles of stress-susceptible and normal pigs and found that, in the former, muscle fibre hypertrophy was associated with enlargement of motor end-plates, increased complexity of terminal ramification, increased ultraterminal sprouting, and more double end-plates. Growth of end-plates in the muscle of stress-susceptible pigs of the Poland China breed was found to be proportional to muscle fibre cross-sectional area during the early phases of muscle fibre hypertrophy only.

There are similarities in the distribution of muscle fibre types, and also in the terminal innervation of muscle (Swatland, Kauffman and Kieffer, 1972; Swatland, 1973) between the muscles of stress-susceptible pigs and those of cattle with 'double muscling'. The latter also tend to be susceptible to a stress syndrome involving myopathic changes.

The investigations carried out by Cheah and Cheah (1976) suggest that the 'trigger' in the biochemical changes leading to pale, soft exudative pork is efflux of mitochondrial Ca^{++}. These authors found significant differences between breeds in the rate of Ca^{++} efflux from mitochondria during anaerobiosis; the rate for stress-susceptible breeds was abnormally high. The excess Ca^{++} is free to activate myofibrillar ATPase and phosphorylase kinase. This leads to rapid glycolysis. The result, under anaerobic conditions, is a high rate of lactic acid production, an increase in heat production, and a rapid fall in the pH of muscle. Low pH depresses the ability of the sarcoplasmic reticulum to take up Ca^{++} and leads to a cascade effect of increasing concentration of calcium in the sarcoplasm, and further glycolysis.

When these changes occur at slaughter, the pH of muscle falls while the temperature is still high. The result is denaturation of sarcoplasmic and myofibrillar proteins, and a loss of the water-binding capacity of the tissue. These changes are indicated by dripping from the carcase, and pallor caused by changes in surface reflectance.

If the muscle glycogen reserves of stress-susceptible pigs are depleted by prolonged but non-fatal stress before slaughter, the ultimate pH of the meat is high and the meat appears dark, firm and dry, and has poor keeping qualities.

While it may be possible to determine a tendency to stress-susceptibility *ante* or *post mortem* using the criteria of histochemical profiles, muscle cell diameter, and the morphology of terminal motor innervation, confirmation of death due to PSS is more simply achieved by the histological demonstration of characteristic contraction bands (Fig. 24.12) in affected muscle. These occur typically in the longissimus dorsi and semitendinosus muscles. The contraction bands are demonstrated particularly well in formalin-fixed paraffin sections stained with Heidenhain's iron haematoxylin.

Myocardial lesions in pigs killed while suffering from the stress syndrome have been described by Johansson and Jönsson (1977). These authors attributed the lesions to the action of cardiotoxic catecholamines.

There is a general opinion that susceptibility to the stress syndrome is influenced by heritable factors; there has been a corresponding interest in diagnostic tests for stress susceptibility, with the aim of removing susceptible animals during the selection of breeding stock. Exposure to halothane anaesthesia is a reliable test (Eikelenboom and Minkema, 1974; Webb and Jordan, 1978) because susceptible pigs develop spasms and muscular rigidity within a few minutes. Halothane sensitivity may be inherited; a single autosomal recessive gene is thought to be responsible (Smith and Bampton, 1977). The induced metabolic reaction is likely, however, to be more simply inherited than either the PSS or PSE syndromes because the stress stimulus will be variable in practice. The degree of genetic association between the halothane test, PSS and production traits is difficult to assess (Webb and Jordan, 1978). There is also evidence that stress susceptibility is associated with blood type in the H system (a complex system of blood groups controlled by several alleles) of red blood cell antigens in pigs. It may prove possible to predict PSS susceptibility by blood typing for H-system factors (Rasmusen and Christian, 1976). Furthermore, there appears to be a close association between the gene responsible for halothane sensitivity, and the phosphohexose isomerase allele, the latter being closely linked with the locus of the H blood group system. Jørgensen, Hyldgaard-Jensen, Moustgaard and

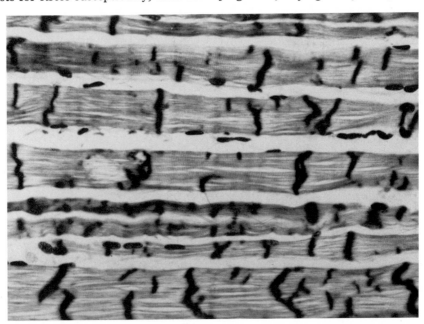

Fig. 24.12 Porcine stress syndrome. *M. longissimus dorsi* of a pig dying as a result of stress and showing extensive contraction band necrosis. Heidenhain's iron haematoxylin, ×275

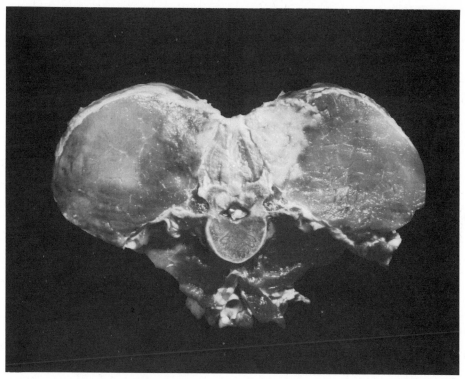

Fig. 24.13 Acute back-muscle necrosis. Section through the back of a pig at the level of the last rib showing pale areas of necrosis in *Mm. longissimus dorsi* and *multifidi*

Eikelenboom (1976) found that all halothane-sensitive pigs (and a considerable number of others) in their test groups had the same phosphohexose isomerase phenotype, and they suggested that this observation could provide the basis for one of a combined series of non-destructive tests for stress-susceptible pigs.

Back-muscle necrosis of pigs is well recognised in parts of the European mainland but has only recently been reported in Britain (Bradley, Wells and Gray, 1979). Clinical signs appear suddenly; affected pigs are reluctant to rise, and have bilateral or unilateral swellings on the back. Skin sensation is lost over the affected areas. In severe cases, if the animal does not die, repair of affected muscles leads to atrophy, giving a 'dished' appearance to affected areas. Bickhardt, Chevalier and Tuch (1975) found that back-muscle necrosis was likely to occur in stress-susceptible animals, and that a likely cause of death was lactic acidosis. They suggested that back-muscle necrosis is a

particular manifestation of the porcine stress syndrome.

Gross lesions consistently appear in *Mm. longissimus dorsi* and *multifidi* (Fig. 24.13) and in acute cases, consist of haemorrhages between muscle fascicles, with variable pallor of muscles. In chronic cases there may be atrophy of muscle cells and fibrosis. The histological features form a spectrum of non-specific changes ranging from acute to chronic. They consist of separation, necrosis and rounding of muscle cells, hyaline change, haemorrhage, cellular infiltration, phagocytosis and fibrosis, with variable attempts at regeneration.

MYODEGENERATION DUE TO NUTRITIONAL DEFICIENCIES

Nutritional myodegeneration (nutritional myopathy; nutritional muscular dystrophy; white muscle disease). Interpretation of the mechanism of this disease, which until recently seemed to have a relatively well-defined and well-understood aetiology, has in some respects regressed into uncertainty. Notable advances have been made in the elucidation of the biochemical mechanisms but experimental reproduction of the disease under controlled conditions has not always been possible, while the triggering mechanisms of some outbreaks in the field have defied precise definition. We suggest that, at present, it should be regarded as myodegeneration with an aetiology principally involving nutritional deficiency of vitamin E and/or selenium, but also involving metabolic and non-nutritional environmental factors. The disease, which has been thoroughly discussed and documented by Sir Kenneth Blaxter in earlier editions of this book, and by other authors elsewhere (Hadlow, 1962, 1973; Hulland, 1970; Bradley, 1975; Lannek and Lindberg, 1975), is a primary myopathy, not a dystrophy. It is a degenerative disease of striated muscle, usually acute and sometimes, especially in adults, accompanied by myoglobinuria. In the surviving animal, muscle cell regeneration is a constant feature. Because of losses through death, and growth retardation in non-fatal cases, the condition is of considerable economic importance to the farming industries of Europe, North America and New Zealand. Its occurrence has been reported in species of farm and domesticated animals, laboratory and captive wild animals, and birds. Susceptibility varies considerably with the species. Herbivores are highly susceptible; the guinea pig and rabbit are very suitable subjects for the experimental reproduction of the disease, while rats and mice are relatively resistant. Nutritional myodegeneration is not hereditary although it is possible that the clinical manifestations are mediated by genetic susceptibility. Environmental factors other than nutritional deficiencies may be involved in precipitating clinical signs.

The principal cause is dietary deficiency of selenium or vitamin E (α-tocopherol), or both, and the disease responds to supplementation, each factor having a partial sparing effect on the other. The pathological effects of selenium or vitamin E deficiency can be exacerbated in chickens by deficiencies of sulphur-containing amino acids and, in several species, by an excessive intake of polyunsaturated fats. Vitamin E-responsive lesions are particularly associated with the latter type of diet.

This discussion is restricted to muscle; it should be noted, however, that nutritional deficiencies of vitamin E and selenium cause a number of important disease syndromes in pigs, poultry, rodents and mink. The topic of vitamin E and selenium-responsive deficiency diseases has been reviewed by Lannek and Lindberg (1975).

In general, it appears that the incidence of selenium-responsive diseases in livestock is higher in areas where the selenium content of the soil and crops is low. There are, however, exceptions; Lannek and Lindberg (1975) suggest that high levels of dietary vitamin E due to long grazing seasons can compensate for lack of selenium in some deficient areas. The counterpart of this is the hazard of vitamin E deficiency in livestock fed on crops which have been harvested or stored under unfavourable conditions.

In recent years, in Britain, there has been an apparent increase in nutritional myodegeneration of yearling, young adult and pregnant cattle (Bradley, 1977). Most of the outbreaks investigated have been shown to be associated with nutritional deficiencies of vitamin E and selenium. This trend may be attributed, in selenium-deficient areas, to the increased consumption of home-grown feeds, to selenium deficiency caused by the replacement of proteins with urea in ruminant feeds, and to low dietary intakes of vitamin E caused by feeding with propionic acid-treated cereals (Allen, Parr, Bradley, Swannack, Barton and Tyler, 1974). The tocopherol content of grain which has been treated with propionic acid falls considerably during storage (Madsen, Mortensen, Hjarde, Leerbeck and Leth, 1973; Allen et al., 1974).

In New Zealand the disease in sheep is likely to appear when housed, pregnant ewes are fed on a diet of hay, legumes and grain, and also when ewes are grazing irrigated legume pastures. Congenital white muscle disease may occur (Hartley and Dodd, 1957). In Scandinavia the disease in pigs appears particularly in the autumn, and coincides with the feeding of newly harvested grain when this has been subjected to heavy rainfall during growth.

Calves are notoriously susceptible but yearlings, pregnant heifers and adult cows may also be affected. Calves may be at risk *in utero* when pregnant cows are fed a diet deficient in selenium; fetal or congenital disease, however, is rarely reported. After birth, disease can occur when calves are fed on diets rich in polyunsaturated fat and possibly also deficient in vitamin E. Fur-bearing animals are also particularly liable to develop vitamin E deficiency because they consume large amounts of unsaturated fatty acids in the fish content of their customary diet.

In Britain there is a marked seasonal increase in the incidence of nutritional myopathy in the spring, when calves are turned out to graze. There is a strong association between the onset of the disease and the sudden increase in exercise, the exposure to inclement weather, and the change in diet. Clinical outbreaks of the disease in New Zealand sheep have been reported after droving or transportation, while the disease in lambs may be precipitated by bad weather (Talos and Roth, 1974). These observations suggest that the development of nutritional myopathy may be triggered by sudden physical activity. However, in trials conducted with calves to investigate this aspect of the disease, Hidiroglou and Jenkins (1968) found that calves that had been allowed to exercise before being turned on to pasture showed an increased rather than decreased incidence of the disease.

An important functioning form of selenium in the body is the selenoprotein glutathione per-oxidase (GSHPx), which catalyses the reduction of membrane-damaging peroxides in the tissues. The activity of this enzyme in the blood and tissues indicates the selenium status of the animal and of the diet in the preceding few weeks (Underwood, 1977 (review); Anderson, Berrett and Patterson, 1978).

The protective effect of both selenium compounds and vitamin E appears to depend on their ability to protect membranes from oxidation. Noguchi, Cantor and Scott (1973) put forward the hypothesis that GSHPx is of primary importance in that it can destroy peroxides within the cytosol before they can attack the cellular membranes, while vitamin E acts as an antioxidant within the membrane itself and so prevents chain-reactive autoxidation of membrane lipids. This hypothesis was advanced to explain the pathology of the capillary cell in the selenium- and vitamin E-responsive exudative diathesis in chicks. The same authors showed that dietary vitamin E and selenium are both necessary for protection of hepatic mitochondrial and microsomal membranes from ascorbic acid-induced lipid peroxidation *in vitro*.

In this connection a specific syndrome, within the disease complex occurring in pigs, is of particular interest. We refer to the acute myodegeneration that occurs among the progeny of sows of reduced vitamin E status, when the very young piglets are given parenteral injections of iron-dextrose in order to prevent anaemia. Amounts of iron that are normally well tolerated cause acute illness and severe, acute myodegeneration which may be fatal within a few hours. The cause is iron-catalysed lipid peroxidation with membrane damage; the concentration of peroxides in muscle is more than doubled. There also appears to be lysosomal damage, as there is a release of acid phosphatase and β-glucuronidase into the plasma. Potassium is released from the damaged cells; its level in the plasma rises sharply and may cause death from cardiac failure (Patterson, Allen, Berrett, Sweasey, Thurley and Done, 1969; Patterson, Allen, Berrett, Sweasey and Done, 1971).

It is clear that the syndrome of nutritional myopathy may be of complex aetiology. It is possible that under some circumstances it is precipitated by dietary deficiency of copper, mediated through depletion of the copper-containing enzyme superoxide dismutase. This possibility is being investigated by our colleague, Dr J.R. Arthur. The coincidence of enzootic ataxia, a disease of the central nervous system of newborn lambs attributed to copper deficiency, and white muscle disease, has been reported in the field (Sheriff and Rankin, 1973).

The clinical muscular disease typically takes the form of stiffness, weakness, difficulties in rising, and tremor. Cardiac involvement, which is common in calves but not in older animals, frequently results in arrhythmia, dyspnoea and high mortality. When the intercostal muscles are affected the clinical appearance may simulate pneumonia (Morgan and Bradley, 1978).

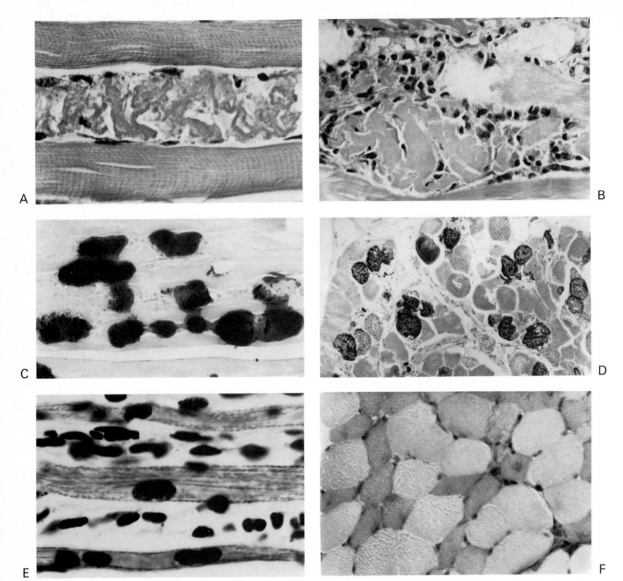

Fig. 24.14 Myodegeneration with an aetiology principally involving nutritional deficiency of vitamin E and/or selenium, but involving metabolic and non-nutritional environmental factors. A. Floccular change. H & E, ×280. B. Phagocytosis of necrotic cell contents. H & E, ×180. C. Cellular calcification. Nuclear fast red, ×70. D. Mitochondrial calcification. Notice that the distribution of necrotic cells is similar to the distribution of type I cells in normal muscle. H & E, ×70.
E. Regeneration showing myotubes with central nuclei and peripheral myofibrils. Loyez's haematoxylin, ×480.
F. Regeneration showing darkly staining small cells, many of which have internal nuclei. These are regenerating cells rich in RNA. Quinolic phthalocyanin, ×220

The gross pathology is of whitish-yellow areas in affected muscles. The lesions may be widespread in calves, but in older cattle the proximal part of the *M. biceps femoris* appears to be primarily affected. Extensive and severe lesions can occur in pigs, but are relatively uncommon in the United Kingdom. The histopathological process is myodegeneration (Fig. 24.14); type I (β, red; slow, oxidative) fibres are preferentially attacked and the sequelae include a change in the histochemical profiles of affected muscles. The hyperacute phase is characterised by floccular, granular and hyaline change. Sometimes mitochondrial and cellular calcification are prominent. These changes are followed by phagocytosis of necrotic fibres, and regeneration. The acute phase of myodegeneration is accompanied by a rise in serum CK and GOT activities.

The studies of Noguchi and his colleagues (1973), and the tendency for the lesions of nutritional myopathy to involve particularly type I muscle fibres, focus attention on the muscle cell mitochondrion as an organelle likely to be involved at an early stage of pathogenesis. In a number of tissues, vitamin E deficiency is accompanied by loss of electron-microscopic positive contrast in osmium-fixed cell membranes. In mitochondrial membranes isolated from the liver of vitamin E-deficient ducklings, this change appears to be caused by a critical loss of specific polyunsaturated membrane-bound fatty acids (Vos, Molenaar, Searle-Van Leeuwen and Hommes, 1973).

The effects of a vitamin E-deficient diet on the ultrastructure of skeletal muscle in the rat have been described by Howes, Price and Blumberg (1964). Changes included thickening of the membrane of the sarcoplasmic reticulum, and mitochondrial degeneration with the appearance of myelin-like forms. The degenerative changes were accompanied by the appearance of lysosomes and dense bodies, some of which appeared to contain mitochondrial remnants. There was streaming of Z-line material and disintegration of myofilaments. The inclusion bodies, the membranous transformation of sarcoplasm, and the many myelin-like figures appeared to contribute to the appearance of a ceroid-like pigment that was a conspicuous histopathological feature of the affected muscle (see Senile myopathy of rats).

Ultrastructural studies also revealed early changes in the mitochondria of skeletal muscle fibres of vitamin E-deficient rabbits. The changes consisted of swelling, fragmentation of cristae, and formation of intramitochondrial myelin figure-like membranous arrays (Van Vleet, 1967; Van Vleet, Hall and Simon, 1967, 1968). Van Vleet considered that the mitochondrial lesions were the primary intracellular changes. Degeneration of contractile elements followed, and there was a sequence of intramitochondrial calcification in degenerate fibres. A very similar type of pathological sequence was later found in the pectoral muscles of chickens deficient in selenium and

vitamin E, with lesions of both myodegeneration and an exudative diathesis (Van Vleet and Ferrans, 1976). There was also widespread endothelial damage in the vasculature of affected muscles. Prominent lesions in the vascular endothelium were disrupted mitochondria and increased numbers of lysosomes.

Sweeny, Buchanan-Smith, de Mille, Pettit and Moran (1972) compared the ultrastructural changes occurring in the muscles of chickens and lambs deficient in selenium and vitamin E. They reported that, in both species, the earliest changes found were lesions of vascular endothelium, fibroblasts and neuromuscular junctions. Mitochondrial lesions were conspicuous in these elements. They suggested that the pathogenesis of nutritional myopathy is influenced by vascular insufficiency and physiological anoxia, complicated by atrophic muscle changes due to nonfunctional junctional complexes. Further support for the concept that mitochondrial changes occur early in the pathogenesis of nutritional myopathy comes from the investigations of Godwin, Kuchel and Fuss (1974) and Godwin, Edwardly and Fuss (1975). These workers found that one of the first demonstrable effects of selenium deficiency on the skeletal muscle of lambs, was abnormal mitochondrial retention of calcium and impairment of the respiratory properties of muscle cell mitochondria.

It is well established that structural and enzymic changes occur during the development of muscle, apparently as adaptive responses to changes in functional activity. These normal developmental processes appear to be reversed, not only in some types of muscular dystrophy of genetic origin but also in rabbits affected by nutritional myodegeneration due to deprivation of α-tocopherol (Lobley, Perry and Stone, 1971). Lobley and his colleagues found that, as the myopathy progressed, the 3-methyl histidine content, ATPase activity and low molecular weight components of myosin isolated from the muscle of affected animals were reduced in amount, becoming similar to those of the neonatal rabbit. They suggested that these changes represented an increased synthesis of the fetal type of myosin, which contains no 3-methyl histidine. No significant change was found in the 3-methyl histidine content of actin; the same authors inferred that the structure of myosin changes as the myopathy progresses, while that of actin does not.

Nutritional myodegeneration of guinea pigs.

Goettsch and Pappenheimer (1931) were the first workers to describe a primary degeneration of skeletal muscle caused by nutritional deficiency. They observed fatal myodegeneration in guinea pigs and rabbits but were unable to prevent it with vitamin E supplementation. Ward, Johnsen, Kovatch and Peace (1977) described a nutritional myopathy, with skeletal and cardiac myodegeneration, in a colony of guinea pigs. An intramuscular injection of α-tocopherol and sodium selenite brought prompt remission of clinical signs. A similar disease in guinea pigs, with clinical signs of hind-leg weakness, was described by Howell and Buxton (1975). This was largely, but not entirely, responsive to vitamin E supplementation. The diet was markedly deficient in vitamins A and E, although overt signs of vitamin A deficiency were not detected.

Cobalt deficiency in sheep.

Cobalt deficiency in ruminants is, in effect, deficiency of vitamin B_{12}; there is a rapid response to B_{12} therapy. The pathological changes in sheep, which are still being evaluated, include atrophic and degenerative changes in the heart, diaphragm and other skeletal muscles (Fell, Wilson and Duncan, unpublished). The lesions are probably of complex origin, involving changes due to cachexia and denervation atrophy. Central nervous system neuronal damage and demyelination are conspicuous lesions.

It is possible, however, that there is also a direct effect on muscle metabolism mediated through depression of methylmalonyl-CoA mutase, resulting in a breakdown of propionic acid metabolism, interference with acetate metabolism, and aberrations of fatty acid synthesis. An alternative mechanism could possibly be depressed activity of 5-methyl-tetrahydrofolate: homocysteine methyltransferase, which catalyses the reformation of methionine from homocysteine, thus permitting the recycling of methionine following the loss of its labile group. Such a mechanism could lead to a loss of available methionine (see Choline deficiency).

Zinc deficiency in sheep.

In squirrel monkeys, the specific lesions of zinc deficiency include atrophy of the muscle fibres of the tongue (Barney, Macapinlac, Pearson and Darby, 1967). Similar lesions in the tongue of sheep deficient in zinc were described by Mann, Fell and Dalgarno (1974), who attributed them to denervation atrophy, possibly complicated by vascular changes due to degeneration of arteriovenous shunts. Fell, Wilson and Leigh (unpublished), using histological, histochemical and electron-microscopic methods, failed to detect lesions of skeletal muscle in zinc-deficient sheep and rats.

Choline deficiency in pigs.

There is evidence, reviewed by Ward (1978), that deficiency of choline in the diet of pregnant sows may be one of the factors which predispose to 'splayleg' in the newborn pig. Interest in the possible relationship between the levels of choline and methionine in the maternal diet, and 'splayleg' in the offspring, was revived by Cunha (1968). Consistent effects, however, have not been found in feeding trials carried out by others. Supplementary choline has been found to improve reproductive performance in sows fed supplemented diets (NRC-42 Committee on Swine Nutrition, 1973) but the precise effect of choline on the occurrence of 'splayleg' remains unclear.

Patterson and Allen (1972) found no evidence of depressed phospholipid synthesis, such as might result from choline deficiency, in the muscles of 'splayleg' piglets. They concluded that the abnormal permeability of muscle cell membranes found in this condition could not be explained by abnormalities of lipoprotein membrane constituents, unless these were of a patchy character not detectable by biochemical assay of total phospholipid.

MYOPATHIES OF COMPLEX OR UNRESOLVED AETIOLOGY

Myodegeneration and steatitis of horse and donkey foals has been recognised in young foals in New Zealand (Dodd, Blakely, Thornbury and Dewes, 1960), in Holland (Kroneman and Wensvoort, 1968), in Sweden (Lannek and Lindberg, 1975), in Japan and America (Hadlow, 1973) and in Britain (Baker, 1969; Platt and Whitwell, 1971). A congenital form can occur (Teige, 1969) but more commonly the disease appears between a few days and three months *post partum*. The condition may be fatal within a few hours of the onset of clinical signs. Affected animals become generally weak and stiff, and have a rapid heart rate. Sometimes the lesions occur in the masticatory muscles and tongue, in which case the foals are unable to suck. Myoglobinuria commonly occurs, and serum CK activity is raised.

Some animals develop steatitis, which causes painful swellings in the subcutaneous fat of the nuchal crest, abdominal wall and gluteal region. This lesion has been observed (Bradley, unpublished) in donkey foals.

Macroscopically and histologically the lesions in cardiac and skeletal muscle resemble those of vitamin E- and/or selenium-responsive myopathy and the disease is usually attributed to this cause. The aetiology, however, has not been definitely established. The steatitis is characterised histologically by necrosis, infiltration with neutrophil polymorphonuclear leucocytes, and mineralisation.

'Spastic paresis'. This form of lameness affects many breeds of cattle, but most reports have concerned certain strains of Friesians (Götze, 1932; Formston and Jones, 1956; Baird, Johnston and Hartley, 1974). It is not a partial paralysis, as one might infer, neither does it conform to the neurological definition of spasticity (Palmer, 1976). The condition has been reported from many countries, and appears to be increasing in frequency and importance (De Ley and De Moor, 1977). It has been reviewed and documented by Baird *et al.* (1974).

Lameness usually begins when the calves are aged between 6 weeks and 8 months; however, clinical signs may be earlier, or delayed for up to two years. The condition affects one or both hind legs, which become progressively more straight. Locomotion is progressively impaired until the more severely affected leg is held clear of the ground and is moved in 'pendulum' fashion.

The nature and site of the lesion have not been established, although the disability can be cor-

rected by tenotomy, by tibial neurectomy, or by surgical deafferentation of the gastrocnemius muscle by section of spinal dorsal roots. Various causes have been suggested, including tendon contracture, primary muscle disorders, aberrant innervation of the vastus lateralis muscle, nutritional deficiency or a central nervous system defect. Several investigators have reported increased values for serum enzymes of muscular origin but significant lesions have not been found in the gastrocnemius muscle (Baird *et al.*, 1974; De Ley and De Moor, 1976).

Dawson (1975) conducted sire–daughter matings in order to investigate the reputed hereditary nature of the condition. He concluded that it is not transmitted by a simple recessive gene, and that it is unlikely that the condition can be controlled by withdrawing the sires of affected calves. He suggested that some calves may have an inherited predisposition to spastic paresis which becomes clinically observable only under certain environmental conditions.

Muscular steatosis. There is little to add to the account by Hadlow (1962) of this condition, which usually attracts the attention of the meat inspector rather than of the pathologist. It is not a clinical condition. Fatty replacement of muscle cells is a non-specific feature of many muscle diseases, and particularly so when these follow a chronic course. Usually, however, there is evidence of inflammatory or degenerative changes in the myofibres. In muscular steatosis there is no such evidence and no sign of myofibre regeneration, and the cause is unknown. The condition may result from occasional trauma causing local myofibre denervation and degeneration in animals feeding on high-energy diets at the time of injury (Swatland, 1974). It has been observed in sheep recovering from a period of vitamin B_{12} deficiency induced by cobalt deprivation (Fell, Wilson and Duncan, unpublished). Though occasionally the lesions may be widespread, they are usually localised in a small group of muscles of the neck, back or upper limbs. The extent of lesions within a muscle can vary considerably. They are usually most prominent close to the epimysium, and may be bilaterally symmetrical. Although severely affected muscle

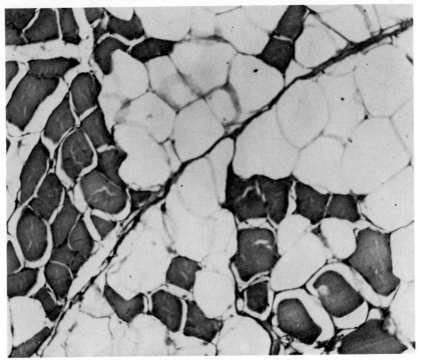

Fig. 24.15 Muscular steatosis. Hind-quarter muscle of a beef carcass showing high proportion of fat cells within muscle fascicles of normal architecture. Lillie's allochrome, ×85

may float in formalin fixative, the normal architecture of fascicles is retained, and normal muscle cells occur in groups between normal fat cells (Fig. 24.15). The condition is relatively rare; it occurs in cattle but is probably more common in pigs (Hulland, 1970). It should be noted, however, that while fat cells are usually found in the perimysium of adult meat-producing animals, under some circumstances pigs have intrafascicular fat cells which are either solitary or in small groups. Care should be taken to distinguish these from muscle cells with artefactual loss of myofibrillar content during histological processing. Some of these intrafascicular fat cells may result from replacement of focal degenerating cells; alternatively they may be normal features of some types of fat pig.

Xanthosis. This condition, which occurs in cattle, is not accompanied by myopathic changes. The term is used to indicate the occurrence of a brownish pigment which is deposited close to cell nuclei, or as rows of granular material between the myofibrils of muscle cells (Fig. 24.16). It appears to be restricted to the heart and skeletal muscles,

the renal cortex and the zona glomerulosa of the adrenal gland. It is usually noticed incidentally during the inspection of otherwise normal carcases, and is important because the discoloured meat is considered, on aesthetic grounds, to be unfit for human consumption.

The pigment is a lipochrome, tinctorially similar to lipofuscin or wear-and-tear pigment; the extent of pigmentation, however, greatly exceeds that seen in senile brown atrophy. It is acid-fast but not birefringent. The diaphragm and masseter muscles are affected most frequently but sometimes the pigment is generalised throughout the muscles of the carcase. Duffell and Edwardson (1978) found 26 cases, three of which were generalised, in 291 Ayrshires (8.9 per cent) while only 12 of 3153 cattle of other breeds (0.38 per cent) were affected, none of these being generalised.

Myopathy associated with hydrocephalus in cattle. A congenital hydrocephalus in Hereford cattle, which is inherited as an autosomal recessive trait, is associated with a progressive dystrophy-like myopathy (Fig. 24.17). A detailed description

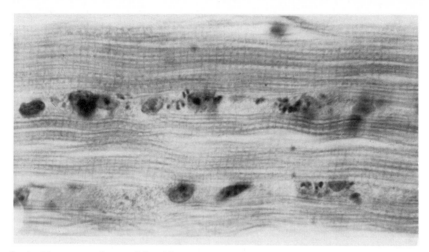

Fig. 24.16 Xanthosis. *M. masseter* of an aged Ayrshire cow. There is an accumulation of lipofuscin-like pigment close to the nuclear poles. H & E, ×675

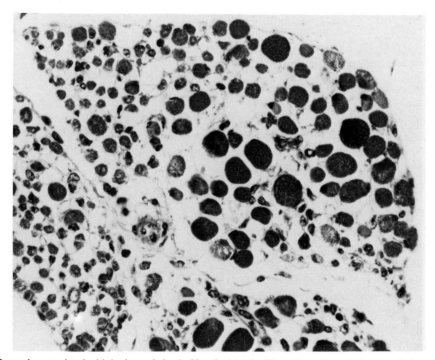

Fig. 24.17 Myopathy associated with hydrocephalus in Hereford cattle. There is a wide variation in cell size and many cells are hypotrophic. H & E, ×275 (section supplied by courtesy of Dr W. J. Hadlow)

of the syndrome appears in the review by Hadlow (1973), with the suggestion that the myopathic changes are of a primary character. The syndrome was discussed by Swatland (1974), who pointed out that brain defects may affect muscle differentiation, and that the myopathic changes may be secondary effects.

Transport myopathy. Long journeys, prolonged droving, chasing or struggling may cause an acute myopathy with a high mortality rate (Hadlow, 1962). Cattle appear to be most susceptible to the disease; in mixed consignments they alone may be affected (Donaldson, 1970).

The clinical signs vary from transitory abnor-

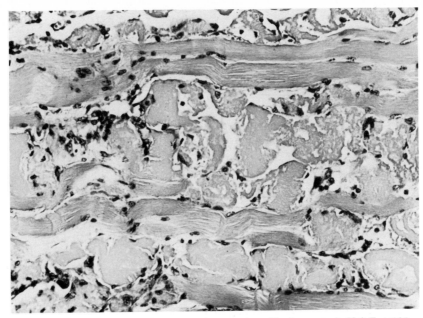

Fig. 24.18   Capture myopathy. There is a severe acute myodegeneration with phagocytosis. H & E, ×125

malities of gait to sudden death. The lesions, and the increased serum enzyme activities, are indistinguishable from those occurring in nutritional myopathy (white muscle disease). Van Logtestijn and van der Linden (1971) reported rail transport myopathy of the longissimus dorsi muscle of adult steers.

In an outbreak reported by Donaldson (1970), 102 out of 355 cattle died while being transported by sea. Subsequent consignments of cattle from the same source were not fully protected by prophylactic treatment with selenium, but combined prophylaxis with selenium and vitamin E was effective. The blood concentrations of selenium and total tocopherols were, however, within the normal range before the animals received these treatments. Donaldson suggested that a key factor may have been low water intake; this was restricted in the earlier voyages, and later given freely.

The disease has been reported in New Zealand in sheep subjected to droving in cold and wet conditions, and after long distance transportation by road or rail (Hartley and Dodd, 1957).

Capture myopathy of wild animals. Among the range of degenerative myopathies of wild animals there is one rather consistent syndrome which may develop during the chase, or during struggling after capture. The syndrome has been discussed by Mugera and Wandera (1967), Young and Bronkhorst (1971), Young (1972), Hofmeyr, Louw and du Preez (1973) and Harthoorn and Young (1974). As pointed out by Hadlow (1973), the condition has been reported most frequently in wild ruminants, especially in African antelope and gazelle.

The animals develop muscular stiffness and respiratory embarrassment and may die quickly, or several days later. The cause of death appears to be severe, metabolic acidosis and profound acidaemia due to excessive muscular effort (Harthoorn and Young, 1974). Myoglobinuria may occur, and may result in renal damage. This may be a contributory cause of death in animals which survive for a few days only.

Gross lesions, appearing as white streaks, occur in the myocardium and in the muscles of the hind legs; these appear histologically as zones of acute myodegeneration (Fig. 24.18). It is possible that a predisposing factor may be subclinical myopathy due to earlier exposure to plant toxins, or to nutritional deficiency.

Free-living and captive wild animals are frequently found to have lesions in the skeletal muscle and myocardium. Myodegeneration is commonly found in ruminants, but similar lesions have also been found in zebra foals (Higginson, Julian and van Dreumel, 1973), tree kangaroos, Rottnest quokka (Kakulas and Adams, 1966; *see also* Ch. 11), and wallabies in captivity (Bradley, unpublished). Many of these lesions are very probably due to nutritional deficiencies of vitamin E or selenium. The quokka appears to have a high requirement for vitamin E and, when captive, is subject to a spontaneously occurring vitamin E-responsive primary myopathy.

Polymyopathy of adult sheep. A myopathic condition in adult sheep, many of which were suffering from scrapie, was described by Bosanquet, Daniel and Parry (1956). These investigators suggested that scrapie was a manifestation of a more widely occurring myopathy. The lesions consisted of severe primary muscle degeneration and, although non-inflammatory, these were considered to have features in common with the lesions of dermatomyositis and muscular dystrophy in man. The disease was slowly progressive and usually fatal. In many of its pathological features the disease described by Bosanquet and her colleagues appears to be very similar to nutritional myopathy.

It is now known that scrapie cannot be considered to be a primary disease of muscle; it is likely that the association between the myopathy and scrapie was fortuitous, and that many of the clinical manifestations of the condition studied by Bosanquet *et al.* (1956) were attributable to scrapie rather than to the myopathy. Nevertheless, the disease differed from typical nutritional myopathy in that sheep were affected when fully mature rather than when young and growing rapidly, and in that clinically affected ewes gave birth to normal lambs.

The situation is possibly clarified a little by the observation by Stamp (1960) that adult sheep may have asymptomatic degenerative myopathy. Stamp found extensive lesions of this type in clinically normal ewes; they were not related either to scrapie or to nutritional deprivation of vitamin E.

It is not easy to interpret these reports, which concern sheep from widely separated areas; the myopathies may have been of complex origin, involving nutritional and other environmental factors. The selenium intake of affected animals was unknown.

Myopathy of the abdominal muscles of pregnant sheep. Muscle cell hypertrophy, with splitting and necrosis of type I (slow, oxidative) fibres was observed by Wilson, Duncan, Wrottesley and Fell (1978) in the *M. obliquus abdominis internus* of sheep subjected to intensive breeding (Fig. 24.19). There was histochemical evidence of increased respiratory activity in slowly degenerating muscle cells. In older sheep there were signs of muscle fibre replacement with fibrous tissue and fat cells. Wilson *et al.* (1978) suggested that the hypertrophy was a response to stretching or increased work load, while the fibre splitting was probably a physiological device to improve nutrition and gaseous exchange. The aetiology of the pathological changes appeared to be complex; there was circumstantial evidence that it involved nerve damage with collateral reinnervation and fibre-type grouping. In general, there appeared to be cycles of cell hypertrophy, atrophy and necrosis which were geared to the reproductive cycles of the ewes.

Cachexia in sheep. Changes in muscle due to cachexia may be superimposed on other pathological effects, particularly when animals are disabled, unable to eat or show anorexia due to nutritional deficiencies or other causes. The main features described by Suzuki (1969; 1973a, b, c; 1974) in severely starved sheep were first, in some muscles, transformation of muscle cells from one type to another; second, progressive atrophy of his type B cells that are roughly equated with type II cells; third, an increase in cellular triglyceride in A, C, D and E cells (type I and intermediate cells). Some C and D cells had a targetoid appearance. The atrophic process involved a reduction in the number of myofibrils within a fibre, reduction in fibre diameter and an increase in interfibre spaces. There was a striking loss of glycogen from the muscle cells during the longer periods of starvation, but no decrease in myofibrillar ATPase activity.

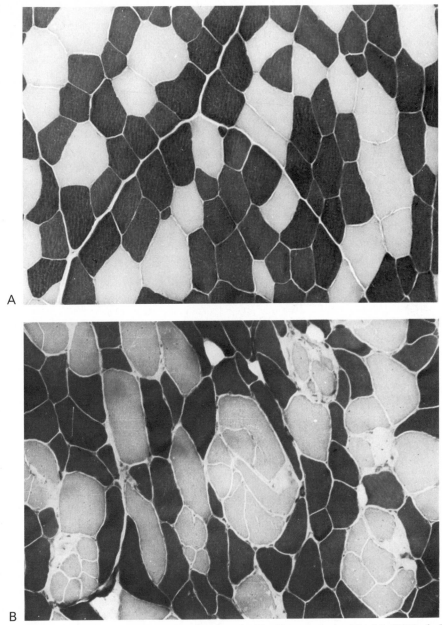

Fig. 24.19 Myopathy of abdominal muscles of pregnant sheep. A: *M. obliquus internus abdominis* (OIA) of a Finnish Landrace × Dorset Horn ewe after two pregnancies at pasture. B: *M.OIA* of Finn × Dorset ewe after 7 pregnancies of intensive breeding. Type I cells show variable cross sectional areas, cell splitting and focal necrosis. Alkali-stable myosin ATPase, ×120

Degeneration and necrosis of muscle fibres was detected when sheep had been starved for 20 days or longer; finally, such fibres lost all contractile material and only the sarcolemma and nuclei remained. There was an increase in the number of muscle cell nuclei, but these showed a high incidence of pyknosis and other degenerative changes.

Bradley (unpublished) also found atrophy of type II cells (Fig. 24.20) in the muscles of stunted

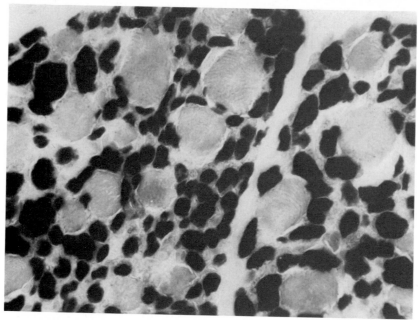

Fig. 24.20   Cachectic atrophy in a lamb. Type I (low-reacting) cells are of about normal size but type II (high-reacting) cells are severely atrophic. Alkali-stable myosin ATPase, ×325

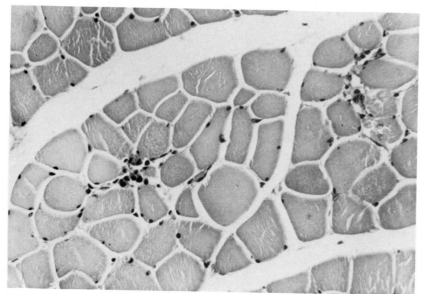

Fig. 24.21   Focal myopathy. Myodegeneration and phagocytosis occur focally within 2 fascicles. H & E, ×125

lambs. These were the offspring of malnourished ewes which almost certainly had a poor milk yield.

Focal myopathy. The Pietrain pig is a breed susceptible to the porcine stress syndrome. Muir (1970) examined the structure of skeletal muscle of Pietrain pigs to determine whether any histological features might be related to a genetically determined muscular abnormality. He found none, but described small foci of degenerating and regenerating muscle fibres (Fig. 24.21) which appeared to be a sign of a continuous process of cell turnover. The significance of the focal myopathy is not clear; Muir suggested that the changes could not be attributed to known nutritional or cytotoxic factors, but pointed out that certain idiopathic or genetic dystrophies cause similar regenerative patterns. Similar foci have since been observed by others in clinically normal pigs (Bradley and Wells, 1978) and, to a lesser extent, in clinically normal cattle and sheep.

Chronic myopathy, with cytoplasmic bodies, in pigs. Scarlato and Meola (1978) used stress-susceptible (Landrace) and stress-resistant (Large White) pigs to conduct breeding trials aimed at producing a back-cross of pigs that would not be susceptible to the porcine stress syndrome but which would preserve the superior carcase characteristics of stress-susceptible pigs. The project was partly successful in that the F_2 animals did not produce pale, soft and exudative pork and had good carcase quality; there was evidence, however, of hind-leg weakness in these animals.

Histological examination of the longissimus dorsi muscle revealed no abnormality except for the presence of cytoplasmic bodies in single muscle cells. The bodies appeared round in cross-section, but extended through the length of the muscle cell for many sarcomeres. They were confined to type II cells and gave strongly positive reactions with the PAS method; after diastase digestion they gave positive histochemical reactions for enzymes concerned with the synthesis and degradation of glycogen (glycogen synthetase; phosphorylase, α-glucan-phosphorylase). The bodies appeared to lack myofibrillar ATPase activity. They occurred in almost all type II muscle cells of F_2 pigs with 75 per cent Landrace but in only about 33 per cent of type II cells in F_2 pigs with 75 per cent Large White.

It was suggested by Scarlato and Meola (1978) that the presence of cytoplasmic bodies in F_2 pigs, in percentages which varied with the cross, probably indicates a metabolic impairment of the muscle of such pigs. The impairment, however, is usually subclinical and is not enough to cause more than a slight structural change in the muscle cells.

Dystrophy-like myopathies of the dog and cat. Generally, muscular dystrophy in the dog is rare; it may affect adult animals of either sex. It is accompanied by weakness, loss of condition and atrophy of proximal limb muscles.

Innes (1951) described a solitary case of progressive pseudohypertrophic muscular dystrophy in a 9-year-old Retriever dog. The gastrocnemius muscles of both hind limbs were pallid, and the muscle fibres were extensively replaced with fat cells. Other isolated cases of progressive muscular dystrophy in dogs were described by Meier (1958) and Whitney (1958), and a general account is given by Hulland (1970). Conspicuous histological features are atrophy and hypertrophy of muscle cells, cell splitting, myodegeneration and replacement with fat cells. Regeneration is not a conspicuous feature. In some cases there is an increase in the number of muscle cell nuclei.

Where muscle fibres have been extensively replaced with adipose tissue, the terminal boutons of the redundant motor innervation may occur on the surface of fat cells (Hulland, 1970).

A possible case of familial dystrophy-like myopathy in Siamese kittens was described by Hulland (1970). Clinically, there was progressive weakness leading to postural collapse; attempts at sternal locomotion led to a peculiar, laborious, back-humping progression. Terminally, there was severe muscle atrophy but there was hypertrophy of groups of cells in some muscles.

Abnormal development of the pectineus muscle of dogs. While developing investigative techniques to study the mechanism of hip dysplasia, Cardinet, Wallace, Fedde, Guffy and Bardens (1969) encountered a developmental abnormality of the pectineus muscle in young dogs. The condition was recognised in both pure-bred Alsatians (German Shepherds) and in mongrels. In some animals, during the postnatal development of this muscle, there was retardation of the growth of type II muscle fibres, with compensatory hypertrophy of type I fibres. The condition was classified as type II cell hypotrophy. It was usually bilateral, affecting between 25 and 75 per cent of the muscle cross-sectional area. In a small number of animals the lesions were unilateral and affected less than 25 per cent of the area of one muscle. No lesions were observed in other adductor muscles innervated by the obturator nerve.

It is possible that the developmental abnormality may play a part in the pathogenesis of hip dysplasia; section or removal of this muscle has been advocated as a corrective measure. A critical evaluation of the results of this surgical technique was made by Vaughan, Clayton Jones and Lane (1975).

Laryngeal myopathy of dogs. O'Brien, Harvey, Kelly and Tuckers (1973) performed histological examinations of resected laryngeal tissues from dogs suffering from a clinical syndrome of abnormal laryngeal function, laryngitis and oedema of the vocal cords. They found neurogenic atrophy of the laryngeal muscles.

The mechanism of laryngeal myopathy (laryngeal hemiplegia) in Bouvier dogs in Holland is less easy to interpret. Dr S.A. Goedegebuure of Utrecht reports that dogs of this breed may lose their ability to bark when aged between 3 and 18 months. A similar condition occurs in another large breed, the Leonberger, but the age of onset is between 1 and 5 years.

Laryngoscopy reveals paralysis of one vocal cord—usually the left. The EMG pattern is that associated with denervation atrophy, but lesions have not been found in either the recurrent laryngeal nerve or the nucleus ambiguus.

There are lesions in the extrinsic muscles of the larynx except in the *M. crico-thyroideus*. These do not conform with the clinical and EMG findings, consisting mainly of fibrosis round the branches of intramuscular nerves, atrophy of type I and type II muscle cells, muscle-cell splitting, an increase in the number of nuclei and fibre-type grouping. Further work is required to resolve these apparently paradoxical findings.

Myopathy with unstructured cores and mitochondrial abnormality in a dog. Through the courtesy of Dr N. Edington of the Royal Veterinary College, London, one of us (R.B.) examined a hitherto undescribed myopathy in a 4-year-old West Highland terrier. Clinical signs were progressive weakness, muscle tremors, ataxia and muscle atrophy. The histological lesions were dramatic. There were extreme variations in muscle cell diameter, replacement of muscle fibres with fat cells, an apparent proliferation of capillaries and nerve fibres, and alterations in the internal structure of muscle cells (Fig. 24.22). The last-mentioned change took the form of darkly stained central areas which were particularly well demonstrated with trichrome stains and with Heidenhain's iron haematoxylin. These had the appearance of central unstructured cores; ultrastructurally, they consisted of disarrayed actin and myosin filaments, and Z-disc material. The mitochondria contained bar-like inclusions.

Myositis of masticatory muscles in dogs. Diseases in this category form a spectrum of inflammatory and atrophic changes. They have been described in some detail by Hulland (1970), and are of unknown aetiology. One case was examined in detail by Oghiso, Kubokawa, Lee and Fujiwara (1976). Expressions of the disease complex appear to vary with the breed and with the stage of progression. The disease appearing in Alsatians as eosinophilic myositis may be the same as that which is manifested in other breeds as progressive atrophy and fibrosis of the temporal (Fig. 24.23) and other masticatory muscles. Other muscles, particularly those of the neck and shoulder, are irregularly and inconsistently involved.

Acute myopathy and Haffkrankheit in man, cats and other animals. Gardner (1967) reported an acute myopathy in a 3-year-old cat following a febrile disease of 10 days' duration. The cat was fed mainly on raw mutton and milk. Although the cause was not determined, selenium deficiency was suspected. The skeletal muscles contained bilaterally symmetrical pale areas which microscopically appeared as areas of severe myodegeneration with extensive calcification.

Earlier knowledge of the features of Haffkrankheit (Germany and Sweden) and Minimata disease (Japan) was summarised by Innes and Saunders (1962). These diseases were associated with the regular consumption of raw or cooked fish, and occurred in man, pigs, cats, dogs, foxes and birds. Minimata disease has since been shown to be due to alkyl-mercury toxicity, and is essentially a disease of the nervous system. In cattle, however, this disease is accompanied by

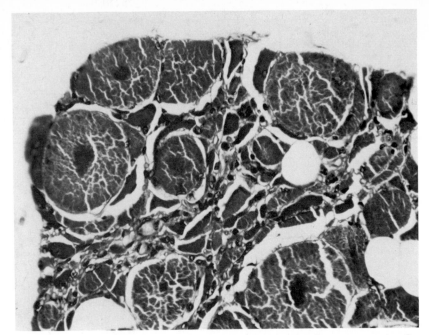

Fig. 24.22 Canine myopathy with unstructured cores. *M. semimembranosus* showing severe atrophy of muscle cells, increase in intrafascicular fat cells and central cores in some of the larger muscle cells. Picro-Mallory, ×275 (section supplied by courtesy of Dr N. Edington)

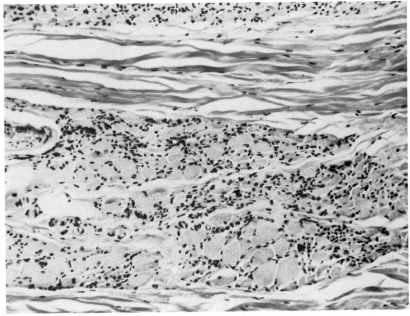

Fig. 24.23 Myositis of the masticatory muscles of dogs. *M. temporalis* showing severe atrophy of muscle cells and fibrosis in the perimysium. H & E, ×85

consistent granular degeneration and calcification of Purkinje cells in the heart.

Haffkrankheit appears to have both neurological and myopathic features. In man, muscle pains occur after exercise; these are accompanied by degenerative changes in skeletal muscle, and myoglobinuria. Possible causes are alkyl–mercurial toxicity, vitamin E deficiency or thiamine deficiency due to the action of thiaminase in the food.

Necrotising myopathy of guinea pigs. Two cases of primary necrotising myopathy were found by Webb (1970) in a group of 24 otherwise healthy and normal young guinea pigs. Macroscopically, the muscles of all four legs and of the trunk were soft, reduced in bulk and darker than normal. They contained purple streaks which gave a mottled appearance to the cut surface. Myodegenerative lesions consisted of muscle cell necrosis, infiltration with mononuclear cells, and regenerative changes. The cause was not established.

Senile myopathy of rats. While studying the ageing process in rats, Berg (1956) observed a myopathy which was an important cause of death in senescent animals. It was rarely seen in animals less than 2 years old.

The disease affected chiefly the gastrocnemius and adductor muscles of the hind legs, and appeared clinically as a waddling gait which, within about eight weeks, progressed to complete postural collapse of the hind quarters. The syndrome rapidly led to loss of body weight, inanition and death. The affected muscles became atrophic, brown and flabby. The histological lesions resembled those of chronic vitamin E deficiency, consisting of myodegeneration with regeneration, and replacement of degenerating fibres with fat cells. A ceroid-like pigment occurred in the sarcoplasm of degenerating muscle cells. (*see* Nutritional myodegeneration p. 845).

The vitamin E content of the diet was thought to be fully adequate, but Berg suggested that the dietary requirement of rats might possibly increase considerably with age.

TOXIC MYOPATHIES

Skeletal muscle is largely resistant to chemical toxins, although certain cytotoxic substances, such as plasmocid (8-(3-diethylaminopropylamino-6-methoxyquinoline) and a dye, Brown FK, selectively damage striated muscle (Hicks, 1950; Grasso, Muir, Goldberg and Batstone, 1968). Very few instances of toxic myopathy due to plant poisons have been recognised; these are briefly discussed here, together with a note of a small number of toxic agents with possible pathological effects on muscle, to which livestock may be exposed.

Because, in some of these toxic syndromes, it may be necessary to consider the simultaneous effects of nerve damage, it should be noted that the main effect of denervation on muscle is atrophy of muscle cells (Tower, 1939). Ultrastructural investigations, however, reveal that an early degenerative autolytic process precedes the 'simple' atrophic process (Pellegrino and Franzini, 1963).

Cassia occidentalis myopathy of cattle. An economically important toxic myopathy occurs in cattle in eastern Texas and Florida (Hadlow, 1973). It is caused by ingestion of an indigenous plant, *Cassia occidentalis*. The plant is eaten most readily after the first frosts and, typically, cattle are affected in early winter. Large numbers of cattle may be poisoned in this way. Early clinical signs include diarrhoea; muscular weakness becomes evident about one week after ingestion of the plant. Affected cattle have a swaying, stumbling gait and fall easily. Animals which become recumbent die after several days; others may die suddenly, two or three days after consuming large amounts of the plant. The cause of death in such acute cases is cardiac myodegeneration. The myocardium is not consistently involved, however, and may be unaffected in less acute forms of the toxicosis.

Affected muscles appear diffusely pale, or have numerous stippled pale foci. The muscles of the hind legs are commonly involved. On histological examination the lesions appear as severe, widespread, acute myodegeneration.

The activities of muscle enzymes in the serum are raised, and myoglobinuria may occur.

Limberleg of sheep and goats (coyotillo poisoning). In south-west Texas a condition known as 'limberleg' occurs in sheep and goats which ingest the mature fruit of the coyotillo plant (*Karwinskia humboldtiana*). The disease is characterised clinically by tremor, progressive leg weakness, incoordination, recumbency, loss of patellar and gastrocnemius reflexes, and death. Earlier investigations revealed widespread myodegeneration in affected goats; the heart, diaphragm and ocular muscles were involved, and a specific myotoxin was thought to be responsible (Dewan,

Henson, Dollahite and Bridges, 1965).

Later studies, using goats poisoned with daily oral doses of the fruits, revealed additional, and possibly primary, lesions in the form of neurological changes specifically involving Schwann cells (Charlton, 1970; Charlton and Pierce, 1970). These investigators reported the occurrence, in poisoned goats, of dystrophic axons in the cerebellum, and peripheral neuropathy with sequential demyelination and Wallerian degeneration of peripheral nerves.

Humpy back of sheep. This is a locomotor disorder of Merino sheep which occurs in western Queensland (O'Sullivan, 1976). It usually occurs in summer, 6 to 10 weeks after substantial rainfall, and usually becomes evident when adult sheep in full fleece are being mustered for shearing. The disease is thought to be caused by ingestion of a toxic plant, which from field evidence may be *Solanum esuriale*. When driven, affected animals fall to the rear of the flock, drag their hind feet, knuckle over at the fetlocks, and finally stop with lowered head and arched back. The principal lesion appears to be Wallerian degeneration of the spinal cord.

O'Sullivan carried out a detailed examination of eight affected sheep and found, in addition, severe myodegeneration in the muscles of the hind leg in three, and milder focal lesions of muscle in another three of the sheep. The myodegeneration was bilateral and was characterised by granular degeneration of fibres with macrophage infiltration. He attributed the muscle lesions to the stress of prolonged muscular exercise associated with transportation. Clearly, if that is the correct interpretation, the muscle lesions are superimposed and are a form of transport myopathy. Possibly the loss of normal innervation by a proportion of the muscle fibres increases the susceptibility of the remainder to the pathological effects of prolonged exertion.

Selenium toxicity occurs in a number of well-defined territories. These are characterised by the presence of highly seleniferous plants which have the ability to convert insoluble selenium compounds to soluble selenates. Acute toxicity may occur in livestock following the ingestion of such unpalatable plants in times of food shortage, or by accidental overdosage with selenium-rich compounds used to combat deficiency states (Bradley, 1975). Shortridge, O'Hara and Marshall (1971) recorded the death of 376 out of 557 calves following the injection of 100 mg instead of 12 mg selenium as sodium selenite. Lesions were present in the liver, kidney, lungs and heart. The last showed focal necrosis and lipofuscinosis of cardiac muscle cells. There was also degeneration of smooth muscle cells in the walls of pulmonary and myocardial arterioles.

The pathology of acute selenium toxicity in piglets, induced by injections of selenite, was described by Van Vleet, Meyer and Olander (1974). Pathological changes, observed grossly and histologically, included pulmonary oedema, skeletal myodegeneration, hepatic degeneration, transudation into body cavities and widespread circulatory disturbances.

Toxic effects of copper and cobalt in sheep. In spite of the drama of the 'haemolytic crisis', which is characteristic of the acute phase of copper poisoning in sheep, neither of us, working independently, has recognised myopathic changes associated with the elevation of the copper content of the blood. Nevertheless, Thompson and Todd (1974), working with Irish sheep, and Howell (1978) with Merinos, reported a rise in serum CK activity when chronic copper poisoning progressed to the haemolytic crisis. These authors suggested that the rise may have been due to a change in the permeability of muscle cell membranes.

Additive cobalt has been incriminated as the cause of epidemics of cardiac failure in beer drinkers (Anon, 1968). The quantities of cobalt consumed were considerably less than amounts used therapeutically for longer periods without untoward effects. In view of this finding it is of some interest that sheep can tolerate relatively large single doses of a soluble cobalt salt (Andrews, 1965) but may exhibit chronic toxicity when exposed to daily doses of a few milligrams over a long period. Toxic signs so produced may be associated with liver cobalt concentrations in the range of $1-10$ parts/10^6. In man, the myocardial lesions consist of diffuse hydropic degeneration in the muscle cells. It is possible that, under some circumstances, lesions of this type may occur in cattle or sheep, and complicate the interpretation of other myopathies.

Molybdenum toxicity in rabbits. During studies of hematopoiesis and epiphyseal growth zones in rabbits with dietary molybdenosis, Valli, McCarter, McSherry and Robinson (1969) observed severe muscular degeneration in the hind legs of three rabbits, and foci of myocardial degeneration in two, from an experimental group of 12 rabbits. They were unable to establish the mechanism of this and other toxic manifestations; they suggested, however, that the primary biochemical lesions were not attributable to the well-known antagonism between molybdenum and copper metabolism.

Iodine toxicity in rats. Oral administration of iodides to rats induces muscular rigidity, motor disturbances and a widespread myopathy which has some clinical and morphological similarities with thyrotoxic myopathy in man (Cantin, 1967). Pronounced lesions are located in the intercostal muscles, and in the quadriceps and triceps brachii muscles. Lesions also occur in the intrinsic muscles of the larynx, resulting in a clinical condition resembling laryngeal paralysis, with gaping mouth and laboured respiration. The lesions are characterised by atrophy, myodegeneration, phagocytosis and fibrous replacement. A distinctive feature of the myopathy is the formation of groups of damaged muscle cell nuclei which form dense, Feulgen-positive aggregates. Such bodies may occur in otherwise normal muscle cells.

MYOPATHY DUE TO STORAGE DISEASE

Glycogen storage disease. A generalised glycogen storage disease occurring in Corriedale sheep has been recognised in New Zealand (Manktelow and Hartley, 1975). When between 6 and 10 months of age, the animals became lethargic and incoordinated, and lost condition. Some collapsed and died on exertion. There was an accumulation of glycogen in skeletal, cardiac and smooth muscle cells, and in nerve cells of the brain stem; Manktelow and Hartley suggested that the disease was comparable with Pompe's disease of man (type II glycogenosis or acid maltase (α-1,4-glucosidase) deficiency).

Richards, Edwards, Cook and White (1977) described the clinical, biochemical and pathological features of hereditary glycogenosis type II in cattle. The affected animals were part of a group of yearling Shorthorn beef cattle in Western Australia. The clinical signs were muscle weakness, inability to rise properly and incoordination of gait. Stored intracytoplasmic glycogen was demonstrated in the central nervous system, heart and skeletal muscle (Fig. 24.24). Richards *et al.* (1977) suggested that the clinical signs and necropsy findings in the affected cattle were similar to those reported in Pompe's disease in man. Pompe's disease is generally considered to be a lysosomal storage disease. It was not possible to obtain evidence of an association between glycogen and lysosomes in the bovine tissues, but in the liver, skeletal muscle and heart there was a deficiency of the lysosomal enzyme α-1,4-glucosidase. Assays of this enzyme in extracts of lymphocytes, coupled with genealogical information, were considered by Jolly, Van-De-Water, Richards and Dorling (1977) to be useful for identifying heterozygous individuals with a reasonably high degree of probability.

Type II glycogenosis has also been recorded in dogs and cats. Rafiquzzaman, Svenkerud, Strande and Hauge (1976) discussed glycogen storage diseases in domestic animals and described, in detail, glycogenosis in four female Alsatian dogs. They considered the disease to be similar to type III glycogenosis (Cori's disease of man). Biochemical investigation of one of these animals by Čeh, Hauge, Svenkerud and Strande (1976) provided further evidence that the disease was similar to Cori's disease and was associated with deficiency of the debranching enzyme amylo-1,6-glucosidase.

Hegreberg and Norby (1973) reported an inherited storage disease of cats, which was accompanied by growth retardation, progressive muscular weakness and atrophy. The changes particularly involved the musculature of the hind

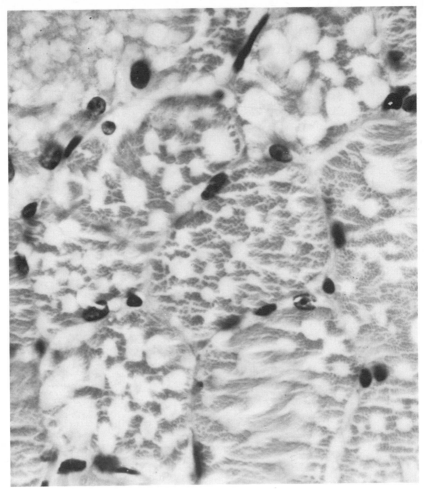

Fig. 24.24 Glycogenosis type II. Skeletal muscle from a yearling Beef Shorthorn showing multiple vacuoles in muscle cells. H & E, ×900 (section supplied by courtesy of Dr R.B. Richards)

limbs. Periodic acid–Schiff positive material occurred in reticuloendothelial cells, liver and muscle cells. There was focal necrosis of muscle and increased serum CK activity.

MYASTHENIA GRAVIS

Myasthenia gravis in dogs. There is now strong evidence that the neuromuscular junction can be selectively injured by antibodies against homologous tissue. The basis for myasthenia gravis appears to be defective function of the thymus, leading to a breakdown of immunological tolerance, and autoimmune damage to acetyl-

choline receptors (Simpson, 1977; *see also* Ch. 16).

For many years, myasthenia gravis was considered to be a disease of man; recently, however, it was passively transferred to mice by injection of pooled immunoglobulin from human patients (Toyka, Drachman, Pestronk and Kao, 1975). Furthermore, a closely similar disease was produced in rabbits by immunising them against nicotinic acetylcholine receptor protein isolated from the electric organ of *Torpedo marmorata* (Thornell, Sjöström, Mattsson and Heilbronn, 1976).

In recent years the disease has been recognised in dogs (Fraser, Palmer, Senior, Parkes and Yealland, 1970; Palmer and Barker, 1974; Darke,

McCullagh and Geldart, 1975) and in a cat (Dawson, 1970). In three dogs, myasthenia gravis was associated with thymoma (Darke *et al.*, 1975).

Most of the cases have occurred in the larger breeds, such as Alsatian, and Golden and Labrador Retrievers, but the disease has also been noted in Jack Russell terriers. Clinical manifestations are fatigue and considerably reduced tolerance to exercise. The fore legs appear to be primarily involved; affected animals take shorter and shorter strides and fall forwards if forced to go on. The bark may become hoarse or high-pitched, and diarrhoea and vomiting may occur. The latter is attributed to dilatation of the oesophagus which, in the dog, contains a high proportion of striated muscle cells.

It is unusual to find histological lesions in the muscle of affected dogs (Palmer and Barker, 1974), although Darke *et al.* (1975) reported the occurrence of sporadic, non-specific degenerative and atrophic changes in the muscles of the head and larynx. These were associated with isolated foci of lymphocyte infiltration. Ultrastructural examination shows widening and atrophy of the secondary synaptic clefts of the motor end-plates.

CONCLUDING REMARKS

We have restricted the coverage of this review to the primary myopathies of non-primate mammals and, in so doing, have excluded birds and fish. A very much longer review would be required if we were to attempt an adequate and comprehensive description of all the animal myopathies.

We have also excluded a number of diseases, in spite of their scientific interest, on the grounds that they are neurogenic, for example Haloxon (organophosphorus) delayed neurotoxicity in pigs and femoral nerve degeneration and neurogenic atrophy of the quadriceps femoris muscle in calves. Other myopathies, such as eosinophilic myositis, have been omitted because they have an inflammatory character. An adequate description of eosinophilic myositis in cattle is available in the text of Jubb and Kennedy (1970), while Harcourt and Bradley (1973) have described the condition in sheep.

Our attempts to classify the animal myopathies

have highlighted the frequent overlap apparent in their aetiologies, particularly with regard to the impact of nutritional and other environmental factors. It is likely that, with further progression in knowledge, some of the syndromes which we have described as separate entities will be found to have common factors that can be identified with precision, and will coalesce.

In contrast to the diverse aetiologies is the relative uniformity of morphological change, which draws attention to the limited repertoire of the muscle cell in its reaction to injury. In general, the description of a syndrome is insufficient to warrant attribution of cause. Nevertheless there are marked differences between species in their reactions to a particular causal factor, as exemplified by differing species' susceptibility to nutritional myopathy. There are also differences within a species; young, rapidly growing animals are generally most susceptible to nutritional deficiencies.

In addition to the relative uniformity of the visible responses to injury, it is possible to discern certain functional defects that occur repeatedly within a range of genetically determined muscular dystrophies and other myopathies. These are: myotonic effects, which may be related to defects in the sarcolemma associated with impaired chloride conductance; mitochondrial calcium overload associated with energy deficiency; and possibly a general reversion of sarcoplasmic enzymes and structural components of myosin to the relative amounts and forms that normally characterise the fetal or immature muscle. The central theme presumably concerns the muscle cell rather than the aetiology. The corollary is that particular care is required to elucidate the pathogenesis of muscle disease, because primary and secondary effects, whether these are morphological or biochemical, may quickly overlap. Such investigations should be supported with parallel studies on possible changes in muscle fibre type distribution since type I and type II cells, and regenerating cells, differ in their biochemical characteristics.

Much has been said about the interest and potential value to science and medicine of comparative pathology. Animal models provide an opportunity for the experimental investigation of causal agents such as toxicological, nutritional and genetic factors, and for sequential studies that may allow the identification of primary morphological and biochemical changes. Indeed, it is evident that some of the conditions in this review have counterparts in man, and may prove of value as models for research. We endorse, however, the view put forward in a different context by Done (1976). That is, it is unrealistic to look for an exact replica of a disease in man, which could clarify all the problems of the human condition. We agree with his opinion that 'a less simplistic view recognises the potential of animal models for the study of *mechanisms* and appreciates that the very genetic diversity of the animal population contributes to the scope of the model system'.

ACKNOWLEDGEMENTS

We are indebted to numerous colleagues in our respective Institutes and around the world. We are particularly grateful for the generous gifts of tissues and sections which enabled us to study unfamiliar diseases at first hand. Special acknowledgement has been given under the respective figures. At the Central Veterinary Laboratory we thank particularly Dr P.H. Anderson, Mr M. Gitter, Mr L.M. Markson, Dr S. Terlecki, Dr P.S. Ward and Mr G.A.H. Wells for provision of material and access to data, Mr J. Bailey and Miss M. Hanton for assistance in preparing the work for publication, and Mr R. Sayer for skilled photographic advice and for the preparation of the prints. It is also a pleasure to thank Sir Kenneth Blaxter and Dr J.T. Done for their critical comments on the script, and Miss Gwyneth Alexander for secretarial work. All the illustrations included in this Chapter are Crown Copyright, and we are grateful to the Ministry of Agriculture, Fisheries and Food for permission to reproduce them here.

REFERENCES

Adrian, R.H. & Bryant, S.H. (1974) On the repetitive discharge in myotonic muscle fibres. *Journal of Physiology*. **240**, 505.

Allen, W.M., Parr, W.H., Bradley, R., Swannack, K., Barton, C.R.Q. & Tyler, R. (1974) Loss of vitamin E in stored cereals in relation to a myopathy of yearling cattle. *Veterinary Record*, **94**, 373.

Anderson, P.H., Berrett, S. & Patterson, D.S.P. (1976) The significance of elevated plasma creatine phosphokinase activity in muscle disease of cattle. *Journal of Comparative Pathology*, **86**, 531.

Anderson, P.H., Berrett, S. & Patterson, D.S.P. (1978) Glutathione peroxidase activity in erythrocytes and muscle of cattle and sheep and its relationship to selenium. *Journal of Comparative Pathology*, **88**, 181.

Anderson, P.H., Bradley, R., Berrett, S. & Patterson, D.S.P. (1977) The sequence of myodegeneration in nutritional myopathy of the older calf. *British Veterinary Journal*, **133**, 160.

Andrews, E.D. (1965) Cobalt poisoning in sheep. *New Zealand Veterinary Journal*, **13**, 101.

Anon. (1968) Epidemic cardiac failure in beer drinkers. *Nutrition Reviews*, **26**, 173.

Baird, J.D., Johnston, K.G. & Hartley, W.J. (1974) Spastic paresis in Friesian calves. *Australian Veterinary Journal*, **50**, 239.

Baker, J.R. (1969) Muscular dystrophy in the horse. *Veterinary Record*, **84**, 488.

Ball, V. (1936) Le syndrome des raideurs congénitales multiples à type quadriplégique dans les deux médecines. *Revue vétérinaire, Toulouse*, **88**, 121.

Banker, B.Q. (1967) A phase and electron microscopic study of dystrophic muscle. 1. The pathological changes in the two-week-old Bar Harbor 129 dystrophic mouse. *Journal of Neuropathology and Experimental Neurology*, **26**, 259.

Barney, G.H., Macapinlac, M.P., Pearson, W.N. & Darby, W.J. (1967) Parakeratosis of the tongue—a unique histopathologic lesion in the zinc-deficient squirrel monkey. *Journal of Nutrition*, **93**, 511.

Berg, B.N. (1956) Muscular dystrophy in aging rats. *Journal of Gerontology*, **11**, 134.

Bergmann, V. (1976a) Licht-und elektronmikroskopische Untersuchungen zur Pathogenese der Grätschstellung neugeborener Ferkel. *Monatshefte für Veterinärmedizin*, **31**, 129.

Bergmann, V. (1976b) Elektronenmikroskopische Befunde an der skelettmuskulatur von neugeborenen Ferkeln mit Grätschstellung. *Archives of Experimental Veterinary Medicine*, **30**, 239.

Bickhardt, K., Chevalier, H.J. & Tuch, K. (1975) Zur Ätiologie und Pathogenese der Akuten Rückenmuskelnekrose des Schweines. *Deutsche Tierärztliche Wochenschrift*, **82**, 475.

Bickhardt, K., Ueberschär, S. & Giese, W. (1967) Protrahierte Atrophie der caudelan Oberschenkelmuskulator beim Schwein. *Deutsche Tierärztliche Wochenschrift*, **74**, 324.

Blaxter, K.L. (1964) Protein metabolism and requirements in pregnancy and lactation. In *Mammalian Protein Metabolism*, Eds H.N. Munro & J.B. Allison, Vol. 2. pp. 173–223 (Academic Press: New York).

Bone, J.F. (1963) The 'tying-up' syndrome. In *Equine*

medicine and surgery, Eds J.F. Bone, E.J. Catcott, A.A. Gabel, L.E. Johnson & W.F. Riley, Jr., pp. 475–476 (American Veterinary Publications Inc.: Santa Barbara, California).

Bosanquet, F.D., Daniel, P.M. & Parry, H.B. (1956) Myopathy in sheep. Its relationship to scrapie and to dermatomyositis and muscular dystrophy. *Lancet*, **2**, 737.

Boyd, J.W. (1976) Creatine phosphokinase in normal sheep and in sheep with nutritional muscular dystrophy. *Journal of Comparative Pathology*, **86**, 23.

Bradley, R. (1975) Selenium deficiency and bovine myopathy. *The Veterinary Annual*, 15th issue, Eds C.S.G. Grunsell, & F.W.G. Hill, pp. 27–35 (Wright–Scientechnica: Bristol).

Bradley, R. (1977) Nutritional myodegeneration (White muscle disease) of yearling and adult cattle. In *Proceedings of the third International Conference on Production Disease in Farm Animals*. Wageningen, The Netherlands, September 13–16, 1976. Section I, pp. 132–134 (Centre for Agricultural Publishing and Documentation: Wageningen).

Bradley, R. (1978a) Double-muscling in cattle, boon or bane? *The Veterinary Annual*, 18th issue. Eds C.S.G. Grunsell & F.W.G. Hill, pp. 51–59 (Wright–Scientechnica: Bristol).

Bradley, R. (1978b) Hereditary 'Daft lamb' disease of Border Leicester sheep: the ultrastructural pathology of the skeletal muscles. *Journal of Pathology*, **125**, 205.

Bradley, R. (1979) A primary bovine skeletal myopathy with absence of Z discs, sarcoplasmic inclusions, myofibrillar hypoplasia and nuclear abnormality. *Journal of Comparative Pathology*, **89**, 381.

Bradley, R. & Terlecki, S. (1977) Muscle lesions in hereditary 'Daft lamb' disease of Border Leicester sheep. *Journal of Pathology*, **123**, 225.

Bradley, R. & Wells, G.A.H. (1978) Developmental muscle disorders in the pig. *The Veterinary Annual*. 18th issue. Eds. C.S.G. Grunsell & F.W.G. Hill, pp. 144–157 (Wright-Scientechnica: Bristol).

Bradley, R., Wells, G.A.H. & Gray, L.J. (1979) Back muscle necrosis of pigs. *Veterinary Record*, **104**, 183.

Bradley, W.G. & Jenkison, M. (1975) Neural abnormalities in the dystrophic mouse. *Journal of the Neurological Sciences*, **25**, 249.

Bray, G.M. & Banker, B.Q. (1970) An ultrastructural study of degeneration and necrosis of muscle in the dystrophic mouse. *Acta Neuropathologica (Berlin)*, **15**, 34.

Brown, G.L. & Harvey, A.M. (1939) Congenital myotonia in the goat. *Brain*, **62**, 341.

Bryant, S.H. & Morales-Aguilera, A. (1971) Chloride conductance in normal and myotonic muscle fibres and the action of monocarboxylic aromatic acids. *Journal of Physiology*, **219**, 367.

Bryant, S.H., Lipicky, R.J. & Herzog, W.H. (1968) Variability of myotonic signs in myotonic goats. *American Journal of Veterinary Research*, **29**, 2371.

Cantin, M. (1967) Skeletal muscle lesions in iodine-treated rats. *Archives of Pathology*, **83**, 500.

Cardinet, G.H. III, Wallace, L.J., Feede, M.R., Guffy, M.M. & Bardens, J.W. (1969) Developmental myopathy in the canine with type II muscle fibre hypotrophy. *Archives of Neurology*, **21**, 620.

Caulfield, J.B. (1966) Electron microscopic observations on the dystrophic hamster muscle. *Annals of the New York Academy of Sciences*, **138**, 151.

Caulfield, J.B. (1972) Striated muscle lesions in dystrophic hamsters. *Progress in Experimental Tumor Research*, **16**, 274.

Čeh, L., Hauge, J.G., Svenkerud, R. & Strande, A. (1976) Glycogenosis type III in the dog. *Acta Veterinaria Scandinavica*, **17**, 210.

Charlton, K.M. (1970) A study of the pathogenesis of the peripheral neuropathy of the experimental coyotillo (*Karwinskia humboldtiana*) poisoning in goats. *Dissertation Abstracts International*, **31B**, 2790.

Charlton, K.M. & Pierce, K.R. (1970) A neuropathy in goats caused by experimental coyotillo (*Karwinskia humboldtiana*) poisoning. II. Lesions in the peripheral nervous system—teased fiber and acid phosphatase studies. III. Distribution of lesions in peripheral nerves. IV. Light and electron microscopic lesions in peripheral nerves. *Pathologia Veterinaria*, **7**, 385, 408 and 420.

Cheah, K.S. & Cheah, A.M. (1976) The trigger for PSE condition in stress-susceptible pigs. *Journal of the Science of Food and Agriculture*, **27**, 1137.

Coetzer, J.A.W. & Barnard, B.J.H. (1977) Hydrops amnii in sheep associated with hydranencephaly and arthrogryposis with Wesselsbron disease and Rift Valley fever viruses as aetiological agents. *Onderstepoort Journal of Veterinary Research*, **44**, 119.

Cunha, T.J. (1968) Spraddled hind legs may be a result of choline deficiency. *Feedstuffs, Minneapolis*, **40**, No. 10, 25.

Darke, P.G.G., McCullagh, K.G. & Geldart, P.H. (1975) Myasthenia gravis, thymoma and myositis in a dog. *Veterinary Record*, **97**, 392.

Davies, A.S. & Gunn, H.M. (1972) Histochemical fibre types in the mammalian diaphragm. *Journal of Anatomy*, **112**, 41.

Dawson, J.R.B. (1970) Myasthenia gravis in a cat. *Veterinary Record*, **86**, 562.

Dawson, P.L.L. (1975) The economic aspect of spastic paresis of the hind legs of Friesian cattle. *Veterinary Record*, **97**, 432.

De Ley, G. & De Moor, A. (1976) Bovine spastic paralysis. A comparative study of serum enzymes and biopsies of the gastrocnemius muscle. *Zentralblatt für Veterinärmedizin*, **23A**, 89.

De Ley, G. & De Moor, A. (1977) Seizoen-invloeden in het voorkomen van spastische parese bij het rund. *Vlaams Diergeneeskundig Tijdschrift*, **46**, 179.

Deutsch, K. & Done, J.T. (1971) Congenital myofibrillar hypoplasia of piglets: ultrastructure of affected fibres. *Research in Veterinary Science*, **12**, 176.

Dewan, M.L., Henson, J.B., Dollahite, J.W. & Bridges, C.H. (1965) Toxic myodegeneration in goats produced by feeding mature fruits from the coyotillo plant (*Karwinskia humboldtiana*). *American Journal of Pathology*, **46**, 215.

Dodd, D.C., Blakely, A.A., Thornbury, R.S. & Dewes, H.F. (1960) Muscle degeneration and yellow fat disease in foals. *New Zealand Veterinary Journal*, **8**, 45.

Donaldson, L.E. (1970) Muscular dystrophy in cattle suffering heavy mortalities during transport by sea. *Australian Veterinary Journal*, **46**, 405.

Done, J.T. (1976) Developmental disorders of the nervous system in animals. *Advances in Veterinary Science and Comparative Medicine*, **20**, 69.

Done, J.T., Allen, W.M., Bailey, J., De Gruchy, P.H. & Curran, M.K. (1975) Asymmetric hindquarter syndrome (AHQS) in the pig. *Veterinary Record*, **96**, 482.

Dubowitz, V. & Brooke, M.H. (1973) *Muscle Biopsy: a modern approach* (Saunders: London).

Duchen, L.W. (1975a) 'Sprawling': A new mutant mouse

with failure of myelination of sensory axons and a deficiency of muscle spindles. *Neuropathology and Applied Neurobiology*, **1**, 89.

Duchen, L.W. (1975b) Pathology of the innervation of skeletal muscle. In *Recent Advances in Pathology, No. 9*, Eds C.V. Harrison & K. Weinbren, pp. 217–248 (Churchill-Livingstone: Edinburgh).

Duchen, L.W., Searle, A.G. & Strich, S.J. (1967) An hereditary motor end plate disease in the mouse. *Journal of Physiology*, **189**, 4P.

Duchen, L.W., Strich, S.J. & Falconer, D.S. (1964) Clinical and pathological studies of an hereditary neuropathy in mice (dystonia musculorum). *Brain*, **87**, 367.

Duffell, S.J. & Edwardson, R. (1978) Xanthosis in cattle. *Veterinary Record*, **102**, 269.

Duncan, I.D., Griffiths, I.R. & McQueen, A. (1975) A myopathy associated with myotonia in the dog. *Acta Neuropathologica*, **31**, 297.

Duncan, I.D., Griffiths, I.R. & Nash, A.S. (1977) Myotonia in canine Cushing's disease. *Veterinary Record*, **100**, 30.

Eikelenboom, G. & Minkema, D. (1974) Prediction of pale, soft, exudative muscle with non-lethal test for the halothane-induced porcine malignant hyperthermia syndrome. *Tijdschrift voor Diergeneeskunde*, **99**, 421.

Formston, C. & Jones, E.W. (1956) A spastic form of lameness in Friesian cattle. *Veterinary Record*, **68**, 624.

Fraser, D.C., Palmer, A.C., Senior, J.E.B., Parkes, J.D. & Yealland, M.F.T. (1970) Myasthenia gravis in the dog. *Journal of Neurology, Neurosurgery and Psychiatry*, **33**, 431.

Fraser Roberts, J.A. (1929) The inheritance of a lethal muscle contracture in the sheep. *Journal of Genetics*, **21**, 57.

Gardner, D.E. (1967) Skeletal myonecrosis in a cat. *New Zealand Veterinary Journal*, **15**, 211.

Godwin, K.O., Edwardly, J. & Fuss, C.N. (1975) Retention of ⁴⁵Ca in rats and lambs associated with the onset of nutritional muscular dystrophy. *Australian Journal of Biological Sciences*, **28**, 457.

Godwin, K.O., Kuchel, R.E. & Fuss, C.N. (1974) Some biochemical features of white muscle disease in lambs, and the influence of selenium. *Australian Journal of Biological Sciences*, **27**, 633.

Goedegebuure, S.A. & Hoebe, H.P. (1976) Zwerchfells-myopathie bei MRY-Rindern. Vortag für die *25 Tagung der Europäischen Gesellschaft für Veterinärpathologie*: Freiburg. 8 June, 1976.

Goettsch, M. & Pappenheimer, A.M. (1931) Nutritional muscular dystrophy in the guinea pig and rabbit. *Journal of Experimental Medicine*, **54**, 145.

Götze, R. (1932) Spastische Parese der hinteren Extremität bei Kälbern un Jungrindern. *Deutsche tierärztliche Wochenschrift*, **40**, 197.

Grasso, P., Muir, A., Goldberg, L. & Batstone, E. (1968). Brown FK. IV Cytopathic effects of Brown FK on cardiac and skeletal muscle in the rat. *Food and Cosmetics Toxicology*, **6**, 13.

Greenough, P.R., MacCallum, F.J. & Weaver, A.D. (1972) In *Lameness in Cattle*, p. 357 (Oiver and Boyd: Edinburgh).

Griffiths, I.R. & Duncan, I.D. (1973) Myotonia in the dog: a report of four cases. *Veterinary Record*, **93**, 184.

Gunn, H.M. (1975) Adaptations of skeletal muscle that favour athletic ability. *New Zealand Veterinary Journal*, **23**, 249.

Gunn, H.M. (1976) Morphological aspects of the deep digital flexor muscle in horses having rigid flexion of their distal forelimb joints at birth. *Irish Veterinary Journal*, **30**, 145.

Guth, L. & Samaha, F.J. (1970) Procedure for the histochemical demonstration of actomyosin ATPase. *Experimental Neurology*, **28**, 365.

Hadlow, W.J. (1962) Diseases of skeletal muscle. In *Comparative Neuropathology*. Eds J.R.M. Innes & L.Z. Saunders, pp. 147–243 (Academic Press: New York).

Hadlow, W.J. (1973) Myopathies of animals. In *The Striated Muscle*, ed. Pearson, C.M. & Mostofi, F.K. pp. 364–409. International Academy of Pathology. Monograph No. 12. (Williams & Wilkins: Baltimore.)

Hamilton, M.J., Hegreberg, G.A. & Gorham, J.R. (1974) Histochemical muscle fibre typing in inherited muscular dystrophy of mink. *American Journal of Veterinary Research*, **35**, 1321.

Harcourt, R.A. & Bradley, R. (1973) Eosinophilic myositis in sheep. *Veterinary Record*, **92**, 233.

Harman, P.J., Tassoni, J.P., Curtis, R.L. & Hollinshead, M.B. (1963) Muscular dystrophy in the mouse. In *Muscular Dystrophy in Man and Animals*, Eds. G.H. Bourne & M.N. Golarz, pp. 407–456 (Hafner Publishing Co.: New York).

Harris, C.I. & Milne, G. (1977) The unreliability of urinary 3-methyl-histidine excretion as a measure of muscle protein degradation in sheep. *Proceedings of the Nutrition Society*, **36**, 138A.

Harris, C.I. & Milne, G. (1978) Urinary excretion of 3-methyl histidine in cattle as a measure of muscle protein degradation. *Proceedings of the Nutrition Society*, **38**, 11A.

Harris, C.I., Milne, G., Lobley, G.E. & Nicholas, G.A. (1977) 3-methyl histidine as a measure of skeletal-muscle protein catabolism in the adult New Zealand white rabbit. *Biochemical Society Transactions*, **5**, 706.

Harthoorn, A.M. & Young, E. (1974) A relationship between acid–base balance and capture myopathy in zebra (*Equus burchelli*) and an apparent therapy. *Veterinary Record*, **95**, 337.

Hartley, W.J. & Dodd, D.C. (1957) Muscular dystrophy in New Zealand livestock. *New Zealand Veterinary Journal*, **5**, 61.

Hartley, W.J., Wanner, R.A., Della-Porta, A.J. & Snowdon, W.A. (1975) Serological evidence for the association of Akabane virus with epizootic bovine congenital arthrogryposis and hydranencephaly syndromes in New South Wales. *Australian Veterinary Journal*, **51**, 103.

Hegreberg, G.A. & Norby, D.E. (1973) An inherited storage disease of cats. *Federation Proceedings. Federation of American Societies for Experimental Biology*, **32**, 821.

Hegreberg, G.A., Comacho, Z. & Gorham, J.R. (1974) Histopathologic description of muscular dystrophy of mink. *Archives of Pathology*, **97**, 225.

Hegreberg, G.A., Hamilton, M.J., Comacho, Z. & Gorham, J.R. (1974) Biochemical changes of a muscular dystrophy of mink. *Clinical Biochemistry*, **7**, 313.

Hicks, S.P. (1950) Brain metabolism in vivo. II. The distribution of lesions caused by azide, malononitrile, plasmocid and dinitrophenol poisoning in rats. *Archives of Pathology*, **50**, 545.

Hidiroglou, M. & Jenkins, K.J. (1968) Factors affecting the development of nutritional muscular dystrophy in northern Ontario. *Canadian Journal of Animal Science*, **48**, 7.

Higginson, J.A., Julian, R.J. & Van Dreumel, A.A. (1973) Muscular dystrophy in zebra foals. *Journal of Zoo Animal Medicine*, **4**, 24.

Hoebe, H.P. (1975) Diaphragm myopathy in Meuse-Rhine-Ijssel cattle. *Tijdschrift voor diergeneeskunde*, **100**, 1201.

Hofmeyer, J.M., Louw, G.N. & du Preez, J.S. (1973) Incipient capture myopathy as revealed by blood chemistry of chased zebras. *Madoqua, Ser. 1*, No. 7, 45.

Holmes, J.H.G. & Ashmore, C.R. (1972) A histochemical study of development of muscle fiber type and size in normal and 'double muscled' cattle. *Growth*, **36**, 351.

Homburger, F. (1972) Disease models in Syrian hamsters. *Progress in Experimental Tumor Research*, **16**, 69.

Homburger, F., Baker, J.R., Nixon, C.W. & Wilgram, G. (1962) New hereditary disease of Syrian hamsters. Primary, generalised polymyopathy and cardiac necrosis. *Archives of Internal Medicine*, **110**, 660.

Homburger, F., Baker, J.R., Nixon, C.W., Wilgram, G. & Harrop, J. (1965) The early histopathological lesion of muscular dystrophy in the Syrian golden hamster. *Journal of Pathology and Bacteriology*, **89**, 133.

Homburger, F., Baker, J.R., Wilgram, G., Caulfield, J.B. & Nixon, C.W. (1966) Hereditary dystrophy-like myopathy. The histopathology of hereditary dystrophy-like myopathy in Syrian hamsters. *Archives of Pathology*, **81**, 302.

Homburger, F., Nixon, C.W., Harrop, J., Wilgram, G. & Baker, J.R. (1963) Further morphologic and genetic studies on dystrophy-like primary myopathy of Syrian hamsters. *Federation Proceedings. Federation of American Societies for Experimental Biology*, **22**, 195.

Hoorens, J. & Oyaert, W. (1970) Degenerative spieveraderingen bij het varken. *Vlaams Diergeneeskundig Tijdschrift*, **39**, 246.

Howell, J. McC. (1978) The pathology of chronic copper poisoning in sheep. In *Trace Element Metabolism in Man and Animals—3*. Ed. M. Kirchgessner, p. 536 (Arbeitskreis für Tierernährungsforschung Weihenstephan).

Howell, J. McC. & Buxton, P.H. (1975) α-tocopherol responsive muscular dystrophy in guinea pigs. *Neuropathology and Applied Neurobiology*, **1**, 49.

Howes, E.L., Price, H.M. & Blumberg, J.M. (1964) The effects of a diet producing lipochrome pigment (ceroid) on the ultrastructure of skeletal muscle in the rat. *American Journal of Pathology*, **45**, 599.

Hulland, T.J. (1970) Muscle. In *Pathology of Domestic Animals* 2nd edition. Eds K.V.F. Jubb & P.C. Kennedy, vol. 2, pp. 453–494 (Academic Press: New York).

Innes, J.R.M. (1951) Myopathies in animals. *British Veterinary Journal*, **107**, 131.

Innes, J.R.M. & Saunders, L.Z. (1962) *Comparative Neuropathology* (Academic Press: New York).

Innes, J.R.M., Rowlands, W.T. & Parry, H.B. (1949) An inherited form of cortical cerebellar atrophy in ('Daft') lambs in Great Britain. *Veterinary Record*, **61**, 225.

Jackson, A.E. (1978) Congenital arthrogryposis in Charolais calves. *Veterinary Record*, **102**, 149.

James, N.T. & Meek, G.A. (1975) Ultrastructure of muscle spindles in dystrophic mice. *Nature*, **254**, 612.

Johansson, G. & Jönsson, L. (1977) Myocardial cell damage in the porcine stress syndrome. *Journal of Comparative Pathology*, **87**, 67.

Jolly, R.D., Van-De-Water, N.S., Richards, R.B. & Dorling, P.R. (1977) Generalized glycogenosis in beef Shorthorn cattle—heterozygote detection. *Australian Journal of Experimental Biology and Medical Science*, **55**, 141.

Jørgensen, P.F., Hyldgaard-Jensen, J., Moustgaard, J. & Eikelenboom, G. (1976) Phosphohexose isomerase (PHI) and porcine halothane sensitivity. *Acta Veterinaria Scandinavica*, **17**, 370.

Jubb, K.V.F. & Kennedy, P.C. (1970) *Pathology of Domestic Animals*. 2nd edition, vol. 2, pp. 454–491 (Academic Press: New York).

Kakulas, B.A. & Adams, R.A. (1966) Principles of myopathology as illustrated in the nutritional myopathy of the Rottnest quokka (*Setonix brachyurus*). *Annals of the New York Academy of Sciences*, **138**, 90.

Keller, P. (1971) Serumenzyme beim Rind: Organanalysen und Normalwerte. *Schweizer Archiv für Tierheilkunde*, **113**, 615.

Kohler, E.M., Cross, R.F. & Ferguson, L.C. (1969) Experimental induction of spraddled-legs in newborn pigs. *Journal of the American Veterinary Medical Association*, **155**, 139.

Kramer, J. W., Hegreberg, G.A., Bryan, G.M., Meyers, K. & Ott, R.L. (1976) A muscle disorder of Labrador retrievers characterized by deficiency of type II muscle fibers. *Journal of the American Veterinary Medical Association*, **169**, 817.

Kroneman, J. & Wensvoort, P. (1968) Muscular dystrophy and yellow fat disease in Shetland pony foals. *Netherlands Journal of Veterinary Science*, **1**, 42.

Lamb, R.C., Arave, C.W. & Shupe, J.L. (1976) Inheritance of limber legs in Jersey cattle. *Journal of Heredity*, **67**, 241.

Lannek, N. & Lindberg, P. (1975) Vitamin E and selenium deficiencies (VESD) of domestic animals. *Advances in Veterinary Science and Comparative Medicine*, **19**, 127.

Lax, T. (1971) Hereditary splayleg in pigs. *Journal of Heredity*, **62**, 250.

Leipold, H.W., Blaugh, B., Huston, K., Edgerly, C.G.M. & Hibbs, C.M. (1973) Weaver syndrome in Brown Swiss Cattle: clinical signs and pathology. *Veterinary Medicine/Small Animal Clinician*, **68**, 645.

Lipicky, R.J., Bryant, S.H. & Salmon, J.H. (1971) Cable parameters, sodium, potassium, chloride and water content, and potassium efflux in isolated external intercostal muscle of normal volunteers and patients with myotonia congenita. *Journal of Clinical Investigation*, **50**, 2091.

Lobley, G.E., Perry, S.V. & Stone, D. (1971) Structural changes in myosin induced by vitamin E dystrophy. *Nature*, **231**, 317.

McGavin, M.D. (1974) Progressive ovine muscular dystrophy. *Comparative Pathology Bulletin*, **VI**, 3.

McGavin, M.D. & Baynes, I.D. (1969) A congenital progressive ovine muscular dystrophy. *Pathologia Veterinaria*, **6**, 513.

Madsen, A., Mortensen, H.P., Hjarde, W., Leerbeck, E. & Leth, T. (1973) Vitamin E in barley treated with propionic acid with special reference to the feeding of bacon pigs. *Acta Agriculturae Scandinavica*, Suppl. 19, 169.

Manktelow, B.W. & Hartley, W.J. (1975) Generalized glycogen storage disease in sheep. *Journal of Comparative Pathology*, **85**, 139.

Mann, S.O., Fell, B.F. & Dalgarno, A.C. (1974) Observations on the bacterial flora and pathology of the tongue of sheep deficient in zinc. *Research in Veterinary Science*, **17**, 91.

Meier, H. (1958) Myopathies in the dog. *Cornell Veterinarian*, **48**, 313.

Meier, H. & MacPike, A.D. (1973) Pleiotropic gene effects on muscle ultrastructure of normal and dystrophic mice. *Experimental Neurology*, **40**, 258.

Meier, H. & Southard, J.L. (1970) Muscular dystrophy in

the mouse caused by an allele at the *dy*-locus. *Life Sciences*, **9**, II, 137.

Meier, H., West, W.T. & Hoag, W.G. (1965) Preclinical histopathology of mouse muscular dystrophy. *Archives of Pathology*, **80**, 165.

Mercer, D.W. (1974) Separation of tissue and serum creatine kinase isoenzymes by ion-exchange column chromatography. *Clinical Chemistry*, **20**, 36.

Miller, J.K., Hacking, A., Harrison, J. & Gross, V.J. (1973) Stillbirths, neonatal mortality and small litters in pigs associated with the ingestion of *Fusarium* toxin by pregnant sows. *Veterinary Record*, **93**, 555.

Milne, G. & Harris, C.I. (1978) The inadequacy of urinary 3-methylhistidine excretion as an index of muscle protein degradation in the pig. *Proceedings of the Nutrition Society*, **37**, 18A.

Morgan, G. & Bradley, R. (1978) White muscle disease in the differential diagnosis of clinical pneumonia. *Veterinary Record*, **102**, 449.

Morley, F.H.W. (1954) A new lethal factor in Australian Merino sheep. *Australian Veterinary Journal*, **30**, 237.

Mugera, G.M. & Wandera, J.G. (1967) Degenerative polymyopathies in East African domestic and wild animals. *Veterinary Record*, **80**, 410.

Muir, A. R. (1970) Normal and regenerating skeletal muscle fibres in Pietrain pigs. *Journal of Comparative Pathology*, **80**, 137.

Nieberle, K. & Cohrs, P. (1967) *Textbook of the Special Pathological Anatomy of Domestic Animals*, 1st English Edn. pp. 881–906 (Pergamon Press: Oxford).

Nisbet, D.I. & Renwick, C.C. (1961) Congenital myopathy in lambs. *Journal of Comparative Pathology and Therapeutics*, **71**, 177.

Noguchi, T., Cantor, A.H. & Scott, M.L. (1973) Mode of action of selenium and vitamin E in prevention of exudative diathesis in chicks. *Journal of Nutrition*, **103**, 1502.

NRC-42 Committee on Swine Nutrition (1973) Effect of supplemental choline on reproductive performance of sows. *Journal of Animal Science*, **37**, 281 (abstract).

O'Brien, J.A., Harvey, C.E., Kelly, A.M. & Tuckers, J.A. (1973) Neurogenic atrophy of the laryngeal muscles of the dog. *Journal of Small Animal Practice*, **14**, 521.

Oghiso, Y., Kubokawa, K., Lee, Y.-S. & Fujiwara, K. (1976) Clinical and pathological studies on a spontaneous case of canine systemic atrophic myositis. *Japanese Journal of Veterinary Science*, **38**, 553.

O'Sullivan, B.M. (1976) Humpy back of sheep, clinical and pathological observations. *Australian Veterinary Journal*, **52**, 414.

Pai, A.C. (1965a) Developmental genetics of a lethal mutation, muscular dysgenesis (mdg), in the mouse. I. Genetic analysis and gross morphology. *Developmental Biology*, **11**, 82.

Pai, A.C. (1965b) Developmental genetics of a lethal mutation, muscular dysgenesis (mdg) in the mouse. II. Developmental analysis. *Developmental Biology*, **11**, 93.

Palmer, A.C. (1976) *Introduction to Animal Neurology*. 2nd edition (Blackwell Scientific Publications: Oxford).

Palmer, A.C. & Barker, J. (1974) Myasthenia in the dog. *Veterinary Record*, **95**, 452.

Parsonson, I.M., Della-Porta, A.J. & Snowdon, W.A. (1977) Congenital abnormalities in newborn lambs after infection of pregnant sheep with Akabane virus. *Infection and Immunity*, **15**, 254.

Patterson, D.S.P. & Allen, W.M. (1972) Biochemical aspects of some pig muscle disorders. *British Veterinary Journal*, **128**, 101.

Patterson, D.S.P., Allen, W.M., Berrett, S., Sweasey, D. & Done, J.T. (1971) The toxicity of parenteral iron preparations in the rabbit and pig with a comparison of the clinical and biochemical responses to iron-dextrose in 2-day-old and 8-day-old piglets. *Zentralblatt für Veterinärmedizin*, **18A**, 453.

Patterson, D.S.P., Sweasey, D., Allen, W.M., Berrett, S. & Thurley, D.C. (1969) The chemical composition of neonatal piglet muscle and some observations on the biochemistry of myofibrillar hypoplasia occurring in otherwise normal litters. *Zentralblatt für Veterinärmedizin*, **16A**, 741.

Patterson, D.S.P., Allen, W.M., Berrett, S., Sweasey, D., Thurley, D.C. & Done, J.T. (1969) A biochemical study of the pathogenesis of iron-induced myodegeneration of piglets. *Zentralblatt für Veterinärmedizin*, **16A**, 199.

Pearce, G.W. & Walton, J.N. (1963) A histological study of muscle from the Bar Harbor strain of dystrophic mice. *Journal of Pathology and Bacteriology*, **86**, 25.

Pellegrino, C. & Franzini, C. (1963) An electron microscope study of denervation atrophy in red and white skeletal muscle fibres. *Journal of Cell Biology*, **17**, 327.

Platt, H. & Whitwell, K.E. (1971) Clinical and pathological observations on generalised steatitis in foals. *Journal of Comparative Pathology*, **81**, 499.

Platzer, A.C. (1971) The ultrastructure of embryonic skeletal muscle in normal and dystrophic mice. *Dissertation Abstracts International*, **32**, 3708B.

Rafiquzzaman, M., Svenkerud, R., Strande, A. & Hauge, J.G. (1976) Glycogenosis in the dog. *Acta Veterinaria Scandinavica*, **17**, 196.

Rasmusen, B.A. & Christian, L.L. (1976) H blood types in pigs as predictors of stress susceptibility. *Science*, **191**, 947.

Richards, R.B., Edwards, J.R., Cook, R.D. & White, R.R. (1977) Bovine generalized glycogenosis. *Neuropathology and Applied Neurobiology*, **3**, 45.

Rings, D.M., Hoffsis, G.F. & Donham, J.C. (1976) A myotonia-like syndrome in sheep. *Speculum*, **28**, 13.

Rooney, J.R. (1966) Contracted foals. *Cornell Veterinarian*, **56**, 172.

Rüdel, R. & Senges, J. (1972) Experimental myotonia in mammalian skeletal muscle: changes in membrane properties. *Pflügers Archiv. European Journal of Physiology*, **331**, 324.

Rudert, C.P., Lawrence, J.A., Foggin, C. & Barlow, R.M. (1978) A rigid lamb syndrome in sheep in Rhodesia. *Veterinary Record*, **102**, 374.

Scarlato, G. & Meola, G. (1978) Chronic myopathy with cytoplasmic bodies in the pig. *Journal of Comparative Pathology*, **88**, 31.

Sheriff, D. & Rankin, G.J. (1973) Concurrent enzootic ataxia and white muscle disease in a flock of lambs. *Veterinary Record*, **92**, 89.

Shimshony, A. (1978) Rigid lamb syndrome. *Veterinary Record*, **103**, 409.

Shortridge, E.H., O'Hara, P.J. & Marshall, P.M. (1971) Acute selenium poisoning in cattle. *New Zealand Veterinary Journal*, **19**, 47.

Shupe, J.L., Binns, W., James, L.F. & Keeler, R.F. (1967) Lupine, a cause of crooked calf disease. *Journal of the American Veterinary Medical Association*, **151**, 198.

Simpson, J.A. (1977) Myasthenia gravis—validation of a

Drug-induced neuromuscular disorders in man

INTRODUCTION

An increasing number of drugs have been re-cognised to have effects on the neuromuscular system when used therapeutically in man. Some have a selective effect on the structure and function of muscle (Lane and Mastaglia, 1978), while others interfere with neuromuscular transmission or are neurotoxic. Certain drugs such as vincris-tine and chloroquine are both myotoxic and neurotoxic.

The frequency of drug-induced neuromuscular disorders in clinical practice is difficult to establish because the association with drug therapy is not always recognised, and subclinical forms are probably commoner than is generally appreciated. The recognition of such iatrogenic forms of neuromuscular disease is important, because early withdrawal of the offending agent often results in complete reversal of symptoms, while failure to do so may lead to serious disability. Awareness of the possibility of drug effects on the neuromuscular system is also of importance as the range of therapeutic agents introduced into clinical practice continues to expand. The increasing recognition of neuromuscular effects of drugs in widespread clinical use also has important implications with regard to the adequacy of laboratory testing of new therapeutic agents before they are released for general use.

MYOPATHIES

Muscle damage may result from the local effects of drugs administered by intramuscular injection, or from a more widespread effect on the skeletal muscles. The resulting clinical syndromes vary in severity, mode of onset and rate of progression. Some are acute or subacute and are associated with muscle pain, while others are more protracted and painless (Table 25.1). Muscle involvement is usually widespread and symmetrical, the proximal muscles often being most severely affected, while those innervated by the cranial nerves are usually spared.

Focal myopathy

Intramuscular injections produce localised areas of muscle damage as a result of needle insertion ('needle myopathy') and local effects of the agent injected. Creatine kinase (CK) levels in the serum may be raised after injection of a variety of drugs including diazepam, lidocaine and digoxin; his-tological examination of the injection site in animals has shown extensive necrosis after in-jection of these drugs, but not after injection of saline (Steiness, Rasmussen, Svendsen and Niel-sen, 1978). Other drugs which have a local toxic effect include chloroquine (Aguayo and Hudgson, 1970), and the opiates and chlorpromazine which

Table 25.1   Features of drug-induced myopathies

Disorder	Drugs implicated	Clinical features	Serum† enzymes	Myoglobin- uria	Electro- myography findings	Pathology
Focal myopathy	IM injections of various drugs	–	may be ↑	–	–	Focal necrosis
Muscle fibrosis and contractures	antibiotics pethidine pentazocine heroin	Induration and contracture of injected muscles	Normal	–	BSAPPs; variable spontaneous activity	Marked fibrosis and myopathic changes in injected areas
Acute/subacute painful proximal myopathy						
Toxic effect	clofibrate EACA emetine heroin	Muscle pain, tenderness, proximal or general- ised weakness; reflexes usually preserved	↑ ↑	+/−	BSAPPs; spon- taneous potentials may be prominent	Necrosis/ regeneration
	vincristine	Proximal pain, atrophy, weakness, absent reflexes	?	–	?	
	clofibrids isoetherine danazol cimetidine metolazone bumetadine lithium salbutamol cytotoxics	Myalgia/cramps/ myokymia/weakness	?	?	?	?
Hypokalaemia	diuretics purgatives liquorice carbenoxolone amphotericin B	Weakness may be periodic; reflexes may be depressed or absent	↑ ↑	+/−	BSAPPs	Vacuolar myopathy ± necrosis/ regeneration
Inflammatory myopathy	D-Penicillamine procainamide levodopa	Proximal muscle pain, weakness ± skin changes	↑ ↑	–	Myopathic features	Necrosis/ regeneration/ inflammation
Acute rhabdo- myolysis	heroin methadone amphetamine barbiturates diazepam meprobamate isoniazid amphotericin B phenformin/ fenfluramine carbenoxolone	Severe muscle pain, swelling, flaccid quadriparesis, areflexia, renal failure	↑ ↑ ↑	+++	BSAPPs; prominent spontaneous discharges	Severe necrosis; regeneration
Chronic painless proximal myopathy	corticosteroids	Predominantly proximal, atrophy and weakness	Normal	–	BSAPPs	Type II fibre atrophy
	chloroquine	Reflexes may be lost due to associated neuropathy	Normal	–	Myopathic/ neuropathic features; spontaneous discharges may be prominent	Vacuolar myopathy
	heroin perhexiline					Nonspecific myopathic changes
	*Drugs causing ↓K+		*Vide supra*			

Disorder	Drugs implicated	Clinical features	Serum† enzymes	Myoglobin-uria	Electro-myography findings	Pathology
Myotonic syndrome	20,25 diaza-cholesterol and analogues	Muscle cramps, weakness, myotonia			Myotonic and other spontan-eous discharges	
	suxamethonium propranolol (? other beta blockers) }	May aggravate myotonia	Normal	–		
Malignant hyperpyrexia	suxamethonium halothane diethyl ether cyclopropane chloroform methoxyflurane ketamine enflurane psychotropics	Rigidity, hyperpyrexia, acidosis, hyper-kalaemia, disseminated intra-vascular coagulation, renal failure	↑ ↑ ↑ (↑ in some cases at risk)	+++	Variable myopathic changes in survivors and family members at risk	Necrosis (variable abnormalities in cases at risk)

★Creatine kinase, aldolase, aspartate transaminase
BSAPPs: brief duration, small amplitude, polyphasic ('myopathic') motor unit action potentials

are thought to cause damage by inducing his-tamine release (Cohen, 1972). Some drugs such as paraldehyde and cephalothin sodium, which are particularly irritant, may cause more severe tissue damage leading to abscess formation (Lane and Mastaglia, 1978; Greenblatt and Allen, 1978). These focal forms of muscle damage are usually of little clinical consequence apart from the fact that the finding of elevated serum enzyme levels may be misleading in patients with suspected myocardial infarction, unless isoenzyme studies are performed (Marmor, Alpan, Keider, Grenadier and Palant, 1978).

Marked muscle fibrosis leading to progressive induration and contractures may occur as a result of repeated intramuscular injections. This com-plication has occurred particularly in children who have had intramuscular injections of antibiotics (Saunders, Hoefnagel and Staples, 1965; Bat-tacharrya, 1966; Hagen, 1968), and in adults addicted to pethidine (Mastaglia, Gardner-Medwin and Hudgson, 1971), or pentazocine (Steiner, Winkelman and de Jesus, 1973; Levin and Engel, 1975). The quadriceps femoris and

deltoid muscles have been most commonly affected but more widespread involvement has been reported in some drug addicts (Aberfeld, Beinenstock, Shapiro, Namba and Grob, 1968; Mastaglia et al., 1971; Steiner et al., 1973). Repeated needle trauma, toxic effects of the drug, haemorrhage and low-grade infection may all be contributory factors.

Acute or subacute painful proximal myopathy

A number of drugs may cause a rapidly evolving syndrome characterised by muscle pain, tender-ness and weakness involving the proximal limb and axial muscles most severely. This may be due to a direct toxic effect of the drug on muscle or to the development of hypokalaemia or of an in-flammatory myopathy. The tendon reflexes are usually preserved unless the myopathy is pro-found or is associated with a peripheral neurop-athy. Serum levels of CK and other enzymes are usually considerably raised and myoglobinuria may occur. Electromyography (EMG) shows the typical changes of primary muscle disease (*see* Ch. 28) and spontaneous potentials may be prominent (Lane, McLelland, Martin and Mastaglia, 1979).

Toxic myopathy. The drugs which most frequently produce this syndrome as a result of a direct toxic effect are clofibrate, epsilon-aminocaproic acid (EACA) and emetine, all of which cause a necrotising myopathy (Fig. 25.1a). An identical syndrome has also been reported in heroin addicts (Richter, Challenor, Pearson, Kagen, Hamilton and Ramsey, 1971) and alcoholics (Perkoff, Hardy and Velez-Garcia, 1966).

Clofibrate. In the case of clofibrate, the myopathy appears to be dose-dependent; it is uncommon when the drug is administered in conventional therapeutic doses but is more likely to develop in patients with renal failure (Pierides, Alvarez-Ude, Kerr and Skillen, 1975), the nephrotic syndrome (Bridgeman, Rosen and Thorp, 1972) or hypothyroidism, probably because plasma levels of the unbound drug are high in these conditions (Rumpf, Albers and Scheler, 1976). Symptoms develop quite abruptly, possibly when the concentration of the drug in the blood reaches a critical level (Teräväinen, Larsen and Hillbom, 1977). The mechanism whereby clofibrate causes muscle necrosis is uncertain, but the observation that the drug causes a significant increase in muscle lipoprotein-lipase activity may be relevant (Lithell, Boberg, Hellsing, Lundqvist and Vessby, 1978).

Epsilon aminocaproic acid. The myopathy attributable to EACA usually develops abruptly after 4–6 weeks of treatment with daily doses of 18–30 g, suggesting that it is due to a cumulative dose-related effect of the drug (Lane *et al.*, 1979). It has been reported most frequently in patients with hereditary angioneurotic oedema (Korsan-Bengsten, Ysander, Blohme and Tibblin, 1969) or subarachnoid haemorrhage (Lane *et al.*, 1979), and it has been suggested that complement abnormalities and lysine deficiency may possibly be predisposing factors. Active muscle regeneration occurs and complete recovery over a period of weeks is the rule (Lane *et al.*, 1979).

Emetine. Patients treated with the anti-amoebic agent emetine hydrochloride frequently develop generalised muscle weakness during (Klatskin and Friedman, 1948) or after a course of treatment (Young and Tudhope, 1926). This is usually reversible, but the outcome may be fatal, particularly when there is an associated cardio-myopathy (Fewings, Burns and Kakulas, 1973). Early clinical reports suggested that there were both 'neuritic' and 'myositic' forms of emetine toxicity. However, experimental studies have shown a pure myotoxic effect with mitochondrial and myofibrillar changes followed by necrosis and regeneration (Duane and Engel, 1970; Bradley, Fewings, Harris and Johnson, 1976), and no evidence of damage to intramuscular nerves or motor end-plates.

Vincristine. A painful proximal necrotising myopathy may occur in some patients treated with vincristine in association with the severe poly-neuropathy caused by the drug (Bradley, Lassman, Pearce and Walton, 1970). Electron-microscopic studies in man (Bradley *et al.*, 1970) and in the experimental animal (Anderson, Song and Slotwiner, 1967; Bradley, 1970) have shown that the drug has a profound effect on membrane systems and causes severe autophagic degeneration of muscle fibres.

Other drugs. A number of other drugs including lithium carbonate (Ghose, 1977), cimetidine (Wade, 1977), clofibride, danazol, isoetherine, metolazone, bumetanide, cytotoxic agents (Dukes, 1977) and salbutamol (Palmer, 1978) have been reported to cause myalgia, muscle cramps, myokymia or weakness in some patients. The mechanisms involved have not been investigated.

Myositis. A painful inflammatory myopathy develops in some patients treated with D-penicillamine or procainamide. In the case of procainamide an interstitial form of myositis occurs (Fig. 25.1b), usually as part of a lupus-like syndrome and may be a manifestation of an arteritic process (Dubois, 1969; Blomgren, Condemi and Vaughan, 1972). A similar type of myopathy has been described in a patient on long-term levodopa therapy for parkinsonism (Wolf,

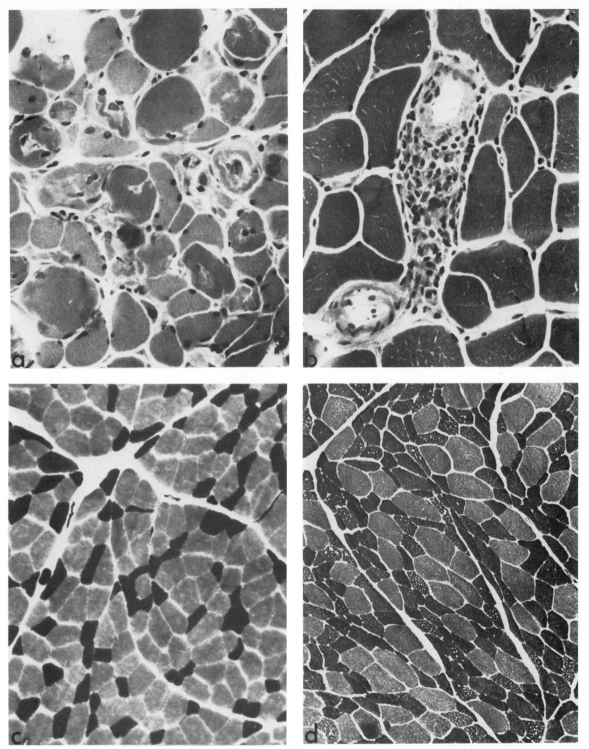

Fig. 25.1 (a) Severe necrotising myopathy due to epsilon-amino caproic acid in a 67-year-old female. Quadriceps femoris biopsy; H & E, ×320. (b) Interstitial perivascular mononuclear cell infiltrate in a 54-year-old man with a procainamide-induced lupus-like syndrome. Quadriceps femoris biopsy; H & E, ×320. (c) Type II fibre atrophy in a 26-year-old female treated with corticosteroids for systemic lupus erythematosus (SLE). Quadriceps femoris biopsy; myofibrillar ATPase (pH 9.4), ×125. (d) Vacuolar myopathy with predominant involvement of intermediate and type II fibres in a 55-year-old female with suspected SLE who was treated with chloroquine. Quadriceps femoris biopsy; myofibrillar ATPase (pH 7.2), ×160

Goldberg and Verity, 1976). A number of patients with rheumatoid arthritis or Wilson's disease treated with D-penicillamine in daily doses of up to 700 mg have developed acute or subacute polymyositis (Schraeder, Peters and Dahl, 1972; Bettendorf and Neuhaus, 1974; Cucher and Goldman, 1976) or dermatomyositis (Fernandes, Swinson and Hamilton, 1977). Two of the reported cases, one fatal, have had associated myocardial involvement (Bettendorf and Neuhaus, 1974; Cucher and Goldman, 1976). Spontaneous recovery occurred after withdrawal of the drug in another case (Schraeder et al., 1972). This complication has been reported less frequently than the immunologically mediated myasthenic syndrome which develops in some patients treated with penicillamine. It remains to be determined whether these two disorders have a related pathogenesis.

Hypokalaemic myopathy. Widespread muscle weakness, which may be painful, and which may be associated with depressed or absent tendon reflexes and marked elevation of serum CK levels and myoglobinuria, may result from hypokalaemia in patients taking diuretics (Jensen, Mosdal and Reske-Nielsen, 1977), purgatives (Basser, 1979), liquorice (Gross, Dexter and Roth, 1966), carbenoxolone (Mohamed, Chapman and Crooks, 1966), or amphotericin B which causes renal tubular damage (Drutz, Fan, Tai, Cheng and Hsieh, 1970). Histological studies in such cases usually show a vacuolar myopathy but, in severe cases, necrosis and regeneration may be present.

Acute rhabdomyolysis

Although a number of drugs already discussed may cause a severe necrotising myopathy and myoglobinuria, the features of the potentially fatal condition referred to as acute rhabdomyolysis are sufficiently distinctive to merit special consideration. It is characterised by the abrupt onset of severe generalised muscle pain, tenderness and flaccid areflexic paralysis, often with severe muscle swelling which may require fasciotomy. Gross myoglobinuria usually leads to acute oliguric renal failure which may be responsible for death. Serum levels of CK and of other enzymes are markedly

raised and the EMG reveals myopathic changes, often with prominent spontaneous discharges. Muscle biopsy shows widespread necrosis with mild reactive inflammatory changes, and regenerative activity may be profuse. Recovery usually occurs over a period of weeks, but full muscle power may not be restored for several months.

Acute rhabdomyolysis has occurred in association with amphotericin B (Drutz et al., 1970) and carbenoxolone therapy (Mohamed et al., 1966), intoxication with barbiturates, meprobamate and diazepam (Nicolas, Baron, Dixneuf, Visset and Dubigeon, 1970; Penn, Rowland and Fraser, 1972; Wattel, Chopin, Durocher and Berzin, 1978) and phencyclidine (Cogen, Rigg, Simmons and Domino, 1978), amphetamine poisoning (Grossman, Hamilton, Morse, Penn and Goldberg, 1974), combined overdosage with phenformin and fenfluramine (Palmucci, Bertolotto and Schiffer, 1978), alcoholism (Perkoff et al., 1966) and heroin and methadone addiction (Richter et al., 1971). The mechanisms of myotoxicity in these situations have not been investigated and it remains to be determined whether a direct toxic drug effect is involved, or whether individual idiosyncrasy or other predisposing factors play a part.

Less severe forms of rhabdomyolysis have been recognised in apparently normal individuals (Gibbs, 1978) and in patients with Duchenne muscular dystrophy (Watters, Karpati and Kaplan, 1977) following administration of suxamethonium during anaesthesia.

Chronic painless proximal myopathy

This is probably the commonest form of drug-induced myopathy encountered in clinical practice and occurs most frequently in patients on long-term corticosteroid therapy.

Corticosteroids. Myopathy occurs particularly in patients treated with the fluorinated steroids triamcinalone (Williams, 1959), betamethasone and dexamethasone (Golding and Begg, 1960), but has also been associated with cortisone, prednisone, prednisolone and methylprednisolone therapy (Askari, Vignos and Moskowitz, 1976). Myopathy is more likely to develop in patients maintained on high doses of these drugs for prolonged periods (Askari *et al.*, 1976) and is unlikely to occur if the daily dose of steroid is kept down to 10 mg or less of prednisone or its equivalent (Yates, 1970). Severe myopathy may occasionally follow parenteral treatment with high doses of hydrocortisone (MacFarlane and Rosenthal, 1977), and may even complicate topical steroid therapy (Rawlins, personal communication). Severe myopathy is uncommon but the true frequency of the condition is difficult to determine because mild forms may be overlooked, particularly in patients with an underlying disorder such as rheumatoid arthritis, which also may cause muscle weakness and wasting. Electromyographic findings indicate that subclinical myopathy is common (Coomes, 1965a; Yates, 1970).

In the typical case there is symmetrical involvement of proximal limb muscles, particularly those of the pelvic girdle, and atrophy and weakness of the quadriceps femoris are prominent. Muscle pain is not a feature and the tendon reflexes are usually preserved. Serum enzyme levels are normal and, if found to be elevated, should suggest the possibility of active inflammatory muscle disease. Creatinuria occurs and urinary creatine levels have been held to be useful in diagnosis and in monitoring progress (Askari *et al.*, 1976). The EMG shows the typical changes of primary muscle disease particularly in proximal groups, spontaneous discharges usually being absent. In contrast to experimental corticosteroid myopathy (*see* Ch. 11), the histological changes in steroid myopathy in man are relatively inconspicuous. Muscle biopsy shows an atrophic process with particular involvement of the type II fibres (Fig. 25.1c), and necrosis, regeneration and vacuolar change are not usually found. The myopathy is usually reversible on stopping the drug or, to some extent, on substituting prednisone for the offending steroid (Williams, 1959; Walton, 1977). Anabolic agents do not prevent the development of the myopathy (Coomes, 1965b).

The mechanism of steroid-induced myopathy has been clarified by experimental studies, which have shown that specific steroid receptor proteins are present in muscle (Shoji and Pennington, 1977a), and that steroids interfere with oxidative metabolism (Koski, Rifenberick and Max, 1974), enhance glycogen synthesis (Shoji, Takagi, Sugita and Toyokura, 1974), and inhibit protein synthesis (Shoji and Pennington, 1977b).

Chloroquine. A severe myopathy may result from the prolonged administration of chloroquine (Whisnant, Espinosa, Kierland and Lambert, 1963). It may be indistinguishable clinically from steroid myopathy and there may be difficulty in deciding which drug is responsible, in patients receiving both chloroquine and corticosteroids (Mastaglia, Papadimitriou, Dawkins and Beveridge, 1977). As the drug may also cause a mild peripheral neuropathy, sensory changes, reflex depression and abnormal nerve conduction may be found (Whisnant *et al.*, 1963). In contrast to steroid myopathy, spontaneous potentials, including myotonic discharges, are commonly found in the EMG, in addition to the typical changes of primary muscle disease (Mastaglia *et al.*, 1977). Biopsy shows a vacuolar myopathy, type I fibres usually being more severely affected, although in some cases there is predominant involvement of intermediate or type II fibres (Fig. 25.1d) (Mastaglia *et al.*, 1977). Electron-microscopic studies of human and experimental animal material have shown that the drug has a profound effect on intracellular membrane systems, leading to the formation of a variety of membranous bodies and to autophagic degeneration of muscle fibres (MacDonald and Engel, 1970; Mastaglia *et al.*, 1977). The myopathy is reversible after withdrawal of the drug, but recovery may be protracted (Mastaglia *et al.*, 1977).

Other drugs. Some of the drugs already mentioned, such as heroin and those causing hypokalaemia, may also produce a painless proximal or generalised myopathy. Such a syndrome has also been ascribed to other drugs, including perhexiline (Tomlinson and Rosenthal, 1977), but such cases have not usually been investigated fully.

Myotonia

The classic example of a drug-induced myotonic syndrome was that produced by the hypocholesterolaemic agent 20,25-diazacholesterol

(Somers and Winer, 1966). Patients taking the drug in daily doses of 25–50 mg developed muscle spasms and weakness with clinical and EMG evidence of myotonia. Complete recovery occurred over a period of 2–3 months after withdrawal of the drug. A comparable syndrome occurs in rats and goats after administration of the drug or of its analogues. Accumulation of desmosterol has been demonstrated in the serum and sarcolemma (Winer, Klachko, Baer, Langley and Burns, 1966) and the altered sterol composition and enzyme activity of the sarcolemma are thought to be the basis for the myotonia (Peter and Fiehn, 1973).

A number of drugs may precipitate or exacerbate myotonia in patients with dystrophia myotonica or other myotonic disorders. These include propranolol (Blessing and Walsh, 1977), and the depolarising muscle relaxant suxamethonium (Mitchell, Ali and Savarese, 1978). In contrast, non-depolarising muscle relaxants do not have this effect in patients with dystrophia myotonica (Mitchell et al., 1978).

Myotonic discharges may be found, together with other high frequency ('pseudomyotonic') discharges, in some of the drug-induced syndromes already discussed, such as chloroquine neuromyopathy (Mastaglia et al., 1977) and EACA myopathy (Lane et al., 1978), and may rarely be associated with clinical myotonia (Blomberg, 1965).

Malignant hyperpyrexia

In this serious condition, various anaesthetic agents and other drugs may precipitate a potentially fatal state characterised by generalised muscular rigidity, severe hyperpyrexia, metabolic acidosis and myoglobinuria (King and Denborough, 1973a). The condition is usually familial, being inherited by an autosomal dominant mechanism, and susceptible individuals have either a clinically apparent or, more frequently, a subclinical myopathy (King, Denborough and Zapf, 1972; Harriman, Sumner and Ellis, 1973). Those who are clinically normal may be identified by the finding of elevated serum CK levels (King et al., 1972; Ellis, Clarke, Modgill, Currie and Harriman, 1975), focal myopathic changes in the EMG (Mastaglia, unpublished observations), or,

most reliably, by the demonstration of abnormal sensitivity of muscle tissue to anaesthetic agents in vitro (Ellis, Keaney, Harriman, Sumner, Kyei-Mensah, Tyrrell, Hargreaves, Parikh and Mulrooney, 1972). A second group of individuals with this susceptibility are young males of short stature with a progressive congenital myopathy, skeletal abnormalities and other dysmorphic features similar to those seen in the Noonan syndrome, and in whom an autosomal recessive mechanism of inheritance is probably involved (King and Denborough, 1973b; Kaplan, Bergeson, Gregg and Curless, 1977). Others have had myotonia congenita (Morley, Lambert and Kakulas, 1973) or central core disease (Denborough, Dennett and Anderson, 1973; Eng, Epstein, Engel, McKay and McKay, 1978).

The drugs which may precipitate malignant hyperpyrexia in susceptible individuals include suxamethonium, halothane, diethyl ether, cyclopropane, chloroform, methoxyflurane (Newson, 1972), ketamine (Page, Morgan and Loh, 1972) and enflurane (Knape, 1977). Tricyclic antidepressants and monoamine oxidase inhibitors have also been reported to precipitate a similar syndrome (Newson, 1972). A safe anaesthetic regime for muscle biopsy in susceptible individuals comprises oral premedication with diazepam followed by thiopentone, fentanyl citrate and nitrous oxide (Ellis et al., 1975). Althesin, D-tubocurarine, and local, regional or spinal anaesthesia and neuroleptanalgesia may also be used with safety (Denborough, 1977).

The mechanism of the reaction to anaesthetic agents has been clarified by studies in man and in certain inbred strains of swine which suffer from an apparently identical syndrome (Hall, Woolf, Bradley and Jolly, 1966). On the basis of such studies it has been concluded that, in susceptible individuals, there is an intrinsic abnormality of the excitation–contraction coupling mechanism in muscle, exposure to these agents causing excessive release of Ca^{++} ions into the myoplasm and sustained myofibrillar contraction (Denborough, 1977). The possibility of a primary disorder of catecholamine metabolism has also been suggested (Williams, Hoech and Roberts, 1978).

Various drugs have been used in the treatment of the acute fulminant hyperpyrexia syndrome with the aim of reducing myoplasmic Ca^{++} levels. These include procaine, procainamide, hydrocortisone, dexamethasone, and dantrolene sodium (Denborough, 1977). The latter drug, which blocks excitation–contraction coupling and enhances Ca^{++} uptake by the sarcoplasmic reticulum, is probably the drug of choice (Austin and Denborough, 1977; Nelson and Denborough, 1977).

DISORDERS OF NEUROMUSCULAR TRANSMISSION

A variety of drugs, in addition to the neuromuscular blocking agents used in anaesthesia, may interfere with neuromuscular transmission in man (Argov and Mastaglia, 1979a). Drug-induced neuromuscular block may manifest clinically in the following ways.

Clinical presentations

Drug-induced myasthenic syndrome. As shown in Table 25.2, a number of drugs have been implicated in causing a myasthenic syndrome in patients with no evidence of pre-existing myasthenia gravis (MG). The disorder has usually developed within a short period of starting treatment and has been reversible after withdrawal of the drug. In spite of this, the possibility remains that, in at least some of these cases, a subclinical disorder of neuromuscular transmission was unmasked by the effects of the drug. This is a relatively uncommon complication of treatment with these drugs, probably because of the high safety factor for neuromuscular transmission which exists under normal circumstances (Desmedt, 1973; Stälberg, Schiller and Schwartz, 1975). Clinically manifest neuromuscular block probably occurs only when this safety margin is reduced, as in hypocalcaemia or other electrolyte

Table 25.2 Clinical syndromes of drug-induced neuromuscular blockade and drugs implicated

Clinical presentation	Antibiotics	Antirheumatic drugs	Cardio-vascular drugs	Anticonvulsants	Psychotropic drugs	Anaesthetics	Other drugs
Drug-induced myasthenic syndrome	neomycin streptomycin kanamycin gentamycin polymyxin B colistins	D-penicillamine	oxprenolol practolol	trimethadione phenytoin			busulfan (?) oral contraceptive (?)
Aggravation or unmasking of myasthenia gravis	streptomycin kanamycin colistin rolitetracycline oxytetracycline	chloroquine (?)	quinidine procainamide propranolol	phenytoin	lithium chlorpromazine		methoxyflurane ACTH corticosteroids thyroid hormones ACh-esterase inhibitors
Postoperative respiratory depression							
Antibiotic-induced respiratory arrest syndrome	neomycin streptomycin kanamycin colistin lincomycin clindamycin						
Potentiation of muscle relaxants		chloroquine	quinidine		lithium promazine phenelzine	diazepam ketamine propanidid ether	oxytocin Trasylol cholinesterase inhibitors procaine lidocaine

disturbances (Katz, 1966), or when high blood levels of the drug develop, as in patients with renal failure (Lindesmith, Baines, Bigelow and Petty, 1968).

With drugs such as the antibiotics, which have a direct effect at the neuromuscular junction, the onset is relatively acute and respiratory paralysis with variable involvement of other muscle groups is the rule. On the other hand, in the case of D-penicillamine, which induces neuromuscular block through an immunological mechanism, symptoms usually develop only after a period of months or years, are generally less acute in onset, and the resulting clinical syndrome resembles more closely classical MG.

Aggravation or unmasking of myasthenia gravis. It is well known that certain drugs may lead to clinical deterioration when administered to previously stable myasthenic patients (Table 25.2). This is probably caused by a further reduction in the already lowered safety margin for transmission in such patients (Desmedt, 1973), because of the effects of the drug at the neuromuscular junction. In patients in whom an irreversible myasthenic syndrome develops it is likely that the drug has unmasked previously undeclared MG.

Postoperative respiratory depression. This is perhaps the commonest manifestation of drug-induced neuromuscular blockade. As shown in Table 25.2, a number of drugs may cause respiratory depression, during or after anaesthesia, through an effect on neuromuscular transmission. This may be due to a direct effect of the drug itself, or to enhancement of the blockade induced by muscle relaxants, or to a combination of these effects. The commonest example is the respiratory depression which may occur in patients given certain antibiotics in the preoperative period or during operation. In addition, some patients are unduly susceptible to the neuromuscular blocking action of certain drugs administered in the immediate postoperative period. For example, respiratory depression may occur following the administration of quinidine in patients who have recovered from the effects of muscle relaxants and have already been extubated,

a phenomenon which has been referred to as 'recurarisation' (Way, Katzung and Larson, 1967).

Mechanisms of drug-induced neuromuscular block

Drugs may interfere with neuromuscular transmission through a presynaptic local anaesthetic-like action at the nerve terminal, a postsynaptic curariform action, a combined pre- and postsynaptic action, or by a separate effect on the muscle fibre membrane (Fig. 25.2). The mechanism of action of some of the drugs to be discussed has been determined by experimental studies, while that of others is still conjectural.

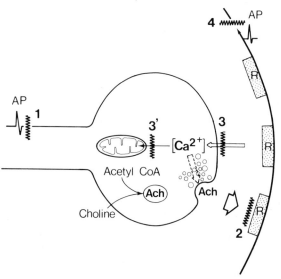

Fig. 25.2 Schematic representation of neuromuscular junction showing the possible sites of action of the drugs discussed. 1—Presynaptic local anaesthetic-like effect on propagation of nerve action potential (AP); 2—Postsynaptic receptor (R) blockade; 3,3'-interference with acetylcholine (ACh) release through inhibition of entry of Ca⁺⁺ ions into the nerve terminal (3) and into mitochondria (3'); 4—Impairment of muscle action potential propagation

Presynaptic local anaesthetic-like action. A number of drugs with local anaesthetic properties are suspected to reduce transmitter release by interfering with the generation of the nerve terminal action potential (Table 25.3). Confirmation of such an action would require simultaneous extracellular recording of the nerve terminal potential and the end-plate current

Table 25.3 Mechanisms of action of drugs which cause neuromuscular blockade

Mechanism	Antibiotics	Antirheumatic drugs	Cardio-vascular drugs	Anticonvulsants	Psychotropic drugs	Anaesthetics	Other drugs
Presynaptic local anaesthetic-like action (1)★	clindamycin lincomycin	chloroquine	propranolol		lithium imipramine		
Postsynaptic curare-like action (2)★	polymyxin B rolitetracycline lincomycin clindamycin	chloroquine	propranolol procainamide		ampheta-mines	ketamine ether halothane	emetine
Pre- and post-synaptic membrane stabilising action (2,3)★	neomycin streptomycin gentamycin polymyxins			phenytoin	chlorprom-azine amitripty-line droperidol haloperidol barbiturates	methoxy-flurane	ACTH (?) diphen-hydramine
Inhibition of muscle membrane conductance (4)★	polymyxin B (?)				imipramine		amantadine
Other mechanisms	colistin		ajmaline				
Immunological		D-penicillamine		trimethadione			busulfan (?)

★Refer to Figure 25.2

produced by nerve stimulation (Katz and Miledi, 1965).

Postsynaptic curariform block. A number of drugs exert their effect by competing for acetylcholine (ACh) receptor binding sites on the postsynaptic membrane (Table 25.3). Some of these drugs possess an ionised ammonium group which is thought to be the active binding site to the receptor (Koelle, 1975). Such an effect has been demonstrated *in vitro* by the finding of a reduced end-plate electrical response to iontophoretically applied ACh (Werman and Wislicki, 1971), or of a rapid reduction in miniature end-plate potential (mepp) amplitude after addition of the drug (Gissen, Karis and Nastuk, 1966). The *in vivo* demonstration of potentiation of neuromuscular block by D-tubocurarine and reversal by neostigmine, though less conclusive, has been the basis for establishing a curare-like action of certain drugs such as the amphetamines (Skau and Gerald, 1978), and procainamide (Galzigna, Manani, Mammano, Gasparetto and Deana, 1972).

The neuromuscular block which occurs in patients who develop myasthenia during treatment with D-penicillamine is also postsynaptic in nature. ACh receptor antibodies have been demonstrated in the serum of such patients (Masters, Dawkins, Zilko, Simpson, Leedman and Lindstrom, 1977; Vincent, Newsom Davis and Martin, 1978; Russell and Lindstrom, 1978) and mepp amplitude is reduced (Vincent *et al.*, 1978), presumably because of binding of antibody to the receptor such as that which occurs in classical MG (Shibuya, Mori and Nakazawa, 1978).

Combined pre- and postsynaptic block. A number of drugs have been shown to have both a presynaptic inhibitory effect on transmitter release and a postsynaptic curariform action. In the case of drugs with so-called 'membrane-stabilising' properties, the presynaptic effect has been shown to be due to interference with the movement of Ca^{++} ions into and within the nerve terminal (Fig. 25.2). These include phenytoin (Yaari, Pincus and

Argov, 1977), chlorpromazine (Argov and Yaari, 1979), and the aminoglycoside antibiotics (Elmqvist and Josefsson, 1962; Dretchen, Sokoll, Gergis and Long, 1973).

Interference with muscle membrane conductance. Certain drugs, such as amantadine, imipramine and possibly polymyxin B, produce a postsynaptic block by interfering directly with ionic conductance across the muscle end-plate membrane rather than by binding to receptor sites. This has been demonstrated conclusively in the case of amantadine using the voltage clamp technique (Albuquerque, Eldefrawi, Eldefrawi, Mansour and Tsai, 1978).

Specific drugs

Antibiotics

Aminoglycosides. Various antibiotics may interfere with neuromuscular transmission (Pittinger, Eryasa and Adamson, 1970). The most severe forms of neuromuscular block have occurred in patients treated with the aminoglycosides neomycin (Pridgeon, 1956), kanamycin (Mullet and Keats, 1961), streptomycin (Bodley and Brett, 1962) and gentamycin (Warner and Sanders, 1971). This complication has developed either following introduction of one of these drugs into the peritoneal or pleural cavities during surgery, or after oral or parenteral administration of the drug, leading to postoperative respiratory depression. This has usually been seen as a delay in recovery of spontaneous respiration, both in patients in whom muscle relaxants had been administered and in some in whom inhalational anaesthetics alone were used (Pridgeon, 1956; Bennetts, 1964). In some cases, respiratory depression has occurred some time after apparently complete recovery from the effects of muscle relaxants (Pinkerton and Munro, 1964). Involvement of the respiratory muscles has been the only, or predominant, manifestation of the neuromuscular block in some cases, while in others there was more generalised weakness. Some patients have had associated pupillary dilatation, blurring of vision, depression of corneal reflexes and paraesthesiae (McQuillen, Cantor and O'Rourke, 1968).

Neomycin (Percy and Saef, 1967), streptomycin (Loder and Walker, 1959) and kanamycin (Ream, 1963) may also produce a myasthenic syndrome unrelated to surgery, or may lead to transient deterioration in patients with MG (Hokkanen, 1964). Streptomycin and neomycin have been shown to interfere with neuromuscular transmission by a combined pre- and postsynaptic effect (Elmqvist and Josefsson, 1962; Tamaki, 1978) and it is likely that the other closely related drugs act in a similar way. Treatment of the severe postoperative neuromuscular block produced by these drugs involves assisted respiration and other supportive measures, the infusion of calcium gluconate to overcome the presynaptic component of the block, and the use of parenteral neostigmine to antagonise the curare-like effect of the drugs (Pittinger *et al.*, 1970).

Polypeptide antibiotics. Polymyxin B (Lindesmith *et al.*, 1968), colistin (Hokkanen, 1964) and colistin methosulphonate (Perkins, 1964; Zaunder, Barton, Benetts and Lore, 1966) may have similar effects to the aminoglycosides, but their mechanism of action has not been as well clarified. Colistin has been shown to reduce mepp amplitude and it has been suggested that this is due to a reduction in quantum size (McQuillen and Engbaek, 1975). However, as these drugs have an ionised ammonium group at physiological pH, a postsynaptic effect seems more likely (Wright and Collier, 1976a). Indeed, a recent study has shown that these drugs have predominantly a postsynaptic action with an additional presynaptic effect (Viswanath and Jenkins, 1978).

Other antibiotics. Oxytetracycline and rolitetracycline have been reported to aggravate MG in some patients (Gibbels, 1967; Wullen, Kast and Bruck, 1967). The mechanism of action has been studied in the case of rolitetracycline, which has been shown to have a postsynaptic curare-like effect (Wright and Collier, 1976a). Lincomycin (Duignan, Andrews and Williams, 1973; Samuelson, Giesecke, Kallus and Stanley, 1975) and its derivative clindamycin (Fogdall and Miller, 1974) have been shown to prolong the action of muscle relaxants in some patients. These drugs have been shown to have a postsynaptic effect and also a presynaptic local anaesthetic-like action in higher concentrations (Wright and Collier, 1976b; Rubbo, Gergis and Sokoll, 1977). It has been suggested that ampicillin and erythromycin may produce an Eaton-Lambert type of disorder of neuromuscular transmission on the basis of an electromyographic and repetitive nerve stimulation study (Herishanu and Taustein, 1971). If it is confirmed, this finding is important because ampicillin is one of the drugs of choice in the treatment of infections in patients with MG.

Antirheumatic drugs

D-penicillamine. A syndrome resembling classical MG may develop in patients with rheumatoid arthritis or Wilson's disease on long-term D-penicillamine therapy; this is now a well-recognised complication of treatment with the drug (Seitz, Hopf, Janzen and Meyer, 1976; Bucknall, 1977). Involvement of the ocular muscles has usually been an early manifestation in such cases, and some have subsequently developed more widespread involvement. The duration of treatment before the appearance of myasthenic symptoms in the cases reported was between 4 months and 5 years. In about two-thirds of affected patients, spontaneous recovery has occurred after withdrawal of the drug, while the remainder have required continuing anticholinesterase therapy or thymectomy, and one death has been recorded (Delrieu, Menkes, Sainte-Croix, Babinet, Chesneau and Delbarre, 1976).

It has been suggested that this complication may be more likely to develop in patients with rheumatoid arthritis, because most of the cases reported have been in patients with this condition (Bucknall, 1977). That an immunological mechanism is involved has been shown by the finding of raised ACh receptor antibody levels in the serum in most patients who have been studied in this way (Masters *et al.*, 1977; Russell and Lindstrom, 1978; Vincent *et al.*, 1978). In addition, antibody levels have been shown to fall with clinical improvement after withdrawal of the drug, suggesting that the antibody is directly involved in the pathogenesis of the disorder (Vincent *et al.*, 1978). The typical association with HLA A1 and B8

found in classical MG has been found in some patients with the drug-induced disorder (Bucknall, 1977; Russell and Lindstrom, 1978), but an association with thymoma has not been reported. It has been suggested that the development of myasthenia may be due to an independent effect of the drug on the immune system rather than to unmasking of subclinical MG. It remains to be determined why it is that this complication develops in only a small proportion of patients treated with the drug.

Chloroquine has also been reported to aggravate or unmask MG (Robinson, 1959). In addition, respiratory depression has occurred in the immediate postoperative period in 14 per cent of a series of 67 patients in whom the drug was introduced into the peritoneal cavity during abdominal surgery to prevent the formation of adhesions (Jui-Yen, 1971). Experimental studies have shown that the drug may have both a presynaptic local anaesthetic-like effect (Vartanian and Chinyanga, 1972) and a postsynaptic curariform action (Jui-Yen, 1971).

Cardiovascular drugs. Quinidine, procainamide and a number of the β-adrenergic blocking drugs possess neuromuscular blocking properties. Quinidine has been reported to aggravate or to unmask MG in some patients (Weisman, 1949; Kornfeld, Horowitz, Genkins and Papatestas, 1976). In addition, this drug may interact with muscle relaxants and has been reported to cause delayed respiratory depression in the postoperative period (Grogono, 1963; Schmidt, Vick and Sadove, 1963; Way *et al.*, 1967). The mechanism of action of the drug has not been fully investigated. Procainamide, which has been shown to have a postsynaptic blocking effect on neuromuscular transmission (Galzigna *et al.*, 1972), has also been reported to aggravate MG (Drachman and Skom, 1965; Kornfeld *et al.*, 1976).

Propranolol, oxprenolol and practolol have been reported to induce a myasthenic syndrome or to unmask MG (Herishanu and Rosenberg, 1975; Hughes and Zacharias, 1976). Experimental studies with propranolol (Werman and Wislicki, 1971) have shown that, in concentrations comparable to those achieved during therapy, the drug has a postsynaptic curariform action, while at higher concentrations it has an additional presynaptic anaesthetic-like effect. Pindolol has both a pre- and postsynaptic action (Larsen, 1978).

Anticonvulsants. Phenytoin and trimethadione have been reported to induce myasthenia, probably through different mechanisms. In the case of trimethadione, this was associated with an SLE-like syndrome and high titres of antimuscle antibodies and antinuclear factor in the peripheral blood, suggesting that the myasthenia may have been part of a drug-induced autoimmune disorder (Peterson, 1966; Booker, Chun and Sanguino, 1970). A myasthenic syndrome has been reported in patients with evidence of phenytoin intoxication and it is not clear whether or not this complication may also occur with well-controlled therapy (Norris, Colella and McFarlin, 1964; Regli and Guggenheim, 1965; Brumlik and Jacobs, 1974). The effects of phenytoin on neuromuscular transmission have been studied in detail and the drug has been shown to have both a postsynaptic curariform and a presynaptic action, the latter being thought to predominate (Yaari, Pincus and Argov, 1977, 1979).

Psychotropic drugs. Lithium carbonate may unmask MG (Neil, Himmelhoch and Licata, 1976; Granacher, 1977) and has also been shown to prolong the neuromuscular blockade produced by pancuronium (Borden, Clarke and Katz, 1974) and suxamethonium (Hill, Wong and Hodges, 1976). The action of the drug is probably mainly a presynaptic one, resulting from substitution of Li^+ for Na^+ ions at the nerve terminal (Crawford, 1975), but a postsynaptic effect has also been demonstrated (Onodera and Yamakawa, 1966). Chlorpromazine, which has been shown in experimental studies to interfere with transmitter release and to have a lesser postsynaptic curare-like effect (Argov and Yaari, 1979), may also aggravate MG (McQuillen, Gross and Johns, 1963). Promazine (Regan and Aldrete, 1967) and phenelzine (Bodley, Halwax and Potts, 1969) may potentiate the effect of suxamethonium. In the case of phenelzine this has been shown to be associated with reduced blood pseudocholinesterase levels.

Anaesthetic agents. Methoxyflurane has been reported to unmask subclinical MG (Elder, Beal, DeWald and Cobb, 1971) and has been shown experimentally to have a combined pre- and postsynaptic action, the latter predominating (Kennedy and Galindo, 1975). Ketamine and propanidid have been shown to potentiate the neuromuscular blocking effect of suxamethonium (Clarke, Dundee and Hamilton, 1967; Bovill, Dundee, Coppel and Moore, 1971), and diazepam that of gallamine (Feldman and Crawley, 1970).

Other drugs. A number of other drugs have been shown to have an effect on neuromuscular transmission when used therapeutically. These include oxytocin (Hodges, Bennett and Tunstall, 1959), Trasylol (aprotinin) (kallikrein—trypsin inactivator) (Chasapakis and Dimas, 1966), procaine and lidocaine (Usubiaga, Wikinski, Morales and Usubiaga, 1967) and eye drops containing potent anticholinesterases (Gesztes, 1966), all of which have been reported to cause postoperative respiratory depression through potentiation of muscle relaxants. There have been single reports of the development of myasthenic syndromes in patients taking the oral contraceptive pill Bickerstaff, 1975) or busuphan (Djaldetti, Pinkhas, De Vries, Kott, Joshua and Dollberg, 1968) but these are difficult to evaluate. Thyroid hormones in doses affecting the basal metabolic rate may also aggravate MG (Engel, 1961; Drachman, 1962). It is well known that corticosteroids, ACTH and the anticholinesterases which are used in the treatment of MG may interfere with neuromuscular transmission in their own right and lead to exacerbation of the myasthenic state. This is discussed further in Chapter 16.

A number of other drugs which have not been implicated clinically, have been shown to interfere with neuromuscular transmission in experimental studies. The inhalational anaesthetics halothane and ether have been shown to have a postsynaptic curariform action (Watland, Long, Pittinger and Cullen, 1957; Gissen et al., 1966). The barbiturates (Procter and Weakly, 1976), amitriptyline (Lermer, Avni and Bruderman, 1971), haloperidol and droperidol (Sokoll, Gergis, Post, Cronnelly and Long, 1974; Boucher and Katz, 1977) and certain of the antihistamines (Abdel-Aziz and

Bakry, 1973) have been shown to have combined pre- and postsynaptic blocking properties while the amphetamines (Skau and Gerald, 1978) and emetine (Salako, 1970) have a postsynaptic curariform action. Imipramine is thought to have a presynaptic anaesthetic-like effect (Chang and Chuang, 1972). Amantadine has been shown to interfere with muscle membrane conductance (Albuquerque *et al.*, 1978), and ajmaline is thought to interfere with neuromuscular transmission by combining with ACh (Manani, Gasparetto, Bettini, Caldesi Valeri and Galzigna, 1970).

PERIPHERAL NEUROPATHIES

Over 50 drugs used in clinical practice have been reported over the past 30 years to cause peripheral nerve damage in man (Le Quesne, 1970 and 1975). Some, such as thalidomide and clioquinol which led to severe forms of neuropathy, have been withdrawn from clinical use, while a variety of other drugs which cause peripheral neuropathy only infrequently are still freely prescribed (Argov

and Mastaglia, 1979b). Prompt recognition of this complication of drug therapy is clearly of importance if severe neurological deficits are to be avoided. Mild forms of neuropathy are easily overlooked and subclinical involvement is not uncommon, particularly in the case of certain drugs such as nitrofurantoin and perhexiline.

Clinical presentations

The common clinical forms of drug-induced neuropathy are shown in Table 25.4. While in most instances specific drugs produce fairly consistent and characteristic syndromes, this is not always the case and some drugs may cause either a sensorimotor neuropathy or a pure motor or sensory neuropathy.

Paraesthesiae and sensory neuropathy. A variety of drugs cause acroparaesthesiae suggesting a disturbance of sensory nerve function, but clinical examination and electrophysiological studies fail to show objective evidence of peripheral nerve damage (Table 25.4). Some, such as acetazolamide and cytosine arabinoside, cause

Table 25.4 Drug-induced peripheral neuropathies (clinical syndromes and drugs implicated)

Clinical presentation	Antimicrobial drugs	Antineoplastic drugs	Antirheumatic drugs	Hypnotics and psychotropics	Cardio-vascular drugs	Other drugs
Sensory neuropathy	ethionamide chloramphenicol thiamphenicol diamines	procarbazine nitrofurazone				calcium carbimide sulfoxone ergotamine propylthiouracil
paraesthesiae only	colistin streptomycin nalidixic acid	cytosine arabinoside		phenelzine	propranolol	sulthiame chlorpropamide methysergide acetazolamide
Sensorimotor neuropathy	isoniazid ethambutol streptomycin nitrofurantoin clioquinol metronidazole	vincristine podophyllin chlorambucil	gold indomethacin colchicine chloroquine phenylbutazone	thalidomide methaqualone glutethimide amitriptyline	perhexiline hydrallazine amiodarone disopyramide clofibrate	phenytoin disulfiram carbutamide tolbutamide chlorpropamide methimazole methylthiouracil
Predominantly motor	sulphonamides amphotericin B			imipramine		dapsone
Localised neuropathies	amphotericin B penicillin	nitrogen mustard ethoglucid				anticoagulants

unpleasant and even painful paraesthesiae. Others, such as streptomycin and stilbamidine, cause facial paraesthesiae or other unpleasant sensations in the upper part of the body (Collard and Hargreaves, 1947; Janssen, 1960).

A number of other drugs produce a sensory neuropathy with clinical and electrophysiological evidence of damage to sensory nerve fibres (Table 25.4). The resulting clinical syndrome is that of a symmetrical distal sensory disturbance, initially with paraesthesiae, and subsequently impairment, particularly of superficial sensory modalities, with relative sparing of vibration and proprioceptive sensation. The tendon reflexes are usually preserved but may be depressed or absent in some cases, presumably due to involvement of afferent fibres from the muscle spindles.

Sensorimotor neuropathy. Most cases of drug-induced neuropathy fall into this category (Table 25.4). Sensory manifestations usually appear first and are followed by motor involvement at a later stage only if the drug is not stopped. The onset and clinical progression of the disorder is usually gradual, but may be relatively acute in some cases, and may even resemble the Guillain-Barré form of post-infective polyneuropathy. Sensory and motor involvement is usually distal and symmetrical and, with occasional exceptions in which there is predominant involvement of the upper limbs (Bruun and Herman, 1942), the lower limbs are usually involved first and most severely. Muscle pain and cramps may be prominent in some cases (Le Quesne, 1975). The tendon reflexes are usually depressed or absent even when motor involvement is absent or inconspicuous (Casey, Jellife, Le Quesne and Millett, 1973). Exaggerated tendon reflexes in some cases suggest concomitant involvement of central motor pathways (Le Quesne, 1975).

Some drugs such as dapsone cause a motor neuropathy with absent or inconspicuous sensory abnormalities (Saquenton, Lorinz, Vick and Hamer, 1969; Epstein and Bohm, 1976), while others such as nitrofurantoin, which usually produce a sensorimotor neuropathy, may rarely cause a pure motor neuropathy (Toole and Parrish, 1973).

Localised neuropathies. Involvement of peripheral nerve trunks may occur as a complication of intramuscular injections of drugs, attributable either to direct needle trauma or to a local toxic effect of the drug itself. The best-known example is the sciatic nerve damage which may occur with injections into the buttock. Peripheral nerve involvement may also occur as a result of haemorrhage into confined spaces in patients on poorly controlled oral anticoagulant therapy. The femoral nerve trunk and the lumbosacral roots are most frequently affected in this way when the haemorrhage is retroperitoneal, but other peripheral nerves such as the median may also be involved (Dhaliwal, Schlagenhauff and Megahed, 1976). Localised forms of neuropathy may also occur after intra-arterial perfusion of cytotoxic agents such as nitrogen mustard or ethoglucid in the treatment of malignancy (Scholes, 1960; Westbury, 1962; Bond, Clark and Neal, 1964). In addition, local damage to nerves in the cubital fossa may occur as a result of intravenous infusions of certain drugs (Utz, Louria, Feder, Emmons and McCullough, 1957). Of particular interest is the occasional occurrence of brachial plexus neuropathy following penicillin injections into the buttock (Kolb and Gray, 1946), presumably on an 'allergic' basis.

Cranial neuropathies. Certain cranial nerves may be involved, either selectively or as part of a more generalised drug-induced neuropathy. A variety of drugs may cause an optic neuropathy (Leibold, 1971). Of the drugs which also cause peripheral neuropathy, chloramphenicol (Joy and Scalettar, 1960), clioquinol (Sobue, Ando, Iida, Takayanagi, Yamamura and Matsuoka, 1971) and perhexiline (Geraud, Caussanel, Jauzac, Arbus and Bes, 1978) are most likely to be associated with optic nerve damage. Stilbamidine and other diamines cause a trigeminal neuropathy (Cohen, 1970). Eighth nerve involvement occurs with a number of drugs but particularly with the aminoglycoside antibiotics. Streptomycin, gentamycin, tobramycin and sissomycin are primarily vestibulotoxic, while neomycin, kanamycin, framycetin and amikacin cause hearing loss which is thought to be due to a toxic effect on the cochlea (Noone, 1978).

Pathogenesis

The mechanisms involved in the production of drug-induced neuropathies are, in general, not well understood. Experimental animal studies have clarified the mechanism of action of certain drugs such as vincristine (Bradley, 1970) and nitrofurantoin (Klinghardt, 1967), while that of others remains to be determined. Few histological studies of peripheral nerve have been performed in patients with drug-induced neuropathy, but axonal degeneration appears to be the principal process in most cases. A predominantly de-myelinating process has been described in some patients with neuropathy due to perhexiline (Said, 1978) or amiodarone (Aronson, 1978), but this is uncommon.

In general, the drugs which cause peripheral neuropathy do so either by interfering with axonal or Schwann cell metabolism or through a vascular effect. The neuropathy in which the nature of the metabolic disturbance is best understood is probably that caused by isoniazid in which peripheral nerve damage is thought to be secondary to an effect of the drug on pyridoxine metabolism (Biehl and Vilter, 1954; McCormick and Snell, 1959). Vitamin deficiency may also play a part in other drug-induced neuropathies. For example, it has been shown that prolonged administration of chloramphenicol in the rat may lead to vitamin B_{12} deficiency, which may play a part in causing the neuropathy which occasionally develops in patients treated with the drug (Satoyoshi and Wakata, 1978). Thalidomide is thought to inhibit riboflavine (Leck and Millar, 1962) and to interfere with pyruvate metabolism (Buckle, 1963), while the nitrofurans interfere with pyruvate oxidation by competing with thiamine pyrophosphate (Paul, Paul, Kopko, Bryson and Harrington, 1954). Preliminary work has suggested that a disturbance of lipid metabolism may underlie the neuropathy caused by perhexiline (Pollet, Hauw, Escourolle and Baumann, 1977). Vincristine and colchicine are neurotubular toxins (Schochet, Usar and Lampert, 1968; Rasmussen, 1970).

Some drugs cause peripheral nerve damage by an effect on neural blood vessels. This may result either from severe vasospasm, as occurs in chronic ergotism (Merhoff and Porter, 1974), or from a vasculitic process (Stafford, Bogdanoff, Green and Spector, 1975). The possibility that certain drugs such as streptomycin may produce a true 'allergic' polyneuropathy has been considered (Janssen, 1960; Cohen, 1970) but the evidence for this is tenuous.

Predisposing factors

Some drugs such as amitriptyline, clofibrate and disopyramide cause peripheral neuropathy only rarely and the possibility therefore arises that certain individuals are unduly susceptible to the effects of such drugs. By contrast, other drugs such as vincristine are highly neurotoxic and will consistently cause peripheral nerve damage if administered for long enough in high enough doses (Bradley et al., 1970).

The best-known example of a genetic predisposition is the striking susceptibility of the Japanese to clioquinol neurotoxicity. The syndrome of subacute myelo-opticoneuropathy (SMON) developed in 17 per cent of Japanese patients who took the drug (Tsubaki, Honma and Hoshi, 1971), whereas very few cases were reported from other parts of the world where the drug was also freely used (Selby, 1972; Le Quesne, 1975). Variations in the pharmacokinetics of certain drugs may also modify the susceptibility to neurotoxic effects. Impaired renal function may lead to toxic blood levels of drugs such as nitrofurantoin which are excreted through the kidneys, and thereby increase the likelihood of neuropathy developing (Ellis, 1962). Similarly, it is well known that slow acetylators of isoniazid are more likely to develop peripheral neuropathy if pyridoxine supplements are not given (Hughes, Biehl, Jones and Schmidt, 1954). Strenuous exercise was thought to predispose to the development of neuropathy in patients treated with the older sulphonamides (Bruun and Hermann, 1942).

The underlying disease process may itself modify the susceptibility to drug-induced neuropathy. For example, patients with lymphoma develop neuropathy more frequently when treated with vincristine than those with other forms of malignancy (Watkins and Griffin, 1978). Whether or not drug-induced neuropathy is more likely to occur in patients with cancer, diabetes, vitamin deficiency or alcoholism, situations in which the peripheral nervous system may already be affected, remains to be determined.

Specific drugs

Antimicrobial agents. Over a dozen drugs used in the treatment of bacterial and protozoal infections over the past 35 years have been recognised to cause peripheral neuropathy.

Isoniazid. The occurrence of peripheral neuropathy in patients treated with this antituberculous agent was first recognised soon after its introduction (Gammon, Burge and King, 1953). The incidence of neuropathy was found to be dose-dependent, being as high as 17 per cent in patients taking 400 mg of the drug per day, and 35 per cent during a second course of treatment (Mandel, 1959). As indicated previously, the neuropathy has been shown to be due to the development of pyridoxine deficiency (Biehl and Vilter, 1954), being more likely to occur in individuals who inactivate the drug at slow rates in the liver, and being preventable when adequate supplements of vitamin B_6 are administered with the drug (10 mg per 100 mg of isoniazid) (Cohen, 1970; Le Quesne, 1975). It is not clear how the drug causes pyridoxine deficiency but this may be due to the formation of an inactive hydrazone complex by interaction between the drug and the vitamin (Le Quesne, 1970).

The initial symptoms consist of distal limb paraesthesiae which may be painful, and which usually resolve if the drug is stopped (Biehl and Nimitz, 1954). If, on the other hand, the drug is continued, impairment of superficial and to a lesser extent of deep sensory modalities, tenderness and weakness of distal muscles, and depression of tendon reflexes supervene (Le Quesne, 1970). Nerve conduction velocities are only mildly reduced and histological studies have shown axonal degeneration affecting both myelinated and unmyelinated nerve fibres (Ochoa, 1970). Recovery in the more severely affected patients is gradual but usually complete, and is not hastened by the administration of vitamin B_6 (Gammon *et al.*, 1953; Le Quesne, 1975).

Other anti-tuberculous agents. Ethambutol may also cause a sensorimotor neuropathy (Cohen, 1970; Tugwell and James, 1972) which responds favourably to withdrawal of the drug. Some of the reported cases were on combined chemotherapy but withdrawal of ethambutol alone led to improvement. The occurrence of a predominantly sensory neuropathy (Tugwell and James, 1972) and of optic neuropathy in some patients treated with ethambutol (Leibold, 1966) leave no doubt that it too is neurotoxic. Ethionamide, which is structurally similar to isoniazid, is also known to cause a mild sensory neuropathy (Poole and Schneeweiss, 1961) and to have other neurotoxic effects (Brouet, Marche, Rist, Chevallier and Le Meur, 1959). Whether or not the drug has a similar effect to that of isoniazid on pyridoxine metabolism is not known. Streptomycin has been reported to cause a peripheral neuropathy (Janssen, 1960), but this is much less common than its ototoxic effects.

Nitrofurantoin. Peripheral neuropathy is a relatively frequent complication of treatment with this drug. A review of the literature by Toole and Parrish in 1973 disclosed 137 reported cases. The important features of the neuropathy were documented in this study. It was found that it occurred not only in patients taking the drug orally but also following local instillation into the bladder. Symptoms usually appeared within the first 45 days of treatment, although in 16 per cent of cases symptoms developed only during the month after the drug was withdrawn. The daily dose in affected patients varied from 100 to 800 mg, with no evidence of a cumulative effect, and no clear relationship between the dose of the drug and the severity of the resulting clinical syndrome. With the exception of two patients who had a pure motor neuropathy (Morris, 1966), the majority of cases presented with distal sensory symptoms followed after a few days by pain and muscle weakness, the latter being profound in some cases and contributing to a fatal outcome (Rubenstein, 1964). Of the series of patients reviewed by Toole and Parish (1973) the prognosis for recovery was found to be related to the severity of the condition, 63 per cent of mildly affected cases recovering completely while only 10 per cent of severely affected cases made a full recovery.

Neuropathy is more frequent in patients with renal insufficiency (Ellis, 1962) but may also occur with normal renal function. In a clinical and EMG study of 48 non-uraemic patients on the drug, only five (10 per cent) showed clinical signs of peripheral nerve involvement while the electrical studies showed evidence of nerve damage in 62 per cent of cases (Lindholm, 1967). Motor and sensory conduction velocities were found to be reduced in a group of healthy volunteers who took the drug in therapeutic doses for a period of two weeks (Toole, Gergen, Hayes and Felts, 1968).

Few histological studies have been reported in man. Evidence of axonal degeneration in peripheral nerves and of associated spinal cord damage was found in a case at post-mortem examination (Le Quesne, 1975). Observations in the experimental animal have shown evidence of a 'dying-back' neuropathy (Klinghardt, 1967). The pathogenesis of the neuropathy may be related to that of beri-beri and isoniazid neuropathy as the nitrofurans have been shown to interfere with pyruvate oxidation by competing with thiamine pyrophosphate (Paul et al., 1954).

Sulphonamides. Peripheral neuropathy was a well-recognised complication of treatment with sulphonamides in the 1940s. The clinical features were well documented in two Scandinavian reviews of over 100 patients, most of whom were treated with sulfanyldimethylsulfanilamide (Uliron) (Bruun and Herman, 1942; Müller, 1945). Although transient paraesthesiae occurred in some cases, the neuropathy was predominantly motor and usually developed 1–3 weeks after completion of treatment. The mechanism of the neuropathy remains uncertain, but it has been suggested that in some cases it is due to a toxic effect of the drug, while in others it may be allergic in nature (Le Quesne, 1970). None of the sulphonamides in current clinical use are known to have toxic effects on the peripheral nervous system (Weinstein, Madoff and Samet, 1974).

Other antibiotics. Thiamphenicol, a derivative of chloramphenicol has also been reported to cause a sensory peripheral neuropathy (Manten, 1975). A number of other antibiotics may cause peripheral

paraesthesiae without objective evidence of peripheral nerve damage (Table 25.4).

Clioquinol. The SMON syndrome which was characterised by abdominal pain and the subsequent development of a neurological disorder involving the optic nerves, spinal cord and peripheral nerves, was prevalent in Japan during the 1950s and 60s. Kono reviewed a total of 7856 probable cases of this syndrome in 1971. The association with clioquinol was recognised in 1971 (Tsubaki et al., 1971), when it was found that 96 per cent of a series of 969 affected patients had taken the drug before the onset of neurological symptoms. The incidence among individuals treated with clioquinol was found to be 17 per cent and was even higher in those who took the drug for longer than two weeks. Sobue et al. (1971) summarised the clinical and laboratory manifestations in a series of 752 patients. Initial symptoms included peripheral numbness, paraesthesiae and pain. Symmetrical distal impairment of superficial and deep sensory modalities was present in 95 per cent, weakness in 53 per cent, and depression of tendon reflexes in 40 per cent of cases. Histological studies of nerve biopsies did not clearly establish the nature of the nerve damage, but a recent electrophysiological study has shown evidence of a primarily axonal neuropathy (Gourie-Devi, 1978). As indicated previously, the low incidence of SMON in other parts of the world where clioquinol has also been used widely (Selby, 1972; Gourie-Devi, 1978) suggests a racial predisposition to the neurotoxic effects of this drug, or the contribution of some additional factor such as a viral agent (Nakamura and Inoue, 1972).

Metronidazole. There have been a number of reports of a sensory neuropathy developing in patients with various conditions who were treated with this drug for prolonged periods (Ramsay, 1968; Ingham, Selkon and Hale, 1975; Ursing and Kamme, 1975; Coxon and Pallis, 1976; Bradley, Karlsson and Rasool, 1977). Motor involvement has not been apparent clinically, but mild prolongation of distal motor latencies was found in one case (Bradley et al., 1977). A sural nerve biopsy from this patient showed evidence of axonal degeneration involving both small and large

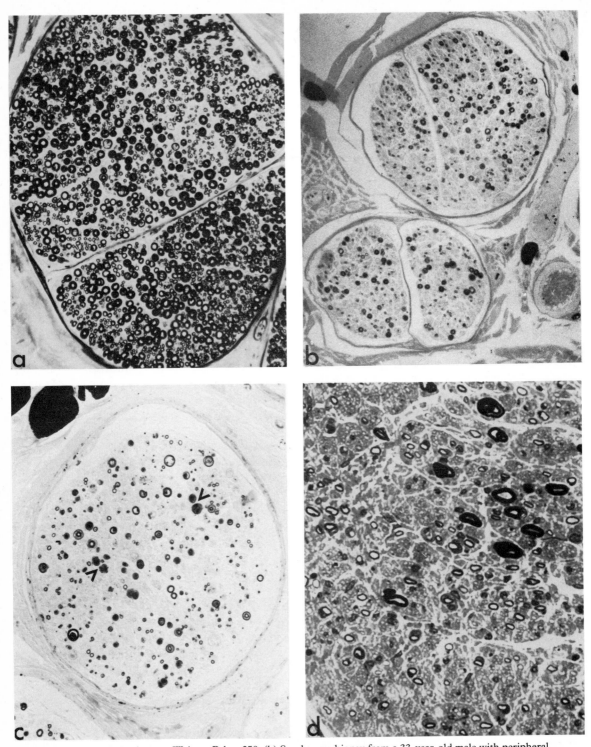

Fig. 25.3 (a) Normal sural nerve. Weigert-Pal, ×250. (b) Sural nerve biopsy from a 33-year-old male with peripheral neuropathy due to metronidazole, showing depletion of myelinated fibres of all sizes. Weigert-Pal, ×100. (c) Marked loss of myelinated fibres from the sural nerve of a 26-year-old male with peripheral neuropathy due to disulfiram. A number of fibres are undergoing Wallerian-type degeneration (arrowheads). Weigert-Pal, ×224. (d) Severe loss of small and large-diameter myelinated fibres from the sural nerve of a 68-year-old male with a demyelinating peripheral neuropathy due to perhexiline maleate. Osmium/toluidine blue, ×500

diameter fibres (Fig. 25.3b). The patient made a good recovery over a period of seven months after withdrawal of the drug.

Other antimicrobial agents. Stilbamidine and other diamines, which have been used in the treatment of leishmaniasis and trypanosomiasis, have been recognised to cause a trigeminal sensory neuropathy in as many as 50 per cent of patients on prolonged therapy (Snapper, 1947; Cohen, 1970). In 22 out of 24 patients treated with stilbamidine who were reported by Collard and Hargreaves (1947), a trigeminal sensory disturbance was associated with paraesthesiae and sensory impairment over the neck and chest. Gradual improvement occurred over a period of up to two years after withdrawal of the drug. So specific was the effect of stilbamidine on the trigeminal nerve that it was, at one stage, used in the treatment of trigeminal neuralgia (Cohen, 1970).

Amphotericin B also has neurotoxic effects. Evidence of a demyelinating process was found at post-mortem examination in the peripheral nerves of a patient who had developed a peripheral neuropathy and myelopathy during the course of treatment with the drug (Haber and Joseph, 1962). Other cases with a predominantly motor neuropathy (Cohen, 1970), or with localised forms of nerve damage after intravenous infusion of the drug (Utz *et al.*, 1957) have also been reported.

Anti-neoplastic agents

Vinca alkaloids. These drugs, which have been used in the treatment of various malignancies, are extremely neurotoxic. Vincristine is particularly toxic and most patients who are on the drug for long enough will develop signs of peripheral nerve damage. The clinical features of vincristine neuropathy are well documented (Warot, Goudemand and Habay, 1965; Bradley *et al.*, 1970; Casey *et al.*, 1973). Distal paraesthesiae, which are usually the earliest symptoms, may involve the hands before the feet and may antedate sensory or motor deficits for long periods. Muscle cramps may be a prominent symptom which accompanies the onset of motor involvement. The latter shows a predilection for the forearm extensor muscles in some cases (Casey *et al.*, 1973). The tendon

reflexes are lost at an early stage, particularly in the lower limbs. Autonomic involvement may also occur and postural hypotension and constipation may be early symptoms (Warot *et al.*, 1965). Recovery may occur if the drug is stopped or even if the dose is reduced, but mild sensory impairment and reflex depression often persist. Electrophysiological studies have shown evidence of severe axonal damage involving both motor and sensory fibres (Hildebrand and Coërs, 1965; Bradley *et al.*, 1970; Casey *et al.*, 1973), and have shown that the early loss of tendon reflexes is probably due to involvement of afferent fibres from the muscle spindles (McLeod and Penny, 1969). Histological observations on sural nerve biopsies have confirmed that axonal degeneration is the predominant process with only minor segmental demyelination (Bradley *et al.*, 1970) (Fig. 25.3c).

Other cytotoxic drugs. A number of other drugs used in the treatment of malignancy may cause neuropathy. Procarbazine, which is structurally similar to isoniazid, has occasionally been associated with a sensory neuropathy (Weiss, Walker and Wiernik, 1974) as have nitrofurazone, a congener of nitrofurantoin which was used in the treatment of testicular carcinoma (Le Quesne, 1975) and cytosine arabinoside (Russell and Powles, 1974). Podophyllin derivatives, which have been used in the treatment of disseminated malignancies, and which are also constituents of certain laxative preparations, may cause a mild peripheral neuropathy (Falkson, van Dyk, van Eden, van der Merwe, van der Bergh and Falkson, 1975; Langman, 1975). Chlorambucil has also been reported to cause a sensorimotor neuropathy occasionally (Sandler and Gonsalkorale, 1977).

Anti-rheumatic drugs

Gold. Peripheral neuropathy is a well-recognised complication of gold therapy in rheumatoid arthritis (Endtz, 1958), occurring in 0.5–1 per cent of patients treated in this way (Hartfall, Garland and Goldie, 1937; Doyle and Cannon, 1950). Motor involvement is usually prominent and may be asymmetrical, and sensory signs may be inconspicuous. The onset may be abrupt and

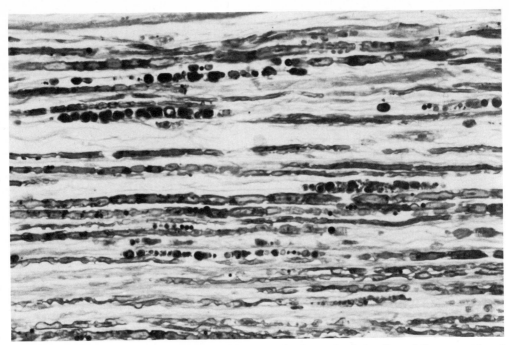

Fig. 25.4   Sural nerve biopsy from a 28-year-old male with neuropathy due to vincristine. Several fibres are undergoing Wallerian-type degeneration. Weigert-Pal, ×320

progression rapid, mimicking the Guillain-Barré form of postinfective polyneuropathy, particularly in some patients who also develop facial diplegia and have considerably elevated cerebrospinal fluid protein levels (Le Quesne, 1970). Fever and a skin rash may be associated with the neuropathy, indicating a more generalised reaction in some cases (Doyle and Cannon, 1950). The few electrophysiological and pathological studies performed have shown that axonal degeneration is the major process (Walsh, 1970).

Chloroquine. Evidence of peripheral nerve involvement has been found in some patients who developed a vacuolar myopathy while being treated with chloroquine (Loftus, 1963; Whisnant *et al.*, 1963; Hicklin, 1968). Examination of a sural nerve biopsy in one patient showed evidence of primary axonal degeneration and prominent multilamellar inclusion bodies in the cytoplasm of Schwann cells (Bischoff, 1978).

Other anti-inflammatory drugs. Indomethacin has also been implicated in causing a neuropathy.

Eade, Acheson, Cuthbert and Hawkes (1975) reported four patients with a mixed sensorimotor neuropathy and two with only sensory symptoms in the hands, in whom it was felt that the drug was responsible. Nerve biopsy was not carried out, but electrophysiological studies in one case showed considerable slowing of motor conduction velocities. Further studies are needed to determine how often this commonly used drug causes peripheral nerve damage.

There are occasional reports of peripheral neuropathy developing in patients treated with colchicine (Prescott, 1975) or D-penicillamine (Meyboom, 1977), the latter drug being known to have an antipyridoxine effect (Jaffe, Altman and Merryman, 1964). Paraesthesiae and muscle weakness have also been reported occasionally in patients treated with phenylbutazone (Arden, 1964) but the significance of these symptoms is uncertain.

Hypnotics and psychotropic drugs

Thalidomide. This drug was first reported to

cause neuropathy in 1960, five years after it was introduced into clinical use (Florence, 1960). Although the drug was withdrawn from the market two years later, victims of its teratogenic and neurotoxic effects are still seen. The characteristics of thalidomide neuropathy were reviewed by Fullerton and Kremer (1961) and Fullerton and O'Sullivan (1968). Sensory involvement was prominent in all cases and sensory deficits were still present in 50 per cent of cases re-examined after an interval of six years. The finding of exaggerated tendon reflexes and extensor plantar responses in some cases suggested that there was additional spinal cord involvement. Cerebrospinal fluid protein levels were frequently elevated (Le Quesne, 1975). Electrophysiological (Fullerton and Kremer, 1961) and nerve biopsy studies (Klinghardt, 1965) have shown that the primary process is one of axonal degeneration.

Methaqualone. A number of reports have raised suspicion that methaqualone may be neurotoxic. Some patients experience transient acroparaesthesiae or numbness shortly after taking the drug before the onset of sleep (McQuaker and Bruggen, 1963). At least 11 cases of a sensorimotor neuropathy have now been reported in patients taking 200–600 mg of methaqualone nightly for periods of a few days to two years, either alone or with diphenhydramine, diazepam, meprobamate or promazine (Finke and Spiegelberg, 1973; Hoaken, 1975; Marks and Sloggen, 1976). Improvement occurred in most cases after stopping methaqualone and was rapid and complete in those with recent onset of symptoms. In another study of 232 patients taking the drug, 44 of whom had EMG studies, only a single case of peripheral neuropathy was found (Kunze, Noelle and Prüll, 1967). Few cases of neuropathy have been reported and further clinical and EMG studies of regular consumers of the drug are required to determine the frequency of this complication.

Glutethimide. Reports of two patients with sensory symptoms and areflexia after prolonged high-dose treatment with this drug (Bartholomew, 1961), and of a suspected case of neuropathy in a glutethimide addict (Lingle, 1966) raised suspicion that the drug, which has structural similar-

ities to thalidomide, may be neurotoxic. Nover (1967) reported the development of sensory symptoms, areflexia and ataxia in another glutethimide addict in whom EMG studies confirmed the diagnosis of a sensorimotor polyneuropathy. The sensory symptoms disappeared when the drug was stopped but the ataxia and areflexia persisted. Three similar cases have been studied by Haas and Marasigan (1968).

Other drugs. There have been occasional reports of a predominantly motor neuropathy developing in patients treated with imipramine (Collier and Martin, 1960; Miller, 1963; Cohen, 1970) and amitriptyline (Isaacs and Carlish, 1963) but none of these cases were studied in detail. Reports of 'neuritis' developing in four patients on chlorprothixene (Cohen, 1970), and of peripheral paraesthesiae in patients treated with phenelzine, are difficult to evaluate (Davies, 1968).

Cardiovascular drugs

Perhexiline. The occurrence of neuropathy in patients treated with this coronary vasodilator has been reported only recently but is now well recognised (Bousser, Bouche, Brochard and Herreman, 1976; Lhermitte, Fardeau, Chedru and Mallecourt, 1976; Fraser, Campbell and Miller, 1977; Sebille, 1978). It has been claimed that clinically manifest neuropathy occurs in about 0.1 per cent of patients treated with the drug and that subclinical involvement is even commoner (Sebille, 1978). Thus, in a study of 35 asymptomatic patients taking the drug, 30 per cent were found to have prolonged distal motor latencies and 65 per cent had abnormal H-reflex studies (Sebille, 1978). Sensory symptoms, which are usually prominent, may appear as early as three weeks after commencement of treatment (Robinson, 1978) and are followed by distal motor involvement in the limbs. In most cases, symptoms usually occur only after several months of treatment with daily doses of 200–300 mg (Geraud *et al.*, 1978). Some of the reported cases have also had papilloedema, deafness (Geraud *et al.*, 1978), dysgeusia, pupillary abnormalities (Nick, Dudognon, Escourolle, Bakouche, Nicolle, Reignier, Hauw, Ermidou, Pollet, Baumann, Singlas and

Lévy, 1978), autonomic involvement (Fraser *et al.*, 1977), and elevated cerebrospinal fluid protein levels (Geraud *et al.*, 1978). Complete recovery occurs over a period of several months in most cases (Geraud *et al.*, 1978). Electrophysiological and histological studies have shown evidence of both segmental demyelination and axonal degeneration, the former being the predominant process (Mussini, Hauw and Escourolle, 1977; Said, 1978) (Fig. 25.3d). Electron microscopy has shown prominent membranous and paracrystalline inclusions in Schwann cells (Mussini *et al.*, 1977), and biochemical studies have demonstrated an increased ganglioside content in peripheral nerves (Pollet *et al.*, 1977). The available evidence suggests that the neuropathy is due primarily to an effect of the drug on the metabolism of the Schwann cell.

Amiodarone. This drug, which is also used in the treatment of angina pectoris, has recently been reported to cause a mixed sensorimotor neuropathy which is demyelinating in nature (Robinson, 1975; Aronson, 1978).

Hydrallazine. A number of cases of a mixed but predominantly sensory peripheral neuropathy have been reported in patients treated with this drug (Kirkendall and Page, 1958; Le Quesne, 1970; Perry, 1973) and it has been suggested that mild or subclinical neuropathy may occur in as many as 15 per cent of patients taking the drug (Le Quesne, 1970). As hydrallazine is structurally similar to isoniazid it has been suggested that the neuropathy may be due to an effect on pyridoxine metabolism (Raskin and Fishman, 1965). The neuropathy appears to be unrelated to the lupus-like syndrome induced by the drug.

Disopyramide. Patients treated with this anti-arrhythmic drug occasionally complain of peripheral paraesthesiae (Jennings, Jones, Besterman, Model, Turner and Kidner, 1976). There has also been a recent report of a sensorimotor neuropathy developing in a patient who had been on the drug for six months (Dawkins and Gibson, 1978).

Clofibrate. Clinical and electrophysiological evidence of peripheral nerve involvement was found in two patients with clofibrate myopathy (Gabriel and Pearce, 1976; Pokroy, Ress and Gregory, 1977). However, there is some doubt as to the cause of the neuropathy in these cases and further evidence is required before accepting that the drug is neurotoxic.

Digitalis. Painful paraesthesiae, mainly in trigeminal distribution but also in the limbs, may occur in patients intoxicated with digitalis leaf preparations (Batterman and Gutner, 1948).

Other drugs

Phenytoin. The occurrence of a mild peripheral neuropathy in patients on long-term phenytoin treatment is well recognised (Finkleman and Arieff, 1942; Lovelace and Horwitz, 1968). Sensory symptoms are present in some patients but most are asymptomatic, being found to have reflex depression or sensory impairment on clinical examination (Lovelace and Horwitz, 1968). The frequency of polyneuropathy appears to increase with the duration of therapy (Lovelace and Horwitz, 1968; Eisen, Woods and Sherwin, 1974). Electrophysiological studies have shown mild slowing of conduction in motor and sensory nerve fibres, and evidence of denervation in distal muscles, particularly in the lower limbs. Such findings were often subclinical and were more frequent in patients who had consumed the largest quantities of the drug (Eisen *et al.*, 1974). The electrophysiological studies point to a primary axonal degeneration of the 'dying-back' type but, to our knowledge, histological studies have not been reported.

It has been suggested that phenytoin may cause two basic types of peripheral nerve dysfunction, the first being a reversible phenomenon associated with acute drug toxicity, and the second being the form of peripheral neuropathy associated with long-term therapy described above (Eisen *et al.*, 1974). Evidence for acute reversible depression of nerve function has come from the following two studies. In a study of patients at the beginning of phenytoin treatment it was found that, after only one week on the drug, there was slowing of conduction in slow-conducting motor nerve fibres, whereas maximal motor conduction velocities were normal (Hopf, 1968). In the second study, of epileptic patients with serum phenytoin levels greater than 20 μg/ml, it was found that there was a significant improvement in motor nerve conduction velocities when the serum phenytoin level was reduced (Birket-Smith and Krogh, 1971). There is also experimental evidence that phenytoin has acute depressant effects on peripheral nerve excitability (Toman, 1949; Morell, Bradley and Ptashne, 1958).

Other anticonvulsants. Peripheral paraesthesiae have been reported in patients treated with sulthiame, but electrophysiological studies have not been performed in such patients. Although some of the patients on phenytoin who developed peripheral neuropathy were also taking other anticonvulsants (Lovelace and Horwitz, 1968), there is no convincing evidence that any of the other commonly used anticonvulsants interfere with peripheral nerve function.

Disulfiram. The occurrence of a sensorimotor polyneuropathy in alcoholics treated with this drug is well established (Hayman and Wilkins, 1956; Bradley and Hewer, 1966; Gardner-Thorpe and Benjamin, 1971), although in some cases it has been difficult to be certain of the extent to which alcohol or nutritional deficiencies may have contributed to the neuropathy. Electrophysiological studies have shown evidence primarily of axonal degeneration with involvement of both motor and sensory fibres (Bradley and Hewer, 1966; Gardner-Thorpe and Benjamin, 1971) and this has recently been confirmed by a histological study of the sural nerve in one patient (Moddel, Bilbao, Payne and Ashby, 1978). One of the metabolites of disulfiram is carbon disulphide (Prickett and Johnston, 1953) which is neurotoxic and is known to cause peripheral neuropathy (Vigiliani, 1954).

Citrated calcium carbamide, which has also been used in the treatment of alcoholics, has recently been reported to induce a reversible form of sensory neuropathy (Reilly, 1976).

Dapsone. This drug, which has been used in the treatment of leprosy and of a number of dermatological conditions, is known to cause an almost exclusively motor form of peripheral neuropathy (Saquenton et al., 1969; Epstein and Bohm, 1976; Gehlmann, Koller and Malkinson, 1977). This has usually developed after prolonged high-dose therapy but has also occurred with lower doses of the drug (Rapoport and Guss, 1972). Electrophysiological studies have shown mild impairment of motor conduction (Saquenton et al., 1969; Fredericks, Kugelman and Kirsch, 1976) with normal sensory conduction (Wyatt and Stevens, 1972; Fredericks et al., 1976). Sulfoxone sodium, another of the sulphones, has on the other hand been reported to cause a sensory neuropathy (Volden, 1977).

Oral hypoglycaemic agents. There is some evidence that the sulphonylureas may cause peripheral neuropathy in some diabetics, although in this situation also, it is difficult to be certain of the relative extent to which the drug and the underlying disease are responsible. Nevertheless, four cases of peripheral neuropathy have been attributed to carbutamine (Cohen, 1970), and three to tolbutamide (Ellenberg, 1959). In addition, chlorpropamide has been reported to cause peripheral paraesthesiae (Davies, 1968) and has been implicated in a patient with a rapidly evolving Guillain-Barré-like syndrome (Ince, 1962).

Ergotamine. As mentioned previously, this drug may cause severe vasospasm and secondary peripheral nerve damage when consumed in large doses. In a group of 19 chronic ergotamine users, four had symptoms suggestive of a sensory neuropathy and other vasospastic phenomena, which resolved on withdrawal of the drug (Horton and Peters, 1963). Methysergide, which also has a vasospastic effect, has been reported to cause paraesthesiae (Davies, 1968).

Antithyroid agents. Several drugs which were used in the treatment of thyrotoxicosis have been associated with neurotoxic side effects. Methimazole was reported to cause acute motor neuropathy (Accetta, Fitzmorris and Wettingfeld, 1954) or sensory neuropathy (Roldan and Nigrin, 1972) in single case records. Propylthiouracil caused sensory neuropathy (Crile, 1947; Frawley and

Koeppe, 1950), while methylthiouracil was claimed to be responsible for widespread sensori-motor neuropathy in a case report (Barfred, 1947). Loss of taste and smell was also recorded with these drugs (Leys, 1945; Hallman and Hurst, 1953).

CONCLUSIONS

It will be seen from the present review that drugs used in various clinical situations may interfere with neuromuscular function. The possibility of such a complication should be considered in any patient who complains of muscle pain, weakness, fatiguability or sensory disturbances while on drug therapy: patients complaining of such symptoms should be subjected to a careful neurological examination and EMG study. In view of their potentially reversible nature, drug-induced disorders should enter into the differential diagnosis in any patient presenting with a myopathy, neuropathy or myasthenic syndrome and full details of drug therapy should be obtained in all such patients. The possibility of drug effects should be considered, particularly in patients with a pre-existing neuromuscular disorder, who may be more susceptible to, and less able to compensate for, such effects.

In addition to their diagnostic role, electro-physiological and pathological studies of patients with drug-induced neuromuscular disorders will help to provide a clearer indication of the true incidence of such complications. In addition, they will contribute to the understanding of the pathogenesis and pathophysiology of toxic forms of neuropathy and myopathy and of the basic pathological reactions of peripheral nerve and muscle.

Experimental studies *in vivo* and *in vitro* have elucidated the mechanisms whereby a number of drugs interfere with neuromuscular function. However, because of various differences between the experimental and human situation, the results of such studies have not always been directly applicable to man. Thus, in the case of certain drugs such as amantadine, an effect on neuromuscular transmission has been identified in *in vitro* studies but has not been manifest clinically. Nevertheless, such studies are clearly of importance for the screening of newly introduced therapeutic agents and will serve to alert the clinician to possible effects on neuromuscular function.

ACKNOWLEDGEMENTS

The authors are grateful to Miss M. Jenkison who prepared the photomicrographs and provided technical assistance, and to Mrs I. Gibbs for secretarial assistance.

REFERENCES

Abdel-Aziz, A. & Bakry, N. (1973) The action and interaction of diphenhydramine (Benadryl) hydrochloride at the neuromuscular junction. *European Journal of Pharmacology*, **22**, 169.

Aberfeld, D.C., Bienenstock, H., Shapiro, M.S., Namba, T. & Grob, D. (1968) Diffuse myopathy related to meperidine addiction in a mother and daughter. *Archives of Neurology*, **19**, 384.

Accetta, G.S., Fitzmorris, A.O. & Wettingfeld, R.F. (1954) Toxicity of methimazole. *Journal of the American Medical Association*, **155**, 253.

Aguayo, A.J. & Hudgson, P. (1970) The short-term effects of chloroquine on skeletal muscle: an experimental study in the rabbit. *Journal of the Neurological Sciences*, **11**, 301.

Albuquerque, E.X., Eldefrawi, A.T., Eldefrawi, M.E., Mansour, N. & Tsai, M.C. (1978) Amantadine: neuromuscular blockade by suppression of ionic conductance of the acetylcholine receptor. *Science*, **199**, 788.

Anderson, P.J., Song, S.K. & Slotwiner, P. (1967) The fine structure of spheromembranous degeneration of skeletal muscle induced by vincristine. *Journal of Neuropathology and Experimental Neurology*, **26**, 15.

Arden, G.P. (1954) The value of phenylbutazone in orthopaedic conditions. *Rheumatism*, **10**, 44.

Argov, Z. & Mastaglia, F.L. (1979a) Drug-induced disorders of neuromuscular transmission. *Adverse Drug Reaction Bulletin*, **74**, 264.

Argov, Z. & Mastaglia, F.L. (1979b) Drug-induced peripheral neuropathies. *British Medical Journal*, **1**, 663.

Argov, Z. & Yaari, Y. (1979) The action of chlorpromazine at an isolated cholinergic synapse. *Brain Research*, **164**, 227.

Aronson, J.K. (1978) Cardiac glycosides and drugs used in dysrhythmias. In Dukes, M.N.G. *Side Effects of Drugs* (Excerpta Medica, Amsterdam), II, 163.

Askari, A., Vignos, P.J. & Moskowitz, R.W. (1976) Steroid myopathy in connective tissue disease. *American Journal of Medicine*, **61**, 485.

Austin, K.L. & Denborough, M.A. (1977) Drug treatment of malignant hyperpyrexia. *Anaesthesia and Intensive Care*, **5**, 207.

Barfred, A. (1947) Methylthiouracil in the treatment of thyrotoxicosis. *American Journal of Medical Sciences*, **214**, 349.

Bartholomew, A.A. (1961) in correspondence, *British Medical Journal*, **2**, 1570.

Basser, L.S. (1979) Purgatives and periodic paralysis. *Medical Journal of Australia*, **1**, 47.

Battacharrya, S. (1966) Abduction contracture of the shoulder from contracture of the intermediate part of the deltoid. Report of three cases. *Journal of Bone and Joint Surgery*, **46B**, 127.

Batterman, R.C. & Gutner, L.B. (1948) Hitherto undescribed neurological manifestations of digitalis toxicity. *American Heart Journal*, **36**, 582.

Bennetts, F.E. (1964) Muscular paralysis due to streptomycin following inhalation anaesthesia. *Anaesthesia*, **19**, 93.

Bettendorf, U. & Neuhaus, R. (1974) Penicillamin-induzierte polymyositis. *Deutsche Medizinische Wochenschrift*, **99**, 2522.

Bickerstaff, E.R. (1975) *Neurological Complications of Oral Contraceptives*, p. 93 (Clarendon Press: Oxford).

Biehl, J.P. & Nimitz, H.J. (1954) Studies on the use of a high dose of isoniazid. *American Review of Tuberculosis*, **70**, 430.

Biehl, J.P. & Vilter, R.W. (1954) Effects of isoniazid on pyridoxine metabolism. *Journal of the American Medical Association*, **156**, 1549.

Birket-Smith, E. & Krogh, E. (1971) Motor nerve conduction velocity during diphenylhydantoin intoxication. *Acta Neurologica Scandinavica*, **47**, 265.

Bischoff, A. (1978) Peripheral neuropathy following chloroquine therapy. *4th International Congress on Neuromuscular Diseases*. Montreal: Canada. Abstract 149.

Blessing, W. & Walsh, J.C. (1977) Myotonia precipitated by propranolol therapy. *Lancet*, **1**, 73.

Blomberg, L.H. (1965) Dystrophia myotonica probably caused by chloroquine. *Acta Neurologica Scandinavica*, Suppl. 13, part II, p. 647.

Blomgren, S.E., Condemi, J.J. & Vaughan, J.H. (1972) Procainamide-induced lupus erythematosus. *American Journal of Medicine*, **52**, 338.

Bodley, P.O. & Brett, J.E. (1962) Post-operative respiratory inadequacy and the part played by antibiotics. *Anaesthesia*, **17**, 438.

Bodley, P.O., Halwax, K. & Potts, L. (1969) Low pseudocholinesterase levels complicating treatment with phenelzine. *British Medical Journal*, **3**, 510.

Bond, M.R., Clark, S.D. & Neal, F.E. (1964) Use of ethoglucid in treatment of advanced malignant disease. *British Medical Journal*, **1**, 951.

Booker, H.E., Chun, R.W.M. & Sanguino, M. (1970) Myasthenia gravis syndrome associated with trimethadione. *Journal of the American Medical Association*, **212**, 2262.

Borden, H., Clarke, M.T. & Katz, H. (1974) The use of pancuronium bromide in patients receiving lithium carbonate. *Canadian Anaesthetic Society Journal*, **21**, 79.

Boucher, S.D. & Katz, N.L. (1977) Effects of several 'membrane stabilizing' agents on frog neuromuscular junction. *European Journal of Pharmacology*, **42**, 139.

Bousser, M.G., Bouche, P., Brochard, C. & Herreman, G. (1976) Sept neuropathies peripheriques apres traitment par maleate de perhexiline. *La Nouvelle Presse Médicale*, **5**, 652.

Bovill, J.G., Dundee, J.W., Coppel, D.L. & Moore, J. (1971) Current status of ketamine anaesthesia. *Lancet*, **1**, 1285.

Bradley, W.G. (1970) The neuropathy of vincristine in the guinea pig. An electrophysiological and pathological study. *Journal of the Neurological Sciences*, **10**, 133.

Bradley, W.G. & Hewer, R.L. (1966) Peripheral neuropathy due to disulfiram. *British Medical Journal*, **1**, 449.

Bradley, W.G., Karlsson, I.J. & Rasool, C.G. (1977) Metronidazole neuropathy. *British Medical Journal*, **2**, 610.

Bradley, W.G., Fewings, J.D., Harris, J.B. & Johnson, M.A. (1976) Emetine myopathy in the rat. *British Journal of Pharmacology*, **57**, 29.

Bradley, W.G., Lassman, L.P., Pearce, G.W. & Walton, J.N. (1970) The neuromyopathy of vincristine in man. Clinical, electrophysiological and pathological studies. *Journal of the Neurological Sciences*, **10**, 107.

Bridgeman, J.F., Rosen, A.M. & Thorp, J.M. (1972) Complications during clofibrate treatment of nephrotic syndrome hyperlipoproteinaemia. *Lancet*, **2**, 502.

Brouet, G., Marche, J., Rist, N., Chevallier, J. & Le Meur, G. (1959) Observation on the antituberculous effectiveness of alpha-ethyl-thioisonicotinamide in tuberculosis in humans. *American Review of Tuberculosis*, **79**, 6.

Brumlik, J. & Jacobs, R.S. (1974) Myasthenia gravis associated with diphenylhydantoin therapy for epilepsy. *Canadian Journal of Neurological Sciences*, **1**, 127.

Bruun, E. & Hermann, K. (1942) Polyneuritis after treatment with sulfonamide preparations. *Acta Medica Scandinavica*, **111**, 261.

Buckle, R.M. (1963) Blood pyruvic acid in thalidomide neuropathy. *British Medical Journal*, **2**, 973.

Bucknall, R.C. (1977) Myasthenia associated with D-penicillamine therapy in rheumatoid arthritis. *Proceedings of the Royal Society of Medicine*, **70** (Supp. 3), 114.

Casey, E.B., Jellife, A.M., Le Quesne, P.M. & Millett, Y.L. (1973) Vincristine neuropathy, clinical and electrophysiological observations. *Brain*, **96**, 69.

Chang, C.C. & Chuang, S.T. (1972) Effects of desipramine and imipramine on the nerve, muscle and synaptic transmission of rat diaphragms. *Neuropharmacology*, **11**, 777.

Chasapakis, G. & Dimas, C. (1966) Possible interaction between muscle relaxants and the kallikrein-trypsin inactivator Trasylol. *British Journal of Anaesthesia*, **38**, 838.

Clarke, R.S.J., Dundee, J.W. & Hamilton, R.C. (1967) Interaction between induction agents and muscle relaxants. *Anaesthesia*, **22**, 235.

Cogen, F.C., Rigg, G., Simmons, J.L. & Domino, E.F. (1978) Phencyclidine-associated acute rhabdomyolysis. *Annals of Internal Medicine*, **88**, 210.

Cohen, L. (1972) CPK test—Effect of intramuscular injection in myocardial infarction. *Journal of the American Medical Association*, **219**, 625.

Cohen, M.M. (1970) Toxic neuropathies. In *Handbook of Clinical Neurology*, Vol. 7, Eds P.J. Vinken & G.W. Bruyn, p. 527 (North Holland: Amsterdam).

Collard, P.J. & Hargreaves, W.H. (1947) Neuropathy after stilbamidine treatment of kala-azar. *Lancet*, **2**, 686.

Collier, G. & Martin, A. (1960) Les effects secondaires du tofranil. Revue générale a propos de trois cas de polynévrite des membres inferieurs. *Annales Medico-psychologiques*, **118**, 719.

Coomes, E.N. (1965a) Corticosteroid myopathy. *Annals of Rheumatic Diseases*, **24**, 465.

Coomes, E.N. (1965b) The rate of recovery of reversible myopathies and the effects of anabolic agents.

Neurology (Minneapolis), **15**, 523.

Coxon, A. & Pallis, C.A. (1976) Metronidazole neuropathy. *Journal of Neurology, Neurosurgery and Psychiatry*, **39**, 403.

Crawford, A.C. (1975) Lithium ions and the release of transmitter at the frog neuromuscular junction. *Journal of Physiology*, **246**, 109.

Crile, G. (1947) Treatment of hyperthyroidism. *Canadian Medical Association Journal*, **57**, 359.

Cucher, B.G. & Goldman, A.L. (1976) D-penicillamine-induced polymyositis in rheumatoid arthritis. *Annals of Internal Medicine*, **85**, 615.

Davies, D.M. (1968) *Adverse Drug Reaction Bulletin*, **9**, 19.

Dawkins, K.D. & Gibson, J. (1978) Peripheral neuropathy with disopyramide. *Lancet*, **1**, 329.

Delrieu, F., Menkes, C.J., Sainte-Croix, A., Babinet, P., Chesneau, A.M. & Delbarre, F. (1976) Myasthenie et thyroidite auto-immune au cours du traitement de la polyarthrite rhumatoide par la D-penicillamine. *Annales Medicine Interne*, **127**, 739.

Denborough, M.A. (1977) Malignant hyperpyrexia. *Medical Journal of Australia*, **2**, 757.

Denborough, M.A., Dennett, X. & Anderson, R. McD. (1973) Central-core disease and malignant hyperpyrexia. *British Medical Journal*, **1**, 272.

Desmedt, J.E. (1973) The neuromuscular disorder in myastenia gravis. In *New Developments in Electromyography and Clinical Neurophysiology*, Ed. J.E. Desmedt, Vol. 1, p. 305 (Karger: Basel).

Dhaliwal, G.S., Schlagenhauff, R.E. & Megahed, S.M. (1976) Acute femoral neuropathy induced by oral anticoagulation. *Diseases of the Nervous System*, **37**, 539.

Djaldetti, M., Pinkhas, J., De Vries, A., Kott, E., Joshua, H. & Dollberg, L. (1968) Myasthenia gravis in a patient with chronic myeloid leukemia treated by busulfan. *Blood*, **32**, 336.

Doyle, J.B. & Cannon, E.F. (1950) Severe polyneuritis following gold therapy for rheumatoid arthritis. *Annals of Internal Medicine*, **33**, 1468.

Drachman, D.A. & Skom, J.H. (1965) Procainamide—a hazard in myasthenia gravis. *Archives of Neurology*, **13**, 316.

Drachman, D.B. (1962) Myasthenia gravis and the thyriod gland. *New England Journal of Medicine*, **266**, 330.

Dretchen, K.L., Sokoll, M.D., Gergis, S.D. & Long, J.P. (1973) Relative effects of streptomycin on motor nerve terminal and endplate. *European Journal of Pharmacology*, **22**, 10.

Drutz, D.J., Fan, J.H., Tai, T.Y., Cheng, J.T. & Hsieh, W.C. (1970) Hypokalaemic rhabdomyolysis and myoglobinuria following amphotericin B therapy. *Journal of the American Medical Association*, **211**, 824.

Duane, D.D. & Engel, A.G. (1970) Emetine myopathy. *Neurology (Minneapolis)*, **20**, 733.

Dubois, E.L. (1969) Procainamide induction of a systemic lupus erythematosus-like syndrome. *Medicine (Baltimore)*, **48**, 217.

Duignan, N., Andrews, J. & Williams, J.D. (1973) Pharmacological studies with lincomycin in late pregnancy. *British Medical Journal*, **3**, 75.

Dukes, M.N.G. (1977) *Side Effects of Drugs*; Annual 1, pp. 118, 181, 292, 331, 339 (Excerpta Medica: Amsterdam).

Eade, O.E., Acheson, E.D., Cuthbert, M.F. & Hawkes, C.H. (1975) Peripheral neuropathy and indomethacin. *British Medical Journal*, **2**, 66.

Eisen, A.A., Woods, J.F. & Sherwin, A.L. (1974) Peripheral nerve function in long-term therapy with diphenylhydantoin. *Neurology (Minneapolis)*, **24**, 411.

Elder, B.F., Beal, H., DeWald, W. & Cobb, S. (1971) Exacerbation of subclinical myasthenia by occupational exposure to an anesthetic. *Anesthesia and Analgesia Current Researches*, **50**, 383.

Ellenberg, M. (1959) Diabetic neuropathy precipitated by diabetic control with tolbutamide. *Journal of the American Medical Assocition*, **169**, 1755.

Ellis, F.G. (1962) Acute polyneuritis after nitrofurantoin therapy. *Lancet*, **2**, 1136.

Ellis, F.R., Clarke, I.M.C., Modgill, M., Currie, S. & Harriman, D.G.F. (1975) Evaluation of creatine phosphokinase in screening patients for malignant hyperpyrexia. *British Medical Journal*, **3**, 511.

Ellis, F.R., Keaney, N.P., Harriman, D.G.F., Sumner, D.W., Kyei-Mensah, K., Tyrrell, J.H., Hargreaves, J.B., Parikh, R.K. & Mulrooney, P.L. (1972) Screening for malignant hyperpyrexia. *British Medical Journal*, **3**, 559.

Elmqvist, D. & Josefsson, J.O. (1962) The nature of the neuromuscular block produced by neomycin. *Acta Physiologica Scandinavica*, **54**, 105.

Endtz, L.J. (1958) Complications nerveuses du traitement aurique. *Revue Neurologique*, **99**, 395.

Eng, G.D., Epstein, B.S., Engel, W.K., McKay, D.W. & McKay, R. (1978) Malignant hyperthermia and central core disease in a child with congenital dislocating hips. *Archives of Neurology*, **35**, 189.

Engel, A.G. (1961) Thyroid function and myasthenia gravis. *Archives of Neurology*, **4**, 663.

Epstein, F.W. & Bohm, M. (1976) Dapsone-induced peripheral neuropathy. *Archives of Dermatology*, **112**, 1761.

Falkson, G., van Dyk, J.J., van Eden, E.B., van der Merwe, A.M., van der Bergh, J.A. & Falkson, H.C. (1975) A clinical trial of the oral form of 4′-demethyl-epipodophyllotoxin-β-D ethylidene glucoside (NSC 141540) VP 16-213. *Cancer*, **35**, 1141.

Feldman, S.A. & Crawley, B.E. (1970) Interaction of diazepam with the muscle-relaxant drugs. *British Medical Journal*, **2**, 336.

Fernandes, L., Swinson, D.R. & Hamilton, E.B.D. (1977) Dermatomyositis complicating penicillamine treatment. *Annals of Rheumatic Diseases*, **36**, 94.

Fewings, J.D., Burns, R.J. & Kakulas, B.A. (1973) A case of acute emetine myopathy. In *Clinical Studies in Myology*, Ed. B.A. Kakulas, p. 594 (Exerpta Medica: Amsterdam).

Finke, J. & Spiegelberg, U. (1973) Polyneuropathy nach methaqualone. *Nervenarzt*, **44**, 104.

Finkelman, I. & Arieff, A.J. (1942) Untoward effects of phenytoin sodium in epilepsy. *Journal of the American Medical Association*, **118**, 1209.

Florence, A.L. (1960) Is thalidomide to blame? *British Medical Journal*, **2**, 1954.

Fogdall, R.P. & Miller, R.D. (1974) Prolongation of pancuronium induced neuromuscular block by clindamycin. *Anesthesiology*, **41**, 407.

Fraser, D.M., Campbell, I.W. & Miller, H.C. (1977) Peripheral and autonomic neuropathy after treatment with perhexiline maleate. *British Medical Journal*, **2**, 75.

Frawley, T.F. & Koeppe, G.F. (1950) Neurotoxicity due to thiouracil and thiourea derivatives. *Journal of Clinical Endocrinology*, **10**, 623.

Fredericks, E.J., Kugelman, T.P. & Kirsch, N. (1976) Dapsone-induced motor polyneuropathy

Archives of Dermatology, **112**, 1158.

Fullerton, P.M. & Kremer, M. (1961) Neuropathy after intake of thalidomide (Distaval). *British Medical Journal*, **2**, 855.

Fullerton, P.M. & O'Sullivan, D.J. (1968) Thalidomide neuropathy: a clinical, electrophysiological, and histological follow-up study. *Journal of Neurology, Neurosurgery and Psychiatry*, **31**, 543.

Gabriel, R. & Pearce, J.M.S. (1976) Clofibrate-induced myopathy and neuropathy. *Lancet*, **2**, 906.

Galzigna, L., Manani, G., Mammano, S., Gasparetto, A. & Deana, R. (1972) Experimental study on the neuromuscular blocking action of procain amide. *Agressologie*, **13**, 107.

Gammon, G.D., Burge, F.W. & King, G. (1953) Neural toxicity in tuberculous patients treated with isoniazid (isonicotinic acid hydrazine). *Archives of Neurology and Psychiatry*, **70**, 64.

Gardner-Thorpe, C. & Benjamin, S. (1971) Peripheral neuropathy after disulfiram administration. *Journal of Neurology, Neurosurgery and Psychiatry*, **34**, 253.

Gehlmann, L.K., Koller, W.C. & Malkinson, F.D. (1977) Dapsone-induced neuropathy. *Archives of Dermatology*, **113**, 845.

Geraud, G., Caussanel, J.P., Jauzac, P.H., Arbus, L. & Bes, A. (1978) Peripheral neuropathy after perhexiline maleate therapy. *4th International Congress on Neuromuscular Diseases*. Montreal: Canada. Abstract 81.

Gesztes, T. (1966) Prolonged apnoea after suxamethonium injection associated with eye drops containing an anticholinesterase agent. *British Journal of Anaesthesia*, **38**, 408.

Ghose, K. (1977) Lithium salts: therapeutic and unwanted effects. *British Journal of Hospital Medicine*, **18**, 578.

Gibbels, E. (1967) Weitere beobachtungen zur nebenwirkung intravenöser reverin-gaben bei myasthenia gravis pseudoparalytica. *Deutsche Medizinische Wochenschrift*, **92**, 1153.

Gibbs, J.M. (1978) A case of rhabdomyolysis associated with suxamethonium. *Anaesthesia and Intensive Care*, **6**, 141.

Gissen, A.J., Karis, J.H. & Nastuk, W.L. (1966) Effect of halothane on neuromuscular transmission. *Journal of the American Medical Association*, **197**, 116.

Golding, D.N. & Begg, T.B. (1960) Dexamethasone myopathy. *British Medical Journal*, **2**, 1129.

Gourie-Devi, M. (1978) Effect of clioquinol on peripheral nerves in humans in Delhi—an electrophysiological study. *4th International Congress on Neuromuscular Diseases*. Montreal: Canada. Abstract 85.

Granacher, R.P. (1977) Neuromuscular problems associated with lithium. *American Journal of Psychiatry*, **134**, 702.

Greenblatt, D.J. & Allen, D. (1978) Intramuscular injection-site complications. *Journal of the American Medical Association*, **240**, 542.

Grongono, A.W. (1963) Anaesthesia for atrial defibrillation. Effects of quinidine on muscular relaxation. *Lancet*, **2**, 1039.

Gross, E.G., Dexter, J.D. & Roth, R.G. (1966) Hypokalemic myopathy with myoglobinuria associated with licorice ingestion. *New England Journal of Medicine*, **274**, 602.

Grossman, R.A., Hamilton, R.W., Morse, B.M., Penn, A.S. & Goldberg, M. (1974) Nontraumatic rhabdomyolysis and acute renal failure. *New England Journal of Medicine*, **291**, 807.

Haas, D.C. & Marasigan, A. (1968) Neurological effects of glutethimide. *Journal of Neurology, Neurosurgery and Psychiatry*, **31**, 561.

Haber, R.W. & Joseph, M. (1962) Neurological manifestations after amphotericin B therapy. *British Medical Journal*, **1**, 230.

Hagen, R. (1968) Contracture of the quadriceps muscle. A report of 12 cases. *Acta Orthopaedica Scandinavica*, **39**, 565.

Hall, L.W., Woolf, N., Bradley, J.W.P. & Jolly, D.W. (1966) Unusual reaction to suxamethonium chloride. *British Medical Journal*, **2**, 1305.

Hallman, B.L. & Hurst, J.W. (1953) Loss of taste as a toxic effect of methimazole (Tapazole) therapy: report of three cases. *Journal of the American Medical Association*, **152**, 322.

Harriman, D.G.F., Sumner, D.W. & Ellis, F.R. (1973) Malignant hyperpyrexia myopathy. *Quarterly Journal of Medicine*, **42**, 639.

Hartfall, S.J., Garland, H.G. & Goldie, W. (1937) Gold treatment of arthritis. A review of 900 cases. *Lancet*, **2**, 838.

Hayman, M. & Wilkins, P.A. (1956) Polyneuropathy as a complication of disulfiram therapy of alcoholism. *Quarterary Journal of Studies in Alcohol*, **17**, 601.

Herishanu, Y. & Rosenberg, P. (1975) β-blockers and myasthenia gravis. *Annals of Internal Medicine*, **83**, 834.

Herishanu, Y. & Taustein, I. (1971) The electromyographic changes induced by antibiotics. A preliminary study. *Confinia Neurologica*, **33**, 41.

Hicklin, J.A. (1968) Chloroquine neuromyopathy. *Annals of Physical Medicine*, **9**, 189.

Hildebrand, J. & Coërs, S. (1965) Etude clinique, histologique et électrophysiologique des neuropathies associées au traitement par la vincristine. *European Journal of Cancer*, **1**, 51.

Hill, G., Wong, K.C. & Hodges, M.R. (1976) Potentiation of succinylcholine neuromuscular blockage by lithium carbonate. *Anesthesiology*, **44**, 439.

Hoaken, P.C.S. (1975) Adverse effect of methaqualone. *Canadian Medical Association Journal*, **112**, 685.

Hodges, R.J.H., Bennett, J.R. & Tunstall, M.E. (1959) Effects of oxytocin on the response to suxamethonium. *British Medical Journal*, **1**, 413.

Hokkanen, E. (1964) The aggravating effect of some antibiotics on the neuromuscular blockade in myasthenia gravis. *Acta Neurologica Scandinavica*, **40**, 346.

Hopf, H.C. (1968) Effect of diphenylhydantoin on peripheral nerves in man. *Electroencephalography and Clinical Neurophysiology*, **25**, 411.

Horton, B.T. & Peters, G.A. (1963) Clinical manifestations of excessive use of ergotamine preparation and management of withdrawal effect. Report of 52 cases. *Headache*, **2**, 214.

Hughes, H.B., Biehl, J.P., Jones, A.P. & Schmidt, L.H. (1954) Metabolism of isoniazid in man as related to the occurrence of peripheral neuritis. *American Review of Tuberculosis*, **70**, 266.

Hughes, R.O. & Zacharias, F.J. (1976) Myasthenic syndrome during treatment with practolol. *British Medical Journal*, **1**, 460.

Ince, W.E. (1962) Peripheral neuropathy following chlorpropamide. *British Journal of Clinical Practice*, **16**, 607.

Ingham, H.R., Selkon, J.B. & Hale, J.H. (1975) The antibacterial activity of metronidazole. *Journal of*

Antimicrobial Chemotherapy, **1**, 355.

Isaacs, A.D. & Carlish, S. (1963) Peripheral neuropathy after amitriptyline. *British Medical Journal*, **1**, 1739.

Jaffe, I.A., Altman, K. & Merryman, P. (1964) Antipyridoxine effect of penicillamine in man. *Journal of Clinical Investigation*, **43**, 1869.

Janssen, P.J. (1960) Peripheral neuritis due to streptomycin. *American Review of Respiratory Diseases*, **81**, 726.

Jennings, G., Jones, M.B.S., Besterman, E.M.M., Model, D.G., Turner, P.P. & Kidner, P.H. (1976) Oral disopyramide in prophylaxis of arrhythmias following myocardial infarction. *Lancet*, **1**, 51.

Jensen, O.B., Mosdal, C. & Reske-Nielsen, E. (1977) Hypokalaemic myopathy during treatment with diuretics. *Acta Neurologica Scandinavica*, **55**, 465.

Joy, R.J.T. & Scalettar, R. (1960) Optic and peripheral neuritis, probable effect of prolonged chloramphenicol therapy. *Journal of the American Medical Association*, **173**, 1731.

Jui-Yen, T. (1971) Clinical and experimental studies on mechanisms of neuromuscular blockade by chloroquine cliorotate. *Japanese Journal of Anesthesia*, **20**, 491.

Kaplan, A.M., Bergeson, P.S., Gregg, S.A. & Curless, R.G. (1977) Malignant hyperthermia associated with myopathy and normal muscle enzymes. *Journal of Pediatrics*, **91**, 431.

Katz, B. (1966) *Nerve, Muscle and Synapse* (McGraw-Hill: New York).

Katz, B. & Miledi, R. (1965) Propagation of electric activity in motor nerve terminals. *Proceedings of the Royal Society*, B, **161**, 453.

Kennedy, R.D. & Galindo, A.D. (1975) Comparative site of action of various anaesthetic agents at the mammalian myoneural junction. *British Journal of Anaesthesia*, **47**, 533.

King, J.O. & Denborough, M.A. (1973a) Malignant hyperpyrexia in Australia and New Zealand. *Medical Journal of Australia*, **1**, 525.

King, J.O. & Denborough, M.A. (1973b) Anesthetic-induced malignant hyperpyrexia in children. *Journal of Pediatrics*, **83**, 37.

King, J.O., Denborough, M.A. & Zapf, P.W. (1972) Inheritance of malignant hyperpyrexia. *Lancet*, **1**, 365.

Kirkendall, W.M. & Page, E.B. (1958) Polyneuritis occurring during hydralazine therapy. *Journal of the American Medical Association*, **167**, 427.

Klatskin, G. & Friedman, H. (1948) Emetine toxicity in man: studies on the nature of early toxic manifestations, their relation to the dose level, and their significance in determining safe dosage. *Annals of Internal Medicine*, **28**, 892.

Klinghardt, G.W. (1965) Ein Beitrag der experimentellen Neuropathologie zur Toxizitätsprüfung neuer chemotherapeutica. *Mitteilungen Max-Planck-Gesellschaft*, **3**, 142.

Klinghardt, G.W. (1967) Schadigungen des nervensystems durch nitrofurane bei der ratte. *Acta Neuropathologica (Berlin)*, **9**, 18.

Knape, H. (1977) In *Side Effects of Drugs*, Ed. M.N.G. Dukes. Vol. I, p. 103 (Excerpta Medica: Amsterdam).

Koelle, G.B. (1975) Neuromuscular blocking agents. In *The Pharmocological Basis of Therapeutics*, 5th ed. Eds L.S. Goodman & A. Gilman, p. 577 (Macmillan: New York).

Kolb, L.C. & Gray, S.J. (1946) Peripheral neuritis as a complication of penicillin therapy. *Journal of the American Medical Association*, **132**, 323.

Kono, R. (1971) Subacute myelo-optico-neuropathy, a new neurological disease prevailing in Japan. *Japanese Journal of Medical Science and Biology*, **24**, 195.

Kornfeld, P., Horowitz, S.H., Genkins, G. & Papatestas, A.E. (1976) Myasthenia gravis unmasked by antiarrhythmic agents. *Mount Sinai Journal of Medicine*, **43**, 10.

Korsan-Bengsten, K., Ysander, L., Blohme, G. & Tibblin, E. (1969) Extensive muscle necrosis after long-term treatment with amino-caproic acid (EACA) in a case of hereditary periodic oedema. *Acta Medica Scandinavica*, **185**, 341.

Koski, C.L., Rifenberick, D.H. & Max, S.R. (1974) Oxidative metabolism of skeletal muscle in steroid atrophy. *Archives of Neurology*, **31**, 407.

Kunze, K., Noelle, H. & Prüll, G. (1967) Untersuchungen uber die wirkung and vertraglisch von methaqualone bei neurologischen Krankheiten. *Arneimittel-Forsch Drug Research*, **17**, 1052.

Lane, R.J.M. & Mastaglia, F.L. (1978) Drug-induced myopathies in man. *Lancet*, **2**, 562.

Lane, R.J.M., McLelland, N.J., Martin, A.M. & Mastaglia, F.L. (1979) Epsilon aminocaproic acid (EACA) myopathy. *Postgraduate Medical Journal*, **55**, 282.

Langman, M.J.S. (1975) Gastrointestinal drugs. In *Meyler's Side-Effects of Drugs*, Ed. M.N.G. Dukes, Vol. 8, p. 795 (Excerpta Medica: Amsterdam).

Larsen, A. (1978) On the neuromuscular effects of pindolol and sotalol in the rat. *Acta Physiologica Scandinavica*, **102**, 35.

Leck, I.M. & Millar, E.L.M. (1962) Incidence of malformation since the introduction of thalidomide. *British Medical Journal*, **1**, 16.

Leibold, J.E. (1966) The ocular toxicity of ethambutol and its relation to dose. *Annals of the New York Academy of Sciences*, **135**, 904.

Leibold, J.E. (1971) Drugs having a toxic effect on the optic nerve. *International Ophthalmological Clinic*, **11**, 137.

Le Quesne, P.M. (1970) Iatrogenic neuropathies. In *Handbook of Clinical Neurology*, Eds P.J. Vinken & G.W. Bruyn, pp. 527–551 (North Holland: Amsterdam).

Le Quesne, P.M. (1975) Neuropathy due to drugs. In *Peripheral Neuropathy*, Eds P.J. Dyck, P.K. Thomas & E.H. Lambert, pp. 1263–1280 (Saunders: Philadelphia).

Lermer, H., Avni, J. & Bruderman, I. (1970) Neuromuscular blocking action of amitriptyline. *European Journal of Pharmacology*, **13**, 266.

Levin, B.E. & Engel, W.K. (1975) Iatrogenic muscle fibrosis. Arm levitation as an initial sign. *Journal of the American Medical Association*, **234**, 621.

Leys, D. (1945) Hyperthyroidism treated with methylthiouracil. *Lancet*, **1**, 461.

Lhermitte, F., Fardeau, M., Chedru, F. & Mallecourt, J. (1976) Polyneuropathy after perhexiline maleate therapy. *British Medical Journal*, **1**, 1256.

Lindesmith, L.A., Baines, R.D., Bigelow, D.B. & Petty, T.L. (1968) Reversible respiratory paralysis associated with polymyxin therapy. *Annals of Internal Medicine*, **68**, 318.

Lindholm, T. (1967) Electromyographic changes after nitrofurantoin (Furadantin) therapy in nonuremic patients. *Neurology (Minneapolis)*, **17**, 1017.

Lingle, F.A. (1966) Irreversible effects of glutethimide addiction. *Journal of Psychiatry*, **123**, 349.

Lithell, H., Boberg, J., Hellsing, K., Lundqvist, G. &

Vessby, B. (1978) Increase in the lipoprotein-lipase activity in human skeletal muscle during clofibrate administration. *European Journal of Clinical Investigation*, **8**, 67.

Loder, R.E. & Walker, G.F. (1959) Neuromuscular-blocking action of streptomycin. *Lancet*, **1**, 812.

Loftus, L.R. (1963) Peripheral neuropathy following chloroquine therapy. *Canadian Medical Association Journal*, **89**, 917.

Lovelace, R.E. & Horwitz, S.J. (1968) Peripheral neuropathy in long-term diphenylhydantoin therapy. *Archives of Neurology*, **18**, 69.

MacDonald, R.D. & Engel, A.G. (1970) Experimental chloroquine myopathy. *Journal of Neuropathology and Experimental Neurology*, **29**, 479.

MacFarlane, I.A. & Rosenthal, F.D. (1977) Severe myopathy after status asthmaticus. *Lancet*, **2**, 615.

Manani, G., Gasparetto, A., Bettini, V., Caldesi Valeri, V. & Galzigna, G.L. (1970) Mechanism of action of ajmaline on neuromuscular junction. *Agressologie*, **11**, 275.

Mandel, W. (1959) Pyridoxine and the isoniazid induced neuropathy. *Diseases of the Chest*, **36**, 293.

Manten, A. (1975) Antibiotic drugs. In *Meyler's Side Effects of Drugs*, Ed. M.N.G. Dukes, Vol. 8, p. 610 (Excerpta Medica: Amsterdam).

Markes, P. & Sloggen, J. (1976) Peripheral neuropathy caused by methaqualone. *American Journal of the Medical Sciences*, **272**, 323.

Marmor, A., Alpan, G., Keider, S., Grenadier, E. & Palant, A. (1978) The MB isoenzyme of creatine kinase as an indicator of severity of myocardial infarction. *Lancet*, **2**, 812.

Mastaglia, F.L., Gardner-Medwin, D. & Hudgson, P. (1971) Muscle fibrosis and contractures in a pethidine addict. *British Medical Journal*, **4**, 532.

Mastaglia, F.L., Papadimitriou, J.M., Dawkins, R.L. & Beveridge, B. (1977) Vacuolar myopathy associated with chloroquine, lupus erythematosus and thymoma. *Journal of the Neurological Sciences*, **34**, 315.

Masters, C.L., Dawkins, R.L., Zilko, P.J., Simpson, J.A., Leedman, R.J. & Lindstrom, J. (1977) Penicillamine-associated myasthenia gravis, antiacetylcholine receptor and antistriatal antibodies. *American Journal of Medicine*, **63**, 689.

McCormick, D.B. & Snell, E.E. (1959) Pyridoxal kinase of human brain and its inhibition by hydrazine derivatives. *Proceedings of the National Academy of Sciences (U.S.A.)*, **45**, 1371.

McLeod, J.G. & Penny, R. (1969) Vincristine neuropathy: an electrophysiological and histological study. *Journal of Neurology, Neurosurgery and Psychiatry*, **32**, 297.

McQuaker, W. & Bruggen, P. (1963) Side-effects of methaqualone. *British Medical Journal*, **1**, 749.

McQuillen, M.P. & Engbaek, L. (1975) Mechanism of colistin-induced neuromuscular depression. *Archives of Neurology*, **32**, 235.

McQuillen, M.P., Cantor, H.E. & O'Rourke, J.R. (1968) Myasthenic syndrome associated with antibiotics. *Archives of Neurology*, **18**, 402.

McQuillen, M.P., Gross, M. & Johns, R.J. (1963) Chlorpromazine-induced weakness in myasthenia gravis. *Archives of Neurology*, **8**, 286.

Merhoff, G.C. & Porter, J.M. (1974) Ergot intoxication: Historical review and description of unusual clinical manifestation. *Annals of Surgery*, **180**, 773.

Meyboom, R.H.B. (1977) Heavy metal antagonists. In *Side Effects of Drugs*, Ed. M.N.G. Dukes, Vol. I, p. 192 (Excerpta Medica: Amsterdam).

Miller, M. (1963) Neuropathy, agranulocytosis and hepatotoxicity following imipramine therapy. *American Journal of Psychiatry*, **120**, 185.

Mitchell, M.M., Ali, H.H. & Savarese, J.J. (1978) Myotonia and neuromuscular blocking agents. *Anesthesiology*, **49**, 44.

Moddel, G., Bilbao, J.M., Payne, D. & Ashby, P. (1978) Disulfiram neuropathy. *Archives of Neurology*, **35**, 658.

Mohamed, S.D., Chapman, R.S. & Crooks, J. (1966) Hypokalaemia, flaccid quadriparesis, and myoglobinuria with carbenoxolone (Biogastrone). *British Medical Journal*, **1**, 1581.

Morell, F., Bradley, W. & Ptashne, M. (1958) Effect of diphenylhydantoin on peripheral nerve. *Neurology (Minneapolis)*, **8**, 140.

Morley, J.B., Lambert, T.F. & Kakulas, B.A. (1973) A case of hyperpyrexia with myotonia congenita. In *Clinical Studies in Myology*, Ed. B.A. Kakulus, p. 543 (Excerpta Medica: Amsterdam).

Morris, J.S. (1966) Nitrofurantoin and peripheral neuropathy with megaloblastic anemia. *Journal of Neurology, Neurosurgery and Psychiatry*, **29**, 224.

Müller, R. (1945) Polyneuritis following sulfanilamide therapy. *Acta Medica Scandinavica*, **121**, 95.

Mullet, R.D. & Keats, A.S. (1961) Apnea and respiratory insufficiency after intraperitoneal administration of kanamycin. *Surgery*, **49**, 530.

Mussini, J.M., Hauw, J.J. & Escourolle, R. (1977) Etude en microscopie electronique des lesions nerveuses, musculaires et cutanées determinées par le maléate perhexiline. *Acta Neuropathologica (Berlin)*, **38**, 53.

Nakamura, Y. & Inoue, Y.K. (1972) Pathogenicity of virus associated with subacute myelo-neuropathy. *Lancet*, **1**, 223.

Neil, J.F., Himmelhoch, J.M. & Licata, S. (1976) Emergence of myasthenia gravis during treatment with lithium carbonate. *Archives of General Psychiatry*, **33**, 1090.

Nelson, T.E. & Denborough, M.A. (1977) Studies on normal human skeletal muscle in relation to the pathopharmacology of malignant hyperpyrexia. *Clinical and Experimental Pharmacology and Physiology*, **4**, 315.

Newson, A.J. (1972) Malignant hyperthermia: Three case reports. *New England Journal of Medicine*, **75**, 138.

Nick, J., Dudognon, P., Escourolle, R., Bakouche, P., Nicolle, M.H., Reignier, A., Hauw, J.J., Ermidou, S., Pollet, S., Baumann, N., Singlas, E. & Lévy, J. (1978) Manifestations neurologiques en rapport avec le traitement par le maléate de perhexiline. *Revue Neurologique*, **134**, 103.

Nicolas, F., Baron, D., Dixneuf, B., Visset, J. & Dubigeon, P. (1970) Les nécroses musculaires au cours des intoxications aiguës. *Presse Médicale*, **78**, 751.

Noone, P. (1978) Use of antibiotics. Aminoglycosides. *British Medical Journal*, **2**, 549.

Norris, F.H., Colella, J. & McFarlin, D. (1964) Effect of diphenylhydantoin on neuromuscular synapse. *Neurology (Minneapolis)*, **14**, 869.

Nover, R. (1967) Persistent neuropathy following chronic use of glutethimide. *Clinical Pharmacology and Therapeutics*, **8**, 283.

Ochoa, J. (1970) Isoniazid neuropathy in man: Quantitative electron microscope study. *Brain*, **93**, 831.

Onodera, K. & Yamakawa, K. (1966) The effects of lithium on the neuromuscular junction of the frog. *Japanese*

Journal of Physiology, **16**, 541.

Page, P., Morgan, M. & Loh, L. (1972) Ketamine anaesthesia in paediatric procedures. *Acta Anaesthesiologica Scandinavica*, **16**, 155.

Palmer, K.N.V. (1978) Muscle cramp and oral salbutamol. *British Medical Journal*, **3**, 833.

Palmucci, L., Bertolotto, A. & Schiffer, D. (1978) Acute muscle necrosis after chronic overdosage of phenformin and fenfluramine. *Muscle and Nerve*, **1**, 245.

Paul, M.F., Paul, H.E., Kopko, F., Bryson, M.J. & Harrington, C. (1954) Inhibition by furacin of citrate formation in testis preparations. *Journal of Biological Chemistry*, **206**, 491.

Penn, A.S., Rowland, L.P. & Fraser, D.W. (1972) Drugs, coma and myoglobinuria. *Archives of Neurology*, **26**, 336.

Percy, A.K. & Saef, E.C. (1967) An unusual complication of retrograde pyelography: neuromuscular blockade. *Pediatrics*, **39**, 603.

Perkins, R.L. (1964) Apnea with intramuscular colistin therapy. *Journal of the American Medical Association*, **190**, 421.

Perkoff, G.T., Hardy, P. & Velez-Garcia, E. (1966) Reversible acute muscular syndrome in chronic alcoholism. *New England Journal of Medicine*, **274**, 1277.

Perry, H.M. (1973) Late toxicity to hydralazine resembling systemic lupus erythematosus or rheumatoid arthritis. *American Journal of Medicine*, **54**, 58.

Peter, J.B. & Fiehn, W. (1973) Diazacholesterol myotonia: Accumulation of desmosterol and increased adenosine triphosphatase activity of sarcolemma. *Science*, **179**, 910.

Peterson, H.C. (1966) Association of trimethadione therapy and myasthenia gravis. *New England Journal of Medicine*, **274**, 506.

Pierides, A.M., Alvarez-Ude, F., Kerr, D.N.S. & Skillen, A.W. (1975) Clofibrate-induced muscle damage in patients with renal failure. *Lancet*, **2**, 1279.

Pinkerton, H.A. & Munro, J.R. (1964) Respiratory insufficiency associated with the use of streptomycin. *Scottish Medical Journal*, **9**, 256.

Pittinger, C.B., Eryasa, Y. & Adamson, R. (1970) Antibiotic-induced paralysis. *Anesthesia and Analgesia Current Researches*, **49**, 487.

Pokroy, N., Ress, S. & Gregory, M.C. (1977) Clofibrate-induced complications in renal disease. *South African Medical Journal*, **52**, 806.

Pollet, S., Hauw, J.J., Escourolle, R. & Baumann, N. (1977) Peripheral-nerve lipid abnormalities in patients on perhexiline maleate. *Lancet*, **1**, 1258.

Poole, G.W. & Schneeweiss, J. (1961) Peripheral neuropathy due to ethionamide. *American Review of Respiratory Diseases*, **84**, 890.

Prescott, L.F. (1975) Anti-inflammatory analgesics and drugs used in rheumatoid arthritis and gout. In *Meyler's Side Effects of Drugs*. Ed. M.N.G. Dukes, Vol. 8, p. 228 (Excerpta Medica: Amsterdam).

Prickett, C.S. & Johnston, C.D. (1953) The *in vivo* production of carbon disulfide from tetraethyllhiuram disulfide (Antabuse). *Biochimica and Biophysica Acta*, **12**, 542.

Pridgeon, J.E. (1956) Respiratory arrest thought to be due to intraperitoneal neomycin. *Surgery*, **40**, 571.

Proctor, W.R. & Weakly, J.N. (1976) A comparison of the presynaptic and post-synaptic actions of pentobarbitone and phenobarbitone in the neuromuscular junction of the frog. *Journal of Physiology*, **258**, 257.

Ramsay, I.D. (1968) Endocrine ophthalmopathy. *British Medical Journal*, **4**, 706.

Rapoport, A.M. & Guss, S.B. (1972) Dapsone-induced peripheral neuropathy. *Archives of Neurology*, **27**, 184.

Raskin, N.H. & Fishman, R.A. (1965) Pyridoxine-deficiency neuropathy due to hydralazine. *New England Journal of Medicine*, **273**, 1182.

Rasmussen, H. (1970) Cell communication, calcium ion and cyclic adenosine monophosphate. *Science*, **170**, 404.

Ream, C.R. (1963) Respiratory and cardiac arrest after intravenous administration of kanamycin with reversal of toxic effects by neostigmine. *Annals of Internal Medicine*, **59**, 384.

Regan, A.G. & Aldrete, J.A. (1967) Prolonged apnea after administration of promazine hydrochloride following succinylcholine infusion. *Anesthesia and Analgesia Current Researches*, **46**, 315.

Regli, F. & Guggenheim, P. (1965) Myasthenisches syndrom als seltene komplikation unter hydantoinbehandlung. *Nervenartz*, **36**, 315.

Reilly, T.M. (1976) Peripheral neuropathy associated with citrated-calcium carbimide. *Lancet*, **1**, 911.

Richter, R.W., Challenor, Y.B., Pearson, J., Kagen, L.J., Hamilton, L.L. & Ramsey, W.H. (1971) Acute myoglobinuria associated with heroin addiction. *Journal of the American Medical Association*, **216**, 1172.

Robinson, B.F. (1975) Drugs acting on the cardiovascular system. In *Meyler's Side Effects of Drugs*. Ed. M.N.G. Dukes, Vol. 8, p. 447 (Excerpta Medica: Amsterdam).

Robinson, B.F. (1978) Anti-anginal and beta adreno-receptor blocking drugs. In *Meyler's Side Effects of Drugs*. Ed. M.N.G. Dukes, Vol. 2, p. 173 (Excerpta Medica: Amsterdam).

Robinson, R.G. (1959) Leucotrichia totalis from chloroquine. *Medical Journal of Australia*, **2**, 460.

Roldan, E.C. & Nigrin, G. (1972) Peripheral neuritis after methimazole therapy. *New York State Journal of Medicine*, **72**, 2898.

Rubbo, J.T., Gergis, S.D. & Sokoll, M.D. (1977) Comparative neuromuscular effects of lincomycin and clindamycin. *Anesthesia and Analgesia Current Researches*, **56**, 329.

Rubenstein, C.J. (1964) Peripheral neuropathy caused by nitrofurantoin. *Journal of the American Medical Association*, **187**, 647.

Rumpf, K.W., Albers, R. & Scheler, F. (1976) Clofibrate-induced myopathy syndrome. *Lancet*, **1**, 249.

Russell, A.S. & Lindstrom, J.M. (1978) Penicillamine-induced myasthenia gravis associated with antibodies to acetylcholine receptor. *Neurology (Minneapolis)*, **28**, 847.

Russell, J.A. & Powles, R.L. (1974) Neuropathy due to cytosine arabinosine. *British Medical Journal*, **4**, 652.

Said, G. (1978) Perhexiline neuropathy: A clinicopathological study. *Annals of Neurology*, **3**, 259.

Salako, L.A. (1970) Inhibition of neuromuscular transmission in the intact rat by emetine. *Journal of Pharmaceutics and Pharmacology*, **22**, 69.

Samuelson, R.J., Giesecke, A.H., Kallus, F.T. & Stanley, V.F. (1975) Lincomycin-curare interaction. *Anesthesia and Analgesia Current Researches*, **54**, 103.

Sandler, R.M. & Gonsalkorale, M. (1977) Chronic lymphatic leukemia, chlorambucil, and sensorimotor peripheral neuropathy. *British Medical Journal*, **2**, 1265.

Saquenton, A.C., Lorinz, A.L., Vick, N.A. & Hamer, R.D. (1969) Dapsone and peripheral motor neuropathy. *Archives* of *Dermatology*, **100**, 214.

Satoyoshi, E. & Wakata, N. (1978) Chloramphenicol neuropathy and vitamin B_{12} deficiency. *International Congress on Neuromuscular Diseases*. Montreal, Canada. Abstract 89.

Saunders, F.P., Hoefnagel, D. & Staples, O.S. (1965) Progressive fibrosis of the quadriceps muscle. *Journal of Bone and Joint Surgery*, **47A**, 380.

Schmidt, J.L., Vick, N.A. & Sadove, M.S. (1963) The effect of quinidine on the action of muscle relaxants. *Journal of the American Medical Association*, **183**, 669.

Schochet, S.S., Usar, M.C. & Lampert, P.W. (1968) Neuronal changes induced by intrathecal vincristine sulfate. *Journal of Neuropathology and Experimental Neurology*, **27**, 645.

Scholes, D.M. (1960) Pelvic perfusion with nitrogen mustard for cancer: a neurological complication. *American Journal of Obstetrics and Gynecology*, **80**, 481.

Schraeder, P.L., Peters, H.A. & Dahl, D.S. (1972) Polymyositis and penicillamine. *Archives of Neurology*, **27**, 456.

Sebille, A. (1978) Prevalence of latent perhexiline neuropathy. *British Medical Journal*, **1**, 1321.

Seitz, D., Hopf, H.C., Janzen, R.C.W. & Meyer, W. (1976) Penicillamin induzierte myasthenie bei chronischer polyarthritis. *Deutsche Medizinische Wochenschrift*, **101**, 1153.

Selby, G. (1972) Subacute myelo-optic neuropathy in Australia. *Lancet*, **1**, 123.

Shibuya, N., Mori, K. & Nakazawa, Y. (1978) Serum factor blocks neuromuscular transmission in myasthenia gravis: electrophysiologic study with intracellular microelectrodes. *Neurology (Minneapolis)*, **28**, 804.

Shoji, S. & Pennington, R.J.T. (1977a) Binding of dexamethasone and cortisol to cytosol receptors in rat extensor digitorum longus and soleus muscles. *Experimental Neurology*, **57**, 342.

Shoji, S. & Pennington, R.J.T. (1977b) The effect of cortisone on protein breakdown and synthesis in rat skeletal muscle. *Molecular and Cellular Endocrinology*, **6**, 159.

Shoji, S., Takagi, A., Sugita, H. & Toyokura, Y. (1974) Muscle glycogen metabolism in steroid-induced myopathy of rabbits. *Experimental Neurology*, **45**, 1.

Skau, K.A. & Gerald, M.C. (1978) Curare-like effects of the amphetamine isomers on neuromuscular transmission. *Neuropharmacology*, **17**, 271.

Snapper, I. (1947) Stilbamidine and pentamidine in multiple myeloma. *Journal of the American Medical Association*, **133**, 157.

Sobue, I., Ando, K., Iida, M., Takayanagi, T., Yamamura, Y. & Matsuoka, Y. (1971) Myeloneuropathy with abdominal disorders in Japan. *Neurology (Minneapolis)*, **21**, 168.

Sokoll, M.D., Gergis, S.D., Post, E.L., Cronnelly, R. & Long, J.P. (1974) Effects of droperidol on neuromuscular transmission and muscle membrane. *European Journal of Pharmacology*, **28**, 209.

Somers, J.E. & Winer, N. (1966) Reversible myopathy and myotonia following administration of a hypocholesterolaemic agent. *Neurology (Minneapolis)*, **16**, 761.

Stafford, C.R., Bogdanoff, B.M., Green, L. & Spector, H.B. (1975) Mononeuropathy multiplex as a complication of amphetamine angiitis. *Neurology (Minneapolis)*, **25**, 570.

Stålberg, E., Schiller, H.H. & Schwartz, M.S. (1975) Safety factor in single human motor end-plates studied *in vivo* with single fibre electromyography. *Journal of Neurology, Neurosurgery and Psychiatry*, **38**, 799.

Steiner, J.C., Winkelman, A.C. & De Jesus, P.V. (1973) Pentazocine-induced myopathy. *Archives of Neurology* **28**, 408.

Steiness, E., Rasmussen, F., Svendsen, O. & Nielsen, P. (1978) A comparative study of serum creatine phosphokinase (CPK) activity in rabbits, pigs and humans after intramuscular injection of local damaging drugs. *Acta Pharmacologica et Toxicologica*, **42**, 357.

Tamaki, M. (1978) The effect of streptomycin on the neuromuscular junction of the frog. *4th International Congress on Neuromuscular Diseases*. Montreal: Canada. Abstract 48.

Teräväinen, H., Larsen, A. & Hillbom, M. (1977) Clofibrate-induced myopathy in the rat. *Acta Neuropathologica (Berlin)*, **39**, 135.

Toman, J.E.P. (1949) The neuropharmacology of antiepileptics. *Electroencephalography and Clinical Neurophysiology*, **17**, 314.

Tomlinson, I.W. & Rosenthal, F.D. (1977) Proximal myopathy after perhexiline maleate treatment. *British Medical Journal*, **2**, 1319.

Toole, J.F. & Parrish, M.L. (1973) Nitrofurantoin polyneuropathy. *Neurology (Minneapolis)*, **23**, 554.

Toole, J.F., Gergen, J.A., Hayes, D.M. & Felts, J.H. (1968) Neural effects of nitrofurantoin. *Archives of Neurology* **18**, 680.

Tsubaki, T., Honma, Y. & Hoshi, M. (1971) Neurological syndrome associated with clioquinol. *Lancet*, **1**, 696.

Tugwell, P. & James, S.L. (1972) Peripheral neuropathy with ethambutol. *Postgraduate Medical Journal*, **48**, 667.

Ursing, B. & Kamme, C. (1975) Metronidazole for Crohn's disease. *Lancet*, **1**, 775.

Usubiaga, J.E., Wikinski, J.A., Morales, R.L. & Usubiaga, L.E.J. (1967) Interaction of intravenously administered procaine, lidocaine and succinylcholine in anesthetized subjects. *Anesthesia and Analgesia Current Researches*, **46**, 39.

Utz, J.P., Louria, D.B., Feder, N., Emmons, C.W. & McCullough, N.B. (1957) A report of clinical studies on the use of amphotericin in patients with systemic fungal diseases. *Antibiotics Annals*, **65**.

Vartanian, G.A. & Chinyanga, H.M. (1972) The mechanism of acute neuromuscular weakness induced by chloroquine. *Canadian Journal of Physiology and Pharmacology*, **50**, 1099.

Vigliani, E.C. (1954) Carbon disulphide poisoning in viscose rayon factories. *British Journal of Industrial Medicine*, **11**, 235.

Vincent, A., Newsom Davis, J. & Martin, V. (1978) Anti-acetylcholine receptor antibodies in D-penicillamine-associated myasthenia gravis. *Lancet*, **1**, 1254.

Viswanath, D.V. & Jenkins, H.J. (1978) Neuromuscular block of the polymyxin group of antibiotics. *Journal of Pharmaceutical Sciences*, **67**, 1275.

Volden, G. (1977) Peripheral neuropathy: A side-effect of sulphones. *British Medical Journal*, **1**, 1193.

Wade, A. (1977) *Martindale—The Extra Pharmacopoeia*. 27th Edn. p. 1295 (The Pharmaceutical Press: London).

Walsh, J.C. (1970) Gold neuropathy. *Neurology (Minneapolis)*, **20**, 455.

Walton, J.N. (1977) *Brain's Diseases of the Nervous System*, 8th Edn., p. 1032 (Oxford University Press: Oxford).

Warner, W.A. & Sanders, E. (1971) Neuromuscular blockage associated with gentamycin therapy. *Journal of the American Medical Association*, **215**, 1153.

Warot, P., Goudemand, M. & Habay, D. (1965) Troubles neurologiques provoques par les alcaloides de Vinca rosea (la polynevrite de la pervenche). *Revue Neurologique*, **113**, 464.

Watkins, S.M. & Griffin, J.P. (1978) High incidence of vincristine-induced neuropathy in lymphomas. *British Medical Journal*, **1**, 610.

Watland, D.C., Long, J.P., Pittinger, C.B. & Cullen, S.C. (1957) Neuromuscular effects of ether, cyclopropane, chloroform and fluothane. *Anesthesiology*, **18**, 883.

Wattel, F., Chopin, C., Durocher, A. & Berzin, B. (1978) Rhabdomylyses au cours des intoxications aiguës. *La Nouvelle Presse Médicale*, **7**, 2253.

Watters, G., Karpati, G. & Kaplan, B. (1977) Post-anesthetic augmentation of muscle damage as a presenting sign in three patients with Duchenne muscular dystrophy. *Canadian Journal of Neurological Sciences*, **4**, 228.

Way, W.L., Katzung, B.G. & Larson, C.P. (1967) Recurarization with quinidine. *Journal of the American Medical Association*, **200**, 163.

Weinstein, L., Madoff, M.A. & Samet, C.M. (1974) The sulfonamides. *New England Journal of Medicine*, **291**, 793.

Weiss, H.D., Walker, M.D. & Wiernik, P.H. (1974) Neurotoxicity of commonly used antineoplastic agents. *New England Journal of Medicine*, **291**, 127.

Werman, R. & Wislicki, L. (1971) Propranolol, a curariform and cholinomimetic agent at the frog neuromuscular junction. *Comparative General Pharmacology*, **2**, 69.

Weisman, S.J. (1949) Masked myasthenia gravis. *Journal of the American Medical Association*, **141**, 917.

Westbury, G. (1962) Treatment of advanced cancer by extracorporeal perfusion and continuous intra-arterial infusion. *Proceedings of the Royal Society of Medicine*, **55**, 643.

Whisnant, J.P., Espinosa, R.E., Kierland, R.R. & Lambert, E.H. (1963) Chloroquine neuromyopathy. *Proceedings of the Mayo Clinic*, **38**, 501.

Williams, C.H., Hoech, G.P. & Roberts, J.T. (1978)

Experimental malignant hyperthermia. *Anesthesiology*, **49**, 58.

Williams, R.S. (1959) Triamcinoline myopathy. *Lancet*, **1**, 698.

Winer, N., Klachko, D.M., Baer, R.D., Langley, P.L. & Burns, T.W. (1966) Myotonic response induced by inhibitors of cholesterol biosynthesis. *Science*, **153**, 312.

Wolf, S., Goldberg, L.S. & Verity, A. (1976) Neuromyopathy and periarteriolitis in a patient receiving levadopa. *Archives of Internal Medicine*, **136**, 1055.

Wright, J.M. & Collier, B. (1976a) The site of the neuromuscular block produced by polymyxin B and rolitetracycline. *Canadian Journal of Physiology and Pharmacology*, **54**, 937.

Wright, J.M. & Collier, B. (1976b) Characterization of the neuromuscular block produced by clindamycin and lincomycin. *Canadian Journal of Physiology and Pharmacology*, **54**, 937.

Wullen, F., Kast, G. & Bruck, A. (1967) Uber nebenwirkungen bei tetracyclinverabreichung an myastheniker. *Deutsche Medizinische Wochenschrift*, **92**, 667.

Wyatt, E.H. & Stevens, C. (1972) Dapsone induced peripheral neuropathy. *British Journal of Dermatology*, **86**, 521.

Yaari, Y., Pincus, J.H. & Argov, Z. (1977) Depression of synaptic transmission by diphenlyhydantoin. *Annals of Neurology*, **1**, 334.

Yaari, Y., Pincus, J.H. & Argov, Z. (1979) Phenytoin and transmitter release at the neuromuscular junction of the frog. *Brain Research*, **160**, 479.

Yates, D.A.H. (1970) Steroid myopathy. In *Muscle Diseases*. Eds J.N. Walton, N. Canal & G. Scarlato, p. 482 (Excerpta Medica: Amsterdam).

Young, W.A. & Tudhope, G.R. (1926) The pathology of prolonged emetine administration. *Transactions of the Royal Society of Tropical Medicine and Hygiene*, **20**, 93.

Zaunder, H.L., Barton, N., Benetts, E.J. & Lore, J. (1966) Colistimethate as a cause of post-operative apnoea. *Canadian Anaesthetic Society Journal*, **13**, 607.

Neuromuscular stimulation and transmission

INTRODUCTION

Neuromuscular stimulation refers to techniques whereby electrical impulses are delivered to peripheral nerves and the action potentials generated in muscles supplied by such nerves are recorded. Repetitive nerve stimulation has been used for a long time in the study of myasthenia gravis. The technique has certain pitfalls and its value is considered to be limited; in consequence, it is often omitted in routine electrodiagnosis. It is, however, of value not only in distinguishing different types of myasthenic disorder, some of which are not evident upon clinical assessment, but also in showing changes in other neuromuscular disorders where concentric needle electromyography may be unhelpful. Initially, some of the earlier methods of studying neuromuscular stimulation will be described.

The conduction of the nerve impulse and the subsequent contraction of muscle are associated with changes in membrane polarity which can be measured accurately by electrical methods. Similarly, nerve and muscle are excitable by electric currents and the study of the excitability response was the earliest technique of electrodiagnosis to be used in clinical practice. The use of stimulation techniques to study the state of innervation of the lower motor neurone dates back to the late nineteenth century, when Erb (1883) described the faradic–galvanic test. Together with this test, the polar formula, voltage capacity curves and the changes in chronaxie with denervation and reinnervation became widely employed as aids to clinical diagnosis. The many peripheral nerve injuries in the 1939–1945 war demanded more sensitive techniques and with the advent of accurate electronic stimulators, strength–duration (SD) curves gradually supplanted the faradic–galvanic test in the specialist centres. However, it was Adrian (1916) who first demonstrated the value of SD curves in clinical practice and published serial curves showing the changes which occur in denervation and reinnervation. While SD curves were being developed, many workers experimented with allied techniques, including strength–frequency and strength–interval curves, and the response of nerve and muscle to progressive currents.

The advent of electromyography and, later, of methods of measuring nerve conduction velocity, have diverted interest from these methods of neuromuscular stimulation. Indeed, many workers in electrodiagnosis no longer use SD curves, while others use abbreviated methods. But we believe that there is still a place for the use of SD curves and simple tests of nerve conduction. Hence the various techniques still in use will be reviewed critically, their value in modern electrodiagnosis will be examined and an attempt will be made to place them in perspective by suggesting which are of value in routine electrodiagnosis.

OLDER TECHNIQUES

Faradic–galvanic test

In early editions of this book, this test was described in detail. Its inadequacies have at last been appreciated and it is no longer, or very rarely used.

Physiotherapists in Great Britain are still taught the rationale and technique of SD curves and variable pulse stimulators are available in modern departments. However, the plotting of SD curves is useful enough in routine practice to make it advisable for electrophysiologists also to master the technique, which is simple and quickly learnt.

Voltage capacity curves, strength–interval curves, strength–frequency curves and measurements of accommodation are all now obsolete and will not be described.

Rheobase

The rheobase of a tissue is defined as the amount of current passing for infinite duration, required to cause a minimal detectable response. For practical purposes, infinite duration is taken to be any value of 100 ms or more.

In denervated muscle, the rheobase represents the excitability threshold of muscle tissue, while in normally innervated muscle the rheobase represents the excitability threshold of the intramuscular nerve fibres. The rheobase varies for different muscles. Facial muscles have a low rheobase (1–2 volts), proximal limb muscles average 30 volts, and the small muscles of the hand 40–60 volts. Although changes in rheobase value occur with changes in the innervation of muscle—falling in denervation and rising with reinnervation, it is now known that these are too variable to be of any diagnostic value (Wynn Parry, 1953).

Chronaxie

This is a measure of excitability, defined as the

minimum time required to excite the tissue with a stimulus twice the rheobase. In the past, chronaximeters were used to assess changes in innervation. Chronaxie of muscle is long—about 10 ms—while that for nerve is short (0.06 ms) and a change from long to short was taken to herald recovery while lengthening of chronaxie indicated degeneration.

It is now known that chronaxie is too variable to be a reliable guide, being dependent on many factors such as temperature, blood supply, skin resistance and oedema (Harris, 1962). Low values may be present when the full SD curve indicates an element of denervation (see Fig. 26.2).

STRENGTH–DURATION CURVES

Rationale

This method allows the expression of the characteristic excitability response of the tissue under test, in graphical form.

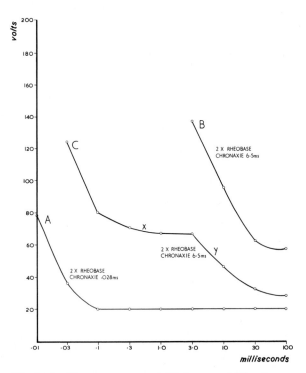

Fig. 26.1 SD curves on normal (A) denervated (B) and partially denervated (C) muscle. In curve (C) that part of the curve marked X represents the response of normally innervated fibres and that part marked Y the response of denervated fibres. The curve thus expresses the ratio of denervated to innervated fibres

A long-duration square wave electrical impulse of instantaneous rise time is applied to the muscle under test and the amount of current (or voltage) required to elicit minimal contraction (rheobase) is measured and expressed in milliamps or volts. The duration of the impulse is progressively shortened and the intensity of current required to produce minimal contraction is measured for each duration. A curve relating strength of current and duration of impulse can now be drawn. In normally innervated muscle the intensity of current for minimal contraction is the same over a wide range of pulse durations and has to be increased only when very short pulse durations are used. This is because of the greater excitability of nerve which has a short chronaxie (0.06 ms or less for constant-voltage stimulators). When muscle alone is being stimulated (i.e. denervated muscle) the curve is no longer a horizontal straight line but a steeply rising parabola and no response is elicited at the shorter pulse durations. This is attributable to the much lower excitability of muscle compared with that of nerve (chronaxie 3 ms or more). In partially innervated muscle the curve is broken, showing elements of both excitable tissues—muscle and nerve. This break is known as a kink or a discontinuity. Figure 26.1 shows the three curves of normal, denervated and partially innervated muscle.

It can be seen from Figure 26.1 that the excitability curve of muscle is the same shape as that of nerve, but is shifted to the right. If the muscle curve were prolonged to the right it would be horizontal, as the point obtained by using a pulse of 100 ms duration is, by definition, the rheobase and represents the threshold of the tissue.

Mathematically, the shape of the SD curve is described by the following formula (Katz, 1939):

$$\frac{I}{I_o} = \frac{1}{(1 - e^{-t/k})}$$

where I = intensity of pulse
t = duration of pulse
I_o = rheobase
k = constant (time factor)
e = 2.178

The double curve of partial innervation cannot as easily be expressed mathematically.

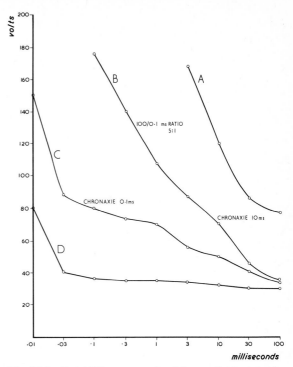

Fig. 26.2 Serial SD curves on the abductor digiti minimi in a patient with a recovering nerve lesion. Curve (A) 3 months after suture at the wrist—complete denervation. Curve (B) 3 weeks later—a kink in the curve indicates regeneration—clinically no contraction was detectable. Curve (C) 6 weeks later—an obvious double curve indicating further reinnervation. Curve (D) 2 months later—the curve is almost normal

The earliest signs of reinnervation are, first, a kink in a previously steeply rising curve, and second, the appearance of more points on the curve, giving a shift of the curve to the left. As reinnervation progresses so the kink broadens, the curve moves further to the left and the slope becomes less steep (Fig. 26.2), provided that regeneration proceeds satisfactorily. Should recovery be halted, then the curve will show no change at repeated intervals. In progressive denervation the curve will show gradually increasing abnormality with the appearance of kinks, a rise in slope and a shift to the right (Fig. 26.3).

As mentioned above, Adrian (1916) was the first to describe the use of SD curves in patients with polyneuritis and peripheral nerve lesions. Discontinuities were seen in the recovering stage and these appeared with longer pulse durations as recovery progressed. At this time there was much debate on the nature of the double curve of partial

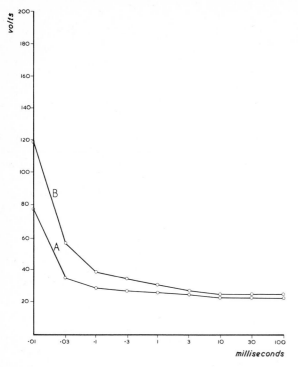

Fig. 26.3 SD curves on right abductor pollicis brevis in a patient with symptoms of a carpal tunnel syndrome. Curve (A) 4 weeks after onset of symptoms indicating mild denervation. Curve (B) 3 weeks later showing progressive denervation

However, 27 per cent of patients showed voluntary contraction before discontinuities were seen. It now seems that they used stimulators with an insufficient number of pulse durations and also that they disregarded slight discontinuities. Modern stimulators are so accurate that, provided the operator is experienced and the technique good, even minor changes are significant.

The accuracy of this technique is well illustrated when comparing curves on muscles which remain in the same state of innervation over many months or years. Figure 26.4 shows curves recorded at an interval of 9 months on the same muscle in a patient with poliomyelitis. As already indicated, the shape of the curve is all-important and will give a rough idea of the amount of denervation present, because the SD curve is an expression of the ratio of denervated to innervated fibres.

Some workers use an abbreviated test in which the responses to pulses of 100 ms and of 1 ms duration are measured and the ratio of the current required to produce contraction with the shorter pulse to that needed with the larger one is innervation. Adrian suggested that either this was due to the fact that there were two groups of muscle fibres in different stages of recovery, or else it indicated different effects of the current on normal and denervated muscle. In 1930 Rushton performed his classical experiments on frog muscle and described the alpha and gamma excitabilities which Keith Lucas had mentioned 20 years earlier. Two years later he was able to prove that the alpha excitability was isochronous (i.e. having the same time relations) with muscle and corresponded to the right-hand portion of the double curve, while the gamma excitability was isochronous with nerve and corresponded to the left-hand portion of the double curve.

The first detailed report of the use of SD curves in nerve injuries was made by Pollock, Golseth and Arieff (1944) who showed that discontinuities in the curve preceded recovery by many weeks. Newman and Livingstone (1974) found that in 54 per cent of patients, such discontinuities preceded clinical recovery by an average time of 97 days.

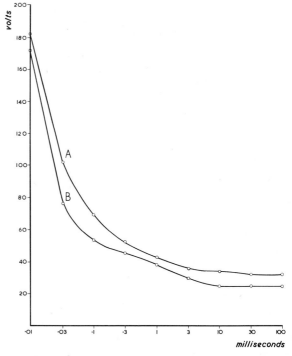

Fig. 26.4 Two curves at 6-month intervals on the right quadriceps in a patient with poliomyelitis, showing virtually no change

calculated. Clearly, if this ratio is unity the curve is flat, and will be that of normally innervated muscle. If the ratio is high (4 or more) then the curve will be the steep one of denervation. Intermediate values suggest partial innervation. Although theoretically attractive, this technique is liable to error and it is possible to have ratios suggestive of denervation when the full curve shows undoubted signs of reinnervation. Similarly, the ratio may be low, suggesting normality, when the curve shows a definite kink. Amick and Hickey (1959) investigated the 1–100 ms ratios in a series of normal, partially innervated and denervated muscles and compared their results with those obtained by doing full SD curves using both constant-current and constant-voltage stimulators and also with the findings of electromyography (EMG). In normal muscle, the ratio was always lower than 2.2, but some partially denervated muscles gave similar ratios. No denervated muscle had a ratio below 2.5 and it was usually much higher. Taking the ratio 2 as the significant level with a constant-current stimulator, 5 per cent of normally innervated muscle gave figures outside normal limits, while 8 per cent of partially denervated muscles would be considered normal. Using the constant-voltage stimulator, 3 per cent of normal muscle would be regarded as denervated and 7 per cent of muscles showing partial denervation would be regarded as normal. Harris (1962) put the whole position admirably when he stated: 'The kind of cases in which electrodiagnostic tests are of greatest value are those with minimal or partial denervation and in such cases the abbreviated technique has an undesirably high error'.

Fallacies

The SD curve will show only the state of innervation of the fibres stimulated. In small muscles such as the intrinsics of the hand, the curve is likely to give a true picture of the state of the whole muscle. However, in a very large one such as quadriceps, glutei or hamstrings, the superficial fibres which are most easy to stimulate may be in a different state of innervation from the deeper ones and the SD curve will not, therefore, give a true indication of the state of the whole muscle.

In motor neurone disease a muscle may be severely wasted and weak and yet the SD curve can be surprisingly normal. In the same case the EMG may show little or no fibrillation. It seems that this occurs in states of chronic denervation when denervated fibres are incorporated into a surviving motor unit, being reinnervated and 'adopted' by sprouts from normal axons. Thus there are few denervated muscle fibres left to give their characteristic electrical response in the SD curve or in the EMG.

Technique

The muscle under examination must be well lit and warm. The skin should be clean but elaborate precautions to lower skin resistance are not needed. Experiments on various methods of lowering skin resistance were carried out by Wynn Parry (1962) and showed that since the maximum difference in threshold of curves before and after lowering skin resistance was 10 volts, this question need cause no concern.

Two techniques, unipolar and bipolar, are available. In the unipolar method a large electrode is placed, either behind the neck and upper back when testing arm muscles, or behind the lumbar spine when testing lower limb muscles; a small active electrode is used to stimulate the muscle. In the bipolar technique, two similar electrodes are used and are placed on either side of, and equidistant from, the 'motor point' of the muscle to be tested. In both techniques the active electrodes must be kept moist. With the unipolar technique, the active electrode is placed over the motor point. A convenient diameter for active electrodes is 1 cm. The rheobase is first determined with the 100 ms pulse by observing by eye the voltage at which the minimum response occurs. When muscles insert by easily palpable tendons such as, for example, the dorsiflexors of the foot, movement of the tendon may be felt and this can help to determine the end-point.

As soon as the rheobase has been determined, the pulse selector switch is turned to the next shortest pulse duration, and the amount of current required for minimal contraction is again determined. This is repeated for each pulse duration down to the 0.01 ms pulse or as far as a response can be elicited. With practice, a curve should take no more than a few minutes to obtain.

Choice of apparatus

There are two main types of apparatus available. One is the constant-current stimulator, in which the current is stabilised for a wide range of voltage, and the other is the constant-voltage stimulator, in which the voltage is stabilised for a wide range of current. The constant-voltage stimulator should have an output impedance at maximum output of less than 500 ohms. The constant-current stimulator should have an output impedance of more than 100 000 ohms. The only difference in design between the two stimulators is in the output circuit. The effect of the stimulus output from these two stimulators in the tissues is different (Brennand, 1959).

However, in practice both stimulators give identical shapes for the SD curve, the main difference being that the curve for the constant-voltage stimulator is shifted to the left and the chronaxie of both nerve and muscle is much shorter. Full details of the recommended design of these two types of stimulator are given in the MRC Nerve Injuries Committee Report (1958).

The choice of stimulator will be governed by the experience and training of the operator. Those who have had much experience with one stimulator will not readily change to the other. In general, however, the constant-voltage stimulator is preferred, because it is more comfortable for the patient and a larger number of points are obtained on the curve. Whatever type of stimulator is used, nine pulse durations are necessary, namely 100, 30, 10, 3, 1, 0.3, 0.1, 0.03 and 0.01 ms. The output should give a maximum of 200 volts for constant-voltage stimulators and 50 milliamps for constant-current stimulators. The apparatus should be checked at frequent intervals because component failures may not be obvious in practice and false curves may be obtained without the operator realising that the fault lies in the stimulator.

Appraisal

The SD curve offers a simple, reliable, quick and cheap method of assessing the state of innervation of the muscle and it is a reliable method of detecting slight signs of denervation; the presence of a kink or discontinuity in the curve is the salient feature. Trojaborg (1962) showed that there is a good correlation between abnormalities in SD curves and reduced conduction velocity in neuropathies. The SD curves were normal in over two-thirds of 44 patients in whom conduction velocity was normal. He pointed out that in some partial traumatic lesions the fast-conducting motor fibres may survive, giving a normal conduction latency, yet the SD curve is clearly abnormal. Moody (1965) in a study of carcinomatous neuromyopathy stated 'In the present study an abnormal SD curve was always associated with slowed motor conduction in the nerve to the muscle and in every case in which motor conduction was reduced, there was an abnormality in the SD curve; this correlation suggests that all the large diameter fast-conducting fibres of the nerve are affected early in the disorder.' He concluded that the SD curve is a rapid and accurate method of detecting early denervation in patients with malignant neoplasms.

It is, however, possible that in a large muscle, the superficial fibres may be normally innervated and deep fibres may show abnormality, in which case the EMG may reveal fibrillation or abnormalities of conduction velocity. Thus a normal curve in a large muscle, such as the quadriceps, may not preclude denervation in the deeper parts of the muscle, though an abnormal SD curve in the superficial fibres clearly indicates denervation. The same remarks apply to the detection of the earliest signs of reinnervation. Despite this difficulty, the time lag between the appearance of nascent polyphasic ('recovery') units in the EMG and a kink in an SD curve previously typical of total denervation is usually only 10–14 days and unless there is urgent need to settle the issue, either for medicolegal reasons or because surgical treatment is proposed, electromyography is not always necessary in the routine follow-up of peripheral nerve injuries. The SD curve is a fairly accurate and quick means of assessing the proportion of denervated to innervated fibres and can be used as a guide to the severity of denervation; it can also be helpful in following the progress of a case when serial curves are plotted. This is particularly useful when a rapid survey of many muscles is required, as in a brachial plexus palsy with multiple root or cord involvement, or in diffuse weakness due to polyneuropathy, when multiple EMG needling may be both painful and unnecessary.

Clinical application

It must be emphasised that SD curves offer information only on the presence or absence of denervation and an approximate index of its extent. They give no guide to the localisation of the lesion. This can be obtained only from a study of the type and amount of motor unit activity observed in the EMG and from a consideration of conduction velocities in the peripheral nerves at various levels. It may therefore be unnecessary to plot SD curves in a case where there is obvious wasting and weakness and the problem is to determine the level of the lesion in the lower motor neurone or the site of compression of a peripheral nerve.

In young children, it is better to study the EMG first and only subsequently to plot an SD curve, as the procedure may be distressing and general anaesthesia may be necessary in the very young. On the other hand, if serial examinations are likely to be made, it is often better to plot SD curves as they afford a more reliable method of comparing the state of innervation of a muscle over a period of time.

There are some situations in which examining the response of muscle to nerve conduction and plotting SD curves are all that are required and in which EMG adds nothing of value. Some examples may help to illustrate this fundamental point.

Facial palsy. Most cases of facial palsy referred for electrodiagnosis are cases of Bell's palsy seen within a few days of the onset. The problem is to be able to give an opinion as soon as possible as to whether the lesion is neurapraxial, in which case full recovery will take place in a few days or weeks, or whether nerve fibre degeneration has occurred, in which case the prognosis is less good. Fibrillation potentials are not often detectable in facial muscles before 10 days after the onset and it is on their detection that the EMG diagnosis of denervation depends. Moreover, the detection of fibrillation potentials merely means that some

fibres have degenerated, not necessarily all. In fact, it is rare to find a pure neurapraxial lesion—if careful SD curves and EMG studies are made in patients with facial palsy, most will be found eventually to show mild abnormalities of the curve and some fibrillation. However, such mild electrical abnormalities are consistent with rapid recovery and complete clinical normality. Thus the EMG may suggest a falsely bad prognosis. The retention of nerve conduction in the facial nerve and a normal SD curve, however, give clear evidence that little or no degeneration has occurred and a good prognosis can be given. Collier (1959) showed that complete paralysis without degeneration can persist for up to 11 weeks with retention of nerve excitability. The critical point is, at what time interval can the prognosis be accurately established? Campbell, Hickey, Nixon and Richardson (1962) showed that if nerve excitability is retained at 72 h after the onset, the prognosis is excellent. Moldaver (1964), Taverner (1965) and Laumanns (1965) also confirmed the value of studies of nerve excitability and of the SD curve in cases of facial palsy, but the latter author drew attention to the development of late denervation in some cases. Similarly, King and Wynn Parry (1977) found that, in a small proportion of patients with Bell's palsy, conduction may be retained for some days yet denervation can develop later—as much as 10 days after onset in some cases. It is therefore wise to repeat conduction studies and SD curves at intervals up to 3 weeks after paralysis develops in order not to miss those few patients who show late denervation. These authors also showed that surgical decompression of the facial nerve in such cases led to a better functional result than in those treated conservatively. Therefore, electrical studies can be most helpful in long-term management.

In assessing reinnervation after a degenerative lesion, SD curves show kinks long before nerve excitability returns and within a few days of the development of typical EMG signs; here again, therefore, electromyography is rarely necessary. Later, when enough time has lapsed for reinnervation to be well advanced, it occasionally happens that the SD curves may be nearly normal, yet clinical function is poor. Ritchie (1944) cautioned against attempts to equate improvement in the SD curve with functional recovery in cases of facial palsy. Cross-innervation and mass movements are complicating features peculiar to this nerve. Thus the SD curve will be a reliable guide to the situation at 7 days, but is less reliable at 3 days after the onset, when nerve conduction tests will be the most valuable diagnostic aid.

Assessment of peripheral nerve lesions. Although SD curves offer a reliable method of assessing the extent of a peripheral nerve injury, if the question of exploratory surgery is at stake, it is wise to carry out electromyography as well, because a few surviving motor units indicate at least partial continuity of the nerve, which may not respond in an SD curve or to nerve stimulation. In the case of an extensive lesion, such as a brachial plexus palsy, excitability tests are of great value. Oedema, pain and stiffness in the early stages all make the clinical assessment of a brachial plexus lesion extremely difficult. SD curves carried out on a muscle supplied by each root will show whether the lesion is partial or complete and will also indicate its extent.

Electromyography often adds little, except possibly in the case of deep muscles, in which motor unit potentials may be detected when the response of superficial fibres suggests a complete lesion.

Hysteria. In a suspected hysterical palsy, the detection of a normal SD curve and normal excitability responses in the presence of paralysis without wasting will be conclusive. Electromyography will not reveal motor units, as volitional activity will be absent; the absence of fibrillation is too unreliable and negative a piece of evidence to be of value.

NERVE CONDUCTION

This refers to the technique of stimulating peripheral nerves at accessible points by a short-duration (1 ms) pulse and observing the muscular response. This should be the first investigation in electrodiagnosis and failure to carry it out may lead to serious error. The most obvious reason is to determine if there is anomalous innervation. For instance, 20 per cent of all normal subjects show deviations from the text-book description of innervation of the intrinsic muscles of the hand. The opponens is frequently supplied by the ulnar nerve, the flexor pollicis brevis either by the ulnar nerve entirely or the median nerve entirely, while the third lumbrical may be supplied by the median nerve or the second by the ulnar nerve. In a suspected median or ulnar nerve lesion it is thus important to determine the anatomical distribution in order not to confuse an unusual pattern of motor supply with a partial nerve lesion.

In a neurapraxial lesion, stimulation below the site of the block may result in muscle contraction, whereas stimulation above the block will not; this both establishes the temporary nature of the lesion and determines its level.

This technique is particularly valuable in facial palsy, as discussed fully above. In some cases, a session of facial nerve stimulation will result in some return of voluntary power so that the technique can have some limited therapeutic value.

One of the earliest signs of neurological disturbance is an increase in threshold to the response of nerve to stimulation, and serial comparisons between the threshold on the affected and on the normal side can be helpful in indicating progress.

In a brachial plexus lesion, stimulation at Erb's point in the anterior triangle of the neck will show which muscles contract, and will therefore afford a quick survey of the extent of the lesion. In multiple injuries, when several peripheral nerves are suspected of being damaged at different levels in the limbs, conduction studies will soon reveal the various sites of damage and indicate which further procedures, such as SD curves and electromyography, should be used.

Conduction studies will speedily reveal the normality of nerve behaviour in patients with hysterical palsies.

It must, however, be remembered that in reinnervation, nerve conduction may not return until well after recovery of voluntary movement and significant changes in strength duration curves and in the EMG findings. Although the loss of conduction or an increase in threshold is a sensitive index of denervation, the regenerating nerve apparently has a much higher threshold to artificial electrical stimulation than to a voluntary impulse; this is frequently seen in regenerating facial nerves. No reliance should therefore be placed on nerve conduction as an index of reinnervation, the SD curve and the EMG being the methods of choice.

Thus stimulation techniques still have definite indications, and it is a mistake to believe that electromyography has entirely superseded their use. It would be a pity if the considerable information they offer simply and quickly were to be ignored for the sake of a few minutes' extra effort.

REPETITIVE STIMULATION TECHNIQUES

Site

The study requires stimulation of an accessible peripheral nerve with immobilisation of both the stimulating electrode and of the limb used. Isometric contraction of the relevant muscle must be guaranteed by mechanical fixation.

In the upper limb, a satisfactory stimulus site is the ulnar nerve at the wrist, recordings being made from the abductor digiti minimi. The median nerve is accessible to stimulation but the prevention of movement of the thumb, with consequent distortion of the muscle action potential (MAP) recording, requires more elaborate fixation. Where myasthenia gravis is suspected, stimulation and recording from a more proximal site may be desirable (Ozdemir and Young, 1971). In the lower limb, the anterior tibial nerve may be stimulated at the ankle and recording made from the extensor digitorum brevis.

Using ulnar nerve stimulation as an example of the technique, the arm is immobilised on a splint to which the fingers are strapped or otherwise held firm. An earth electrode is placed between the stimulating and recording sites.

Stimulation

The stimulating equipment must be capable of generating trains of electrical stimuli of variable duration, of which the pulse frequency, intensity and width can also be varied. A pulse width of 0.2 ms is usually satisfactory.

A suitable type of stimulating electrode is that used by Harvey and Masland (1941). A frame encircles the wrist, the anode, a silver–silver chloride plate measuring 5 × 2 cm being attached to the dorsal aspect of this frame. The cathode, a silver–silver chloride rod with a rounded tip of 5 mm diameter, can be moved freely over the wrist until the optimal site for stimulation is found, the site at which the lowest stimulus intensity evokes the entire MAP. The stimulator is then as close as possible to the underlying nerve and in this position is attached to the volar aspect of the frame.

Failure to locate this stimulating site accurately will result in the use of an unduly high stimulus intensity to guarantee that all fibres in the underlying nerve are, in fact, being stimulated. During rapid repetitive stimulation, slight movement of the wrist in relation to the stimulating electrode is inevitable. For this reason the stimulus intensity should be increased to 150 per cent of that required to evoke the entire MAP. Such stimulation is unpleasant and, if a high stimulus intensity is required, it may be difficult for the patient to tolerate. It is for this reason that the initial accurate localisation of the optimal site is so crucial.

Preliminary abrasion by scratching the skin with a needle and cleansing with spirit will improve conductance and lower slightly the stimulus intensity required. Should marked obesity or hyperkeratosis necessitate the use of a high stimulus, intensity, needle stimulating electrodes may be needed. Slomic, Rosenfalck and Buchthal (1968) used stainless steel needles coated with teflon except for the 3 mm at the tip, inserted 25 mm apart along the ulnar nerve at the wrist with the cathode distal. Alternatively, proximal local anaesthetic block may be used. However, as there is a slight risk of nerve injury, this is not recommended routinely.

Recording

Surface electrodes are preferable to intramuscular needle electrodes because they record the response of the entire muscle (compound MAP). Silver disc electrodes 1 cm in diameter are satisfactory, one situated over the belly of the abductor digiti minimi and the other as a reference electrode at the base of the fifth finger. Slomic *et al.* (1968)

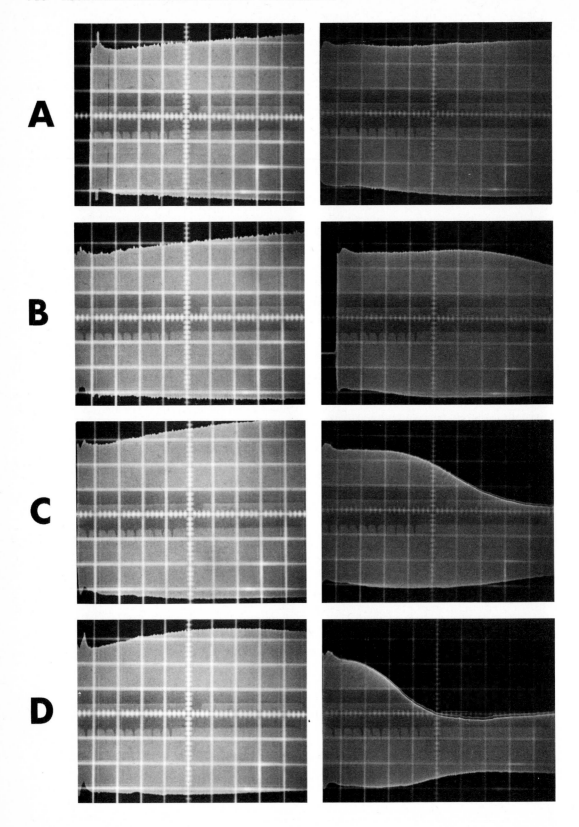

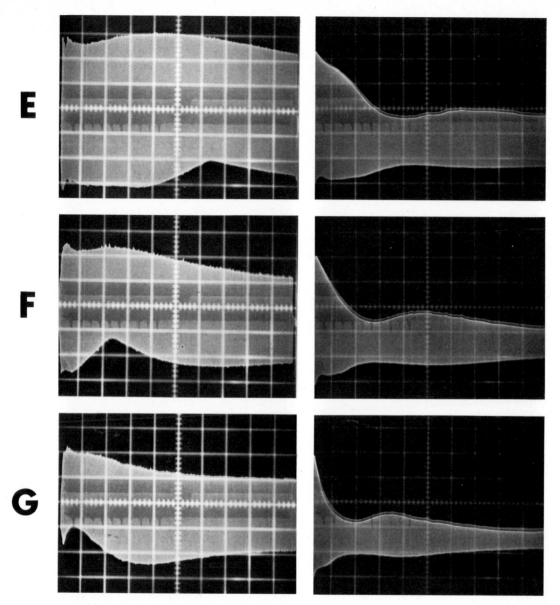

Fig. 26.5 Compound action potential of abductor digiti minimi muscle evoked by rapid repetitive stimulation of the ulnar nerve at stimulus frequencies of A, 40 Hz; B, 50 Hz; C, 60 Hz; D, 70 Hz; E, 80 Hz; F, 90 Hz; and G, 100 Hz. At each frequency, the recording on the left is from a normal subject and that on the right from a subject where disuse of the hand and arm have resulted from a painful shoulder.

preferred subcutaneous recording electrodes because they produce less artefact. After suitable amplification, the MAP is displayed on a storage oscilloscope, the sweep of which is triggered by the stimulating unit.

A series of stimulus frequencies should be used, because different frequencies may be required to reveal different abnormalities. In many instances, stimulation for a long as 10 s may be required before changes in MAP amplitude are seen. The precise technique employed will, however, depend upon the clinical problem (Table 26.1).

During stimulation at rapid rates, there is shortening of the muscle fibres and improved synchronisation. A shorter action potential results and thus the peak-to-peak amplitude increases. This does not represent an increase in the overall MAP. This change may be fallaciously interpreted as indicating such growth of the MAP, unless potentials are superimposed on the oscilloscope so that changes in duration and shape may also be noted. However, after the recording of such a train of superimposed potentials, neither the sequence of changes nor their rate will be apparent and, if a permanent record is required, then the potentials

Table 26.1. Suggested techniques which may be used in the clinical study of neuromuscular transmission

Procedure	Remarks
Evoke single MAP by ulnar nerve stimulation as described in text.	Substantially reduced in the Eaton–Lambert syndrome, antibiotic-induced weakness or particularly severe myasthenia gravis.
Deliver 10 s stimulus trains at frequencies of 1, 3, 10 and 30 per s.	Changes in generalised myasthenia gravis (Fig. 26.6) likely only if limb is weak but invariable in Eaton–Lambert syndrome (Fig. 26.7).
Evoke MAP before and after 10 s of voluntary effort.	Slight decline or no change in myasthenia gravis. Marked growth in Eaton–Lambert syndrome.
Evoke MAP before and after 2 s of tetanic nerve stimulation.	Post-tetanic facilitation in myasthenia gravis if the limb is weak and in the Eaton–Lambert syndrome.
Deliver stimulus trains after repeated tetanisation or voluntary effort.	May bring out latent defect in myasthenia gravis.
Deliver stimulus trains with limb rendered ischaemic.	
Look for staircase phenomenon using mechanical responses.	Present in normal subjects. Usually absent in myasthenia gravis.
Compare MAP before and after 10 mg of edrophonium	Growth of MAP usual in myasthenia gravis and the Eaton–Lambert syndrome.
Record from other (more proximal) sites.	Movement artefact difficulties arise but may show with ulnar nerve stimulation in myasthenia gravis.

must also be recorded sequentially with a slow sweep speed (*see* Fig. 26.7).

In addition to observing the effect of an anticholinesterase drug such as edrophonium upon the evoked MAP, a competitive neuromuscular blocking agent, such as D-tubocurarine may be used. While the systemic use of such a drug is hazardous, regional techniques, temporarily isolating the circulation to a hand and forearm, may enable neuromuscular stimulation to reveal alterations in neuromuscular transmission not evident using conventional methods (Brown, Charlton and White, 1975; Brown and Charlton, 1975a; Brown and Charlton, 1975b).

Finally, techniques recording single muscle fibre action potentials (Eksedt, 1964) and the measurement of the 'jitter' phenomenon, provide a more sensitive method of revealing disordered neuromuscular transmission (*see* Ch. 29) than do most repetitive stimulation techniques.

NORMAL SUBJECTS

Harvey and Masland (1941) noted that the MAP of normal subjects showed little change in size or character during stimulation at frequencies below 50 Hz. Above this rate, there is usually a slow progressive decline in the size of the response. The duration of the stimulus train is important: Simpson (1966) noted a 50 per cent decline in amplitude after stimulating at 50 Hz for 30 s.

At 60 Hz this decline rarely commences before some 7 s of stimulation, an indication of the remarkable functional reserve of neuromuscular transmission, because the frequency of depolarisation of the motor nerve during voluntary effort is only about half this rate. As the stimulus frequently is increased above 60 Hz, the decrement in MAP response starts earlier and is more profound. Even when allowance is made for muscle shortening, in the majority of normal subjects there is a transient increase in MAP amplitude during stimulation between 20 and 40 Hz.

In many systemic and neuromuscular disorders, a decline in evoked MAP amplitude occurs with stimulus frequencies lower than 60 Hz. Even disuse results in the decline in MAP amplitude occurring at slower stimulus frequencies than in healthy normal subjects (Fig. 26.5). At slow stimulus rates, this change in amplitude is usually indicative of a defect of neuromuscular transmission. At more rapid rates, muscle or nerve fibre latency may also be determining factors.

MYASTHENIC DISORDERS

Myasthenia gravis

The decline in evoked MAP amplitude during repetitive nerve stimulation in subjects with myasthenia gravis was studied by Harvey and Masland (1941); the techniques and observations have since been elaborated by Johns, Grob and Harvey (1955; 1956), Simpson and Lenman (1959), Preswick (1965), Simpson (1966) and Slomic *et al.* (1968).

Botelho, Deaterly, Austin and Comroe (1952) pointed out that the characteristic changes could be shown only in a proportion of myasthenic muscles tested, usually where they are clinically weak. Thus, a normal response may occur in the apparently unaffected muscle of a patient with myasthenia gravis, while such muscle exhibits

abnormal pharmacological responses (to curare or decamethonium). Ozdemir and Young (1971) obtained characteristic changes in only 13 patients out of 30 with generalised myasthenia gravis, when responses were recorded from the abductor digiti minimi. However, when recording from the deltoid, an MAP evoked by stimulating at Erb's point, characteristic changes were obtained in 23 patients. While movement artefact presents more of a problem at the latter site, these authors maintain that repetition of the recording will easily distinguish random alterations of MAP amplitude caused by movement, from the reproducible alterations reflecting defective neuromuscular transmission. It is, nonetheless, unfortunate that the muscles most accessible to neuromuscular transmission studies are those which are rarely weak early in myasthenia and may never be involved.

There are considerable variations in the types of response seen in myasthenia gravis, reflecting no doubt the different facets of neuromuscular transmission which may be impaired. The amplitude of a single evoked MAP may be slightly depressed: indeed, the only abnormality of neuromuscular transmission in clinically uninvolved muscles of

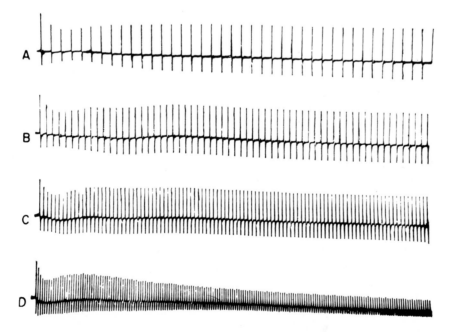

Fig. 26.6 Action potential response to repetitive nerve stimulation in generalised myasthenia gravis. Stimulation at rates of A, 5 Hz; B, 10 Hz; C, 25 Hz and D, 50 Hz (reproduced by courtesy of Dr R.J. Johns, from Johns *et al.*, 1955)

patients with oculobulbar myasthenia is a reduction in this potential in response to a single nerve stimulus. However, in the individual subject this is still usually within the normal range and only in particularly severe myasthenia gravis or in other myasthenic disorders is this depression likely to be of diagnostic help.

The most usual response to repetitive nerve stimulation, illustrated in Figure 26.6, consists of an initial decrease in evoked MAP amplitude followed by a transient increase, after which there is a slower progressive decrease, more striking at rapid stimulus rates (Johns et al., 1955). However, sometimes this decline is more evident at slow stimulus rates. Indeed, Slomic et al. (1968) found that a frequency of 3 Hz gave the best diagnostic yield in myasthenia gravis.

This decline is less marked after slight cooling: this also has the effect of increasing the amplitude both of a single evoked MAP and of the maximum force induced by tetanic stimulation (Ricker, Hertel and Stodieck, 1977).

The types of response at rapid stimulus rates (over 20 Hz) have been summarised by Simpson (1966). The most common is an initial decline followed by a maintained amplitude. However, there may also be a progressive steady decline, a decline, rise and then further decline, or finally a brief decline followed by an increase in the amplitude to as much as 150 per cent of the initial value. This latter phenomenon is usually transitory and is thought to indicate that an intermittent defect in the acetylcholine release mechanism is present (Takamore, 1971), though guanidine (which enhances acetylcholine release) has no lasting therapeutic value in such patients (Brown and Johns, 1969). Mayer and Williams (1974) noted this incrementing response at some time in the course of their disorder in 8 out of 22 patients with myasthenia gravis. It was most often seen while patients were in relapse.

The phenomenon of post-tetanic facilitation is sometimes helpful in the diagnosis of myasthenic disorders. In myasthenia gravis, after a brief train of tetanic stimulation (above 20 Hz), the amplitude of a single evoked MAP will be greater than that evoked immediately before the train (see Ch. 16): this becomes evident within a second of the termination of the train and persists for about 10–20 s. The degree of this facilitation is related to the duration and frequency of the tetanic stimulation and is at the expense of the myasthenic patient's ability to transmit subsequent impulses: indeed, a prolonged depression of the evoked MAP amplitude follows long periods of nerve stimulation in patients with even mild generalised myasthenia gravis (Johns et al., 1956). Facilitation of acetylcholine release is the probable explanation for this transient enhancement of neuromuscular transmission which follows the tetanic train and, as it does not occur in normal subjects, it provides further evidence that there is a degree of block of neuromuscular transmission in rested myasthenic muscle, for unstimulated muscle fibres must be available for recruitment during post-tetanic facilitation.

While tetanic stimulation results in facilitation of the subsequent evoked MAP, it is little altered immediately after voluntary effort (Slomic et al., 1968).

In mild myasthenia gravis the decremental response may become evident only after prolonged or repeated nerve stimulation or voluntary effort. If the myasthenic limb is rendered ischaemic, the decline in MAP amplitude during stimulation is accentuated and the latent defect of neuromuscular transmission in the limb can then be revealed in oculobulbar myasthenia (Borenstein and Desmedt, 1966). Growth of the MAP during the intravenous injection of 10 mg of edrophonium is another feature which may enable the diagnosis of myasthenia to be made.

The slight increase in latency and prolongation of the MAP that are seen at the end of tetanic stimulation in normal subjects are more striking in myasthenia. In some severe cases there is a significant slowing of motor velocity during the tetanus (Preswick, 1965) and the distal latency of the MAP may be prolonged in the rested state (Slomic et al., 1968).

Using a single-fibre preparation, Schwartz and Stalberg (1975b) have shown that submaximal nerve stimulation at 2 Hz induces both impulse-blocking and facilitation in all patients with myasthenia gravis, even in the purely ocular form. Similar results were obtained from the extensor digitorum brevis muscle in myasthenia by Boiardi, Bussone and Caccia (1976).

The measurement of mechanical responses to nerve stimulation, used in early studies of myasthenia gravis, has largely given way to the recording of the MAP. Nevertheless, useful information can be obtained from this procedure and, where possible, it should be combined with MAP recording. The staircase phenomenon is of particular interest: during slow rates of nerve stimulation (optimal at a frequency of 2 Hz) in normal subjects, after a brief decrement there is a gradual increase in the force of the twitch response unaccompanied by any change in MAP amplitude. This increase is related to the number of stimuli delivered, rather than to the stimulus frequency, and usually reaches about 40 per cent of the initial twitch response after 90 s of stimulation. In myasthenia gravis the incremental staircase phenomenon is absent, even in mild cases, providing a valuable aid to early diagnosis (Slomic et al., 1968).

The myasthenic syndrome of bronchogenic carcinoma (Eaton–Lambert syndrome)

This syndrome is, after myasthenia gravis, the commonest naturally occurring myasthenic disorder, the block in neuromuscular transmission being due to a defect in the acetylcholine release mechanism, thus resembling that of magnesium ion excess (del Castillo and Katz, 1954). The co-existence of carcinoma is, in fact, by no means inevitable. Neuromuscular stimulation is required to establish the diagnosis. There is a marked reduction in the amplitude of the MAP evoked by a single nerve stimulus. At slow rates of stimulation (1–3 Hz) this becomes still further reduced. At rapid rates of stimulation (10–50 Hz) there is a remarkable growth (Fig. 26.7): the amplitude may reach 4–20 times that of its initial low value, although it may take over 10 s to do so.

Voluntary effort results in a similar facilitatory effect; this can be shown by evoking a single MAP before and after contraction of the relevant muscle against resistance. The block in transmission is thus greatest in the rested muscle. After tetanic stimulation or voluntary effort are discontinued, the amplitude of the MAP rapidly falls to its initial level and then decreases still further for a few minutes. Unlike the situation in myasthenia gravis, these changes can be shown in peripheral muscles which are not weak (Eaton and Lambert, 1956: Lambert, Rooke, Eaton and Hodgson, 1961; Lambert, Okihiro and Rooke, 1965; Lambert, 1966).

These studies clearly distinguish this condition from myasthenia gravis, in which the facilitation occasionally seen at rapid stimulus rates is never as great nor the initial evoked MAP as reduced. Furthermore, there are significant clinical differences between the two disorders. The symmetrical proximal muscle weakness of this syndrome, in which oculobulbar involvement is mild or absent, results in a clinical resemblance to primary myopathy. In addition, the defect of neuromuscular transmission leads to a reduction of both amplitude and duration of the MAP recorded with concentric needle electrodes, with an excess of polyphasic activity. These changes characteristic of myopathic disorders, may be reversed by the administration of guanidine (Joong, 1972) and explain why an erroneous diagnosis of a primary myopathy may be made in this condition. Indeed, the characteristic changes of facilitation may be seen on neuromuscular stimulation, yet failure to realise that this syndrome is not inevitably associated with carcinoma may lead to this facilitation being either disregarded or wrongly attributed to a myopathy. In view of the usual clinical response to guanidine in this syndrome (Brown and Johns, 1967; McQuillen and Johns, 1967), this point requires emphasis.

Nonetheless, there is in fact considerable variation in clinical presentation of this disorder (Brown and Johns, 1974). Henriksson, Nialsson, Roseni and Schiller (1977) have described initial symptoms of fits and dysarthria and of dry mouth and urinary difficulties in patients with the electrophysiological features of the disorder. The variable weakness in a 13-year-old boy described by Dahl and Sato (1974) was also associated with such electrophysiological features. In addition, Schwartz and Stalberg (1975a) reported a case with the clinical features of mild myasthenia gravis, yet after muscle contraction or tetanic stimulation the amplitude of the single evoked MAP more than doubled. It is still not clear whether such cases merely represent an unusual presentation of myasthenia gravis or are a separate clinical entity.

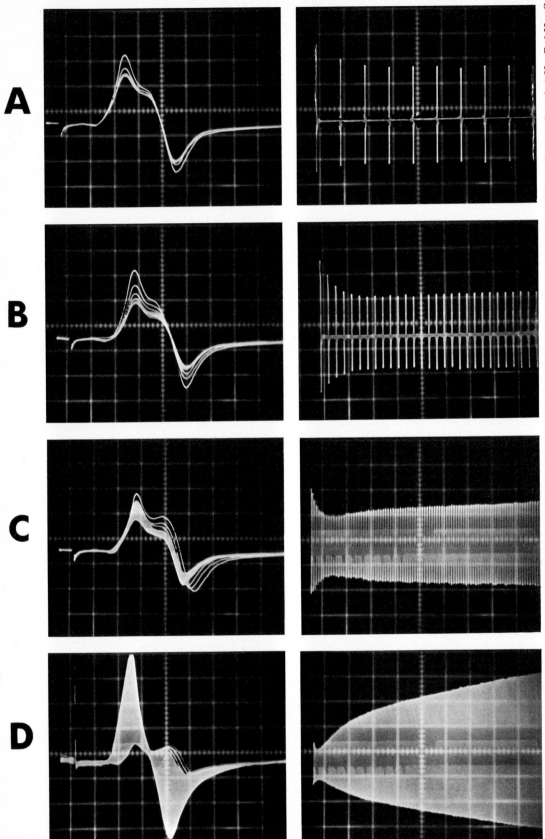

Fig. 26.7 Eaton–Lambert syndrome. Compound action potential of abductor digiti minimi muscle evoked by ulnar nerve stimulation at different frequencies—A, 1 Hz; B, 3 Hz; C, 10 Hz; D, 30 Hz. At each frequency; left, superimposed responses, 2 ms per horizontal division; right, sequential responses, 1 s per horizontal division. Vertical scale, A–C, 1 mV per division; D, 5 mV per division.

Using the single muscle fibre recording technique, Schwartz and Stalberg (1975b) have shown excessive jitter, leading to blocking of neuromuscular transmission. This was always worse in the rested muscle.

Myasthenic weakness induced by antibiotics and other drugs

While many antibiotics may cause worsening in patients with myasthenia, on occasion, profound flaccid weakness with pupillary and visual changes follow the administration of certain antibiotics to patients with no previous evidence of neuromuscular disorder. Neomycin has received the most attention, but other antibiotics may also be responsible (McQuillen, 1968, 1970). Pittinger (1972) noted that some 18 different antibiotics had been incriminated experimentally: the neomycin, kanamycin, colistin and streptomycin group were responsible for the majority of cases, although tetracyclines and polymyxin might also impair neuromuscular transmission. Subclinical alterations in neuromuscular transmission can, in fact, be shown after therapeutic doses of kanamycin in normal subjects (Wright and McQuillen, 1971).

Neuromuscular stimulation shows this block; where weakness has been induced there may be slowing of terminal nerve conduction and the amplitude of a single evoked MAP is reduced. This declines further during repetitive stimulation at all frequencies, particularly at slow rates. Post-tetanic facilitation is inconstant. These physiological features distinguish the block from that both of myasthenia gravis and of the myasthenic syndrome of bronchogenic carcinoma. Significant improvement in neuromuscular transmission occurs during intravenous calcium infusion; there is slight improvement with neostigmine but guanidine has no effect. The mechanism of this block is still in dispute: inhibition of acetylcholine release has been postulated, yet the above physiological changes would be better explained by a defect in aacetylcholine mobilisation (Wright and McQuillen, 1971).

In experimental studies of neuromuscular function, a very large number of drugs have been found to alter transmission. Occasionally such a drug in either therapeutic or excessive dosage may induce myasthenic weakness in man. Thus Norris, Colella and McFarlin (1964) found that the MAP declined at stimulus frequencies between 10–30 Hz in two patients taking diphenylhydantoin, and Brumlik and Jacobs (1974) described myasthenic features appearing in patients taking this drug. In each case, a decline in the MAP amplitude appeared at rapid stimulus frequencies. Peterson (1966) and Booker (1968) noted myasthenic features in patients taking trimethadione, and penicillamine has also been so incriminated (Bucknall, Dixon and Glick, 1975; Czlonkowske, 1975).

Botulism

There is some variation in the findings upon neuromuscular stimulation in patients with this condition. Cherington and Ryan (1968) obtained a decremental response with stimulus frequencies below 20 Hz, while de Jesus, Slater, Spitz and Penn (1973) and Hagenah and Muller-Jensen (1978) obtained an incremental response with rapid stimulus frequencies.

Gutman and Pratt (1976), after studying six patients, felt able to distinguish the neuromuscular transmission block from that of the Eaton–Lambert syndrome on the following grounds: the post-tetanic facilitation was less in the more severe cases and lasted several minutes; there was no post-tetanic depression; no decremental responses occurred at slow rates of stimulation and an incremental response during tetanic stimulation occurred in less than half of their cases. On this evidence alone, it seems likely that the neuromuscular block is attributable to more than a defect of the acetylcholine release mechanism.

Schiller and Stalberg (1978) have studied two mild cases of botulism using single muscle fibre recordings: only one showed any abnormality with repetitive stimulation, but an abnormal 'jitter' phenomenon revealed defective neuromuscular transmission in both.

OTHER NEUROMUSCULAR DISORDERS

Neuropathies and central nervous system disorders

Repetitive nerve stimulation may show changes in evoked MAP amplitude in disorders of the lower motor neurone. In both neuropathies and myopathies there may be random variation in MAP amplitude even when the stimulus is clearly supramaximal. Hodes (1948) showed that a decremental response might occur in poliomyelitis.

In certain peripheral neuropathies, the decline in MAP amplitude at rapid rates of stimulation is greater than that in normal subjects (Miglietta, 1969, 1971) and a myasthenic-like decrement may occur (Baginsky, 1968).

In a proportion of patients with motor neurone disease, extensive collateral branching of motor neurones results in a secondary myasthenic defect; neuromuscular stimulation may then reveal changes identical to those seen in myasthenia gravis (Mulder, Lambert and Eaton, 1959).

Similarly, upper motor neurone disorders result in a more rapid MAP decrement than normal: in a personal study of 16 hemiplegic patients there was, in each case, a greater decrement in the hemiplegic than in the normal limb. Similar changes were also noted in parkinsonism.

Three patients studied by Patten, Hart and Lovelace (1972) had defective neuromuscular transmission in association with multiple sclerosis; myasthenic fatigue was accompanied by a decremental response at 2 and 5 stimuli per second while an incremental response occurred at 10 and 20 Hz. A patient with multiple sclerosis studied by Cendrowski (1975), however, showed no decline at slow frequencies but a decrement of 70 per cent at a frequency of 35 Hz.

Eison, Yufe, Trop and Campbell (1978) have used a regional technique to show a delay in the recovery of the evoked MAP amplitude after D-tubocurarine administration in patients with multiple sclerosis. From this they infer that the neuromuscular transmission safety factor must be reduced in this condition.

Myopathies

Decremental responses at rapid stimulus rates occur also in many disorders of muscle (Mertens and Ruedas, 1961; Ricker and Mertens, 1968). Using stimulus frequencies of up to 30 Hz McComas, Sica and Currie (1970) were able to show a decline in the action potential of the extensor digitorum brevis when this muscle was

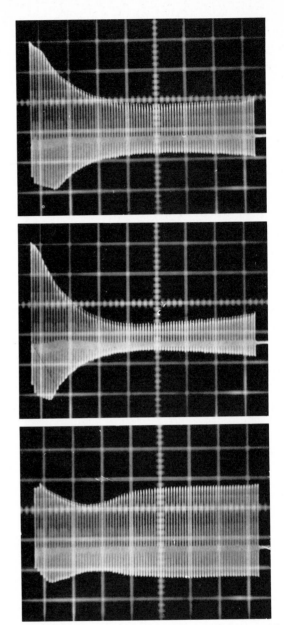

Fig. 26.8   Myotonia congenita. Compound action potential of abductor digiti minimi muscle evoked by ulnar nerve stimulation at rate of 10 Hz. A, initial response; B, response after 5 min rest (note decline is greater); C, response immediately after conditioning train (note first responses are smaller but no subsequent decline). Scale, vertical: 1 mV per division; horizontal: 1 s per division

clinically unaffected in some patients with Duchenne muscular dystrophy. This decline occurred in the majority of patients with limb-girdle and facioscapulohumeral muscular dystrophy (Sica and McComas, 1971). Myotonic disorders are distinctive in that the decremental response which they show, often at frequencies as low as 5 Hz, is present in the rested muscle only and may not be evident if the stimuli are delivered immediately after a previous conditioning stimulus train (Fig. 26.8). This phenomenon is most evident in myotonia congenita but can usually be elicited in dystrophia myotonica also. It is not attributable to defective neuromuscular transmission but the same phenomenon can be obtained by direct muscle fibre stimulation (Brown, 1974).

In McArdle's disease (myophosphorylase deficiency) a significant decremental response at a stimulus frequency of 19 Hz accompanying the cramp after exercise was noted by Dyken, Smith and Peak (1967). Delwaide, Lemaire and Reznik (1968) reported that, even in the absence of cramp, a decrement occurred provided the stimulus train was continued for over 4 s.

Systemic disorders

In thyroid disease, weakness due to defective neuromuscular transmission is an occasional occurrence. A decremental response similar to that of myasthenia gravis is most common, the association between these disorders being well recognised. However, Norris (1966) noted marked facilitation at rapid stimulus rates in a patient with thyrotoxicosis. Takamore (1972) also noted the characteristic changes of the Eaton–Lambert syndrome in a patient with myxoedema, and Drechsler and Lastoukay (1969) noted a decremental response in patients with both thyroto-

xicosis and myxoedema who were not clinically weak. More recently, the physiological features of both the myasthenic syndrome and of myasthenia gravis have been obtained from different sites in a patient with hyperthyroidism (Mori and Takamori, 1976).

Using stimulus frequencies of up to 500 Hz, Miglietta (1973) showed that a decline in MAP amplitude occurred earlier, and was more marked, in patients with diabetes mellitus than in normal subjects, even where there was no clinical evidence of a neuropathy. However, in view of the high frequencies used and the segmental demyelination of peripheral nerve in this condition, such findings do not necessarily indicate defective neuromuscular transmission. Basomba, Permuy, Pelaez, Campos and Villalmenzo (1976) reported a significant decremental response to repetitive stimulation, particularly at rates of 20–30 Hz in a proportion of patients with intrinsic asthma, and Schiller, Schwartz and Friman (1977) used single-fibre electromyography to show an increase in the 'jitter' phenomenon in patients in both the acute and convalescent phases of virus illnesses.

The considerable functional reserve of the neuromuscular junction must ensure that transmission is unaffected in the majority of systemic illnesses. Remembering that even disuse of muscle leads to a more rapid decline in MAP at rapid stimulus frequencies, it is not always possible to infer that such changes are a direct consequence of systemic illness on the neuromuscular junction. Nevertheless, the application of these techniques to other neuromuscular and systemic disorders could be of considerable interest.

REFERENCES

Adrian, E.D. (1916) The electrical reactions of muscles before and after nerve injury. *Brain*, **39**, 1.

Amick, L.D. & Hickey, R.P. (1959) Abbreviated electrodiagnostic tests of denervation. *Annals of Physical Medicine*, **5**, 48.

Baginsky, R.G. (1968) A case of peripheral neuropathy displaying myasthenic E.M.G. patterns. *Electroencephalography and Clinical Neurophysiology*, **25**, 397.

Basomba, A., Permuy, J., Pelaez, A., Campos, A. & Villalmanzo, I.G. (1976) Myasthenic-like electrophysiological response in intrinsic bronchial asthma. *Lancet*, **2**, 968.

Boiardi, A., Bussone, G. & Caccia, M.R. (1976) Effect of

threshold, low frequency, long lasting stimulation on single motor unit electrical responses from the extensor digitorum brevis muscle in normal and myasthenic subjects. *Journal of Neurology*, **212**, 41.

Booker, H.E. (1968) Myasthenic syndrome associated with trimethadione. *Neurology (Minneapolis)*, **18**, 274.

Borenstein, S. & Desmedt, J.E. (1966) Sensibilisation par l'ischeamie de la réaction de l'épuisement de post-activation dans la myasthenie humaine. *Comptes Rendus Hebdomadaire des Séances de l'Academie des Sciences*, **262**, 1472.

Botelho, S.Y., Deaterly, C.F., Austin, S. & Comroe, J.A. (1952) Evaluation of the electromyogram and patients with myasthenia gravis. *Archives of Neurology and Psychiatry*, **67**, 441.

Brennand, R. (1959) Recommendations for medical electronic instrumentation. *Journal of the British Institution of Radio Engineers*, **19**, 245.

Brown, J.C. (1974) Muscle weakness after rest in myotonic disorders: an electrophysiological study. *Journal of Neurology, Neurosurgery and Psychiatry*, **37**, 1336.

Brown, J.C. & Charlton, J.E. (1975a) A study of sensitivity to curare in myasthenic disorders using a regional technique. *Journal of Neurology, Neurosurgery and Psychiatry*, **38**, 27.

Brown, J.C. & Charlton, J.E. (1975b) A study of sensitivity to curare in certain neurological disorders using a regional technique. *Journal of Neurology, Neurosurgery and Psychiatry*, **38**, 34.

Brown, J.C. & Johns, R.J. (1967) The Eaton-Lambert syndrome masquerading as proximal myopathy. *Transactions of the American Clinical and Climatological Association*, **79**, 134.

Brown, J.C. & Johns, R.J. (1969) Clinical and physiological studies of the effect of guanidine on patients with myasthenia gravis. *Johns Hopkins Medical Journal*, **124**, 1.

Brown, J.C. & Johns, R.J. (1974) Diagnostic difficulties encountered in a myasthenic syndrome sometimes associated with carcinoma. *Journal of Neurology, Neurosurgery and Psychiatry*, **37**, 1214.

Brown, J.C., Charlton, J.E. & White, D.J.K. (1975) A regional technique for the study of sensitivity to curare in human muscle. *Journal of Neurology, Neurosurgery and Psychiatry*, **38**, 18.

Brumlik, J. & Jacobs, R. (1974) Myasthenia gravis associated with diphenylhydantoin therapy for epilepsy. *Canadian Journal of Neurological Sciences*, **1**, 127.

Bucknall, R.C., Dixon, A.St.J. & Glick, E.N. (1975) Myasthenia gravis associated with penicillamine treatment for rheumatoid arthritis. *British Medical Journal*, **1**, 600.

Campbell, E.D.R., Hickey, R.P., Nixon, K.H. & Richardson, A.T. (1962) Value of nerve excitability measurements in prognosis of facial palsy. *British Medical Journal* **2**, 7.

Cendrowski, M.D.W. (1975) A case of multiple sclerosis associated with defective neuromuscular transmission. *Acta Neurologica Belgica*, **75**, 11.

Cherington, M. & Ryan, D.W. (1968) Botulism and guanidine. *New England Journal of Medicine*, **278**, 931.

Collier, J. (1959) Rationale for operative treatment in facial palsy. *Proceedings of the Royal Society of Medicine*, **52**, 1075.

Czlonkowske, A. (1975) Myasthenic syndrome during penicillamine treatment. *British Medical Journal*, **2**, 726.

Dahl, D.S. & Sato, S. (1974) Unusual myasthenic state in a teenage boy. *Neurology (Minneapolis)*, **24**, 897.

de Jesus, P.V., Slater, R., Spitz, L.K. & Penn, A.S. (1973) Neuromuscular physiology of wound botulism. *Archives of Neurology*, **29**, 425.

Del Castillo, J. & Katz, B. (1954) The effect of magnesium on the activity of motor nerve endings. *Journal of Physiology*, **124**, 553.

Delwaide, P.J., Lemaire, R. & Reznik, M. (1968) EMG findings in a case of McArdle's myopathy. *Electroencephalography and Clinical Neurophysiology*, **25**, 414.

Drechsler, B. & Lastoukay, M. (1969) An electrophysiological study of patients with thyreopathy. *Electroencephalography and Clinical Neurophysiology*, **26**, 234.

Dyken, M.L., Smith, D.M. & Peak, R.L. (1967) An electromyographic diagnostic screening test in McArdle's

disease and a case report. *Neurology (Minneapolis)*, **17**, 45.

Eaton, L.M. & Lambert, E.H. (1956) Electromyography and electric stimulation of nerves in diseases of motor unit. Observations on myasthenic syndrome associated with malignant tumours. *Journal of the American Medical Association*, **163**, 1117.

Eisen, A., Yufe, R., Trop, D. & Campbell, I. (1978) Reduction of neuromuscular transmission safety factor in multiple sclerosis. *Neurology (Minneapolis)*, **28**, 598.

Ekstedt, J. (1964) Human single muscle fibre action potentials. *Acta Physiologica Scandinavica*, **61**, Supplement 266, 1.

Erb, W. (1883) *Handbook of Electrotherapeutics*, trans. by A. Putzel (William Wood: New York).

Gutman, L. & Pratt, L. (1976) Pathophysiological aspects of human botulism. *Archives of Neurology*, **33**, 175.

Hagenah, R. & Muller-Jensen, A. (1978) Botulism: clinical neurophysical findings. *Journal of Neurology*, **217**, 159.

Harris, R. (1962) In *Electrodiagnosis and Electromyography* Ed. S. Licht (Licht: Connecticut, U.S.A.).

Harvey, A.M. & Masland, R.L. (1941) A method for the study of neuromuscular transmission in human subjects. *Bulletin of the Johns Hopkins Hospital*, **68**, 81.

Henriksson, K.G., Nialsson, O., Roseni, I. & Schiller, H.H. (1977) Clinical, neurophysiological and morphological findings in Eaton-Lambert syndrome. *Acta Neurologica Scandinavica*, **56**, 117.

Hodes, R. (1948) Electromyographic study of defects of neuromuscular transmission in human poliomyelitis. *Archives of Neurology and Psychiatry*, **60**, 457.

Johns, R.J. Grob, D. & Harvey, A.M. (1955) Electromyographic changes in myasthenia gravis. *American Journal of Medicine*, **19**, 679.

Johns, R.J., Grob, D. & Harvey, A.M. (1956) Studies in neuromuscular function 11. Effects of nerve stimulation in normal subjects and in patients with myasthenia gravis. *Bulletin of the Johns Hopkins Hospital*, **99**, 125.

Joong, S. (1972) The Eaton-Lambert syndrome. *Archives of Neurology*, **27**, 91.

Katz, B. (1939) *Electric Excitation of Nerve* (Oxford University Press: London).

King, P. & Wynn Parry, C.B. (1977) Results of treatment in peripheral facial paralysis—a 25 years' study. *Journal of Laryngology & Otology*, **91**, 551.

Lambert, E.H. (1966) Defects of neuromuscular transmission in syndromes other than myasthenia gravis. *Annals of the New York Academy of Science*, **135**, 367.

Lambert, E.H., Okihiro, M. & Rooke, E.D. (1965) Clinical physiology of the neuromuscular junction. In *Muscle*. Eds. W.M. Paul, E.E. Daniel, C.M. Kay & G. Monckton (Pergamon Press: New York).

Lambert, E.H., Rooke, E.D., Eaton, L.M. & Hodgson, C.H. (1961) Myasthenic syndrome occasionally associated with bronchial neoplasm: neurophysiologic studies. In *Myasthenia Gravis* Ed. H.R. Viets, *2nd International Symposium Proceedings* (Thomas: Springfield, Illinois).

Mayer, R.F. & Williams, I.R. (1974) Incrementing responses to myasthenia gravis. *Archives of Neurology*, **31**, 24.

McComas, A.J., Sica, R.E.P. & Currie, S. (1970) Evidence for a neural factor in muscular dystrophy. *Nature*, **226**, 1263.

McQuillen, M.P. (1968) Myasthenic syndrome associated with antibiotics. *Archives of Neurology*, **18**, 402.

McQuillen, M.P. (1970) Hazard from antibiotics in myasthenia gravis. *Annals of Internal Medicine*, **73**, 487.

McQuillen, M.P. & Johns, R.J. (1967) The nature of the defect in the Eaton-Lambert syndrome. *Neurology (Minneapolis)*, **17**, 527.

Medical Research Council Sub-committee Report (1958) Electro-diagnostic stimulators. *British Medical Journal*, **2**, 714.

Mertens, H.G. & Ruedas, G. (1961) Electromyographic studies in electrical nerve irritation, 1. Frequency stress capacity of neuromuscular transmission in myopathies. *Deutsche Zeitschrift für Nervenheilkunde*, **182**, 577

Miglietta, O.E. (1969) Myasthenic-like responses in patients with neuropathy. *Electroencephalography and Clinical Neurophysiology*, **27**, 713.

Miglietta, O.E. (1971) Myasthenic-like response in patients with neuropathy. *American Journal of Physical Medicine*, **50**, 1.

Miglietta, O.E. (1973) Neuromuscular junction defect in diabetes. *Diabetes*, **22**, 719.

Moldaver, J. (1964) Facial nerve rehabilitation. *Transactions of the American Society of Opthalmology and Otolaryngology*, **68**, 1045.

Moody, J.F. (1965) Neurological complications of cancer. *Brain*, **88**, 1023.

Mori, M. & Takimori, M. (1976) Hyperthyroidism and myasthenia gravis with features of Eaton-Lambert syndrome. *Neurology (Minneapolis)*, **26**, 882.

Mulder, D.W., Lambert, E.H. & Eaton, L.M. (1959) Myasthenic syndrome in patients with amyotrophic lateral sclerosis. *Neurology (Minneapolis)*, **9**, 627.

Newman, H.W. & Livingstone, W.K. (1947) Electrical aids in prognosis of nerve injuries. *Journal of Neurology, Neurosurgery and Psychiatry*, **10**, 118.

Norris, F.H. (1966) Neuromuscular transmission in thyroid disease. *Annals of Internal Medicine*, **64**, 81.

Norris, F.H., Colella, J. & McFarlin, D. (1964) Effect of diphenylhydantoin on neuromuscular synapse. *Neurology (Minneapolis)*, **14**, 869.

Ozdemir, C. & Young, R.R. (1971) Electrical testing on myasthenia gravis. *Annals of the New York Academy of Sciences*, **183**, 287.

Patten, B.M., Hart, A. & Lovelace, R. (1972) Multiple sclerosis associated with defects in neuromuscular transmission. *Journal of Neurology, Neurosurgery and Psychiatry*, **35**, 385.

Peterson, H. (1966) Association of trimethadione therapy and myasthenia gravis. *New England Journal of Medicine*, **274**, 506.

Pittinger, C. (1972) Antibiotic blockade of neuromuscular function. *Annual Review of Pharmacology*, **12**, 169.

Pollock, L.J., Golseth, J.G. & Arieff, A.J. (1944) The use of discontinuity of strength duration curves in muscle in diagnosis of peripheral nerve lesions. *Surgery, Gynecology, and Obstetrics*, **79**, 133.

Preswick, G. (1965) The myasthenic syndromes and their reactions. *Proceedings of the Australian Association of Neurologists*, **3**, 61.

Ricker, K. & Mertens, H.G. (1968) Myasthenic reaction in primary muscle fibre disease. *Electroencephalography and Clinical Neurophysiology*, **25**, 413.

Ricker, K., Hertel, G. & Stodieck, S. (1977) Influence of temperature on neuromuscular transmission in myasthenia gravis. *Journal of Neurology*, **216**, 273.

Ritchie, A.E. (1944) The electrical diagnosis of peripheral nerve injury. *Brain*, **67**, 314.

Rushton, W.A.H. (1930) Excitable substances in the nerve muscle complex. *Journal of Physiology*, **70**, 317.

Schiller, H.H. & Stalberg, E. (1978) Human botulism studied with single-fibre electromyography. *Archives of Neurology*, **35**, 346.

Schiller, H.H., Schwartz, M.S. & Friman, G. (1977) Disturbed neuromuscular transmission in viral infection. *New England Journal of Medicine*, **296**, 884.

Schwartz, M.S. & Stalberg, E. (1975a) Myasthenia gravis with features of the myasthenic syndrome. *Neurology (Minneapolis)*, **25**, 80.

Schwartz, M.S. & Stalberg, E. (1975b) Myasthenic syndrome studied with single-fibre electromyography. *Archives of Neurology*, **32**, 815.

Schwartz, M.S. & Stalberg, E. (1975c) Single-fibre electromyographic studies in myasthenia gravis with repetitive nerve stimulation. *Journal of Neurology, Neurosurgery and Psychiatry*, **38**, 678.

Sica, R.E.P. & McComas, A.J. (1971) An electrophysiological investigation of limb-girdle and facioscapulohumeral dystrophy. *Journal of Neurology, Neurosurgery and Psychiatry*, **34**, 469.

Simpson, J.A. (1966) Disorders of neuromuscular transmission. *Proceedings of the Royal Society of Medicine*, **59**, 993.

Simpson, J.A. & Lenman, J.A.R. (1959) Electromyography of neuromuscular transmission. The effect of frequency of stimulation in neuromuscular disease. *Electroencephalography and Clinical Neurophysiology*, **2**, 604.

Slomic, A., Rosenfalck, A. & Buchthal, F. (1968) Electrical and mechanical responses of normal and myasthenic muscle. *Brain Research (Special Issue)*, **10**, 8.

Takamore, M. (1971) Intermittent defect of acetylcholine release in myasthenia gravis. *Neurology (Minneapolis)*, **21**, 47.

Takamore, M. (1972) Myasthenic syndromes in hypothyroidism. Electrophysiological study of neuromuscular transmission and muscle contraction in two patients. *Archives of Neurology*, **26**, 326.

Taverner, D. (1965) Electrodiagnosis in facial palsy. *Archives of Otolaryngology*, **81**, 470.

Trojaborg, W. (1962) Correlation between motor nerve conduction velocity, electromyography and strength duration curves. *Danish Medical Bulletin*, **9**, 23.

Wright, E. & McQuillen, M.P. (1971) Antibiotic-induced neuromuscular blockade. *Annals of the New York Academy of Sciences*, **183**, 358.

Wynn Parry, C.B. (1953) Electrical methods in diagnosis and prognosis of peripheral nerve injuries and poliomyelitis. *Brain*, **76**, 229.

Wynn Parry, C.B. (1962) In *Electrodiagnosis and Electromyography*. Ed. S. Licht (Licht: Newhaven, Connecticut).

Studies in nerve conduction

INTRODUCTION

The study of nerve conduction velocity in peripheral nerves is now a well-established clinical tool in the investigation of various forms of neuromuscular disease. Hodes, Larrabee and German (1948) introduced motor nerve conduction studies into clinical medicine. They examined the median, ulnar, tibial and peroneal nerves, evoking muscle responses to percutaneous supramaximal stimulation. By stimulating at least two points along the course of a single nerve and measuring the differences in latency values obtained, it was possible to calculate the velocity along the nerve trunk. The subsequent developments and results of the application of this technique will be discussed below.

Although motor conduction velocities are useful, they give no indication of conduction in sensory fibres. Dawson and Scott (1949) showed that it was possible to detect nerve potentials in the median and ulnar nerves, evoked by distal percutaneous electrical stimulation of these nerves at the wrist. The evoked response was picked up by bipolar surface electrodes over the nerve at the elbow. The response was made up of contributions from sensory fibres conducting orthodromically and motor fibres conducting antidromically. In 1956, utilising the fact that the digital nerves of the fingers contain no motor fibres, Dawson recorded pure sensory action potentials at the wrist from the median and ulnar nerves on electrical stimulation of the index and little fingers. The now widespread application of sensory nerve studies has largely been a function of improved instrumentation which enables small signals to be readily extracted from background noise.

TECHNIQUE

Apparatus

Stimulator. There are two types of stimulator: (1) constant voltage, which should be capable of delivering up to 250 V; (2) constant current, which should provide a current output of up to 100 mA (Guld, Rosenfalck and Willison, 1970). Buchthal and Rosenfalck (1966) prefer the latter type, because constant monitoring of the current allows changes in electrode and tissue impedance to be detected. The most common form of stimulus is a rectangular pulse, the duration of which may be varied between 0.05–1.0 ms. It is essential that the stimulator is isolated in order to reduce stimulus artefact and this is most conveniently achieved using a shielded isolation transformer (Guld, 1960).

The oscilloscope sweep should be triggered either simultaneously by the stimulator or just before the actual stimulus is delivered to the patient, allowing the stimulus artefact to be displayed for measurement purposes.

A wide range of stimulus frequencies (0.5–100 Hz) should be available, but for nerve conduction studies a frequency of 1 Hz is usually employed and is well tolerated by the patient.

Stimulating electrodes. Various kinds of ring electrodes may be used to evoke sensory potentials by stimulation of digital nerves. Dawson (1956) recommends silver strip electrodes 2–4 mm wide covered in salinated lint. Pipe-cleaners soaked in saline perform equally well. When stimulating nerve trunks, bipolar or monopolar methods may be used, although the bipolar method is preferable, particularly if stimulating above the elbow with recording electrodes in the axilla. A convenient type of electrode consists of silver discs of 0.6 mm diameter covered with salinated felt pads mounted 2.5 mm apart in a perspex holder, which may either be hand-held or strapped to the skin.

One type of electrode consists of bare rods covered at the tips with discs of salinated lint and fixed in a plastic holder which contains a variable voltage control from the stimulator. Bare metal electrodes should be avoided because they require electrode paste, which may become spread over the skin and short-circuit the stimulator when the electrodes are moved in search of optimal placement. The size of the stimulating electrode is probably not crucial, as Henriksen (1956) has shown that the effective stimulus point is the centre of the circular electrode. Needle electrodes may be necessary occasionally where the nerve to be stimulated lies deeply (e.g. the sciatic) or where skin resistance is high due to hyperkeratosis.

Recording electrodes. For motor conduction, either surface or concentric needle electrodes may be used. The former usually consist of 0.5–1 cm diameter silver plates attached to the skin with adhesive tape. Surface electrodes avoid the need for needle puncture and may pick up from a wider and more representative area, an advantage when some muscle fibres may be atrophied. Needle electrodes have the advantage of being more selective, enabling the motor response to be isolated to a single muscle. In addition, the muscle response generally has a sharper take-off point, making it easier to measure the latency. However, because the needle electrode records from a restricted area within the muscle, it is possible that the recorded activity may not arise from motor units supplied by the fastest-conducting motor fibres. For recording evoked nerve potentials silver disc electrodes 1 cm in diameter mounted in a perspex holder with a fixed interelectrode distance of 2.5–3 cm are most suitable, and may be conveniently applied in line with the underlying nerve trunk. In this situation Gilliatt, Melville, Velate and Willison (1965) have shown that the interelectrode distance significantly affects the amplitude and duration of the potential. It is therefore important that each laboratory should standardise on one type of recording electrode. Buchthal and Rosenfalck (1966) prefer needle electrodes inserted close to the nerve, and use a system of unipolar recording which gives rather shorter latency values than those obtained by bipolar recording. They also use an input transformer to improve the signal:noise ratio of the potentials. Needle electrodes may be necessary for the recording of evoked potentials which are small, as in the common peroneal and radial nerves, but their use is not without risk as minor injury may be caused to the nerve and may result in unpleasant persisting paraesthesiae.

Recording apparatus. A large variety of high-quality apparatus is now available commercially to suit varying needs and budgets and will not be discussed here in detail. Readily mobile units allow recording of routine electromyography (EMG), strength–duration curves, motor conduction and the simpler nerve action potential examinations. For most purposes, amplification so that a 10 μV signal produces at least a 1 cm deflection of the oscilloscope trace is adequate. Considerable filtering of high frequency 'noise' is permissible but may produce slight changes in apparent latency, so that allowance for this may have to be made in establishing control values. Instability of the baseline when working at high amplification may be troublesome and may result from many factors. Suitable low-frequency filters and careful attention to relaxation of the patient will usually avoid this difficulty. Reduction of skin resistance by preliminary cleaning with acetone is advisable, but mild abrasion with sandpaper or light scratching is necessary only if the skin is unusually thick or dry. Adequate calibration of the sweep is also necessary and can be attained by a variety of means. A time-marker with 1 ms divisions, which can be readily checked against the 50 or 60 Hz AC mains supply and can be superimposed on the trace, is convenient.

A vertical step deflection or separate marker, which can be moved along the horizontal axis of the oscilloscope trace to coincide with any point which has to be measured and whose distance from the beginning of the trace is indicated on a digital counter down to tenths of a millisecond, is a valuable addition to a commercial instrument. For clinical work it largely obviates the need to photograph in order to make accurate measurements.

Signal averaging. The size of sensory action potentials from normal and pathological nerves may be of the order of 5 μV or less and, as such, may be difficult to distinguish from noise. Dawson and Scott (1949) originally introduced the technique of photographic superimposition of 10–100 responses as a means of improving the signal:noise ratio to record small sensory potentials percutaneously. More recently, the use of the powerful electronic averaging technique has greatly improved the isolation of very small signals from noise (Buchthal and Rosenfalck, 1966; Mavor and Atcheson, 1966) and many of the currently available EMG instruments have this facility. The method is based on the principle that stimulus-linked events will enhance as successive traces summate algebraically, while randomly occurring activity will cancel out. The improvement of the signal:noise ratio is a function of the square root of the number of sweeps. Signals as low as 0.03 μV may be detected by averaging 1000 sweeps or more (Singh, Behse and Buchthal, 1974), but such large numbers of stimuli may be unpleasant for the patient, and usually 32–128 sweeps are satisfactory.

Permanent records. Photography of traces, apart from providing a permanent record, also allows photographic superimposition which, as mentioned earlier, is one means of improving the signal:noise ratio. A Polaroid camera is convenient for rapid availability of results, although the ability to project film allows more accurate measurement. A number of commercial instruments provide recording facilities which are adequate for most purposes.

Methods

General. Adequate earthing of the patient is essential, using a plate or strap-type electrode placed where possible between the stimulating and recording electrodes to minimise stimulus artefact. Ideally, the patient and machine should be placed in a screened environment to reduce extraneous electrical interference to a minimum, but satisfactory recordings can often be obtained without these precautions.

Motor conduction. The motor conduction velocity may be most satisfactorily measured in the median, ulnar, radial, peroneal and posterior tibial nerves which are accessible for stimulation at two or more points along their course. The optimal site for stimulation of the nerve at a distal point is found by using a submaximal stimulus (usually 3–5 mA at 0.1 ms) and moving the stimulating electrode until a maximal response for that stimulus is obtained. The stimulus is then increased until the muscle response is maximal, following which the stimulus is further increased by about 25 per cent to ensure that the nerve is being stimulated supramaximally. The response thus produced is observed on the oscilloscope and a permanent record obtained. The procedure is repeated at two or more proximal sites so that the latency between the these separate responses can be measured. The distance between the two points of stimulation is then measured and divided by the latency difference to give the conduction velocity. Dawson (1956) pointed out that, when a motor nerve is stimulated with only a threshold stimulus, the first response recorded from the muscle often has a longer latency than the response recorded with a maximal stimulus. This unexpected finding may be an artefact, however, caused by spread of the effective stimulus point away from the stimulating cathode towards the recording electrode at high stimulus intensities (Wiederholt, 1970). This is a cogent reason for using as standardised a stimulus as possible, preferably one which is just

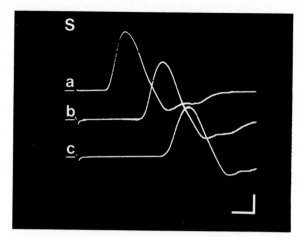

Fig. 27.1 Evoked muscle responses recorded with surface electrodes from abductor pollicis brevis following stimulation of the median nerve at (a) wrist, (b) elbow and (c) axilla in a control subject. S=stimulus. Calibration: 2ms; 5mV

supramaximal, before attempting to measure conduction rate in the fastest-conducting fibres.

Upper limbs. For the median and ulnar nerves, the active recording electrode is placed over the muscle belly of abductor pollicis brevis and abductor digiti minimi respectively, with the reference electrode over the tendon of insertion at the base of the appropriate digit. The nerves may be stimulated at the wrist, elbow, axilla and Erb's point, and the conduction velocity measured over each intervening segment (Fig. 27.1). Spread of stimulus from median to ulnar nerve and *vice versa* when stimulating at the wrist and axilla may give rise to misleading responses when recording from the small muscles of the hand. The shape of the muscle response, however, is helpful in avoiding any error of interpretation (Mavor and Libman, 1962). Other errors may arise from the anomalous innervation of the small muscles of the hand (Gassel, 1964a).

Motor conduction in the radial nerve has been studied by Gassel and Diamantopoulos (1964) by stimulating the nerve above the clavicle and in the mid-arm. Trojaborg and Sindrup (1969) used stimulus points over the nerve in the axilla and 6 cm proximal to the lateral epicondyle of the humerus, recording the muscle response from brachioradialis or other forearm muscles innervated by the radial nerve. The latency from

application of a stimulus to one distal point on a nerve to the resulting muscle contraction (terminal latency) cannot be converted into a true nerve conduction rate, but it is nevertheless sufficiently constant in healthy subjects to be of value. Gassel (1964b) has also studied terminal latency measurement to the muscles of the shoulder girdle following stimulation at Erb's point.

Lower limbs. Conduction rates in fibres supplying the small muscles of the foot may be tested in the distribution of the common peroneal and posterior tibial nerves. The distal stimulus is applied to the deep peroneal or posterior tibial nerve at the ankle, and the proximal stimulus at the head of the fibula or in the lower popliteal fossa respectively. The muscle action potential is usually recorded from the extensor digitorum brevis or abductor hallucis (Mavor and Atcheson, 1966). Conduction rate in the sciatic nerve can also be estimated (Gassel and Trojaborg, 1964) using needle electrodes placed deeply in the gluteal region to provide the proximal stimulus; Gassel (1963) reported a method for estimating conduction in the femoral nerve, based on the measurement of latencies to two points within the quadriceps femoris.

'F' wave conduction technique. Supramaximal stimulation of the peripheral nerve as well as producing a direct 'M' response often results in a small-amplitude late response of variable latency and configuration, which Magladery and McDougal (1950) separated from the 'H' reflex and called the 'F' wave (Fig. 27.2). It is best obtained from the distal muscles of the hand and foot and, in contrast to the latency of the 'M' response, that of the 'F' wave decreases as the stimulus is applied more proximally, indicating a centripetal conduction of the impulse before distal transmission. Controversy has surrounded its origins, some believing it to be a reflex (Magladery, Porter, Park and Teasdall, 1951; Hagbarth, 1962), others a recurrent discharge of a few antidromically excited motor neurones (Dawson and Merton, 1956). That it can be elicited in a deafferented limb (Mayer and Feldman, 1967) confirms its recurrent nature in part, while single motor unit studies (Thorne, 1965) and single-fibre electromyography (Trontelj and Trontelj, 1973; Schiller and Stålberg, 1978) have shown it to occur only when preceded by an identical direct motor-unit response. Although reflex components cannot be excluded completely, it can be assumed that in the resting state, most, if not all, of the late responses are 'F' waves. Recently, a number of authors have used the fact that the 'F' wave traverses the central portion of the nerve, to examine the motor conduction velocity in this segment which, hitherto, has been inaccessible to conventional nerve conduction methods. The technique, first described by Kimura (1974), depends upon measuring the latencies of the direct 'M' response and that of the 'F' wave, taking the shortest latency obtained from a number of trials (usually 10–20), following stimulation of the nerve at a suitable proximal site. The 'F' wave conduction time in the central segment related to the upper limb may be calculated using the following simple formula:

'F' wave conduction time (ms) =

$$\frac{('F' \text{ latency} - 'M' \text{ latency}) - 1 \text{ ms}\star}{2}$$

and the conduction velocity:

'F' wave velocity (m/s) =

$$\frac{\text{Distance from stimulus point to C7 spine} \times 2 \text{ (mm)}}{('F' \text{ latency} - 'M' \text{ latency}) - 1 \text{ ms}\star}$$

The technique assumes that: (1) the 'F' wave with the shortest latency is being conducted in the largest-diameter fibres; (2) that the corresponding motor unit is also the first to be activated in the 'M' response; and (3) that the central delay due to turnabout of the impulse is 1 ms. It also requires measurement of the segment between C7 and the arm, which may introduce considerable in-accuracies. Young and Shahani (1978) have cast doubt on a number of these assumptions and argue against the need to calculate 'F' wave conduction velocity, preferring to use the shortest 'F' wave latency which they relate to a nomogram comparing 'F' wave latency and arm length. Despite these differences of opinion, the 'F' wave has proved to be of considerable value in the examination of the

★Time allowed for turnabout at the cell body★

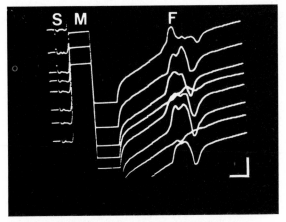

Fig. 27.2 Recordings from abductor pollicis brevis following supramaximal stimulation of the median nerve at the wrist in a control subject. Note the initial large direct muscle responses which are followed by small late 'F' waves which show variation of latency and configuration. S=stimulus; M=direct response; F='F' wave. Calibration: 5ms; 500μV

proximal nerve segment (Kimura and Butzer, 1975; King and Ashby, 1976; Eisen, Schomer and Melmed, 1977a and b) and in various peripheral neuropathies (Lefebre-D'Amour, Shahani, Young and Bird, 1976; Panayiotopoulos and Scarpalezos, 1977).

Evoked nerve action potential techniques. An example of normal nerve action potentials in the median and ulnar nerves is seen in Figure 27.3.

Upper limbs—distal segments. By applying the stimulus through ring electrodes wrapped around the base and middle of the index or little finger, an evoked nerve action potential can be elicited from electrodes placed over the median or ulnar nerves at the wrist (Dawson, 1956). This pure sensory potential is formed from the summated action potentials of larger fibres in the digital nerves. Reversal of the position of the stimulating and the recording electrodes produces a similar response, although of higher amplitude, and represents antidromic conduction (Sears, 1959). A higher-amplitude response can also be obtained ortho-dromically by placing the stimulating electrodes at the base of adjacent fingers, e.g. index and middle (for median nerve) (Fig. 27.4).

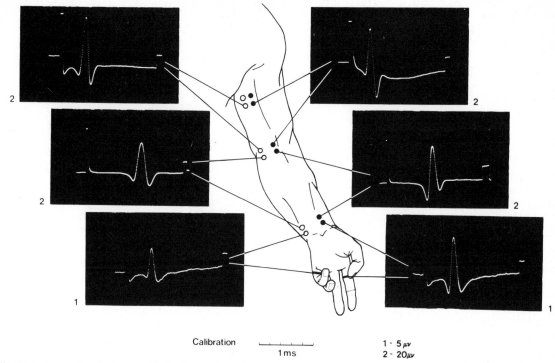

Calibration |___|___| 1 - 5 μν
                1 ms   2 - 20μν

Fig. 27.3 Normal evoked potentials in ulnar and median nerves. In each case the stimulus was applied distally, and the response was recorded proximally

Upper limbs—proximal segments. When the median or ulnar nerve is stimulated at the wrist, the compound action potential elicited above the elbow is formed by orthodromic conduction in

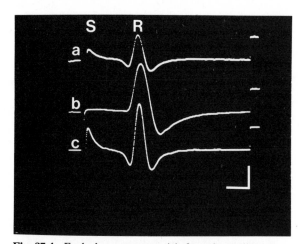

Fig. 27.4 Evoked sensory potentials from the median nerve in a control subject, elicited by three techniques; (a) stimulus to index, recording at wrist; (b) stimulus at wrist, recording from index; and (c) stimulus at base of index and medius, recording from wrist. S=stimulus; R=response. Calibration: lms; 20μV

sensory fibres and antidromic conduction in the motor fibres. Dawson (1956) showed that the sensory fibres have a lower threshold and slightly faster conduction rate than the motor ones, but Buchthal and Rosenfalck (1966) found no consistent variation in threshold, and variable findings with regard to conduction velocity depended upon the age of the patient and the nerve tested. In some pathological situations, for instance, severe anterior horn cell disease, it is likely that the residual evoked potential seen at the elbow originates in sensory fibres only. Conduction rate above the elbow may be tested in a similar way by placing the recording electrode over the median nerve at the elbow. Replacement of the earth electrode to a position between stimulating and recording electrodes is essential here, but even with this safeguard, stimulus artefact may still be troublesome. By rotation of the position of the stimulating anode while keeping the cathode fixed over the nerve, a critical point is reached at which artefact is minimal. Relaxation of the patient is particularly important when examining these segments. Occasionally, in suitable subjects, it is possible to record potentials above the clavicle from the upper part of the brachial plexus by stimulation of the median, ulnar or radial nerve at the wrist or near the elbow.

Radial nerve. The radial nerve is accessible for stimulation or recording from the sensory fibres in several sites: (a) at the proximal phalanx of the thumb (digital nerves); (b) at the wrist, or just distally where the superficial branches can be felt as they cross the tendon of extensor pollicis brevis; (c) along the course of the cephalic vein in the lower third of the forearm; (d) about 6 cm above the lateral epicondyle of the humerus where it is now a mixed nerve; or (e) in the axilla. Spread of stimulus from the radial to other nerves may readily occur at (a) and (e) and, to a lesser extent, at (b), and may cause problems in interpretation. Antidromic stimulation of sensory fibres at (c) with recording distally through surface electrodes (Downie and Scott, 1967) normally provides a potential of considerable amplitude (20–50 μV) which is free from contamination from cross-stimulation (Fig. 27.5). Further detailed studies of radial nerve function have been carried out by Trojaborg (1970) using needle electrodes and, in some instances, electronic averaging.

Lower limbs. Gilliatt, Goodman and Willison (1961) developed a technique with which, by

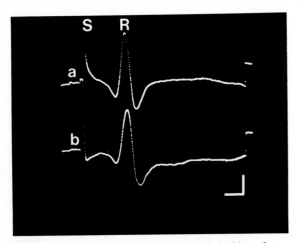

Fig. 27.5 Evoked sensory potentials recorded with surface electrodes from the radial nerve over the hand-to-forearm segment; (a) antidromic and (b) orthodromic conduction. S = stimulus; R = response. Calibration: 1ms; 10μV

stimulation of the deep peroneal nerve at the ankle, an evoked potential could be recorded from the common peroneal nerve at the head of the fibula. The amplitude of this potential using surface electrodes was small, and better results were obtained using needle electrodes placed 3–4 cm apart and inserted subcutaneously near the nerve at the head of the fibula. The stimulus necessary to obtain a maximal response was somewhat higher than that necessary in the upper limbs. This potential is not a pure sensory potential but is formed partly by antidromic conduction in motor fibres travelling to the extensor digitorum brevis. Where evoked potentials are small, as in this instance, there is a possibility that failure to elicit them may be due to anatomical rather than pathological variations. Furthermore, only slight temporal dispersion of individual fibre potentials from very minor nerve damage may make them disappear. This somewhat reduces their value in assessing the extent of the injury to a nerve.

Sensory nerve action potentials in the lower limbs may be recorded from the posterior tibial, including the medial plantar (Mavor and Atcheson, 1966; Guiloff and Sherratt, 1977), sural (Di Benedetto, 1970; Burke, Skuse and Lethlean, 1974) and superficial peroneal nerves (Di Benedetto, 1970) but, because the potentials are often buried in noise, averaging techniques are usually necessary for their retrieval. The above authors have found the use of surface recording electrodes to be quite satisfactory, but Behse and Buchthal (1971) prefer needle recording electrodes and have reported their extensive findings on all these nerves using this technique. Di Benedetto (1970) and Burke *et al.* (1974) suggested that measurement of the sensory action potential in the sural nerve may be a more sensitive index of peripheral neuropathy than the sensory potentials in the upper limbs. However, Guiloff and Sherratt (1977) found that alterations of the median plantar sensory action potentials were an even more sensitive test of peripheral nerve damage.

Measurement and sources of errors. Problems of measurement and possible sources of errors in the estimation of nerve conduction velocities are well discussed by Mavor and Libman (1962), Gassel (1964) and Simpson (1964a).

Measurement of the distance between two points of stimulation on the surface can be only an approximation of the true length of the underlying nerve, accounting for one of the most significant sources of error. Nevertheless, comparison of surface and true nerve measurement in cadavers has shown a close correlation between the two (Carpendale, 1956). This relationship is less certain when the course of the nerve is not straight and, in this situation, measurement by obstetric calipers may be more accurate than with a surface tape (Jebsen, 1967; London, 1975). The error of measurement is more significant for shorter distances, and care should be taken to ensure that the segment of nerve examined is as long as possible. In motor nerve conduction tests, measurement has to be made between the two points of the active stimulating electrode (cathode). In circumstances where it is not possible to stimulate the nerve at two sites (e.g. proximal limb muscles) the terminal latency may be used as an estimate of conduction time, and this may be related to the distance between the stimulating cathode and the recording electrode in order to allow for variations in the length of the limb (Gassel, 1964b). The terminal latency is the time interval between the departure of the impulse from the cathode and the take-off point of the muscle response. It represents not only the time lag necessary for the passage of the impulse along the terminal nerve fibres distal to the point stimulated but also conduction in the fine intramuscular terminal branches and across the motor end-plate. When measuring the latency, the initial take-off point of the evoked muscle action potential is used and, as a result, the conduction velocity is calculated for the fastest-conducting motor fibres. The same amplification gain should be used for recording the latency at each site, because altering the gain may result in apparent changes of latency (Goodgold and Eberstein, 1977). Gassel (1964a) has also pointed out that volume conduction of a

Table 27.1 Normal values for conduction rate in motor fibres

Nerve and segment	No. of Examinations	Conduction rate (ms)	Terminal latency (ms)	Reference
Ulnar				
axilla to elbow	47	63.8		Trojaborg (1977)
axilla to wrist	50	58.3		Norris, Shock & Wagman (1953)
elbow to wrist	225	59.9	2.7	Mulder, Lambert, Bastron & Sprague (1961)
elbow to wrist	188	60.0 Range 47.0–73.0		Thomas & Lambert (1960)
Erb's point to above elbow	30	58.9 Range 50.0–67.7		London (1975)
Erb's point to above elbow		61.3 Range 52.0–78.0		Jebsen (1967)
Median				
axilla to elbow	15	71.1 Range 60.3–86.4 ⎫	3.3	Mavor & Libman (1962)
axilla to wrist	15	64.3 Range 59.8–70.4 ⎭		
elbow to wrist	145	58.8	3.5	Mulder, Lambert, Bastron & Sprague (1961)
Radial				
axilla to elbow	9	70.0 SD ± 4.9	2.5 (to brachioradialis)	Trojaborg & Sindrup (1969)
Sciatic	20	56.0 SD ± 5.5	5.4 (to soleus)	Gassel & Trojaborg (1964)
Femoral	42		3.7 (at 14 cm from stim. point)	Gassel (1963)
Posterior tibial	12	48.7 SD ± 3.5	5.0	Mavor & Atcheson (1966)
	30	43.2 SD ± 4.9		Thomas, Sears & Gilliatt (1959)
Lateral popliteal	41	50.2 Range 30.0–60.0	5.0	Mulder, Lambert, Bastron & Sprague (1961)
	172	50.1 SD ± 7.2		Johnson & Olsen (1960)

distant muscle response may obscure the true take-off point and lead to significant miscalculation of the conduction rate. Activity from distant muscles may usually be recognised by the characteristic, initially positive-going deflection of the potential.

Measurement of the latency of evoked nerve action potentials depends upon the method of recording. For bipolar recording, Gilliatt et al. (1965) suggest that latency measurements should be made to the onset of the initial positive deflection, as this represents the arrival of the action potential in the fastest-conducting fibres. With exceedingly small potentials it may not be possible to identify the onset clearly and, for this reason, measurement to the peak of the response has been advocated. However, with currently available averaging techniques, satisfactory definition of the evoked potential should be possible, allowing accurate measurement of the latency to onset. For the 'monopolar' form of recording preferred by Buchthal and Rosenfalck (1966) the latency should be measured to the point where the initial positive deflection crosses the baseline. Gilliatt et al. (1965) observed that an accurate estimate of the conduction velocity can be obtained in the segment between the stimulating cathode and active recording electrode, provided that the stimulus is not more than 25 per cent supramaximal. The velocity may also be calculated by the subtraction method, after recording the potential at two sites.

NORMAL FINDINGS

General

Because of variations in technique, it is highly desirable that each laboratory should define its own control value for each nerve and segment of nerve. Tables 27.1 and 27.2 give a representative sample of results obtained by different authors, and this is sufficient to show the considerable

Table 27.2 Nerve conduction rates as judged from evoked nerve action potentials*†

Nerve and segment	No. of Examinations	Age (years)	Conduction rate (m/s)
Ulnar			
Vth finger to wrist	9	18–25	51.9 SD±5.6
Vth finger to wrist	10	70–89	50.2 SD±3.7
wrist to elbow	9	18–25	63.9 SD±5.1
elbow to axilla	9	18–25	62.5 SD±7.3
Median			
1st finger to wrist	13	18–25	50.2 SD±5.2
1st finger to wrist	10	70–88	44.1 SD±3.6
wrist to elbow	20	18–25	64.1 SD±4.7
elbow to axilla	20	18–25	70.3 SD±6.3
Radial			
1st finger to wrist	12	18–25	5.6–5.3
Superficial peroneal			
big toe to above extensor retinaculum	19	15–25	46.1 SD±4.1
big toe to above extensor retinaculum	17	40–65	42.2 SD±6.3
extensor retinaculum to head of fibula	24	15–33	55.9 SD±3.8
extensor retinaculum to head of fibula	23	40–65	52.9 SD±3.7
Sural			
dorsum of foot to lateral malleolus	16	15·30	51.2 SD±4.5
	15	40–65	48.3 SD±5.3
Posterior tibial			
big toe to medial malleolus	23	15–30	46.1 SD±3.5
	10	40–65	43.4 SD±3.8

*From Buchthal and Rosenfalck (1966) and Behse and Buchthal (1971)
†Conduction velocity measured to the initial positive peak of the evoked potential and recorded with a monopolar technique as in this Table gives rates substantially higher than when recorded with bipolar electrodes and to the negative peak of the potential

variation from segment to segment and the wide range of values even within one segment in normal subjects. Variations from one segment to another can, to large extent, be explained by fibre size. Hursch (1939) proposes a factor of six in correlating diameter (in μm) with conduction velocity (in m/s). Magladery and McDougal (1950) showed that, at least in motor fibres, tapering and branching occur distally, while Buchthal and Rosenfalck (1966) found evidence of similar changes in sensory fibres below the wrist.

Variations due to age

Gamstorp (1963) has shown that the conduction rate in motor fibres at birth is only about half of that in adults. Furthermore, the conduction rate increases at different rates in different nerves, reaching a maximum by early adolescence. Slowing of conduction velocity in motor fibres with increasing age in adult life has been demonstrated by several authors including Norris, Shock and Wagman (1953) and Mulder, Lambert, Bastron and Sprague (1961). Buchthal and Rosenfalck (1966) observed a significant decrease in sensory conduction velocity in upper arm and forearm segments and also an increase in distal latency with advancing age; in addition, they noted a reduction of the amplitude and increase in duration of the evoked sensory response.

Effects of temperature

Studies by Henriksen (1956) and Johnson and Olsen (1960) in motor fibres, and by Buchthal and Rosenfalck (1966) in the larger sensory fibres, show that conduction rate slows with cooling by 2–2.4 ms/°C. Coolness of the limbs may account for the slight degree of slowing seen in conditions such as poliomyelitis, and may add to the slowing due to nerve fibre damage in peripheral neuropathies such as peroneal muscular atrophy. In routine clinical recordings it is generally found impracticable to control temperature accurately. Provided, however, that the room temperature is maintained within a limited range and patients are allowed to become equilibrated, the range of variation will seldom cause confusion. If, however, one is following the course of a progressive or recovering neuropathy by repeated measurements in the same patient at different times, then temperature control is essential.

ABNORMAL NERVE CONDUCTION

General considerations

Abnormalities in nerve conduction rate, as shown by the techniques already described, will depend not only on the site of the lesion within the lower motor neurone or first sensory neurone, but also upon the degree of damage and the time relationship to the onset of injury. Gilliatt and Taylor (1959) have shown that, after surgical section of the facial nerve, no significant slowing of conduction in motor nerve fibres occurs for several days, after which conduction fails abruptly. If damage to a segment of nerve occurs without discontinuity of the axon, conduction distal to the block is variably disturbed. One major difference between conduction rates estimated in motor fibres only, and by the evaluation of evoked nerve potentials, must be stated. In the former, as long as one normally functioning motor fibre remains, then normal values for nerve conduction rate may be obtained, provided that one uses the take-off point of the muscle response as the sole criterion. Hodes et al. (1948) also took into consideration the amplitude and duration of the muscle potentials, but this depends upon several factors, such as the strength of the stimulus and the type and position of the recording electrodes, so that evaluation is difficult. Even when all fibres are involved to some degree, some motor conduction may remain and conduction rates as low as 7 m/s may be recorded. With evoked nerve potentials, however, a lesser degree of damage with variable degrees of slowing in different fibres may so spread out the summated action potential and lower its amplitude that it is no longer discernible. This can occur when the degree of disturbance, as judged clinically, is minimal or not even detectable. Conduction rates slower than 20 m/s are seldom seen when judged by evoked nerve potentials because, beyond this point, the amplitude of the evoked potential is usually too small to be registered. In this situation, Desmedt and Noel (1974) have shown that somatosensory cortical evoked responses may still be recorded, and they have used this technique to assess the sensory conduction velocity in a number of patients with severe neuropathy where the sensory nerve potential was not seen. Examination of the nerve action potential is, therefore, likely to uncover evidence of peripheral nerve lesions at an earlier stage than would the use of simple motor conduction techniques. On the other hand, the latter give measurable data in a more advanced stage of a neuropathy before conduction fails completely. Attempts have been made to elicit more information from motor conduction studies, and ingenious techniques have been devised to estimate the range of conduction velocities in different sizes of α-fibres within the normal and damaged nerves (Thomas, Sears and Gilliatt, 1959; Hopf, 1963). These techniques require two independently variable stimuli applied to the nerve at two points, the first stimulus being applied distally and resulting in a partial block of the descending volley initiated by the proximal stimulus. The effects of varying the distal stimulus intensity in one technique or the interval between two stimuli in the second are noted. Gilliatt, Hopf, Rudge and Baraitser (1976) have slightly modified the technique of Thomas et al. (1959), stimulating at two sites in the proximal part of the limb instead of one, the conduction velocity being calculated by subtraction in the usual way. The theoretical considerations on which these techniques are based are not entirely beyond dispute, but they do give a reflection of a spectrum of fibre size.

More recently, two methods have been reported for estimating the nerve fibre conduction velocity distributions by computer analysis of the compound action potential recorded from nerve trunks. Barker, Brown and Fressdon (1978) base their technique on the analyses of the dispersion components present in two compound action potentials recorded from a single site following stimulation at two points along the nerve. Cummins, Dorfman and Perkel (1978) have developed a model of the compound action potential in terms of constituent single-fibre action potentials. They have applied this to the study of two compound action potentials separated by a known distance along the nerve, from which they are able to derive an estimate of the distribution of fibre conduction velocities. Both these techniques are extremely complex, requiring sophisticated computer analysis and, as such, they may remain in the sphere of the research worker for some considerable time.

Median nerve lesions

Carpal tunnel syndrome (Fig. 27.6). The median nerve is subject to entrapment at a number of sites, by far the most common of which is at the

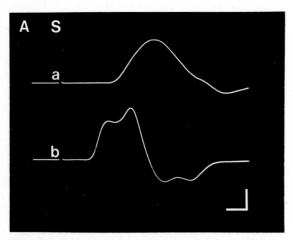

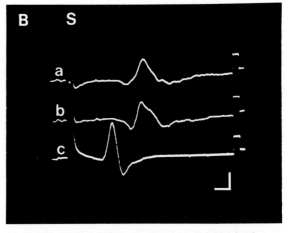

Fig. 27.6 Patient with carpal tunnel syndrome. A. Evoked muscle responses recorded from (a) abductor pollicis brevis and (b) abductor digiti minimi, following stimulation of the median and ulnar nerves respectively at the wrist. Terminal latency: median, 5.5 ms; ulnar, 2.9 ms. B. Evoked sensory potentials recorded at the wrist following stimulation of (a) digit II, (b) digit III (median) and (c) digit V (ulnar). Note that the median motor terminal latency is prolonged and the median digit sensory potentials are delayed, reduced in amplitude and dispersed. S=stimulus. Calibration: A, 2 ms; 5 mV. B, 1 ms; 5 μV

wrist within the carpal tunnel. Early studies by Simpson (1956) and Thomas (1960) showed prolongation of the terminal motor latency to abductor pollicis brevis in most cases of carpal tunnel syndrome, and Gilliatt and Sears (1958) demonstrated slowing of conduction in the median sensory fibres between the appropriate digits and the wrist. In a comprehensive study of 300 patients, combining motor and sensory techniques, Thomas, Lambert and Cseuz (1967) found motor abnormalities in 67 per cent and sensory changes in 85 per cent of clinically affected hands. Motor changes comprised: (a) increased terminal latency of more than 4.7 ms (60 per cent); (b) absence of an evoked muscle response (4.4 per cent); and (c) a difference of more than 1 ms between the terminal latencies of affected and unaffected hands, despite both values being within normal limits (2.7 per cent). The principal sensory findings were absence of a sensory action potential at the wrist (50 per cent) and an increase in latency of the sensory potential above 3.5 ms at the wrist (35 per cent). While most lesions may be demonstrable by the above techniques, a substantial number of symptomatic patients remain in whom the motor and sensory findings lie within the normal range. In an attempt to improve the diagnostic sensitivity of the investigations, Loong and Seah (1971) compared the amplitudes of digital nerve action potentials from the index (median) and little (ulnar) fingers. Normally this ratio is greater than one, but in 20 of 22 affected hands the ratio was reversed. However, concurrent ulnar nerve lesions may be present in up to 15–30 per cent of patients with a carpal tunnel syndrome (Buchthal, Rosenfalck and Trojaborg, 1974; Sedal, McLeod and Walsh, 1973) and a normal ratio may not, therefore, exclude the diagnosis of carpal tunnel compression. Buchthal et al. (1974) have shown significant slowing of sensory conduction from palm to wrist in patients in whom conduction between digit and wrist was normal, and they conclude that this is the most sensitive method for demonstrating a mild lesion. Kimura (1978) has recently reported localised slowing of motor conduction across the wrist in such cases.

Mild slowing of motor conduction in the forearm segment has been reported by several authors (Thomas, 1960; Thomas et al., 1967; Buchthal et al., 1974) but no relationship between the degree of slowing and the increase in terminal latency was noted. Hence, proximal slowing of motor conduction does not exclude a carpal tunnel syndrome.

Anatomical variations of the median nerve in the forearm may give rise to considerable confusion if their presence is not appreciated. Communication between the median and ulnar nerves in the forearm exists in 15–31 per cent of the normal population (Buchthal et al., 1974; Gutman, 1977) and, when associated with a carpal tunnel syndrome, will result in the unexpected finding of a prolonged distal latency and a paradoxically normal proximal latency (Iyer and Fenichel, 1976). This discrepancy is caused by the proximally evoked muscle potential arising from the thenar muscles supplied by axons which have taken an aberrant course via the anastomosis and the ulnar nerve, thereby escaping compression in the carpal tunnel. The presence of such an anomaly may be recognised by the spuriously high apparent motor conduction velocity in the forearm, and an initial positive deflection of the muscle action potential attributable to volume conduction of the muscle potential derived from the first dorsal interosseous or other thenar muscles, whose motor points are distant to the recording electrode.

Pronator syndrome. Less commonly, the median nerve may be entrapped at the elbow as it passes between the two heads of pronator teres, giving rise to the pronator syndrome (Seyffarth, 1951). Nerve conduction studies may help to localise the lesion by showing normal distal motor and sensory latencies at the wrist, and slowing of conduction in the forearm segment (Morris and Peters, 1976).

Ulnar nerve lesions

Ulnar nerve lesions in the hand may give rise to a variable combination of muscle and sensory involvement depending upon the exact site of the lesion. In most cases the deep palmar branch is affected distal to the branches supplying the hypothenar muscles, thus producing weakness of the remaining ulnar-innervated muscles but no sensory impairment. In such cases the motor terminal latency to the first dorsal interosseous or adductor pollicis may be markedly prolonged in contrast to the normal latency to abductor digiti minimi, and the sensory action potential from the little finger will be preserved at the wrist (Simpson, 1956; Ebeling, Gilliatt and Thomas, 1960). More proximally situated lesions will involve the hypothenar muscles but may still spare the sensory fibres; however, a lesion in Guyon's canal at the level of the wrist will affect both sensory and motor fibres, producing prolonged motor latencies to all the muscles, and impaired sensory conduction. Care must be taken to distinguish lesions at this site from others in the nerve, for example at the elbow, which may give rise to similar electrophysiological changes.

Ulnar nerve lesions at the elbow. The ulnar nerve is particularly vulnerable to damage by repeated trauma or entrapment as it traverses the groove behind the medial epicondyle. Simpson (1956) originally showed slowing of motor conduction in this affected segment in such a case, and further studies by Gilliatt and Thomas (1960) revealed decreased motor conduction velocities in the elbow-to-wrist segment in 12–13 patients with chronic traumatic ulnar neuropathy. They also observed a slight increase in the terminal latencies between the wrist and ulnar-supplied muscles, but conduction in the proximal segment between the elbow and axilla was normal, or only slightly slowed. Sensory nerve action potentials were unrecordable at the wrist following stimulation of the fifth finger in nine patients, and in eight of these no mixed nerve action potential could be recorded above the elbow after stimulation of the nerve trunk at the wrist. However, in six patients in whom the nerve was stimulated above the elbow, satisfactory responses were recorded in the axilla, indicating normal proximal function and thereby excluding the possibility of a lower brachial plexus lesion, which may be clinically indistinguishable from a disturbance of the ulnar nerve.

A number of authors have examined motor conduction across the elbow, where it might be expected to be maximally slowed (Jebsen, 1967; Payan, 1970; Eisen, 1974). However, it is difficult to measure accurately the length of nerve in this segment because of its curved course and, as Eisen stresses, it is important to ensure a distance of at least 10 cm to obtain a reliable value. Because slight slowing in the elbow segment may be present in asymptomatic controls, Eisen (1974) suggests that a decrease of at least 10 m/s or more, compared with the velocities in adjacent segments, should be taken to indicate a significant lesion at this site. Of a number of parameters examined by Eisen (1974), the most sensitive indices of mild ulnar nerve dysfunction were an increase in the motor latency from above elbow to muscle greater than 8.7 ms and a latency from wrist to muscle of more than 3.4 ms. In our experience we have seen patients with borderline normal motor and sensory values, in whom a reduced and dispersed mixed nerve action potential, evoked at the wrist and recorded above the elbow, pointed to the existence of a lesion. Nevertheless, some patients with very mild sensory symptoms have completely normal findings.

Apart from localising a lesion, the severity of conduction velocity changes may provide a useful guide to the necessity for surgical decompression or transposition of the ulnar nerve at the elbow (Payan, 1970; Eisen and Danan, 1974).

Radial nerve lesions

The radial nerve is frequently injured in the region of the spiral groove, either in association with fractures of the humerus or due to prolonged pressure, producing the familiar syndrome of 'Saturday night palsy'. Lesions at this site spare triceps but usually involve brachioradialis and the other extensor muscles in the forearm, producing variable sensory impairment in the hand and fingers. Several studies on patients with pressure palsy have shown normal motor conduction in the distal segment below the site of compression, as judged by latencies to the forearm muscles (Gassel and Diamantopoulos, 1964; Downie and Scott, 1964; Trojaborg, 1970). Sensory conduction in the distal forearm segment was usually well preserved. However, slowing or, in more severe cases, complete block of motor and sensory conduction, was demonstrated in the axilla-to-elbow segment containing the compressed portion of the nerve. Full recovery was observed to occur within six to eight weeks (Trojaborg, 1970) and, with the electrophysiological findings, suggested local demyelination as the cause of the palsy. In lesions due to traction or associated with fractures of the humerus, Trojaborg (1970) found evidence of axonal disruption, with either absence of motor and sensory responses or with normal velocities in the surviving axons. Recovery in this group was more protracted and less complete because of the slow outgrowth of nerve fibres, which he estimated to be about 1 mm/day.

As the radial nerve is less likely than the median or ulnar nerve to be affected by clinically unrecognised compressive neuropathy, it is a useful nerve in which to observe evoked sensory potentials when early neuropathy is suspected. Furthermore, one of the distal superficial branches in which conduction has been measured can be biopsied readily without causing troublesome sensory loss.

Brachial plexus lesions

Compression of the lower portion of the brachial plexus by a cervical rib or band produces the characteristic clinical picture of wasting of the hand and selective sensory impairment. Gilliatt, Le Quesne, Logue and Summer (1970) showed either normal or only mild alterations or motor conduction in the distal segments of the median and ulnar nerves, helping to exclude the more common compressive lesions seen in these nerves at the wrist and elbow. Demonstration of slowed conduction in the ulnar nerve across the thoracic outlet (Jebsen, 1967; London, 1975; Trojaborg, 1977) may further localise the site of the disturbance. Gilliatt et al. (1970) also observed loss, or significant reduction, of the sensory action potential in the ulnar nerve from the little finger, without any significant increase in latency. More extensive lesions affecting the brachial plexus, caused by traction injuries or neuralgic amyotrophy, may result in the loss of evoked potentials in one or more of the median, ulnar and radial nerves due to distal neuronal degeneration. In two cases of pressure palsy of the brachial plexus, Trojaborg (1977) found attenuation of the muscle responses following stimulation at the supraclavicular fossa, and slowing of the motor and sensory conduction through the damaged region.

Root lesions

As peripheral nerves, such as the median and ulnar, contain fibres derived from more than one nerve root, a lesion of a single root is unlikely to modify either the motor or sensory conduction rate. Furthermore, lesions of the sensory root proximal to the posterior root ganglion will leave the first sensory neurone intact: hence, evoked sensory potentials will be preserved, even when several roots are involved at this level. This is helpful in patients presenting with mild sensory symptoms in the hand, where confusion with distal median or ulnar nerve lesions might occur. The presence of normal evoked sensory potentials in this situation strongly favours a root, rather than a peripheral, nerve lesion. Boney and Gilliatt (1958) cite a case in which the presence of normal evoked sensory potentials in the median and ulnar nerves was used as evidence to indicate that the roots had been avulsed from the cord. Nevertheless, lesions of the root distal to the posterior root ganglion may result in reduction or loss of the sensory potential (Eisen et al., 1977a).

Conventional motor conduction techniques are generally unrewarding in the examination of radicular lesions. A number of recent reports have described the application of the 'H' reflex and 'F' wave studies in this situation. Drechsler, Lastovka and Kalvodova (1966) found that the 'H' reflex latency was significantly prolonged in both legs in patients with L5 and S1 root lesions while Braddom and Johnson (1974) observed that the 'H' reflex was delayed or absent on the affected side in 25 patients with unilateral S1 radiculopathy. A difference of 1.5 ms in the 'H' reflex latency of both legs was taken to indicate an S1 root lesion. Proximal entrapment in the upper and lower limb has been examined by Eisen et al. (1977a and b) using the 'F' wave technique to calculate the motor velocity over the segment. They found a significant reduction of the velocity over the proximal when compared with the distal segment. Because of the inherent inaccuracy in measuring the distance to the C7 spinous process, they suggested that estimation of the conduction time between elbow and cord is more reliable and should not be greater than 9.0 ms for the ulnar nerve or 8.5 ms for the median.

Lower limbs

Motor and sensory conduction studies on the lower limb nerves have revealed significantly slower velocities and very much smaller evoked responses than in the nerves of the upper limbs (Thomas *et al.*, 1959; Mavor and Atcheson, 1966; Behse and Buchthal, 1971). However, the advent of modern averaging techniques has greatly facilitated the recording of small sensory potentials in the distal segments of these nerves, and alterations in these responses may be the earliest indication of a mild peripheral neuropathy. In more profound peripheral neuropathies or nerve lesions, severe wasting of the distal (foot) muscles may result in failure to elicit a muscle response and preclude the estimation of motor conduction velocity.

Dropped foot caused by either a common peroneal nerve palsy or a root lesion is a frequent clinical problem, and in severe cases where there is no recordable evoked response from extensor digitorum brevis, motor conduction rates will be unobtainable and therefore of no diagnostic value. In mild peroneal palsies, the motor velocity between the popliteal fossa and the ankle may be within the normal range. In this situation, Gilliatt *et al.* (1961) found that alterations of the mixed nerve action potential, evoked at the ankle and recorded at the neck of the fibula, were helpful. In a large series of cases of peroneal palsy, Singh *et al.* (1974) noted that slowing of motor conduction across the capitulum fibulae was helpful in localising the lesion in one-third of cases, and a significant drop in the size of the muscle response evoked above in comparison with that evoked below the neck of the fibula identified the lesion in about 15 per cent. The most helpful localising feature was slowing of sensory conduction in the segment across the capitulum, which was present in 64 per cent of patients. It is evident that great care is required in this situation for correct interpretation of nerve conduction studies, which should be combined with an electromyographic examination of appropriate muscles.

Measurement of motor terminal latency in the posterior tibial nerve and the sensory action potential in the medial plantar nerve may help in the diagnosis of the tarsal tunnel syndrome (Mayor and Atcheson, 1966; Guiloff and Sherratt, 1977).

Diseases of the spinal cord

Muscle atrophy secondary to disturbances of the anterior horn cell due to motor neurone disease or syringomyelia may often begin in a focal manner and, while the clinical findings may point to a central lesion, patients are seen occasionally in whom it is not possible to exclude a disturbance of the peripheral nerves on clinical grounds. It is therefore of importance to known whether diseases involving the anterior horn cell have any effect on peripheral nerve function. Early workers did suggest that the conduction rate in the leg involved by poliomyelitis might be slowed, but Henriksen (1956) found only minor degrees of slowing (amounting to no more than 10 per cent) in such cases, provided that allowance was made for the lower temperature in the paretic limb. Similarly, Lambert and Mulder (1957), Willison (1962) and Ertekin (1967) found that motor conduction velocity was within the normal range in most patients with motor neurone disease. However, Miglietta (1968) and Chaco (1970) have found, using the Hopf technique, that the range of conduction velocities is narrowed, suggesting an early loss of the slower-conducting fibres.

Several studies have shown normal evoked sensory potentials and mixed nerve action potentials in motor neurone disease (Willison, 1962; Fincham and Van Allen, 1964; Ertekin, 1967) and this finding will help to exclude a peripheral nerve lesion in patients presenting with muscle wasting. Despite the profound sensory disturbances seen in syringomyelia, evoked sensory potentials are normal (Gilliatt, 1961; Fincham and Cape, 1968), indicating a disruption of the sensory pathway central to the posterior root ganglion.

Polyneuropathy

General considerations. Slowing of the conduction rate in motor fibres in patients with polyneuropathy was first described by Henriksen (1956), while Gilliatt and Sears (1958) and Kaeser (1965) confirmed this finding and also described absence or delay in the appearance of evoked sensory potentials. It has become apparent that peripheral neuropathies can, in most instances, be divided into two main groups by the nerve conduction findings. In the first, only a slight degree of slowing of the rate in motor or sensory fibres is seen, accompanied by lowering of the amplitude of evoked nerve potentials or occasional loss where these are normally of low amplitude. The degree of slowing may be so slight that it is still within the normal range, and its significance then can be determined only by serial studies, or by comparison of a group of patients against normal controls. Slight slowing may, to some extent, anticipate clinical abnormalities, but as the neuropathy progresses, the slowing of conduction rate deteriorates over a limited range. This is seen in the neuropathies associated with alcoholism and uraemia.

In the second group, nerve conduction is grossly disturbed. Evoked nerve action potentials are absent and motor responses may not be obtained at all. When motor conduction rates can be estimated, they are slowed by more than 30 per cent of their normal value and may be as low as 7 m/s. Terminal latencies are often strikingly prolonged up to 35 ms. This pattern is most frequently seen in acute polyneuropathies of Guillain-Barré type. Here, clinical recovery may considerably antedate recovery in nerve conduction findings and, indeed, in some instances marked permanent residual slowing may remain, despite good clinical function. Gilliatt (1966) has suggested that these two groups can be correlated pathologically with primary axonal degeneration and with segmental demyelination respectively. However, recent evidence from histopathological studies of peripheral neuropathies indicates that division into these two groups may not be as sharply defined as was originally suggested (Thomas, 1971). It has become increasingly clear that a combination of axonal degeneration and segmental demyelination may be present in most neuropathies, reflecting a close functional relationship between axons and Schwann cells. Nevertheless, one or other process may predominate, giving rise to the changes in nerve conduction described above.

Certainly, it is not safe to assume, on the basis of relatively normal findings at one stage of the illness, that a given case of peripheral neuropathy falls into the first group rather than the second, and the temporal profile of these disorders from the nerve conduction point of view has to be considered. A discussion of the findings in different neuropathies follows.

Neuropathy associated with diabetes mellitus. Diabetic neuropathy may present in a variety of forms, with either mild distal sensory impairment beginning in the legs or evidence of diffuse motor and sensory involvement, or as a mononeuropathy or mononeuritis multiplex. Several studies have revealed slowing of motor and sensory conduction in those with, and to a lesser extent those without, clinical evidence of neuropathy (Downie and Newell, 1961; Lawrence and Locke, 1961; Mulder et al., 1961; Gilliatt and Willison, 1962). The abnormalities tended to be more marked in the common peroneal nerve, but similar changes were found in median and ulnar nerves even in the absence of clinical signs. Nevertheless, in patients with a mononeuropathy, examination of the remaining clinically normal nerves revealed either normal or borderline conduction rates (Mulder et al., 1961; Gilliatt and Willison, 1962). In a comparative electrophysiological and clinical study, Lamontagne and Buchthal (1970) found abnormalities of the sensory potential to be the most sensitive indicator of sub-clinical involvement, with the presence of fibrillation potentials during electromyography of distal muscles as the next most sensitive parameter. However, the only electrophysiological change which correlated with the degree of clinical neuropathy was slowing of motor conduction in the common peroneal nerve. Histopathological studies have shown segmental demyelination and remyelination to be the predominant abnormality (Thomas and Lascelles, 1966; Chopra, Hurwitz and Montgomery, 1969; Behse, Buchthal and Carlsen, 1977) accounting for the slowing of conduction. Axonal loss or dysfunction has also been reported (Thomas and Lascelles, 1966; Behse et al., 1977; Hansen and Ballantyne, 1977), particularly in severe and chronic cases, and the considerable decrease or loss of the evoked potentials in these patients may be explained on this basis. The cause of the peripheral neuropathy in diabetes remains obscure, but current evidence suggests a metabolic disturbance rather than an underlying microangiopathy of the vasa nervorum. However, mononeuritis multiplex in such cases is probably due to small infarcts in the nerve, while many cases of mononeuropathy may be related to an undue sensitivity of the nerves to local trauma or compression. Nevertheless, Gregersen (1968) has demonstrated a relative insensitivity of diabetic nerves to the effects of ischaemia.

Neuropathy associated with uraemia. Peripheral neuropathy associated with chronic renal failure is well recognised, and has been reported in up to 50 per cent of patients, who generally present with mild sensory symptoms or signs of a mixed sensorimotor neuropathy. Numerous electrophysiological studies have shown slowing of nerve conduction, which may be present in clinically unaffected patients (Preswick and Jeremy, 1964; Jennekens, Dorhout Mees and van der Most van Spijk, 1971; Nielsen, 1973b). Nielsen (1973a) found almost uniform impairment of conduction in upper and lower limb nerves, involving equally motor and sensory fibres in proximal and distal nerve segments. The degree of slowing and severity of the clinical features correlated best with a reducing creatinine clearance and the duration of renal failure (Jennekens *et al.*, 1971; Nielsen, 1973b). The institution of 'adequate' haemodialysis usually results in a fairly rapid clinical improvement, not always accompanied by improved nerve conduction, which may remain impaired for many months before slowly recovering (Konatey-Ahulu, Baillod, Comty, Heron, Shaldon and Thomas, 1965; Tenckhoff, Boen, Jebsen and Spiegler, 1965; Nielsen, 1974b). In contrast, renal transplantation may be quickly followed by considerable clinical and electrophysiological improvement (Funck-Bretano, Chaumont, Mery, Vantelon and Zingaff-Kok, 1964; Nielsen, 1974a). Nielsen found significant increases of nerve conduction velocity within weeks of transplantation, and suggests that this rapid change may reflect a restoration of the normal axon membrane potential, although early remyelination could not be excluded. A secondary, more protracted, phase of recovery was thought to be due to axonal regeneration, correlating with the main histological findings in uraemic neuropathy of axonal damage with secondary segmental demyelination (Dyck, Johnson, Lambert and

O'Brien, 1971; Thomas, Hollinrake, Lascelles, O'Sullivan, Baillod, Moorhead and Mackenzie, 1971).

Neuropathy associated with rheumatoid arthritis. As in the two previous conditions, a variety of clinical types of neuropathy occur in rheumatoid arthritis. Apart from compression neuropathies, predominantly sensory but occasionally mixed sensorimotor disturbances are seen. Weller, Bruckner and Chamberlain (1970) suggest that the milder degrees of neuropathy, seemingly paradoxically, show more slowing in motor conduction rates, possibly because of demyelination, while some of the more severely involved patients show EMG evidence of denervation but little slowing of conduction, this being due to axonal degeneration more than to demyelination.

Alcoholic neuropathy. Mild to moderate slowing of motor and sensory conduction has been demonstrated in alcoholic patients with and without clinical features of peripheral nerve disease (Mawdsley and Mayer, 1965; Walsh and McLeod, 1970; Behse and Buchthal, 1977). Changes are present in upper and lower limb nerves, but tend to be more pronounced in the lower extremities. Mawdsley and Mayer (1965) and Casey and Le Quesne (1972) found evidence of greater involvement of the distal portions of the nerve, while Behse and Buchthal (1977) reported equal affection of distal and intermediate segments. Blackstock, Rushworth and Gath (1972) concluded from their study using the Hopf technique, that smaller-calibre motor fibres may be preferentially affected in patients without clinical evidence of neuropathy, although histological findings from sural nerve biopsy material indicate a more uniform involvement of large and small sensory fibres (Walsh and McLeod, 1970; Behse and Buchthal, 1977). The most significant electrophysiological abnormality in these latter studies was reduction of the sensory potential amplitude with only slight slowing of the maximal conduction velocity. These changes suggested axonal loss and correlated closely with the histological evidence of predominantly axonal damage, contrasting with earlier proposals that the primary disturbance in alcoholic neuropathy was segmental demyelination with secondary axonal changes (Denny-Brown, 1958). Behse and Buchthal (1977) were unable to find any evidence of vitamin deficiency in their patients and suggested that the neuropathy was the result of a direct neurotoxic effect of alcohol.

Peripheral neuropathy in chronic liver disease. While clinical signs of peripheral neuropathy in chronic liver disease may be slight, histological and electrophysiological studies have revealed evidence of peripheral nerve damage in a large proportion of patients. Dayan and Williams (1967) originally reported the presence of segmental demyelination in 10 patients and this finding was later confirmed by Knill-Jones, Goodwill, Dayan and Williams (1972). Mild slowing of motor conduction and increased distal motor latencies were reported by the latter authors in a small number of cases. Changes in sensory conduction have been observed more frequently (Seneviratne and Peiris, 1970; Kardel and Nielsen, 1974) consisting of increased latency or reduced amplitude of the sensory action potential recorded in the distal segment of the median nerve. These abnormalities were found as frequently in those without as in those with evidence of underlying alcoholism or carbohydrate intolerance, suggesting a causal relationship between hepatic failure and the neuropathy. Nevertheless, the aetiology remains obscure, although the increased frequency of collateral venous (porto-systemic) shunting in patients with neuropathy, and the improvement noted in one patient during protein restriction, point to a toxic agent(s) normally removed by the liver (Knill-Jones et al., 1972). It is interesting that Seneviratne and Peiris (1970) and Kardel and Nielsen (1974) report a relative resistance to the effects of ischaemia on peripheral nerve function in these patients, similar to that observed in diabetes.

Vitamin B$_{12}$ deficiency. Mayer (1965) found a rather poor correlation between the clinical picture and nerve conduction findings in a group of 53 patients with past or present deficiency. Patients without neurological abnormalities had normal nerve conduction, but patients with sensory loss

and areflexia had either normal conduction or mild slowing. In cases with relatively normal conduction, the pathological changes might be in the spinal cord rather than in the peripheral nerve. Some focal involvement of particular nerves subject to compression was also found.

Paraneoplastic neuropathy. A variety of neuromuscular disturbances, including peripheral neuropathy, has been described as remote manifestations of underlying neoplastic disease (Brain and Norris, 1965; Henson, Russell and Wilkinson, 1954). Moody (1965) found evidence of impaired sensory and motor conduction in about 17 per cent of patients with various neoplasms. Trojaborg, Frantzen and Andersen (1969) recorded fibrillation potentials during electromyography in 33 per cent of cases, implying a diffuse axonal polyneuropathy despite normal conduction rates. Of 30 patients with carcinoma of the lung who were neurologically normal, Campbell and Paty (1974) observed mild slowing of conduction in only four, but found evidence of loss of motor and sensory axons in nine. More pronounced slowing of conduction was seen in some patients with clinical signs of neuropathy, but others in this group had normal conduction rates. The electrophysiological findings indicated principally axonal degeneration with secondary segmental demyelination occurring only at a late stage. Similar observations have been reported by Walsh (1971) in 62 patients with lymphoma, 35 per cent of whom had impairment of conduction. Histological studies on the sural nerves in five of these patients revealed axonal degeneration and segmental demyelination.

Drug-induced neuropathy. A large number of drugs has been implicated as the cause of peripheral neuropathy, and the reader is referred to Chapter 25 which deals with this topic in detail. In most drug-induced neuropathies in which nerve conduction studies have been performed, mild to moderate slowing of motor and sensory conduction has been observed, consistent with axonal damage, e.g. nitrofurantoin (Toole, Gergen, Hayes and Felts, 1968); metronidazole (Bradley, Karlsson and Rasool, 1977); disulfiram (Bradley and Hewer, 1966); vincristine (Bradley,

Lassman, Pearce and Walton, 1970); phenytoin (Lovelace and Horowitz, 1968; Eisen, Woods and Sherwin, 1974; Chokroverty and Sayeed, 1975). Conversely, the neuropathy produced by perhexilene maleate is associated with moderate to severe slowing of motor conduction and reduction or loss of sensory evoked potentials (Said, 1978, and personal observations) indicative of demyelination.

Acute or sub-acute polyneuropathy (the Guillain-Barré syndrome). The pattern of nerve conduction changes may show considerable variation in patients presenting with this disorder. The finding is usually that of slowing of motor conduction velocity to about 60–70 per cent of normal in one or more nerves. Proximal and distal segments may be affected to roughly the same extent (Kimura and Butzer, 1975; King and Ashby, 1976) although in some patients, slowing may be patchy (Isch, Isch-Treussard, Buchheit, Delgado and Kircher, 1964) or most pronounced in common sites of nerve compression such as the carpal or cubital tunnel (Lambert and Mulder, 1964; Eisen and Humphreys, 1974). Prolonged distal motor latencies in the presence of normal or only slightly reduced conduction velocities may be the only abnormality in a further 20 per cent of patients. While slowing may be present early in the illness, it may not be apparent for two to three weeks after onset, or until after the condition has reached its peak. A number of studies (Lambert and Mulder, 1964; McQuillen, 1971; Eisen and Humphreys, 1974) have shown normal motor conduction in the distal segments in about 10–20 per cent of cases. However, using the 'F' wave conduction technique to examine the velocity over the proximal segments including the roots, Kimura and Butzer (1975) and King and Ashby (1976) showed significant slowing restricted to this segment in a number of patients. The electrophysiological finding of reduced conduction velocity correlates well with the predominantly demyelinating nature of the defect (Arnason, 1974), but in addition a significant proportion of patients have EMG evidence of denervation indicating axonal damage. Sensory conduction is usually normal or only slightly altered in milder cases, but distal slowing or loss of evoked sensory potentials has been reported in more severely affected patients (Bannister and Sears, 1962; Eisen and Humphreys, 1974; Raman and Taori, 1976).

The electrophysiological features may have a predictive value, for those patients with no conduction abnormalities tend to recover rapidly within about four weeks (Eisen and Humphreys, 1974) while those with only slowing of conduction generally take longer. Recovery in the presence of fibrillations is more protracted and often incomplete, pronounced residual deficits being more common (Eisen and Humphreys, 1974; Raman and Taori, 1976).

Chronic polyneuropathy

Peroneal muscular atrophy. Early studies of motor nerve conduction velocity in this disorder revealed considerable slowing to about half the normal value or less (Gilliatt and Thomas, 1957; Amick and Lemmi, 1963; Dyck, Lambert and Mulder, 1963). However, later reports on patients with a similar clinical picture showed some to have normal or only slightly reduced motor conduction rates (Gilliatt et al., 1961; Earl and Johnson, 1963). This was confirmed by Dyck and Lambert (1968), who separated two main groups on the basis of clinical, genetic, electrophysiological and histological findings—a hypertrophic group with slowed conduction, and a neuronal group with virtually normal conduction. Thomas and Calne (1974) also found that their patients displayed a bimodal distribution with respect to motor conduction velocity, with a cut-off point at about 40 m/s. By contrast, others have observed a wide spectrum of motor conduction velocity (Salisachs, 1974; Brust, Lovelace and Devi, 1978) or have found evidence of an intermediate group (Bradley, Madrid and Davis, 1977). Nevertheless, the findings of Buchthal and Behse (1977) support the presence of two main types of this disorder and they suggest that measurement of the sensory conduction velocity in the sural nerve may be of better discriminatory value than motor conduction. A small group of patients has also been described in whom the peripheral nerves appeared to be normal, implying a primary disturbance of the anterior horn cell (Buchthal and Behse, 1977).

Measurement of the conduction velocity may

help to identify clinically normal carriers in a family (Dyck *et al.*, 1963) and can also be of prognostic value as the illness seems to progress more rapidly in the hypertrophic than in the neuronal variety. Hypertrophic polyneuropathy may occur in several disorders such as Refsum's disease and Dejerine-Sottas' disease. It also occurs in some cases of recurrent or chronic non-specific and non-familial polyneuropathy. It is to be expected that nerve conduction might be profoundly disturbed in this condition and this, indeed, was confirmed by Thomas and Lascelles (1967) in six cases which they studied.

Metachromatic leucodystrophy (sulphatide lipidosis) has been shown to involve the peripheral nerves as well as the central nervous system. Fullerton (1964) showed that nerve conduction studies might be a valuable aid in the early screening of patients in whom this was a possible diagnosis, definite confirmation then being given by nerve biopsy. She found that conduction rates in six out of seven patients were slowed by more than 50 per cent.

Globoid leucodystrophy (Krabbe). As in metachromatic leucodystrophy, slowing of conduction rate in peripheral nerves has been demonstrated (Hogan, Guttman and Chou, 1969).

Friedreich's ataxia is also usually regarded as a disorder of the central nervous system, but Preswick (1968) found abnormalities in motor and sensory conduction in seven consecutive apparently 'pure' cases. These findings were confirmed by McLeod (1969) and Oh and Halse (1973), who observed that the sensory potentials were more seriously affected than the motor conduction velocities.

USE OF NERVE CONDUCTION TECHNIQUES IN CHILDREN

Gamstorp and Shelburne (1965) have shown that evoked sensory potentials may be reliably measured in children over the age of three months, while motor conduction can be estimated even in the newborn (Gamstorp, 1963). The established normal control values show that rates in the median and ulnar nerves at birth are about half those of the adult (Thomas and Lambert, 1960). The increasing conduction velocity with age varies with different nerves, but in all, adult values are reached by adolescence. While the size of the hand makes the calculation of conduction rate difficult in very young children, these tests are still of great help at a time when the clinical assessment of motor function, and more particularly of sensation, is so difficult.

The use of nerve conduction tests in screening for metachromatic and globoid leucodystrophy has already been discussed.

NERVE CONDUCTION IN FUNCTIONAL DISORDERS

Preservation of normal conduction in sensory and motor fibres is of occasional help in functional disorders and in medico-legal situations, for instance when hysterical glove and stocking anaesthesia may suggest a peripheral neuropathy. It must be remembered that, in root or in cord lesions, nerve conduction will usually be normal despite organic motor or sensory disturbance.

REFERENCES

Amick, L.D. & Lemmi, H. (1963) Electromyographic studies in peroneal muscular atrophy. *Archives of Neurology*, **9**, 273–284.

Arnason, B.G.W. (1974) Inflammatory polyradiculo-neuropathies. In *Peripheral Neuropathy*, Eds P.J. Dyck, P.K. Thomas & E.H. Lambert, Vol. II, p. 1110 (Saunders: Philadelphia).

Bannister, R.G. & Sears, J.A. (1962) The changes in nerve conduction in acute idiopathic polyneuritis. *Journal of Neurology, Neurosurgery and Psychiatry*, **25**, 321–328.

Barker, A.T., Brown, B.H. & Fressdon, I.L. (1978) Determination of the distribution of conduction velocities in peripheral nerve trunks. Abstracts: *International Evoked Potentials Symposium*, Nottingham.

Behse, F. & Buchthal, F. (1971) Normal sensory conduction in the nerves of the leg in man. *Journal of Neurology, Neurosurgery and Psychiatry*, **34**, 404–414.

Behse, F. & Buchthal, F. (1977) Alcoholic neuropathy: clinical, electrophysiological and biopsy findings. *Annals of Neurology*, **2**, 95–110.

Behse, F., Buchthal F. & Carlsen, F. (1977) Nerve biopsy and conduction studies in diabetic neuropathy. *Journal of Neurology, Neurosurgery and Psychiatry*, **40**, 1072–1082.

Blackstock, E., Rushworth, G. & Gath, P. (1972) Electrophysiological studies in alcoholism. *Journal of Neurology, Neurosurgery and Psychiatry*, **35**, 326–334.

Boney, G. & Gilliatt, R.W. (1958) Sensory nerve conduction of the traction lesion of the brachial plexus. *Proceedings of the Royal Society of Medicine*, **56**, 365.

Braddom, R.L. & Johnson, E.W. (1974) 'H' reflex: Review and classification with suggested clinical uses. *Archives of Physical Medicine and Rehabilitation*, **55**, 412–417.

Bradley, W.G. & Hewer, R.L. (1966) Peripheral neuropathy due to Disulfiram. *British Medical Journal*, **2**, 449–450.

Bradley, W.G., Karlsson, I.J. & Rasool, C.G. (1977) Metronidazole neuropathy. *British Medical Journal*, **2**, 610.

Bradley, W.G., Madrid, R. & Davis, C.J.F. (1977) The peroneal muscular atrophy syndrome. Clinical, genetic, electrophysiological and nerve biopsy studies. Part 3. Clinical, electrophysiological and pathological correlations. *Journal of the Neurological Sciences*, **32**, 123–136.

Bradley, W.G., Lassman, L.P., Pearce, G.W. & Walton, J.N. (1970) The neuropathy of Vincristine in man. Clinical, electrophysiological and pathological studies. *Journal of the Neurological Sciences*, **10**, 107–131.

Brain, W.R. & Norris, F. (1965) *The Remote Effects of Cancer on the Nervous System* (Grune and Stratton: New York).

Brust, J.C.M., Lovelace, R.E. & Devi, S. (1978) Clinical and electrophysiological features of C.M.T. syndrome. *Acta Neurologica Scandinavica*, Supp. **68**, 58.

Buchthal, F. & Behse, F. (1977) Peroneal muscular atrophy (P.M.A.) and related disorders. 1. Clinical manifestations as related to biopsy findings, nerve conduction and electromyography. *Brain*, **100**, 41–66.

Buchthal, F. & Rosenfalck, A. (1966) Evoked action potentials and conduction velocity in human sensory nerves. *Brain Research*, **3**, 1–22.

Buchthal, F., Rosenfalck, A. & Trojaborg, W. (1974) Electrophysiological findings in entrapment of the median nerve at the wrist and elbow. *Journal of Neurology, Neurosurgery and Psychiatry*, **37**, 340–360.

Burke, D., Skuse, N.F. & Lethlean, A.K. (1974) Sensory conduction of the sural nerve in polyneuropathy. *Journal of Neurology, Neurosurgery and Psychiatry*, **37**, 647–652.

Campbell, M.J. & Paty, D.W. (1974) Carcinomatous neuropathy: 1. Electrophysiological studies. An electrophysiological and immunological study of patients with carcinoma of the lung. *Journal of Neurology, Neurosurgery and Psychiatry*, **37**, 131–141.

Carpendale, M.T.F. (1956) Conduction time in the terminal portion of the motor fibres of the ulnar, median and peroneal nerves in healthy subjects and in patients with neuropathy. M.S. (Physical Medicine) Thesis. University of Minnesota.

Casey, E.B. & Le Quesne, P.M. (1972) Electrophysiological evidence for a distal lesion in alcoholic neuropathy. *Journal of Neurology, Neurosurgery and Psychiatry*, **35**, 624–630.

Chaco, J. (1970) Conduction velocity of motor nerve fibres in progressive spinal atrophy. *Acta Neurologica Scandinavica*, **46**, 119–122.

Chokroverty, S. & Sayeed, Z.A. (1975) Motor conduction study in patients on diphenyl hydantoin therapy. *Journal of Neurology, Neurosurgery and Psychiatry*, **38**, 1235–1239.

Chopra, J.S., Hurwitz, L.J. & Montgomery, D.A.D. (1969) The pathogenesis of sural nerve changes in diabetes mellitus. *Brain*, **92**, 391–418.

Cummins, K.L., Dorfman, L.J. & Perkel, D.H. (1978) Nerve-fiber conduction velocity distributions: A new clinically applicable method for estimation based on compound nerve action potentials. Abstracts: *IVth International Congress on Neuromuscular Disease*. Montreal.

Dawson, G.D. (1956) The relative excitability and conduction velocity of sensory and motor nerve fibres in man. *Journal of Physiology*, **131**, 436.

Dawson, G.D. & Merton, P.A. (1956) 'Recurrent' discharges from motor neurones. Abstract: *20th International Congress of Physiology*, Bruxelles, pp. 221–222.

Dawson, G.D. & Scott, J.W. (1949) The recording of nerve action potentials through the skin in man. *Journal of Neurology, Neurosurgery and Psychiatry*, **12**, 259.

Dayan, A.D. & Williams, R. (1967) Demyelinating peripheral neuropathy and liver disease. *Lancet*, **2**, 133–134.

Denny-Brown, D.E. (1958) The neurological aspects of thiamine deficiency. *Federation Proceedings*, **17**, Suppl. 2, 35–39.

Desmedt, J.E. & Noel, P. (1974) Cerebral evoked potentials. In *Peripheral Neuropathy*, Eds P.J. Dyck, P.K. Thomas, & E.H. Lambert, Vol. I, p. 480 (Saunders: Philadelphia).

Di Benedetto, M. (1970) Sensory nerve conduction in the lower extremities. *Archives of Physical Medicine*, **51**, 253.

Downie, A.W. & Newell, D.J. (1961) Sensory nerve conduction in patients with diabetes mellitus and controls. *Neurology (Minneapolis)*, **14**, 839–843.

Downie, A.W. & Scott, T.R. (1964) Radial nerve conduction studies. *Neurology (Minneapolis)*, **14**, 839–843.

Downie, A.W. & Scott, T.R. (1967) An improved technique for radial nerve conduction studies. *Journal of Neurology, Neurosurgery and Psychiatry*, **30**, 332–336.

Drechsler, D., Lastovka, M. & Kalvodova, E. (1966) Electrophysiological study of patients with herniated intervertebral discs. *Electromyography*, **6**, 187–204.

Dyck, P.J. & Lambert, E.H. (1968) Lower motor and primary sensory neurone disease with peroneal muscular atrophy. 1. Neurologic, genetic and electrophysiologic findings in hereditary polyneuropathies. *Archives of Neurology*, **18**, 603–618.

Dyck, P.J., Lambert, E.H. & Mulder, D.W. (1963) Charcot-Marie-Tooth disease: nerve conduction and clinical studies of a large kinship. *Neurology (Minneapolis)*, **13**, 1–11.

Dyck, P.J., Johnson, W.J., Lambert, E.H. & O'Brien, P.C. (1971) Uraemic polyneuropathy—segmental demyelination secondary to axonal degeneration. *Mayo Clinic Proceedings*, **46**, 400–429.

Earl, W.C. & Johnson, E.W. (1963) Motor nerve conduction velocity in CMT disease. *Archives of Physical Medicine*, **44**, 247–252.

Ebeling, P., Gilliatt, R.W. & Thomas, P.K. (1960) A clinical and electrical study of ulnar nerve lesions in the hand. *Journal of Neurology, Neurosurgery and Psychiatry*, **23**, 1.

Eisen, A. (1974) Early diagnosis of ulnar nerve palsy. *Neurology (Minneapolis)*, **24**, 256–262.

Eisen, A. & Danan, J. (1974) The mild cubital tunnel syndrome. *Neurology (Minneapolis)*, **24**, 608–613.

Eisen, A. & Humphreys, P. (1974) The Guillain-Barré syndrome. A clinical and electrodiagnostic study. *Archives of Neurology*, **30**, 438–443.

Eisen, A., Schomer, D. & Melmed, C. (1977a) The application of 'F' wave measurements in the differentiation of proximal and distal upper limb entrapments. *Neurology*

(*Minneapolis*), **27**, 662–668.

Eisen, A., Schomer, D. & Melmed, C. (1977b) An electrophysiological method for examining lumbosacral root compression. *The Canadian Journal of the Neurological Sciences*, **4**, 117–123.

Eisen, A., Woods, J.F. & Sherwin, A.L. (1974) Peripheral nerve function in long term therapy with diphenyl hydantoin. *Neurology (Minneapolis)*, **24**, 411–417.

Ertekin, C. (1967) Sensory and motor conduction in motor neurone disease. *Acta Neurologica Scandinavica*, **43**, 499–512.

Fincham, R.W. & Cape, C.A. (1968) Sensory nerve conduction in syringomyelia. *Neurology (Minneapolis)*, **18**, 200–201.

Fincham, R.W. & Van Allen, M.W. (1964) Sensory nerve conduction in amyotrophic lateral sclerosis. *Neurology (Minneapolis)*, **14**, 31–33.

Fullerton, P.M. (1964) Peripheral nerve conduction in metachromatic leucodystrophy (sulphatide lipidosis). *Journal of Neurology, Neurosurgery and Psychiatry*, **27**, 100.

Funck-Bretano, J.L., Chaumont, P., Mery, J.P., Vantelon, J. & Zingaff-Kok, J. (1964) Intéret de la mésure de la vitesse de conduction aveuse soumis ner des hémodialyses répetées. *Proceedings of the European Dialysis and Transplant Association*, **1**, 23.

Gamstorp, I. (1963) Normal conduction velocity of ulnar, median and peroneal nerves in infancy, childhood and adolescence. *Acta Paediatrica Scandinavica* (Supplement 146), 68.

Gamstorp, I. & Shelburne, S.A. (1965) Peripheral sensory conduction in ulnar and median nerves of normal infants. *Acta Paediatrica Scandinavica*, **54**, 309.

Gassel, M.M. (1963) A study of femoral nerve conduction time. *Archives of Neurology*, **9**, 607.

Gassel, M.M. (1964a) Sources of error in motor nerve conduction studies. *Neurology (Minneapolis)*, **14**, 825–835.

Gassel, M.M. (1964b) A test of nerve conduction to muscles of the shoulder girdle as an aid in the diagnosis of proximal neurogenic and muscular disease. *Journal of Neurology, Neurosurgery and Psychiatry*, **27**, 200–205.

Gassel, M.M. & Diamantopoulos, E. (1964) Pattern of conduction times in the distribution of the radial nerve. *Neurology (Minneapolis)*, **14**, 222–231.

Gassel, M.M. & Trojaborg, W. (1964) Clinical and electrophysiological study of the pattern of conduction times in the distribution of the sciatic nerve. *Journal of Neurology, Neurosurgery and Psychiatry*, **27**, 351.

Gilliatt, R.W. (1961) *Electrodiagnosis and Electromyography*, Ed. Elizabeth Licht (Licht: Newhaven, Connecticut).

Gilliatt, R.W. (1966) Applied electrophysiology in nerve and muscle disease. *Proceedings of the Royal Society of Medicine*, **59**, 989.

Gilliatt, R.W. & Sears, T.A. (1958) Sensory nerve action potentials in patients with peripheral nerve lesions. *Journal of Neurology, Neurosurgery and Psychiatry*, **21**, 109.

Gilliatt, R.W. & Taylor, J.C. (1959) Electrical changes following section of the facial nerve. *Proceedings of the Royal Society of Medicine*, **52**, 1080.

Gilliatt, R.W. & Thomas, P.K. (1957) Extreme slowing of nerve conduction in peroneal muscular atrophy. *Annals of Physical Medicine*, **4**, 104–106.

Gilliatt, R.W. & Thomas, P.K. (1960) Changes in nerve conduction with ulnar nerve lesions at the elbow. *Journal of Neurology, Neurosurgery and Psychiatry*, **23**, 312.

Gilliatt, R.W. & Willison, R.G. (1962) Peripheral nerve conduction in diabetic neuropathy. *Journal of Neurology, Neurosurgery and Psychiatry*, **25**, 11–18.

Gilliatt, R.W., Goodman, H.V. & Willison, R.G. (1961) The recording of lateral popliteal nerve action potentials in man. *Journal of Neurology, Neurosurgery and Psychiatry*, **24**, 305–318.

Gilliatt, R.W., Hopf, H.C., Rudge, P. & Baraitser, M. (1976) Axonal velocities of motor units in the hand and foot muscles of the baboon. *Journal of the Neurological Sciences*, **29**, 249–258.

Gilliatt, R.W., Le Quesne, P.M., Logue, V. & Sumner, A.J. (1970) Wasting of the hand associated with a cervical rib or band. *Journal of Neurology, Neurosurgery and Psychiatry*, **33**, 615–624.

Gilliatt, R.W., Melville, I.D., Velate, A.S. & Willison, R.G. (1965) A study of normal nerve action potentials using an averaging technique (barrier grid storage tube). *Journal of Neurology, Neurosurgery and Psychiatry*, **28**, 191.

Goodgold, J. & Eberstein, A. (1977) *Electrodiagnosis of Neuromuscular Diseases* (Williams and Wilkins: Baltimore).

Gregersen, G. (1968) A study of the peripheral nerves in diabetic subjects during ischaemia. *Journal of Neurology, Neurosurgery and Psychiatry*, **31**, 175.

Guiloff, R.J. & Sherratt, R.M. (1977) Sensory conduction in medial plantar nerve. *Journal of Neurology, Neurosurgery and Psychiatry*, **40**, 1168–1181.

Guld, C.E. (1960) Use of screened power transformers and output transformers to reduce stimulus artefacts. In *Medical Electronics* (Thomas: Springfield, Ill.).

Guld, C., Rosenfalck, A. & Willison, R.G. (1970) Report of the committee on E.M.G. instrumentation. *Electroencephalography and Clinical Neurophysiology*, **28**, 399–413.

Gutman, L. (1977) Median-ulnar nerve communications and carpal tunnel syndrome. *Journal of Neurology, Neurosurgery and Psychiatry*, **40**, 982–986.

Hagbarth, E.E. (1962) Post-tetanic potentiation of myotonic reflexes in man. *Journal of Neurology, Neurosurgery and Psychiatry*, **25**, 1.

Hansen, S. & Ballantyne, J.P. (1977) Axonal dysfunction in the neuropathy of diabetes mellitus: quantitative electrophysiological study. *Journal of Neurology, Neurosurgery and Psychiatry*, **40**, 555–564.

Henriksen, J.D. (1956) Conduction velocities of motor nerves in normal subjects and patients with neuromuscular disorders. M.S. (Physical Medicine) Thesis: University of Minnesota.

Henson, R.A., Russell, D.S. & Wilkinson, M. (1954) Carcinomatous neuropathy and myopathy. A clinical and pathological study. *Brain*, **77**, 82.

Hodes, R., Larrabee, M.G. & German, W. (1948) The human electromyogram in response to nerve stimulation and the conduction velocity of motor axons. *Archives of Neurology and Psychiatry*, **60**, 340.

Hogan, G.R., Guttman, L. & Chou, S.M. (1969) The peripheral neuropathy of Krabbe's (globoid) leukodystrophy. *Neurology (Minneapolis)*, **19**, 1094.

Hopf, H.C. (1963) Electromyographic study on so-called mononeuritis. *Archives of Neurology*, **9**, 307.

Hursch, J.B. (1939) Conduction velocity and diameter of nerve fibres. *American Journal of Physiology*, **127**, 131.

Isch, F., Isch-Treussard, C., Buchheit, F., Delgado, V. & Kircher, J.P. (1964) Measurement of conduction velocity of motor nerve fibres in polyneuritis and polyradiculoneuritis. (Abstracted). *Electroencephalography* and Clinical Neurophysiology, **16**, 416.

Iyer, V. & Fenichel, G.M. (1976) Normal median nerve proximal latency in carpal tunnel syndrome: a. due to co-existing Martin-Gruber anastomosis. *Journal of Neurology, Neurosurgery and Psychiatry*, **39**, 449–452.

Jebsen, R.H. (1967) Motor conduction velocities in the median and ulnar nerves. *Archives of Physical Medicine and Rehabilitation*, **48**, 185–194.

Jennekens, F.G.I., Dorhout Mees, E.J. & van der Most van Spijk, D. (1971) Clinical aspects of uraemic polyneuropathy. *Nephron*, **8**, 414–426.

Johnson, E.W. & Olsen, K.J. (1960) Clinical value of motor nerve conduction velocity determination. *Journal of the American Medical Association*, **172**, 2030.

Kaeser, H.E. (1965) Changes in the conduction velocity in neuropathies and neuritides. *Fortschritte der Neurologie und Psychiatrie und ihrer Grinzgebiete*, **33**, 221.

Kardel, T. & Nielsen, V.K. (1974) Hepatic neuropathy (a clinical and electrophysiological study). *Acta Neurologica Scandinavica* **50**, 513–526.

Kimura, J. (1974) 'F' wave velocity in the central segment of the median and ulnar nerve. A study in normal subjects and in patients with Charcot-Marie-Tooth disease. *Neurology (Minneapolis)*, **24**, 539–546.

Kimura, J. (1978) A method for determining median nerve conduction velocity across the carpal tunnel. *Journal of the Neurological Sciences*, **38**, 1–10.

Kimura, J. & Butzer, J.F. (1975) 'F' wave conduction velocity in Guillain-Barré syndrome. *Archives of Neurology* **32**, 524–529.

King, D. & Ashby, P. (1976) Conduction velocity in the proximal segments of a motor nerve in the Guillain-Barré syndrome. *Journal of Neurology, Neurosurgery and Psychiatry*, **39**, 538–544.

Knill-Jones, R.P., Goodwill, C.J., Dayan, A.D. & Williams, R. (1972) Peripheral neuropathy in chronic liver disease: clinical electrophysiological and nerve biopsy findings. *Journal of Neurology, Neurosurgery and Psychiatry*, **35**, 22–30.

Konotey-Ahulu, F.I.D., Baillod, R., Comty, C.M., Heron, J.R., Shaldon, S. & Thomas, P.K. (1965) Effect of periodic dialysis on the peripheral neuropathy of end-stage and renal failure. *British Medical Journal*, **2**, 1212–1215.

Lambert, E.H. & Mulder, D.W. (1957) Electromyographic studies in amyotrophic lateral sclerosis. *Proceedings of the Staff Meetings of the Mayo Clinic*, **32**, 441.

Lambert, E.H. & Mulder, D.W. (1964) Nerve conduction in the Guillain-Barré syndrome. *Electroencephalography and Clinical Neurophysiology*, **17**, 86.

Lamontagne, A. & Buchthal, F. (1970) Electrophysiological studies in diabetic neuropathy. *Journal of Neurology, Neurosurgery and Psychiatry*, **33**, 442–452.

Lawrence, D.G. & Locke, S. (1961) Motor nerve conduction velocity in diabetes. *Archives of Neurology*, **5**, 483–489.

Lefebre-d'Amour, M., Shahani, B.T., Young, R.R. & Bird, K.T. (1976) Importance of studying sural conduction and late responses in the evaluation of alcoholic subjects. *Neurology (Minneapolis)*, **26**, 368.

London, G.W. (1975) Normal ulnar nerve conduction velocity across the thoracic outlet: comparison of two measuring techniques. *Journal of Neurology, Neurosurgery and Psychiatry*, **38**, 756–760.

Loong, S.C. & Seah, C.S. (1971) Comparison of median and ulnar sensory nerve action potentials in the diagnosis of the carpal tunnel syndrome. *Journal of Neurology,*

Neurosurgery and Psychiatry, **34**, 750.

Lovelace, R.E. & Horowitz, S.J. (1968) Peripheral neuropathy in long term diphenyl hydantoin therapy. *Archives of Neurology*, **18**, 69–77.

Magladery, J.W. & McDougal, D.D. Jr. (1950) Electrophysiological studies of nerve and reflex activity in normal man. 1. Identification of certain reflexes in the electromyogram and the conduction velocity of peripheral nerve fibres. *Bulletin of the Johns Hopkins Hospital*, **86**, 265–290.

Magladery, J.W., Porter, W.E., Park, A.M. & Teasdall, R.D. (1951) Electrophysiological studies of nerve and reflex activity in normal man. IV. The two-neurone reflex and identification of certain action potentials from spinal roots and cord. *Bulletin of the Johns Hopkins Hospital*, **88**, 499–519.

Mavor, H. & Atcheson, J.B. (1966) Posterior tibial nerve conduction. *Archives of Neurology*, **14**, 661–669.

Mavor, H. & Libman, I. (1962) Motor nerve conduction velocity measurement as a diagnostic tool. *Neurology (Minneapolis)*, **12**, 733.

Mawdsley, C. & Mayer, R.F. (1965) Nerve conduction in alcoholic polyneuropathy. *Brain*, **88**, 335–356.

Mayer, R.F. (1965) Peripheral nerve function in Vitamin B_{12} deficiency. *Archives of Neurology*, **13**, 355–362.

Mayer, R.F. & Feldman, R.G. (1967) Observations on the nature of the 'F' wave in man. *Neurology (Minneapolis)*, **17**, 147–156.

McLeod, J.G. (1969) Electrophysiological and histological studies in patients with Friedreich's ataxia. *Electroencephalography and Clinical Neurophysiology*, **27**, 723.

McQuillen, M.P. (1971) Idiopathic polyneuritis: serial studies of nerve and immune functions. *Journal of Neurology, Neurosurgery and Psychiatry*, **34**, 607–615.

Miglietta, O. (1968) Motor nerve fibres in amyotrophic lateral sclerosis. *American Journal of Physical Medicine*, **47**, 118–124.

Moody, J. (1965) Electrophysiological investigation into the neurological complications of carcinoma. *Brain*, **88**, 1023–1036.

Morris, H.H. & Peters, B.H. (1976) Pronator syndrome: clinical and electrophysiological features in seven cases. *Journal of Neurology, Neurosurgery and Psychiatry*, **39**, 461–464.

Mulder, D.W., Lambert, E.H., Bastron, J.A. & Sprague, R.G. (1961) The neuropathies associated with diabetes mellitus. *Neurology (Minneapolis)*, **11**, 275–284.

Nielsen, V.K. (1973a) The peripheral nerve function in chronic renal failure. V. Sensory and motor conduction velocity. *Acta Medica Scandinavica*, **194**, 445–454.

Nielsen, V.K. (1973b) The peripheral nerve function in chronic renal failure. VI. The relationship between sensory and motor nerve conduction and kidney function, azotaemia, age, sex and clinical neuropathy. *Acta Medica Scandinavica*, **194**, 455–462.

Nielsen, V.K. (1974a) The peripheral nerve function in chronic renal failure. IX. Recovery after renal transplantation. Electrophysiological aspects (sensory and motor conduction). *Acta Medica Scandinavica*, **195**, 171.

Nielsen, V.K. (1974b) The peripheral nerve function in chronic renal failure—(a survey). *Acta Medica Scandinavica* (Supplement), 573.

Norris, A.H., Shock, N.W. & Wagman, I.H. (1953) Age changes in the maximum conduction velocity of motor fibres of human ulnar nerves. *Journal of Applied Physiology*, **5**, 589–593.

Oh, S.J. & Halse, J.H. (1973) Abnormality in nerve potentials in Friedreich's ataxia. *Neurology (Minneapolis)*, **23**, 52–54.

Panayiotopoulos, C.P. & Scarpalezos, S. (1977) 'F' wave studies on the deep peroneal nerve. Part 2–1. Chronic renal failure. 2. Limb-girdle muscular dystrophy. *Journal of the Neurological Sciences*, **31**, 331–341.

Payan, J. (1970) Anterior transposition of the ulnar nerve, an electrophysiological study. *Journal of Neurology, Neurosurgery and Psychiatry*, **33**, 157.

Preswick, G. (1968) The peripheral neuropathy of Friedreich's ataxia. (Abstract) *Electroencephalography and Clinical Neurophysiology*, **25**, 399.

Preswick, G. & Jeremy, D. (1964) Subclinical polyneuropathy in renal insufficiency. *Lancet*, **2**, 731.

Raman, P.T. & Taori, G.M. (1976) Prognostic significance of electrodiagnostic studies in the Guillain-Barré syndrome. *Journal of Neurology, Neurosurgery and Psychiatry*, **39**, 163–170.

Said, G. (1978) Perhexiline neuropathy: A clinico-pathological study. *Annals of Neurology*, **3**, 252–266.

Salisachs, P. (1974) Wide spectrum of motor conduction velocity in Charcot-Marie-Tooth disease. An anatomic-physiological interpretation. *Journal of the Neurological Sciences*, **23**, 25–31.

Schiller, H.H. & Stålberg, E. (1978) 'F' responses studied with single fibre E.M.G. in normal subjects and spastic patients. *Journal of Neurology, Neurosurgery and Psychiatry*, **41**, 45–53.

Sears, T.A. (1959) Action potentials evoked in digital nerves by stimulation of the mechano receptors in the human finger. *Journal of Physiology*, **148**, 30–31.

Sedal, L., McLeod, J.G. & Walsh, J.C. (1973) Ulnar nerve lesions associated with carpal tunnel syndrome. *Journal of Neurology, Neurosurgery and Psychiatry*, **36**, 118–123.

Seneviratne, K.N. & Peiris, O.A. (1970) Peripheral nerve function in chronic liver disease. *Journal of Neurology, Neurosurgery and Psychiatry*, **33**, 609–614.

Seyffarth, H. (1951) Primary myoses in the m. pronator teres as a cause of lesion of the n. medianus (the pronator syndrome). *Acta Psychiatrica et Neurologica Scandinavica*, (Supplement 74), 251.

Simpson, J.A. (1956) Electrical signs in the diagnosis of carpal tunnel and related syndromes. *Journal of Neurology, Neurosurgery and Psychiatry*, **19**, 275.

Simpson, J.A. (1964) Fact and fallacy in measurement of conduction velocity in motor nerves. *Journal of Neurology, Neurosurgery and Psychiatry*, **27**, 381.

Singh, N., Behse, F. & Buchthal, F. (1974) Electrophysiological study of peroneal palsy. *Journal of Neurology, Neurosurgery and Psychiatry*, **37**, 1202–1213.

Tenckhoff, H.A., Boen, F.S.T., Jebsen, R.H. & Spiegler, J.H. (1965) Polyneuropathy in chronic renal insufficiency. *Journal of the American Medical Association*, **192**, 1121.

Thomas, J.E. & Lambert, E.H. (1960) Ulnar nerve conduction velocity and 'H' reflex in infants and children. *Journal of Applied Physiology*, **15**, 1–9.

Thomas, J.E., Lambert, E.H. & Cseuz, K.A. (1967) Electrodiagnostic aspects of the carpal tunnel syndrome. *Archives of Neurology*, **16**, 635.

Thomas, P.K. (1960) Motor nerve conduction in the carpal tunnel syndrome. *Neurology (Minneapolis)*, **10**, 1045.

Thomas, P.K. (1971) The morphological basis for alterations in nerve conduction in peripheral neuropathy. *Proceedings of the Royal Society of Medicine*, **64**, 295–298.

Thomas, P.K. & Calne, D.B. (1974) Motor nerve conduction velocity in peroneal muscular atrophy: evidence for genetic heterogeneity. *Journal of Neurology, Neurosurgery and Psychiatry*, **37**, 68–75.

Thomas, P.K. & Lascelles, R.G. (1966) The pathology of diabetic neuropathy. *Quarterly Journal of Medicine*, **35**, 489–509.

Thomas, P.K. & Lascelles, R.G. (1967) Hypertrophic neuropathy. *Quarterly Journal of Medicine*, **36**, 223.

Thomas, P.K., Sears, T.A. & Gilliatt, R.W. (1959) The range of conduction velocity in normal motor nerve fibres to the small muscles of the hand and foot. *Journal of Neurology, Neurosurgery and Psychiatry*, **22**, 175–181.

Thomas, P.K., Hollinrake, K., Lascelles, R.G., O'Sullivan, D.J., Baillod, R.A., Moorhead, J.F. & Mackenzie, J.C. (1971) The polyneuropathy of chronic renal failure. *Brain*, **94**, 761–780.

Thorne, J. (1965) Central responses to electrical activation of the peripheral nerves supplying the intrinsic hand muscles. *Journal of Neurology, Neurosurgery and Psychiatry*, **28**, 482.

Toole, J.F., Gergen, J.A., Hayes, D.M. & Felts, J.H. (1968) Neural effects of nitrofurantoin. *Archives of Neurology*, **18**, 180–687.

Trojaborg, W. (1970) Rate of recovery in motor and sensory fibres of the radial nerve: clinical and electrophysiological aspects. *Journal of Neurology, Neurosurgery and Psychiatry*, **33**, 625–638.

Trojaborg, W. (1977) Electrophysiological findings in pressure palsy of the brachial plexus. *Journal of Neurology, Neurosurgery and Psychiatry*, **40**, 1160–1167.

Trojaborg, W. & Sindrup, E.H. (1969) Motor and sensory conduction in different segments of the radial nerve in normal subjects. *Journal of Neurology, Neurosurgery and Psychiatry*, **32**, 354–359.

Trojaborg, W., Frantzen, E. & Andersen, I. (1969) Peripheral neuropathy and myopathy associated with carcinoma of the lung. *Brain*, **92**, 71–82.

Trontelj, J.V. & Trontelj, M. (1973) 'F' responses of human facial muscles. A single motor neurone study. *Journal of the Neurological Sciences*, **20**, 211–222.

Walsh, J.C. (1971) Neuropathy associated with lymphoma. *Journal of Neurology, Neurosurgery and Psychiatry*, **34**, 42–50.

Walsh, J.C. & McLeod, J.G. (1970) Alcoholic neuropathy. An electrophysiological and histological study. *Journal of the Neurological Sciences*, **10**, 457–469.

Weller, P.O., Bruckner, F.E. & Chamberlain, M.A. (1970) Rheumatoid neuropathy: a histological and electrophysiological study. *Journal of Neurology, Neurosurgery and Psychiatry*, **33**, 592.

Wiederholt, W.R. (1970) Stimulus intensity and site of excitation in human median nerve sensory fibres. *Journal of Neurology, Neurosurgery and Psychiatry*, **33**, 438–441.

Willison, R.G. (1962) Electrodiagnosis in motor neurone disease. *Proceedings of the Royal Society of Medicine*, **55**, 1024.

Young, R.R. & Shahani, B.T. (1978) Clinical value and limitations of 'F' wave determination. *Muscle and Nerve*, **1**, 248–249.

Clinical electromyography

INTRODUCTION

Clinical electromyography (EMG) may be defined as the study for diagnostic purposes of the electrical activity of skeletal muscle. It may indicate whether the lower motor neurone and/or muscle fibre is the site of a lesion and whether any interruption of lower motor neurone function is complete or partial.

Adequate electrophysiological delineation of lower motor neurone and muscle fibre disorders requires more than the electromyographic techniques that we describe here; in particular, the techniques described in the two preceding and in the subsequent chapter must be intelligently combined with the EMG, in the planned investigation of a clinical problem.

TECHNIQUE OF CLINICAL ELECTROMYOGRAPHY

Modern EMG technique consists of the sampling of several areas of muscle with an intramuscular electrode in order to localise, amplify, identify and measure any electrical activity present. Voluntary muscles are numerous, dispersed and subject to diseases which affect them patchily, precluding the sampling of muscle fibre potentials by means of standard recording electrode positions. Activation of voluntary muscle is accompanied by potentials of low voltage, fluctuating rapidly and interfering with each other in an irregular manner. Such electrical activity is difficult to analyse unless electrodes with a limited recording range are used, coupled to a high-gain, wide frequency-response amplifier and inertia-free recording.

Exploring electrodes may be of various types; that most widely used in clinical work is the concentric (co-axial) needle electrode. Variations in voltage are measured between the bare tip of an insulated wire (the exploring electrode), usually stainless steel, silver or platinum, and the bare shaft of a steel cannula (the reference electrode) through which it is inserted. Less commonly used is the monopolar electrode consisting of a solid wire, usually of stainless steel, insulated except at its tip. Variations in voltage between the tip (exploring electrode) within the muscle and the metal plate on the skin surface or a second bare needle in subcutaneous tissue at a distance are measured. Bipolar (bifilar) needle electrodes record the variations in voltage between the bare tips of two insulated wires cemented side by side in a steel cannula which may be earthed. Multilead electrodes, where three or more insulated wires are inserted into a cannula, may also be used. One such multilead electrode has been used extensively by Buchthal (1961) and his school. More recently, Ekstedt and Stålberg (1965) have introduced a more selective multilead electrode. Microelectrodes for intracellular recording will be described elsewhere in this volume. Surface (skin) electrodes are unsuitable for qualitative clinical EMG because they produce an integration of the potentials which precludes accurate study of their individual form.

The technical details of amplifiers suitable for EMG recording are featured in a report by the Special Committee on EMG Instrumentation (Guld, Rosenfalck and Willison, 1970). The principles of the electrophysiological recording and instrumentation have also been featured in the *Handbook of Electroencephalography and Clinical Neurophysiology* (pp. 10–19). The recording system, including the electrodes, should be flat over a frequency range with -3db points at 2–$10\,000$ Hz and should allow faithful reproduction of the potentials in the amplitude range from $10\,\mu V$ to 20 mV. The noise level for the above band-width should be below $5\,\mu V$ peak-to-peak with the input short-circuited. A high discrimination ratio, e.g. $1000\!:\!1$ between in-phase and out-of-phase signals is also necessary. Finally, the input impedance should well exceed the highest impedance of the electrode at any frequency, in order that the voltage change across the electrodes can be faithfully reproduced, on an oscilloscope. For single-fibre EMG and the study of jitter (see Ch. 29 and below) a time resolution in microseconds rather than milliseconds is also necessary. The use of a delay line greatly facilitates the study of spontaneous activity and motor unit potentials occurring during voluntary effort. Permanent records may be made of the electrical phenomena on FM electromagnetic tape, on a moving or still film, or with special proprietary systems (UVL or fibre-optic recording).

There are no muscle action potentials pathognomonic of specific diseases, and it is impossible to sample every muscle in a patient nor, indeed, more than a few, if due regard is paid to the patient's comfort. Thus, the clinician must select for examination those muscles most likely to provide the information required and for this reason clinical EMG has often been described as an extension of the clinical examination.

THE PHYSIOLOGICAL BASIS OF ELECTROMYOGRAPHY

Adequate description of the physiological basis of the EMG is impossible in the available space. Readers are referred to Chapter 1 for a fuller description of the anatomical and physiological factors of importance.

The action potentials of skeletal muscle are defined by shape (particularly the number of phases), amplitude (microvolts (μV) or millivolts (mV)), duration (milliseconds (ms)) and rate of discharge (frequency per second (Hz)). The origin of these potentials is the movement of ions across the polarised cell membrane of nerve and muscle fibres. Such potentials are normally propagated along the nerve fibres (the nerve impulse) and along the muscle fibre immediately preceding contraction. The configuration of a potential led off from a single nerve or muscle fibre depends on its propagation and particularly on the position of the active electrode in relation to the area of initiation of that potential. Potentials have a diphasic or triphasic form if conducted across the electrode and have an initial positive wave unless the active electrode is at the point of initiation when the initial deflection is negative (Buchthal, Guld and Rosenfalck, 1955). A potential of more than four phases (a polyphasic potential) is derived from the summation of more than one potential source. The action potentials of skeletal muscle are, for the most part, derived from more than one potential source, and are derived from individual muscle fibres acting singly or in groups. The action potential of a normal muscle fibre is initiated at the motor end-plate by the summation of sub-threshold end-plate potentials and is propagated down the fibres in both directions from the end-plate. The end-plate potentials result from the release of acetylcholine, a process which is greatly accelerated by the arrival of the nerve impulse. The physiological grouping of the muscle fibres that give rise to a summated action potential is that of the motor unit.

The motor unit

The motor unit consists of a single lower motor neurone and the muscle fibres innervated by its branches. It is the smallest unit that can be activated by a volitional effort in which all the constituent muscle fibres are fired off synchronously. The number of muscle fibres innervated by a single neurone varies from about 30 in the extraocular muscles to some 400 to 17 000 in normal limb muscles (Christensen, 1959). Buchthal (1957, 1961) suggested that, in limb muscles, the fibres of the motor unit were arranged in groups of sub-units, each comprising an average of 10–30 closely packed fibres. This view was challenged both on electrophysiological grounds by Ekstedt (1964) and, in experimental animals, histochemically by Edstrom and Kugelberg (1968). It now appears that the fibres of individual motor units are dispersed widely, either in isolation or in small groups of 2–4 fibres and the sub-unit hypothesis has been abandoned (Buchthal and Rosenfalck, 1973). The active (central) wire of a concentric needle electrode may be in contact with 5–10 muscle fibres. Other fibres within 0.5 mm of the electrode contribute a much lower amplitude to the electrical activity recorded. The amplitude of the spike of an isolated muscle fibre recorded extracellularly in saline decreases rectilinearly with the logarithm of the distance of the fibre from the recording electrode and increases in proportion to the fibre diameter and the amplitude of the resting membrane potential (Hakkansson, 1957). In intact muscle, the situation is complicated by the inhomogeneity of the tissues, the resistivity and anisotropy (*Handbook of Electroencephalography and Clinical Neurophysiology, Volume 16B*, pp. 20–29).

THE POTENTIALS STUDIED IN CLINICAL ELECTROMYOGRAPHY

The most useful EMG classification of muscle action potentials is into those occurring spontaneously and those occurring on volition. This accords with the technique of inserting the needle electrode into a muscle in several areas, each time studying the activity accompanying electrode movement and that which continues in the absence of such movement (spontaneous activity), before studying potentials accompanying a minimal and then a maximal volitional effort.

Movement of the intramuscular electrode may, by injury to the muscle, evoke potentials called insertion activity (Kugelberg and Petersen, 1949). The distinction between the end of the insertion activity and the beginning of spontaneous activity is at best arbitrary. In this account, therefore, insertional activity is not classified separately but is included with spontaneous forms. Where a form of electrical activity is particularly provoked by electrode movement, this will be noted. Reduced insertional activity is noticeable in atrophied muscle where fibrous replacement has occurred (the toughness of such tissue to electrode movement is also a useful physical sign), and in conditions of acute inexcitability of muscle fibres, e.g. familial periodic paralysis.

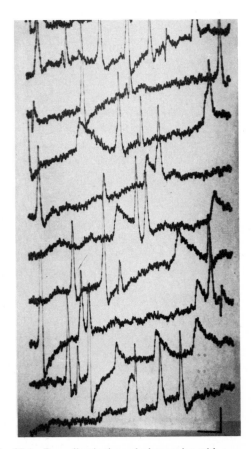

Fig. 28.1 Recording in the end-plate region with a concentric needle electrode. Numerous miniature end-plate potentials. Calibration: 10 ms; 25 μV

End-plate potentials

When a concentric needle electrode, either by accident or design, is placed in the end-plate zone of the muscle, spontaneous activity may be recorded (Fig. 28.1). Monophasic negative potentials of amplitude up to 100 μV and of 0.5–2 ms duration occur at high frequency somewhat irregularly (Rosenfalck and Buchthal, 1962). Buchthal and Rosenfalck (1966) and Weiderholt (1970) suggest that these spontaneous negative discharges correspond to minature end-plate potentials recorded with an intracellular microelectrode. In the same region, spontaneous diphasic potentials having an amplitude of 100–200 μV and a duration of 3–5 ms with an initial negative deflection may also be recorded (Jones, Lambert and Sayre, 1955). It was suggested that these potentials may originate from small bundles of intramuscular nerve fibres but Buchthal and Rosenfalck (1966) suggest that they are caused by the synchronised firing of several muscle fibres due to the mechanical irritation of the electrode; the nerve action potentials which can very occasionally be recorded in the end-plate zone have a much smaller amplitude.

Spontaneous muscle fibre potentials

Positive sharp waves. Figure 28.2 illustrates positive sharp waves, previously also called positive potentials, V waves or saw-tooth waves. Described independently by Kugelberg and Petersen (1949) and by Jasper and Ballem (1949), positive potentials exhibit greatly variable voltages in the range of 50–400 μV and durations between 10–100 ms or more. Evoked by needle movement, they are considered to arise in a damaged region of a muscle fibre where they are led off from the action currents spreading from the inside of the fibres to the surrounding conducting tissue. They discharge at a rate of 2–50/s and are recognised by their abrupt initial positive deflection followed by a long almost exponential decaying phase in a negative direction which may continue into a prolonged negative phase of lower amplitude. Such potentials have not been recorded from normal muscle (Buchthal and Rosenfalck, 1966) and are an important sign of abnormality. They are particularly associated with fibrillation potentials.

Fibrillation potentials. Spontaneous fibrillation potentials (Fig. 28.2) are of di- or triphasic wave form and between 20–300 μV in amplitude. Their duration is short, often less than 2 ms and not more than 5 ms, and their rate of discharge is of the order of 2–20/s. Electrode insertion into the muscle may produce profuse fibrillation which settles with the electrode at rest. The presence of a needle in the muscle is unnecessary for the production of fibrillation as such potentials can be recorded subcutaneously (Rosenfalck and Buchthal, 1966) indicating that mechanical stimulation of the fibres is not necessary for their production.

Fibrillation potentials usually arise in the end-plate region, where they show an initial negative phase if led off from that region (Buchthal and Rosenfalck, 1976). Fibrillations may be recorded from the end-plate regions in normal individuals and an isolated fibrillation potential outside of the end-plate zone may occasionally occur in an

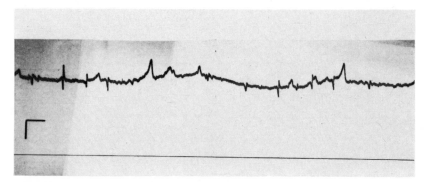

Fig. 28.2 Positive sharp waves and fibrillation potentials. Calibration: 10 ms; 100 μV

apparently normal subject (Buchthal and Rosenfalck, 1966). Denny-Brown and Pennybacker (1938) concluded in their original paper that fibrillation was due to the periodic rhythmical twitching of single muscle fibres sensitised by neural atrophy to the small amount of circulating acetylcholine. In denervation, fibrillation potentials appear on an average 10–21 days after nerve section, persisting as long as there are viable muscle fibres. Warmth, muscular activity or the injection of neostigmine or one of its analogues aids detection of these potentials, but they are unaffected by curare (Thesleff, 1963). Fibrillation and positive sharp-wave activity are particularly widespread and easy to detect in recently denervated muscle but also occur in other situations. Action potentials of identical dimensions, and therefore presumably also derived in the same manner, occur in the absence of lower motor neurone degeneration, e.g. in hyperkalaemic familial periodic paralysis (Morrison, 1960), in botulism (Josefsson, 1960) and in a variety of hereditary and acquired myopathies. Fibrillation rapidly vanishes following the resolution of an attack of hyperkalaemic familial periodic paralysis, suggesting that, in this condition at least, all the abnormalities may be explained on the basis of hyperexcitability of the muscle fibre, probably due to electrolyte changes occurring in relation to the fibre membrane.

It has long been known that denervated muscle shows an abnormal sensitivity to acetylcholine (Brown, 1937) although the mechanism of production of fibrillation in denervated muscle remains ill understood. Denny-Brown and Pennybacker (1938) suggested that circulating acetylcholine might excite the abnormally sensitive denervated fibre. Axelson and Thesleff (1959) have demonstrated that the whole of the muscle fibre membrane becomes sensitive to acetylcholine following denervation of the muscle. Further support for a humoral factor comes from the observations of Hnik and Scorpil (1962) that fibrillation disappears after occlusion of the blood supply to the muscle examined, and that of Thesleff (1963) that fibrillation cannot be recorded in isolated muscles. However, fibrillation potentials appear always to arise in the end-plate zone and continue to occur in the presence of curare (Thesleff, 1963; Belmar and Eyzaguirre, 1966). Other factors of possible importance are alterations in the muscle fibre membrane following denervation (Nicholls, 1956) and lowering of the resting membrane potential (Lenman, 1965). The Li hypothesis (Li, Shy and Wells, 1957) suggests that fibrillation potentials are due to metabolically initiated slow rhythmical changes of the resting potential of the denervated muscle fibre, at times reaching amplitudes sufficient to evoke a propagated spike.

Fasciculation potentials. Fasciculation is the visible muscle twitching accompanying the spontaneous contraction of the constituent fibres of motor units (Fig. 28.3): such activity may occur in healthy subjects and is not uncommon in debilitat-

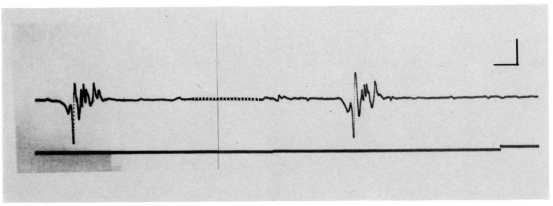

Fig. 28.3 Fasciculation potentials in the quadriceps of a 44-year-old male with motor neurone disease. Calibration: 10 ms; 250 μV

ing disorders which are not clearly associated with diseases of the lower motor neurone. It occurs in advancing destruction of motor (anterior horn) cells, e.g. motor neurone disease or intramedullary spinal cord tumours (Abbruzzese, del Conte, Pastorino and Sacco, 1971). The EMG may aid in its detection by sometimes revealing the accompanying potentials deep in muscle or by finding them unexpectedly in obese patients. The form of the fasciculation potential is variable, and the variation is similar to that seen in the configuration of randomly recorded motor unit action potentials. Fasciculation in motor neurone disease was first studied by Denny-Brown and Pennybacker (1938), who observed it occurring at intervals of 2–10s, apparently involving motor units which were still under voluntary control. Forster and Alpers (1944) claimed that it was not abolished by procaine block of the peripheral nerve and later Forster, Borkowski and Alpers (1946) said that it persisted for 3–5 days after section of the nerve. This fact, combined with the enhancement of fasciculation of motor neurone disease by neostigmine then suggested an origin at the motor endplate with subsequent intraneural, antidromic excitation. Denny-Brown (1949), re-investigating the problem, described only reduction of fasciculation after nerve block, deducing both a central and a peripheral neuronal origin for the fasciculation of motor neurone disease. Synchronous fasciculation in different muscles innervated by the same spinal segment has been reported in advanced motor neurone disease (Norris, 1965), suggesting a central origin. Despite early attempts to relate the wave form of fasciculation to its site of origin and its clinical significance (Denny-Brown, 1953; Weddell, Feinstein and Pattle, 1944) further investigation (Trojaborg and Buchthal, 1975) suggests that, in an individual case, it is usually impossible to decide whether fasciculations are 'benign' or 'malignant'. These investigators found that only 10–20 per cent of fasciculations were polyphasic and were unable to confirm that a fasciculating bundle could be activated by weak or moderate effort or by stretch. Fasciculation in normal muscle differed only from that of motor neurone disease in the shorter interval between successive potentials. The average intervals between successive fasciculation potentials in motor neurone disease were 3.5 s (SD $\pm$ 2.5 s), whereas in benign fasciculation the average interval was 0.8 s with a standard deviation of 0.8 s. There was no evidence of any synchronous discharge in the neighbouring or contralateral muscles. The 'benign' fasciculations studied by Trojaborg and Buchthal were not recorded in patients with myokymia or other relatively benign disorders in which fasciculation may be a gross or striking feature. The 'benign' fasciculations of myokymia, observable clinically as undulating muscle contractions, may produce a distinctive form of activity (Gamstorp and Wohlfart, 1959). This consists of repetitive (grouped) bursts of some 2–200 identical motor unit potentials occurring at a rate of about 50/s. They form grouped or 'iterative' motor unit discharges or 'multiplets'. They are at first accentuated, and later abolished, by ischaemia (Mertens and Zschocke, 1965) and are blocked by neuromuscular blocking agents (Harman and Richardson, 1954). The associated symptoms are helped by hydantoin and carbamazepine. Isaacs (1957) believed that there was an excessive release of acetylcholine at the motor endplate and coined the term 'quantal squander'. Gardner-Medwin and Walton (1969) described a second type of EMG abnormality consisting of irregular continuous synchronous firing of two or three different motor units in any one area of the explored muscle.

Another form of spontaneous motor unit activity of uncertain neurological significance has been described by Buchthal and Olsen (1970) as the most consistent finding in the single-fibre EMG in the investigation of infantile spinal muscular atrophy. The units discharged regularly at rates from 5–51/s even during sleep, but the same units could be activated during voluntary contraction. Double discharges (doublets) consisting of two action potentials of the same form and similar amplitude, occurring consistently in the same relation to one another, and triple discharges (triplets) consisting of three action potentials of the same form and nearly the same amplitude, occurring consistently in the same relation to one another, when the interval between the second and third potential often exceeds that between the first two, may be seen in this situation. Similar discharges occur with tetany, uraemia, thyrotoxicosis and nerve compression, and they are not unknown in normal persons. The status of the myokymia syndrome is still subject to debate (Greenhouse, Bicknell, Pesch and Seelinger, 1967; Gardner-Medwin and Walton, 1969; Hughes and Matthews, 1969), and there have been conflicting views on the mechanism of the production of the spontaneous activity sometimes seen in this condition (DeJong, Matzner and Unger, 1951; Harman and Richardson, 1954), whether it be 'primary' or symptomatic. Attempts to distinguish between benign fasciculation and that associated with progressive motor cell lesions by study of the form of the fasciculation potentials remain difficult and controversial. The significance of fasciculation is best determined by its distribution and by the co-existence of fibrillation potentials or other signs of denervation.

The myotonic response

Myotonia is a delayed relaxation of the muscle following a maintained contraction or a twitch. The phenomenon may be elicited by movement of the needle electrode within the muscles as well as by percussion of the muscle. In the myotonias (dystrophia myotonica, paramyotonia and myotonia congenita) prolonged trains of potentials occur in great profusion in response to electrode movement (Fig. 28.4). Their frequency may reach 150/s, dropping subsequently to 20 or 13/s. They may resemble fibrillation potentials, positive sharp potentials or may be larger and more complex. An initial increase in frequency and amplitude is rapidly followed by a diminution in both, giving rise to a characteristic sound increasing and decreasing in pitch, which has been likened to the

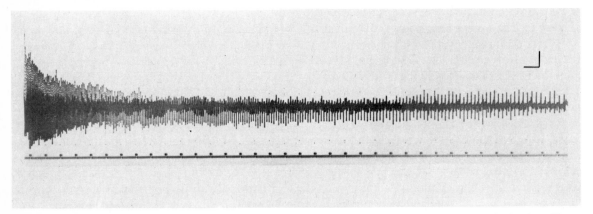

Fig. 28.4   Myotonic discharge from the thenar muscles of a 50-year-old male with dystrophia myotonica. Calibration: 25 ms; 250 μV

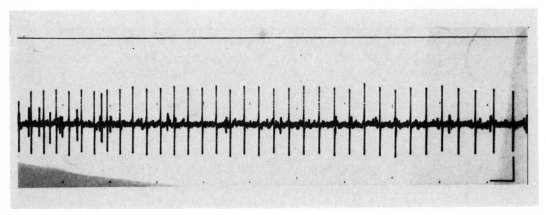

Fig. 28.5   Bizarre high-frequency discharge in brachial biceps of a 28-year-old woman with polymyositis. Calibration: 25 ms; 100 μV

noise of a dive-bomber. Myotonic discharges are presumed to arise from the repetitive activity of single fibres or groups of muscle fibres; in the latter instance, the grouping is not necessarily determined by neuronal linkage as evinced by the persistence of myotonia after curarisation (Landau, 1952).

Bizarre high-frequency discharges

Rapid discharges of constant frequency, amplitude and wave form (usually polyphasic) may occur in other primary disorders of muscle and also neurogenic atrophy, especially in anterior horn cell disease where the discharges may be particularly persistent (Eisen and Karpati, 1971). They frequently are also evoked by needle movement, sometimes accompanying rather than following volitional activity, and generally start and stop abruptly. They are often referred to as 'pseudo-myotonic discharges' (Fig. 28.5).

Volitional action potentials

Dimensions of normal motor unit potentials have been measured by several groups of workers (Kugelberg, 1947; Jasper and Ballem, 1949). The most comprehensive studies have emanated from Buchthal's laboratory in Copenhagen. Only those recruiting on minimal voluntary effort are studied using a concentric needle electrode of the ordinary clinical EMG laboratory. To be acceptable for measurement, the action potential from an individual motor unit must be recorded, free from distortion by more distant activity, at least three times. This condition can more easily be fulfilled when using a delay line, when the action potential being studied triggers the oscilloscope sweep and appears delayed, so that its dimensions can be readily studied.

The dimensions of the motor unit potential remain constant for a single needle position. Concentric needle electrodes have fairly marked directional properties (Nakao, Nakanishi and Tsubaki, 1965). Amplitude is the most, and duration the least, variable with changes of needle position in relation to the single motor unit potential. Most such potentials have a diphasic or triphasic form of 300 μV to 2 mV in amplitude

and a duration of 4–10 ms. In normal limb muscles up to 10 per cent of units may be polyphasic (Caruso and Buchthal, 1965). The effects of various physical and physiological variables upon the normal motor unit potentials have been studied by Buchthal, Guld and Rosenfalck (1954) and Buchthal, Pinelli and Rosenfalck (1954). In addition to the characteristics of the amplifying and recording system used, the type of electrode is also critical in determining the characteristics of the motor unit (Ekstedt and Stålberg, 1973). The high-voltage spikes of an action potential are probably due to the activity of one, or occasionally more, fibres lying close (within 0.5 mm) to the tip of the inner core of a concentric needle electrode. The onset and termination of the action potential is then related to the volume conduction of more distant fibres which make up the same motor unit. Using bipolar electrodes these distant contributions tend to arise simultaneously at both pick-up points and to some extent cancel each other out—the action potential duration recorded with bipolar needles tends to be shorter than that of unipolar recording. When a concentric needle lies deep within the muscle, the outer cannula receives numerous potential changes from all those motor units through which it has passed, becoming in effect a 'reference' electrode; thus the central insulated cannula acts as a unipolar electrode. Nearer the surface of the muscle, the rim of the cannula and the tip of the concentric electrode come to resemble a bipolar electrode. This may explain why the mean duration of units sampled deep within the muscle tends to be longer than those recorded at, or nearer, the surface (Buchthal, Guld and Rosenfalck, 1954).

Another factor of importance in determining the dimensions of a motor unit potential is the anatomy of the muscle explored. The mean action potential duration of limb muscle is much larger than that of facial muscles, and this difference appears to depend upon the width of the innervation zone. Scattering the time of arrival at the electrode of the individual muscle fibre potential of a normal motor unit (Fig. 28.6) is mainly dependent upon the distribution of the motor endplates. Normally these are distributed in one or sometimes in two zones (Coërs and Woolf, 1959), extending for about 10 per cent of the total length

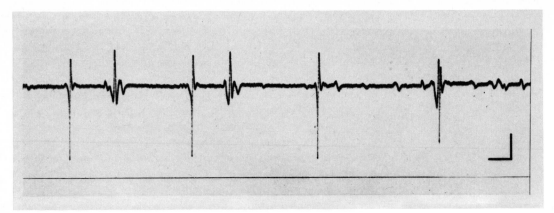

Fig. 28.6 Normal gentle volitional contraction in the brachioradialis of a 45-year-old male. Calibration: 20 ms; 100 μV

of the muscle. In the biceps muscle there is a 20–30 mm longitudinal spread of the site of the end-plates and therefore of the origin of muscle fibre potentials. Assuming that the propagation velocity along the muscle fibre lies between the 4.7 m/s of Buchthal (1961) and the 3.37 m/s of Stålberg (1966) there would be a difference in the time of arrival of the volume-conducted elements going to make up a summated motor unit action potential; this would be sufficient to account for the duration of a motor unit action potential of the order of 6 ms. In most muscles, the mean action potential duration increases with age and is also increased by cooling.

INTERPRETATION OF THE EMG

In general terms, even minimal lower motor neurone lesions may produce distinctive EMG signs, but muscle fibre lesions may be more difficult to distinguish from the normal.

In healthy muscle at rest, with the exploring electrode outside the end-plate zone, no electrical activity can be detected. In the end-plate zone a variety of activities already described may be seen, including miniature end-plate potentials and the occasional fibrillation potential. Electrical activity accompanying the insertion and movement of the needle electrode is brief. The initiation of volitional activity is accompanied by the discharge of a small number of motor unit action potentials firing at low frequency with asynchrony between each separate unit. The development of increased tension in the muscle is associated with recruitment of a larger number of motor units and with a rise in the firing rate of those units already present. When recording with a concentric needle electrode, this results in the development of an 'inter-

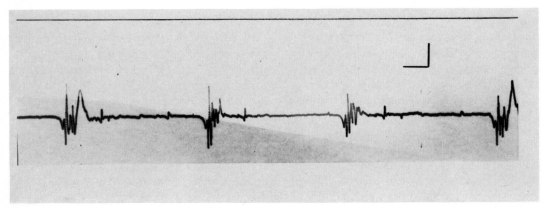

Fig. 28.7 Long-duration polyphasic motor units and infrequent fibrillation potentials in the biceps femoris of a 44-year-old male with motor neurone disease. Calibration: 20 ms; 500 μV

ference pattern' of motor unit potentials, within which individual deflections can no longer be distinguished (Fig. 28.7). Isolated motor units produce a thumping sound in the speaker, the build-up and interference pattern being accompanied by a low rumbling noise (the 'Piper' rhythm). 'Double discharges' may occur when a motor unit is newly recruited (Gordon and Holbourn, 1949). Kugelberg and Skoglung (1946a and b) demonstrated that small motor unit potentials accompany the initiation of volitional contraction, and Norris and Gasteiger (1955) confirmed that the units producing large potentials appeared later, being recruited only at high tensions. Factors concerned in the gradation of muscular contraction are discussed more fully in Section VI of Volume 16B of the *Handbook of Electroencephalography and Clinical Neurophysiology* (1973).

In physiological hypertrophy of muscle and the wasting of disuse the EMG recorded with concentric needles remains normal, apart from some increase in polyphasic potentials reported in the latter condition by Pinelli and Buchthal (1953).

THE EMG IN LOWER MOTOR NEURONE LESIONS

Following complete nerve section, total electrical silence of the denervated muscle ensues. About 10 days later, fibrillation activity is seen, at first in response to the mechanical stimulation of electrode movement and later spontaneously. By three weeks, fibrillation potentials, almost always associated with positive sharp wave discharges, are easily detectable. Volitional potentials are, of course, absent from the onset of the injury.

Fibrillation potentials may be difficult to detect in slowly progressive lesions such as motor neurone disease, in the early recovery phase of acute denervation and in long-standing lesions—the absence of fibrillation may be presumed only after an exacting search. The distribution of the fibrillation activity in several muscles can be helpful in localising the lesion to a peripheral nerve or root.

The retention of some motor unit activity in a muscle affected by a lower motor neurone lesion indicates that the lesion is incomplete, a finding of considerable importance in peripheral nerve injuries. Absence of the motor unit potential indicates no more than total dysfunction of the nerve or, in the absence of demonstrable nerve excitability peripheral to the lesion, complete degeneration of the nerve. This does not necessarily indicate complete section of the nerve, in that the sheath may remain intact with complete degeneration of the axonal content. In this event, evidence of continuity may have to await the return of motor unit activity following axonal regeneration at approximately one inch a month. The widespread use of nerve conduction velocity measurements has limited the value of the EMG in neuropathic conditions.

In addition to the presence of spontaneous activity, the other feature common to incomplete

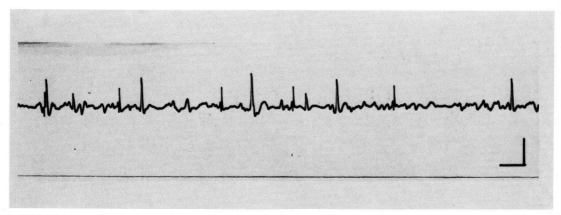

Fig. 28.8 Large-amplitude motor units and reduced recruitment in the brachioradialis of a 47-year-old female with motor neurone disease. Calibration: 20 ms; 10 μV

lower motor neurone lesions is the fact that they cause a loss of motor unit activity on volition. This may preclude the build-up of a full interference pattern on full volition (Fig. 28.8). In advanced motor neurone disease, this may be so extreme that a single potential recurring at rates of up to 50/s may represent maximum effort (Willison, 1962). The presence of fibrillation and positive sharp waves in distal muscles may be a useful early sign of axonal involvement in peripheral neuropathy (Thage, Trojaborg and Buchthal, 1963; Trojaborg, Franzen and Anderson, 1969) and may appear before motor conduction is affected. In demyelinating neuropathy of severe degree, the slowing of conduction velocity may be indistinguishable from that found in remyelinating fibres or in fibres regenerating after axonal degeneration. The EMG may aid in resolving the nature of the process. Long-duration (15–30 ms) polyphasic motor unit potentials, consisting of many short spikes, appear to be a feature of regeneration rather than remyelination (Buchthal, 1970).

A variety of changes may occur in the morphology of the surviving motor units when partial denervation has been present for any length of time. Collateral sprouting and re-innervation of denervated muscle fibres tends to occur in this situation. Borenstein and Desmedt (1973) have described late components of motor units revealed by the use of the delay line and multiple superimpositions of single potentials. These small potentials, often occurring as late as 40 ms after the main spike, would be overlooked without the delay line and have been seen in chronic spinal muscular atrophy and in traumatic lesions of the peripheral nerves. In the early stages of re-innervation, increased jitter (see below) and intermittent blocking were observed, but the connections between the re-innervating axon and muscle became more stable at a later stage. The 'parasite' potential described by Denny-Brown (1949) is similar but shows a much shorter latency which allowed its detection.

Chronic partial denervation often results in the presence of large potentials of increased duration (giant units) (Fig. 28.8): this is believed to be due to the incorporation into an enlarged motor unit of large numbers of denervated muscle fibres by collateral sprouts from axons of surviving anterior horn cells (Kugelberg, 1973). This ability of a motor neurone to increase the number of fibres it controls appears to have been an important property of the healthy motor neurone (McComas, Sica and Campbell, 1971). The widening of the innervation zone consequent upon collateral re-innervation leads to an increased temporal dispersion of fibre action potentials, in turn leading to an increased motor unit action potential duration or to a polyphasic action potential of long duration (Buchthal and Clemmesen, 1941). It is not clear to what extent the increased muscle fibre content of the motor unit contributes to the size of the recorded action potential by summation of action potentials, or to what extent the probability that the recording needle has an increased likelihood of being very close to one of the fibres of the unit contributes to the recording of a 'giant' unit.

SYNCHRONISATION OF MOTOR UNIT ACTIVITY

Studying the muscles in acute anterior poliomyelitis, Buchthal and Clemmesen (1941) described synchronous activity of motor unit potentials, attributing this to central (spinal cord) lesions. Clinical techniques based on the detection of synchronously discharging motor unit potentials recorded by two needle electrodes placed at separate points transversely across a muscle were then introduced and this sign was regarded as indicative of a cord lesion (myelopathy). Denny-Brown (1949) attributed the apparent synchronisation of motor unit potentials to the uncovering of motor units producing large potentials due to loss by disease of those motor units which produce small potentials and which normally initiate contraction. Kugelberg and Taverner (1950) demonstrated that synchronous activity could be produced by stimulation of the motor nerve peripherally. When motor unit action potentials consistently occur on volition simultaneously or nearly so at two or more electrodes, spaced more than 2 cm apart and placed transversely across the long axis of the muscle fibres, or in separate muscles, synchronisation of motor unit action potentials may be said to occur. In a single muscle such a finding might be due to some central mechanism causing synchronisation of the activity of different anterior horn cells, particularly if some disease process had resulted in a marked reduction in the motor neurone pool (Norris, 1965; Simpson, 1962, 1966). Alternatively, peripheral sprouting from surviving intramuscular filaments may re-innervate denervated nerve fibres and incorporate them into the motor unit. Under these circumstances, such potentials might well be detectable over a larger than normal area, i.e. they might show an increased motor unit territory (Erminio, Buchthal and Rosenfalck, 1959). Buchthal and Clemmesen (1941) and Simpson (1962) raise the possibility that the apparent large size of synchronised potentials may be due to a central mechanism, for example, that each Renshaw interneurone receives fewer recurrent collateral fibres in the presence of a reduced anterior horn cell population. The case for and against collateral sprouting and synchronisation accounting for 'giant' units has been discussed by Lambert (1969) and Stålberg and Trontelj (1970). In normal individuals and in patients with chronic ulnar nerve lesions (Fullerton and Gilliatt, 1965) axonal branching may occur more proximally, although usually distal to the site of a chronic compressive lesion, producing another form of synchronisation. Esslen (1960) demonstrated synchronous 'volitional' motor unit discharges in different muscles following aberrant re-innervation in a variety of recovering peripheral nerve lesions. Synchronisation cannot be recorded in a normal muscle

under the conditions described above. It is apparent that the finding of synchronous motor unit action potentials is not diagnostic of any particular condition. Synchronisation of large-amplitude potentials has been found in a high percentage of cases of benign spinal muscular atrophy arising in childhood and adolescence (Kugelberg-Welander syndrome) and may be a useful screening procedure in cases where the presence of a family history and the clinical picture may suggest a dystrophy (Gardner-Medwin, Hudgson and Walton, 1967; Mastaglia and Walton, 1971).

THE EMG IN MUSCLE FIBRE LESIONS

High-frequency discharges and fibrillation potentials may occur in muscles which are the site of primary muscle fibre disease (Fig. 28.9). The dimensions of these abnormal muscle action potentials have already been described, and reference has also been made to the profuse occurrence of high-frequency discharges in the myotonias. In myotonia congenita such discharges may occur in the absence of clinical signs and are useful in the detection of the disease, for example in the infants of affected mothers. In these instances, the potentials have all the characteristics of the myotonic discharge. Similar high-frequency discharges, usually with abrupt onset and termination and constant firing frequency, also occur in the myotonic disorders but may also be seen in

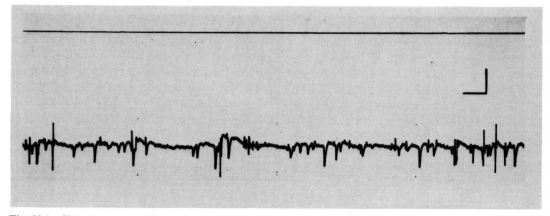

Fig. 28.9 Short-duration, small-amplitude potentials with some positive sharp waves during gentle contraction of the brachial biceps in a 28-year-old female with polymyositis. Calibration: 20 ms; 250 μV

polymyositis (dermatomyositis), muscular dystrophy of various types, myxoedema and hyperkalaemic periodic paralysis. In the hyperkalaemic periodic paralysis–paramyotonia syndrome, both types of discharge may be seen. The presence of fibrillation in primary muscle lesions was thought by McComas and Mrozek (1968) to be related to the functional denervation which occurs when segmental necrosis of the fibres separates a viable portion of the muscle from its end-plate. The frequent presence of fibrillation potentials in polymyositis (especially in the acute or subacute cases) has led to the suggestion that secondary involvement of the terminal branches of the lower motor neurone by the inflammatory process may be responsible. With the possible exception of thyrotoxic myopathy, spontaneous fasciculation of single or grouped motor unit potentials occurs no more frequently in the myopathies than in normal individuals.

The general EMG features seen in myopathy have been recently discussed in the *Handbook of Electroencephalography and Clinical Neurophysiology* (Volume 16 pp. 80–84). These are, first, reduction in the mean duration of motor unit action potentials. This is regarded as the most characteristic feature and, to be considered significant, this reduction should be by more than 20 per cent of that seen in the corresponding muscle of a normal subject of a similar age. A second feature may be an increase in the number of polyphasic potentials and, when this increase is combined with the presence of shortening of the action potential duration, the probability of myopathy is very high. More difficult to assess is a reduction in the maximum amplitude among the potentials recorded, because the major determinant of spike amplitude is the proximity of the nearest active muscle fibre. Because of the fall-out of individual fibres within a unit contributing to the contractile process, many more units are recruited at low tensions so that this may lead to the development of a full interference pattern at less than maximum contraction, but the average amplitude of this interference pattern is reduced.

Measurements of motor unit territory require special electrodes and the results vary according to the type of electrode used. The presence of small, brief, polyphasic action potentials recruiting in large numbers in degenerative myopathy may be strikingly different from the activity seen in chronic neurogenic disorders, where small numbers of action potentials of large amplitude and often of long duration may be seen (Fig. 28.7). In the Duchenne form of muscular dystrophy the decrease in mean action potential, voltage and duration most typical of a myopathy occurs, and this may well derive mainly from the reduced membrane potential of the individual fibre, as well as from a reduced motor unit territory accompanying thinning out of the component muscle fibres of the motor unit (Buchthal, Rosenfalck and Erminio, 1960). As in normal muscle, the polyphasic potentials seen in myopathy tend to be of longer duration than the more simple forms, but both may show a reduction in duration compared with normal muscle.

The motor unit action potentials in myotonia congenita appear to be normal, but in dystrophia myotonica in the forearm and leg muscles, although not usually in the small muscles of the hand and foot, there is an increase in the number of polyphasic potentials together with a shortening of the mean action potential duration. Electrophysiological evidence of a 'myopathic disorder' has now been obtained in a variety of endocrine and metabolic disorders. Thyrotoxic myopathy (Sanderson and Adey, 1952) is an infrequent clinical presentation of thyrotoxicosis but quantitative electromyography showed shortening of the mean action potential duration to be a constant feature of the disorder (Ramsay, 1965; Buchthal, 1970). Hypothyroidism may less constantly be complicated by muscular manifestations and EMG abnormalities (Åström, Kugelberg and Muller, 1961). When present, the abnormalities are abolished following appropriate treatment (Norris and Panner, 1966); unlike the percussion dimple produced in the myotonias, the myoidema of hypothyroid myopathy is electrically silent (Salick and Pearson, 1967) but both contraction and relaxation are slowed (pseudomyotonia). However, a recent single case report describes the presence of clinical myotonia and typical myotonic activity in the EMG in a case of hypothyroidism, and its disappearance following adequate thyroid replacement therapy (Venables, Bates and Shaw, 1978). There are no striking associated histological changes. A proximal myopathy with associated EMG changes may be a prominent feature of Cushing's syndrome (Muller and Kugelberg, 1959). Similar changes are produced by synthetic corticosteroids, especially triamcinolone (Williams, 1959; Yates, 1963; Coomes, 1965). Addison's disease (Buchthal, 1970) is characterised by generalised muscular weakness and this may be associated with shortening of the mean action potential duration. A rare endocrine myopathy is that associated with increasing cutaneous pigmentation in patients previously subject to adrenalectomy for Cushing's syndrome. The development of pigmentation and muscular weakness may be due to high circulating ACTH levels, and shortening of the mean action potential duration can be demonstrated (Prineas, Hall, Barwick and Watson, 1968).

Despite their formidable appearance, patients with acromegaly often complain of weakness and this is accompanied by electrophysiological evidence of myopathy (Mastaglia, Barwick and Hall, 1970; Lundberg, Osterman and Stålberg, 1970).

Vicale (1949) drew attention to the mild proximal weakness present in some patients with hyperparathyroidism. Other workers (Bischoff and Esslen, 1965; Frame, Heinze, Block and Manson, 1968) confirmed these observations and showed that electrical abnormalities appropriate to a myopathy were present in such cases. Hudson, Cholod and Haust (1970) described a familial incidence of this myopathic disorder. Many other disorders in which osteomalacia may develop are often complicated by proximal muscular weakness and myopathic changes in the EMG (Smith and Stern, 1967).

Although neuropathy is well recognised in chronic renal failure and in patients receiving regular haemodialysis, there are some in whom gross proximal weakness is evidently due to a myopathy (Lindholm, 1968; Floyd, Ayyar, Hudgson and Kerr, 1969) with appropriate EMG changes. There is some suggestion that renal transplantation may reverse the myopathic disorder. Hed, Lundmark, Fahlgren and Orell (1962) described a syndrome occurring in chronic alcoholics and characterised by acute muscular necrosis following the cessation of a heavy drinking bout. There are no EMG findings specific to any of these toxic or metabolic disorders but the technique may be of particular value when, as in alcoholism or uraemia, a neuropathy may be thought initially to be the cause of the patient's symptoms.

Both generalised and localised scleroderma may be associated with shortening of the action potential duration and increase in the percentage of polyphasic potentials. In the localised form of scleroderma the abnormalities are most striking adjacent to the sclerodermatous area but occasionally may be more widespread (Hausmanowa-Petrusewicz and Kozinska, 1961).

In polymyalgia rheumatica, characterised by widespread muscular pain, restricted movements of proximal joints, a high sedimentation rate and rapid resolution on treatment with steroids, although qualitative electromyography appears to be normal, Buchthal (1970) using quantitative techniques has shown evidence of a mild myopathy in six elderly women with the disorder. Buchthal (1970) also reported a high incidence of myopathic EMG changes in patients with established lupus erythematosus even in the absense of clinical signs suggestive of myopathic involvement.

Systematic EMG examination of groups of patients with a condition known to be variably associated with a clinically obvious myopathy may aid in deciding on the nature of the association. In thyrotoxicosis a myopathy is a constant accompaniment of the endocrinopathy (Ramsay, 1965). From the studies of Moody (1965) and Shy and Silverstein (1965) it would appear that myopathy occurring as a remote complication of malignant disease is distinctly uncommon and that the so-called myopathic–myasthenic (Eaton-Lambert syndrome) is rare.

MUSCLE ACTION POTENTIAL VARIATION WITH REPETITION

Normal fatigue during voluntary contraction is accompanied by the drop-out of motor unit potentials rather than by any change in their form. In contrast, Lindsley (1935) found that the characteristic fatigue of myasthenic muscle was accompanied by a marked fluctuation in the

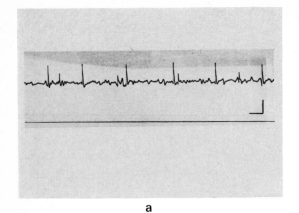

a

Fig. 28.10 (a)   Normal volitional activity on weak contraction. Calibration: 20 ms; 500 μV

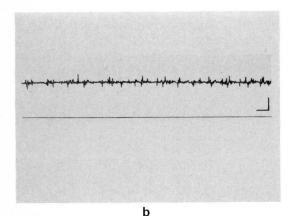

b

Fig. 28.10 (b)   Excessive recruitment of low-voltage short-duration potentials on weak contraction in myopathy. Calibration: 20 ms; 500 μV

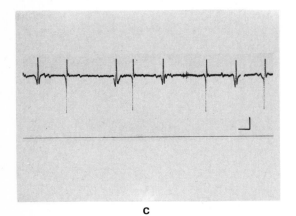

c

Fig. 28.10 (c)   Reduced recruitment of large units on weak contraction in neuropathy. Calibration: 20 ms; 500 μV

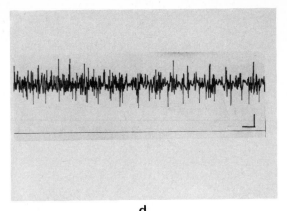

d

Fig. 28.10 (d)   Normal recruitment on forceful contraction. Calibration: 25 ms; 500 μV

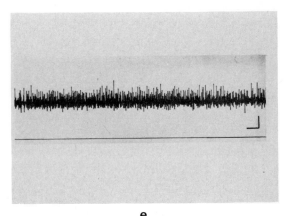

e

Fig. 28.10 (e)   Very full recruitment on full volitional contraction of a weak muscle in myopathy. Calibration: 25 ms; 500 μV

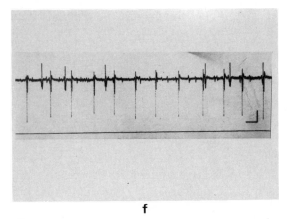

f

Fig. 28.10 (f)   Reduced recruitment on full volitional contraction of a weak muscle in chronic neurogenic disease. Calibration: 25 ms; 500 μV

amplitude of the individual motor unit potentials. Mean action potential duration is significantly reduced in myasthenia gravis (Oosterhuis, Hoostmans, Veenhuyzen and Van Zadelhoff, 1972), especially in clinically weak muscles. Measurements of the progressive diminution in the amplitude of the summated action potentials of myasthenic muscle obtained in response to supramaximal stimulation of a motor nerve at a rate of 3–25/s recorded with surface electrodes may be useful in diagnosis (Harvey and Masland, 1941). Subcutaneous electrodes inserted over the muscle, however, give rise to less artefact (Slomic, Rosenfalck and Buchthal, 1968; Desmedt, 1973). The response is not, however, found in all muscles consistently (Bothelho, Deaterly, Austin and Comroe, 1952). The diminution is due to the production of progressive neuromuscular block which depends on the frequency and the duration of the stimulation and may be reversed by prostigimine or edrophonium (Tensilon). A number of other conditions including poliomyelitis (Buchthal and Honke, 1944; Desmedt, 1973) and polymyositis (Vasilescu, Bucur, Petrovici and Florescu, 1978) may show peripheral fatigue and also some improvement with prostigmine or edrophonium. Another phenomenon in myasthenic and in normal muscles is that the amplitude of the action potentials is increased immediately following a series of tetanic stimuli delivered by a motor nerve, i.e. post-tetanic facilitation. In myasthenic muscle this is followed by a further decrease in amplitude which reaches its maximum a few minutes after tetanic stimulation, i.e. post-tetanic exhaustion (Desmedt, 1959). This response is similar to that seen in some animals after the administration of hemicholinium 3 and originally led to the suggestion that the defect in myasthenia is one of failure of acetylcholine release (Elmqvist and Quastel, 1965; Elmqvist, Hoffmann, Kugelberg and Quastel, 1964). The number of quanta of acetylcholine released in response to nerve stimulation seemed normal but there appeared to be a reduced amount of transmitter substance in each quantum and the amplitude of the end-plate potentials was reduced. Much of this evidence is now difficult to correlate with the known facts relating to an antibody reaction to acetylcholine receptor being responsible for myasthenia gravis. Although there is evidence that the excitability of the muscle fibre membrane is unimpaired in myasthenia gravis (Van der Most Van Spijk, 1964) in that the refractory period is normal, there is other evidence to suggest that the muscle fibre is abnormal and that there may be a disorder of excitation–contraction coupling (Slomic et al., 1968). Recent improvements in technique have been directed towards the detection of a conduction defect in muscles which are apparently unaffected clinically. The increased jitter found with the single-fibre technique has already been mentioned and is described below. Desmedt (1973) in a series of papers has carefully examined the various factors which influence the diagnostic yield in testing myasthenic subjects and has stressed the importance of careful temperature control. He suggests that a 'double step' test be employed in which post-activation exhaustion is assessed after a first exercise carried out with normal circulation to the tested limb, then after a second exercise period under ischaemia. The stimulation rate is 3/s. This test appears to have considerable sensitivity, approaching that of the single-fibre technique, but requires much less special apparatus.

In the myasthenic syndrome associated with malignant tumours, a single stimulus may provoke a low-amplitude action potential response in contrast with the usual finding in myasthenia gravis, where it is normal or nearly so. In the myasthenic syndrome, repetitive stimulation at tetanic rates may produce a marked facilitation in the response up to 10 times the initial amplitude (Lambert, Rooke, Eaton and Hodgson, 1961). Similar, although less striking, findings have been reported by Simpson (1960) to occur at times in patients with myasthenia gravis. McQuillen and Johns (1967) have suggested that the curious response in the myasthenic syndrome associated with carcinoma (Eaton-Lambert syndrome) is due to an abnormality of the end-plate resulting in a defect in the release of acetylcholine. The evidence is that the defect appears on nerve stimulation but not on direct stimulation of the muscle fibre. Guanidine, which promotes the release of acetylcholine from the nerve endings, corrects the electrical abnormality, as it also does in botulism.

It has been suggested (Dyken, Smith and Peake, 1967) that supramaximal stimulation of peripheral nerves is a useful test in McArdle's disease, in which a rapid decrement of the evoked response and the development of an electrically silent physiological contracture would be evidence of the presence of the condition. However, I have failed to observe this response in two proven cases of McArdle's syndrome.

In recent years the traditional distinction between pathological processes affecting the lower motor neurone and the muscles have been challenged. Based on a method of counting motor units in the extensor digitorum brevis (McComas, Fawcett, Campbell and Sica, 1971), which will be described in detail in Chapter 29, Campbell, McComas and Petito (1973) demonstrated that the preservation of distal innervation in the elderly relates to physical activity. In a series of papers, McComas and various co-workers studied Duchenne dystrophy, limb-girdle and facioscapulohumeral dystrophy, dystrophia myotonica and myasthenia gravis. In all of these they found evidence which suggested to them a functional loss of motor units and a failure to the normal trophic influences which maintain healthy fibres. They suggested that, in classical denervation, the influence of the motor unit on a muscle is suddenly and totally withdrawn, whereas in a 'hereditary myopathy' withdrawal may be a more gradual process. A healthy motor neurone, as well as transmitting impulses, exerts a normal 'trophic' influence on muscle fibres and has the capacity to grow new axonal branches and to re-innervate previously denervated muscle. A 'sick' motor neurone has difficulty in maintaining proper connections with its muscle fibres. This may be manifest in impaired neuromuscular transmission (as in myasthenia gravis). Such a motor neurone will be unable to maintain all the fibres it innervates in a healthy state and will be unable to produce an effective axonal sprout. These concepts emphasise the functional integrity of a motor unit, but both the techniques and the conclusions of the McComas school have been challenged. This hypothesis will be discussed more fully in the following chapter but as far as clinical electromyography is concerned the major disadvantage of the McComas technique and the results it has produced so far is that, in suggesting that all processes are 'neurogenic', it fails to make clinically useful distinctions between the processes of neurogenic atrophy and muscular dystrophy, and therefore affords little help in differential diagnosis of individual clinical problems.

It is recognised that there are considerable difficulties in the diagnosis of advanced neuromuscular disease (Garth, Sjaastad and Løken, 1969). It has now become apparent that both histological and electrophysiological changes suggestive of myopathy may occur in long-standing partial denervation (Drachman, Murphy, Nigam and Hill, 1967). In other instances, in what appears to be a myopathic process, changes suggestive of denervation may be seen and may be regarded as secondary neuropathic change (Guy, Lefebre, Lerique and Scherrer, 1950). In the late stages of myopathy or denervation it may be virtually impossible to decide in the presence of mixed evidence of both myopathic and neurogenic change as to which of these processes is primary. The presence of defects in neuromuscular transmission in certain neuropathic disorders and the appearance of myotonic activity in the EMG of others becomes less difficult to account for if we accept that some of these motor neurones may show a gradual rather than a sudden failure.

SINGLE-FIBRE ELECTROMYOGRAPHY

The use of a fine multilead electrode, with a needle diameter of 0.5 mm and with round leading-off surfaces of 25 μm together with a suitable amplification and display system (Ekstedt, 1964) has allowed the recording of single-fibre action potentials during volitional activity. Many subsequent studies have shed considerable light on the microphysiology of the motor units. Although the use of this electrode has shown that individual muscle fibres in motor units are usually dispersed and that there is no evidence that subunits exist, it remains possible on occasions to record from two muscle fibres belonging to the same motor unit. On doing so, a variation in the time interval in the arrival of the two action potentials is seen. This variability in the time interval is called jitter. In normal subjects, this appears to be caused by a variability in neuromuscular conduction time and also in the propagation time of the action potentials and of nerve and muscle fibres. In normal muscles, the jitter expressed as 'mean consecutive difference' (MCD) lies between 5–50 µs in normal muscles. Variability in muscle fibre and nerve fibre conduction probably contributes in only a minor fashion to the jitter. The jitter is increased with lowering of muscle temperature and is decreased slightly by warming (Stålberg, Ekstedt and Broman, 1971). Ischaemia (Dahlback, Ekstedt and Stålberg, 1970) has a profound effect on the jitter, which increases rapidly with partial and later with total block of conduction to one or other action potential in the pair. Restoration of the circulation soon results in a reappearance of the blocked potential with an initially increased jitter which returns to normal over a further few minutes. The effects of regional anaesthesia are described by Stålberg and Ekstedt (1973), who demonstrated a variety of actions dependent upon the concentration and distribution in the muscle of the local anaesthetic. While a pair of potentials could show increased jitter going on to partial and complete block, it was common to find the sudden disappearance of a single motor unit potential without any preceding increase in jitter. On other occasions when it was possible to record from three single fibres, it was shown that simultaneous blockage to two potentials would occur, suggesting a block proximal to the end-plate, perhaps at a neuronal branching point. Ekstedt and Stålberg (1969a) studied the effect on jitter of small doses of D-tubocurarine. With a dose of 15 µg/kg the jitter increased by 5–15 µs from normal. As the dose was increased the jitter rose to more than 70 µs and occasional blocking occurred. Thus, increased jitter could be expected in the presence of minor disturbances of neuromuscular transmission.

Applying the technique to myasthenia gravis (Ekstedt and Stålberg, 1965; Stålberg and Ekstedt, 1973) it was apparent that in myasthenia gravis increased jitter occurs with or without partial neuromuscular blocking. In the same muscle, some motor end-plates may have a normal jitter and, indeed, within the same motor unit there may be considerable variations between the jitter at different motor end-plates. Blom and Ringqvist (1971) showed that jitter was likely to be grossly abnormal and blocking was present if the muscle explored was clinically weak or fatiguable, but that there was an increased jitter without blocking even in the apparently unaffected muscles of individuals with myasthenia. On exercise, jitter increases in myasthenic muscle as does blocking. This is related to the phenomenon of post-activation exhaustion (Desmedt, 1957): although edrophonium injections and neostigime treatment decrease the jitter in myasthenics, it does not return to normal unless and until the myasthenia has remitted.

The single-fibre electrode also allows estimation of motor unit territory and fibre density, giving results which differ from those of Buchthal and Rosenfalck (1957). In muscular dystrophy Stålberg and Ekstedt (1973) found that the fibre density is increased and the increase is greater when moderate atrophy is present than when the wasting is only slight. In more advanced cases some decreases in the fibre density were detected. In the dystrophies, there was some increase in jitter and the degree of disturbance was most marked in patients with severe disease. In myotonia congenita the jitter is normal but it is increased in dystrophia myotonica where the fibre density is also increased. In some individuals with dystrophy, an abnormally small jitter between two action potentials may be found (2–3 µs), suggesting that the two fibres share a common end-plate and that fibre splitting may be contributing to the apparent increase in fibre density (Ekstedt and Stålberg, 1973; Swash and Schwartz, 1977).

A wide spectrum of neurogenic disorders have in common a marked increase in jitter. The action potentials are often more complex than in normal muscle, due to increased fibre density, and individual spikes show occasional blockings in addition. Neurogenic blocking of impulses (Stålberg and Thiele, 1972) is the term given to the presence of simultaneous blocking of two or more components, similar to that found with the administration of local anaesthetics (vide supra). The phenomenon is easiest to find in post-traumatic re-innervation during the first months after injury. It is held to indicate the presence of immature connections between nerve and muscle and it may be more easily detected at high innervation rates.

Schwartz, Stålberg, Schiller and Thiele (1976) have studied motor unit potentials in patients with motor neurone disease and polyneuropathy. Clear evidence of abnormal grouping of single fibres with increased fibre density was found in both groups of patients, the abnormalities being evident even in apparently clinically normal muscles.

Patients with motor neurone disease had complex, unstable motor unit action potentials. The fasciculation potentials of active motor neurone disease are also revealed by single-fibre electromyography to be unstable and complex, contrasting with the stability of fasciculation in non-progressive disorders (Stålberg and Trontelj, 1979). Evidence of regeneration after preceding denervation, consisting of increased fibre density, increased jitter and blocking and potentials of increased duration are found in the axonal neuropathy of alcoholism but not in segmental demyelination occurring in diabetics (Thiele and Stålberg, 1975).

In myopathies there is also evidence of instability of the motor unit when the disease process is active, and in polymyositis there is evidence suggesting involvement of the terminal innervation (Stålberg and Trontelj, 1979). At present it appears that single-fibre studies are more useful to indicate the activity of the disease processes than to differentiate between various pathological processes. Evidence suggesting fibre splitting does appear to be rare in neurogenic disorders but is quite frequent in dystrophy and is occasionally seen in polymyositis (Stålberg and Trontelj, 1979).

The technique of single-fibre recording has been applied to other disorders of neuromuscular transmission, as well as to myasthenia gravis. In the myasthenic syndrome (Schwartz and Stålberg, 1975) despite minimal involvement of the muscle examined, all but one of the potential pairs examined showed increased jitter. Neuromuscular transmission improved at high rates of innervation and worsened on resting. Human botulism was studied in two mildly affected patients (Schiller and Stålberg, 1978). Increased jitter improving with high innervation rates was present and persisted for some time after full clinical recovery. Schwartz and Stålberg (1975) reported an interesting single patient with myasthenia gravis, in

whom features of both myasthenia gravis and the myasthenic syndrome co-existed.

Single-fibre EMG has already thrown considerable light upon the applied physiology of many disorders. Over the next few years its relationship to concentric needle electromyography should be clearer, as should the theoretical basis of electromyography.

ELECTROMYOGRAPHY IN CARRIER DETECTION IN THE DUCHENNE TYPE OF MUSCULAR DYSTROPHY

Since 1963, when it was suggested by Van der Bosch and by Barwick that the female carrier of the gene responsible for Duchenne muscular dystrophy showed EMG abnormalities, there has been considerable interest in the detection of minor changes in such individuals. Davey and Woolf (1964), using the biceps muscle and a technique similar to, though not identical with, that of Van den Bosch, were unable to confirm his results. Observer bias may be a considerable problem in assessments of this sort (Barwick and Gardner-Medwin, 1967). In 1965 Davey and Woolf, reporting a larger series, showed that the carriers had small but statistically significant abnormalities and tended to have more polyphasic potentials than the 33 control subjects. Caruso and Buchthal (1965) used measurements of action potential duration and of the absolute refractory period of muscle. In their series there were probably only three definite carriers of the Duchenne gene and 13 possible carriers. The three carriers all had significantly short refractory periods and five of the 13 possible carriers also showed shortening of the refractory period. Alterations in the mean action potential duration were not sufficiently marked in any individual case to allow carrier identification. Emery, Teasdall and Coomes (1966) studied 22 definite or probable carriers and 12 controls. They found that the mean number of polyphasic potentials was higher in the carriers than in the controls, but the differences were not significant. Smith, Amick and Johnson (1966), in a semi-quantitative study, showed the presence of some patchy EMG abnormalities correlating well with serum enzyme and biopsy results. Gardner-

Medwin (1968) reported that the mean action potential duration, the number of phases per potential or the proportion of polyphasic potentials were abnormal in many carriers and, of 26 known carriers in this study, 17 could be identified by a combination of these measurements. Moosa and Brown (1972) described a similar technique and Moosa, Brown and Dubowitz (1972) reported its application to carrier detection. Other sophisticated techniques of automatic analysis of EMG activity, including the extraction of the dimensions of a single motor neurone from the full interference pattern, have been described (Magora and Gonen, 1970; Lang, Nurrkanen and Vaahtoranta, 1971; Prochazka and Kornhuber, 1973). Methods of measuring motor unit activity in human muscle initially by mechanical and subsequently by electronic analysis have been developed by Willison (1963; 1964; 1965; 1966). These, and other methods of EMG analysis, will be discussed in detail in the following chapter.

REFERENCES

Abbruzzese, M., Del Conte, I., Pastorino, P. & Sacco, G. (1971) Electromyographic findings in intraspinal tumours. Proceedings of the Fourth International Congress of Electromyography (Abstracts). Unpublished.

Astròm, K.E., Kugelberg, E. & Muller, R. (1961) Hypothyroid myopathy. Archives of Neurology, 5, 472–482.

Axelson, J. & Thesleff, F.A. (1959) A study of supersensitivity in denervated mammalian skeletal muscle. Journal of Physiology, 147, 178–193.

Barwick, D.D. (1963) Investigations of the carrier state in the Duchenne type dystrophy. In Proceedings of the 2nd Symposium on Research in Muscular Dystrophy, pp. 10–19 (Pitman: London).

Barwick, D.D. & Gardner-Medwin, D. (1967) Observer bias in the measurement of motor unit action potentials. Electroencephalography and Clinical Neurophysiology, 23, 490.

Belmar, J. & Eyzaguirre, C. (1966) Pacemaker site of fibrillation potentials in denervated mammalian muscle. Journal of Neurophysiology, 29, 425–441.

Bischoff, A. & Esslen, E. (1965) Myopathy with primary hyperparathyroidism. Neurology (Minneapolis), 15, 64–68.

Blom, S. & Ringqvist, I. (1971) Neurophysiological findings in myasthenia gravis single muscle fibre activity in relation to muscular fatiguability and response to anticholine esterase. Electroencephalography and Clinical Neurophysiology, 30, 477–487.

Borenstein, S. & Desmedt, J.E. (1973) Electromyographical signs of collateral reinnervation. New Developments in Electromyography and Clinical Neurophysiology. Ed. J.E. Desmedt, Vol. 1, pp. 130–140 (Karger: Basel).

Bothelho, S.Y., Deaterly, C.F., Austin, S. & Comroe, J.H. (1952) Evaluation of the electromyogram of patients with myasthenia gravis. Archives of Neurology, 67, 441.

Brown, G.L. (1937) The actions of acetyl choline on denervated mammalian and frog's muscle. Journal of Physiology, 89, 438–461.

Buchthal, F. (1957) The functional organisation of the motor unit. American Journal of Physical Medicine, 38, 125–128.

Buchthal, F. (1961) The general concept of the motor unit. Research Publications of the Association of Nervous and Mental Diseases, 38, 3–30.

Buchthal, F. (1970) Electrophysiological abnormalities in metabolic myopathies and neuropathies. Acta Neurologica Scandinavica, Supplement 43, 129–176.

Buchthal, F. & Clemmesen, S. (1941) On the differentiation of muscle atrophy by electromyography. Acta Psychiatrica Neurologica, 16, 143–181.

Buchthal, F. & Honke, P. (1944) Electromyographic examination of patients suffering from poliomyelitis. Acta Medica Scandinavica, 116, 148–164.

Buchthal, F. & Olsen, P.Z. (1970) Electromyography and muscle biopsy in infantile spinal muscular atrophy. Brain, 93, 15–30.

Buchthal, F. & Rosenfalck, P. (1966) Spontaneous electrical activity of human muscles. Electroencephalography and Clinical Neurophysiology, 20, 321–336.

Buchthal, F. & Rosenfalck, P. (1973) On the structure of motor units. New Developments in Electromyography and Clinical Neurophysiology. Ed. J.E. Desmedt, Vol. 1, pp. 71–85 (Karger: Basel).

Buchthal, F., Guld, C. & Rosenfalck, P. (1954) Action potential parameters in normal human muscle and their dependence on physical variable. Acta Physiologica Scandinavica, 32, 200–18.

Buchthal, F., Guld, C. & Rosenfalck, P. (1955) Innervation zone and propagation velocity in human muscle. Acta Physiologica Scandinavica, 35, 174–190.

Buchthal, F., Guld, C. & Rosenfalck, P. (1957) Volume conduction of the spike of the motor unit potential investigated with a new type of multielectrode. Acta Physiologica Scandinavica, 38, 331–354.

Buchthal, F., Pinelli, P. & Rosenfalck, P. (1954) Action potential parameters in normal human muscle and their physiological determinants. Acta Physiologica Scandinavica, 32, 219–229.

Buchthal, F., Rosenfalck, P. & Erminio, P. (1960) Motor unit territory and fibre density in myopathies. Neurology (Minneapolis), 10, 398–408.

Campbell, M.J., McComas, A.J. & Petito, F. (1973) Physiological changes in ageing muscles. Journal of Neurology, Neurosurgery and Psychiatry, 36, 174–182.

Caruso, G. & Buchthal, F. (1965) Refractory period of muscle and electromyographic findings in relatives of patients with muscular dystrophy. Brain, 88, 29–50.

Christensen, E. (1959) Topography of terminal motor innervation in striated muscles from stillborn infants. American Journal of Physical Medicine, 38, 17–30.

Cöers, C. & Woolf, A.L. (1959) The Innervation of Muscle, p. 149 (Blackwell: Oxford).

Coomes, E.N. (1965) Cortico-steroid myopathy. Annals of the Rheumatic Diseases, 24, 465–472.

Dahlback, L.-O., Ekstedt, J. & Stålberg, E. (1970) Ischaemic effects on impulse transmission to muscle fibres in man. *Electroencephalography and Clinical Neurophysiology*, **29**, 579–591.

Davey, M.R. & Woolf, A.L. (1964) The electromyographic detection of carriers of muscular dystrophy. *Electroencephalography and Clinical Neurophysiology*, **17**, 705.

Davey, M.R. & Woolf, A.L. (1965) An electromyographic study of carriers of muscular dystrophy. *Proceedings of the 6th International Congress of Electroencephalography and Clinical Neurophysiology*, pp. 653–658 (Weiner Medizinische Akademie: Vienna).

De Jong, H.H., Matzner, I.A. & Unger, A.A. (1951) Clinical and physiological studies in a case of myokymia. *Archives of Neurology and Psychiatry*, **65**, 181.

Denny-Brown, D. (1949) Interpretation of the electromyogram. *Archives of Neurology and Psychiatry*, **61**, 97–128.

Denny-Brown, D. (1953) Clinical problems in neuromuscular physiology. *American Journal of Medicine*, **15**, 368.

Denny-Brown, D. and Pennybacker, J.B. (1938) Fibrillation and fasciculation in voluntary muscle. *Brain*, **61**, 311–334.

Desmedt, J.E. (1957) Nature of the defect of neuromuscular transmission in myasthenic patients: 'post-tetanic exhaustion'. *Nature*, **179**, 156–157.

Desmedt, J.E. (1959) The physio-pathology of neuromuscular transmission and the trophic influence of motor innervation. *American Journal of Physical Medicine*, **38**, 248–261.

Desmedt, J.E. (1973) The neuromuscular disorder in myasthenia gravis. In *New Developments in Electromyography and Clinical Neurophysiology*. Ed. J.E. Desmedt, Vol. 1, pp. 241–304 (Karger: Basel).

Drachman, D.B., Murphy, S.R., Nigam, M.P. & Hill, J.R. (1967) 'Myopathic' changes in chronically denervated muscles. *Archives of Neurology*, **16**, 14–24.

Dyken, M.C., Smith, O.M. & Peake, R.C. (1967) An electromyographic diagnostic screening test and a case report. *Neurology (Minneapolis)*, **17**, 45–50.

Edstrom, J. & Kugelberg, E. (1968) Histochemical composition, distribution of fibres and fatiguability of single motor units. *Journal of Neurology, Neurosurgery and Psychiatry*, **31**, 424–433.

Eisen, A.A. & Karpati, G. (1971) Spontaneous electrical activity in muscle. Description of two patients with motor neurone disease. *Journal of the Neurological Sciences*, **12**, 137.

Ekstedt, J. (1964) Human single muscle fibre action potentials. *Acta Physiologica Scandinavica*, **61**, Supplement 226, 1–91.

Ekstedt, J. & Stålberg, E. (1965) The diagnostic use of single muscle fiber recording and the neuromuscular jitter in myasthenia gravis. In *The 6th International Congress of Electroencephalography and Clinical Neurophysiology Communications*, pp. 669–672 (Wiener Medizinische Akademie: Vienna).

Ekstedt, J. & Stålberg, E. (1969a) The effect of non-paralytic doses of d-tubocurarine on individual motor end-plate in man, studied with a new electrophysiological method. *Electroencephalography and Clinical Neurophysiology*, **27**, 557–562.

Ekstedt, J. & Stålberg, E. (1969b) Abnormal connections between skeletal muscle fibres. *Electroencephalography and Clinical Neurophysiology*, **27**, 607–609.

Ekstedt, J. & Stålberg, E. (1973) Single fibre electromyography for the study of the microphysiology of the human muscle. In *New Developments in Electromyography and Clinical Neurophysiology*, Ed. J.E. Desmedt, Vol. 1, 89–112 (Karger: Basel).

Elmquist, D. & Quastel, D.M.J. (1965) Presynaptic action of hemicholinium at the neuromuscular junction. *Journal of Physiology*, **117**, 463–482.

Emery, A.E.H., Teasdall, R.D. & Coomes, E.N. (1966) Electromyographic studies in carriers of Duchenne muscular dystrophy. *Bulletin of the Johns Hopkins Hospital*, **118**, 439.

Erminio, F., Buchthal, F. & Rosenfalck, P. (1959) Motor unit territory and muscle fiber concentration in paresis due to peripheral nerve injury and anterior horn cell involvement. *Neurology (Minneapolis)*, **9**, 657–671.

Esslen, E. (1960) Electromyographic findings in two types of misdirection of regenerating axons. *Electroencephalography and Clinical Neurophysiology*, **12**, 738–741.

Floyd, M., Ayyar, D.R., Hudgson, P. & Kerr, D.N.S. (1969) Myopathy in chronic renal failure. *Proceedings of the European Dialysis and Transplant Association*, **6**, 203–214.

Forster, F.M. & Alpers, B.J. (1944) The site of origin of fasciculation in voluntary muscle. *Archives of Neurology and Psychiatry*, **51**, 254.

Forster, F.M., Borkowski, W.J. & Alpers, B.J. (1946) Effects of denervation on fasciculation in human muscle. *Archives of Neurology*, **56**, 276.

Frame, B., Heinze, E.G. Jr., Block, M.A. & Manson, G.A. (1968) Myopathy in primary hyperparathyroidism. Observations in three patients. *Annals of Internal Medicine*, **68**, 1022.

Fullerton, P.M. & Gilliatt, R.W. (1965) Axonal reflexes in human motor nerve fibres. *Journal of Neurology, Neurosurgery and Psychiatry*, **28**, 1–11.

Gamstorp, I. & Wohlfart, G. (1959) A syndrome characterised by myokymia, myotonia, muscular wasting and increased perspiration. *Acta Psychiatrica Scandinavica*, **34**, 181–194.

Gardner-Medwin, D. (1968) Studies on the carrier state of the Duchenne type of muscular dystrophy. 2. Quantitative electromyography as a method of carrier detection. *Journal of Neurology, Neurosurgery and Psychiatry*, **31**, 124.

Gardner-Medwin, D. & Walton, J.N. (1969) Myokymia with impaired muscular relaxation. *Lancet*, **1**, 127–130.

Gardner-Medwin, D., Hudgson, P. & Walton, J.N. (1967) Benign spinal muscular atrophy arising in childhood and adolescence. *Journal of the Neurological Sciences*, **5**, 121–158.

Garth, I., Sjaastad, O., & Løken, A.C. (1969) Myopathic electromyographic changes correlated with histopathy in Wohlfart-Kugelberg-Welander disease. *Neurology (Minneapolis)*, **19**, 344–352.

Gordon, G. & Holbourn, A.H.S. (1949) The mechanical activity of single motor units in reflex contraction of skeletal muscle. *Journal of Physiology*, **110**, 26–35.

Greenhouse, A.H., Bicknell, J.M., Pesch, R.N. & Seelinger, D.F. (1967) Myotonia, myokymia, hyperhidrosis and wasting of muscle. *Neurology (Minneapolis)*, **17**, 263–268.

Guld, C., Rosenfalck, A. & Willison, R.G. (1970) Technical factors in recording electrical activity of muscle and nerve in man. *Electroencephalography and Clinical Neurophysiology*, **28**, 399–413.

Guy, E., Lefebre, J., Lerique, J. & Scherrer, J. (1950) Le signes electromyographiques des dermatomyosites. Etude de 9 cas. *Revue Neurologique*, **83**, 278–279.

Hakkansson, C.H. (1957) Action potentials recorded intra- and extracellularly from the isolated frog muscle fibre in Ringer's solution and in air. *Acta Physiologica Scandinavica*, **39**, 291–312.

Handbook of Electroencephalography and Clinical Neurophysiology (1973) Editor-in-chief A. Remond; Vol. 16: *Electromyography*. Ed. F. Buchthal; Part B: *Neuromuscular diseases*. Ed. J.A. Simpson (Elsevier: Amsterdam).

Harman, J.B. & Richardson, A.T. (1954) Generalised myokymia in thyrotoxicosis. Report of a case. *Lancet*, **2**, 473–474.

Harvey, A.M. & Masland, R.L. (1941) A method for the study of neuromuscular transmission in human subjects. *Bulletin of the Johns Hopkins Hospital*, **69**, 1.

Hausmanowa-Petrusewicz, I. & Kozinska, A. (1961) Electromyographic findings in scleroderma. *Archives of Neurology*, **4**, 281–287.

Hed, R., Lundmark, C., Fahlgren, H. & Orell, S. (1962) Acute muscular syndrome in chronic alcoholism. *Acta Medica Scandinavica*, **171**, 585–599.

Hnik, P. & Scorpil, V. (1962) Fibrillation activity in denervated muscle. In *The Denervated Muscle*. Ed. E. Gutman (Czech Academy of Science: Prague).

Hudson, A.J., Cholod, E.J. & Haust, M.D. (1970) Familial hyperparathyroid myopathy. In *Muscle Diseases*, Eds J.N. Walton, N. Canal & G. Scarlato. pp. 526–530 (Excerpta Medica: Amsterdam).

Hughes, R.C. & Matthews, W.B. (1969) Pseudomyotonia and myokymia. *Journal of Neurology, Neurosurgery and Psychiatry*, **32**, 11–14.

Isaacs, H. (1961) A syndrome of continuous muscle-fibre activity. *Journal of Neurology, Neurosurgery and Psychiatry*, **24**, 319–325.

Jasper, H. & Ballem, G. (1949) Unipolar electromyograms of normal and denervated human muscle. *Journal of Neurophysiology*, **12**, 231–244.

Jones, R.V., Lambert, E.H. & Sayre, G.P. (1955) Source of a type of 'insertion activity' in electromyography with evaluation of a histologic method of localisation. *Archives of Physical Medicine*, **36**, 301–310.

Josefsson, I.O. (1960) An electromyographic study of botulism intoxicated skeletal muscle. *Acta Physiologica Scandinavica*, **49** Supplement, 172.

Kugelberg, E. (1947) Electromyogram in muscular disorders. *Journal of Neurology, Neurosurgery and Psychiatry*, **10**, 122–133.

Kugelberg, E. (1973) Properties of the rat hind-limb motor units. *New Developments in Electromyography and Clinical Neurophysiology*. Ed. J.E. Desmedt, Vol. 1, pp. 2–13 (Karger: Basel).

Kugelberg, E. & Petersen, I. (1949) 'Insertion activity' in electromyography. *Journal of Neurology, Neurosurgery and Psychiatry*, **12**, 268–273.

Kugelberg, E. & Skoglund, C.R. (1946a) Responses of a single human motor unit to electrical stimulation. *Journal of Neurophysiology*, **9**, 391–398.

Kugelberg, E. & Skoglund, C.R. (1946b) Natural and artificial activation of motor units, a comparison. *Journal of Neurophysiology*, **9**, 399–412.

Kugelberg, E. & Taverner, D. (1950) A comparison between the voluntary and electrical activation of motor units in anterior horn cell disease. *Electroencephalography and Clinical Neurophysiology*, **2**, 125–132.

Lambert, E.H. (1969) Electromyography in amyotrophic lateral sclerosis. In *Motor Neurone Disease*, Eds F.H. Norris and L.T. Kurland, pp. 135–153 (Grune and Stratton: New York).

Lambert, E.H., Rooke, E.D., Eaton, L.M. & Hodgson, C.H. (1961) Myasthenic syndrome occasionally associated with bronchial neoplasm—neurophysiologic studies. In *Myasthenia Gravis*, Ed. H.R. Vieto, pp. 362–410 (Thomas: Springfield, Illinois).

Landau, W.M. (1952) The essential mechanism in myotonia. *Neurology (Minneapolis)*, **2**, 369–388.

Lang, A.H., Nurkkanen, P. & Vaahtoranta, K.M. (1971) Automatic sampling and averaging of electromyographic unit potentials. *Electroencephalography and Clinical Neurophysiology*, **31**, 404.

Lenman, J.A.R. (1965) Effect of denervation on the resting membrane potential of healthy and dystrophic muscle. *Journal of Neurology, Neurosurgery and Psychiatry*, **28**, 525–528.

Li, C-Y, Shy, G.M. & Wells, J. (1957) Some properties of mammalian skeletal muscle fibres with particular reference to fibrillation potentials. *Journal of Physiology*, **135**, 522–535.

Lindholm, T. (1968) The influence of uraemia and electrolyte disturbances on muscle action potentials and motor nerve conduction in man. *Acta Medica Scandinavica*, Supplement 491, 81.

Lindsley, D.B. (1935) Electrical activity of human motor units during voluntary contraction. *American Journal of Physiology*, **114**, 90–99.

Lundberg, P.O., Osterman, P.O. & Stålberg, E. (1970) Neuromuscular signs and symptoms in acromegaly. In *Muscle Diseases*, Eds J.N. Walton, N. Canal & G. Scarlato, pp. 531–534 (Excerpta Medica: Amsterdam).

McComas, A.J. & Mrozek, K. (1968) The electrical properties of muscle fibre membranes in dystrophia myotonica and myotonia congenita. *Journal of Neurology, Neurosurgery and Psychiatry*, **31**, 441–447.

McComas, A.J., Sica, R.E.P. & Campbell, M.J. (1971) 'Sick motor neurones', a unifying concept of muscle disease. *Lancet*, **1**, 321–325.

McComas, A.J., Fawcett, P.R.W., Campbell, M.J. & Sica, R.E.P. (1971) Electrophysiological estimation of the number of motor units within a human muscle. *Journal of Neurology, Neurosurgery and Psychiatry*, **34**, 121–131.

McQuillen, M.P. & Johns, R.J. (1967) The nature of the defect in Eaton-Lambert syndrome. *Neurology (Minneapolis)*, **17**, 527–536.

Magora, A. & Cohen, B. (1970) A new technique for the extraction of the activity of single motor units from the electromyogram of maximal contraction. *Electromyography*, **2**, 155.

Mastaglia, F.L., Barwick, D.D. & Hall, R. (1970) Myopathy in acromegalics. *Lancet*, **2**, 907–909.

Mastaglia, F.L. & Walton, J.N. (1971) Histological and histochemical changes in skeletal muscle from cases of chronic juvenile and early adult spinal muscular atrophy (the Kugelberg-Welander syndrome). *Journal of the Neurological Sciences*, 12–15.

Mertens, H.G. & Zschocke, S. (1965) Neuromyotonia. *Klinische Wochenschrift*, **43**, 917–925.

Moody, J.F. (1965) Electrophysiological investigations into the neurological complications of carcinoma. *Brain*, **88**, 1023–1035.

Moosa, A. & Brown, B.H. (1972) Quantitative electromyography: a new analogue technique for detecting changes in action potential duration. *Journal of Neurology, Neurosurgery and Psychiatry*, **35**, 216–220.

Moosa, A., Brown, B.H. & Dubowitz, V. (1972) Quantitative electromyography: carrier detection in Duchenne type muscular dystrophy using a new automatic technique. *Journal of Neurology, Neurosurgery and Psychiatry*, **35**, 841–844.

Morrison, J.B. (1960) The electromyographic changes in hyperkalaemic familial periodic paralysis. *Annals of Physical Medicine*, **5**, 153–155.

Muller, R. & Kugelberg, E. (1959) Myopathy in Cushing's syndrome. *Journal of Neurology, Neurosurgery and Psychiatry*, **22**, 314–319.

Nakao, K., Nakanishi, T. & Tsubaki, T. (1965) Action potentials recorded by co-axial needle electrodes in Ringer's solution. *Electroencephalography and Clinical Neurophysiology*, **18**, 412–414.

Nicholls, J.G. (1956) The electrical properties of denervated skeletal muscle. *Journal of Physiology*, **131**, 1–12.

Norris, F.H. Jr. (1965) Central mechanisms of fasciculations. *Proceedings of the 6th International Congress of Electro-encephalography and Clinical Neurophysiology*, p. 715 (Wiener Med. Zinische Akademie: Vienna).

Norris, F.H. Jr. & Gasteiger, E.L. (1955) Action potentials of single motor units in normal muscle. *Electro-encephalography and Clinical Neurophysiology*, **7**, 115–126.

Norris, F.H. Jr. & Panner, B.J. (1966) Hypothyroid myopathy, clinical electromyographic and ultrastructural observations. *Archives of Neurology*, **14**, 574–589.

Oosterhuis, H.J.G.H., Hoostmans, W.J.M., Veenhuyzen, H.B. & Van Zadelhoff, I.V. (1972) The mean duration of motor unit potentials in patients with myasthenia gravis. *Electroencephalography and Clinical Neurophysiology*, **32**, 697–700.

Pinelli, P. & Buchthal, F. (1953) Muscle action potentials in myopathies with special regard to progressive muscular dystrophy. *Neurology (Minneapolis)*, **3**, 347–359.

Prineas, J.W., Hall, R., Barwick, D.D. & Watson, A.J. (1968) Myopathy associated with pigmentation following adrenalectomy for Cushing's syndrome. *Quarterly Journal of Medicine*, **37**, 63–77.

Prochazka, V.J. & Kornhuber, H.H. (1973) On line multiunits sorting with resolution of superimposed potentials. *Electroencephalography and Clinical Neurophysiology*, **34**, 91.

Ramsay, I.D. (1965) Electromyography in thyrotoxicosis. *Quarterly Journal of Medicine*, **34**, 225–267.

Rosenfalck, P. & Buchthal, F. (1962) Studies on the fibrillation potentials of denervated human muscle. *Electroencephalography and Clinical Neurophysiology*, Supplement 22, 130–132.

Salick, A.I. & Pearson, C.M. (1967) The electrical silence of myoidema. *Neurology (Minneapolis)*, **17**, 899–901.

Sanderson, K.V. & Adey, W.R. (1952) Electromyographic and endocrine studies in chronic thyrotoxic myopathy. *Journal of Neurology, Neurosurgery and Psychiatry*, **15**, 200–205.

Schiller, H.H. & Stålberg, E. (1978) Human botulism studied with single fiber electromyography. *Archives of Neurology*, **35**, 346–349.

Schwartz, M.S. & Stålberg, E. (1975) Myasthenia gravis with features of the myasthenic syndrome. *Neurology (Minneapolis)*, **25**, 80–84.

Schwartz, M.S., Stålberg, E., Schiller, H.H. & Thiele, B. (1976) The reinnervated motor unit in man. A single fibre

EMG multi-electrode investigation. *Journal of the Neurological Sciences*, **27**, 303–312.

Shy, G.M. & Silverstein, I. (1965) A study of the effects on the motor unit by remote malignancy. *Brain*, **86**, 515–528.

Simpson, J.A. (1960) Myasthenia gravis: a new hypothesis. *Scottish Medical Journal*, **5**, 419–436.

Simpson, J.A. (1962) Recent studies on the physiology of the human spinal cord and its disturbance in poliomyelitis. *Proceedings of the 8th Symposium of the European Association for Poliomyelitis*, pp. 347–360 (Masson: Paris).

Simpson, J.A. (1966) Control of muscle in health and disease. *Control and Innervation of Skeletal Muscle*, Ed. B.L. Andrew, pp. 171–180 (E. and S. Livingstone: Edinburgh).

Slomic, A., Rosenfalck, A. & Buchthal, F. (1968) Electrical and mechanical responses of normal and myasthenic muscle. *Brain Research*, **10**, 1–78.

Smith, H.L., Amick, L.D. & Johnson, W.W. (1966) Detection of subclinical and carrier state in Duchenne muscular dystrophy. *Journal of Paediatrics*, **69**, 67.

Smith, R. & Stern, G. (1967) Myopathy, osteomalacia and hyperparathyroidism. *Brain*, **90**, 593–602.

Stålberg, E. (1966) Propagation velocity in human muscle fibres in situ. *Acta Physiologica Scandinavica*, **70**, Supplement 287, 1–111.

Stålberg, E. & Ekstedt, J. (1973) Single fibre EMG and microphysiology of the motor unit in normal and diseased muscle. In *New Developments in Electromyography and Clinical Neurophysiology*, Ed. J.E. Desmedt, Vol. 1, pp. 113–129 (Karger: Basel).

Stålberg, E. & Thiele, B. (1972) Transmission block in terminal nerve twigs. A single fibre electromyographic finding in man. *Journal of Neurology, Neurosurgery and Psychiatry*, **35**, 52–59.

Stålberg, E. & Trontelj, J.V. (1970) Demonstration of axon reflexes in human motor nerve fibres. *Journal of Neurology, Neurosurgery and Psychiatry*, **33**, 571–579.

Stålberg, E. & Trontelj, J.V. (1979) *Single fibre electromyography* (The Mirvalle Press: Old Woking, Surrey).

Stålberg, E., Ekstedt, J. & Broman, A. (1971) The electromyographic jitter in normal human muscles. *Electroencephalography and Clinical Neurophysiology*, **31**, 429–438.

Swash, M. & Schwartz, M.S. (1977) Implications of longitudinal muscle fibre splitting in neurogenic and myopathic disorders. *Journal of Neurology, Neurosurgery and Psychiatry*, **40**, 1152–1159.

Thage, O., Trojaborg, W. & Buchthal, F. (1963) Electromyographic findings in polyneuropathy. *Neurology (Minneapolis)*, **13**, 273–278.

Thesleff, S. (1962) Spontaneous electrical activity in denervated rat skeletal muscle. *Proceedings of a Symposium on the Effects of Use and Disuse of Neuromuscular Junctions*, Eds E. Gutman & P. Hnik, pp. 41–51 (Elsevier: Amsterdam).

Thiele, B. & Stålberg, E. (1975) Single fibre EMG findings in polyneuropathies of different aetiology. *Journal of Neurology, Neurosurgery and Psychiatry*, **38**, 881–887.

Trojaborg, W. & Buchthal, F. (1965) Malignant and benign fasciculations. *Acta Neurologica Scandinavica*, **41**, Supplement 13, 251–254.

Trojaborg, W., Franzen, E. & Andersen, I. (1969) Peripheral neuropathy associated with carcinoma of the lung. *Brain*, **92**, 71–82.

Van Den Bosch, J. (1963) Investigation of the carrier state in the Duchenne type dystrophy. In *Proceedings of the 2nd Symposium on Research in Muscular Dystrophy*, pp. 23–30 (Pitman: London).

Van Der Most Van Spijk, D. (1964) Refractory and irresponsive period of muscle in myasthenia gravis. *Electroencephalography and Clinical Neurophysiology*, **17**, 103.

Vasilescu, C., Bucur, G., Petrovici, A. & Florescu, A. (1978) Myasthenia in patients with dermatomyositis. Clinical, electrophysiological and ultrastructural studies. *Journal of the Neurological Sciences*, **38**, 129–144.

Venables, G.S., Bates, D. & Shaw, D.A. (1978) Hypothyroidism with true myotonia. *Journal of Neurology, Neurosurgery and Psychiatry*, **41**, 1013–1015.

Vicale, C.T. (1949) The diagnostic features of a muscular syndrome resulting from hyperparathyroidism, osteomalacia owing to renal tubular acidosis, and perhaps to related disorders of calcium metabolism. *Transactions of the American Neurological Association*, **74**, 143–147.

Weddell, G., Feinstein, B. & Pattle, R.E. (1944) The electrical activity of voluntary muscle in man under normal and pathological conditions. *Brain*, **67**, 178–257.

Weiderholt, W.C. (1970) 'End-plate noise' in electromyography. *Neurology (Minneapolis)*, **20**, 214–224.

Williams, R.S. (1959) Triamcinolone myopathy. *Lancet*, **1**, 698–701.

Willison, R.G. (1962) Electrodiagnosis in motor neurone disease. *Proceedings of the Royal Society of Medicine*, **55**, 1024.

Willison, R.G. (1963) A method of measuring motor unit activity in human muscle. *Journal of Physiology*, **168**, 35.

Willison, R.G. (1964) Analysis of electrical activity in healthy and dystrophic muscle in man. *Journal of Neurology, Neurosurgery and Psychiatry*, **27**, 386.

Willison, R.G. (1965) A method of measuring motor unit activity in human muscle. *Proceedings of the 3rd Symposium on Research in Muscular Dystrophy*, p. 285 (Pitman: London).

Willison, R.G. (1966) Some problems in the diagnosis of primary muscle disease. *Proceedings of the Royal Society of Medicine*, **59**, 998.

Yates, D.A.H. (1963) The estimation of mean potential duration in endocrine myopathy. *Journal of Neurology, Neurosurgery and Psychiatry*, **26**, 458–461.

Integration and analysis of the electromyogram and related techniques

INTRODUCTION

Although the electrical activity of human muscle has been studied for many years, and Piper's work with surface electrodes was an important landmark (Piper, 1912), it was not until the introduction of the concentric needle electrode (Adrian and Bronk, 1929) that individual motor unit action potentials could be studied and electromyography could develop into a useful method of clinical investigation. Early work was hindered by limitations of recording technique but increasing technical refinement has enabled electromyography to become a practical diagnostic method. Modern equipment will display the electromyogram (EMG) on the screen of a cathode ray tube for visual analysis and provide a simultaneous auditory record through a loudspeaker. At the same time a permanent record can be made by photography or on magnetic tape.

In this way the direct examination of muscle action potentials in disorders affecting muscle and nerve is possible. Under normal circumstances the potentials seen are motor unit action potentials which are the summated action potentials derived from groups of fibres supplied by the same motor neurone. In healthy muscle they occur only in volitional activity but in neuromuscular disease they can occur spontaneously, and abnormal discharges representing the contraction of single fibres may also occur spontaneously or on mechanical stimulation. The frequency and shape of motor unit potentials may be greatly modified by disease.

While the recognition of different patterns of motor unit or muscle fibre activity has a ready clinical application, the quantitative application of electromyography has been relatively slow to develop. Although it has provided much information of physiological interest, and some of diagnostic value, it has advanced only gradually to the extent of providing clinically standardised techniques. An important exception is the measurement of nerve conduction velocity now firmly established as a routine test (Ch. 27). Other methods which have been studied are the measurement of integrated electrical activity during voluntary contraction, and the analysis of action potential dimensions and distribution by direct measurement or electronic techniques. The measurement of refractory period has provided a method of studying indirectly the properties both of individual muscle fibres and of peripheral nerves. In a number of instances the development of computer programmes has made it possible to extend the information provided by direct examination and, by providing automatic methods of analysis, to lessen the amount of time-consuming measurement which may be necessary. The study of muscle action potentials after electrical or mechanical stimulation of normal muscle has provided a means of examining reflex action and of measuring the excitability of the motor neurone pool. In this chapter consideration will be given to the application of quantitative methods for the integration and analysis of the EMG and the study of reflex activity.

THE INTEGRATION OF THE ELECTROMYOGRAM

Introduction

During an electromyographic examination the number of action potentials appearing on the oscilloscope screen increases with the force of the contraction until, at near maximal effort, it is no longer possible to distinguish individual potentials and the continuous wave-form is referred to as an 'interference pattern'. The increase in electrical activity which occurs as a muscle contracts more powerfully has provided an important means of studying how far different muscles are implicated in movements about particular joints (Dempster and Finerty, 1947). Recently, the quantitative analysis of the relationship between tension and electrical activity has been used to study the physiology of motor unit activity in health and disease.

Because motor unit action potentials have a complex form with both positive and negative components, some form of integration in terms of mean voltage is necessary before quantitation of the EMG becomes possible. In the study of motor unit potentials for diagnostic purposes it is desirable to study a small portion of muscle, so that concentric needle electrodes, which record the potential differences between closely adjacent points, are generally employed. Where electrodes are widely separated the potential difference between them will be affected by changes in potential arising in comparatively distant fibres (Adrian and Bronk, 1929). In integration studies, therefore, where it is important to sample a large part of the muscle, it is more satisfactory to use surface electrodes placed on the overlying skin.

The EMG recorded from surface electrodes, particularly if these are large and widely separated, is already to some extent integrated in that it appears as a continuous positive and negative variation in potential, in which the action potentials of individual units can no longer be clearly distinguished. The mean voltage of the EMG recorded in this way can readily be measured by rectifying the voltage after amplification and by passing the rectified voltage into a meter. More elaborate methods of integration are now available.

Methods of integration

In 1950 Bayer and Flechtenmayer showed that the mean voltage recorded through surface electrodes over biceps was approximately proportional to the force of contraction. They measured the voltage on a meter while the muscle contracted isometrically; the subject held weights of differing magnitude.

The relation of muscle tension and length to the integrated EMG has been studied in amputees with cineplastic muscle tunnels (Inman, Ralston, Saunders, Feinstein and Wright, 1952). The EMG was recorded both with surface and needle electrodes while the muscle tension during effort was measured with a strain gauge dynamometer. The electrical activity was rectified and the rectified voltage recorded simultaneously with the tension. Provided that the muscular contraction was isometric the integrated EMG increased in parallel with the tension, but no quantitative relationship between the two could be demonstrated if the muscle were allowed to change in length. There was no quantitative relationship between the EMG and muscle power.

Lippold has studied the relationship between the integrated EMG recorded through surface electrodes over the calf muscle and the tension of voluntary contraction recorded isometrically (Lippold, 1952). The mean voltage of the EMG was originally determined by measurement of the area of the photographed action potentials with a planimeter. When isometric tension was plotted against mean voltage a linear relationship was found between the two. As the force of a contraction depends on the number of motor units which are taking part and on their frequency of activation, it is reasonable to conclude that the integrated EMG gives an index of the number and activity of the motor units participating.

In later studies a more elaborate technique was employed (Bigland and Lippold, 1954a; Edwards and Lippold, 1956; Scherrer and Bourguignon, 1959; Lenman, 1959a). The EMG was first amplified and then fed into a circuit which rectified the record and gave out pulses proportional to the rectified voltage. It can be shown that the number of pulses given off per unit time by this electrical method is proportional to the area of the action potentials when determined by planimetry (Bigland and Lippold, 1954a). The frequency of the pulses may be measured directly after recording on paper or they may be counted electronically. Voltage and tension may be expressed in arbitrary units but can, if necessary, be calibrated appropriately (Lenman, 1959a). A method which avoids the necessity for computing voltage–tension curves is to apply the voltage representing tension to the X plates of an oscilloscope and the rectified mean voltage of the EMG to the Y plates. If this is done throughout a series of graded contractions the voltage–tension curve is obtained automatically (Simpson and Sanderson, 1965; Stephens and Taylor, 1972, 1973; Zuniga and Simons, 1969).

Not everybody has found a strictly linear relationship between muscle tension and the integrated EMG. Thus Zuniga and Simons (1969), working with the biceps brachii, found a curvilinear relationship between EMG and tension, recording progressively increasing values of electrical activity with increasing tension. Similarly, Kuroda, Klissouras and Milsum (1970), studying the movement of extension of the knee and recording from the rectus femoris, found the relationship between force and EMG to be linear throughout the greater part of the force range, but when the tension approached that of maximum voluntary contraction there was a steep increase in electrical activity. Possible reasons for this non-linearity include the possibility that there may be increased synchronisation at high values of tension where fatigue may also be a modifying factor. Where movement at a joint such as the elbow is studied, the situation may be further complicated by the action of other forearm flexors apart from

the muscle from which recordings are made. Stephens and Taylor (1973) however have found a strictly linear relationship between integrated electrical activity and tension when recording from the first dorsal interosseus muscle. Technical considerations in the recording and integration of EMG signals have been discussed by Zuniga, Truong and Simons (1969) and McLeod (1973).

Discharge frequency and the grading of muscular contraction

The linear relationship between isometric tension and electrical activity of voluntary muscle makes it clear that the integrated EMG provides a quantitative measure of the level of excitation in a muscle. Electromyographic studies during isotonic contractions have further clarified the relationship. If a muscle is allowed to shorten there is still a linear relationship between integrated electrical activity and tension provided that the velocity of shortening is not allowed to change. Likewise, if a muscle is allowed to shorten at a constant tension then the integrated electrical activity is proportional to the velocity of shortening (Bigland and Lippold, 1954a).

How far the integrated EMG reflects the number of fibres taking part and how far it is a measure of their frequency of activation is an important question which bears closely on the matter of how the force of a voluntary contraction is graded. The frequency of nerve impulse transmission in motor nerves has a range of approximately 5–100 Hz (Adrian and Bronk, 1929) but under ordinary circumstances it is doubtful whether the higher frequencies often occur, at least in the limb muscles. If a muscle is stimulated through its motor nerve at different rates of stimulation, the tension developed by the muscle increases in linear fashion with stimulus frequency, until a frequency in the region of 50 Hz is attained. With higher frequencies there is relatively little increase in tension (Adrian and Bronk, 1929). Marsden, Meadows and Merton (1971) monitored action potentials from an aberrant unit supplied by the median nerve in adductor pollicis when the ulnar nerve was blocked, and recorded potentials which had a peak frequency of 150 Hz at maximal effort.

During powerful contractions, the frequency of discharge of motor units is not easy to measure by ordinary electromyographic techniques because of the difficulty of observing single units when many are firing at once. Lindsley (1935) used fine wire electrodes to explore a number of muscles in human subjects and never observed a frequency of motor unit responses exceeding 40–50 Hz; generally the action potentials fell within the range of 5–30 Hz. The study of paretic muscles has been helpful because, when the number of available units is decreased, it may be less difficult to follow the frequency of discharge of a single unit throughout the entire range of a contraction. Thus Seyffarth (1941a, b) recorded maximal discharge rates of 55–60 Hz in healthy muscles but in a number of paretic muscles he recorded frequencies of 90 Hz with maximal effort. In certain muscles which are able to subserve exceptionally rapid movements, very much faster rates may occur, as in the external ocular muscles where action potential frequencies of 200 Hz have been recorded (Björk and Kugelberg, 1953).

Bigland and Lippold (1954b) studied the rate of firing of single units in the hand muscles. They recorded with pairs of fine wire electrodes during different grades of contraction, but partially blocked conduction in the ulnar nerve to reduce the number of units firing during maximal effort. When a single unit potential was observed throughout different grades of contraction it was seen that, although the discharge frequency increased as did tension, it did so through a restricted range and not in a linear manner. Frequencies above 50 Hz were never observed and frequencies of 40–50 Hz occurred only during very strong contractions. It was often found that a particular unit would always start firing at a definite tension and cease to fire when a certain level of tension was reached (Fig. 29.1). When a unit appeared in this manner during a limited part of the range of a contraction, its discharge rate often remained relatively constant. When the average frequency of all the units observed at different tensions was plotted against the force of contraction, it was seen that the relationship between frequency and tension was given by an S-shaped curve.

Motor units with a characteristic range of discharge frequency appearing at particular levels

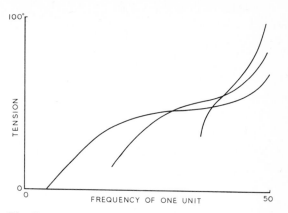

Fig. 29.1 Scheme illustrating possible mode of behaviour of individual motor units during the voluntary contraction of a muscle. A particular unit starts firing when the tension in the muscle reaches a certain level, its frequency increasing with tension over a comparatively small range except at low and high tensions (from Bigland and Lippold, 1954b)

of tension were also observed by Norris and Gasteiger (1955). Their study, using microelectrodes of fine wire which recorded from a very restricted area, was carried out principally on the gastrocnemius and rectus femoris. They were able to record units which fired at a rate of more than 100 Hz during brief bursts at maximal effort, and they observed a small number of large motor units which appeared only during powerful contractions and fired at a rate of less than 5 Hz.

It might be concluded that an important, if not the major, factor in grading the force of a muscular contraction is the recruitment and dropping out of motor units as the tension rises and falls, variations in the frequency of motor unit discharge serving to provide fine adjustments of muscular tension. However, it is evident from studies of motor unit recruitment and firing frequency at different tensions that the majority of motor units are recruited at relatively low tension, nearly half reaching activation before the tension attains 20 per cent of maximum and relatively little recruitment occurring at tensions greater than 50 per cent of maximum. In general, the discharge frequency of single units increases with the force of contraction, although the relationship between the firing rate of single units and force is dependent on the rate of increasing or decreasing voluntary force. It would appear, therefore, that the contribution of motor unit recruitment to the increase in voluntary force is greatest at low levels of tension, at higher levels changes in firing frequency becoming increasingly important (Milner-Brown, Stein and Yemm, 1973a, b; Tanji and Kato, 1973a, b). It is of interest that, in these studies, motor unit recruitment is seen to occur in an orderly manner, larger units tending to be recruited at higher tensions. This is consistent with the size principle (Henneman, Somjen and Carpenter, 1965), according to which the smallest motor neurones have the lowest threshold of excitation. Further evidence that this principle applies to human muscle is provided by the observation of Freund, Dietz, Wita and Kapp (1973), that the conduction velocity of nerve fibres innervating high threshold units is faster than that of fibres innervating low threshold units.

Milner-Brown and Stein (1975) have reviewed the studies which have been carried out to explain the theoretical basis for a relation between EMG and muscular force. These, in general, suggest that electrical activity should increase with the square root of the tension rather than linearly, which would give a change in slope in the opposite direction to that observed by workers who have found a non-linear relationship experimentally. To try to clarify the relationship between surface EMG and muscular force, and how this depends on motor unit activity, these authors have studied the recruitment of motor units in the first dorsal interosseous muscle, using an averaging technique to determine the waveform contributed by each motor unit to the surface EMG. By this means they found that the amplitude of the waveform of the surface EMG contributed by a single unit tended to increase according to the threshold force at which the unit was recruited, but not in a linear manner, the increase being proportional to the square root of the threshold force. Recruitment of motor units, however, was found to be less important at higher force levels where firing frequency contributed predominantly to tension. The non-linear effect on the surface EMG of motor unit recruitment could be compensated for if the tension increment derived from increased firing frequency were also non-linear: it is likely that this may, indeed, be the case because the firing rates of some units may be high enough to give rise to a fused tetanus. The observed linear re-lationship between EMG and tension may, therefore, depend on a balance between non-linear summation of EMG potentials and contractile responses at higher levels of tension.

The integrated electromyogram in fatigue

In 1923 Cobb and Forbes commented that 'The study of muscular fatigue is so complicated by psychological factors that a method of accurately recording any of its concomitant phenomena may be of value'. They studied fatigue in the flexors of the wrist, using surface electrodes and a string galvanometer to record action potentials from the muscles while fatiguing contractions were carried out. They confirmed the earlier observation of Piper, that the rhythm of the action potentials slowed during fatigue (Piper, 1912). They also noted that the amplitude of the potentials increased.

Although these observations have been confirmed repeatedly, their interpretation has been hindered by lack of understanding of the underlying mechanisms of fatigue, and methods for its quantitative measurement have been slow to develop. In myasthenia gravis, where there is abnormal fatiguability of muscle, a rapid decline occurs in the amplitude of the action potentials which may be evoked by repetitive stimulation of a muscle through its nerve and this procedure has been used as a diagnostic test (Harvey and Masland, 1941). A similar fatigue of evoked potentials has been observed in some forms of neurogenic atrophy, particularly poliomyelitis (Hodes, 1948) and motor neurone disease (Mulder, Lambert and Eaton, 1959; Simpson and Lenman, 1959). In healthy mammalian muscle, exhaustion at the motor end-plate occurs less readily and is probably but one aspect of fatigue, less important than exhaustion of the contractile substance of the fibre (Brown and Burns, 1949; Merton, 1954; Naess and Storm-Mathison, 1955).

In 1956, Edwards and Lippold suggested that, if a voluntary contraction is maintained for a period at a constant tension, it might be expected that more units would be recruited as the tension developed by the fatigued muscle fibres declined. This would alter the proportionality which has been shown to exist between electrical activity and

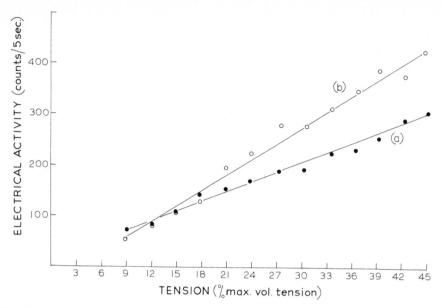

Fig. 29.2 Comparison of relation between integrated electrical activity and tension in soleus muscle (a) before and (b) after a 4-minute fatiguing contraction. Tension values are given as a percentage of maximum voluntary tension; electrical activity in counts of integrator pulses/5 seconds (from Edwards and Lippold, 1956)

tension (Lippold, 1952). They measured the tension of the calf muscles simultaneously with the integrated EMG throughout a range of tensions before and after a prolonged fatiguing contraction. When a muscle is fatigued in this way the relationship between tension and the integrated EMG remains linear but the slope of the curve alters, so that a given tension is associated with more electrical activity (Fig. 29.2) (Edwards and Lippold, 1956). Similar observations have been made on the human biceps and triceps (Lenman, 1959b). If the integrated EMG is recorded during sustained contractions of different magnitude, but of less than maximal tension, the rate of increase in electrical activity as fatigue develops is greater the more powerful the contraction (Eason, 1960). Analysis of the potentials recorded through surface electrodes shows that, with increasing loads, while both the amplitude and frequency of the potentials alter progressively, the decrease in frequency becomes particularly prominent as the load is increased (Person, 1960).

These studies have been carried out under isometric conditions and it is important to know how far the changes result from fatigue developing in the contracting fibres, and how far they relate to the ischaemia which may develop during an isometric contraction. However, a similar increase in electrical activity associated with fatigue occurs during exercise in an ergometer in which the muscle is allowed to shorten (Scherrer, Samson and Soula, 1954).

These observations are consistent with the view that the fatigue of a voluntary muscular contraction is generally due to exhaustion of the contractile substance of the muscle fibres, and there seems to be little doubt that this is the case, at least during the later stages of voluntary contraction. There is less certainty regarding the mechanism of fatigue in the early stages of a maximal contraction. Merton's observation (1954) that, in fatigue produced by a sustained voluntary contraction, the tension could not be restored by an electrical stimulus and that the action potentials in an electrically evoked contraction did not change in amplitude as the muscle tension declined, suggested that contractile-element fatigue was the main, if not the sole, mechanism. However, Stephens and Taylor (1972) found that, during the first minute of a maximal contraction of the first dorsal interosseus muscle, force declined by about 50 per cent; during this phase the relationship between tension and the integrated EMG remained unchanged and only later did force fall faster than electrical activity. In addition they found that if they evoked the muscle contraction by stimulation of the ulnar nerve, the action potential would fall to about 65 per cent of normal. They concluded that, in the early stage of maximal voluntary contraction, neuromuscular-junction fatigue was the main factor, contractile-element fatigue developing only later. Bigland-Ritchie, Hosking and Jones (1975) found that, during sustained maximal voluntary contractions of the quadriceps muscle, the subject could produce temporary increases in tension by a brief 'super effort', which he was unable to maintain; they concluded that, during the early phase of a maximal contraction, some of the loss of force is the result of a reduction in central drive. A similar conclusion has been reached by Dietz (1978), who studied fatigue in contractions in the wrist flexors, using the automatic method of spike-counting analysis described by Rose and Willison (1967); he concluded that, in the first phase of muscle fatigue, the decline in force was related to a slowing of discharge rates. Slowing of discharge rates during maximal effort has also been noted by Marsden, Meadows and Merton (1971) in a study of motor units in the adductor pollicis supplied by aberrant fibres of the median nerve. Stephens and Usher-wood (1975) have found that high-threshold motor units tend to fatigue earlier than low-threshold units; this finding suggests that the smaller motor units which are recruited earlier correspond to the motor units which are associated with tonic contraction, and which are less susceptible to fatigue.

The aspect of fatigue which is measured by the change in the ratio of mean voltage to tension during contraction would appear to be mainly that element of fatigue which affects the contractile substance of the muscle fibre. In neuromuscular block one would not anticipate any change in the ratio. Observations have been made of the integrated EMG during sustained effort in myasthenia gravis. In this condition there may be little or no increase in mean voltage during a sustained contraction of an affected muscle, and often there is an early decline in electrical activity associated with a fall in tension (Scherrer and Bourguignon,

1959; Lenman, 1966). Comparative studies of the rate of change in the voltage–tension relationship during fatiguing contractions have been made in patients with rheumatoid arthritis, and suggest that the electrical changes associated with fatigue may be prominent during the phase of morning stiffness (Lenman and Potter, 1966).

The effect of muscle training on the electromyogram

Inman and his colleagues reported that there is no correlation between the integrated EMG and muscle power (Inman et al., 1952). Nevertheless, it is possible that the alteration in power which follows a period of training may be accompanied by an alteration in the relationship between integrated mean voltage and muscular tension. Repeated exercise results in an increase in muscle strength, but this is not always associated with hypertrophy (MacQueen, 1954). Although structural changes in the muscle fibres are undoubtedly important in the development of strength, a neuromuscular adaptation leading to a more efficient use of the available motor units may be equally significant (Lenman, 1959a).

If a change in the efficiency of the individual fibres were the more important factor, one would expect a muscular contraction in the trained subject to be associated with less electrical activity than in the untrained, the reverse of the situation in fatigue. Stepanov (1959) recorded the EMG through surface electrodes from the muscles of athletes during training in heavy weight lifting. It was found that both the mean amplitude and the frequency of the action potentials decreased as the training proceeded. De Vries (1968) has used the slope of the voltage–tension relationship to measure what he terms efficiency of electrical activity (EEA) in subjects of differing strength, and before and after muscle training. He found that, in subjects of differing strength, the slope of the voltage–tension relationship corresponded to less electrical activity for a given muscle tension in strong, as opposed to weak, individuals; this change in slope, which is the reverse of that which occurs in fatigued muscle, became more pronounced as the strength of a muscle was increased by training. After immobilisation in a plaster cast the reverse effect occurred, so that more electrical activity corresponded to a given tension.

The integrated electromyogram in muscular weakness

In 1949 Kugelberg showed that, in many cases of muscular dystrophy, there is a full interference pattern on maximal effort, although the individual motor unit potentials are highly broken-up and polyphasic. He concluded that, in a dystrophic muscle, the strength represented by an action potential must be greatly reduced when compared with normal muscle. An important consideration here is that dystrophic units contain fewer muscle fibres than healthy ones—one effect of the dystrophic process. There is evidence also that the contractile force which many dystrophic fibres can exert is significantly diminished (Sandow and Brust, 1958; Botelho, Beckett and Bendler, 1960).

In a sense this is comparable to the state of affairs which may exist in fatigued muscle. If one regards the slope of the curve relating voltage to tension as a measure of the efficiency (or more precisely the reciprocal of efficiency) of the muscle, it would be reasonable to expect a disease process affecting the structure of the individual muscle fibres to affect the efficiency of the muscle in a manner similar to fatigue. It could be predicted that the slope of the curve relating voltage to tension would be shifted in the same direction as in fatigued muscle, so that more voltage would be associated with a given tension than in the healthy state.

A different state of affairs is to be expected in muscular weakness of neurogenic origin, where a muscle is weak because of impairment of its nerve supply, so that the full number of motor units can no longer be activated. One would predict no alteration in the ratio of voltage to tension. During a maximal contraction there would be a reduction both in the tension exerted and in the accompanying mean voltage, but both would be affected strictly in proportion. Factors which might affect the proportionality are alterations in the structure or mode of action of the units; there is evidence that such changes may occur in disease affecting the lower motor neurone. Thus in long-standing peripheral nerve lesions, irregular regeneration may affect the synchrony of contraction of the elements of the motor unit. In disease of the anterior horn cells, the surviving motor neurones may innervate greatly enlarged units through the mechanism of collateral sprouting and re-innervation of denervated fibres (Coërs, 1955; Wohlfart, 1955). It is not clear how important true synchronous firing of motor units is as a factor in spinal cord disease, or how it affects the voltage–tension relationship.

Lenman (1959b) studied the relationship between isometric tension and the integrated EMG in the biceps and triceps of healthy subjects and of patients with weakness of neurogenic and myopathic origin. In patients with neurogenic weakness due to spinal cord or peripheral nerve lesions, the mean slope of the voltage–tension curves did not differ significantly from that of healthy subjects. On the other hand, myopathic weakness caused by muscular dystrophy or polymyositis, was associated with a significant shift in the slope of the curve in the direction of reduced efficiency, i.e. in the same direction as the shift which occurs in fatigued muscle (Fig. 29.3). In patients with weakness resulting from old poliomyelitis the results differed from those in other patients with neurogenic weakness. Here, the slope of the curves showed a shift in the direction of reduced efficiency; in addition, the absolute values obtained for mean voltage were considerably higher than those obtained in healthy subjects, a finding which was previously reported by Knowlton, Hines, Keever and Bennett (1956). It is likely that these curves reflect the alterations in motor unit structure which follow recovery from poliomyelitis, in particular the increase in size of the motor units. Histologically, many of the collateral sprouts which give rise to this increase are immature and poorly differentiated (Wohlfart, 1959b) and this may have a significant bearing on the efficiency of the enlarged units. The use of the voltage–tension relationship to study the effects of therapy in muscle disease has been discussed by Simpson and Sanderson (1965).

THE ANALYSIS OF ACTION POTENTIAL CHARACTERISTICS

Introduction

The technique of electromyography, in which

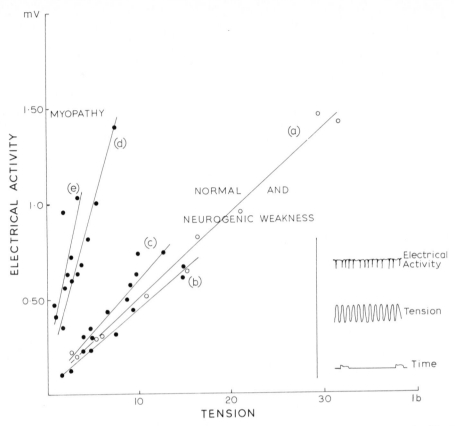

Fig. 29.3 Regression lines for relationship between mean voltage and isometric tension of biceps muscle of healthy subject and patients with neurogenic and myopathic weakness: (a) healthy subject; (b) peripheral neuritis; (c) motor neurone disease; (d) polymyositis; (e) pseudohypertrophic muscular dystrophy. Insert shows specimen of ink writer recording from subject (a) in which time (seconds), tension (amplitude of sine wave) and integrated electrical activity (number of pulses) are recorded simultaneously (Lenman, 1959b)

muscles are explored with concentric needle electrodes and in which action potentials are recorded from discrete areas within the muscle, is now well established, so that the appearance of the action potentials in disorders of the lower motor neurone and of muscle provides reliable information of diagnostic value.

Insertion of the needle electrode into healthy muscle evokes an outburst of action potentials (Weddell, Feinstein and Pattle, 1944). These are known as insertion activity and are made up of a high-frequency discharge of potentials of slightly shorter duration and smaller amplitude than motor unit action potentials; they last only a brief period longer than the needle movement (Kugelberg and Petersén, 1949). With the needle in position, if the muscle is relaxed it is electrically silent (Adrian and Bronk, 1929). During a weak contraction the electrode picks up discharges from the fibres of the motor units in its immediate vicinity. A motor unit consists of an 'individual motor nerve fibre with the bunch of muscle fibres it activates' (Sherrington, 1929). The contraction of these muscle fibres is not synchronous and their individual action potentials summate to form the motor unit action potential. This may be monophasic, diphasic or triphasic and is generally of 5–10 ms duration and 100 μV–2.0 mV in amplitude. As the contraction becomes more powerful the number of motor unit potentials increases, until they can no longer be distinguished separately in the interference pattern.

Action potentials from single muscle fibres are not normally seen, but occur spontaneously in denervated muscle as fibrillation potentials (Denny-Brown and Pennybacker, 1938). The cause of this activity is unknown, but there is evidence that fibrillation potentials originate in the denervated end-plate area (Belmar and Eyzaguirre, 1966). Fibrillation potentials recorded from the end-plate zone are diphasic with an initial negative deflection; elsewhere in the muscle the initial deflection is positive (Buchthal and Rosenfalck, 1966b). They occur characteristically at a regular rate of from 2 to 10 Hz, are of less than 2.0 ms duration and have an average amplitude of about 100 μV (Weddell et al., 1944). The occasional occurrence of fibrillation potentials of large size suggests that some are due to the spontaneous discharge of more than a single fibre (Buchthal and Rosenfalck, 1966b). Fibrillation potentials are not confined to denervated muscle but also occur in certain forms of myopathy, particularly polymyositis (Walton and Adams, 1958). Fibrillation potentials may be associated with a marked increase in insertion activity. In denervated muscle this consists of discharges of brief potentials which may be indistinguishable from fibrillation, and sometimes also of large positive potentials, known as 'positive saw-tooth potentials'. The origin of these is not known, but they rarely occur in healthy muscle (Jasper and Ballem, 1949; Kugelberg and Petersén, 1949).

During a voluntary contraction in disease of the lower motor neurone there is generally a reduction in the interference pattern, because the number of functioning motor units is diminished. In severe cases the needle electrode may record only the activity from isolated surviving units, the 'single oscillation' of Buchthal and Clemmeson (1941).

In primary muscle disease, which includes the inherited forms of muscular dystrophy and the acquired myopathies, there is degeneration and atrophy of individual muscle fibres. Except in the terminal stages (Kugelberg, 1949) this does not lead to a reduction in the number of available motor units, but brings about a disruption of their structure. Because in a given unit many of the constituent muscle fibres will have ceased to function, the action potentials of the surviving fibres will not summate smoothly as in the healthy motor unit, but will give rise to a motor unit action potential which has a highly polyphasic and broken-up appearance. Although there may be no reduction in the interference pattern during a voluntary contraction, there is now evidence from studies of the recruitment of motor units during electrically evoked contractions that, at least in certain muscles, there may be a reduction in the total number of motor units in addition to loss of fibres within the units (McComas, Sica and Currie, 1970).

Dimensions of the motor unit potential

Many studies have been carried out to try to establish values for the duration and amplitude of motor unit action potentials, in healthy subjects and in patients with neuromuscular disorders. The range of values obtained depends to some extent on recording technique. Thus, the mean amplitude of the potentials is higher when unipolar electrodes are used than with concentric electrodes, although both types of electrode give similar values for mean action potential duration. With bipolar electrodes, the potentials recorded have a shorter duration than when recorded by concentric electrodes, and the duration depends both on the distance apart of the electrodes and on the plane of insertion. Different concentric electrodes of the same batch may give different values for mean duration and amplitude, even though the electrodes have the same dimensions (Buchthal, Guld and Rosenfalck, 1954).

In the normal individual there is considerable variation in action potential duration between different muscles. Thus, for the biceps brachii the mean duration has been found to be 7.56 ± 0.14 ms compared with 2.28 ± 0.03 ms in the facial muscles (Petersén and Kugelberg, 1949), and 1.60 ± 0.06 ms in the external ocular muscles (Björk and Kugelberg, 1953). In infants the mean duration is significantly shorter than that in adults, and in the elderly it is significantly prolonged. These changes have been attributed, in the change from infancy to adult life, to an increase in width of the end-plate zone which occurs with growth, and, in the changes with advancing age, to the increase in fibre density which may be caused by a reduction in muscle volume (Sacco, Buchthal and Rosenfalck, 1962).

Buchthal, Erminio and Rosenfalck (1959) and Buchthal (1960) attempted to measure the extent of the territory in which the muscle fibres giving rise to a motor unit action potential can be identified. The fibres of motor units extend lengthwise in bundles along the muscles but in cross-section there is considerable overlap between units. Hence it is difficult to measure, anatomically, the distribution of units across a muscle. Measurements of motor unit dispersion were made using a stainless steel multi-electrode containing 12 independent leads, each recording from separate points at intervals along its length. When this electrode, or preferably two such electrodes at right angles to one another, were inserted transversely across a muscle it was possible to measure the dispersion of the potentials arising from a single unit. By this means it was shown that the territory of a motor unit in the human biceps brachii in terms of muscle cross-section is approximately circular and has an average extent of 5.0 mm.

Kugelberg (1949) found that the mean duration of action potentials in patients with lesions of the lower motor neurone was increased, and he also found an increase in the amplitude of the potentials. Buchthal and Pinelli (1952, 1953b) found that, in peripheral nerve lesions, this increase in duration was often accompanied by a normal or diminished amplitude, in contrast to atrophies of spinal origin where, in addition to an increase in the mean duration of the action potentials, which frequently exceeded 12.0 ms there was an increase in their mean amplitude. Measurement of the territory of motor units in patients with lower motor neurone lesions, using a multilead electrode, showed that in patients with long-standing weakness due to peripheral nerve injury, the motor unit territory may be increased by 15–40 per cent, and in patients with weakness due to anterior horn cell involvement, by 80–140 per cent (Erminio, Buchthal and Rosenfalck, 1959). The reasons for this increase in the size of units, which accounts in large measure for the altered dimensions of the action potentials, are probably complex, but an important factor must be collateral sprouting from the distal branches of the nerve fibres in disease of the lower motor neurone; this is a particularly prominent feature in poliomyelitis

and motor neurone disease (Wohlfart, 1958; Coërs and Woolf, 1959).

In the myopathies, not only are the action potentials often polyphasic in appearance but there is a reduction both in their mean duration and also to a lesser extent in their amplitude. Kugelberg (1949) found that in muscles such as the biceps, where in healthy subjects the mean duration is comparatively prolonged, many potentials may have a duration of less than 3.0 ms. He did, however, observe that even in patients where muscular weakness was considerable it was not unusual to find potentials of normal magnitude. Buchthal and Pinelli (1952, 1953a) and Pinelli and Buchthal (1953) found that, although in many patients with muscular dystrophy there was a decrease in the mean duration of action potentials, this was not invariable and in some patients the potentials showed a normal or increased duration and an increase in amplitude. In polymyositis, on the other hand, nearly every patient studied showed a significant reduction in their mean duration (Fig. 29.4).

A suggested explanation of the shortened duration of motor unit potentials in myopathy is that the conduction velocity of the action potential over the fibres may be more rapid in dystrophic than in healthy muscle. However, measurement of conduction velocity in muscle fibres in muscular dystrophy has shown that it is within the normal range (Buchthal, Guld and Rosenfalck, 1955; Buchthal, Rosenfalck and Erminio, 1960). Motor unit territory, as measured with a multilead electrode, is reduced in many, but not all, cases of muscular dystrophy and also in cases of polymyositis. This reduction of motor unit territory has been ascribed to the loss of muscle fibres through degeneration which occurs in the myopathies, and it is probably this reduction in the number of fibres comprising them which leads to a reduction in the duration of the action potential of a proportion of the motor units in this disease (Buchthal et al., 1960).

The measurement of action potential duration readily lends itself to computer analysis and a number of systems have been developed for the automatic determination of mean action potential duration (Kopec, Hausmanowa-Petrusewicz, Rawski and Wolynski, 1973; Lee and White,

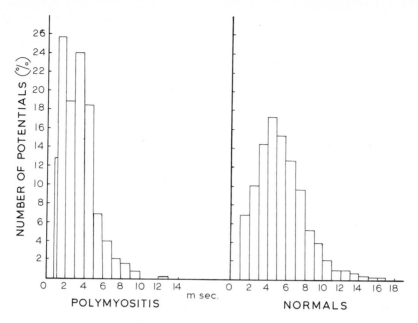

Fig. 29.4 Histograms showing the distribution of action potential duration in the muscles of patients with polymyositis and normal subjects (adapted from Buchthal and Pinelli, 1952)

1973; Pinelli, 1975). This allows much more rapid handling of data than can be achieved by direct measurement and has the advantage that the computer can be programmed to adopt rigid criteria of measurement.

Muscle fibre density

Ekstedt (1964) has developed a multi-electrode capable of recording potentials from single muscle fibres. This consists of a cannula which contains either two or 14 platinum wires, which reach the surface through a hole in the side of the electrode, to provide a series of leading-off surfaces 25 μm in diameter. These leading-off surfaces can record potentials from single muscle fibres during a voluntary contraction. If the potential recorded from a single fibre is used to trigger the sweep of the oscilloscope, potentials from other fibres in the same unit may appear on the same sweep, time-locked to the initial potential. The slight variation in the time interval separating the first and a subsequent potential is known as 'jitter'. As jitter is markedly increased if there is neuromuscular block, this technique has provided a useful method for recognising neuromuscular block in conditions such as myasthenia gravis. In the healthy subject

only a small number of muscle fibres are likely to lie within the uptake area of an electrode, which will record only one or two action potentials during a single sweep. However, if the number of muscle fibres within a single motor unit is increased, as may occur in peripheral neuropathy where there is reinnervation, a larger number of muscle fibre potentials may be recorded. This measure of muscle fibre density within a motor unit has been of value in distinguishing poly-neuropathy where the main process is one of segmental demyelination, from a neuropathy where the changes affect mainly the axons and where reinnervation may be more prominent (Stålberg and Thiele, 1975; Thiele and Stålberg, 1975).

Synchronous motor unit activity

Although the smoothness of a muscular contraction is largely brought about by the asynchronous discharge of motor units, there is some apparent grouping of the action potentials. This grouping occurs characteristically at a frequency of about 9 Hz and is more striking during fatigue. It has been suggested that it is due to oscillation in the stretch reflex servo-loop, and that it accounts in part for physiological tremor (Lippold, Redfearn and Vuco, 1957). Apparent grouping of motor unit activity, however, may occur even in de-afferented muscle, so that not all grouping is necessarily a reflex phenomenon and there is evidence that, under normal conditions, a significant amount of grouping is a purely random occurrence (Taylor, 1962).

In patients who have muscular weakness as a result of disease of the anterior horn cells, such as poliomyelitis, action potentials can be recorded simultaneously from widely separated electrodes in the same muscle (Buchthal and Clemmeson, 1943). These synchronised potentials are more frequent in muscles affected by anterior horn cell disease than in muscles affected by peripheral nerve pathology (Buchthal and Madsen, 1950). While this may be interpreted as indicating that in anterior horn cell disease there is some interaction between motor neurones, leading to synchronous firing, Denny-Brown (1949) suggested that apparent synchronisation is the result of separate needle electrodes recording from the same abnormally large motor unit. In motor neurone disease and poliomyelitis many of the motor units are abnormally large as a result of collateral sprouting (Wohlfart, 1958; Coërs and Woolf, 1959). Likewise, the motor unit territory, determined electrically, is enlarged in anterior horn cell disease (Erminio et al., 1959).

It is not certain how far collateral sprouting with re-innervation can account for synchronisation or the enlargement of motor unit size. Wohlfart (1959a) suggested that collateral regeneration may take place as far proximally as the axons of the ventral horn cells, to establish contact between them and, if this were the case, it would provide a possible anatomical basis for interaction between motor neurones. A further possibility is that, where the size of the motor neurone pool has been reduced by disease of the spinal grey matter, one action of the Renshaw inhibitory loop is to promote synchronous firing (Simpson, 1966).

Frequency analysis of the electromyogram

In clinical practice it is frequently possible, by means of careful electromyographic examination, to reach an exact diagnosis of the pathological process giving rise to muscular weakness. In the early stages of disease, however, recognition of characteristic action potential patterns may be difficult, and this is particularly the case in the myopathies, where the large range in shape and size of the action potentials may make a shift in configuration and size difficult to recognise. Minor abnormalities may also be present in clinically unaffected carriers of muscular dystrophy, and these may be difficult to distinguish from the normal pattern without quantitative analysis.

One method of analysis is to study the distribution curves for action potential duration. This has the limitation that action potentials can be measured only during weak voluntary contractions, which may not give a representative sample of the motor unit population in the muscle. Methods which are capable of analysing the interference pattern may be expected, therefore, to give additional quantitative information.

One method for studying the interference pattern is to subject it to Fourier analysis; this can be done by feeding the EMG into a system of tuned circuits which will display the frequency analysis of the oscilloscope simultaneously with the interference pattern (Richardson, 1951). If this analysis is applied to the interference pattern obtained by recording the EMG during maximal effort against resistance, the dominant frequency in normal subjects is 100–200 Hz tailing off to zero at 800 Hz (Fig. 29.5). In the facial muscles the frequency pattern may extend to about 1250 Hz. In patients with myopathy the analysis may show a dominant frequency of over 400 Hz (Walton, 1952). In patients with weakness following poliomyelitis and motor neurone disease, the shift in frequency may be towards the lower end of the spectrum, in keeping with the extended action potential duration which may be found in these conditions (Fex and Krakau, 1957).

Gerston, Cenkovich and Jones (1965) have also found high peak frequencies in myopathic patients and lower than normal frequencies in patients with neuropathic weakness. The use of the digital computer in data processing has extended the capacity for frequency analysis by the use of digital techniques for power spectral analysis and autocorrelation; this subject has been reviewed by Basmajian, Clifford, McLeod and Nunnally

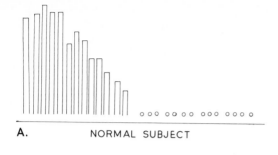

A.   NORMAL SUBJECT

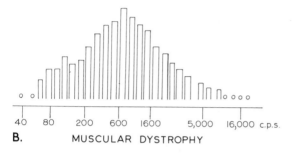

B.   MUSCULAR DYSTROPHY

Fig. 29.5 Histograms showing the frequency distribution of the electromyogram represented on the screen of an oscilloscope by means of an audio-frequency spectrometer; A. healthy subject; B. patient with facio-scapulo-humeral dystrophy showing a shift toward the high frequency end of the spectrum (adapted from Walton, 1952)

(1975). Kwatny, Thomas and Kwatny (1970) have found a shift in power spectral densities in fatigued muscle, towards the lower end of the frequency spectrum.

The analysis of spike distribution and frequency

A further development in the quantitative analysis of the EMG has been to measure the number of spikes occurring in the interference pattern during isometric contractions. This has been of interest in muscle disease because it takes into account both the polyphasic character of the motor units in muscular dystrophy and the considerable amount of electrical activity which can be recorded from the muscles even at low tensions. The method represents a useful advance because the necessary procedures can be carried out automatically and the data presented in a form suitable for computer analysis.

Van den Bosch (1963) studied the quadriceps during conditions of minimum voluntary contraction. The EMG was recorded through concentric electrodes and photographed. Polyphasic potentials were defined as potentials having more than three phases, and the number of phases in each polyphasic potential was counted so that the mean number of phases could be determined. From this value, taken together with the mean duration, the result could be expressed in terms of a mean frequency per response in Hz (ϕ). In patients with muscular dystrophy there was an increase in the number of phases per potential and in the mean frequency of the waveform of each potential, while carriers of muscular dystrophy gave values intermediate between those of the controls and affected patients. Gardner-Medwin (1968) derived ϕ from the ratio of the mean number of phases per potential to the mean action potential duration, calculating the value from all potentials measured regardless of whether they were polyphasic. He also included a correction factor for age and found ϕ to be a sensitive index for the detection of carriers of muscular dystrophy. Moosa and Brown (1972) developed an automatic analogue method to derive an index which is closely related to ϕ. As small action potentials may be difficult to distinguish from noise, they introduced a correction to weight the mean duration according to the amplitude of the deflections. The index ψ obtained in this way is the reciprocal of the mean phase duration weighted for amplitude; in their study of a series of patients with myopathic disorders it was outside the normal range in 75 per cent of cases studied.

A difficulty with any method of spike counting is to reach an objective definition of the size of potential change to be regarded as a spike. Willison (1964) therefore counted as spikes all changes in phase of greater than 100 μV and carried out the analysis at known tensions. It was found that counts of up to three times the maximum encountered in normal subjects could be recorded in patients with muscle disease (Willison, 1964). Later, automatic analysis was carried out by passing the EMG into an analyser which gives out two sets of pulses (Fitch, 1967). The first set of pulses refers to changes of voltage regardless of phase and without reference to any baseline, each pulse representing an increment of 100 μV. The

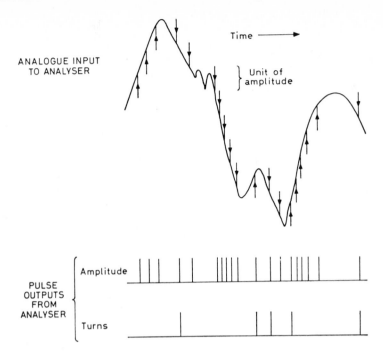

Fig. 29.6   Analysis of a typical waveform to show pulses derived from the analyser each of which represent increments of voltage and changes of phase (from Fitch, 1967)

second refers to changes in phase; pulses occur whenever the waveform changes from positive to negative or vice versa, provided that the change in phase is greater than $100 \mu V$ (Fig. 29.6). This second set of pulses corresponds to the spike count obtained by visual analysis.

In this way a 'read-out' is obtained of the number of spikes in the record per unit time and also of the total voltage change in the record. A further stage in the analysis may be carried out by digital computer. This can register the interval between pulses and the amplitude of the individual potentials: the distributions may be expressed in the form of a histogram.

Using this automatic method of analysis it is possible to study several muscles in any patient and, when this is done, the overlap between values found in healthy subjects and in mildly affected patients is reduced. The significance of the computer analysis is that, in a patient with muscular dystrophy, the interval between spikes may be reduced even where the total spike count is normal. In partly denervated muscle the number of spikes or turns may be increased if there is an excess of polyphasic units, but the most consistent finding in chronic denervation is an increase in mean amplitude: this may be the result of increased fibre density in motor units, caused by reinnervation (Rose and Willison, 1967; Willison, personal communication, 1967; Hayward and Willison, 1977).

Refractory period

The refractory period of a nerve or muscle depends on the recovery time of the fibre membrane after it has been depolarised. For a short interval after a stimulus the fibre will not respond to a second stimulus, however powerful; this is the absolute refractory period. The relative refractory period follows, in which a second stimulus of sufficient magnitude is effective. Finally, there may be a supernormal phase in which the tissue is hyperexcitable. The refractory period of nerve is shorter than that of muscle. In human peripheral nerve the absolute refractory period is 0.6–0.7 ms (Gilliatt and Willison, 1963), whereas in healthy human muscle it ranges from 2.2–4.6 ms (Farmer,

Buchthal and Rosenfalck, 1960). While the refractory period is defined as the shortest interval between two effective stimuli, the shortest time between two evoked potentials is known as the irresponsive period (Lucas, 1910). The irresponsive period may differ from the refractory period, and one explanation of this may be that the conduction velocity in a fibre may be reduced during the relative refractory period. This reduction in conduction velocity has been demonstrated in human nerve (Buchthal and Rosenfalck, 1966a) and in frog muscle (Buchthal and Engbaek, 1963) but has not been shown to be present in human muscle.

The refractory period of muscle fibres is of interest because it gives information regarding the membrane properties of individual fibres. In the human subject the study of refractory period is limited by the fact that different fibres do not have the same refractory period and, even when using small electrodes to stimulate and record from a muscle, it is not possible to measure the refractory period of single fibres. In the frog this was done using intracellular electrodes and the absolute refractory period of a single fibre corresponded to the duration of the action potential measured to the time of onset of the negative after-potential (Buchthal and Engbaek, 1963). In man, using fine electrodes to stimulate small bundles of muscle fibres, it was found that the average refractory period is reduced in dystrophic muscle and lengthened in partially denervated muscle (Farmer, Buchthal and Rosenfalck, 1959). This corresponds to observations in dystrophic (Conrad and Glaser, 1961) and denervated (Lenman, 1965) muscle in the mouse. An important observation was that the average refractory period of muscle fibres is frequently shorter than normal in clinically unaffected carriers of muscular dystrophy (Caruso and Buchthal, 1965).

Measurements of refractory period in peripheral nerve suggest that in certain types of peripheral neuropathy, such as may occur in association with diabetes, alcoholism and uraemia, the refractory period may be increased when nerve conduction velocity remains normal (Lowitzsch and Hopf, 1975; Tackmann, Ullerich and Lehmann, 1975). Lithium has been found to give rise to a marginal lengthening of refractory period, and a marked increase has been recorded in patients who have taken rubidium (Betts, Paschalis, Jarratt and Jenner, 1978). Measurement of refractory period in motor nerves is not readily carried out by direct measurement, but methods have been described which use collision techniques (Hopf and Lowitzsch, 1975; Kimura, Yamada and Rodnitzky, 1978), and Kopec, Delbeke and McComas (1978) have developed a subtraction technique by which the refractory period of the distal motor nerve branches and the muscle fibres can be determined.

Propagation velocity

The technical arrangements used to determine refractory period in human muscle may also be used to measure the propagation velocity along the muscle fibre. The stimulus is applied through a bipolar electrode in the distal end of the muscle, as far from the innervation zone as possible, and evoked potentials are recorded from three concentric electrodes inserted for a short distance proximally into the fibre bundle. With this method a mean propagation velocity of 4.1 ± 0.13 m/s has been found in the biceps brachii following electrical stimulation, compared with 4.7 ± 0.1 m/s with voluntary activation (Buchthal et al., 1955). In denervated muscles a 50–80 per cent reduction in conduction velocity has been found (Buchthal and Rosenfalck, 1958) but in dystrophic muscle normal values have been obtained (Farmer et al., 1959).

A different method was adopted by Stålberg (1966). This makes use of a concentric multielectrode which contains 14 platinum wires, the tips of which are exposed through an opening in the shaft of the electrode to form a row of adjacent recording points. When this electrode is aligned close to a muscle fibre the action potential can be recorded at different points, separated by a known distance, along the same fibre. Using this method to record the propagation velocity of voluntarily evoked potentials, a mean propagation velocity of 3.37 ± 0.67 ms was recorded in the biceps brachii. If the same electrode is used to record from two adjacent muscle fibres, so that the potential from one fibre triggers the oscilloscope sweep, the potential from the second fibre is seen to show jitter as previously described (Ekstedt and Stålberg, 1969).

Contraction time

Observations of tension changes in muscle made in association with electromyographic studies have shown that the contraction time may be altered in different conditions. Thus, in myxoedema, muscular contraction is slow, particularly in Hoffmann's syndrome (Wilson and Walton, 1959) and delay in relaxation is characteristic of myotonia. A slow build-up of tension during voluntary contraction has been noted in rheumatoid arthritis (Lenman and Potter, 1966) and rarely in myopathy (Lenman, 1959a). Botelho and her associates (1960) found that, in the small hand muscles of patients with muscular dystrophy, muscular weakness was associated with prolongation of all phases of muscular contraction, and Sandow and Brust (1958) recorded a prolonged relaxation time in the muscles of the dystrophic mouse. It is not clear how far these changes relate to alterations in the contractile property of the muscle fibres, and how far to changes in the interstitial tissue. In rheumatoid arthritis, connective tissue changes are probably important, but in muscular dystrophy Botelho et al. found a decrease rather than an increase in muscle stiffness, so it is likely that in this condition the changes lie in the muscle fibres. McComas and Thomas (1968) demonstrated a prolongation of all phases of muscle twitch in the first dorsal interosseus muscle of patients with Duchenne muscular dystrophy and suggested that the change may represent reversion of the muscle to the conditions of neonatal muscle, where the contraction time is slow, due to lack of a trophic factor.

Buchthal and Schmalbruch (1969) developed a method for measuring the contraction time of small fibre bundles in the biceps and triceps muscles, and they correlated the spectrum of contraction time in these muscles with the distribution of fibre types found on histochemical staining. In Duchenne dystrophy they found that the mean contraction times were prolonged, and with histochemical techniques they showed an increase in the proportion of type C fibres rich in mitochondrial enzymes. They also studied patients with neurogenic weakness due to lesions of the brachial plexus, motor neurone disease or poliomyelitis, and in each of these groups they also found a preponderance of extended contraction times and of type C fibres on histochemical staining (Buchthal, Schmalbruch and Kamieniecka, 1971a, b).

Tokizane and his associates have related the proportion of slow and fast fibres in a muscle to the pattern of motor unit activity. Normally, during a weak contraction, motor unit potentials appear not only at a slower, but at a more variable rate. They plotted the mean interval between individual spikes against the standard deviation of the spike intervals and found that the units fell into two groups, represented by two distinct curves. In the first curve there was marked variability in spike frequency at low discharge rates: they termed this the K or kinetic curve. In the second, or tonic (T), curve there was much less variation. In the muscles of the hand, face and tongue and in extraocular muscles, analysis showed a predominance of K type units. In the muscles of the foot and calf and in sphincter ani there was a relative predominance of T type units. They suggested that these K and T type units correspond to the fast white and slow red muscle fibres respectively (Tokizane and Shimazu, 1964). They also considered that the variability of discharge frequency was related in part to the activity of the muscle spindles and observed that, in parkinsonism, there was a decreased variation in discharge frequency at low tensions (Shimazu, Hongo, Kubota, and Narabayashi, 1962).

Bergamini (1959) found that, in patients with muscular dystrophy, motor unit potentials were disposed along the K curves, and he suggested that in muscular dystrophy there is a selective loss of motor units having a postural function. This observation is difficult to reconcile with the finding of a slow contraction time in muscular dystrophy (Botelho et al., 1960; McComas and Thomas, 1968). Das Gupta (1963) was not able to identify two distinct groups of tonic and kinetic motor units in normal muscle. He found an increased variability in discharge frequency in weak muscles, occurring both in myopathy and in neuropathic conditions, and he concluded that this was related to the inability of the weak muscles to develop tension, and not to any selective disorder affecting a particular type of unit.

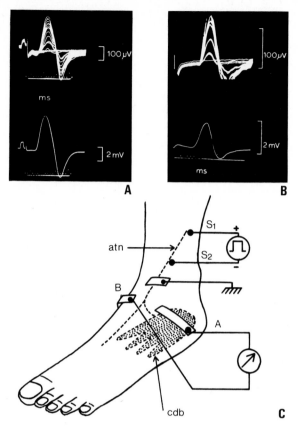

Fig. 29.7 Action potentials in extensor digitorum brevis evoked by stimulation of deep peroneal nerve in (A) control subject and (B) a 16-year-old boy with Duchenne dystrophy. The recording arrangements are illustrated in (C) (from McComas et al., 1970)

ESTIMATION OF MOTOR UNIT POPULATION

The quantitative methods which have been described for the integration and analysis of the EMG have provided information regarding the recruitment of motor units during voluntary contraction of a muscle, and also of the characteristics and territory occupied by motor units in different disorders of nerve and muscle. A different approach has been to measure the number of motor units in a muscle which can be excited by graded stimuli. If the twitch tension is measured at the same time, it is not only possible to estimate the number of motor units and their average size, but also to estimate mechanical efficiency of the units in terms of their ability to develop tension. In partly denervated muscle the number of surviving units in the muscle is a measure of the degree of denervation, and the size of the surviving units and their ability to develop tension provides information regarding the capacity of the muscle to compensate functionally.

McComas, Fawcett, Campbell and Sica (1971) described a method whereby an estimate can be made of the number of functioning units in extensor digitorum brevis (EDB). The method is illustrated in Figure 29.7. Recording is carried out by means of three strips of silver foil which form the stigmatic electrode over the end-plate zone of the muscle, the reference electrode on the sole of the foot and the earth electrode between the stigmatic electrode and the stimulating cathode. The stimulating electrodes are placed over the deep peroneal nerve above the ankle. If gradually increasing stimuli are applied to the nerve, evoked potentials are recorded from the muscle and increase in size by discrete increments, each of which may be considered to represent the recruitment of an additional motor unit. The average amplitude of the incremental potentials can be obtained by measuring the amplitude of the first group of increments recorded. If the amplitude of the potential obtained by a supramaximal stimulus is measured, this value divided by the mean amplitude of the incremental values will provide an estimate of the number of units in the muscle. In this study, the EDB was chosen as the most suitable muscle because its anatomical situation is such that there is relatively little interference from other muscles, it has a single end-plate zone and its flattened muscle belly makes it relatively simple to study. A further advantage is that the twitch tension can readily be measured.

Using this method, McComas, Sica, Campbell and Upton (1971) studied the numbers of surviving units together with the twitch tension developed by EDB in a group of patients with a variety of chronic denervating disorders. In the patients studied there was a marked reduction in the number of functioning units in EDB compared with controls, but in many patients the average amplitude of the incremental responses was markedly increased and the twitch tension remained in the normal range until the number of motor units had fallen to about 10 per cent of normal. The evidence suggested that this functional compensation is largely the result of enlargement of motor units by collateral sprouting from surviving axons. Particular interest attaches to the motor unit population of EDB in muscular dystrophy (McComas *et al.*, 1970). In Duchenne dystrophy (McComas, Sica and Currie, 1971), dystrophia myotonica (McComas, Campbell and Sica, 1971) and limb-girdle and facioscapulohumeral dystrophy (Sica and McComas, 1971), a significant reduction in the number of functioning units in EDB was found in comparison with controls, but the patients with limb-girdle and facioscapulohumeral dystrophy differed from those in the other two groups in that many of the motor units were abnormally large. McComas and his associates suggested on the basis of these findings that the primary disturbance in muscular dystrophy may lie in the motor neurones. On this hypothesis, the absence of abnormally large units in Duchenne dystrophy and in dystrophia myotonica could be due to the presence in these patients of a large proportion of 'sick' neurones which had lost the capacity to generate peripheral sprouts in response to denervation. In a further study of a group of patients rendered hemiplegic by a cerebrovascular accident, McComas, Sica, Upton, Aguilera and Currie (1971) found evidence of loss of motor units in the EDB on the affected side. They suggested that this provides evidence that wasting in hemiplegia may be due, not to disuse but to degeneration of anterior horn cells following deprivation of 'trophic' influences from cortical sources.

Ballantyne and Hansen (1974a, b, c) extended this technique by using a digital computer to measure, not only the change in amplitude produced by each increment of stimulus, but also the latency, duration and area of the potentials comprising the summated response. The motor unit potentials were each stored in digital form in a separate computer memory trace or template. If the second template contained the summated potentials of the first and second evoked responses, and the third template that of the first, second and third evoked responses, subtraction of the first template potential from the second will yield the second evoked response in isolation; similarly subtraction of the third template from the second

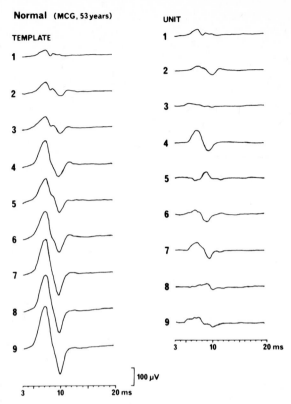

Fig. 29.8 Computer printout of templates and units obtained by template subtraction (from Ballantyne and Hansen, 1974)

will yield the third evoked response in isolation. In this way the configuration of any of the stored motor unit potentials can be derived by template subtraction (Fig. 29.8). If the motor unit potential (MUP) derived from supramaximal stimulation is stored in the final template of the series the number of motor unit potentials in the EDB can be calculated from the formula

$$MUC = n \times \frac{A(M)}{A(n)}$$

where MUC = motor unit count
   A(M) = area of supramaximal evoked MUP
   A(n) = area of compound muscle action potential containing n MUPs

In healthy subjects this method gave broadly similar motor unit counts to those obtained by the amplitude summation technique. Reduced motor unit counts were found in myotonic muscular dystrophy but in patients with Duchenne, limb-girdle or facioscapulohumeral muscular dystrophy and with myasthenia gravis, motor unit counts within the normal range were obtained. The authors also used this method of measuring motor unit loss from a muscle as a means of evaluating the relative preponderance of axonal degeneration and segmental demyelination in different varieties of peripheral neuropathy (Ballantyne and Hansen, 1974a, b, c; Hansen and Ballantyne, 1977).

Other workers have stressed the technical problems which may affect the accuracy of motor unit estimation. Thus Panayiotopoulos, Scarpalezos and Papapetropoulos (1974), who obtained similar motor unit counts in patients with Duchenne dystrophy and controls by the amplitude summation method, commented that the noise level of the recording system may obscure low amplitude potential changes and they used enlarged superimposed photographs to identify incremental responses. Milner-Brown and Brown (1976) found that fluctuations in response and overlapping firing levels of motor axons may lead to over-estimation of the number of motor units. In addition, they pointed out that the presence of large motor units with a high threshold of excitation may signify that the motor units which give rise to the potentials from which the mean motor unit action potential is derived, may not always be representative of the motor unit population in the muscle. Peyronnard and Lamarre (1977) compared motor unit counts by the amplitude summation method in monkeys with anatomical counts of the numbers of alpha motor fibres supplying the EDB. The findings were broadly similar, but in one animal where the muscle was partially denervated the electrophysiological method underestimated the number of units.

THE STUDY OF REFLEX ACTION

Introduction

Reflexes which are studied in clinical practice include the phasic stretch reflex—of which a widely studied example is the tendon jerk—the tonic stretch reflex and a variety of nociceptive responses to cutaneous stimulation. All these reflexes are routinely studied in the clinical examination, and the character of response may give information regarding both the integrity of the reflex arc and the integrity of the suprasegmental pathways which regulate reflex excitability. Many of these reflexes can now also be precisely recorded by electrophysiological means using the EMG and sometimes a tension recorder to register the reflex response, the reflex being evoked by a precisely timed electrical or mechanical stimulus. By this means it is possible not only to measure the precise time course of the reflex, which is useful in studying the peripheral reflex pathway, but also to measure the effects of conditioning stimuli and to study factors such as sensitisation and habituation which may be relevant to the study of suprasegmental functions.

The time course of a tendon reflex can be readily measured with simple apparatus and requires only an arrangement whereby the impact of a tendon hammer triggers the sweep of an oscilloscope, and a device for recording the muscular contraction. This can be done mechanically and also by recording the action potentials from the contracting muscle. This simple technique has been of value in connection with thyroid disease, where the prolonged relaxation period of the tendon reflex which is seen in myxoedema is a reliable diagnostic sign (Ord, 1884; Chaney, 1924; Lambert, Underdahl, Beckett and Mederos, 1951; Bowers, Gordon and Segaloff, 1955).

Particular interest attaches to reflexes and to delayed responses which may be elicited by electrical excitation of nerves; two such responses which have been studied extensively are the H and F waves. Tonic stretch reflexes, as distinct from phasic reflexes, can be studied by the application of manual stretch to a muscle while action potentials are recorded from surface or intramuscular electrodes, and this method has been used to study the changes in muscle evoked by passive stretch in patients with spasticity, rigidity or torsion dystonia. A particularly useful technique for studying the tonic stretch reflex has been the application of vibration, because a vibrator with appropriate characteristics is capable of applying a controlled stimulus that will activate the dynamic stretch receptors in the muscle spindles, which activate the tonic stretch reflex.

Cutaneous reflexes can be evoked by nociceptive stimuli: particularly useful among these are the plantar response, the abdominal reflexes and the blink reflex. The blink reflex in particular has proved suitable for quantitative study.

The H reflex

If the posterior tibial nerve is stimulated in the popliteal fossa, an evoked muscle action potential may be recorded from the triceps surae muscle. If a weak stimulating pulse is employed a second action potential may be seen, appearing about 20 ms after the first. This late potential has a relatively low threshold, requiring a smaller stimulus to evoke it than the first, and disappears as the stimulus increases (Fig. 29.9). The latency of this second potential is long enough to suggest that it represents a spinal reflex. This is supported by the fact that the latency is increased if the

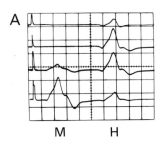

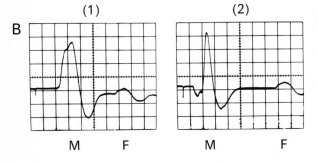

Fig. 29.9A H wave evoked from triceps surae muscle following stimulation of medial popliteal nerve with stimuli of increasing intensity (uppermost trace, weakest stimulus). When stimulus is adequate to evoke direct muscle response (M wave), amplitude of H wave is diminished

B F wave evoked from abd. dig. min. following stimulation of ulnar nerve at elbow (1), and at wrist (2). Latency of F wave diminished as stimulation cathode is moved proximally. Squares on horizontal axis of graticule represent 5 ms, on vertical axis 2 mV

stimulus site is moved distally. This late potential, first described by Hoffmann (1918), is called the H wave. The first potential due to direct stimulation of the muscle through its nerve is known as the M wave.

The reflex nature of the H wave was established by Magladery and his associates. They stimulated the posterior tibial nerve in the popliteal fossa, recording spinal root potentials from intrathecally placed electrodes. When these electrodes were placed close to the cord at L 1, the time interval between anterior and posterior root potentials was only 1.5 ms. Allowing for the conduction time in the afferent and efferent arcs of the reflex, this is sufficient time for passage through a single cord synapse. With increasing strength of stimulus an antidromic potential was recorded on the anterior roots which, with strong stimuli, occluded the anterior root potential (Magladery, Porter, Park and Teasdall, 1951). Conduction velocity studies showed that the afferent arc of the reflex is subserved by low-threshold, rapidly conducting group I fibres, and it seems that the H reflex represents the electrical equivalent of the ankle jerk elicited by stimulation proximal to the muscle spindle. The monosynaptic character of the ankle jerk has been shown by Lloyd (1943).

Under normal circumstances the H reflex can be elicited only from the calf muscles (Magladery and McDougal, 1950) and, at present, it is the only spinal monosynaptic reflex that can readily be elicited by electrical stimulation. It has been widely studied as a measure of motor neurone excitability. If the H wave is elicited by paired stimuli there is a period of up to several seconds after the conditioning stimulus when the excitability to the test stimulus is altered (Magladery, Teasdall, Park and Languth, 1952). The shape of the recovery curve depends on a variety of factors, among them the strength of the conditioning stimulus. If a stimulus of slightly above threshold is employed the test reflex may be evoked during the 10 ms following the conditioning stimulus ('early facilitation'). After that, until about 80 ms after the conditioning stimulus, the reflex cannot be obtained. From 100 to 300 ms after the conditioning stimulus the H wave builds up to reach a maximum at about 250 ms, 'the second facilitation'. There is then a second period of

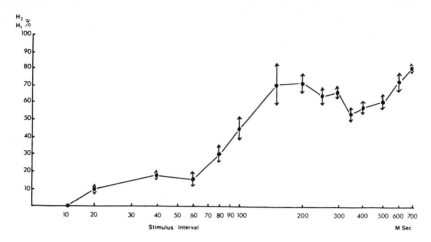

Fig. 29.10 H reflex recovery cycle obtained from 10 healthy adults. Ratio of test to conditioning H reflex plotting against stimulus intervals. Conditioning and test stimuli of equal magnitude, stimulus strength selected to give maximum H response. Vertical bars represent standard error of means

depression when the H reflex following the test stimulus is again reduced in size. This late depression is most marked at about 600 ms. Thereafter the test response gradually returns to normal (Fig. 29.10).

Magladery *et al.* (1952) found that, in patients with upper motor neurone lesions, the shape of the recovery curve was altered in that, throughout the cycle, the H wave was more readily elicited by the test stimulus. In subsequent studies the increased excitability associated with spasticity was confirmed (Takamori, 1967) and increased excitability was also demonstrated in Parkinson's disease (Matsuoka, Waltz, Terada, Ikeda and Cooper, 1966; Olsen and Diamantopoulos, 1967; Yap, 1967). In spinal shock the recovery cycle of the H reflex is depressed (Diamantopoulos and Olsen, 1966) and this is also the case in patients with the Holmes–Adie syndrome (McComas and Payan, 1966). In a study of evolving hemiplegia, Garcia-Mullin and Mayer (1972) found that the level of motoneurone excitability, judged by the H/M ratio and the H wave recovery cycle, may be depressed in acute hemiplegia but enhanced in chronic hemiplegia, when the H reflex may also be elicited in the upper limbs. McLeod and Walsh (1972), using paired stimuli of near-threshold intensity in patients with Parkinson's disease, found that the initial irresponsive period was significantly shorter in patients than in controls, but lengthened after treatment with levodopa.

A major difficulty in the use of the H reflex as a measure of motor neurone excitability is the variability of the response and its liability to be influenced by peripheral factors. Thus it is facilitated by active contraction or by passive stretch of the muscle and depressed by contraction of the antagonist (Mayer and Mawdsley, 1965). It may show post-tetanic facilitation (Hagbarth, 1962) and is abolished by vibration applied to the muscle or to its tendon (Hagbarth and Eklund, 1966). Clearly, if the recovery curve is to have any meaning it must be recorded using a technique that will avoid peripheral modifying factors as far as possible. McLeod and Van Der Meulen (1967) studied the significance of these factors in the cat by comparing the recovery curve of the H reflex with that of the monosynaptic reflex recorded from the ventral root, before and after section of the posterior tibial nerve. There was no difference in the duration of the irresponsive period but the first and second periods of facilitation were reduced after section. The irresponsive period is, therefore, a valid measurement of the excitability of the motor neurone pool, but the two periods of facilitation may be related to spindle activation determined by the reflex muscle contraction. Táboriková and Sax (1969) reduced the influence of peripheral factors in the human subject by using a sub-threshold conditioning stimulus which is too small to elicit an H response. With this technique a full-sized H reflex is obtained following the test stimulus, at stimulus intervals of up to 25 ms. This is followed by successive stages of early depression, intercurrent facilitation, late depression and then a gradual recovery. They suggest that the depression of the H reflex, after the test stimulus, can be accounted for by depletion of transmitter output following the conditioning stimulus. The intercurrent facilitation which occurs after a latent period of 50–300 ms could be explained by a long-loop reflex acting through brain-stem and cerebellar pathways. For a review of the methodology for eliciting an H reflex the reader is referred to the recommendations of Hugon, Delwaide, Pierrot-Deseilligny and Desmedt (1973).

The amplitude of the H reflex may have some significance as representing the proportion of the motor neurone pool which can be excited. Unfortunately, the size of the reflex depends on many variables, such as site of electrode placement, stimulus strength and state of relaxation of the muscle. Angel and Hofmann (1963) have suggested that these variables will affect the H and M waves equally and they have studied the ratio of the largest obtainable H wave divided by the largest obtainable M wave. They found this ratio to be higher than normal in spastic limbs, but to be little affected in parkinsonian rigidity. McComas and Payan (1966) found that the ratio was reduced in patients with the Holmes–Adie syndrome. Matthews (1966) studied the effect of relaxant drugs on this ratio in spastic patients but found that diazepam, while it reduced the size of the ankle jerk, had little effect on that of the H reflex. Táborikova and Sax (1968) have commented that estimation of the size of the motor neurone pool from the ratio of the H and M waves is inaccurate. One possible reason is that a stimulus capable of evoking an H wave without evoking an M wave may be too weak to excite a maximum Ia volley. They describe a method whereby a stimulus large enough to evoke a maximal M wave is given after a previous stimulus has evoked a large H wave. If the second stimulus is given at an interval after the first, so that the M wave occurs when the muscle fibres are still refractory following the H wave, the M wave will be reduced in size in proportion to that fraction of the muscle fibres which was activated by the H reflex.

Studies on the effect of reinforcement on the H reflex have not yielded wholly consistent results. Sommer (1940) observed that, while the Jendrassik manoeuvre augments the ankle jerk, it may have little effect on the H reflex, and argued that reinforcement must proceed through motor nerves acting on spindles. These observations were confirmed by Buller and Dornhorst (1957) and by Paillard (1959) but Landau and Clare (1964) and Gassel and Diamantopoulos (1964) found it possible to augment the H reflex by reinforcement, provided that the H reflex is submaximal. Others have found the situation variable (Mayer and Mawdsley, 1965; McComas and Payan, 1966) and it remains uncertain to what extent the Jendrassik manoeuvre depends on fusimotor activity, and how far on excitation of α-neurones in the motor neurone pool.

If the H reflex is elicited by stimulation of the posterior tibial nerve during a voluntary contraction, it may be facilitated (Cerrie and Harden, 1964; Takamori, 1967). If the median nerve is excited during a voluntary contraction, two late responses can be recorded in the abductor pollicis brevis. One occurs about 2–3 ms after the F wave (*see below*) and the second has a latency of between 48–60 ms. These two potentials have been termed V_1 and V_2, and V_1 has the characteristics of a potentiated H reflex. The origin of V_2 is unknown, but it may represent a polysynaptic reflex. If V_1 is elicited in patients with hemiparesis, it has been found that the potentiation produced by a voluntary contraction is less than in healthy subjects; it has been suggested that a background facilitatory mechanism, which is normally present, is reduced (Sica, McComas and Upton, 1971).

It is possible to measure the conduction velocity of both the afferent and efferent segments of the H reflex arc, but results have differed in different laboratories (Diamantopoulos and Gassel, 1965; Mayer and Mawdsley, 1965). In healthy adults the latency varies between 26–32 ms. In peripheral neuropathy this latency may be substantially prolonged (Mayer and Mawdsley, 1965).

The F wave

While the H reflex, in the absence of facilitation, can be obtained only from the calf muscles, a late evoked response, having rather different characteristics, can be elicited elsewhere following nerve stimulation. If the ulnar or median nerve is stimulated, and evoked potentials are then recorded from the hand muscles, the M wave may be followed by a late response, of relatively high threshold, with a latency of up to about 30 ms. Increasing the strength of the stimulus increases the size of the response up to a certain level, but it is not blocked by supramaximal stimuli. If the stimulating electrode is moved distally, the latency increases (Fig. 29.9). This late response appears irregularly, shows occasional variations in latency and has been designated the F wave (Magladery and McDougal, 1950).

Subsequent studies have shown that the F wave may be elicited from small muscles in the hand or foot, and it has been recorded from the calf muscles of patients with tabes dorsalis, the Holmes-Adie syndrome and patients with congenital sensory neuropathy associated with loss of reflexes. It does not show post-tetanic potentiation and, following a conditioning stimulus, there is no consistent long-lasting depression (Thorne, 1965).

Magladery and McDougal considered the F wave to be a reflex response, possibly with polysynaptic connections. Other workers, however, have suggested that it represents the discharge of motor neurones in the cord following antidromic activation (Dawson and Merton, 1956; Thorne, 1965; Gassel and Wiesendanger, 1965). This view was supported by studies carried out by McLeod and Wray (1966) on the baboon; they obtained a response with the characteristics of the F wave in the small muscles of the hand, following section of all the dorsal roots derived from the forelimb. Single-fibre electrode studies have confirmed the recurrent nature of the F response in man, because it can be recorded only from single fibres after a preceding M response and the jitter is too short to be compatible with synaptic transmission (Trontelj, 1973).

In some patients with chronic partial denervation of the small hand muscles, stimulation of the ulnar or median nerve at the wrist may evoke a response with a latency between that of the M and F waves. This has been shown to be an axon reflex. It is not found in healthy muscle and may be related to branching of recovering nerve fibres (Fullerton and Gilliatt, 1965).

The tonic contraction evoked by vibration

The tendon reflexes are mediated by the phasic stretch reflex, as distinct from the tonic stretch reflex which gives rise to muscle tone in the clinical sense. Probably these two types of reflex are subserved by specific receptors in the muscle spindles, which have been termed static and dynamic respectively. The phasic tendon reflexes are widely used clinically and the electrical equivalent of the ankle jerk, the H reflex, has been extensively studied.

Hagbarth and Eklund (1966) have shown that, if a muscle tendon is exposed to vibration at about 100/s a tonic contraction gradually develops and persists as long as the vibration is maintained. If the vibrator is applied to the Achilles tendon there is marked depression of those H reflexes in the calf muscles which are elicited by shocks to the posterior tibial nerve.

The characteristics of this tonic contraction have been studied by Lance and his associates. They found that vibration-induced tonic contraction was markedly diminished below the level of spinal cord transection or of a cerebellar lesion and was inhibited by drugs such as thiopentone or diazepam which depress polysynaptic reflexes. Not only did vibration depress the tendon jerks and the H reflex, but withdrawal of vibration was followed by a long-lasting depression of the H reflex similar to that produced by a conditioning stimulus to the posterior tibial nerve. They concluded that vibration excites the dynamic stretch receptors in the muscle spindles, and that the reflex must have a polysynaptic component dependent on supraspinal centres such as the cerebellum (de Gail, Lance and Neilson, 1966).

The tonic contraction produced by vibration can, however, be potentiated following a tetanus to the affected muscle and this favours the view that tonic contraction is mediated in part through a monosynaptic reflex. The reason why phasic reflexes are suppressed when the tonic reflex is evoked by vibration is uncertain, but an occlusion effect on the afferent fibres by the impulses evoked by vibration would appear to meet the existing evidence (Lance, de Gail and Neilson, 1966). While the principal value of this reflex may be in the analysis of tonic reflexes in man, a further possible application may be to study how far spasticity may be affected by applying vibration to the antagonists of affected muscles (Hagbarth and Eklund, 1966).

The blink reflex

The blink reflex, which occurs following a light tap to the forehead, can be studied by recording the electrical responses of the orbicularis oculi following a glabellar tap or electrical stimulation of the supra-orbital nerve. The reflex response has two components, comprising an initial response, R1 with a latency of 10–15 ms and a more prolonged late response, R2 with a relatively variable latency of 25–40 ms (Kugelberg, 1952; Rushworth, 1962). If the reflex is evoked by a tap on the forehead, both components of the reflex occur bilaterally. However, if the reflex is elicited by an electrical

stimulus, only R2 will be recorded bilaterally, R1 appearing on the ipsilateral side. The afferent arc of the reflex is the sensory route of the trigeminal nerve, the efferent is through the facial nerve. R2 has a more complex central pathway than R1 which includes the spinal tract to the trigeminal nerve. On repeated stimulation R1 persists relatively unchanged but, in the healthy subject, R2 habituates rapidly. It is generally recognised that R2 is a polysynaptic nociceptive response from the skin but R1 was originally considered to be a proprioceptive reflex. However, R1 can be evoked by cutaneous stimulation over a wide area of the face, its latency is not absolutely constant and it may be concluded that it is more likely to be an oligosynaptic response of cutaneous origin (Shahani, 1970). If the blink reflex is evoked by paired stimuli, recovery curves can be obtained for both the R1 and R2 components. The R1 recovery cycle

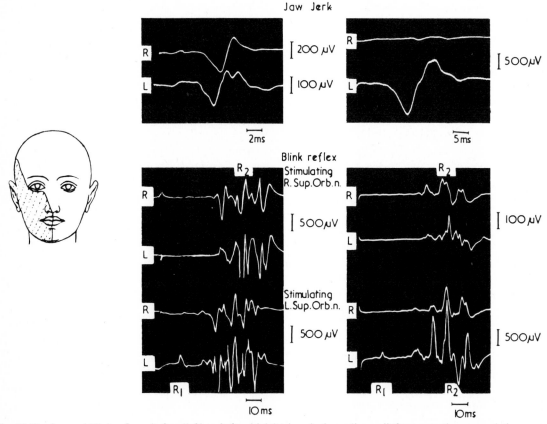

Fig. 29.11   Jaw and blink reflexes before (left) and after (right) trigeminal ganglion radiofrequency thermoregulation. Diagram of the face indicates minimal hypaesthesia of right maxillary and mandibular divisions. Note absent early blink response (R1) when stimulating the right supraorbital nerve and absent jaw jerk after operation (from Ferguson, 1978)

is shorter than that of the H reflex being complete in about 300 ms. There is an initial phase of increased excitability, lasting about 10 ms which is followed by a short phase of depression and then by a phase of potentiation, which persists for about 50 ms and is followed by another phase of depression, which may last for up to 200 ms. In contrast with R2 a conditioning shock to the face is followed by complete inhibition lasting 150–200 ms (Penders and Delwaide, 1973).

Abnormalities in the blink reflex response may be seen both in peripheral lesions affecting the trigeminal or facial nerve or their central connections and in the presence of suprasegmental disturbances of function. In lesions of the trigeminal nerve the first component may be small or absent or have a prolonged latency (Fig. 29.11), whereas in lesions of the facial nerve both components may occur late. In disease of the brain stem, if a lesion is confined to the pons the early component may be delayed but in a medullary lesion, such as the lateral medullary syndrome, R2 may be late or absent (Kimura and Lyon, 1972; Ongeboer de Visser and Kuypers, 1978). In coma caused by supratentorial lesions, R2 may be lost but R1 can generally be obtained unless the brain stem is also affected, whereas in sleep R2 can generally be obtained if strong enough stimuli are used, even in stages II, III and IV (Lyon, Kimura and McCormick, 1972; Kimura, 1973). In hemiplegia, R2 may be small or absent or have a long latency (Kimura, 1974) and in multiple sclerosis the latency of R1 may be prolonged (Kimura, 1975).

The habituation of the second component of the blink reflex, which generally occurs in healthy subjects, is frequently modified in diseases of the central nervous system. Thus, in Parkinson's disease R2 consistently fails to habituate (Penders and Delwaide, 1971) and failure to habituate is also seen in dementia (Gregoric, 1973; Ferguson, Lenman and Johnston, 1978). Conversely, in Huntington's chorea habituation may occur abnormally rapidly (Esteban and Gimenez-Roldan, 1975). As a quantitative measure of habituation, Penders and Delwaide (1971) have described a habituation index to indicate the stimulus frequency at which the blink reflex fails to habituate.

The jaw jerk

The jaw jerk is a reflex which is routinely elicited clinically by applying a brisk tap to the chin with a tendon hammer, and it is generally accepted that a lively jaw jerk is indicative of a suprasegmental lesion above the fifth nerve nucleus. It can be recorded electrically by using a tendon hammer which has a microswitch to trigger the oscilloscope sweep, and by recording evoked potentials from the masseter muscles with surface electrodes.

This reflex is of physiological interest in that early animal work suggested that the afferent and efferent fibres shared a common pathway in the motor root of the fifth cranial nerve (Szentagothai, 1948; McIntyre, 1951), and McIntyre and Robinson (1959) believed that this arrangement also existed in man. However, Ferguson (1978) in a study of 32 patients who had undergone surgery for trigeminal neuralgia found that an abnormal jaw jerk could be obtained in patients with no evidence of motor root involvement (Fig. 29.11).

Although on clinical testing the jaw jerk is frequently difficult to obtain in healthy adults, it can always be demonstrated electrically, except in the very old. Its latency varies from 6–9 ms. In the presence of trigeminal nerve lesions it may be absent, and it may be useful in discriminating between idiopathic and symptomatic facial pain as the reflex may be absent or of prolonged latency if there is localised pressure on the trigeminal nerve (Ongeboer de Visser and Goor, 1974).

ACKNOWLEDGEMENTS

I am grateful for permission to publish illustrations included in this article to Dr O.C.J. Lippold, Professor F. Buchthal, Mr P. Fitch, Dr A.J. McComas and Professor Sir John Walton and to the editors of the journals in which they originally appeared. I am indebted to Dr J.W. Lance and Dr R.G. Willison for access to unpublished material. Figures 29.8 and 29.11 are reproduced from the *Journal of Neurology, Neurosurgery and Psychiatry* and I am grateful to Dr J.P. Ballantyne, Dr S. Hansen and Dr I.T. Ferguson and to the editor and publisher of the journal for permission.

REFERENCES

Adrian, E.D. & Bronk, D.W. (1929) The discharge of impulses in motor nerve fibres, Part II. *Journal of Physiology*, **67**, 119.

Angel, R.W. & Hofmann, W.W. (1963) The H reflex in normal, spastic and rigid subjects. *Archives of Neurology*, **8**, 591.

Ballantyne, J.P. & Hansen, S. (1974a) A new method for the estimation of the number of motor units in a muscle. 1. Control subjects and patients with myasthenia gravis. *Journal of Neurology, Neurosurgery and Psychiatry*, **37**, 907.

Ballantyne, J.P. & Hansen, S. (1974b) Computer method for the analysis of evoked motor unit potentials. 1. Control subjects and patients with myasthenia gravis. *Journal of Neurology, Neurosurgery and Psychiatry*, **37**, 1187.

Ballantyne, J.P. & Hansen, S. (1974c) A new method for the estimation of the number of motor units in a muscle. 2. Duchenne, limb-girdle and facioscapulohumeral, and myotonic muscular dystrophies. *Journal of Neurology, Neurosurgery and Psychiatry*, **37**, 1195.

Basmajian, J.V., Clifford, H.C., McLeod, W.D. & Nunnally, H.N. (1975) *Computers in Electromyography* (Butterworth: London).

Bayer, H. & Flechtenmayer, C. (1950) Ermüding und Aktionspannung bei der isometrischen Muskelkontraktion des Menschen. *Arbeitsphysiologie*, **14**, 261.

Belmar, J. & Eyzaguirre, C. (1966) Pacemaker site of fibrillation potentials in denervated mammalian muscle. *Journal of Neurophysiology*, **29**, 425.

Bergamini, V. (1959) Studi elettromiografici nell distrofia muscolare progressiva. *Rivista di Patologia Nervosa e Mentale (Florence)*, **80**, 708.

Betts, R.P., Paschalis, C., Jarratt, J.A. & Jenner, F.A. (1978) Nerve fibre refractory period in patients treated with rubidium and lithium. *Journal of Neurology, Neurosurgery and Psychiatry*, **41**, 791.

Bigland, B. & Lippold, O.C.J. (1954a) The relation between force, velocity and integrated electrical activity in human muscles. *Journal of Physiology*, **123**, 214.

Bigland, B. & Lippold, O.C.J. ((1954b) Motor unit activity in the voluntary contraction of human muscle. *Journal of Physiology*, **125**, 322.

Bigland-Ritchie, B., Hosking, G.P. & Jones, D.A. (1975) The site of fatigue in sustained maximal contractions of the quadriceps muscle. *Journal of Physiology*, **250**, 45P.

Björk, A. & Kugelberg, E. (1953) Motor unit activity in the human extraocular muscles. *Electroencephalography and Clinical Neurophysiology*, **5**, 271.

Botelho, S.Y., Beckett, S.B. & Bendler, E. (1960) Mechanical and electrical responses of intact thenar muscles to indirect stimuli. *Neurology (Minneapolis)*, **10**, 601.

Bowers, C.Y., Gordon, D.L. & Segaloff, A. (1955) The myxedema reflex in infants and children with hypothyroidism. *Journal of Paediatrics*, **54**, 46.

Brown, G.L. & Burns, B.D. (1949) Fatigue and neuromuscular block in mammalian skeletal muscle. *Proceedings of the Royal Society of London. Series B*, **36**, 182.

Buchthal, F. (1960) The general concept of the motor unit in neuromuscular disorders. *Proceedings of the Association for Research in Nervous and Mental Diseases*, **38** (The Williams and Wilkins Company: Baltimore).

Buchthal, F. & Clemmeson, S. (1941) On the differentiation of muscle atrophy by electromyography. *Acta Psychiatrica et Neurologia*, **16**, 143.

Buchthal, F. & Clemmeson, S. (1943) The electromyogram of atrophic muscles in cases of intramedullary affections. *Acta Psychiatrica et Neurologica*, **18**, 377.

Buchthal, F. & Engbaek, L. (1963) Refractory period and conduction velocity of the striated muscle fibre. *Acta Physiologica Scandinavica*, **59**, 199.

Buchthal, F. & Madsen, A. (1950) Synchronous activity in normal and atrophic muscle. *Electroencephalography and Clinical Neurophysiology*, **2**, 425.

Buchthal, F. & Pinelli, P. (1952) Analysis of muscle action potentials as a diagnostic aid in neuro-muscular disorders. *Acta Medica Scandinavica*, **142**, suppl. 266, 315.

Buchthal, F. & Pinelli, P. (1953a) Muscle action potentials in polymyositis. *Neurology (Minneapolis)*, **3**, 424.

Buchthal, F. & Pinelli, P. (1953b) Action potentials in muscular atrophy of neurogenic origin. *Neurology (Minneapolis)*, **3**, 591.

Buchthal, F. & Rosenfalck, P. (1958) Rate of impulse conduction in denervated human muscle. *Electroencephalography and Clinical Neurophysiology*, **10**, 521.

Buchthal, F. & Rosenfalck, A. (1966b) Sensory action potentials evoked by supramaximal paired stimuli and by trains of stimuli. *Brain Research*, **3**, 56.

Buchthal, F. & Rosenfalck, P. (1966a) Spontaneous electrical activity of human muscle. *Electroencephalography and Clinical Neurophysiology*, **20**, 321.

Buchthal, F. & Schmalbruch, H. (1969) Spectrum of contraction times of different fibre bundles in the brachial biceps and triceps muscles of man. *Nature*, **222**, 89.

Buchthal, F., Erminio, F. & Rosenfalck, P. (1959) Motor unit territory in different human muscles. *Acta Physiologica Scandinavica*, **45**, 72.

Buchthal, F., Guld, C. & Rosenfalck, P. (1954) Action potential parameters in normal muscle and their dependence on physical variables. *Acta Physiologica Scandinavica*, **32**, 200.

Buchthal, F., Guld, C. & Rosenfalck, P. (1955) The innervation and propagation velocity in human muscle. *Acta Physiologica Scandinavica*, **35**, 174.

Buchthal, F., Rosenfalck, P. & Erminio, F. (1960) Motor unit territory and fibre density in myopathies. *Neurology (Minneapolis)*, **10**, 398.

Buchthal, F., Schmalbruch, H. & Kamieniecka, Z. (1971a) Contraction times and fiber types in neurogenic paresis. *Neurology (Minneapolis)*, **21**, 58.

Buchthal, F., Schmalbruch, H. & Kamieniecka, Z. (1971b) Contraction times and fiber types in patients with progressive muscular dystrophy. *Neurology (Minneapolis)*, **21**, 131.

Buller, A.J. & Dornhorst, A.C. (1957) The reinforcement of tendon reflexes. *Lancet*, **2**, 1260.

Caruso, G. & Buchthal, F. (1965) Refractory period of muscle and electromyographic findings in relatives of patients with muscular dystrophy. *Brain*, **88**, 29.

Chaney, W.C. (1924) Tendon reflexes in myxedema: a valuable aid in diagnosis. *Journal of the American Medical Association*, **82**, 2013.

Cobb, S. & Forbes, A. (1923) Electromyographic studies of muscular fatigue in man. *American Journal of Physiology*, **65**, 234.

Coërs, C. (1955) *Les variations structurelles normales et*

pathologiques de la jonction musculaire. Thèse de Bruxelles, 1950.

Coërs, C. & Woolf, A.L. (1959) *The Innervation of Muscle, a Biopsy Study* (Blackwell: Oxford).

Conrad, J.T. & Glaser, G.H. (1961) Bioelectric properties of dystrophic mammalian muscle. *Archives of Neurology*, **5**, 46.

Corrie, W.S. & Hardin, W.B. Jr. (1964) Post-tetanic potentiation of H reflex in normal man. *Archives of Neurology*, **11**, 317.

Das Gupta, A. (1963) The possibility of selective involvement of motor units in muscular dystrophy. In *Research in Muscular Dystrophy. Proceedings of Second Symposium on Current Research in Muscular Dystrophy*, p. 256 (Pitman: London).

Dawson, G.D. & Merton, P.A. (1956) 'Recurrent' discharges from motoneurones. *XX. International Congress on Physiology, Brussels*: Abstracts of Communications, pp. 221–222.

De Gail, P., Lance, J.W. & Neilson, P.O. (1966) Differential effects on tonic and phasic reflex mechanisms produced by vibration of muscles in man. *Journal of Neurology, Neurosurgery and Psychiatry*, **29**, 1.

Dempster, W.T. & Finerty, J.C. (1947) The relative activity of wrist-moving muscles in static support of the wrist joint; an electromyographic study. *American Journal of Physiology*, **150**, 596.

Denny-Brown, D. (1949) The interpretation of the electromyogram. *Archives of Neurology and Psychiatry*, **61**, 99.

Denny-Brown, D. & Pennybacker, J.B. (1938) Fibrillation and fasciculation in voluntary muscle. *Brain*, **61**, 311.

De Vries, H.A. (1968) 'Efficiency of electrical activity' as a physiological measure of the functional state of muscle tissue. *American Journal of Physical Medicine*, **47**, 10.

Diamantopoulous, E. & Gassel, M.M. (1965) Electrically-induced monosynaptic reflexes in man. *Journal of Neurology, Neurosurgery and Psychiatry*, **28**, 496.

Diamantopoulos, E. & Olsen, P. Zander (1966) Motoneurone excitability in patients with abnormal reflex activity. In *Muscular Afferents and Motor Control. Proceedings of the First Nobel Symposium, Stockholm*, Ed. Ragnar Granit (Almqvist and Wiksell: Stockholm).

Dietz, V. (1978) Analysis of the electrical muscle activity during maximal contraction and the influence of ischaemia. *Journal of the Neurological Sciences*, **37**, 187.

Eason, R.G. (1960) Electromyographic study of local and generalised muscular impairment. *Journal of Applied Physiology*, **15**, 479.

Edwards, R.G. & Lippold, O.C.J. (1956) The relationship between force and integrated electrical activity in fatigued muscle. *Journal of Physiology*, **132**, 677.

Ekstedt, S. (1964) Human muscle fiber action potentials. Extracellular recording during voluntary and chemical activation. With some comments on end-plate physiology and on the fiber arrangement of the motor unit. *Acta Physiologica Scandinavica*, **61**, suppl. 226. 1–91.

Ekstedt, J. & Stålberg, E. (1969) The effect of non-paralytic doses of D-tubocurarine on individual motor end-plates in man studied with a new electrophysiological method. *Electroencephalography and Clinical Neurophysiology*, **27**, 557.

Erminio, F., Buchthal, F. & Rosenfalck, P. (1959) Motor unit territory and muscle fibre concentration in paresis due to peripheral nerve injury and anterior horn cell involvement.

Neurology (Minneapolis), **10**, 657.

Esteban, A. & Gimenez-Roldan, S. (1975) Blink reflexes in Huntington's chorea and Parkinson's disease. *Acta Neurologica Scandinavica*, **52**, 145.

Farmer, T.W., Buchthal, F. & Rosenfalck, P. (1959) Refractory and irresponsive periods of muscle in progressive muscular dystrophy and paresis due to lower motor neurone involvement. *Neurology (Minneapolis)*, **9**, 747.

Farmer, T.W., Buchthal, F. & Rosenfalck, P. (1960) Refractory period of human muscle after the passage of a propagated action potential. *Electroencephalography and Clinical Neurophysiology*, **12**, 455.

Ferguson, I.T. (1978) Electrical study of jaw and orbicularis oculi reflexes after trigeminal nerve surgery. *Journal of Neurology, Neurosurgery and Psychiatry*, **41**, 819.

Ferguson, I.T., Lenman, J.A.R. & Johnston, B.B. (1978) Habituation of the orbicularis oculi reflex in dementia and dyskinetic states. *Journal of Neurology, Neurosurgery and Psychiatry*, **41**, 824.

Fex, J. & Krakau, C.E.T. (1957) Some experiences with Walton's frequency analysis of the electromyogram. *Journal of Neurology, Neurosurgery and Psychiatry*, **20**, 178.

Fitch, P. (1967) An analyser for use in human electromyography. *Electronic Engineering*, **39**, 240.

Freund, H.J., Dietz, V., Wita, C.W. & Kapp, H. (1973) Discharge characteristics of single motor units in normal subjects and patients with supraspinal motor disturbances. In *New Developments in Electromyography and Clinical Neurophysiology*, Ed. J.E. Desmedt, Vol. 3, pp. 242–250 (Karger: Basel).

Fullerton, P. & Gilliatt, R.W., (1965) Axon reflexes in human motor nerve fibres. *Journal of Neurology, Neurosurgery and Psychiatry*, **28**, 1.

Garcia-Mullin, R. & Mayer, R.F. (1972) H reflexes in acute and chronic hemiplegia. *Brain*, **95**, 559.

Gardner-Medwin, D. (1968) Studies of the carrier state in the Duchenne type of muscular dystrophy. 2. Quantitative electromyography as a method of carrier detection. *Journal of Neurology, Neurosurgery and Psychiatry*, **31**, 124.

Gassel, M.M. & Diamantopoulos, E. (1964) The Jendrassik maneuver. I. The pattern of reinforcement of monosynaptic reflexes in normal subjects and patients with spasticity or rigidity. *Neurology (Minneapolis)*, **14**, 555.

Gassel, M.M. & Wiesendanger, M. (1965) Recurrent and reflex discharges in plantar muscles of the cat. *Acta Physiologica Scandanavica*, **65**, 138.

Gerston, J.W., Cenkovich, F.S. & Jones, B.S. (1965) Harmonic analysis of normal and abnormal electromyograms. *American Journal of Physical Medicine*, ·**44**, 235.

Gilliatt, R.W. & Willison, R.G. (1963) The refractory and supernormal periods of the human median nerve. *Journal of Neurology, Neurosurgery and Psychiatry*, **26**, 136.

Gregoric, M. (1973) Habituation of the blink reflex. In *New Developments in Electromyography and Clinical Neurophysiology*, Ed. J.E. Desmedt, Vol. 3, pp. 673–677 (Karger: Basel).

Hagbarth, K.E. (1962) Post-tetanic potentiation of myotatic reflexes in man. *Journal of Neurology, Neurosurgery and Psychiatry*, **25**, 1.

Hagbarth, K.E. & Eklund, G. (1966) Motor effects of vibratory muscle stimuli in man. In *Muscular Afferents and Motor Control. Proceedings of the First Nobel Symposium, Stockholm* Ed. Ragnar Granit, p. 177 (Almqvist and Wiksell: Stockholm).

Hansen, S. & Ballantyne, J.P. (1977) Axonal degeneration in the neuropathy of diabetes mellitus: a quantitative electromyographic study. *Journal of Neurology, Neurosurgery and Psychiatry*, **40**, 555.

Harvey, A.M. & Masland, R.L. (1941) The electromyogram in myasthenia gravis. *Bulletin of the Johns Hopkins Hospital*, **69**, 1.

Hayward, M. & Willison, R.G. (1977) Automatic analysis of the electromyogram in patients with chronic partial denervation. *Journal of the Neurological Sciences*, **33**, 415.

Henneman, E., Somjen, G. & Carpenter, D.O. (1965) Functional significance of cell size in spinal motoneurones. *Journal of Neurophysiology*, **28**, 560.

Hodes, R. (1948) Electromyographic study of neuromuscular transmission in human poliomyelitis. *Archives of Neurology and Psychiatry*, **60**, 457.

Hoffmann, P. (1918) Über die Beziehungen der Sehnenreflex zur willkürlichen Bewegung und zum Tonus. *Zeitschrift für Biologie*, **68**, 351.

Hopf, H.C. & Lowitzsch, K. (1975) Relative refractory period of motor nerves. In *Studies on Neuromuscular Diseases. Proceedings of an International Symposium, Giessen, 1973*, Eds K. Kunze & J.E. Desmedt, pp. 264–267 (Karger: Basel).

Hugon, M., Delwaide, P., Pierrot-Deseilligny, E. & Desmedt, J.E. (1973) A discussion of the methodology of the triceps sural T- and H-reflexes. In *New Developments in Electromyography and Clinical Neurophysiology*, Ed. J.E. Desmedt, Vol. 3, pp. 773–780 (Karger: Basel).

Inman, V.T., Ralston, H.J., Saunders, J.B. de C.M., Feinstein, B. & Wright, E.W. (1952) Relation of human electromyogram to muscular tension. *Electroencephalography and Clinical Neurophysiology*, **4**, 187.

Jasper, H. & Ballem, G. (1940) Unipolar electromyograms of normal and denervated human muscle. *Journal of Neurophysiology*, **12**, 231.

Kimura, J. (1973) The blink reflex as a test for brain-stem and higher nervous system function. In *New Developments in Electromyography and Clinical Neurophysiology*, Ed. J.E. Desmedt, Vol. 3, pp. 682–691 (Karger: Basel).

Kimura, J. (1974) Effect of hemispheral lesions on the contralateral blink reflex. *Neurology (Minneapolis)*, **24**, 168.

Kimura, J. (1975) Electrically elicited blink reflex in diagnosis of multiple sclerosis (review of 260 patients over a seven year period). *Brain*, **98**, 413.

Kimura, J. & Lyon, L.W. (1972) Obicularis oculi reflex in the Wallenberg syndrome: alteration of the late reflex by lesions of the spinal tract and nucleus of the trigeminal nerve. *Journal of Neurology, Neurosurgery and Psychiatry*, **35**, 228.

Kimura, J., Yamada, T. & Rodnitzky, R.L. (1978) Refractory period of human motor nerve fibres. *Journal of Neurology, Neurosurgery and Psychiatry*, **41**, 784.

Knowlton, G.C., Hines, T.F., Keever, K.W. & Bennett, R.L. (1956) Relation between electromyographic voltage and load. *Journal of Applied Physiology*, **9**, 473.

Kopec, J., Delbeke, J. & McComas, A.J. (1978) Refractory period studies in a human neuromuscular preparation. *Journal of Neurology, Neurosurgery and Psychiatry*, **41**, 54.

Kopec, J., Hausmanowa-Petrusewicz, I., Rawski, M. & Woynski, M. (1973) Automatic analysis in electromyography. In *New Developments in Electromyography and Clinical Neurophysiology*, Ed. J.E. Desmedt, Vol. 2, pp. 477–481 (Karger: Basel).

Kugelberg, E. (1949) Electromyography in muscular dystrophies. *Journal of Neurology, Neurosurgery and Psychiatry*, **12**, 129.

Kugelberg, E. (1952) Facial reflexes. *Brain*, **75**, 385.

Kugelberg, E. & Petersén, I. (1949) 'Insertion activity' in electromyography. *Journal of Neurology, Neurosurgery and Psychiatry*, **12**, 268.

Kuroda, V., Klissouras, V. & Milsum, J.H. (1970) Electrical and mechanical activities and fatigue in human isometric contraction. *Journal of Applied Physiology*, **29**, 358.

Kwatny, E., Thomas, D.A. & Kwatny, H.G. (1970) An application of signal processing techniques to the study of myoelectric signals. *IEEE trans. on Biomedical Engineering* BME-17, 303.

Lambert, E.H., Underdahl, L.O., Beckett, S. & Mederos, L.O. (1951) A study of the ankle jerk in myxedema. *Journal of Clinical Endocrinology*, **11**, 1186.

Lance, J.W., De Gail, P. & Nielson, P.D. (1966) Tonic and phasic spinal cord mechanisms in man. *Journal of Neurology, Neurosurgery and Psychiatry*, **29**, 535.

Landau, W.M. & Clare, M.H. (1964) Fusimotor function, Part IV. Reinforcement of the H reflex in normal subjects. *Archives of Neurology*, **10**, 117.

Lee, R.G. & White, D.G. (1973) Computer analysis of motor unit action potentials in routine clinical electromyography. In *New Developments in Electromyography and Clinical Neurophysiology*. Ed. J.E. Desmedt, Vol. 2, pp. 454–461 (Karger: Basel).

Lenman, J.A.R. (1959a) A clinical and experimental study of the effects of exercise on motor weakness in neurological disease. *Journal of Neurology, Neurosurgery and Psychiatry*, **22**, 182.

Lenman, J.A.R. (1959b) Quantitative electromyographic changes associated with muscular weakness. *Journal of Neurology, Neurosurgery and Psychiatry*, **22**, 306.

Lenman, J.A.R. (1965) Observations on the refractory period of denervated muscle. In *Neuromuscular Diseases. Proceedings of 8th International Congress of Neurology (Vienna)*, Vol. 2, 395.

Lenman, J.A.R. (1966) Quantitative aspects of electromyography. In *Control and Innervation of Skeletal Muscle*, Ed. B.L. Andrew, p. 64 (E. & S. Livingstone: Edinburgh).

Lenman, J.A.R. & Potter, J.L. (1966) Electromyographic measurement of fatigue in rheumatoid arthritis and neuromuscular disease. *Annals of the Rheumatic Diseases (London)*, **25**, 76.

Lindsley, D.B. (1935) Electrical activity of human motor units during voluntary contraction. *American Journal of Physiology*, **114**, 90.

Lippold, O.C.J. (1952) The relation between integrated action potentials in a human muscle and its isometric tension. *Journal of Physiology*, **117**, 492.

Lippold, O.C.J., Redfearn, J.W.T. & Vuco, J. (1957) The rhythmical activity of groups of motor units in the voluntary contraction of muscle. *Journal of Physiology*, **137**, 473.

Lloyd, D.P.C. (1943) Conduction and synaptic transmission of the reflex response to stretch in spinal cats. *Journal of Neurophysiology*, **6**, 317.

Lowitzsch, K. & Hopf, H.C. (1975) Propagation of compound action potentials of the mixed peripheral nerves in man at high stimulus frequencies. In *Studies on Neuromuscular Diseases. Proceedings of an International Symposium, Giessen, 1973*. Eds K. Kunze & J.E. Desmedt

(Karger: Basel).

Lucas, K. (1910) On the refractory period of muscle and nerve. *Journal of Physiology*, **39**, 331.

Lyon, L.W., Kimura, J. & McCormick, W.F. (1972) Orbicularis oculi reflex in coma: clinical, electrophysiological, pathological correlations. *Journal of Neurology, Neurosurgery and Psychiatry*, **35**, 582–588.

McComas, A.J., & Payan, J. (1966) Motoneurone excitability in the Holmes-Adie syndrome. In *Control and Innervation of Skeletal Muscle* Ed. B.L. Andrew, p. 182 (E. & S. Livingstone: Edinburgh).

McComas, A.J. & Thomas, H.C. (1968) A study of the muscle twitch in the Duchenne type muscular dystrophy. *Journal of the Neurological Sciences*, **7**, 309.

McComas, A.J., Campbell, M.J. & Sica, R.E.P. (1971) Electrophysiological study of dystrophia myotonica. *Journal of Neurology and Psychiatry*, **34**, 132.

McComas, A.J., Sica, R.E.P. & Currie, S. (1970) Muscular dystrophy: evidence for a neural factor. *Nature*, **226**, 1263.

McComas, A.J., Sica, R.E.P. & Currie, S. (1971) An electrophysiological study of Duchenne dystrophy. *Journal of Neurology, Neurosurgery and Psychiatry*, **34**, 461.

McComas, A.J., Fawcett, P.R.W., Campbell, M.J. & Sica, R.E.P. (1971) Electrophysiological estimation of the number of motor units within a human muscle. *Journal of Neurology, Neurosurgery and Psychiatry*, **34**, 121.

McComas, A.J., Sica, R.E.P., Campbell, M.J. & Upton, A.R.M. (1971) Functional compensation in partially denervated muscles. *Journal of Neurology, Neurosurgery and Psychiatry*, **34**, 453.

McComas, A.J., Sica, R.E.P., Upton, A.R.M., Aguilera, N. & Currie, S. (1971) Motoneurone dysfunction in patients with hemiplegic atrophy. *Nature*, **233**, 21.

McIntyre, A.K. (1951) Afferent limb of the myotatic reflex arc. *Nature*, **168**, 168.

McIntyre, A.K. & Robinson, R.G. (1959) Pathway for the jaw jerk in man. *Brain*, **82**, 468.

McLeod, J.G. & Van Der Meulen, J.P. (1967) Effect of cerebrellar ablation on the H reflex of the cat. *Archives of Neurology*, **16**, 421.

McLeod, J.G. & Walsh, J.C. (1972) H reflex studies in patients with Parkinson's disease. *Journal of Neurology, Neurosurgery and Psychiatry*, **35**, 77.

McLeod, J.G. & Wray, S.H. (1966) An experimental study of the F wave in the baboon. *Journal of Neurology, Neurosurgery and Psychiatry*, **29**, 196.

McLeod, W.D. (1973) EMG instrumentation in biochemical studies: amplifiers, recorders and integrators. In *New Developments in Electromyography and Clinical Neurophysiology*, Ed. J.E. Desmedt, Vol. 2, pp. 511–518 (Karger: Basel).

MacQueen, I.J. (1954) Recent advances in the technique of progressive resistance exercises. *British Medical Journal*, **2**, 1193.

Magladery, J.W. & McDougal, D.B. (1950) Electrophysiological studies of nerve and reflex activity in normal man. *Bulletin of the Johns Hopkins Hospital*, **86**, 265.

Magladery, J.W., Porter, W.E., Park, A.M. & Teasdall, R.D. (1951) Electrophysiological studies of nerve and reflex activity in normal man. *Bulletin of the Johns Hopkins Hospital*, **88**, 499.

Magladery, J.W., Teasdall, R.D., Park, A.M. & Languth, H.W. (1952) Electrophysiological studies of reflex activity

in patients with lesions of the nervous system. *Bulletin of the Johns Hopkins Hospital*, **91**, 219.

Marsden, C.D., Meadows, J.C. & Merton, P.A. (1971) Isolated single motor units in human muscle and their rate of discharge during maximal voluntary effort. *Journal of Physiology*, **217**, 12–13.

Matsuoka, S., Waltz, J.M., Terada, C., Ikeda, T. & Cooper, I.S. (1966) A computer technique for evaluation of recovery cycle of the H reflex in the abnormal movement disorders. *Electroencephalography and Clinical Neurophysiology*, **21**, 496.

Matthews, W.B. (1966) Ratio of maximum H reflex to minimum M response as a measure of spasticity. *Journal of Neurology, Neurosurgery and Psychiatry*, **29**, 201.

Mayer, R.F. & Mawdsley, C. (1965) Studies in man and cat of the significance of the H reflex. *Journal of Neurology, Neurosurgery and Psychiatry*, **28**, 201.

Merton, P.A. (1954) Voluntary strength and fatigue. *Journal of Physiology*, **123**, 553.

Milner-Brown, H.S. & Brown, W.F. (1976) New methods of estimating the number of motor units in a muscle. *Journal of Neurology, Neurosurgery and Psychiatry*, **39**, 258.

Milner-Brown, H.S. & Stein, R.B. (1975) the relation between the surface electromyogram and muscular force. *Journal of Physiology*, **246**, 549.

Milner-Brown, H.S., Stein, R.B. & Yemm, R. (1973a) The orderly recruitment of human motor units during voluntary isometric contractions. *Journal of Physiology*, **230**, 359.

Milner-Brown, H.S., Stein, R.B. & Yemm, R. (1973b) Changes in firing rate of human motor units during linearly changing voluntary contractions. *Journal of Physiology*, **230**, 371.

Moosa, A. & Brown, B.H. (1972) Quantitative electromyography: a new analogue technique for detecting changes in action potential duration. *Journal of Neurology, Neurosurgery and Psychiatry*, **35**, 216.

Mulder, D.W., Lambert, E.H. & Eaton, L.M. (1959) Myasthenic syndrome in patients with amyotrophic lateral sclerosis. *Neurology (Minneapolis)*, **9**, 627.

Naess, K. & Storm-Mathison, A. (1955) Fatigue of sustained tetanic contractions. *Acta Physiologica Scandinavica*, **34**, 351.

Norris, F.H. Jr. & Gasteiger, E.L. (1955) Action potentials of single motor units in normal muscle. *Electroencephalography and Clinical Neurophysiology*, **7**, 115.

Olsen, P. Zander & Diamantopoulos, E. (1967) Excitability of spinal motor neurones in normal subjects and patients with spasticity. Parkinsonian rigidity, and cerebellar hypotonia. *Journal of Neurology, Neurosurgery and Psychiatry*, **30**, 325.

Ongeboer de Visser, B.W. & Goor, C. (1974) Electromyographic and reflex study in idiopathic and symptomatic trigeminal neuralgias: latency of the jaw and blink reflexes. *Journal of Neurology, Neurosurgery and Psychiatry*, **37**, 1225.

Ongeboer de Visser, B.W. & Kuypers, H.G.J.M. (1978) Late blink reflex changes in lateral medullary lesions. *Brain*, **101**, 285.

Ord, W.M. (1884) On some disorders of nutrition related with affections of the nervous system. *British Medical Journal*, **2**, 205.

Paillard, J. (1959) Functional organization of afferent innervation of muscle studied in man by monosynaptic testing. *American Journal of Physical Medicine*, **38**, 239.

Panayiotopoulos, C.P., Scarpalezos, S. & Papapetropoulos, Th. (1974) Electrophysiological estimation of motor units in Duchenne muscular dystrophy. *Journal of the Neurological Sciences*, **23**, 89.

Penders, C.A. & Delwaide, P.L. (1971) Blink reflex studies in patients with Parkinsonism before and during therapy. *Journal of Neurology, Neurosurgery and Psychiatry*, **34**, 674.

Penders, C.A. & Delwaide, P.L. (1973) Physiologic approach to the human blink reflex. In *New Developments in Electromyography and Clinical Neurophysiology*, Ed. J.E. Desmedt, Vol. 3, pp. 649–657 (Karger: Basel).

Person, R.S. (1960) Electrophysiological study of the activity of the motor apparatus of man in fatigue. *Fiziologicheskiĭ Zhurnal (Moscow)*, **36**, 810.

Petersén, I. & Kugelberg, E. (1949) Duration and form of action potentials in the normal human muscle. *Journal of Neurology, Neurosurgery and Psychiatry*, **12**, 124.

Peyronnard, Jean-Marie & Lamarre, Y. (1977) Electrophysiological and anatomical estimation of the number of motor units in the monkey extensor digitorum brevis. *Journal of Neurology, Neurosurgery and Psychiatry*, **40**, 756.

Pinelli, P. (1975) Action potential parameters of motor units. In *Studies on Neuromuscular Diseases. Proceedings of an International Symposium, Giessen 1973*. Eds K. Kunze & J.E. Desmedt, pp. 92–93 (Karger: Basel).

Pinelli, P. & Buchthal, F. (1953) Muscle action potentials in myopathies with special regard to progressive muscular dystrophy. *Neurology (Minneapolis)*, **3**, 347.

Piper, H. (1912) *Elektrophysiologie menschlicher Muskeln* (Julius Springer: Berlin).

Richardson, A.T. (1951) Newer concepts of electrodiagnosis. *St. Thomas's Hospital Reports*, **7**, 164.

Rose, A.L. & Willison, R.G. (1967) Quantitative electromyography using automatic analysis. Studies in healthy subjects and patients with primary muscle disease. *Journal of Neurology, Neurosurgery and Psychiatry*, **30**, 403.

Rushworth, G. (1962) Observation on blink reflexes. *Journal of Neurology, Neurosurgery and Psychiatry*, **25**, 93.

Sacco, G., Buchthal, F. & Rosenfalck, P. (1962) Motor unit potentials at different ages. *Archives of Neurology*, **6**, 366.

Sandow, A. & Brust, M. (1958) Contractility of dystrophic mouse muscle. *American Journal of Physiology*, **194**, 557.

Scherrer, J. & Bourguignon, A. (1959) Changes in the electromyogram produced by fatigue in man. *American Journal of Physical Medicine*, **38**, 148.

Scherrer, J., Samson, M. & Soula, C. (1954) Étude électromyographique de la fatigue musculaire normale. *Journal de Physiologie*, **46**, 517–520.

Seyffarth, H. (1941a) The behaviour of motor units in healthy and paretic muscles in man. I. *Acta Psychiatrica et Neurologica*, **16**, 79.

Seyffarth, H. (1941b) The behaviour of motor units in healthy and paretic muscles in man, II. *Acta Psychiatrica et Neurologica*, **16**, 261.

Shahani, B. (1968) Effects of sleep on human reflexes with a double component. *Journal of Neurology, Neurosurgery and Psychiatry*, **31**, 574.

Shahani, B. (1970) The human blink reflex. *Journal of Neurology, Neurosurgery and Psychiatry*, **33**, 792.

Sherrington, C.S. (1929) Some functional problems attaching to convergence. *Proceedings of Royal Society, Series B*, **105**, 332.

Shimazu, H., Hongo, T., Kubota, K. & Narabayashi, H. (1962) Rigidity and spasticity in man. *Archives of Neurology*, **6**, 10.

Sica, R.E.P. & McComas, A.J. (1971) An electrophysiological investigation of limb-girdle and facioscapulohumeral dystrophy. *Journal of Neurology, Neurosurgery and Psychiatry*, **34**, 469.

Sica, R.E.P., McComas, A.J. & Upton, A.R.M. (1971) Impaired potentiation of H-reflexes in patients with upper motor neurone lesions. *Journal of Neurology, Neurosurgery and Psychiatry*, **34**, 712.

Simpson, J.A. (1966) Control of muscle in health and disease. In *Control and Innervation of Skeletal Muscle*, Ed. B.L. Andrew (E. & S. Livingstone: Edinburgh).

Simpson, J.A. & Lenman, J.A.R. (1959) The effect of frequency of stimulation in neuromuscular disease. *Electroencephalography and Clinical Neurophysiology*, **11**, 604.

Simpson, J.A. & Sanderson, I.D. (1965) Experimental studies of the effect of 'Laevadosin' in muscular dystrophy. In *Research in Muscular Dystrophy. Proceedings of the Third Symposium on Current Research in Muscular Dystrophy*, p. 342 (Pitman: London).

Sommer, J. (1940) Periphere Bahnung von Muskeleigenreflexen als Wesen des Jendrassiksen Phänomens. *Deutsche Zeitschrift für Nervenheilkunde*, **150**, 249.

Stålberg, E. (1966) Propagation velocity in human muscle fibres in situ. *Acta Physiologica Scandinavica*, **70**, suppl. 287.

Stålberg, E. & Thiele, B. (1975) Motor unit fibre density in the extensor digitorum communis muscle. *Journal of Neurology, Neurosurgery and Psychiatry*, **38**, 874.

Stepanov, A.S. (1959) Electromyogram changes produced by training in weight lifting. *Fiziologicheskiĭ Zhurnal (Moscow)*, **45**, 129.

Stephens, J.A. & Taylor A. (1972) Fatigue of maintained voluntary muscle contraction in man. *Journal of Physiology*, **220**, 1.

Stephens, J.A. & Taylor, A. (1973) The relationship between integrated electrical activity and force in normal and fatiguing human voluntary muscle contractions. In *New Developments in Electromyography and Clinical Neurophysiology*, Ed. J.E. Desmedt, Vol. 1, pp. 623–627 (Karger: Basel).

Stephens, J.A. & Usherwood, T.P. (1975) The fatiguability of human motor units. *Journal of Physiology*, **250**, 37P.

Szentagothai, J. (1948) Anatomical considerations of monosynaptic reflex arcs. *Journal of Neurophysiology*, **11**, 445.

Taborikova, H. & Sax, D.S. (1968) Motoneurone pool and the H-reflex. *Journal of Neurology and Psychiatry*, **31**, 354.

Táborikova, H. & Sax, D.S. (1969) Conditioning of H-reflexes by a preceding subthreshold H-reflex stimulus. *Brain*, **92**, 203.

Tackmann, W., Ullerich, D. & Lehmann, H.J. (1975) Impulse series neuropathy and paired stimuli in early stages of human polyneuropathy. In *Studies on Neuromuscular Disease. Proceedings of an International Symposium, Giessen, 1973*, Eds K. Kunze & J.E. Desmedt, pp. 251–257 (Karger: Basel).

Takamori, M. (1967) H reflex study in upper motoneuron diseases. *Neurology (Minneapolis)*, **17**, 32.

Tanji, J. & Kato, M. (1973a) Recruitment of motor units in voluntary contraction of a finger muscle in man. *Experimental Neurology*, **40**, 759.

Tanji, J. & Kato, M. (1973b) Firing rate of individual motor units in voluntary contraction of abductor digiti minimi muscle in man. *Experimental Neurology*, **40**, 771.

Taylor, A. (1962) The significance of grouping of motor unit activity. *Journal of Physiology*, **162**, 259.

Thiele, B. & Stålberg E. (1975) Single fibre EMG findings in polyneuropathies of different aetiology. *Journal of Neurology, Neurosurgery and Psychiatry*, **38**, 881.

Thorne, J. (1965) Central responses to electrical activation of the peripheral nerves supplying the intrinsic hand muscles. *Journal of Neurology, Neurosurgery and Psychiatry*, **28**, 482.

Tokizane, T. & Shimazu, H. (1964) *Functional Differentiation of Human Skeletal muscle. Corticalization and Spinalization of Movement* (Charles C. Thomas: Springfield, Illinois).

Trontelj, J.V. (1973) A study of the F response by single fibre electromyography. In *New Developments in Electromyography and Clinical Neurophysiology*, Ed. J.E. Desmedt. Vol. 3, pp. 318–322 (Karger: Basel).

Upton, A.R.M., McComas, A.J. & Sica, R.E.P. (1971) Potentiation of late responses evoked in muscle during effort. *Journal of Neurology, Neurosurgery and Psychiatry*, **34**, 699.

Van den Bosch, J. (1963) Investigations of the carrier state in the Duchenne type dystrophy. In *Research in Muscular Dystrophy. Proceedings of Second Symposium on Current Research in Muscular Dystrophy*, p. 23 (Pitman: London).

Walton, J.N. (1952) The electromyogram in myopathy: analysis with the audio frequency spectrometer. *Journal of Neurology, Neurosurgery and Psychiatry*, **15**, 219.

Walton, J.N. & Adams, R.D. (1958) *Polymyositis* (E. & S. Livingstone: Edinburgh).

Weddell, B.G., Feinstein, B. & Pattle, R.E. (1944) The electrical activity of voluntary muscle in man under normal and pathological conditions. *Brain*, **67**, 178.

Willison, R.G. (1964) Analysis of electrical activity in healthy and dystrophic muscle in man. *Journal of Neurology, Neurosurgery and Psychiatry*, **27**, 386.

Wilson, J. & Walton, J.N. (1959) Some muscular manifestations of hypothyroidism. *Journal of Neurology, Neurosurgery and Psychiatry*, **22**, 320.

Wohlfart, G. (1955) Aktuelle Probleme der Muskelpathologie. *Deutsche Zeitschrift für Nervenheilkunde*, **173**, 426.

Wohlfart, G. (1958) Collateral regeneration in partially denervated muscles. *Neurology (Minneapolis)*, **8**, 175.

Wohlfart, G. (1959a) Degenerative and regenerative axonal changes in the ventral horns, brain stem and cerebral cortex in amyotrophic lateral sclerosis. *Lunds Universitets Arsskrift* 56, No. 2, *Transactions of the Royal Physiographic Society*, **71**, No. 2.

Wohlfart, G. (1959b) Clinical considerations on innervation of skeletal muscle. *American Journal of Physical Medicine*, **37**, 223.

Yap, C-B. (1967) Spinal segmental and long-loop reflexes in spinal motoneurone excitability in spasticity and rigidity. *Brain*, **80**, 887.

Zuniga, N.E. & Simons, D.G. (1969) Non linear relationship between averaged electromyogram potential and muscle tension in normal subjects. *Archives of Physical Medicine and Rehabilitation*, **50**, 613.

Zuniga, E.N., Truong, X.T. & Simons, D.G. (1969) Effects of skin electrode position on averaged electromyographic potentials. *Archives of Physical Medicine and Rehabilitation*, **51**, 264.

Potential changes in the normal and diseased muscle cell

INTRODUCTION

One of the characteristic physiological features of a muscle fibre is the maintenance of a potential difference across its cell membrane. This resting membrane potential is altered by activity of the muscle cell. The phasic change in membrane potential in the end-plate region of the muscle membrane, produced by the liberation of acetylcholine from the nerve terminal, is the end-plate potential, while the propagation of a potential change along the surface of the muscle fibre is the muscle action potential. Thus, the potential difference across the membrane may vary from time to time, and from position to position along the membrane.

The membrane potential at any given time and position depends upon two factors: first, the ionic concentrations on either side of the membrane, and second, the ease with which these ions pass through the membrane at that point. It is the aim of this chapter to consider the relationship between ionic concentrations, ionic permeabilities and the membrane potential. A description of

methods for measuring membrane potential will follow. Finally, examples will be presented showing how measurements of membrane potential may help in the investigation of disease of the muscle cell.

THEORETICAL CONSIDERATIONS

The following section is intended to give the reader an outline of the factors influencing potential differences across the muscle cell membrane and to allow him to predict the direction and order of magnitude of changes. It does not pretend to delve into the physical chemistry of ionic fluxes through semi-permeable membranes. The physical relationships are neither rigorously proved nor derived. For these, reference should be made to Goldman (1943), Hodgkin (1951) and Hodgkin and Huxley (1952). Detailed citation of the experimental evidence is given in the reviews of Shanes (1961) and Tower, Luse and Grundfest (1962), while the monographs by Hodgkin (1964) and Katz (1966) are especially recommended.

Equilibrium potentials

First, let us consider a cell with a membrane permeable to one species of ion, potassium. Let us further assume that its internal concentration is 150 mEq/l, while the external concentration is 5 mEq/l. We shall assume that other ions are present so that the total internal and the total external ionic concentrations are equal. Thus, the cell is in osmotic equilibrium and electro-neutrality is preserved.

Potassium ions will move both inward and

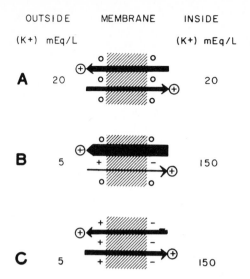

OUTSIDE   MEMBRANE   INSIDE

(K+) mEq/L   (K+) mEq/L

Fig. 30.1 Diagrammatic representation of the equilibrium potential. The magnitudes of the potassium ion fluxes are indicated by the breadth of the arrows. A. With equal ionic concentrations, fluxes are equal in both directions. There is no net transfer of charged ion, and the membrane is not polarised. B. Initially, with unequal ionic concentrations, the flux away from the side of higher concentrations exceeds that toward it. This net efflux of positive ions begins to polarise the membrane as indicated. C. At equilibrium the polarisation of the membrane reduces the efflux of positive ion and increases the influx. Thus, the fluxes are equalised, there is no net flux, and a potential difference is established across the membrane

outward through the cell membrane (Fig. 30.1). As the potassium ions are in higher concentration at the inner surface of the membrane, initially the efflux of potassium ions will exceed their influx. But for the fact that these ions are charged, this net outward movement of potassium down the chemical potential gradient would continue until the internal and external concentrations approached equality.

However, the initial net efflux of positively charged potassium ions leaves a dearth of positive charge inside and excess of positive charge outside the cell membrane. Thus, the membrane becomes electrically polarised, its internal surface becoming negative with respect to its external surface. This electrical potential gradient tends to retard the efflux of positive ions and to augment their influx. At equilibrium, then, the enhanced potassium influx equals the efflux, there is no net flux, and the membrane is polarised with the internal surface negative. This last could also be stated as

the external surface positive with respect to the internal, but by convention it is usual to consider charge with reference to the external surface.

It is apparent that the magnitude of this membrane potential at equilibrium will depend upon the magnitude of the chemical potential difference, that is, upon the difference in concentration of the diffusible ion on either side of the membrane. Furthermore, the sign of the equilibrium potential (E) will depend upon which side of the membrane has the higher concentration and also upon the charge of the ion. These parameters are related quantitatively in the Nernst equation:

$$E_{K+} = -\frac{RT}{F} \ln \frac{(K^+)_i}{(K^+)_e}$$

Where E is the membrane potential in millivolts (mV), $(K^+)_i$ is the internal and $(K^+)_e$ the external potassium ion concentration. R, T and F are constants, namely the gas constant, absolute temperature, and the faraday. At body temperature, this expression may be simplified to:

$$E_{K+} = -60 \log \frac{(K^+)_i}{(K^+)_e}$$

In our example:

$$E_{K+} = -60 \log \frac{150}{5}$$

$$= -60 \log 30$$

$$= -60 \times 1.48$$

$$= -89 \, \text{mV}.$$

If a muscle fibre is either *in situ*, or alternatively *in vitro* using a plasma medium (Kernan, 1963), the agreement between the resting potential and the potassium equilibrium potential is within the limits of experimental error. Nevertheless, in applying the Nernst equation to the muscle fibre membrane, two important assumptions have been made. The membrane has been considered, first, as if it were in thermodynamic equilibrium and second, as being selectively permeable to potassium. While there is no certainty about the first point, the second assumption is clearly incorrect because the resting membrane is actually rather more permeable to chloride than to potassium (Hutter and Noble, 1960). Furthermore, although the resting membrane is not significantly permeable to sodium this is no longer the case under conditions of excitation. It is therefore necessary to calculate the equilibrium potentials for sodium and chloride ions, using equation (2), and to see how these potentials are related to the potassium equilibrium potential in determining the muscle membrane potential. Perhaps the most effective way of achieving this is to consider an electrical analogue of the membrane.

Electrical analogue

In Figure 30.2A the potassium equilibrium potential has been represented as a battery with a potential difference of 89 mV across its terminals; the negative terminal is connected to the inner surface of the membrane and the positive terminal to the outer surface. The sodium and chloride equilibrium potentials may be represented similarly. Although chloride is more concentrated outside the fibre than inside, the polarity of the chloride battery is identical to that of the potassium one, as chloride is an anion. On the other hand, sodium is a cation which is more concentrated on the outside of the fibre and its equilibrium potential is therefore opposite in sign to that of potassium; this is shown diagrammatically by the positive terminal of the sodium battery being connected to the inner surface of the membrane.

An indication of the permeability of the membrane for each species of ion must be added to the electrical analogue. The ionic permeability of the membrane will also determine its *conductance*, that is, the ease with which electrical charges (in this instance ions) flow through the membrane. Furthermore, the conductance (G) of an electronic device can be described in terms of its reciprocal, resistance (R), since $G = 1/R$. Thus, the higher the permeability (and conductance) of the membrane to an ion, the lower is its electrical resistance. The ionic permeability of the membrane has been given the dimensions of a resistance in the electrical analogue (Fig. 30.2A). For each of the ion species, sodium, potassium and chloride, there is a battery (the equilibrium potential) in series with its

resistance. Furthermore, the elements (battery and resistance) for one species of ion are shown in parallel with those of the other two species. This analogue represents a small part of the muscle membrane. The entire membrane should be conceived as containing many of these elements connected in parallel.

At this stage, the potential difference across the muscle fibre membrane can be readily deduced from inspection of the analogue circuits, B, C, D in Figure 30.2. It can be seen that, if the resistance of the membrane for an ion is very high (conductance low), that ion will not influence the membrane potential. On the other hand, if the resistance for an ion decreases (conductance increases) the membrane potential will approach the equilibrium potential for that ion.

Resting membrane potential

The observed resting membrane potential ($ca-85$ mV) can be compared with the equilibrium potentials calculated from intra- and extracellular ionic concentrations. As there is close agreement with the potassium and chloride potential, we conclude from our analogue that the membrane conductance for sodium is low while that for chloride and potassium is high. This supposition, that the resting potential is determined only by the equilibrium potentials and relative conductances for potassium and chloride (Fig. 30.2B) may be tested experimentally.

First, we would anticipate that alterations in the equilibrium potential for either potassium or chloride would effect a change in membrane potential. The most convenient method of varying the equilibrium potential is to alter the concentration of ions in the extracellular fluid (i.e. K_e^+, Cl_e^-, in the Nernst equation). The results are informative. When the potassium concentration is changed, the membrane potential alters in accord with the calculated potassium equilibrium potential (within the limits of experimental error). When the chloride equilibrium potential is altered, a change in membrane potential also results. In this instance, however, the effect on membrane potential is transient because chloride ions are redistributed across the membrane until the membrane potential once again reaches the potassium

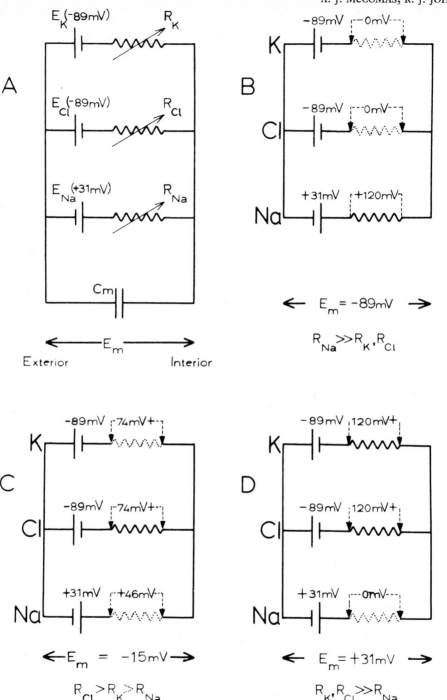

Fig. 30.2 A. Electrical analogue of membrane. E_K, E_{Cl} and E_{Na} are equilibrium potentials for the three species of ion (values in brackets) while R_K, R_{Cl} and R_{Na} represent the corresponding membrane resistances; C^N is membrane capacitance. B, C and D show, in a simplified and approximate manner, how membrane potential is determined at rest, B, during the end-plate potential, C, and during the action potential, D. A relatively small membrane resistance for an ion (i.e. high conductance) is shown by a dotted line; a heavy line indicates a large resistance (low conductance). The distribution of potentials across the three ionic resistances is shown for each condition of the membrane; the resulting potential between the internal and external surfaces of the membrane (E_m) is the membrane potential

equilibrium potential (Hodgkin and Horowicz, 1959). In other words, although the resting membrane is permeable to both potassium and chloride, it is the potassium conductance and the potassium equilibrium potential which ultimately set the level of the resting potential.

We may also test the analogue in another way by measuring the membrane resistance. The simplest way of doing this is to pass a known current through the muscle fibre membrane from an intracellular electrode and to record the potential difference developed across the membrane resistance. The recording may be made with a second intracellular electrode close to the stimulating electrode or, alternatively, the same electrode may be employed for both purposes by means of a Wheatstone bridge circuit. In the record of Figure 30.3, the smallest current, 5.3×10^{-8} A, produced a steady drop in potential (*or depolarisation*) of 7 mV. By Ohm's law,

$$\text{Resistance} = \frac{\text{Potential Difference}}{\text{Current}} ;$$

therefore the membrane resistance ('input resistance') =

$$\frac{7 \times 10^{-3} \text{ V}}{5.3 \times 10^{-8} \text{ A}} = 1.3 \times 10^5 \ \Omega.$$

The corresponding membrane conductance will be the reciprocal of this resistance, i.e.

$$\frac{1}{1.3 \times 10^5 \Omega} = 7.7 \times 10^{-6} \text{ mho.}\star$$

Not only can the total membrane conductance be measured in this way, but the component conductances can also be determined. For example, the chloride conductance can be abolished by replacing the external chloride with an impermeant anion such as methylsulphate or ethanesulphate; the same amount of current flowing through the membrane as before will now produce a larger depolarisation because the membrane resistance has been increased.

An inspection of the depolarisation produced by a rectangular current pulse flowing through the membrane reveals an interesting fact (Fig. 30.3).

*If the fibre radius is known the conductance may be expressed not only as an absolute value, but also in terms of unit area of membrane.

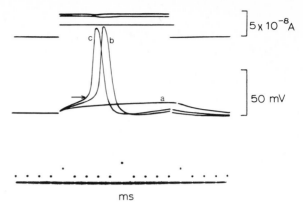

$$]5 \times 10^{-8} \text{A}$$

$$] 50 \text{ mV}$$

ms

Fig. 30.3 Depolarisations of membrane (superimposed lower traces) produced by two 10 ms rectangular current pulses (upper traces). The separation of the upper and lower traces, before the onset of the current pulses, represents the resting potential; dotted lines indicate baselines from which measurements of current and evoked potential are made. In this muscle fibre the smallest current, 5.3×10^{-8} A, produced an electrotonic potential (a) which had a maximum amplitude of approximately 7 mV. A larger current, of 7.9×10^{-8} A, evoked a depolarisation (b) which reached the critical membrane potential for the initiation of an action potential (at level of arrow). In this fibre the resting potential was −83 mV and the critical membrane potential −72 mV; the critical membrane depolarisation (i.e. the depolarisation required to bring the membrane from the resting potential to the critical membrane potential) was 11 mV. The action potential had an amplitude of 111 mV (spike retouched)

The depolarisation is not instantaneously achieved, as would be anticipated if the membrane were a pure resistance; instead, the membrane depolarisation increases exponentially to a plateau. This behaviour is attributable to the capacitance of the membrane—as indeed would be expected of a lipoprotein structure separating two electrolyte solutions. The velocity with which the final depolarisation is attained is, in fact, a function of the product of the specific membrane resistance (R_m, measured in Ω cm^2) and the membrane capacitance (C_m, Fig. 30.2) in parallel with it; this product is the *time constant* of the membrane.

The action potential

What happens if a larger depolarising current is passed through the membrane? Inspection of Figure 30.3 shows that a *critical membrane depolarisation* takes place and the fibre fires an action potential. To understand the ionic basis of this

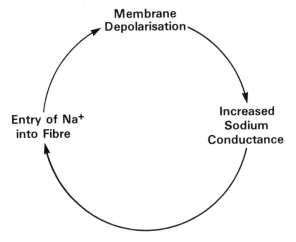

Fig. 30.4 The regenerative cycle of events which increases the sodium conductance of the membrane during the action potential (see text)

potential we must return to the electrical analogue. As already stated, the sodium conductance of the resting membrane is insignificant (Fig. 30.2B). As the membrane depolarises, however, the sodium conductance increases rapidly and this, in turn, leads to further depolarisation, as explained below. The *critical membrane potential* represents the point at which this depolarisation process becomes irreversible. Thus, from Figure 30.2 it is seen that an increase in sodium conductance will cause the membrane potential to move towards the sodium equilibrium potential, i.e. to depolarise. Furthermore, the increased sodium conductance allows sodium ions to flow passively into the fibre down their concentration gradient and also down their electrical gradient (being positive ions they are attracted to the negative interior of the cell). This entry of positive charge depolarises the membrane further, resulting in further increase in sodium conductance, more sodium ion entry, and so on (Fig. 30.4); the increase in the sodium conductance of the membrane is thus regenerative.

So great is the sodium conductance during the action potential that the membrane potential approaches the sodium equilibrium potential and reverses its polarity (Fig. 30.2C). The action potential is terminated after a millisecond or so by an increase in potassium conductance which, together with the now declining sodium conductance, restores the membrane potential to the potassium equilibrium potential; potassium ions

are lost from the intracellular compartment during this phase. Thus, at the end of the action potential, the muscle fibre has gained some sodium and lost some potassium. The sodium ions are now expelled by a metabolically driven pump, in exchange for potassium ions.

Neuromuscular transmission

Under physiological circumstances, muscle action potentials are initiated only at the neuromuscular junction and then propagate smoothly towards the two ends of the fibre with a velocity of 3.5 to 5 m/s. Although the evolving sequence of events culminating in the action potential is similar to that described above, the initial depolarisation of the membrane is produced by acetylcholine (ACh). This substance is formed in the nerve terminals and is packed into small vesicles some 50 nm in diameter. Even in the absence of motor nerve impulses there is a random release of ACh from individual vesicles, resulting in small depolarisations of the muscle fibre membrane; these are the *miniature end-plate potentials* (Fig. 30.5). The arrival of an action potential at the motor nerve terminals causes the synchronous release of ACh from possibly several hundred vesicles at each neuromuscular junction. The ACh diffuses across the narrow (20 nm) synaptic cleft separating the nerve and muscle fibre membranes and combines with receptors on the surface of the

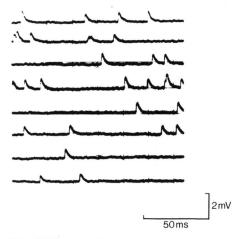

2 mV

50 ms

Fig. 30.5 Miniature end-plate potentials recorded with an intracellular micro-electrode in mouse gracilis muscle (McComas and Mossawy, unpublished data)

latter. This chemical reaction increases both the sodium and potassium conductances of the membrane (Fig. 30.2D). As a consequence of the increased sodium conductance, the membrane begins to depolarise until the critical membrane potential for the initiation of an action potential is reached; this chemically induced depolarisation following a motor nerve impulse is the *end-plate potential*.

METHODS

The membrane potential can be measured directly by inserting an electrode inside the muscle cell and measuring the potential difference between it and an electrode outside the cell. Such measurements are accurate if the electrodes themselves generate no spurious potentials, if the measuring device draws no current, and if the insertion of the electrode produces no damage to the cell or its membrane. This last factor prevented direct measurements of membrane potential in muscle fibres until electrolyte-filled micropipettes were introduced as intracellular electrodes (Ling and Gerard, 1949).

The essential components of the system used to measure membrane potential are illustrated in Figure 30.6. The muscle fibre is surrounded by the extracellular solution, which may be extracellular fluid *in situ* or an artificial electrolyte solution *in vitro*. The indifferent, or reference, electrode is connected to the extracellular solution. The micro-electrode penetrates the cell wall and connects at its tip with the intracellular fluid of the fibre. The membrane potential, E_m, appears between these two electrodes.

The potential difference between the electrodes is applied to the two input terminals of the input coupler. A potential equal or proportional to the input signal appears at its output terminals. The measuring device transforms this output voltage into a measurable form, either meter deflection, strip chart record, or oscilloscope tracing. The final portion of the system is the mechanical device which supports the micro-electrode assembly. This must at the same time provide for rigid support and micromanipulation of the electrode tip.

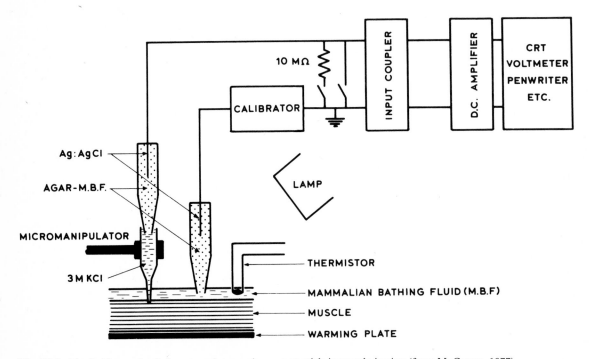

Fig. 30.6   Typical input circuit for measuring membrane potentials in muscle *in vitro* (from McComas, 1977)

Micro-electrodes

Micro-electrodes are made of capillary glass tubing drawn to a fine hollow point and filled with an electrolyte solution. The micropipettes are most easily and reproducibly made by a semi-automatic glass melting and pulling device (e.g. Alexander and Nastuk, 1953). Initial adjustments are made by trial and error. The tip diameter must be so small that it penetrates the cell membrane with minimal damage. Tip diameters of 0.5 μm or less are considered to be suitable for mammalian muscle fibres.

A potential difference may develop across the interface between different solutions, such as obtains at the tip of the micro-electrode, for the anion may diffuse out with greater rapidity than the cation, or *vice versa*. Potassium chloride solution is usually used to fill the micropipettes because the mobilities of the potassium and chloride ions are similar. The sodium ion, in contrast, has a much lower mobility than chloride. Metallic micro-electrodes are unsuitable for membrane potential measurements because of their large and variable junction potentials.

For a given micro-electrode tip diameter it is advantageous that the electrode resistance should be as low as possible. Hence, the filling solution should have a high conductivity. Using a 3-molar (saturated) solution of potassium chloride, electrode resistances of 10 to 50 MΩ are obtained with external tip diameters of less than 0.5 μm. Because these diameters are beyond the resolution of light microscopy, resistance measurements are used to determine whether an electrode is of appropriate size.

Some electrodes which are satisfactory from the standpoint of size develop an anomalous potential across their tips, called 'tip potential' (Adrian, 1956). Unfortunately, the tip potential is inconstant and varies with the ionic composition and concentration of the media surrounding the tip. As tip potentials cannot be completely nullified by subtraction, electrodes exhibiting potentials greater than 5 mV should be discarded.

Thus, satisfactory micro-electrodes should have resistances of 10–50 MΩ, and tip potentials of less than 5 mV.

Techniques for filling the micropipettes with electrolyte solution vary. It is now possible to purchase capillary glass tubing containing a fine glass fibre. A piece of this glass is drawn out in the usual way and the filling solution is introduced by inserting the needle of a hypodermic syringe into the shank of the electrode. The effect of the glass fibre is to increase the capillary attractive force so that the filling solution penetrates to the tip of the electrode within a few seconds, dislodging the remaining pocket of air as it does so.

Input circuitry

It is the function of the input circuit to transmit the potential difference between the micro-electrode and indifferent electrode to the measuring device with fidelity. The input circuit consists of the muscle fibre (when a fibre is impaled), the electrodes, the electrolyte solutions (termed salt-bridges) connecting them to their metallic terminals, and the input portion of the input coupler (Fig. 30.6). This circuit should not draw current from (nor permit external currents to leak through) the muscle membrane. It should not introduce spurious potentials, or, if it does, they should be balanced out. When transient phenomena such as end-plate potentials and action potentials are recorded, this circuit must compensate for the poor high-frequency response of the micro-electrode.

Ideally, no current should flow in the input circuit. Practically, the current need be reduced only to the point where it does not produce significant errors in voltage measurements and where the current flowing through the muscle membrane near the micro-electrode tip does not produce significant changes in its polarisation. The only site in the external part of the input circuit at which the current might cause a significant error in the measurement of voltage is the micro-electrode tip, as this constitutes the only appreciable resistance. If a 1 per cent error in measuring 100 mV is acceptable, the potential difference across the micro-electrode tip should be less than 1 mV. By Ohm's law it can be calculated that for an electrode of 50 MΩ resistance the maximum permissible current would be 2×10^{-11} A. However, in order to avoid local changes in membrane polarisation it is considered good practice to reduce the input circuit current still further, to less than 10^{-12} A; this is achieved by using a coupling device with a very high input impedance (e.g. 10^{12} Ω) and low leakage current.

Spurious junction potentials can be avoided by seeing that the junctions in the input circuit are symmetrically disposed with respect to the micro-electrode. This situation is achieved in Figure 30.6, where the following sequence of junctions is present: silver; silver chloride; bathing fluid; potassium chloride (in micro-electrode); bathing fluid; silver chloride; silver.

The input coupling device itself will be discussed in no further detail. Several excellent devices are available commercially; they include such features as bridge circuitry for intracellular stimulation (see below), capacitance neutralisation for accurate recording of fast transient signals, micro-electrode resistance determination and signal voltage calibration.

Potential measuring

The potential-measuring devices will not be discussed in great detail. Their purpose is to indicate the magnitude of the signal from the input device and, hence, the potential between the electrodes. The choice depends upon the degree of precision required, and upon whether a written record is desired. Ordinary meter movements can be read to 5 per cent of full scale, cathode ray oscilloscope traces to 2 per cent of the nominal tube diameter, and self-balancing potentiometers to 1 per cent of the chart width. When higher precision is necessary, zero suppression can be used. The accuracy of any measuring device should be verified periodically by reference to a standard cell.

Intracellular stimulation myography

A further development has enabled a muscle fibre to be stimulated directly through an intracellular micro-electrode, and the evoked change in membrane potential to be recorded simultaneously with the same electrode. With this technique it is possible to obtain additional information about the muscle fibre membrane, such as the membrane time constant (equal to the product of the specific membrane resistance and capacitance), the critical membrane depolarisation (the depolarisation required to initiate an action potential) and the threshold stimulating current (see above). The method depends on the use of a Wheatstone bridge circuit to eliminate the stimulus artefact (cf. Araki and Otani, 1955; Frank and Fuortes, 1956); its application to muscle physiology has been described by Beranek (1964) and by McComas and Mossawy (1966).

Types of muscle preparation used in human studies

Three different techniques have been used to examine human muscle: they are (1) the in vitro method, (2) the in situ cannula method, (3) the in situ 'open' method. All three methods have advantages and disadvantages and one's choice must ultimately depend on the type of information which is required.

The in vitro method. A piece of excised muscle is mounted in a bath containing a physiological bathing solution and the fibres are impaled under direct vision. The fibres must be intact, because injury will result in electrolyte changes associated with membrane depolarisation. For this reason, intercostal muscle is ideal, as the fibres are relatively short and can therefore be easily excised intact (Dillon, Fields, Gumas, Jenden and Taylor, 1955). This method has several advantages. First, the muscle preparation can be transilluminated and fine details of its structure, such as the disposition of small nerve branches, are more easily observed. Second, the effect of ionic changes on the membrane can be readily investigated by altering the composition of the bathing fluid. A third advantage of an in vitro recording system is its high mechanical stability. This is important because human skeletal muscle fibres are only 20–70 μm in diameter, and small movements occurring between fibre and electrode may easily dislodge the tip. The one disadvantage of the method is the inevitable uncertainty regarding the relevance of in vitro findings to the in situ condition. For example, the resting potential will be significantly lower in vitro than in situ (McComas and Mossawy, 1965) unless protein is added to the fluid bathing the excised muscle (Kernan, 1963). In addition there is a marked tendency for 'spontaneous' electrical activity such as fibrillation potentials (Thesleff, 1962) and myotonic discharges (Hofmann, Alston and Rowe, 1967) to disappear *in vitro*.

The *in situ* cannula method. In this system a rigidly held metal cannula is used to puncture the skin, subcutaneous tissue and muscle fascia; an internal micro-electrode is then gently driven down to sample the muscle fibres lying below the tip of the cannula (Beranek, 1964). Cutaneous anaesthesia is desirable if repeated electrode penetrations are contemplated. The advantages of the method are that it is *in situ*, and that there is minimal inconvenience both for patients and for control subjects. The disadvantage is that the first few fibres encountered by the exploring electrode will have been damaged by the cannula and selection of the results is therefore necessary. In addition, artefacts caused by changes in micro-electrode tip potential are likely to occur with deeper penetrations (*see below* and also Nastuk and Hodgkin, 1950; Del Castillo and Katz, 1955).

The *in situ* open method. This technique may be performed under general or local anaesthesia. However, it is important that the local anaesthetic should not be allowed to reach the muscle because it may affect the properties of the fibre membranes (*cf*. Draper, Friebel and Karzel, 1959; Draper and Karzel, 1961). For this reason a cutaneous nerve block at a distance from the site of the experiment is preferable to a local injection. The skin is incised, the subcutaneous fatty tissue retracted and the fascial sheath of the muscle gently reflected. The surface of the muscle is then covered with a physiological bathing solution such as that described by Liley (Na, 150; K, 5.0; Ca, 2.0; Mg, 1.0; HCO_3, 12.0; H_2PO_4, 1.0; values in mM; Liley, 1956). The muscle fibres may then be impaled under direct vision through a dissecting microscope. This method, although otherwise inconvenient, may readily be undertaken just before a muscle biopsy; unlike the cannula method, all the fibres should be in good condition, so that there is no need to select results. A disadvantage of this, and of the *in situ* cannula

technique, is the poor mechanical stabilisation of the muscle so that only transient impalements of fibres are usually possible. Because the muscle movements take place in a mainly lateral direction there is an obvious advantage to be gained in making the electrode assembly compliant laterally while remaining rigid in the axis of penetration. This can be accomplished by thrusting the butt of the micro-electrode into agar gel (Johns, 1958) or by inserting a segment of latex tubing into the micro-electrode shaft (Vaughan Williams, 1959). The lateral compliance of this system now allows the micro-electrode to follow small lateral displacements of the muscle without breakage of the tip.

Errors and artefacts

Erroneous measurements of membrane potential may occur through physiological, electrical or interpretative problems.

Virtually every form of physical or chemical injury to the muscle cell causes a reduction in the membrane potential. As this is one of the most sensitive indicators of injury, there is usually no direct means of verifying whether or not a given measurement was obtained from a fibre injured by anoxia or minor trauma. Care must therefore be exercised in exposing the fibres and in maintaining them during the course of an experiment. Some experimenters arbitrarily discard low values of membrane potential, assuming that they have been obtained from damaged fibres. As will be mentioned later, such data selection *per se* introduces a systematic error.

Traumatic impalement is a common form of membrane injury. As pressure from the micro-electrode tip indents the membrane, a negative-going potential is recorded. With a clean impalement there is then an abrupt negative shift in potential as the tip penetrates the membrane. The further negative change in the micro-electrode potential which occurs over the next 10–30 s has been ascribed to protoplasmic sealing about the micro-electrode tip. The potential will then remain constant for many minutes until the tip is withdrawn. With traumatic impalements the abrupt drop may not occur, and there is a gradual reduction in membrane potential following impalement. Potentials exhibiting these features may justifiably be discarded. Artefacts introduced by the micro-electrode have been mentioned. Electrodes whose resistances are too low will be of large diameter and may damage the fibres. Those exhibiting significant tip potentials will also introduce errors. While the tip potential can be balanced out when the tip is in the extracellular fluid, the potential is not the same when the tip is intracellular. Furthermore, it is possible that the tip potential may change if the micro-electrode is pushed beyond the first few superficial fibres. Thus, a substantial steady potential can be regularly observed in between penetrations of deeper fibres, and is invariably associated with an increased impedance at the electrode tip. The effect of this change is to introduce uncertainty as to the correct reference potential to use for the measurement of membrane potential. In practice, however, the change in tip potential is presumed to be negligible when the latter is less than 5 mV and only superficial fibres are sampled.

Either electrode may introduce spurious potentials if symmetry is not preserved or if the potential due to asymmetry is not carefully balanced out. Any element in the system may be responsible for drift or temporal instability in the reference level. If, for example, the recorded output level drifts from zero to +5 mV, a membrane potential of −86 mV would be recorded at that time as −81 mV. The input coupler is the least stable element in the system. Frequent reference to the zero level by short-circuiting the electrode terminals permits detection of all drifts except those arising from the electrodes.

Any element may produce inaccurate amplification of the membrane potential before its display. Although this is much less of a problem than drift, periodic verification of accuracy by referring the electrode terminals to a standard potential source is recommended. The resistance of the input circuit will reduce the apparent membrane potential unless it exceeds the micro-electrode resistance by a hundredfold. Dirt and moisture on input circuit elements may considerably reduce the input resistance. It is common practice to use hermetic sealing and non-hygroscopic insulating materials in critical parts of the circuit.

Measurements of membrane potential of muscle fibres vary about a mean. If data from otherwise satisfactory impalements are discarded because they are low, the mean value obtained will be spuriously high, as pointed out by Harvey and Zierler (1958).

RESULTS IN NORMAL SUBJECTS

In the pioneering investigation by Johns (1958) the mean resting membrane potential of human muscle, examined by the *in situ* open technique, was −77.8 ± 2.4 mV. In the many studies which have followed, the mean values reported have ranged from −68.5 mV (Brooks and Hongdalarom, 1968) to −87.2 mV (Riecker, Dobbelstein, Rohl and Bolte, 1964); most values, irrespective of the recording method employed, have been between −75 and −80 mV (*see below* for references).

From determinations of the amounts of water and potassium in human muscle it is possible to calculate the intracellular potassium concentration, provided that the total water can be allocated between intra- and extra-cellular compartments. This is usually done by measuring some substance whose distribution is assumed to be limited to the extracellular fluid. Chloride and inulin are commonly used. Values for intracellular potassium ion concentration, based on chloride space, range from 140 to 160 mEq/l (Barnes, Gordon and Cope, 1957; Johns, 1958; Flear and Florence, 1961). While there is reasonable agreement between the membrane potential calculated from these data using Equation 2 and the observed membrane potential, two reservations must be made. First, a 15 mV range in the observed membrane potential encompasses a +36 and −25 mEq/l change in the intracellular potassium ion concentration; it is thus difficult to escape reasonable agreement. Second, correlation between membrane potential and potassium equilibrium potential must be demonstrated at several ranges of potassium concentrations and not at one range only.

In rat muscle *in vitro* it has been shown that the resting membrane potential may be lower than the calculated potassium equilibrium potential if a conventional protein-free physiological bathing solution is used; on the other hand there is good agreement between these two values if plasma is substituted (Kernan, 1963). The relationship between potassium equilibrium potential and resting membrane potential has been investigated in excised human intercostal muscle by Ludin (1969); although the intracellular potassium concentration was not measured, the resting membrane potential varied inversely with the logarithm of the extracellular potassium concentration, as would be expected from the Nernst equation.

In a few studies some of the passive electrical ('cable') properties of the membrane have been determined. As with the resting potential, however, the results have shown considerable differences. For example, a membrane time constant of 18.9 ms was found by Elmqvist, Hofmann, Kugelberg and Quastel (1964) in intercostal muscle *in vitro* while Lipicky, Bryant and Salmon (1971), using the same preparation, obtained a value of 12.8 ms. Even this last result is considerably greater than the figure of 6.3 ms determined by McComas, Mrozek, Gardner-Medwin and Stanton (1968) for limb muscles. From the first two studies cited it is evident that differences in experimental technique must have accounted for a considerable part of the discrepancy between the results. However, the two values for intercostal muscle reported above are not only greater than that of McComas *et al.* (1968) for limb muscle but are also larger than those given for limb muscles in other species (Boyd and Martin, 1959; McComas and Mossawy, 1966). As the membrane time constant is equal to the product of the specific membrane resistance and capacity, the results must indicate that either, or both, of these values are higher in intercostal than in limb muscle. In addition, Lipicky *et al.* (1971) were able to demonstrate a species difference for the same type of muscle fibre, for they found that the specific membrane resistance of intercostal muscle fibres was significantly greater in man than in the goat. These findings raise the possibility that there may be subtle differences in membrane structure between various types of muscle in the same species and between the same type of muscle in different species.

The critical membrane depolarisation required for the initiation of an action potential may also depend on the human muscle preparation used. In excised intercostal muscle fibres, critical membrane depolarisations greater than 28–33 mV were noted by Hofmann *et al.* (1967) while Brooks and Hongdalarom (1968) derived a mean value of approximately 20 mV for tibialis anterior muscle *in situ*. In contrast, McComas *et al.* (1968) found that action potentials could be elicited by much smaller depolarisations and that their mean value was only 11.8 mV.

RESULTS IN DISEASE STATES

Familial periodic paralysis

Hypokalaemic type. It has long been known that one type of familial periodic paralysis (FPP) is associated with hypokalaemia and that potassium is not lost from the body (Allott and McArdle, 1938; Gammon, Austin, Blithe and Reid, 1939). It was assumed that the hypokalaemia resulted from a shift of potassium from the extra- to the intracellular compartment. Subsequently, this was confirmed by measurements of the arterio-venous differences in potassium concentration (Zierler and Andres, 1957; Grob, Johns and Liljestrand, 1957b). The large fall in extracellular concentration, together with the presumed slight rise in intracellular concentration would increase the potassium equilibrium potential. It was assumed that this would be associated with an increase in membrane potential or hyperpolarisation. The paralysis was shown to be associated with block of neuromuscular transmission and also with a failure of spread of electrical excitation along the fibre (Grob, Liljestrand and Johns, 1957a). Recently Sica and Aguilera (1972) have been able to demonstrate that some motor units are especially susceptible to paralysis.

In view of the paralysis and of the possibility that this could stem from hyperpolarisation of the fibre membrane, the results of micro-electrode studies of hypokalaemic FPP are of great interest. So far six patients have been observed. In the first, 37 fibre impalements during attacks of paresis were compared with 45 impalements when not paretic and no difference was found (Shy, Wanko, Rowley and Engel, 1961). The mean potential ($\pm$

standard deviation) during attacks was -71.2 ± 11.6 mV, which was within the control range.

Control studies in the second patient were obtained when he was minimally weak from an attempt to precipitate an attack by exercise and a late meal (Creutzfeldt, Abbott, Fowler and Pearson, 1963). Mild weakness was produced by the further administration of glucose and insulin, and the studies were repeated. The serum potassium concentration fell from 4.25 to 3.17 mEq/l. The mean membrane potential in the control period was -85.6 ± 6.1 mV (SE) while during the induced attack the corresponding values were -77.1 ± 8.2 mV. While this reduction in potential was found to be statistically significant, the authors felt that it was due, in part at least, to cooling and drying of the superficial fibres.

In a third patient, investigated by Riecker and Bolte (1966), a markedly reduced membrane potential of -49.1 mV was observed during an induced attack in which the serum potassium concentration fell from 4.5 to 2.0 mEq/l. The remaining three patients were studied by Hofmann and Smith (1970) using specimens of external intercostal muscle *in vitro*. These authors also noted a depolarisation of the muscle fibre membranes and, significantly, this persisted in the presence of a normal potassium concentration (5 mM) in the bathing solution.

As it is clearly established that potassium enters the cell during an attack of FPP and that its extracellular concentration falls to half or one-third normal, why is it that the membrane potential either shows little change or actually depolarises? Three mechanisms seem possible. First, the effective intracellular potassium ion concentration could be simultaneously reduced to one-half by some binding mechanism. The concentration ratio would thus remain constant and the potential unchanged. At first sight, the ability of muscle to bind some 70 mEq of ion per litre of fibre water seems unlikely. However, the dilated sarcoplasmic vacuoles demonstrated during an attack of FPP by Shy *et al*. (1961) (*see also* Engel, 1970) could conceivably provide such a mechanism by keeping the extra potassium in an intracellular compartment where it was unable to influence the polarisation of the surface membrane. The transport system responsible for this net inward flux of potassium would remain to be elucidated.

Second, a concomitant influx of water into the fibre, such that the intracellular potassium concentration is halved, would preserve the concentration unchanged; this would require that fibre water be doubled. While Shy *et al*. (1961) have found an increase in muscle water of 111 ml/Kg, this is inadequate to produce the necessary reduction in intracellular potassium even if the increase in water were entirely intracellular.

Third, an associated increase in sodium conductance would serve to lower the membrane potential and would compensate for the potassium-induced rise (Fig. 30.2). In keeping with this possibility is the finding by Hofmann and Smith (1970) that the depolarisation could be abolished *in vitro* if 90 per cent of the external sodium was replaced by choline.

To summarise, although an increase in potential was anticipated in FPP, studies in six patients have revealed a normal or reduced resting membrane potential. If these results are confirmed by further observations, studies on membrane conductance will be needed to explain why the potential does not rise in the face of the sharp reduction in the extracellular potassium concentration. It will also be necessary to determine why neuromuscular transmission is blocked and the action potential fails to spread if hyperpolarisation is not present.

Although much uncertainty remains, there is increasing agreement that the inexcitability of the fibre surface membrane is sufficient to account for the paralysis observed. Crucial evidence on this issue came from the ingenious experiment of Engel and Lambert (1969). These authors obtained specimens of intercostal muscle during an attack of paralysis and then removed the sarcolemma of single fibres, using the desheathing technique of Natori (1954). They were then able to demonstrate that the myofibrils could be made to contract by the direct application of calcium ions to the skinned fibres.

Hyperkalaemic type (adynamia episodica hereditaria). The paralysis in this condition occurs in association with a modest rise in serum potassium concentration (Tyler, Stephens, Gunn and Perkoff, 1951; Stevens, 1954; Sagild and Helweg-Larsen, 1955; Gamstorp, 1956; Creutzfeldt, 1961; McArdle, 1962). This factor alone cannot account for the paralysis, for hyperkalaemia of this degree is not normally associated with demonstrable weakness (Winkler, Hoff and Smith, 1941; Keith, Osterberg and Burchell, 1942; Grob et al., 1957a).

It is assumed that the rise in serum concentration is caused by potassium moving out of cells, for there is no reduction in the renal execretion of potassium before or during an attack (Gamstorp, 1956; Egan and Klein, 1959; Klein, Egan and Usher, 1960). Such a shift would produce a negligible fall in the intracellular potassium concentration. It is unlikely that the rise in extracellular potassium concentration together with the slight fall in intracellular potassium concentration could produce a significant reduction in the resting membrane potential, unless the intracellular potassium concentration was low initially.

The intracellular potassium content has been studied in eight patients by measurement of their total exchangeable potassium. In six, the total exchangeable potassium was within normal limits (Sagild, 1958; McArdle, 1962), in one it was high (McArdle, 1962) and in one it was low (Liljestrand, 1957). Direct measurement of total muscle potassium showed that the content was slightly low (Liljestrand, 1957; Klein et al., 1960; Creutzfeldt, 1961). Thus, it is difficult to explain the paralysis on the basis of depolarisation and inexcitability of the muscle membrane caused by intracellular potassium depletion.

The direct measurement of membrane potential in a patient with adynamia episodica has been reported by Creutzfeldt et al. (1963). These authors found that, during a spontaneous episode of paralysis, the mean membrane potential fell to -51.5 mV from a value of -68.5 mV measured in an attack-free period. In an induced attack the depolarisation was even greater, the mean potential reaching -46.3 mV. A second patient with this condition was studied in detail by Brooks (1969). This patient also exhibited marked cold-sensitive myotonia, thereby indicating the close functional relationship between hyperkalaemic periodic paralysis and paramyotonia congenita (von Eulenburg's syndrome). Using the in situ cannula technique, Brooks was able to show, not only that the mean membrane potential fell during an induced attack of paralysis (from -75.5 mV to -47.3 mV), but that the fibres could not respond to currents passed through the intracellular microelectrode. It is of interest that in Brooks' patient the resting membrane potential was normal between attacks whereas, in the case of Creutzfeldt et al. (1963) a partial depolarisation persisted. In the four subjects studied, between attacks, by McComas, Mrozek and Bradley (1968), a persisting depolarisation was also observed, together with raised thresholds of the fibres to direct stimulation.

A partial depolarisation of the muscle membrane is compatible with many of the known electrophysiological abnormalities in adynamia episodica. These include spontaneous firing of fibres, increased mechanical irritability, and increased sensitivity to intra-arterially injected acetylcholine (Liljestrand, 1957; Buchthal, Engbaek and Gamstorp, 1958a, b; Morrison, 1960; Creutzfeldt, 1961). Other findings, such as the reduction in the number of motor units responding during maximal effort and a reduction in the number of muscle fibres contributing to a motor unit potential, may be attributed to a partial block in neuromuscular transmission caused by endplate depolarisation (Buchthal et al., 1958a, b).

Nevertheless, the mechanism of the partial depolarisation remains to be explained. Creutzfeldt et al. (1963) have calculated from their membrane potential data (Equation 2) that the intracellular potassium concentration must be reduced to 51 mEq/l before, and 38 to 41 mEq/l during, an attack if an alteration in the distribution of potassium is the sole defect. That such reductions in intracellular potassium have not been found suggests that a primary abnormality of potassium cannot account for the depolarisation.

The explanation favoured by Creutzfeldt et al. (1963) and by McComas et al. (1968) is that the underlying membrane abnormality is a sudden increase in sodium permeability, caused by some precipitating factor as yet undetermined. Once the sodium permeability rises the membrane potential will drop, as indicated in the electrical analogue of the membrane (Fig. 30.2). At the same time, sodium ions will enter the fibre down their electrochemical gradient and, by replacing potassium as intracellular cations, will enable a net outward flux of potassium to take place. The extracellular potassium concentration will now rise. However, the new membrane potential remains lower than the potassium equilibrium potential because the sodium–potassium pump maintains an active inward movement of potassium. Indirect evidence for a rise in sodium permeability is the reduced membrane time constant and input resistance observed by McComas *et al.* (1968). If the membrane potential drops sufficiently quickly myotonia may occur as the threshold for impulse initiation is reached (*see also* Jenerick and Gerard, 1953). Subsequently, the fibres become inexcitable because of depolarisation block; the regenerative sodium conductance system remains inactive and can no longer participate in the generation of an action potential ('refractoriness').

As with hypokalaemic periodic paralysis, it is clear that more experimental observations are needed, preferably using a combination of sensitive electrophysiological and biochemical techniques.

Normokalaemic type. The normokalaemic variant of FPP (Tyler *et al.*, 1951; Poskanzer and Kerr, 1961) has been the least studied. In one patient with this condition, who was investigated between attacks of paralysis by McComas *et al.* (1968), a fall in resting potential was observed together with a reduction in membrane time constant. It is possible that this type of periodic paralysis is an example of the hyperkalaemic type in which the clinical data have been insufficient to demonstrate the potassium shift. Alternatively, it may represent an underlying increase in sodium permeability of the muscle fibre membranes.

The myotonias

Myotonia is best defined as a sustained contraction of muscle fibres caused by repetitive depolarisation of their membranes. This physiological definition serves to exclude from consideration other types of sustained contraction or slow relaxation of muscle. Myotonia may be seen in various clinical conditions, including dystrophia myotonica, myotonia congenita, paramyotonia congenita and hyperkalaemic familial periodic paralysis (FPP), as well as in the hereditary myotonia of goats and in hereditary mouse dystrophy.

The electromyographic findings are similar in all of these conditions. Characteristically there are bursts of action potentials which decrease in amplitude and frequency following contraction, percussion or needle electrode movement. An intracellular recording of repetitive impulse activity in a patient with myotonia congenita is shown in Figure 30.7; similar recordings in human myotonia have been published by Norris (1962) and Hofmann *et al.* (1967). The fact that this electrical activity withstands curarisation indicates that it does not depend on motor nerve activity or, indeed, upon the presence of ACh (Brown and Harvey, 1939; Floyd, Kent and Page, 1955; McComas and Mossawy, 1965); instead, the evidence indicates that it is the muscle fibre membrane itself which is hyperexcitable.

There is no *a priori* reason for supposing that the abnormality causing the hyperexcitability is the

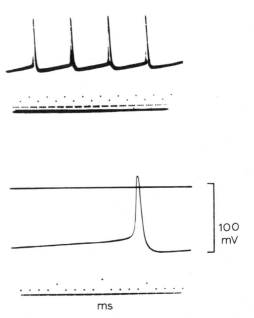

Fig. 30.7 Myotonic activity recorded *in situ* with an intracellular microelectrode from two fibres of a patient with myotonia congenita. Note that the upper recording was made with a slower sweep of the oscilloscope time-base (from McComas and Mrożek, 1968)

same in all types of myotonic disorder and, indeed, the evidence which has accumulated to date indicates that there are at least two possible mechanisms. One of these, that responsible for the myotonia of hyperkalaemic FPP and the closely related condition of paramyotonia congenita, has already been considered. It has been shown that, in these diseases, the muscle fibre membrane depolarises, probably as a result of an increased permeability to sodium. When the membrane reaches the critical level for impulse initiation, myotonic discharges will occur.

The second myotonic mechanism involves a reduction in the permeability of the resting membrane to chloride. From a series of careful studies by Bryant and Lipicky it now seems likely that this abnormality underlies the membrane hyperexcitability of human myotonia congenita and that of goats with hereditary myotonia. In his initial study, Bryant (1962) noted that normal mammalian muscle fibres developed myotonic features if chloride was removed from the extracellular fluid. Lipicky and Bryant (1966) were then able to show that in myotonic goats the membrane permeability for chloride was naturally reduced, and a similar defect was subsequently demonstrated in biopsy specimens of intercostal muscle taken from patients with myotonia congenita (Lipicky, Bryant and Salmon, 1971; Lipicky and Bryant, 1973). In addition to the marked change in chloride permeability in myotonia congenita, it now appears that there is a smaller but significant reduction in the permeability of the membrane to potassium (Lipicky, 1977). In contrast to the situation in myotonia congenita, the muscle fibres of patients with myotonic dystrophy show relatively small and variable reductions in chloride permeability with little change in potassium permeability (Lipicky, 1977).

Bryant and Morales-Aguilera (1971) and Rüdel and Sanges (1972), among others, have investigated the action on normal mammalian muscle fibre membranes of certain compounds which can cause myotonia. One type of substance used in these studies is 20, 25-diazocholesterol, while another class consists of the monocarboxylic aromatic acids. In view of the findings described above in hereditary myotonia, it is of the greatest interest that the chloride permeability of the fibre membranes is also reduced in these pharmacological models of myotonia.

The mechanism by which a reduction in chloride permeability can cause electrical instability of the membrane is now well understood (Adrian and Bryant, 1974; Adrian and Marshall, 1976). It is known that at the conclusion of an action potential there will have been a net flux of potassium ions into the T-tubular system from the interior of the fibre. Because the narrow dimensions of the tubules retard the diffusion of these ions from the vicinity of the cell, the tubular concentration of potassium rises, thereby lowering the potassium equilibrium potential (see Nernst equation, page 1009). The tendency of the membrane potential to follow the declining potassium equilibrium potential is normally minimised by the relatively large chloride permeability; the latter has the effect of keeping the membrane potential closer to the equilibrium potential for chloride than that for potassium (see Fig. 30.2). In the myotonic fibre, however, the stabilising effect of the chloride permeability is diminished and the efflux of potassium can cause appreciable depolarisation after a small number of impulses have been conducted. This depolarisation of the fibre in turn triggers off further action potentials by activating the sodium permeability mechanism and the cycle of events can then be repeated many times, producing the characteristic myotonic train of impulses. Mathematical models of the membrane, based on a low chloride permeability, have been shown to produce regenerative impulse activity of this type (Bretag, 1973; Barchi, 1975; Adrian and Marshall, 1976).

Muscular dystrophy

The type of muscular dystrophy which has been studied most frequently in man is the myotonic variety. In the patients of Norris (1962) and Haynes (1971) the mean resting membrane potentials were judged to be normal though the latter author gives reasons for minimising the significance of this observation. In the studies of Hofmann et al. (1967) and of McComas and Mrozek (1968), however, substantial reductions were observed. McComas and Mrozek noted that, not only was the mean resting potential some 15 per cent lower than normal, but the individual measurements exhibited a large scatter. This last finding is hardly surprising in view of the marked variations in pathological severity which can be observed among a population of fibres within the same muscle. It is not known to what extent the fall in resting potential is a factor in the induction of myotonia and, indeed, the unequal pathological involvement of fibres in myotonic dystrophy makes this latter condition ill-suited to an examination of the myotonic mechanism.

As far as other forms of human dystrophy are concerned, Ludin (1970) has investigated two patients with limb-girdle dystrophy and one with the facioscapulohumeral form (see also Haynes, 1971). Ludin not only measured the resting membrane potential of intercostal fibres in vitro but also observed the effects of changing the external potassium concentration. He showed that, in these conditions, the resting potential was also reduced; from the slope of the curve relating resting potential to external potassium concentration he deduced that this resulted from a reduction in intracellular potassium. This suggestion is supported by biochemical studies of mice with a hereditary form of muscular dystrophy (Bar Harbor 129 strain) in which the sodium concentration is raised, and that of potassium depressed (Baker, Blahd and Hart, 1958; Young, Young and Edelman, 1959; Mossawy, 1966). In these animals there is also a significant fall in resting membrane potential (Lenman, 1963; McComas and Mossawy, 1965), especially of small diameter fibres (Kleeman, Partridge and Glaser, 1961). In Duchenne dystrophy, Sakakibara, Engel and Lambert (1977) have examined external intercostal muscle biopsy specimens from three patients. In this condition, too, the resting membrane potential was commonly reduced; the same authors also showed that neuromuscular transmission remained unimpaired.

Myasthenia gravis

The resting membrane potential in myasthenia gravis was reported to be normal (Dahlback, Elmqvist, Johns, Radner and Thesleff, 1961). These in vitro measurements were incidental to a study of miniature end-plate potentials. These potentials, which are depolarisations produced by the release of small packets of acetylcholine (ACh) from the nerve endings (Fig. 30.5), were at first reported as being normal in amplitude but reduced in frequency. Subsequently, however, it was shown by Elmqvist et al. (1964) that the frequency was, in fact, normal because the majority of the myasthenic miniature end-plate potentials were unusually small and had not therefore been observed in the initial study. The presence of unusually small miniature end-plate potentials in myasthenic muscle has been confirmed in biopsy specimens of limb muscle (Haynes, 1971) and of external intercostal muscle (Ito, Miledi, Vincent and Newsom Davis, 1978). An important application of the micro-electrode technique has been to test the sensitivity of the myasthenic end-plates to ACh, the latter being ejected from a micropipette in small but controlled amounts by iontophoresis. In contrast to the earlier report by Dahlback et al. (1961) it is now accepted that the ACh sensitivity of the end-plate is markedly reduced (see Albuquerque, Rash, Mayer and Satterfield, 1976). This last conclusion has been supported by the findings of reduced numbers of ACh receptors, as revealed by α-bungarotoxin (Fambrough, Drachman and Satyamurti, 1973; Engel, Lindstrom, Lambert and Lennon, 1977), and of severe destruction of the postsynaptic array of secondary clefts (Santa, Engel and Lambert, 1972). As far as the axon terminals are concerned, it was previously thought that these contained reduced amounts of ACh. Electron microscopy has since revealed that, in contrast to the underlying muscle fibre surface, the structure of the terminals is well preserved (Santa et al., 1972); furthermore, the total amount of ACh in myasthenic muscle, measured by gas chromatography and mass spectrometry, is significantly increased rather than reduced (Ito, Miledi, Molenaar, Vincent, Polak, Van Gelder and Davis, 1976).

Pseudomyasthenic syndromes

In the pseudomyasthenic syndrome of Eaton and Lambert (1957) there is a characteristic type of weakness which can usually be shown to be a remote complication of malignant disease. In this condition there is a defect in neuromuscular transmission; unlike myasthenia gravis, however, muscle strength improves with continued exercise and may also be enhanced by guanidine. Micro-electrode studies of this syndrome have been undertaken by Lambert and Elmqvist (1971; 12 patients) and by Hofmann, Kundin and Farrell (1967; 2 patients); the investigations were conducted *in vitro* using specimens of external intercostal muscle. In both instances it was found that the resting membrane potentials were normal and that the miniature end-plate potentials had normal amplitudes and discharge frequencies. When the intercostal nerve twigs were stimulated, however, the end-plate potentials were severely reduced because insufficient quanta of ACh appeared to be discharged from the axon terminals. Electron microscopic studies by Santa *et al.* (1972) revealed that the axon terminals were of normal size and contained abundant synaptic vesicles (i.e. ACh quanta). Lambert and Elmqvist (1971) demonstrated that the release of ACh could be facilitated by either raising the concentration of calcium ions in the bathing solution, adding guanidine to the latter, or stimulating the nerve fibres repetitively (post-tetanic potentiation).

Mention may also be made of a newly recognised pseudomyasthenic syndrome which differs from that described above in that the terminal axonic expansions are small and contain reduced numbers of synaptic vesicles. Although the miniature end-plate potentials are of normal size, too few quanta are available for release and the end-plate potentials are consequently small (Engel, Lambert and Gomez, 1977).

Denervated muscle

A loss of motor innervation not only causes well-marked morphological changes in the muscle fibres but also alters the functional properties of the fibre membranes in several important respects (Thesleff, 1974). These changes are attributable to the withdrawal of a 'trophic' influence normally exerted by motor neurones on muscle fibres. The nature of this trophic influence has aroused much interest and a full account of the relevant experimental observations is beyond the scope of this chapter (*see* McComas, 1977). It is sufficient to state that trophic effects appear to be mediated

both by impulses and by chemical substances manufactured in the motor neurone and transported along the motor axon to the muscle fibre. The importance of impulse activity has recently been confirmed by Lømo and Rosenthal (1972) who found that they were able to prevent the development of some features of denervation by direct electrical stimulation of muscle. On the other hand there are a number of studies which show that the onset of certain denervation phenomena in muscle fibres is related to the distance from the muscle at which the nerve is cut (*see* Harris and Thesleff, 1972). If impulse activity were the only trophic mechanism, the onset should be independent of the site of nerve section. The fact that it is not, suggests that the muscle fibres continue to use up trophic substances contained in the distal nerve stump. Irrespective of the relative importance of impulses and trophic substances, there is now increasing evidence that these factors may act by controlling regulator genes in the fibre (Samaha, Guth and Albers, 1970; Grampp, Harris and Thesleff, 1972). The special characteristics of denervated muscle fibre membranes which can be detected by microelectrodes are as follows.

Increased chemosensitivity. The sensitivity of the muscle fibre membrane to ACh may be tested in a very precise manner by recording the membrane depolarisations evoked by the release of small amounts of the chemical from a micropipette. It has been shown by Axelsson and Thesleff (1959) that a few days after denervation has occurred the sensitivity of the muscle fibre membrane to ACh begins to spread out from the end-plate until ultimately the whole fibre is involved. Katz and Miledi (1964) have shown that this ability to form new ACh receptors is inherent in the muscle membrane.

Decreased membrane conductance. Following denervation the membrane conductance falls (Nicholls, 1956). Because the membrane at rest has significant permeability only for potassium and chloride, either, or both, of these component conductances could be altered. It is possible to resolve this problem by measuring the membrane conductance after chloride has been replaced with an impermeant anion such as methylsulphate or ethanesulphate. It appears that, in frog muscles, the potassium conductance only is reduced (Hubbard, 1963) while in mammalian muscle both the potassium and chloride conductances are probably diminished (Thesleff, 1962). The reduction in potassium conductance has several important consequences for the membrane potential; as these are not entirely similar in frog and mammalian muscle, only the latter situation will be described. First, a fall in potassium conductance produces a depolarisation by allowing the resting membrane potential to fall below the potassium equilibrium potential (Ware, Bennett, and McIntyre, 1954; Thesleff, 1962; Lenman, 1965). Second, because the resting membrane potential is low, the critical membrane depolarisation required to initiate an action potential will be proportionately reduced. Finally, the increase in potassium conductance which serves to terminate the action potential has the effect of temporarily bringing the membrane potential back to the potassium equilibrium potential; this causes a large positive after-potential (Lüllmann, 1960).

Tetrodotoxin-resistant action potentials. The initiation of action potentials in a muscle fibre is normally prevented by minute concentrations of tetrodotoxin (TTX), a poison obtained from the Japanese puffer fish. Within a few hours of denervation, however, it is found that the action potentials which can be evoked by direct electrical stimulation of muscle fibres have become resistant to the application of this substance (Redfern and Thesleff, 1971).

Fibrillation potentials. After denervation a proportion of the muscle fibres begin to discharge in a slow but regular sequence. The suggestion that these potentials depend on the increased sensitivity of the fibre to small amounts of circulating ACh (Denny-Brown and Pennybacker, 1938) seems unlikely in view of the different times of onset of the two phenomena. More convincing evidence against the ACh hypothesis is the fact that the fibrillation potentials are unaffected by curarisation (Rosenblueth and Luco, 1937). The question of the site of origin of the fibrillation potentials is one which has also attracted argument. However, Belmar and Eyzaguirre (1966) used a variety of techniques to demonstrate that fibrillation potentials arise exclusively at the end-plate. Thus, the extracellularly recorded potentials changed polarity only when the micro-electrode reached the end-plate. Furthermore, the frequency of the fibrillation potentials could readily be altered by passing current through the fibre membrane in the end-plate region, but nowhere else along its surface. Finally, the intracellular recording in the end-plate region showed that the action potentials were preceded by prepotentials similar to those found in myotonia (*cf.* Fig. 30.7). The finding of prepotentials is important because it indicates the presence of a depolarising 'generator' mechanism at the denervated end-plate; it further suggests that the electrical properties of this part of the fibre membrane may be different from those elsewhere (*see also* Purves and Sakmann, 1974, and Thesleff and Ward, 1975).

REFERENCES

Adrian, R.H. (1956) The effects of internal and external potassium concentration on the membrane potential of frog muscle. *Journal of Physiology*, **133**, 631.

Adrian, R.H. & Bryant, S.H. (1974) On the repetitive discharge in myotonic muscle fibres. *Journal of Physiology*, **240**, 505–515.

Adrian, R.H. & Marshall, M.W. (1976) Action potentials reconstructed in normal and myotonic muscle fibres. *Journal of Physiology*, **258**, 125–143.

Albuquerque, E.X., Rash, J.E., Mayer, R.F. & Satterfield, J.R. (1976) An electrophysiological and morphological study of the neuromuscular junction in patients with myasthenia gravis. *Experimental Neurology*, **51**, 536–563.

Alexander, J.T. & Nastuk, W.L. (1953) An instrument for the production of microelectrodes used in electrophysiological studies. *Review of Science Instruments*, **24**, 528.

Allott, E.N. & McArdle, B. (1938) Further observations on familial periodic paralysis. *Clinical Science*, **3**, 229.

Araki, T. & Otani, T. (1955) Response of single motoneurones to direct stimulation in toad's spinal cord. *Journal of Neurophysiology*, **18**, 472.

Axelsson, J. & Thesleff, S. (1959) A study of supersensitivity in denervated mammalian skeletal muscle. *Journal of Physiology*, **149**, 178.

Baker, N., Blahd, W.H. & Hart, P. (1958) Concentration of K and Na in skeletal muscle of mice with a hereditary myopathy (Dystrophia muscularis). *American Journal of Physiology*, **193**, 530.

Barnes, B.A., Gordon, E.B. & Cope, O. (1957) Skeletal muscle analysis in health and in certain metabolic disorders. I. The method of analysis and the values in normal muscle. *Journal of Clinical Investigation*, **36**, 1239.

Belmar, J. & Eyzaguirre, C. (1966) Pacemaker site of fibrillation potentials in denervated mammalian muscle. *Journal of Neurophysiology*, **29**, 425.

Beranek, R. (1964) Intracellular stimulation myography in man. *Electroencephalography and Clinical Neurophysiology*, **16**, 301.

Boyd, I.A. & Martin, A.R. (1959) Membrane constants of mammalian muscle fibres. *Journal of Physiology*, **147**, 450.

Bretag, A.H. (1973) Mathematical modelling of the myotonic action potential. In *New Developments in Electromyography and Clinical Neurophysiology*. Ed. J.E. Desmedt, Vol. 1, pp. 464–482 (Karger: Basel).

Brooks, J.E. (1969) Hyperkalaemic periodic paralysis. Intracellular electromyographic studies. *Archives of Neurology*, **20**, 13.

Brooks, J.E. & Hongdalarom, T. (1968) Intracellular electromyography. *Archives of Neurology*, **18**, 291.

Brown, G.L. & Harvey, A.M. (1939) Congenital myotonia in the goat. *Brain*, **62**, 341.

Bryant, S.H. (1962) Muscle membrane of normal and myotonic goats in normal and low external chloride. *Federation Proceedings*, **11**, 312.

Bryant, S.H. & Morales-Aguilera, A. (1971) Chloride conductance in normal and myotonic muscle fibres and the action of monocarboxylic aromatic acids. *Journal of Physiology*, **219**, 367.

Buchthal, F., Engbaek, L. & Gamstorp, I. (1958a) Paresis and hyperexcitability in adynamia episcodica hereditaria. *Neurology (Minneapolis)*, **8**, 347.

Buchthal, F., Engbaek, L. & Gamstorp, I. (1958b) Some aspects of the pathophysiology of adynamia episodica hereditaria. *Danish Medical Bulletin*, **5**, 167.

Creutzfeldt, O.D. (1961) Die episodiche Adynamie (Adnamia episodica hereditaria Gamstorp) eine familiäre hyperkalämische Lähmung. *Fortschritte der Neurologie, Psychiatric und ihrer Grinzgebiete*, **10**, 529.

Creutzfeldt, O.D., Abbott, B.C., Fowler, W.M. & Pearson, C.M. (1963) Muscle membrane potentials in episodic adynamia. *Electroencephalography and Clinical Neurophysiology*, **15**, 508.

Dahlback, O., Elmqvist, D., Johns, T.R., Radner, S. & Thesleff, S. (1961) An electrophysiologic study of the neuromuscular junction in myasthenia gravis. *Journal of Physiology*, **156**, 336.

del Castillo, J. & Katz, B. (1955) Local activity at a depolarized nerve-muscle junction. *Journal of Physiology*, **128**, 396.

Denny-Brown, D. & Pennybacker, J.B. (1938) Fibrillation and fasciculation in voluntary muscle. *Brain*, **61**, 311.

Dillon, J.B., Fields, J., Gumas, T., Jenden, D.J. & Taylor, D.B. (1955) An isolated human voluntary muscle preparation. *Proceedings of the Society for Experimental Biology and Medicine*, **90**, 409.

Draper, M.H., Friebel, H. & Karzel, K. (1959) Some actions of cocaine on frog sartorius muscle. *Journal of Physiology*, **148**, 61P.

Draper, M.H. & Karzel, K. (1961) The action of local anaesthetics on the action potential of frog sartorius muscle fibres. *Journal of Physiology*, **155**, 27P.

Eaton, L.M. & Lambert, E.H. (1957) Electromyography and electric stimulation of nerves in diseases of motor unit: observations on the myasthenic syndrome associated with malignant tumours. *Journal of the American Medical Association*, **613**, 1117–1124.

Egan, T.J. & Klein, R. (1959) Hyperkalaemic familial periodic paralysis. *Paediatrics*, **24**, 761.

Elmqvist, D., Hofmann, W.W., Kugelberg, J. & Quastel, D.M.J. (1964) An electrophysiological investigation of neuromuscular transmission in myasthenia gravis. *Journal of Physiology*, **174**, 417.

Engel, A.G. (1970) Evolution and content of vacuoles in primary hypokalaemic periodic paralysis. *Mayo Clinic Proceedings*, **45**, 774–814.

Engel, A.G. & Lambert, E.H. (1969) Calcium activation of electrically inexcitable muscle fibres in primary hypokalemic periodic paralysis. *Neurology (Minneapolis)*, **19**, 85.

Engel, A.G., Lambert, E.H. & Gomez, M.R. (1977) A new myasthenic syndrome with end-plate acetylcholinesterase deficiency, small nerve terminals, and reduced acetylcholine release. *Annals of Neurology*, **1**, 315–330.

Engel, A.G., Lindstrom, J.M., Lambert, E.H. & Lennon, J.A. (1977) Ultrastructural localization of the acetylcholine receptor in myasthenia gravis and in the experimental autoimmune model. *Neurology (Minneapolis)*, **27**, 307–315.

Fambrough, D.M., Drachman, D.B. & Satyamurti, S. (1973) Neuromuscular function in myasthenia gravis: decreased acetylcholine receptors. *Science (New York)*, **182**, 293–295.

Flear, C.T.G. & Florence, I. (1961) A rapid and micro method for the analysis of skeletal muscle for water, sodium, potassium, chloride, and fat. *Clinica Chimica Acta*, **6**, 129.

Floyd, W.F., Kent, P. & Page, F. (1955) An electromyographic study of myotonia. *Electroencephalography and Clinical Neurophysiology*, **7**, 621.

Frank, K. & Fuortes, M.G.F. (1956) Stimulation of spinal motoneurones with intracellular electrodes. *Journal of Physiology*, **134**, 451.

Gammon, G.D., Austin, J.H., Blithe, M.D. & Reid, C.G. (1939) The relation of potassium to periodic family paralysis. *American Journal of Medical Sciences*, **197**, 326.

Gamstorp, I. (1956) Adynamia episodica hereditaria. *Acta Paediatrica*, **45**, Supplement 108, 1.

Goldman, D.E. (1943) Potential, impedance and rectification in membrane. *Journal of General Physiology*, **27**, 37.

Grampp, W., Harris, J.B. & Thesleff, S. (1972) Inhibition of denervation changes in skeletal muscle by blockers of *protein synthesis*. *Journal of Physiology*, **221**, 743–754.

Grob, D., Johns, R.J. & Liljestrand, A. (1957b) Potassium movement in patients with familial periodic paralysis. *American Journal of Medicine*, **23**, 356.

Grob, D., Liljestrand, A. & Johns, R.J. (1957a) Potassium movement in normal subjects. *American Journal of Medicine*, **23**, 340.

Harris, J.B. & Thesleff, S. (1972) Nerve stump length and membrane changes in denervated skeletal muscle. *Nature*, **236**, 60.

Harvey, A.M. & Zierler, K.L. (1958) The production of very high extracellular potassium concentration in the intact rat and its effect on muscle membrane potential. *Physiologist*, **1**, 35.

Haynes, J. (1971) Miniature end-plate potentials in neuromuscular disease: an electrophysiological investigation of motor-point muscle biopsies. *Journal of Neurology, Neurosurgery and Psychiatry*, **34**, 521.

Hodgkin, A.L. (1951) The ionic basis of electrical activity in nerve and muscle. *Biological Reviews of the Cambridge*

Philosophical Society, **26**, 339.

Hodgkin, A.L. (1964) *The Conduction of the Nervous Impulse* (Liverpool University Press: Liverpool).

Hodgkin, A.L. & Horowicz, P. (1959) The influence of potassium and chloride ions on the membrane potential of single muscle fibres. *Journal of Physiology*, **148**, 127.

Hodgkin, A.L. & Huxley, A.F. (1952) A quantitative description of membrane current and its application to conduction and excitation in nerve. *Journal of Physiology*, **117**, 500.

Hofmann, W.W. & Smith, R.A. (1970) Hypokalaemic periodic paralysis studies *in vitro*. *Brain*, **93**, 445–474.

Hofmann, W.W., Alston, W. & Rowe, G. (1967) A study of individual neuromuscular junctions in myotonia. *Electroencephalography and Clinical Neurophysiology*, **21**, 521.

Hofmann, W.W., Kundin, J.E. & Farrell, D.F. (1967) The pseudomyasthenic syndrome of Eaton and Lambert: An electrophysiological study. *Electroencephalography and Clinical Neurophysiology*, **23**, 214.

Hubbard, S.J. (1963) The electrical constants and component conductances of frog skeletal muscle after denervation. *Journal of Physiology*, **165**, 443.

Hutter, O.F. & Noble, D. (1960) The chloride conductance of frog skeletal muscle. *Journal of Physiology*, **151**, 89.

Ito, Y., Miledi, R., Vincent, A. & Newsom Davis, J. (1978) Acetylcholine receptors and end-plate electrophysiology in myasthenia gravis. *Brain*, **101**, 345–368.

Ito, Y., Miledi, R., Molenaar, P.C., Vincent, A. Polak, R.L., Van Gelder, M. & Davis, J.N. (1976) Acetylcholine in human muscle. *Proceedings of the Royal Society (series B)*, **192**, 475.

Jenerick, H.P. & Gerard, R.W. (1953) Membrane potential and threshold of single muscle fibres. *Journal of Cellular and Comparative Physiology*, **42**, 79.

Johns, R.J. (1958) Microelectrode studies of muscle membrane potentials in man. *Research Publications of the Association for Research in Nervous and Mental Disease*, **38**, 704.

Katz, B. (1966) *Nerve, Muscle and Synapse* (McGraw-Hill: New York).

Katz, B. & Miledi, R. (1964) The development of actylcholine sensitivity in nerve-free segments of skeletal muscle. *Journal of Physiology*, **170**, 389.

Keith, N.M., Osterberg, A.E. & Burchell, H.B. (1942) Some effects of potassium salts in man. *Annals of Internal Medicine*, **16**, 879.

Kernan, R.P. (1963) Resting potential of isolated rat muscles measured in plasma. *Nature*, **200**, 474.

Kleeman, F.J., Partridge, L.D. & Glaser, G.H. (1961) Resting potential and muscle fibre size in hereditary mouse dystrophy. *American Journal of Physical Medicine*, **40**, 219.

Klein, R., Egan, T. & Usher, P. (1960) Changes in sodium, potassium and water in hyperkalaemic familial paralysis. *Metabolism*, **9**, 1005.

Lambert, E.H. & Elmqvist, D. (1971) Quantal components of end-plate potentials in the myasthenic syndrome. In *Myasthenia Gravis*, Ed. W.S. Fields, *Annals of the New York Academy of Sciences*, **183**, 183–199.

Lenman, J.A.R. (1963) Micro-electrode studies in muscle disease. In *Research in Muscular Dystrophy. Proceedings of the Second Symposium of the Muscular Dystrophy Group* (Pitman Medical: London).

Lenman, J.A.R. (1965) Effect of denervation on the resting membrane potential of healthy and dystrophic mice.

Journal of Neurology, Neurosurgery and Psychiatry, **28**, 525.

Liley, A.W. (1956) An investigation of spontaneous activity at the neuromuscular junction of the rat. *Journal of Physiology*, **132**, 650.

Liljestrand, A. (1957) Fall av adynamia episodica hereditaria. *Opuscular Medicana*, **7**, 183.

Ling, G. & Gerard, R.W. (1949) Normal membrane potential of frog sartorius fibres. *Journal for Cellular and Comparative Physiology*, **34**, 383.

Lipicky, R.J. (1977) Studies in human myotonic dystrophy. In *Pathogenesis of Human Muscular Dystrophies*, Ed. L.P. Rowland, pp. 729–738 (Excerpta Medica: Amsterdam).

Lipicky, R.J. & Bryant, S.H. (1966) Sodium, potassium and chloride fluxes in intercostal muscle from normal goats with hereditary myotonia. *Journal of General Physiology*, **50**, 89.

Lipicky, R.J. & Bryant, S.H. (1973) A biophysical study of the human myotonias. In *New Developments in Electromyography and Clinical Neurophysiology*, Ed. J.E. Desmedt, pp. 451–463 (Karger: Basel).

Lipicky, R.J., Bryant, S.H. & Salmon, J.H. (1971) Cable parameters, sodium, potassium, chloride, and water content, and potassium efflux in isolated external intercostal muscle of normal volunteers and patients with myotonia congenita. *Journal of Clinical Investigation*, **50**, 2091.

Lømo, T. & Rosenthal, J. (1972) Control of ACh sensitivity by muscle activity in the rat. *Journal of Physiology* **221**, 493.

Ludin, H.P. (1969) Microelectrode study of normal human skeletal muscle. *European Neurology*, **2**, 340.

Ludin, H.P. (1970) Microelectrode study of dystrophic human skeletal muscle. *European Neurology*, **3**, 116.

Lüllmann, H. (1960) Über die ursache spontaner fibrillationen denervierter skeletmuskulatur. *Klinische Wochenschrift*, **38**, 1169.

McArdle, B. (1962) Adynamia episodica hereditaria and its treatment. *Brain*, **85**, 121.

McComas, A.J. (1977) *Neuromuscular Function and Disorders*. p. 364 (Butterworths: London).

McComas, A.J. & Mossawy, S.J. (1965) Electrophysiological investigation of normal and dystrophic muscles in mice. In *Research in Muscular Dystrophy. Proc. Third Symposium of the Muscular Dystrophy Group* (Pitman: London).

McComas, A.J. & Mossawy, S.J. (1966) Excitability of muscle fibre membranes in dystrophic mice. *Journal of Neurology, Neurosurgery and Psychiatry*, **29**, 440.

McComas, A.J. & Mrozek, K. (1967) Denervated muscle fibres in hereditary mouse dystrophy. *Journal of Neurology, Neurosurgery and Psychiatry*, **30**, 526.

McComas, A.J. & Mrozek, K. (1968) The electrical properties of muscle fibre membranes in dystrophia myotonica and myotonia congenita. *Journal of Neurology, Neurosurgery and Psychiatry*, **31**, 441.

McComas, A.J., Mrozek, K. & Bradley, W.G. (1968) The nature of the electrophysiological disorder in adynamia episodica. *Journal of Neurology, Neurosurgery and Psychiatry*, **31**, 448.

McComas, A.J., Mrozek, K., Gardner-Medwin, D. & Stanton, W.H. (1968) Electrical properties of muscle fibre membranes in man. *Journal of Neurology, Neurosurgery and Psychiatry*, **31**, 434.

Morrison, J.B. (1960) The electromyographic changes in hyperlakaemic familial periodic paralysis. *Annals of*

Physical Medicine, **5**, 153.

Mossawy, S.J. (1966) An electrophysiological study of dystrophic muscle in the mouse. *Ph.D. Thesis:* University of Newcastle upon Tyne.

Nastuk, W.L. & Hodgkin, A.L. (1950) The electrical activity of single muscle fibres. *Journal of Cellular and Comparative Physiology*, **35**, 39.

Natori, R. (1954) The property and contraction process of isolated myofibrils. *Jikeikai Medical Journal*, **1**, 119.

Nicholls, J.G. (1956) The electrical properties of denervated skeletal muscle. *Journal of Physiology*, **131**, 1.

Norris, F.H. Jnr. (1962) Unstable membrane potential in human myotonic muscle. *Electroencephalography and Clinical Neurophysiology*, **14**, 197.

Poskanzer, D.C. & Kerr, D.N.S. (1961) A third type of periodic paralysis with normokalemia and favorable response to sodium chloride. *American Journal of Medicine*, **31**, 328.

Purves, D. & Sakmann, B. (1974) Membrane properties underlying spontaneous activity of denervated muscle fibres. *Journal of Physiology*, **239**, 125–153.

Redfern, P. & Thesleff, S. (1971) Action potential generation in denervated rat skeletal muscle. I. Quantitative aspects. *Acta Physiologica Scandinavica*, **81**, 557.

Riecker, G. & Bolte, H.D. (1966) Membranpotentiale einzelner Skeletmuskelzellen bei hypokaliamischer periodischer Muskelparalyse. *Klinische Wochenschrift*, **44**, 804.

Riecker, G., Dobbelstein, H., Rohl, D. & Bolte, H.D. (1964) Messungen des Membranepotentials einzelner quergestreifter Muskelzellen bei Myotonia congenita (Thomsen). *Klinische Wochenschrift*, **42**, 519.

Rosenblueth, A. & Luco, J.V. (1937) A study of denervated mammalian skeletal muscle. *American Journal of Physiology*, **120**, 781.

Rüdel, R. & Senges, J. (1972) Experimental myotonia in mammalian skeletal muscle: Changes in membrane properties. *Pflügers Archiv für die gesamte Physiologie des Menschen und der Tiere*, **331**, 324.

Sagild, V. (1958) Cited in Buchthal, Engbaek and Gamstorp (1958a, b).

Sagild, V. & Helweg-Larsen, H.F. (1955) Det Kliniske billede ved arvelige transitoriske muskellammelser. *Nordist Medicia*, **53**, 981.

Sakakibara, H., Engel, A.G. & Lambert, E.H. (1977) Duchenne dystrophy: ultrastructural localization of the acetylcholine receptor and intracellular microelectrode studies of neuromuscular transmission. *Neurology (Minneapolis)*, **27**, 741–745.

Samaha, F.J., Guth, L. & Albers, R.W. (1970) The neural regulation of gene expression in the muscle cell. *Experimental Neurology*, **27**, 276.

Santa, T., Engel, A.G. & Lambert, E.H. (1972) Histometric study of neuromuscular junction ultrastructure. I. Myasthenia gravis. *Neurology (Minneapolis)*, **22**, 71.

Shanes, A.M. (1961) In *Biophysics of Physiological and Pharmacological Actions* Ed. A.M. Shanes (American Association for the Advancement of Science: Washington).

Shy, G.M., Wanko, T., Rowley, P.T. & Engel, A.G. (1961) Studies in familial periodic paralysis. *Experimental Neurology*, **3**, 53.

Sica, R.E.P. & Aguilera, N. (1972) Electrophysiological properties in hypokalemic periodic paralysis. *Medicina*, **32**, 93.

Stevens, J.R. (1954) Familial periodic paralysis, myotonia, progressive amyotrophy, and pes cavus in members of a single family. *Archives of Neurology and Psychiatry (Chicago)*, **72**, 726.

Thesleff, S. (1962) Spontaneous electrical activity in denervated rat skeletal muscle. In *The Effect of Use and Disuse on Neuromuscular Functions*. Eds E. Gutmann and P. Hnik (Elsevier: Amsterdam).

Thesleff, S. (1974) Physiological effects of denervation of muscle. In *Trophic Functions of the Neuron*, Ed. D.B. Drachman, *Annals of the New York Academy of Sciences*, **228**, 89–103.

Thesleff, S. & Ward, M.R. (1975) Studies on the mechanism of fibrillation potentials in denervated muscle. *Journal of Physiology*, **244**, 313–323.

Tower, D.B., Luse, S.A. & Grundfest, H. (1962) *Properties of Membranes and Disease of the Nervous System* (Springer: New York).

Tyler, F.H., Stephens, F.E., Gunn, F.D. & Perkoff, G.T. (1951) Studies in disorder of muscle; clinical manifestations and inheritance of type of periodic paralysis without hypopotassaemia. *Journal of Clinical Investigation*, **30**, 492.

Vaughan Williams, E.M. (1959) A method of mounting micro-electrodes for intracellular recording from contracting muscle. *Journal of Physiology*, **147**, 3.

Ware, F. Jnr., Bennett, A.L. & McIntyre, A.R. (1954) Membrane resting potentials of denervated mammalian skeletal muscle measured *in vivo*. *American Journal of Physiology*, **117**, 115.

Winkler, A.W., Hoff, H.E. & Smith, P.K. (1941) The toxicity of orally administered potassium salts in renal insufficiency. *Journal of Clinical Investigation*, **20**, 119.

Young, H.L., Young, W. & Edelman, I.S. (1959) Electrolyte and lipid composition of skeletal and cardiac muscle in mice with hereditary muscular dystrophy. *American Journal of Physiology*, **197**, 487.

Zierler, K.L. & Andres, R. (1957) Movement of potassium into skeletal muscle during spontaneous attack in family periodic paralysis. *Journal of Clinical Investigation*, **36**, 730.

Index